Contents in Brief

BRUNNER & SUDDARTH'S

Textbook of Medical-Surgical Nursing

VOLUME 1

Edition
13

BRUNNER & SUDDARTH'S

Textbook of Medical-Surgical Nursing

Janice L. Hinkle, PhD, RN, CNRN
Associate Professor
The Catholic University of America
Washington, DC

Kerry H. Cheever, PhD, RN
Professor and Chairperson
Department of Nursing
Moravian College
Bethlehem, Pennsylvania

Edition
13

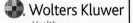

Wolters Kluwer | Lippincott Williams & Wilkins
Health

Philadelphia • Baltimore • New York • London
Buenos Aires • Hong Kong • Sydney • Tokyo

Publisher: Lisa McAllister
Executive Editor: Sherry Dickinson
Supervisor, Product Development: Betsy Gentzler
Editorial Assistant: Dan Reilly
Design Coordinator: Joan Wendt
Art Director, Illustration: Jennifer Clements
Illustrator, 13th edition: Wendy Beth Jackelow
Production Project Manager: Cynthia Rudy
Manufacturing Coordinator: Karin Duffield
Prepress Vendor: Aptara, Inc.

13th Edition

9 8 7 6 5 4 3 2 1

Printed in China.

Library of Congress Cataloging-in-Publication Data

Hinkle, Janice L., author.
  Brunner & Suddarth's textbook of medical-surgical nursing / Janice L. Hinkle, Kerry H. Cheever. –
Thirteenth edition.
      p. ; cm.
  Brunner and Suddarth's textbook of medical-surgical nursing
  Textbook of medical-surgical nursing
  Preceded by Brunner & Suddarth's textbook of medical-surgical nursing / Suzanne C. Smeltzer ...
[et al.]. 12th ed. c2010.
  Includes bibliographical references and index.
  Summary: "This textbook has been a favorite resource for students, instructors, and practicing nurses for almost a half-century. Its comprehensive yet accessible approach covers a broad scope of medical conditions while focusing strongly on the nurse's role in caring for, educating, and assisting patients and families"–Provided by publisher.
  ISBN 978-1-4511-3060-7 (1-volume American edition : hardback : alk. paper) –
  ISBN 978-1-4511-4666-0 (2-volume American edition : hardback : alk. paper)
  I. Cheever, Kerry H., author.   II. Title.   III. Title: Brunner and Suddarth's textbook of medical-surgical nursing.   IV. Title: Textbook of medical-surgical nursing.
  [DNLM: 1. Nursing Care.   2. Perioperative Nursing.   WY 150]
  RT41
  617'.0231–dc23
                                                                                                    2013028429

CCS1013

Contributors

Christina M. Amidei, PhD, RN, CNRN, CCRN, FAAN
Research Scientist
Neuro-Oncology Research
University of Chicago
Chicago, Illinois

Chapter 65: Assessment of Neurologic Function
Chapter 70: Management of Patients With Oncologic or
Degenerative Neurologic Disorders

Janice M. Beitz, PhD, RN, CS, CNOR, CWOCN, CRNP
Professor
School of Nursing
Rutgers University
Camden, New Jersey

Chapter 48: Management of Patients With Intestinal and Rectal Disorders

Elizabeth Blunt, PhD, RN, FNP-BC
Assistant Professor
Coordinator Nurse Practitioner Programs
College of Nursing
Villanova University
Villanova, Pennsylvania

Chapter 38: Assessment and Management of Patients With
Allergic Disorders

Lisa Bowman, MSN, RN, CRNP, CNRN
Nurse Practitioner
Division of Cerebrovascular Disease and Neurological
Critical Care
Thomas Jefferson University Hospital
Philadelphia, Pennsylvania

Chapter 67: Management of Patients With Cerebrovascular Disorders

Jo Ann Brooks, PhD, RN, FAAN, FCCP
Adjunct Assistant Professor
Indiana University
Indianapolis, Indiana

Chapter 23: Management of Patients With Chest and Lower
Respiratory Tract Disorders
Chapter 24: Management of Patients With Chronic Pulmonary Disease

Kim Cantwell-Gab, MN, ARNP, CVN, RVT, RDMS
Acute Care Advanced Registered Nurse Practitioner
Thoracic and Vascular Surgery, Southwest Medical Center
Vancouver, Washington

Chapter 30: Assessment and Management of Patients With Vascular
Disorders and Problems of Peripheral Circulation

Patricia E. Casey, MSN, RN, CPHQ
Associate Director
NCDR Training and Orientation
American College of Cardiology
Washington, DC

Chapter 26: Management of Patients With Dysrhythmias and
Conduction Problems

Jill Cash, MSN, RN, APN
Family Nurse Practitioner
Southern Illinois Rheumatology
Herrin, Illinois

Chapter 64: Assessment and Management of Patients With Hearing
and Balance Disorders

Kerry H. Cheever, PhD, RN
Professor and Chairperson
Department of Nursing
Moravian College
Bethlehem, Pennsylvania

Chapter 43: Management of Patients With Musculoskeletal Trauma

Odette Y. Comeau, MS, RN
Clinical Nurse Specialist
Adult Critical Care
University of Texas Medical Branch
Galveston, Texas

Chapter 62: Management of Patients With Burn Injury

Linda Carman Copel, PhD, RN, PMHCNS, BC, CNE,
NCC, FAPA
Professor
College of Nursing
Villanova University
Villanova, Pennsylvania

Chapter 4: Health Education and Promotion
Chapter 6: Individual and Family Homeostasis, Stress,
and Adaptation
Chapter 59: Assessment and Management of Problems Related to
Male Reproductive Processes

Carolyn Cosentino, RN, ANP-BC
Memorial Sloan-Kettering Cancer Center
New York, New York

Chapter 58: Assessment and Management of Patients With
Breast Disorders

Susanna Garner Cunningham, PhD, BSN, MA, FAAN
Professor
Biobehavioral Nursing and Health Systems
University of Washington
Seattle, Washington

Chapter 31: Assessment and Management of Patients
With Hypertension

Nancy Donegan, MPH, RN
Director, Infection Control
MedStar Washington Hospital
Washington, DC

Chapter 71: Management of Patients With Infectious
Diseases

Diane K. Dressler, MSN, RN, CNRN, CCNS
Clinical Assistant Professor
College of Nursing
Marquette University
Milwaukee, Wisconsin

Chapter 27: Management of Patients With Coronary Vascular Disorders
*Chapter 29: Management of Patients With Complications From
   Heart Disease*

Phyllis Dubendorf, MSN, RN, CNRN, CCNS
Clinical Nurse Specialist
Hospital of the University of Pennsylvania
Philadelphia, Pennsylvania

Chapter 66: Management of Patients With Neurologic Dysfunction

Susan M. Fallone, MS, RN, CNN
Clinical Nurse Specialist Adult and Pediatric Dialysis
Albany Medical Center Hospital
Albany, New York

Chapter 53: Assessment of Kidney and Urinary Function

Eleanor Fitzpatrick, MSN, RN, CCRN
Clinical Nurse Specialist
Surgical Intensive Care Unit and Intermediate Surgical
   Intensive Care Unit
Thomas Jefferson University Hospital
Philadelphia, Pennsylvania

*Chapter 49: Assessment and Management of Patients With
   Hepatic Disorders*
*Chapter 50: Assessment and Management of Patients With
   Biliary Disorders*

Kathleen Kelleher Furniss, APN-C, DMH, CBCM, DVS
Women's Health Nurse Practitioner
Chilton Memorial Hospital
Pompton Plains, New Jersey

*Chapter 57: Management of Patients With Female
   Reproductive Disorders*

Catherine Glynn-Milley, RN, CPHQ, CRNO
Ophthalmology Clinical/Research Coordinator
VA Palo Alto Health Care System
Palo Alto, California

*Chapter 63: Assessment and Management of Patients With Eye and
   Vision Disorders*

Dawn M. Goodolf, PhD, RN
RN to BS Program Coordinator, Assistant Professor
Department of Nursing
Moravian College
Bethlehem, Pennsylvania

Chapter 40: Assessment of Musculoskeletal Function

Theresa Green, PhD, RN
Assistant Professor
Faculty of Nursing
University of Calgary
Calgary, Alberta, Canada

Chapter 10: Principles and Practices of Rehabilitation

Jamie Moore Heffernan, BSN, RN, CCRN
Manager
Blocker Burn Unit
The University of Texas Medical Branch
Galveston, Texas

Chapter 62: Management of Patients With Burn Injury

Melissa Hladek, MSN, RN, FNP-BC
Family Nurse Practitioner Program Coordinator
Assistant Clinical Professor
The Catholic University of America
Washington, DC

*Chapter 39: Assessment and Management of Patients With
   Rheumatic Disorders*

Joyce Young Johnson, PhD, MSN, RN
Dean and Professor
College of Sciences and Health Professions
Albany State University
Albany, Georgia

*Chapter 1: Health Care Delivery and Evidence-Based
   Nursing Practice*
Chapter 2: Community-Based Nursing Practice
*Chapter 3: Critical Thinking, Ethical Decision Making, and the
   Nursing Process*
Chapter 7: Overview of Transcultural Nursing

Tamara M. Kear, PhD, RN, CNN
Assistant Professor of Nursing
College of Nursing
Villanova University
Villanova, Pennsylvania

*Chapter 54: Management of Patients With
   Kidney Disorders*
*Chapter 55: Management of Patients With
   Urinary Disorders*

Elizabeth K. Keech, PhD, RN
Assistant Professor
College of Nursing
Villanova University
Villanova, Pennsylvania

Chapter 11: Health Care of the Older Adult

Lynne Kennedy, PhD, MSN, RN, CNOR, CHPN
Program Coordinator
Minimally Invasive Gynecologic Surgery and
   Palliative Care
Inova Fair Oaks Hospital
Fairfax, Virginia

Chapter 17: Preoperative Nursing Management
Chapter 18: Intraoperative Nursing Management
Chapter 19: Postoperative Nursing Management

Mary Theresa Lau, MS, APN, CNSN, CRNI
Nutrition Support/PICC Clinical Nurse Specialist
Edward Hines Jr. VA Hospital
Hines, Illinois

*Chapter 45: Digestive and Gastrointestinal Treatment
   Modalities*

Dale Halsey Lea, MPH, RN, CGC, FAAN
Consultant
Maine Genetics Program
Cumberland Foreside, Maine

Chapter 8: Overview of Genetics and Genomics in Nursing Genetics in Nursing Practice Charts

Linda M. Lord, MS, RN, CNSC, NP
Nurse Practitioner
Ambulatory Nursing-Nutrition Support Clinic
University of Rochester Medical Center
Rochester, New York

Chapter 45: Digestive and Gastrointestinal Treatment Modalities

Mary Beth Flynn Makic, PhD, RN, CNS
Associate Professor
College of Nursing
University of Colorado Medical Campus
Research Nurse Scientist, Critical Care
University of Colorado Hospital
Aurora, Colorado

Chapter 14: Shock and Multiple Organ Dysfunction Syndrome

Elizabeth Petit de Mange, PhD, MSN, RN
Assistant Professor
College of Nursing
Villanova University
Villanova, Pennsylvania

Chapter 52: Assessment and Management of Patients With Endocrine Disorders

Barbara J. Maschak-Carey, MSN, RN, CDE
Diabetes Clinical Nurse Specialist
Department of Psychiatry, Center for Weight and Eating Disorders
University of Pennsylvania
Philadelphia, Pennsylvania

Chapter 51: Assessment and Management of Patients With Diabetes

Agnes Masny, BS, MPH, MSN, RN, ANP-BC
Nurse Practitioner
Department of Clinical Genetics
Fox Chase Cancer Center
Philadelphia, Pennsylvania

Chapter 8: Overview of Genetics and Genomics in Nursing

Phyllis J. Mason, MS, RN, ANP
Faculty
Acute and Chronic Care
Johns Hopkins University School of Nursing
Baltimore, Maryland

Chapter 44: Assessment of Digestive and Gastrointestinal Function
Chapter 47: Management of Patients With Gastric and Duodenal Disorders

Jennifer D. McPherson, DNP, CRNA
Clinical Instructor
Uniformed Services University of Health Sciences
Bethesda, Maryland

Chapter 21: Respiratory Care Modalities

Donna M. Molyneaux, PhD, RN
Associate Professor of Nursing
Gwynedd-Mercy College
Gwynedd Valley, Pennsylvania

Chapter 22: Management of Patients With Upper Respiratory Tract Disorders

Barbara Moran, PhD, CNM, RNC, FACCE
Assistant Clinical Professor
The Catholic University of America
Washington, DC

Chapter 56: Assessment and Management of Female Physiologic Processes

Susan Snight Moreland, DNP, CRNP
Nurse Practitioner
The Center for Breast Health
Bethesda, Maryland

Chapter 35: Assessment of Immune Function
Chapter 36: Management of Patients With Immunodeficiency Disorders

Martha A. Mulvey, MSN, ANP-BC
Adult Nurse Practitioner
Department of Neurosciences
University of Medicine and Dentistry of New Jersey—University Hospital
Newark, New Jersey

Chapter 13: Fluid and Electrolytes: Balance and Disturbance

Donna A. Nayduch, MSN, RN, ACNP, CAIS
Trauma Consultant
K-Force
Evans, Colorado

Chapter 72: Emergency Nursing
Chapter 73: Terrorism, Mass Casualty, and Disaster Nursing

Kathleen M. Nokes, PhD, RN, FAAN
Professor and Director of Graduate Program
City University of New York, Hunter College of Nursing
Hunter College
New York, New York

Chapter 37: Management of Patients With HIV Infection and AIDS

Kristen J. Overbaugh, MSN, RN, ACNS-BC
Clinical Assistant Professor
Health Restoration and Care Systems Management
University of Texas at San Antonio Health Science Center
San Antonio, Texas

Chapter 20: Assessment of Respiratory Function

Janet A. Parkosewich, DNSc, RN, FAHA
Nurse Researcher
Patient Services
Yale-New Haven Hospital
New Haven, Connecticut

Chapter 25: Assessment of Cardiovascular Function

Chris Pasero, MS, RN-BC, FAAN
Pain Management Educator and Clinical Consultant
El Dorado Hills, California

Chapter 12: Pain Management

Mae Ann Pasquale, PhD, RN
Assistant Professor of Nursing
Cedar Crest College
Allentown, Pennsylvania

Chapter 41: Musculoskeletal Care Modalities

Sue Baron Pugh, MSN, RN, CNS-BC, CRRN, CNRN, CBIS, FAHA
Clinical Nurse Specialist
Brain and Spine Institute
Sinai Hospital of Baltimore
Baltimore, Maryland

Chapter 69: Management of Patients With Neurologic Infections, Autoimmune Disorders, and Neuropathies

Kimberly L. Quinn, BSN, MSN, RN, CRNP, ANP, ACNP, CCRN
Senior Nurse Practitioner
Department of Oncology
University of Maryland
Baltimore, Maryland

Chapter 46: Management of Patients With Oral and Esophageal Disorders

JoAnne Reifsnyder, PhD, APRN, BC-PCM
Research Assistant Professor
Division Director, Health Policy and Health Services Research
Department of Health Policy
Thomas Jefferson University
Philadelphia, Pennsylvania

Chapter 16: End-of-Life Care

Marylou V. Robinson, PhD, FNP-C
Assistant Professor
College of Nursing
University of Colorado
Aurora, Colorado

Chapter 42: Management of Patients With Musculoskeletal Disorders

Linda Schakenbach, MSN, RN, CNS, CCRN, CWCN, ACNS-BC
Clinical Nurse Specialist
Cardiac Critical Care Services
Inova Fairfax Hospital
Falls Church, Virginia

Chapter 28: Management of Patients With Structural, Infectious, and Inflammatory Cardiac Disorders

Suzanne C. Smeltzer, EdD, RN, FAAN
Professor and Director
Center for Nursing Research
Villanova University College of Nursing
Villanova, Pennsylvania

Chapter 9: Chronic Illness and Disability

Anthelyn Jean Smith-Temple, DNS, MSN, BSN
Former Assistant Dean and Associate Professor
College of Nursing
Valdosta State University
Valdosta, Georgia

Chapter 1: Health Care Delivery and Evidence-Based Nursing Practice
Chapter 2: Community-Based Nursing Practice
Chapter 3: Critical Thinking, Ethical Decision Making, and the Nursing Process
Chapter 7: Overview of Transcultural Nursing

Jennifer A. Specht, PhD, RN
Assistant Professor
Department of Nursing
Moravian College
Bethlehem, Pennsylvania

Chapter 5: Adult Health and Nutritional Assessment

Karen A. Steffen-Albert, MSN, RN
Clinical Nurse Specialist
Performance Improvement
Thomas Jefferson University Hospital
Philadelphia, Pennsylvania

Chapter 68: Management of Patients With Neurologic Trauma

Cindy L. Stern, MSN, RN, CCRP
Cancer Network Administrator
Abramson Cancer Center
University of Pennsylvania
Philadelphia, Pennsylvania

Chapter 15: Oncology: Nursing Management in Cancer Care

Candice Jean Sullivan, MSN, RNC, LCCE
Education Coordinator
Inova Learning Network
Inova Health System
Falls Church, Virginia

Chapter 56: Assessment and Management of Female Physiologic Processes

Mary Laudon Thomas, MS, RN
Associate Clinical Professor
Physiological Nursing
University of California
San Francisco, California

Chapter 32: Assessment of Hematologic Function and Treatment Modalities
Chapter 33: Management of Patients With Nonmalignant Hematologic Disorders
Chapter 34: Management of Patients With Hematologic Neoplasms

Lauren M. Weaver, MS, RN, CNS, ACNP, CCRN, CCNS
Advanced Heart Failure Nurse Practitioner
MedStar Washington Hospital Center
Washington, DC

Chapter 28: Management of Patients With Structural, Infectious, and Inflammatory Cardiac Disorders

Kristin Weitmann, MSN, RN, ACNP
Acute Care Nurse Practitioner
Cardiovascular Surgery
Aurora St. Luke's Medical Center
Milwaukee, Wisconsin

Chapter 27: Management of Patients With Coronary Vascular Disorders
Chapter 29: Management of Patients With Complications From
*   Heart Disease*

Iris Woodard, BSN, RN-CS, ANP
Nurse Practitioner
Department of Dermatology
Kaiser Permanente Mid-Atlantic States
Rockville, Maryland

Chapter 60: Assessment of Integumentary Function
Chapter 61: Management of Patients With Dermatologic Problems

Reviewers

Joyette L. Aiken, MScN, RN, ORN, RM
Lecturer
University of the West Indies, Mona
Kingston, Jamaica, West Indies

Terra Baughman, MSN, RN
Assistant Professor of Nursing
Ivy Tech Community College,
    Greencastle
Greencastle, Indiana

Jane Benedict, MSN, RN, CNE
Associate Professor of Nursing
Pennsylvania College of Technology
Williamsport, Pennsylvania

Jean S. Bernard, MSN, RN
Associate Professor, Fort Sanders
    Nursing Department
Tennessee Wesleyan College
Knoxville, Tennessee

Joyel Brule, PhD, MSN, RN, ACNS-BC
Nurse Educator
Bay de Noc Community College
Escanaba, Michigan

Milagros Cartagena-Cook, MSN, RN
Associate Professor, Nursing
Tompkins Cortland Community
    College
Dryden, New York

Erin M. Cattoor, MSN, RN
Clinical Assistant Professor of
    Nursing
Maryville University
Saint Louis, Missouri

Julie C. Chew, PhD, MS, RN
Faculty
Mohave Community College
Colorado City, Arizona

Sandra Croasdell, BBA, BSN,
    MSNE, MSN
Lead Faculty for Advanced Medical
    Surgical Nursing
Bay de Noc Community College
Escanaba, Michigan

Jane F. deLeon, PhD, RN
Assistant Professor
San Francisco State University
San Francisco, California

Lorraine Emeghebo, EdD, RN
Molloy College
Rockville Centre, New York

Susan R. Evancho, DNP, RN
Nursing Faculty
Bridgeport Hospital School of
    Nursing
Bridgeport, Connecticut

Diane M. Evans-Prior, MSN, RN
Nursing Program Director
Central New Mexico Community
    College
Albuquerque, New Mexico

Lisa Foertsch, MSN, RN
Instructor
University of Pittsburgh School of
    Nursing
Pittsburgh, Pennsylvania

Deborah Gielowski, BS, MS
Professor of Nursing
Buffalo, New York

Tammy Greathouse, MSN, RN
Faculty, Health Science Institute
Metropolitan Community
    College–Penn Valley
Kansas City, Missouri

Anne D. Green, MSN, RN
Nursing Instructor
Keiser University
Melbourne, Florida

Sue Greenfield, PhD, MS, CRNA
Associate Professor
Columbia University
New York, New York

Laura Greep, MS, RN
Faculty
Maricopa Community Colleges
Scottsdale, Arizona

Annette L. Griffin, MSN, MBA, RN
Assistant Professor of Nursing
Rhode Island College
Providence, Rhode Island

Anna Gryczman, DNP, RN, AHN-BC
Nurse Educator
Century College
White Bear Lake, Minnesota

Wade Hagan, PhD, RN, PHN, CCRN
Associate Professor of Nursing
Mt. San Jacinto College
Menifee, California

Katherine C. Hall, MSN, RN-BC
Assistant Professor of Nursing
Northeast State Community College
Kingsport, Tennessee

Tamara L. Hall, BSN, MSN, RN
Assistant Professor, Nursing Faculty
Ivy Tech Community College,
    Madison Campus
Madison, Indiana

Anissa Harris-Smith, MSN, RN
Assistant Professor
Broward College, Central Campus
Davie, Florida

Melissa Hladek, APRN, FNP-BC
Family Nurse Practitioner
Unity Health Care, Inc.
Washington, DC

Marie J. Hunter, BSN, MSN
Faculty, Nursing Department
Utah Valley University
Orem, Utah

Catherine Jamaris-Stauts, MSN, RN
Associate Professor
Community College of Baltimore County
Catonsville, Maryland

Karen Jilot-Elick, MSN
Associate Professor, Program Chair in
    Nursing
Ivy Tech Community College,
    Bloomington
Bloomington, Indiana

Heather Johnson, MS, ANP, RN
Director, Associate Degree Program
Helene Fuld College of Nursing
New York, New York

Janice Jones, PhD, RN, CS
Clinical Professor
University at Buffalo, School of Nursing
Buffalo, New York

Barbara Kennedy, MS, AAS, BS
Assistant Professor
Nassau Community College
Garden City, New York

Preface

The 1st edition of *Brunner & Suddarth's Textbook of Medical-Surgical Nursing* was published in 1964 under the leadership of Lillian Sholtis Brunner and Doris Smith Suddarth. Lillian and Doris pioneered a medical-surgical nursing textbook that has become a trusted learning resource. Lillian and Doris chose Suzanne Smeltzer and Brenda Bare as their successors. For several decades, Suzanne and Brenda continued the legacy of medical-surgical nursing excellence established by Lillian and Doris, meticulously supervising all updates and revisions for subsequent editions of this textbook. Suzanne and Brenda, in turn, served as our mentors for the past several editions of this textbook and have passed that legacy of excellence on to us. The result of the seamless and meticulous succession planning for editorship of this textbook is this new 13th edition.

Medical-surgical nursing has significantly advanced since 1964 but continues to be strongly influenced by the expansion of a host of other disciplines and new developments in technology, as well as myriad social, cultural, economic, and environmental changes throughout the world. In today's environment, nurses must be particularly skilled in critical thinking and clinical decision making, as well as in consulting and collaborating with other members of the multidisciplinary health care team.

Along with the challenges that today's nurses confront, there are many opportunities to provide skilled, compassionate nursing care in a variety of health care settings, for patients in the various stages of illness, and for patients across the age continuum. At the same time, there are significant opportunities for fostering health promotion activities for individuals and groups; this is an integral part of providing nursing care.

Continuing the tradition of the first 12 editions, this 13th edition of *Brunner & Suddarth's Textbook of Medical-Surgical Nursing* has evolved to prepare nurses to think critically and practice collaboratively within today's challenging and complex health care delivery system. The textbook focuses on physiologic, pathophysiologic, and psychosocial concepts as they relate to nursing care, and emphasis is placed on integrating a variety of concepts from other disciplines such as nutrition, pharmacology, and gerontology. Content relative to health care needs of people with disabilities, nursing research findings, ethical considerations, evidence-based practice, bariatrics, and prioritization has been expanded to provide opportunities for the nurse to refine clinical decision making skills.

Organization

Brunner & Suddarth's Textbook of Medical-Surgical Nursing, 13th edition, is organized into 17 units. These units mirror those found in previous editions with the incorporation of some changes. Content was streamlined throughout all units, with cross-references to specific chapters included as appropriate. Units 1 through 4 cover core concepts related to

medical-surgical nursing practice. Units 5 through 17 discuss adult health conditions that are treated medically or surgically. The sequential ordering of some of these units was changed so that they dovetailed more logically with each other. For instance, the musculoskeletal unit (Unit 9) follows the immunologic unit (Unit 8) so that coverage of rheumatic disorders precedes coverage of orthopedic disorders. Hematologic disorders are now no longer presented in a chapter within the cardiovascular unit but have been expanded into a separate unit with three chapters organized consistently with other units focused on adult health conditions. Each of these units is structured in the following way to better facilitate comprehension:

- The first chapter in the unit covers assessment and includes a review of normal anatomy and physiology of the body system being discussed.
- Subsequent chapters in the unit cover management of specific disorders. Pathophysiology, clinical manifestations, assessment and diagnostic findings, medical management, and nursing management are presented. Nursing Process sections, provided for selected conditions, clarify and expand on the nurse's role in caring for patients with these conditions.

Special Features

When caring for patients, nurses assume many different roles, including practitioner, educator, advocate, and researcher. Many of the features in this textbook have been developed to help nurses fulfill these varied roles. Key updates to practice-oriented features in the 13th edition include new unit-opening Case Studies and QSEN Competency Focus—a feature that highlights a competency from the Quality and Safety Education for Nurses (QSEN) Institute that is applicable to the case study and poses questions for students to consider about relevant knowledge, skills, and attitudes (KSAs). New Obesity Considerations icons identify content related to obesity or to the nursing care of obese patients. In addition, Quality and Safety Nursing Alerts, Genetics in Nursing Practice charts, and Ethical Dilemma charts offer updated formats and information.

The text also provides pedagogical features developed to help readers engage and learn critical content. New to this edition are Concept Mastery Alerts, which clarify fundamental nursing concepts to improve the reader's understanding of potentially confusing topics, as identified by Misconception Alerts in Lippincott's Adaptive Learning Powered by PrepU. Data from hundreds of actual students using this program in medical-surgical courses across the United States identified common misconceptions for the authors to clarify in this new feature. In addition, prioritization questions have also been added to chapter-ending Critical Thinking Exercises. An enhanced suite of online, interactive multimedia resources is also highlighted with icons placed in text near relevant topics.

Read the User's Guide that follows the Preface for a full explanation and visual representation of all special features.

A Comprehensive Package for Teaching and Learning

To further facilitate teaching and learning, a carefully designed ancillary package has been developed to assist faculty and students.

Instructor Resources

Tools to assist you with teaching your course are available upon adoption of this text on thePoint at http://thePoint.lww.com/Brunner13e.

- A thoroughly revised and augmented **Test Generator** contains more than 2,900 NCLEX-style questions mapped to chapter learning objectives.
- An extensive collection of materials is provided for each book chapter:
  - **Lesson Plans** outline learning objectives and identify relevant resources from the robust instructor and student resource packages to help you prepare for your class.
  - **Pre-Lecture Quizzes** (and answers) allow you to check students' reading.
  - **PowerPoint Presentations** provide an easy way to integrate the textbook with your students' classroom experience; multiple-choice and true/false questions are included to promote class participation.
  - **Guided Lecture Notes** are organized by objective and provide corresponding PowerPoint slide numbers to simplify preparation for lecture.
  - **Discussion Topics** (and suggested answers) can be used in the classroom or in online discussion boards to facilitate interaction with your students.
  - **Assignments** (and suggested answers) include group, written, clinical, and Web assignments to engage students in varied activities and assess their learning.
  - **Case Studies** with related questions (and suggested answers) give students an opportunity to apply their knowledge to a client case similar to one they might encounter in practice.
  - Sample **Syllabi** are provided for one- and two-semester courses.
  - A **QSEN Competency Map** identifies content and special features in the book related to competencies identified by the QSEN Institute.
  - An **Image Bank** lets you use the photographs and illustrations from this textbook in your course materials.
  - **Strategies for Effective Teaching** provides general tips for instructors related to preparing course materials and meeting student needs.
  - Access to all **Student Resources** is provided so that you can understand the student experience and use these resources in your course as well.

Student Resources

An exciting set of free learning resources is available on thePoint to help students review and apply vital concepts in medical-surgical nursing. For the 13th edition, multimedia engines have been optimized so that students can access many of these resources on mobile devices. Students can activate the codes printed in the front of their textbooks at http://thePoint.lww.com/activate to access these resources:

- **NCLEX-Style Review Questions** for each chapter, totaling more than 1,800 questions, help students review important concepts and practice for NCLEX.
- Interactive learning resources appeal to a variety of learning styles. Icons in the text direct readers to relevant resources:
  - **Concepts in Action Animations** bring physiologic and pathophysiologic concepts to life.
  - **Interactive Tutorials** review key information for common or complex medical-surgical conditions. Tutorials include graphics and animations and provide interactive review exercises as well as case-based questions.
  - **Practice & Learn Case Studies** present case scenarios and offer interactive exercises and questions to help students apply what they have learned.
  - **Watch & Learn Video Clips** reinforce skills from the textbook and appeal to visual and auditory learners. With the 13th edition, all content from *Lippincott's Video Series for Brunner & Suddarth's Textbook of Medical-Surgical Nursing* is included!
- A **Spanish–English Audio Glossary** provides helpful terms and phrases for communicating with patients who speak Spanish.
- **Journal Articles** offer access to current articles relevant to each chapter and available in Lippincott Williams & Wilkins journals to familiarize students with nursing literature.

Study Guide

A comprehensive study aid for reviewing key concepts, *Study Guide for Brunner & Suddarth's Textbook of Medical-Surgical Nursing,* 13th edition, has been thoroughly revised and presents a variety of exercises, including case studies and practice NCLEX-style questions, to reinforce textbook content and enhance learning.

Quick Reference Tools

Clinical Handbook for Brunner & Suddarth's Textbook of Medical-Surgical Nursing, 13th edition, presents need-to-know information on nearly 200 commonly encountered disorders in an easy-to-use, alphabetized outline format that is perfect for quick access to vital information in the clinical setting. *Brunner & Suddarth's Handbook of Laboratory and Diagnostic Tests*, 2nd edition, includes a review of specimen collection procedures followed by a concise, alphabetical presentation of tests and their implications. Information for each test includes reference values or normal findings, abnormal findings and related nursing implications, critical values, purpose, description, interfering factors, precautions, and nursing considerations.

Both quick references are available in print or e-book format. An enhanced e-book format is available to facilitate mobile use for on-the-go reference. For more information on these two quick references and available formats, please visit thePoint, http://thePoint.lww.com.

Adaptive Learning Powered by PrepU

Updated to accompany the 13th edition, Lippincott's Adaptive Learning Powered by PrepU helps every student learn more, while giving instructors the data they need to monitor each student's progress, strengths, and weaknesses. The adaptive learning system allows instructors to assign quizzes or students to take quizzes on their own that adapt to each student's individual mastery level. Visit thePoint at http://thePoint.lww.com/PrepU to learn more.

Computer Simulations

Lippincott | Laerdal Computer Simulations for Medical-Surgical Nursing offers innovative scenario-based learning modules consisting of Web-based virtual simulations, course learning materials, and curriculum tools designed to develop critical thinking skills and promote clinical confidence and competence. The Computer Simulations for Medical-Surgical Nursing include 10 virtual simulations based on the National League for Nursing Volume I Complex patient scenarios. Students can progress through suggested readings, pre- and post-simulation assessments, documentation assignments, and guided reflection questions, and will receive an individualized feedback log immediately upon completion of the simulation. Throughout the student learning experience, the product offers remediation back to trusted Lippincott resources, including *Brunner & Suddarth's Textbook of Medical-Surgical Nursing,* as well as Lippincott's Nursing Advisor and Lippincott's Nursing Procedures and Skills—two online, evidence-based, clinical information solutions used in health care facilities throughout the United States. This innovative product provides a comprehensive patient-focused solution for learning and integrating simulation into the classroom.

Contact your Lippincott Williams & Wilkins sales representative or visit thePoint, http://thePoint.lww.com, for options to enhance your medical-surgical nursing course with Computer Simulation.

A Comprehensive, Digital, Integrated Course Solution

Lippincott's CoursePoint is the only integrated digital course solution for nursing education, combining the power of digital course content, interactive resources, Adaptive Learning Powered by PrepU, and Computer Simulation. Pulling these resources together into one solution, the integrated product offers a seamless experience for learning, studying, applying, and remediating.

Lippincott's CoursePoint provides a personalized learning experience that is structured in the way students study. It drives students to immediate remediation in their text; digital course content and interactive course resources like case studies, videos, and journal articles are also immediately available in the same digitally integrated course solution to help expand on concepts and bring them to life. After students complete an adaptive, formative assessment on the reading, the results identify students' specific weaknesses, and at the moment it's identified they don't understand, they can immediately remediate to that content. Instructors also have a powerful and measurable way to assess their students' understanding and to help engage them in the course content. Knowing where students are struggling, instructors can adapt class time as appropriate.

Lippincott's CoursePoint can bring Adaptive Learning Powered by PrepU and Computer Simulations together on the same platform to provide all of the resources that students need to study more effectively, score higher on exams, and prepare for clinical practice. The SmartSense links feature included throughout CoursePoint integrates all of the content, offering immediate remediation and additional learning resources at the click of a mouse. Similarly, in Computer Simulations, students receive feedback with remediation to the digital course content and other trusted Lippincott resources. With Lippincott's CoursePoint, instructors can collaborate with students at any time, identify common misunderstandings, evaluate student comprehension, and differentiate instruction as needed. And students can learn and retain course material in an adaptive, personalized way. This unique offering creates an unparalleled learning experience for students.

Contact your Lippincott Williams & Wilkins sales representative or visit thePoint, http://thePoint.lww.com/course pointbrunner13, for more information about Lippincott's CoursePoint solution.

It is with pleasure that we introduce these resources—the textbook, ancillary resources, and additional supplements and learning tools—to you. One of our primary goals in creating these resources has been to help nurses and nursing students provide quality care to patients and families across health care settings and in the home. We hope that we have succeeded in that goal, and we welcome feedback from our readers.

Janice L. Hinkle, PhD, RN, CNRN
Kerry H. Cheever, PhD, RN

Nursing diagnoses in text are from Herdman, T. H. (Ed.). *Nursing Diagnoses: Definitions and Classification 2012–2014.* Copyright © 2012, 1994–2012 by NANDA International. Used by arrangement with John Wiley & Sons Limited. In order to make safe and effective judgments using NANDA-I nursing diagnoses, it is essential that nurses refer to the definitions and defining characteristics of the diagnoses listed in this work.

User's Guide

Brunner & Suddarth's Textbook of Medical-Surgical Nursing, 13th edition, has been revised and updated to reflect the complex nature of nursing practice today. This textbook includes many features to help you gain and apply the knowledge that you need to pass NCLEX and successfully meet the challenges and opportunities of clinical practice. In addition, features have been developed specifically to help you fulfill the varied roles that nurses assume in practice.

Opening Features That Start With the End in Mind

Unit opening features put the patient first and highlight competent nursing as well as application of the nursing process.

- **New! A Case Study with QSEN Competency Focus** opens each unit and provides discussion points focusing on one competency from the QSEN Institute: patient-centered care, interdisciplinary teamwork and collaboration, evidence-based practice, quality improvement, safety, and informatics. This feature helps you consider the KSAs required for the delivery of safe, quality patient care.

- **Applying Concepts from NANDA-I, NIC, and NOC** offers additional online case study content on nursing classifications and language (NANDA-I, NIC, and NOC) as well as concept maps illustrating the nursing process.

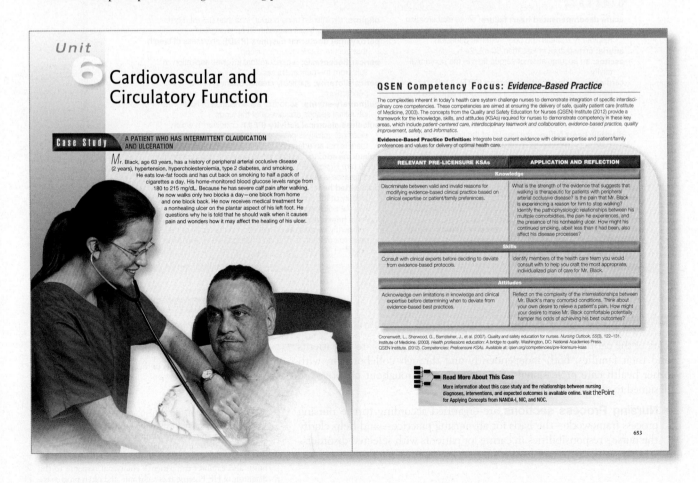

Chapter-opening pedagogical features help organize learning.

- **Learning Objectives** give an overview of each chapter and identify learning goals to help focus reading and studying.

- A **Glossary** provides a list of key terms and definitions at the beginning of each chapter, providing a review of vocabulary words before reading the material and a useful reference and study tool.

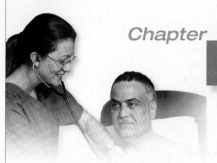

Chapter 29

Management of Patients With Complications From Heart Disease

Learning Objectives

On completion of this chapter, the learner will be able to:

1 Describe the management of patients with heart failure.
2 Use the nursing process as a framework for care of patients with heart failure.
3 Develop an education plan for patients with heart failure.

4 Describe the medical and nursing management of patients with pulmonary edema.
5 Describe the medical and nursing management of patients with thromboembolism, pericardial effusion, and cardiac arrest.

Glossary

acute decompensated heart failure: acute exacerbation of heart failure, with signs and symptoms of severe respiratory distress and poor systemic perfusion

anuria: urine output of less than 50 mL/24 h

ascites: an accumulation of serous fluid in the peritoneal cavity

cardiac resynchronization therapy (CRT): a treatment for heart failure in which a device paces both ventricles to synchronize contractions

congestive heart failure (CHF): a fluid overload condition (congestion) associated with heart failure

diastolic heart failure: the inability of the heart to pump sufficiently because of an alteration in the ability of the heart to fill; term used to describe a type of heart failure

ejection fraction (EF): percentage of blood volume in the ventricles at the end of diastole that is ejected during systole; a measurement of contractility

heart failure (HF): a clinical syndrome resulting from structural or functional cardiac disorders that impair the ability of a ventricle to fill or eject blood

left-sided heart failure (left ventricular failure): inability of the left ventricle to fill or eject sufficient blood into the systemic circulation

oliguria: diminished urine output; less than 0.5 mL/kg/hr

orthopnea: shortness of breath when laying flat

paroxysmal nocturnal dyspnea (PND): shortness of breath that occurs suddenly during sleep

pericardiocentesis: procedure that involves aspiration of fluid from the pericardial sac

pericardiotomy: surgically created opening of the pericardium

pulmonary edema: abnormal accumulation of fluid in the interstitial spaces and alveoli of the lungs

pulseless electrical activity (PEA): condition in which electrical activity is present on an electrocardiogram, but there is not an adequate pulse or blood pressure

pulsus paradoxus: systolic blood pressure that is more than 10 mm Hg lower during inhalation than during exhalation; difference is normally less than 10 mm Hg

right-sided heart failure (right ventricular failure): inability of the right ventricle to fill or eject sufficient blood into the pulmonary circulation

systolic heart failure: inability of the heart to pump sufficiently because of an alteration in the ability of the heart to contract; term used to describe a type of heart failure

Features to Develop the Nurse as Practitioner

One of the central roles of the nurse is to provide holistic care to patients and their families, both independently and through collaboration with other health care professionals. Special features throughout chapters are designed to assist readers with clinical practice.

- **Nursing Process sections** are organized according to the nursing process framework—the basis for all nursing practice—and help clarify the nurse's responsibilities in caring for patients with selected disorders.

NURSING PROCESS

The Patient With Heart Failure

Despite advances in treatment of HF, morbidity and mortality remain high. Nurses have a major impact on outcomes for patients with HF, especially in the areas of patient education and monitoring.

Assessment

Nursing assessment for the patient with HF focuses on observing for effectiveness of therapy and for the patient's ability to understand and implement self-management strategies. Signs and symptoms of increasing HF are analyzed and reported to the patient's provider so that therapy can be adjusted. The nurse also explores the patient's emotional response to the diagnosis of HF, because it is a chronic and often progressive condition that is commonly associated with depression and other psychosocial issues (Pressler, Subramanian, Perkins, et al., 2011; Sherwood, Blumenthal, Hinderliter, et al., 2011).

- **Plans of Nursing Care**, provided for selected disorders, illustrate how the nursing process is applied to meet the patient's health care and nursing needs.

Chart 27-11

PLAN OF NURSING CARE
Care of the Patient With an Uncomplicated Myocardial Infarction

NURSING DIAGNOSIS: Ineffective cardiac tissue perfusion related to reduced coronary blood flow
GOAL: Relief of chest pain/discomfort

Nursing Interventions	Rationale	Expected Outcomes

1. Initially assess, document, and report to the physician the following:
 	
a. The patient's description of chest discomfort, including location, intensity, radiation, duration, and factors that affect it; other symptoms such as nausea, diaphoresis, or complaints of unusual fatigue
b. The effect of coronary ischemia on perfusion to the heart (e.g., change in blood pressure, heart rhythm), to the brain (e.g., changes in level of consciousness), to the kidneys (e.g., decrease in urine output), and to the skin (e.g., color, temperature)
2. Obtain a 12-lead ECG recording during symptomatic events, as prescribed, to assess for ongoing ischemia.
3. Administer oxygen as prescribed.
 	
4. Administer medication therapy as prescribed, and evaluate the patient's response continuously.
 	
5. Ensure physical rest: head of bed elevated to promote comfort; diet as tolerated; the use of bedside commode; the use of stool softener to prevent straining at stool. Provide a restful environment, and allay fears and anxiety by being calm and supportive. Individualize visitation, based on patient response.
	1. These data assist in determining the cause and effect of the chest discomfort and provide a baseline with which post-therapy symptoms can be compared.
	a. There are many conditions associated with chest discomfort. There are characteristic clinical findings of ischemic pain and symptoms.
	
	b. Myocardial infarction (MI) decreases myocardial contractility and ventricular compliance and may produce dysrhythmias. Cardiac output is reduced, resulting in reduced blood pressure and decreased organ perfusion.
	
	2. An ECG during symptoms may be useful in the diagnosis of ongoing ischemia.
	3. Oxygen therapy increases the oxygen supply to the myocardium.
	4. Medication therapy (nitroglycerin, morphine, beta-blocker, aspirin) is the first line of defense in preserving myocardial tissue.
	5. Physical rest reduces myocardial oxygen consumption. Fear and anxiety precipitate the stress response; this results in increased levels of endogenous catecholamines, which increase myocardial oxygen consumption.
		• Reports beginning relief of chest discomfort and symptoms
		• Appears comfortable and is free of pain and other signs or symptoms
		• Respiratory rate, cardiac rate, and blood pressure return to prediscomfort level
		• Skin warm and dry
		• Adequate cardiac output as evidenced by:
		  • Stable/improving electrocardiogram (ECG)
		  • Heart rate and rhythm
		  • Blood pressure
		  • Mentation
		  • Urine output
		  • Serum blood urea nitrogen (BUN) and creatinine
		  • Skin color and temperature
		• No adverse effects from medications

- **Assessment charts** focus on data that should be collected as part of the assessment step of the nursing process.

- **Risk Factors charts** outline factors that can impair health.

Chart 29-1

ASSESSMENT
Heart Failure

Be alert for the following signs and symptoms:

Congestion

- Dyspnea
- Orthopnea
- Paroxysmal nocturnal dyspnea
- Cough (recumbent or exertional)
- Pulmonary crackles that do not clear with cough
- Weight gain (rapid)
- Dependent edema
- Abdominal bloating or discomfort
- Ascites
- Jugular venous distention
- Sleep disturbance (anxiety or air hunger)
- Fatigue

Chart 27-1

RISK FACTORS
Coronary Artery Disease

A nonmodifiable risk factor is a circumstance over which a person has no control. A modifiable risk factor is one over which a person may exercise control, such as by changing a lifestyle or personal habit or by using medication. A risk factor may operate independently or in tandem with other risk factors. The more risk factors a person has, the greater the likelihood of coronary artery disease (CAD). Those at risk are advised to seek regular medical examinations and to engage in heart-healthy behavior (a deliberate effort to reduce the number and extent of risks).

Nonmodifiable Risk Factors

Family history of CAD (first-degree relative with cardiovascular disease at 55 years of age or younger for men and at 65 years of age or younger for women)

Increasing age (more than 45 years for men; more than 55 years for women)

• **Guidelines charts** review key nursing interventions and rationales for specific patient care situations.

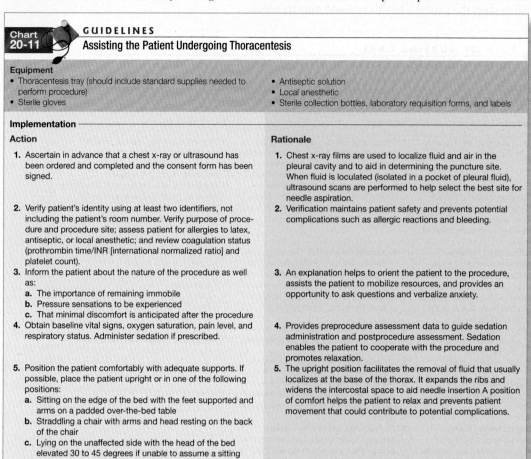

Chart 20-11

GUIDELINES

Assisting the Patient Undergoing Thoracentesis

Equipment
• Thoracentesis tray (should include standard supplies needed to perform procedure)
• Sterile gloves
• Antiseptic solution
• Local anesthetic
• Sterile collection bottles, laboratory requisition forms, and labels

Implementation

Action	Rationale
1. Ascertain in advance that a chest x-ray or ultrasound has been ordered and completed and the consent form has been signed.	1. Chest x-ray films are used to localize fluid and air in the pleural cavity and to aid in determining the puncture site. When fluid is loculated (isolated in a pocket of pleural fluid), ultrasound scans are performed to help select the best site for needle aspiration.
2. Verify patient's identity using at least two identifiers, not including the patient's room number. Verify purpose of procedure and procedure site; assess patient for allergies to latex, antiseptic, or local anesthetic; and review coagulation status (prothrombin time/INR [international normalized ratio] and platelet count).	2. Verification maintains patient safety and prevents potential complications such as allergic reactions and bleeding.
3. Inform the patient about the nature of the procedure as well as: a. The importance of remaining immobile b. Pressure sensations to be experienced c. That minimal discomfort is anticipated after the procedure	3. An explanation helps to orient the patient to the procedure, assists the patient to mobilize resources, and provides an opportunity to ask questions and verbalize anxiety.
4. Obtain baseline vital signs, oxygen saturation, pain level, and respiratory status. Administer sedation if prescribed.	4. Provides preprocedure assessment data to guide sedation administration and postprocedure assessment. Sedation enables the patient to cooperate with the procedure and promotes relaxation.
5. Position the patient comfortably with adequate supports. If possible, place the patient upright or in one of the following positions: a. Sitting on the edge of the bed with the feet supported and arms on a padded over-the-bed table b. Straddling a chair with arms and head resting on the back of the chair c. Lying on the unaffected side with the head of the bed elevated 30 to 45 degrees if unable to assume a sitting position	5. The upright position facilitates the removal of fluid that usually localizes at the base of the thorax. It expands the ribs and widens the intercostal space to aid needle insertion A position of comfort helps the patient to relax and prevents patient movement that could contribute to potential complications.

• **Pharmacology charts and tables** display important considerations related to administering medications and monitoring drug therapy.

TABLE 29-3   Common Medications Used to Treat Heart Failure

Medication	Therapeutic Effects	Key Nursing Conside
Angiotensin-Converting Enzyme Inhibitors		
Lisinopril (Prinivil) Enalapril (Vasotec)	↓ BP and ↓ afterload Relieves signs and symptoms of HF Prevents progression of HF	Observe for symptoma and worsening rena
Angiotensin Receptor Blockers		
Valsartan (Diovan) Losartan (Cozaar)	↓ BP and ↓ afterload Relieves signs and symptoms of HF Prevents progression of HF	Observe for symptoma worsening renal fun
Hydralazine and Isosorbide Dinitrate (Dilatrate)	Dilates blood vessels ↓ BP and ↓ afterload	Observe for symptoma
Beta-Adrenergic Blocking Agents (Beta-Blockers)		
Metoprolol (Lopressor) Carvedilol (Coreg)	Dilates blood vessels and ↓ afterload ↓ Signs and symptoms of HF Improves exercise capacity	Observe for decreased dizziness, and fatigu

Chart 29-2

PHARMACOLOGY

Administering and Monitoring Diuretic Therapy

When nursing care involves diuretic therapy for conditions such as heart failure, the nurse needs to administer the medication and monitor the patient's response carefully, as follows:

• Prior to administration of the diuretic, check laboratory results for electrolyte depletion, especially potassium, sodium, and magnesium.
• Prior to administration of the diuretic, check for signs and symptoms of volume depletion, such as postural hypotension, lightheadedness, and dizziness.
• Administer the diuretic at a time conducive to the patient's lifestyle—for example, early in the day to avoid nocturia.
• Monitor urine output during the hours after administration, and analyze intake, output, and daily weights to assess response.
• Continue to monitor serum electrolytes for depletion. Replace potassium with increased oral intake of food rich in potassium or potassium supplements. Replace magnesium as needed.
• Monitor for hyperkalemia in patients receiving potassium-sparing diuretics.
• Continue to assess for signs of volume depletion.
• Monitor creatinine for increased levels indicative of renal dysfunction.
• Monitor for elevated uric acid level and signs and symptoms of gout.
• Assess lungs sounds and edema to evaluate response to therapy.
• Monitor for adverse reactions such as gastrointestinal distress and dysrhythmias.
• Encourage supine position after dose is given to facilitate effects of the diuretic.
• Assist patients to manage urinary frequency and urgency associated with diuretic therapy.

• *Updated!* **Quality and Safety Nursing Alerts** offer tips for best clinical practice and red-flag safety warnings to help avoid common mistakes.

 Quality and Safety Nursing Alert

Patients placed on continuous ECG monitoring must be informed of its purpose and cautioned that it does not detect shortness of breath, chest pain, or other ACS symptoms. Thus, patients are instructed to report new or worsening symptoms immediately.

• **Critical Care icons** identify nursing considerations for the critically ill patient.

 Surgical Procedures: Coronary Artery Revascularization

Advances in diagnostics, medical management, and surgical and anesthesia techniques, as well as the care provided in critical care and surgical units, home care, and rehabilitation programs, have continued to make surgery an effective treatment option for patients with CAD. CAD has been treated by myocardial revascularization since the 1960s, and the most common CABG techniques have been performed for more than 40 years. **Coronary artery bypass graft (CABG)** is a surgical procedure in which a blood vessel is grafted to an

• **Genetics in Nursing Practice charts** summarize and highlight nursing assessments and management issues related to the role of genetics in selected disorders.

Chart 25-1 **GENETICS IN NURSING PRACTICE**
Cardiovascular Disorders

Several cardiovascular disorders are associated with genetic abnormalities. Some examples are:
• Familial hypercholesterolemia
• Hypertrophic cardiomyopathy
• Long QT syndrome
• Hereditary hemochromatosis
• Elevated homocysteine levels

Nursing Assessments

Family History Assessment
• Assess all patients with cardiovascular symptoms for coronary artery disease (CAD), regardless of age (early-onset CAD occurs).
• Assess family history of sudden death in people who may or may not have been diagnosed with CAD (especially of early onset).
• Ask about sudden death in a previously asymptomatic child, adolescent, or adult.
• Ask about other family members with biochemical or neuromuscular conditions (e.g., hemochromatosis or muscular dystrophy).

• Assess whether DNA mutation or other genetic testing has been performed on an affected family member.

Patient Assessment
• Assess for signs and symptoms of hyperlipidemias (xanthomas, corneal arcus, abdominal pain of unexplained origin).
• Assess for muscular weakness.

Management Issues Sp
• If indicated, refer for further g so that the family can discus members, and availability of based interventions.
• Offer appropriate genetic inf Genetic Alliance Web site, A
• Provide support to families n related cardiovascular diseas

Genetics Resources
See Chapter 8, Chart 8-6 for g

• **New! Obesity Considerations icons** identify content related to obesity or to the nursing care of patients who are obese.

 Bariatric Patients

Bariatrics has to do with patients who are obese. Like age, obesity increases the risk and severity of complications associated with surgery. During surgery, fatty tissues are especially susceptible to infection. Wound infections are more common in the obese patient (Haupt & Reed, 2010). Obesity also increases technical and mechanical problems related to surgery, such as dehiscence (wound separation). It may be more challenging to provide care for the patient who is obese owing

• **Gerontologic Considerations**, identified with an icon applied to headings, charts, and tables, highlight information that pertains specifically to the care of the older adult patient. In the United States, older adults comprise the fastest-growing segment of the population.

Chart 14-1 **Recognizing Shock in Older Patients**

The physiologic changes associated with aging, coupled with pathologic and chronic disease states, place older people at increased risk for developing a state of shock and possibly multiple organ dysfunction syndrome. Older adults can recover from shock if it is detected and treated early with aggressive and supportive therapies. Nurses play an essential role in assessing and interpreting subtle changes in older patients' responses to illness.
• Medications such as beta-blocking agents (metoprolol [Lopressor]) used to treat hypertension may mask tachycardia, a primary compensatory mechanism to increase cardiac output, during hypovolemic states.
• The aging immune system may not mount a truly febrile response (temperature greater than 38°C [100.4°F]); however, a lack of a febrile response (temperature less than 37°C [98.6°F]) or an increasing trend in body temperature should be addressed. The patient may also report increased fatigue and malaise in the absence of a febrile response.
• The heart does not function well in hypoxemic states, and the aging heart may respond to decreased myocardial oxygenation with dysrhythmias that may be misinterpreted as a normal part of the aging process.
• There is a progressive decline in respiratory muscle strength, maximal ventilation, and response to hypoxia. Older patients have a decreased respiratory reserve and decompensate more quickly.
• Changes in mentation may be inappropriately misinterpreted as dementia. Older people with a sudden change in mentation should be aggressively assessed for acute delirium and treated for the presence of infection and organ hypoperfusion.

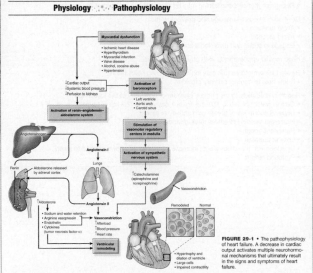

FIGURE 29-1 • The pathophysiology of heart failure. A decrease in cardiac output activates multiple neurohormonal mechanisms that ultimately result in the signs and symptoms of heart failure.

• **Physiology/Pathophysiology figures** include illustrations and algorithms describing normal physiologic and pathophysiologic processes.

Features to Develop the Nurse as Educator

Health education is a primary responsibility of the nursing profession. Nursing care is directed toward promoting, maintaining, and restoring health; preventing illness; and helping patients and families adapt to the residual effects of illness. Patient education and health promotion are central to all of these nursing activities.

- **Patient Education charts** help the nurse prepare the patient and family for procedures, assist them in understanding the patient's condition, and explain to them how to provide self-care.

PATIENT EDUCATION

Chart 25-6

Self-Management After Cardiac Catheterization

After discharge from the hospital for cardiac catheterization, patients should follow these guidelines for self-care:

- *If the artery in your arm or wrist artery was used:* For the next 48 hours, avoid lifting anything heavier than 5 pounds and avoid repetitive movement of your affected hand and wrist.
- *If the artery in your groin was used:* For the next 24 hours, do not bend at the waist, strain, or lift heavy objects.
- Do not submerge the puncture site in water. Avoid tub baths, but shower as desired.
- Talk with your primary provider about when you may return to work, drive, or resume strenuous activities.
- If bleeding occurs, sit (arm or wrist approach) or lie down (groin approach) and apply firm pressure to the puncture site for 10 minutes. Notify your primary provider as soon as possible and follow instructions. If there is a large amount of bleeding, call 911. Do not drive to the hospital.

- Call your primary provider if any of the following occur: swelling, new bruising or pain from your procedure puncture site, temperature of 101°F or more.
- If test results show that you have coronary artery disease, talk with your primary provider about options for treatment, including cardiac rehabilitation programs in your community.
- Talk with your primary provider about lifestyle changes to reduce your risk for further or future heart problems, such as quitting smoking, lowering your cholesterol level, initiating dietary changes, beginning an exercise program, or losing weight.
- Your primary provider may prescribe one or more new medications depending on your risk factors (medications to lower your blood pressure or cholesterol; aspirin or clopidogrel to prevent blood clots). Take all of your medications as instructed. If you feel that any of them are causing side effects, call your primary provider immediately. Do not stop taking any medications before talking to your primary provider.

Adapted from Durham, K. A. (2012). Cardiac catheterization through the radial artery. *American Journal of Nursing, 112*(1), 49–56; and Woods, S. L., Froelicher, E. S., Motzer, S. A., et al. (2009). *Cardiac nursing* (6th ed.). Philadelphia: Lippincott Williams & Wilkins.

- **Home Care Checklists** review points that should be covered as part of home care education prior to discharge from the health care facility.

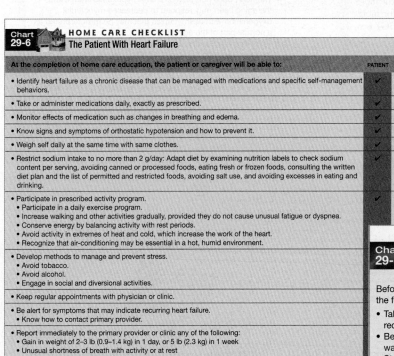

HOME CARE CHECKLIST

Chart 29-6

The Patient With Heart Failure

At the completion of home care education, the patient or caregiver will be able to:	PATIENT	CAREGIVER
• Identify heart failure as a chronic disease that can be managed with medications and specific self-management behaviors.	✓	✓
• Take or administer medications daily, exactly as prescribed.	✓	✓
• Monitor effects of medication such as changes in breathing and edema.	✓	✓
• Know signs and symptoms of orthostatic hypotension and how to prevent it.	✓	✓
• Weigh self daily at the same time with same clothes.	✓	
• Restrict sodium intake to no more than 2 g/day: Adapt diet by examining nutrition labels to check sodium content per serving, avoiding canned or processed foods, eating fresh or frozen foods, consulting the written diet plan and the list of permitted and restricted foods, avoiding salt use, and avoiding excesses in eating and drinking.	✓	
• Participate in prescribed activity program. • Participate in a daily exercise program. • Increase walking and other activities gradually, provided they do not cause unusual fatigue or dyspnea. • Conserve energy by balancing activity with rest periods. • Avoid activity in extremes of heat and cold, which increase the work of the heart. • Recognize that air-conditioning may be essential in a hot, humid environment.	✓	
• Develop methods to manage and prevent stress. • Avoid tobacco. • Avoid alcohol. • Engage in social and diversional activities.		
• Keep regular appointments with physician or clinic.		
• Be alert for symptoms that may indicate recurring heart failure. • Know how to contact primary provider.		
• Report immediately to the primary provider or clinic any of the following: • Gain in weight of 2–3 lb (0.9–1.4 kg) in 1 day, or 5 lb (2.3 kg) in 1 week • Unusual shortness of breath with activity or at rest • Increased swelling of ankles, feet, or abdomen • Persistent cough • Loss of appetite • Development of restless sleep; increase in number of pillows needed to sleep • Profound fatigue		

HEALTH PROMOTION

Chart 29-4

An Exercise Program for Patients With Heart Failure

Before undertaking physical activity, the patient should be given the following guidelines:

- Talk with your primary provider for specific exercise program recommendations.
- Begin with low-impact activities such as walking, cycling, or water exercises.
- Start with warm-up activity followed by sessions that gradually build up to about 30 minutes.
- Follow your exercise period with cool-down activities.
- Avoid performing physical activities outside in extreme hot, cold, or humid weather.
- Wait 2 hours after eating a meal before performing the physical activity.
- Ensure that you are able to talk during the physical activity; if you cannot do so, decrease the intensity of activity.
- Stop the activity if severe shortness of breath, pain, or dizziness develops.

Adapted from Andreuzzi, R. (2010). Does aerobic exercise have a role in the treatment plan of a patient with heart failure. *Internet Journal of American Physician Assistants, 7*(2), 1–29; and Flynn, K. E., Piña, I. L., Whellan, D. J., et al. (2009). Effects of exercise training on health status in patients with chronic heart failure: HF-ACTION randomized controlled trial. *Journal of the American Medical Association, 301*(14), 1451–1459.

- **Health Promotion charts** review important points that the nurse should discuss with the patient to prevent common health problems from developing.

Features to Develop the Nurse as Patient Advocate

Nurses advocate for patients by protecting their rights (including the right to health care) and assisting patients and their families in making informed decisions about health care.

- *Updated!* **Ethical Dilemma charts** provide a clinical scenario, discussion points, and questions to help analyze fundamental ethical principles related to the dilemma.

ETHICAL DILEMMA

Chart 27-9

Should Invasive Therapy Be Recommended for Older Adults With Acute Coronary Syndrome?

Case Scenario

An 80-year-old woman is hospitalized with acute coronary syndrome (ACS). When discussing the situation with her two adult sons, the cardiologist recommends emergent cardiac catheterization with a possible percutaneous coronary intervention (PCI). The patient has full capacity to make her own decisions but wishes to defer decision making to her sons regarding treatment decisions. One son worries that she will be subjected to an invasive procedure that is potentially high risk, painful, expensive, and possibly futile. The second son feels that if there is hope of success, then she should have the procedure.

Discussion

Many patients who present with ACS are older adults. They often have chronic conditions such as diabetes or arthritis. Older patients have traditionally been managed conservatively with medications. Currently, however, invasive interventions such as cardiac catheterization and PCI may be recommended. Indeed, studies suggest that older patients may benefit as much, if not more, than younger patients from coronary reperfusion procedures in terms of reduction of death or myocardial infarction (Ionescu, Amuchastegui, Ionescu, et al., 2010).

Analysis

- Describe the ethical principles that are in conflict in this case (see Chart 3-3). Which principle should have preeminence in recommending the best treatment plan for the patient?
- One son apparently wishes that the patient not be subjected to a procedure that may be futile and painful (wishes to ensure nonmaleficence), whereas the other hopes that the patient has the opportunity for a positive outcome (wishes to assure beneficence). Are these two ethical principles necessarily in conflict with each other in this case? How would you approach the patient and her sons to ensure that they receive the information needed to help them reach consensus regarding the decision that is most consistent in preserving the patient's autonomy?
- What resources are available to help you facilitate this discussion with the patient and her sons?

Reference

Ionescu, C. N., Amuchastegui, M., Ionescu, S., et al. (2010) Treatment and outcomes of nonagenarians with ST-elevation. *Journal of Invasive Cardiology, 22*(10), 479–480.

Resources

See Chapter 3, Chart 3-6 for ethics resources.

Features to Develop the Nurse as Researcher

Nurses identify potential research problems and questions to increase nursing knowledge and improve patient care. The use and evaluation of research findings in nursing practice are essential to further the science of nursing.

- **Nursing Research Profiles** identify the implications and applications of nursing research findings for evidence-based nursing practice.

NURSING RESEARCH PROFILE

Chart 27-14

Aspiration Prevention Protocol: Decreasing Postoperative Pneumonia in Heart Surgery Patients

Starks, B., & Harbert, C. (2011). Aspiration prevention protocol: Decreasing postoperative pneumonia in heart surgery patients. *Critical Care Nurse, 31*(5), 38–45.

Purpose

Postoperative pulmonary dysfunction (including atelectasis and pneumonia) is a frequent cause of morbidity and mortality in patients who have open heart surgery. The purpose of this study was to determine if implementation of an aspiration prevention protocol in patients after cardiac surgery would decrease the incidence of postoperative pneumonia.

Design

An aspiration prevention protocol was developed and implemented in a 24-bed intensive care unit using the Plan-Do-Study-Act Model for quality improvement advocated by the Institute for Healthcare Improvement (IHI). The protocol incorporated extending the time that patients received nothing by mouth from 2 hours to at least 6 hours preoperatively and incorporating a postoperative bedside swallowing evaluation by a speech therapist. After the swallow evaluation was completed, nurses implemented a progressive oral intake protocol. A convenience sample of 79

adult patients who had cardiothoracic surgery from April 2008 through October 2008 were enrolled in the study. Historical controls were used to compare rates of pneumonia.

Findings

The interdisciplinary team of nurses, physicians, administrators, and speech therapists who developed and implemented this protocol set a goal that no patients who participated in this protocol would develop postoperative pneumonia. This goal was met; no study participants (*n* = 79) developed pneumonia. However, 11% of historical controls (*n* = 65) developed postoperative pneumonia.

Nursing Implications

The Plan-Do-Study-Act Model encourages team collaboration between nurses and their interdisciplinary colleagues and results in rapid cycle improvement. These rapid cycle improvements enhance quality patient outcomes and ensure patient safety. The development and implementation of this aspiration prevention protocol expeditiously met an ambitious aim to reduce the rate of postoperative pneumonia in patients who had cardiothoracic surgery to nil.

2 **ebp** You are caring for an 88-year-old man who is hospitalized with a diagnosis of syncope. After ambulating in the hall, he tells you that he is having some chest pain and mild shortness of breath. Based on your knowledge of evidence-based guidelines, identify the initial interventions and diagnostic testing that are indicated for patients with these symptoms. Describe how the diagnosis of acute MI is made. If a diagnosis of STEMI is made, which treatment options may be considered?

- **Evidence-Based Practice questions**, included in the Critical Thinking Exercises sections, encourage you to think about the evidence base for specific nursing interventions.

Features to Facilitate Learning

In addition to practice-oriented features, special features have been developed to help readers learn key information.

- **New! Concept Mastery Alerts** highlight and clarify fundamental nursing concepts to improve understanding of difficult topics, as identified by Misconception Alerts in Lippincott's Adaptive Learning Powered by PrepU, an adaptive quizzing platform. Data from hundreds of actual students using this program in medical-surgical courses across the United States identified common misconceptions for the authors to clarify in this new feature.

 Concept Mastery Alert

Left-sided HF refers to failure of the left ventricle; it results in pulmonary congestion. Right-sided HF, failure of the right ventricle, results in congestion in the peripheral tissues and the viscera.

- Interactive learning tools available online enrich learning and are identified with icons in the text:

  - **Concepts in Action Animations** bring physiologic and pathophysiologic concepts to life.

  - **Interactive Tutorials** review key information for common or complex medical-surgical conditions. Tutorials include graphics and animations and provide interactive review exercises as well as case-based questions.

  - **Practice & Learn Case Studies** present case scenarios and offer interactive exercises and questions to help students apply what they have learned.

  - **Watch & Learn Video Clips** reinforce skills from the textbook and appeal to visual and auditory learners. With the 13th edition, all content from Lippincott's Video Series for Brunner & Suddarth's Textbook of Medical-Surgical Nursing is included!

Cardiac Cycle

The cardiac cycle refers to the events that occur in the heart from the beginning of one heartbeat to the next. The

- **Critical Thinking Exercises** foster critical thinking and challenge you to apply textbook knowledge to clinical scenarios. In addition to the Evidence-Based Practice questions mentioned earlier, Prioritization (PQ) questions ask you to consider the priorities for nursing care for specific patients and conditions.

Critical Thinking Exercises

1 **PQ** A 67-year-old patient has just been diagnosed with metabolic syndrome with hypertension, obesity, dyslipidemia, and insulin resistance. She is asking for more information about this syndrome and what she can do about it. How will you define metabolic syndrome for this patient? What does this diagnosis mean for her future health and health care needs? Knowing that multiple lifestyle changes are recommended, what is your first priority for patient education?

2 **ebp** You are caring for an 88-year-old man who is hospitalized with a diagnosis of syncope. After ambulating in the hall, he tells you that he is having some chest pain and mild shortness of breath. Based on your knowledge of evidence-based guidelines, identify the initial interventions and diagnostic testing that are indicated for patients with these symptoms. Describe how the diagnosis of acute

MI is made. If a diagnosis of STEMI is made, which treatment options may be considered?

3 A 60-year-old woman has just returned to your unit following a heart catheterization and PCI. She appears restless and uncomfortable. What should be included in your initial assessment? What type of monitoring is indicated? Identify serious complications that you should watch for in patients following PCI.

4 You are caring for a 72-year-old man who was recently admitted to the ICU following CABG. His current vital signs are as follows: heart rate, 114 bpm; blood pressure, 88/60 mmHg; CVP, 2 mm Hg. Which other assessment parameters will you evaluate? What type of postoperative interventions do you expect?

- **References** cited are listed at the end of each chapter and include updated, current sources.

- **Resources** lists at the end of each chapter include sources of additional information, Web sites, agencies, and patient education materials.

References

*Asterisk indicates nursing research.

Books

Aschenbrenner, D. S., & Venable, S. J. (2012). *Drug therapy in nursing* (4th ed.). Philadelphia: Wolters Kluwer.

Bickley, L. S., & Szilagyi, P. G. (2009). *Bates' guide to physical examination and history taking* (10th ed.). Philadelphia: Lippincott Williams & Wilkins.

Doenges, M. E., Moorhouse, M. F., & Murr, A. C. (2010). *Nursing care plans. Guidelines for individualizing client care across the life span* (8th ed.). Philadelphia: F. A. Davis.

McCance, K. L., Huether, S. E., Brashers, V. L., et al. (2010). *Pathophysiology. The biologic basis for disease in adults and children* (6th ed.). Maryland Heights, MO: Mosby Elsevier.

Porth, C. M. (2011). *Essentials of pathophysiology* (3rd ed.). Philadelphia: Wolters Kluwer.

Journals and Electronic Documents

*Albert, N., Trochelman, K., Li, J., et al. (2010). Signs and symptoms of heart failure: Are you asking the right questions? *American Journal of Critical Care, 19*(5), 443–453.

Colucci, W. S. (2011). *Treatment of acute decompensated heart failure: Components of therapy.* Available at: www.uptodate.com/contents/treatment-of-acute-decompensated-heart-failure-components-of-therapy?source=search_result&search=acute+decompensated+heart+failure&selectedTitle=1%7E150

Damman, K., Voors, A. A., Navis, G., et al. (2011). The cardiorenal syndrome in heart failure. *Progress in Cardiovascular Diseases, 54*(3), 144–153.

Downing, J., & Balady, G. J. (2011). The role of exercise training in heart failure. *Journal of the American College of Cardiology, 58*(6), 561–569.

Fiaccadori, E., Regolisti, G., Maggiore, U., et al. (2011). Ultrafiltration in heart failure. *American Heart Journal, 161*(3), 439–449.

Field, J. M., Hazinski, M. F., Sayre, M. F... mary: 2010 American Heart Associat...

Resources

American Heart Association, www.americanheart.org
Heart Failure Society of America (HFSA), www.hfsa.org
National Heart, Lung, and Blood Institute, www.nhlbi.nih.gov

- **Brunner Suite Resources** highlighted at the end of each chapter identify additional resources available for further review, application, and clinical reference.

Brunner Suite Resources
Explore these additional resources to enhance learning for this chapter:
- NCLEX-Style Questions and Other Resources on thePoint, http://thePoint.lww.com/Brunner13e
- Study Guide
- PrepU
- Clinical Handbook
- Handbook of Laboratory and Diagnostic Tests

Contents

BRUNNER & SUDDARTH'S

Textbook of Medical-Surgical Nursing

Edition
13

Unit
1
Basic Concepts in Nursing

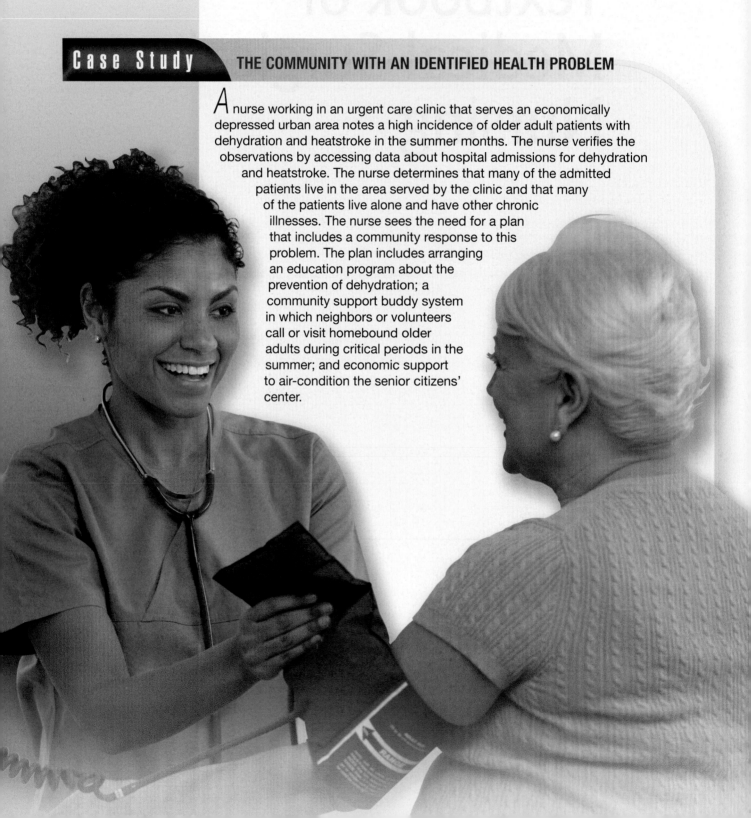

Case Study THE COMMUNITY WITH AN IDENTIFIED HEALTH PROBLEM

A nurse working in an urgent care clinic that serves an economically depressed urban area notes a high incidence of older adult patients with dehydration and heatstroke in the summer months. The nurse verifies the observations by accessing data about hospital admissions for dehydration and heatstroke. The nurse determines that many of the admitted patients live in the area served by the clinic and that many of the patients live alone and have other chronic illnesses. The nurse sees the need for a plan that includes a community response to this problem. The plan includes arranging an education program about the prevention of dehydration; a community support buddy system in which neighbors or volunteers call or visit homebound older adults during critical periods in the summer; and economic support to air-condition the senior citizens' center.

QSEN Competency Focus: *Quality Improvement*

The complexities inherent in today's health care system challenge nurses to demonstrate integration of specific interdisciplinary core competencies. These competencies are aimed at ensuring the delivery of safe, quality patient care (Institute of Medicine, 2003). The concepts from the Quality and Safety Education for Nurses (QSEN) Institute (2012) provide a framework for the knowledge, skills, and attitudes (KSAs) required for nurses to demonstrate competency in these key areas, which include *patient-centered care, interdisciplinary teamwork and collaboration, evidence-based practice, quality improvement, safety,* and *informatics.*

Quality Improvement (QI) Definition: Use data to monitor the outcomes of care processes and use improvement methods to design and test changes to continuously improve the quality and safety of health care systems.

SELECTED PRE-LICENSURE KSAs	APPLICATION AND REFLECTION
Knowledge	
Explain the importance of variation and measurement in assessing quality of care.	Describe how the nurse's observation of seasonal variations in a specific population was then linked to data-derived measures that verified a need to plan a quality improvement initiative.
Skills	
Use quality measures to understand performance. Use tools (such as control charts and run charts) that are helpful for understanding variation.	What tools might the nurse use to gain buy-in from key constituents in the community? What benchmarks of quality might he or she wish to use for community-based constituents?
Attitudes	
Appreciate how unwanted variation affects care. Value measurement and its role in good patient care.	Reflect on what you learned from this case study. Do you appreciate that seasonal variations may occur in specific populations (e.g., in this case, older adults within this community were identified as at-risk of dehydration and heat stroke during the summer)? If you practiced within the same setting, do you think you could have made the same observations and analyses? What is required for you to make these types of complex interconnections?

Cronenwett, L., Sherwood, G., Barnsteiner, J., et al. (2007). Quality and safety education for nurses. *Nursing Outlook, 55*(3), 122–131.
Institute of Medicine. (2003). *Health professions education: A bridge to quality.* Washington, DC: National Academies Press.
QSEN Institute (2012). *Competencies: Prelicensure KSAs.* Available at: qsen.org/competencies/pre-licensure-ksas

Read More About This Case

More information about this case study and the relationships between nursing diagnoses, interventions, and expected outcomes is available online. Visit thePoint for Applying Concepts From NANDA-I, NIC, and NOC.

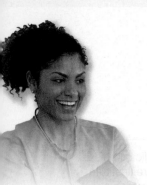
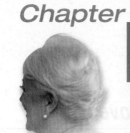

Chapter

1

Health Care Delivery and Evidence-Based Nursing Practice

Learning Objectives

On completion of this chapter, the learner will be able to:

1 Define nursing, health, and wellness.
2 Describe factors causing significant changes in the health care delivery system and their impact on health care and the nursing profession.
3 Describe care planning tools and nursing roles that are useful in coordinating patient care.

4 Discuss behavioral competencies and characteristics of professional nursing practice.
5 Compare and contrast the advanced practice registered nurse roles most relevant to medical-surgical nursing practice.
6 Describe models that foster interdisciplinary collaborative practice and promote safety and quality outcomes in the practice of health care.

Glossary

advanced practice registered nurse (APRN): a title that encompasses certified nurse practitioners (CNPs), clinical nurse specialists (CNSs), certified nurse-midwives (CNMs), and certified registered nurse anesthetists (CRNAs)
bundle: a set of three to five evidence-based practices that, when implemented appropriately, can measurably improve patients' outcomes
clinical nurse leader (CNL): a title conferred upon a certified master's-prepared nurse generalist who supervises the care coordination of a group of patients while assuring implementation of evidence-based practices and evaluation of quality outcomes
core measures: benchmark standards of best practices used to gauge how well a hospital gives care to its patients who are admitted to seek treatment for a specific disease (e.g., heart failure) or who need a specific treatment (e.g., an immunization)
evidence-based practice (EBP): a best practice derived from valid and reliable research studies that also considers the health care setting, patient preferences and values, and clinical judgment
health: according to the World Health Organization (2006), a "state of complete physical, mental, and social well-being and not merely the absence of disease and infirmity" (p. 1); often viewed as equivalent to wellness
health–illness continuum: description of a person's health status as a range with anchors that include poor health or imminent death on one end of the continuum to high-level wellness on the other end
interprofessional collaborative practice: employing multiple health professionals to work together with

patients, families, and communities to deliver best practices, thus ensuring best patient outcomes
Joint Commission: a nonprofit organization that accredits hospitals and health care organizations
National Patient Safety Goals (NPSGs): areas of patient safety concern identified annually by the Joint Commission that, if rectified, may have the most positive impact on improving patient care and outcomes
nursing: according to the American Nurses Association (2010b), "the protection, promotion, and optimization of health and abilities, prevention of illness and injury, alleviation of suffering through the diagnosis and treatment of human response, and advocacy in the care of individuals, families, communities, and populations" (p. 3)
patient: a traditional term used to identify someone who is a recipient of health care
pay for performance: a health insurance model that reimburses health care provider groups, hospitals, and health care agencies for either meeting or exceeding metrics that demonstrate that the care and treatments rendered are both cost-efficient and of best quality; also known as *value-based purchasing*
Quality and Safety Education for Nurses (QSEN): a project whose aim is to develop curricula that prepare future nurses with the knowledge, skills, and attitudes (KSAs) required to continuously improve the quality and safety of the health care system through demonstrating competency in patient-centered care, teamwork and collaboration, evidence-based practice, quality improvement, safety, and informatics

As American society has undergone changes, so has the nation's health care system. Sweeping health care legislation, such as the 2010 Affordable Care Act (ACA) and the comprehensive study of health care delivery reported by the

Robert Wood Johnson Foundation (RWJF) and the Institute of Medicine (IOM), ensure that health care and its delivery will continue to change for years to come (IOM, 2011). Nursing, as the health care profession with the greatest number of employees and a major contributor to the health care delivery system, has been significantly affected by these changes. Nursing has played an important role in the health care system and will continue to do so. This chapter provides an overview of the nature of the practice of nursing in the United States today.

The Nursing Profession and the Health Care Industry

Nursing Defined

Since the time of Florence Nightingale, who wrote in 1858 that the goal of nursing was "to put the patient in the best condition for nature to act upon him," nursing leaders have described nursing as both an art and a science. However, the definition of nursing has evolved over time. In the American Nurses Association (ANA) Social Policy Statement (2010b, p. 3) and Scope and Standards of Practice (2010a, p. 1), **nursing** is defined as "the protection, promotion, and optimization of health and abilities, prevention of illness and injury, alleviation of suffering through the diagnosis and treatment of human response, and advocacy in the care of individuals, families, communities, and populations." Chart 1-1 identifies the phenomena that are the foci for nursing care, education, and research. Nurses have a responsibility to carry out their role as described in the Social Policy Statement (ANA, 2010b) to comply with the nurse practice act of the state in which they practice, and to comply with the Code of Ethics for Nurses as spelled out by the ANA (2001) and the International Council of Nurses (ICN, 2006). To have a foundation for examining the delivery of nursing care, it is necessary to understand the needs of health care consumers and the health care delivery system, including the forces that affect nursing and health care delivery.

The Patient: Consumer of Nursing and Health Care

The central figure in health care services is the patient. The term **patient**, derived from a Latin verb meaning "to suffer," has traditionally been used to describe a person who is a recipient of care. The connotation commonly attached to the word is one of dependence. For this reason, many nurses prefer to use the term *client*, which is derived from a Latin verb meaning "to lean," connoting alliance and interdependence. The term *patient* is used throughout this book, with the understanding that either term is acceptable.

The patient who seeks care for a health problem or problems (increasing numbers of people have multiple health problems) is also an individual person, a member of a family, and a citizen of the community. Patients' needs vary depending on their problems, associated circumstances, and past experiences. Many patients, who as consumers of health care have become more knowledgeable about health care options, are assuming a collaborative approach with the nurse in the quest for optimal health (Naik, Dyer, Kunik, et al., 2009). Among the nurse's important functions in health care delivery are identifying the patient's immediate needs and working in concert with the patient to address them.

The Patient's Basic Needs

Certain needs are basic to all people. Some of these needs are more important than others. Once an essential need is met, people often experience a need on a higher level of priority. Addressing needs by priority reflects Maslow's hierarchy of needs (Fig. 1-1).

Maslow's Hierarchy of Needs

Maslow ranked human needs as follows: physiologic needs; safety and security; sense of belonging and affection; esteem and self-respect; and self-actualization. Self-actualization includes

Chart 1-1	The Focal Points for Nursing Care, Education, and Research

Promotion of health and wellness
Promotion of safety and quality of care
Care, self-care processes, and care coordination
Physical, emotional, and spiritual comfort, discomfort, and pain
Adaptation to physiological and pathophysiological processes
Emotions related to the experience of birth, growth and development, health, illness, disease, and death
Meanings ascribed to health, illnesses, and other concepts
Linguistic and cultural sensitivity
Health literacy
Decision making and the ability to make choices
Relationships, role performance, and change processes within relationships
Social policies and their effects on health
Health care systems and their relationships to access, cost, and quality of health care
The environment and the prevention of disease and injury

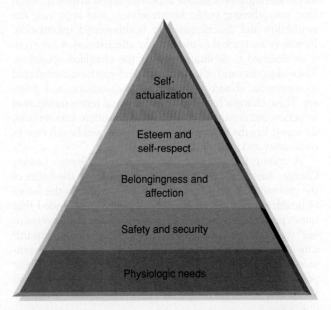

FIGURE 1-1 • This scheme of Maslow's hierarchy of needs shows how a person moves from fulfillment of basic needs to higher levels of needs, with the ultimate goal being integrated human functioning and health.

self-fulfillment, desire to know and understand, and aesthetic needs. Lower-level needs always remain; however, a person's ability to pursue higher-level needs indicates movement toward psychological health and well-being (Maslow, 1954). Such a hierarchy of needs is a useful framework that can be applied to many nursing models for assessment of a patient's strengths, limitations, and need for nursing interventions.

 Concept Mastery Alert

Physiologic needs *always* take priority over other higher-level needs in any given situation. These needs must be met first before addressing higher-level needs.

Health Care and Nursing in Transition

Changes occurring in health care delivery and nursing are the result of societal, economic, technologic, scientific, and political forces that have evolved throughout the past century. Among the most significant changes are shifts in population demographics, particularly the increase in the aging population and the cultural diversity of the population; changing patterns of diseases; increased technology; increased consumer expectations; higher costs of health care and changes in health care financing; and major health care reform efforts.

The *Healthy People* initiatives, which began with *Healthy People 1990* after the 1979 Surgeon General's report, *Healthy People: The Surgeon General's Report on Health Promotion and Disease Prevention*, identified important periodic goals that, if reached, could have major impacts on improving the nation's health (U.S. Department of Health and Human Services [HHS], 2011). *Healthy People 2020* (HHS, 2011), the most recent of these initiatives, set several goals that are aimed at reducing or eliminating illness, disability, and premature death among individuals and communities. Other health care objectives focus on broader issues such as eliminating health disparities, addressing social determinants of health, improving access to quality health care, strengthening public health services, and improving the availability and dissemination of health-related information. Indicators are tracked to measure the effectiveness of interventions designed to facilitate meeting the identified objectives. These objectives and other health care reforms have contributed to continuous change in health care organization and delivery. These changes have led to institutional restructuring, staff reduction and cross-training, increased outpatient care services, decreased lengths of hospital stay, and increased health care in community and home settings.

A recent IOM report, *The Future of Nursing: Leading Change, Advancing Health* (2010), identified that the future of the profession of nursing was inextricably tied into the future of health care in the nation. This report recommended that nurses practice, "to the full extent of their education and training" (p. 1), to meet the growing primary care needs of health care consumers. This recommendation and other IOM recommendations and key messages are included in Chart 1-2. These proposed changes reflect society's changing views of health and illness and will dramatically influence where and how nurses practice.

As the proportion of the population reaching age 65 years has increased, and with the shift from acute illnesses to chronic illnesses, the traditional focus on episodic acute care disease management has shifted (Conway, Goodrich, Machlin, et al., 2011). Emerging infectious diseases, trauma, obesity, and bioterrorism also raise concerns. Thus, health care must focus more on disease prevention, health promotion, and management of chronic conditions and disability than in previous times. This shift in focus coincides with President Obama's signing of H.R. 3590: *The Patient Protection and Affordable Care Act*, also known as the ACA. The ACA seeks to reform the current U.S. health care system so that all Americans have access to quality, affordable health care; improved access to innovative and preventive health care programs and therapies; and expanded insurance coverage. In addition, the ACA seeks to establish a more integrated health care system (Responsible Reform for the Middle Class, 2010).

Health, Wellness, and Health Promotion

The U.S. health care system, which traditionally has been disease oriented, is placing increasing emphasis on health and its promotion. Similarly, a significant number of nurses in past decades focused on the care of patients with acute conditions; however, many are now directing efforts toward health promotion and illness prevention.

Health

How health is perceived depends on how health is defined. The World Health Organization (WHO, 2006) defines **health** in the preamble to its constitution as a "state of complete physical, mental, and social well-being and not merely the absence of disease and infirmity" (p. 1). Although this definition of health does not allow for any variation in degrees of wellness or illness, the concept of a **health–illness continuum** allows for a greater range in describing a person's health status. By viewing health and illness on a continuum, it is possible to consider a person as being neither completely healthy nor completely ill. Instead, a person's state of health is ever-changing and has the potential to range from high-level wellness to extremely poor health and imminent death. The use of the health–illness continuum makes it possible to regard a person as simultaneously possessing degrees of both health and illness. On the health–illness continuum, even people with a chronic illness or disability may attain a high level of wellness if they are successful in meeting their health potential within the limits of their chronic illness or disability (Manderscheid, Ryff, Freeman, et al., 2010).

Wellness

Wellness has been defined as being equivalent to health. Wellness involves being proactive and being involved in self-care activities aimed toward a state of physical, psychological, and spiritual well-being. Hood and Leddy (2010) consider that wellness has four components: (1) the capacity to perform to the best of one's ability, (2) the ability to adjust and adapt to varying situations, (3) a reported feeling of well-being, and (4) a feeling that "everything is together" and harmonious. With this in mind, health care providers must aim to promote positive changes that are directed toward health and well-being. The sense of wellness has a subjective aspect that addresses the importance of recognizing

Chart 1-2	The Institute of Medicine's Key Messages and Recommendations for the Future of Nursing
Key Message I	Nurses should practice to the full extent of their education and training.
Key Message II	Nurses should achieve higher levels of education and training through an improved education system that promotes seamless academic progression.
Key Message III	Nurses should be full partners, with physicians and other health professionals, in redesigning health care in the United States.
Key Message IV	Effective workforce planning and policy making require better data collection and an improved information infrastructure.
Recommendation 1: Remove scope-of-practice barriers.	Advanced practice registered nurses should be able to practice to the full extent of their education and training.
Recommendation 2: Expand opportunities for nurses to lead and diffuse collaborative improvement efforts.	Private and public funders, health care organizations, nursing education programs, and nursing associations should expand opportunities for nurses to lead and manage collaborative efforts with physicians and other members of the health care team to conduct research and to redesign and improve practice environments and health systems. These entities should also provide opportunities to diffuse successful practices.
Recommendation 3: Implement nurse residency programs.	State boards of nursing, accrediting bodies, the federal government, and health care organizations should take actions to support nurses' completion of a transition-to-practice program (nurse residency) after they have completed a prelicensure or advance practice degree program or when they are transitioning into new clinical practice areas.
Recommendation 4: Increase the proportion of nurses with a baccalaureate degree to 80 percent by 2020.	Academic nurse leaders across all schools of nursing should work together to increase the proportion of nurses with a baccalaureate degree from 50 to 80 percent by 2020. These leaders should partner with education accrediting bodies, private and public funders, and employers to ensure funding, monitor progress, and increase the diversity of students to create a workforce prepared to meet the demands of diverse populations across the lifespan.
Recommendation 5: Double the number of nurses with a doctorate by 2020.	Schools of nursing, with support from private and public funders, academic administrators and university trustees, and accrediting bodies, should double the number of nurses with a doctorate by 2020 to add to the cadre of nurse faculty and researchers, with attention to increasing diversity.
Recommendation 6: Ensure that nurses engage in lifelong learning.	Accrediting bodies, schools of nursing, health care organizations, and continuing competency educators from multiple health professions should collaborate to ensure that nurses and nursing students and faculty continue their education and engage in lifelong learning to gain the competencies needed to provide care for diverse populations across the lifespan.
Recommendation 7: Prepare and enable nurses to lead change to advance health.	Nurses, nursing education programs, and nursing associations should prepare the nursing workforce to assume leadership positions across all levels, while public, private, and governmental health care decision makers should ensure that leadership positions are available to and filled by nurses.
Recommendation 8: Build an infrastructure for the collection and analysis of interprofessional health care workforce data.	The National Health Care Workforce Commission, with oversight from the Government Accountability Office and the Health Resources and Services Administration, should lead a collaborative effort to improve research and the collection and analysis of data on health care workforce requirements. The Workforce Commission and the Health Resources and Services Administration should collaborate with state licensing boards, state nursing workforce centers, and the Department of Labor in this effort to ensure that the data are timely and publicly accessible.

Reprinted with permission from the Institute of Medicine. (2010). *The future of nursing: Leading change, advancing health.* Washington, DC: National Academies Press.

and responding to patient individuality and diversity in health care and nursing.

Health Promotion

Today, increasing emphasis is placed on health, health promotion, wellness, and self-care. Health is seen as resulting from a lifestyle oriented toward wellness. The result has been the evolution of a wide range of health promotion strategies, including multiphasic screening, genetic testing, lifetime health monitoring, environmental and mental health programs, risk reduction, and nutrition and health education. A growing interest in self-care skills is reflected by the many health-related publications, conferences, and workshops designed for the lay public.

People are increasingly knowledgeable about their health and take more interest in and responsibility for their health and well-being. Organized self-care education programs emphasize health promotion, disease prevention, management of illness, self-care, and collaborative use of the professional health care system. In addition, numerous Web sites and chat groups promote sharing of experiences and information about self-care with others who have similar conditions, chronic diseases, or disabling conditions (Pender, Murdaugh, & Parsons, 2011).

Special efforts are being made by health care professionals to reach members of various cultural and socioeconomic groups and educate them about lifestyle and health practices. Stress, unhealthy diet, lack of exercise, smoking, use of illicit drugs, high-risk behaviors (including risky sexual practices), and poor hygiene are all lifestyle behaviors known to affect health negatively. The goal is to motivate people to improve the way they live, to modify risky behaviors, and to adopt healthy behaviors. (See Chapter 4 for further discussion of health promotion and health promotion models.)

Influences on Health Care Delivery

The health care delivery system is constantly adapting to changes in health care needs and expectations. For example, shifting population demographics, increases in chronic illnesses and disability, technologic advances, and greater emphasis on health care quality, costs, and reform efforts have impacted health care delivery and nursing.

Population Demographics

Changes in the population in general are affecting the need for and the delivery of health care. The U.S. Bureau of the Census (Mackun & Wilson, 2011) estimated that nearly 309 million people reside in the country. Population growth is attributed in part to improved public health services.

Not only is the population increasing, but its composition is also changing. The decline in birth rate and the increase in lifespan owing to improved health care have resulted in fewer school-age children and more senior citizens, many of whom are women. Much of the population resides in highly congested urban areas, with a steady migration of members of ethnic minorities to the inner cities and a migration of members of the middle class to suburban areas. The number of homeless people, including entire families, has increased significantly. The population has become more culturally diverse as increasing numbers of people from different national backgrounds enter the country.

Because of population changes, the health care needs of people of specific ages, of women, and of diverse groups of people in specific geographic locations are altering the effectiveness of traditional means of providing health care. As a result, far-reaching changes in the overall health care delivery system are necessary.

Aging Population

The older adult population in the United States has increased significantly and will continue to grow in future years. In 2010, 40.3 million adults were 65 years of age and older, constituting 13% of the U.S. population (Vincent & Velkoff, 2010). The population of those 45 to 64 years of age grew at a higher rate (31.5%) than any age range over the past 10 years. This aging of the baby boomer generation accounts for the significant aging of the U.S. population. By the year 2030, 20% of the U.S. population is expected to be older than 65 years. From 2000 to 2010, the number of people older than 65 years grew at a higher rate (15.1%) than the number of people younger than 45 years (less than 4%) (Howden & Meyer, 2011). In addition, over the past century, people 85 years of age and older constituted one of the fastest-growing segments of the population; the number was 34 times larger in 1999 than in 1900. It is projected that people older than 85 years (currently 14% of the older adult population) will comprise 21% of the total population of older adults (i.e., those older than 65 years) in the year 2050 (Vincent & Velkoff, 2010).

The health care needs of older adults are complex and demand significant investments, both professional and finan-cial, by the health care industry. Many older adults suffer from multiple chronic conditions that are exacerbated by acute episodes. In particular, older women, whose conditions are frequently underdiagnosed and undertreated, are of concern. In the 2010 census, there were 96.7 males per 100 females. Although older women continue to outnumber older men, the overall number of older men has also increased over the past decade (Howden & Meyer, 2011). (See Chapter 11 for further discussion of health care of the older adult.)

Cultural Diversity

An appreciation for the diverse characteristics and needs of people from varied ethnic and cultural backgrounds is important in health care and nursing. Some projections indicate that by 2030, racial and ethnic minority populations in the United States will triple. The 2010 census classified five distinct races (White, Black, Asian, Native American, and Native Hawaiian/Pacific Islander). The Asian race showed the largest growth rate among the five groups. The Hispanic population, classified primarily under the White race, was noted to account for more than half of the increased growth in the United States. With increased immigration, both legal and illegal, this figure could approach 50% by the year 2030 (Humes, Jones, & Ramerez, 2011). As the cultural composition of the population changes, it is increasingly important to address cultural considerations in the delivery of health care. Patients from diverse sociocultural groups not only bring various health care beliefs, values, and practices to the health care setting but also have various risk factors for some disease conditions and unique reactions to treatment. These factors significantly affect a person's responses to health care problems or illnesses, to caregivers, and to the care itself. Unless these factors are assessed, understood, and respected by health care providers, the care delivered may be ineffective, and health care outcomes may be negatively affected. (See Chapter 7 for further discussion of transcultural nursing.)

Changing Patterns of Disease

During the past 50 years, the health problems of the American people have changed significantly. Although some infectious diseases have been controlled or eradicated, others, such as tuberculosis, acquired immunodeficiency syndrome (AIDS), and sexually transmitted infections, are on the rise. An increasing number of infectious agents are becoming resistant to antibiotic therapy as a result of widespread and inappropriate use of antibiotics. Obesity has become a major health concern, and the multiple comorbidities that accompany it, such as hypertension, heart disease, diabetes, and cancer, add significantly to its associated mortality.

The prevalence of chronic illnesses and disability is increasing because of the lengthening lifespan in the United States and the advances in care and treatment options for conditions such as cancer, human immunodeficiency virus (HIV) infection, and cystic fibrosis. In addition, improvements in care for trauma and other serious acute health problems have meant that many people with these conditions live decades longer than in the past. People with chronic illness are the largest group of health care consumers in the United States. Because most health problems seen today are chronic in nature, many people are learning to maximize their health within the constraints of chronic illness and disability.

As chronic conditions increase, health care broadens from a focus on cure and eradication of disease to include the prevention or rapid treatment of exacerbations of chronic conditions. Nursing, which has always encouraged patients to take control of their health and wellness, has a prominent role in the current focus on management of chronic illness and disability. (See Chapter 9 for further discussion on chronic illness and disability.)

Advances in Technology and Genetics

Advances in technology and genetics have occurred more rapidly during the past several decades compared with other time periods. Sophisticated techniques and devices have revolutionized surgery and diagnostic testing, making it possible to perform many procedures and tests on an outpatient basis. Increased knowledge and understanding of genetics have resulted in expanded screening, diagnostic testing, and treatments for a variety of conditions. The sophisticated communication systems that connect most parts of the world, with the capability of rapid storage, retrieval, and dissemination of information, have stimulated brisk change as well as swift obsolescence in health care delivery strategies. Advances in genetics and technology have also resulted in many ethical issues for the health care system, health care providers, patients, families, and society. (See Chapter 8 for further discussion on genetics.)

Demand for Quality Health Care

Nurses in acute care settings must work with other health care team members to maintain quality care while facing pressures to care for patients who are hospitalized for relatively few days. Nurses in the community care for patients who need high-technology acute care services as well as long-term care in the home. The importance of effective discharge planning and quality improvement cannot be overstated. Acute care nurses must also work with community-based nurses and others in community settings to ensure continuity of care.

The general public has become increasingly interested in and knowledgeable about health care and health promotion through television, newspapers, magazines, the Internet, and other communications media. Health care is a topic of political debate. The public has also become very health conscious and subscribes to the belief that health and quality health care constitute a basic right, rather than a privilege for a chosen few.

Quality, Safety, and Evidence-Based Practice

In the 1980s, hospitals and other health care agencies implemented ongoing quality assurance programs that provided the foundation for the establishment of continuous quality improvement (CQI) programs in the 1990s. Despite these efforts to ensure the provision of quality health care, the IOM (2000) reported an alarming breakdown in quality control in the American health care system. The IOM report *To Err Is Human: Building a Safer Health System* (2000) noted that nearly 100,000 Americans died annually from preventable errors in hospitals, and many more suffered nonfatal injuries from errors. A subsequent IOM report, *Crossing the Quality Chasm: A New Health System*

for the 21st Century (2001), envisioned a reformed health care system that is evidence based and systems oriented. Its proposed six aims for improvement included ensuring that patient care is safe, effective, patient centered, timely, efficient, and equitable (IOM, 2001).

As a result of these landmark reports (IOM, 2000; IOM, 2001) and because of provisions within the ACA (Responsible Reform for the Middle Class, 2010), the landscape of health care is rapidly changing to ensure that quality benchmarks are established. Whether or not hospitals, health care agencies, and health care providers meet these benchmarks may then be publicly reported to health care consumers. Many health insurance companies are adopting pay for performance measures, also known as *value-based purchasing*. **Pay for performance** is a health insurance model that reimburses health care provider groups, hospitals, and health care agencies for either meeting or exceeding metrics that demonstrate that the care and treatments rendered are both cost-efficient and of best quality. By the same token, these same insurance companies may disallow reimbursement for care or treatment that either does not meet a predetermined quality metric or for care that is necessary because of provider error (i.e., iatrogenic).

The **Joint Commission** is a nonprofit organization that accredits hospitals and health care organizations. Over the past decade, it has annually updated and published its **National Patient Safety Goals (NPSGs)**—selected NPSGs include areas of patient safety concern that, if rectified, may have the most positive impact on improving patient care and outcomes. Recently adopted NPSGs revolve around identifying patients correctly, improving staff communication, using medications safely, preventing infections, identifying patient safety risks, and preventing surgery-related mistakes (Joint Commission, 2011). Each NPSG has implications for scrutinizing and perhaps changing and improving nursing practices. In addition, the Joint Commission provides evidence-based practice solutions for these NPSGs. An **evidence-based practice (EBP)** is a best practice derived from valid and reliable research studies that also considers the health care setting, patient preferences and values, and clinical judgment. The facilitation of EBP involves identifying and evaluating current literature and research findings, and then incorporating these findings into patient care as a means of ensuring quality care (Stichler, Fields, Kim, et al., 2011).

In addition to the NPSGs, the Joint Commission, in cooperation with the Centers for Medicare and Medicaid Services (CMS), has developed sets of performance measures for hospitals called *core measures*. The **core measures** are used to gauge how well a hospital gives care to its patients who are admitted to seek treatment for a specific disease (e.g., heart failure) or who need a specific treatment (e.g., an immunization) as compared to evidence-based guidelines and standards of care. Benchmark standards of quality are used to compare the care or treatment that patients receive as compared to the best practice standards (Joint Commission, 2010). The percentage of the patients who receive the best care or treatment as specified at a given hospital is then calculated and reported so that hospitals can use those results to continue to improve their processes and performance until they consistently meet best practice standards 100% of the time.

Patients' satisfaction with the care they receive when hospitalized is also an important quality metric for hospitals to consider. CMS partnered with the Agency for Healthcare Research and Quality (AHRQ) to launch the Hospital Consumer Assessment of Healthcare Providers and Systems (HCAHPS) survey. HCAHPS is a survey that is administered to a random sample of recently hospitalized patients within 6 weeks of discharge. Most items on the HCAHPS survey measure patients' satisfaction with the quality of the nursing care they receive, including their satisfaction with their communication with the nurses, the responsiveness of the hospital staff, the quietness of the environment, their pain management, communication about their medications, and their discharge information. Discharged patients are also asked to provide an overall rating of the hospital and whether or not they would recommend the hospital. Hospitals' HCAHPS scores are calculated and publicly reported on the HCAHPS Web site (CAHPS Hospital Survey, 2010).

The Institute for Healthcare Improvement (IHI) is a nonprofit organization whose mission is adapted from the IOM's six aims for improvement; namely, ensuring that patient care is safe, effective, patient centered, timely, efficient, and equitable (IOM, 2001). The IHI launched its 5 Million Lives Campaign in 2007, anticipating that if evidence-based guidelines it advocated were voluntarily implemented by U.S. hospitals, 5 million lives would be saved from either harm or death over a 2-year period (IHI, 2011b). Although the data are not fully analyzed as of this time, the credibility of IHI's quality improvement methods has encouraged hospitals to change their quality improvement processes and nursing practices. For instance, many hospitals have adopted the IHI's change model (sometimes called the *rapid cycle testing* model) to more rapidly integrate proven performance improvement processes. The principles and steps that guide the Model for Improvement are shown in Chart 1-3 (IHI, 2011c). This model is commonly used by nurses and other health care professionals to monitor quality and performance improvement processes in U.S. hospitals.

The IHI has developed numerous sets of readily implemented EBP sets for use by hospitals. These **bundles** include a set of three to five EBPs that, when implemented appropriately, can measurably improve patients' outcomes. Many of these practices are within the scope of independent nursing practice. For instance, the IHI Ventilator Bundle advocates that the head of the bed should be elevated and that oral care should be provided using chlorhexidine for all patients on ventilators (IHI, 2011a; see Chapter 23 for further discussion of ventilator-associated pneumonia). Throughout this book, key bundles advocated by the IHI will be noted, and their implications for implementing best nursing practices will be discussed as appropriate.

EBP tools used for planning patient care may include not only bundles but also clinical guidelines, algorithms, care mapping, multidisciplinary action plans (MAPs), and clinical pathways. These tools are used to move patients toward predetermined outcomes. Algorithms are used more often in acute situations to determine a particular treatment based on patient information or response. Care maps, clinical guidelines, and MAPs (the most detailed of these tools) help to facilitate coordination of care and education throughout hospitalization and after discharge. Nurses who provide direct care have an important role in the development and use of these tools through their participation in researching the literature and then developing, piloting, implementing, and revising them as needed.

Care Coordination

Coordination of care for patients from the time of hospital admission to discharge—and in many cases after discharge to the home care and community settings—is vitally important to ensure that they continue to achieve benchmarks of quality. Care coordination failure occurs when a patient is readmitted to the hospital shortly after discharge with the same condition for which he or she had been originally hospitalized. Health insurance plans are increasingly holding hospitals accountable for readmissions to the hospital within 30 days of hospital discharge, and many times the plans will not reimburse hospitals for costs associated with these readmissions. Therefore, patient care must be coordinated seamlessly from the inpatient hospital environment through the community care system. However, the current U.S. health care system has been frequently criticized for its fragmented system of delivery. Two roles have evolved to provide improved care coordination: the case manager and the clinical nurse leader (CNL).

Case management is a system of coordinating health care services to ensure cost-effectiveness, accountability, and quality care. Under this system, the responsibility for meeting patient needs rests with one person or a team whose goals are to provide the patient and family with access to required services, to ensure coordination of these services, and to evaluate how effectively these services are delivered. Case managers may be nurses or may have backgrounds in other health professions, such as social work. The case manager coordinates the care of a caseload of patients through facilitating communication between nurses, other health care personnel who provide care, and insurance companies. In some settings, particularly the community setting, the case manager focuses on managing the treatment plan of the patient with complex conditions. The case manager may follow the patient throughout hospitalization and at home after discharge in an effort to coordinate health care services that will avert or delay rehospitalization. The caseload is usually limited in scope to patients with similar diagnoses, needs, and therapies (Case Management Society of America, 2011).

The CNL is a new role launched within the past decade, and the first new role in the profession of nursing in more than 35 years. A **clinical nurse leader (CNL)** is a certified nurse generalist with a master's degree in nursing and a special background in clinical leadership, educated to help patients navigate the complex health care system (American Association of Colleges of Nursing [AACN], 2007). According to the AACN (2007): "The CNL provides and manages care at the point of care to individuals, clinical populations and communities.... In order to impact care, the CNL has the knowledge and authority to delegate tasks to other health care personnel, as well as supervise and evaluate these personnel and the outcomes of care.... The CNL is accountable for improving individual care outcomes and processes in a quality, cost-effective manner" (p. 11). CNLs are being utilized in hospital-based environments as well as community health settings.

Professional Nursing Practice

Novice, entry-level registered nurses, as well as those with advanced degrees who work in highly specialized settings, all

Chart 1-3 **Model for Improvement (Known as Rapid Cycle Testing)**

Forming the Team

Including the right people on a process improvement team is critical to a successful improvement effort. Teams vary in size and composition. Each organization builds teams to suit its own needs.

Setting Aims

Improvement requires setting aims. The aim should be time-specific and measurable; it should also define the specific population of patients or other system that will be affected.

Establishing Measures

Teams use quantitative measures to determine if a specific change actually leads to an improvement.

Selecting Changes

Ideas for change may come from the insights of those who work in the system, from change concepts or other creative thinking techniques, or by borrowing from the experience of others who have successfully improved.

Testing Changes

The Plan-Do-Study-Act (PDSA) cycle is shorthand for testing a change in the real work setting—by planning it, trying it, observing the results, and acting on what is learned. This is the scientific method adapted for action-oriented learning (see Figure on right side).

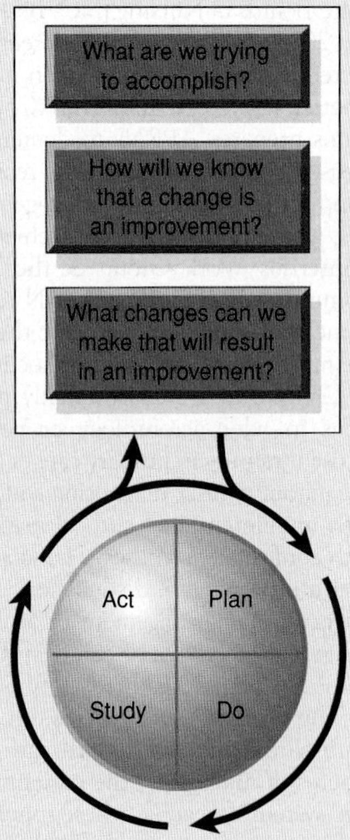

Implementing Changes

After testing a change on a small scale, learning from each test, and refining the change through several PDSA cycles, the team may implement the change on a broader scale—for example, for an entire pilot population or on an entire unit.

Spreading Changes

After successful implementation of a change or package of changes for a pilot population or an entire unit, the team can spread the changes to other parts of the organization or in other organizations.

What are we trying to accomplish?

How will we know that a change is an improvement?

What changes can we make that will result in an improvement?

Act | Plan
Study | Do

Reprinted with permission from Institute for Healthcare Improvement. (2011c). *Science of improvement: How to improve.* Available at: http://www.ihi.org/knowledge/Pages/HowtoImprove/ScienceofImprovementHowtoImprove.aspx; Langley, G. L., Nolan, K. M., Nolan, T. W., et al. (2009). *The improvement guide: A practical approach to enhancing organizational performance* (2nd ed.). San Francisco: Jossey-Bass.

engage in the practice of nursing. The ANA (2010a) notes that "the profession of nursing has one scope of practice that encompasses the full range of nursing practice, pertinent to general and specialty practice. The depth and breadth in which individual registered nurses engage in the total scope of nursing practice are dependent on their education, experience, role, and the population served" (p. 2). The ANA (2010a, p. 4) also identifies the following tenets characteristic of all nursing practice:

- Nursing practice is individualized.
- Nurses coordinate care by establishing partnerships.
- Caring is central to the practice of the registered nurse.
- Registered nurses use the nursing process to plan and provide individualized care to their health care consumers. (See Chapter 2 for further discussion of the nursing process.)
- A strong link exists between the professional work environment and the registered nurse's ability to provide quality health care and achieve optimal outcomes.

The profession of nursing has its own distinct disciplinary body of knowledge, education and specialty standards of practice, social contract (ANA, 2010b), and code of ethics (ANA, 2001). Nursing's Standards of Practice describe basic competencies in delivering nursing care using the nursing process (see Chapter 2), whereas the Standards of Professional Performance describe expectations for behavioral competencies (ANA, 2010a, p. 11), which include that the nurse:

- Practices ethically
- Attains knowledge and competence that reflects current nursing practice
- Integrates evidence and research findings into practice
- Communicates effectively in all areas of practice
- Demonstrates leadership in the professional practice setting and the profession
- Collaborates with health care consumers, families, and others in the conduct of nursing practice
- Evaluates her or his own practice
- Utilizes appropriate resources to plan and provide nursing services that are safe, effective, and financially responsible
- Practices in an environmentally safe and healthy manner

Advanced Practice Nursing Roles

Nurses may pursue generalist master's degrees in nursing that prepare them to practice as CNLs, as described previously. Alternatively, they may enroll in specialized graduate nursing education programs and pursue role preparation as certified nurse practitioners (CNPs), clinical nurse specialists (CNSs), certified nurse-midwives (CNMs), and certified registered nurse anesthetists (CRNAs), all of whom are collectively identified as **advanced practice registered nurses (APRNs)** (APRN Consensus Work Group & the National Council of State Boards of Nursing [NCSBN] APRN Advisory Committee, 2008). This educational preparation may occur in either accredited master's programs in nursing or doctor of nursing practice (DNP) programs (AACN, 2006). Each of these programs prepares APRNs to demonstrate competence with a focused population that is the recipient of care. The population foci include family, adult-gerontology, neonatal, pediatrics, women's health, and psychiatric-mental health (APRN Consensus Work Group & the NCSBN APRN Advisory Committee, 2008). The APRN roles that are most relevant to medical-surgical nursing are the CNP and CNS roles, and the most relevant population focus is adult-gerontology.

CNPs who are educationally prepared with a population focus in adult-gerontology or pediatrics receive additional focused training in primary care or acute care. CNPs may practice autonomously, diagnosing and treating individual patients with undifferentiated clinical manifestations as well as those with confirmed diagnoses. The scope of CNP practice includes health promotion and education, disease prevention, and the diagnosis and management of acute and chronic diseases for individual recipients of care (APRN Consensus Work Group & the NCSBN APRN Advisory Committee, 2008).

The primary role of CNSs, on the other hand, is to integrate care across the health care continuum through three spheres of influence—the patient, the nurse, and the health care system. In each of these spheres of influence, the goal of CNS practice is to continuously monitor and improve aggregate patient outcomes and nursing care (APRN Consensus Work Group & the NCSBN APRN Advisory Committee, 2008). CNSs define their role as having five major components: clinical practice, education, management, consultation, and research. CNSs practice in various settings, including the community and the home, although most practice in acute care settings (Hamric, Spross, & Hanson, 2009).

Historically, the scope of practice for APRNs and the professional titles conferred upon them have varied considerably from state to state. For instance, in some states, CNPs use the title *advanced nurse practitioner* (ANP), whereas in other states, CNPs use the title *certified registered nurse practitioner* (CRNP). CNSs have prescriptive authority in some states but not in others. This occurs because individual states have devised their own distinct state boards of nursing (and sometimes state boards of medicine) regulations that govern APRN practice. The Consensus Model for APRN Regulation (APRN Consensus Work Group & the NCSBN APRN Advisory Committee, 2008) promotes a new APRN regulatory model that addresses the essential elements of APRN licensure, accreditation, certification, and education (LACE). The goals of the APRN LACE model are to provide for national consistency in APRN regulations and standards of practice while promoting quality APRN education and patient outcomes (APRN Consensus Work Group & the NCSBN APRN Advisory Committee, 2008).

APRN roles enable nurses to function interdependently and to establish more collegial relationships with physicians and other health care professionals. As noted previously, a key recommendation from the IOM's *Future of Nursing* report (2010) is to fully utilize the skills and knowledge of the APRN to help to meet national health care needs. The role of APRNs is expected to continue to increase in terms of scope, responsibility, and recognition.

Professional Nursing and Collaborative Practice

This chapter has explored the changing role of nursing. Many references have been made to the significance of nurses as members of the health care team. As the unique competencies of nurses have become clearly articulated, it is now evident that nurses provide distinct and necessary health care services. However, the IOM (2001) recommended across-the-board reform of all health professions education, including nursing education programs, to improve the delivery of quality and safe patient care practices. A 2003 IOM report, *Health Professions Education: A Bridge to Quality*, challenged health professions education programs to integrate interdisciplinary core competencies into their respective curricula to include patient-centered care, interdisciplinary teamwork and collaboration, EBP, quality improvement, safety, and informatics.

Quality and Safety Education for Nurses

The **Quality and Safety Education for Nurses (QSEN)** project was funded by the nonprofit RWJF to develop curricula that prepare future nurses with the knowledge, skills, and attitudes (KSAs) required to continuously improve the quality and safety of the health care system. In particular, nurses educated under QSEN concepts demonstrate the KSAs consonant with competency in patient-centered care, teamwork and collaboration, EBP, quality improvement, safety, and informatics (QSEN, 2011). Table 1-1 highlights the QSEN definition of quality improvement and its associated KSAs.

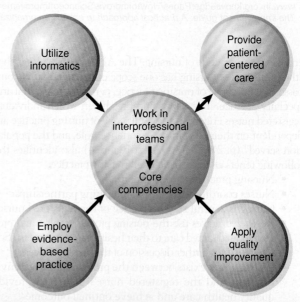

FIGURE 1-2 • Interprofessional teamwork and Institute of Medicine core competencies. From Interprofessional Education Collaborative Expert Panel. (2011). *Core competencies for interprofessional collaborative practice: Report of an expert panel.* Washington, DC: Author, p. 14. © 2011 Association of American Medical Colleges. All rights reserved. Reproduced with permission.

TABLE 1-1   Quality and Safety Education for Nurses (QSEN) Definition of Quality Improvement and Knowledge, Skills, and Attitudes (KSAs) for Pre-Licensure Nursing Students

Quality Improvement
Definition: Use data to monitor the outcomes of care processes and use improvement methods to design and test changes to continuously improve the quality of safety of health care systems.

Knowledge	Skills	Attitudes
Describe strategies for learning about the outcomes of care in the setting in which one is engaged in clinical practice.	Seek information about outcomes of care for populations served in the care setting. Seek information about quality improvement projects in the care setting.	Appreciate that continuous quality improvement is an essential part of the daily work of all health professionals.
Recognize that nursing and other health professions students are parts of systems of care and care processes that affect outcomes for patients and families. Give examples of the tension between professional autonomy and system functioning.	Use tools (such as flow charts, cause–effect diagrams) to make processes of care explicit. Participate in a root cause analysis of a sentinel event.	Value own and others' contributions to outcomes of care in local care settings.
Explain the importance of variation and measurement in assessing quality of care.	Use quality measures to understand performance. Use tools (such as control charts and run charts) that are helpful for understanding variation. Identify gaps between local and best practice.	Appreciate how unwanted variation affects care. Value measurement and its role in good patient care.
Describe approaches for changing processes of care.	Design a small test of change in daily work (using an experiential learning method such as Plan-Do-Study-Act). Practice aligning the aims, measures, and changes involved in improving care. Use measures to evaluate the effect of change.	Value local change (in individual practice or team practice on a unit) and its role in creating joy in work. Appreciate the value of what individuals and teams can do to improve care.

Reprinted with permission from Cronenwett, L., Sherwood, G., Barnsteiner, J., et al. (2007). Quality and safety education for nurses. *Nursing Outlook, 55*(3), 122–131; QSEN Institute (2012). Competencies: Prelicensure KSAs. Available at: http://qsen.org/competencies/pre-licensure-ksas

Interprofessional Collaborative Practice

As a response to the 2003 IOM report, the Interprofessional Education Collaborative Expert Panel (IPEC) published *Core Competencies for Interprofessional Collaborative Practice* (IPEC, 2011) with the goal to "prepare all health professions students for deliberately working together with the common goal of building a safer and better patient-centered and community/population oriented U.S. health care system" (p. 3). **Interprofessional collaborative practice** involves employing multiple health professionals to work together with patients, families, and communities to deliver best practices, thus assuring best patient outcomes. Interprofessional teamwork is viewed as central to this model, which incorporates the interdisciplinary core competencies identified in the 2003 IOM report as displayed in Figure 1-2. The IPEC devised four collaborative practice competency domains, which include values/ethics for interprofessional practice, roles and responsibilities for collaborative practice, interprofessional communication practices, and interprofessional teamwork and team-based practice. The interplay between these competency domains, practice settings, and professional learning trajectories is displayed in Figure 1-3. Implementation of the IPEC model should not only result in improved collaborative practice between nurses, physicians, and other health professions, but it should also promote safe, quality care, and best practices.

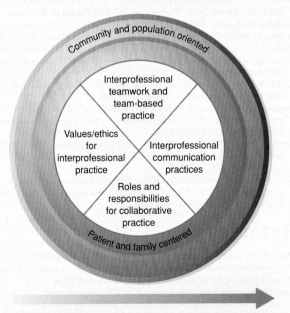

The learning continuum pre-licensure through practice trajectory

FIGURE 1-3 • Interprofessional collaborative practice domains. From Interprofessional Education Collaborative Expert Panel. (2011). *Core competencies for interprofessional collaborative practice: Report of an expert panel.* Washington, DC: Author, p. 15. © 2011 Association of American Medical Colleges. All rights reserved. Reproduced with permission.

Critical Thinking Exercises

1 Your clinical assignment is in a hospital step-down cardiac care unit. Identify a patient care issue (e.g., post-op activity progression plan) that could be improved. Identify processes that are available within hospitals to address such quality improvement issues. Describe how you might collaborate with your interdisciplinary colleagues to ensure best outcomes for this patient population.

2 [pcs] You are planning the discharge of a young adult patient who has been newly diagnosed with diabetes. The patient is uninsured and has no regular income. He is given instructions to obtain health teaching at the local health center. What would be the first three priority issues a case manager should examine on the first visit with this patient? How should the role of the case manager be explained to the patient and family?

3 [ebp] You are assigned to care for an older hospitalized patient with a new diagnosis of heart failure. A CNL is assigned to provide consistent, quality care for this patient from hospital admission to discharge. Identify the evidence that supports the effectiveness of CNLs in supervising care of patients with heart failure and promoting positive outcomes. What is the strength of the evidence? How might this patient's care be affected?

Brunner Suite Resources
Explore these additional resources to enhance learning for this chapter:
• NCLEX-Style Questions and Other Resources on thePoint, http://thePoint.lww.com/Brunner13e
• Study Guide
• PrepU
• Clinical Handbook
• Handbook of Laboratory and Diagnostic Tests

References

**Double asterisk indicates classic reference.

Books

American Association of Colleges of Nursing. (2006). *The essentials of doctoral education for advanced nursing practice.* Washington, DC: Author.

American Association of Colleges of Nursing. (2007). *White paper on the education and role of the clinical nurse leader.* Washington, DC: Author.

American Nurses Association. (2001). *Code of ethics for nurses with interpretive statements.* Washington, DC: Author.

American Nurses Association. (2010a). *Nursing: Scope and standards of practice* (2nd ed.). Silver Springs, MD: Author.

American Nurses Association. (2010b). *Nursing's social policy statement* (3rd ed.). Silver Springs, MD: Author.

Hamric, A. B., Spross, J. A., & Hanson, C. M. (2009). *Advanced practice nursing: An integrative approach* (4th ed.). St. Louis: Elsevier.

Hood, L., & Leddy, S. K. (2010). *Leddy & Pepper's conceptual bases of professional nursing* (6th ed.). Philadelphia: Lippincott Williams & Wilkins.

**Institute of Medicine. (2000). *To err is human: Building a safer health system.* Washington, DC: National Academies Press.

**Institute of Medicine. (2001). *Crossing the quality chasm: A new health system for the 21st century.* Washington, DC: National Academies Press.

**Institute of Medicine. (2003). *Health professions education: A bridge to quality.* Washington, DC: National Academies Press.

Institute of Medicine. (2010). *The future of nursing: Leading change, advancing health.* Washington, DC: National Academies Press.

Interprofessional Education Collaborative Expert Panel. (2011). *Core competencies for interprofessional collaborative practice: Report of an expert panel.* Washington, DC: Author.

**Maslow, A. (1954). *Motivation and personality.* New York: Harper.

Pender, N., Murdaugh, C., & Parsons, M. (2011). *Health promotion in nursing practice* (6th ed.). Upper Saddle River, NJ: Pearson Education.

U.S. Department of Health and Human Services, Office of Disease Prevention and Health Promotion. (2011). *Healthy People 2020.* Washington, DC: Author.

**World Health Organization. (2006). *Constitution of the World Health Organization* (45th ed.). New York: Author.

Journals and Electronic Documents

APRN Consensus Work Group, & the National Council of State Boards of Nursing APRN Advisory Council. (2008). *Consensus model for APRN regulation: Licensure, accreditation, certification & education.* Available at: www.aacn.nche.edu/education-resources/APRNReport.pdf

CAHPS Hospital Survey. (2010). *HCAHPS fact sheet.* Available at: www.hcahpsonline.org/facts.aspx

Case Management Society of America. (2011). *What is a case manager?* Available at: www.cmsa.org/Consumer/FindaCaseManager/WhatisaCaseManager/tabid/276/Default.aspx

Conway, P., Goodrich, K., Machlin, S., et al. (2011). Patient-centered care categorization of U.S. health care expenditures. *Health Services Research, 46*(2), 479–490.

Howden, L. A., & Meyer, J. A. (2011). Age and sex composition. *2010 Census Briefs.* Washington, DC: U.S. Bureau of the Census.

Humes, K. R., Jones, N. A., & Ramerez, R. R. (2011). Overview of race and Hispanic origin: 2010. *2010 Census Briefs.* Washington, DC: U.S. Bureau of the Census.

Institute for Healthcare Improvement. (2011a). *Implement the IHI ventilator bundle.* Available at: www.ihi.org/knowledge/Pages/Changes/ImplementtheVentilatorBundle.aspx

Institute for Healthcare Improvement. (2011b). *Protecting 5 million lives from harm.* Available at: www.ihi.org/offerings/Initiatives/PastStrategicInitiatives/

Institute for Healthcare Improvement. (2011c). *Science of improvement: How to improve.* Available at: www.ihi.org/knowledge/Pages/HowtoImprove/ScienceofImprovementHowtoImprove.aspx

Institute of Medicine. (2011). Leading health indicators for Healthy People 2020: Letter report. Available at: www.nap.edu/catalog.php?record_id=13088

International Council of Nurses. (2006). *The ICN code of ethics for nurses.* Available at: www.icn.ch/images/stories/documents/about/icncode_english.pdf

Joint Commission. (2010). *Core measure sets.* Available at: www.jointcommission.org/core_measure_sets.aspx

Joint Commission. (2011). *National Patient Safety Goals effective July 1, 2011.* Available at: www.jointcommission.org/assets/1/6/NPSG_EPs_Scoring_HAP_20110706.pdf

Mackun, P., & Wilson, S. (2011). Population distribution and change: 2000 to 2010. *2010 Census Briefs.* Washington, DC: U.S. Bureau of the Census.

Manderscheid, R. W., Ryff, C. D., Freeman, E. J., et al. (2010). Evolving definitions of mental illness and wellness. *Preventing Chronic Disease, 7*(1), 1–6.

Naik, A. D., Dyer, C. B., Kunik, M. E., et al. (2009). Patient autonomy for the management of chronic conditions: A two-component re-conceptualization. *American Journal of Bioethics, 9*(2), 23–30.

QSEN Institute (2012). Competencies: Prelicensure KSAs. Available at: http://qsen.org/competencies/pre-licensure-ksas

Responsible Reform for the Middle Class. (2010). *The Patient Protection and Affordable Care Act:* Detailed summary. Available at: dpc.senate.gov/healthreformbill/healthbill04.pdf

Stichler, J. Fields, W., Kim, S. C., et al. (2011). Faculty knowledge, attitudes, and perceived barriers to teaching evidence-based nursing. *Journal of Professional Nursing, 27*(2), 92–100.

Vincent, G. K., & Velkoff, V. A. (2010). The next four decades: The older population in the U.S.: 2010-2050. *Current Population Reports, P25-1138.* Washington, DC: U.S. Bureau of the Census.

Resources

Agency for Healthcare Research and Quality (AHRQ), www.ahrq.gov
American Association of Colleges of Nursing (AACN), www.aacn.nche.edu
American Nurses Association (ANA), www.nursingworld.org
Case Management Society of America (CMSA), www.cmsa.org
Centers for Medicare and Medicaid Services (CMS), www.cms.gov
Clinical Nurse Leader Association (CNLA), www.cnlassociation.org
Institute for Healthcare Improvement (IHI), www.ihi.org
Institute of Medicine (IOM), www.iom.edu
International Council of Nurses (ICN), www.icn.ch
Joint Commission, www.jointcommission.org
National Council of State Boards of Nursing (NCSBN), www.ncsbn.org/index.htm
QSEN Institute: Quality and Safety Education for Nurses, www.qsen.org
World Health Organization (WHO), www.who.int/en

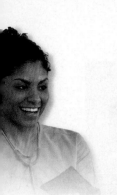

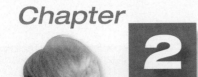

Community-Based Nursing Practice

Learning Objectives

On completion of this chapter, the learner will be able to:

1 Discuss the multiple roles and various settings in which nurses practice in the community.
2 Compare the differences and similarities between community- and hospital-based nursing.
3 Describe the discharge planning process.

4 Explain methods for identifying community resources and making referrals.
5 Discuss how to prepare for a home health care visit and how to conduct the visit.

Glossary

community-based nursing: nursing care of individuals and families that is designed to promote and maintain health and prevent disease. It is provided as patients transition through the health care system to health-related services outside of the hospital setting

community hub: centralized networks with infrastructure focused on coordinating health care and social services to reduce health risks in a given community

primary prevention: health care delivery focused on health promotion and prevention of illness or disease

secondary prevention: health care delivery centered on health maintenance and aimed at early detection of

disease, with prompt intervention to prevent or minimize loss of function and independence

tele-health: the use of technology such as telephones, computers, video or imaging transmissions, and links to health care instruments that remove the barriers of time and space to provide improved access to health care services for community-dwelling patients

tertiary prevention: health care delivery focused on minimizing deterioration associated with disease and improving quality of life through rehabilitation measures

third-party payor: an organization or insurance company that provides reimbursement for services covered by a health plan

---

The role of nurses in community settings is ever expanding. The shift in health care delivery from inpatient to outpatient is a result of multiple factors, including new population trends (the growing number of older adults), changes in federal legislation, tighter insurance regulations, and decreasing hospital revenues. Transitions in the health care industry, the nursing profession, and changing patterns of disease have also affected the community setting (see Chapter 1).

On an increasing basis, hospitals and other health care organizations and providers are held accountable for providing health care using best practices, as evidenced by meeting performance benchmarks for quality and efficiency, known as pay for performance or value-based purchasing (see Chapter 1 for further discussion). Under this system, hospitals and other health care organizations and providers can reduce costs and earn additional income by carefully monitoring the types of services they provide, discharging patients as soon as possible, and keeping patients who are discharged from the hospital from being readmitted. Consequently, patients are discharged from acute care facilities to their homes or to residential or long-term care facilities in the early stages of recovery.

Nurses work in various community-based settings, including public health departments, ambulatory health

clinics, long-term care facilities, schools, hospice centers, industrial environments (as occupational nurses), homeless shelters and clinics, nursing centers, home health agencies, urgent care centers, same-day surgical centers, short-stay facilities, and patients' homes. In these settings, nurses often deliver care without the direct on-site supervision or support of other health care personnel that is present in the hospital setting. Nurses practicing in the community must be self-directed, flexible, adaptable, and accepting of various lifestyles and living conditions. To function effectively, nurses in these settings must have expertise in independent decision making, critical thinking, assessment, health education, and competence in basic nursing care (Stanhope & Lancaster, 2012).

In addition, nurses in community settings must be culturally competent, as culture plays a role in the delivery of care in all settings. This is particularly important in a setting in which most community members share a cultural heritage that is unfamiliar to the nurse. To provide optimal care, the nurse should practice cultural sensitivity within the context of care through the utilization of a theoretical framework involving cultural competence (Clark, Calvillo, Dela Cruz, et al., 2011; Dayer-Berenson, 2011).

Key Components of Community-Based Care

Community-based nursing is a philosophy of care in which the care is provided as patients and their families move among various service providers outside of hospitals. It focuses on promoting and maintaining the health of individuals and families, preventing and minimizing the progression of disease, and improving quality of life (Stanhope & Lancaster, 2012). Community health nurses provide direct care to patients and families and use political advocacy to secure resources for aggregate populations (e.g., the older adult population). Community health nurses have many roles, including epidemiologist, case manager, coordinator of services provided to a group of patients, occupational health nurse, school nurse, visiting nurse, hospice nurse, or parish nurse. (In parish nursing, also called *faith community nursing,* the members of a faith-based community, typically the parish or the community the parish serves, are the recipients of care.) These roles have one element in common: a focus on community needs as well as the needs of individual patients. The primary concepts of community-based nursing care are preventive care and self-care within the context of culture and community.

Prevention

The ideal approach to community-based health care is to address potential issues with a client and family using upstream thinking (prior to disease or illness, or in the early stage of the development of a health issue) instead of focusing on health restoration or chronic illness management later, after the health issue has progressed. Upstream thinking focuses on the root cause of a given problem, whereas downstream thinking focuses on treating a health issue once it becomes problematic. Downstream thinking is the traditional mode of thinking used by health professionals. This approach has done little to reduce the prevalence of chronic illnesses and has not improved the health status of communities (Nies & McEwen, 2011).

Nurses in community-based practice provide preventive care at three levels: primary, secondary, and tertiary. **Primary prevention** focuses on health promotion and prevention of illness or disease, including interventions such as teaching about healthy lifestyles. **Secondary prevention** centers on health maintenance and is aimed at early detection, with prompt intervention to prevent or minimize loss of function and independence, including interventions such as health screening (Fig. 2-1) and health risk appraisal. **Tertiary prevention** focuses on minimizing deterioration and improving quality of life, including rehabilitation to assist patients in achieving their maximum potential by working through their physical or psychological challenges. Home care nurses often focus on tertiary preventive nursing care, although they also address primary and secondary prevention.

Discharge Planning for Transition to the Community or Home Care Setting

Discharge planning is an essential component of facilitating the transition of the patient from the acute care to the community or home care setting, or for facilitating the transfer of the patient from one health care setting to another. A documented discharge plan is mandatory for patients who receive Medicare or

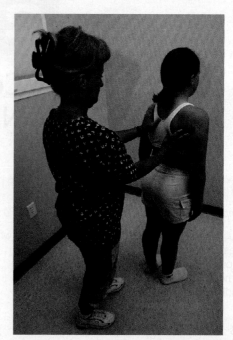

FIGURE 2-1 • Community-based nursing takes many forms and focuses. Here, the school nurse performs screening for scoliosis. This is an example of secondary prevention.

Medicaid health insurance benefits. Discharge planning begins with the patient's admission to the hospital or health care setting and must consider the potential for necessary follow-up care in the home or another community setting. Several different personnel (e.g., social workers, home care nurses, case managers) or agencies may be involved in the planning process.

The development of a comprehensive discharge plan requires collaboration between professionals at the referring agency and the home care agency, as well as other community agencies that provide specific resources upon discharge. The process involves identifying the patient's needs and developing a thorough plan to meet them. It is essential to have open lines of communication with family members to ensure their understanding and cooperation.

Community Resources and Referrals

As case managers and discharge planners, community-based nurses often make referrals to other team members, such as home health aides and social workers. These nurses work collaboratively with the health care team and the referring agency or person. Continuous coordinated care among all health care providers involved in a patient's care is essential to avoid duplication of effort by the various personnel caring for the patient.

A community-based nurse must be knowledgeable about community resources available to patients, as well as services provided by local agencies, eligibility requirements for those services, and any possible charges for the services. Most communities have directories or resource booklets that list local health and social service agencies and their offerings. The telephone book and the Internet are often useful in helping patients identify the location and accessibility of grocery and drug stores, banks, health care facilities, ambulances, physicians, dentists, pharmacists, social service agencies, and senior citizens' programs. In addition, a patient's place of worship or parish may be an important resource for services.

The community-based nurse is responsible for informing the patient and family about the community resources available to meet their needs. When appropriate, nurses may make the initial contact.

Home Health Care

Home care nursing is a unique component of community-based nursing. Home care visits are made by nurses who work for home care agencies, public health agencies, and visiting nurse associations; by nurses employed by hospitals; and by parish nurses or faith community nurses who work with the members or vulnerable populations. Such visits may also be part of the responsibilities of school nurses, clinic nurses, or occupational health nurses.

Holistic care is provided in the home through the collaboration of an interdisciplinary team that includes professional nurses; home health aides; social workers; physical, speech, and occupational therapists; and physicians. An interdisciplinary approach is used to provide health and social services with oversight of the total health care plan by a case manager, clinical nurse specialist, or nurse practitioner. Interdisciplinary collaboration is required if a home health agency is to receive Medicare certification (Stanhope & Lancaster, 2012).

Most home health agencies are reimbursed by various sources, including Medicare and Medicaid programs, private insurance, and direct patient payment. Older adults are the most frequent users of home care expenditures financed by Medicare, which allows nurses to manage and evaluate care of seriously ill patients who have complex, labile conditions and are at high risk for rehospitalization. Each funding source has its own requirements for services rendered, number of visits allowed, and amount of reimbursement the agency receives. The Omaha System's care documentation referred to as the Outcome and Assessment Information Set (OASIS) has been required for more than a decade to ensure that outcome-based care is provided for all care reimbursed by Medicare. This system uses six major domains—sociodemographic, environment, support system, health status, functional status, and behavioral status—and addresses selected health service utilization (Martin, Monsen, & Bowles, 2011; Tullai-McGuinness, Madigan, & Fortinsky, 2009).

Services Provided

The type of nursing services provided to patients in their homes varies from agency to agency. Clinic nurses may conduct home visits as part of patient follow-up. Public health, parish, and school nurses may make visits to provide anticipatory guidance to high-risk families and follow-up care to patients with communicable diseases. Many home care patients are acutely ill, and many have chronic health problems or disabilities, requiring that nurses provide more education and monitoring to patients and families. Nurses from home care or hospice agencies make home visits to provide skilled nursing care, follow-up care, and teaching to promote health and prevent complications. Hospice nursing is a specialty area of nursing practice in which nurses provide palliative care in patients' homes or within hospice centers, thus promoting comfort, peace, and dignity to patients who are dying.

Home health care visits may be intermittent or periodic, and case management via telephone or Internet may be used

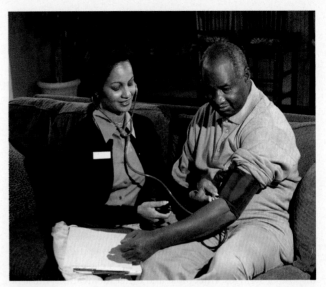

FIGURE 2-2 • Assessment is an important part of any home health visit.

to promote communication with home care consumers. The nurse instructs the patient and family about skills, self-care strategies, and health maintenance and promotion activities (e.g., nutritional counseling, exercise programs, stress management). Nursing care includes skilled assessment of the patient's physical, psychological, social, and environmental status (Fig. 2-2). Nursing interventions may include intravenous (IV) therapy and injections, parenteral nutrition, venipuncture, catheter insertion, pressure ulcer treatment, wound care, ostomy care, and patient and family teaching. Complex technical equipment, such as dialysis machines and ventilators, may be involved in home health care (Stanhope & Lancaster, 2012). Nurses have a role in evaluating the safety and effectiveness of technology in the home setting. In addition, **tele-health** is an emerging trend in home health care that facilitates exchange of information via telephone or computers between patients and nurses regarding health information such as blood glucose readings, vital signs, and cardiac parameters (Stanhope & Lancaster, 2012). The use of a broad spectrum of computer and Internet resources, such as webcams, also facilitates exchange of information.

The Home Setting

The home care nurse is a guest in the patient's home and must have permission to visit and give care. The nurse has minimal control over the lifestyle, living situation, and health practices of the visited patients. This lack of full decision-making authority can create a conflict for the nurse and lead to problems in the nurse–patient relationship. To work successfully with patients in any setting, the nurse must be nonjudgmental and convey respect for patients' beliefs, even if they differ sharply from those of the nurse. This can be difficult when a patient's lifestyle involves activities that a nurse considers harmful or unacceptable, such as smoking, the use of alcohol, drug abuse, or overeating.

The cleanliness of a patient's home may not meet the standards of a hospital. Although the nurse can provide teaching points about maintaining clean surroundings, the patient and family decide if they will implement the nurse's suggestions.

The nurse must accept their decisions and deliver the care required regardless of the conditions of the setting.

The kind of equipment and the supplies or resources that usually are available in acute care settings are often unavailable in the patient's home. The nurse has to learn to improvise when providing care, such as when changing a dressing or catheterizing a patient in a regular bed that is not adjustable and lacks a bedside table (Smith-Temple & Johnson, 2010).

Infection control is as important in the home as it is in the hospital; however, it can be more challenging in the home and requires creative approaches. As in any situation, it is important to clean one's hands before and after giving direct patient care, even in a home that does not have running water. If aseptic technique is required, the nurse must have a plan for implementing this technique before going to the home. This applies to universal precautions, transmission-based precautions, and disposal of bodily secretions and excretions. If injections are given, the nurse must use a closed container to dispose of syringes. Injectable and other medications must be kept out of the reach of children during visits and stored in a safe place if the medications will remain in the home.

> ◤ *Quality and Safety Nursing Alert*
>
> Friends, neighbors, or family members may ask the nurse about the patient's condition. The patient has a right to confidentiality, and information should be shared only with the patient's permission. If the nurse carries a patient's medical record into the home, it must be put in a secure place to prevent it from being misplaced or picked up by others.

Home Health Visits

Most agencies have a policy manual that identifies the agency's philosophy and procedures and defines the services provided. Becoming familiar with these policies is essential before initiating a home visit. It is also important to know the state laws regarding what actions to take if the nurse finds a patient dead, suspects abuse, determines that a patient cannot safely remain at home, or observes a situation that possibly indicates malicious harm to the community at large.

Preparing for a Home Visit

Before making a home visit, the nurse should review the patient's referral form and other pertinent data. It may be necessary to contact the referring agency if the purpose for the referral is unclear or important information is missing. The nurse calls the patient to obtain permission to visit, schedules a time for the visit, and verifies the address. This initial phone conversation provides an opportunity to introduce oneself, identify the agency, and explain the reason for the visit. If the patient does not have a telephone, the nurse should see if the person who made the referral is able to contact the patient regarding the visit. If an unannounced visit to a patient's home must be made, the nurse should ask permission to come in before entering the house. Explaining the purpose of the referral at the outset and setting up the times for future visits before leaving are also recommended.

Most agencies provide nurses with bags that contain standard supplies and equipment needed during home visits. It is important to keep the bag properly supplied and to bring any additional items that might be needed for the visit. Patients rarely have the medical supplies needed for treatment.

Conducting a Home Visit

Personal Safety Precautions

Community nurses must pay attention to personal safety, because they often practice in unknown environments. Based on the principle of due diligence, agencies should investigate at-risk working environments prior to making the assignment and must inform employees accordingly. Agencies have policies and procedures concerning the promotion of safety for clinical staff, and training is provided to facilitate personal safety. Environments must be proactively assessed for safety by the individual nurse and agency. Suggested precautions to take when making a home visit are presented in Chart 2-1.

Initial Home Visit

The first visit sets the tone for subsequent visits and is crucial in establishing the nurse–patient relationship. The situations encountered depend on numerous factors. Patients may be in pain and have additional factors that make them unable to care for themselves. Family members may be overwhelmed and doubt their ability to care for their loved ones. They may not understand why the patient was sent home from the hospital before being totally rehabilitated. They may not comprehend what home care is or why they cannot have 24-hour nursing services. It is critical that the nurse conveys

Chart 2-1 Safety Precautions in Home Health Care

- Learn, or preprogram a phone with, the telephone numbers of the agency, police, and emergency services. Most agencies provide phones for their nurses so that the agency can contact the nurse and the nurse can easily contact the agency.
- Carry agency identification and a charged phone to make telephone calls if you become lost or have problems.
- Let the agency know your daily schedule and the telephone numbers of your patients so that you can be located if you do not return when expected.
- Know where the patient lives before leaving to make the visit, and carry a map or global positioning device for quick referral.
- Keep your car in good working order, and have sufficient gas in the tank.
- Park the car near the patient's home, and lock the car during the visit.
- Do not drive an expensive car or wear expensive jewelry when making visits.
- Know the regular bus schedule, and know the routes when using public transportation or walking to the patient's house.
- When making visits in high-crime areas, visit with another person rather than alone (if possible).
- Try to schedule visits during daylight hours (when possible).
- Never walk into a patient's home uninvited.
- If you do not feel safe entering a patient's home, leave the area.
- Become familiar with the layout of the house, including exits from the house.
- If a patient or family member is intoxicated or hostile, leave and reschedule the visit.
- If a family is having a serious argument or abusing the patient or anyone else in the household, leave, reschedule the visit, contact your supervisor, and report the abuse to the appropriate authorities.

an understanding of what patients and families are experiencing and how the illness is affecting their lives.

During the initial home visit, which usually lasts less than an hour, the patient is evaluated and a plan of care is established that may be modified on subsequent visits. The nurse informs the patient of the agency's practices, policies, and hours of operation. If the agency is to be reimbursed for the visit, the nurse asks for insurance information, such as a Medicare or Medicaid card. The initial assessment includes evaluating the patient, the home environment (Chart 2-2),

the patient's self-care abilities or the family's ability to provide care, and the patient's need for additional resources.

Determining the Need for Future Visits

While conducting an assessment of a patient's situation, the home care nurse evaluates and clearly documents the need for future visits and the frequency with which those visits may need to be made. To make these judgments, the nurse should consider the questions listed in Chart 2-3. With each subsequent visit, these same factors are evaluated to determine the

---

Chart 2-2 **Assessing the Home Environment**

Physical Facilities (check all that apply)

Exterior

☐ Steps
☐ Unsafe steps
☐ Porch
☐ Litter
☐ Noise
☐ Adequate lighting
☐ Other _____

Interior

☐ Accessible bathroom
☐ Level, safe floor surface
☐ Number of rooms
☐ Privacy
☐ Sleeping arrangements
☐ Refrigeration
☐ Trash management
☐ Animals
☐ Adequate lighting
☐ Steps/stairs
☐ Other _____

Safety Hazards (check all that apply)

☐ None
☐ Inadequate floor, roof, or windows
☐ Inadequate lighting
☐ Unsafe gas/electric appliances
☐ Inadequate heating
☐ Inadequate cooling
☐ Lack of fire safety devices
☐ Unsafe floor coverings
☐ Inadequate stair rails
☐ Lead-based paint
☐ Improperly stored hazardous material
☐ Improper wiring/electrical cords
☐ Other _____

Safety Factors (check all that apply)

☐ Fire/smoke detectors
☐ Working telephone
☐ Placement of electrical cords
☐ Emergency plan
☐ Emergency phone numbers displayed
☐ Safe portable heaters
☐ Oxygen in use
☐ Obstacle-free paths
☐ Other _____

Chart 2-3 **Assessing the Need for Home Visits**

Current Health Status

- How well is the patient progressing?
- How serious are the present signs and symptoms?
- Has the patient shown signs of progressing as expected, or does it seem that recovery will be delayed?

Home Environment

- Are safety concerns apparent?
- Are family or friends available to provide care, or is the patient alone?

Level of Self-Care Ability

- Is the patient capable of self-care?
- What is the patient's level of independence?
- Is the patient ambulatory or bedridden?
- Does the patient have sufficient energy, or is he or she frail and easily fatigued?
- Does the patient need and use assistive devices?

Level of Nursing Care Needed

- What level of nursing care does the patient require?
- Does the care require basic skills or more complex interventions?

Prognosis

- What is the expectation for recovery in this particular instance?
- What are the chances that complications may develop if nursing care is not provided?

Educational Needs

- How well has the patient or family grasped the teaching points made?
- Is there a need for further follow-up and retraining?
- What level of proficiency does the patient or family show in carrying out the necessary care?

Mental Status

- How alert is the patient?
- Are there signs of confusion or thinking difficulties?
- Does the patient tend to be forgetful or have a limited attention span?

Level of Adherence

- Is the patient following the instructions provided?
- Does the patient seem capable of following the instructions?
- Are the family members helpful, or are they unwilling or unable to assist in caring for the patient as expected?

continuing health needs of the patient. As progress is made and the patient—with or without the help of significant others—becomes more capable of self-care and more independent, the need for home visits may decline.

Ending the Visit

As the visit comes to a close, it is important to summarize the main points of the visit for the patient and family and to identify expectations for future visits or patient achievements. The following points should be considered at the end of each visit:

- What are the main points the patient or family should remember from the visit?
- What positive attributes have been noted about the patient and the family that will give them a sense of accomplishment?
- What were the main points of the teaching plan or the treatments needed to ensure that the patient and family understand what they must do? A written set of instructions should be left with the patient or family, provided they can read and see (alternative formats include video or audio recordings). Printed material must be in the patient's primary language and in large print when indicated.
- Whom should the patient or family call if someone needs to be contacted immediately? Are current emergency telephone numbers readily available? Is telephone service available, or can an emergency phone service be provided?
- What signs of complications should be reported immediately?
- How frequently will visits be made? How long will they last (approximately)?
- What is the day and time of the next visit? Will a different nurse make the visit?

Documenting the Visit

Documentation considerations for home visits follow fairly specific regulations. The patient's needs and the nursing care provided must be documented to ensure that the agency qualifies for payment for the visit. Medicare, Medicaid, and other **third-party payors** (i.e., organizations that provide reimbursement for services covered under a health care insurance plan) require documentation of the patient's homebound status and the need for skilled professional nursing care. The medical diagnosis and specific detailed information on the functional limitations of the patient are usually part of the documentation. The goals and the actions appropriate for attaining those goals must be identified. Expected outcomes of the nursing interventions must be stated in terms of patient behaviors and must be realistic and measurable. In addition, the goals must reflect the nursing diagnosis or the patient's problems and must specify those actions that address the patient's problems. Inadequate documentation may result in nonpayment for the visit and care services.

Other Community-Based Health Care

Hospice Care

Community-based nurses may serve a population that is not moving toward restoration of health but instead toward death. During this terminal stage, hospice nurses provide education

---

Chart 2-4

Hospice Services Provided to Enhance Palliative Care

- Nursing care
- Medical social worker services
- Physician services
- Counseling (including dietary, pastoral, and other)
- Inpatient care (including respite care and short-term inpatient care for procedures necessary for pain control and acute and chronic symptom management)
- Hospice aide and homemaker services
- Medical appliances and supplies (including drugs and biologicals)
- Physical and occupational therapies
- Speech-language pathology services
- Bereavement services for families (up to 13 months following a patient's death)

Adapted from National Association for Home Care and Hospice. (2010). *Hospice facts and statistics.* Available at: www.nahc.org/facts/HospiceStats10.pdf

---

and support and also coordinate care between various health care and social service agencies. Hospice care can be provided in the home or in specialized facilities designed to assist the patient and family through the death experience. Patients are eligible for hospice care services if they are determined to be within the final 6 months of life. Many hospice services are covered by third-party payors for terminal patients and their families during the final stages of an illness and after death with bereavement support for family members. Beneficiaries must be re-certified by the hospice medical director as terminally ill at the beginning of each benefit period (National Association for Home Care and Hospice, 2010). Chart 2-4 displays the services that may be covered by hospice care. Chart 2-5 summarizes nursing research findings that patients in rural communities have limited access to hospice services.

Ambulatory Settings

Ambulatory health care is provided for patients in community- or hospital-based settings. The types of agencies that provide such care are medical clinics, ambulatory care units, urgent care centers, cardiac rehabilitation programs, mental health centers, student health centers, community outreach programs, and nursing centers. Some ambulatory centers provide care to a specific population, such as migrant workers or Native Americans. Neighborhood community health centers provide services to patients who live in a geographically defined area. These centers collectively provide affordable, accessible health care services to more than 20 million people in the United States, most of whom are impoverished (Hawkins & Groves, 2011). The centers may operate in freestanding buildings, storefronts, or mobile units. Agencies may provide ambulatory health care in addition to other services, such as an adult day care or health program. The kinds of services offered and the patients served depend on the agency's mission.

Nursing responsibilities in ambulatory health care settings include providing direct patient care, conducting patient intake screenings, treating patients with acute or chronic illnesses or emergency conditions, referring patients to other agencies for additional services, teaching patients self-care activities, and offering health education programs that promote health maintenance. Constraints imposed by federal legislation and ambulatory payment classifications require

| **Chart 2-5** | **NURSING RESEARCH PROFILE** |
| **Hospice Care in Rural Settings** | |

Campbell, C. L., Merwin, E., & Yan, G. (2009). Factors that influence the presence of a hospice in a rural community. *Journal of Nursing Scholarship, 41*(4), 420–428.

Purpose

Utilization of hospice services has generally increased over the past decade. However, terminally ill patients who live in rural communities, are ethnic minorities, and use Medicare services are less likely to die at home than patients who do not share this profile. The purpose of this study was to find socioeconomic, physician, and geographic and demographic factors that influence whether or not a Medicare-certified hospice was present in a given rural–urban area.

Design

This study performed secondary analyses of variables available in a database called the 2005 Area Resource File (ARF). The ARF contains more than 6,000 variables for each of the 3,225 counties in the United States and its territories. Each county was classified on a rural–urban continuum. Variables analyzed by county included median age, percentage of those older than 65 years, percentage of residents living in poverty, percentages of ethnic minorities (African Americans, Asian Americans, Native Americans, and Hispanics), and numbers of physicians per 10,000 residents. Logistic regression was performed to find if there was an association between any of these variables and the presence of a Medicare-certified hospice.

Findings

Those counties that were classified as most rural, had the greatest ethnic diversity, and had the lowest numbers of physicians per 10,000 residents were least likely to have a Medicare-certified hospice. The factor that was most predictive of the presence of a Medicare-certified hospice was the percentage of physicians living in a given county. The less the "rate" of physicians, the less likely there was a hospice present in a given county.

Nursing Implications

Hospices are valuable community resources that improve the delivery of palliative care services to terminally ill patients. Furthermore, they provide valuable social support to the families of terminally ill patients, improving their quality of life and decreasing their financial burden. Advanced practice nurses could fill the gap in providing this important service in rural communities, where access to physicians may limit access to hospice services.

efficient and effective management of patients in ambulatory settings. A useful tool in these settings is the classification scheme developed by the Visiting Nurses Association of Omaha, which contains three fully integrated patient-focused components: a problem classification scheme that requires assessment of the patient and family; an intervention scheme that includes the plan of care setup to deliver service in the safest, most effective, and high-quality manner; and a problem rating scale to judge the effectiveness of the plan and implementation based upon outcomes (Martin et al., 2011).

Nurses may work as clinic managers, direct the operation of clinics, and supervise other health team members. Nurses can play an important part in facilitating the function of the varied types of ambulatory care facilities. For instance, primary care nurse practitioners often practice in ambulatory care settings that focus on gerontology, pediatrics, family or adult health, or women's health. Some nurse practitioner faculty provide care in nurse-managed clinics as a part of their faculty practice appointments. Support for the full utilization of nurse practitioners is addressed in the *Future of Nursing* report produced by the Institute of Medicine (IOM) and the Robert Wood Johnson Foundation (RWJF) (IOM, 2010; see Chapter 1 for full discussion).

Occupational Health Programs

Federal legislation, especially the Occupational Safety and Health Act (OSHA), has been enacted to ensure safe and healthy work conditions. A safe working environment results in decreased employee absenteeism, hospitalization, and disability, as well as reduced costs.

Occupational nurses may work in solo units in industrial settings, or they may serve as consultants on a limited or part-time basis. They may be members of an interdisciplinary team composed of various personnel such as nurses, physicians, exercise physiologists, health educators, counselors, nutritionists, safety engineers, and industrial hygienists. Occupational health nurses may provide direct care to employees who become ill or injured; conduct health education programs for company staff members; set up programs aimed at establishing specific health outcomes, such as healthy eating and regular exercise; monitor employees' hearing, vision, blood pressure, or blood glucose; and track exposure to radiation, infectious diseases, and toxic substances, reporting results to government agencies as necessary.

Occupational health nurses must be knowledgeable about federal regulations pertaining to occupational health and familiar with other pertinent legislation, such as the Americans With Disabilities Act.

School Health Programs

School health programs provide services to students and may also serve the school's community. Ideally, school health programs have an interdisciplinary health team consisting of physicians, nurses, dentists, social workers, counselors, school administrators, parents, and students. The school may serve as the site for a family health clinic that offers primary health and mental health services to all family members in the community. Advanced practice nurses perform physical examinations and diagnose and treat students and families for acute and chronic illnesses within the scope of their practice. These clinics are cost-effective and benefit students from low-income families who lack access to traditional health care or have no health insurance.

School nurses play several roles, including care provider, health educator, consultant, and counselor. They collaborate with students, parents, administrators, and other health and social service professionals regarding student health problems. School nurses perform health screenings, provide basic care for minor injuries and complaints, administer medications, monitor the immunization status of students and families, identify children with health problems, provide teaching related to health maintenance and safety, and monitor the weight of children to facilitate prevention and treatment of obesity. They need to be knowledgeable about state and local regulations affecting school-age children, such as ordinances for excluding students from school because of communicable diseases or parasites such as lice or scabies.

School nurses are also health education consultants for teachers. In addition to providing information on health practices, teaching health classes, and participating in the development of the health education curriculum, school nurses educate teachers and classes when a student has a special problem, a disability, or a disease such as hemophilia, asthma, or human immunodeficiency virus (HIV) infection.

Community Nurse–Managed Centers

Community nurse–managed centers are another component of community-based care. Frequently sponsored by academic institutions, these centers typically are designed for the delivery of primary health care and serve people who are vulnerable, underinsured or uninsured, and without access to health services. Community nurse–managed centers, which are usually run by advanced practice nurses, serve numerous patients who are poor, members of minority groups, women, older adults, or homeless. The nurses provide health teaching, wellness and illness care, case management services, and psychosocial counseling (Coddington & Sands, 2008). In some areas, various community partnership models facilitate care for the growing number of migrant workers. The concept of **community hubs** to address vulnerable populations is gaining acceptance. These hubs contain the infrastructure to identify those at risk, treat using evidence-based practice, and evaluate benchmarks and outcomes to determine the effectiveness of care (Agency for Healthcare Research and Quality, 2011).

Care for Those Who Are Homeless

The homeless population is increasing in the United States. It is heterogeneous and includes members of both dysfunctional and intact families, the unemployed, and those who cannot find affordable housing. In addition, increasing numbers of women with children (often victims of domestic abuse), older adults, and veterans are homeless. Some people are homeless because of the nation's economic struggles or are temporarily homeless as a result of catastrophic natural disasters (National Coalition for the Homeless, 2009b).

Those who are homeless are often underinsured or uninsured and have limited or no access to health care. Because of numerous barriers, they often seek health care late in the course of a disease and deteriorate more quickly than patients who are not homeless. Many of their health problems are related in large part to their living situation. Street life exposes people to the extremes of hot and cold environments, and it compounds their health risks. This population has high rates of trauma, tuberculosis, upper respiratory tract infections, poor nutrition and anemia, lice, scabies, peripheral vascular disorders, sexually transmitted infections (STIs), dental problems, arthritis, hypothermia, skin disorders, and foot problems. Common chronic health problems also include diabetes, hypertension, heart disease, acquired immunodeficiency syndrome (AIDS), mental illness, and abuse of alcohol or other drugs (National Coalition for the Homeless, 2009a). These problems are made more difficult by living on the streets or discharge to a transitory homeless situation in which follow-up care is unlikely. Shelters frequently are overcrowded and unventilated, promoting the spread of communicable diseases such as tuberculosis. Those

who are homeless also tend to have a lower life expectancy of between 42 and 52 years of age compared to the average population life expectancy of 78 years (National Coalition for the Homeless, 2009a).

Community-based nurses who work with the homeless population must be nonjudgmental, patient, and understanding. They must be skilled in dealing with people who have various health problems and needs and must recognize that individualized treatment strategies are required in highly unpredictable environments. Nursing interventions are aimed at evaluating the health care needs of people who live in shelters and attempting to obtain health care services for those who are homeless.

Nurses serve in many capacities in the community setting. As varied as the service settings and roles might be, the common thread lies in the nurse's provision and coordination of evidence-based and outcome-driven care. The focus of nursing care in any community setting is to support the patient, family, and community to live the healthiest life possible.

Critical Thinking Exercises

1 **pq** You are a nurse employed at a college student health clinic. You have noted that many students have a history of type 1 diabetes. After a student loses consciousness on the football field, which is attributed to low blood glucose, you decide to form a specialty hub to support this population. What are your priorities as you begin to organize this hub, and what support would you request from your college administrators? How might health fairs fit into the hub you are developing? Name the top five areas of concern that you will address.

2 **ebp** A 77-year-old man with new diagnosis of heart failure is being referred for home care after discharge from the hospital, and he needs regular monitoring and teaching. He has several family members at home; however, they all work. You are concerned about his ability to manage his activities of daily living (ADLs) because of severe decreased activity tolerance and his need for assistance with self-care activities. What resources could you use to assist him to remain in his home for as long as possible? How would you go about obtaining this information? What is needed to ensure appropriate home care follow-up and facilitate maximum independent self-care measures within the limits of activity intolerance owing to decreased cardiac function? What is the strength of the evidence?

Brunner Suite Resources
Explore these additional resources to enhance learning for this chapter:
• NCLEX-Style Questions and Other Resources on **thePoint**, http://thePoint.lww.com/Brunner13e
• Study Guide
• PrepU
• Clinical Handbook
• Handbook of Laboratory and Diagnostic Tests

References

*Asterisk indicates nursing research.

Books

Dayer-Berenson, L. (2011). *Cultural competencies for nurses.* Boston: Jones & Bartlett.

Institute of Medicine. (2010). *The future of nursing: Leading change, advancing health.* Washington, DC: Author.

Nies, M. A., & McEwen, M. (2011). *Community/public health nursing.* St Louis: Elsevier.

Smith-Temple, A. J., & Johnson, J. Y. (2010). *Nurses' guide to clinical procedures.* Philadelphia: Lippincott Williams & Wilkins.

Stanhope, M., & Lancaster, J. (2012). *Public health nursing* (8th ed). St. Louis: Mosby.

Journals and Electronic Documents

Agency for Healthcare Research and Quality, U.S. Department of Health and Human Services. (2011). *Community hubs ensure better care for the most vulnerable.* Available at: www.ahrq.gov/research/jun11/0611RA1.htm

*Campbell, C. L., Merwin, E., & Yan, G. (2009). Factors that influence the presence of a hospice in a rural community. *Journal of Nursing Scholarship, 41*(4), 420–428.

Clark, L., Calvillo, E., Dela Cruz, F., et al. (2011). Cultural competencies for graduate nursing education. *Journal of Professional Nursing, 27*(3), 133–139.

Coddington, J. A., & Sands, L. P. (2008). Cost of health care and quality outcomes of patients at nurse-managed clinics. *Nursing Economics, 26*(2), 75–84.

Hawkins, D., & Groves, D. (2011). The future role of community health centers in a changing health care landscape. *Journal of Ambulatory Care Management, 34*(1), 90–99.

Martin, K. S., Monsen, K. A., & Bowles, K. H. (2011). The Omaha System and meaningful use: Applications for practice, education and research. *Computers, Informatics, Nursing, 29*(1), 52–58.

National Association for Home Care and Hospice. (2010). *Hospice facts and statistics.* Available at: www.nahc.org

National Coalition for the Homeless. (2009a). *Healthcare and homelessness.* Available at: www.nationalhomeless.org

National Coalition for the Homeless. (2009b). *Why are people homeless? NCH fact sheet #1.* Available at: www.nationalhomeless.org/publications/facts/Why.pdf

Tullai-McGuinness, S., Madigan, E. A., & Fortinsky, R. H. (2009). Validity testing the Outcomes and Assessment Information Set (OASIS). *Home Health Care Service Quarterly, 28*(1), 45–57.

Resources

Case Management Society of America (CMSA), www.cmsa.org
Centers for Disease Control and Prevention (CDC), www.cdc.gov
Centers for Medicare and Medicaid Services (CMS), www.cms.hhs.gov
Literacy Information and Communication System (LINCS), http://lincs.ed.gov/
National Association for Home Care and Hospice (NAHC), www.nahc.org
National Association of School Nurses (NASN), www.nasn.org
National Guideline Clearinghouse (NGC), www.guideline.gov
NurseLinx.com (MDLinx Inc.), www.sitealytics.com/nurselinx.com
Parish Nursing Health Information Resource, www.hshsl.umaryland.edu/faith/
U.S. Department of Health and Human Services, Office of Disease Prevention and Health Promotion, *Healthy People 2020,* http://healthypeople.gov/2020/
Urban Institute, www.urban.org

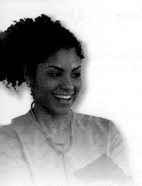

3

Critical Thinking, Ethical Decision Making, and the Nursing Process

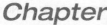
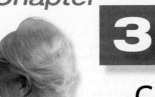

Learning Objectives

On completion of this chapter, the learner will be able to:

1 Define the characteristics of critical thinking, critical thinkers, and the critical thinking process.
2 Define ethics and nursing ethics.
3 Identify several ethical dilemmas common to the medical-surgical area of nursing practice.

4 Specify strategies that can aid nurses in ethical decision making.
5 Describe the components of the nursing process.
6 Develop a plan of nursing care for a patient using strategies of critical thinking.

Glossary

assessment: the systematic collection of data to determine the patient's health status and any actual or potential health problems

collaborative problems: specific pathophysiologic manifestations that nurses monitor to detect onset of complications or changes in status

critical thinking: a process of insightful thinking that utilizes multiple dimensions of one's cognition to develop conclusions, solutions, and alternatives that are appropriate for the given situation

deontologic or formalist theory: an ethical theory maintaining that ethical standards or principles exist independently of the ends or consequences

ethics: the formal, systematic study of moral beliefs

evaluation: determination of the patient's responses to the nursing interventions and the extent to which the outcomes have been achieved

implementation: actualization or carrying out of the plan of care through nursing interventions

moral dilemma: situation in which a clear conflict exists between two or more moral principles or competing moral claims

moral distress: conflict that arises within oneself when a person is aware of the correct course of action but institutional constraints stand in the way of pursuing the correct action

moral problem: competing moral claim or principle; one claim or principle is clearly dominant

moral uncertainty: conflict that arises within a person when he or she cannot accurately define what the moral situation is or what moral principles apply but has a strong feeling that something is not right

morality: the adherence to informal personal values

nursing diagnoses: actual or potential health problems that can be managed by independent nursing interventions

nursing process: a deliberate problem-solving approach for meeting people's health care and nursing needs; common components are assessment, diagnosis, planning, implementation, and evaluation

planning: development of goals and outcomes, as well as a plan of care designed to assist the patient in resolving the diagnosed problems and achieving the identified goals and desired outcomes

teleologic theory or consequentialism: the theoretical basis of ethics, which focuses on the ends or consequences of actions, such as utilitarianism

utilitarianism: a teleologic theory of ethics based on the concept of "the greatest good for the greatest number"

In today's health care arena, nurses face increasingly complex issues and situations resulting from advanced technology, greater acuity of patients in both hospital and community settings, an aging population, and complex disease processes, as well as ethical issues and cultural factors. The decision-making part of nurses' problem-solving activities has become increasingly multifaceted and requires critical thinking.

Critical Thinking

Critical thinking is a multidimensional skill, a cognitive or mental process or set of procedures. It involves reasoning and purposeful, systematic, reflective, rational, outcome-directed thinking based on a body of knowledge, as well as examination and analysis of all available information and ideas. Critical thinking leads to the formulation of conclusions and alternatives that are the most appropriate for the situation. Although many definitions of critical thinking have been offered in various disciplines, some consistent themes within those definitions are (1) a strong formal and informal foundation of knowledge; (2) willingness to pursue or ask questions; and (3) ability to develop solutions that are new, even those that do not fit the standard or current state of knowledge or attitudes. Willingness and openness to various viewpoints are inherent in critical thinking, and it is also important to reflect on the current situation (Brubakken, Grant, Johnson, et al., 2011). Critical thinking includes metacognition—the examination of one's own reasoning or thought processes—to help refine thinking skills. Independent judgments and decisions evolve from a sound knowledge base and the ability to synthesize information within the context in which it is presented. Nursing practice in today's society requires the use of high-level critical thinking skills. Critical thinking enhances clinical decision making, helping to identify patient needs and the best nursing actions that will assist patients in meeting those needs.

Because critical thinking is a conscious, outcome-oriented activity, it is systematic and organized, not erratic. Critical thinkers are inquisitive truth seekers who are open to the alternative solutions that might surface. Alfaro-LeFevre (2009) identified critical thinkers as people who ideally are active thinkers, fair minded, open minded, persistent, empathic, independent in thought, good communicators, honest, organized and systematic, proactive, flexible, realistic, humble, cognizant of the rules of logic, curious and insightful, and creative and committed to excellence. The skills involved in critical thinking are developed over time through effort, practice, and experience.

Rationality and Insight

Skills needed in critical thinking include interpretation, analysis, inference, explanation, evaluation, and self-regulation. Critical thinking requires background knowledge and knowledge of key concepts as well as logical thinking. Nurses use this disciplined process to validate the accuracy of data and the reliability of any assumptions they have made, and they then carefully evaluate the effectiveness of what they have identified as the necessary actions to take. Nurses also evaluate the reliability of sources, being mindful of and questioning inconsistencies. Nurses use interpretation to determine the significance of data that are gathered, analysis to identify patient problems suggested by the data, and inference to draw conclusions. Explanation is the justification of actions or interventions used to address patient problems and to help patients move toward desired outcomes. Evaluation is the process of determining whether outcomes have been or are being met. Self-regulation is the process of examining the care provided and adjusting the interventions as needed.

Critical thinking is also reflective, involving metacognition, active evaluation, and refinement of the thinking process. Nurses engaged in critical thinking consider the possibility of cultural differences and personal bias when interpreting data and determining appropriate actions (see Chapter 7). Critical thinkers must be insightful and have a sense of fairness and integrity, the courage to question personal ethics, and the perseverance to strive continuously to minimize the effects of egocentricity, ethnocentricity, and other biases on the decision-making process (Alfaro-LeFevre, 2009).

Components of Critical Thinking

Certain cognitive or mental activities are key components of critical thinking. Critical thinkers:

- Ask questions to determine why certain developments have occurred and to see whether more information is needed to understand the situation accurately.
- Gather as much relevant information as possible to consider as many factors as possible.
- Validate the information presented to make sure that it is accurate (not just supposition or opinion), that it makes sense, and that it is based on fact and evidence.
- Analyze the information to determine what it means and to see whether it forms clusters or patterns that point to certain conclusions.
- Draw on past clinical experience and knowledge to explain what is happening and to anticipate what might happen next, acknowledging personal bias and cultural influences.
- Maintain a flexible attitude that allows the facts to guide thinking and take into account all possibilities.
- Consider available options and examine each in terms of its advantages and disadvantages.
- Formulate decisions that reflect creativity and independent decision making.

Critical thinking requires going beyond basic problem solving into a realm of inquisitive exploration, looking for all relevant factors that affect the issue, and being an "out-of-the-box" thinker. It includes questioning all findings until a comprehensive picture emerges that explains the phenomenon, possible solutions, and creative methods for proceeding (Wilkinson, 2011). Critical thinking in nursing practice results in a comprehensive plan of care with maximized potential for success.

Critical Thinking and Clinical Reasoning in Nursing Practice

Critical thinking and decision making are thought to be associated with improved clinical expertise. Critical thinking is at the center of the process of clinical reasoning and clinical judgment (Arafeh, Hansen, & Nichols, 2010). Using critical thinking to develop a plan of nursing care requires considering the human factors that might influence the plan. Nurses interact with patients, families, and other health care providers in the process of providing appropriate, individualized nursing care. The culture, attitude, and thought processes of nurses, patients, and others affect the critical thinking process from the data-gathering stage through the decision-making stage; therefore, aspects of the nurse–patient interaction must be considered (Wilkinson, 2011).

Nurses must use critical thinking skills in all practice settings—acute care, ambulatory care, extended care, and the home and community—and must view each patient situation as unique and dynamic. Key components of critical thinking behavior are withholding judgment and being open to options and explanations from one patient to another in similar circumstances (Brubakken et al., 2011). The unique factors that patients and nurses bring to the health care situation are considered, studied, analyzed, and interpreted. Interpretation of the information then allows nurses to focus on those factors that are most relevant and most significant to the clinical situation. Decisions about what to do and how to do it are then developed into a plan of action.

In decision making related to the nursing process, nurses use intellectual skills in critical thinking. These skills include systematic and comprehensive assessment, recognition of assumptions and inconsistencies, verification of reliability and accuracy, identification of missing information, distinguishing relevant from irrelevant information, support of the evidence with facts and conclusions, priority setting with timely decision making, determination of patient-specific outcomes, and reassessment of responses and outcomes (Alfaro-LeFevre, 2009). For example, nurses use critical thinking and decision-making skills in providing genetics-related nursing care when they:

- Assess and analyze family history data for genetic risk factors.
- Identify those individuals and families in need of referral for genetic testing or counseling.
- Ensure the privacy and confidentiality of genetic information.

To depict the process of "thinking like a nurse," Tanner (2006, 2009) developed the Clinical Judgment Model, which supports the idea that nurses engage in a complex process of clinical reasoning when caring for patients. Nurses draw on personal knowledge and experience from various situations and consider the contextual background of the clinical culture. As nursing students develop their clinical reasoning skills and become professional nurses, their ability to reason clinically and to make sound clinical nursing judgments becomes more refined. Research findings by Jenkins (2011) imply that many common critical thinking skills develop over time among nursing students from different cultural backgrounds and countries. This suggests that critical thinking skills that are requisite to competent nursing practice transcend cultural and societal boundaries (Chart 3-1).

Because developing the skill of critical thinking takes time and practice, critical thinking exercises are offered at the end of each chapter as a means of honing the reader's ability to think critically. Some exercises include questions that stimulate the reader to seek information about evidence-based practice relative to the clinical situation described, whereas others challenge the reader to identify priority assessments and interventions. Additional exercises may be found in the study guide that accompanies the text. The questions listed in Chart 3-2 can serve as a guide in working through the exercises. It is important to remember that each clinical situation is unique and calls for an individualized approach that fits its unique set of circumstances. As critical thinking may require consideration of ethical principles and cultural contexts, discussion of these concepts are discussed in this chapter and in Chapter 7.

Ethical Nursing Care

In the complex modern world, we are surrounded by ethical issues in all facets of our lives. Consequently, there has been a

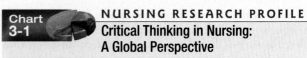

Chart 3-1

NURSING RESEARCH PROFILE
Critical Thinking in Nursing: A Global Perspective

Jenkins, S. D. (2011). Cross-cultural perspectives on critical thinking. *Journal of Nursing Education, 50*(5), 268–274.

Purpose

Although it is widely asserted that schools of nursing foster the development of critical thinking in nursing students, few studies support this assertion. Furthermore, the conceptual definition of critical thinking in nursing may differ from its definition in other disciplines and may differ from definitions within the discipline of nursing, based upon culture. The purpose of this study was to elicit definitions of critical thinking from seasoned faculty at schools of nursing in the United States and Thailand to find both common and dissimilar constructs that may define critical thinking in nursing.

Design

Five seasoned nursing educators from the United States and five from Thailand were purposively selected for this study. Each of them participated in individual taped interviews that lasted 45 to 60 minutes. The data from these interviews were coded and analyzed until themes emerged.

Findings

American and Thai participants expressed many common constructs that they felt characterized critical thinking. For example, educators from both countries felt that students who were critical thinkers were able to analyze, synthesize, question, evaluate, investigate, flex, and reflect. Of note, both American and Thai participants believed that students' ability to stay calm when stressed also characterized critical thinking, a construct not noted as essential within other disciplines. Only Thai participants felt that another key construct that defined critical thinking was that it led to happiness. Both American and Thai participants felt that a universal definition of critical thinking in nursing would help to guide and advance both nursing practice and research.

Nursing Implications

Findings from this research suggest that there are many common constructs that define the acquisition of critical thinking skills in nursing across cultures. Furthermore, these findings suggest that there may be at least one characteristic of critical thinking in nursing that is unique to nursing (i.e., the ability to stay calm when stressed).

heightened interest in the field of ethics in an attempt to gain a better understanding of how these issues influence us. Specifically, the focus on ethics in health care has intensified in response to controversial developments, including advances in technology and genetics, as well as diminished health care and financial resources.

Today, sophisticated technology can prolong life well beyond the time when death would have occurred in the past. Expensive experimental procedures, medications, equipment, and devices are available for attempting to preserve life, even when such attempts are likely to fail. The development of technologic support has influenced the quality and delivery of nursing care at all stages of life and also has contributed to an increase in average life expectancy. For example, the

Chart 3-2 The Inquiring Mind: Critical Thinking in Action

Throughout the critical thinking process, a continuous flow of questions evolves in the thinker's mind. Although the questions will vary according to the particular clinical situation, certain general inquiries can serve as a basis for reaching conclusions and determining a course of action.

When faced with a patient situation, seeking answers to some or all of the following questions may help to determine those actions that are most appropriate:

- What relevant assessment information do I need, and how do I interpret this information? What does this information tell me? What contextual factors must be considered when gathering this information? What are the priority assessments?
- To what problems does this information point? Have I identified the most important ones? Does the information point to any other problems that I should consider?
- Have I gathered all of the necessary information (signs and symptoms, laboratory values, medication history, emotional factors, mental status)? Is anything missing?
- Is there anything that needs to be reported immediately? Do I need to seek additional assistance?
- Does this patient have any special risk factors? Which ones are most significant? What must I do to minimize these risks?
- What possible complications must I anticipate?
- What are the most important problems in this situation? Do the patient and the patient's family recognize the same problems?
- What are the desired outcomes for this patient? Which have the highest priority? Do the patient and I agree on these points?
- What is going to be my first action in this situation? Why is this action a priority?
- How can I construct a plan of care to achieve the goals?
- Are there any age-related factors involved, and will they require some special approach? Will I need to make some change in the plan of care to take these factors into account?
- How do the family dynamics affect this situation, and will they affect my actions or the plan of care?
- Are there cultural factors that I must address and consider?
- Am I dealing with an ethical issue here? If so, how am I going to resolve it?
- Has any nursing research been conducted on this subject? What are the nursing implications of this research for care of this patient? What is the strength of the evidence found from research?

prenatal period has been influenced by genetic screening, in vitro fertilization, the harvesting and freezing of embryos, and prenatal surgery. Premature infants who once would have died early in life now may survive because of advances in technology. Patients who would have died of organ failure are living longer because of organ transplantation.

These advances in technology have been a mixed blessing. Questions have been raised about whether it is appropriate to use such technology and, if so, under what circumstances. Although many patients do achieve a good quality of life, others face extended suffering as a result of efforts to prolong life, usually at great expense. Ethical issues also surround those practices or policies that seem to allocate health care resources unjustly on the basis of age, race, gender, disability, or social mores.

The ethical dilemmas that nurses may encounter in the medical-surgical nursing arena are numerous and diverse

and occur in all settings. An awareness of underlying philosophical concepts helps nurses use reason to work through these dilemmas. Basic concepts related to moral philosophy, such as ethics and its terminology, theories, and approaches, are included in this chapter. Understanding the role of the professional nurse in ethical decision making not only helps nurses articulate their ethical positions and develop the skills needed to make ethical decisions but also helps them use the nursing process to develop plans of care from an ethical perspective.

Ethics Versus Morality

The terms *ethics* and *morality* are used to describe beliefs about right and wrong and to suggest appropriate guidelines for action. In essence, **ethics** is the formal, systematic study of moral beliefs, whereas **morality** is the adherence to informal personal values. Because the distinction between ethics and morality is slight, the terms are often used interchangeably.

Ethics Theories

One classic theory in ethics is **teleologic theory or consequentialism**, which focuses on the ends or consequences of actions. The best-known form of this theory, **utilitarianism**, is based on the concept of "the greatest good for the greatest number." The choice of action is clear under this theory, because the action that maximizes good over bad is the correct one. The theory poses difficulty when one must judge intrinsic values and determine whose good is the greatest. In addition, it is important to ask whether good consequences can justify any amoral actions that might be used to achieve them.

Another theory in ethics is the **deontologic or formalist theory**, which argues that ethical standards or principles exist independently of the ends or consequences. In a given situation, one or more ethical principles may apply. Nurses have a duty to act based on the one relevant principle, or the most relevant of several ethical principles. Problems arise with this theory when personal and cultural biases influence the choice of the most primary ethical principle.

Approaches to Ethics

Two approaches to ethics are meta-ethics and applied ethics. An example of meta-ethics (understanding the concepts and linguistic terminology used in ethics) in the health care environment is analysis of the concept of informed consent. Nurses are aware that patients must give consent before surgery; however, sometimes a question arises as to whether a patient is truly informed. Delving more deeply into the concept of informed consent would be a meta-ethical inquiry. (See Chapter 17 for more information about informed consent before surgery.)

Applied ethics refers to identification of ethical problems relevant to a specific discipline and that discipline's practice. Various disciplines use the frameworks of general ethical theories and principles and apply them to specific problems within their domain. Nursing ethics may be considered a form of applied ethics because it addresses moral situations that are specific to the nursing profession and patient care. Common ethical principles that can be used to validate moral claims in clinical practice include autonomy, beneficence and nonmaleficence, double effect, and distributive justice. Brief definitions of these important principles can be found in Chart 3-3.

Chart 3-3 **Common Ethical Principles**

The following common ethical principles may be used to validate moral claims.

Autonomy

This word *autonomy* is derived from the Greek words *autos* ("self") and *nomos* ("rule" or "law") and therefore refers to self-rule. In contemporary discourse, it has broad meanings, including individual rights, privacy, and choice. The principle of autonomy entails the right of patients to receive adequate and accurate information so that they have the ability to make a choice free from external constraints.

Beneficence and Nonmaleficence

Beneficence is the duty to do good and the active promotion of benevolent acts (e.g., goodness, kindness, charity). It also entails taking positive action to prevent patients from harming themselves or others, including society as a whole. Nonmaleficence is the duty to not inflict harm. The only time when it is considered morally permissible to exercise power over a competent person against his or her will is when by doing so, harm to others is prevented.

Double Effect

The double effect is a principle that may morally justify some actions that produce both good and evil effects.
    All four of the following criteria must be fulfilled:

1. The action itself is good or morally neutral.
2. The agent sincerely intends the good and not the evil effect (the evil effect may be foreseen but is not intended).
3. The good effect is not achieved by means of the evil effect.
4. There is proportionate or favorable balance of good over evil.

Distributive Justice

From a broad perspective, justice states that like cases should be treated alike. More specifically, distributive justice is an ethical principle commonly applicable to clinical situations. This principle is upheld when benefits and burdens are distributed equitably and fairly without consideration of age, gender, socioeconomic status, religion, ethnicity, or sexual orientation.

Moral Situations

Many situations exist in which ethical analysis is needed. Some are **moral dilemmas,** or situations in which a clear conflict exists between two or more moral principles or competing moral claims, and nurses must choose the lesser of two evils. Other situations represent **moral problems,** in which there may be competing moral claims or principles, although one claim or principle is clearly dominant. Some situations result in **moral uncertainty,** when one cannot accurately define what the moral situation is or what moral principles apply but has a strong feeling that something is not right. Still other situations may result in **moral distress,** in which one is aware of the correct course of action but constraints stand in the way of pursuing the correct action.

For example, an older adult patient with emphysema falls and is admitted to the hospital with a fractured hip. Although she has been advised to have surgery to repair her hip, she tells the nurse that she would rather be discharged home. She is cognitively competent and says, "I have walked long enough and am tired of walking. I'd rather just go home, stay in bed, and see what happens." The surgeon and the patient's adult daughter feel differently and do not support the patient's wishes to go home and not have surgery. The nurse believes that the patient should be able to make autonomous decisions about her treatment options. However, the surgeon and the patient's daughter are concerned that if she is discharged home unable to walk, the patient will likely become even sicker and could die. Thus, the ethical principles of autonomy and nonmaleficence are at odds with each other—a moral problem exists because of the competing moral claims of the patient's daughter and physician, who wish to pursue what is ordinarily considered a best treatment option, and the nurse, who desires to uphold the wishes of the patient. If the patient's competency were questionable, a moral dilemma would exist because no dominant principle would be evident.

It is essential that nurses freely engage in dialogue concerning moral situations, even though such dialogue is difficult for everyone involved. Improved interdisciplinary communication is supported when all members of the health care team can voice their concerns and come to an understanding of the moral situation. Consultation with an ethics committee could be helpful to assist the health care team, patient, and family to identify the moral dilemma and possible approaches to the dilemma (see the Ethics Committees section). Nurses should be familiar with agency policy supporting patient self-determination and resolution of ethical issues.

Types of Ethical Problems in Nursing

As a profession, nursing is accountable to society. Nursing has identified its standards of accountability through formal codes of ethics that explicitly state the profession's values and goals. The International Council of Nurses (ICN) has endorsed a globally applicable *Code of Ethics for Nurses* (ICN, 2006). Likewise, the American Nurses Association (ANA) established a code of ethics that includes ethical standards, each with its own interpretive statements (ANA, 2001a; Fowler, 2008) (Chart 3-4). The interpretive statements provide guidance to address and resolve ethical dilemmas by incorporating universal moral principles. In addition, the ANA sponsors a Center for Ethics and Human Rights that contains a repository of position statements that can be used to guide nursing practice (Chart 3-5).

Ethical issues have always affected the role of professional nurses. The accepted definition of professional nursing supports the advocacy role for nurses. The ANA, in *Nursing's Social Policy Statement* (2010a), defines *nursing* as "the protection, promotion, and optimization of health and abilities, prevention of illness and injury, alleviation of suffering through the diagnosis and treatment of human response, and advocacy in the care of individuals, families, communities, and populations" (p. 9). This definition supports the claim that nurses must be actively involved in the decision-making process regarding ethical concerns surrounding health care and human responses. Nurses are morally obligated to present ethical conflicts within a logical, systematic framework. Health care settings in which nurses are valued members of the team promote interdisciplinary communication and may

---

Chart 3-4   American Nurses Association Code of Ethics for Nurses

1. The nurse, in all professional relationships, practices with compassion and respect for the inherent dignity, worth, and uniqueness of every individual, unrestricted by considerations of social or economic status, personal attributes, or the nature of health problems.
2. The nurse's primary commitment is to the patient, whether an individual, family, group, or community.
3. The nurse promotes, advocates for, and strives to protect the health, safety, and rights of the patient.
4. The nurse is responsible and accountable for individual nursing practice and determines the appropriate delegation of tasks consistent with the nurse's obligation to provide optimum patient care.
5. The nurse owes the same duties to self as to others, including the responsibility to preserve integrity and safety, to maintain competence, and to continue personal and professional growth.
6. The nurse participates in establishing, maintaining, and improving health care environments and conditions of employment conducive to the provision of quality health care and consistent with the values of the profession through individual and collective action.
7. The nurse participates in the advancement of the profession through contributions to practice, education, administration, and knowledge development.
8. The nurse collaborates with other health professionals and the public in promoting community, national, and international efforts to meet health needs.
9. The profession of nursing, as represented by associations and their members, is responsible for articulating nursing values, for maintaining the integrity of the profession and its practice, and for shaping social policy.

Reprinted with permission from the American Nurses Association, *Code of Ethics for Nurses with Interpretive Statements,* © 2001, American Nurses Publishing, American Nurses Foundation/American Nurses Association, Washington, DC.

Chart 3-5   Position Statements from the American Nurses Association Center for Ethics and Human Rights

Position Statement	Latest Approval/ Revision Date
Foregoing Nutrition and Hydration	Revised 3/11/11
Registered Nurses' Roles and Responsibilities in Providing Expert Care and Counseling at the End of Life	Approved 6/14/10
The Nurses' Role in Ethics and Human Rights: Protecting and Promoting Individual Worth, Dignity, and Human Rights in Practice Setting	Approved 6/14/10
Nurses' Role in Capital Punishment	Approved 1/28/10
In Support of Patients' Safe Access to Therapeutic Marijuana	Approved 12/12/08
Stem Cell Research	Approved 1/10/07
Privacy and Confidentiality	Approved 12/8/06
Assuring Patient Safety: The Employers' Role in Promoting Healthy Nursing Work Hours for Registered Nurses in All Roles and Settings to Guard Against Working When Fatigued	Approved 12/8/06
Risk and Responsibility in Providing Nursing Care	Approved 6/21/06
Nursing Care and Do Not Resuscitate Decisions	Approved 12/1/03
Reduction of Patient Restraint and Seclusion in Health Care Settings	Approved 10/17/01
Assisted Suicide	Approved 12/08/94
Active Euthanasia	Approved 12/08/94
Cultural Diversity in Nursing Practice	Approved 10/22/91

---

enhance patient care. To practice effectively in these settings, nurses must be aware of ethical issues and assist patients in voicing their moral concerns.

Nursing theories that incorporate the biopsychosocial–spiritual dimensions emphasize a holistic viewpoint, with humanism or caring at the core. *Caring* is often cited as the moral foundation for professional nursing practice. For nurses to embrace this professional ethos, they must be aware not only of major ethical dilemmas but also of those daily interactions with health care consumers that frequently give rise to less easily identifiable ethical challenges. Although technologic advances and diminished resources have been instrumental in raising numerous ethical questions and controversies, including life-and-death issues, nurses should not ignore the many routine situations that involve ethical considerations. Some of the most common issues faced by nurses today include confidentiality, the use of restraints, trust, refusing care, and end-of-life concerns.

Confidentiality

All nurses should be aware of the confidential nature of information obtained in daily practice. If information is not pertinent, nurses should question whether it is prudent to document it in a patient's record. In the practice setting, discussion of patients with other members of the health care team is often necessary. However, these discussions should occur in a private area where it is unlikely that the conversation will be overheard. Nurses should also be aware that the use of family members as interpreters for patients who are not fluent in the English language or who are deaf violates patients' rights of confidentiality. Translation services should be provided for non–English-speaking patients, and interpreters should be provided for those who use sign language.

Another threat to confidentiality is the widespread use of computer-based technologies and people's easy access to them. The growing demand for tele-health innovations and the increasing use of this method can result in unchecked access to health information. In addition, personal and health information is often made available to numerous individuals and corporate stakeholders, which may increase the potential for misuse of health care information. Because of these possibilities of maleficence, sensitivity to the principle of confidentiality is essential. The ANA (1999) published a position statement that addresses patients' rights to privacy and confidentiality of their health information.

Federal legislation has been developed to protect the right of confidentiality. According to the Health Insurance Portability and Accountability Act (HIPAA) (U.S. Department of Health and Human Services [HHS], 2003), efforts must be made to protect each patient's private information, whether it is transmitted by verbal, written, or electronic means of communication. Communication should be confined to the appropriate settings and with appropriate individuals and should occur for the appropriate purposes of facilitating patient care. Violations of protection of any patient's privacy could result in criminal or civil litigation (HHS, 2003).

Restraints

The use of restraints (including physical and pharmacologic measures) is another issue with ethical overtones because of the limits on a person's autonomy when restraints are used. It is important to weigh carefully the risks of limiting autonomy and increasing the risks of injury by using restraints against the risks of injury if not using restraints, which have been documented as resulting in physical harm and death. The ANA (2001b) advocates that "only when no other viable option is available should restraint be employed" (p. 1). The Joint Commission and the Centers for Medicare and Medicaid Services (CMS) have designated standards for the use of restraints. (See the Joint Commission and CMS Web sites listed in the Resources section.)

Trust Issues

Telling the truth (veracity) is one of the basic principles of our culture. Three ethical dilemmas in clinical practice that can directly conflict with this principle are the use of placebos (nonactive substances used for treatment), not revealing a diagnosis to a patient, and revealing a diagnosis to people other than the patient with the diagnosis. All involve the issue of trust, which is an essential element in the nurse–patient relationship.

Placebos may be used in experimental research, in which a patient is involved in the decision-making process and is aware that placebos are being used in the treatment regimen. However, the use of a placebo as a substitute for an active drug to show that a patient does not have actual symptoms of a disease is deceptive, has both ethical and legal implications, and severely undermines the nurse–patient relationship.

Informing a patient of his or her diagnosis when the family and physician have chosen to delay full disclosure of pertinent information is an ethical situation that can occur in nursing practice. The nursing staff may often use evasive comments with the patient in these situations. This area is indeed complex, because it challenges a nurse's integrity. Nurses could consider the following strategies:

- Avoid lying to the patient.
- Provide all information related to nursing procedures and diagnoses.
- Communicate the patient's requests for information to the family and physician. The family is often unaware of the patient's repeated questions to the nurse. With a better understanding of the situation, the family members may change their perspective.

Although providing the information may be the morally appropriate behavior, the manner in which the patient is told is important. Nurses must be compassionate and caring when informing patients; disclosure of information merely for the sake of patient autonomy does not convey respect for others and in some circumstances may result in emotional distress.

Family support or the support of a spiritual advisor (e.g., chaplain) may be needed to reduce the impact of distressing information or a poor prognosis.

Disclosing the patient's diagnosis to others without the patient's consent is a HIPAA violation and therefore is not only unethical but also illegal. Although family members and friends who request the information may be well-intentioned, the nurse must be firm in explaining that the patient's permission must be obtained before any information can be shared with anyone else (Wielawski, 2009).

Refusing to Provide Care

Any nurse who feels compelled to refuse to provide care for a particular type of patient faces an ethical dilemma. Reasons for refusal range from a conflict of personal values to a fear of personal injury. Feelings related to care of people of different cultures also surface as changes emerge in the cultural makeup of the U.S. population. The ethical obligation to care for all patients is clearly identified in the first statement of the *Code of Ethics for Nurses* (ANA, 2001a). Lachman (2009) asserts, "As a professional, the nurse is expected to reflect and move beyond feelings to provide the same level of care to every patient, regardless of diagnosis, skin color, ethnic origin, or economic status" (p. 55). To avoid facing ethical dilemmas, nurses can follow certain strategies. For example, when applying for a job, a nurse should ask questions regarding the patient population. If a nurse is uncomfortable with a particular situation, then not accepting the position would be an option. Denial of care, or providing substandard nursing care to some members of society, is not acceptable nursing practice.

End-of-Life Issues

Dilemmas that center on death and dying are prevalent in medical-surgical nursing practice. With the availability of increasingly sophisticated and advanced technology, it may be difficult to accept that nothing more can be done to prolong life or that technology may prolong life but at the expense of the patient's comfort and quality of life. Nurses face increasingly controversial dilemmas concerning patients' desires to avoid prolongation of life (Burns, Jacobs, & Jacobs, 2011). Many people who are terminally ill seek legal options for a peaceful and dignified death.

End-of-life issues shift the focus from curative care to palliative and end-of-life care. Focusing on the caring as well as the curing role may help nurses deal with these difficult moral situations. Needs of patients and families require holistic and interdisciplinary approaches. End-of-life issues that often involve ethical dilemmas include pain control, "do not resuscitate" orders, life support measures, and administration of food and fluids. These issues are discussed in detail in Chapter 16.

Preventive Ethics

When a nurse is faced with two conflicting alternatives, it is his or her moral responsibility to choose the lesser of the two evils. Various preventive strategies are available to help nurses anticipate or avoid certain kinds of ethical dilemmas, address the moral distress that is stimulated, and act with courage to do what is ethically sound (Callister & Sudia-Robinson, 2011).

Patient Self-Determination

Frequently, dilemmas occur when health care practitioners are unsure of the patient's wishes because the patient is unconscious or cognitively impaired and cannot communicate. The Patient Self-Determination Act, enacted in December 1991, encourages people to prepare advance directives in which they indicate their wishes concerning the degree of supportive care they wish if they become incapacitated. This legislation requires that patients be informed about advance directives by the staff of the health care facility.

Advance directives are legal documents that specify a person's wishes before hospitalization and provide valuable information that may assist health care providers in decision making. A living will is one type of advance directive. Typically, living wills are limited to situations in which the patient's medical condition is deemed terminal. Because it is difficult to define *terminal* accurately, living wills are not always honored. Another potential drawback is that living wills are frequently written while people are in good health. It is not unusual for people to change their minds as an illness progresses; therefore, patients retain the option to nullify these documents.

Durable power of attorney for health care, in which one person identifies another person to make health care decisions on his or her behalf, is another type of advance directive. Patients may have clarified their wishes concerning various medical situations. The power of attorney for health care is a less restrictive type of advance directive. Laws concerning advance directives vary among state jurisdictions. However, even in states where these documents are not legally binding, they provide helpful information to determine the patient's prior expressed wishes in situations in which this information can no longer be obtained. (See Chapter 16 for further discussion of end-of-life care.)

Advance directives are limited in scope to hospital and long-term care facility environments. Emergency medical system (EMS) personnel (e.g., paramedics) therefore cannot legally follow advance directives. Yet, there are many patients with debilitating long-term chronic and eventually fatal illnesses who reside at home. Some of these patients may not wish to have invasive, life-sustaining emergency interventions should their status rapidly deteriorate. To protect the wishes of these patients to forego life-sustaining treatments, a document titled Physician Orders for Life-Sustaining Treatment (POLST) has been legally endorsed by many states. POLST gives EMS personnel the ability to rapidly determine whether a patient wishes to have cardiopulmonary resuscitation (CPR) or receive any type of emergency interventions that may sustain life in the event the patient suddenly becomes incapacitated (Fromme, Zive, Schmidt, et al., 2012; Hickman, Sabatino, Moss, et al., 2008).

Ethics Committees

Institutional ethics committees exist in many hospitals to assist clinicians with ethical dilemmas. The purpose of these multidisciplinary committees varies among institutions. In some hospitals, the committees exist solely for the purpose of developing policies, whereas in others, they may have a strong educational or consultation focus. These committees usually are composed of people with some advanced training in ethics and are important resources for the health care team, patient, and family. Nurses with a particular interest or expertise in the area of ethics can serve as members of these committees, which are valuable resources for staff nurses.

Ethical Decision Making

Ethical dilemmas are common and diverse in nursing practice. Situations vary, and experience indicates that there are no clear solutions to these dilemmas. However, the fundamental philosophical principles are the same, and the process of moral reflection helps nurses justify their actions. The approach to ethical decision making can follow the steps of the nursing process. Ethics charts contained in all units within this text present case scenarios that challenge the reader to identify the ethical principles involved that may or may not be in conflict (see Chart 3-3). Chart 3-6 outlines the steps of an ethical analysis that may be used to resolve the moral dilemmas presented in these charts.

The Nursing Process

Definition

The **nursing process** is a deliberate problem-solving approach for meeting people's health care and nursing needs. Although the steps of the nursing process have been stated in various ways by different writers, the common components cited are assessment, diagnosis, planning, implementation, and evaluation (Carpenito, 2013). The ANA's *Standards of Clinical Nursing Practice* (2010b) includes an additional component entitled outcome identification and establishes the sequence of steps in the following order: **assessment**, diagnosis, outcome identification, **planning**, **implementation**, and **evaluation**. For the purposes of this text, the nursing process is based on the traditional five steps and delineates two components in the diagnosis step: **nursing diagnoses** and **collaborative problems**. After the diagnoses or problems have been determined, the desired outcomes are often evident. The traditional steps are defined as follows:

1. *Assessment:* The systematic collection of data that will be used in the next step of the nursing process to determine the patient's health status and any actual or potential health problems (Analysis of data is included as part of the assessment. Analysis may also be identified as a separate step of the nursing process.)
2. *Diagnosis:* Identification of the following two types of patient problems:
   - *Nursing diagnoses:* Actual or potential health problems that can be managed by independent nursing interventions
   - *Collaborative problems:* According to Carpentino (2013), "Certain physiologic complications that nurses monitor to detect onset or changes in status. Nurses manage collaborative problems using physician-prescribed and nurse-prescribed interventions to minimize the complications of the events" (p. 23).
3. *Planning:* Development of goals and outcomes as well as a plan of care designed to assist the patient in resolving the diagnosed problems and achieving the identified goals and desired outcomes

Chart 3-6   Steps of an Ethical Analysis

The following guidelines reflect an active process in decision making, similar to the nursing process detailed in this chapter. Nurse can use these guidelines to engage in ethical decision making. Key resources that may assist in ethical decision making are also included.

Assessment

1. Assess the ethical/moral situations of the problem. This step entails recognition of the ethical, legal, and professional dimensions involved.
   a. Does the situation entail substantive moral problems (conflicts among ethical principles or professional obligations)?
   b. Are there procedural conflicts? (For example, who should make the decisions? Any conflicts among the patient, health care providers, family, and guardians?)
   c. Identify the significant people involved and those affected by the decision.
   d. Identify agency or hospital policy or protocol to use when a conflict exists. Is there an ethics committee or council? How is an ethics consult made, and who may request this consultation? What other resources are available to help resolve this conflict?

Planning

2. Collect information.
   a. Include the following information: the medical facts, treatment options, nursing diagnoses, legal data, and the values, beliefs, cultures, and religious components.
   b. Make a distinction between the factual information and the values/beliefs.
   c. Validate the patient's capacity, or lack of capacity, to make decisions.
   d. Identify any other relevant information that should be elicited.
   e. Identify the ethical/moral issues and the competing claims.

Implementation

3. List the alternatives. Compare alternatives with applicable ethical principles and professional code of ethics. Choose either of the frameworks that follow, or other frameworks, and compare outcomes.
   a. *Utilitarian approach:* Predict the consequences of the alternatives; assign a positive or negative value to each consequence; choose the consequence that predicts the highest positive value or "the greatest good for the greatest number."
   b. *Deontologic approach:* Identify the relevant moral principles; compare alternatives with moral principles; appeal to the "higher-level" moral principle if there is a conflict.

Evaluation

4. Decide and evaluate the decision.
   a. What is the best or morally correct action?
   b. Give the ethical reasons for your decision.
   c. What are the ethical reasons against your decision?
   d. How do you respond to the reasons against your decision?

Resources

American Nurses Association, Center for Ethics and Human Rights: An online resource that contains a repository of positions papers, codes, and other materials aimed at improving the ethical competence of nurses, www.nursingworld.org/ethics

The Hastings Center: A nonprofit, nonpartisan research institute dedicated to interdisciplinary bioethics, www.thehastingscenter.org

National Center for Ethics in Health Care: Provides key analysis of topics in health care ethics, publishes ethics-related news, and posts seminal national reports in ethics, www.ethics.va.gov/ETHICS/pubs/index.asp

---

4. *Implementation:* Actualization or carrying out of the plan of care through nursing interventions
5. *Evaluation:* Determination of the patient's responses to the nursing interventions and the extent to which the outcomes have been achieved

Dividing the nursing process into distinct steps serves to emphasize the essential nursing actions that must be taken to address the patient's nursing diagnoses and manage any collaborative problems or complications. However, dividing the process into separate steps is artificial: The process functions as an integrated whole, with the steps being interrelated, interdependent, and recurrent (Fig. 3-1). Chart 3-7 presents an overview of the nursing activities involved in applying the nursing process. Note that the use of the nursing process requires critical thinking and consideration of common ethical principles to ensure that a truly comprehensive plan of care is developed.

Using the Nursing Process

Assessment

Assessment data are gathered through the health history and the physical assessment. In addition, ongoing monitoring is crucial to remain aware of changing patient needs and the effectiveness of nursing care.

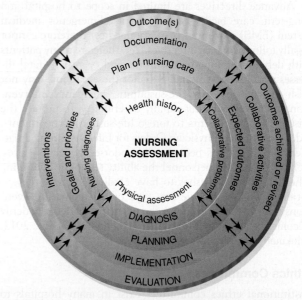

FIGURE 3-1 • The nursing process is depicted schematically in this circle. Starting from the innermost circle, nursing assessment, the process moves outward through the formulation of nursing diagnoses and collaborative problems; planning, with setting of goals and priorities in the nursing plan of care; implementation and documentation; and, finally, the ongoing process of evaluation and outcomes.

Chart 3-7 Steps of the Nursing Process

Assessment

1. Conduct the health history.
2. Perform the physical assessment.
3. Interview the patient's family or significant others.
4. Study the health record.
5. Organize, analyze, synthesize, and summarize the collected data.

Diagnosis

Nursing Diagnoses

1. Identify the patient's nursing problems.
2. Identify the defining characteristics of the nursing problems.
3. Identify the etiology of the nursing problems.
4. State nursing diagnoses concisely and precisely.

Collaborative Problems

1. Identify potential problems or complications that require collaborative interventions.
2. Identify health care members with whom collaboration is essential.

Planning

1. Assign priority to the nursing diagnoses.
2. Specify the goals.
   a. Develop immediate, intermediate, and long-term goals.
   b. State the goals in realistic and measurable terms.
3. Identify nursing interventions appropriate for goal attainment.
4. Establish expected outcomes.
   a. Make sure that the outcomes are realistic and measurable.
   b. Identify critical times for the attainment of outcomes.

5. Develop the written plan of nursing care.
   a. Include nursing diagnoses, goals, nursing interventions, expected outcomes, and critical times.
   b. Write all entries precisely, concisely, and systematically.
   c. Keep the plan current and flexible to meet the patient's changing problems and needs.
6. Involve the patient, family or significant others, nursing team members, and other health care team members in all aspects of planning.

Implementation

1. Put the plan of nursing care into action.
2. Coordinate the activities of the patient, family or significant others, nursing team members, and other health care team members.
3. Record the patient's responses to the nursing actions.

Evaluation

1. Collect data.
2. Compare the patient's actual outcomes with the expected outcomes. Determine the extent to which the expected outcomes were achieved.
3. Include the patient, family or significant others, nursing team members, and other health care team members in the evaluation.
4. Identify alterations that need to be made in the nursing diagnoses, collaborative problems, goals, nursing interventions, and expected outcomes.
5. Continue all steps of the nursing process: assessment, diagnosis, planning, implementation, and evaluation.

Health History

The health history is conducted to determine a person's state of wellness or illness and is best accomplished as part of a planned interview. The interview is a personal dialogue between a patient and a nurse that is conducted to obtain information. The nurse's approach to the patient largely determines the amount and quality of the information received. To achieve a relationship of mutual trust and respect, the nurse must communicate a sincere interest in the patient. Examples of effective therapeutic communication techniques that can be used to achieve this goal are found in Table 3-1.

A health history guide may help in obtaining pertinent information and directing the course of the interview. Various health history formats designed to guide the interview are available; however, they must be adapted to the responses, problems, and needs of the person. (See Chapter 5 for more information about the health history.)

Physical Assessment

A physical assessment may be carried out before, during, or after the health history, depending on a patient's physical and emotional status and the immediate priorities of the situation. The purpose of the physical assessment is to identify those aspects of a patient's physical, psychological, and emotional state that indicate a need for nursing care. It requires

the use of sight, hearing, touch, and smell, as well as appropriate interview skills and techniques. Physical examination techniques, as well as techniques and strategies for assessing behaviors and role changes, are presented in Chapter 5 and in the first chapter of each unit of this book.

Other Components of the Assessment

Additional relevant information should be obtained from the patient's family or significant others, from other members of the health care team, and from the patient's health record or chart. Depending on the patient's immediate needs, this information may have been completed before the health history and the physical assessment were obtained. Whatever the sequence of events, the nurse should use all available sources of pertinent data to complete the nursing assessment.

Recording the Data

After the health history and physical assessment are completed, the information obtained is recorded in the patient's permanent record. These records are more commonly becoming electronic (i.e., electronic health records [EHRs]). The ANA (2009) advocates that when EHRs are used, that they be "designed to facilitate and support critical thinking and decision making, such as in the nursing process, and the associated documentation activities" (p. 1). Regardless of whether the record is in a traditional paper

TABLE 3-1 Therapeutic Communication Techniques		
Technique	**Definition**	**Therapeutic Value**
Listening	Active process of receiving information and examining one's reactions to the messages received	Nonverbally communicates nurse's interest in patient
Silence	Periods of no verbal communication among participants for therapeutic reasons	Gives patient time to think and gain insights, slows the pace of the interaction, and encourages the patient to initiate conversation while conveying the nurse's support, understanding, and acceptance
Restating	Repeating to the patient what the nurse believes is the main thought or idea expressed	Demonstrates that the nurse is listening and validates, reinforces, or calls attention to something important that has been said
Reflection	Directing back to the patient his or her feelings, ideas, questions, or content	Validates the nurse's understanding of what the patient is saying and signifies empathy, interest, and respect for the patient
Clarification	Asking the patient to explain what he or she means or attempting to verbalize vague ideas or unclear thoughts of the patient to enhance the nurse's understanding	Helps to clarify the patient's feelings, ideas, and perceptions and to provide an explicit correlation between them and the patient's actions
Focusing	Questions or statements to help the patient develop or expand an idea or verbalize feelings	Allows the patient to discuss central issues and keeps communication goal directed
Broad openings	Encouraging the patient to select topics for discussion	Indicates acceptance by the nurse and the value of the patient's initiative
Humor	Discharge of energy through the comic enjoyment of the imperfect	Promotes insight by bringing repressed material to consciousness, resolving paradoxes, tempering aggression, and revealing new options; a socially acceptable form of sublimation
Informing	Providing information	Helpful in health teaching or patient education about relevant aspects of the patient's well-being and self-care
Sharing perceptions	Asking the patient to verify the nurse's understanding of what the patient is thinking or feeling	Conveys the nurse's understanding to the patient and has the potential to clarify confusing communication
Theme identification	Underlying issues or problems experienced by the patient that emerge repeatedly during the course of the nurse–patient relationship	Allows the nurse to best promote the patient's exploration and understanding of important problems
Suggesting	Presentation of alternative ideas for the patient's consideration relative to problem solving	Increases the patient's perceived options or choices

Adapted from Stuart, G. W. (2009). *Principles and practice of psychiatric nursing* (9th ed.). St. Louis: CV Mosby.

format or an EHR, it must provide a means of communication among members of the health care team and facilitate coordinated planning and continuity of care. The record fulfills other functions as well:

- It serves as the legal and business record for a health care agency and for the professional staff members who are responsible for the patient's care. Various systems are used for documenting patient care, and each health care agency selects the system that best meets its needs.
- It serves as a basis for evaluating the quality and appropriateness of care and for reviewing the effective use of patient care services.
- It provides data that are useful in research, education, and short- and long-range planning.

Diagnosis

The assessment component of the nursing process serves as the basis for identifying nursing diagnoses and collaborative problems. Soon after the completion of the health history and the physical assessment, nurses organize, analyze, synthesize, and summarize the data collected and determine the patient's need for nursing care.

Nursing Diagnoses

Nursing diagnoses, the first taxonomy created in nursing, have fostered autonomy and accountability in nursing and have helped to delineate the scope of practice. Many state nurse

practice acts include nursing diagnosis as a nursing function, and nursing diagnosis is included in the ANA's *Standards of Clinical Nursing Practice* (2010b) and the standards of nursing specialty organizations.

NANDA International (NANDA-I; formerly known as the North American Nursing Diagnosis Association) is the official organization responsible for developing the taxonomy of nursing diagnoses and formulating nursing diagnoses that are acceptable for study. Approved nursing diagnoses are compiled and categorized by NANDA-I in a taxonomy that is updated to maintain currency. The diagnostic labels identified by NANDA-I (2012) have been generally accepted; however, ongoing validation, refinement, and expansion based on clinical use and research are encouraged.

Choosing a Nursing Diagnosis

When choosing the nursing diagnoses for a particular patient, nurses must first identify the commonalities among the assessment data collected. These common features lead to the categorization of related data that reveal the existence of a problem and the need for nursing intervention. The identified problems are then defined as specific nursing diagnoses. Nursing diagnoses represent actual or potential health problems that can be managed by independent nursing actions.

It is important to remember that nursing diagnoses are not medical diagnoses; they are not medical treatments prescribed by the physician, and they are not diagnostic studies. Rather, they are succinct statements in terms of specific patient problems that guide nurses in the development of the plan of nursing care.

To give additional meaning to the nursing diagnosis, the characteristics and etiology of the problem are identified and included as part of the diagnosis. For example, the nursing diagnoses and their defining characteristics and etiology for a patient who has anemia may include the following:

- Activity intolerance related to weakness and fatigue
- Ineffective peripheral tissue perfusion related to decreased hemoglobin
- Imbalanced nutrition: less than body requirements related to fatigue and inadequate intake of essential nutrients

Collaborative Problems

In addition to nursing diagnoses and their related nursing interventions, nursing practice involves certain situations and interventions that do not fall within the definition of nursing diagnoses. These activities pertain to potential problems or complications that are medical in origin and require collaborative interventions with the physician and other members of the health care team. The term *collaborative problem* is used to identify these situations.

Collaborative problems are certain physiologic complications that nurses monitor to detect changes in status or onset of complications. Nurses manage collaborative problems using physician-prescribed and nurse-prescribed interventions to minimize complications (Carpenito, 2013). When treating collaborative problems, a primary nursing focus is monitoring patients for the onset of complications or changes in the status of existing complications. The complications are usually related to the disease process, treatments, medications, or diagnostic studies. The nurse recommends nursing interventions that are appropriate for managing the complications and implements the treatments prescribed by the physician. The algorithm in Figure 3-2 depicts the differences between nursing diagnoses and collaborative problems. After the nursing diagnoses and collaborative problems have been identified, they are recorded on the plan of nursing care.

Planning

Once the nursing diagnoses have been identified, the planning component of the nursing process begins. This phase involves the following steps:

1. Assigning priorities to the nursing diagnoses and collaborative problems
2. Specifying expected outcomes
3. Specifying the immediate, intermediate, and long-term goals of nursing action
4. Identifying specific nursing interventions appropriate for attaining the outcomes
5. Identifying interdependent interventions
6. Documenting the nursing diagnoses, collaborative problems, expected outcomes, nursing goals, and nursing interventions on the plan of nursing care
7. Communicating to appropriate personnel any assessment data that point to health care needs that can best be met by other members of the health care team

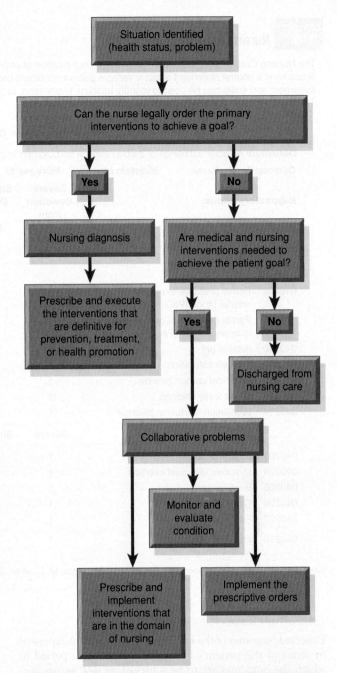

FIGURE 3-2 • Differentiating nursing diagnoses and collaborative problems. Redrawn from Carpenito, L. J. (2013). *Nursing diagnosis: Application to clinical practice* (14th ed., p. 27). Philadelphia: Lippincott Williams & Wilkins.

Setting Priorities

Assigning priorities to the nursing diagnoses and collaborative problems is a joint effort by the nurse and the patient or family members. Any disagreement about priorities is resolved in a way that is mutually acceptable. Consideration must be given to the urgency of the problems, with the most critical problems receiving the highest priority. Maslow's hierarchy of needs provides one framework for prioritizing problems, with importance being given first to physical needs; once those basic needs are met, higher-level needs can be addressed. (See Chapter 1 for a discussion of Maslow's hierarchy of needs.)

Nursing Outcomes Classification

The Nursing Outcomes Classification (NOC) is a classification of patient outcomes that is sensitive to nursing interventions. Each outcome is a neutral statement about a variable patient condition, behavior, or perception, coupled with a rating scale. The outcome statement and scale can be used to identify baseline functioning, expected outcomes, and actual outcomes for individual patients. The following table is an example of a nursing-sensitive outcome.

Respiratory Status: Gas Exchange (0402)

Definition: Alveolar exchange of carbon dioxide and oxygen to maintain arterial blood gas concentrations.

OUTCOME TARGET RATING   *Maintain at* _____   *Increase to* _____

Respiratory Status: **Gas Exchange** **Overall Rating**	**Severe Deviation from Normal Range** **1**	**Substantial Deviation from Normal Range** **2**	**Moderate Deviation from Normal Range** **3**	**Mild Deviation from Normal Range** **4**	**No Deviation from Normal Range** **5**	
Indicators						
040208 Partial pressure of oxygen in arterial blood (PaO$_2$)	1	2	3	4	5	NA
040209 Partial pressure of carbon dioxide in arterial blood (PaCO$_2$)	1	2	3	4	5	NA
040210 Arterial pH	1	2	3	4	5	NA
040211 Oxygen saturation	1	2	3	4	5	NA
040212 End-tidal carbon dioxide	1	2	3	4	5	NA
040213 Chest x-ray findings	1	2	3	4	5	NA
040214 Ventilation–perfusion balance	1	2	3	4	5	NA
	Severe	**Substantial**	**Moderate**	**Mild**	**None**	
040203 Dyspnea at rest	1	2	3	4	5	NA
040204 Dyspnea with mild exertion	1	2	3	4	5	NA
040205 Restlessness	1	2	3	4	5	NA
040206 Cyanosis	1	2	3	4	5	NA
040207 Somnolence	1	2	3	4	5	NA
040216 Impaired cognition	1	2	3	4	5	NA

Used with permission from Moorhead, S., Johnson, M., Maas, M. L., et al. (Eds.). (2013). *Nursing outcomes classification (NOC)* (5th ed.). St. Louis: Mosby-Elsevier.

Establishing Expected Outcomes

Expected outcomes of the nursing interventions are expressed in terms of the patient's behaviors and the time period in which the outcomes are to be achieved, as well as any special circumstances related to achieving the outcome (Smith-Temple & Johnson, 2010). These outcomes must be realistic and measurable. Resources for identifying appropriate expected outcomes include the Nursing Outcomes Classification (NOC) (Chart 3-8) and standard outcome criteria established by health care agencies for people with specific health problems. These outcomes can be associated with nursing diagnoses and interventions and can be used when appropriate. However, the NOC may need to be adapted to establish realistic criteria for the specific patient involved.

The expected outcomes that define the patient's desired behavior are used to measure the progress made toward resolving the problem. The expected outcomes also serve as the basis for evaluating the effectiveness of the nursing interventions and for deciding whether additional nursing care is needed or whether the plan of care needs to be revised.

Establishing Goals

After the priorities of the nursing diagnoses and expected outcomes have been established, goals (immediate, intermediate, and long-term) and the nursing actions appropriate for attaining the goals are identified. The patient and family are included in establishing goals for the nursing actions. Immediate goals are those that can be attained within a short period. Intermediate and long-term goals require a longer time to be achieved and usually involve preventing complications and other health problems and promoting self-care and rehabilitation. For example, goals for a patient with a nursing diagnosis of impaired physical mobility related to pain and edema following total knee replacement may be stated as follows:

- Immediate goal: Stands at bedside for 5 minutes 6 to 12 hours after surgery
- Intermediate goal: Ambulates with walker or crutches in hospital and home
- Long-term goal: Ambulates independently 1 to 2 miles each day

Chart 3-9 Nursing Interventions Classification

The Nursing Interventions Classification (NIC) is a standardized classification of nursing treatments (interventions) that includes independent and collaborative interventions. Intervention labels are terms such as *hemorrhage control, medication administration,* or *pain management.* Listed under each intervention are multiple discrete nursing actions that together constitute a comprehensive approach to the treatment of a particular condition. Not all actions are applicable to every patient; nursing judgment will determine which actions to implement. The following is an example of a nursing intervention:

Ventilation Assistance

Definition

Promotion of an optimal spontaneous breathing pattern that maximizes oxygen and carbon dioxide exchange in the lungs

Activities

Maintain a patent airway.
Position to alleviate dyspnea.
Position to facilitate ventilation–perfusion matching ("good lung down"), as appropriate.
Assist with frequent position changes, as appropriate.

Position to minimize respiratory efforts (e.g., elevate head of bed and provide overbed table for patient to lean on).
Monitor the effects of position change on oxygenation (e.g., arterial blood gases, SaO_2, $S\bar{v}\text{-}O_2$).
Encourage slow deep breathing, turning, and coughing.
Assist with incentive spirometer, as appropriate.
Auscultate breath sounds, noting areas of decreased or absent ventilation and presence of adventitious sounds.
Monitor for respiratory muscle fatigue.
Initiate and maintain supplemental oxygen, as prescribed.
Administer appropriate pain medication to prevent hypoventilation.
Ambulate three to four times per day, as appropriate.
Monitor respiratory and oxygenation status.
Administer medications (e.g., bronchodilators and inhalers) that promote airway patency and gas exchange.
Teach pursed lips breathing techniques, as appropriate.
Teach breathing techniques, as appropriate.
Initiate a program of respiratory muscle strength and/or endurance training, as appropriate.
Initiate resuscitation efforts, as appropriate.

Used with permission from Bulechek, G. M., Butcher, H. K., & Dochterman, J. M. (Eds.). (2013). *Nursing interventions classification (NIC)* (6th ed.). St. Louis: Mosby-Elsevier.

Determining Nursing Actions

In planning appropriate nursing actions to achieve the desired goals and outcomes, the nurse, with input from the patient and significant others, identifies individualized interventions based on the patient's circumstances and preferences that address each outcome. Interventions should identify the activities needed and who will implement them. Determination of interdisciplinary activities is made in collaboration with other health care providers as needed. The patient's medications and other prescribed treatments should be integrated into the plan of care to assist the nurse in determining how all interventions contribute to resolution of the identified problems.

The nurse identifies and plans patient education and demonstration as needed to assist the patient in learning certain self-care activities. Planned interventions should be ethical and appropriate to the patient's culture, age, and gender. Standardized interventions, such as those found on standardized care plans or in the Nursing Interventions Classification (NIC) (Bulechek, Butcher, & Dochterman, 2013) can be used. Chart 3-9 describes the NIC system and provides an example of an NIC system intervention. It is important to individualize prewritten interventions to promote optimal effectiveness for each patient. Actions of nurses should be based on established standards.

Implementation

The implementation phase of the nursing process involves carrying out the proposed plan of nursing care. The nurse assumes responsibility for the implementation and coordinates the activities of all those involved in implementation, including the patient and family, and other members of the health care team so that the schedule of activities facilitates the patient's recovery. The plan of nursing care serves as the basis for implementation as such:

- The immediate, intermediate, and long-term goals are used as a focus for the implementation of the designated nursing interventions.
- While implementing nursing care, the nurse continually assesses the patient and his or her response to the nursing care.
- Revisions are made in the plan of care as the patient's condition, problems, and responses change and when reordering of priorities is required.

Implementation includes direct or indirect execution of the planned interventions. It is focused on resolving the patient's nursing diagnoses and collaborative problems and achieving expected outcomes, thus meeting the patient's health needs. The following are examples of nursing interventions:

- Assist with hygiene care
- Promote physical and psychological comfort
- Support respiratory and elimination functions
- Facilitate the ingestion of food, fluids, and nutrients
- Manage the patient's immediate surroundings
- Provide health education
- Promote a therapeutic relationship
- Carry out various therapeutic nursing activities

Judgment, critical thinking, and good decision-making skills are essential in the selection of appropriate evidence-based and ethical nursing interventions. All nursing interventions are patient focused and outcome directed and are implemented with compassion, confidence, and a willingness to accept and understand the patient's responses.

 Concept Mastery Alert

Implementation is nursing action. Therefore, statements involving implementation always start with a verb.

Although many nursing actions are independent, others are interdependent, such as carrying out prescribed treatments, administering medications and therapies, and collaborating with other health care team members to accomplish specific expected outcomes and to monitor and manage potential complications. Such interdependent functioning is just that—interdependent. Requests or orders from other health care team members should not be followed blindly but should be assessed critically and questioned when necessary. The implementation phase of the nursing process ends when the nursing interventions have been completed.

Evaluation

Evaluation, the final step of the nursing process, allows the nurse to determine the patient's response to the nursing interventions and the extent to which the objectives have been achieved. The plan of nursing care is the basis for evaluation. The nursing diagnoses, collaborative problems, priorities, nursing interventions, and expected outcomes provide the specific guidelines that dictate the focus of the evaluation. Through evaluation, the nurse can answer the following questions:

- Were the nursing diagnoses and collaborative problems accurate?
- Did the patient achieve the expected outcomes within the critical time periods?
- Have the patient's nursing diagnoses been resolved?
- Have the collaborative problems been resolved?
- Do priorities need to be reordered?
- Have the patient's nursing needs been met?
- Should the nursing interventions be continued, revised, or discontinued?
- Have new problems evolved for which nursing interventions have not been planned or implemented?
- What factors influenced the achievement or lack of achievement of the objectives?
- Should changes be made to the expected outcomes and outcome criteria?

Objective data that provide answers to these questions are collected from all available sources (e.g., patients, families, significant others, health care team members). These data are included in patients' records and must be substantiated by direct patient observation before the outcomes are documented.

Documentation of Outcomes and Revision of the Plan

Outcomes are documented concisely and objectively. Documentation should relate outcomes to the nursing diagnoses and collaborative problems, describe the patient's responses to the interventions, indicate whether the outcomes were met, and include any additional pertinent data. As noted previously, the nurse individualizes a plan of care for each patient's particular circumstances. Chart 3-10 gives an example of a plan of nursing care that has been developed for a 52-year-old overweight woman admitted with acute cholecystitis.

The plan of care is subject to change as a patient's needs change, as the priorities of needs shift, as needs are resolved, and as additional information about a patient's state of health is collected. As the nursing interventions are implemented, the patient's responses are evaluated and documented, and the plan of care is revised accordingly. A well-developed, continuously updated plan of care is the greatest assurance that the patient's nursing diagnoses and collaborative problems are addressed and his or her basic needs are met.

Framework for a Common Nursing Language: Combining NANDA-I, NIC, and NOC

Various frameworks or taxonomies can be used for determining nursing diagnoses (e.g., NANDA-I), establishing outcomes (e.g., NOC), and designing interventions (e.g., NIC). Ultimately, a framework that uses a language common to all aspects of nursing, regardless of the classification system, is desirable. In 2001, a taxonomy of nursing practice was developed for the harmonization of NANDA-I, NIC, and NOC. This three-part combination links nursing diagnoses, accompanying interventions, and outcomes, organizing them in the same way. Such organization of concepts in a common language may facilitate the process of critical thinking, because interventions and outcomes are more accurately matched with appropriately developed nursing diagnoses (Johnson, Bulechek, Butcher, et al., 2012). The final taxonomic scheme identifies four clinical domains (functional, physiologic, psychosocial, and environmental) that contain numerous classes of diagnoses, outcomes, and interventions. Chart 3-11 presents the taxonomy of nursing practice.

Chart 3-10 **PLAN OF NURSING CARE**

Example of a Plan of Nursing Care for a Patient With Acute Cholecystitis

NURSING DIAGNOSIS: Acute pain
GOAL: Relief of pain and discomfort

Nursing Interventions	Rationale	Expected Outcomes
1. When taking vital signs, use pain scale to assess pain and discomfort characteristics: location, quality, frequency, durations, etc., at baseline and on an ongoing basis.	1. Provides baseline data	• Reports decreased level of pain and discomfort on pain scale
2. Assure the patient that you know that pain is real and will assist in reducing it.	2. Fear that pain will not be considered real increases anxiety and reduces pain tolerance	• Reports less disruption in activity and quality of life from pain and discomfort
3. Assess other factors contributing to patient's pain: fear, fatigue, other symptoms, psychosocial distress, etc.	3. Provides data about factors that decrease patient's ability to tolerate pain and increase pain level	• Reports decrease in other symptoms and psychosocial distress

Chart 3-10

PLAN OF NURSING CARE

Example of a Plan of Nursing Care for a Patient With Acute Cholecystitis (continued)

Nursing Interventions	Rationale	Expected Outcomes
4. Administer prescribed analgesic regimen, and provide education to patient and family regarding regimen.	4. Analgesics tend to be more effective when administered early in pain cycle, around the clock at regular intervals, or when administered in long-acting forms; breaks the pain cycle; premedication with analgesics is used for activities that cause increased pain or breakthrough pain.	• Adheres to analgesic regimen as prescribed
5. Address myths or misconceptions and lack of knowledge about use of opioid analgesics.	5. Barriers to adequate pain management involve patients' fear of side effects, fatalism about the possibility of achieving pain control, fear of distracting providers from treating the cholecystitis, belief that pain is indicative of progressive disease, and fears about addiction. Professional health providers also have demonstrated limited knowledge about pain management, potential analgesic side effects, and management and risk of addiction.	• Barriers to adequately addressing pain do not interfere with strategies for managing pain
6. Collaborate with patient, primary provider, and other health care team members when changes in pain management are necessary.	6. New methods of administering analgesia must be acceptable to the patient, primary provider, and health care team to be effective; patient's participation decreases sense of powerlessness.	• Takes an active role in administration of analgesia • Identifies additional effective pain relief strategies
7. Encourage strategies of pain relief that patient has used successfully in previous pain experience.	7. Encourages success of pain relief strategies accepted by patient and family	• Uses previously employed successful pain relief strategies appropriately
8. Offer nonpharmacologic strategies to relieve pain and discomfort: distraction, imagery, relaxation, cutaneous stimulation, etc.	8. Increases options and strategies available to patient that serve as adjuncts to pharmacologic interventions	• Reports effective use of nonpharmacologic pain relief strategies and decrease in pain • Reports that decreased level of pain permits participation in other activities and events and quality of life

NURSING DIAGNOSIS: Risk for electrolyte imbalance
GOAL: Fluid and electrolyte balance within normal limits

Nursing Interventions	Rationale	Expected Outcomes

1. Monitor and support fluid and electrolyte status:
  a. Monitor weight.
  b. Monitor intake and output (I&O).
  c. Monitor skin turgor and temperature.
  d. Monitor serum electrolytes.
  e. Monitor color and consistency or urine and stool output.
	1. Monitoring and noting trends in fluid and electrolyte status provides information about disease progression as well as patient's response to therapy.
	  a. Weight is best indicator of fluid balance; sudden weight loss indicates fluid deficit, whereas a gain over a short period of time indicates fluid excess.
	  b. I&O is a good indicator of fluid status.
	  c. Dry skin indicates fluid deficit, whereas moist skin can indicate fluid excess.
	  d. Provides baseline for later evaluation
	  e. Indicates fluid and electrolyte imbalances
		• Fluid balance maintained
		• Urinary output adequate in relation to oral and intravenous intake
		• Skin warm and supple; good recoil
		• Electrolytes in normal range

NURSING DIAGNOSIS: Activity intolerance related to fatigue
GOAL: Participation in activity within tolerance

Nursing Interventions	Rationale	Expected Outcomes

1. Assess factors contributing to activity intolerance and fatigue
2. Promote atmosphere conducive to physical and mental rest:
  a. Encourage alternation of rest and activity.
  b. Encourage limitation of visitors and stress-producing interactions.
	1. Indicates factors contributing to severity of fatigue
	2. Promotes rest, activity tolerance, and decreased overall stress
		• Identifies factors contributing to severity of fatigue
		• Alternates periods of rest and activity
		• Limits visitors to family in the evenings
		• Avoids stress-producing interactions
		• Accurately describes relationship between stress, sedentary lifestyle, and obesity

(continues on page 40)

Chart 3-10

PLAN OF NURSING CARE

Example of a Plan of Nursing Care for a Patient With Acute Cholecystitis (continued)

NURSING DIAGNOSIS: Deficient knowledge regarding condition and treatment
GOAL: Increased knowledge about condition and related treatment

Nursing Interventions	Rationale	Expected Outcomes
1. Assess understanding of cause of acute cholecystitis, its consequences, and its treatment: a. Cause of patient's cholecystitis. b. Meaning of cholecystitis. 2. Provide education about the importance of maintaining low-fat liquid diet and progression toward long-term low-fat diet. 3. Provide education about food and menus choices low in fat. 4. Request consultation with dietitian and reinforce instructions given.	1. Provides baseline for further explanations and education. 2. Identifies harmful effects of increased weight and high-fat foods and makes plans for preplanned meals. 3. Identifies foods/menu choices low in fat. 4. Dietitian may provide additional strategies and education to assist with maintaining low-fat liquid diet and progression toward long-term low-fat diet.	• Verbalizes relationship of cause of cholecystitis to consequences • Accurately describes effects of obesity and intake of high-fat foods on overall physical health and well-being • Plans to attend Weight Watchers; has had success with this program in the past • Identifies that preparing low-fat lunches at home the night before work is a good preplanning option

Chart 3-11

Hierarchy of Taxonomy in Nursing Practice: A Unified Structure of Nursing Language

I. The Functional Domain
The functional domain includes diagnoses, outcomes, and interventions that promote basic needs and includes the following eight classes:
Activity/exercise: physical activity, including energy conservation and expenditure
Comfort: a sense of emotional, physical, and spiritual well-being and relative freedom from distress
Growth/development: physical, emotional, and social growth and developmental milestones
Nutrition: processes related to taking in, assimilating, and using nutrients
Self-care: ability to accomplish basic and instrumental activities of daily living
Sexuality: maintenance or modification of sexual identity and patterns
Sleep/rest: the quantity and quality of sleep, rest, and relaxation patterns
Values/beliefs: ideas, goals, perceptions, and spiritual and other beliefs that influence choices or decisions

II. The Physiologic Domain
The physiologic domain includes diagnoses, outcomes, and interventions to promote optimal biophysical health and includes the following 10 classes:
Cardiac function: cardiac mechanisms used to maintain tissue perfusion
Elimination: processes related to secretion and excretion of body wastes
Fluid/electrolyte: regulation of fluid/electrolytes and acid–base balance
Neurocognition: mechanisms related to the nervous system and neurocognitive functioning, including memory, thinking, and judgment
Pharmacologic function: effects (therapeutic and adverse) of medications or drugs and other pharmacologically active products
Physical regulation: body temperature, endocrine, and immune system responses to regulate cellular processes

Reproduction: processes related to human procreation and birth
Respiratory function: ventilation adequate to maintain arterial blood gases within normal limits
Sensation/perception: intake and interpretation of information through the senses, including seeing, hearing, touching, tasting, and smelling
Tissue integrity: skin and mucous membrane protection to support secretion, excretion, and healing

III. The Psychosocial Domain
The psychosocial domain includes diagnoses, outcomes, and interventions to promote optimal mental and emotional health and social functioning and includes the following seven classes:
Behavior: actions that promote, maintain, or restore health
Communication: receiving, interpreting, and expressing spoken, written, and nonverbal messages
Coping: adjusting or adapting to stressful events
Emotional: a mental state of feeling that may influence perceptions of the world
Knowledge: understanding and skill in applying information to promote, maintain, and restore health
Roles/relationships: maintenance and/or modification of expected social behaviors and emotional connectedness with others
Self-perception: awareness of one's body and personal identity

IV. The Environmental Domain
The environmental domain includes diagnoses, outcomes, and interventions that promote and protect the environmental health and safety of individuals, systems, and communities and includes the following three classes:
Health care system: social, political, and economic structures and processes for delivery of health care services
Populations: aggregates of individuals or communities having characteristics in common
Risk management: avoidance or control of identifiable health threats

Adapted from Herdman, T. H. (2012). *Nursing diagnoses: Definitions & classification 2012–2014*. Oxford: Wiley-Blackwell.

Critical Thinking Exercises

1 `pq` A 20-year-old man who is morbidly obese is admitted to your unit with severe chest pain. He is complaining of extreme shortness of breath with sternal chest pain. What are your priorities for assessing this patient's current condition? How would these priorities change if the patient shows you a bruise on his chest from being involved in a motor vehicle crash 2 days ago?

2 You are at the bedside of a 53-year-old patient whose mother is designated as his power of attorney for health care. The patient has been comatose for 3 days, and the physician has indicated that the likelihood of recovery is very poor. The mother wants to discuss removing life support; however, the patient's wife, whom he recently married, wants "everything done" and protests against any actions that would "kill him." The patient's three adult children from a previous marriage are divided in their opinions, with two supporting the patient's mother and one supporting the patient's wife. The physician indicates that he will hold a meeting with the family and put the decision to a vote. What actions should be taken in this situation? What ethical and legal dilemmas exist? What other health professionals could be helpful in satisfactorily resolving these issues?

3 `ebp` You are assigned to care for an 80-year-old man admitted to the hospital yesterday with acute coronary syndrome who had an emergent percutaneous coronary intervention with a stent placement. When you walk into his room, he states, "That last nurse gave me a medication I don't think I was supposed to have. She told me it was metoprolol, but it looked different from the metoprolol I got yesterday." You note that the patient's heart rate is now 56 beats per minute (bpm), although the previous day it had been between 72 and 88 bpm. According to the patient's chart, he received the prescribed dose of metoprolol 4 hours ago. The prescribed dosage of this medication was not changed; it was the same yesterday. What actions should be taken? Should this information be communicated to your supervisor? What is the care priority for the patient? What evidence supports or does not support disclosure of medication administration errors to patients? What steps would you take and in what order?

Brunner Suite Resources
Explore these additional resources to enhance learning for this chapter:
• NCLEX-Style Questions and Other Resources
on **thePoint**, http://thePoint.lww.com/Brunner13e
• Study Guide
• PrepU
• Clinical Handbook
• Handbook of Laboratory and Diagnostic Tests

References

*Asterisk indicates nursing research.
**Double asterisk indicates classic reference.

Books

Alfaro-LeFevre, R. (2009). *Critical thinking and clinical judgment: A practical approach to outcome focused thinking* (4th ed.). Philadelphia: Saunders.
**American Nurses Association. (2001a). *Code of ethics for nurses with interpretive statements*. Washington, DC: American Nurses Publishing.
American Nurses Association. (2010a). *Nursing's social policy statement* (3rd ed.). Washington, DC: Nursebooks.org.
American Nurses Association. (2010b). *Standards of clinical nursing practice* (3rd ed.). Washington, DC: Author.
Bulechek, G. H., Butcher, H. K. & Dochterman, J. M. (Eds.). (2013). *Nursing interventions classification (NIC)* (6th ed.). St. Louis: Mosby-Elsevier.
Carpenito, L. J. (2013). *Nursing diagnosis: Application to clinical practice* (14th ed.). Philadelphia: Lippincott Williams & Wilkins.
Fowler, M. D. (2008). *Guide to the code of ethics for nurses: Interpretation and application*. Silver Springs, MD: American Nurses Association.
**International Council of Nurses. (2006). *Code of ethics for nurses*. Geneva: Author.
Johnson, M., Bulechek, G., Butcher, H., et al. (2012). *NANDA, NOC, and NIC linkages: Nursing diagnoses, outcomes, and interventions* (3rd ed.). St. Louis: Mosby-Elsevier.
NANDA International. (2012). *Nursing diagnoses: Definitions & classification 2012–2014*. Oxford: Wiley-Blackwell.
Smith-Temple, J., & Johnson, J. Y. (2010). *Nurses' guide to clinical procedures* (6th ed.). Philadelphia: Lippincott Williams & Wilkins.
Wilkinson, J. M. (2011). *Nursing process and critical thinking* (5th ed.). Upper Saddle River, NJ: Prentice-Hall.

Journals and Electronic Documents

**American Nurses Association. (1999). *Position statement on privacy and confidentiality*. Available at: gm6.nursingworld.org/MainMenuCategories/Policy-Advocacy/Positions-and-Resolutions/ANAPositionStatements/Position-Statements-Alphabetically/PrivacyandConfidentiality.html
**American Nurses Association. (2001b). *Position statement on reduction of patient restraint and seclusion in health care settings*. Available at: www.nursingworld.org/restraintposition
American Nurses Association. (2009). *Position statement on electronic health record*. Available at: gm6.nursingworld.org/MainMenuCategories/Policy-Advocacy/Positions-and-Resolutions/ANAPositionStatements/Position-Statements-Alphabetically/Electronic-Health-Record.html
Arafeh, J. M., Hansen, S. S., & Nichols, A. (2010). Debriefing in simulated-based learning facilitating a reflective discussion. *Journal of Perinatal Neonatal Nursing, 24*(4), 302–309.
Brubakken, K., Grant, S., Johnson, M. K., et al. (2011). Reflective practice: A framework for case manager development. *Professional Case Management, 16*(4), 170–179.
Burns, K. J., Jacobs, B. B., & Jacobs, L. M. (2011). A time for trauma end-of-life optimum support: The TELOS best-practice model. *Journal of Trauma Nursing, 18*(2), 97–101.
Callister, L. C., & Sudia-Robinson, T. (2011). Overview of ethics in maternal-child nursing. *Maternal/Child Nursing, 36*(3), 154–159.
Fromme, E. K., Zive, D., Schmidt, T. A., et al. (2012). POLST registry do-not-resuscitate orders and other patient treatment preferences. *Journal of the American Medical Association, 307*(1), 34–35.
Hickman, S. E., Sabatino, C. P., Moss, A. H., et al. (2008). The POLST (Physician Orders for Life-Sustaining Treatment) paradigm to improve end-of-life care: Potential state legal barriers to implementation. *Journal of Law, Medicine, and Ethics, 36*(1), 119–140.
*Jenkins, S. D. (2011). Cross-cultural perspectives on critical thinking. *Journal of Nursing Education, 50*(5), 268–274.
Lachman, V. D. (2009). Practical use of the Nursing Code of Ethics: Part I. *MEDSURG Nursing, 18*(1), 55–57.
Tanner, C. (2006). Thinking like a nurse: A research based model of clinical judgment. *Journal of Nursing Education, 45*(6), 204–211.
Tanner, C. A. (2009). The case for cases: A pedagogy for developing habits of thought. *Journal of Nursing Education, 48*(6), 299–300.

**U.S. Department of Health and Human Services. (2003). *Summary of the HIPAA privacy rule*. Available at: www.hhs.gov/ocr/privacy/hipaa/understanding/summary/privacysummary.pdf

Wielawski, I. M. (2009). HIPAA: Not so bad after all? *American Journal of Nursing, 109*(7), 22–24.

Resources

American Nurses Association Center for Ethics and Human Rights, www.nursingworld.org/ethics

Centers for Medicare and Medicaid Services (CMS), www.cms.hhs.gov

The Hastings Center, www.thehastingscenter.org

Joint Commission, www.jointcommission.org

NANDA International, www.nanda.org

National Center for Ethics in Health Care (NCEHC), www.ethics.va.gov/ETHICS/pubs/index.asp

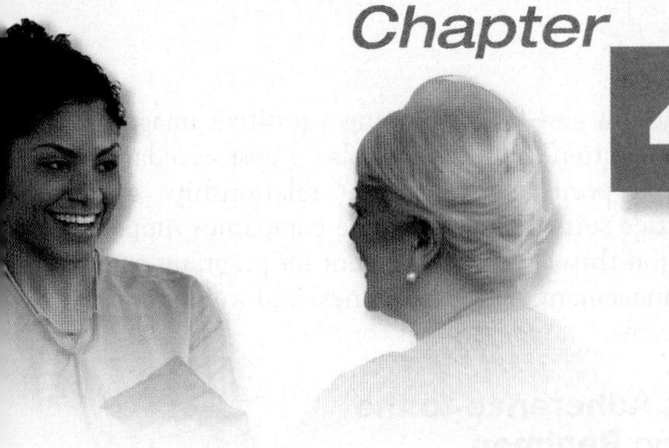

Chapter 4

Health Education and Health Promotion

Learning Objectives

On completion of this chapter, the learner will be able to:

1 Describe the purposes and significance of health education.
2 Describe the concept of adherence to a therapeutic regimen.
3 Identify variables that affect learning readiness and adult learning abilities.
4 Describe the relationship of the teaching–learning process to the nursing process.
5 Develop an individualized teaching plan for a patient.
6 Define health promotion and discuss major health promotion models.
7 Describe the components of health promotion: self-responsibility, nutritional awareness, stress reduction and management, and physical fitness.
8 Specify the variables that affect health promotion activities for adolescents, young and middle-aged adults, and older adults.
9 Describe the role of the nurse in health promotion.

Glossary

adherence: the process of faithfully following guidelines or directions
community: an interacting population of individuals living together within a larger society
feedback: the return of information about the results of input given to a person or a system
health education: various learning experiences designed to promote behaviors that facilitate health
health promotion: the art and science of assisting people to change their lifestyle toward a higher state of wellness
learning: the act of acquiring knowledge, attitudes, or skills
learning readiness: the optimum time for learning to occur; usually corresponds to the learner's perceived need and desire to obtain specific knowledge
nutrition: the science that deals with food and nourishment in humans
physical fitness: the condition of being physically healthy as a result of proper exercise and nutrition
reinforcement: the process of strengthening a given response or behavior to increase the likelihood that the behavior will continue
self-responsibility: personal accountability for one's actions or behavior
stress management: behaviors and techniques used to strengthen a person's resources against stress
teaching: helping another person learn
therapeutic regimen: a routine that promotes health and healing

Effective **health education** lays a solid foundation for individual and **community** wellness. All nurses use teaching as a tool to assist patients and families in developing effective health behaviors and altering lifestyle patterns that predispose people to health risks. Health education is an influential factor directly related to positive health outcomes.

Purpose of Health Education

Today's health care environment mandates the use of an organized approach to **health education** so that patients can meet their specific health care needs. There are many reasons for providing health education.

Meeting Nursing Standards

Teaching, as a function of nursing, is included in all state nurse practice acts and in the American Nurses Association's (ANA) *Scope and Standards of Practice* (ANA, 2010). Health education is an independent function of nursing practice and a primary nursing responsibility. All nursing care is directed toward promoting, maintaining, and restoring health; preventing illness; and helping people adapt to the residual effects of illness. Many of these nursing activities are accomplished through patient education. Nurses in their role as teachers are challenged to focus on the educational needs of communities and to provide specific patient and family education. Health education is important to nursing care because it affects the abilities of people and families to perform important self-care activities.

Every contact a nurse has with a health care consumer, whether or not that person is ill or has a disability, should be considered an opportunity for health education. Although people have a right to decide whether or not to learn, nurses have the responsibility to present information that motivates people to recognize the need to learn. Therefore, nurses must use opportunities in all health care settings to promote wellness. Educational environments may include homes, hospitals, community health centers, schools, places of business, service agencies, shelters, and consumer action or support groups.

Supporting Informed Decision Making and Self-Care

The emphasis on health education stems in part from the public's right to comprehensive health care, which includes up-to-date health information. It also reflects the emergence of an informed public that is asking more significant questions about health and health care. Because of the importance that American society places on health and the responsibility that each person has to maintain and promote his or her own health, members of the health care team, specifically nurses, are obligated to make health education available. Significant factors to consider when planning patient education include the availability of health care outside the hospital setting, the use of diverse health care providers to accomplish care management goals, and the increased use of complementary and alternative strategies rather than traditional approaches to care. Without adequate knowledge and training in self-care skills, consumers cannot make informed decisions about their health. Guidance from nurses may assist consumers to obtain health information from trustworthy, credible, and timely Internet resources (McInnes, Gifford, Kazis, et al., 2010). People with chronic illnesses and disabilities are among those most in need of health education. As the lifespan of the population increases, the number of people with such illnesses also increases. Health information targeted at identifying and managing the exacerbations or issues commonly associated with having a chronic illness or disability is a major focus of health education. People with chronic illness need health care information to participate actively in and assume responsibility for self-care. Health education can help those with chronic illness adapt to their illness, prevent complications, carry out prescribed therapy, and solve problems when confronted with new situations. It can also help to prevent crisis situations and reduce the potential for rehospitalization resulting from inadequate information about self-care. The goal of health education is to teach people to live life to its healthiest—that is, to strive toward achieving their maximum health potential.

 Concept Mastery Alert

Chronic illnesses are ongoing, and patients often face many ups and downs related to their condition. Therefore, health education—important for all persons—is of the utmost importance for those with chronic illnesses so that they can achieve the best possible outcomes for health and self-care.

In addition to the public's right to and desire for health education, patient education is also a strategy for promoting self-care at home and in the community, reducing health care costs by preventing illness, effectively managing necessary therapies, avoiding expensive medical interventions, decreasing lengths of hospital stay, and facilitating earlier discharge. For health care agencies, offering community wellness programs is a public relations tool for increasing patient satisfaction and for developing a positive image of the institution. Patient education is also a cost-avoidance strategy in that positive staff–patient relationships may avert malpractice suits. Some insurance companies support health education through reimbursement for programs such as diabetic management classes and fitness and weight management programs.

Promoting Adherence to the Therapeutic Regimen

One of the goals of patient education is to encourage people to adhere to their **therapeutic regimen**. **Adherence** to treatment usually requires that a person make one or more lifestyle changes to carry out specific activities that promote and maintain health. Common examples of behaviors facilitating health include taking prescribed medications, maintaining a healthy diet, increasing daily activities and exercise, self-monitoring for signs and symptoms of illness and changes in baseline health status, practicing specific hygiene measures, seeking recommended health evaluations and screening, and performing other therapeutic and preventive measures. When using nursing diagnosis language, the term *compliance* is used to discuss patient adherence.

Factors Affecting Adherence

Many people do not adhere to their prescribed regimens; rates of adherence are generally low, especially when the regimens are complex or of long duration (e.g., therapy for tuberculosis, multiple sclerosis, and human immunodeficiency virus [HIV] infection and hemodialysis). Nonadherence to prescribed therapy has been the subject of many studies (Cook, Emiliozzi, El-Hajj, et al., 2010; Daleboudt, Broadbent, McQueen, et al., 2011; Garcia Rodriquez, Cea Soriano, Hill, et al., 2011; Malee, Williams, Montepiedra, et al., 2011; Sherman & Koelmeyer, 2011). For the most part, findings have been inconclusive, and no one predominant causative factor has been identified. Instead, a wide range of variables appears to influence the degree of adherence, including the following:

- Demographic variables, such as age, gender, race, socioeconomic status, and level of education
- Illness variables, such as the severity of the illness and the relief of symptoms afforded by the therapy
- Therapeutic regimen variables, such as the complexity of the regimen and uncomfortable side effects
- Psychosocial variables, such as intelligence, motivation, availability of significant and supportive people (especially family members), competing or conflicting demands, attitudes toward health professionals, acceptance or denial of illness, substance abuse, and religious or cultural beliefs
- Financial variables, especially the direct and indirect costs associated with a prescribed regimen

Nurses' success with health education is determined by ongoing assessment of the variables that affect patients' ability to adopt specific behaviors, obtain resources, and maintain a healthy social environment (Edelman & Mandle, 2009). Teaching programs are more likely to succeed if the variables affecting patient adherence are identified and considered in the teaching plan. Teaching strategies are discussed later in the chapter.

Motivation

The problem of nonadherence to therapeutic regimens is substantial and must be addressed before patients can achieve their maximum health potential. Patients' need for knowledge has not been found to be a sufficient stimulus for acquiring knowledge and thereby enabling complete adherence to a health regimen. Teaching directed toward stimulating patient motivation results in varying degrees of adherence. Research suggests that factors such as medication costs, perceived control, and type of health problem must also be considered (Eskridge, 2010; Girard & Murray, 2010; Hayman, Helden, Chyun, et al., 2011; Mazer, Bisgaier, Dailey, et al., 2011; Schneider, Hess, & Gosselin, 2011). The variables of choice, establishment of mutual goals, and quality of the patient–provider relationship also influence the behavioral changes that can result from patient education. Many factors are linked to motivation for learning.

Using a learning contract or agreement can also be a motivator for learning. Such a contract is based on assessment of patient needs; health care data; and specific, measurable goals (Miller & Stoeckel, 2011). The learning contract is recorded in writing and contains methods for ongoing evaluation. A well-designed learning contract is realistic and positive. In a typical learning contract, a series of measurable goals is established, beginning with small, easily attainable objectives and progressing to more advanced goals. Frequent, positive **reinforcement** is provided as the person moves from one goal to the next. For example, incremental goals such as weight loss of 1 to 2 pounds per week are more appropriate in a weight reduction program than a general goal such as a 30-pound weight loss.

 ### Gerontologic Considerations

Nonadherence to therapeutic regimens is a significant problem for older adults, leading to increased morbidity, mortality, and cost of treatment (U.S. Public Health Service, 2010). Many admissions to nursing homes and hospitals are associated with nonadherence.

Older adults frequently have one or more chronic illnesses that are managed with numerous medications and complicated by periodic acute episodes. Older adults may also have other problems that affect adherence to therapeutic regimens, such as increased sensitivity to medications and their side effects, difficulty in adjusting to change and stress, financial constraints, forgetfulness, inadequate support systems, lifetime habits of self-treatment with over-the-counter medications, visual and hearing impairments, and mobility limitations. To promote adherence among older adults, all variables that may affect health behavior should be assessed (Fig. 4-1). Nurses must also consider that cognitive impairment may be manifested by the older adult's inability to draw inferences, apply information, or understand the major teaching points (Mauk, 2009; Tabloski, 2009; Touhy & Jett, 2010). The person's strengths and limitations must be assessed to encourage the use of existing strengths to compensate for limitations. Above all, health care professionals must work together to provide continuous, coordinated care; otherwise, the efforts of one health care professional may be negated by those of another.

The Nature of Teaching and Learning

Learning can be defined as acquiring knowledge, attitudes, or skills. **Teaching** is defined as helping another person learn.

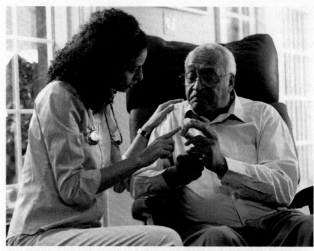

FIGURE 4-1 • Taking time to teach patients about their medication and treatment program promotes interest and cooperation. Older adults who are actively involved in learning about their medication and treatment program and the expected effects may be more likely to adhere to the therapeutic regimen.

These definitions indicate that the teaching–learning process is an active one, requiring the involvement of both teacher and learner in the effort to reach the desired outcome—a change in behavior. The teacher does not simply give knowledge to the learner but instead serves as a facilitator of learning. Although learning can take place without teachers, most people who are attempting to learn new or altered health behaviors benefit from contact with a nurse. The interpersonal interaction between the person and the nurse who is attempting to meet the person's learning needs may be formal or informal, depending on the method and techniques of teaching.

In general, there is no definitive theory about how learning occurs and how it is affected by teaching. However, learning can be affected by factors such as readiness to learn, the learning environment, and the teaching techniques used (Miller & Stoeckel, 2011).

Learning Readiness

One of the most significant factors influencing learning is a person's **learning readiness**. For adults, readiness is based on culture, personal values, physical and emotional status, and past experiences in learning (Schumacher, 2011). The "teachable moment" occurs when the content and skills being taught are congruent with the task to be accomplished (Miller & Stoeckel, 2011).

Culture encompasses values, ideals, and behaviors, and the traditions within each culture provide the framework for solving the issues and concerns of daily living. Because people with different cultural backgrounds have different values and lifestyles, choices about health care vary. Culture is a major variable influencing readiness to learn because it affects how people learn and what information can be learned. Sometimes people do not accept health teaching because it conflicts with culturally mediated values. Before beginning health teaching, nurses must conduct an individual cultural assessment instead of relying only on generalized assumptions about a particular culture. A patient's social and cultural patterns must be appropriately incorporated into the teaching–learning interaction. (See Chapter 7, Chart 7-4, which describes cultural assessment components to consider when formulating a teaching plan.)

A person's values include beliefs about behaviors that are desirable and undesirable. The nurse must know what value the patient places on health and health care. In clinical situations, patients express their values through their actions and the level of knowledge pursued (Ray, 2009). When the nurse is unaware of the patient's values (cultural and personal), misunderstanding, lack of cooperation, and negative health outcomes may occur (Leininger & McFarland, 2006). A person's values and behaviors can be either an asset or a deterrent to readiness to learn. Therefore, patients are unlikely to accept health education unless their values and beliefs about health and illness are respected (Dayer-Berenson, 2011).

Physical readiness is of vital importance, because until the person is physically capable of learning, attempts at teaching and learning may be both futile and frustrating. For example, a person in acute pain is unable to focus attention away from the pain long enough to concentrate on learning. Likewise, a person who is short of breath concentrates on breathing rather than on learning.

Emotional readiness also affects the motivation to learn. A person who has not accepted an existing illness or the threat of illness is not motivated to learn. A person who does not accept a therapeutic regimen, or who views it as conflicting with his or her present lifestyle, may consciously avoid learning about it. Until the person recognizes the need to learn and demonstrates an ability to learn, teaching efforts may be thwarted. However, it is not always wise to wait for the person to become emotionally ready to learn, because that time may never come unless the nurse makes an effort to stimulate the person's motivation. For example, a person with colon cancer who has a fasting blood sugar twice the expected normal value may focus only on the cancer diagnosis and exclude or deny the health consequences of an abnormal blood sugar.

Illness and the threat of illness are usually accompanied by anxiety and stress. Nurses who recognize such reactions can use simple explanations and instructions to alleviate these anxieties and provide further motivation to learn. Because learning involves behavior change, it often produces mild anxiety, which can be a useful motivating factor.

Emotional readiness can be promoted by creating a warm, accepting, positive atmosphere and by establishing realistic learning goals. When learners achieve success and a feeling of accomplishment, they are often motivated to participate in additional learning opportunities. **Feedback** about progress also motivates learning. Such feedback should be presented in the form of positive reinforcement when the learner is successful, and in the form of constructive suggestions for improvement when the learner is unsuccessful.

 Concept Mastery Alert

Learning should be a "positive" experience. So, when promoting learning, nurses need to be "positive" in their approach to giving feedback to patients.

Experiential readiness refers to past experiences that influence a person's ability to learn. Previous educational experiences and life experiences in general are significant determinants of a person's approach to learning. People with little or no formal education may not be able to understand the instructional materials presented. People who have had difficulty learning in the past may be hesitant to try again. Many behaviors required for reaching maximum health potential require knowledge, physical skills, and positive attitudes. In their absence, learning may be very difficult and very slow. For example, a person who does not understand the basics of normal nutrition may not be able to understand the restrictions of a specific diet. A person who does not view the desired learning as personally meaningful may reject teaching efforts. A person who is not future oriented may be unable to appreciate many aspects of preventive health teaching. Experiential readiness is closely related to emotional readiness, because motivation tends to be stimulated by an appreciation for the need to learn and by those learning tasks that are familiar, interesting, and meaningful.

The Learning Environment

Learning may be optimized by minimizing factors that interfere with the learning process. For example, the room temperature, lighting, noise levels, and other environmental conditions should be appropriate to the learning situation. In addition, the time selected for teaching should be suited to the needs of the individual person. Scheduling a teaching session at a time of day when a patient is fatigued, uncomfortable, or anxious about a pending diagnostic or therapeutic procedure, or when visitors are present, is not conducive to learning. However, if the family is to participate in providing care, the sessions should be scheduled when family members are present so that they can learn any necessary skills or techniques.

Teaching Techniques

Teaching techniques and methods enhance learning if they are appropriate to the patient's needs. Numerous techniques are available, including the following:

- *Lectures:* Lectures are explanation methods of teaching and should be accompanied by discussion, because discussion affords learners opportunities to express their feelings and concerns, ask questions, and receive clarification.
- *Group teaching:* Group teaching allows people not only to receive needed information but also to feel secure as members of a group (promoting moral support). Assessment and follow-up are imperative to ensure that each person has gained sufficient knowledge and skills. Not all patients relate or learn well in groups.
- *Demonstration and practice:* Demonstration and practice are especially important when teaching skills. It is best to demonstrate the skill and then give the learner ample opportunity for practice. When special equipment is involved, such as syringes or colostomy bags, it is important to teach with the same equipment that will be used in the home setting to avoid confusion, frustration, and mistakes.
- *Teaching aids:* Teaching aids include books, pamphlets, pictures, films, slides, audiotapes, models, programmed instruction, other visual aids (e.g., charts), and

TABLE 4-1	Educating People With Disabilities
Type of Disability	**Educational Strategy**
Physical, Emotional, or Cognitive Disability	Adapt information to accommodate the person's cognitive, perceptual, and behavioral disabilities. Give clear written and oral information. Highlight significant information for easy reference. Avoid medical terminology or "jargon."
Hearing Impairment	Use slow, directed, deliberate speech. Use sign language or interpreter services if appropriate. Position yourself so that the person can see your mouth if speech reading. Use telecommunication devices (TTY or TDD) for the person with hearing impairment. Use written materials and visual aids, such as models and diagrams. Use captioned videos, films, and computer-generated materials. Speak on the side of the "good ear" if unilateral deafness is present.
Visual Impairment	Use optical devices such as a magnifying lens. Use proper lighting and proper contrast of colors on materials and equipment. Use or convert information to auditory and tactile formats if appropriate (e.g., Braille or large-print materials). Obtain audiotapes and talking books. Explain noises associated with procedures, equipment, and treatments. Arrange materials in clockwise pattern.
Learning Disabilities Input disability	If visual perceptual disorder: • Explain information verbally; repeat and reinforce frequently. • Use audiotapes. • Encourage learner to verbalize information received. If auditory perceptual disorder: • Speak slowly with as few words as possible; repeat and reinforce frequently. • Use direct eye contact to focus person on task. • Use demonstration and return demonstration such as modeling, role-playing, and hands-on experiences. • Use visual tools, written materials, and computers.
Output disability	Use all senses as appropriate. Use written, audiotape, and computer information. Review information, and give time verbally to interact and ask questions. Use hand gestures and motions.
Developmental disability	Base information and teaching on developmental stage, not chronologic age. Use nonverbal cues, gestures, signing, and symbols as needed. Use simple explanations and concrete examples with repetition. Encourage active participation. Demonstrate information, and have person perform return demonstrations.

computer-assisted learning modules. They are invaluable when used appropriately and can save a significant amount of personnel time and related cost. However, all such aids should be reviewed before use to ensure that they meet the person's learning needs and are free of advertisements that may confuse the patient.

• *Reinforcement and follow-up:* It is important to allow ample time to learn and provide reinforcement. Follow-up sessions are imperative to promote the learner's confidence in his or her abilities and to plan for additional teaching sessions.

• *Motivational interviewing:* Pilot research suggests that using motivational interviewing as an enhanced educational method in an acute inpatient setting can increase both patient and caregiver knowledge as well as patient satisfaction following discharge from the acute care setting (Byers, Lamanna, & Rosenburg, 2010).

The chance of success is maximized when nurses, families, and other health care professionals work collaboratively to facilitate learning. Successful learning should result in improved self-care management skills, enhanced self-esteem, confidence, and a willingness to learn in the future. There are specific considerations for teaching special populations. Table 4-1 outlines some of the teaching strategies to use when teaching people with disabilities. (See Chapters 9 and 11 for additional teaching strategies for people with disabilities and older adults.)

The Nursing Process in Patient Education

The nurse relies on the steps of the nursing process when constructing an individualized teaching plan to meet the patient's teaching and learning needs (Chart 4-1).

Assessment

Assessment in the teaching–learning process is directed toward the systematic collection of data about the person and family's learning needs and readiness to learn. The nurse identifies all internal and external variables that affect the patient's readiness to learn. There are learning assessment guides available. Some guides are directed toward the collection of general health information (e.g., healthy eating), whereas others are specific to medication regimens or disease processes (e.g., stroke risk assessments). Such guides facilitate assessment but must be adapted to the responses, problems,

Chart 4-1 Summary of the Nursing Process for Individualized Patient Education

Assessment

1. Assess the person's readiness for health education.
   a. What are the person's health beliefs and behaviors?
   b. What physical and psychosocial adaptations does the person need to make?
   c. Is the learner ready to learn?
   d. Is the person able to learn these behaviors?
   e. What additional information about the person is needed?
   f. Are there any variables (e.g., hearing or visual impairment, cognitive issues, literacy issues) that will affect the choice of teaching strategy or approach?
   g. What are the person's expectations?
   h. What does the person want to learn?
2. Organize, analyze, synthesize, and summarize the collected data.

Nursing Diagnosis

1. Formulate the nursing diagnoses that relate to the person's learning needs.
2. Identify the learning needs, their characteristics, and their etiology.

Planning

1. Assign priority to the nursing diagnoses that relate to the individual's learning needs.
2. Specify the immediate, intermediate, and long-term learning goals established by teacher and learner together.
3. Identify teaching strategies appropriate for goal attainment.
4. Establish expected outcomes.
5. Develop the written teaching plan.
   a. Include diagnoses, goals, teaching strategies, and expected outcomes.
   b. Put the information to be taught in logical sequence.
   c. Write down the key points.
   d. Select appropriate teaching aids.
   e. Keep the plan current and flexible to meet the person's changing learning needs.
6. Involve the learner, family or significant others, nursing team members, and other health care team members in all aspects of planning.

Implementation

1. Put the teaching plan into action.
2. Use language that the person can understand.
3. Use appropriate teaching aids and provide Internet resources if appropriate.
4. Use the same equipment that the person will use after discharge.
5. Encourage the person to participate actively in learning.
6. Record the learner's responses to the teaching actions.
7. Provide feedback.

Evaluation

1. Collect objective data.
   a. Observe the person.
   b. Ask questions to determine whether the person understands.
   c. Use rating scales, checklists, anecdotal notes, and written tests when appropriate.
2. Compare the person's behavioral responses with the expected outcomes. Determine the extent to which the goals were achieved.
3. Include the person, family or significant others, nursing team members, and other health care team members in the evaluation.
4. Identify alterations that need to be made in the teaching plan.
5. Make referrals to appropriate sources or agencies for reinforcement of learning after discharge.
6. Continue all steps of the teaching process: assessment, diagnosis, planning, implementation, and evaluation.

and needs of each person. The nurse organizes, analyzes, synthesizes, and summarizes the assessment data collected and determines the patient's need for teaching.

Nursing Diagnosis

The process of formulating nursing diagnoses makes educational goals and evaluations of progress more specific and meaningful. Teaching is an integral intervention implied by all nursing diagnoses, and for some diagnoses, education is the primary intervention. Examples of nursing diagnoses that help in planning for educational needs are ineffective therapeutic regimen management, impaired or ineffective home maintenance, health-seeking behaviors (specify), and decisional conflict (specify). The diagnosis "Deficient knowledge" should be used cautiously, because knowledge deficit is not a human response but a factor relating to or causing the diagnosis. For example, "Ineffective health maintenance related to a lack of information about wound care" is a more appropriate nursing diagnosis than "Deficient knowledge" (Carpenito-Moyet, 2009; Herdman, 2012). A nursing diagnosis that relates specifically to a patient's and family's learning needs serves as a guide in the development of the teaching plan.

Planning

Once the nursing diagnoses have been identified, the planning component of the teaching–learning process is established in accordance with the steps of the nursing process:
1. Assigning priorities to the diagnoses
2. Specifying the immediate, intermediate, and long-term goals of learning
3. Identifying specific teaching strategies appropriate for attaining goals
4. Specifying the expected outcomes
5. Documenting the diagnoses, goals, teaching strategies, and expected outcomes of the teaching plan

The assignment of priorities to the diagnoses should be a collaborative effort by the nurse and the patient or family members. Consideration must be given to the urgency of the patient's learning needs; the most critical needs should receive the highest priority.

After the diagnostic priorities have been mutually established, it is important to identify the immediate and long-term goals and the teaching strategies appropriate for attaining the goals. Teaching is most effective when the objectives of both the patient and nurse are in agreement (Bastable, Gramet, Jacobs, et al., 2012). Learning begins with the establishment of goals that are appropriate to the situation and realistic in terms of the patient's ability and desire to achieve them. Involving the patient and family in establishing goals and in planning teaching strategies promotes their cooperation in the implementation of the teaching plan.

Outcomes of teaching strategies can be stated in terms of expected behaviors of patients, families, or both. Outcomes should be realistic and measurable, and the critical time periods for attaining them should be identified. The desired outcomes and the critical time periods serve as a basis for evaluating the effectiveness of the teaching strategies.

During the planning phase, the nurse must consider the sequence in which the subject matter is presented. Critical information (e.g., survival skills for a patient with diabetes) and material that the person or family identifies to be of particular importance must receive high priority. An outline is often helpful for arranging the subject matter and for ensuring that all necessary information is included. In addition, appropriate teaching aids to be used in implementing teaching strategies are prepared or selected at this time. Patient Education charts throughout this textbook guide teaching about self-care.

The entire planning phase concludes with the formulation of the teaching plan. This teaching plan communicates the following information to all members of the nursing team:

- The nursing diagnoses that specifically relate to the patient's learning needs and the priorities of these diagnoses
- The goals of the teaching strategies
- The teaching strategies that are appropriate for goal attainment
- The expected outcomes, which identify the desired behavioral responses of the learner
- The critical time period within which each outcome is expected to be met
- The patient's behavioral responses (which are documented on the teaching plan)

The same rules that apply to writing and revising the plan of nursing care apply to the teaching plan.

Implementation

In the implementation phase of the teaching–learning process, the patient, family, and other members of the nursing and health care team carry out the activities outlined in the teaching plan. The nurse coordinates these activities.

Flexibility during the implementation phase of the teaching–learning process and ongoing assessment of patient responses to the teaching strategies support modification of the teaching plan as necessary. Creativity in promoting and sustaining the patient's motivation to learn is essential. New learning needs that may arise after discharge from the hospital or after home care visits have ended should also be taken into account.

The implementation phase ends when the teaching strategies have been completed and when the patient's responses to the actions have been recorded. This serves as the basis for evaluating how well the defined goals and expected outcomes have been achieved.

Evaluation

Evaluation of the teaching–learning process determines how effectively the patient has responded to teaching and to what extent the goals have been achieved. An evaluation must be made to determine what was effective and what needs to be changed or reinforced. It cannot be assumed that patients have learned just because teaching has occurred; learning does not automatically follow teaching. An important part of the evaluation phase addresses the question, "What can be done to improve teaching and enhance learning?" Answers to this question direct the changes to be made in the teaching plan.

Various measurement techniques can be used to identify changes in patient behavior as evidence that learning has taken place. These techniques include directly observing the behavior; using rating scales, checklists, or anecdotal notes to document the behavior; and indirectly measuring results using oral questioning and written tests. All direct measurements should be supplemented with indirect measurements whenever possible. Using more than one measuring technique enhances the reliability of the resulting data and decreases the potential for error from a measurement strategy.

In many situations, measurement of actual behavior is the most accurate and appropriate evaluation technique. Nurses often perform comparative analyses using patient admission data as the baseline: Selected data points observed when nursing care is given and self-care is initiated are compared with the patient's baseline data. In other cases, indirect measurement may be used. Some examples of indirect measurement are patient satisfaction surveys, attitude surveys, and instruments that evaluate specific health status variables.

Measurement is only the beginning of evaluation, which must be followed by data interpretation and judgments about learning and teaching. These aspects of evaluation should be conducted periodically throughout the teaching–learning program, at its conclusion, and at varying periods after the teaching has ended.

Evaluation of learning after teaching that occurs in any setting (e.g., clinics, offices, nursing centers, hospitals) is essential, because the analysis of teaching outcomes must extend into aftercare. With shortened lengths of hospital stay and with short-stay and same-day surgical procedures, follow-up evaluation is especially important. Coordination of efforts and sharing of information between hospital- and community-based nursing personnel facilitate postdischarge teaching and home care evaluation.

Evaluation is not the final step in the teaching–learning process but is the beginning of a new patient assessment. The information gathered during evaluation should be used to redirect teaching actions, with the goal of improving the patient's responses and outcomes.

Health Promotion

Health teaching and **health promotion** are linked by a common goal—to encourage people to achieve as high a level of wellness as possible so that they can live maximally healthy lives and avoid preventable illnesses. The call for health promotion has become a cornerstone in health policy because of the need to control costs and reduce unnecessary sickness and death.

Health goals for the nation are established in the publication *Healthy People 2020*. The priorities from this initiative were identified as health promotion, health protection, and

Selected Topics for Objectives of *Healthy People 2020*

Access to Health Services
Adolescent Health
Arthritis, Osteoporosis, and Chronic Back Conditions
Blood Disorders and Blood Safety
Cancer
Chronic Kidney Disease
Dementias, including Alzheimer's Disease
Diabetes
Disability and Health
Educational and Community-Based Programs

the use of preventive services. *Healthy People 2020* defines the current national health promotion and disease prevention initiative for the nation. Measurable goals for key health topics for the nation are shown in Chart 4-2. The overall goals are to (1) increase the quality and years of healthy life for people and (2) eliminate health disparities among various segments of the population (U.S. Department of Health and Human Services, 2010).

Definition

Health promotion may be defined as those activities that assist people in developing resources that maintain or enhance well-being and improve their quality of life. These activities involve people's efforts to remain healthy in the absence of symptoms, may not require the assistance of a health care team member, and occur within or outside of the health system (Chenoweth, 2011; Haber, 2011).

The purpose of health promotion is to focus on the person's potential for wellness and to encourage appropriate alterations in personal habits, lifestyle, and environment in ways that reduce risks and enhance health and well-being. As discussed in Chapter 1, health is viewed as a dynamic, ever-changing condition that enables people to function at an optimal potential at any given time, whereas wellness, a reflection of health, involves a conscious and deliberate attempt to maximize one's health. Health promotion is an active process—that is, it is not something that can be prescribed or dictated. It is up to each person to decide whether to make changes to promote a higher level of wellness. Only the individual can make these choices.

A significant amount of research has shown that people, by virtue of what they do or fail to do, influence their own health. Today, many of the major causes of illness are chronic diseases that have been closely related to lifestyle behaviors (e.g., diabetes, coronary artery disease, lung and colon cancer, chronic obstructive pulmonary diseases, hypertension, cirrhosis, traumatic injury, and HIV infection). To a large extent, a person's health status may be reflective of his or her lifestyle. Chart 4-3 summarizes a research study exploring self-care practices among individuals living with rheumatic arthritis.

Health Promotion Models

Several health promotion models identify health-protecting behaviors and seek to explain what makes people engage in preventive behaviors. A health-protecting behavior is defined as any behavior performed by people, regardless of

NURSING RESEARCH PROFILE

Chart 4-3
Health Promotion in People With Rheumatic Disease

Arvidsson, S., Bergman, S., Arvidsson, B, et al. (2011). Experiences of health-promoting self-care in people living with rheumatic disease. *Journal of Advanced Nursing, 67*(6), 1264–1272.

Purpose

The purpose of this study was to describe the experience of health-promoting self-care for people living with rheumatic diseases and to identify the process they use to manage their disease and their lives.

Design

The study used a Husserlian phenomenologic approach to capture and describe the experience of self-care. The researchers sought to understand the meaning of self-care as a process used to manage their disease and their lives. Researchers interviewed 12 participants living in Sweden—6 women and 6 men—in a private place on rheumatology units or the participant's homes. The interviews lasted from 80 to 135 minutes and were tape recorded.

Findings

The qualitative findings of this study revealed that patients living with rheumatic diseases engage in self-care from a framework of continual hope and a belief that they can influence their health in a positive manner. Self-care is a way of life that focuses on the need to interpret, understand, and respond to signals from the body. Three constituent factors—dialogue, power struggle, and choice—characterized the essence of the participants' experience. Participants believed that they were in constant dialogue with their bodies to identity what was happening to them and to evaluate their bodies' signals to decide the self-care course of action. In managing the body's signals, power struggles occurred in the participants' effort to fight their disease. During this process of assessing and evaluating the body's signals, the participants made choices about their self-care priorities and beliefs about their ability to select self-care activities that promoted health and well-being.

Nursing Implications

Nurses need to consider the unique health-promoting, self-care perspective of people with rheumatic diseases. These patients manage their lives from a framework of continual hope and a strong belief that they can influence their health in a positive manner. Health care providers can use this information to support and educate both patients and their significant others. Additionally, the nurse must recognize the patient's need for both internal and external dialogue about aspects of self-care and allocate time for teaching activities so that this dialogue may occur. The patient is better able to make informed, self-care choices with specific and clear teaching about rheumatic disease.

their actual or perceived health condition, for the purpose of promoting or maintaining their health, whether or not the behavior produces the desired outcome (Pender, Murdaugh, & Parsons, 2011).

The Health Belief Model was designed to foster understanding of why some healthy people choose actions to prevent illness while others do not. Developed by Becker (1974), the model is based on the premise that four variables influence the selection and use of health promotion behaviors. Demographic and disease factors, the first variable, include patient characteristics such as age, gender, education, employment, severity of illness or disability, and length of illness. Barriers, the second variable, are defined as factors leading to unavailability or difficulty in gaining access to a specific health promotion alternative. Resources, the third variable, encompass such factors as financial and social support. Perceptual factors, the fourth variable, consist of how the person views his or her health status, self-efficacy, and the perceived demands of the illness. Further research has demonstrated that these four variables have a positive correlation with a person's quality of life (Becker, Stuifbergen, Oh, et al., 1993).

Another model, the Resource Model of Preventive Health Behavior, addresses the ways in which people use resources to promote health (Pender et al., 2011). It is based on social learning theory and emphasizes the importance of motivational factors in acquiring and sustaining health promotion behaviors. This model explores how cognitive-perceptual factors affect the person's view of the importance of health. It also examines perceived control of health, self-efficacy, health status, and the benefits and barriers to health-promoting behaviors. Nurse educators can use this model to assess how demographic variables, health behaviors, and social and health resources influence health promotion.

The Canadian health promotion initiative, Achieving Health for All, builds on the work of Lalonde (1977), in which four determinants of health—human biology, environment, lifestyle, and the health care delivery system—were identified. Determinants of health were defined as factors and conditions that have an influence on the health of individuals and communities. Since the 1970s, a total of 12 health determinants have been identified, and this number will continue to increase as population health research progresses. Determinants of health provide a framework for assessing and evaluating the population's health.

The Transtheoretical Model of Change, also known as the Stages of Change Model, is a framework that focuses on the motivation of a person to make decisions that promote healthy behavior change (DiClemente, 2007). Table 4-2 shows the six stages in the model. Research indicates that people seeking assistance from professionals or self-help

groups progress through these stages of change (Hoke & Timmerman, 2011; Sealy & Farmer, 2011). Any of the models can serve as an organizing framework for clinical work and research that support the enhancement of health. Research suggests the application of health promotion models, concepts, and frameworks increase the nurse's understanding of the health promotion behaviors of families and communities (Hudson & Macdonald, 2010; Tresdale-Kennedy, Taggart, & McIlfatrick, 2011; Vallance, Murray, Johnson, et al., 2011; Van Achterberg, Huism-De Waal, Ketelaar, et al., 2010; Wang, Lin, & Hsieh, 2011).

Components of Health Promotion

There are several components of health promotion as an active process: self-responsibility, nutritional awareness, stress reduction and management, and physical fitness.

Self-Responsibility

Taking responsibility for oneself is the key to successful health promotion. The concept of **self-responsibility** is based on the understanding that the individual controls his or her life. Each person alone must make the choices that determine the health of his or her lifestyle. As more people recognize that lifestyle and behavior significantly affect health, they may assume responsibility for avoiding high-risk behaviors such as smoking, alcohol and drug abuse, overeating, driving while intoxicated, risky sexual practices, and other unhealthy habits. They may also assume responsibility for adopting routines that have been found to have a positive influence on health, such as engaging in regular exercise, wearing seat belts, and eating a healthy diet.

Various techniques have been used to encourage people to accept responsibility for their health, including public service announcements, educational programs, and reward systems. No one technique has been found to be superior to any other. Instead, self-responsibility for health promotion is individualized and depends on a person's desires and inner motivations. Health promotion programs are important tools for encouraging people to assume responsibility for their health and to develop behaviors that improve health.

Nutritional Awareness

Nutrition, as a component of health promotion, has become the focus of considerable attention and publicity with the growing epidemic of obesity in the United States. A vast array of books and magazine articles address the topics of special diets; natural foods; and the hazards associated with certain substances, such as sugar, salt, cholesterol, trans fats, carbohydrates, artificial colors, and food additives. It has been suggested that good nutrition is the single most significant factor in determining health status, longevity, and weight control.

Nutritional awareness involves an understanding of the importance of a healthy diet that supplies all essential nutrients. Understanding the relationship between diet and disease is an important facet of a person's self-care. Some clinicians believe that a healthy diet is one that substitutes "natural" foods for processed and refined ones and reduces the intake of sugar, salt, fat, cholesterol, caffeine, alcohol, food additives, and preservatives.

Chapter 5 contains further information about the assessment of a person's nutritional status. It describes the physical

TABLE 4-2	Stages in the Transtheoretical Model of Change
Stage	**Description**
1. Precontemplative	The person is not thinking about making a change.
2. Contemplative	The person is only thinking about change in the near future.
3. Decision making	The person constructs a plan to change behavior.
4. Action	The person takes steps to operationalize the plan of action.
5. Maintenance	The person works to prevent relapse and to sustain the gains made from the actions taken.
6. Termination	The person has the ability to resist relapse back to unhealthy behavior(s).

Adapted from DiClemente, C. (2007). The transtheoretical model of intentional behavior change. *Drugs & Alcohol Today, 7*(1), 29–33; Miller, C. A. (2009). *Nursing wellness in older adults* (5th ed.). Philadelphia: Lippincott Williams & Wilkins.

signs indicating nutritional status, assessment of food intake (food record, 24-hour recall), the dietary guidelines presented in the MyPlate plan, and calculation of ideal body weight.

Stress Reduction and Management

Stress management and stress reduction are important aspects of health promotion. Studies suggest the negative effects of stress on health and a cause-and-effect relationship between stress and infectious diseases, traumatic injuries (e.g., motor vehicle crashes), and some chronic illnesses. Stress has become inevitable in contemporary societies in which demands for productivity have become excessive. More and more emphasis is placed on encouraging people to manage stress appropriately and to reduce the pressures that are counterproductive. Research suggests that including techniques such as relaxation training, exercise, and modification of stressful situations in health promotion programs assists patients in dealing with stress (Jefferson, 2010). Further information on stress management, including health risk appraisal and stress reduction methods such as the Benson Relaxation Response, can be found in Chapter 6.

Physical Fitness

Physical fitness and exercise are important components of health promotion. Clinicians and researchers (Krol-Zielinska, Kusy, Zielinska, et al., 2010; Wittink, Engelbert, & Takken, 2011) who have examined the relationship between health and physical fitness have found that a regular exercise program can promote health in the following ways:

- Improve the function of the circulatory system and the lungs
- Decrease cholesterol and low-density lipoprotein levels
- Decrease body weight by increasing calorie expenditure
- Delay degenerative changes such as osteoporosis
- Improve flexibility and overall muscle strength and endurance

An appropriate exercise program can have a positive effect on a person's performance capacity, appearance, and level of stress and fatigue, as well as his or her general state of physical, mental, and emotional health (Smith, Griffin, & Fitpatrick, 2011). An exercise program should be designed specifically for a given person, with consideration to age, physical condition, and any known cardiovascular or other risk factors. Exercise can be harmful if it is not started gradually and increased slowly in accordance with a person's response.

Health Promotion Strategies Throughout the Lifespan

Health promotion is a concept and a process that extends throughout the lifespan. The health of a child can be affected either positively or negatively by the health practices of the mother during the prenatal period. Therefore, health promotion starts before birth and extends through childhood, adolescence, adulthood, and old age (Haber, 2011).

Health promotion includes health screening, counseling, immunizations, and preventive medications. The U.S. Preventive Services Task Force (2010) evaluates clinical research to assess the merits of preventive measures. Table 4-3 presents general population guidelines including adult immunization

recommendations (Centers for Disease Control and Prevention [CDC], 2011; U.S. Preventive Services Task Force, 2010).

Adolescents

Health screening has traditionally been an important aspect of adolescent health care. The goal has been to detect health problems at an early age so that they can be treated at that time. Today, health promotion goes beyond the mere screening for illnesses and disabilities and includes extensive efforts to promote positive health practices at an early age. Because health habits and practices are formed early in life, adolescents should be encouraged to develop positive health attitudes. For this reason, more programs are being offered to adolescents to help them develop good health habits. Although the negative results of practices such as smoking, risky sex, alcohol and drug abuse, and poor nutrition are explained in these educational programs, emphasis is also placed on values training, self-esteem, and healthy lifestyle practices. The projects are designed to appeal to a particular age group, with emphasis on learning experiences that are fun, interesting, and relevant.

Young and Middle-Aged Adults

Young and middle-aged adults represent an age group that not only expresses an interest in health and health promotion but also responds enthusiastically to suggestions that show how lifestyle practices can improve health. Adults are frequently motivated to change their lifestyles in ways that are believed to enhance their health and wellness. Many adults who wish to improve their health turn to health promotion programs to help them make the desired changes in their lifestyles. Many have responded to programs that focus on topics such as general wellness, smoking cessation, exercise, physical conditioning, weight control, conflict resolution, and stress management. Because of the nationwide emphasis on health during the reproductive years, young adults actively seek programs that address prenatal health, parenting, family planning, and women's or men's health issues.

Programs that provide health screening, such as those that screen for cancer, high cholesterol, hypertension, diabetes, abdominal aneurysm, and visual and hearing impairments, are quite popular with young and middle-aged adults. Programs that involve health promotion for people with specific chronic illnesses such as cancer, diabetes, heart disease, and pulmonary disease are also popular. Chronic disease and disability do not preclude health and wellness; rather, positive health attitudes and practices can promote optimal health for people who must live with the limitations imposed by their chronic illnesses and disabilities.

Health promotion programs can be offered almost anywhere in the community. Common sites include local clinics, schools, colleges, recreation centers, churches, and even private homes. Health fairs are frequently held in civic centers and shopping malls. The outreach idea for health promotion programs has served to meet the needs of many adults who otherwise would not avail themselves of opportunities to strive toward a healthier lifestyle.

The workplace has become a center for health promotion activity for several reasons. Employers have become increasingly concerned about the rising costs of health care insurance

TABLE 4-3   Routine Health Promotion Screening for Adults

Type of Screening	Suggested Time Frame
Routine health examination	Yearly
Blood chemistry profile	Baseline at age 20 years, then as mutually determined by patient and clinician
Complete blood count	Baseline at age 20 years, then as mutually determined by patient and clinician
Lipid profile	Baseline at age 20 years, then as mutually determined by patient and clinician
Hemoccult screening	Yearly after age 50 years
Electrocardiogram	Baseline at age 40 years, then as mutually determined by patient and clinician
Blood pressure	Yearly, then as mutually determined by patient and clinician
Tuberculosis skin test	Every 2 years or as mutually determined by patient and clinician
Chest x-ray film	For positive PPD results
Breast self-examination	Monthly
Mammogram	Every other year for women older than 50 years, or earlier or more often as indicated
Clinical breast examination	Yearly
Gynecologic examination	Yearly
Papanicolaou (Pap) test	Yearly
Bone density screening	Based on identification of primary and secondary risk factors (prior to onset of menopause, if indicated)
Nutritional screening	As mutually determined by patient and clinician
Digital rectal examination	Yearly
Colonoscopy	Every 3–5 years after age 50 years or as mutually determined by patient and clinician
Prostate examination	Yearly
Prostate-specific antigen	Every 1–2 years after age 50 years
Testicular examination	Monthly
Skin examination	Yearly or as mutually determined by patient and clinician
Vision screening: Glaucoma	Every 2–3 years
	Baseline at age 40 years, then every 2–3 years until age 70 years, then yearly
Dental screening	Every 6 months
Hearing screening	As needed
Health risk appraisal	As needed
Adult Immunizations	
Hepatitis B (if not received as a child)	Series of three doses (now, 1 month later, then 5 months after the second date)
Human papillomavirus (HPV)	3 doses for females between 19 and 26 years if lacking documentation of prior immunization
Influenza vaccine	Yearly
Meningococcal	1 or more doses after 19 years old
Tetanus	Every 10 years
Zoster	After age 60 years

Note: Any of these screenings may be performed more frequently if deemed necessary by the patient or recommended by the health care provider.
Adapted from Advisory Committee on Immunization Practices. (2010). Recommended adult immunization schedule: United States, 2010. *Annals of Internal Medicine, 152*(1), 36–39; U.S. Preventive Services Task Force. (2010). *Recommendations.* Available at: www.uspreventiveservicestaskforce.org/recommendations.htm

to treat illnesses related to lifestyle behaviors, and they are also concerned about increased absenteeism and lost productivity. Some employers use health promotion specialists to develop and implement these programs, and others purchase packaged programs that have already been developed by health care agencies or private health promotion corporations.

Programs offered at the workplace usually include employee health screening and counseling, physical fitness, nutritional awareness, work safety, and stress management and stress reduction. In addition, efforts are made to promote a safe and healthy work environment. Many large businesses provide exercise facilities for their employees and offer their health promotion programs to retirees.

 Gerontologic Considerations

Health promotion is as important for older adults as it is for others. Although 80% of people older than 65 years have one or more chronic illnesses and many are limited in their activity, the older adult population experiences significant gains from health promotion. Older adults are very health conscious, and most view their health positively and are willing to adopt practices that will improve their health and well-being (Tabloski, 2009; Touhy & Jett, 2010). Although their chronic illnesses and disabilities cannot be

eliminated, these adults can benefit from activities and education that help them maintain independence and achieve an optimal level of health (Lanier & Buffum, 2011; Pierce, 2009; Rigdon, 2010).

Various health promotion programs have been developed to meet the needs of older Americans. Both public and private organizations continue to be responsive to health promotion, and more programs that serve this population are emerging. Many of these programs are offered by health care agencies, churches, community centers, senior citizen residences, and various other organizations. The activities directed toward health promotion for older adults are the same as those for other age groups: physical fitness and exercise, nutrition, safety, and stress management (Fig. 4-2).

Nursing Implications of Health Promotion

By virtue of their expertise in health and health care and their long-established credibility with consumers, nurses play a vital role in health promotion. In many instances, they initiate health promotion and health screening programs or participate with other health care personnel in developing and providing wellness services in various settings.

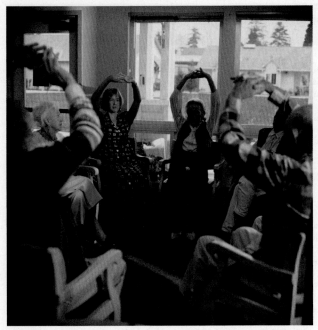

FIGURE 4-2 • Health promotion for older adults includes physical fitness. Here, a nurse teaches simple exercises at a senior center.

As health care professionals, nurses have a responsibility to promote activities that foster well-being, self-actualization, and personal fulfillment. Every interaction with consumers of health care must be viewed as an opportunity to promote positive health attitudes and behaviors. Health Promotion charts and tables throughout this textbook identify opportunities for promoting health.

Critical Thinking Exercises

1 **ebp** A male college student with a long history of asthma makes an appointment with the nurse practitioner at the college health center. The student states, "I have taken up smoking to fit in with the guys I am living with this year. I've been using my inhaler several times a day." What health promotion components guide the nurse in assessing the student's situation? What is the evidence base for offering information and health programs to help this young adult make appropriate health decisions and establish positive health behaviors? Identify the criteria used to evaluate the strength of the evidence for this practice.

2 Following a fall on ice, a 40-year-old woman is recuperating at home after two surgeries to repair her fractured leg. A home health nurse visits three times a week to perform wound care. During a visit, the woman complains that she misses her daily exercise routine and asks when she will be able to resume exercising. Determine the factors that influence her ability to engage in exercise. Identify the factors that support the overall relationship between fitness and health. Develop an exercise plan to assist the woman to maintain muscle tone and promote well-being.

3 A 76-year-old man is attending a local health fair with his granddaughter. When the nurse coordinator asks the man if he would like to participate in the screening events and other informational activities, he replies, "No, thank you. I'm too old to think about health promotion. I just need to take care of the health problems that I already have." What are the priorities to consider when selecting health promotion strategies for use with this older adult? What specific information should you include in a discussion with this man about promoting health in older adults? What type of information, available at various booths at the health fair, would be appropriate for this man to obtain?

Brunner Suite Resources
Explore these additional resources to enhance learning for this chapter:
• NCLEX-Style Questions and Other Resources on thePoint, http://thePoint.lww.com/Brunner13e
• Study Guide
• PrepU
• Clinical Handbook
• Handbook of Laboratory and Diagnostic Tests

References

*Asterisk indicates nursing research.
**Double asterisk indicates classic reference.

Books

American Nurses Association. (2010). *Nursing: Scope and standards of practice*. Washington, DC: Author.

Bastable, S., Gramet, P., Jacobs, K., et al. (2012). *Health professional as educator: Principles of teaching and learning*. Sudbury, MA: Jones & Bartlett.

**Becker, M. H. (Ed.). (1974). *The health belief model and personal health behavior*. Thorofare, NJ: Charles B. Slack.

Carpenito-Moyet, L. J. (2009). *Handbook of nursing diagnosis* (13th ed.). Philadelphia: Lippincott Williams & Wilkins.

Chenoweth, D. H. (2011). *Worksite health promotion* (3rd ed.). Champaign, IL: Human Kinetics.

Dayer-Berenson, L. (2011). *Cultural competencies for nurses: Impact on health and illness*. Sudbury, MA: Jones & Bartlett.

Edelman, C. L., & Mandle, C. L. (2009). *Health promotion throughout the life span* (7th ed.). Philadelphia: Elsevier Health Sciences.

Haber, D. (2011). *Health promotion and aging: Practical application for health professionals* (4th ed.). New York: Springer.

Herdman, T. H. (Ed.). (2012). *NANDA International nursing diagnoses: Definitions and classification 2012–2014*. Oxford: Wiley-Blackwell.

**Lalonde, M. (1977). *New perspectives on the health of Canadians: A working document*. Ottawa, Canada: Minister of Supply and Services.

Leininger, M. M., & McFarland, M. (2006). *Culture care diversity and universality: A worldwide nursing theory* (2nd ed.). Sudbury, MA: Jones & Bartlett.

Mauk, K. L. (2009). *Gerontological nursing: Competencies for care*. Sudbury, MA: Jones & Bartlett.

Miller, M. A., & Stoeckel, P. R. (2011). *Client education: Theory and practice*. Sudbury, MA: Jones & Bartlett.

Pender, N. J., Murdaugh, C. L., & Parsons, M. A. (Eds.). (2011). *Health promotion in nursing practice* (6th ed.). Upper Saddle River, NJ: Prentice-Hall Health.

Ray, M. A. (2009). *Transcultural caring: The dynamics of contemporary nursing*. Philadelphia: F. A. Davis.

Tabloski, P. (2009). *Gerontological nursing: The essential guide to clinical practice* (2nd ed.). New York: Pearson.

Touhy, T. A., & Jett, K. F. (2010). *Ebersole and Hess' gerontological nursing and healthy aging* (3rd ed.). St. Louis: Mosby.

Journals and Electronic Documents

*Arvidsson, S., Bergman, S., Arvidsson, B., et al. (2011). Experiences of health-promoting self-care in people living with rheumatic disease. *Journal of Advanced Nursing, 67*(6), 1264–1272.

**Becker, H. A., Stuifbergen, A. K., Oh, H., et al. (1993). The self-rated abilities for health practices scale: A health self-efficacy measure. *Health Values, 17*, 42–50.

*Byers, A.M., Lamanna, L., & Rosenburg, A. (2010). The effect of motivational interviewing after ischemic stroke on patient knowledge and patient satisfaction with care: Pilot study. *Journal of Neuroscience Nursing, 42*(6), 312–322.

Centers for Disease Control and Prevention. (2011). Recommended adult immunization schedule—United States, 2011. *Morbidity Mortality Weekly Report, 60*(4), 1–4. Available at: www.cdc.gov/mmwr/preview/mmwrhtml/mm6004a10.htm?s_cid=mm6004a10_w

*Cook, P. F., Emiliozzi, S., El-Hajj, D., et al. (2010). Telephone nurse counseling for medication adherence in ulcerative colitis: A preliminary study. *Patient Education & Counseling, 81*(2), 182–186.

*Daleboudt, G. M. N., Broadbent, E., McQueen, F., et al. (2011). Intentional and unintentional treatment nonadherence in patients with systemic lupus erythematosus. *Arthritis Care and Research, 63*(3), 342–350.

**DiClemente, C. (2007). The transtheoretical model of intentional behavior change. *Drugs & Alcohol Today, 7*(1), 29–33.

Eskridge, M. S. (2010). Hypertension and chronic kidney disease: The role of lifestyle modification and medication management. *Nephrology Nursing Journal, 37*(1), 55–60, 99.

*Garcia Rodriquez, L. A., Cea Soriano, L., Hill, C., et al. (2011). Increased risk of stroke after discrimination of acetylsalicylic acid: A UK primary care study. *Neurology, 76*(8), 740–746.

*Girard, B. R., & Murray, T. (2010). Perceived control: A construct to guide patient education. *Canadian Journal of Cardiovascular Nursing, 20*(3), 18–26.

Hayman, L. L., Helden, L., Chyun, D., et al. (2011). A life course approach to cardiovascular disease prevention. *Journal of Cardiovascular Nursing, 26*(4S), S22–S34.

*Hoke, M. M., & Timmerman, G. M. (2011). Transtheoretical model: Potential usefulness with overweight rural Mexican American women. *Hispanic Health Care International, 9*(1), 41–49.

Hudson, S., & Macdonald, M. (2010). Hemodialysis arteriovenous fistula self-cannulation: Moving theory to practice in developing patient-teaching resources. *Clinical Nurse Specialist: The Journal of Advanced Nursing Practice, 24*(6), 304–312.

*Jefferson, L. L. (2010). Exploring effects of therapeutic massage and patient teaching in the practice of diaphragmatic breathing on blood pressure, stress, and anxiety in hypertensive African-American women: An intervention study. *Journal of National Black Nurses Association, 21*(1), 17–24.

*Krol-Zielinska, M., Kusy, K., Zielinski, J., et al. (2010). Physical activity and functional fitness in institutional vs. independently living elderly: A comparison of 70-80-year-old city dwellers. *Archives of Gerontology and Geriatrics, 53*(11), 10–16.

*Lanier, E. M., & Buffum, M. D. (2011). What are neuroscience nurses teaching Parkinson's patients and families before deep brain stimulation? *Journal of Neuroscience Nursing, 43*(1), 1–7.

*Malee, K., Williams, P., Montepiedra, G., et al. (2011). Medication adherence in children and adolescents with HIV infection: Associations with behavioral impairments. *AIDS Patient Care, 25*(3), 191–200.

*Mazer, M., Bisgaier, J., Dailey, E., et al. (2011). Risk for cost-related medication nonadherence among emergency department patients. *Academic Emergency Medicine, 18*(3), 267–272.

*McInnes, D. K., Gifford, A. L., Kazis, L. E., et al. (2010). Disparities in health-related Internet use by US veterans: Results from a national survey. *Informatics in Primary Care, 18*(1), 59–68.

Pierce, D. N. (2009). Breast health education: Postradiation. *Journal of Radiology Nursing, 28*(3), 83–86.

Rigdon, A. S. (2010). Development of patient education for older adults receiving chemotherapy. *Clinical Journal of Oncology Nursing, 14*(4), 433–441.

Schneider, S. M., Hess, K., & Gosselin, T. (2011). Interventions to promote adherence with oral agents. *Seminars in Oncology Nursing, 27*(2), 133–141.

*Schumacher, G. (2011). Culture care meanings, beliefs, and practices in rural Dominican Republic. *Journal of Transcultural Nursing, 21*(2), 93–103.

*Sealy, Y. M., & Farmer, G. L. (2011). Parents' stage of change for diet and physical activity: Influence on childhood obesity. *Social Work in Health Care, 50*(4), 274–291.

*Sherman, K. A., & Koelmeyer, L. (2011). The role of information sources and objective risk status on lymphedema risk minimization behaviors in women recently diagnosed with breast cancer. *Oncology Nursing Forum, 38*(1), 27–36.

*Smith, D. W., Griffin, Q., & Fitpatrick, J. (2011). Exercise and exercise intentions among obese and overweight individuals. *Journal of the American Academy of Nurse Practitioners, 23*(2), 92–100.

*Tresdale-Kennedy, M., Taggart, L., & McIlfatrick, S. (2011). Breast cancer knowledge among women with intellectual disabilities and their experiences of receiving breast mammography. *Journal of Advanced Nursing, 67*(6), 1294–1304.

U.S. Department of Health and Human Services, Office of Disease Prevention and Health Promotion. (2010). *Healthy People 2020.* Available at: www.healthypeople.gov/2020/about/disparitiesAbout.aspx

U.S. Preventive Services Task Force. (2010). *Recommendations.* Available at: www.uspreventiveservicestaskforce.org/recommendations.htm

Vallance, J., Murray, T., Johnson, S., et al. (2011). Understanding physical activity intentions and behavior in postmenopausal women: An application of the theory of planned behavior. *International Journal of Behavioral Medicine, 18*(2), 139–149.

*Van Achterberg, T., Huism-De Waal, G. G. J., Ketelaar, N. A. B. M., et al. (2010). How to promote healthy behaviors in patients? An overview of evidence for behavior change techniques. *Health Promotion International, 26*(2), 148–162.

*Wang, J., Lin, Y., & Hsieh, L. (2011). Effects of gerotranscendence support group on gerotranscendence perspective, depression, and life satisfaction of institutionalized elders. *Aging and Mental Health, 15*(5), 580–586.

Wittink, H., Engelbert, R., & Takken, T. (2011). The dangers of inactivity; exercise and inactivity physiology for the manual therapist. *Manual Therapy, 16*(3), 209–216.

Resources

Centers for Disease Control and Prevention (CDC), www.cdc.gov/nccdphp/dnpao/hwi/resources/preventative_screening.htm

Health Education Resource Exchange, Washington State Department of Health, here.doh.wa.gov

Health Promotion for Women With Disabilities, Villanova University College of Nursing, www.nurseweb.villanova.edu/WomenWithDisabilities/welcome.htm

Healthy People 2020, www.healthypeople.gov/2020/about/default.aspx

Take Charge of Your Life by Making Healthy Choices, helpguide.org

U.S. Army Public Health Command (USAPHC), phc.amedd.army.mil/topics/healthyliving/Pages/default.aspx

U.S. Department of Agriculture (USDA), www.choosemyplate.gov/

U.S. Department of Health and Human Services, National Institutes of Health, www.nih.gov/icd/

U.S. Department of Health and Human Services, Office of Disease Prevention and Health Promotion, www.odphp.osophs.dhhs.gov

World Health Organization, www.who.int/hpr/

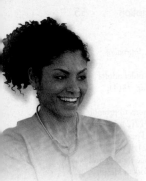

5

Adult Health and Nutritional Assessment

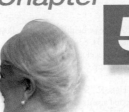

Learning Objectives

On completion of this chapter, the learner will be able to:

1 Identify ethical considerations necessary for protecting a person's rights related to data collected in the health history and physical assessment.
2 Describe the components of a holistic health history.
3 Explore the concept of spirituality and the assessment of spiritual needs of patients.
4 Apply culturally sensitive interviewing skills and techniques to conduct a successful health history, physical examination, and nutritional assessment.
5 Identify genetic aspects that nurses should incorporate into the health history and physical assessment.

6 Identify modifications needed to obtain a health history and conduct a physical assessment for a person with a disability.
7 Describe the techniques of inspection, palpation, percussion, and auscultation to perform a basic physical assessment.
8 Discuss the techniques of measurement of body mass index, biochemical assessment, clinical examination, and assessment of food intake to assess a person's nutritional status.
9 Describe factors that may contribute to altered nutritional status in high-risk groups such as adolescents and older adults.

Glossary

auscultation: listening to sounds produced within different body structures created by the movement of air or fluid

body mass index (BMI): a calculation done to estimate the amount of body fat of a person

electronic medical record (EMR): computerization of medical records

faith: trust in God, belief in a higher power or something that a person cannot see

health history: the collection of subjective data, most often a series of questions that provides an overview of the patient's current health status

inspection: visual assessment of different aspects of the patient

palpation: examination of different organs of the body using the sense of touch

percussion: the use of sound to examine different organs of the body

physical examination: collection of objective data about the patient's health status

self-concept: a person's view of himself or herself

spirituality: connectedness with self, others, a life force, or God that allows people to find meaning in life

substance abuse: a maladaptive pattern of drug use that causes physical and emotional harm with the potential for disruption of daily life

The ability to assess patients in a holistic manner is a skill integral to nursing, regardless of the practice setting. Eliciting a complete health history and using appropriate physical assessment skills are critical to identifying physical and psychological problems and concerns experienced by the patient. As the first step in the nursing process, a holistic patient assessment is necessary to obtain data that enable the nurse to make an accurate nursing diagnosis, identify and implement appropriate interventions, and assess their effectiveness. This chapter covers health assessment, including the complete health history and basic physical assessment techniques. Because a patient's nutritional status is an important factor in overall health and well-being, nutritional assessment is addressed.

Considerations for Conducting a Health Assessment

The Role of the Nurse

All members of the health care team collaborate and use their unique skills and knowledge to contribute to the resolution of patient problems by first obtaining some level of history and assessment (Weber & Kelley, 2010). Various formats for obtaining the **health history** (the collection of subjective data about the patient's health status) and performing the **physical examination** (the collection of objective data about the patient's health status) have been developed because the focus of each member of the health care team is unique. Regardless of the format, the information obtained by the nurse complements the data obtained by other members of the health care team and focuses on nursing's unique concerns for the patient. In health assessment, the nurse obtains the patient's health history and performs a physical assessment, which can be carried out in a variety of settings, including the acute care setting, clinic or outpatient office, school, long-term care facility, or home. A nursing diagnosis is used to determine the appropriate plan of care for the patient and drives interventions and patient outcomes. Nursing diagnoses also provide a standard nomenclature for use in the **electronic medical record (EMR)**, enabling clear communication among care team members and the collection of data for continuous improvement in patient care (NANDA International, 2011).

Effective Communication

People who seek health care for a specific problem are often anxious. Their anxiety may be increased by fear about potential diagnoses, possible disruption of lifestyle, and other concerns. With this in mind, the nurse attempts to establish rapport, put the patient at ease, encourage honest communication, make eye contact, and listen carefully to the patient's responses to questions about health issues (Fig. 5-1).

When obtaining a health history or performing a physical examination, the nurse must be aware of his or her own nonverbal communication, as well as that of the patient. The nurse should take into consideration the patient's educational and cultural background and language proficiency. Questions and instructions to the patient should be phrased in a way that is easily understandable. Technical terms and medical jargon are avoided. In addition, the nurse must consider the patient's disabilities or impairments (hearing, vision, cognitive, and physical limitations). At the end of the assessment, the nurse may summarize and clarify the information obtained and ask the patient if he or she has any questions; this gives the nurse the opportunity to correct misinformation and add facts that may have been omitted.

Ethical Use of Health Assessment Data

Whenever information is elicited from a person through a health history or physical examination, the person has the right to know why the information is sought and how it will be used. For this reason, it is important to explain the purpose of the health history and physical examination, how the information will be obtained, and how it will be used (Bickley, 2009; Weber & Kelley, 2010). It is also important that the person knows that the decision to participate is voluntary. A private setting for the history interview and physical examination promotes trust and encourages open, honest communication. After the history and examination are completed, the nurse selectively records the data pertinent to the patient's health status. This written record of the patient's history and physical examination findings is then maintained in a secure place and made available only to those health professionals directly involved in the care of the patient. The Health Insurance Portability and Accountability Act (HIPAA), passed in 1996, established national standards to protect individuals' medical records and other personal health information and applies to health plans, health care clearinghouses, and those health care providers that conduct certain health care transactions electronically. The act requires appropriate safeguards to protect the privacy of personal health information and sets limits and conditions on the uses and disclosures that may be made of such information without patient authorization. HIPAA outlines patients' rights over their health information, including rights to examine and obtain a copy of their health records and to request corrections (U.S. Department of Health and Human Services [HHS], 2003).

The Role of Technology

The use of technology to augment the information-gathering process through the use of EMRs has become an increasingly important aspect of obtaining a health history and physical examination. An EMR serves to guide standardization of medical terms and to prevent duplication and transcription errors, promoting the accuracy of the documentation. Continuity of care between disciplines is also enhanced because all health providers are able to access patient information simultaneously and even remotely. Because information in EMRs is standardized, the data can be categorized and sorted, enabling nurses to easily measure patient outcomes related to nursing interventions, providing evidence of quality care, and identifying opportunities for improvement (Kutz, 2010). Nurses must be sensitive to the needs of older adults and others who may not be comfortable with computer technology. Nurses may need to allow extra time and provide detailed instructions or assistance. It is important to establish and maintain eye contact with the patient during the health history and to not focus solely on the computer screen for data entry.

Health History

The health history is a series of questions used to provide an overview of the patient's current health status. Many nurses are responsible for obtaining a detailed history of the person's current health problems, past medical history and family history, and a review of the person's functional status. This results in a total health profile that focuses on health as well as illness.

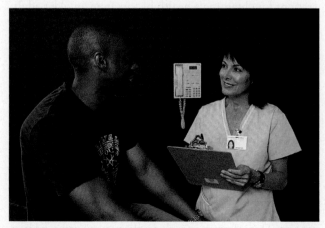

FIGURE 5-1 • A comfortable, relaxed atmosphere and an attentive interviewer are essential for a successful clinical interview.

When obtaining the health history, attention is focused on the impact of psychosocial, ethnic, and cultural background on a person's health, illness, and health promotion behaviors. The interpersonal and physical environments, as well as the person's lifestyle and activities of daily living, are explored in depth.

The format of the health history traditionally combines the medical history and the nursing assessment. Both the review of systems and the patient profile are expanded to include individual and family relationships, lifestyle patterns, health practices and nutritional assessment, and coping strategies. These components of the health history are the basis of nursing assessment and can be easily adapted to address the needs of any patient population in any setting, institution, or agency (Bickley, 2009; Weber & Kelley, 2010).

The health history format discussed in this chapter is only one approach that is useful in obtaining and organizing information about a person's health status. Some experts consider this traditional format to be inappropriate for nurses, because it does not focus exclusively on the assessment of human responses to actual or potential health problems. Several attempts have been made to develop an assessment format and database with this focus in mind. One example is a nursing database based on the North American Nursing Diagnosis Association (currently known as NANDA International) and its 13 domains: health promotion, nutrition, elimination/exchange, activity/rest, perception/cognition, self-perception, role relationship, sexuality, coping/stress tolerance, life principles, safety/protection, comfort, and growth/development (NANDA International, 2011). Although there is support in nursing for using this approach, no consensus for its use has been reached.

The National Information Center on Health Services Research and Health Care Technology (NICHSR) and other groups from the public and private sectors have focused on assessing not only biologic health but also other dimensions of health. These dimensions include physical, functional, emotional, mental, and social health. Efforts to assess health status have focused on the manner in which disease or disability affects a patient's functional status—that is, the ability of the person to function normally and perform his or her usual physical, mental, and social activities. An emphasis on functional assessment is viewed as more holistic than the traditional health or medical history. Instruments to assess health status in these ways may be used by nurses along with their own clinical assessment skills to determine the impact of illness, disease, disability, and health problems on functional status.

Regardless of the assessment format used, the focus of nurses during data collection is different from that of physicians and other health care team members. Combining the information obtained by the physician and the nurse into one health history prevents duplication of information and minimizes efforts on the part of the patient to provide this information repeatedly. This also encourages collaboration among members of the health care team who share in the collection and interpretation of the data.

The Informant

The informant, or the person providing the health history, may not always be the patient, as in the case of a

---

Chart 5-1   Health Assessment in the Older Adult

A health history should be obtained from older patients in a calm, unrushed manner. Because of the increased incidence of impaired vision and hearing in the older adult, lighting should be adequate but not glaring, and distracting noises should be kept to a minimum. The interviewer should assume a position that enables the person to read lips and facial expressions. Sometimes sitting at a 90-degree angle to the patient is helpful because some visual impairments, such as macular degeneration, can limit the patient's vision to only peripheral vision (Sharts-Hopko, 2009). It is best to ask the patient where the interviewer should sit in relation to the patient to optimize the patient's view of the interviewer. People who normally use a hearing aid are asked to use it during the interview.

Older adults often assume that new physical problems are a result of age rather than a treatable illness. In addition, the signs and symptoms of illness in older adults are often more subtle than those in younger people and may go unreported. Therefore, a question such as "What interferes most in your daily activities?" may be useful in focusing the clinical evaluation (Soriano, Fernandes, Cassel, et al., 2007). Special care is taken in obtaining a complete history of medications used, because many older people take many different kinds of prescription and over-the-counter medications. Although older people may experience a decline in mental function, it should not be assumed that they are unable to provide an adequate history (Soriano et al., 2007). Nevertheless, including a member of the family in the interview process (e.g., spouse, adult child, sibling, caretaker) may validate information and provide missing details. However, this should be done after obtaining the patient's permission. (Further details about assessment of the older adult are provided in Chapter 11.)

---

developmentally delayed, mentally impaired, disoriented, confused, unconscious, or comatose patient. The interviewer assesses the reliability of the informant and the usefulness of the information provided. For example, a disoriented patient is often unable to provide reliable information; people who use alcohol and illicit drugs often deny using these substances. The interviewer must make a clinical judgment about the reliability of the information (based on the context of the entire interview) and include this assessment in the record. Chart 5-1 provides special considerations for obtaining a health history from an older adult.

Components of the Health History

When a patient is seen for the first time by a member of the health care team, the first requirement is that baseline information be obtained (except in emergency situations). The sequence and format of obtaining data about a patient may vary; however, the content, regardless of format, usually addresses the same general topics. A traditional health history includes the following: biographical data, chief complaint, present health concern (or history of present illness), past history, family history, review of systems, and patient profile.

Biographical Data

Biographical information puts the patient's health history into context. This information includes the person's name, address, age, gender, marital status, occupation, and ethnic origins. Some interviewers prefer to ask more personal questions at this part of the interview, whereas others wait until more trust and confidence have been established or until a patient's immediate or urgent needs are first addressed. A patient who is in severe pain or has another urgent problem is unlikely to have a great deal of patience for an interviewer who is more concerned about marital or occupational status than with quickly addressing the problem at hand.

Chief Complaint

The chief complaint is the issue that caused the patient to seek the care of the health care provider. Questions such as "Why have you come to the health center today?" or "Why were you admitted to the hospital?" usually elicit the chief complaint. However, a statement such as "My doctor sent me" should be followed up with questions that identify and clarify the chief complaint (Bickley, 2009; Weber & Kelley, 2010). In the home setting, the initial question might be, "What is bothering you most today?" When a problem is identified, the person's exact words are usually recorded in quotation marks.

Present Health Concern or Illness

The history of the present health concern or illness is the single most important factor in helping the health care team arrive at a diagnosis or determine the patient's current needs. The physical examination is also helpful and often validates the information obtained from the history. A careful history and physical examination assist in the correct selection of appropriate diagnostic tests. Although diagnostic test results can be helpful, they often support rather than establish the diagnosis.

If the present illness is only one episode in a series of episodes, the nurse records the entire sequence of events. For example, a history from a patient whose chief complaint is an episode of insulin shock describes the entire course of the diabetes to put the current episode in context. The history of the present illness or problem includes such information as the date and onset (sudden or gradual) in which the problem occurred, the setting in which the problem occurred (at home, at work, after an argument, after exercise), manifestations of the problem, and the course of the illness or problem. This includes self-treatment (including complementary and alternative therapies), medical interventions, progress and effects of treatment, and the patient's perceptions of the cause or meaning of the problem.

Specific symptoms such as headaches, fever, or changes in bowel habits are described in detail. The interviewer also asks whether the symptom is persistent or intermittent, what factors aggravate or alleviate it, and whether any associated manifestations exist. If the patient complains of pain, the location, quality, severity, and duration of the pain are determined. (See Chapter 12 for a more detailed discussion of pain.)

Associated manifestations are symptoms that occur simultaneously with the chief complaint. The presence or absence of such symptoms may help to determine the origin or extent of the problem, as well as the diagnosis. These symptoms are referred to as significant positive or negative findings and are obtained from a review of systems directly related to the chief complaint. For example, if a patient reports a vague symptom such as fatigue or weight loss, all body systems are reviewed and included in this section of the history. On the other hand, if a patient's chief complaint is something specific, such as chest pain, then the cardiopulmonary and gastrointestinal systems will be the focus of the history of the present illness. In either situation, both positive and negative findings are recorded to further define the issue.

Past Health History

A detailed summary of a person's past health is an important part of the health history. After determining the general health status, the interviewer should inquire about immunization status according to the recommendations of the adult immunization schedule and record the dates of immunization (if known). The Advisory Committee on Immunization Practices (ACIP) General Recommendations Work Group (GRWG) updates its general recommendations on immunization every 3 to 5 years (Kroger, Sumaya, Pickering, et al., 2011). The interviewer should also inquire about any known allergies to medications or other substances, along with the nature of the allergy and adverse reactions. Other relevant material includes information, if known, about the patient's last physical examination, chest x-ray, electrocardiogram, eye examination, hearing test, dental checkup, Papanicolaou (Pap) smear and mammogram (if female), digital rectal examination of the prostate gland (if male), bone density testing, colon cancer screening, and any other pertinent tests.

The interviewer discusses previous illnesses and records negative as well as positive responses to a list of specific diseases. Dates of illness, or the age of the patient at the time, as well as the names of the primary health care provider and hospital, the diagnosis, and the treatment are noted. The interviewer elicits a history of the following areas:

- Childhood illnesses—rubeola, rubella, polio, whooping cough, mumps, measles, chickenpox, scarlet fever, rheumatic fever, strep throat
- Adult illnesses
- Psychiatric illnesses
- Injuries—burns, fractures, head injuries
- Hospitalizations
- Surgical and diagnostic procedures

If a particular hospitalization or major medical intervention is related to the present illness, the account of it is not repeated here; rather, the report refers to the appropriate part of the record, such as "See history of present illness" on the data sheet.

Family History

To identify diseases that may be genetic, communicable, or possibly environmental in origin, the interviewer asks about the age and health status, or the age and cause of death, of first-order relatives (parents, siblings, spouse, children) and second-order relatives (grandparents, cousins). In general, the following conditions are included: cancer, hypertension, heart disease, diabetes, epilepsy, mental illness, tuberculosis, kidney disease, arthritis, allergies, asthma, alcoholism, and obesity. One of the easiest methods of recording such data is by using the family tree, genogram, or pedigree (Fig. 5-2). The results of genetic testing or screening, if known, are recorded. Chart 5-2 provides genetic considerations related to health assessment. (See Chapter 8 for a detailed discussion of genetics.)

Review of Systems

The review of systems includes an overview of general health as well as symptoms related to each body system. Questions

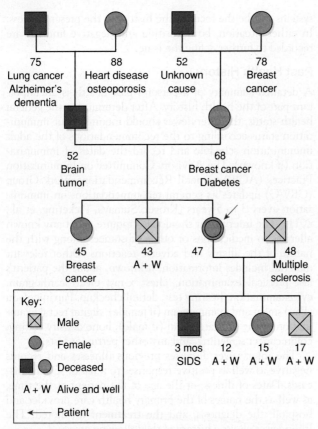

FIGURE 5-2 • Diagram (called a *genogram*) used to record history of family members, including their age and cause of death or, if living, their current health status.

Key:
- Male
- Female
- Deceased
- A + W Alive and well
- ← Patient

are asked about each of the major body systems for information about past and present symptoms. Negative and positive answers are recorded. If a patient responds positively to questions about a particular system, the information is analyzed carefully. If any illnesses were previously mentioned or recorded, it is not necessary to repeat them in this part of the history.

A review of systems can be organized in a formal checklist, which becomes part of the health history. One advantage of

a checklist is that it can be easily audited and is less subject to error than a system that relies heavily on the interviewer's memory.

Patient Profile

In the patient profile, more biographical information is gathered. A complete composite, or profile, of the patient is critical to analysis of the chief complaint and of the person's ability to deal with the problem. A complete patient profile is summarized in Chart 5-3.

At this point in the interview, the information elicited is highly personal and subjective. People are encouraged to express feelings honestly and to discuss personal experiences. It is best to begin with general, open-ended questions and to move to direct questioning when specific facts are needed. Interviews that progress from information that is less personal (birthplace, occupation, education) to information that is more personal (sexuality, body image, coping abilities) often reduce anxiety.

A general patient profile consists of the following content areas: past life events related to health, education and occupation, financial resources, environment (physical, spiritual, cultural, family relationships, support system), lifestyle (patterns and habits), presence of a physical or mental disability, self-concept, sexuality, risk for abuse, and stress and coping response.

Past Life Events Related to Health

The patient profile begins with a brief life history. Questions about place of birth and past places of residence help focus attention on the earlier years of life. Personal experiences during childhood or adolescence that have special significance may be elicited by asking a question such as, "Was there anything that you experienced as a child or adolescent that would be helpful for me to know about?" The interviewer's intent is to encourage the patient to make a quick review of his or her earlier life, highlighting information of particular significance. Although many patients may not recall anything significant, others may share information such as a personal achievement, a failure, a developmental crisis, or an instance of physical, emotional, or sexual abuse. The life history should include a brief medication history as appropriate for the patient.

GENETICS IN NURSING PRACTICE

Chart 5-2

Genetics Aspects of Health Assessment

Nursing Assessments

Family History Assessment
- Obtain information about maternal and paternal sides of family for three generations.
- Obtain history of known diseases or disorders for at least three generations.
- Look for clustering of diseases or disorders that occur at young ages and two or more close relatives with the same type of disease or disorder.
- Cultural, social, and spiritual assessment—assess for individual and family perceptions and beliefs around genetics topics.

Patient Assessment
- Assess physical findings that may suggest a genetic condition (e.g., unusually tall stature—Marfan syndrome).

Management Issues Specific to Genetics
- Assess patient's understanding of genetic factors related to his or her health risks.
- Refer for risk assessment when a hereditary disease or disorder is suspected so that patient and family can discuss inheritance risk with other family members and availability of genetic testing.
- Offer appropriate genetic information and resources.
- Assess patient's understanding of genetic information.
- Provide support to patients and families with known genetic test results for hereditary disease or disorders.

Genetics Resources

See Chapter 8, Chart 8-6 for genetics resources.

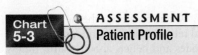

Chart
5-3

ASSESSMENT
Patient Profile

Past Events Related to Health

Place of birth
Places lived
Significant childhood/adolescent experiences

Current Medications

Prescription, over-the-counter, home remedies, complementary
   and alternative therapies

Education and Occupation

Jobs held in past
Current position/job
Length of time at position
Educational preparation
Work satisfaction and career goals

Financial Resources

Income
Insurance coverage

Environment

Physical—living arrangements (type of housing, neighborhood,
   presence of hazards)
Spiritual—extent to which religion is a part of individual's life;
   religious beliefs related to perception of health and illness;
   religious practices
Interpersonal—ethnic background (language spoken, customs
   and values held, folk practices used to maintain health or
   cure illness); family relationships (family structure, roles,
   communication patterns, support system); friendships (quality
   of relationship)

Lifestyle Patterns

Sleep (time person retires, hours per night, comfort measures,
   awakens rested)
Exercise (type, frequency, time spent)
Nutrition (24-hour diet recall, idiosyncrasies, restrictions)

Recreation (type of activity, time spent)
Caffeine (type: coffee, tea, cola, chocolate), amount
Smoking (type: cigarette, pipe, cigar, marijuana; amount per day;
   number of years; desire to quit)
Alcohol (type, amount, pattern over past year)
Drugs (type, amount, route of administration)

Physical or Mental Disability

Presence of a disability (physical or mental)
Effect of disability on function and health access
Accommodations needed to support functioning

Self-Concept

View of self in present
View of self in future
Body image (level of satisfaction, concerns)

Sexuality

Perception of self as a man or woman
Quality of sexual relationships
Concerns related to sexuality or sexual functioning

Risk for Abuse

Physical injury in past
Afraid of partner, caregiver, or family member
Refusal of caregiver to provide necessary equipment or
   assistance

Stress and Coping Response

Major concerns or problems at present
Daily "hassles"
Past experiences with similar problems
Past coping patterns and outcomes
Present coping strategies and anticipated outcomes
Individual's expectations of family/friends and health care team in
   problem resolution

Education and Occupation

Inquiring about current occupation can reveal much about
a person's economic status and educational preparation.
A statement such as "Tell me about your job" often elicits information about role, job tasks, and satisfaction with
the position. Direct questions about past employment and
career goals may be asked if the person does not provide this
information.

It is important to learn about a person's educational background. Asking a person what kind of educational requirements were necessary to attain his or her present job is a more
sensitive approach than asking whether he or she graduated
from high school.

Financial Resources

Information about the patient's general financial status may
be obtained by questions such as "Do you have any financial concerns at this time?" or "Many people are struggling in
the current economic situation. Has it affected you or your
family?" Inquiries about the person's insurance coverage and
plans for health care payment are also appropriate.

Environment

The concept of environment includes a person's physical
environment and its potential hazards. It also includes a person's spiritual awareness, cultural background, family relationships, and support system.

Physical Environment. Information is elicited about the
type of housing (apartment, duplex, single family) in which
the person lives, its location, the level of safety and comfort within the home and neighborhood, and the presence
of environmental hazards (e.g., isolation, potential fire risks,
inadequate sanitation). If the patient is homeless, details
about available resources are important to ascertain.

Spirituality and Spiritual Environment. **Spirituality** is
defined as connectedness with self, others, a life force, or
God that allows people to experience self-transcendence and
find meaning in life. Spirituality helps people discover a purpose in life, understand the ever-changing qualities of life,
and develop their relationship with God or a higher power.
Within the framework of spirituality, people may discover
truths about the self, about the world, and about concepts

such as love, compassion, wisdom, honesty, commitment, imagination, reverence, and morality. Sacred texts for the major religious traditions offer guidelines for personal conduct and social and spiritual behavior (O'Brien, 2011).

Spiritual behavior can be expressed through devotion, sacrifice, self-discipline, and spending time in activities that focus on the inner self or the soul. Although religion and nature are two vehicles that people use to connect themselves with God or a higher power, bonds to religious institutions, beliefs, or dogma are not required to experience the spiritual sense of self. **Faith**, considered the foundation of spirituality, is trust in God, belief in a higher power or something that a person cannot see. The spiritual part of a person views life as a mystery that unfolds over one's lifetime, encompassing questions about meaning, hope, relatedness to God or a higher power, acceptance or forgiveness, and transcendence. A strong sense of spirituality or religious faith can have a positive impact on health. Spirituality is also a component of hope, and, especially during chronic, serious, or terminal illness, patients and their families often find comfort and emotional strength in their religious traditions or spiritual beliefs. At other times, illness and loss can cause a loss of faith or meaning in life and a spiritual crisis.

The term *spiritual environment* refers to the degree to which a person thinks about or contemplates his or her existence, accepts challenges in life, and seeks and finds answers to personal questions. Spirituality may be expressed through identification with a particular religion. Spiritual values and beliefs often direct a person's behavior and approach to health problems and can influence responses to sickness. Illness may create a spiritual crisis and can place considerable stress on a person's internal resources and beliefs. It is important that the spiritual beliefs of people and families be acknowledged, valued, and respected for the comfort and guidance they provide. Inquiring about spirituality can identify possible support systems as well as beliefs and customs that need to be considered in planning care. Information is gathered about the extent to which religion is a part of the person's life as well as religious beliefs and practices related to health and illness.

A spiritual assessment may involve asking the following questions:

- Is religion or God important to you?
- If yes, in what way?
- If no, what is the most important thing in your life?
- Are there any religious practices that are important to you?
- Do you have any spiritual concerns because of your present health problem?

The nurse assesses spiritual strength further by inquiring about the patient's sense of spiritual well-being, hope, and peacefulness and assesses whether spiritual beliefs and values have changed in response to illness or loss. In addition, the nurse assesses current and past participation in religious or spiritual practices and notes the patient's responses to questions regarding spiritual needs—grief, anger, guilt, depression, doubt, anxiety, or calmness—to help determine the patient's need for spiritual care. Researchers have developed both English and Spanish versions of a spiritual coping strategies scale that measures how frequently religious and nonreligious strategies are used to cope with a stressful situation (Hawthorne, Youngblut, & Brooten, 2011). Another simple assessment technique is to inquire about the patient's and family's desire for spiritual support.

Cultural Environment. When obtaining the health history, the person's cultural and religious backgrounds are taken into account. Cultural attitudes and beliefs about health, illness, health care, hospitalization, the use of medications, and the use of complementary and alternative therapies, which are derived from personal experiences, vary according to ethnic, cultural, and religious background. A person from another culture may have different views of personal health practices from those of the health care practitioner (Bickley, 2009; Weber & Kelley, 2010). (See Chapter 7 for more cultural considerations.)

The beliefs and practices that have been shared from generation to generation are known as cultural or ethnic patterns. They are expressed through language, dress, dietary choices, and role behaviors; in perceptions of health and illness; and in health-related behaviors. The influence of these beliefs and customs on how a person reacts to health problems and interacts with health care providers cannot be underestimated. The following questions may assist in obtaining relevant information:

- Where did your parents or ancestors come from? When?
- What language do you speak at home?
- Are there certain customs or values that are important to you?
- Do you do anything special to keep in good health?
- Do you have any specific practices for treating illness?

Family Relationships and Support System. An assessment of family structure (members, ages, and roles), patterns of communication, and the presence or absence of a support system is an integral part of the patient profile. Although the traditional family is recognized as a mother, a father, and children, many different types of living arrangements exist within our society. "Family" may mean two or more people bound by emotional ties or commitments, such as those shared by gay or lesbian partners. Live-in companions, roommates, and close friends can also play a significant role in a person's support system.

Lifestyle

The lifestyle section of the patient profile provides information about health-related behaviors. These behaviors include patterns of sleep, exercise, nutrition, and recreation, as well as personal habits such as smoking and the use of illicit drugs, alcohol, and caffeine. Although most people readily describe their exercise patterns or recreational activities, many are unwilling to report their smoking, alcohol use, and illicit drug use, and many deny or understate the degree to which they use such substances. Questions such as "What kind of alcohol do you enjoy drinking at a party?" may elicit more accurate information than "Do you drink?" Determining the specific type of alcohol (e.g., wine, liquor, beer) the patient drinks and the last time he or she had a drink are important aspects of the assessment (Bickley, 2009).

The lifestyle of some people includes the use of mood-altering substances. People who engage in **substance abuse** use illegally obtained drugs, prescribed or over-the-counter (OTC) medications, and alcohol alone or in combination with other drugs in ineffective attempts to cope with the pressures, strains, and burdens of life. Over time, physiologic, emotional, cognitive, and behavioral problems develop as a result of continuous substance abuse.

ASSESSMENT
Chart 5-4 Assessing for Alcohol or Drug Use

CAGE Questions
Adapted to Include Drugs (CAGE-AID)*
Have you felt you ought to cut down on your drinking *(or drug use)*?
_____Yes _____No

Have people annoyed you by criticizing your drinking *(or drug use)*?
_____Yes _____No

Have you felt bad or guilty about your drinking *(or drug use)*?
_____Yes _____No

Have you ever had a drink *(or used drugs)* **first thing in the morning to steady your nerves or get rid of a hangover** *(or to get the day started)*?
_____Yes _____No

*Boldface text shows the original CAGE questions; boldface italic text shows modifications of the CAGE questions used to screen for drug disorders. In a general population, two or more positive answers indicate a need for more in-depth assessment.
Fleming, M. F., & Barry, K. L. (1992). *Addictive disorders*. St. Louis: Mosby; Ewing, J. A. (1984). Detecting alcoholism: The CAGE questionnaire. *Journal of the American Medical Association, 252*(14), 1905–1907. Reprinted with permission from Elsevier.

If alcohol abuse is suspected, additional information may be obtained by using common alcohol screening questionnaires such as the CAGE (Cutting down, Annoyance by criticism, Guilty feeling, and Eye-openers) (Ewing, 1984), AUDIT (Alcohol Use Disorders Identification Test), TWEAK (Tolerance, Worry about drinking, Eye-opener, Amnesia, Kut down on drinking) (Chan, Pristach, Welte, et al., 1993), or SMAST (Short Michigan Alcohol Screening Test). Chart 5-4 shows CAGE Adapted to Include Drugs (CAGE-AID). The MAST (Michigan Alcohol Screening Test) has been updated to include drug use and has a geriatric version (New York State Office of Alcoholism and Substance Abuse Services [OASAS], 2007).

Similar questions can be used to elicit information about smoking and caffeine consumption. Questions about illicit drug use follow naturally after questions about smoking, caffeine consumption, and alcohol use. A nonjudgmental approach makes it easier for a person to respond truthfully and factually. If street names or unfamiliar terms are used to describe drugs, the person is asked to define the terms used.

Investigation of lifestyle should also include questions about complementary and alternative therapies. It is estimated that there are more than 1,800 types of complementary and alternative therapies, including special diets, prayer, visualization or guided imagery, massage, meditation, herbal products, and many others (Snyder & Lindquist, 2010). Marijuana is used for management of symptoms, especially pain, in several chronic conditions.

Lifestyle also includes questions about continuing health promotion and screening practices. If the person has not been involved in these practices in the past, he or she should be educated about their importance and referred to appropriate health care providers. It has been established that older adults can benefit from health promotion behaviors such as improving and maintaining activity levels. Nurses should recognize health promotion as part of their role in working with older people (Goodman, Davies, Dinan, et al., 2011).

Disability

The general patient profile needs to contain questions about any hearing, vision, or other type of physical disability (Chart 5-5). In addition, mental, sensory, or cognitive disabilities need to be addressed. The presence of an obvious physical limitation (e.g., using crutches to walk or using a wheelchair to get around) necessitates further investigation. The initial cause or onset of the disability, as well as the impact on functional ability, should be established. Although patients are always the most valuable source of information about their condition and care, family members or caregivers of patients with disabilities can be utilized as a resource if cognitive

NURSING RESEARCH PROFILE
Chart 5-5 Health Care Experiences of the Visually Impaired

Sharts-Hopko, N. C., Smeltzer, S., Ott, B. B., et al. (2010). Healthcare experiences of women with visual impairment. *Clinical Nurse Specialist, 24*(3), 149–153.

Purpose

Nurses utilize a holistic focus when performing health assessment and providing care. The main purpose of this investigation was to address the question of how women with low vision or blindness have experienced health care.

Design

This study was a secondary analysis of qualitative data that was performed on transcripts from two focus groups that were conducted at an agency serving people with visual impairment. The two focus groups included 7 and 11 women, respectively, having low vision or blindness, who had been part of an original study of hard-to-reach women with disabilities. Content analysis for the identification of thematic clusters was performed on transcriptions of the focus group data.

Findings

Findings were consistent with existing research on the health needs of women with disabilities but added specific understanding related to visual impairment. Six thematic categories were identified: health professionals' awareness, information access, health care access, isolation, the need for self-advocacy, and perception by others. Patients noted that many of their needs relating to visual impairment were not met.

Nursing Implications

Nurses and other health professionals need to increase their sensitivity to the challenges faced by women with visual impairment, planning and providing care accordingly. Nurses must accurately identify the needs of patients with low vision or blindness and advocate for them so they receive the resources they need (e.g., talking prescription bottles, reliable transportation for health care–related appointments, nonvisual teaching aids). Furthermore, students need to be prepared by sensitized faculty to interact appropriately with people who are visually impaired, and health care settings need to respond to their needs.

Chart
5-6

ASSESSMENT

Assessing the Health of People With Disabilities

Overview

People with disabilities are entitled to the same level of health assessment and physical examination as people without disabilities. The nurse needs to be aware of the patient's disabilities or impairments (hearing, vision, cognitive, and physical limitations) and take these into consideration when obtaining a health history and conducting a physical assessment (Futcher, 2011). It is appropriate to ask the patient what assistance he or she needs rather than assuming that help is needed for all activities or that, if assistance is needed, the patient will ask for it.

Health History

Communication between the nurse and the patient is essential. To ensure that the patient is able to respond to assessment questions and provide needed information, interpreters, assistive listening devices, or other alternative formats (e.g., Braille, large-print forms) may be required.

When interpreters are needed, interpretation services should be arranged. Health care facilities have a responsibility to provide these services without charge to the patient. Family members (especially children) should *not* be used as interpreters, because doing so violates the patient's right to privacy and confidentiality.

The nurse should speak directly to the patient and not to family members or others who have accompanied the patient. If the patient has vision or hearing loss, normal tone and volume of the voice should be used when conducting the assessment. The patient should be able to see the nurse's face clearly during the health history so that speech reading and nonverbal clues can be used to aid communication.

The health history should address general health issues that are important to all patients, including sexual history and risk for abuse. It should also address the impact of the patient's disability on health issues and access to care, as well as the effect of the patient's current health problem on his or her disability.

The nurse should verify what the patient has said; if the patient has difficulty communicating verbally, the nurse should ask for clarification rather than assume that it is too difficult for the patient to do so. Most people would rather be asked to explain again than run the risk of being misunderstood (Smeltzer, Sharts-Hopko, Ott, et al., 2007).

Physical Examination

Inaccessible facilities remain a major barrier to health care for people with disabilities. Barriers include lack of ramps and grab bars, inaccessible restrooms, small examination rooms, and examination tables that cannot be lowered to allow the patient to move himself or herself onto, or be transferred easily and safely to, the examination table. The patient may need help getting undressed for the physical examination (and dressed

again), moving on and off the examination table, and maintaining positions usually required during physical examination maneuvers. It is important to ask the patient what assistance is needed.

If the patient has impaired sensory function (e.g., lack of sensation, hearing or vision loss), it is important to inform the patient that you will be touching him or her. Furthermore, it is important to explain all procedures and maneuvers.

Gynecologic examinations should *not* be deferred because a patient has a disability or is assumed to be sexually inactive. Explanations of the examination are important for all women, and even more so for women with disabilities, because they may have had previous negative experiences. Slow, gentle moving and positioning of the patient for the gynecologic examination and warming the speculum before attempting insertion often minimize spasticity in women with neurologically related disabilities.

Health Screening and Testing

Many people with disabilities report that they have not been weighed for years or even decades because they are unable to stand for this measurement. Alternative methods (e.g., use of wheelchair scales) are needed to monitor weight and body mass index. This is particularly important because of the increased incidence of obesity and its effects on health status and transfer of persons with disabilities.

Patients with disabilities may require special assistance if urine specimens are to be obtained as part of the visit. They are often able to suggest strategies to obtain urine specimens based on previous experience.

If it is necessary for the nurse to wear a mask during a procedure or if the patient is unable to see the face of the nurse during a procedure, it is important to explain the procedure and the expected role of the patient ahead of time. If the patient is unable to hear or communicate with the nurse or other health care provider verbally during an examination or diagnostic test, a method of communication (e.g., signaling the patient by tapping the arm, signaling the nurse by using a bell) should be established beforehand.

People with disabilities experience difficulties related to obtaining care, challenges accessing health care facilities, perceptions that health professionals are insensitive to their needs, and concerns about the quality of care they receive (Sharts-Hopko, 2009; Sharts-Hopko, Smeltzer, Ott, et al., 2010). Therefore, it is important to ask about health screening and recommendations for screening. In addition, people with disabilities should be asked about their participation in health promotion activities, because inaccessible environments and other barriers may limit their participation in exercise, health programs, and other health promotion efforts.

---

disabilities are present for effective planning and provision of patients' care (Dinsmore & Higgins, 2011). Chart 5-6 presents specific issues that the nurse should consider when obtaining health histories and conducting physical assessments of patients with disabilities.

Self-Concept

Self-concept, a person's view of himself or herself, is an image that develops over many years. To assess self-concept, the

interviewer might ask how a person views life, using a question such as "How do you feel about your life in general?" A person's self-concept can be threatened very easily by changes in physical function or appearance or other threats to health. The impact of certain medical conditions or surgical interventions, such as a colostomy or a mastectomy, can threaten body image. The question, "Do you have any particular concerns about your body?" may elicit useful information about self-image.

Sexuality

The sexual history is an extremely personal area of assessment. Interviewers are frequently uncomfortable with such questions and ignore this area of the patient profile or conduct a very cursory interview about this subject. It is the nurse's professional and clinical responsibility to discuss issues of sexuality with patients. Lack of knowledge about sexuality, preconceived notions (e.g., assuming all people are heterosexual or assuming people with disabilities are asexual), and anxiety about one's own sexuality may hamper the interviewer's effectiveness in dealing with this subject (Saunamaki, Anderson, & Engstrom, 2010; Futcher, 2011).

Sexual assessment can be approached at the end of the interview or at the time interpersonal or lifestyle factors are assessed; otherwise, it may be easier to discuss sexuality as a part of the genitourinary history within the review of systems. In female patients, a discussion of sexuality would follow questions about menstruation. In male patients, a similar discussion would follow questions about the urinary system.

Obtaining the sexual history provides an opportunity to discuss sexual matters openly and gives the person permission to express sexual concerns to an informed professional. The interviewer must be nonjudgmental and must use language appropriate to the patient's age, background, and cognitive level (Futcher, 2011). The assessment begins with an orienting sentence such as "Next, I would like to ask about your sexual health and practices." This type of opening may lead to a discussion of concerns related to sexual expression or the quality of a relationship, or to questions about contraception, risky sexual behaviors, and safer sex practices. Examples of other questions include "Do you have one or more sexual partners?" and "Are you satisfied with your sexual relationships?"

Determining whether a person is sexually active should precede any attempts to explore issues related to sexuality and sexual function. Care should be taken to initiate conversations about sexuality with older adult patients and patients with disabilities and not to treat them as asexual people. Questions are worded in such a way that the person feels free to discuss his or her sexuality regardless of marital status or sexual preference. Direct questions are usually less threatening when prefaced with such statements as "Some people feel that..." or "Many people worry about...." This suggests the normalcy of such feelings or behavior and encourages the person to share information that might otherwise be omitted because of fear of seeming "different."

If a person answers abruptly or does not wish to carry the discussion any further, then the interviewer should move to the next topic. However, introducing the subject of sexuality indicates to the person that a discussion of sexual concerns is acceptable and can be approached again in the future if so desired. (Further discussion of the sexual history is presented in Chapters 56 and 59.)

Risk for Abuse

Physical, sexual, and psychological abuse affects people of both genders, of all ages, and from all socioeconomic, ethnic, and cultural groups. Patients rarely discuss this topic unless specifically asked about it. In fact, research shows that most women in an abusive relationship have never told a health

care provider. Therefore, it is important to ask direct questions, such as:

- Is anyone physically hurting you or forcing you to engage in sexual activities?
- Has anyone ever hurt you physically or threatened to do so?
- Are you ever afraid of anyone close to you (your partner, caregiver, or other family members)?

Patients who are older or have disabilities are at increased risk for abuse and should be asked about it as a routine part of assessment. However, when older patients are questioned directly, they rarely admit to abuse. Health care professionals should assess for risk factors, such as high levels of stress or alcoholism in caregivers, evidence of violence, and emotional outbursts, as well as financial, emotional, or physical dependency.

Two additional questions have been found to be effective in uncovering specific types of abuse that may occur only in people with disabilities:

- Does anyone prevent you from using a wheelchair, cane, respirator, or other assistive device?
- Does anyone you depend on refuse to help you with an important personal need, such as taking your medicine, getting to the bathroom, getting in or out of bed, bathing, dressing, or getting food or drink?

If a person's response indicates that abuse is a risk, further assessment is warranted, and efforts are made to ensure the patient's safety and provide access to appropriate community and professional resources and support systems. (Further discussion of domestic violence and abuse is presented in Chapter 56.)

Stress and Coping Responses

Each person handles stress differently. How well people adapt to stress depends on their ability to cope. During a health history, past coping patterns and perceptions of current stresses and anticipated outcomes are explored to identify the person's overall ability to handle stress. It is especially important to identify the expectations that a person may have related to family, friends, and caregivers in terms of providing financial, emotional, or physical support. (Further discussion of stress and coping is presented in Chapter 6.)

Physical Assessment

Physical assessment, or the physical examination (collection of objective data about the patient's health status), is an integral part of nursing assessment. The basic techniques and tools used in performing a physical examination are described in general in this chapter. The examinations of specific systems, including special maneuvers, are described in the appropriate chapters throughout the book.

Examination Considerations

The physical examination is usually performed after the health history is obtained. It is carried out in a well-lighted, warm area. The patient is asked to (or helped to) undress and is draped appropriately so that only the area to be examined is exposed. The person's physical and psychological comfort are considered at all times. It is necessary to describe procedures to the patient and explain what sensations to expect before each part of the examination. The examiner washes his or her hands before and immediately after the examination. Fingernails are kept short to avoid injuring the patient. If there is a possibility of coming into contact with blood or other body secretions during the physical examination, gloves should be worn.

An organized and systematic examination is the key to obtaining appropriate data in the shortest time. Such an approach encourages cooperation and trust on the part of the patient. The person's health history provides the examiner with a health profile that guides all aspects of the physical examination.

A "complete" physical examination is not routine. Many of the body systems are selectively assessed on the basis of the presenting problem. For example, if a healthy 20-year-old college student requires an examination to study abroad and reports no history of neurologic abnormality, the neurologic assessment is brief. Conversely, a history of transient numbness and diplopia (double vision) usually necessitates a complete neurologic investigation. Similarly, a patient with chest pain receives a much more intensive examination of the chest and heart than one with an earache. In general, the health history guides the examiner in obtaining additional data for a complete picture of the patient's health.

The process of learning to perform a physical examination requires repetition and reinforcement in a simulated or clinical setting. Only after basic physical assessment techniques are mastered can the examiner tailor the routine screening examination to include thorough assessments of particular systems, including special maneuvers (Bickley, 2009; Weber & Kelley, 2010).

Components of the Physical Examination

The components of a physical examination include general observations and then a more focused assessment of the pertinent body systems. The tools of the physical examination are the human senses of vision, hearing, touch, and smell. These may be augmented by special tools (e.g., stethoscope, ophthalmoscope, reflex hammer) that are extensions of the human senses; they are simple tools that anyone can learn to use well. Expertise comes with practice, and sophistication comes with the interpretation of what is seen and heard.

Initial Observations

General inspection begins with the first contact with the patient. Introducing oneself and shaking hands provide opportunities for making initial observations: Is the person old or young? How old? How young? Does the person appear to be his or her stated age? Is the person thin or obese? Does the person appear anxious or depressed? Is the person's body structure normal or abnormal—in what way and how different from normal? It is essential to pay attention to the details in observation. Vague, general statements are not a substitute for specific descriptions based on careful observation. Consider the following examples:

- "The person appears sick." In what way does he or she appear sick? Is the skin clammy, pale, jaundiced, or cyanotic? Is the person grimacing in pain or having difficulty breathing? Does he or she have edema? What specific physical features or behavioral manifestations indicate that the person is "sick"?

- "The person appears chronically ill." In what way does he or she appear chronically ill? Does the person appear to have lost weight? People who lose weight secondary to muscle-wasting diseases (e.g., acquired immunodeficiency syndrome [AIDS], malignancy) have a different appearance than those who are merely thin, and weight loss may be accompanied by loss of muscle mass or atrophy. Does the skin have the appearance of chronic illness (i.e., is it pale, or does it give the appearance of dehydration or loss of subcutaneous tissue)?

These important specific observations are documented in the patient's chart or health record. Among general observations that should be noted in the initial examination of the patient are posture, body movements, nutritional status, speech pattern, and vital signs.

Posture

The posture that a person assumes often provides valuable information. Patients who have breathing difficulties (dyspnea) secondary to cardiac disease prefer to sit and may report feeling short of breath when lying flat for even a brief time. Patients with abdominal pain owing to peritonitis prefer to lie perfectly still; even slight jarring of the bed or examination table causes agonizing pain. In contrast, patients with abdominal pain owing to renal or biliary colic are often restless and may pace the room.

Body Movements

There are two kinds of abnormalities of body movement: generalized disruption of voluntary or involuntary movement and asymmetry of movement. The first category includes various tremors; some tremors may occur at rest (Parkinson's disease), whereas others occur only on voluntary movement (cerebellar ataxia). Other tremors may exist during both rest and activity (alcohol withdrawal syndrome, thyrotoxicosis). Some voluntary or involuntary movements are fine, and others are quite coarse. Extreme examples include the convulsive movements of generalized grand mal seizures or tetanus and the choreiform (involuntary and irregular) movements of patients with rheumatic fever or Huntington disease.

Asymmetry of movement, in which only one side of the body is affected, may occur with disorders of the central nervous system (CNS), primarily in those patients who have had a cerebrovascular accident (stroke). Patients may have drooping of one side of the face, weakness or paralysis of the extremities on one side of the body, or a foot-dragging gait.

Nutritional Status

Nutritional status is important to note. Obesity may be generalized as a result of excessive intake of calories, or it may be specifically localized to the trunk in patients who have an endocrine disorder (Cushing disease) or who have been taking corticosteroids for long periods. Loss of weight may be generalized as a result of inadequate caloric intake, or it may be seen in loss of muscle mass with disorders that affect protein synthesis. Nutritional assessment is discussed in more detail later in this chapter.

Speech Pattern

Speech may be slurred because of CNS disease or because of damage to cranial nerves. Recurrent damage to the laryngeal nerve results in hoarseness, as do disorders that produce edema or swelling of the vocal cords. Speech may be halting, slurred, or interrupted in flow in patients with some CNS disorders (e.g., multiple sclerosis, stroke).

Vital Signs

The recording of vital signs is a part of every physical examination (Bickley, 2009). Blood pressure, pulse rate, respiratory rate, and body temperature measurements are obtained and recorded. Acute changes and trends over time are documented, and unexpected changes and values that deviate significantly from a patient's normal values are brought to the attention of the patient's primary health care provider. The "fifth vital sign," pain, is also assessed and documented, if indicated.

Focused Assessment

Following the general inspection, a more focused assessment is conducted. Although the sequence of physical examination depends on the circumstances and the patient's reason for seeking health care, the complete examination usually proceeds as follows:

- Skin
- Head and neck
- Thorax and lungs
- Breasts
- Cardiovascular system
- Abdomen
- Rectum
- Genitalia
- Neurologic system
- Musculoskeletal system

In clinical practice, all relevant body systems are tested throughout the physical examination, not necessarily in the sequence described (Weber & Kelley, 2010). For example, when the face is examined, it is appropriate to check for facial asymmetry and, thus, for the integrity of the fifth and seventh cranial nerves; the examiner does not need to repeat this as part of a neurologic examination. When systems are combined in this manner, the patient does not need to change positions repeatedly, which can be exhausting and time-consuming.

The traditional technique sequence in the focused portion of the examination is inspection, palpation, percussion, and then auscultation, except in the case of an abdominal examination (where auscultation precedes palpation and percussion).

Inspection

The first fundamental technique is **inspection**, or observation of each relevant body system in more detail as indicated from the health history or the general inspection. Characteristics such as skin color, presence and size of lesions, edema, erythema, symmetry, and pulsations are noted. Specific body movements that are noted on inspection include spasticity, muscle spasms, and an abnormal gait (Porth & Matfin, 2009).

Palpation

Palpation is a vital part of the physical examination. Many structures of the body, although not visible, may be assessed through the techniques of light and deep palpation (Fig. 5-3). Examples include the superficial blood vessels, lymph nodes,

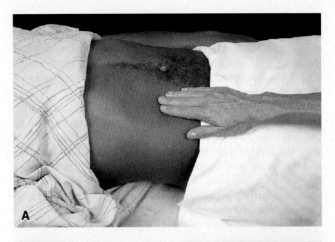

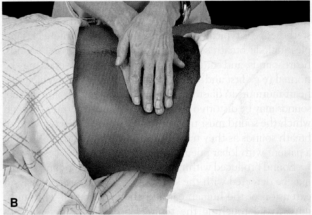

FIGURE 5-3 • **A.** Light palpation. **B.** Deep palpation.

thyroid gland, organs of the abdomen and pelvis, and rectum. When the abdomen is examined, auscultation is performed before palpation and percussion to avoid altering bowel sounds (Bickley, 2009; Weber & Kelley, 2010).

Some sounds generated within the body, if within specified frequency ranges, may also be detected through touch. For example, certain murmurs generated in the heart or within blood vessels (thrills) may be detected. Thrills cause a sensation to the hand much like the purring of a cat. Voice sounds are transmitted along the bronchi to the periphery of the lung. These may be perceived by touch and may be altered by disorders affecting the lungs. The phenomenon is called *tactile fremitus* and is useful in assessing diseases of the chest. The significance of these findings is discussed in Chapters 20 and 25.

Percussion

The technique of **percussion** translates the application of physical force into sound. It is a skill requiring practice that yields much information about disease processes in the chest and abdomen (Bickley, 2009; Weber & Kelley, 2010). The principle is to set the chest wall or abdominal wall into vibration by striking it with a firm object. The sound produced reflects the density of the underlying structure. Certain densities produce sounds as percussion notes. These sounds, listed in a sequence that proceeds from the least to the densest, are tympany, hyperresonance, resonance, dullness, and flatness.

Tympany is the drumlike sound produced by percussing the air-filled stomach. Hyperresonance is audible when one percusses over inflated lung tissue in a person with emphysema. Resonance is the sound elicited over air-filled lungs. Percussion of the liver produces a dull sound, whereas percussion of the thigh produces a flat sound.

Percussion allows the examiner to assess such normal anatomic details as the borders of the heart and the movement of the diaphragm during inspiration. It is also possible to determine the level of a pleural effusion (fluid in the pleural cavity) and the location of a consolidated area caused by pneumonia or atelectasis (collapse of alveoli). The use of percussion is described further with disorders of the thorax and abdomen. (See Chapters 20 and 44.)

Auscultation

Auscultation is the skill of listening to sounds produced within the body created by the movement of air or fluid (Fig. 5-4). A stethoscope is typically used to enhance this technique. Examples include breath sounds, the spoken voice, bowel sounds, heart sounds, and cardiac murmurs. Physiologic sounds may be normal (e.g., first and second heart sounds) or pathologic (e.g., heart murmurs in diastole, crackles in the lung). Some normal sounds may be distorted by abnormalities of structures through which the sound must travel (e.g., changes in the character of breath sounds as they travel through the consolidated lung of a patient with lobar pneumonia).

Sound produced within the body, if of sufficient amplitude, may be detected with the stethoscope, which functions as an extension of the human ear and channels sound. The nurse must avoid touching the tubing or rubbing other surfaces (hair, clothing) during auscultation to minimize extraneous noises. Sounds detected by auscultation are classified according to their intensity (loud or soft), pitch (high or low), duration (length), and quality (musical, raspy, crackling) (Bickley, 2009; Weber & Kelley, 2010).

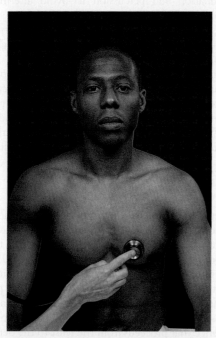

FIGURE 5-4 • Auscultation of the heart in forward sitting position.

Nutritional Assessment

Nutrition is important to maintain health and to prevent disease and death. When illness or injury occurs, optimal nutrition is essential for healing and for resisting infection and other complications. An in-depth nutritional assessment is often integrated into the health history and physical examination. Assessment of nutritional status provides information about obesity, undernutrition, and malnutrition.

Certain signs and symptoms that suggest possible nutritional deficiency, such as muscle wasting, poor skin integrity, loss of subcutaneous tissue, and obesity, are easy to note because they are specific; these should be pursued further. Other physical signs may be subtle and must be carefully assessed. For example, certain signs that appear to indicate nutritional deficiency may actually reflect other systemic conditions (e.g., endocrine disorders, infectious disease). Others may result from impaired digestion, absorption, excretion, or storage of nutrients in the body (Porth & Matfin, 2009; Weber & Kelley, 2010).

Disorders caused by nutritional deficiency, overeating, or eating unhealthy meals are among the leading causes of illness and death in the United States today. Examples of health problems associated with poor nutrition include obesity, osteoporosis, cirrhosis, diverticulitis, and eating disorders.

Obesity is a major concern for children, adolescents, and adults in the United States and globally. The World Health Organization (WHO) defines obesity as abnormal or excessive fat accumulation that may impair health. Obesity and being overweight are the fifth leading risk factors for global deaths. Additionally, diabetes, coronary artery disease, and certain cancers can be attributable to obesity (WHO, 2011).

Lifespan Considerations

Adolescence is a time of critical growth and when lifelong eating habits are established. Nutritional assessment is particularly important during this time period. It is vital to assess for obesity in adolescents to prevent complications from obesity as they enter adulthood.

Adolescent girls are at particular nutritional risk, because iron, folate, and calcium intakes are below recommended levels and they are a less physically active group compared to adolescent males. Adolescents with other nutritional disorders, such as anorexia and bulimia, have a better chance of recovery if these disorders are identified and treated in the adolescent years rather than in adulthood.

Older adults are also at risk for altered nutrition. Special considerations for nutritional assessment in older adults are presented in Chart 5-7.

Components of Nutritional Assessment

The sequence of assessment of parameters may vary; however, evaluation of nutritional status includes one or more of the following methods: measurement of **body mass index (BMI)** and waist circumference, biochemical assessment, clinical examination findings, and dietary data. Measurement of BMI and waist circumference is recommended to determine if a patient is obese (Reilly, 2010).

Chart 5-7 Nutritional Assessment in the Older Adult

Nutritional screening in the older adult is a first step in maintaining adequate nutrition and replacing nutrient losses to maintain the individual's health and well-being. Aging is associated with increases in the incidence of weight loss, being underweight, and having protein-energy malnutrition (Soriano et al., 2007).

Inadequate dietary intake in older adults may result from physiologic changes in the gastrointestinal tract, socioeconomic factors, drug interactions, disease, excessive use of alcohol, and poor dentition or missing teeth. Malnutrition is a common consequence of these factors and in turn leads to illness and frailty of older persons. Important aspects of care of older adults in the hospital, home, outpatient setting, or extended care facility include recognizing risk factors and identifying those who are at risk for inadequate nutrition (Soriano et al., 2007). Older adult residents of nursing homes or other institutions may have malnutrition caused by factors such as changes in appetite, smell and taste, dentition, eating ability, or swallowing. These factors can often be associated with multimorbidity, multiple treatments, and the social situation (Lammes, Torner, & Akner, 2009). Even well older adults may be nutritionally at risk because of decreased odor perception, poor dental health, limited ability to shop and cook, financial hardship, and the fact that they often eat alone. In addition, reduction in exercise with age without concomitant changes in carbohydrate intake places the older adult at risk for obesity.

Many older people take excessive and inappropriate medications; this is referred to as polypharmacy. The number of adverse reactions increases proportionately with the number of prescribed and over-the-counter medications taken. Age-related physiologic and pathophysiologic changes may alter the metabolism and elimination of many medications. Medications can influence food intake by producing side effects such as nausea, vomiting, decreased appetite, and changes in sensorium. They may also interfere with the distribution, utilization, and storage of nutrients. Disorders affecting any part of the gastrointestinal tract can alter nutritional requirements and health status in people of any age; however, they are likely to occur more quickly and more frequently in older persons. Nutritional problems in older adults often occur with or are precipitated by such illnesses as pneumonia and urinary tract infections. Acute and chronic diseases may affect the metabolism and utilization of nutrients, which already are altered by the aging process.

Chart 5-8 Calculating Ideal Body Weight

Women

- Allow 100 lb for 5 feet of height.
- Add 5 lb for each additional inch over 5 feet.
- Subtract 10% for small frame; add 10% for large frame.

Men

- Allow 106 lb for 5 feet of height.
- Add 6 lb for each additional inch over 5 feet.
- Subtract 10% for small frame; add 10% for large frame.

Example: Ideal body weight for a 5'6" adult:

	Female	Male
5' of height	100 lb	106 lb
Per additional inch	6" × 5 lb/inch = 30 lb	6" × 6 lb/inch = 36 lb
Ideal body weight	130 lb ± 13 lb depending on frame size	142 lb ± 14 lb depending on frame size

It is important to assess for usual body weight and height and to compare these values with ideal weight (Chart 5-8). Current weight does not provide information about recent changes in weight; therefore, patients are asked about their usual body weight. Loss of height may be attributable to osteoporosis—an important problem related to nutrition, especially in postmenopausal women (Bickley, 2009; Weber & Kelley, 2010).

In addition to the calculation of BMI, waist circumference measurement is a useful assessment tool. To measure waist circumference, a tape measure is placed in a horizontal plane around the abdomen at the level of the iliac crest. A waist circumference greater than 40 inches for men or 35 inches for women indicates excess abdominal fat. Those with a high waist circumference are at an increased risk for diabetes, dyslipidemias, hypertension, heart attack, and stroke (Bickley, 2009; Weber & Kelley, 2010).

Biochemical Assessment

Biochemical assessment reflects both the tissue level of a given nutrient and any abnormality of metabolism in the utilization of nutrients. Values applicable to Ch. 5 (Serum: albumin, transferrin, retinol-binding protein, electrolytes, hemoglobin, vitamin A, carotene, vitamin C, and total lymphocyte count; Urine: creatinine, thiamine, riboflavin, niacin, and iodine) are within acceptable range. Some of these tests, while reflecting recent intake of the elements detected, can also identify below-normal levels when there are no clinical symptoms of deficiency.

Low serum albumin and prealbumin levels are most often used as measures of protein deficit in adults. Albumin synthesis depends on normal liver function and an adequate supply of amino acids. Because the body stores a large amount of albumin, the serum albumin level may not decrease until malnutrition is severe; therefore, its usefulness in detecting recent protein depletion is limited. Decreased albumin levels may be

Body Mass Index, Ideal Weight, and Waist Circumference

BMI is a ratio based on body weight and height. The obtained value is compared to the established standards; however, trends or changes in values over time are considered more useful than isolated or one-time measurements. BMI (Fig. 5-5) is highly correlated with body fat, although increased lean body mass or a large body frame can also increase the BMI. People who have a BMI lower than 18.5 (or who are 80% or less of their desirable body weight for height) are at increased risk for problems associated with poor nutritional status. In addition, a low BMI is associated with a higher mortality rate among hospitalized patients and community-dwelling older adults. Those who have a BMI between 25 and 29.9 are considered overweight. Obesity is defined as a BMI of greater than 30 (WHO, 2011). In analyzing BMI, the nurse must be aware that cutoff scores for normal, overweight, and obese may vary for different ethnic groups.

Body Mass Index

The body mass index (BMI) is used to determine who is overweight.

$$BMI = \frac{703 \times \text{weight in pounds}}{(\text{height in inches})^2} \quad OR \quad \frac{\text{weight in kilograms}}{(\text{height in meters})^2}$$

BMI score is at the intersection of height and weight. A body mass index score of 25 or more is considered overweight and 30 or more is considered obese.

[25] Overweight Limit   Overweight

Weight	100	105	110	115	120	125	130	135	140	145	150	155	160	165	170	175	180	185	190	195	200	205
Height																						
5'0"	20	21	21	22	23	24	**25**	26	27	28	29	30	31	32	33	34	35	36	37	38	39	40
5'1"	19	20	21	22	23	24	**25**	26	26	27	28	29	30	31	32	33	34	35	36	37	38	39
5'2"	18	19	20	21	22	23	24	**25**	26	27	27	28	29	30	31	32	33	34	35	36	37	37
5'3"	18	19	19	20	21	22	23	24	**25**	26	27	27	28	29	30	31	32	33	34	35	35	36
5'4"	17	18	19	20	21	21	22	23	24	**25**	26	27	27	28	29	30	31	32	33	33	34	35
5'5"	17	17	18	19	20	21	22	22	23	24	**25**	26	27	27	28	29	30	31	32	32	33	34
5'6"	16	17	18	19	19	20	21	22	23	23	24	**25**	26	27	27	28	29	30	31	31	32	33
5'7"	16	16	17	18	19	20	20	21	22	23	23	24	**25**	26	27	27	28	29	30	31	31	32
5'8"	15	16	17	17	18	19	20	21	21	22	23	24	24	**25**	26	27	27	28	29	30	30	31
5'9"	15	16	16	17	18	18	19	20	21	21	22	23	24	24	**25**	26	27	27	28	29	30	30
5'10"	14	15	16	17	17	18	19	19	20	21	22	22	23	24	24	**25**	26	27	27	28	29	29
5'11"	14	15	15	16	17	17	18	19	20	20	21	22	22	23	24	24	**25**	26	26	27	28	29
6'0"	14	14	15	16	16	17	18	18	19	20	20	21	22	22	23	24	24	**25**	26	26	27	28
6'1"	13	14	15	15	16	16	17	18	18	19	20	20	21	22	22	23	24	24	**25**	26	26	27
6'2"	13	13	14	15	15	16	17	17	18	19	19	20	21	21	22	22	23	24	24	**25**	26	26
6'3"	12	13	14	14	15	16	16	17	17	18	19	19	20	21	21	22	22	23	24	24	**25**	26
6'4"	12	13	13	14	15	15	16	16	17	18	18	19	19	20	21	21	22	23	23	24	24	**25**

Source: Shape Up America. National Institutes of Health

FIGURE 5-5 • Body mass index.

caused by overhydration, liver or renal disease, or excessive protein loss owing to burns, major surgery, infection, or cancer. Serial measurements of prealbumin levels are also used to assess the results of nutritional therapy.

Additional laboratory data, such as levels of transferrin and retinol-binding protein, anergy panels, and lymphocyte and electrolyte counts, are used in many institutions. Transferrin is a protein that binds and carries iron from the intestine through the serum. Because of its short half-life, transferrin levels decrease more quickly than albumin levels in response to protein depletion. Although measurement of retinol-binding protein is not available from many laboratories, it may be a useful means of monitoring acute, short-term changes in protein status. The total lymphocyte count may be reduced in people who are acutely malnourished as a result of stress and low-calorie feeding and in those with impaired cellular immunity. Anergy, or the absence of an immune response to injection of small concentrations of recall antigen under the skin, may also indicate malnutrition because of delayed antibody synthesis and response. Serum electrolyte levels provide information about fluid and electrolyte balance and kidney function. The creatinine/height index calculated over a 24-hour period assesses the metabolically active tissue and indicates the degree of protein depletion, comparing expected body mass for height with actual body cell mass. A 24-hour urine sample is obtained, and the amount of creatinine is measured and compared to normal ranges based on the patient's height and gender. Values lower than normal may indicate loss of lean body mass and protein malnutrition.

Clinical Examination

The state of nutrition is often reflected in a person's appearance. Although the most obvious physical sign of good nutrition is a normal body weight with respect to height, body frame, and age, other tissues can serve as indicators of general nutritional status and adequate intake of specific nutrients; these include the hair, skin, teeth, gums, mucous membranes, mouth and tongue, skeletal muscles, abdomen, lower extremities, and thyroid gland (Table 5-1).

Dietary Data

Commonly used methods of determining individual eating patterns include the food record, the 24-hour food recall, and a dietary interview. Each of these methods helps to estimate whether food intake is adequate and appropriate. If these methods are used to obtain the dietary history, instructions must be given to the patient about measuring and recording food intake.

Methods of Collecting Data

Food Record. The food record is used most often in nutritional status studies. A person is instructed to keep a record of food consumed over a period of time, varying from 3 to 7 days, and to accurately estimate and describe the specific

TABLE 5-1	Physical Indicators of Nutritional Status	
Indicator	**Signs of Good Nutrition**	**Signs of Poor Nutrition**
General appearance	Alert, responsive	Listless, appears acutely or chronically ill
Hair	Shiny, lustrous; firm, healthy scalp	Dull and dry, brittle, depigmented, easily plucked; thin and sparse
Face	Skin color uniform; healthy appearance	Skin dark over cheeks and under eyes, skin flaky, face swollen or hollow/sunken cheeks
Eyes	Bright, clear, moist	Eye membranes pale, dry (xerophthalmia); increased vascularity, cornea soft (keratomalacia)
Lips	Good color (pink), smooth	Swollen and puffy; angular lesion at corners of mouth (cheilosis)
Tongue	Deep red in appearance; surface papillae present	Smooth appearance, swollen, beefy-red, sores, atrophic papillae
Teeth	Straight, no crowding, no dental caries, bright	Dental caries, mottled appearance (fluorosis), malpositioned
Gums	Firm, good color (pink)	Spongy, bleed easily, marginal redness, recession
Thyroid	No enlargement of the thyroid	Thyroid enlargement (simple goiter)
Skin	Smooth, good color, moist	Rough, dry, flaky, swollen, pale, pigmented; lack of fat under skin
Nails	Firm, pink	Spoon shaped, ridged, brittle
Skeleton	Good posture, no malformation	Poor posture, beading of ribs, bowed legs or knock knees
Muscles	Well developed, firm	Flaccid, poor tone, wasted, underdeveloped
Extremities	No tenderness	Weak and tender; edematous
Abdomen	Flat	Swollen
Nervous system	Normal reflexes	Decreased or absent ankle and knee reflexes
Weight	Normal for height, age, and body build	Overweight or underweight

foods consumed. Food records are fairly accurate if the person is willing to provide factual information and is able to estimate food quantities.

24-Hour Recall. As the name implies, the 24-hour recall method is a recall of food intake over a 24-hour period. A person is asked to recall all foods eaten during the previous day and to estimate the quantities of each food consumed. Because information does not always represent usual intake, at the end of the interview the patient is asked whether the previous day's food intake was typical. To obtain supplementary information about the typical diet, it is also necessary to ask how frequently the person eats foods from the major food groups.

Dietary Interview. The success of the interviewer in obtaining information for dietary assessment depends on effective communication, which requires that good rapport be established to promote respect and trust. The interview is conducted in a nondirective and exploratory way, allowing the respondent to express feelings and thoughts while encouraging him or her to answer specific questions. The manner in which questions are asked influences the respondent's cooperation. The interviewer must be nonjudgmental and avoid expressing disapproval by verbal comments or facial expression.

Several questions may be necessary to elicit the information needed. When attempting to elicit information about the type and quantity of food eaten at a particular time, leading questions such as "Do you use sugar or cream in your coffee?" should be avoided. In addition, assumptions should not be made about the size of servings; instead, questions are phrased to clearly determine the quantities. For example, to help determine the size of one hamburger, the patient may be asked, "How many servings were prepared with the pound of meat you bought?" Another approach to determining quantities is to use food models of known sizes in estimating portions of meat, cake, or pie, or to record quantities in common measurements, such as cups or spoonfuls (or the size of containers when discussing intake of bottled beverages).

In recording a particular combination dish, such as a casserole, it is useful to ask about the ingredients, recording the largest quantities first. When recording quantities of ingredients, the interviewer notes whether the food item was raw or cooked and the number of servings provided by the recipe. When a patient lists the foods for the recall questionnaire, it may help to read back the list of foods and ask whether anything was forgotten, such as fruit, cake, candy, between-meal snacks, or alcoholic beverages.

An individual's culture determines to a large extent which foods are eaten and how they are prepared and served. Culture and religious practices together often determine whether certain foods are prohibited and whether certain foods and spices are eaten on certain holidays or at specific family gatherings. Because of the importance of culture and religious beliefs to many individuals, it is important to be sensitive to these factors when obtaining a dietary history. It is, however, equally important not to stereotype individuals and assume that because they are from a certain culture or religious group, they adhere to specific dietary customs. One particular area of consideration is the presence of fish and shellfish in the diet, where they come from (farmed vs. wild), and the method of preparation. Certain methods may put certain populations at risk for toxicity owing to contaminants. Culturally sensitive materials, such as the food pagoda and the Mediterranean Diet Pyramid, are available for making appropriate dietary recommendations (U.S. Department of Agriculture & U.S. Department of Health and Human Services, 2010).

Evaluating Dietary Information

After obtaining basic dietary information, the nurse evaluates the patient's dietary intake and communicates the information to the dietitian and the rest of the health care team for more detailed assessment and clinical nutrition intervention. If the goal is to determine whether the patient generally eats a healthful diet, his or her food intake may be compared with the dietary guidelines outlined in the U.S. Department of Agriculture's MyPlate (Fig. 5-6). The pyramid divides foods into five major groups (grains, vegetables, fruits, dairy, and

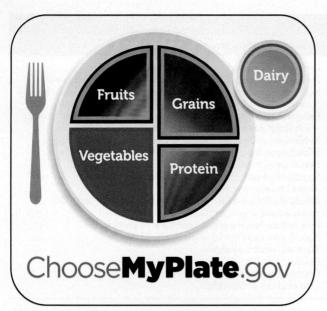

FIGURE 5-6 • MyPlate, a simple reminder for healthy eating. From the U.S. Department of Agriculture. Available at: www.choosemyplate.gov

protein), plus fats and oils. Recommendations are provided for variety in the diet, proportion of food from each food group, and moderation in eating fats, oils, and sweets. A person's food intake is compared with recommendations based on various food groups for different age groups and activity levels (Weber & Kelley, 2010).

If nurses or dietitians are interested in knowing about the intake of specific nutrients, such as vitamin A, iron, or calcium, the patient's food intake is analyzed by consulting a list of foods and their composition and nutrient content. The diet is analyzed in terms of grams and milligrams of specific nutrients. The total nutritive value is then compared with the recommended dietary allowances specific for the patient's age category, gender, and special circumstances such as pregnancy or lactation.

Fat intake and cholesterol levels are additional aspects of the nutritional assessment. Trans fats are produced when hydrogen atoms are added to monounsaturated or polyunsaturated fats to produce a semisolid product, such as margarine. Trans fats, which are contained in many baked goods and restaurant foods, are a concern because increased amounts of trans fats have been associated with increased risk for heart disease and stroke. Since 2006, the U.S. Food and Drug Administration has required the inclusion of trans fats information on food labels.

Factors Influencing Nutritional Status in Various Situations

One sensitive indicator of the body's gain or loss of protein is its nitrogen balance. An adult is said to be in nitrogen equilibrium when the nitrogen intake (from food) equals the nitrogen output (in urine, feces, and perspiration); it is a sign of health. A positive nitrogen balance exists when nitrogen intake exceeds nitrogen output and indicates tissue growth, such as occurs during pregnancy, childhood, recovery from surgery, and rebuilding of wasted tissue. A negative nitrogen

balance indicates that tissue is breaking down faster than it is being replaced. In the absence of an adequate intake of protein, the body converts protein to glucose for energy. This can occur with fever, starvation, surgery, burns, and debilitating diseases. Each gram of nitrogen loss in excess of intake represents the depletion of 6.25 g of protein or 25 g of muscle tissue. Therefore, a negative nitrogen balance of 10 g/day for 10 days could mean the wasting of 2.5 kg (5.5 pounds) of muscle tissue as it is converted to glucose for energy (Dudek, 2010).

Patients who are hospitalized may have an inadequate dietary intake because of the illness or disorder that necessitated the hospital stay or because the hospital's food is unfamiliar or unappealing (Dudek, 2010). Patients who are at home may feel too sick or fatigued to shop and prepare food, or they may be unable to eat because of other physical problems or limitations. Limited or fixed incomes or the high costs of medications may result in insufficient money to buy nutritious foods. Because complex treatments (e.g., mechanical ventilation, intravenous infusions, chemotherapy) once used only in the hospital setting are now being provided in the home and outpatient settings, nutritional assessment of patients in these settings is an important aspect of home and community-based care.

Many medications influence nutritional status by suppressing the appetite, irritating the oral or gastric mucosa, or causing nausea and vomiting. Others may influence bacterial flora in the intestine or directly affect nutrient absorption so that secondary malnutrition results. People who must take many medications in a single day often report feeling too full to eat. A patient's use of prescription and OTC medications and their effects on appetite and dietary intake are assessed. Many of the factors that contribute to poor nutritional status are identified in Table 5-2.

Analysis of Nutritional Status

Physical measurements (BMI, waist circumference) and biochemical, clinical, and dietary data are used in combination to determine a patient's nutritional status. Often, these data provide more information about the patient's nutritional status than the clinical examination, which may not detect subclinical deficiencies unless they become so advanced that overt signs develop. A low intake of nutrients over a long period may lead to low biochemical levels and, without nutritional intervention, may result in characteristic and observable signs and symptoms (see Table 5-2). A plan of action for nutritional intervention is based on the results of the dietary assessment and the patient's clinical profile. To be effective, the plan must meet the patient's need for a healthy diet, maintain (or control) weight, and compensate for increased nutritional needs.

Assessment in the Home or Community

Assessment of people in community settings, including the home, consists of collecting information specific to existing health problems, including data on the patient's physiologic and emotional status, the community and home environment, the adequacy of support systems or care given by family and other care providers, and the availability of needed resources. In addition, it is important to evaluate the ability of the individual and family to cope with and address their

TABLE 5-2   Factors Associated With Potential Nutritional Deficits

Factor	Possible Consequences
Dental and oral problems (missing teeth, ill-fitting dentures, impaired swallowing or chewing)	Inadequate intake of high-fiber foods
Nothing by mouth (NPO) for diagnostic testing	Inadequate caloric and protein intake; dehydration
Prolonged use of glucose and saline intravenous fluids	Inadequate caloric and protein intake
Nausea and vomiting	Inadequate caloric and protein intake; loss of fluid, electrolytes, and minerals
Stress of illness, surgery, and/or hospitalization	Increased protein and caloric requirement; increased catabolism
Wound drainage	Loss of protein, fluid, electrolytes, and minerals
Pain	Loss of appetite; inability to shop, cook, eat
Fever	Increased caloric and fluid requirement; increased catabolism
Gastrointestinal intubation	Loss of protein, fluid, and minerals
Tube feedings	Inadequate amounts; various nutrients in each formula
Gastrointestinal disease	Inadequate intake and malabsorption of nutrients
Alcoholism	Inadequate intake of nutrients; increased consumption of calories without other nutrients; vitamin deficiencies
Depression	Loss of appetite; inability to shop, cook, eat
Eating disorders (anorexia, bulimia)	Inadequate caloric and protein intake; loss of fluid, electrolytes, and minerals
Medications	Inadequate intake owing to medication side effects, such as dry mouth, loss of appetite, decreased taste perception, difficulty swallowing, nausea and vomiting, physical problems that limit shopping, cooking, eating; malabsorption of nutrients
Restricted ambulation or disability	Inability to help self to food, liquids, other nutrients

respective needs. The physical assessment in the community and home consists of similar techniques to those used in the hospital, outpatient clinic, or office setting. Privacy is provided, and the person is made as comfortable as possible. (See Chapter 2 for more information on community-based nursing practice.)

Critical Thinking Exercises

1 **ebp** Your health history and physical examination of a young adult female patient alerts you to the possibility of alcohol abuse. Explain how you would pursue this. What is the evidence base for available assessments to assist in a more comprehensive evaluation of substance abuse? Identify the criteria used to evaluate the strength of the evidence for this practice.

2 You are conducting a health assessment of an older adult man who has recently moved to an assisted living facility owing to his worsening dementia. His current diet consists of high fat and carbohydrate foods, high sodium intake, and minimal nonstarchy vegetable consumption. He does not exercise and has smoked one pack of cigarettes a day since he was in his early 20s. Generate a list of possible nursing diagnoses for this patient. Identify the nursing interventions that would be most appropriate for each of the possible nursing diagnoses and evaluation criteria for these interventions.

3 **pq** Identify the priorities, approach, and techniques you would use to perform a comprehensive admission assessment on a 45-year-old woman with metastatic liver cancer. How would your priorities, approach, and techniques differ if the patient has metastatic lesions to the brain and is disoriented? If the patient has a visual impairment or is hard of hearing? If the patient is from a culture with very different values from your own?

Brunner Suite Resources
Explore these additional resources to enhance learning for this chapter:
• NCLEX-Style Questions and Other Resources on thePoint, http://thePoint.lww.com/Brunner13e
• Study Guide
• PrepU
• Clinical Handbook
• Handbook of Laboratory and Diagnostic Tests

References

*Asterisk indicates nursing research.
**Double asterisk indicates classic reference.

Books

Bickley, L. S. (2009). *Bates' guide to physical examination and history taking* (10th ed.). Philadelphia: Lippincott Williams & Wilkins.
Dudek, S. G. (2010). *Nutrition essentials for nursing practice* (6th ed.). Philadelphia: Lippincott Williams & Wilkins.
**Fleming, M. F., & Barry, K. L. (1992). *Addictive disorders*. St. Louis: Mosby.
O'Brien, M. E. (2011). *Servant leadership in nursing: Spirituality and practice in contemporary health care*. Sudbury, MA: Jones & Bartlett.
Porth, C. M., & Matfin, G. (2009). *Pathophysiology: Concepts of altered health states* (8th ed.). Philadelphia: Lippincott Williams & Wilkins.
Soriano, R. P., Fernandes, H. M., Cassel, C. K., et al. (2007). *Fundamentals of geriatric medicine: A case-based approach*. New York: Springer.
Snyder, M., & Lindquist, R. (2010). *Complementary & alternative therapies in nursing* (6th ed.). New York: Springer.
Weber, J., & Kelley, J. (2010). *Health assessment in nursing* (4th ed.). Philadelphia: Lippincott Williams & Wilkins.

Journals and Electronic Documents

General Assessment
**Chan, A. W. K., Pristach, E. A., Welte, J. W., et al. (1993). Use of the TWEAK test in screening for alcoholism/heavy drinking in three populations. *Alcoholism: Clinical and Experimental Research, 17*(6), 1188–1192.
*Dinsmore, A., & Higgins, L. (2011). Study of patients' experiences of treatment by hospital staff. *Learning Disability Practice, 14*(5), 18–22.
**Ewing, J. A. (1984). Detecting alcoholism: The CAGE questionnaire. *Journal of the American Medical Association, 252*(14), 1905–1907.
Futcher, S. (2011). Attitudes to sexuality of patients with learning disabilities: A review. *British Journal of Nursing, 20*(1), 8–13.

*Goodman, C., Davies, S. L., Dinan, S., et al. (2011). Activity promotion for community-dwelling older people: A survey of the contribution of primary care nurses. *British Journal of Community Nursing, 16*(1), 12–17.

*Hawthorne, D., Youngblut, J. M., & Brooten, D. (2011). Psychometric evaluation of the English and Spanish versions of the spiritual coping strategies scale. *Journal of Nursing Measurement, 19*(1), 46–54.

Kroger, A. T., Sumaya, C. V., Pickering, L. K., et al. (2011). *General recommendations on immunization*. Recommendations of the Advisory Committee on Immunization Practices (ACIP). Available at: www.cdc.gov/mmwr/preview/mmwrhtml/rr6002a1.htm?s_cid=rr6002a1_e

Kutz, M. K. (2010). Embracing the electronic medical record: Helping nurses overcome possible barriers. *Nursing for Women's Health, 14*(4), 292–300.

NANDA International. (2011). *Nursing diagnosis frequently-asked questions*. Available at: www.nanda.org/NursingDiagnosisFAQ.aspx#NDxBasics

New York State Office of Alcoholism and Substance Abuse Services (OASAS). (2007). *Elderly alcohol and substance abuse*. Available at: www.oasas.ny.gov/AdMed/FYI/FYIInDepth-Elderly.cfm

*Saunamaki, N., Anderson, M., & Engstrom, M. (2010). Discussing sexuality with patients: Nurses' attitudes and beliefs. *Journal of Advanced Nursing, 66*(6), 1308–1316.

Sharts-Hopko, N. (2009). Low vision and blindness among midlife and older adults. *Holistic Nursing Practice, 23*(2), 94–100.

*Sharts-Hopko, N. C., Smeltzer, S., Ott, B. B., et al. (2010). Healthcare experiences of women with visual impairment. *Clinical Nurse Specialist, 24*(3), 149–153.

*Smeltzer, S. C., Sharts-Hopko, N., Ott, B., et al. (2007). Perspectives of women with disabilities on reaching those who are hard to reach. *Journal of Neuroscience Nursing, 39*(3), 163–171.

Nutritional Assessment

*Lammes, E., Torner, A., & Akner, G. (2009). Nutrient density and variation in nutrient intake with changing energy intake in multimorbid nursing home residents. *Journal of Human Nutrition and Dietetics, 22*(3), 210–218.

Reilly, J. J. (2010). Assessment of obesity in children and adolescents: Synthesis of recent systematic reviews and clinical guidelines. *Journal of Human Nutrition and Dietetics, 23*(3), 205–211.

U.S. Department of Agriculture, Center for Nutrition Policy and Promotion. (2005). *Your Personal Path to Health: Steps to a Healthier You!* Available at: www.choosemyplate.gov/food-groups/downloads/resource/MyPyramid BrochurebyIFIC.pdf

U.S. Department of Agriculture & U.S. Department of Health and Human Services. (2010). *Dietary guidelines for Americans 2010*. Available at: health.gov/dietaryguidelines/dga2010/DietaryGuidelines2010.pdf

**U.S. Department of Health and Human Services. (2003). *Summary of the HIPAA privacy rule*. Available at: www.hhs.gov/ocr/privacy/hipaa/understanding/summary/privacysummary.pdf

World Health Organization. (2011). *Obesity and overweight*. Available at: www.who.int/mediacentre/factsheets/fs311/en/

Resources

Academy of Nutrition and Dietetics, www.eatright.org

Advisory Committee on Immunization Practices (ACIP), Centers for Disease Control and Prevention, National Immunization Program, Division of Epidemiology and Surveillance, www.cdc.gov/vaccines/acip/index.html

Alliance for Cannabis Therapeutics, marijuana-as-medicine.org/alliance.htm

American Heart Association, www.heart.org/HEARTORG/

Healthcare Information and Management Systems Society (HIMSS), www.himss.org/ASP/index.asp

National Cancer Institute, Cancer Information Service, www.nci.nih.gov or www.cancer.gov

Substance Abuse

Adult Children of Alcoholics World Service Organization, www.adultchildren.org

Al-Anon Family Groups, www.al-anon.alateen.org

Alcoholics Anonymous, www.alcoholics-anonymous.org

Center for Substance Abuse Treatment (CSAT), www.samhsa.gov/about/csat.aspx

Center on Addiction and the Family, www.phoenixhouse.org

Co-Anon Family Groups, www.co-anon.org

Cocaine Anonymous, www.ca.org

Dual Recovery Anonymous World Network Central Office, www.draonline.org

Narcotics Anonymous World Services, www.na.org

National Council on Alcoholism and Drug Dependence Hope Line, 1-800-NCA-CALL (1-800-622-2255)

National Cocaine Hotline, 1-800-COCAINE (1-800-262-2463)

Rational Recovery Systems, www.rational.org

Substance Abuse and Mental Health Services Administration (SAMHSA), Division of Workplace Programs, www.drugfreeworkplace.gov

Genetics Resources for Nurses and Patients

GeneTests, www.ncbi.nlm.nih.gov/sites/GeneTests/

Genetic Alliance, www.geneticalliance.org

National Organization for Rare Disorders (NORD), www.rarediseases.org/

Online Mendelian Inheritance in Man (OMIM), www.ncbi.nlm.nih.gov/Omim/mimstats.html

Unit 2

Biophysical and Psychosocial Concepts in Nursing Practice

Case Study

A PATIENT WITH A DISABILITY

Ms. Hannah Tupolov is a 24-year-old woman admitted to the hospital for an emergency appendectomy. She is admitted to a general surgery unit postoperatively. Ms. Tupolov has not had any previous surgery, nor ever been admitted to a hospital prior to this episode, and has been blind since birth. She resides with both of her parents, is a college graduate, and works for a local accounting firm as a certified public accountant.

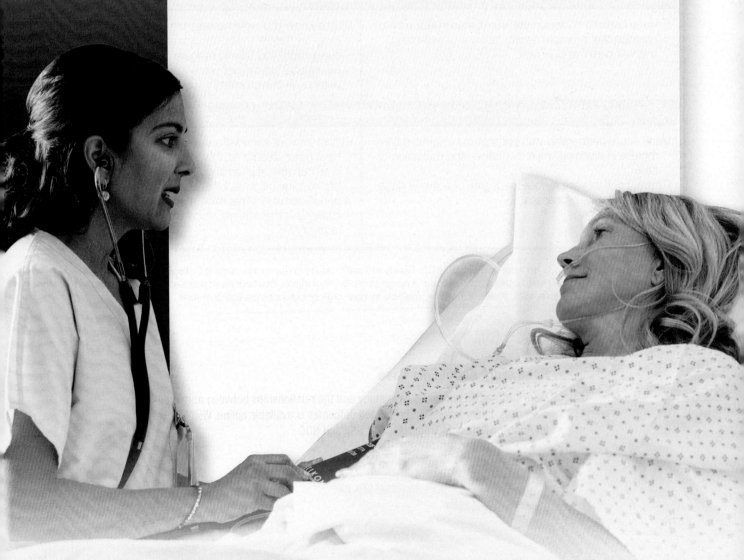

QSEN Competency Focus: *Patient-Centered Care*

The complexities inherent in today's health care system challenge nurses to demonstrate integration of specific interdisciplinary core competencies. These competencies are aimed at ensuring the delivery of safe, quality patient care (Institute of Medicine, 2003). The concepts from the Quality and Safety Education for Nurses (QSEN) Institute (2012) provide a framework for the knowledge, skills, and attitudes (KSAs) required for nurses to demonstrate competency in these key areas, which include *patient-centered care, interdisciplinary teamwork and collaboration, evidence-based practice, quality improvement, safety,* and *informatics.*

Patient-Centered Care Definition: Recognize the patient or designee as the source of control and full partner in providing compassionate and coordinated care based on respect for patient's preferences, values, and needs.

SELECTED PRE-LICENSURE KSAS	APPLICATION AND REFLECTION
Knowledge	
Describe strategies to empower patients or families in all aspects of the health care process.	Describe strategies you would use to ensure that Ms. Tupolov is fully engaged in all aspects of her postoperative recovery. How might this empower her?
Skills	
Engage patients or designated surrogates in active partnerships that promote health, safety and well-being, and self-care management.	Discuss how you would assess the unit-based environment for threats to Ms. Tupolov's safety. What measures might you take to mitigate potential threats to her safety? How might you engage her, as well as her parents, in this process?
Attitudes	
Value active partnership with patients or designated surrogates in planning, implementation, and evaluation of care. Respect patient preferences for degree of active engagement with care processes.	Reflect on your attitudes toward people who are blind or have other disabilities. Do you believe that Ms. Tupolov is as capable of attending to her self-care needs during her hospitalization as other patients who have appendectomies? What might be some of the unique challenges that she may face in her postoperative recovery?

Cronenwett, L., Sherwood, G., Barnsteiner, J., et al. (2007). Quality and safety education for nurses. *Nursing Outlook, 55*(3), 122–131.
Institute of Medicine. (2003). *Health professions education: A bridge to quality.* Washington, DC: National Academies Press.
QSEN Institute (2012). *Competencies: Prelicensure KSAs.* Available at: qsen.org/competencies/pre-licensure-ksas

Read More About This Case

More information about this case study and the relationships between nursing diagnoses, interventions, and expected outcomes is available online. Visit thePoint for Applying Concepts From NANDA-I, NIC, and NOC.

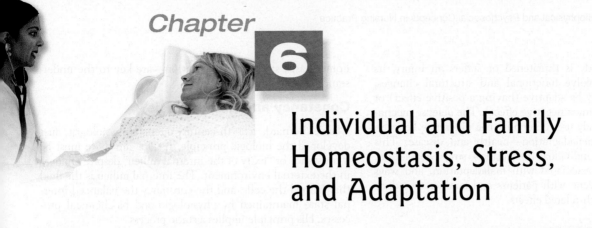

Individual and Family Homeostasis, Stress, and Adaptation

Learning Objectives

On completion of this chapter, the learner will be able to:

1 Relate the principles of internal constancy, homeostasis, stress, and adaptation to the concept of steady state.
2 Identify the significance of the body's compensatory mechanisms in promoting adaptation and maintaining the steady state.
3 Compare physical, physiologic, and psychosocial stressors.
4 Describe the general adaptation syndrome as a theory of adaptation to biologic stress.
5 Compare the sympathetic-adrenal-medullary and hypothalamic-pituitary responses to stress.

6 Identify ways in which maladaptive responses to stress can increase the risk of illness and cause disease.
7 Describe the relationship of the process of negative feedback to the maintenance of the steady state.
8 Compare the adaptive processes of hypertrophy, atrophy, hyperplasia, dysplasia, and metaplasia.
9 Describe the inflammatory and reparative processes.
10 Assess the health patterns of a person and families; determine their effects on maintenance of the steady state.
11 Identify individual, family, and group measures that are useful in reducing stress.

Glossary

adaptation: a change or alteration designed to assist in adjusting to a new situation or environment
adrenocorticotropic hormone (ACTH): a hormone produced by the anterior lobe of the pituitary gland that stimulates the secretion of cortisol and other hormones by the adrenal cortex
antidiuretic hormone (ADH): a hormone secreted by the posterior lobe of the pituitary gland that constricts blood vessels, elevates blood pressure, and reduces the excretion of urine
catecholamines: any of the group of amines (such as epinephrine, norepinephrine, or dopamine) that serve as neurotransmitters
coping: the cognitive and behavioral strategies used to manage the stressors that tax a person's resources
disease: an abnormal variation in the structure or function of any part of the body that disrupts function and therefore can limit freedom of action
dysplasia: bizarre cell growth resulting in cells that differ in size, shape, or arrangement from other cells of the same tissue type
family: a group whose members are related by reciprocal caring, mutual responsibilities, and loyalties
fight-or-flight response: the alarm stage in the general adaptation syndrome described by Selye
glucocorticoids: the group of steroid hormones, such as cortisol, that are produced by the adrenal cortex; they are involved in carbohydrate, protein, and fat metabolism and have anti-inflammatory properties

gluconeogenesis: the formation of glucose by the liver from noncarbohydrate sources, such as amino acids and the glycerol portion of fats
guided imagery: the mindful use of a word, phrase, or visual image to achieve relaxation or direct attention away from uncomfortable sensations or situations
homeostasis: a steady state within the body; the stability of the internal environment
hyperplasia: an increase in the number of new cells in an organ or tissue
hypoxia: inadequate supply of oxygen to the cell
inflammation: a localized reaction of tissue to injury, irritation, or infection that is manifested by pain, redness, heat, swelling, and sometimes loss of function
metaplasia: a cell transformation in which there is conversion of one type of mature cell into another type of cell
negative feedback: response that decreases the output of a system
positive feedback: reaction that increases the output of a system
steady state: a stable condition that does not change over time, or when change in one direction is balanced by change in an opposite direction
stress: a disruptive condition that occurs in response to adverse influences from the internal or external environments
stressor: an internal or external event or situation that creates the potential for physiologic, emotional, cognitive, or behavioral changes

When the body is threatened or suffers an injury, its response may involve functional and structural changes; these changes may be adaptive (having a positive effect) or maladaptive (having a negative effect). The defense mechanisms that the body uses determine the difference between adaptation and maladaptation—health and disease. This chapter discusses individual homeostasis, stress, adaptation, health problems associated with maladaptation, and ways that nurses intervene with patients and families to reduce stress and its health-related effects.

Fundamental Concepts

Each body system performs specific functions to sustain optimal life for an organism. Compensatory mechanisms for adjusting internal conditions promote the steady state of the organism, ensure its survival, and restore balance in the body. Pathophysiologic processes result when cellular injury occurs at such a rapid rate that the body's compensatory mechanisms can no longer make the adaptive changes necessary to remain healthy.

Physiologic mechanisms must be understood in the context of the body as a whole. Each person has both an internal and external environment, between which information and matter are continuously exchanged. Within the internal environment, each organ, tissue, and cell is also a system or subsystem of the whole, each with its own internal and external environment, each exchanging information and matter (Fig. 6-1). The goal of the interaction of the body's subsystems is to produce a dynamic balance or **steady state** (even in the presence of change) so that all subsystems are in harmony with each other. Four concepts—constancy,

homeostasis, stress, and adaptation—are key to the understanding of steady state.

Constancy and Homeostasis

Claude Bernard, a 19th-century French physiologist, first developed the biologic principle that for life there must be a constancy or "fixity of the internal milieu" despite changes in the external environment. The internal milieu is the fluid that bathed the cells, and the constancy the balanced internal state maintained by physiologic and biochemical processes. His principle implies a static process.

Bernard's principle of "constancy" underpins the concept of **homeostasis**, which refers to a steady state within the body. When a change or stress occurs that causes a body function to deviate from its stable range, processes are initiated to restore and maintain dynamic balance. An example of this restorative effort is the development of rapid breathing (hyperpnea) after intense exercise in an attempt to compensate for an oxygen deficit and excess lactic acid accumulated in the muscle tissue. When these adjustment processes or compensatory mechanisms are not adequate, steady state is threatened, function becomes disordered, and dysfunctional responses occur. For example, in heart failure, the body reacts by retaining sodium and water and increasing venous pressure, which worsens the condition. Dysfunctional responses can lead to **disease**, which is a threat to steady state.

Stress and Adaptation

Stress is a state produced by a change in the environment that is perceived as challenging, threatening, or damaging to a person's dynamic balance or equilibrium. The person may feel unable to meet the demands of the new situation. The change or stimulus that evokes this state is the stressor. A person appraises and copes with changing situations. The desired goal is **adaptation**, or adjustment to the change so that the person is again in equilibrium and has the energy and ability to meet new demands. This is the process of **coping** with the stress, a compensatory process that has physiologic and psychological components.

Because both stress and adaptation may exist at different levels of a system, it is possible to study these reactions at the cellular, tissue, and organ levels. Biologists are concerned mainly with subcellular components or with subsystems of the total body. Behavioral scientists, including many nurse researchers, study stress and adaptation in individuals, families, groups, and societies; they focus on how a group's organizational features are modified to meet the requirements of the social and physical environment in which the group exists. In any system, the desired goals of adaptation are survival, growth, and reproduction.

Overview of Stress

Each person operates at a certain level of adaptation and regularly encounters a certain amount of change. Such change is expected; it contributes to growth and enhances life. A stressor can upset this equilibrium. A **stressor** may be defined as an internal or external event or situation that creates the potential for physiologic, emotional, cognitive, or behavioral changes.

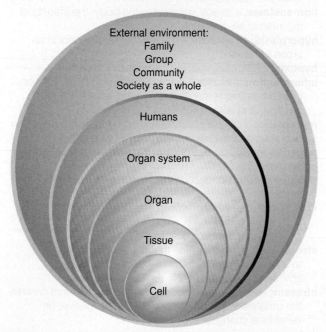

FIGURE 6-1 • Constellation of systems. Each system is a subsystem of the larger system (suprasystem) of which it is a part. The cells represent the smallest system and are a subsystem of all other systems.

External environment:
Family
Group
Community
Society as a whole

Humans

Organ system

Organ

Tissue

Cell

Types of Stressors

Stressors exist in many forms and categories. They may be described as physical, physiologic, or psychosocial. Physical stressors include cold, heat, and chemical agents; physiologic stressors include pain and fatigue. An example of a psychosocial stressor is fear (e.g., fear of failing an examination, losing a job, and waiting for a diagnostic test result). Stressors can also occur as normal life transitions that require some adjustment, such as going from childhood into puberty, getting married, or giving birth.

Stressors have also been classified as day-to-day frustrations or hassles, major complex occurrences involving large groups, and stressors that occur less frequently and involve fewer people. Day-to-day stressors include common occurrences as getting caught in a traffic jam, experiencing computer downtime, and having an argument with a spouse or roommate. These experiences vary in effect. For example, encountering a rainstorm while you are vacationing at the beach will most likely evoke a more negative response than it might at another time. These daily hassles have been shown to have a greater health impact than major life events because of the cumulative effect they have over time. They can lead to high blood pressure, palpitations, or other physiologic problems (Rice, 2011).

Major stressors influence larger groups of individuals, families, and sometimes even entire nations. These include events of history, such as terrorism and war, experienced either directly in the war zone or indirectly through live news coverage. The demographic, economic, and technologic changes occurring in society also serve as stressors. The tension produced by any stressor is sometimes a result not only of the change itself but also of the speed with which change occurs.

Stressors concerning relatively infrequent situations that directly affect people have been studied extensively. This category includes the influence of life events such as death, birth, marriage, divorce, and retirement. It also includes the psychosocial crises that occur in the life cycle stages of the human experience. More enduring chronic stressors may include having a permanent disability or coping with the need to provide long-term care to a frail older parent.

Duration may also be used to categorize stressors, as in the following:

- An acute, time-limited stressor, such as studying for final examinations
- A stressor sequence—a series of stressful events that result from an initial event such as job loss or divorce
- A chronic intermittent stressor, such as daily hassles
- A chronic enduring stressor that persists over time, such as chronic illness, a disability, or poverty

Stress as a Stimulus for Disease

Relating life events to illness (the theoretical approach that defines stress as a stimulus) has been a major focus of psychosocial studies. Research suggests that people under constant stress have a high incidence of psychosomatic disease.

Holmes and Rahe (1967) developed life events scales that assign numerical values, called *life-change units*, to typical life events. Because the items in the scales reflect events that require a change in a person's life pattern, and stress is viewed

as an accumulation of changes in one's life that require psychological adaptation, one can theoretically predict the likelihood of illness by checking off the number of recent events and deriving a total score. The Recent Life Changes Questionnaire (Tausig, 1982) contains 118 items such as death, birth, marriage, divorce, promotions, serious arguments, and vacations. The items include both desirable and undesirable events.

Sources of stress for people have been well researched (Dow, 2011; Mair, Cutchin, & Peek, 2011; Pierce, Lewandowski-Romps, & Silverschanz, 2011). People typically experience distress related to alterations in their physical and emotional health status, changes in their level of daily functioning, and decreased social support or the loss of significant others (Berendes, Keefe, & Somers, 2010; Bertoni, Burke, Owusu, et al., 2010). Fears of immobilization, isolation, loneliness, sensory changes, financial problems, and death or disability increase a person's anxiety level. Loss of one's role or perceived purpose in life can cause intense discomfort. Any of these identified variables, plus myriad other conditions or overwhelming demands, are likely to cause ineffective coping, and a lack of effective coping skills is often a source of additional distress for the person. When a person endures prolonged or unrelenting suffering, the outcome is frequently the development of a stress-related illness. Nurses have the skills to assist people to alter their distressing circumstances and manage their responses to stress, as discussed later in the chapter.

Psychological Responses to Stress

After recognizing a stressor, a person consciously or unconsciously reacts to manage the situation. This is termed the *mediating process*. A theory developed by Lazarus (1991a) emphasizes cognitive appraisal and coping as important mediators of stress. Appraisal and coping are influenced by antecedent variables, including the internal and external resources of the individual person.

Appraisal of the Stressful Event

Cognitive appraisal (Lazarus, 1991a; Lazarus & Folkman, 1984) is a process by which an event is evaluated with respect to what is at stake (primary appraisal) and what might and can be done (secondary appraisal). What a person sees as being at stake is influenced by his or her personal goals, commitments, or motivations. Important factors include how important or relevant the event is to the person, whether the event conflicts with what the person wants or desires, and whether the situation threatens the person's own sense of strength and ego identity.

Primary appraisal results in the situation being identified as either nonstressful or stressful. Secondary appraisal is an evaluation of what might and can be done about the situation. Reappraisal—a change of opinion based on new information—may occur. The appraisal process is not necessarily sequential; primary and secondary appraisal and reappraisal may occur simultaneously.

The appraisal process contributes to the development of an emotion. Negative emotions such as fear and anger accompany harm/loss appraisals, and positive emotions accompany challenge. In addition to the subjective component or feeling that accompanies a particular emotion, each emotion also includes a tendency to act in a certain way. For example, unprepared students may view an unexpected quiz as threatening. They might feel fear, anger, and resentment and might express these emotions through hostile behavior or comments.

Lazarus (1991a) expanded his initial ideas about stress, appraisal, and coping into a more complex model relating emotion to adaptation. He called this model a "cognitive-motivational-relational theory," with the term *relational* "standing for a focus on negotiation with a physical and social world" (p. 13). A theory of emotion was proposed as the bridge to connect psychology, physiology, and sociology: "More than any other arena of psychological thought, emotion is an integrative, organismic concept that subsumes psychological stress and coping within itself and unites motivation, cognition, and adaptation in a complex configuration" (p. 40).

Coping With the Stressful Event

Coping consists of the cognitive and behavioral efforts made to manage the specific external or internal demands that tax a person's resources and may be emotion focused or problem focused. Emotion-focused coping seeks to make the person feel better by lessening the emotional distress. Problem-focused coping aims to make direct changes in the environment so that the situation can be managed more effectively. Both types of coping usually occur in a stressful situation. Even if the situation is viewed as challenging or beneficial, coping efforts may be required to develop and sustain the challenge—that is, to maintain the positive benefits of the challenge and to ward off any threats. In harmful or threatening situations, successful coping reduces or eliminates the source of stress and relieves the emotion generated.

Appraisal and coping are affected by internal characteristics such as health, energy, personal belief systems, commitments or life goals, self-esteem, control, mastery, knowledge, problem-solving skills, and social skills. The characteristics that have been studied in nursing research are health-promoting lifestyles and resilience (Neenan, 2009; Reich, Zautra, & Hall, 2010). Resilience is considered both a personal trait and a process. Researchers have defined resilience as the ability of a person to function well in stressful situations such as traumatic events and other types of adverse situations (Johnson, 2010). A resilient individual maintains flexibility even in difficult circumstances and controls strong emotional reactions using appropriate communication and problem-solving skills. Factors that play a role in building a person's resilience are having strong, supportive relationships with family members and other individuals, and being exposed to positive role models. A resilient individual knows when to take action, when to step back and rely on others, and when to stop to re-energize and nurture the self. Researchers have found positive support for resilience as a significant variable that positively influences rehabilitation and overall improvement after a challenging or traumatic experience (Chen, Shiu, Simoni, et al., 2011; Hahn, Cichy, Almeida, et al., 2011; Herrman, Stewart, Diaz-Granados, et al., 2011; Pierini & Stuifbergen, 2010).

A health-promoting lifestyle buffers the effect of stressors. From a nursing practice standpoint, this outcome—buffering the effect of stressors—supports nursing's goal of promoting health. In many circumstances, promoting a healthy lifestyle is more achievable than altering the stressors.

Physiologic Response to Stress

The physiologic response to a stressor, whether it is physical, psychological, or psychosocial, is a protective and adaptive mechanism to maintain the body's homeostatic balance. When a stress response occurs, it activates a series of neurologic and hormonal processes within the brain and body systems. The duration and intensity of the stress can cause both short- and long-term effects.

Selye's Theory of Adaptation

Hans Selye (1976) developed a theory of adaptation to biologic stress that profoundly influenced the scientific study of stress.

General Adaptation Syndrome

Selye's theory, called the *general adaptation syndrome* (GAS), has three phases: alarm, resistance, and exhaustion. During the alarm phase, the sympathetic **fight-or-flight response** is activated with release of **catecholamines** and the onset of the **adrenocorticotropic hormone (ACTH)**–adrenal cortical response. The alarm reaction is defensive and anti-inflammatory but self-limited. Because living in a continuous state of alarm would result in death, people move into the second stage—resistance. During the resistance stage, adaptation to the noxious stressor occurs, and cortisol activity is still increased. If exposure to the stressor is prolonged, the third stage—exhaustion—occurs. During the exhaustion stage, endocrine activity increases, which has negative effects on the body systems (especially the circulatory, digestive, and immune systems) that can lead to death. Stages one and two of this syndrome are repeated, in different degrees, throughout life as the person encounters stressors.

Selye compared the GAS with the life process. During childhood, too few encounters with stress occur to promote the development of adaptive functioning, and children are vulnerable. During adulthood, numerous stressful events occur, and people develop resistance or adaptation. During the later years, the accumulation of life's stressors and wear and tear on the organism again decrease people's ability to adapt, resistance falls, and eventually death occurs.

Local Adaptation Syndrome

According to Selye, a local adaptation syndrome also occurs. This syndrome includes the inflammatory response and repair processes that occur at the local site of tissue injury. The local adaptation syndrome occurs in small, topical injuries, such as contact dermatitis. If the local injury is severe enough, the GAS is activated as well.

Selye emphasized that stress is the nonspecific response common to all stressors, regardless of whether they are physiologic, psychological, or psychosocial. The many conditioning factors in each person's environment account for why different demands are experienced by different people as stressors. Conditioning factors also account for differences in the tolerance of different people for stress: Some people may develop diseases of adaptation, such as hypertension and migraine headaches, whereas others are unaffected.

Interpretation of Stressful Stimuli by the Brain

Physiologic responses to stress are mediated by the brain through a complex network of chemical and electrical messages. The neural and hormonal actions that maintain

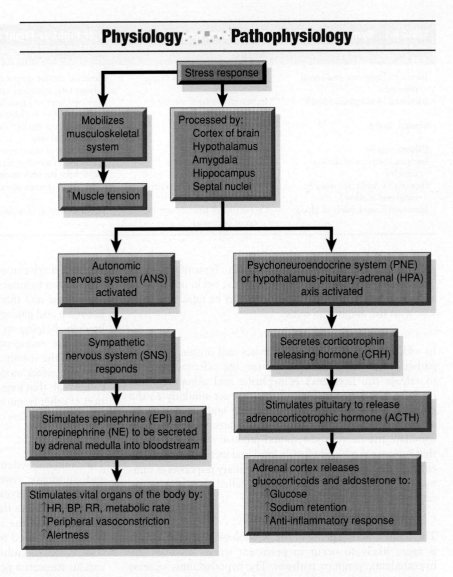

Physiology · · · · Pathophysiology

Stress response

Mobilizes musculoskeletal system → ↑Muscle tension

Processed by:
Cortex of brain
Hypothalamus
Amygdala
Hippocampus
Septal nuclei

Autonomic nervous system (ANS) activated

↓

Sympathetic nervous system (SNS) responds

↓

Stimulates epinephrine (EPI) and norepinephrine (NE) to be secreted by adrenal medulla into bloodstream

↓

Stimulates vital organs of the body by:
↑HR, BP, RR, metabolic rate
↑Peripheral vasoconstriction
↑Alertness

Psychoneuroendocrine system (PNE) or hypothalamus-pituitary-adrenal (HPA) axis activated

↓

Secretes corticotrophin releasing hormone (CRH)

↓

Stimulates pituitary to release adrenocorticotrophic hormone (ACTH)

↓

Adrenal cortex releases glucocorticoids and aldosterone to:
↑Glucose
↑Sodium retention
↑Anti-inflammatory response

FIGURE 6-2 • The physiologic response to stress. The body is prepared through brain activation of the autonomic nervous system and psychoneuroendocrine system commonly referred to as the hypothalamus-pituitary-adrenal axis to cope with stress.

homeostatic balance are integrated by the hypothalamus, which is located in the center of the brain, surrounded by the limbic system and the cerebral hemispheres. The hypothalamus is made up of a number of nuclei and integrates autonomic nervous system mechanisms that maintain the chemical constancy of the internal environment of the body. Together with the limbic system, which contains the amygdala, hippocampus, and septal nuclei, along with other structures, the hypothalamus regulates emotions and many visceral behaviors necessary for survival (e.g., eating, drinking, temperature control, reproduction, defense, aggression).

Each of the brain structures responds differently to stimuli. The cerebral hemispheres are concerned with cognitive functions: thought processes, learning, and memory. The limbic system has connections with both the cerebral hemispheres and the brain stem. In addition, the reticular activating system (RAS), a network of cells that forms a two-way communication system, extends from the brain stem into the midbrain and limbic system. This network controls the alert or waking state of the body.

In the stress response, afferent impulses are carried from sensory organs (eye, ear, nose, skin) and internal sensors (baroreceptors, chemoreceptors) to nerve centers in the brain. The response to the perception of stress is integrated in the hypothalamus, which coordinates the adjustments necessary to return to homeostatic balance. The degree and duration of the response vary; initially, there is a sympathetic nervous system discharge, followed by a sympathetic-adrenal-medullary discharge. If the stress persists, the hypothalamic-pituitary system is activated (Fig. 6-2).

Sympathetic Nervous System Response

The sympathetic nervous system response is rapid and short-lived. Norepinephrine is released at nerve endings that are in direct contact with their respective end organs to cause an increase in function of the vital organs and a state of general body arousal (Porth & Matfin, 2009). Heart rate increases and peripheral vasoconstriction occurs, raising the blood pressure. Blood is also shunted away from abdominal organs. The purpose of these responses is to provide better perfusion of vital organs (brain, heart, skeletal muscles). Blood glucose is increased, supplying more readily available energy. The pupils dilate, and mental activity increases; a greater sense of awareness exists. Constriction of the blood vessels of the skin limits bleeding in the event of trauma. The person is likely to experience cold feet, clammy skin and hands, chills,

TABLE 6-1	Sympathetic-Adrenal-Medullary Response to Stress or Fight-or-Flight Reaction	
Effect	**Purpose**	**Mechanism**
Increased heart rate and blood pressure	More perfusion to vital organs	Increased cardiac output owing to increased myocardial contractility and heart rate; increased venous return (peripheral vasoconstriction)
Increased blood glucose level	Increased available energy	Increased liver and muscle glycogen breakdown; increased breakdown of adipose tissue triglycerides
Mental acuity	Alert state	Increase in amount of blood shunted to the brain from the abdominal viscera and skin
Dilated pupils	Increased awareness	Contraction of radial muscle of iris
Increased tension of skeletal muscles	Preparedness for activity, decreased fatigue	Excitation of muscles; increase in amount of blood shunted to the muscles from the abdominal viscera and skin
Increased ventilation (may be rapid and shallow)	Provision of oxygen for energy	Stimulation of respiratory center in medulla; bronchodilation
Increased coagulability of blood	Prevention of hemorrhage in event of trauma	Vasoconstriction of surface vessels

palpitations, and "knots" in the stomach. Typically, the person appears tense, with the muscles of the neck, upper back, and shoulders tightened; respirations may be rapid and shallow, with the diaphragm tense.

Sympathetic-Adrenal-Medullary Response

In addition to directly affecting major end organs, the sympathetic nervous system stimulates the adrenal medulla to release the hormones epinephrine and norepinephrine into the bloodstream. These hormones act similarly to the sympathetic nervous system, sustaining and prolonging its actions. Because these hormones are catecholamines, they stimulate the nervous system and produce metabolic effects that increase the blood glucose level and metabolic rate. The effect of the sympathetic-adrenal-medullary responses is summarized in Table 6-1. This effect is called the *fight-or-flight response* (Porth & Matfin, 2009).

Hypothalamic-Pituitary Response

The longest-acting phase of the physiologic response, which is more likely to occur in persistent stress, involves the hypothalamic-pituitary pathway. The hypothalamus secretes corticotropin-releasing factor, which stimulates the anterior pituitary to produce ACTH, which in turn stimulates the adrenal cortex to produce **glucocorticoids**, primarily cortisol (Porth & Matfin, 2009). Cortisol stimulates protein catabolism, releasing amino acids; stimulates liver uptake of amino acids and their conversion to glucose (**gluconeogenesis**); and inhibits glucose uptake (anti-insulin action) by many body cells, but not those of the brain and heart (Porth & Matfin, 2009). These cortisol-induced metabolic effects provide the body with a ready source of energy during a stressful situation. This effect has some important implications. For example, a person with diabetes who is under stress, such as that caused by an infection, needs more insulin than usual. Any patient who is under stress (e.g., illness, surgery, trauma, or prolonged psychological stress) catabolizes body protein and needs supplements.

The actions of the catecholamines (epinephrine and norepinephrine) and cortisol are the most important in the general response to stress. Other hormones that play a role are **antidiuretic hormone (ADH)** released from the posterior pituitary and aldosterone released from the adrenal cortex. ADH and aldosterone promote sodium and water retention, which is an adaptive mechanism in the event of hemorrhage

or loss of fluids through excessive perspiration. ADH has also been shown to influence learning and may thus facilitate coping in new and threatening situations. Secretion of growth hormone and glucagon stimulates the uptake of amino acids by cells, helping to mobilize energy resources. Endorphins, which are endogenous opioids, increase during stress and enhance the threshold for tolerance of painful stimuli. They may also affect mood and have been implicated in the so-called high that long-distance runners experience. The secretion of other hormones is also affected; however, their adaptive function is less clear.

Immunologic Response

The immune system is connected to the neuroendocrine and autonomic systems. Lymphoid tissue is richly supplied by autonomic nerves capable of releasing a number of different neuropeptides that can have a direct effect on leukocyte regulation and the inflammatory response. Neuroendocrine hormones released by the central nervous system and endocrine tissues can inhibit or stimulate leukocyte function. The various stressors a person experiences may result in different alterations in autonomic activity and subtle variations in neurohormone and neuropeptide synthesis. All of these possible autonomic and neuroendocrine responses can interact to initiate, weaken, enhance, or terminate an immune response.

The study of the relationships among the neuroendocrine system, the central and autonomic nervous systems, and the immune system and the effects of these relationships on overall health outcomes is called *psychoneuroimmunology*. Because one's perception of events and one's coping styles determine whether, and to what extent, an event activates the stress response system, and because the stress response affects immune activity, one's perceptions, ideas, and thoughts can have profound neurochemical and immunologic consequences. Studies have demonstrated altered immune function in people who are under stress (Dunser & Hasibeder, 2009; Gill, Saligan, Woods, et al., 2009; Thoma, 2011; Weston, 2010). Other studies have identified certain personality traits, such as agreeableness and emotional stability, as having positive effects on health (Cosci, Corlando, Fornai, et al., 2009; Erlen, Stilley, Bender, et al., 2011; Welch & Poulton, 2009). As research continues, this field of study will likely uncover to what extent and by what mechanisms people can consciously influence their immunity.

Maladaptive Responses to Stress

The stress response, as indicated earlier, facilitates adaptation to threatening situations and is retained from humans' evolutionary past. The fight-or-flight response, for example, is an anticipatory response that mobilized the bodily resources of our ancestors to deal with predators and other harsh factors in their environment. This same mobilization comes into play in response to emotional stimuli unrelated to danger. For example, a person may get an "adrenaline rush" when competing over a decisive point in a ball game or when excited about attending a party.

When responses to stress are ineffective, they are referred to as *maladaptive*. Maladaptive responses are chronic, recurrent responses or patterns of response that do not promote the goals of adaptation. The goals of adaptation are somatic or physical health (optimal wellness); psychological health or having a sense of well-being (happiness, satisfaction with life, morale); and enhanced social functioning, which includes work, social life, and family (positive relationships). Maladaptive responses that threaten these goals include faulty appraisals and inappropriate coping (Lazarus, 1991a).

The frequency, intensity, and duration of stressful situations contribute to the development of emotions and subsequent patterns of neurochemical discharge. By appraising situations adequately and coping appropriately, it is possible to anticipate and defuse some of these situations. For example, frequent stressful encounters (e.g., marital discord) might be avoided with better communication and problem solving, or a pattern of procrastination (e.g., delaying work on tasks) could be corrected to reduce stress when deadlines approach.

Coping processes that include the use of alcohol or drugs to reduce stress increase the risk of illness. Other inappropriate coping patterns may increase the risk of illness less directly. For example, people who demonstrate "type A" behaviors, including impatience, competitiveness, and achievement orientation, have an underlying aggressive approach to life and are more prone than others to develop stress-related illnesses. Type A behaviors increase the output of catecholamines, the adrenal-medullary hormones, with their attendant effects on the body. Additional forms of inappropriate coping include denial, avoidance, and distancing.

Models of illness frequently include stress and maladaptation as precursors to disease. A general model of illness, based on Selye's theory, suggests that any stressor elicits a state of disturbed physiologic equilibrium. If this state is prolonged or the response is excessive, it increases the susceptibility of the person to illness. This susceptibility, coupled with a predisposition in the person (from genetic traits, health, or age), leads to illness. If the sympathetic-adrenal-medullary response is prolonged or excessive, a state of chronic arousal develops that may lead to high blood pressure, arteriosclerotic changes, and cardiovascular disease. If the production of ACTH is prolonged or excessive, behavior patterns of withdrawal and depression are seen. In addition, the immune response is decreased, and infections and tumors may develop.

Selye (1976) proposed a list of disorders known as diseases of maladaptation: high blood pressure (including hypertension of pregnancy), diseases of the heart and blood vessels, diseases of the kidney, rheumatic and rheumatoid arthritis, inflammatory diseases of the skin and eyes, infections, allergic and hypersensitivity diseases, nervous and mental diseases, sexual dysfunction, digestive diseases, metabolic diseases, and cancer. Research continues on the complex interconnections between stress, coping (adaptive and maladaptive), and disease (Bertoni et al., 2010; Hang, Weaver, Park, et al., 2009; Rousseau, Hassan, Moreau, et al., 2011; Rzucidlo & Campbell, 2009).

Indicators of Stress

Indicators of stress and the stress response include both subjective and objective measures. Chart 6-1 lists signs and symptoms that may be observed directly or reported by a person. They are psychological, physiologic, or behavioral and reflect social behaviors and thought processes. Some of these reactions may be coping behaviors. Over time, each person tends to develop a characteristic pattern of behavior during stress to warn that the system is out of balance.

Laboratory measurements of indicators of stress have helped in understanding this complex process. Blood and urine analyses can be used to demonstrate changes in hormonal levels and hormonal breakdown products. Blood levels of catecholamines, glucocorticoids, ACTH, and eosinophils are reliable measures of stress. Serum cholesterol and free fatty acid levels can be used to measure stress. When the body experiences distress,

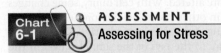

Chart 6-1

ASSESSMENT

Assessing for Stress

Be alert for the following signs and symptoms:

- Restlessness
- Dry mouth
- Overpowering urge to act out
- Fatigue
- Loss of interest in life activities
- Intense periods of anxiety
- Strong startle response
- Hyperactivity
- Gastrointestinal distress
- Diarrhea
- Nausea or vomiting
- Changes in menstrual cycle
- Change in appetite
- Prone to injury
- Palpitations
- Impulsive behaviors
- Emotional lability
- Concentration difficulties
- Feeling weak or dizzy
- Increased body tension
- Tremors
- Nervous habits
- Nervous laughter
- Bruxism (grinding of teeth)
- Difficulty sleeping
- Excessive perspiration
- Urinary frequency
- Headaches
- Pain in back, neck, or other parts of the body
- Increased use of tobacco
- Substance use or abuse
- Unintentional weight loss or gain

there are changes in adrenal hormones such as cortisol and aldosterone. As the levels of these chemicals increase, additional cholesterol is released simultaneously into the general circulation. Both physical and psychological distress can trigger an elevated cholesterol level. In addition, the results of immunoglobulin assays are increased when a person is exposed to various stressors, especially infections and immunodeficiency conditions. With greater attention to the field of neuroimmunology, improved laboratory measures are likely to follow.

In addition to using laboratory tests, researchers have developed questionnaires to identify and assess stressors, stress, and coping strategies. The work of Rice (2011) includes a compilation of information gained from research on stress, coping, and health, and includes some of these questionnaires.

Stress at the Cellular Level

The cell exists on a continuum of function and structure, ranging from the normal cell, to the adapted cell, to the injured or diseased cell, to the dead cell (Fig. 6-3). Changes from one state to another may occur rapidly and may not be readily detectable, because each state does not have discrete boundaries, and disease represents disruption of normal processes. The earliest changes occur at the molecular or subcellular level and are not perceptible until steady-state functions or structures are altered. With cell injury, some changes may be reversible; in other instances, the injuries are lethal. For example, tanning of the skin is an adaptive, morphologic response to exposure to the rays of the sun. However, if the exposure is continued, sunburn and injury occur, and some cells may die, as evidenced by desquamation ("peeling").

Different cells and tissues respond to stimuli with different patterns and rates of response, and some cells are more vulnerable to one type of stimulus or stressor than others. The cell involved, its ability to adapt, and its physiologic state are determinants of the response. For example, cardiac muscle cells respond to **hypoxia** (inadequate oxygenation) more quickly than do smooth muscle cells.

Other determinants of cellular response are the type or nature of the stimulus, its duration, and its severity. For example, neurons that control respiration can develop a tolerance to regular, small amounts of a barbiturate; however, one large dose may result in respiratory depression and death.

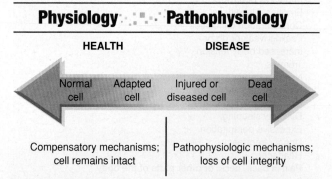

FIGURE 6-3 • The cell on a continuum of function and structure. Changes in the cell are not as easily discerned as the diagram depicts, and the point at which compensation subsides and pathophysiology begins is not clearly defined.

Control of the Steady State

The concept of the cell as existing on a continuum of function and structure includes the relationship of the cell to compensatory mechanisms, which occur continuously in the body to maintain the steady state. Compensatory processes are regulated primarily by the autonomic nervous system and the endocrine system, with control achieved through negative feedback.

Negative Feedback

Negative feedback mechanisms throughout the body monitor the internal environment and restore homeostasis when conditions shift out of the normal range. These mechanisms sense deviations from a predetermined set point or range of adaptability and trigger a response to offset the deviation. Functions regulated through such compensatory mechanisms include blood pressure, acid–base balance, blood glucose level, body temperature, and fluid and electrolyte balance.

Most of the human body's control systems are integrated by the brain with feedback from the nervous and endocrine systems. Control activities involve detecting deviations from the predetermined reference point and stimulating compensatory responses in the muscles and glands of the body. The major organs affected are the heart, lungs, kidneys, liver, gastrointestinal tract, and skin. When stimulated, these organs alter their rate of activity or the amount of secretions they produce. Because of this, these major organs are considered the "organs of homeostasis or adjustment" (Porth & Matfin, 2009).

In addition to the responses influenced by the nervous and endocrine systems, local responses consisting of small feedback loops in a group of cells or tissues occur. The cells detect a change in their immediate environment and initiate an action to counteract its effect. For example, the accumulation of lactic acid in an exercised muscle stimulates dilation of blood vessels in the area to increase blood flow and improve the delivery of oxygen and removal of waste products.

The net result of negative feedback loops is homeostasis. A steady state is achieved by the continuous, variable action of the organs involved in making the adjustments and by the continuous exchange of chemical substances among cells, interstitial fluid, and blood. For example, an increase in the carbon dioxide (CO_2) concentration of the extracellular fluid leads to increased pulmonary ventilation, which decreases the CO_2 level. On a cellular level, increased CO_2 raises the hydrogen ion concentration of the blood. This is detected by chemosensitive receptors in the brain's medullary respiratory control center. The chemoreceptors then stimulate an increase in the rate of discharge of the neurons that innervate the diaphragm and intercostal muscles, which increases the respiratory rate. Excess CO_2 is exhaled, the hydrogen ion concentration returns to normal, and the chemically sensitive neurons are no longer stimulated (Porth & Matfin, 2009).

Positive Feedback

Another type of feedback, **positive feedback**, perpetuates the chain of events set in motion by the original disturbance instead of compensating for it. As the system becomes more unbalanced, disorder and disintegration occur. There are some exceptions to this; blood clotting in humans, for example, is an important positive feedback mechanism.

Cellular Adaptation

Cells are complex units that dynamically respond to the changing demands and stresses of daily life. They possess a maintenance function and a specialized function. The maintenance function refers to the activities that the cell performs with respect to itself; specialized functions are those that the cell performs in relation to the tissues and organs of which it is a part. Individual cells may cease to function without posing a threat to the organism. However, as the number of dead cells increases, the specialized functions of the tissues are altered, and health is threatened.

Cells can adapt to environmental stress through structural and functional changes. Some of these adaptations include cellular hypertrophy, atrophy, hyperplasia, dysplasia, and metaplasia. Such adaptations reflect changes in the normal cell in response to stress. If the stress is unrelenting, cellular injury and death may occur.

Hypertrophy and atrophy lead to changes in the size of cells and hence the size of the organs they form. Compensatory hypertrophy is the result of an enlarged muscle mass and commonly occurs in skeletal and cardiac muscle that experiences a prolonged, increased workload. One example is the bulging muscles of the athlete who engages in bodybuilding.

Atrophy can be the consequence of disease, decreased use, decreased blood supply, loss of nerve supply, or inadequate nutrition. Disuse of a body part is often associated with the aging process and immobilization. Cell size and organ size decrease, and the structures principally affected are the skeletal muscles, the secondary sex organs, the heart, and the brain.

Hyperplasia is an increase in the number of new cells in an organ or tissue. As cells multiply and are subjected to increased stimulation, the tissue mass enlarges. This mitotic response (a change occurring with mitosis) is reversible when the stimulus is removed. This distinguishes hyperplasia from neoplasia or malignant growth, which continues after the stimulus is removed. Hyperplasia may be hormonally induced. An example is the increased size of the thyroid gland caused by thyroid-stimulating hormone (secreted from the pituitary gland) when a deficit in thyroid hormone occurs.

Dysplasia is bizarre cell growth resulting in cells that differ in size, shape, or arrangement from other cells of the same tissue type. Dysplastic cells have a tendency to become malignant; dysplasia is seen commonly in epithelial cells in the bronchi of people who smoke.

Metaplasia is a cell transformation in which there is conversion of one type of mature cell into another type of cell. This serves a protective function, because less-transformed cells are more resistant to the stress that stimulated the change. For example, the ciliated columnar epithelium lining the bronchi of people who smoke is replaced by squamous epithelium. The squamous cells can survive; loss of the cilia and protective mucus, however, can have damaging consequences.

Cellular Injury

Injury is defined as a disorder in steady-state regulation. Any stressor that alters the ability of the cell or system to maintain

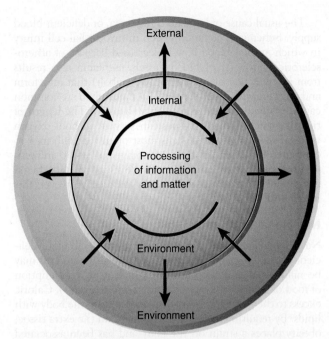

FIGURE 6-4 • Influences leading to disorder may arise from the internal and external environments of the system. Excesses or deficits of information and matter may occur, or there may be faulty regulation of processing.

optimal balance of its adjustment processes leads to injury. Structural and functional damage then occurs, which may be reversible (permitting recovery) or irreversible (leading to disability or death). Homeostatic adjustments are concerned with the small changes within the body's systems. With adaptive changes, compensation occurs and a new steady state may be achieved. With injury, steady-state regulation is lost, and changes in functioning ensue.

Causes of disorder and injury in the system (cell, tissue, organ, body) may arise from the external or internal environment (Fig. 6-4) and include hypoxia, nutritional imbalance, physical agents, chemical agents, infectious agents, immune mechanisms, and genetic defects. The most common causes are hypoxia (oxygen deficiency), chemical injury, and infectious agents. In addition, the presence of one injury makes the system more susceptible to another injury. For example, inadequate oxygenation and nutritional deficiencies make the system vulnerable to infectious agents. These agents damage or destroy the integrity of the cell membrane (necessary for ionic balance) as well as the cell's ability to:

- Transform energy (aerobic respiration, production of adenosine triphosphate)
- Synthesize enzymes and other necessary proteins
- Grow and reproduce (genetic integrity)

Hypoxia

Inadequate cellular oxygenation (hypoxia) interferes with the cell's ability to transform energy. Hypoxia may be caused by a decrease in blood supply to an area, a decrease in the oxygen-carrying capacity of the blood (decreased hemoglobin), a ventilation–perfusion or respiratory problem that reduces the amount of arterial oxygen available, or a problem in the cell's enzyme system that makes it unable to use oxygen.

The usual cause of hypoxia is ischemia, or deficient blood supply. Ischemia is commonly seen in myocardial cell injury in which arterial blood flow is decreased because of atherosclerotic narrowing of blood vessels. Ischemia also results from intravascular clots (thrombi or emboli) that may form and interfere with blood supply. Thromboemboli are common causes of cerebrovascular accidents (strokes). The length of time in which different tissues can survive without oxygen varies. For example, brain cells most often succumb in 3 to 6 minutes. If the condition leading to hypoxia is slow and progressive, collateral circulation may develop, whereby blood is supplied by other blood vessels in the area. However, this mechanism is not highly reliable.

Nutritional Imbalance

Nutritional imbalance refers to a relative or absolute deficiency or excess of one or more essential nutrients. This may be manifested as undernutrition (inadequate consumption of food or calories) or overnutrition (caloric excess). Caloric excess to the point of obesity overloads cells in the body with lipids. By requiring more energy to maintain the extra tissue, obesity places a strain on the body and has been associated with the development of disease, especially pulmonary and cardiovascular disease.

Specific deficiencies arise when an essential nutrient is deficient or when a nutrient imbalance exists. Protein deficiencies and avitaminosis (deficiency of vitamins) are typical examples. An energy deficit leading to cell injury can occur if there is insufficient glucose, or insufficient oxygen to transform the glucose into energy. A lack of insulin, or the inability to use insulin, may also prevent glucose from entering the cell from the blood. This occurs in diabetes, a metabolic disorder that can lead to nutritional deficiency, as well as a host of short- and long-term life-threatening complications.

Physical Agents

Physical agents, including temperature extremes, radiation, electrical shock, and mechanical trauma, can cause injury to the cells or to the entire body. The duration of exposure and the intensity of the stressor determine the severity of damage.

Temperature

When a person's temperature is elevated, hypermetabolism occurs and the respiratory rate, heart rate, and basal metabolic rate increase. With fever induced by infections, the hypothalamic thermostat may be reset at a higher temperature and then return to normal when the fever abates. The increase in body temperature is achieved through physiologic mechanisms. Body temperatures greater than 41°C (106°F) indicate hyperthermia, because the physiologic function of the thermoregulatory center breaks down and the temperature soars (Porth & Matfin, 2009). This physiologic condition occurs in people who have heat stroke. Eventually, the high temperature causes coagulation of cell proteins, and cells die.

The local response to burn injury is similar. Increased metabolic activity occurs, and, as heat increases, proteins coagulate and enzyme systems are destroyed. In extreme situations, charring or carbonization occurs. (See Chapter 62 for more information about burn injuries.)

Extremes of low temperature, or cold, cause vasoconstriction. Blood flow becomes sluggish and clots form, leading to ischemic damage in the involved tissues. With still lower temperatures, ice crystals may form, and cells may burst.

Radiation and Electrical Shock

Radiation is used for diagnosis and treatment of diseases. Ionizing forms of radiation may cause injury by their destructive action. Radiation decreases the protective inflammatory response of the cell, creating a favorable environment for opportunistic infections. Electrical shock produces burns as a result of the heat generated when electrical current travels through the body. It may also abnormally stimulate nerves, leading, for example, to fibrillation of the heart.

Mechanical Trauma

Mechanical trauma can result in wounds that disrupt the cells and tissues of the body. The severity of the wound, amount of blood loss, and extent of nerve damage are significant factors in determining the extent of injury.

Chemical Agents

Chemical injuries are caused by poisons, such as lye, that have a corrosive action on epithelial tissue, or by heavy metals, such as mercury, arsenic, and lead, each of which has its own specific destructive action. Many other chemicals are toxic in certain amounts, in certain people, and in specific tissues. For example, excessive secretion of hydrochloric acid can damage the stomach lining; large amounts of glucose can cause osmotic shifts, affecting the fluid and electrolyte balance; and too much insulin can cause subnormal levels of glucose in the blood (hypoglycemia) and can lead to coma.

Drugs, including prescribed medications, can also cause chemical poisoning. Some people are less tolerant of medications than others and manifest toxic reactions at the usual or customary dosages. Aging tends to decrease tolerance to medications. Polypharmacy (taking many medications at one time) occurs frequently in the aging population, and the unpredictable effects of the resulting medication interactions can cause injury.

Alcohol (ethanol) is also a chemical irritant. In the body, alcohol is broken down into acetaldehyde, which has a direct toxic effect on liver cells that leads to various liver abnormalities, including cirrhosis in susceptible people. Disordered liver cell function leads to complications in other organs of the body.

Infectious Agents

Biologic agents known to cause disease in humans are viruses, bacteria, rickettsiae, mycoplasmas, fungi, protozoa, and nematodes. The severity of the infectious disease depends on the number of microorganisms entering the body, their virulence, and the host's defenses (e.g., health, age, immune responses).

An infection exists when the infectious agent is living, growing, and multiplying in the tissues and is able to overcome the body's normal defenses. Some bacteria, such as those that cause tetanus and diphtheria, produce exotoxins that circulate and create cell damage. Others, such as gram-negative bacteria, produce endotoxins when they die. Tubercle bacilli induce an immune reaction.

Viruses are among the smallest living organisms known and survive as parasites of the living cells they invade. Viruses infect specific cells. Through a complex mechanism, viruses replicate within cells and then invade other cells, where they continue to replicate. As the body mounts an immune response to eliminate the viruses, cells harboring the viruses can be injured in the process. Typically, an inflammatory response and immune reaction are the body's physiologic responses to viral infection.

Disordered Immune Responses

The immune system is an exceedingly complex system, the purpose of which is to defend the body from invasion by any foreign object or foreign cell type, such as cancerous cells. This is a steady-state mechanism; however, like other adjustment processes, it can become disordered, and cellular injury results. The immune response detects foreign bodies by distinguishing non-self substances from self substances and destroying the non-self entities. The entrance of an antigen (foreign substance) into the body evokes the production of antibodies that attack and destroy the antigen (antigen–antibody reaction).

The immune system may function normally, or it may be hypoactive or hyperactive. When it is hypoactive, immunodeficiency diseases occur; when it is hyperactive, hypersensitivity disorders occur. A disorder of the immune system can result in damage to the body's own tissues. Such disorders are labeled autoimmune diseases (see Unit 8).

Genetic Disorders

There is intense interest in genetic defects as causes of disease and modifiers of genetic structure. Many of these defects produce mutations that have no recognizable effect, such as lack of a single enzyme; others contribute to more obvious congenital abnormalities, such as Down syndrome. (For further information on genetics, see Chapter 8.)

Cellular Response to Injury: Inflammation

Cells or tissues of the body may be injured or killed by any of the agents (physical, chemical, infectious) described earlier. When this happens, an inflammatory response (or inflammation) naturally occurs in the healthy tissues adjacent to the site of injury. **Inflammation** is a localized reaction intended to neutralize, control, or eliminate the offending agent to prepare the site for repair. It is a nonspecific response (not dependent on a particular cause) that is meant to serve a protective function. For example, inflammation may be observed at the site of a bee sting, in a sore throat, in a surgical incision, and at the site of a burn. Inflammation also occurs in cell injury events, such as stroke, deep vein thrombosis, and myocardial infarction.

Inflammation is not the same as infection. An infectious agent is only one of several agents that may trigger an inflammatory response. Regardless of the cause, a general sequence of events occurs in the local inflammatory response. This sequence involves changes in the microcirculation, including vasodilation, increased vascular permeability, and leukocytic cellular infiltration (Fig. 6-5). As these changes take place, five cardinal signs of inflammation are produced: redness, warmth, swelling, pain, and loss of function.

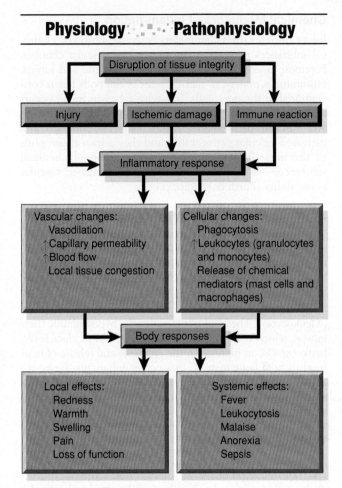

FIGURE 6-5 • Inflammatory response.

The transient vasoconstriction that occurs immediately after injury is followed by vasodilation and an increased rate of blood flow through the microcirculation to the area of tissue damage. Local warmth and redness result. Next, the structure of the microvascular system changes to accommodate the movement of plasma protein from the blood into the tissues. Following this increase in vascular permeability, plasma fluids (including proteins and solutes) leak into the inflamed tissues, producing swelling. Leukocytes migrate through the endothelium and accumulate in the tissue at the site of the injury. The pain that occurs is attributed to the pressure of fluids or swelling on nerve endings and to the irritation of nerve endings by chemical mediators released at the site. Bradykinin is one of the chemical mediators suspected of causing pain. Loss of function is most likely related to the pain and swelling; however, the exact mechanism is not completely known.

As blood flow increases and fluid leaks into the surrounding tissues, the formed elements (red blood cells, white blood cells, and platelets) remain in the blood, causing it to become more viscous. Leukocytes (white blood cells) collect in the vessels, exit, and migrate to the site of injury to engulf offending organisms and to remove cellular debris in a process called *phagocytosis*. Fibrinogen in the leaked plasma fluid coagulates, forming fibrin for clot formation, which serves to wall off the injured area and prevent the spread of infection.

Chemical Mediators of Inflammation

Injury initiates the inflammatory response; however, chemical substances released at the site induce vascular changes. Foremost among these chemicals are histamine and kinins. Histamine is present in many tissues of the body but is concentrated in the mast cells. It is released when injury occurs and is responsible for the early changes in vasodilation and vascular permeability. Kinins cause vasodilation and increased vascular permeability, and they attract neutrophils to the area. Prostaglandins—another group of chemical substances—are also suspected of causing increased vascular permeability (Porth & Matfin, 2009).

Systemic Response to Inflammation

The inflammatory response is often confined to the site, causing only local signs and symptoms. However, systemic responses can also occur. Fever is the most common sign of a systemic response to injury, and it is most likely caused by endogenous pyrogens (internal substances that cause fever) released from neutrophils and macrophages (specialized forms of leukocytes). These substances reset the hypothalamic thermostat, which controls body temperature, and produce fever. Leukocytosis, an increase in the synthesis and release of neutrophils from bone marrow, may occur, enhancing the body's ability to fight infection. During this process, general, nonspecific symptoms develop, including malaise, loss of appetite, aching, and weakness.

Types of Inflammation

Inflammation is categorized primarily by its duration and the type of exudate produced. It is most often acute or chronic. Acute inflammation is characterized by the local vascular and exudative changes described previously and usually lasts less than 2 weeks. An acute inflammatory response is immediate and serves a protective function. After the causative agent is removed, the inflammation subsides and healing takes place with the return of normal or near-normal structure and function.

Chronic inflammation develops if the injurious agent persists and the acute response is perpetuated. Symptoms are present for many months or years. Chronic inflammation may also begin insidiously and never have an acute phase. The chronic response does not serve a beneficial and protective function; on the contrary, it is debilitating and can produce long-lasting effects. As the inflammation becomes chronic, changes occur at the site of injury and the nature of the exudate becomes proliferative. A cycle of cellular infiltration, necrosis, and fibrosis begins, with repair and breakdown occurring simultaneously. Considerable scarring may occur, resulting in permanent tissue damage.

Cellular Healing

The reparative process begins at approximately the same time as the injury. Healing proceeds after the inflammatory debris has been removed. Healing may occur by regeneration, in which the defect is gradually repaired by proliferation of the same type of cells as those destroyed, or by replacement, in which cells of another type, usually connective tissue, fill in the tissue defect and result in scar formation.

Regeneration

The ability of cells to regenerate depends on whether they are labile, permanent, or stable. Labile cells multiply constantly to replace cells worn out by normal physiologic processes; these include epithelial cells of the skin and those lining the gastrointestinal tract. Permanent cells include neurons—the nerve cell bodies, not their axons. Destruction of neurons is permanent; however, axons may regenerate. If normal activity is to return, tissue regeneration must occur in a functional pattern, especially in the growth of several axons. Stable cells in some organ systems have a latent ability to regenerate. Under normal physiologic processes, they are not shed and do not need replacement; if they are damaged or destroyed, they are able to regenerate. Examples include functional cells of the kidney, liver, and pancreas. Cells in other organs, such as the brain, for example, do not regenerate.

Replacement

The condition of the host, the environment, and the nature and severity of the injury affect the processes of inflammation, repair, and replacement. Depending on the extent of damage, repair and replacement may occur by first-, second-, or third-intention healing. In first-intention healing, the wound edges are approximated, as in a surgical wound (see Chapter 19). Little scar formation occurs, and the wound healing occurs without granulation. In second-intention healing, the edges are not approximated and the wound fills with granulation tissue. The process of repair takes longer and may result in scar formation, with loss of specialized function. For example, people who have recovered from myocardial infarction have abnormal electrocardiographic tracings because the electrical signal cannot be conducted through the connective tissue that has replaced the infarcted area. In third-intention healing, the wound edges are not approximated and healing is delayed.

Nursing Management

Stress or the potential for stress is ubiquitous—that is, it is both everywhere and anywhere. Anxiety, frustration, anger, and feelings of inadequacy, helplessness, or powerlessness are emotions often associated with stress. In the presence of these emotions, the customary activities of daily living may be disrupted—for example, a sleep disturbance may occur, eating and activity patterns may be altered, and family processes or role performance may be disrupted.

It is important for nurses to know that the optimal point of intervention to promote health is during the stage when a person's own compensatory processes are still functioning effectively. A major role of nurses is the early identification of both physiologic and psychological stressors. Nurses should be able to relate the presenting signs and symptoms of distress to the physiology they represent and identify a person's position on the continuum of function, from health and compensation to pathophysiology and disease.

In the assessment of people who seek health care, both objective signs and subjective symptoms are the primary indicators of existing physiologic processes. The following questions are addressed:

- Are the heart rate, respiratory rate, and temperature normal?
- What emotional distress may be contributing to the patient's health problems?
- Are there other indicators of steady-state deviation?
- What are the patient's blood pressure, height, and weight?
- Are there any problems in movement or sensation?
- Are there any problems with affect, behavior, speech, cognitive ability, orientation, or memory?
- Are there obvious impairments, lesions, or deformities?

Objective evidence can be obtained from laboratory data, such as electrolytes, blood urea nitrogen, blood glucose, and urinalysis results. Further signs of injury are seen in diagnostic studies such as computed tomography (CT) scanning, magnetic resonance imaging (MRI), and positron emission tomography (PET). Further information on diagnostic evaluation can be found in assessment chapters of each unit of this book. Many nursing diagnoses are possible for patients suffering from stress. One nursing diagnosis related to stress is Anxiety, which is defined as a vague, uneasy feeling, the source of which may be nonspecific or not known to the person. Stress may also be manifested as ineffective coping patterns, impaired thought processes, or disrupted relationships. These human responses are reflected in the nursing diagnoses of Anxiety, Ineffective coping, Defensive coping, and Ineffective denial, all of which indicate poor adaptive responses (Herdman, 2012). Other possible nursing diagnoses include Social isolation, Risk for spiritual distress, Readiness for enhanced family processes, Decisional conflict, Risk for compromised resilience, Impaired individual resilience, Readiness for enhanced resilience, and Risk for powerlessness, among others. Because human responses to stress are varied, as are the sources of stress, arriving at an accurate diagnosis allows interventions and goals to be more specific and leads to improved outcomes.

Stress management is directed toward reducing and controlling stress and improving coping. The need to prevent illness, improve the quality of life, and decrease the cost of health care makes efforts to promote health essential, and stress control is a significant health promotion goal. Stress reduction methods and coping enhancements can derive from either internal or external sources. For example, healthy eating habits and relaxation techniques are internal resources that help reduce stress, and a broad social network is an external resource that helps reduce stress. Goods and services that can be purchased are also external resources for stress management. It may be easier for people with adequate financial resources to cope with constraints in the environment, because their sense of vulnerability to threat is decreased compared to those without adequate financial resources.

Promoting a Healthy Lifestyle

A health-promoting lifestyle provides internal resources that aid in coping, and it buffers or cushions the impact of stressors. Lifestyles or habits that contribute to the risk of illness can be identified through a health risk appraisal, which is an assessment method designed to promote health by examining a person's habits and recommending changes when a health risk is identified.

Chart 6-2 Information Addressed in Health Risk Questionnaires

Demographic data: age, gender, race, ethnic background
Personal and family history of diseases and health problems
Lifestyle choices:

- Eating, sleeping, exercise, smoking, drinking, sexual activity, recreation activity, and driving habits
- Stressors at home and on the job
- Roles, role relationships, and associated stressors
- Living and family situation
- Social and family supports

Physical measurements:

- Blood pressure
- Height, weight, body mass index
- Laboratory analyses of blood and urine

Participation in high-risk behaviors

Health risk appraisals involve the use of health risk questionnaires to estimate the likelihood that people with a given set of characteristics will become ill. It is hoped that if people are provided with this information, they will adopt healthy behaviors (e.g., stop smoking, have periodic screening examinations) to improve their health. Questionnaires typically address the information presented in Chart 6-2.

The personal information is compared with average population risk data, and the risk factors are identified and weighted. From this analysis, a person's risks and major health hazards are identified. Further comparisons with population data can estimate how many years will be added to a person's lifespan if the suggested changes are made. However, research has not yet demonstrated that providing people with such information ensures that they will change their behaviors. The single most important factor for determining health status is social class, and within a social class, research suggests that the major factor influencing health is level of education (Bastable, Gramet, Jacobs, et al., 2012).

Enhancing Coping Strategies

Bulechek, Butcher, and McCloskey Dochterman (2008) identified "coping enhancement" as a nursing intervention and defined it as "assisting a patient to adapt to perceived stressors, changes, or threats that interfere with meeting life demands and roles" (p. 228) (Chart 6-3). The nurse can build on the patient's existing coping strategies, as identified in the health appraisal, or teach new strategies for coping if necessary.

The five predominant ways of coping with illness identified in a review of 57 nursing research studies were as follows (Jalowiec, 1993):

- Trying to be optimistic about the outcome
- Using social support
- Using spiritual resources
- Trying to maintain control either over the situation or over feelings
- Trying to accept the situation

Other ways of coping included seeking information, reprioritizing needs and roles, lowering expectations, making compromises, comparing oneself to others, planning activities to

---

Chart 6-3 Coping Enhancement: Nursing Interventions

Definition

Facilitation of cognitive and behavioral efforts to manage perceived stressors, changes, or threats that interfere with meeting life demands and roles.

Selected Activities

Assist the patient in identifying appropriate short- and long-term goals.

Assist the patient to solve problems in a constructive manner.

Provide factual information concerning diagnosis, treatment, and prognosis.

Encourage an attitude of realistic hope as a way of dealing with feelings of helplessness.

Acknowledge the patient's spiritual/cultural background, and encourage the use of spiritual resources if desired.

Foster constructive outlets for anger and hostility.

Assist the patient in examining available resources to meet goals.

Appraise the needs and desires for social support, and assist the patient to identify available support systems.

Assist the patient to identify positive strategies to deal with limitations, manage needed lifestyle or role changes, and work through the losses of chronic illness and/or disability if appropriate.

Adapted from Bulechek, G. M., Butcher, H. K., Dochterman, J. C. & Wagner, C. M. (Eds.). (2013). *Nursing interventions classification (NIC)* (6th ed.). St. Louis: Elsevier.

Chart 6-4 The Benson Relaxation Response

1. Pick a brief phrase or word that reflects your basic belief system.
2. Choose a comfortable position.
3. Close your eyes.
4. Relax your muscles.
5. Become aware of your breathing, and start using your selected focus word.
6. Maintain a passive demeanor.
7. Continue for a set period of time.
8. Practice the technique twice daily.

Adapted from Benson, H. (1993). The relaxation response. In D. Goleman & J. Gurin (Eds.), *Mind-body medicine: How to use your mind for better health*. Yonkers, NY: Consumer Reports Books.

---

conserve energy, taking things one step at a time, listening to one's body, and using self-talk for encouragement.

Relaxation Techniques

Relaxation techniques are a major method used to relieve stress. The goal of relaxation training is to produce a response that counters the stress response. When this goal is achieved, the action of the hypothalamus adjusts, decreasing sympathetic and parasympathetic nervous system activity. The sequence of physiologic effects and their signs and symptoms are then interrupted, thus reducing psychological stress. This is a learned response and requires practice to achieve. Commonly used techniques include progressive muscle relaxation, the Benson relaxation response, and relaxation with guided imagery (all discussed later). Other relaxation techniques include meditation, breathing techniques, massage, Reiki, music therapy, biofeedback, and the use of humor.

The different relaxation techniques share four similar elements: (1) a quiet environment, (2) a comfortable position, (3) a passive attitude, and (4) a mental device (something on which to focus one's attention, such as a word, phrase, or sound).

Progressive Muscle Relaxation

Progressive muscle relaxation involves tensing and releasing the muscles of the body in sequence and sensing the difference in feeling. It is best if the person lies on a soft cushion in a quiet room, breathing easily. Someone usually reads the instructions in a low tone in a slow and relaxed

manner, or a recording of the instructions may be played. The person tenses the muscles in the entire body (one muscle group at a time), holds, senses the tension, and then relaxes. As each muscle group is tensed, the person keeps the rest of the body relaxed. Each time the focus is on feeling the tension and relaxation. When the exercise is completed, the entire body should be relaxed (Benson, 1993; Benson & Stark, 1996).

The Benson Relaxation Response

The Benson relaxation response (Chart 6-4) combines meditation with relaxation. Along with the repeated word or phrase, a passive demeanor is essential. If other thoughts or distractions (noises, pain) occur, Benson recommends not fighting the distraction but simply continuing to repeat the focus phrase. Time of day is not important; however, the exercise works best on an empty stomach (Benson, 1993; Benson & Proctor, 1984; Benson & Stark, 1996).

Guided Imagery

Simple **guided imagery** is the mindful use of a word, phrase, or visual image for the purpose of distracting oneself from distressing situations or consciously taking time to relax or re-energize. A nurse can help a person select a pleasant scene or experience, such as watching the ocean or dabbling the feet in a cool stream. The image serves as the mental device in this technique. As the person sits comfortably and quietly, the nurse guides the person to review the scene, trying to feel and relive the imagery with all of the senses. A recording may be made of the description of the image, or commercial recordings for guided imagery and relaxation can be used.

Educating About Stress Management

Two commonly prescribed nursing educational interventions—providing sensory information and providing procedural information (e.g., preoperative education)—aim to reduce stress and improve the patient's coping ability. This preparatory education includes giving structured content, such as a lesson in childbirth preparation to expectant parents, a review of how an implantable cardioverter defibrillator works to a cardiac patient, or a description of sensations a patient will experience during cardiac catheterization. These techniques may alter the person–environment relationship such that something that might have been viewed as harmful or a threat will now be perceived more positively (Chart 6-5). Giving patients information also reduces

NURSING RESEARCH PROFILE

Chart 6-5

Experiences of Implantable Cardioverter Defibrillators

Palacios-Cena, D., Losa-Iglesias, M., Alvarez-Lopez, C., et al. (2011). Patients, intimate partners, and family experiences of implantable cardioverter defibrillators: Qualitative systematic review. *Journal of Advanced Nursing, 67*(12), 2537–2550.

Purpose

The main purpose of this study was to describe the experiences of patients, intimate partners, and family members related to how an implantable cardioverter defibrillator (ICD) influenced both the physical and psychosocial aspects of a person's life. An additional purpose was to determine what measures health care professionals could perform to assist patients and significant others in coping with this device.

Design

The study used a thematic analysis to extract data from qualitative research studies that met the criteria for inclusion. Published qualitative research studies from the databases of CINAHL (Cumulative Index to Nursing and Allied Health), PubMed, Medline, and ISI Web of Knowledge were used. Specific search methods included the use of the following terms: internal defibrillators, implantable defibrillator, implantable cardioverter defibrillator, qualitative research, nursing, and sudden death. All studies were published during the period from 1999 to 2009 in either the English or Spanish language. A total of 22 studies met the inclusion criteria. The specific data obtained from each study included sample size, methodology, data analysis, and significant findings.

Findings

Seven types of qualitative research methods were identified, including Ethnography, Grounded Theory, Phenomenology, Focus Groups, Biographies, Case Studies, and Action Research. The analysis revealed nine major findings from the following categories: (1) the challenges of daily life with an ICD; (2) a change in their life and world views; (3) the effects of the spontaneous shocks; (4) the complexity of making decisions related to the use of the ICD; (5) the time period need for adjustment to the ICD; (6) the effects of the ICD on personal, intimate, and sexual relationships; (7) the need and benefits of external support mechanisms; (8) the need for quality patient care after discharge; and (9) the lack of qualitative research on women patients with ICDs.

Nursing Implications

Nurses must recognize the physiological and psychosocial challenges, struggles, and dilemmas experienced by people with ICDs. This recognition must be the focus of interactions between the patient, significant others, and the nurse with the intention of building resources to process the various types of changes occurring. Education targeting readjustment during the postimplantation period is an essential part of care. Introduction to and development of support mechanisms including face-to-face and Internet support groups can assist in the establishment of communication, adjustment, and overall coping with the ICD experience. Nurses must become involved in establishing educational venues that support the transitions experienced by patients, intimate partners, and families. The need for nurses to engage in research studies on the needs of women with ICDs is the first step for establishing evidence-based care.

the emotional response so that they can concentrate and solve problems more effectively (Miller & Smith, 1993; Miller & Stoeckel, 2011; Palacios-Cena, Losa-Iglesias, Alvarez-Lopez, et al., 2011).

Promoting Family Health

In addition to individual concepts of homeostasis, stress, adaptation, and health problems associated with maladaptation, the concept of family is also important. Nurses can intervene with both individuals and families to reduce stress and its health-related effects. The **family** plays a central role in the life of the patient and is a major part of the context of the patient's life. It is within families that people grow, are nurtured, acquire a sense of self, develop beliefs and values about life, and progress through life's developmental stages (Fig. 6-6). Families are also the first source for socialization and teaching about health and illness.

Ideally, the health care team conducts a careful and comprehensive family assessment (including coping style), develops interventions tailored to handle the stressors, implements the specified treatment protocols, and facilitates the construction of social support systems. The use of existing family strengths, resources, and education is augmented by therapeutic family interventions. The primary goals of the nurse are to maintain and improve the patient's present level of health and to prevent physical and emotional deterioration. Next, the nurse intervenes in the cycle that the illness

creates: patient illness, stress for other family members, new illness in other family members, and additional patient stress.

Helping the family members manage the myriad stressors that bombard them daily involves working with family members to develop coping skills. Seven traits that enhance coping of family members under stress have been identified (Burr, Klein, Burr, et al., 1994). Communication skills and spirituality were frequently useful traits. Cognitive abilities, emotional strengths, relationship capabilities, willingness to

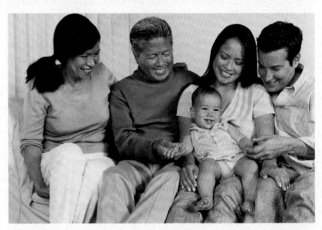

FIGURE 6-6 • Within families, individuals progress through life's developmental stages.

use community resources, and individual strengths and talents were also associated with effective coping. As nurses work with families, they must not underestimate the impact of their therapeutic interactions, educational information, positive role modeling, provision of direct care, and education on promoting health. Maladaptive coping may result if health care team members are not perceived as actively supporting family members. Often, denial and blaming of others occur. Sometimes, physiologic illness, emotional withdrawal, and physical distancing are the results of severe family conflict, violent behavior, or addiction to drugs and alcohol. Substance abuse may develop in family members who feel unable to cope or solve problems. People may engage in these dysfunctional behaviors when faced with difficult or problematic situations.

Enhancing Social Support

The nature of social support and its influence on coping have been studied extensively. Social support has been demonstrated to be an effective moderator of life stress. Such support has been found to provide people with several different types of emotional information (Maisel & Gable, 2010). The first type of information leads people to believe that they are cared for and loved. This emotional support appears most often in a relationship between two people in which mutual trust and attachment are expressed by helping one another meet their emotional needs. The second type of information leads people to believe that they are esteemed and valued. This is most effective when there is recognition demonstrating a person's favorable position in the group. Known as esteem support, this elevates the person's sense of self-worth. The third type of information leads people to feel that they belong to a network of communication and mutual obligation. Members of this network share information and make goods and services available to the members as needed.

Social support also facilitates a person's coping behaviors; however, this depends on the nature of the social support. People can have extensive relationships and interact frequently; however, the necessary support comes only when there is a deep level of involvement and concern, not when people merely touch the surface of each other's lives. The critical qualities within a social network are the exchange of intimate communications and the presence of solidarity and trust.

Emotional support from family and significant others provides love and a sense of sharing the burden. The emotions that accompany stress are unpleasant and often increase in a spiraling fashion if relief is not provided. Being able to talk with someone and express feelings openly may help a person gain mastery of the situation. Nurses can provide this support, but it is important to identify the person's social support system and encourage its use. People who are "loners," who are isolated, or who withdraw in times of stress have a high risk of coping failure.

Because anxiety can also distort a person's ability to process information, it helps to seek information and advice from others who can assist with analyzing the threat and developing a strategy to manage it. Again, this use of others helps people maintain mastery of a situation and self-esteem.

Thus, social networks assist with management of stress by providing people with:
- A positive social identity
- Emotional support
- Material aid and tangible services
- Access to information
- Access to new social contacts and new social roles

Recommending Support and Therapy Groups

Support groups exist especially for people in similar stressful situations. Groups have been formed by people with ostomies; women who have had mastectomies; and people with cancer or other serious diseases, chronic illnesses, and disabilities. There are groups for single parents, substance abusers and their family members, homicide bereavement, and victims of child abuse. Professional, civic, and religious support groups are active in many communities (Burke, Neimeyer, & McDevitt-Murphy, 2010). There are also encounter groups, assertiveness training programs, and consciousness-raising groups to help people modify their usual behaviors in their transactions with their environment. Many find that being a member of a group with similar problems or goals has a releasing effect that promotes freedom of expression and exchange of ideas.

The Role of Stress in Health Patterns

As noted previously, a person's psychological and biologic health, internal and external sources of stress management, and relationships with the environment are predictors of health outcomes. These factors are directly related to the person's health patterns. The nurse has a significant role and responsibility in identifying the health patterns of patients receiving care as well as those of their families. If those patterns are not achieving physiologic, psychological, and social balance, the nurse is obligated, with the assistance and agreement of the patient, to seek ways to promote individual and family balance.

Although this chapter has presented some physiologic mechanisms and perspectives on health and disease, the way that one copes with stress, the way that one relates to others, and the values and goals held are also interwoven into those physiologic patterns. To evaluate a patient's health patterns and to intervene if a disorder exists requires a total assessment of the person. Specific disorders and their nursing management are addressed in greater depth in other chapters.

Critical Thinking Exercises

1 **ebp** A male college student with a 3-year history of irritable bowel syndrome makes an appointment to speak with the nurse at the health center to discuss his increased use of antidiarrheal medication. The student states, "I've been very stressed. I've been going out with my friends a lot and I haven't been eating right." What is the evidence base for offering information on stress reduction and health programs to help this young adult make appropriate health decisions and establish positive health behaviors?

Identify the criteria used to evaluate the strength of the evidence for this practice.

2 A 45-year-old woman who is homeless is in a hospital emergency department for treatment of severe lacerations following a hurricane. She tells the nurse she is fearful that her spouse, who was already admitted to the hospital with a fractured hip, is alone and suffering. She states, "I am nervous about his condition and that he will go to surgery before I see him. I know that he will be better if he knows that I am all right, too. Please, let me see him!" Generate a list of possible nursing diagnoses for this patient. Identify the nursing interventions that would be most appropriate for each of the possible nursing diagnoses and the evaluation criteria for these interventions.

3 **pq** A 78-year-old man recently moved to a retirement community where he lives semi-independently. The family health history reveals that his mother had diabetes and thyroid disease, and his father had hypertension and coronary artery disease. This patient has limited resources and support networks for making necessary lifestyle changes. Identify the priorities, approach, and techniques that you would use to assess this patient's health promotion needs.

Brunner Suite Resources

Explore these additional resources to enhance learning for this chapter:
• NCLEX-Style Questions and Other Resources on thePoint, http://thePoint.lww.com/Brunner13e
• Study Guide
• PrepU
• Clinical Handbook
• Handbook of Laboratory and Diagnostic Tests

References

*Asterisk indicates nursing research.
**Double asterisk indicates classic reference.

Books

Bastable, S., Gramet, P., Jacobs, K., et al. (2012). *Health professional as educator: Principles of teaching and learning.* Sudbury, MA: Jones & Bartlett.

**Benson, H. (1993). The relaxation response. In D. Goleman & J. Gurin (Eds.), *Mind-body medicine: How to use your mind for better health.* Yonkers, NY: Consumer Reports Books.

**Benson, H., & Proctor, W. (1984). *Beyond the relaxation response.* New York: Berkley Books.

**Benson, H., & Stark, M. (1996). *Timeless healing.* New York: Scribner.

Bulechek, G. M., Butcher, H. K., Dochterman, J. C. & Wagner, C. M. (Eds.). (2013). *Nursing interventions classification (NIC)* (6th ed.). St. Louis: Elsevier.

**Burr, W., Klein, S., Burr, R., et al. (1994). *Reexamining family stress: New theory and research.* Thousand Oaks, CA: Sage.

Herdman, T. H. (2012). *NANDA International nursing diagnoses: Definitions and classification 2012–2014.* Oxford: Wiley-Blackwell.

**Jalowiec, A. (1993). Coping with illness: Synthesis and critique of the nursing literature from 1980–1990. In J. D. Barnfather & B. L. Lyon (Eds.), *Stress and coping: State of the science and implications for nursing theory, research, and practice.* Indianapolis: Sigma Theta Tau International.

**Lazarus, R. S. (1991a). *Emotion and adaptation.* New York: Oxford University Press.

**Lazarus, R. S. (1993). Why we should think of stress as a subset of emotion. In L. Goldberger & S. Breznitz (Eds.), *Handbook of stress: Theoretical and clinical aspects* (2nd ed.). New York: Free Press.

**Lazarus, R. S., & Folkman, S. (1984). *Stress, appraisal, and coping.* New York: Springer.

**Miller, L. H., & Smith, A. D. (1993). *The stress solution.* New York: Pocket Books.

Miller, M. A., & Stoeckel, P. R. (2011). *Client education: Theory and practice.* Sudbury, MA: Jones & Bartlett.

Neenan, M. (2009). *Developing resilience: A cognitive behavioral approach.* New York: Routledge.

**Pearsall, P. (2003). *The Beethoven factor: The new positive psychology of hardiness, happiness, healing, and hope.* Charlottesville, VA: Hampton Roads Publishing Company.

Porth, C. M., & Matfin G. (2009). *Pathophysiology. Concepts of altered health status* (8th ed.). Philadelphia: Lippincott Williams & Wilkins.

Reich, J. W., Zautra, A. J., & Hall, J. S. (2010). *Handbook of adult resilience.* New York: Guilford Press.

*Rice, V. H. (Ed.). (2011). *Handbook of stress, coping, and health: Implications for theory, research, and practice* (2nd ed.). Bern, Germany: Huber Publishing.

**Selye, H. (1976). *The stress of life* (Rev. ed.). New York: McGraw-Hill.

Journals and Electronic Documents

*Berendes, D., Keefe, F. J., & Somers, T. J. (2010). Hope in the context of lung cancer: Relationships of hope to symptoms. *Journal of Pain and Symptom Management, 40*(2), 174–182.

*Bertoni, A. G., Burke, G. L., Owusu, J. A., et al. (2010). Inflammation and the incidence of type 2 diabetes: The Multi-Ethnic Study of Atherosclerosis (MESA). *Diabetes Care, 33*(4), 804–810.

*Burke, L. A., Neimeyer, R. A., & McDevitt-Murphy, M. E. (2010). African American homicide bereavement: aspects of social support that predict complicated grief, PTSD, and depression. *Omega: Journal of Death and Dying, 61*(1), 1–24.

*Chen, W., Shiu, C., Simoni, J. M., et al. (2011). In sickness and in health: A qualitative study of how Chinese women with HIV navigate stigma and negotiate disclosure within their marriages/partnerships. *AIDS Care, 23*(Suppl. 1), 120–125.

*Cosci, F., Corlando, A., Fornai, E., et al. (2009). Nicotine dependence, psychological distress and personality traits as possible predictors of smoking cessation: Results of a double-blind study with nicotine patch. *Addictive Behaviors, 34*(1), 28–35.

Dow, H. D. (2011). An overview of stressors faced by immigrants and refugees: A guide for mental health practitioners. *Home Health Care Management & Practice, 23*(3), 210–217.

Dunser, M. W., & Hasibeder, W. R. (2009). Sympathetic overstimulation during critical illness: Adverse effects of adrenergic stress. *Journal of Intensive Care Medicine, 24*(5), 293–316.

*Erlen, J. A., Stilley, C. S., Bender, A., et al. (2011). Personality traits and chronic illness: A comparison of individuals with psychiatric, coronary heart disease, and HIV/AIDS diagnoses. *Applied Nursing Research, 24*(2), 74–81.

Gill, J. M., Saligan, L., Woods, S., et al. (2009). PTSD associated with an excess of inflammatory immune activities. *Perspectives in Psychiatric Care, 45*(4), 262–277.

*Hahn, E. A., Cichy, K. E., Almeida, D. M., et al. (2011). Time use and well-being in older widows: Adaptation and resilience. *Journal of Women and Aging, 23*(2), 149–159.

*Hang, D., Weaver, M. T., Park, N., et al. (2009). Significant impairment in immune recovery after cancer treatment. *Nursing Research, 58*(2), 105–114.

Herman, H., Stewart, D. E., Diaz-Granados, N., et al. (2011). What is reliance? *Canadian Journal of Psychiatry, 56*(5), 258–264.

*Hickman, R. L., Daly, B. J., Douglas, S. L., & Clochesy, J. M. (2010). Informational coping style and depressive symptoms in family decision makers. *American Journal of Critical Care, 19*(5), 410–420.

**Holmes, T. H., & Rahe, R. H. (1967). The social readjustment rating scale. *Journal of Psychosomatic Research, 11*, 213–218.

Johnson, C. M. (2010). African-American teens girls grieve the loss of friends to homicide: Meaning making and resilience. *Omega: Journal of Death & Dying, 61*(2), 121–143.

**Lazarus, R. S. (1991b). Cognition and motivation in emotion. *American Psychologist, 46*(4), 352–367.

**Lazarus, R. S. (1991c). Progress on a cognitive-motivational-relational theory of emotion. *American Psychologist, 46*(8), 819–834.

*Mair, C. A., Cutchin, M. P., & Peek, M. K. (2011). Allostatic load in an environmental riskscape: The role of stress and gender. *Health & Place, 17*(4), 978–987.

Maisel, N. C., & Gable, S. L. (2010). The paradox of received social support: The importance of responsiveness. *Psychological Science, 20*(8), 928–932.

*Motl, R. W., McAuley, E., Snook, E. M., et al. (2009). Physical activity and quality of life in multiple sclerosis: Intermediary roles of disability, fatigue, mood, pain, self-efficacy and social support. *Psychological Health Medicine, 14*(1), 111–124.

*Palacios-Cena, D., Losa-Iglesias, M., Alvarez-Lopez, C., et al. (2011). Patients, intimate partners, and family experiences of implantable cardioverter defibrillators: Qualitative systematic review. *Journal of Advanced Nursing, 67*(12), 2537–2550.

*Pierce, P. F, Lewandowski-Romps, L., & Silverschanz, P. (2011). War-related stressors as predictors of post-deployment health of Air Force women. *Women's Health Issues, 21*(4), S152–S159.

*Pierini, D., & Stuifbergen, A. K. (2010). Psychological resilience and depressive symptoms in older adults diagnosed with post-polio syndrome. *Rehabilitation Nursing, 35*(4), 167–175.

*Rousseau, C., Hassan, G., Moreau, N., et al. (2011). Perceived discrimination and its association with psychological distress among newly arrived immigrants before and after September 11, 2001. *American Journal of Public Health, 101*(5), 909–915.

Rzucidlo, S. E., & Campbell, M. (2009). Beyond the physical injuries: Parent and child coping with medical traumatic stress after pediatric trauma. *Journal of Trauma Nursing, 16*(3), 130–135.

**Tausig, M. (1982). Measuring life events. *Journal of Health and Social Behavior, 23*(1), 52–64.

Thoma, A. G. (2011). Immune system impairment in response to chronic anxiety. *Integrative Medicine, 10*(1), 20.

*Thornton, M., Parry, M., Gill, P., et al. (2011). Hard choices: A qualitative study of influences on the treatment decisions made by advanced lung cancer patients. *International Journal of Palliative Care, 17*(2), 68–74.

*Van Dyke, C. J., Glenwick, D. S., Cecero, J. J., et al. (2009). The relationship of religious coping and spirituality to adjustment and psychological distress in urban early adolescents. *Mental Health, Religion and Culture, 12*(4), 369–383.

*Watson, R., Gardiner, E., Hogston, R., et al. (2009). A longitudinal study of stress and psychological distress in nurses and nursing students. *Journal of Clinical Nursing, 18*(2), 270–278.

*Weider, G., Zahn, D., Mendell, N. R., et al. (2011). Patients' sex and emotional support as predictors of death and clinical deterioration in the waiting for a new heart study: Results from the 1-year follow-up. *Progress in Transplantation, 21*(2), 106–114.

*Welch, D., & Poulton, R. (2009). Personality influences on change in smoking behavior. *Health Psychology, 28*(3), 292–299.

Weston, D. (2010). The pathogenesis of infection and immune response. *British Journal of Nursing, 19*(16), S4–S11.

*Yermal, S. J., Witek-Janusek, L., Peterson, J., et al. (2010). Perioperative pain, psychological distress, and immune function in men undergoing prostatectomy for cancer of the prostate. *Biological Research for Nursing, 11*(4), 351–362.

Resources

General
A.D.A.M. Inc.: Stress, http://adam.about.com/reports/Stress.htm
American Holistic Nurses Association (AHNA), www.ahna.org
Centre for Stress Management, www.managingstress.com/articles/definition.htm
Grief Recovery Institute, www.griefrecoverymethod.com
Inflammation—The Key to Chronic Disease, www.womentowomen.com/inflammation/default.aspx
Institute of HeartMath: Connecting Hearts and Minds, www.heartmath.org
Learnthat: How to Cope with Stress—Stress Management Tutorial and Exercises, learnthat.com/2004/11/stress-management-and-relief
National Hospice and Palliative Care Organization (NHPCO), www.nhpco.org
Physiological Stress Response: Its Effects on the Body, www.stressfocus.com/stress_focus_article/physiological-stress-effects.htm
The Psychology of "Stress," www.guidetopsychology.com/stress.htm
Stress: The Silent Killer, http://holisticonline.com/stress/stress_GAS.htm

Anxiety
Anxiety and Depression Association of America (ADAA), www.adaa.org

Bereavement
The Compassionate Friends, www.compassionatefriends.org
Widowed Persons Service, 3950 Ferrara Dr, Silver Spring, MD; 1-301-949-7398

7

Overview of Transcultural Nursing

Learning Objectives

On completion of this chapter, the learner will be able to:

1 Identify key components of cultural assessment.
2 Apply transcultural nursing principles, concepts, and theories when providing nursing care to individuals, families, groups, and communities.
3 Develop strategies for planning, providing, and evaluating culturally competent nursing care for patients from diverse backgrounds.

4 Critically analyze the influence of culture on nursing care decisions and actions for patients.
5 Discuss the impact of diversity and health care disparities on health care delivery.

Glossary

culture: the knowledge, belief, art, morals, laws, customs, and any other capabilities and habits acquired by humans as members of society

cultural awareness or sensitivity: being alert to and having knowledge of cultural preferences, aspects, or perspectives that may impact the health care experience, including communication, personal choices, or other elements

cultural humility: acknowledging one's cultural knowledge deficits using self-reflection, continuous self-evaluation, and consultation with others (including patients) to detect barriers to culturally competent care and address bias, or lack of knowledge or skills related to a culture other than one's own, to provide culturally appropriate care

cultural nursing assessment: a systematic appraisal or examination of individuals, families, groups, and communities in terms of their cultural beliefs, values, and practices

culturally competent nursing care: effective, individualized care that demonstrates respect for the dignity, personal rights, preferences, beliefs, and practices of the person receiving care while acknowledging the biases of the caregiver and preventing these biases from interfering with the care provided

ethnocentrism: making a value judgment on another culture from the vantage point of one's own culture

minority: a group of people whose physical or cultural characteristics differ from the dominant culture or majority of people in a society

subculture: relatively large groups of people who share characteristics that identify them as a distinct entity

transcultural nursing: nursing care to clients and families across cultural variations

In the health care delivery system, as in society, nurses interact with people of similar as well as diverse cultural backgrounds. People may have different frames of reference and varied preferences regarding their health and health care needs, depending on their cultures. Nurses must often practice **transcultural nursing**, which is defined as providing care to clients and families across cultural variations. Acknowledging, respecting, and adapting to the cultural needs of patients, families, and communities are important components of nursing care. In addition, facilitating access to culturally appropriate health care is critical to ensure holistic nursing care. To plan and deliver culturally appropriate and competent care, nurses must understand the language of culture, culturally appropriate care, and cultural competence and the various aspects of culture that should be explored for each patient.

Cultural Concepts

The concept of culture and its relationship to the health care beliefs and practices of the patient and his or her family or significant others provide the foundation for transcultural nursing. This awareness of culture in the delivery of nursing care has been described in different terms and phrases, including respect for cultural diversity or cultural humility; cultural awareness or sensitivity; comprehensive care; and culturally competent, appropriate care (Giger, Davidhizar, Purnell, et al., 2007), or culturally congruent nursing care (Higginbottom, Magdelena, Richter, et al., 2011; Leininger, 2002).

Culture is commonly defined as the knowledge, belief, art, morals, laws, customs, and any other capabilities and habits acquired by humans as members of society. During the past century, and especially during recent decades, hundreds of definitions of culture have been offered that integrate these themes as well as the themes of ethnic variations of a population based on race, nationality, religion, language, physical characteristics, and geography (Higginbottom et al., 2011). To fully appreciate the broad impact of culture, factors such as disabilities, gender, social class, physical appearance (e.g., weight, height), ideologies (political views), or sexual orientation also must be integrated into the definition of culture (Dayer-Berenson, 2011).

Madeleine Leininger (2002), founder of the specialty known as transcultural nursing, writes that culture involves learned and transmitted knowledge about values, beliefs, rules of behavior, and lifestyle practices that guide designated groups in their thinking and actions in patterned ways. Culture develops over time as a result of exposure to social and religious structures and intellectual and artistic manifestations, and each individual person, including each nurse, is culturally unique (Giger & Davidhizar, 2012).

Ethnic culture has four basic characteristics:
- It is learned from birth through language and socialization.
- It is shared by members of the same cultural group, and it includes an internal sense and external perception of distinctiveness.
- It is influenced by specific conditions related to environmental and technical factors and to the availability of resources.
- It is dynamic and ever changing.

With the exception of the first characteristic, culture related to age, physical appearance, and lifestyle, as well as other less frequently acknowledged aspects, also shares these characteristics.

Cultural diversity has also been defined in several ways. Often, differences in skin color, religion, and geographic area are the only elements used to identify diversity, with ethnic minorities being considered the primary sources of cultural diversity. However, many other sources of cultural diversity exist. To truly acknowledge the cultural differences that may influence health care delivery, the nurse must confront bias and recognize the influence of his or her own culture and cultural heritage on the care provided to patients (Dayer-Berenson, 2011).

Cultural humility—addressing one's cultural knowledge deficit(s) by exploring the patient's needs from the patient's cultural perspective and exploring one's own cultural beliefs and how they might conflict with the patient's beliefs—is a critical step toward becoming culturally competent (Giger & Davidhizar, 2012). Understanding the diversity within cultures, such as subcultures, is also important. In addition, culturally competent care involves facilitating patient access to culturally appropriate resources (Dayer-Berenson, 2011; Williamson & Harrison, 2010).

Subcultures

Although culture is a universal phenomenon, it takes on specific and distinctive features for a particular group because it encompasses all of the knowledge, beliefs, customs, and skills acquired by the members of that group. When such groups function within a larger cultural group, they are referred to as subcultures.

The term **subculture** is used for relatively large groups of people who share characteristics that identify them as a distinct entity. Examples of American subcultures based on ethnicity (i.e., subcultures with common traits such as physical characteristics, language, or ancestry) include African Americans, Hispanic/Latino Americans, Asian/Pacific Islanders, and Native Americans. Each of these subcultures may be further divided; for example, Native Americans consist of American Indians and Alaska Natives, who represent more than 500 federally and state-recognized tribes in addition to an unknown number of tribes that are not officially recognized.

Subcultures may also be based on religion (more than 1,200 religions exist in the United States), occupation (e.g., nurses, physicians, other members of the health care team), disability (e.g., the deaf community), or illness (e.g., heart disease, cerebrovascular disease). In addition, subcultures may be based on age (e.g., infants, children, adolescents, adults, older adults), gender (e.g., male, female), sexual orientation (e.g., homosexual, bisexual, heterosexual), or geographic location (e.g., Texan, Southern, Appalachian).

Nurses should also be sensitive to interracial differences when providing care to individuals of cultures with which the nurse is unfamiliar. Differences between individuals in subcultures in a designated group add to the challenge to plan and provide culturally competent care. Focusing on cultural "norms" while ignoring individual uniqueness could offend or anger patients and result in stereotyped care that is not truly culturally appropriate for that patient (Lowes & Archibald, 2009). Nurses must refrain from culturally stereotyping patients. Instead, nurses should consult patients or significant others regarding personal values, beliefs, preferences, and cultural identification. This strategy is also applicable for members of nonethnic subcultures.

Minorities

The term **minority** refers to a group of people whose physical or cultural characteristics differ from the dominant culture or majority of people in a society. Minorities may be singled out or isolated from others in society or treated in different or unequal ways. The 2010 census identified four racial groups, as "other than White," including Blacks/African Americans, Asians, Native Hawaiian or Other Pacific Islanders, and Native Americans–American Indian or Alaska Natives (Humes, Jones, & Ramerez, 2011). In addition, ethnicity in Hispanic or Latino origin was assessed separately from race in the 2010 census (Enis, Rios-Vargas, & Albert, 2011). Generally, persons belonging to these non-White racial groups listed or who identified themselves as of Hispanic or Latino origin are considered minorities in the United States. However, the concept of "minority" varies widely and must be understood in a cultural context. For example, men may be considered a minority in the nursing profession but constitute a majority in other fields, such as engineering. Because the term *minority* often connotes inferiority, members of many racial and ethnic groups object to being identified as minorities.

Whites/Caucasians may be in the minority in some communities; however, they are the majority group in the United States. Because most health care providers are members of this majority/Caucasian culture, health care tends to be provided from that perspective and services are often biased toward the majority group, with health care disparities noted in many minority populations. Although it has been projected that by the middle to late 21st century Caucasians may no longer represent the majority of Americans (Sullivan Commission, 2004), there is no evidence that this shift will change the perspective from which care is delivered or that disparities in care will be reduced.

Health Disparities

Health disparities—higher rates of morbidity, mortality, and burden of disease in a population or community than found in the overall population—are significant in ethnic and racial minorities. Key health indicators in the United States reveal a significant gap in health status between the overall American population and people of specific ethnic backgrounds (U.S. Department of Health and Human Services [HHS], 2012). Ethnic and racial minorities are disproportionately burdened with cancer, heart disease, diabetes, human immunodeficiency virus (HIV) infection/acquired immunodeficiency syndrome (AIDS), and other conditions. They receive a lower quality of health care than nonminorities and are at greater risk for declining health. Health disparities also occur with women, gay, lesbian, and transgender people, as well as with people who have disabilities (HHS, 2012). Many reasons are cited for these disparities, including low socioeconomic status, health behaviors, limited access to health care because of poverty or disability, environmental factors, and direct and indirect manifestations of discrimination. Other causes include lack of health insurance; overdependence on publicly funded facilities; and barriers to health care such as insufficient transportation, geographic location (not enough providers in an area), cost of services, and the low numbers of minority health care providers (Institute of Medicine, 2003; HHS, 2012; Sullivan Commission, 2004).

Transcultural Nursing

The term *transcultural nursing* is used interchangeably with cross-cultural, intercultural, or multicultural nursing and refers to research-focused practice that focuses on patient-centered, culturally competent nursing (Giger & Davidhizar, 2012). Transcultural nursing addresses the differences and similarities among cultures in relation to health, health care, and illness. Furthermore, it incorporates the care (caring) values, beliefs, and practices of people and groups from a particular culture without imposing the nurse's cultural perspective on the patient. The underlying focus of transcultural nursing is to provide culture-specific and culture-universal care that promotes the well-being or health of individuals, families, groups, communities, and institutions (Giger & Davidhizar, 2012; Leininger, 2002). All people, as well as the community or institution at large, benefit when culturally competent care is provided. When the care is delivered beyond a nurse's national boundaries, the term *international* or *transnational nursing* is often used.

Although many nurses, anthropologists, and others have written about the cultural aspects of nursing and health care,

Leininger (2002) developed a comprehensive research-based theory—Culture Care Diversity and Universality—to promote culturally congruent nursing for people of different or similar cultures. This means promoting recovery from illness, preventing conditions that would limit the patient's health or well-being, or facilitating a peaceful death in ways that are culturally meaningful and appropriate.

Leininger's theory stresses the importance of providing culturally congruent nursing care (meaningful and beneficial health care tailored to fit the patient's cultural values, beliefs, and lifestyles) through culture care accommodation and culture care restructuring. *Culture care accommodation* refers to professional actions and decisions that nurses make on behalf of those in their care to help people of a designated culture achieve a beneficial or satisfying health outcome. *Culture care restructuring* or repatterning refers to professional actions and decisions that help patients reorder, change, or modify their lifestyles toward new, different, or more beneficial health care patterns (Fig. 7-1). At the same time, the patient's cultural values and beliefs are respected and a better or healthier lifestyle results. Other terms and definitions that provide further insight into culture and health care include the following:

- *Acculturation:* the process by which members of a cultural group adapt to or take on the behaviors of another group
- *Cultural blindness:* the inability of people to recognize their own values, beliefs, and practices and those of others because of strong ethnocentric tendencies (the tendency to judge others based on one's own culture)
- *Cultural imposition:* the tendency to impose one's cultural beliefs, values, and patterns of behavior on a person or people from a different culture
- *Cultural taboos:* activities or behaviors that are avoided or prohibited by a particular cultural group

Culturally Competent Nursing Care

Culturally competent nursing care is defined as effective, individualized care that demonstrates respect for the dignity, personal rights, preferences, beliefs, and practices of the person receiving care while acknowledging the biases of the caregiver and preventing these biases from interfering with the care provided. **Cultural awareness or sensitivity**, on the other hand, implies an awareness of cultural differences that might be present in the health care delivery process. The nurse should go beyond sensitivity to leverage awareness of these differences to plan appropriate culturally competent nursing care.

Culturally competent nursing care is a dynamic process that requires comprehensive knowledge of culture-specific information and an awareness of, and sensitivity to, the effect that culture has on the care situation. It requires that the nurse integrate cultural knowledge, awareness of his or her own cultural perspective, and the patient's cultural perspectives when preparing and implementing a plan of care (Giger & Davidhizar, 2012). Culturally competent nursing care also incorporates the delivery of interventions that are congruent with a given culture. It involves a complex integration of attitudes, knowledge, and skills (including assessment, decision making, judgments, critical thinking, and evaluation) that enables nurses to provide culturally appropriate care.

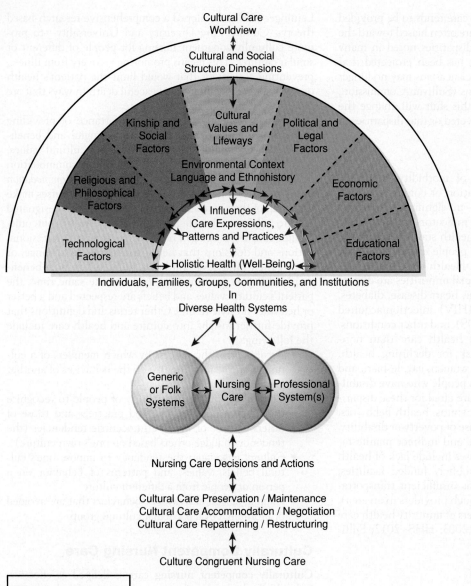

Cultural Care
Worldview

Cultural and Social
Structure Dimensions

Cultural
Values and
Lifeways

Kinship and
Social
Factors

Political and
Legal
Factors

Environmental Context
Language and Ethnohistory

Religious and
Philosophical
Factors

Economic
Factors

Influences
Care Expressions,
Patterns and Practices

Technological
Factors

Educational
Factors

Holistic Health (Well-Being)

Individuals, Families, Groups, Communities, and Institutions
In
Diverse Health Systems

Generic
or Folk
Systems

Nursing
Care

Professional
System(s)

Nursing Care Decisions and Actions

Cultural Care Preservation / Maintenance
Cultural Care Accommodation / Negotiation
Cultural Care Repatterning / Restructuring

Culture Congruent Nursing Care

Code ⟷ Influences

FIGURE 7-1 • Leininger's Sunrise Model depicts her theory of cultural care diversity and universality. From Leininger, M. M. (Ed.). (2001). *Culture care diversity and university: A theory of nursing.* New York: National League for Nursing Press.

Agency policies are important to achieve culturally competent care. Policies that promote culturally competent care establish flexible regulations pertaining to visitors (number, frequency, and length of visits), provide translation services for non–English-speaking patients, and train staff to provide care for patients with different cultural values (Dayer-Berenson, 2011). Culturally competent policies are developed to promote an environment in which the traditional healing, spiritual, and religious practices of patients are respected and encouraged and to recognize the special dietary practices of patients from selected cultural groups.

Giger and Davidhizar (2012) created an assessment model to guide nurses in exploring cultural phenomena that might affect nursing care. They identified communication, space, time orientation, social organization, environmental control, and biologic variations as relevant phenomena. This model has been used in various patient care settings to

provide data that is essential to the provision of culturally competent care.

Cross-Cultural Communication

Establishment of an environment of culturally congruent care and respect begins with effective communication, which occurs not only through words but also through body language and other cues, such as voice, tone, and loudness. Nurse–patient interactions, as well as communication among members of a multicultural health care team, depend on the ability to understand and be understood.

Approximately 150 different languages are spoken in the United States, with Spanish most common after English. Obviously, nurses cannot become fluent in all languages; however, certain strategies for fostering effective cross-cultural communication are necessary when providing care for patients who are not fluent in English. Cultural needs should be considered when choosing an interpreter; for instance, fluency in varied dialects is beneficial (Dayer-Berenson, 2011). The interpreter's voice quality, pronunciation, use of silence, use of touch, and use of nonverbal communication should also be considered (Giger & Davidhizar, 2012). The interpreter should not be a member of the patient's family, because that violates the patient's right to privacy and causes undue stress on the family member.

During illness, patients of all ages tend to regress, and the regression often involves language skills. Chart 7-1 summarizes strategies for overcoming language barriers. Nurses should also assess how well patients and families have

Chart 7-1 | Overcoming Language Barriers

- Greet the patient using the last or complete name. Avoid being too casual or familiar. Point to yourself and say your name. Smile.
- Proceed in an unhurried manner. Pay attention to any effort by the patient or family to communicate.
- Speak in a low, moderate voice. Avoid talking loudly. Remember that there is a tendency to raise the volume and pitch of your voice when the listener appears not to understand. The listener may perceive that you are shouting or angry.
- Organize your thoughts. Repeat and summarize frequently. Use audiovisual aids when feasible.
- Use short, simple sentence structure, and speak in the active voice.
- Use simple words, such as "pain" rather than "discomfort." Avoid medical jargon, idioms, and slang. Avoid using contractions, such as don't, can't, won't.
- Use nouns repeatedly instead of pronouns. *Example:* Do not say: "He has been taking his medicine, hasn't he?" Do say: "Does Juan take his medicine?"
- Pantomime words (use gestures) and simple actions while verbalizing them.
- Give instructions in the proper sequence. *Example:* Do not say: "Before you rinse the bottle, sterilize it." Do say: "First, wash the bottle. Second, rinse the bottle."
- Discuss one topic at a time, and avoid giving too much information in a single conversation. Avoid using conjunctions. *Example:* Do not say: "Are you cold and in pain?" Do say (while pantomiming/gesturing): "Are you cold?" "Are you in pain?"
- Talk directly to the patient rather than to the person who accompanied him or her.
- Validate whether the person understands by having him or her repeat instructions, demonstrate the procedure, or act out the meaning.
- Use any words that you know in the person's language. This indicates that you are aware of and respect the patient's primary means of communicating.
- Try a third language. Many Indo-Chinese speak French. Europeans often know three or four languages. Try Latin words or phrases, if you are familiar with the language.
- Be aware of culturally based gender and age differences and diverse socioeconomic, educational, and tribal or regional differences when choosing an interpreter.
- Obtain phrase books from a library or bookstore, make or purchase flash cards, contact hospitals for a list of interpreters, and use both formal and informal networking to locate a suitable interpreter. Although they are costly, some telecommunication companies provide translation services.

understood what has been said. The following cues may signify a lack of effective communication:

- *Efforts to change the subject:* This could indicate that the listener does not understand what was said and is attempting to talk about something more familiar.
- *Absence of questions:* Paradoxically, this often means that the listener is not grasping the message and therefore has difficulty formulating questions to ask.
- *Inappropriate laughter:* A self-conscious giggle may signal poor comprehension and may be an attempt to disguise embarrassment.
- *Nonverbal cues:* A blank expression may signal poor understanding. However, among some Asian Americans, it may reflect a desire to avoid overt expression of emotion. Avoidance of eye contact may be a cultural expression of respect for the speaker among some Native Americans and Asian Americans.

Culturally Mediated Characteristics

Nurses should be aware that patients act and behave in various ways, in part because of the influence of culture on behaviors and attitudes. However, although certain attributes and attitudes are frequently associated with particular cultural groups, as described in this chapter, it is important to remember that not all people from the same cultural background share the same behaviors and views. Although nurses who fail to consider patients' cultural preferences and beliefs are considered insensitive and possibly indifferent, nurses who assume that all members of any one culture act and behave in the same way run the risk of stereotyping people. As stated previously, the best way to avoid stereotyping is to view each patient as an individual and to assess the patient's cultural preferences. A thorough culture assessment using a culture assessment tool or questionnaire (see later discussion) is very beneficial.

Information Disclosure

Many aspects of care may be influenced by the diverse cultural perspectives held by health care providers, patients, families, or significant others. One example is the issue of communication and full disclosure. In general, nurses may argue that patients have the right to full disclosure concerning their disease and prognosis and may believe that advocacy means working to provide that disclosure. However, family members in some cultural backgrounds may believe that it is their responsibility to protect and spare the patient (their loved one) knowledge about a terminal illness. In some cultures, the head of the family group, elder, or husband is expected to receive all information and make decisions. Patients may in fact not want to know about their condition and may expect their family members to "take the burden" of that knowledge and related decision making. Nurses should not decide that a family or patient is simply wrong or that a patient must know all of the details of his or her illness regardless of the patient's preference. Similar concerns may be noted when patients refuse pain medication or treatment because of cultural beliefs regarding pain or beliefs in divine intervention or faith healing.

Determining the most appropriate and ethical approach to patient care requires an exploration of the cultural aspects of these situations. Self-examination and recognition of one's own cultural bias and worldview, as discussed earlier, play a major part in helping the nurse resolve cultural and ethical conflicts. Nurses must promote open dialogue and work with patients, families, physicians, and other health care providers to reach the culturally appropriate solution for the individual patient.

Space and Distance

People tend to regard the space in their immediate vicinity as an extension of themselves. The amount of space that they need between themselves and others to feel comfortable is a culturally determined phenomenon.

Because nurses and patients usually are not consciously aware of their personal space requirements, they frequently have difficulty understanding different behaviors. For example, one patient may perceive the nurse sitting close to him or her as an expression of warmth and care; another patient may perceive the nurse's act as a threatening invasion of personal space. Research reveals that people from the United States, Canada, and Great Britain require the most personal space between themselves and others, whereas those from Latin America, Japan, and the Middle East need the least amount of space and feel comfortable standing close to others (Giger & Davidhizar, 2012).

If the patient appears to position himself or herself too close or too far away, the nurse should consider cultural preferences for space and distance. Ideally, the patient should be permitted to assume a position that is comfortable to him or her in terms of personal space and distance. The nurse should be aware that the wheelchair of a person with a disability is considered an extension of the person; therefore, the nurse should ask the person's permission before moving or touching the wheelchair. Because a significant amount of communication during nursing care requires close physical contact, the nurse should be aware of these important cultural differences and consider them when providing care (Smith-Temple & Johnson, 2010).

Eye Contact

Eye contact is also a culturally determined behavior. Although most nurses have been taught to maintain eye contact when speaking with patients, some people from certain cultural backgrounds may interpret this behavior differently. For example, some Asians, Native Americans, Indo-Chinese, Arabs, and Appalachians may consider direct eye contact impolite or aggressive, and they may avert their own eyes when talking with nurses and others whom they perceive to be in positions of authority. Some Native Americans stare at the floor during conversations—a cultural behavior conveying respect and indicating that the listener is paying close attention to the speaker. Some Hispanic patients maintain downcast eyes as a sign of culturally appropriate deferential behavior toward others on the basis of age, gender, social position, economic status, and position of authority (Giger & Davidhizar, 2012). The nurse who is aware that eye contact may be culturally determined can better understand the patient's behavior and provide an atmosphere in which the patient can feel comfortable.

Time

Attitudes about time vary widely among cultures and can be a barrier to effective communication between nurses and patients. Views about punctuality and the use of time are culturally determined, as is the concept of waiting. Symbols of time, such as watches, sunrises, and sunsets, represent methods for measuring the duration and passage of time (Giger & Davidhizar, 2012).

For most health care providers, time and promptness are extremely important. For example, nurses frequently expect patients to arrive at an exact time for an appointment, although patients are often kept waiting by health care providers who are running late. Health care providers are likely to function according to an appointment system in which there are short intervals of perhaps only a few minutes. However, for patients from some cultures, time is a relative phenomenon, with little attention paid to the exact hour or minute. For example, some Hispanic people consider time in a wider frame of reference and make the primary distinction between day and night. Time may also be determined according to traditional times for meals, sleep, and other activities or events. For people from some cultures, the present is of the greatest importance, and time is viewed in broad ranges rather than in terms of a fixed hour. Being flexible in regard to schedules is the best way to accommodate these differences.

Value differences also may influence a person's sense of priority when it comes to time. For example, responding to a family matter may be more important to a patient than meeting a scheduled health care appointment. Allowing for these different views is essential in maintaining an effective nurse–patient relationship. Scolding or acting annoyed at patients for being late undermines their confidence and may result in further missed appointments or indifference to health care suggestions.

Touch

The meaning that people associate with touching is culturally determined to a great degree. In some cultures (e.g., Hispanic, Arab), male health care providers may be prohibited from touching or examining certain parts of the female body. Similarly, it may be inappropriate for females to care for males. Among many Asians, it is impolite to touch a person's head because the spirit is believed to reside there. Therefore, assessment of the head or evaluation of a head injury requires permission of the patient or a family member, if the patient is not able to give permission.

The patient's culturally defined sense of modesty must also be considered when providing nursing care. For example, some Jewish and Muslim women believe that modesty requires covering their head, arms, and legs with clothing.

Observance of Holidays

People from all cultures observe certain civil and religious holidays. Nurses should familiarize themselves with major observances for members of the cultural groups they serve. Information about these observances is available from various sources, including religious organizations, hospital chaplains, and patients themselves. Routine health appointments, diagnostic tests, surgery, and other major procedures should be scheduled to avoid observances that patients identify as significant. If not contraindicated, efforts should also be made to accommodate patients and families or significant others who wish to perform cultural and religious rituals in the health care setting.

Diet

The cultural context of food varies widely but usually includes one or more of the following: relief of hunger; promotion of health and healing; prevention of disease or illness; expression of caring for another; promotion of interpersonal closeness among individual people, families, groups, communities, or nations; and promotion of kinship and family alliances. Food is also associated with strengthening of social ties; celebration of life events (e.g., birthdays, marriages, funerals); expression of gratitude or appreciation; recognition of achievement or accomplishment; validation of social, cultural, or religious ceremonial functions; facilitation of business negotiations; and expression of affluence, wealth, or social status.

Culture determines which foods are served and when they are served, the number and frequency of meals, who eats with whom, and who receives the choicest portions. Culture also determines how foods are prepared and served, how they are eaten (with chopsticks, hands, or fork, knife, and spoon), and where people shop (e.g., ethnic grocery stores, specialty food markets). Culture also determines the impact of excess weight and obesity on self-esteem and social standing. In some cultures, physical bulk is viewed as a sign of affluence and health (e.g., a chubby baby is a healthy baby).

Religious practices may include fasting (e.g., Mormons, Catholics, Buddhists, Jews, Muslims) and abstaining from selected foods at particular times (e.g., Catholics abstain from meat on Ash Wednesday and on Fridays during Lent). Practices may also include the ritualistic use of food and beverages (e.g., Passover dinner, consumption of bread and wine during religious ceremonies). Chart 7-2 summarizes some prohibited foods and beverages of selected religious groups.

Most groups feast, often in the company of family and friends, on selected holidays. For example, many Christians eat large dinners on Christmas and Easter and consume other traditional high-calorie, high-fat foods, such as seasonal cookies, pastries, and candies. These culturally based dietary practices are especially significant in the care of patients with diabetes, hypertension, gastrointestinal disorders, obesity, and other conditions in which diet plays a key role in the treatment and health maintenance regimen.

Biologic Variations

Along with psychosocial adaptations, nurses must also consider the physiologic impact of culture on patients' response to treatment, particularly medications. Data have been collected for many years regarding differences in the effect that some medications have on people of diverse ethnic or cultural origins. Genetic predispositions to different rates of metabolism cause some patients to be prone to adverse reactions to the standard dose of a medication, whereas other patients are likely to experience a greatly reduced benefit from the standard dose of the medication. For example, an antihypertensive agent may work well at reducing blood pressure to acceptable levels for a Caucasian man within a 4-week time

---

Chart 7-2 **Prohibited Foods and Beverages of Selected Religious Groups**

Hinduism

All meats
Animal shortenings/fats

Islam

Pork
Alcoholic products and beverages (including extracts, such as vanilla and lemon)
Animal shortenings
Gelatin made from pork, marshmallow, and other confections made with gelatin
Note: Halal is lawful food that may be consumed according to tenets of the Koran, whereas *Haram* is food that is unlawful to consume.

Judaism

Pork
Predatory fowl
Shellfish and scavenger fish (e.g., shrimp, crab, lobster, escargot, catfish). Fish with fins and scales are permissible.
Mixing milk and meat dishes at same meal
Blood by ingestion (e.g., blood sausage, raw meat).
Note: Packaged foods will contain labels identifying kosher ("properly preserved" or "fitting") and pareve (made without meat or milk) items.

Mormonism (Church of Jesus Christ of Latter-Day Saints)

Alcohol
Beverages containing caffeine stimulants (coffee, tea, colas, and selected carbonated soft drinks)

Seventh-Day Adventism

Alcohol
Beverages containing caffeine stimulants (coffee, tea, colas, and selected carbonated soft drinks)
Pork
Certain seafood, including shellfish
Fermented beverages
Note: Optional vegetarianism is encouraged.

---

span but may take much longer to work or not work at all for an African American man with hypertension. General polymorphism—biologic variation in response to medications resulting from patient age, gender, size, and body composition—has long been acknowledged by the health care community (Rugnetta & Desai, 2011). Nurses must be aware that ethnicity and related factors such as values and beliefs regarding the use of herbal supplements, dietary intake, and genetic factors can affect the effectiveness of treatment and adherence to the treatment regimen (Giger & Davidhizar, 2012).

Complementary and Alternative Therapies

Interventions for alterations in health and wellness vary among cultures. Interventions most commonly used in the United States have been labeled as *conventional medicine* by the National Institutes of Health (National Center for Complementary and Alternative Medicine [NCCAM], 2012). Other names for conventional medicine are allopathy, Western medicine, regular medicine, mainstream medicine, and biomedicine. Therapy used to replace or supplement conventional medicine may be referred to as *complementary or alternative therapy*. Interest in interventions that are not an integral part of conventional medicine prompted the National Institutes of Health to create the Office of Alternative Medicine and then to establish NCCAM.

According to a nationwide survey, 38% of adults in the United States use some form of complementary and alternative medicine. This percentage increases to 75% when prayer specifically for health reasons is included in the definition. Complementary and alternative interventions are classified into five main categories: alternative medical systems, mind–body interventions, biologically based therapies, manipulative and body-based methods, and energy therapies (NCCAM, 2012):

- *Alternative medical systems* are defined as complete systems of theory and practice that are different from conventional medicine. Some examples are traditional Eastern medicine (including acupuncture, herbal medicine, Oriental massage, and Qi gong); India's traditional medicine, Ayurveda (including diet, exercise, meditation, herbal medicine, massage, exposure to sunlight, and controlled breathing to restore harmony of a person's body, mind, and spirit); homeopathic medicine (including the use of herbal medicine and minerals); and naturopathic medicine (including diet, acupuncture, herbal medicine, hydrotherapy, spinal and soft tissue manipulation, electrical currents, ultrasound and light therapy, therapeutic counseling, and pharmacology).
- *Mind–body interventions* are defined as techniques to facilitate the mind's ability to affect symptoms and bodily functions. Some examples are meditation, dance, music, art therapy, prayer, and mental healing.
- *Biologically based therapies* are defined as natural and biologically based practices, interventions, and products. Some examples are herbal therapies (a plant or plant part that produces and contains chemical substances that act on the body), special diet therapies (such as those of Drs. Atkins, Ornish, and Pritikin), orthomolecular therapies (magnesium, melatonin, megadoses of vitamins), and biologic therapies (shark cartilage, bee pollen).
- *Manipulative and body-based methods* are defined as interventions based on body movement. Some examples are chiropractic (primarily manipulation of the spine), osteopathic manipulation, massage therapy (soft tissue manipulation), and reflexology.
- *Energy therapies* are defined as interventions that focus on energy fields within the body (biofields) or externally (electromagnetic fields). Some examples are Qi gong, Reiki, therapeutic touch, pulsed electromagnetic fields, magnetic fields, alternating electrical current, and direct electrical current.

Patients may choose to seek an alternative to conventional medical or surgical therapies. Many of these alternative therapies are becoming widely accepted as feasible treatment options. Therapies such as acupuncture and herbal treatments may be recommended by health care providers to address aspects of a condition that are unresponsive to conventional medical treatment or to minimize the side effects associated with conventional medical therapy. Primary providers may work in collaboration with herbalists or with spiritualists or shamans to provide a comprehensive treatment plan. Out of respect for the way of life and beliefs of patients from different cultures, it is often necessary that healers and health care providers respect the strengths of each approach (NCCAM, 2012).

Complementary therapy is becoming more common as health care consumers learn what information is available in printed media and on the Internet. As patients become more informed, they are more likely to participate in various therapies in conjunction with their conventional medical treatments (NCCAM, 2012). Nurses must assess all patients for the use of complementary therapies, be alert to the danger of herb–drug interactions or conflicting treatments, and be prepared to provide information to patients about treatments that may be harmful. However, nurses must be accepting of patients' beliefs and right to autonomy—that is, to control their own care. As patient advocates, nurses facilitate the integration of conventional medical, complementary, and alternative therapies.

Causes of Illness

People may view illness differently. Three major views, or paradigms, attempt to explain the causes of disease and illness: the biomedical or scientific view, the naturalistic or holistic perspective, and the magico-religious view.

Biomedical or Scientific View

The biomedical or scientific worldview prevails in most health care settings and is embraced by most nurses and other health care providers. The basic assumptions underlying the biomedical perspective are that all events in life have a cause and effect, that the human body functions much like a machine, and that all of reality can be observed and measured (e.g., blood pressures, partial pressure of arterial oxygen [PaO_2] levels, intelligence tests). One example of the biomedical or scientific view is the bacterial or viral explanation of communicable diseases.

Naturalistic or Holistic Perspective

The naturalistic or holistic perspective is another viewpoint that explains the cause of illness and is commonly embraced by many Native Americans, Asians, and others. According to this view, the forces of nature must be kept in natural balance or harmony.

One example of a naturalistic belief, held by many Asian groups, is the yin/yang theory, in which health is believed to exist when all aspects of a person are in perfect balance or harmony. Rooted in the ancient Chinese philosophy of Taoism (which translates as "The Way"), the yin/yang theory proposes that all organisms and objects in the universe consist of yin and yang energy. The seat of the energy forces is within the autonomic nervous system, where balance between the opposing forces is maintained during health.

Yin energy represents the female and negative forces, such as emptiness, darkness, and cold, whereas the yang forces are male and positive, emitting warmth and fullness. Foods are classified as cold (yin) or hot (yang) in this theory and are transformed into yin and yang energy when metabolized by the body. Cold foods are eaten when a person has a hot illness (e.g., fever, rash, sore throat, ulcer, infection), and hot foods are eaten when a person has a cold illness (e.g., cancer, headache, stomach cramps, "a cold"). The yin/yang theory is the basis for Eastern or Chinese medicine and is embraced by some Asian Americans.

Many Hispanic, African American, and Arab groups also embrace the hot/cold theory of health and illness. The four humors of the body—blood, phlegm, black bile, and yellow bile—are believed to regulate basic bodily functions and are described in terms of temperature and moisture. The treatment of disease consists of adding or subtracting cold, heat, dryness, or wetness to restore the balance of these humors. Beverages, foods, herbs, medicines, and diseases are classified as hot or cold according to their perceived effects on the body, not their physical characteristics. According to the hot/cold theory, the person as a whole, not just a particular ailment, is significant. People who embrace the hot/cold theory maintain that health consists of a positive state of total well-being, including physical, psychological, spiritual, and social aspects of the person.

According to the naturalistic worldview, breaking the laws of nature creates imbalances, chaos, and disease. People who embrace the naturalistic paradigm use metaphors such as "the healing power of nature." For example, from the perspective of many Chinese people, illness is viewed not as an intruding agent but as a part of life's rhythmic course and an outward sign of disharmony within.

Magico-Religious View

Another major way in which people view the world and explain the causes of illness is the magico-religious worldview. This view's basic premise is that the world is an arena in which supernatural forces dominate, and that the fate of the world and those in it depends on the action of supernatural forces for good or evil. Examples of magical causes of illness include belief in voodoo or witchcraft among some African Americans and people from Caribbean countries. Faith healing is based on religious beliefs and is most prevalent among selected Christian religions, including Christian Science, whereas various healing rituals may be found in many other religions, such as Roman Catholicism and Mormonism (Church of Jesus Christ of Latter-Day Saints).

Of course, it is possible to hold a combination of worldviews, and many patients offer more than one explanation for the cause of their illness. As a profession, nursing largely embraces the scientific or biomedical worldview; however, some aspects of holism have begun to gain popularity, including various techniques for managing chronic pain, such as hypnosis, therapeutic touch, and biofeedback. Belief in spiritual power is also held by many nurses who credit supernatural forces with various unexplained phenomena related to patients' health and illness states. Regardless of the view held and whether the nurse agrees with the patient's beliefs in this regard, it is important to be aware of how the person views

illness and health and to work within this framework to promote patient care and well-being.

Folk Healers

People of some cultures believe in folk or indigenous healers. For example, nurses may find that some Hispanic patients may seek help from a *curandero* or *curandera* (spiritual healer, folk doctor, shaman), *espiritualista* (spiritualist), *yuyero* (herbalist), or *sanador* (healer who manipulates bones and muscles). Some African American patients may seek assistance from a *hougan* (voodoo priest or priestess), spiritualist, root doctor (usually a woman who uses magic rituals to treat diseases), or "old lady" (an older woman who has successfully raised a family and who specializes in child care and folk remedies). Native American patients may seek assistance from a shaman or medicine man or woman. Asian patients may mention that they have visited herbalists, acupuncturists, or bone setters. Several cultures have their own healers, most of whom speak the native tongue of that culture, make house calls, and charge significantly less than healers practicing in the conventional medical health care system.

People seeking complementary and alternative therapies have expanded the practices of folk healers beyond their traditional populations; therefore, the nurse should ask the patient about use of folk healers regardless of the patient's cultural background. Nurses should not disregard the patient's belief in folk healers or try to undermine trust in the healers, because doing so may alienate the patient and drive him or her away from receiving the prescribed care. Instead, nurses should try to accommodate the patient's beliefs while advocating the treatment proposed by health science (Chart 7-3).

Cultural Nursing Assessment

Cultural nursing assessment refers to a systematic appraisal or examination of individuals, families, groups, and communities in terms of their cultural beliefs, values, and practices. The purpose of such an assessment is to provide culturally competent care (Higginbottom et al., 2011). In an effort to establish a database for determining a patient's cultural background, nurses have developed cultural assessment tools or modified existing assessment tools (Leininger, 2002) to ensure that transcultural considerations are included in the plan of care. Giger and Davidhizar's model has been used to design nursing care from health promotion to nursing skills activities (Giger & Davidhizar, 2012; Smith-Temple & Johnson, 2010). The information presented in this chapter and the general guidelines presented in Chart 7-4 can be used to direct nursing assessment of culture and its influence on a patient's health beliefs and practices.

Additional Cultural Considerations: Know Thyself

Because the nurse–patient interaction is the focal point of nursing, nurses must consider their own cultural orientation when conducting assessments of patients and their families

ETHICAL DILEMMA

Chart 7-3

When May Folk Remedies Be Considered Harmful or Complementary?

Case Scenario

You are working in an urban neighborhood health clinic. An 80-year-old woman who is a Hmong immigrant presents with a 7-day history of chills, loss of appetite, fatigue, dizziness, and an unintended weight loss of 5 pounds. The woman's adult daughter has brought her to the clinic, and they both insist to be present during assessment. When you begin to listen to the woman's lung sounds, you incidentally note that she has tracks of petechiae across both scapular regions of her back in a symmetric pattern. You ask her how this happened, and her daughter interjects, "That is from *cao gio,* but it didn't seem to work right this time, because she is still very sick. That is the reason we are here now." You have heard that in some Hmong communities, *cao gio,* or coin rubbing, is practiced as a folk remedy and that the intent of this treatment is to "rub out bad winds."

Discussion

There are many folk remedies that recent immigrants to the United States may continue to use to treat various ailments. Some of these may be complementary to traditional Western medicine, whereas others may be considered harmful therapies in that they may result in delays to seek traditional routes to treatment or may otherwise result in harm to the patient. The American Nurses Association (1991) advises the professional nurse to be cognizant when his or her own ethnocentrism is present during interactions with patients of a different culture—that is, a belief that the nurse's culturally accepted way of practicing health care is inherently superior to another culturally acceptable health care practice.

Analysis

- Describe the ethical principles that are in conflict in this case (see Chart 3-3). Which principle should have preeminence as you proceed with your assessment of this patient?
- Describe any concerns that you may have regarding preservation of the patient's autonomy. What steps might you take to assure that her autonomy is preserved?
- Coin rubbing is a relatively common folk remedy among many people from southeastern Asian cultures. How can you determine whether the marks you find on this patient signify that she may be a victim of elder abuse rather than a willing recipient of a folk remedy? How do you ensure that the patient is not harmed (i.e., ensure nonmaleficence)?
- Assume that you find that the patient has full capacity to make competent decisions and that she does indeed value the traditional practice of *cao gio.* How do you professionally reconcile that she has sought to treat her illness with a folk remedy before seeking traditional care? Does her right to make an autonomous decision over her health care trump your desire that she seek traditional health care sooner (or, in this case, does the principle of autonomy outweigh the dual principles of beneficence and nonmaleficence)?

Reference

American Nurses Association. (1991). *Cultural diversity in nursing practice.* Available at: www.nursingworld.org/MainMenuCategories/Policy-Advocacy/Positions-and-Resolutions/ANAPositionStatements/Position-Statements-Alphabetically/prtetcldv14444.html

Resources

See Chapter 3, Chart 3-6 for ethics resources.

ASSESSMENT

Chart 7-4

Assessing for Patients' Cultural Beliefs

- What is the patient's country of origin? How long has the patient lived in this country? What is the patient's primary language and education level*?
- What is the patient's ethnic background? Does he or she identify strongly with others from the same cultural background?
- What is the patient's religion, and how important is it to his or her daily life?
- Does the patient participate in cultural activities such as dressing in traditional clothing and observing traditional holidays and festivals?
- Does the patient have any food preferences or restrictions?
- What are the patient's communication styles? Is eye contact avoided? How much physical distance is maintained? Is the patient open and verbal about symptoms?
- Who is the head of the family, and is he or she involved in decision making about the patient?
- What does the patient do to maintain his or her health?
- What does the patient think caused the current problem?
- Has the advice of traditional healers been sought?
- Have complementary and alternative therapies been used?
- What kind of treatment does the patient think will help? What are the most important results that he or she hopes to get from this treatment?
- Does the patient observe cultural or religious rituals related to health, sickness, or death?

*Note that education level may or may not correspond with the ability to read and write.

and friends. The following guidelines may prove useful to nurses who want to provide culturally appropriate care:

- Know your own cultural attitudes, values, beliefs, and practices.
- Recognize that despite "good intentions," everyone has cultural "baggage" that ultimately results in **ethnocentrism** (judging another culture based upon standards from one's own culture).
- Acknowledge that it is generally easier to understand those whose cultural heritage is similar to your own, while viewing those who are unlike you as strange and different.
- Maintain a broad, open attitude. Expect the unexpected. Enjoy surprises.
- Avoid seeing all people as alike—that is, avoid cultural stereotypes, such as "all Chinese like rice" or "all Italians eat spaghetti."
- Try to understand the reasons for any behavior by discussing commonalities and differences with representatives of ethnic groups different from your own.
- If a patient has said or done something that you do not understand, ask for clarification. Be a good listener. Most patients will respond positively to questions that arise from a genuine concern for and interest in them.
- If at all possible, speak the patient's language (even simple greetings and social courtesies are appreciated). Avoid feigning an accent or using words that are ordinarily not part of your vocabulary.

- Be yourself. There are no right or wrong ways to learn about cultural diversity.

The Future of Transcultural Nursing Care

By the middle of the 21st century, nearly half of all Americans will trace their ancestry to Africa, Asia, the Pacific Islands, or the Hispanic or Arab worlds, rather than to Europe (Dayer-Berenson, 2011). As indicated previously, the concept of culturally competent care applies to health care institutions, which must develop culturally sensitive policies and provide a climate that fosters the provision of culturally competent care by nurses. Nurses must learn to acknowledge and adapt to diversity among their colleagues in the workplace (Clark, Calvillo, Dela Cruz, et al., 2011).

As the population becomes more culturally diverse, efforts to increase the number of ethnic minority nurses must continue and accelerate (Sullivan Commission, 2004). Today, more than 83% of all nurses are Caucasian (Health Resources and Services Administration [HRSA], 2010). Progress toward increasing the percentage of culturally diverse nurses has been significantly slower than the increasing percentage of ethnic minorities in the United States. Greater efforts must be made to facilitate the recruitment and program completion of nursing students who are members of ethnic minorities. In addition, educational institutions must prepare nurses to deliver culturally competent care and must work to increase the number of ethnic minority providers in the nursing workforce. Nursing programs are exploring creative ways to promote cultural competence and humanistic care in nursing students, including offering multicultural health studies in their curricula. In addition, case studies and simulation modules are being offered in many programs to introduce students to situations that may involve cultural conflicts and facilitate problem solving (McKeon, Norris, Cardell, et al., 2009). Through these pedagogical methods, students may develop the knowledge, skills, and attitudes (KSAs) needed to provide patient-centered care that is consonant with goals set through the Quality and Safety Education for Nurses (QSEN) national nursing education initiative that is funded by the Robert Wood Johnson Foundation (QSEN, 2012).

Cultural diversity remains one of the foremost issues in health care today. Nurses are expected to provide culturally competent care for patients. To do so, nurses must work effectively with the increasing number of patients, nurses, and health care team members whose ancestry reflects the multicultural complexion of contemporary society.

Critical Thinking Exercises

1 **ebp** You are assigned to care for a hospitalized patient who emigrated to the United States from India 5 years ago. You know little about this patient's culture. What is the evidence base for use of a cultural assessment tool to ensure that cultural considerations are included in the nursing plan of care? What best practices and policies located in key organizational books or Internet resources could guide your care for this patient? Explain why it is important to examine your own feelings about the patient's possible cultural beliefs and practices. Is it guaranteed that the common cultural beliefs of persons from India will be the same as this patient's beliefs?

2 A 34-year-old man who was originally from Haiti is hospitalized in the neurosurgical intensive care unit with a traumatic brain injury subsequent to a 30-foot fall from a scaffold. His immediate family members insist on staying with him around the clock, and many extended family members visit each day, staying late into the night. His prognosis is poor, and when his attending physician discusses discontinuing life support therapy with his family members who are his legal next of kin, they acquiesce but request that all family members be allowed to remain present to witness his death. Policies in the intensive care unit do not permit more than three family members to be with a patient at any given time. The staff members complain that they have difficulty completing their tasks with other critically ill patients because of the distractions they face from the multiple family members visiting this man. How can you help the nursing staff explore the meaning of the family's behavior and understand their own negative feelings about this behavior? Devise a strategy that will help resolve this situation.

3 You are a nurse working in a diabetes center. You are assessing a 44-year-old woman newly diagnosed with type 2 diabetes who arrived in United States from Mexico 2 years ago. During your initial assessment of the patient, you note that she has an amulet tied around her neck. When you question her on the meaning of the amulet, she appears reluctant to respond and averts her eyes. What aspects of the patient's background would you want to further assess to determine the best process for continuing assessment and care? Identify culturally sensitive methods that you might use to ensure that the patient receives the care required without violating any cultural practices.

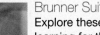

Brunner Suite Resources
Explore these additional resources to enhance learning for this chapter:
- NCLEX-Style Questions and Other Resources on thePoint, http://thePoint.lww.com/Brunner13e
- Study Guide
- PrepU
- Clinical Handbook
- Handbook of Laboratory and Diagnostic Tests

References

*Asterisk indicates classic reference.

Books

Dayer-Berenson, L. (2011). *Cultural competencies for nurses.* Boston: Jones & Bartlett.

Giger, J. N., & Davidhizar, R. E. (2012). *Transcultural nursing: Assessment and intervention* (6th ed.). St. Louis: Elsevier.

*Institute of Medicine. (2003). *Unequal treatment: Confronting racial and ethnic disparities in healthcare*. Washington, DC: National Academies Press.

*Leininger, M. M. (Ed.). (2001). *Culture care diversity and universality: A theory of nursing*. New York: National League for Nursing Press.

Smith-Temple, J., & Johnson, J. Y. (2010). *Nurse's guide to clinical procedures* (6th ed.). Philadelphia: Lippincott Williams & Wilkins.

Journals and Electronic Documents

Clark, L., Calvillo, E., Dela Cruz, F., et al. (2011). Cultural competencies for graduate nursing education. *Journal of Professional Nursing, 27*(3), 133–139.

Enis, S. R., Rios-Vargas, M., & Albert, N. G. (2011). The Hispanic population: 2010. *2010 Census Briefs*. Washington, DC: U.S. Bureau of the Census.

*Giger, J. N., Davidhizar, R., Purnell, L., et al. (2007). Understanding cultural language to enhance cultural competence. American Academy of Nursing Expert Panel Reports. *Nursing Outlook, 55*(4), 100–101.

Health Resources and Services Administration. (2010). *The registered nurse population: Findings from the 2008 National Sample Survey of Registered Nurses*. Available at: http://bhpr.hrsa.gov/healthworkforce/rnsurvey2008.html

Higginbottom, G. M., Magdalena, S., Richter, M. S., et al. (2011). Identification of nursing assessment models/tools validated in clinical practice for use with diverse ethno-cultural groups: An integrative review of the literature. *BMC Nursing, 10*(16).

Humes, K. R., Jones, N. A., & Ramerez, R. R. (2011). Overview of race and Hispanic origin: 2010. *2010 Census Briefs*. Washington, DC: U.S. Bureau of the Census.

*Leininger, M. (2002). Culture care theory: A major contribution to advance transcultural nursing knowledge and practices. *Journal of Transcultural Nursing, 13*(3), 189–192.

Lowes, J., & Archibald, C. (2009). Cultural diversity: The intention of nursing. *Nursing Forum, 44*(1), 11–19.

McKeon, L. M., Norris, T., Cardell, B., et al. (2009). Developing patient-centered care competencies among prelicensure nursing students using simulation. *Journal of Nursing Education, 48*(12), 711–715.

National Institutes of Health, National Center for Complementary and Alternative Medicine. (2012). *What is complementary and alternative medicine?* Available at: nccam.nih.gov

Quality and Safety Education for Nurses. (2012). *Competency KSAs (prelicensure)*. Available at: qsen.org/competencies/pre-licensure-ksas

Rugnetta, M. J., & Desai, K. (2011). *Addressing race and genetics: Health disparities in the age of personalized medicine*. Available at: scienceprogress.org/2011/06/addressing-race-and-genetics-2

*Sullivan Commission. (2004). *Missing persons: Minorities in the health professions*. Available at: www.aacn.nche.edu/media-relations/SullivanReport.pdf

U.S. Department of Health and Human Services, Office of Disease Prevention and Health Promotion. *Healthy People 2020*. Washington, DC. Available at:www.healthypeople.gov/2020/default.aspx

Williamson, M., & Harrison, L. (2010). Providing culturally appropriate care: A literature review. *International Journal of Nursing Studies, 47*(6), 761–769.

Resources

Asian American/Pacific Islander Nurses Association (AAPINA), www.aapina.org/

Council on Nursing and Anthropology (CONAA), www.conaa.org/about.htm

Healthy People 2020, www.healthypeople.gov/2020/default.aspx

LanguageLine Solutions, www.languageline.com/ (Provides written and oral translation in 140 languages.)

National Black Nurses Association (NBNA), www.nbna.org

National Center for Cultural Competence (NCCC), Georgetown University Center for Child and Human Development, nccc.georgetown.edu

National Institutes of Health, National Center for Complementary and Alternative Medicine (NCCAM), nccam.nih.gov

Office of Minority Health (OMH), minorityhealth.hhs.gov

Transcultural Nursing Society, www.tcns.org

Chapter 8

Overview of Genetics and Genomics in Nursing

Learning Objectives

On completion of this chapter, the learner will be able to:

1 Describe the role of the nurse in integrating genetics and genomics in nursing care.
2 Identify the common patterns of inheritance of genetic disorders.
3 Conduct a genetic- and genomic-based assessment.
4 Apply the principles, concepts, and theories of genetics and genomics to individuals, families, groups, and communities.
5 Identify ethical issues in nursing related to genetics and genomics.

Glossary

carrier: a person who is heterozygous; possessing two different alleles of a gene pair

chromosome: microscopic structures in the cell nucleus that contain genetic information and are constant in number in a species (e.g., humans have 46 chromosomes)

deoxyribonucleic acid (DNA): the primary genetic material in humans consisting of nitrogenous bases, a sugar group, and phosphate combined into a double helix

dominant: a genetic trait that is normally expressed when a person has a gene mutation on one of a pair of chromosomes and the "normal" form of the gene is on the other chromosome

genetics: the scientific study of heredity; how specific traits or predispositions are transmitted from parents to offspring

genome: the total genetic complement of an individual genotype

genomics: the study of the human genome, including gene sequencing, mapping, and function

genotype: the genes and the variations therein that a person inherits from his or her parents

Human Genome Project: an international research effort aimed at identifying and characterizing the order of every base in the human genome

mutation: a heritable alteration in a DNA sequence

nondisjunction: the failure of a chromosome pair to separate appropriately during cell division, resulting in abnormal chromosome numbers in daughter cells

pedigree: a diagrammatic representation of a family history

phenotype: a person's entire physical, biochemical, and physiologic makeup, as determined by the person's genotype and environmental factors

predisposition testing: testing that is used to determine the likelihood that a healthy person with or without a family history of a condition will develop a disorder

prenatal screening: testing that is used to identify whether a fetus is at risk for a birth defect such as Down syndrome or spina bifida (e.g., multiple marker maternal serum screening in pregnancy)

presymptomatic testing: genetic testing that is used to determine whether persons with a family history of a disorder, but no current symptoms, have the gene mutation (e.g., testing for Huntington disease)

recessive: a genetic trait that is expressed only when a person has two copies of a mutant autosomal gene or a single copy of a mutant X-linked gene in the absence of another X chromosome

variable expression: variation in the degree to which a trait is manifested; clinical severity

X-linked: located on the X chromosome

The **Human Genome Project** has ushered in a new type of medicine—personalized medicine that includes the influence of both genetic and genomic factors in disease causation, response to treatment, and health outcomes (Lea, 2009). The term **genetics** applies to single genes and their impact on relatively rare single gene disorders (Consensus Panel on Genetic/Genomic Nursing Competencies [Consensus Panel], 2009). The term **genomics** involves "all of the genes in the human **genome** together, including their interactions with each other, the environment, and the influence of other psychosocial and cultural factors" (Consensus Panel, 2009, pp. 8–9). Personalized medicine aims to tailor health care at the individual level by using a patient's genomic information, often called *genetic makeup* or *genomic profile*. Identification of the genetic and genomic factors associated with disease, including gene–gene function and gene–environment interactions, contributes to the development of more effective therapies customized to that particular patient's genetic makeup and the genomic profile of his or her disease. Genetic and genomic profiles allow health care providers to prescribe more specific and effective treatment for each patient, to identify and follow individuals at

TABLE 8-1	Transition from the Medical Era to the Genomic Era of Personalized Medicine	
	Medical Era	**Genomic Era of Personalized Medicine**
Defining Characteristics	• Considers single genes • Waits for disease symptoms to appear • Treats symptoms of presenting disease • Uses trial-and-error approach to treatment	• Considers interaction of genes with each other and the environment • Identifies genetic predisposition and optimize risk reduction to prevent disease • Treats underlying genetic cause of disease • Uses personalized approach tailored to the genetic/genomic profile of the individual and the disease

high risk for disease, and to avoid adverse drug reactions (National Human Genome Research Institute, 2011a). New genomic-based strategies for disease detection, management, and treatment are being utilized, making personalized medicine a reality (Table 8-1).

To meet the challenges of personalized medicine, nurses must understand the new technologies and treatments of genetic- and genomic-based health care. Nurses also must recognize that they are a vital link between the patient and health care services; patients often turn to nurses first with questions about a family history of risk factors, information regarding genetics, and genetic tests and interpretations. The incorporation of genetics and genomics into nursing involves the inclusion of genetics and genomics in health assessments, planning, and interventions that support identification of and response to the changing genetics-related health needs of people (Consensus Panel, 2009). This chapter offers a foundation for the clinical application of genetic and genomic principles in medical-surgical nursing, outlines the nurse's role in genetic counseling and evaluation, addresses important ethical issues, and provides related information and resources for nurses and patients (Consensus Panel, 2009).

Genomic Framework for Nursing Practice

The unique contribution of nursing to genomic medicine is its holistic perspective that takes into account each person's intellectual, physical, spiritual, social, cultural, biopsychologic, ethical, and aesthetic experiences. Because genomics addresses all of the genes of a given individual's human genome working together as a whole, genomics expands nursing's holistic view. Genetics and genomics are the basis of normal and pathophysiologic development, human health and disease, and health outcomes. Knowledge and interpretation of genetic and genomic information, gene-based testing, diagnosis, and treatment broaden the holistic view of nursing. Such expertise in genetics and genomics is basic to nursing practice and its holistic approach to patient care (Consensus Panel, 2009).

The *Essential Nursing Competencies and Curricula Guidelines for Genetics and Genomics* (Consensus Panel, 2009) provides a framework for integrating genetics and genomics into nursing practice (Chart 8-1). This document includes a philosophy of care that recognizes when genetic and genomic factors play a role or could play a role in a person's health. This means assessing predictive genetic and genomic factors using family history and the results of genetic tests

effectively, informing patients about genetics and genomic concepts, understanding the personal and societal impact of genetics and genomic information, and valuing the privacy and confidentiality of genetics and genomic information (Consensus Panel, 2009).

A person's response to genetic and genomic information, genetic testing, or genetics-related conditions may be either empowering or disabling. Genetic and genomic information may stigmatize people if it affects how they view themselves or how others view them. Nurses help individuals and families learn how genetic traits and conditions are passed on within families as well as how genetic and environmental factors influence health and disease (Consensus Panel, 2009). Nurses facilitate communication among family members, the health care system, and community resources, and they offer valuable support to patients and families. All nurses should be able to recognize when a patient is asking a question related to genetic or genomic information and should know how to obtain genetic information by gathering family and health histories and conducting physical and developmental assessments. This enables nurses to provide appropriate genetics resources and support to patients and families (Consensus Panel, 2009).

Chart 8-1

Essential Nursing Competencies for Genetics and Genomics

Professional Responsibilities

1. Recognition of attitudes and beliefs related to genetic and genomic science
2. Advocacy for genetic and genomic services
3. Incorporation of genetic and genomic technologies and information into practice
4. Demonstration of personalizing genetic and genomic information and services
5. Providing autonomous, informed genetics- and genomics-related decision making

Professional Practice

1. Integrate and apply genetic and genomic knowledge to nursing assessment.
2. Identify clients who may benefit from specific genetic and genomic resources, services, or technologies.
3. Facilitate referrals for genetic and genomic services.
4. Provide education, care, and support related to the interpretation of genetic or genomic tests, services, interventions, or treatments.

Adapted from Consensus Panel on Genetic/Genomic Nursing Competencies. (2009). *Essential nursing competencies and curricula guidelines for genetics and genomics.* Silver Spring, MD: American Nurses Association.

For example, when nurses assess patients' cardiovascular risk, they can expand their assessment to include information about family history of hypertension, hypercholesterolemia, and clotting disorders. Knowledge that genes are involved in the control of lipid metabolism, insulin resistance, blood pressure regulation, clotting factors, and vascular lining function helps individualize care based on the patient's genetic and genomic risk profile.

Essential to a genetic and genomic framework in nursing is the awareness of one's attitudes, experience, and assumptions about genetics and genomic concepts and how these are manifested in one's own practice (Consensus Panel, 2009). To develop awareness of these attitudes, experiences, and assumptions, the nurse must examine his or her own:

- Beliefs or values about health as well as family, religious, or cultural beliefs about the cause of illness and how one's values or biases affect understanding of genetic conditions
- Philosophical, theological, cultural, and ethical perspectives related to health and how these perspectives influence one's use of genetic information or services
- Level of expertise about genetics and genomics
- Experiences with birth defects, chronic illnesses, and genetic conditions, along with one's view of such conditions as disabling or empowering
- Attitudes about the right to access and other rights of individuals with genetic disorders
- View and assumptions about DNA and beliefs about the value of information about one's risk for genetic disorders
- Beliefs about reproductive options
- View of genetic testing and engineering
- Approach to patients with disabilities

Integrating Genetic and Genomic Knowledge

Scientific developments and advances in technology have increased understanding of genetics, resulting in better understanding of relatively rare diseases such as phenylketonuria (PKU) or hemophilia that are related to mutations of a single inherited gene. Scientists are able to characterize inherited metabolic variations that interact over time and lead to common diseases such as cancer, heart disease, and dementia. The transition from genetics to genomics has increased understanding of how multiple genes act and control biologic processes. Most diseases are now believed to be the result of a combination of genetic and environmental influences (Feero, Guttmacher, & Collins, 2010).

Genes and Their Role in Human Variation

Genes are central components of human health and disease. The Human Genome Project has linked basic human genetics to human development, health, and disease. Knowledge that specific genes are associated with specific genetic conditions makes diagnosis possible, even in the unborn. Many common conditions have genetic causes, and many more associations between genetics, health, and disease are likely to be identified. Genomics is the study of the interaction of genes and environmental factors.

Genes and Chromosomes

A person's unique genetic constitution, called a **genotype**, is made up of some 30,000 to 40,000 genes (Nussbaum, McInnes, & Willard, 2010). A person's **phenotype**—the observable characteristics of his or her genotype—includes physical appearance and other biologic, physiologic, and molecular traits. Environmental influences modify every person's phenotype, even phenotypes with a major genetic component. This concept of genotype and phenotype applies to a person's total genome and the respective traits of his or her genetic makeup.

The concepts of genotype and phenotype also apply to specific diseases. For example, in hypercholesterolemia, the genotype refers to the genes that control lipid metabolism, and the phenotype may be manifested in various corresponding ways. The genotype involves mutations in low-density lipoprotein (LDL) receptors and in one of the apolipoprotein genes. The phenotype is characterized by early onset of cardiovascular disease, high levels of LDL, skin xanthomas, and a family history of heart disease. An individual's genotype, consisting of normal functioning genes as well as some mutations, is characterized by physical and biologic traits that may predispose to disease.

Human growth, development, and disease occur as a result of both genetic and environmental influences and interactions. The contribution of genetic factors may be large or small. For example, in a person with cystic fibrosis or PKU, the genetic contribution is significant. In contrast, the genetic contribution underlying a person's response to infection may be less applicable.

A single gene is conceptualized as a unit of heredity. A gene is composed of a segment of **deoxyribonucleic acid (DNA)** that contains a specific set of instructions for making the protein or proteins needed by body cells for proper functioning. Genes regulate both the types of proteins made and the rate at which proteins are produced. The structure of the DNA molecule is referred to as a double helix. The essential components of the DNA molecule are sugar–phosphate molecules and pairs of nitrogenous bases. Each nucleotide contains a sugar (deoxyribose), a phosphate group, and one of four nitrogenous bases: adenine (A), cytosine (C), guanine (G), and thymine (T). DNA is composed of two paired strands, each made up of a number of nucleotides. The strands are held together by hydrogen bonds between pairs of bases (Fig. 8-1).

Genes are arranged in a linear order within **chromosomes**, which are located in the cell nucleus. In humans, 46 chromosomes occur in pairs in all body cells except oocytes (eggs) and sperm, which each contain only 23 unpaired chromosomes. Twenty-two pairs of chromosomes, called *autosomes*, are the same in females and males. The 23rd pair is referred to as the sex chromosomes. A female has two X chromosomes, whereas a male has one X and one Y chromosome. At conception, each parent normally gives one chromosome of each pair to his or her child. As a result, children receive half of their chromosomes from their fathers and half from their mothers (Fig. 8-2).

Careful examination of DNA sequences from many people shows that these sequences have multiple versions in a population. The different versions of these sequences are called *alleles*. Sequences found in many forms are said to be

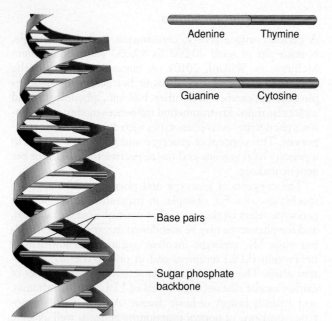

FIGURE 8-1 • DNA is a double helix formed by base pairs attached to a sugar-phosphate backbone. DNA carries the instructions that allow cells to make proteins. DNA is made up of four chemical bases. Redrawn from Genetics Home Reference, ghr.nlm.nih.gov/handbook/illustrations/dnastructure

polymorphic, meaning that there are at least two common forms of a particular gene.

Cell Division

The human body grows and develops as a result of the process of cell division. Mitosis and meiosis are two distinctly different types of cell division.

Mitosis is involved in cell growth, differentiation, and repair. During mitosis, the chromosomes of each cell duplicate. The result is two cells, called *daughter cells,* each of which contains the same number of chromosomes as the parent cell. The daughter cells are said to be diploid because they contain 46 chromosomes in 23 pairs. Mitosis occurs in all cells of the body except oocytes and sperm.

Meiosis, in contrast, occurs only in reproductive cells and is the process by which oocytes and sperm are formed. During meiosis, a reduction in the number of chromosomes takes place, resulting in oocytes or sperm that contain half the usual number, or 23 chromosomes. Oocytes and sperm are referred to as haploid because they contain a single copy of each chromosome, compared to the usual two copies in all other body cells. During meiosis, as the paired chromosomes come together in preparation for cell division, portions cross over, and an exchange of genetic material occurs before the chromosomes separate. This event, called *recombination,* creates greater diversity in the makeup of oocytes and sperm.

During the process of meiosis, a pair of chromosomes may fail to separate completely, creating a sperm or oocyte that contains either two copies or no copy of a particular chromosome. This sporadic event, called **nondisjunction,** can lead to either a trisomy or a monosomy. Down syndrome is an example of trisomy, in which people have three copies of chromosome number 21. Turner syndrome is an example of monosomy, in which girls have a single X chromosome,

causing them to have short stature and infertility (National Human Genome Research Institute, 2011b).

Gene Mutations

Within each cell, many intricate and complex interactions regulate and express human genes. Gene structure and function, transcription and translation, and protein synthesis are all involved. Alterations in gene structure and function and the process of protein synthesis may influence a person's health. Changes in gene structure, called **mutations,** permanently change the sequence of DNA, which in turn can alter the nature and type of proteins made (Fig. 8-3).

Some gene mutations have no significant effect on the protein product, whereas others cause partial or complete changes. How a protein is altered and its importance to body functioning determine the impact of the mutation. Gene mutations may occur in hormones, enzymes, or other important protein products, with significant implications for health and disease. Sickle cell anemia is a genetic condition caused by a small gene mutation that affects protein structure, producing hemoglobin S. A person who inherits two copies of the hemoglobin S gene mutation has sickle cell anemia and experiences the symptoms of severe anemia and thrombotic organ damage resulting from hypoxia (National Human Genome Research Institute, 2011c).

Other gene mutations include deletion (loss), insertion (addition), duplication (multiplication), or rearrangement

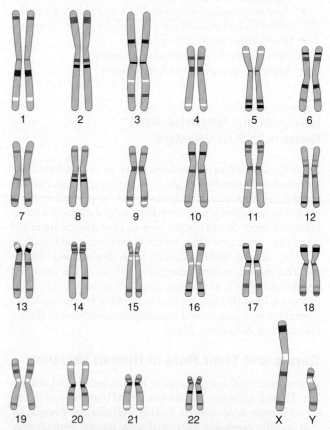

FIGURE 8-2 • Each human cell contains 23 pairs of chromosomes, which can be distinguished by their size and unique banding patterns. This set is from a male, because it contains a Y chromosome. Females have two X chromosomes. Redrawn from Genetics Home Reference, ghr.nlm.nih.gov/handbook/basics/howmanychromosomes

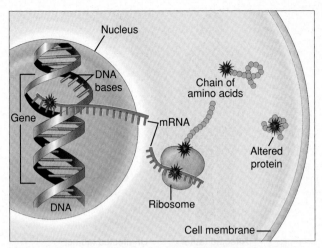

FIGURE 8-3 • When a gene contains a mutation, the protein encoded by that gene is likely to be abnormal. Sometimes the protein is able to function, although it does so imperfectly. In other cases, it is totally disabled. The outcome depends not only on how the mutation alters the protein's function but also on how vital that particular protein is to survival.

(translocation) of a longer DNA segment. Duchenne muscular dystrophy, myotonic dystrophy, Huntington disease, and fragile X syndrome are examples of conditions caused by gene mutations.

Gene mutations may be inherited or acquired. Inherited or germline gene mutations are present in the DNA of all body cells and are passed on in reproductive cells from parent to child. Germline or hereditary mutations are passed on to all daughter cells when body cells replicate (Fig. 8-4). The gene that causes Huntington disease is one example of a germline mutation.

Spontaneous mutations take place in individual oocytes or sperm at the time of conception. A person who carries the

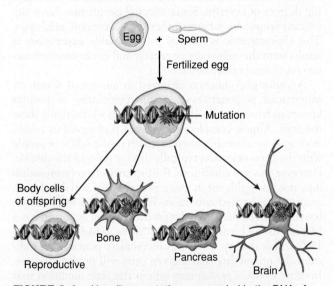

FIGURE 8-4 • Hereditary mutations are carried in the DNA of the reproductive cells. When reproductive cells containing mutations combine to produce offspring, the mutation is present in all of the offspring's body cells. Redrawn from National Cancer Institute, www.cancer.gov/cancertopics/understandingcancer/genetesting/page11

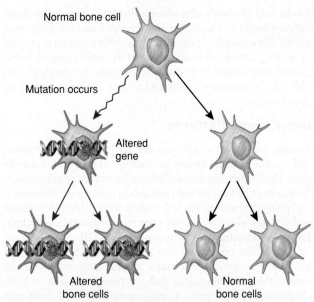

FIGURE 8-5 • Acquired mutations develop in DNA during a person's lifetime. If the mutation arises in a body cell, copies of the mutation will exist only in the descendants of that particular cell. Redrawn from National Cancer Institute, www.cancer.gov/cancertopics/understandingcancer/genetesting/page12

new "spontaneous" mutation may pass on the mutation to his or her children. Achondroplasia, Marfan syndrome, and neurofibromatosis type 1 are examples of genetic conditions that may occur in a single family member as a result of spontaneous mutation.

Acquired mutations take place in somatic cells and involve changes in DNA that occur after conception, during a person's lifetime. Acquired mutations develop as a result of cumulative changes in body cells other than reproductive cells (Fig. 8-5). Somatic gene mutations are passed on to the daughter cells derived from that particular cell line.

Gene mutations occur in the human body all the time. Cells have built-in mechanisms by which they can recognize mutations in DNA, and in most situations, they correct the changes before they are passed on by cell division. However, over time, body cells may lose their ability to repair damage from gene mutations, causing an accumulation of genetic changes that may ultimately result in diseases such as cancer and possibly other conditions of aging, such as Alzheimer's disease (Feero et al., 2010).

Genetic Variation

Genetic variations occur among people of all populations. Single nucleotide polymorphisms (SNPs, referred to as "snips") is the term used to identify common genetic variations that occur most frequently throughout the human genome. SNPs are changes in a single nucleotide (an A, T, C, or G) of the DNA sequence. For example, a normal DNA sequence of AAGGT could change to ATGG; in this case, there is one single nucleotide change from A to T. Most SNPs do not alter normal cell function. Some SNPs do alter gene function and may influence disease development. Knowledge about SNPs that affect biologic function will help pinpoint individuals who may be more prone to common diseases such as cancer, diabetes, and heart disease. Information on SNPs has helped to clarify why some individuals metabolize drugs differently (U.S. Department of Energy Genome Programs, 2008). For example, a polymorphism or SNP can alter protein or enzyme activity of medications. If the SNP causes a variation in drug transport or drug metabolism, the drug's action, half-life, or excretion could lead to lack of drug response or drug toxicity.

Inheritance Patterns

Nursing assessment of the patient's health includes obtaining and recording family history information in the form of a **pedigree**. This is a first step in establishing the pattern of inheritance. Nurses must be familiar with mendelian patterns of inheritance and pedigree construction and analysis to help identify patients and families who may benefit from further genetic counseling, testing, and treatment (Consensus Panel, 2009).

Mendelian conditions are genetic conditions that are inherited in fixed proportions among generations. They result from gene mutations that are present on one or both chromosomes of a pair. A single gene inherited from one or both parents can cause a mendelian condition. Mendelian conditions are classified according to their pattern of inheritance: autosomal dominant, autosomal recessive, and **X-linked**. The terms **dominant** and **recessive** refer to the trait, genetic condition, or phenotype but not to the genes or alleles that cause the observable characteristics (Lea, 2009; Nussbaum et al., 2010).

Autosomal Dominant Inheritance

Autosomal dominant inherited conditions affect female and male family members equally and follow a vertical pattern of inheritance in families (Fig. 8-6). A person who has an autosomal dominant inherited condition carries a gene mutation for that condition on one chromosome of a pair. Each of that person's offspring has a 50% chance of inheriting the gene mutation for the condition and a 50% chance of inheriting the normal version of the gene (Fig. 8-7). Offspring who do not inherit the gene mutation do not develop the condition and do not have an increased chance for having children with

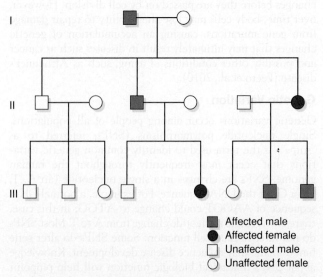

	Affected male
⬤	Affected female
☐	Unaffected male
◯	Unaffected female

FIGURE 8-6 • Three-generation pedigree illustrating autosomal dominant inheritance.

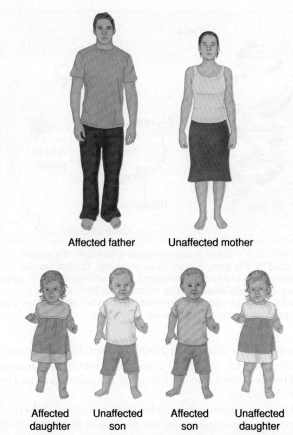

Affected father   Unaffected mother

Affected daughter   Unaffected son   Affected son   Unaffected daughter

FIGURE 8-7 • In dominant genetic disorders, if one affected parent has a disease-causing allele that dominates its normal counterpart, each child in the family has a 50% chance of inheriting the disease allele and the disorder. Redrawn from Genetics Home Reference, ghr.nlm.nih.gov/handbook/illustrations/autodominant

the same condition. Table 8-2 presents characteristics and examples of different patterns of inherited conditions.

Autosomal dominant conditions often manifest with varying degrees of severity. Some affected people may have significant symptoms, whereas others may have only mild ones. This characteristic is referred to as **variable expression**; it results from the influences of genetic and environmental factors on clinical presentation.

Another phenomenon observed in autosomal dominant inheritance is penetrance, or the percentage of persons known to have a particular gene mutation who actually show the trait. Almost complete penetrance is observed in conditions such as achondroplasia, in which nearly 100% of people with the gene mutation typically display traits of the disease. However, in some conditions, the presence of a gene mutation does not invariably mean that a person has or will develop an autosomal inherited condition. For example, a woman who has the *BRCA1* hereditary breast cancer gene mutation has a lifetime risk of breast cancer that can be as high as 80%, not 100%. This quality, known as incomplete penetrance, indicates the probability that a given gene will produce disease. In other words, a person may inherit the gene mutation that causes an autosomal dominant condition but may not have any of the observable physical or developmental features of that condition. However, this person carries the gene mutation and still has a 50% chance of passing the gene for the condition to each of his or her children.

TABLE 8-2   Patterns of Mendelian Inheritance

Characteristics	Examples
Autosomal Dominant Inherited Conditions	
Vertical transmission in families	Hereditary breast/ovarian
Males and females equally affected	cancer syndrome
Variable expression among family members and others with condition	Familial hypercholesterolemia
Reduced penetrance (in some conditions)	Hereditary nonpolyposis colorectal cancer
Advanced paternal age associated with sporadic cases	Huntington disease
	Marfan syndrome
	Neurofibromatosis
Autosomal Recessive Inherited Conditions	
Horizontal pattern of transmission seen in families	Cystic fibrosis
	Galactosemia
Males and females equally affected	Phenylketonuria
Associated with consanguity (genetic relatedness)	Sickle cell anemia
	Tay-Sachs disease
Associated with particular ethnic groups	Canavan disease
X-Linked Recessive Inherited Conditions	
Vertical transmission in families	Duchenne muscular
Males predominantly affected	dystrophy
	Hemophilia A and B
	Wiskott-Aldrich syndrome
	Protan and Deutran forms of color blindness
Multifactorial Inherited Conditions	
Occur as a result of combination of genetic and environmental factors	Congenital heart defects
	Cleft lip and/or palate
May recur in families	Neural tube defects
Inheritance pattern does not demonstrate characteristic pattern of inheritance seen with other mendelian conditions	(anencephaly and spina bifida)
	Diabetes mellitus
	Osteoarthritis
	High blood pressure

Adapted from Jenkins, J., & Lea, D. H. (2005). *Nursing care in the genomic era: A case-based approach.* Sudbury, MA: Jones & Bartlett; Skirton, H., Patch, C., & Williams, J. (2005). *Applied genetics in healthcare: A handbook for specialists.* New York: Taylor & Francis Group.

One of the effects of incomplete penetrance is that the gene appears to "skip" a generation, thus leading to errors in interpreting family history and in genetic counseling. Examples of other genetic conditions with incomplete penetrance include otosclerosis (40%) and retinoblastoma (80%) (Nussbaum et al., 2010).

Autosomal Recessive Inheritance

In contrast to autosomal dominant conditions, autosomal recessive conditions have a pattern that is more horizontal than vertical; relatives of a single generation tend to have the condition (Fig. 8-8). Autosomal recessive conditions are frequently seen among particular ethnic groups and usually occur more often in children of parents who are related by blood, such as first cousins (see Table 8-2).

In autosomal recessive inheritance, each parent carries a gene mutation on one chromosome of the pair and a normal gene on the other chromosome. The parents are said to be **carriers** of the gene mutation. Unlike people with an autosomal dominant condition, carriers of a gene mutation for a recessive condition do not have symptoms of the genetic condition. When carriers have children together, there is a 25% chance that each child may inherit the gene mutation from both parents and have the condition (Fig. 8-9). Gaucher's dis-

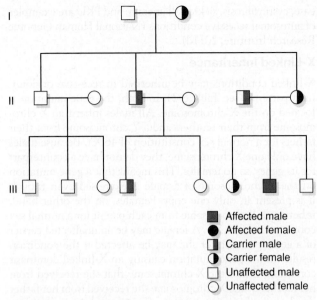

Affected male
Affected female
Carrier male
Carrier female
Unaffected male
Unaffected female

FIGURE 8-8 • Three-generation pedigree illustrating autosomal recessive inheritance.

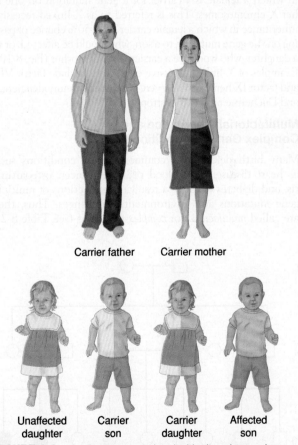

Carrier father   Carrier mother

Unaffected daughter   Carrier son   Carrier daughter   Affected son

FIGURE 8-9 • In diseases associated with altered recessive genes, both parents—although disease free themselves—carry one normal allele and one altered allele. Each child has one chance in four of inheriting two abnormal alleles and developing the disorder; one chance in four of inheriting two normal alleles; and two chances in four of inheriting one normal and one altered allele—therefore being a carrier like both parents. Redrawn from Genetics Home Reference, ghr.nlm.nih.gov/handbook/illustrations/autorecessive

ease, cystic fibrosis, sickle cell anemia, and PKU are examples of autosomal recessive conditions (National Human Genome Research Institute, 2011d).

X-Linked Inheritance

X-linked conditions may be inherited in recessive or dominant patterns (see Table 8-2). In both, the gene mutation is located on the X chromosome. All males inherit an X chromosome from their mothers and a Y chromosome from their fathers for a normal sex constitution of 46,XY. Because males have only one X chromosome, they do not have a counterpart for its genes, as do females. This means that a gene mutation on the X chromosome of a male is expressed even though it is present in only one copy. Females, on the other hand, inherit one X chromosome from each parent for a normal sex constitution of 46,XX. A female may be an unaffected carrier of a gene mutation, or she may be affected if the condition results from a gene mutation causing an X-linked dominant condition. Either the X chromosome that she received from her mother or the X chromosome she received from her father may be passed on to each of her offspring, and this is a random occurrence.

The most common pattern of X-linked inheritance is that in which a female is a carrier for a gene mutation on one of her X chromosomes. This is referred to as X-linked recessive inheritance in which a female carrier has a 50% chance of passing on the gene mutation to a son, who would be affected, or to a daughter, who would be a carrier like her mother (Fig. 8-10). Examples of X-linked recessive conditions include factor VIII and factor IX hemophilia, severe combined immunodeficiency, and Duchenne muscular dystrophy

Multifactorial Inheritance and Complex Genetic Conditions

Many birth defects and common health conditions such as heart disease, high blood pressure, cancer, osteoarthritis, and diabetes occur as a result of interactions of multiple gene mutations and environmental influences. Thus, they are called *multifactorial* or *complex conditions* (see Table 8-2).

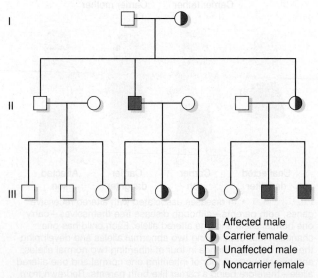

FIGURE 8-10 • Three-generation pedigree illustrating X-linked recessive inheritance.

- ■ Affected male
- ◐ Carrier female
- □ Unaffected male
- ○ Noncarrier female

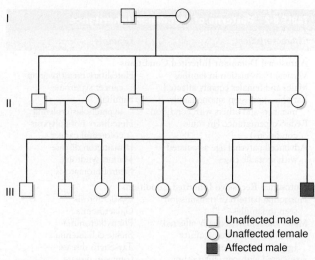

FIGURE 8-11 • Three-generation pedigree illustrating multifactorial conditions.

- □ Unaffected male
- ○ Unaffected female
- ■ Affected male

Other examples of multifactorial genetic conditions include neural tube defects such as spina bifida and anencephaly. Multifactorial conditions may cluster in families; however, they do not always result in the characteristic pattern of inheritance seen in families who have mendelian inherited conditions (Fig. 8-11).

Nontraditional Inheritance

Although mendelian conditions manifest with a specific pattern of inheritance in some families, many diseases and traits do not follow these simple patterns. Various factors influence how a gene performs and is expressed. Different mutations in the same gene can produce variable symptoms in different people, as in cystic fibrosis. Different mutations in several genes can lead to identical outcomes, as in Alzheimer's disease. Some traits involve simultaneous mutation in two or more genes. A recently observed phenomenon—imprinting—can determine which of a pair of genes (that of the mother or the father) is silenced or activated. This form of inheritance has been observed in Angelman syndrome, a severe form of mental retardation and ataxia (National Human Genome Research Institute, 2011e).

Chromosomal Differences and Genetic Conditions

Differences in the number or structure of chromosomes are a major cause of birth defects, mental retardation, and malignancies. Chromosomal differences are present in approximately 1 of every 160 liveborn infants and are the cause of greater than 50% of all spontaneous first-trimester pregnancy losses (Suzumori & Sugiura-Ogasawara, 2010). Chromosomal differences most commonly involve an extra or missing chromosome; this is called *aneuploidy*. Whenever there is an extra or missing chromosome, there is always associated mental or physical disability to some degree.

Down syndrome, or trisomy 21, is a common chromosomal condition that occurs with greater frequency in pregnancies of women who are 35 years of age or older. A person with trisomy 21 has a complete extra chromosome 21, which causes a particular facial appearance and increased risk of congenital heart defects, thyroid and vision problems, and mental retardation. Other examples of chromosomal differences include trisomy 13 and trisomy 18, both more severe than Down syndrome, and conditions involving extra or missing sex chromosomes, such as Turner syndrome (National Human Genome Research Institute, 2011f).

Chromosomal differences may also involve a structural rearrangement within or between chromosomes. These are less common than chromosomal conditions in which there is an extra or missing chromosome, although they still occur in 1 of every 500 newborns (National Human Genome Research Institute, 2011g). People who carry "balanced" chromosome rearrangements have all of their chromosomal material; however, it is rearranged. Women with a "balanced" chromosomal rearrangement have an increased risk of spontaneous pregnancy loss and of having children with an unbalanced chromosomal arrangement that may result in physical or mental disabilities. Known carriers of these chromosomal differences are offered prenatal counseling and testing.

Chromosome studies may be needed at any age, depending on the indication. Two common indications are a suspected diagnosis such as Down syndrome and a history of two or more unexplained pregnancy losses. Chromosome studies are accomplished by obtaining a tissue sample (e.g., blood, skin, and amniotic fluid), preparing and staining the chromosomes, and analyzing them under a microscope. The microscopic study of chromosomes, called *cytogenetics*, is used with molecular techniques such as fluorescent in situ hybridization (FISH), which permits more detailed examination of chromosomes. FISH is useful to detect small abnormalities and to characterize chromosomal rearrangements.

Genetic and Genomic Technologies in Practice

One of the most immediate applications of new genetic and genomic discoveries is the development of genetic tests that can be used to detect a trait, diagnose a genetic condition, and identify people who have a genetic predisposition to a disease such as cancer or heart disease. Another emerging application is pharmacogenetics, which involves the use of genetic testing to identify genetic variations that relate to the safety and efficacy of medications and gene-based treatments so that individualized treatment can be developed. Future applications may include the use of gene chips to map a person's individual genome for genetic variations that may lead to disease. Nurses are involved in caring for patients who are undergoing genetic testing and gene-based treatments. Knowledge of the clinical applications of modern genetic and genomic technologies enables nurses to inform and support patients and to provide high-quality genetics-related health care (Consensus Panel, 2009).

Genetic Testing

Genetic testing is the primary tool used to identify individuals predisposed to specific genetic diseases. Genetic tests provide information leading to the diagnosis of inherited conditions or other conditions with a known genetic contribution.

In genetic testing, approaches may be genotypic or phenotypic. Genotypic methods involve analysis of the chromosomes and genes directly, using specific laboratory techniques to learn whether a genetic alteration related to a specific disease or condition is present. This testing may be DNA based, chromosomal, or biochemical. Phenotypic methods examine the familial or biologic presentation of disease and include assessment of the patient's personal or family history and medical factors influencing his or her disease as well as testing for gene products such as protein markers in body fluids or diseased tissues. The family history, which is considered the first genetic test, is discussed later in this chapter (see the Family History Assessment section). It is expected that all nurses will know how to use this genetic tool.

Another phenotypic approach involves searching for gene products, such as proteins and enzymes that can clinically indicate a genetic abnormality. For example, germline mutations in the repair genes *MLH1, MSH2, MSH6*, and *PMS2* are responsible for hereditary early-onset colorectal cancer. Colorectal tumors are now tested to measure the presence or absence of these proteins using immunohistochemistry, which is a routine type of pathology test. Tumors that stain negative for one of those proteins signify malfunction of the gene whose protein is missing. Patients with absent or negative protein expression in their tumors (e.g., MLH1 protein–negative) can proceed with genetic testing for a germline *MLH1* mutation (Hampel, Frankel, Martin, et al., 2008).

Genetic testing can be used for various purposes in prenatal, pediatric, and adult populations. Prenatal testing is widely used for **prenatal screening** and diagnosis of conditions such as Down syndrome. Carrier testing is used to determine if a person carries a recessive allele for an inherited condition (e.g., cystic fibrosis, sickle cell anemia, Tay-Sachs disease) and therefore risks passing it on to his or her children. Genetic testing is also used widely in newborn screening. In the United States, it is available for an increasing number of genetic conditions (e.g., PKU, galactosemia) (Rare Diseases, 2011).

Diagnostic testing is used to detect the presence or absence of a particular genetic alteration or allele to identify or confirm a diagnosis of a disease or condition (e.g., myotonic dystrophy, fragile X syndrome). Increasingly, genetic tests are being used to predict drug response and to design specific and individualized treatment plans, or personalized medicine. For example, genetic testing is used to identify specific gene variants that can predict the effectiveness of treatments for human immunodeficiency virus (HIV) infection and the use of tacrine for Alzheimer's disease (Weinshilboum & Wang, 2006). Examples of current uses of genetic tests are shown in Table 8-3.

Nurses are increasingly involved in taking family histories and educating the patient about aspects of genetic testing. They contribute by ensuring informed health choices and consent, advocating for privacy and confidentiality with regard to genetic test results, and helping patients understand the complex issues involved (Consensus Panel, 2009).

Genetic Screening

Genetic screening, in contrast to genetic testing, applies to testing of populations or groups independent of a positive

TABLE 8-3 Genetic Tests: Examples of Current Uses	
Purpose of Genetic Test	**Type of Genetic Test**
Carrier Testing	
Cystic fibrosis	DNA analysis
Tay-Sachs disease	Hexosaminidase A activity testing and DNA analysis
Canavan disease	DNA analysis
Sickle cell anemia	Hemoglobin electrophoresis
Thalassemia	Complete blood count and hemoglobin electrophoresis
Prenatal Diagnosis—amniocentesis is often performed when there is a risk for a chromosomal or genetic disorder:	
Risk of Down syndrome	Chromosomal analysis
Risk of cystic fibrosis	DNA analysis
Risk of Tay-Sachs disease	Hexosaminidase A activity testing and/or DNA analysis
Risk of open neural tube defect	Protein analysis
Diagnosis	
Down syndrome	Chromosomal analysis
Fragile X syndrome	DNA analysis
Myotonic dystrophy	DNA analysis
Presymptomatic Testing	
Huntington disease	DNA analysis
Myotonic dystrophy	DNA analysis
Susceptibility Testing	
Hereditary breast/ovarian cancer	DNA analysis
Hereditary nonpolyposis colorectal cancer	DNA analysis

family history or symptom manifestation. Genetic screening, as defined in 1975 by the Committee for the Study of Inborn Errors of Metabolism of the National Academy of Sciences (Secretary's Advisory Committee on Genetics Health and Society, 2009), has several major aims. The first aim is to improve management—that is, to identify people with treatable genetic conditions that could prove dangerous to their health if left untreated. For example, newborns are screened for an increasing number of conditions, including PKU, congenital hypothyroidism, and galactosemia. The second aim is to provide reproductive options to people with a high probability of having children with severe, untreatable diseases and for whom genetic counseling, prenatal diagnosis, and other reproductive options could be helpful

and of interest. For example, people of Ashkenazi Jewish descent (Jews of eastern European origin) are screened for conditions such as Tay-Sachs disease and Canavan disease. The third aim is to screen pregnant women to detect birth defects such as neural tube defects and Down syndrome. Genetic screening may also be used for public health purposes to determine the incidence and prevalence of a birth defect or to investigate the feasibility and value of new genetic testing methods. Most commonly, genetic screening occurs in prenatal and newborn programs. Table 8-4 gives examples of types of genetic screening.

 Concept Mastery Alert

Genetic testing and *genetic screening* are terms that are often confused. Nurses need to remember that testing is individual; screening is population based.

Testing and Screening for Adult-Onset Conditions

Adult-onset conditions with a genetic or genomic basis are manifested in later life. Often, clinical signs or symptoms occur only in late adolescence or adulthood, and disease is clearly observed to run in families. Some of these conditions are attributed to specific genetic mutations and follow either an autosomal dominant or an autosomal recessive inheritance pattern. However, most adult-onset conditions are considered to be genomic or multifactorial—that is, they result from a combination of genes or gene–environment interactions. Examples of multifactorial conditions include heart disease, diabetes, and arthritis. Genomic or multifactorial influences involve interactions among several genes (gene–gene interactions) and between genes and the environment (gene–environment interactions), as well as the individual's lifestyle (Feero et al., 2010).

Nursing assessment for adult-onset conditions is based on family history, personal and medical risk factors, and identification of associated diseases or clinical manifestations (the phenotype). Knowledge of adult-onset conditions and their genetic bases (i.e., mendelian vs. multifactorial conditions) influences the nursing considerations for genetic testing and health promotion. Table 8-5 describes selected adult-onset

TABLE 8-4 Applications for Genetic Screening		
Timing of Screening	**Purpose**	**Examples**
Preconception screening	For autosomal recessive inherited genetic conditions that occur with greater frequency among individuals of certain ethnic groups	Cystic fibrosis—all couples, but especially northern European Caucasian and Ashkenazi Jewish Tay-Sachs disease—Ashkenazi Jewish Sickle cell anemia—African American, Puerto Rican, Mediterranean, Middle Eastern Alpha-thalassemia—Southeast Asian, African American
Prenatal screening	For genetic conditions that are common and for which prenatal diagnosis is available when a pregnancy is identified at increased risk	Neural tube defects—spina bifida, anencephaly Down syndrome Other chromosomal abnormalities—trisomy 18
Newborn screening	For genetic conditions for which there is specific treatment	Phenylketonuria (PKU) Galactosemia Homocystinuria Biotinidase deficiency

TABLE 8-5 Adult-Onset Disorders

Clinical Description	Age of Onset	Genetic Inheritance	Molecular Genetics	Test Availability
Neurologic Conditions				
Early-Onset Familial Alzheimer's Disease (EOFAD) Progressive dementia, memory failure, personality disturbance, loss of intellectual functioning associated with cerebral cortical atrophy, beta-amyloid plaque formation, & intraneuronal neurofibrillary tangles	<60–65 y; often <55 y	A.D.	*PSEN1* (14q24) mutations in presenilin 1 gene; detects 30%–70% of EOFAD cases	Presymptomatic
Late-Onset Familial Alzheimer's Disease Progressive dementia, cognitive decline	>60–65 y		Apolipoprotein E (19q13) Apo E gene product	Presymptomatic
Frontotemporal Dementia With Parkinsonism-17 Dementia &/or parkinsonism: Slowly progressive behavioral changes, language disturbances &/or extrapyramidal signs, rigidity, bradykinesia, & saccadic eye movements	40–60 y	A.D.	*MAPT* gene (linked to 17q21.1)	Diagnostic & Presymptomatic
Huntington Disease Widespread degenerative brain change with progressive motor loss; both voluntary & involuntary disability, cognitive decline, chorea (involuntary movements) at later stage, psychiatric disturbances	Mean age 35–44 y	A.D.	*HD* gene (4p16)	Diagnostic & Presymptomatic
Neuromuscular Disorders				
Spinocerebellar Ataxia Type 6 Slowly progressive cerebellar ataxia, dysarthria & nystagmus	Mean age 43–52 y	A.D.	*CACNA1A* gene (19p13)	Diagnostic & Presymptomatic
Spinocerebellar Ataxia Type 1 Ataxia, dysarthria & bulbar dysfunction	Mean age 30–40 y	A.D.	*ATXN1* gene (6p22-p23)	Diagnostic & Presymptomatic
Spinocerebellar Ataxia Type 2 Slow saccadic eye movement, peripheral neuropathy, decreased deep tendon reflexes, dementia	Mean age 30–40 y	A.D.	*ATXN2* gene (12q24.1)	Diagnostic & Presymptomatic
Spinocerebellar Ataxia Type 3 Progressive cerebellar ataxia & various other neurologic symptoms including dystonic-rigid syndrome, parkinsonian syndrome or combined dystonia & peripheral neuropathy	Mean age onset in 30s	A.D.	*ATXN3* gene (14q21)	Diagnostic & Presymptomatic
Mild Myotonic Muscular Dystrophy Cataracts & myotonia or muscle wasting & weakness, frontal balding & electrocardiogram changes (heart block or dysrhythmia), diabetes mellitus in 5% of all cases	20–70 y	A.D. with variable penetrance	CTG trinucleotide repeat expansion	Diagnostic
Familial Amyotrophic Lateral Sclerosis (ALS) Progressive loss of motor function with predominantly lower motor neuron manifestations	50–70 y	Both A.D. & A.R.	*ALS1 (SOD1)* test for gene product superoxide/dismutase	Diagnostic
Hematologic Conditions				
Hereditary Hemochromatosis (HHC) High absorption of iron by gastrointestinal mucosa resulting in excessive iron storage in liver, skin, pancreas, heart, joints, & testes. Abdominal pain, weakness, lethargy, weight loss are early symptoms. Untreated individuals can present with skin pigmentation, diabetes mellitus, hepatic fibrosis or cirrhosis, congestive heart failure, dysrhythmias, or arthritis.	40–60 y in males; after menopause in females	A.R.	*HFE* gene (6p21) C282Y mutation	Diagnostic & Presymptomatic
Factor V Leiden Thrombophilia Poor anticoagulant response to activated protein C with increased risk for venous thromboembolism & risk for increased fetal loss during pregnancy	30s; during pregnancy in females	A.D.	*F5* (1q23) 1691G>A mutation; abnormal coagulation factor V	Diagnostic & Presymptomatic

(continues on page 118)

TABLE 8-5 **Adult-Onset Disorders** (continued)

Clinical Description	Age of Onset	Genetic Inheritance	Molecular Genetics	Test Availability
Polycystic Kidney Disease Dominant				
Most common genetic disease in humans. Manifests with renal cysts, liver cysts, & occasionally intracranial/aortic aneurysm & hypertension. Loss of glomerular filtration can lead to kidney failure.	Variable onset; all carriers have detectable disease by ultrasound at age 30 y	A.D.	PKD1 (16p13) polycepten; PKD2 (4q21-q23) polycepten2	Diagnostic & Presymptomatic
Diabetes Mellitus Type 2				
Insulin resistance & impaired glucose tolerance	Variable onset most often >30 y	M.F.	Insulin promoter factor 1 (1PF); CAPN10 gene polymorphism (single nucleotide polymorphism)	Research
			Interaction of NIDDM$_1$ chromosome 2 & several candidate genes on chromosomes 1, 2, 3, &15 (CYP19)	Research
Cardiovascular Disease				
Familial hypercholesterolemia; elevated low-density lipoprotein levels leading to coronary artery disease, xanthoma, & corneal arcus.	40–50 y	A.D.	PCSK9 (1p323)	Diagnostic
Hyperlipidemia				
Elevated cholesterol & triglycerides associated with premature coronary disease & peripheral vascular disease	30–40 y	A.R.	APOE gene (19q13)	Clinical testing related to Alzheimer's/ Research
Alpha-1 Antitrypsin Deficiency				
60%–70% small airway & alveolar wall destruction; emphysema, especially at base; chronic obstructive pulmonary disease	35 y/smoker; 45 y/ nonsmoker	M.F. in A.R fashion	PI1 (14q33) alpha-1 antitrypsin	Diagnostic & Presymptomatic
Oncology Conditions				
Multiple Endocrine Neoplasia Familial medullary thyroid cancer: Medullary thyroid cancer, pheochromocytoma, & parathyroid abnormalities	Early adulthood 40–50 y	A.D.	RET gene (10q11)	Presymptomatic
Breast Cancer BRCA1/2 hereditary breast/ovarian cancer: Breast, ovarian, prostate, & colon (BRCA1); breast, ovarian, & other cancer (BRCA2)	30–70 y; often <50 y	A.D.	BRCA1 gene (17q21) BRCA2 (13q12 DNA analysis)	Presymptomatic Presymptomatic
Lynch Syndrome Colorectal, endometrial, bladder, gastric, biliary, & renal cell cancers as well as atypical endometrial hyperplasia & uterine leiomyosarcoma	<50 y	A.D.	MLH1 (3p21) MSH2 (2p22-p21) MSH6 (2p16) PMS1 (2q31-q33) PMS2 (7p22) TGFBR2 (3p22)	Presymptomatic & Diagnostic
Li-Fraumeni Syndrome Soft tissue sarcoma, breast cancer, leukemia, osteosarcoma, melanoma, & other cancers often including colon, pancreas, adrenal cortex, & brain	Often <40 y	A.D.	TP53 gene (17q13); test for protein product	Presymptomatic & Diagnostic
Cowden Syndrome Breast, nonmedullary (papillary or follicular) thyroid cancer; breast fibroadenomas & noncancerous thyroid modules or goiter; multiple buccal mucosa papillomas (cobblestone-line papules), facial trichilemmomas, gastrointestinal polyps; high-arched palate, thickened furrowed tongue, megalencephaly, & pectus excavatum.	40–50 y for cancer; teens–20 y for mucocutaneous lesions	A.D.	PTEN gene (10q23); gene product test	Presymptomatic & Research

A.D., autosomal dominant; A.R., autosomal recessive; M.F., multifactorial.

From Bird, T. D. (2012). *Alzheimer disease overview.* Available at: www.ncbi.nlm.nih.gov/books/NBK1161/; Kohlmann, W. & Gruber, S. B. (2011). *Lynch Syndrome.* Available at: www.ncbi.nlm.nih.gov/books/NBK1161/; Kowdley, K. V., Tait, J. F., Bennett, R. L., et al. (2006). *HFE-associated hereditary hemochromatosis.* Available at: www.ncbi.nlm. nih.gov/books/NBK1440/; Kujovich, J. L. (2010). *Factor V Leiden thrombophilia.* Available at: www.ncbi.nlm.nih.gov/books/NBK1368/#factor-v-leiden.T.selected_f5_allelic_va; Moline, J., & Eng, C. (2010). *Multiple endocrine neoplasia type 2.* Available at: www.ncbi.nlm.nih.gov/books/NBK1257/; OMIM. (2011). Hypercholesterolemia, autosomal dominant, type B. Available at: www.omim.org/entry/144010; Petrucelli, N., Daly, M. B., Bars Culver, J. O., et al. (2011). *BRCA1 and BRCA2 hereditary breast and ovarian cancer.* Available at www.ncbi.nlm.nih.gov/books/NBK1247/; and Warby, S. C., Graham, R. K., & Hayden, M. R. (2010). *Huntington disease.* Available at: www.ncbi.nlm.nih. gov/books/NBK1305/

conditions, their age of onset, pattern of inheritance, molecular genetics, and test availability.

Single Gene Conditions

If a single gene accounts for an adult-onset condition in a symptomatic person, testing is used to confirm a diagnosis to assist in the plan of care and management. Diagnostic testing for adult-onset conditions is most frequently used with autosomal dominant conditions, such as Huntington disease or factor V Leiden thrombophilia, and with autosomal recessive conditions such as hemochromatosis. Other single gene conditions are associated with a confirmed genetic mutation in an affected family member or with a family history suggestive of an inherited pattern of adult-onset disease, such as a particular type of cancer. **Presymptomatic testing** provides asymptomatic people with information about the presence of a genetic mutation and about the likelihood of developing the disease. Presymptomatic testing is considered for people in families with a known adult-onset condition in which either a positive or a negative test result indicates an increased or reduced risk of developing the disease, affects medical management, or allows earlier treatment of a condition.

Huntington disease has long served as the model for presymptomatic testing because the presence of the genetic mutation predicts disease onset and progression. Although preventive measures are not yet available for Huntington disease, the genetic information enables health care providers to develop a clinical, supportive, and psychological plan of care. Indeed, the presence of a single gene mutation has implications for the risk of developing many types of cancer; therefore, presymptomatic testing has become the standard of care so that early planning and implementation of select medical measures may reduce that risk (Ready & Arun, 2010).

Genomic Conditions

The foremost factor that may influence the development and severity of disease is a person's genomic makeup. In the absence of a single disease-causing gene, it is thought that multiple genes and other environmental factors are related to the onset of most adult diseases. For some diseases, the interactions among several genes and other environmental or metabolic events affect disease onset and progression. Specific gene–gene interactions or SNPs can confer susceptibility to disease. Most genomic testing for gene–gene interactions and SNPs is conducted in the research setting to identify candidate genes for diseases such as Alzheimer's disease, psychiatric conditions, heart disease, hypertension, and hypercholesterolemia (Christensen & Murray, 2007). Genomic testing helps distinguish variations within the same disease or response to treatment. For example, no single gene is associated with osteoporosis. Several polymorphisms on candidate genes related to the vitamin D receptor, estrogen and androgen receptors, and regulation of bone mineral density (BMD) have been shown to contribute to osteoporosis and fracture risk. Moreover, diet and exercise have a strong interaction with the polymorphisms regulating BMD (Hosoi, 2010).

Some genomic tests may predict treatment response. For example, people may present with similar clinical signs and symptoms of asthma but have different responses to corticosteroid treatment. Mutations in genes that regulate glucocorticoid (i.e., corticosteroid) receptors help classify people with asthma as sensitive or resistant to treatment with corticosteroids (Masuno, Haldar, Jevaraj, et al., 2011).

Population Screening

Population screening—the use of genetic testing for large groups or entire populations—to identify late-onset conditions is under development. For a test to be considered for population screening, there must be (1) sufficient information about gene distribution within populations, (2) accurate prediction about the development and progression of disease, and (3) appropriate medical management for asymptomatic people with a mutation. Currently, population screening is considered in some ethnic groups to identify cancer-predisposing genes. For example, individuals of Ashkenazi Jewish ancestry have a greater chance of having a specific genetic mutation in the *BRCA1* or *BRCA2* gene. People with one of these *BRCA* mutations have approximately an 80% risk (*BRCA1* carriers) and a 45% risk (*BRCA2* carriers) of breast cancer, a 40% to 65% risk (*BRCA1* carriers) and a 20% risk (*BRCA2* carriers) of ovarian cancer, and a 16% risk of prostate cancer (Chen, Iversen, Friebel, et al., 2006). The identification of one of these mutations gives patients options that may include cancer screening, chemoprevention, or prophylactic mastectomy or oophorectomy. Population screening is also being explored for other adult-onset conditions such as type 2 diabetes, heart disease, and hereditary hemochromatosis (i.e., iron overload disorder).

The Nursing Role in Testing and Screening for Adult-Onset Conditions

Nurses participate in explaining risk and genetic predisposition, supporting informed health decisions and opportunities for prevention and early intervention, and protecting patients' privacy. Nurses assess family histories, which may indicate that multiple generations (autosomal dominant inheritance) or multiple siblings (autosomal recessive inheritance) are affected with the same condition or that onset of disease is earlier than expected (e.g., multiple generations with early-onset hyperlipidemia). Possible adult-onset conditions are discussed with other members of the health care team for appropriate resources and referral. When a family history of disease is identified, a patient is made aware that this is a risk factor for disease; resources and referral are then provided. It is the patient's decision whether or not to pursue a genetic testing workup. For example, if a 45-year-old woman presents for her annual gynecology visit and reports a family history of colon cancer in multiple paternal relatives, including her father, the nurse should discuss the family history with the gynecologist. In addition, the woman should be alerted to the risk of colon cancer based on the family history and given information about possible genetic testing and referral for a colonoscopy.

If the existence of a mutation for an adult-onset condition in a family is identified, at-risk family members can be referred for **predisposition testing**. If the patient is found to carry the mutation, the nurse provides him or her with information and referral for risk-reduction measures and information about the risk to other family members. In that discussion, the nurse assures the patient that the test results are private and confidential and will not be shared with others, including family members, without the patient's permission. If the patient is an unaffected family member, the nurse discusses inheritance and the risk of developing the disease, provides support for the decision-making process, and offers referral for genetics services.

Personalized Genomic Treatments

Information about genes and their variations helps researchers identify genetic differences that predispose certain people to more aggressive diseases and affect their responses to treatment. Genetics and genomics have revolutionized the field of oncology because genetic mutations are the basis for the development and progression of all cancers. Until recently, individuals with cancer faced treatment based on the stage of the cancer, lymph node involvement, and spread to distant organs. Treatments for a particular type of cancer, stage for stage, were similar. However, studies have shown that individuals with the same type and stage of cancer who received the same treatment did not always have the same response or survival rate. The differences in a given cancer are attributable to genetic differences in that cancer (Calzone, Masny, & Jenkins, 2010). For example, women with early-stage breast cancer (i.e., tumor diameter less than 2 cm, estrogen receptor–positive tumors, no lymph node involvement) have often received chemotherapy. In the past, deciding which of these women would benefit the most from chemotherapy was unclear. Currently, a gene tumor profile of these women's tumors can be used to predict which women are more likely to have an aggressive cancer. This genetic test helps clinicians recognize which early breast cancers pose a higher risk for recurrence and should have chemotherapy (Bellcross & Dotson, 2010). Other patients who need treatment are receiving personalized cancer treatment based on the genetic signature of the tumor. This treatment, called *targeted therapy*, tries to match the treatment to the specific malfunctioning genes expressed in the tumor or to selectively inhibit genetic factors that promote cancer growth (Hayden, 2009).

Pharmacogenomics

It has long been known that patients differ in their response to medications. The genetic and genomic variations in drug metabolism account largely for the differences in drug response and drug-related toxicities. Drug metabolism involves genetically controlled protein/enzyme activity for absorption, distribution, drug–cell interaction, inactivation, and excretion—metabolic processes that are known as pharmacokinetics. The cytochrome P450 (CYP) genes play a key role in the pharmacokinetic process of drug metabolism. Once a drug reaches its target cell, other genes such as those regulating cell receptors and cell signaling control the drug's effect. This process is known as pharmacodynamics. Single genes may affect drug response. More commonly, drug response involves the interaction of multiple genes, the host, and the effects of other drugs. Figure 8-12 is a schematic display of the genetic and genomic influences on drug metabolism and treatment effect.

The difference between genetics and genomics, described earlier in this chapter, corresponds to the terms *pharmaco-*

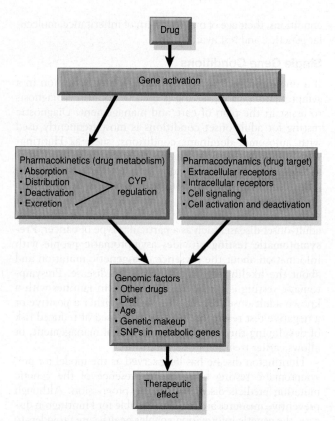

FIGURE 8-12 • Simplified schematic representation of the multiple, complex, genetic-regulated mechanisms involved in pharmacokinetics (cytochrome [CYP] dependent) and pharmacodynamics, along with other genomic and environmental factors affecting drug metabolism and treatment effect. SNP, single nucleotide polymorphism.

genetics and *pharmacogenomics,* which combine pharmacology and genetics/genomics. Pharmacogenetics refers to the study of the effect of variations in a single gene on drug response and toxicity. The field of pharmacogenetics has evolved so that it has become a broader genomic-based approach that recognizes the interaction of multiple genes and the environment on drug response. Pharmacogenomics refers to the study of the combined effect of variations in many genes on drug response and toxicity, and involves methods that rapidly identify which genetic variations influence a drug's effect. Pharmacogenomics involves the search for genetic variations associated with medication metabolism and efficacy, with the goal of tailoring treatment to each individual's genomic makeup (Genetic Home Reference, 2011).

SNPs, described earlier, are common genetic variations that occur most frequently throughout the human genome and often contribute to variations in enzymatic activity that affect drug metabolism. The CYPs, a family of enzymes, play a key role in the pharmacokinetic process of drug metabolism. More than 200 variations (SNPs) of genes that control CYP activation and deactivation have been identified. Researchers have created a catalog of CYP variations because of their role in drug metabolism (Sim & Ingelman-Sundberg, 2010).

Four classes of CYP metabolic activity levels have been identified based on a person's CYP genotype and the corresponding drug response: (1) poor metabolizers, (2) intermediate

TABLE 8-6   Examples of Clinical Effects of Cytochrome P450 Enzyme Variations

Enzyme	Drug	Effects	
		Poor Metabolizer	**Ultrarapid Metabolizer**
CYP2C9	Warfarin (Coumadin)	Bleeding	Longer treatment time to achieve stable dosing
	Phenytoin (Dilantin)	Ataxia	Not established
CYP2C19	Diazepam (Valium)	Sedation	Poor response
	Omeprazole (Prilosec)	Drug-induced side effects (e.g., taste perversion)	
CYP2D6	Tricyclic antidepressants	Cardiotoxicity	No response to recommended dose; need 10-fold increase in dose
	Selective serotonin reuptake inhibitors	Nausea	Not established
	Antipsychotics	Parkinson-like effects	Longer treatment time and higher drug costs

Based on information from Ingelman-Sundberg, M. (2004). Pharmacogenetics of cytochrome P450 and its applications in drug therapy: The past, present and future. *Trends in Pharmacological Science, 25*(4), 193–200.

metabolizers, (3) extensive metabolizers, and (4) ultrarapid metabolizers (Ingelman-Sundberg, 2004). Poor metabolizers have a specific SNP variation in a CYP gene that causes little or no function, resulting in very little or no drug metabolism and higher blood levels of active drug because the drug cannot be absorbed or excreted. Conversely, ultrarapid metabolizers have SNP variations that cause increased enzyme activity, resulting in rapid absorption, distribution, and excretion of a drug. Ultrarapid metabolizers have lower drug blood levels, usually with inadequate therapeutic response or longer treatment time to achieve therapeutic results. Both poor metabolizers and ultrarapid metabolizers are predisposed to adverse drug reactions. Poor metabolizers may have adverse effects or toxicities from high blood levels of drugs and need a lower dose, whereas ultrarapid metabolizers have inadequate treatment response because of lower drug blood levels and may need a higher dose or more frequent dosing. Table 8-6 shows examples of differences in drug response in poor versus ultrarapid metabolizers. Intermediate metabolizers have reduced enzyme activity levels and metabolize drugs at a slower than normal rate. Because intermediate metabolizers have some enzyme activity, they may have differences in treatment response. Extensive metabolizers have normal enzyme activity levels and normal drug metabolism. Differences in metabolism of other medications occur with other genetic variations.

Nurses have traditionally monitored and reported drug response and drug adverse effects. Clinical guidelines for pharmacogenomic testing for several drugs, such as warfarin (Coumadin), vitamin K, and HMG-CoA reductase inhibitors (statins), are being tested, and their implications will likely be incorporated into clinical practice (Kitzmiller, Groen, Phelps, et al., 2011). Pharmacogenomic testing will give patients more information about drug dosage, time to achieve response, and risk of adverse effects. Nurses will provide education about a particular patient's genomic profile for drug metabolism and explain the rationale for the recommended dosage and likelihood of adverse effects. Nurses will continue to incorporate information about gender differences, food interactions, and drug compliance into patient education (Consensus Panel, 2009).

Applications of Genetics and Genomics in Nursing Practice

Nurses who provide genetics- and genomics-related health care blend the principles of human genetics with nursing care in collaboration with other professionals, including genetic specialists, to foster improvement, maintenance, and restoration of patients' health. In all nursing practice settings, nurses have five main tasks (Consensus Panel, 2009): (1) help collect and interpret relevant family and medical histories; (2) identify patients and families who need further genetics evaluation and counseling, and refer them to appropriate genetics services; (3) offer genetic information and resources to patients and families; (4) collaborate with genetic specialists; and (5) participate in the management and coordination of care of patients with genetic conditions. Genetics-related nursing practice involves the care of people who have genetic conditions, those who may be predisposed to develop or pass on genetic conditions, and those who are seeking genetic information and referral for additional genetics services.

Nurses support patients and families with genetics- and genomics-related health concerns by ensuring that their health choices are informed ones and by advocating for the privacy and confidentiality of genetic and genomic information and for equal access to genetic testing and treatments (Consensus Panel, 2009).

Genetics and Genomics in Health Assessment

Assessment of a person's genetic and genomic health status is an ongoing process. Nurses collect information that can help identify individuals and families who have actual or potential genetics- or genomics-related health concerns or who may benefit from further genetic information, counseling, testing, and treatment. This process can begin before conception and continue throughout the lifespan. Nurses evaluate family and past medical histories, including prenatal history, childhood illnesses, developmental history, adult-onset conditions, past surgeries, treatments, and medications; this information may relate to the genetic or genomic condition at hand or to a condition being considered. (See Chapter 5 for more information on assessing past medical history.) Nurses also identify the patient's ethnic background and conduct a physical assessment to gather pertinent genetic information. The assessment also includes information about culture, spiritual beliefs, and ancestry. Health assessment includes determining a patient's or family's understanding of actual or potential genetics- or genomics-related health concerns and awareness of how these issues are communicated within a family (Consensus Panel, 2009).

Family History Assessment

Nurses in any practice setting can assess families' genetics histories to identify a genetic trait, inherited condition, or predisposition. Targeted questions are used to identify genetic and genomic conditions for which further information, education, testing, or treatment can be offered (Chart 8-2). After consultation and collaboration with other health care providers and specialists, further genetic testing and evaluation is offered for

the trait or condition in question. The genetics family history is used to make a diagnosis, identify testing strategies, and establish a pattern of inheritance. It includes at least three generations, as well as information about the current and past health status of all family members, including the age at onset of any illness, cause of death, and age at death. Nurses also can inquire about medical conditions that are known to have a heritable component and for which genetic testing may be available. Information is obtained about the presence of birth defects, mental retardation, familial traits, or similarly affected family members (Consensus Panel, 2009).

Nurses also consider the closeness of the relationship (genetic relatedness or consanguinity) among family members when assessing the risk of genetic conditions in couples or families. For example, when obtaining a preconception or prenatal family history, it is important for the nurse to ask if the prospective parents have common ancestors (i.e., are they first cousins?). This is important because people who are related have more genes in common than those who are unrelated, thus increasing their chance of having children with an autosomal recessive inherited condition such as cystic fibrosis. Ascertaining genetic relatedness provides direction for genetic counseling and evaluation. It may also serve as an explanation for parents who have a child with a rare autosomal recessive inherited condition or for a person who is similarly affected.

When the assessment of family history reveals that a patient has been adopted, genetic- and genomic-based health assessment becomes more challenging. Every effort is made to help the patient obtain as much information as possible about his or her biologic parents, including their ethnic backgrounds.

Questions about previous miscarriage or stillbirth are included in genetics health assessments to identify possible chromosomal conditions. Nurses can also inquire about any history of family members with inherited conditions or birth defects; maternal health conditions such as type 1 diabetes, seizure disorders, or PKU, which may increase the risk for birth defects in children; and about exposure to alcohol or other drugs during pregnancy. Maternal age is also noted; women who are 35 years of age or older who are considering pregnancy and childbearing or who are already pregnant should be offered prenatal diagnosis (e.g., testing through amniocentesis) because of the association between advanced maternal age and chromosomal abnormalities such as Down syndrome.

Physical Assessment

Physical assessment may provide clues that a particular genetic or genomic condition is present in a person and family. Family history assessment may serve as a guide to focus the physical assessment. For example, a history of familial hypercholesterolemia would alert the nurse to assess for symptoms of hyperlipidemias (xanthomas, corneal arcus, and abdominal pain of unexplained origin). As another example, a family history of neurofibromatosis type 1, an inherited condition involving tumors of the central nervous system, would prompt the nurse to carry out a detailed assessment of closely related family members. Skin findings such as *café-au-lait* spots, axillary freckling, or tumors of the skin (neurofibromas) would warrant referral for further evaluation, including

---

Chart 8-2 — Genetics Family History: An Essential Tool for All Nurses

A well-documented family history can be used to:

- Assess risk of certain diseases
- Decide on testing strategies, such as what genetic and other diagnostic tests to order
- Establish a pattern of inheritance
- Identify other family members who are at increased risk
- Identify shared environmental risk factors
- Calculate risks
- Assess risk of passing on conditions to children
- Determine and recommend treatments that modify disease risk
- Make decisions about management or surveillance
- Develop patient rapport
- Educate patients

Key questions to ask about each family member include:

- What is the current age, or what was the age at death?
- What is the ethnic background (some genetic conditions are more common in certain ethnic groups)?
- Is there a history of:
  - Multiple pregnancy losses/stillbirths?
  - Unexplained infertility?
  - Birth defects?
  - Mental retardation or developmental delay?
  - Learning disabilities?
  - Medical problems in children whose parents are closely related (second cousins or closer)?
  - Congenital or juvenile blindness, cataracts, hearing loss or deafness?
  - Very short or very tall stature?
  - Several close relatives with the same or related conditions (e.g., breast or colon cancer, diabetes, heart disease, asthma, stroke, high blood pressure, kidney disease)?
  - Occurrence of a common condition with earlier age of onset than is usual (e.g., breast or colon cancer, hearing loss, dementia, heart disease)?

Adapted from Centers for Disease Control and Prevention (2011). Genomics translation: Family history public health initiative. Available at: www.cdc.gov/genomics/famhistory/famhist.htm; Mayo Clinic. *Medical history: Compiling your medical family tree*. Available at: www.mayoclinic.com/health/medical-history/HQ01707

genetic evaluation and counseling (National Human Genome Research Institute, 2010).

If a genetic or genomic condition is suspected as a result of a family history or physical assessment, the nurse, as a part of his or her role, and in collaboration with the health care team, may initiate further discussion of genetics and genomic information, offering and discussing genetic tests, and suggesting a referral for further genetic evaluation (Chart 8-3).

Ancestry, Cultural, Social, and Spiritual Assessment

Genetics assessment addresses the ancestry of patients and families, as well as their ethnicity. This information helps identify individual patients and groups who could benefit

---

Chart 8-3 Indications for Making a Genetics Referral

Prepregnancy and Prenatal

- Maternal age of 35 years or greater at expected time of delivery
- Previous child with a chromosome problem
- Positive alpha-fetoprotein profile screening test
- Previous child with a birth defect or family history of birth defects
- Pregnancy history of two or more unexplained miscarriages
- Maternal conditions such as diabetes, epilepsy, or alcoholism
- Exposures to certain medications or drugs during pregnancy
- Family history of mental retardation
- Either member of the couple has a birth defect such as cleft lip or palate, spina bifida, or congenital heart defect
- Either member of the couple has a chromosome abnormality

Pediatric

- Positive newborn screening test
- One or more major birth defects
- Unusual (dysmorphic) facial features
- Developmental delay/mental retardation
- Suspicion of a metabolic disorder
- Unusually tall or short stature, or growth delays
- Known chromosomal abnormality

Adult

- Mental retardation without a known cause
- Unexplained infertility or multiple pregnancy losses
- A personal or family history of thrombotic events
- Adult-onset conditions such as hemochromatosis, hearing loss, visual impairment
- Family history of an adult-onset neurodegenerative disorder (e.g., Huntington disease)
- Features of a genetic condition such as neurofibromatosis (café-au-lait spots, neurofibromas on the skin), Marfan syndrome (unusually tall stature, dilation of the aortic root), others
- Personal or family history of cardiovascular disorders known to be associated with genetic factors such as cardiomyopathy or long QT syndrome
- Family history of cancers known to be associated with specific genes such as hereditary breast/ovarian cancer or Lynch syndrome
- Family history of early-onset cancers and familial clustering of related tumors

Adapted from Pletcher, B. A., Toriello, H. V., Noblin, S. J., et al. (2007). Indications for genetic referral: A guide for healthcare providers. *Genetics in Medicine, 9*(6), 385–389.

---

from genetic testing for carrier identification, prenatal diagnosis, and susceptibility testing. For example, carrier testing for sickle cell anemia is routinely offered to people of African American descent, and carrier testing for Tay-Sachs disease and Canavan disease is offered to people of Ashkenazi Jewish descent. The American College of Obstetricians and Gynecologists (ACOG) recommends that members of at-risk racial and ethnic populations be offered carrier testing (ACOG Committee on Genetics, 2009). The ACOG and the American College of Medical Genetics and Genomics (ACMG) recommend that all couples, particularly those of northern European and Ashkenazi Jewish ancestry, be offered carrier screening for cystic fibrosis (ACOG, 2004; Watson, Cutting, Desnick, et al., 2004). Ideally, carrier testing is offered before conception to allow people who are carriers to make decisions about reproduction. Prenatal diagnosis is offered and discussed when both partners of a couple are found to be carriers.

It is important to inquire about the patient's ethnic backgrounds when assessing for susceptibilities to adult-onset conditions such as hereditary breast or ovarian cancer. For example, a *BRCA1* cancer-predisposing gene mutation seems to occur more frequently in women of Ashkenazi Jewish descent. Therefore, asking about ethnicity can help identify people with an increased risk of cancer gene mutations (Calzone et al., 2010).

Nurses also should consider their patients' views about the significance of a genetic condition and its effect on self-concept, as well as patients' perception of the role of genetics in health and illness, reproduction, and disability. Patients' social and cultural backgrounds determine their interpretations and values about information obtained from genetic testing and evaluation and thus influence their perceptions of health, illness, and risk (Chart 8-4). Family structure, decision making, and educational background contribute in the same way (Consensus Panel, 2009).

Assessment of the patients' beliefs, values, and expectations regarding genetic testing and genetic and genomic information helps nurses provide appropriate information about the specific genetics or genomics topic. For example, in some cultures, people believe that health means the absence of symptoms and that the cause of illness is supernatural. Patients with these beliefs may initially reject suggestions for presymptomatic or carrier testing. However, by including resources such as family and cultural and religious community leaders when providing genetics- or genomics-related health care, nurses can help ensure that patients receive information in a way that transcends social, cultural, and economic barriers (Calzone et al., 2010).

Psychosocial Assessment

Psychosocial assessment is an essential nursing component of the genetics health assessment. The assessment findings can help identify the potential impact of new genetic and genomic information on the patient and family and how they may cope with this information (Chart 8-5).

Genetic Counseling and Evaluation Services

People seek genetic counseling for various reasons and at different stages of life. Some are seeking preconception or

NURSING RESEARCH PROFILE

Chart 8-4 Lifestyle Changes and Genetic Risk for Chronic Disease

Taylor, J. Y., & Wu, C. Y. (2009). Effects of genetic counseling for hypertension on changes in lifestyle behaviors among African Americans. *Journal of the National Black Nurses Association*, 20(1), 1–10.

Purpose

African Americans develop more severe hypertension—and at a younger age—compared to other ethnic groups. Lack of exercise, elevated body mass index (BMI), high sodium intake, and family history are contributing risk factors. The purpose of this study was to evaluate lifestyle changes that contribute to the risk of hypertension in African American women after participation in genetic counseling for hypertension risk.

Design

This study used a descriptive correlational research design. A total of 98 African American women were recruited from the Detroit area after they took part in a previous parent study on hypertension risks. Participants' blood pressure, pulse pressure, and lifestyle behaviors were examined at baseline and 6 months after a genetic counseling session with a registered nurse who had specialized training in the genetics of hypertension. During the genetic counseling sessions, participants were provided with information about their risks for hypertension and received

genetic counseling about their family history of heart disease. They also received culturally appropriate education materials about physical activity and dietary sodium recommendations to reduce their risk for hypertension. Paired t-test comparisons were performed to find differences before and after the genetic counseling sessions.

Findings

Six months after the genetic counseling intervention, systolic and diastolic blood pressures and pulse pressures demonstrated a non–statistically significant decrease from baseline. The women reported more physical activity after the intervention; however, their BMIs did not significantly change. Participants' sodium intake decreased from a mean of 3,200 mg/day at baseline to 2,798 mg/day at follow-up ($p < .033$).

Nursing Implications

Nurses with an understanding of the inherited genetic risk for chronic diseases can provide important patient teaching information regarding how risk for diseases such as hypertension can be passed from one generation to the next. Providing appropriate genetic counseling that is coupled with teaching healthy lifestyle behaviors can be cost-effective nursing interventions that may reduce rates of chronic diseases in at-risk populations.

---

prenatal information, others are referred after the birth of a child with a birth defect or suspected genetic condition, and still others are seeking information for themselves or their families because of the presence of, or a family history of, a genetic condition. Regardless of the timing or setting, genetic counseling is offered to all people who have questions about genetics or genomics and their health.

ASSESSMENT

Chart 8-5 Assessing Psychosocial Genetic Health

The nurse's assessment of psychosocial factors impacting a patient's genetic health is based on the nurse's professional responsibility to "demonstrate in practice the importance of tailoring genetic and genomic information and services to clients based on their culture, religion, knowledge level, literacy and preferred language."

The nurse assesses:

- Educational level and understanding of the genetic condition or concern in the family.
- Desired goals and health outcomes in relation to the genetic condition or concern.
- Family rules regarding disclosure of medical information (e.g., some families may not reveal a history of a disease such as cancer or mental illness during the family history assessment).
- Family rules, boundaries, and cultural practices as well as personal preference about knowing genetic information.
- Past coping mechanisms and social support.
- Ability to make an informed decision (e.g., is the patient under stress from family situations, acute or chronic illness, or medications that may impair the patient's ability to make an informed decision?).

Adapted from Consensus Panel on Genetic/Genomic Nursing Competencies. (2009). *Essential nursing competencies and curricula guidelines for genetics and genomics*. Silver Spring, MD: Author, p. 24.

As the contribution of genetics and genomics to the health–illness continuum is recognized, genetic counseling will become a responsibility of all health care professionals in clinical practice. Nurses are in an ideal position to assess the patient's health and genetics family history and to make referrals for specialized diagnosis and treatment. They offer anticipatory guidance by explaining the purpose and goals of a referral. They collaborate with other health care providers in giving supportive and follow-up counseling and coordinating follow-up and case management.

Genetics Services

Genetics services provide genetic information, education, and support to patients and families. Medical geneticists, genetic counselors, and advanced practice nurses in genetics provide specific genetics services to patients and families who are referred by their primary or specialty health care providers. A team approach is often used to obtain and interpret complex family history information, evaluate and diagnose genetic conditions, interpret and discuss complicated genetic test results, support patients throughout the evaluation process, and offer professional and family support. Patients participate as team members and decision makers throughout the process. Genetics services enable patients and their families to learn and understand relevant aspects of genetics and genomics, to make informed health decisions, and to receive support as they integrate personal and family genetic and genomic information into daily living (National Human Genome Research Institute, 2011h).

Genetic counseling may take place over an extended period and may entail more than one counseling session, which may include other family members. The components of genetic counseling are outlined in Chart 8-6. Although genetic counseling may be offered at any point during the lifespan,

| Chart 8-6 | Components of Genetic Counseling |

Information and Assessment Sources

- Reason for referral
- Family history
- Medical history/records
- Relevant test results and other medical evaluations
- Social and emotional concerns
- Relevant cultural, educational, and financial factors

Analysis of Data

- Family history
- Physical examination as needed
- Additional laboratory testing and procedures (e.g., echocardiogram, ophthalmology or neurologic examination)

Communication of Genetic Finding

- Natural history of disorder
- Pattern of inheritance
- Reproductive and family health issues and options
- Testing options
- Management and treatment issues

Counseling and Support

- Identify individual and family questions and concerns.
- Identify existing support systems.
- Provide emotional and social support.
- Refer for additional support and counseling as indicated.

Follow-Up

- Written summary to referring primary care providers and family
- Coordination of care with primary care providers and specialists
- Additional discussions of test results or diagnosis

Genetics Resources

GeneTests: a listing of common genetic disorders with up-to-date clinical summaries and genetic counseling and testing information, www.ncbi.nlm.nih.gov/sites/GeneTests/

Genetic Alliance: a directory of support groups for patients and families with genetic conditions, www.geneticalliance.org

Genetic and Rare Diseases Information Center: provides links with experienced information specialists who can answer questions in English and Spanish to patients, families, and health care providers regarding specific genetic diseases, www.genome.gov/Health/GARD/

Genetics Home Reference: provides a layman's online encyclopedic guide to understanding genetic conditions, ghr.nlm.nih.gov/

National Human Genome Research Institute, Genome Statute and Legislative Database: summarizes each state's legislation on employment and insurance discrimination, www.genome.gov/PolicyEthics/LegDatabase/pubsearch.cfm

National Organization for Rare Disorders (NORD): a directory of support groups and information for patients and families with rare genetic disorders, www.rarediseases.org

Online Mendelian Inheritance in Man (OMIM): a complete listing of inherited genetic conditions, http://www.ncbi.nlm.nih.gov/omim

Adapted from Genetics Home Reference. *Genetic Consultation.* Available at www.ghr.nlm.nih.gov/handbook/consult?show=all#consultation

counseling issues are often relevant to the life stage in which counseling is sought (National Human Genome Research Institute, 2011h). Examples are presented in Chart 8-7.

Advocacy in Genetic and Genomic Decisions

Respecting the patient's right to self-determination—that is, supporting decisions that reflect the patient's personal beliefs, values, and interests—is a central principle in directing how nurses provide genetic and genomic information and counseling. Nurses and others participating in genetic counseling make every attempt to respect the patient's ability to make autonomous decisions. Recognizing one's own values (see Chart 8-1) and how communication of genetic and genomic information may be influenced

| Chart 8-7 | Genetic Counseling Across the Lifespan |

Prenatal Issues

- Understanding prenatal screening and diagnosis testing
- Implications of reproductive choices
- Potential for anxiety and emotional distress
- Effects on partnership, family, and parental–fetal bonding

Newborn Issues

- Understanding newborn screening results
- Potential for disrupted parent–newborn relationship on diagnosis of a genetic condition
- Parental guilt
- Implications for siblings and other family members
- Coordination and continuity of care

Pediatric Issues

- Caring for children with complex medical needs
- Coordination of care

- Potential for impaired parent–child relationship
- Potential for social stigmatization

Adolescent Issues

- Potential for impaired self-image and decreased self-esteem
- Potential for altered perception of family
- Implications for lifestyle and family planning

Adult Issues

- Potential for ambiguous test results
- Identification of a genetic susceptibility or diagnosis without an existing cure
- Effect on marriage, reproduction, parenting, and lifestyle
- Potential impact on insurability and employability

Adapted from Jenkins, J. F., & Lea, D. H. (2005). *Nursing care in the genomic era: A case-based approach.* Boston: Jones & Bartlett.

by those values is a first step toward assuring patients' autonomous decision making.

Confidentiality of genetic and genomic information and respect for privacy are other essential principles underlying genetic counseling. Patients have the right to not have test results divulged to anyone, including insurers, physicians, employers, or family members. Some patients pay for testing themselves so that insurers will not learn of the test, and others use a different name for testing to protect their privacy.

A nurse may want to disclose genetic information to family members who could experience significant harm if they do not know such information. However, the patient may have other views and may wish to keep this information from the family, resulting in an ethical dilemma for both patient and nurse. The nurse must honor the patient's wishes, while explaining to the patient the potential benefit this information may have for other family members (International Society of Nurses in Genetics [ISONG], 2010).

The Health Insurance Portability and Accountability Act (HIPAA) of 1996 prohibits the use of genetic information to establish insurance eligibility. However, HIPAA does not prohibit group plans from increasing premiums, excluding coverage for a specific condition, or imposing a lifetime cap on benefits. The National Human Genome Research Institute, Policy and Program Analysis branch, has a summary of each state's legislation on employment and insurance discrimination (National Human Genome Research Institute, 2011i). (See also the Resources section at the end of this chapter.)

Most lawmakers, scientists, and health advocacy groups strongly believe that there is a need for federal legislation to prevent genetic discrimination. Nurses need to become familiar with the Genetic Information Nondiscrimination Act (GINA), which was signed into law in 2008. Its purpose is to protect Americans against improper use of genetic and genomic information in insurance and employment decisions. The act prohibits health insurers from denying coverage to a healthy person or charging higher insurance rates based on a person's genetic predisposition to a disease (Chart 8-8). The act also prevents employers from using a person's genetic and

---

Chart 8-8

ETHICAL DILEMMA

Are Patients Subject to Genetic Testing at Risk for Discrimination?

Case Scenario

You are employed at a women's health clinic. A woman who is considering *BRCA1/2* genetic testing for hereditary breast/ovarian cancer informs you that she does not wish to bill her insurance company for the testing because she fears that the insurance company will discriminate against her based on her genetic testing results and deny her insurance coverage based on that information.

Discussion

Genetic testing and technologies are increasingly being used for screening, presymptomatic diagnosis, and diagnosis and treatment of both rare and common diseases, thereby providing individuals and their health care providers with previously unavailable genetic information. Genetic information is defined as heritable, biologic information (National Human Genome Research Institute, 2011), and it can be identified at any point throughout a person's lifespan from preconception until after death. In addition to heritable, biologic information, family history, genetic test results, and medical records are also sources of genetic information.

One of the concerns raised by many patients when they are considering having genetic testing is that if their insurance company knows of the genetic testing results that indicate a patient has a genetic condition or is at risk for developing a genetic condition, they will then be denied insurance coverage and discriminated against based on their genetic information. An ethical dilemma arises for nurses and other health care providers when patients choose to pay for their genetic testing out of pocket so that their insurance companies will not have access to their genetic test results.

In 2008, the Genetic Information Nondiscrimination Act (GINA) was signed into law. GINA makes it unlawful for health insurance companies and employers to discriminate against an individual based on his or her genetic profile. GINA has opened the door to allow people to take advantage of personalized medicine based on their individual genetic information without fear of discrimination. GINA, therefore, provides a level of protection against genetic discrimination for all Americans. It is important for nurses

to know what GINA does not do so that they can share this information with patients and families as well. GINA's health care coverage nondiscrimination protections do not include life insurance, disability insurance, and long-term care insurance (Department of Health and Human Services, 2009; National Human Genome Research Institute, 2011). Nurses can turn to the National Human Genome Research Institute and the Department of Health and Human Services to learn more about GINA and what it does and does not do.

Analysis

- Describe the ethical principles that are in conflict in this case (see Chart 3-3). Which principle do you believe should have preeminence in deciding whether or not patients have the right to request to self-pay and withhold information from their insurance company?
- Even after the passage of GINA, what potential ethical concerns about discrimination based on a person's genetic information still exist? How might this affect a patient's ability to make autonomous decisions?
- Are there any professional guidelines that you can turn to for help in determining the ethical issues that still remain around discrimination against an individual based on his or her genetic information? If so, what are they, and how can they help?

References

Department of Health and Human Services. (2009). *"GINA": The Genetic Information Nondiscrimination Act of 2008: Information for researchers and health care professionals.* Available at: www.genome.gov/Pages/PolicyEthics/GeneticDiscrimination/GINAInfoDoc.pdf

National Human Genome Research Institute. (2011). *Genetic Information Nondiscrimination Act (GINA) of 2008.* Available at: www.genome.gov/24519851

Resources

See Chapter 3, Chart 3-6 for ethics resources.

genomic information to make decisions about hiring, job placement, promotion, or firing. As a result, most Americans are free to use genetic and genomic information in health care without the fear of misuse (National Human Genome Research Institute, 2011h). However, GINA does not cover life, disability, or long-term care insurance. Furthermore, GINA and other state and federal protections do not extend to genetic testing of active duty military personnel or genetic information obtained from active military personnel (Hudson, Holohan, & Collins, 2008; Steck & Eggert, 2011).

All genetic specialists, including nurses who participate in the genetic counseling process and those with access to a person's genetic information, must honor a patient's desire for confidentiality. Genetic information should not be revealed to family members, insurance companies, employers, and schools if the patient so desires, even if keeping the information confidential is difficult.

Providing Precounseling Information

Preparing the patient and family, promoting informed decision making, and obtaining informed consent are essential in genetic counseling. Nurses assess the patient's capacity and ability to give voluntary consent. This includes assessment of factors that may interfere with informed consent, such as hearing loss, language differences, cognitive impairment, and the effects of medication. Nurses make sure that a person's decision to undergo testing is not affected by coercion, persuasion, or manipulation. Because information may need to be repeated over time, nurses offer follow-up discussion as needed (Calzone et al., 2010).

The genetics service to which a patient or family is referred for genetic counseling will ask the nurse for background information for evaluation. Genetic specialists need to know the reason for referral, the patient's or family's reason for seeking genetic counseling, and potential genetics-related health concerns. For example, a nurse may refer a family with a new diagnosis of hereditary breast or ovarian cancer for counseling or to discuss the likelihood of developing the disease and the implications for other family members. The family may have concerns about confidentiality and privacy. The nurse and the genetic specialist tailor the genetic counseling to respond to these concerns.

With the patient's permission, genetic specialists will request the relevant test results and medical evaluations. Nurses obtain permission from the patient and, if applicable, from other family members to provide medical records that document the genetic condition of concern. In some situations, evaluation of more than one family member may be necessary to establish a diagnosis of a genetic disorder. Nurses explain that the medical information is needed to ensure that appropriate information and counseling (including risk interpretation) are provided.

The genetics service asks nurses about the emotional and social status of the patient and family. Genetic specialists want to know the coping skills of patients and families who have recently learned of the diagnosis of a genetic disorder as well as what type of genetic information is being sought. Nurses help identify cultural and other issues that may influence how information is provided and by whom. For example, for patients with hearing loss, a sign interpreter's services may have to be arranged. For those with vision loss, alternative forms of communication may be necessary. Genetics professionals prepare for the genetic counseling and evaluation with these relevant issues in mind (Jenkins & Lea, 2005).

Preparing Patients for Genetics Evaluation

Before a genetic counseling appointment, the nurse discusses with the patient and family the type of family history information that will be collected during the consultation. Family history collection and analysis are comprehensive and focus on information that may be relevant to the genetics- or genomics-related concern in question. The genetic analysis always includes assessment for any other potentially inherited conditions for which testing, prevention, and treatment may be possible.

A physical examination may be performed by the medical geneticist to identify specific clinical features commonly associated with a genetic condition. The examination also helps determine if further testing is needed to diagnose a genetic disorder. This examination generally involves assessment of all body systems, with a focus on specific physical characteristics. Nurses describe the diagnostic evaluations that are part of a genetics consultation and explain their purposes.

Communicating Genetic and Genomic Information to Patients

After the family history and physical examination are completed, the genetics team reviews the information gathered before beginning genetic counseling with the patient and family. The genetic specialists meet with the patient and family to discuss their findings. If information gathered confirms a genetic condition in a family, genetic specialists discuss with the patient the natural history of the condition, the pattern of inheritance, and the implications of the condition for reproductive and general health. When appropriate, specialists also discuss relevant testing and management options.

Providing Support

The genetics team provides support throughout the counseling session and identifies personal and family concerns. Genetic specialists use active listening to interpret patient concerns and emotions, seek and provide feedback, and demonstrate understanding of those concerns. They suggest referral for additional social and emotional support. In addition, genetic specialists discuss pertinent patient and family concerns and needs with nurses and primary health care teams so that they can provide additional support and guidance (Jenkins & Lea, 2005; Skirton, Patch, & Williams, 2005). Nurses assess the patient's understanding of the information given during the counseling session, clarify information, answer questions, assess patient reactions, and identify support systems.

Follow-Up After Genetic Evaluation

As a follow-up to genetic evaluation and counseling, genetic specialists prepare a written summary of the evaluation and counseling session for the patient and, with the patient's consent, send this summary to the primary provider as well as other providers identified by the patient as participants in care. The consultation summary outlines the results of the family history and physical and laboratory assessments, provides a discussion of any specific diagnosis made, reviews the inheritance and associated risk of recurrence for the patient and family, presents reproductive and general health options, and makes recommendations for further testing and management. The nurse reviews the summary with the patient and identifies information, education, and counseling for which follow-up genetic counseling may be useful (Skirton et al., 2005).

Follow-up genetic counseling is always offered because some patients and families need more time to understand and discuss the specifics of a genetic test or diagnosis, or they may wish to review reproductive options again later, when pregnancy is being considered. Follow-up counseling is also offered to patients when further evaluation and counseling of extended family members is recommended (Skirton et al., 2005).

During follow-up sessions, nurses can educate patients about sources of information related to genetic and genomic issues. Some resources that provide the most up-to-date and reliable genetic and genomic information are available on the Internet (see the Resources section at the end of this chapter).

Ethical Issues

Nurses must consider their responsibilities in handling genetic and genomic information and potential ethical issues such as informed decision making, privacy and confidentiality of such information, and access to and justice in health care. The ethical principles of autonomy, fidelity, and veracity are also important (American Nurses Association [ANA], 2008).

Ethical questions relating to genetics and genomics occur in all settings and at all levels of nursing practice. At the level of direct patient care, nurses participate in providing genetic information, testing, and gene-based therapeutics. They offer patient care based on the values of self-determination and personal autonomy. To be as fully informed as possible, patients need appropriate, accurate, and complete information given at a level and in a form so that they and their families can make well-informed personal, medical, and reproductive health decisions. Nurses can help patients clarify values and goals, assess understanding of information, protect their rights, and support their decisions. Nurses can advocate for patient autonomy in health decisions. Several resources and position statements have been developed to guide nursing practice (Consensus Panel, 2009). These position statements are listed at the end of this chapter, in Journals and Electronic Documents: International Society of Nurses in Genetics (2010).

Many people are increasingly concerned about threats to their personal privacy and the confidentiality of genetic and genomic information. An ethical foundation provides nurses with a holistic framework for handling these issues with integrity and provides a basis for communicating genetic and genomic information to a patient, a family, other care providers, community agencies and organizations, and society. Ethical principles of beneficence (i.e., to do good) and nonmaleficence (i.e., to do no harm), as well as autonomy, justice, fidelity, and veracity, are used to resolve ethical dilemmas that may arise in clinical care. Respect for people is the ethical principle underlying all nursing care. Using these principles and the values of caring, nurses can promote thoughtful discussions that are useful when patients and families are facing genetics- and genomics-related health and reproductive decisions and con-

sequences (Consensus Panel, 2009; ISONG, 2010). (Further information about ethics is included in Chapter 3.)

Genetics and Genomics Tomorrow

The pace of genetic and genomic research is transforming our understanding of the role of genetics and genomics in health and disease. In addition, it is increasing clinical opportunities for presymptomatic prediction of illness based on a patient's genetic makeup. Genetic research is now focused on identifying the genetic and environmental causes of common diseases such as diabetes, heart disease, and asthma. The studies are opening the doors for many advances in the prevention and treatment of both rare and common diseases (National Human Genome Research Institute, 2011j).

As applications of genetics and genomics to health and disease develop, genetic testing may be used to scan all of a patient's genetic material so that disease risk variants can be identified and early interventions and treatments can be determined. It is projected that the cost of testing a patient's entire genome will be less than $1,000. Personalized medicine will continue to expand, and many treatments and interventions for medical conditions will be chosen based on what genetic testing indicates about a patient's genetic makeup. Nurses will be on the front line in communicating genetic and genomic information to patients, families, and communities. Patients, families, and communities will also expect that health care providers, including nurses, will use new genetic and genomic information and technologies in the provision of care. It is therefore imperative that all nurses become fluent in the language of genetics and genomics so that they can provide effective nursing care (Consensus Panel, 2009).

Critical Thinking Exercises

1 **ebp** A 32-year-old woman has been admitted to your nursing unit after having orthopedic surgery, specifically an open reduction with internal fixation to stabilize a right ankle fracture. Your nursing intervention includes a pain assessment. The patient is already asking questions about when her parenteral opioids for pain will be changed to oral agents. She reports having had poor pain control with oral opioids after a prior fracture; in particular, she describes having to ask more frequently for pain medication than was recommended. During that recovery period, she felt very discouraged because she was accused of "drug-seeking behavior." What pharmacogenomic evidence-based information would you give this patient about her past experience with pain medications? What evidence related to pain medications supports your discussion? How would you determine the strength of that evidence? What pharmacologic measures would you discuss with the surgical team to plan for effective pain control?

2 **ebp** A 42-year-old man has a biopsy that is *positive* for right-sided colon cancer. The pathology report shows a poorly differentiated tumor that is *negative* for MLH1 by immunohistochemistry. This means the MLH1 protein is absent and indicates a potential malfunction of the *MLH1* gene. His father had colon cancer at age 48, and his sister had uterine cancer at age 52. Clinicians present the patient with options for genetic testing and surgical consideration of a colon resection. The patient reports that he does not understand why he should have genetic testing. What evidence about the patient's phenotype (i.e., age and tumor characteristics) is the basis for the recommendation for genetic testing, and what is the strength of that evidence? What information about his family history support genetic testing? What genetic resources or referrals would you suggest for this patient? What professional guidelines support your recommendation for genetic testing?

3 **pq** A 50-year-old woman is seen in the clinic for concerns about recent episodes of forgetfulness. She has a strong family history of early-onset Alzheimer's disease (AD). Her father recently died at the age of 68 after having AD for 10 years. Her physician wants her to see a genetic counselor to discuss the pros and cons of being tested to see if she carries one of the genes for AD. She sees you for patient education and asks how she would cope with knowing that AD may be in her future. In addition, she has concerns about the privacy of genetic information and what that would mean in terms of her health insurance. Identify the priorities, approach, and techniques that you would use to perform a comprehensive genetic assessment for a patient with AD.

Brunner Suite Resources
Explore these additional resources to enhance learning for this chapter:
• NCLEX-Style Questions and Other Resources on **the**Point, http://thePoint.lww.com/Brunner13e
• Study Guide
• PrepU
• Clinical Handbook
• Handbook of Laboratory and Diagnostic Tests

References

*Asterisk indicates nursing research.
**Double asterisk indicates classic reference.

Books

American Nurses Association. (2008). *Guide to the code of ethics for nurses: Interpretation and application*. Washington, DC: Author.

Calzone, K. A., Masny, A., & Jenkins, J. (2010). *Genetics and genomics in oncology nursing practice*. Pittsburgh, PA: Oncology Nursing Society.

Consensus Panel on Genetic/Genomic Nursing Competencies. (2009). *Essentials of genetic and genomic nursing: Competencies, curricular guidelines, and outcome indicators* (2nd ed.). Silver Spring, MD: American Nurses Association.

**Jenkins, J., & Lea, D. H. (2005). *Nursing care in the genomic era: A case-based approach*. Sudbury, MA: Jones & Bartlett.

Nussbaum, R. L., McInnes, R. R., & Willard, H. F. (2010). *Thompson and Thompson's genetics in medicine* (8th ed.). Philadelphia: W. B. Saunders.

**Skirton, H., Patch, C., & Williams J. (2005). *Applied genetics in healthcare: A handbook for specialist practitioners*. New York: Taylor & Francis Group.

Journals and Electronic Documents

American College of Obstetricians and Gynecologists Committee on Genetics. (2004). ACOG committee opinion 298: Prenatal and preconceptional carrier screening for genetic diseases in individuals of eastern European Jewish descent. *Obstetrics & Gynecology, 104*(2), 425–428.

American College of Obstetricians and Gynecologists Committee on Genetics. (2009). ACOG committee opinion 442: Preconception and prenatal carrier screening for genetic diseases in individuals of eastern European Jewish descent. *Obstetrics & Gynecology, 114*(4), 950–953.

Bellcross, C., & Dotson, W. D. (2010). *Tumor gene expression profiling in women with breast cancer*. National Office of Public Health Genomics, CDC, and Office of Public Health Genomics, CDC. Available at: www.ncbi.nlm.nih.gov/pmc/articles/PMC2940139/

Chen, S., Iversen, E. X., Friebel, T., et al. (2006). Characterization of BRCA1 and BRCA2 mutations in a large United States sample. *Journal of Clinical Oncology, 24*(6), 863–871.

Christensen, K., & Murray, J. C. (2007). What genome-wide association studies can do for medicine. *New England Journal of Medicine, 356*(11), 1094–1097.

Feero, W. G., Guttmacher, A. E., & Collins, F. S. (2010). Genomic medicine—an updated primer. *New England Journal of Medicine, 362*(21), 201–211.

Genetic Home Reference. (2011). *What is pharmacogenomics?* Available at: ghr.nlm.nih.gov/handbook/genomicresearch/pharmacogenomics

Hampel, H., Frankel, W. L., Martin, E., et al. (2008). Feasibility of screening for Lynch syndrome among patients with colorectal cancer. *Journal of Clinical Oncology, 26*(35), 5783–5788.

Hayden, E. C. (2009). Personalized cancer therapy gets closer. *Nature, 458*, 131–132.

Hosoi, T. (2010). Genetic aspects of osteoporosis. *Journal of Bone and Mineral Metabolism, 28*(6), 601–607.

Hudson, K., Holohan, J. D., & Collins, F. S. (2008). Keeping pace with the times—the Genetic Information Nondiscrimination Act of 2008. *New England Journal of Medicine, 358*(25), 2661–2663.

**Ingelman-Sundberg, M. (2004). Pharmacogenetics of cytochrome P450 and its applications in drug therapy: The past, present and future. *Trends in Pharmacological Science, 25*(4), 193–200.

International Society of Nurses in Genetics. (2010). *Position statements*. Available at: www.isong.org/ISONG_position_statements.php

Kitzmiller, J. P., Groen, D. K., Phelps, M. A., et al. (2011). Pharmacogenomic testing: Relevance in medical practice: Why drugs work in some patients and others do not. *Cleveland Clinic Journal of Medicine, 78*(4), 243–257.

Lea, D. H. (2009). Basic genetics and genomics: A primer for nurses. *Online Journal of Issues in Nursing, 14*(2). Available at: www.nursingworld.org/MainMenuCategories/ANAMarketplace/ANAPeriodicals/OJIN/TableofContents/Vol142009/No2May09/Articles-Previous-Topics/Basic-Genetics-and-Genomics.aspx

Masuno, K., Haldar, S. M., Jevaraj, D., et al. (2011). Expression profiling identifies Klf15 as glucocorticoid target that regulates airway hyperresponsiveness. *American Journal of Respiratory Cell Molecular Biology, 45*(3), 642–649.

Moline, J., & Eng, C. (2013). Multiple endocrine neoplasia type 2. Available at: www.ncbi.nlm.nih.gov/books/NBK1257

National Human Genome Research Institute. (2010). *Learning about neurofibromatosis*. Available at: www.genome.gov/14514225

National Human Genome Research Institute. (2011a). *NHGRI policy roundtable summary. The future of genomic medicine: Policy implications for research and medicine*. Available at: www.genome.gov/17516574

National Human Genome Research Institute. (2011b). *Learning about Turner syndrome*. Available at: www.genome.gov/19519119

National Human Genome Research Institute. (2011c). *Learning about sickle cell disease*. Available at: www.genome.gov/10001219

National Human Genome Research Institute. (2011d). *Learning about Gaucher disease*. Available at: www.genome.gov/25521505

National Human Genome Research Institute. (2011e). *Genetic imprinting*. Available at: www.genome.gov/Glossary/index.cfm?id=92

National Human Genome Research Institute. (2011f). *Frequently asked questions about genetic and genomic science*. Available at: www.genome.gov/19016904

National Human Genome Research Institute. (2011g). *Frequently asked questions about genetic disorders*. Available at: www.genome.gov/19016930

National Human Genome Research Institute. (2011h). *Frequently asked questions about genetic counseling*. Available at: www.genome.gov/19016905

National Human Genome Research Institute. (2011i). *Genetic Information Nondiscrimination Act (GINA) of 2008*. Available at: www.genome.gov/24519851

National Human Genome Research Institute. (2011j). *New horizons and research activities*. Available at: www.genome.gov/27527636

Rare Diseases. (2011). *Newborn screening for genetic and metabolic disorders*. Available at: rarediseases.about.com/od/geneticdisorders/a/newbornscreen/htm

Ready, K., & Arun, B. (2010). Clinical assessment of breast cancer risk based on family history. *Journal of the National Comprehensive Cancer Network, 8*(10), 1148–1155.

Secretary's Advisory Committee on Genetics Health and Society (2009). SACGHS Documents, Reports and Correspondence. Available at: http://oba.od.nih.gov/SACGHS/sacghs_documents.html#GHSDOC_014

Sim, S. C., & Ingleman-Sundberg, M. (2010). The human cytochrome P450 (CYP) allele nomenclature website: A peer reviewed database of CYP variants and their associated effects. *Human Genomics, 4*(4), 278–281.

Steck, M. B., & Eggert, J. A. (2011). The need to be aware and beware of the Genetic Information Nondiscrimination Act. *Clinical Journal of Oncology Nursing, 15*(3), 34–41.

Suzumori, N., & Sugiura-Ogasawara, M. (2010). Genetic factors as a cause of miscarriage. *Current Medical Chemistry, 17*(29), 3431–3437.

*Taylor, J. Y., & Wu, C. Y. (2009). Effects of genetic counseling for hypertension on changes in lifestyle behaviors among African Americans. *Journal of the National Black Nurses Association, 20*(1), 1–10.

U.S. Department of Energy Genome Programs. (2008). *Genomics and its impact on science and society: The Human Genome Project and beyond*. Available at: www.ornl.gov/sci/techresources/Human_Genome/publicat/primer2001/index.shtml

Watson, M. S., Cutting, G. R., Desnick, R. J., et al. (2004). Cystic fibrosis population screening: 2004 revision of American College of Medical Genetics mutation panel. *Genetics in Medicine, 6*(5), 387–391.

Weinshilboum, R. M., & Wang, L. (2006), Pharmacogenetics and pharmacogenomics: Development, science and translation. *Annual Review of Genomics and Human Genetics, 7*, 223–245.

Resources

Association of Women's Health, Obstetric and Neonatal Nurses (AWHONN), www.awhonn.org/awhonn

GeneTests, www.ncbi.nlm.nih.gov/sites/GeneTests/?db=GeneTests

Genetic Alliance, www.geneticalliance.org.

Genetic Home Reference: Your Guide to Understanding Genetic Conditions, ghr.nlm.nih.gov/

Genetic and Rare Diseases Information Center, www.genome.gov/Health/GARD/

Genetics Nursing Credentialing Commission (GNCC), www.geneticnurse.org

Human Genome Project Information, *SNP Fact Sheet*, www.ornl.gov/sci/techresources/Human_Genome/faq/snps.shtml#snps

International Society of Nurses in Genetics (ISONG), www.isong.org

MedlinePlus Health Topics, www.nlm.nih.gov/medlineplus/healthtopics.html

National Cancer Institute (NCI), www.nci.nih.gov

National Center for Biotechnology Information, www.ncbi.nlm.nih.gov

National Coalition for Health Professional Education in Genetics (NCHPEG), www.nchpeg.org

National Human Genome Research Institute, Genome Statute and Legislative Database (summary of each state's legislation on employment and insurance discrimination), www.genome.gov/PolicyEthics/LegDatabase/pubsearch.cfm

National Organization for Rare Disorders (NORD), www.rarediseases.org

Oncology Nursing Society (ONS), www.ons.org

Chronic Illness and Disability

Learning Objectives

On completion of this chapter, the learner will be able to:

1 Define "chronic conditions."
2 Identify factors related to the increasing incidence of chronic conditions.
3 Describe characteristics of chronic conditions and implications for people with chronic conditions and for their families.

4 Describe advantages and disadvantages of various models of disability.
5 Describe implications of disability for nursing practice.

Glossary

chronic disease: medical or health problems with associated symptoms or disabilities that require long-term management; has also been referred to as noncommunicable disease, chronic condition, or chronic disorder

chronic illness: the experience of living with a chronic disease or condition; the individual's perception of the experience and the individual's and others' responses to the chronic disease or condition

disability: restriction or lack of ability to perform an activity in a normal manner; the consequences of impairment in terms of an individual's functional performance and activity—disabilities represent disturbances at the level

of the person (e.g., bathing, dressing, communication, walking, grooming)

impairment: loss or abnormality of psychological, physiologic, or anatomic structure or function at the organ level (e.g., dysphagia, hemiparesis); an abnormality of body structure, appearance, and organ or system function resulting from any cause

secondary conditions or disorders: any physical, mental, or social disorders resulting directly or indirectly from an initial disabling condition; a condition to which a person with a disability is more susceptible because of having a primary disabling condition

Chronic illness and disability affect people of all ages—the very young, the middle aged, and the very old. Chronic illnesses and disabilities are found in all ethnic, cultural, racial, and socioeconomic groups, although some disorders occur more frequently in some groups than in others. **Chronic diseases** refer to noncommunicable diseases, chronic conditions, or chronic disorders (McKenna & Collins, 2010). In contrast, **chronic illness** refers to the experience of living with a chronic disease or condition. It includes the individual's perception of the experience of having a chronic disease or condition and the individual's and others' responses to it (Lubkin & Larsen, 2013).

Chronic diseases are the most common causes of death in the United States. The most frequently occurring chronic diseases that account for 7 of the 10 leading causes of death and are responsible for more than two thirds of the deaths that occur globally include cardiovascular disease, cancers, diabetes, and chronic lung diseases (Centers for Disease Control and Prevention [CDC], 2010; World Health Organization [WHO], 2011). These diseases or conditions are increasing rapidly in lower-income countries, populations, and communities because of adoption of unhealthy lifestyles. Lack of physical activity, poor nutrition, tobacco use, and excessive

alcohol consumption are modifiable health risk behaviors that are responsible for the high incidence of chronic disease, disability, and early death (CDC, 2010).

Although chronic disease occurs in all socioeconomic groups, people from low-income and disadvantaged backgrounds are more likely to report poor health. Factors such as poverty and inadequate health insurance decrease the likelihood that people with chronic illness or disability receive health care and health screening measures such as mammography, cholesterol testing, and routine checkups (Anderson, 2010). In addition, chronic disease or disability can lead to poverty at the level of the patient and family, a society, or country as a whole because deaths attributable to chronic diseases or disorders occur most often during a person's most productive years (WHO, 2011).

Many people with chronic health conditions and disability function independently with only minor inconvenience to their everyday lives; others, however, require frequent and close monitoring or placement in long-term care facilities. Certain conditions require advanced technology for survival, as in the late stages of chronic obstructive lung disease or end-stage renal disease, or intensive care or mechanical ventilation for periods of weeks or months. People with disorders such as these have been described as being chronically critically ill, although there is no consensus on a definition of chronic critical illness (Daly, Douglas, Gordon, et al., 2009). Some chronic conditions have little effect on quality of life, whereas others have a considerable effect because they result in disability. However, not all disabilities are a result of chronic illness, and not all chronic illnesses cause disability. In this chapter, chronic illness is discussed, followed by a discussion of disability and the implications for nursing practice.

Overview of Chronicity

Although each chronic condition has its own specific physiologic characteristics, chronic conditions share common features. Many chronic conditions, for example, have pain and fatigue as associated symptoms. Some degree of disability is usually present in severe or advanced chronic illness, limiting the patient's participation in many activities. Many chronic conditions require therapeutic regimens to keep them under control. Unlike the term *acute*, which implies a curable and relatively short disease course, the term *chronic* describes a long disease course and conditions that may be incurable. This often makes managing chronic conditions difficult for those who must live with them.

Psychological and emotional reactions of patients to acute and chronic conditions and changes in their health status are described in Chapter 6. People who develop chronic conditions or disabilities may react with shock, disbelief, anger, resentment, or other emotions. How people react to and cope with chronic illness is usually similar to how they react to other events in their lives, depending, in part, on their understanding of the condition and their perceptions of its potential impact on their own and their family's lives. Adjustment to chronic illness (and disability) is affected by various factors:

- Suddenness, extent, and duration of lifestyle changes necessitated by the illness
- Uncertainty related to the course and outcome of chronic illnesses
- Family and individual resources for dealing with stress
- Availability of support from family, friends, and community
- Stages of individual/family life cycle
- Previous experience with illness and crises
- Underlying personality characteristics
- Unresolved anger or grief from the past

Psychological, emotional, and cognitive reactions to chronic conditions are likely to occur at their onset and to recur if symptoms worsen or recur after a period of remission. Symptoms associated with chronic health conditions are often unpredictable and may be perceived as crisis events by patients and their families, who must contend with both the uncertainty of chronic illness and the changes it brings to their lives. These possible effects of chronic conditions can guide nursing assessment and interventions for the patient who has a chronic illness.

Definition of Chronic Diseases or Conditions

Chronic diseases or conditions are often defined as medical conditions or health problems with associated symptoms or disabilities that require long-term management. Some definitions use a duration of 3 months or longer, whereas others use a year or longer to indicate chronic disease. Definitions of chronic disease or chronic illness share the characteristics of being irreversible, having a prolonged course, and unlikely to resolve spontaneously (Lubkin & Larsen, 2013). The specific chronic condition may be a result of illness, genetic factors, or injury; it may be a consequence of conditions or unhealthy behaviors that began during childhood and young adulthood (Johnson & Schoeni, 2011). Management of chronic conditions includes learning to live with symptoms or disabilities and coming to terms with identity changes resulting from having a chronic condition. It also consists of carrying out the lifestyle changes and regimens designed to control symptoms and prevent complications. Although some people assume what might be called a "sick role" identity, most people with chronic conditions do not consider themselves to be sick or ill and try to live as normal a life as possible. Only when complications develop or symptoms interfere with activities of daily living (ADLs) do most people with chronic health conditions think of themselves as being sick or disabled.

 Prevalence and Causes of Chronic Conditions

Chronic conditions occur in people of every age group, socioeconomic level, race, and culture. In 2009, an estimated 145 million people in the United States—almost half the population—had one or more chronic conditions. This number represents an increase of 10 million people since 2002. The proportion of the population with two or more chronic conditions increased from 24% to 28% in that same time period. The percentage of people with five or more chronic conditions has also increased (U.S. Department of Health and Human Services [HHS], 2010a).

It is predicted that by the year 2030, about 167 million people (about half the population) will have a chronic disease or disorder, including 88.5 million people 65 years of age and older (Anderson, 2010). One fifth of those with chronic disease also have an activity limitation. As the incidence of chronic diseases increases, the costs associated with these chronic conditions (i.e., hospital costs, equipment, medications, supportive services) also increase. Expenditures for health care for people with chronic conditions exceed billions of dollars every year; these costs represent four of every five health care dollars expended. Chart 9-1 provides an overview of chronic illness in the United States.

Although some chronic health conditions cause little or no inconvenience, others are severe enough to cause major activity limitations. When people with activity limitations are unable to meet their needs for health care and personal services, they may be unable to carry out their therapeutic regimens or have their prescriptions filled on time, may miss appointments and office visits with their health care providers, and may be unable to carry out ADLs.

Chronic diseases are a global issue that affects both rich and poor nations. Chronic conditions have become the major cause of health-related problems in developed countries as well as in the developing countries, which are also trying to cope with new and emerging infectious diseases. In almost all countries, chronic diseases are the major cause of

Chart 9-1   Overview of Chronic Illness in the United States

- Chronic illness affects people of all ages and all ethnic, cultural, racial, and socioeconomic groups.
- Seven of the 10 leading causes of death are chronic diseases and include cardiovascular disease, cancers, diabetes, and chronic lung diseases.
- In almost all countries, including the United States, chronic conditions are the major cause of health-related problems and deaths; they are also increasing in developing countries.
- The number of people with multiple chronic illness is increasing; the presence of more than one chronic illness increases the costs and complexity of care due to unnecessary hospitalizations, adverse drug events, duplicative tests, conflicting medical advice, and poor functional status and death.
- Chronic disease is associated with 85% of all health care costs in the United States: 96% of home health care, 88% of prescriptions, 72% of physician visits, and 76% of hospital stays.
- Most health care spending through Medicare (96%) and Medicaid (80%) is for treatment of patients with chronic disorders.
- Many people with chronic disorders are of working age and have private health care insurance; their health care accounts for nearly 75% of coverage provided through private insurance.

- The quality and cost of health care for people with chronic diseases vary from one location in the United States to another and from one type of health care setting to another.
- Management of chronic conditions is expensive; out-of-pocket expenses associated with having a chronic health condition are high and increasing.
- Poverty and inadequate health insurance decrease the likelihood that people with chronic illness will receive health care and health screening measures such as mammography, cholesterol testing, and routine checkups.
- Chronic disease can lead to poverty at the level of the patient and family—and society.
- Most chronic diseases and many complications of chronic illness are preventable.
- Having a chronic illness affects the ability to work, quality of life, and participation in community and family activities.
- Chronic illnesses affect the individual with the chronic illness, family members, and society, increasing the risk of stress and caregiver fatigue.
- Although most young adults growing up with a chronic illness graduate from high school and are employed, they are significantly less likely than their healthy peers to achieve important educational and vocational milestones.

Based on data from Anderson, G. (2010). *Chronic care: Making the case for ongoing care*. Princeton, NJ: Robert Wood Johnson Foundation; World Health Organization. (2011). *Global status report on noncommunicable diseases 2010*. Geneva: Author. Available at: http://www.who.int/nmh/publications/ncd_report2010/en/; Dartmouth Atlas of Health Care. (2008). *Executive Summary. The Dartmouth Institute for Health Policy and Clinical Practice*. Dartmouth, NH: Author. Available at: http://www.dartmouthatlas.org/downloads/atlases/2008_Chronic_Care_Atlas.pdf; G. R., Haydon, A. A., Ford, C. A., et al. (2011). Young adult outcomes of children growing up with chronic illness: An analysis of the National Longitudinal Study of Adolescent Health. *Archives of Pediatrics and Adolescent Medicine*, 165(3), 256–261; Parekh, A. K., & Barton, M. B. (2010). The challenge of multiple comorbidity for the US health care system. *Journal of the American Medical Association*, 303(13), 1303–1304.

death among adults. More than 35 million people die annually worldwide because of chronic diseases—a number that is predicted to increase to 52 million people by 2030 (WHO, 2011). Four of every five deaths occurred in countries characterized as low- or middle income, where people tend to develop chronic diseases at younger ages, suffer longer, and die sooner than people in high-income countries. In contrast to common belief, the total number of people dying from chronic disease is twice that of patients dying from infectious (including human immunodeficiency virus [HIV] infection), maternal and perinatal conditions, and nutritional deficiencies combined (WHO, 2011). The number of people worldwide who die because of chronic disease is higher than all other diseases combined. Most of these chronic diseases and complications of chronic illness are preventable, emphasizing the importance of health promotion across the globe (McQueen, 2011). Although chronic diseases or illnesses are common, people have many myths or misunderstandings about them (Table 9-1).

Because of the rapidly increasing prevalence of chronic disease around the world, the WHO (2011), working with partners around the world, developed an action plan focused on prevention and control of chronic diseases (noncommunicable disorders). The six objectives of the action plan are identified in Chart 9-2.

Causes of the increasing number of people with chronic conditions include the following:

- A decrease in mortality from infectious diseases (e.g., smallpox, diphtheria, acquired immunodeficiency syndrome [AIDS]–related infections) and from acute

conditions because of prompt and aggressive management of acute conditions (e.g., myocardial infarction, trauma).

- Lifestyle factors such as smoking, chronic stress, and sedentary lifestyle that increase the risk of chronic health problems such as respiratory disease, hypertension,

Chart 9-2   2008–2013 Action Plan for the Global Strategy for the Prevention and Control of Noncommunicable Diseases

1. To raise the priority accorded to noncommunicable disease in development work at global and national levels, and to integrate prevention and control of such diseases into policies across all government departments
2. To establish and strengthen national policies and plans for the prevention and control of noncommunicable diseases
3. To promote interventions to reduce the main shared modifiable risk factors for noncommunicable diseases: tobacco use, unhealthy diets, physical inactivity, and harmful use of alcohol
4. To promote research for the prevention and control of noncommunicable diseases
5. To promote partnerships for the prevention and control of noncommunicable diseases
6. To monitor noncommunicable diseases and their determinants and evaluate progress at the national, regional, and global levels

Note: The term *noncommunicable diseases* is synonymous in this chart with chronic diseases. Adapted from World Health Organization. (2011). *Global status report on noncommunicable diseases 2010*. Geneva: Author. Available at: http://www.who.int/nmh/publications/ncd_report2010/en/

TABLE 9-1   Myths and Truths About Chronic Disease

Common Misconceptions About Chronic Disease	The Reality About Chronic Disease
1. Everyone has to die of something.	Chronic illnesses typically do not result in sudden death but often result in progressive illness and disability. People with chronic disease often die slowly, painfully, and prematurely.
2. People can live to old age even if they lead unhealthy lives (smoke, are obese).	While there are exceptions (some people who live unhealthy lives live to old age, and some people who live healthy lives develop chronic illnesses), most chronic illnesses can be traced to common risk factors and can be prevented by eliminating these risks.
3. Solutions for chronic disease prevention and control are too expensive to be feasible for low- and middle-income countries.	A full range of chronic disease interventions are very cost-effective for all regions of the world, including the poorest. Many of these interventions are inexpensive to implement. Chronic disease is increasing rapidly around the world, including in low- and middle-income countries.
4. There is nothing that can be done anyway; chronic diseases cannot be prevented.	The major causes of chronic diseases are known, and if these risk factors were eliminated, at least more than 80% of heart disease, stroke, and type 2 diabetes would be prevented, and more than 40% of cancer would be prevented.
5. If individuals develop chronic disease as a result of unhealthy "lifestyles," they have no one to blame but themselves.	Individual responsibility can have its full effect only if individuals have equal access to a healthy life and are supported to make healthy choices. Poor people often have limited choices about the food they eat, their living conditions, and access to education and health care.
6. Certain chronic diseases primarily affect men.	Chronic diseases, including heart disease, affect women and men almost equally. Almost half of all deaths attributed to chronic illness occur in women.
7. Chronic diseases primarily affect old people.	Almost half of chronic disease deaths occur prematurely, in people under 70 years of age.
8. Chronic diseases mainly affect rich (affluent) people.	Poor people are much more likely than the wealthy to develop chronic diseases and as a result are more likely to die. Chronic diseases cause substantial financial burden and result in extreme poverty.
9. The priority of low- and middle-income countries should be on control of infectious diseases.	Although infectious diseases are an issue, low- and middle-income countries are experiencing a dramatic increase in chronic disease risk factors and deaths, especially in urban settings.
10. Chronic diseases affect mostly high-income countries.	80% of deaths attributed to chronic disease are in low- and middle-income countries. The prevalence of chronic diseases in low- and middle-income countries is rapidly growing.

Adapted from World Health Organization. (2005). *Widespread misunderstandings about chronic disease—and the reality*. Facing the Facts #2. Available at: http://www.who.int/chp/chronic_disease_report/media/Factsheet2.pdf

cardiovascular disease, and obesity. Although signs and symptoms of chronic illness often first appear during older age, risks may begin earlier, even during fetal development. Obesity has become a major health issue across the lifespan with one in every three adults and about one in every five persons 6 to 19 years of age being classified as obese (CDC, 2009). The increasing prevalence of obesity has increased the incidence of heart disease, strokes, diabetes, and hypertension. Obesity also affects one's self-esteem, achievement, and emotional state (Galuska & Dietz, 2010).

- Longer lifespans because of advances in technology and pharmacology, improved nutrition, safer working conditions, and greater access (for some people) to health care.
- Improved screening and diagnostic procedures, enabling early detection and treatment of diseases resulting in improved outcomes of management of cancer and other disorders.

Consequences of unhealthy lifestyles include an alarming increase in the incidence of diabetes, hypertension, obesity, and cardiac and chronic respiratory disorders (WHO, 2011). Although most chronic diseases are a result of unhealthy lifestyles, it is important to keep in mind that there are other non-modifiable factors associated with chronic disease, including genetic and physiologic factors (McKenna & Collins, 2010).

Physiologic changes in the body often occur before the appearance of symptoms of chronic disease. Therefore, the goal of emphasizing healthy lifestyles early in life is to improve overall health status and slow the development of such disorders. Major risk factors for chronic disease, which represent a growing challenge to public health, include unhealthy eating habits, decreased energy expenditure associated with a

sedentary lifestyle, increasing age, and tobacco use and alcohol consumption (WHO, 2011). In addition, serious psychiatric or mental illness puts people at greater risk for chronic illness than the general population and leads to higher morbidity and mortality rates of chronic diseases (HHS, 2010a).

Characteristics of Chronic Conditions

Sometimes it is difficult for people who are disease free to understand the profound effect that chronic illness often has on the lives of patients and their families. It is easy for health professionals to focus on the illness or disability itself while overlooking the person who has the disorder. In all illnesses, but even more so with chronic conditions, the illness cannot be separated from the person. People with chronic illness must contend with it daily. To relate to what people must cope with or to plan effective interventions, nurses must understand what it means to have a chronic illness. Characteristics of chronic illness include the following:

- Managing chronic illness involves more than treating medical problems. Associated psychological and social problems must also be addressed, because living for long periods with illness symptoms and disability can threaten identity, bring about role changes, alter body image, and disrupt lifestyles. These changes require continuous adaptation and accommodation, depending on age and situation in life. Each decline in functional ability requires physical, emotional, and social adaptation for patients and their families (Corbin, 2003).
- Chronic conditions usually involve many different phases over the course of a person's lifetime. There can be acute periods, stable and unstable periods, flare-ups,

and remissions. Each phase brings its own set of physical, psychological, and social problems, and each requires its own regimens and types of management.

- Keeping chronic conditions under control requires persistent adherence to therapeutic regimens. Failing to adhere to a treatment plan or to do so consistently increases the risks of developing complications and accelerating the disease process. However, the realities of daily life, including the impact of culture, values, and socioeconomic factors, affect the degree to which people adhere to a treatment regimen. Managing a chronic illness takes time, requires knowledge and planning, and can be uncomfortable and inconvenient. It is not unusual for patients to stop taking medications or alter dosages because of side effects that are more disturbing or disruptive than symptoms of the illness, or to cut back on regimens they consider overly time-consuming, fatiguing, or costly (Corbin, 2003).
- One chronic disease can lead to the development of other chronic conditions. Diabetes, for example, can eventually lead to neurologic and vascular changes that may result in visual, cardiac, and kidney disease and erectile dysfunction. The presence of a chronic illness also contributes to a higher risk of morbidity and mortality in patients admitted to the intensive care unit with acute health conditions as well as greater utilization of clinical services during hospitalization (Anderson, 2010).
- Chronic illness affects the entire family. Family life can be dramatically altered as a result of role reversals, unfilled roles, loss of income, time required to manage the illness, decreases in family socialization activities, and the costs of treatment. Family members often become caregivers for the person with chronic illness while trying to continue to work and keep the family intact. Stress and caretaker fatigue are common with severe chronic conditions, and the entire family rather than just the patient may need care (Anderson, 2010). However, some families are able to master the treatment regimen and changes that accompany chronic illness as well as make the treatment regimen a routine part of life. Furthermore, they are able to keep the chronic illness from becoming the focal point of family life.
- The day-to-day management of illness is largely the responsibility of people with chronic disorders and their families. As a result, the home, rather than the hospital, is the center of care in chronic conditions. Hospitals, clinics, physicians' offices, nursing homes, nursing centers, and community agencies (home care services, social services, and disease-specific associations and societies) are considered adjuncts or backup services to daily home management.
- The management of chronic conditions is a process of discovery. People can be taught how to manage their conditions. However, each person must discover how his or her own body reacts under varying circumstances—for example, what it is like to be hypoglycemic, what activities are likely to bring on angina, and how these or other conditions can best be prevented and managed.
- Managing chronic conditions must be a collaborative process that involves many different health care profes-

sionals working together with patients and their families to provide the full range of services that are often needed for management at home. The medical, social, and psychological aspects of chronic health problems are often complex, especially in severe conditions.
- The management of chronic conditions is expensive. Many of the expenses incurred by an individual patient (e.g., costs for hospital stays, diagnostic tests, equipment, medications, and supportive services) may be covered by health insurance and by federal and state agencies. However, the cost increases affect society as a whole as insurance premiums increase to cover these costs. Cost increases at the government level decrease resources that might benefit society. Many people with chronic disorders, including older adults and those who are working, are uninsured or underinsured and may be unable to afford the high costs of care often associated with chronic illnesses. Absence from work because of chronic disorders may jeopardize job security and lead to loss of household income and financial hardship.

Direct out-of-pocket expenses represent a significant percent of income, especially in low- and middle-income families. These out-of-pocket expenses have risen nearly 30% since 2001 (Anderson, 2010; WHO, 2011). Those with serious chronic disorders may have difficulty paying for care, resulting in bankruptcy or having to rely on family or friends to pay for health care (Anderson, 2010). People from low-income groups who do not receive adequate health care get sicker and die sooner from chronic diseases than those from groups with higher levels of education, greater financial resources, and access to care (WHO, 2011). If a family's primary income earner becomes ill, chronic diseases can result in drastic loss in income with inadequate funds for food, education, and health care. Further, affected families may become unstable and impoverished (WHO, 2011).
- Chronic conditions raise difficult ethical issues for patients, families, health care professionals, and society. Problematic questions include how to establish cost controls, how to allocate scarce resources (e.g., organs for transplantation), and what constitutes quality of life and when life support should be withdrawn.
- Living with chronic illness means living with uncertainty. Although health care providers may be aware of the usual progression of a chronic disease such as Parkinson's disease or multiple sclerosis, no one can predict with certainty a person's illness course because of individual variation. Even when a patient is in remission or symptom free, he or she often fears that the illness will reappear.

Implications of Managing Chronic Conditions

Chronic conditions have implications for everyday living and management for people and their families as well as for society at large. Most importantly, individual efforts should be directed at preventing chronic conditions, because many chronic illnesses or disorders are linked to unhealthy lifestyles or behaviors such as smoking and overeating. Therefore, changes in lifestyle can prevent some chronic disorders or at least delay onset until a later age. Because most people resist change, bringing about alterations in people's lifestyles is a major challenge for nurses today.

Once a chronic condition has occurred, the focus shifts to managing symptoms, avoiding complications (e.g., eye complications in a person with diabetes), and preventing other acute illnesses (e.g., pneumonia in a person with chronic obstructive lung disease). Quality of life—often overlooked by health professionals in their approach to people with chronic conditions—is also important. Health-promoting behaviors, such as exercise, are essential to quality of life even in people who have chronic illnesses or disabilities, because they help to maintain functional status (Lubkin & Larsen, 2013).

Although coworkers, extended family, and health care professionals are affected by chronic illnesses, the problems of living with chronic conditions are most acutely experienced by patients and their immediate families. They experience the greatest impact, with lifestyle changes that directly affect quality of life. Nurses provide direct care, especially during acute episodes, but also provide the education and secure the resources and other supports that enable people to integrate their illness into their lives and to have an acceptable quality of life despite the illness. To understand what nursing care is needed, it is important to recognize and appreciate the issues that people with chronic illness and their families contend with and manage, often on a daily basis (Eggenberger, Meiers, Krumwiede, et al., 2011). The challenges of living with chronic conditions include the need to accomplish the following:

- Alleviate and manage symptoms
- Psychologically adjust to and physically accommodate disabilities
- Prevent and manage crises and complications
- Carry out regimens as prescribed
- Validate individual self-worth and family functioning
- Manage threats to identity
- Normalize personal and family life as much as possible
- Live with altered time, social isolation, and loneliness
- Establish the networks of support and resources that can enhance quality of life
- Return to a satisfactory way of life after an acute debilitating episode (e.g., another myocardial infarction or stroke) or reactivation of a chronic condition
- Die with dignity and comfort

Many people with chronic disease or chronic illness must face an additional challenge: the need to deal with more than one chronic illness or disease at a time (HHS, 2010a). The symptoms or treatment of a second chronic condition may aggravate the first chronic condition. Patients need to be able to deal with their various chronic conditions separately as well as in combination. Some Medicare beneficiaries have five or more chronic conditions, see an average of 13 physicians per year, and fill an average of 50 prescriptions per year (Anderson, 2010). Furthermore, the effects of increasing longevity among Americans are likely to increase health care costs in the future.

Even more challenging for many people with chronic illness is the need to hire and oversee caregivers who come into their homes to assist with ADLs and instrumental activities of daily living (IADLs), such as shopping for food, doing laundry, housekeeping, and handling financial matters. It is difficult for many people to be in a position of hiring, supervising, and sometimes firing people who may provide them with intimate physical care. The need to balance the role of recipient of care and oversight of the person providing care may lead to blurring of role boundaries.

The challenges of living with and managing a chronic illness are well known, and people with chronic illnesses often report receiving inadequate care, information, services, and counseling. This provides an opportunity for nurses to assume a more active role in addressing many of the issues experienced, coordinating care, and serving as an advocate for patients who need additional assistance to manage their illness while maintaining a quality of life that is acceptable to them.

Phases of Chronic Conditions

Several models have been developed and used to describe the continuum or phases of chronic disease and its management. The Trajectory Model of Chronic Illness, a nursing model based on more than 30 years of interdisciplinary research on chronic illness, will be used to describe the phases and the role of nurses in the trajectory of chronic illness. Table 9-2 describes the different phases of chronic illness and the focus of nursing care during different phases. In this model, the term *trajectory* refers to the path or course that the chronic illness follows. The course of an illness can be thought of as a trajectory that can be managed or shaped over time, to some extent, through proper illness management strategies (Corbin, 1998). It is important to keep in mind that the course of a patient's chronic illness may be too uncertain to predict with any degree of accuracy. Further, not all phases occur in all patients; some phases do not occur at all, and some phases may recur. Each phase is characterized by different medical and psychosocial issues. For example, the needs of a patient with a stroke who is a good candidate for rehabilitation are very different from the needs of a patient with terminal cancer. By thinking in terms of phases and individual patients within a phase, nurses can target their care more specifically to each person. Not every chronic condition is necessarily life threatening, and not every patient passes through each possible phase of a chronic condition in the same order.

Using the trajectory model enables the nurse to put the present situation into the context of what might have happened to the patient in the past—that is, the life factors and understandings that might have contributed to the present state of the illness. In this way, the nurse can more readily address the underlying issues and problems.

 Gerontologic Considerations

Changes in the U.S. demographic profile are resulting in an increased number of older adults with chronic illnesses as well as increasing numbers of older adults with multiple chronic illnesses. Individuals with multiple chronic conditions are at increased risk for poor functional status, unnecessary hospitalizations, adverse drug events, unnecessary and duplicative tests, conflicting medical advice, and death (HHS, 2010a).

Nursing Care of Patients With Chronic Conditions

Nursing care of patients with chronic conditions is varied and occurs in a variety of settings. Care may be direct or

TABLE 9-2   Phases in the Trajectory Model of Chronic Illness

Phase	Description	Focus of Nursing Care
Pretrajectory	Genetic factors or lifestyle behaviors that place a person or community at risk for a chronic condition	Refer for genetic testing and counseling if indicated; provide education about prevention of modifiable risk factors and behaviors.
Trajectory onset	Appearance or onset of noticeable symptoms associated with a chronic disorder; includes period of diagnostic workup and announcement of diagnosis; may be accompanied by uncertainty as patient awaits a diagnosis and begins to discover and cope with implications of diagnosis	Provide explanations of diagnostic tests and procedures and reinforce information and explanations given by primary health care provider; provide emotional support to patient and family.
Stable	Illness course and symptoms are under control as symptoms, resulting disability and everyday life activities are being managed within limitations of illness; illness management centered in the home	Reinforce positive behaviors and offer ongoing monitoring; provide education about health promotion, and encourage participation in health promoting activities and health screening.
Unstable	Characterized by an exacerbation of illness symptoms, development of complications, or reactivation of an illness in remission Period of inability to keep symptoms under control or reactivation of illness; difficulty in carrying out everyday life activities May require more diagnostic testing and trial of new treatment regimens or adjustment of current regimen, with care usually taking place at home	Provide guidance and support; reinforce previous patient education
Acute	Severe and unrelieved symptoms or the development of illness complications necessitating hospitalization, bed rest, or interruption of the person's usual activities to bring illness course under control	Provide direct care and emotional support to the patient and family members.
Crisis	Critical or life-threatening situation requiring emergency treatment or care and suspension of everyday life activities until the crisis has passed	Provide direct care, collaborate with other health care team members to stabilize patient's condition.
Comeback	Gradual recovery after an acute period and learning to live with or overcome disabilities and return to an acceptable way of life within the limitations imposed by the chronic condition or disability; involves physical healing, limitations stretching through rehabilitative procedures, psychosocial coming-to-terms, and biographical reengagement with adjustments in everyday life activities	Assist in coordination of care; rehabilitative focus may require care from other health care providers; provide positive reinforcement for goals identified and accomplished.
Downward	Illness course characterized by rapid or gradual worsening of a condition; physical decline accompanied by increasing disability or difficulty in controlling symptoms; requires biographical adjustment and alterations in everyday life activities with each major downward step	Provide home care and other community-based care to help patient and family adjust to changes and come to terms with these changes; assist patient and family to integrate new treatment and management strategies; encourage identification of end-of-life preferences and planning.
Dying	Final days or weeks before death; characterized by gradual or rapid shutting down of body processes, biographical disengagement and closure, and relinquishment of everyday life interests and activities	Provide direct and supportive care to patients and their families through hospice programs.

Adapted from Corbin, J. M. (1998). The Corbin and Strauss Chronic Illness Trajectory Model: An update. *Scholarly Inquiry for Nursing Practice, 12*(1), 33–41.

supportive. Direct care may be provided in the clinic or physician's office, a nurse-managed center or clinic, the hospital, or the patient's home, depending on the status of the illness. Examples of direct care include assessing the patient's physical status, providing wound care, managing and overseeing medication regimens, and performing other technical tasks. The availability of this type of nursing care may allow the patient to remain at home and return to a more normal life after an acute episode of illness. Nurses have also used "telehealth" or "telehomecare" (use of the telephone in health care) to monitor patients with chronic illness, deliver selected nursing interventions (e.g., counseling), and provide ongoing education and support (Bowles, Riegel, Weiner, et al., 2010.)

Because much of the day-to-day responsibility for managing chronic conditions rests with the patient and family, nurses often provide supportive care at home. Supportive care may include ongoing monitoring, education, counseling, serving as an advocate for the patient, making referrals, and

case management. Giving supportive care is just as important as giving technical care. For example, through ongoing monitoring either in the home or in a clinic, a nurse might detect early signs of impending complications and make a referral (e.g., contact the physician or consult the medical protocol in a clinic) for medical evaluation, thereby preventing a lengthy and costly hospitalization.

Working with people with chronic illness requires not only dealing with the medical aspects of their disorder but also working with the whole person—physically, emotionally, and socially. This holistic approach to care requires nurses to draw on their knowledge and skills, including knowledge from the social sciences and psychology in particular. People often respond to illness, health education, and regimens in ways that differ from the expectations of health care providers. Although quality of life is usually affected by chronic illness, especially if the illness is severe, patients' perceptions of what constitutes quality of life often drive their management behaviors or affect how they view advice about health care. Nurses and other health care professionals need to recognize this, even though it may be difficult to see patients make unwise choices and decisions about lifestyles and disease management. People have the right to receive care without fearing ridicule or refusal of treatment, even if their behaviors (e.g., smoking, substance abuse, overeating, and failure to follow health care providers' recommendations) may have contributed to their chronic disorder.

Applying the Nursing Process Using the Phases of the Chronic Illness System

The focus of care for patients with chronic conditions is determined largely by the phase of the illness and is directed by the nursing process, which includes assessment, diagnosis, planning, implementation, and evaluation.

Step 1: Identifying Specific Problems and the Trajectory Phase

The first step is assessment of the patient to determine the specific problems identified by the patient, family, nurse, and other health care providers. Assessment enables the nurse to identify the specific medical, social, and psychological problems likely to be encountered in a phase. For instance, the problems of a patient with early-onset relapsing-remitting multiple sclerosis or emphysema are very different from those likely to occur with the same patient, 15 years later, with advanced multiple sclerosis or end-stage chronic obstructive pulmonary disease. The types of direct care, referrals, education, and emotional support needed in each situation are different as well. Because complementary and alternative therapies are often used by people with chronic illness, it is important to determine whether a patient with a chronic illness is using these regimens.

Step 2: Establishing and Prioritizing Goals

Once the phase of illness has been identified for a specific patient, along with the specific medical problems and related social and psychological problems, the nurse helps prioritize problems and establish the goals of care. Identification of goals must be a collaborative effort, with the patient, family, and nurse working together, and the goals must be consistent with the abilities, desires, motivations, and resources of those involved.

Step 3: Defining the Plan of Action to Achieve Desired Outcomes

Once goals have been established, it is necessary to identify a realistic and mutually agreed-on plan for achieving them, including specific criteria that will be used to assess the patient's progress. Identifying the person responsible for each task in the action plan is also essential, as is identifying the environmental, social, and psychological factors that might interfere with or facilitate achieving the desired outcome.

Step 4: Implementing the Plan and Interventions

This step addresses implementation of the plan. Possible nursing interventions include providing direct care, serving as an advocate for the patient, educating, counseling, making referrals, and case management (e.g., arranging for resources). Nurses can help patients implement the actions that allow

patients to live with the symptoms and therapies associated with chronic conditions, thus helping them to gain independence. The nurse works with each patient and family to identify the best ways to integrate treatment regimens into their ADLs to accomplish two tasks: (1) adhering to regimens to control symptoms and keep the illness stable, and (2) dealing with the psychosocial issues that can hinder illness management and affect quality of life. Helping patients and their families to understand and implement regimens and to carry out ADLs within the limits of the chronic illness or disability is an important aspect of nursing care for patients with chronic disorders and disabilities and their families.

Step 5: Following Up and Evaluating Outcomes

The final step involves following up to determine if the problem is resolving or being managed and if the patient and family are adhering to the plan. This follow-up may uncover the existence of new problems resulting from the intervention, problems that interfere with the ability of the patient and family to carry out the plan, or previously unexpected problems. A primary goal is maintaining the stability of the chronic condition while preserving the patient's sense of control, identity, and accomplishment. Based on the follow-up and evaluation, alternative strategies or revisions to the initial plan may be warranted.

Helping the patient and family to integrate changes into their lifestyle is an important part of the process. Change takes time, patience, and creativity and often requires encouragement from the nurse. Validation by the nurse for each small increment toward goal accomplishment is important for enhancing self-esteem and reinforcing behaviors. Success may be defined as making some progress toward a goal when a patient is unable to implement rapid and dramatic changes in his or her life. If no progress is made, or if progress toward goals seems too slow, it may be necessary to redefine the goals, the intervention, or the time frame. The nurse must realize and accept that some people will not change. Patients share responsibility for management of their conditions, and outcomes are as much related to their ability to accommodate the illness and carry out regimens as they are to nursing intervention.

Home and Community-Based Care

Educating Patients About Self-Care

Because chronic conditions are so costly to people, families, and society, two of the major goals of nursing today should be the prevention of chronic conditions and the care of people with them. This requires promoting healthy lifestyles and encouraging the use of safety and disease prevention measures, such as wearing seat belts and obtaining immunizations. Prevention should also begin early in life and continue throughout life. Education on self-care may need to address interactions among the patient's chronic conditions as well as skills necessary to care for the individual diseases and their interactive effects.

Patient and family education is an important nursing role that may make the difference in the ability of the patient and family to adapt to chronic conditions. Well-informed, educated patients are more likely than uninformed patients to be concerned about their health and do what is necessary to maintain it. They are also more likely to manage symptoms, recognize the onset of complications, and seek health care early. Knowledge is the key to making informed choices and decisions during all phases of the chronic illness trajectory.

Despite the importance of educating the patient and family, the nurse must recognize that patients recently diagnosed with serious chronic conditions and their families may need time to understand the significance of their condition and its effect on their lives. Education must be planned carefully so that it is not overwhelming. Furthermore, it is important to assess the impact of a new diagnosis of chronic illness on a patient's life and the meaning of self-management to the patient (Audulv, Asplund, & Norbergh, 2011; Jones, Mac-Gillivray, Kroll, et al., 2011; Kralik, Price, & Telford, 2010).

The nurse who cares for patients with chronic conditions in the hospital, clinic, home, or any other setting should assess each patient's knowledge about his or her illness and its management; the nurse cannot assume that patients with a long-standing chronic condition have the knowledge necessary to manage the condition. Patients' learning needs change as the trajectory phase and their personal situation change. The nurse must also recognize that patients may know how their body responds under certain conditions and how best to manage their symptoms. Contact with patients in the hospital, clinic, nursing center, home, or long-term care facility offers nurses the ideal opportunity to reassess patients' learning needs and provide additional education about an illness and its management.

Educational strategies and materials should be adapted to the individual patient so that the patient and family can understand and follow recommendations from health care providers. For instance, educational materials should be tailored for people with low literacy levels and available in several languages and in various alternative formats (e.g., Braille, large print, audiotapes). It may be necessary to provide sign language interpreters.

Continuing Care

Chronic illness management is a collaborative process between the patient, family, nurse, and other health care providers. Collaboration extends to all settings and throughout the illness trajectory. Keeping an illness stable over time requires careful monitoring of symptoms and attention to management regimens. Detecting problems early and helping patients develop appropriate management strategies can make a significant difference in outcomes.

Most chronic conditions are managed in the home. Therefore, care and education during hospitalization should focus on essential information about the condition so that management can continue once the patient is discharged home. Nurses in all settings should be aware of the resources and services available in a community and should make the arrangements (before hospital discharge, if the patient is hospitalized) that are necessary to secure those resources and services. When appropriate, home care services are contacted directly. The home care nurse reassesses how the patient and family are adapting to the chronic condition and its treatment and continues or revises the plan of care accordingly.

Because chronic conditions occur worldwide and the world is increasingly interconnected, nurses should think beyond the personal level to the community and global levels. In terms of illness prevention and health promotion, this entails wide-ranging efforts to assess people for risks of chronic illness (e.g., blood pressure and diabetes screening, stroke risk assessments) and group education related to illness prevention and management. Figure 9-1 provides a framework to identify and implement strategies to prevent chronic disease

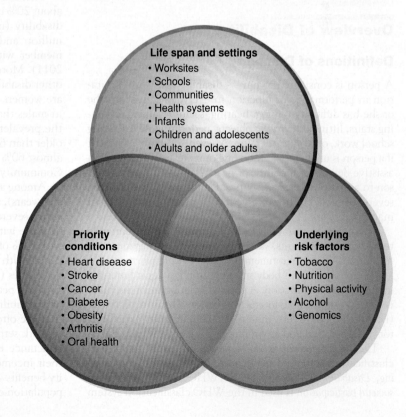

FIGURE 9-1 • Framework for preventing chronic disease and promoting health. Used with permission from Centers for Disease Control and Prevention. (2009). The power to prevent, the call to control: At a glance 2009. Atlanta, GA: Author. Available at www.cdc.gov/chronicdisease/resources/publications/AAG/chronic.htm

Life span and settings
• Worksites
• Schools
• Communities
• Health systems
• Infants
• Children and adolescents
• Adults and older adults

Priority conditions
• Heart disease
• Stroke
• Cancer
• Diabetes
• Obesity
• Arthritis
• Oral health

Underlying risk factors
• Tobacco
• Nutrition
• Physical activity
• Alcohol
• Genomics

and promote health (CDC, 2009). In addition, nurses should remind patients with chronic illnesses or disabilities and their families about the need for ongoing health promotion and screening recommended for all people, because chronic illness and disability are often considered the main concern while other health-related issues are ignored.

Nursing Care for Special Populations With Chronic Illness

When providing care and education, the nurse must consider various factors (e.g., age; gender; culture and ethnicity; cognitive status; the presence of physical, sensory and cognitive limitations) that influence susceptibility to chronic illness and the ways patients respond to chronic disorders. Certain populations, for example, tend to be more susceptible to certain chronic conditions. Populations at high risk for specific conditions can be targeted for special education and monitoring programs; this includes those at risk because of their genetic profile (see Chapter 8 for further discussion of genetics). People of different cultures and genders may respond to illness differently, and being aware of these differences is essential. For cultures in which patients rely heavily on the support of their families, the families must be involved and made part of the nursing plan of care. As the United States becomes more multicultural and ethnically diverse, and as the general population ages, nurses need to be aware of how a person's culture and age affect chronic illness management and be prepared to adapt their care accordingly.

It is also important to consider the effect of a preexisting disability, or a disability associated with recurrence of a chronic condition, on the patient's ability to manage ADLs, self-care, and the therapeutic regimen. These issues are discussed in the following section.

Overview of Disability

Definitions of Disability

A person is considered to have a **disability** such as a limitation in performance or function in everyday activities if he or she has difficulty talking, hearing, seeing, walking, climbing stairs, lifting or carrying objects, performing ADLs, doing school work, or working at a job. A severe disability is present if a person is unable to perform one or more activities, uses an assistive device for mobility, or needs help from another person to accomplish basic activities. People are also considered severely disabled if they receive federal benefits because of an inability to work.

According to the WHO (2001), *disability* is an umbrella term for impairments, activity limitations, participation restrictions, and environmental factors, and **impairment** is a loss or abnormality in body structure or physiologic function, including mental function. A person's functioning or disability is viewed as a dynamic interaction between health conditions (i.e., diseases, disorders, injuries, trauma) and contextual factors (i.e., personal and environmental factors) (WHO, 2001).

The term *handicap* is no longer included in the WHO classification system: *International Classification of Functioning, Disability and Health—ICF* (WHO, 2001). The term *societal participation* is used in the WHO classification system in place of *handicap* to acknowledge the fact that the environment is always interacting with people to either assist or hinder participation in life activities. The 2001 classification system acknowledges that the environment may have a greater impact on the ability of an individual to participate in life activities than does the physical, mental, or emotional condition.

Federal legislation uses more than 50 definitions of disability, which illustrates how difficult it is to define the term. The Americans With Disabilities Act of 1990 (ADA; discussed later) defines a person with a disability as one who (1) has a physical or mental impairment that substantially limits one or more major life activities, (2) has a record of such an impairment, or (3) is regarded as having such an impairment. Other phrases used to describe people with disabilities that are not universally accepted or understood are "people who are physically challenged," and "people with special needs."

Lutz and Bowers (2007) defined *disability* as a multifaceted, complex experience that is integrated into the lives of people with disabilities. The degree of the integration is influenced by three disability-related factors: (1) the effects of the disabling condition, (2) others' perceptions of disability, and (3) the need for and use of resources by the person with a disability.

Prevalence of Disability

An estimated 54 million to 60 million people in the United States have disabilities (American Community Survey, 2011); they compose the nation's third largest minority. The number of people with disabilities is expected to increase over time as people with early-onset disabilities, chronic disorders, and severe trauma survive.

The U.S. Census, last conducted in 2010, indicates that about 20% of people have a disability and 10% have a severe disability (more than 30 million Americans). Between 54 million and 60 million families have at least one family member with a disability (American Community Survey, 2011). More than 46% of people with one disability have other disabilities. More than 50% of people with a disability are women. Although the prevalence of disability is higher in males than in females for people younger than 65 years, the prevalence is higher in women than in men for people older than 65 years. Among people 65 years of age and older, almost 60% of those with disabilities are women (American Community Survey, 2011).

Among all people 21 to 64 years of age (the prime employable years), approximately 54% are employed. Among those with a severe disability the employment rate is 33%, and 77% of those with nonsevere disability are employed, compared with 84% of people without a disability. However, employed people with a disability earn less money than people without disabilities (American Community Survey, 2008, 2011), and 17.5% of people with disabilities live in poverty. Many people with disabilities who are unemployed want to work; however, they are often unable to do so because of the limited access to work settings, lack of accommodations in the workplace, reluctance of employers to hire them, and financial risk if their income exceeds eligibility limits to qualify for disability benefits. Chart 9-3 provides a summary of facts about the population of people with disabilities.

Chart 9-3   Summary of Facts About the Population of People With Disabilities

- Between 54 million and 60 million people in the United States have a disability; this is approximately 20% of the civilian noninstitutionalized population or one in every five people.
- The prevalence of disabilities by age is 5% of children 5 to 17 years of age, 10% percent of people 18 to 64 years, and 38% of adults 65 years of age and older.
- More than 11 million people with disabilities require personal assistance with everyday activities (e.g., getting around inside the home, bathing or showering, preparing meals, and performing light housework).
- Approximately 3.3 million people use a wheelchair; another 10 million use a walking aid such as cane, crutches, or walker.
- More than 1.8 million people report being unable to see printed words because of vision impairment, 1 million are unable to hear conversations because of hearing impairment, and 2.5 million have difficulty with their speech being understood.
- More than 16 million people have limitations in cognitive function or have a mental or emotional illness that interferes with daily activities, including those with Alzheimer's disease and intellectual disabilities.
- Self-reported health status among adults with disabilities differs from that of people without disabilities (see Table 9-3).
- The percentage of people with disabilities who are employed ranges from 17.8% to 23.4%; of those without disabilities, the percent ranges from 63.5% to 66.2%.
- Among all age groups, persons with a disability are much less likely to be employed than those without a disability. People with a disability who work are more likely than those without disability to work part time. People with a disability who were not in the labor force (neither employed nor unemployed) is about 8 in 10, compared with about 3 in 10 of those without a disability.
- Many people with disabilities would like to work but are hampered in doing so by limited access, lack of accommodations in the workplace, lack of transportation, and reluctance of employers to hire them.
- The percentage of people with disabilities below the poverty level is almost twice that of people without disabilities.

From Bureau of Labor Statistics. (2012). *Persons with a disability: Labor force characteristics—2011*. U.S. Department of Labor. Available at: www.bls.gov/news.release/pdf/disabl.pdf; Centers for Disease Control and Prevention. (2010). *Chronic diseases and health promotion*. Atlanta, GA: Author; and American Community Survey. (2008). *U.S. Census Bureau*. Washington, DC. Available at: factfinder2.census.gov/

Characteristics of Disability

Categories and Types of Disability

Disabilities can be categorized as developmental disabilities, acquired disabilities, and age-associated disabilities. Developmental disabilities are those that occur any time from birth to 22 years of age and result in impairment of physical or mental health, cognition, speech, language, or self-care. Examples of developmental disabilities are spina bifida, cerebral palsy, Down syndrome, and muscular dystrophy. Some developmental disabilities occur as a result of birth trauma or severe illness or injury at a very young age, whereas many developmental disabilities are genetic in origin (see Chapter 8). Acquired disabilities may occur as a result of an acute and sudden injury (e.g., traumatic brain injury, spinal cord injury, traumatic amputation), acute

nontraumatic disorders (e.g., stroke, myocardial infarction), or progression of a chronic disorder (e.g., arthritis, multiple sclerosis, chronic obstructive pulmonary disease, blindness due to diabetic retinopathy).

Types of disability include sensory disabilities that affect hearing or vision; learning disabilities that affect the ability to learn, remember, or concentrate; disabilities that affect the ability to speak or communicate; and disabilities that affect the ability to work, shop, care for oneself, or access health care (American Community Survey, 2011). Many disabilities are visible; however, invisible disabilities are often as disabling as those that can be seen. Some disabilities affect only IADLs, whereas others affect ADLs. People can be temporarily disabled because of an injury or acute exacerbation of a chronic disorder but later return to full functioning.

Although different impairments may result from different types of disabilities, there are some similarities across disabilities. People with disabilities are often considered by society to be dependent and needing to be cared for by others; however, many people with disabilities are highly functioning, independent, productive people who are capable of caring for themselves and others, having children and raising families, holding a full-time job, and making significant and major contributions to society (Fig. 9-2). Like other people, those with disabilities often prefer to live in their own homes with family members. Most people with disabilities are able to live at home independently. Some patients live alone in their own homes and use home care services. However, alternative living arrangements may be necessary;

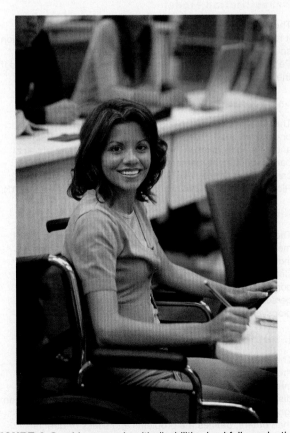

FIGURE 9-2 • Many people with disabilities lead full, productive lives. Here, a woman attends college classes.

these include assisted living facilities, long-term care facilities, and group homes.

Models of Disability

Several models of disability have been used to address or explain the issues encountered by people with disabilities (Drum, 2009; Phelan, 2011; Smeltzer, 2007a). These include the medical and rehabilitation models, the social model, the biopsychosocial model, and the interface model. Chart 9-4 briefly describes these models of disability. Of these, the interface model (Goodall, 1995) may be one of the most appropriate for use by nurses to provide care that is empowering rather than care that promotes dependency.

Chart 9-4   Models of Disability

Medical Model

The medical model equates people who are disabled with their disabilities and views disability as a problem of the person, directly caused by disease, trauma, or other health condition, that requires medical care provided in the form of individual treatment by professionals. Health care providers, rather than people with disabilities, are viewed as the experts or authorities. Management of the disability is aimed at cure or the person's adjustment and behavior change. The model is viewed as promoting passivity and dependency. People with disabilities are viewed as tragic (Goodall, 1995; Scullion, 1999, 2000; WHO, 2001; Lollar & Crews, 2003).

Rehabilitation Model

The rehabilitation model emerged from the medical model. It regards disability as a deficiency that requires a rehabilitation specialist or other helping professional to fix the problem. People with disabilities are often perceived as having failed if they do not overcome the disability (Lollar & Crews, 2003).

Social Model

The social model, which is also referred to as the barriers or disability model, views disability as socially constructed and as a political issue that is a result of social and physical barriers in the environment. Its perspective is that disability can be overcome by removal of these barriers (French, 1992; Richardson, 1997; Shakespeare & Watson, 1997; WHO, 2001).

Biopsychosocial Model

The biopsychosocial model integrates the medical and social models to address perspectives of health from a biologic, individual, and social perspective (HHS, 2005; WHO, 2001). Critiques of this model have suggested that the disabling condition, rather than the person and the experience of the person with a disability, remains the defining construct of the biopsychosocial model (Lutz & Bowers, 2005).

Interface Model

The interface model is based on the life experience of the person with a disability and views disability at the intersection (i.e., interface) of the medical diagnosis of a disability and environmental barriers. It considers rather than ignores the diagnosis. The person with a disability, rather than others, defines the problems and seeks or directs solutions (Goodall, 1995).

The interface model does not ignore the disabling condition or its disabling effects; instead, it promotes the view that people with disabilities are capable, responsible people who are able to function effectively despite having a disability. The interface model can serve as a basis for the role of nurses as advocates for removal of barriers to health care and for examination of how society and health care professionals contribute to discrimination by viewing disability as an abnormal state.

Disability Versus Disabling Disorders

Regardless of which definition or model of disability is adopted, it is important to realize that it is possible to understand the pathophysiology of a disabling condition or injury or be very knowledgeable about the physical changes resulting from a disorder without understanding the concept of disability. The nurse caring for patients with preexisting disabilities or new disabilities must recognize the impact of a disability on current and future health and well-being, ability to participate in self-care or self-management, and ability to obtain required health care and health screening. Nursing management—from assessment through evaluation of the effectiveness of nursing interventions—must be examined to determine whether appropriate modifications have been made to ensure that people with disabilities receive health care equal to that of people without disabilities. Furthermore, nurses as well as other health care providers need to examine their facilities and procedures to ensure that the needs of people with various disabilities can be adequately addressed. Although the health care needs of people with disabilities generally do not differ from those of the general population, some disabilities create special needs and necessitate the use of special accommodations. Chart 9-5 reviews strategies to ensure quality health care for people with disabilities.

Self-Reported Health Status

The self-reported health status among adults with and without a disability differs significantly. Table 9-3 shows how people with disability report their health status compared to people without disabilities (CDC, 2011). These differences are due in part to the lack of accessible health care for people with disabilities.

Federal Legislation

Because of widespread discrimination against people with disabilities, the U.S. Congress enacted legislation to address health care disparities in this population. This legislation includes the Rehabilitation Act of 1973 and the

---

TABLE 9-3   Self-Reported Health Status Among Adults With and Without Disabilities

	With Disabilities	Without Disabilities
Excellent/very good	27.2%	60.2%
Good	32.5%	29.9%
Fair/poor	40.3%	9.9%

From Centers for Disease Control and Prevention. (2011). *What should you know about disability and health?* Atlanta, GA: Author. Available at: www.cdc.gov/ncbddd/disabilityandhealth/index.html

Chart 9-5 | Strategies to Ensure Quality Health Care for People With Disabilities

Communication Strategies

- Does the patient with a disability require or prefer accommodations (e.g., a sign language interpreter) to ensure full participation in conversations about his or her own health care?
- Are appropriate accommodations made to communicate with the patient?
- Are efforts made to direct all conversations to the patient rather than to others who have accompanied the patient to the health care facility?

Accessibility of the Health Care Facility

- Are clinics, hospital rooms, offices, restrooms, laboratories, and imaging facilities accessible to people with disabilities, as legally required by the Americans With Disabilities Act and Rehabilitation Act?
- Has accessibility been verified by a person with a disability?
- Is a sign language interpreter other than a family member available to assist in obtaining a patient's health history and in conducting a physical assessment?
- Does the facility include appropriate equipment to permit people with disabilities to obtain health care (including mammography, gynecologic examination and care, dental care) in a dignified and safe manner?

Assessment

Usual Health Considerations

- Does the health history address the same issues that would be included when obtaining a history from a person without disabilities, including sexuality, sexual function, and reproductive health issues?

Disability-Related Considerations

- Does the health history address the patient's specific disability and the effect of disability on the patient's ability to obtain health care, manage self-care activities, and obtain preventive health screening and follow-up care?
- What physical modifications and positioning are needed to ensure a thorough physical examination, including pelvic or testicular and rectal examination?

Abuse

- Is the increased risk for abuse (physical, emotional, financial, and sexual) by various people (family, paid care providers, strangers) addressed in the assessment?
- If abuse is detected, are men and women with disabilities who are survivors of abuse directed to appropriate resources, including accessible shelters and hotlines?

Depression

- Is the patient experiencing depression? If so, is treatment offered just as it would be to a patient without a disability, without assuming that depression is normal and a result of having a disability?

Aging

- What concerns does the patient have about aging with a preexisting disability?
- What effect has aging had on the patient's disability, and what effect has the disability had on the patient's aging?

Secondary Conditions

- Does the patient have secondary conditions related to his or her disability or its treatment?
- Is the patient at risk for secondary conditions because of environmental barriers or lack of access to health care or health promotion activities?
- Are strategies in place to reduce the risk for secondary conditions or to treat existing secondary conditions?

Accommodations in the Home

- What accommodations does the patient have at home to encourage or permit self-care?
- What additional accommodations does the patient need at home to encourage or permit self-care?

Cognitive Status

- Is it assumed that the patient is able to participate in discussion and conversation rather than assuming that he or she is unable to do so because of a disability?
- Are appropriate modifications made in written and verbal communication strategies?

Modifications in Nursing Care

- Are modifications made during hospital stays, acute illness or injury, and other health care encounters to enable a patient with disability to be as independent as he or she prefers?
- Is "person-first language" used in referring to a patient with disability, and do nurses and other staff talk directly to the patient rather than to those who accompanied the patient?
- Are all staff informed about the activities of daily living for which the patient will require assistance?
- Are accommodations made to enable the patient to use his or her assistive devices (hearing/visual aids, prostheses, limb support devices, ventilators, service animals)?
- If a patient with disability is immobilized because of surgery, illness, injury, or treatments, are risks of immobility addressed and strategies implemented to minimize those risks?
- Is the patient with a disability assessed for other illnesses and health issues (e.g., other acute or chronic illness, depression, psychiatric/mental health and cognitive disorders) not related to his or her primary disability?

Patient Education

- Are accommodations and alternative formats of instructional materials (large print, Braille, visual materials, audiotapes) provided for patients with disabilities?
- Does patient instruction address the modifications (e.g., use of assistive devices) needed by patients with disabilities to enable them to adhere to recommendations?
- Are modifications made in educational strategies to address learning needs, cognitive changes, and communication impairment?

Health Promotion and Disease Prevention

- Are health promotion strategies discussed with people with disabilities along with their potential benefits: improving quality of life and preventing secondary conditions (health problems that result because of preexisting disability)?
- Are patients aware of accessible community-based facilities (e.g., health care facilities, imaging centers, public exercise settings, transportation) to enable them to participate in health promotion?

Independence Versus Dependence

- Is independence, rather than dependence, of the person with a disability the focus of nursing care and interaction?
- Are care and interaction with the patient focused on empowerment rather than promoting dependence of the patient?

Insurance Coverage

- Does the patient have access to the health insurance coverage and other services for which he or she qualifies?
- Is the patient aware of various insurance and other available programs?
- Would the patient benefit from talking to a social worker about eligibility for Medicaid, Medicare, disability insurance, and other services?

ADA. In 2005, the U.S. Surgeon General called for action to improve the health and wellness of people with disabilities (HHS, 2005; Smeltzer, 2007a). Health care in people with disabilities has received further national attention through specific national objectives in *Healthy People 2020* (HHS, 2010b).

The Rehabilitation Act of 1973 protects people from discrimination based on their disability. The act applies to employers and organizations that receive financial assistance from any federal department or agency; this includes many hospitals, long-term care facilities, mental health centers, and human service programs. It forbids organizations from excluding or denying people with disabilities equal access to program benefits and services. It also prohibits discrimination related to availability, accessibility, and delivery of services, including health care services.

The ADA of 1990 mandates that people with disabilities have access to job opportunities and to the community. It requires that employers evaluate an applicant's ability to perform the job and not discriminate on the basis of a disability. According to the ADA, communities must provide public transportation that is accessible to people with disabilities. The ADA also requires that "reasonable accommodations" be provided to facilitate employment of a person with a disability. Facilities used by the public must be accessible and accommodate those with disabilities. Examples of reasonable accommodations in health care settings include accessible facilities and equipment (e.g., accessible restrooms, adjustable examination tables, access ramps, grab bars, elevated toilet seats) and alternative communication methods (e.g., telecommunication devices and sign language interpreters for use by people who are deaf).

Although the ADA took effect in 1992, compliance has been slow, and some facilities continue to be inaccessible although all new construction and modifications of public facilities must address access for people with disabilities. Because courts have interpreted the definition of disability in the ADA so narrowly that few people could meet it, the ADA Amendments Act was signed into law in 2008 and enacted in January 2009. The act broadly defines *disability* to encompass impairments that substantially limit a major life activity. This wording states that effective use of assistive devices, auxiliary aids, accommodations, medical therapies and supplies (other than eyeglasses and contact lenses) does not alter the determination of whether a disability qualifies under the law. The purpose of the amendments to the act was to cover more people and to shift the attention from focusing on who has a disability to making accommodations and avoiding discrimination. Examples of modifications that are needed to provide equal access to health care to people with disabilities are identified in Chart 9-5.

Right of Access to Health Care

People with disabilities have the right of access to health care that is equal in quality to that of other people. For years, people with disabilities have been discriminated against in employment, public accommodations, and public and private services, including health care. The needs of people with disabilities in health care settings present many challenges to health care providers: how to communicate effectively if there are communication deficits, the additional physical requirements for mobility, and time required to provide assistance with self-care routines during hospitalization. Health care providers, including nurses, may not be aware of the specific needs of people with disabilities and may fail to provide appropriate care and services for them. However, it is essential that health care providers, including nurses, realize that people with disabilities have a legally mandated right to accessible health care facilities for all medical care and screening procedures. Furthermore, people with disabilities have the right to health care provided by professionals who are knowledgeable about and sensitive to the effects of disability on access to health care, including care that addresses their reproductive issues and sexuality (Smeltzer, 2007b; Smeltzer & Wetzel-Effinger, 2009). Reasonable accommodations are mandated by law and are the financial responsibility of the health care provider or facility. People with disabilities should not be expected to provide their own accommodations (e.g., sign language interpreters, assistants). Family members should not be expected to serve as interpreters because of concern for the patient's privacy and confidentiality and the risk of errors in interpreting information by either the patient or the health care provider. Chart 9-6 identifies strategies to communicate effectively with people with disabilities.

In response to continued accessibility issues, the U.S. Surgeon General issued *Call to Action to Improve the Health and Wellness of Persons With Disabilities* (HHS, 2005). This report recognized that all persons with disabilities need to have access to comprehensive health care so that they are able to have full, engaged, and productive lives in their own communities. Among strategies to accomplish this, the document stipulated that health care professionals need to become knowledgeable about disability. It further recommended that schools educating health care professionals educate about disability and address the need for increased availability of methods to screen, diagnose, and treat the whole person with a disability with dignity.

Barriers to Health Care

Many people with disabilities encounter barriers to full participation in life, including health care, health screening, and health promotion (HHS, 2005). Some of these barriers are structural and make certain facilities inaccessible. Examples of structural barriers include stairs, lack of ramps, narrow doorways that do not permit entry of a wheelchair, and restroom facilities that cannot be used by people with disabilities (e.g., restrooms that lack grab bars and those that lack larger restroom stalls designed for people using wheelchairs) (Lagu, Hannon, Rothberg et al., 2013).

Structural barriers to accessibility are most easily identified and eliminated. Other less visible barriers include negative and stereotypic attitudes (e.g., believing that all people with disabilities have a poor quality of life and are dependent and nonproductive) on the part of the public. Health care providers with similar negative attitudes make it difficult for people with disabilities to obtain health care equal in quality to that of people without disabilities. The Rehabilitation Act and the ADA were enacted more than 40 and 20 years ago, respectively, to ensure equal access to people with disabilities;

Chart 9-6 Interacting and Communicating With People Who Have Disabilities

Patients will feel most comfortable receiving health care if you consider the following suggestions.

General Considerations

- Do not be afraid to make a mistake when interacting and communicating with someone with a disability or chronic medical condition. Keep in mind that a person with a disability is a person first and is entitled to the dignity, consideration, respect, and rights you expect for yourself.
- Treat adults as adults. Address people with disabilities by their first names only if extending the same familiarity to all others present. Never patronize people by patting them on the head or shoulder.
- Relax. If you do not know what to do, allow the person who has a disability to identify how you may be of assistance and to put you at ease.
- If you offer assistance and the person declines, do not insist. If your offer is accepted, ask how you can best help, and follow directions. Do not take over.
- If someone with a disability is accompanied by another individual, address the person with a disability directly rather than speaking through the accompanying companion.
- Be considerate of the extra time it might take for a person with a disability to get things done or said. Let the person set the pace.
- Do not be embarrassed to use common expressions, such as "See you later" or "Got to be running," that seem to relate to the person's disability.
- Use people-first language: refer to "a person with a disability" rather than "a disabled person," and avoid referring to people by the disability or disorder they have (e.g., "the diabetic").

Mobility Limitations

- Do not make assumptions about what a person can and cannot do.
- Do not push a person's wheelchair or grab the arm of someone walking with difficulty without first asking if you can be of assistance and how you can assist. Personal space includes a person's wheelchair, scooter, crutches, walker, cane, or other mobility aid.
- Never move someone's wheelchair, scooter, crutches, walker, cane, or other mobility aid without permission.
- When speaking for more than a few minutes to a person who is seated in a wheelchair, try to find a seat for yourself so that the two of you are at eye level.
- When giving directions to people with mobility limitations, consider distance, weather conditions, and physical obstacles such as stairs, curbs, and steep hills.
- Shake hands when introduced to a person with a disability. People who have limited hand use or who wear an artificial limb do shake hands.

Vision Loss (Low Vision and Blindness)

- Identify yourself when you approach a person who has low vision or blindness. If a new person approaches, introduce him or her (Sharts-Hopko, Smeltzer, Ott, et al., 2010).
- Touch the person's arm lightly when you speak so that he or she knows to whom you are speaking before you begin.
- Face the person and speak directly to him or her. Use a normal tone of voice.
- Do not leave without saying that you are leaving.

- If you are offering directions, be as specific as possible and point out obstacles in the path of travel. Use specifics such as "Left about twenty feet" or "Right two yards." Use clock cues, such as "The door is at 10 o'clock."
- When you offer to assist someone with vision loss, allow the person to take your arm. This will help you guide rather than propel or lead the person. When offering seating, place the person's hand on the back or arm of the seat.
- Alert people with low vision or blindness to posted information.
- Never pet or otherwise distract a canine companion or service animal unless the owner has given you permission.

Hearing Loss (Hard of Hearing, Deaf, Deaf-Blind)

- Ask the person how he or she prefers to communicate.
- If you are speaking through a sign language interpreter, remember that the interpreter may lag a few words behind—especially if there are names or technical terms to be finger spelled—so pause occasionally to allow the interpreter time to translate completely and accurately.
- Talk directly to the person who has hearing loss, not to the interpreter. However, although it may seem awkward to you, the person who has hearing loss will look at the interpreter and may not make eye contact with you during the conversation.
- Before you start to speak, make sure that you have the attention of the person you are addressing. A wave, a light touch on the arm or shoulder, or other visual or tactile signals are appropriate ways of getting the person's attention.
- Speak in a clear, expressive manner. Do not overenunciate or exaggerate words. Unless you are specifically requested to do so, do not raise your voice. Speak in a normal tone; do not shout.
- To facilitate lip reading, face the person and keep your hands and other objects away from your mouth. Maintain eye contact. Do not turn your back or walk around while talking. If you look away, the person might assume that the conversation is over.
- Avoid talking while you are writing a message for someone with hearing loss, because the person cannot read your note and your lips at the same time.
- Try to eliminate background noise.
- Encourage feedback to assess clear understanding.
- If you do not understand something that is said, ask the person to repeat it or to write it down. The goal is communication; do not pretend to understand if you do not.
- If you know any sign language, try using it. It may help you communicate, and it will at least demonstrate your interest in communicating and your willingness to try.

Speech Disabilities or Speech Difficulties

- Talk to people with speech disabilities as you would talk to anyone else.
- Be friendly; start up a conversation.
- Be patient; it may take the person a while to answer. Allow extra time for communication. Do not speak for the person.
- Give the person your undivided attention.
- Ask the person for help in communicating with him or her. If the person uses a communication device such as a manual or electronic communication board, ask the person the best way to use it.
- Speak in your regular tone of voice.

(continues on page 146)

Chart 9-6 Interacting and Communicating With People Who Have Disabilities (continued)

- Tell the person if you do not understand what he or she is trying to say. Ask the person to repeat the message, spell it, tell you in a different way, or write it down. Use hand gestures and notes.
- Repeat what you understand. The person's reactions will clue you in and guide you to understanding.
- To obtain information quickly, ask short questions that require brief answers or a head nod. Avoid insulting the person's intelligence with oversimplification.
- Keep your manner encouraging rather than correcting.

Intellectual/Cognitive Disabilities

- Treat adults with intellectual/cognitive disabilities as adults.
- Be alert to the individual's responses so that you can adjust your method of communication as necessary. For example, some people may benefit from simple, direct sentences or from supplementary visual forms of communication, such as gestures, diagrams, or demonstrations.
- Use concrete rather than abstract language. Be specific, without being too simplistic. When possible, use words that relate to things you both can see. Avoid using directional terms such as right, left, east, or west.
- Be prepared to give the person the same information more than once in different ways.
- When asking questions, phrase them to elicit accurate information. People with intellectual/cognitive disabilities may be eager to please and may tell you what they think you want to hear. Verify responses by repeating the question in a different way.
- Give exact instructions. For example, "Be back for lab work at 4:30," not "Be back in 15 minutes."
- Avoid giving too many directions at one time, which may be confusing.
- Keep in mind that the person may prefer information provided in written or verbal form. Ask the person how you can best relay the information.
- Using humor is fine, but do not interpret a lack of response as rudeness. Some people may not grasp subtleties of language.
- Know that people with brain injuries may have short-term memory deficits and may repeat themselves or require information to be repeated.
- Recognize that people with auditory perceptual problems may need to have directions repeated and may take notes to help them remember directions or the sequence of tasks. They may benefit from watching a task demonstrated.
- Understand that people with perceptual or "sensory overload" problems may become disoriented or confused if there is too

much to absorb at once. Provide information gradually and clearly. Reduce background noise if possible.
- Repeat information using different wording or a different communication approach if necessary. Allow time for the information to be fully understood.
- Do not pretend to understand if you do not. Ask the person to repeat what was said. Be patient, flexible, and supportive.
- Be aware that some people who have an intellectual disability are easily distracted. Try not to interpret distraction as rudeness.
- Do not expect all people to be able to read well. Some people may not read at all.

Psychiatric/Mental Health Disabilities

- Speak directly to the person. Use clear, simple communication.
- Offer to shake hands when introduced. Use the same good manners in interacting with a person who has a psychiatric/mental health disability that you would with anyone else.
- Make eye contact, and be aware of your own body language. Like others, people with psychiatric/mental health disabilities will sense your discomfort.
- Listen attentively, and wait for the person to finish speaking. If needed, clarify what the person has said. Never pretend to understand.
- Treat adults as adults. Do not patronize, condescend, or threaten. Do not make decisions for the person or assume that you know the person's preferences.
- Do not give unsolicited advice or assistance. Do not panic or summon an ambulance or the police if a person appears to be experiencing a mental health crisis. Calmly ask the person how you can help.
- Do not blame the person. A person with a psychiatric disability has a complex, biomedical condition that is sometimes difficult to control. The person cannot just "shape up." It is rude, insensitive, and ineffective to tell or expect a person to do so.
- Question the accuracy of media stereotypes of psychiatric/mental health disabilities: Movies and media often sensationalize psychiatric/mental health disabilities. Most people never experience symptoms that include violent behavior.
- Relax. Be yourself. Do not be embarrassed if you happen to use common expressions that seem to relate to a psychiatric/mental health disability.
- Recognize that beneath the symptoms and behaviors of psychiatric disabilities is a person who has many of the same wants, needs, dreams, and desires as anyone else. If you are afraid, learn more about psychiatric/mental health disabilities.

This material is adapted and based in part on *Achieving Physical and Communication Accessibility*, a publication of the National Center for Access Unlimited; *Community Access Facts*, an Adaptive Environments Center publication; and *The Ten Commandments of Interacting With People With Mental Health Disabilities*, a publication of the Ability Center of Greater Toledo.

---

however, people with disabilities continue to encounter and report multiple barriers to health care facilities and providers (Smeltzer, Avery, & Haynor, 2012). This legislation and the U.S. Surgeon General's call to improve the health and wellness of people with disabilities (HHS, 2005) and the ADA Amendments Act of 2008 are examples of efforts to eliminate barriers encountered by people with disabilities.

People with disabilities have also reported lack of access to information, transportation difficulties, inability to pay because of limited income, difficulty finding a health care provider knowledgeable about their particular disability, previous negative health care encounters, reliance on caregivers, and the demands of coping with the disability itself (HHS, 2005;

Institute of Medicine [IOM], 2007; Smeltzer, 2007a; Smeltzer et al., 2012). These issues affect both men and women with severe disabilities; however, women appear to be at higher risk for receiving a lower level of health care than men. Women with disabilities are significantly less likely to receive pelvic examinations than women without disabilities; the more severe the disability, the less frequent the examination. In particular, minority women and older women with disabilities are less likely to have regular pelvic examinations and Papanicolaou (Pap) tests. Reasons given by women for not having regular pelvic examinations are difficulty transferring onto the examination table, belief that they do not need pelvic examinations because of their disability, difficulty in accessing the office or clinic, and difficulty finding transportation (HHS, 2005; Smeltzer, 2007a). Health care providers may underestimate the effect of disabilities on women's ability to access health care, including health screening and health promotion, and they may focus on women's disabilities while ignoring women's general health issues and concerns. Furthermore, women with disabilities have also reported lack of knowledge about disability and insensitivity on the part of health care providers (Smeltzer, 2007a).

Because of the persistence of these barriers, it is essential that nurses and other health care providers take steps to ensure that clinics, offices, hospitals, and other health care facilities are accessible to people with disabilities. This includes removal of structural barriers by the addition of ramps, designation of accessible parking spaces, and modification of restrooms to make them usable by people with disabilities. Alternative communication methods (e.g., sign language interpreters, teletypewriter [TTY] devices, assistive listening devices) and types of patient education (e.g., audiotapes, large print, Braille) are essential to provision of appropriate health-related information to people with disabilities (Fig. 9-3). Such accommodations are mandated by the ADA, which requires their provision without cost to the patient.

People with intellectual and developmental disabilities often need assistance in obtaining health care, including preventive health screening. Recent studies indicate that they often lack knowledge about cancer screening, including breast cancer screening. Educational materials and interventions modified to accommodate patients with intellectual and developmental disabilities are needed to enable them to make informed decisions about screening. Major barriers to breast cancer screening by this population of women include fear, anxiety and embarrassment, primarily due to lack of understanding about cancer and the importance of its early detection. (Truesdale-Kennedy, Taggart, & McIlfatrick, 2011).

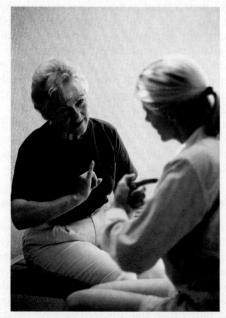

FIGURE 9-3 • Alternative communication methods and types of patient education are essential to provision of appropriate health-related information to people with disabilities. © Will & Deni McIntyre/Photo Researchers, Inc.

Federal Assistance Programs

Lack of financial resources, including health insurance, is an important barrier to health care for people with chronic illness and disabilities. However, several federal assistance programs provide financial assistance for health-related expenses for people with some chronic illnesses, acquired disabling acute and chronic diseases, and childhood disabilities.

Medicare is a federal health insurance program that is available to most people 65 years of age and older, people with permanent renal failure, and qualified people with disabilities. Title II of the Social Security Disability Insurance program pays benefits to those people who meet medical criteria for disability, who have worked long enough (40 quarters of covered employment) to qualify, and who have paid Social Security taxes. Title II also provides benefits to people disabled since childhood (younger than 22 years) who are dependents of a deceased insured parent or a parent entitled to disability or retirement benefits, and disabled widows or widowers, 50 to 60 years of age, if their deceased spouse was insured under Social Security. Title XVI of the Social Security Disability Insurance program provides supplemental security income (SSI) payments to people who are disabled and have limited income and resources.

Medicaid provides home and community-based services to people with disabilities and long-term illnesses to enable them to lead meaningful lives in their families and communities (Bersani & Lyman, 2009). (See the Resources section for more information about these benefits.)

The Affordable Care Act (ACA) is expected to expand insurance options for people with disabilities and make them more affordable. Further, people with pre-existing chronic conditions and disabilities can no longer be dropped by insurance companies (See Chapter 1 and the Resources section at the end of this chapter).

Despite the availability of these federal programs, people with disabilities often have health-related costs and other expenses related to disability that result in low-income status. Furthermore, people must undergo a disability determination process to establish eligibility for benefits, and the process can be prolonged and cumbersome for those who may need assistance in establishing their eligibility.

Nursing Care of Patients With Disabilities

As active members of society, people with disabilities are no longer an invisible minority. An increased awareness of their needs will bring about changes to improve access and accommodations. Modification of the physical environment permits access to public and private facilities and services, including health care, and nurses can serve as advocates for people with disabilities to eliminate discriminatory practices.

Nursing Considerations During Hospitalization

During hospitalization, as well as during periods of acute illness or injury or while recovering from surgery, patients with preexisting disabilities may require assistance with carrying out ADLs that they could otherwise manage at home independently and easily. Patients should be asked preferences about approaches to carrying out their ADLs, and assistive devices they require should be readily available. Careful planning with patients to ensure that the hospital room is arranged with their input enables them to manage as independently as possible. For example, patients who have paraplegia may be able to transfer independently from bed to wheelchair; however, if the bed is left in an elevated position, they may be unable to do so. If patients usually use service animals to assist them with ADLs, it is necessary to make arrangements for the accommodation of these animals. If patients with hearing loss or vision impairment are hospitalized, it is essential to establish effective communication strategies. Alternative methods for these patients to communicate with the health care team must be put in place and used, and all staff members must be aware that some patients are not able to respond to the intercom or telephone. If patients have vision impairment, it is necessary to orient them to the environment and talk to them in a normal tone of voice (Sharts-Hopko, Smeltzer, Ott, et al., 2010).

It may be necessary to obtain a referral with a speech-language therapist or communication specialist to assist in identifying alternative methods (use of sounds, gestures, eye movements) between the nurse and patient when the patient has a severe cognitive disability that affects speech (Ogletree, Bruce, Finch, et al., 2011).

Health Promotion and Prevention

Health care providers often neglect health promotion concerns of people with disabilities, who may be unaware of these concerns. For example, people who have had hearing loss since childhood may lack exposure to information about AIDS through radio and television. People with lifelong disabilities may not have received information about general health issues as children, and people with new-onset as well as lifelong disabilities may not receive encouragement to participate in health promotion activities. Therefore, nurses should take every opportunity to emphasize the importance of participation in health promotion activities (e.g., healthy diet, exercise, social interactions) and preventive health screening.

The management of some disabilities increases the risk of illness, and in some people, health screening (e.g., bone density testing, gynecologic examinations, mammography) may be required earlier in life or more frequently (HHS, 2005). Referrals by nurses to accessible sites for screening may be needed, because many imaging centers are inaccessible. In addition, nursing consultation with physical therapists may be needed to identify creative ways of enabling people with disabilities to exercise safely, because exercise facilities are also often inaccessible for people with disabilities.

General health promotion strategies and health screening recommendations for all men and women also apply to those with disabilities. Although physical limitations, cognitive impairments, and structural and attitudinal barriers existing in clinical facilities may make it difficult for some men and women to obtain health care and preventive health screening, the presence of a disability should not be used as a reason or excuse to defer recommended screening. Rather, the presence of a disability may *increase* the risk of **secondary conditions or disorders** that require screening and follow-up. Just as people

without disabilities should have regular screening tests, such as mammography or testicular and prostate examinations, so should people with disabilities (HHS, 2005). Nurses are often in a position to influence decisions about how equipment and procedures can be adapted to meet the special needs of their patients, whether these needs are cognitive, motor, or communicative.

The effect of the disabling condition on health risks should be considered. For example, the risk of osteoporosis may be increased in women and men whose disabilities limit their ability to participate in weight-bearing exercise or who use medications that contribute to bone loss (Smeltzer, Zimmerman, & Capriotti, 2005). Although people with disabilities have an increased risk of osteoporosis at a younger age than people without disabilities, little attention is given to prevention, detection, and treatment of osteoporosis, despite the increased risk for falls associated with many disabling disorders.

Nurses can provide expert health promotion education classes that are targeted to people with disabilities and refer them to accessible online resources. Classes on nutrition and weight management are extremely important to people who are wheelchair users and need assistance with transfers. Safer sex classes are needed by adolescents and young adults who have spinal cord injury, traumatic brain injury, or developmental disabilities, because the threats of sexually transmitted infections and unplanned pregnancy exist for these populations just as they do for the population in general.

The need for health promotion in the areas of establishing relationships, sex, pregnancy, and childbearing is as great in people with disabilities, including those with intellectual and cognitive disabilities, as people without disabilities. However, societal attitudes and bias against sexual relationships and childbearing in people with disabilities often result in their exclusion from discussions about these issues as well as failure to take their interest and questions seriously. Approaching these topics at the point of interest and knowledge level of a patient with a disability is important for sexual health. Further, addressing sexual issues is important to prepare people with disabilities, who are at risk of sexual and other forms of abuse, to distinguish between healthy and abusive or exploitative sexual interactions and relationships (Swango-Wilson, 2009, 2011).

Other healthy behaviors about which people with neurologic disabilities need education include avoiding alcohol and nonprescription medications while taking antispasmodic and antiseizure medications.

Significance of "People-First" Language

It is important to all people, both those with and those without disabilities, that they not be equated with their illness or physical condition. Therefore, nurses should refer to all people using "people-first" language. That means referring to the person first: "the patient with diabetes" rather than "the diabetic" or "the diabetic patient," "the person with a disability" rather than the "disabled person," "women with disabilities" rather than "disabled women," and "people who are wheelchair users" rather than "the wheelchair bound." This simple use of language conveys the message that the person, rather than the illness or disability, is of greater importance to the nurse.

 Gerontologic Considerations

Changes in the U.S. demographic profile are resulting in an increased number of older people with disabilities. Although disability is often perceived as being associated only with old age, national data demonstrate that disability occurs across the lifespan; however, its incidence increases with age (HHS, 2005). Although many people with intellectual and developmental disabilities (cerebral palsy, Down syndrome) have a shorter lifespan than other people from their age cohort, others live well into adulthood and old age. The number of adults with intellectual and developmental disabilities age 60 years and older is expected to nearly double from 641,860 in 2000 to 1.2 million by 2030 (Heller, Stafford, Davis, et al., 2010).

Age-related disabilities are those that occur in the older adult population and are thought to be attributable to the aging process. Examples of age-related disabilities include osteoarthritis, osteoporosis, and hearing loss. Because people with disabilities, including those with severe developmental disabilities, are surviving longer than ever before, there are a growing number of young, middle-aged, and older adults with disabilities, including developmental disabilities.

Stereotypical thinking may lead to the conclusion that disability is associated only with being older. However, aging is an important issue that affects people with preexisting disabilities. In addition, the process of aging has been described as accelerated in people with disabilities because they often develop changes associated with aging at a younger age than do those without disabilities (IOM, 2007). Therefore, it is important that the nurse consider the effects of aging on a preexisting disability and in turn the effects of disability on aging. The following examples may be useful:

- People who use crutches for ambulation because of polio often experience muscle problems as they age because of long-time overuse of the upper extremities; symptoms may not occur for many years but may cause discomfort and interfere with the person's ability to perform ADLs.
- People who experienced respiratory compromise with the onset of polio decades earlier may experience increasing respiratory symptoms with aging (National Institute of Neurological Disorders and Stroke, 2011).
- Women with long-standing mobility limitations and lack of weight-bearing exercise may experience bone loss and osteoporosis prior to menopause (Smeltzer et al., 2005). Therefore, people with preexisting disability should be evaluated for early onset of changes related to aging.

Concern about what the future holds is common in people aging with preexisting disabilities, who may have questions about what physical, financial, and emotional supports they will have as they age (Nosek, 2000). If their disability becomes more severe in the future, they may be concerned about placement in an assisted living facility or a long-term care facility. The nurse should recognize the concerns of people with disabilities about their future and encourage them to make suitable plans, which may relieve some of their fears and concerns about what will happen to them as they age.

Parents of adult children with developmental disabilities often fear what will happen when they are no longer available and able to care for their children. Limited long-term care resources, increased life expectancy for people with developmental disabilities, changing family patterns, and competition with the older adult population for similar resources increase the fears of these parents. Thus, nurses must identify needed community resources and services. Identifying these issues and concerns and assessing arrangements made by aging parents of adult children with disabilities can help reduce some of parents' fears about their children's futures.

Disability in Medical-Surgical Nursing Practice

Disability is often considered an issue that is specific or confined to rehabilitation nursing or to gerontologic nursing. However, as noted previously, disability can occur across the lifespan and is encountered in all settings. Patients with preexisting disabilities due to conditions that have been present from birth or to illnesses or injuries experienced as an adolescent or young adult often require health care and nursing care in medical-surgical settings. Although in the past many people with lifelong disabilities or adult onset of severe disabilities may have had shortened lifespans, today most can expect to have a normal or near-normal lifespan and to live a productive and meaningful life. They are also at risk for the same acute and chronic illnesses that can affect all people.

Because of unfavorable interactions with health care providers, including negative attitudes, insensitivity, and lack of knowledge, people with disabilities may avoid seeking medical intervention or health care services (Smeltzer et al., 2012). For this reason, and because the number of people with disabilities is increasing, nurses must acquire knowledge and skills and be available to assist them in maintaining a high level of wellness. Nurses are in key positions to influence the architectural design of health care settings and the selection of equipment that promotes ease of access and health. Padded examination tables that can be raised or lowered make transfers easier for people with disabilities. Birthing chairs benefit women with disability during yearly pelvic examinations and Pap smears and during urologic evaluations. Ramps, grab bars, and raised and padded toilet seats benefit many people who have neurologic or musculoskeletal disabilities and need routine physical examination and monitoring (e.g., bone density measurements). When a patient with a disability is admitted to the hospital for any reason, the patient's needs for these modifications should be assessed and addressed (Smeltzer et al., 2012).

Men and women with disabilities may be encountered in hospitals, clinics, offices, and nursing centers when they seek health care to address a problem related to their disability. However, they may also be encountered in these settings when they seek care for a health problem that is not related in any way to their disability. For example, a woman with spina bifida, spinal cord injury, or post-polio syndrome might seek health care related to a gynecologic issue, such as vaginal bleeding. Although her disability should be considered in the course of assessment and delivery of health and nursing care, it should not become the overriding focus or exclusive focus of the assessment or care that she receives. Furthermore, neither a severe physical disability that affects a woman's ability to transfer to an examination table for a gynecologic examination nor a cognitive disability should be a reason to defer a complete health assessment and physical examination, including a pelvic examination. Health care, including preventive health screening and health promotion, is essential to enable people with disabilities to live the highest quality of life within the limitations imposed by their disabling conditions (Todd & Stuifbergen, 2011). Men and women with disabilities have the same needs and same rights for health care and preventive health screening as others, although in some cases, the consequences of their disability increase rather than decrease their need for health screening and participation in health-promoting activities (HHS, 2005). Therefore, it is essential that medical-surgical nurses be knowledgeable about disability and how it affects people across the lifespan (Chart 9-7), as well as how to provide sensitive and quality nursing care for patients with preexisting and new-onset disability. In an effort to address these issues, specific information on health care of people with disabilities has been included throughout this book.

Home and Community-Based Care

Educating Patients About Self-Care

A major and often overlooked issue in educating patients about a health problem, a treatment regimen, or health promotion strategies is the need for alternative formats to accommodate people with various disabilities. Patients with disabilities are in need of the same information as other patients; however, they often require large print, Braille, audiotapes, or the assistance of a sign language interpreter. Materials may be obtained from a variety of sources for patients who need these educational strategies and for patients with cognitive impairments attributable to developmental disabilities or newly acquired disabilities.

Nurses should ensure that all people—whether or not they have disabilities—recognize the warning signs and symptoms of stroke, heart attack, and cancer, as well as how to access help. In addition, nurses should educate all patients who are stroke survivors and those with diabetes how to monitor their own blood pressure or glucose levels.

Continuing Care

When caring for patients with disabilities and helping them plan for discharge and continuing care in the home, it is important to consider how a particular disability affects a patient's ability to adhere to recommended treatment regimens and keep follow-up appointments. Furthermore, it is important to consider how the health issue or treatment regimen affects the disability. Although many people with disabilities are independent and able to make decisions, arrangements for transportation, and appointments to accessible facilities, others may have difficulty doing so, particularly if they are experiencing a health problem. The nurse should recognize the effect that the disability has on the patient's ability to follow up. The nurse should ask the patient whether he or she anticipates having any difficulties arranging for follow-up

Chart 9-7

NURSING RESEARCH PROFILE

Health Promotion in Women With Disabilities

Harrison, T. C., Umberson, D., Lin, L. C., et al. (2010). Timing of impairment and health-promoting lifestyles in women with disabilities. *Qualitative Health Research, 20*(6), 816–829.

Purpose

Research findings indicate that people with disabilities are less likely than those without disabilities to engage in health-promoting activities. There are, however, few explanations for these findings. Further, few studies have focused on behavior change and health promotion needs of people with disabilities. The purpose of this qualitative study was to develop a theory to explain how the timing of the onset of disability in the lives of 45 women with disabilities influenced their health-promoting lifestyles.

Design

A grounded theory approach was used to explore how timing of the onset of disability influenced the health-promoting lifestyles of midlife and older women with disabilities. The life course paradigm served to conceptualize health-promoting lifestyles. The timing of the onset of impairment in the life course was assumed by the researchers to be a developmental milestone. Women were invited to participate in the study if they had a physical or sensory impairment that prevented them from living the life they would have preferred. Women who met the inclusion criteria participated in two to three personal interviews in which they were asked about their disability and its onset, how the disability affected their lives, their perception of changes associated with aging, how these changes affected their ability to function in society and to promote their own health, and how their disability

and social relationships interacted. The sample was comprised of 45 women from 43 to 79 years; more than half had mobility impairments, 19% had either visual or hearing impairments, 18% had both visual and mobility impairments, and 4% had mild cognitive and mobility impairments. Constant comparison was used to analyze the data resulting from the interviews.

Findings

Analysis revealed that women developed a lifestyle after the onset of their disability largely through trial and error in an effort to develop or maintain a perception of themselves. Interactions with others were key in how the women identified meaning and a lifestyle consistent with resources and supports available to them. They experienced changes in their physical abilities over time that allowed them to change their lifestyles depending on what was currently happening in their lives. Timing of the onset of impairment (at an early age vs. later in adulthood) influenced women's skill development and the likelihood that rehabilitation clinicians would offer strategies to promote skill development.

Nursing Implications

Because of the importance of women's perceptions of their own health and disability and the presence of supportive environmental and attitudinal factors to health promotion, nurses and other health care providers can promote healthy lifestyles by considering women's perceptions and the perceptions of changes with aging and using strategies to ensure supportive environments and attitudes for women with disabilities.

care. It is important for the nurse to assist the patient with disabilities to identify unmet needs and to find and use resources (community and social resources, financial and transportation services) that enable the patient to obtain needed services while remaining in his or her home, if preferred. The nurse should have a list of accessible sites and services available and share those resources with the patient and family. In collaboration with other health care providers (occupational and physical therapists, speech therapists), the nurse can identify needed home modifications, including those that are simple and inexpensive, that will enable the patient to participate in self-care at home.

Critical Thinking Exercises

1 A 26-year-old man with who experienced a spinal cord injury (SCI) 2 years ago is a patient on a medical unit for treatment of a pressure ulcer. As a result of his SCI, he has no sensation below the thorax and has loss of bowel and bladder function and mobility. He is able to eat and use a computer with assistive devices. During his hospital stay, he told the nurse caring for him that he really wants to have sex. He reports that he has a new girlfriend and is afraid that if he cannot have sex with her, she will leave him. How will you respond to him? What aspects of assessment are indicated? What suggestions or recommendations can you provide?

2 ebp A 38-year-old man with Down syndrome has been diagnosed with diabetes that requires him to perform daily blood glucose monitoring. He lives in a group home and has had a job washing dishes at a local cafeteria for the past 8 years. What approaches will you use to educate the patient and other significant people in his life about blood glucose monitoring? Identify the evidence base on the use of blood glucose monitoring. Describe the educational strategies that you will use to instruct him about blood glucose monitoring, and identify any modifications that may be needed in your educational strategies and approaches.

3 pq A 48-year-old woman who requires an electric wheelchair because of advanced multiple sclerosis tells you that she has never had a mammography and has not had a gynecologic examination since her children were born 20 years ago. What are the first three priorities for preventive health screening for this woman? How will you prepare her for the barriers she may face in obtaining these services?

Brunner Suite Resources
Explore these additional resources to enhance learning for this chapter:
• NCLEX-Style Questions and Other Resources on thePoint, http://thePoint.lww.com/Brunner13e
• Study Guide
• PrepU
• Clinical Handbook
• Handbook of Laboratory and Diagnostic Tests

References
*Asterisk indicates nursing research.
**Double asterisk indicates classic reference.

Books

Anderson, G. (2010). *Chronic care: Making the case for ongoing care*. Princeton, NJ: Robert Wood Johnson Foundation.

Bersani, H., & Lyman, L. M. (2009). Governmental policies and programs for people with disabilities. In C. E. Drum, G. L. Krahn, & H. Bersani (Eds.). *Disability and public health*. Washington, DC: American Public Health Association.

Centers for Disease Control and Prevention. (2009). *The power to prevent, the call to control: At a glance 2009*. Atlanta, GA: Author.

Centers for Disease Control and Prevention. (2010). *Chronic diseases and health promotion*. Atlanta, GA: Author.

Centers for Disease Control and Prevention. (2011). *What should you know about disability and health?* Atlanta, GA: Author.

Drum, C. E. (2009). Models and approaches to disability. In C. E. Drum, G. L. Krahn, & H. Bersani (Eds.). *Disability and public health*. Washington, DC: American Public Health Association.

Galuska, D. A. & Dietz, W. H. (2010). Obesity and overweight (ICD-10 E66). In P. L. Remington, R. C. Brownson & M. V. Wegner (Eds.). *Chronic disease epidemiology and control*. Washington, DC: American Public Health Association, pp. 269–290.

Institute of Medicine. (2007). *The future of disability in America*. Washington, DC: National Academies Press.

Lubkin, I. M., & Larsen, P. D. (2013). *Chronic illness: Impact and interventions*. Boston: Jones & Bartlett.

Lutz, B. J., & Bowers, B. J. (2007). Understanding how disability is defined and conceptualized in the literature. In A. E. Dell Orto & P. W. Power (Eds.). *The psychological and social impact of illness and disability* (5th ed.). New York: Springer.

McKenna, M., & Collins, J. (2010). Current issues and challenges in chronic disease control. In P. L. Remington, R. C. Brownson, & M. V. Wegner (Eds.). *Chronic disease epidemiology and control*. Washington, DC: American Public Health Association, pp. 1–26.

**U.S. Department of Health and Human Services. (2005). *Surgeon General's call to action to improve the health and wellness of people with disabilities*. Rockville, MD: U.S. Public Health Service, Office of the Surgeon General.

U.S. Department of Health and Human Services. (2010a). *Multiple chronic conditions—A strategic framework: Optimum health and quality of life for individuals with multiple chronic conditions*. Washington, DC: Author.

U.S. Department of Health and Human Services, Office of Disease Prevention and Health Promotion. (2010b). *Healthy People 2020*. Washington, DC: Author.

**World Health Organization. (2001). *International classification of functioning, disability and health. Short version*. Geneva: Author.

Journals and Electronic Documents

American Community Survey. (2008). *U.S. Census Bureau*. Washington, DC. Available at: factfinder2.census.gov/

American Community Survey. (2011). *U.S. Census Bureau*. Washington, DC. Available at: factfinder2.census.gov/

Dartmouth Atlas of Health Care. (2008). *Executive Summary. The Dartmouth Institute for Health Policy and Clinical Practice*. Dartmouth, NH. Available at: http://www.dartmouthatlas.org/downloads/atlases/2008_Chronic_Care_Atlas.pdf

World Health Organization. (2011). *Global status report on noncommunicable diseases 2010*. Geneva: Author. Available at: http://www.who.int/nmh/publications/ncd_report2010/en/

Chronic Illness

*Auduly, A., Asplund, K., & Norbergh, K-G. (2011). The influence of illness perspectives on self-management of chronic disease. *Journal of Nursing and Healthcare of Chronic Illness*, 3(2), 109–118.

*Bowles, K. H., Riegel, B., Weiner, M. G., et al. (2010). The effect of telehomecare on heart failure self care. *AMIA Annual Symposium Proceedings*, 2010, 71–75.

**Corbin, J. M. (1998). The Corbin and Strauss Chronic Illness Trajectory Model: An update. *Scholarly Inquiry for Nursing Practice*, 12(1), 33–41.

**Corbin, J. M. (2003). The body in health and illness. *Qualitative Health Research*, 13(2), 256–267.

*Daly, B. J., Douglas, S. L., Gordon, N. H., et al. (2009). Composite outcomes of chronically critically ill patients 4 months after hospital discharge. *American Journal of Critical Care, 18*(5), 456–464.

*Eggenberger, S. K., Meiers, S. J., Krumwiede, N., et al. (2011). Reintegration within families in the context of chronic illness: A family health promoting process. *Journal of Nursing and Healthcare of Chronic Illness, 3*(3), 283–292.

Johnson, R. C., & Schoeni, R. F. (2011). Early origins of adult disease: National longitudinal population-based study of the United States. *American Journal of Public Health, 101*(12), 2317–2324.

Jones, M. C., MacGillivray, S., Kroll, T., et al. (2011). A thematic analysis of the conceptualization of self-care, self-management and self-management support in the long-term conditions management literature. *Journal of Nursing and Healthcare of Chronic Illness, 3*(3), 174–185.

*Kralik, D., Price, K., & Telford, K. (2010). The meaning of self-care for people with chronic illness. *Journal of Nursing and Healthcare of Chronic Illness, 2*(3), 197–204.

McQueen, D. V. (2011). A challenge for health promotion. *Global Health Promotion, 18*(2), 8–9, 54–67, 90–92.

*Montenegro, H., & Higgins, P. (2009). Composite outcomes of chronically critically ill patients 4 months after hospital discharge. *American Journal of Critical Care, 18*(5), 456–464.

*Todd, A., & Stuifbergen, A. (2011). Barriers and facilitators related to breast cancer screening. A qualitative study of women with multiple sclerosis. *International Journal of MS Care, 13*(2), 49–56.

Disabilities

Americans with Disabilities Act of 1990. Available at: www.ada.gov/pubs/ada.htm

Americans with Disabilities Amendments Act of 2008. Available at: access-board.gov/about/laws/ADA-amendments.htm

Boutin, D. L., & McCarthy, A. K. (2011). Introduction to the special issue on veterans with disabilities. *Journal of Applied Rehabilitation Counseling, 42*(2), 3–4.

**French, S. (1992). Simulation exercises in disability awareness training. *Disability, Handicap and Society, 7*(3), 257–266.

**Goodall, C. J. (1995). Is disability any business of nurse education? *Nurse Education Today, 15*(5), 323–327.

*Harrison, T. C., Umberson, D., Lin, L. C., et al. (2010). Timing of impairment and health-promoting lifestyles in women with disabilities. *Qualitative Health Research, 20*(6), 816–829.

Heller, T., Stafford, P., Davis, L. A., et al. (Eds.). (2010). People with intellectual and developmental disabilities growing old: An overview. *Impact, 23*(1) 2–3.

Lagu, T., Hannon, N. S., Rothberg, M. G., et al. (2013). Access to subspecialty care for patients with mobility impairment: A survey. *Ann Intern Med, 158*(6): 441–446.

*Lollar, D. J., & Crews, J. E. (2003). Redefining the role of public health in disability. *Annual Review of Public Health, 24*, 195–208.

*Lutz, B. J., & Bowers, B. J. (2005). Disability in everyday life. *Qualitative Health Research, 15*(8), 1037–1054.

National Institute of Neurological Disorders and Stroke. (2011). *NINDS post-polio syndrome information page.* National Institutes of Health. Available at: www.ninds.nih.gov/disorders/post_polio/post_polio.htm

**Nosek, M. A. (2000). Overcoming the odds: The health of women with physical disabilities in the United States. *Archives of Physical Medicine and Rehabilitation, 81*(2), 135–138.

Ogletree, B. T., Bruce, S. M., Finch, A., et al. (2011). Recommended communication-based interventions for individuals with severe intellectual disabilities. *Communication Disorders Quarterly, 32*(3), 164–175.

Phelan, S. K. (2011). Constructions of disability: A call for critical reflexivity in occupational therapy. *Canadian Journal of Occupational Therapy, 78*, 164–172.

**Richardson, M. (1997). Addressing barriers: Disabled rights and the implications for nursing of the social construct of disability. *Journal of Advanced Nursing, 25*(6), 1269–1275.

**Scullion, P. (1999). Conceptualizing disability in nursing: Some evidence from students and their teachers. *Journal of Advanced Nursing, 29*(3), 648–657.

**Scullion, P. (2000). Enabling disabled people: Responsibilities of nurse education. *British Journal of Nursing, 9*(15), 1010–1015.

**Shakespeare, T., & Watson, N. (1997). Defending the social model. *Disability and Society, 12*(2), 293–300.

*Sharts-Hopko, N. C., Smeltzer, S., Ott, B. B., et al. (2010). Healthcare experiences of women with visual impairment. *Clinical Nurse Specialist, 24*(3), 149–153.

Smeltzer, S. C. (2007a). Improving the health and wellness of persons with disabilities: A call to action too important for nursing to ignore. *Nursing Outlook, 55*(4), 189–193.

Smeltzer, S. C. (2007b). Pregnancy in women with disabilities. *Journal of Obstetrical, Gynecology, and Neonatal Nursing, 36*(1), 88–96.

*Smeltzer, S. C., Avery, C., & Haynor, P. (2012). Interactions of people with disabilities with nursing staff during hospitalization. *American Journal of Nursing, 112*(4), 30–37.

Smeltzer, S. C., & Wetzel-Effinger, L. (2009). Pregnancy in women with spinal cord injury. *Topics in Spinal Cord Injury Rehabilitation, 15*(1), 29–42.

*Smeltzer, S. C., & Zimmerman, V. (2005). Health promotion interests of women with disabilities. *Journal of Neuroscience Nursing, 37*(2), 80–86.

*Smeltzer, S. C., Zimmerman, V., & Capriotti, T. (2005). Osteoporosis risk and low bone mineral density in women with disabilities. *Archives of Physical Medicine and Rehabilitation, 86*(3), 582–586.

*Swango-Wilson, A. (2009). Perception of sex education for individuals with developmental and cognitive disability: A four cohort study. *Sex and Disability, 27*(4), 223–228.

Swango-Wilson, A. (2011). Meaningful sex education programs for individuals with intellectual/developmental disabilities. *Sex and Disability, 29*(2), 113–118.

*Truesdale-Kennedy, M., Taggart, L., & McIlfatrick, S. (2011). Breast cancer knowledge among women with intellectual disabilities and their experiences of receiving breast mammography. *Journal Advanced Nursing, 67*(6), 1294–1304.

Resources

AbleData, www.abledata.com

American Association of the Deaf-Blind, www.aadb.org

American Association on Intellectual and Developmental Disabilities (formerly American Association on Mental Retardation), www.aaidd.org

American Foundation for the Blind, www.afb.org

American Speech-Language-Hearing Association, www.asha.org

Americans With Disabilities Act National Network, www.adata.org/

Arc of the United States, www.thearc.org

Association of Late-Deafened Adults (ALDA), www.alda.org

Center for Research on Women With Disabilities (CROWD), www.bcm.edu/crowd

Centers for Medicare and Medicaid Services (CMS), www.cms.hhs.gov

ChronicNet, www.chronicnet.org/chronnet/project.htm (Provides local and national data on chronic care issues and populations.)

National Aphasia Association (NAA), www.aphasia.org

National Center for Learning Disabilities, www.ncld.org

North Carolina Office on Disability and Health, www.fpg.unc.edu/~ncodh or www.wch.dhhs.state.nc.us/cay.htm

People with disabilities and the Affordable Care Act (ACA), http://healthcare.gov/law/information-for-you/people-with-disabilities.html

Through the Looking Glass, www.lookingglass.org

United Cerebral Palsy (UCP), www.ucp.org

United Spinal Association, www.unitedspinal.org

Women With Disabilities, Health Promotion for Women With Disabilities Web Site, Villanova University College of Nursing, http://nurseweb.villanova.edu/womenwithdisabilities/welcome.htm

10

Principles and Practices of Rehabilitation

Learning Objectives

On completion of this chapter, the learner will be able to:

1 Describe the goals of rehabilitation.
2 Discuss the interdisciplinary approach to rehabilitation.
3 Describe components of a comprehensive assessment of functional capacity.

4 Use the nursing process as a framework for care of patients with self-care deficits, impaired physical mobility, impaired skin integrity, and altered patterns of elimination.
5 Describe the significance of continuity of care and community reentry from the health care facility to the home or extended care facility for patients who need rehabilitative assistance and services.

Glossary

activities of daily living (ADLs): activities related to personal care (self-care)

adaptive device: a type of assistive technology that is used to change the environment or help the person to modify the environment

assistive device: a type of assistive technology that helps people with disabilities perform a given task

assistive technology: any item, piece of equipment, or product system that is used to improve the functional capabilities of individuals with disabilities; this term encompasses both assistive devices and adaptive devices

habilitation: making able; learning new skills and abilities to meet maximum potential

impairment: loss or abnormality of psychological, physiologic, or anatomic structure or function at the organ level (e.g., dysphagia, hemiparesis); an abnormality of body structure, appearance, an organ, or system function resulting from any cause

instrumental activities of daily living (IADLs): complex skills needed for independent living

orthosis: an external appliance that provides support, prevents or corrects joint deformities, and improves function

pressure ulcer: localized area of skin breakdown due to prolonged pressure and insufficient blood supply, usually at bony prominences

prosthesis: a device used to replace a body part

rehabilitation: making able again; relearning skills or abilities or adjusting existing functions

sinus tract: course or path of tissue destruction occurring in any direction from the surface or edge of a wound; results in dead space with potential for abscess formation; also called *tunneling*

slough: soft, moist avascular (devitalized) tissue; may be white, yellow, tan, grey, or green; may be loose or firmly adherent

undermining: area of destroyed tissue that extends under intact skin along the periphery of a wound; commonly seen in shear injuries; can be distinguished from sinus tract in that there is a significant portion of the wound edge involved, whereas sinus tract involves only a small portion of the wound edge

Rehabilitation is a goal-oriented process that enables people with acute or chronic disorders, including those with physical, mental, or emotional disabilities or impairments, activity limitations, and participation restrictions to (1) identify, reach, and maintain optimal physical, sensory, intellectual, psychological, and/or social functional levels and (2) focus on existing abilities to facilitate independence, self-determination, and social integration (Ackerman, Asindua, Blouin, et al., 2011). During rehabilitation—sometimes called habilitation—patients adjust to disabilities by learning how to use resources and focus on existing abilities. In **habilitation**, abilities, not disabilities, are emphasized.

Rehabilitation is an integral part of nursing because every major illness or injury carries the threat of disability or impairment, which involves a loss of function or an abnormality in body structure or function. Rehabilitation nursing is a specialty that focuses on returning patients to optimal functionality through a holistic approach to care. The principles of rehabilitation are basic to the care of all patients, and rehabilitation efforts should begin during the initial contact with a patient. Ultimately, the goal of rehabilitation nursing is to assist the patient to attain and maintain optimum health as defined by the patient (Hoeman, 2008). If restoring the patient's ability to function independently or at a pre-illness or pre-injury level of functioning is not possible, the aims of rehabilitation are to maximize independence and prevent secondary disability as well as to promote a quality of life acceptable to the patient.

Rehabilitation services are required by more people than ever before because of advances in technology that save or prolong the lives of seriously ill and injured patients and patients with disabilities. Increasing numbers of patients who are recovering from serious illnesses or injuries are returning to their homes and communities with ongoing needs. Significant disability caused by war and terrorism also increases the demand for rehabilitation services. All patients, regardless of age, gender, ethnic group, socioeconomic status, or diagnosis, have a right to rehabilitation services.

A person is considered to have a disability, such as a restriction in performance or function in everyday activities, if he or she has difficulty talking, hearing, seeing, walking, climbing stairs, lifting or carrying objects, performing activities of daily living (ADLs), doing schoolwork, or working at a job. The disability is considered severe if the person cannot perform one or more activities, receives federal benefits because of an inability to work, uses an assistive device for mobility, or needs help from another person to accomplish basic activities. The purpose of **assistive technology** is to incorporate devices to improve the functional capabilities of persons with disabilities; these may include any item, piece of equipment, or product system that may be acquired commercially, off the shelf, modified, or customized. Types of assistive technology may include **adaptive devices**, which help a person with a disability to either modify or change the environment (e.g., an access ramp used in place of steps for a person who uses a wheelchair), and **assistive devices**, which help a person with a disability perform a given task (e.g., a lap board with pictures used to assist a person who cannot talk to communicate). (See Chapter 9 for further discussion on disability.)

The Rehabilitation Team

Rehabilitation is a creative, dynamic process that requires a team of professionals working together with patients and families. The team members represent various disciplines, with each health professional making a unique contribution to the rehabilitation process. In addition to nurses, members of the rehabilitation team may include physicians, nurse practitioners, physiatrists, physical therapists, occupational therapists, recreational therapists, speech-language therapists, psychologists, psychiatric liaison nurses, spiritual advisors, social workers, vocational counselors, orthotists or prosthetists, and sex counselors.

Nurses assume an equal or, depending on the circumstances of the patient, a more critical role than other members of the health care team in the rehabilitation process. The evidence-based plan of care that nurses develop must be approved by the patient and family and is an integral part of the rehabilitation process. (See Chart 10-1 for a Nursing Research Profile on nursing care plan development in a rehabilitation setting.) Principles that undergird the process of rehabilitation-focused care include the following:

- Rehabilitation is a continuous process.
- Rehabilitation requires active patient participation.
- Rehabilitation is goal directed.

Chart 10-1

NURSING RESEARCH PROFILE
Nursing Care Plans in Cardiac Rehabilitation

Zampieron, A., Silla, A., & Marilisa, C. (2011). A retrospective study of nursing diagnoses, outcomes, and interventions for patients admitted to a cardiology rehabilitation unit. *International Journal of Nursing Terminologies and Classifications, 22*(4), 148–156.

Purpose

There is scant information about the most common nursing diagnoses, goals, and interventions used when planning care for patients enrolled in cardiac rehabilitation programs. The purpose of this study was to identify nursing diagnoses, outcomes, and interventions used in care plans for these patients so that areas for improvement in nursing care could be identified.

Design

This was a retrospective study of all patients admitted to a standardized 4-week cardiac rehabilitation outpatient program in northeastern Italy over an 11-month period. Researchers audited nursing care plans in the medical records of these patients.

Findings

Seventy-six patient medical records were audited (87% male; mean age 60 years). These audits revealed the use of a total of 21 NANDA International nursing diagnoses and three collaborative problems, 45 Nursing Outcomes Classification (NOC), and 46 Nursing Interventions Classification (NIC). The average number of nursing diagnoses was 3.8 for each patient. The most common nursing diagnoses were derived from the activity/rest domain (e.g., Decreased cardiac output, activity intolerance) and the nutritional domain (e.g., Imbalanced nutrition: more than body requirements). The average number of nursing outcomes was 7.6 per patient and tended to more commonly be drawn from the physiologic health domain (e.g., cardiac pump effectiveness, circulation status) and the health knowledge and behavior domain (e.g., knowledge: cardiac disease management). The average number of nursing interventions was 13.2 per patient; these tended to revolve around the physiologic: complex domain (e.g., cardiac care: rehabilitative, medication management) and the physiologic: basic domain (e.g., exercise promotion). In general, most nursing diagnoses had two outcomes and four interventions. Although the care plans for this population of patients were indeed individualized, the major focus of nursing interventions revolved around physiologic care. There was little focus on the diagnostic domains of self-perception, role relationships, sexuality, coping, or comfort.

Nursing Implications

Nursing care plans reflect the focused priorities of nursing care. In this particular population of patients enrolled in a cardiac rehabilitation program, it may be presumed that the major focus of nursing interventions revolved around these patients' physiologic needs, which may have been appropriate, given the 4-week time frame of the program. Nonetheless, nurses in these settings should also plan care so that self-care activities and family and community relationships with these patients are fostered and their rehabilitation potential may be reached.

- Rehabilitation requires multiprofessional teamwork (Pryor & O'Connell, 2009).

In working toward maximizing independence, nurses affirm the patient as an active participant and recognize the importance of informal caregivers in the rehabilitation process. The patient is a key member of the rehabilitation team, the focus of the team's effort, and the one who determines the final outcomes of the rehabilitation process. The patient participates in goal setting, in learning to function using his or her remaining abilities, and in adjusting to living with disabilities. The patient's family is also incorporated into the team. Families are dynamic systems; therefore, the disability of one member affects other family members. Only by incorporating the family into the rehabilitation process can the family system adapt to the change in one of its members. The family provides ongoing support, participates in problem solving, and learns to participate in providing ongoing care.

The nurse develops a therapeutic and supportive relationship with the patient and family. The nurse emphasizes the patient's assets and strengths, positively reinforcing the patient's efforts to improve self-concept and self-care abilities. During nurse–patient interactions, the nurse actively listens, encourages, and shares patient and family successes. Using the nursing process, the nurse develops a plan of care designed to facilitate rehabilitation, restore and maintain optimal health, and prevent complications.

Coping with the disability, fostering self-care, identifying mobility limitations, and managing skin care and bowel and bladder training are areas that frequently require nursing care. The nurse acts as a caregiver, educator, counselor, patient advocate, case manager, and consultant. The nurse is often responsible for coordinating the total rehabilitative plan and collaborating with and coordinating the services provided by all members of the health care team, including home care nurses, who are responsible for directing patient care after the patient returns home.

Areas of Specialty Rehabilitation

Although rehabilitation must be a component of every patient's care, specialty rehabilitation programs have been established in general hospitals, free-standing rehabilitation hospitals, and outpatient facilities. The Commission for the Accreditation of Rehabilitation Facilities (CARF) (Centers for Medicare and Medicaid Services, 2011) sets standards for these programs and monitors compliance with the standards.

- *Stroke recovery programs* and *traumatic brain injury rehabilitation* emphasize cognitive remediation, helping patients compensate for memory, perceptual, judgment, and safety deficits as well as teaching self-care and mobility skills. Other goals include helping patients swallow food safely and communicate effectively. Neurologic disorders treated in addition to stroke and brain injury include multiple sclerosis, Parkinson's disease, amyotrophic lateral sclerosis, and nervous system tumors.
- *Spinal cord injury rehabilitation programs* promote understanding of the effects and complications of spinal cord injury; neurogenic bowel and bladder management; sexuality and fertility enhancement; self-care, including prevention of skin breakdown; bed mobility and trans-

fers; and driving with adaptive equipment. The programs also focus on vocational assessment, training, and reentry into employment and the community. There are 23 federally funded spinal cord injury model systems centers across the United States (National Rehabilitation Information Center, 2011).

- *Orthopedic rehabilitation programs* provide comprehensive services to patients with traumatic or nontraumatic amputation, patients undergoing joint replacements, and patients with arthritis. Independence with a prosthesis or new joint is a major goal of these programs. Other goals include pain management, energy conservation, and joint protection.
- *Cardiac rehabilitation* for patients who have had myocardial infarction begins during the acute hospitalization and continues on an outpatient basis. Emphasis is placed on monitored, progressive exercise; nutritional counseling; stress management; sexuality; and risk reduction.
- *Pulmonary rehabilitation programs* may be appropriate for patients with restrictive or chronic obstructive pulmonary disease or ventilator dependency. Respiratory therapists help patients achieve more effective breathing patterns. The programs also teach energy conservation techniques, self-medication, and home ventilatory management.
- *Comprehensive pain management programs* are available for people with chronic pain, especially low back pain. These programs focus on alternative pain treatment modalities, exercise, supportive counseling, and vocational evaluation.
- *Comprehensive burn rehabilitation programs* may serve as step-down units from intensive care burn units. Although rehabilitation strategies are implemented immediately in acute care, a program focused on progressive joint mobility, self-care, and ongoing counseling is imperative for burn patients.
- *Pediatric rehabilitation programs* meet the needs of children with developmental and acquired disabilities, including cerebral palsy, spina bifida, traumatic brain injuries, and spinal cord injuries.

Substance Abuse Issues in Rehabilitation

As in all areas of nursing practice, nurses practicing in the area of rehabilitation must be skilled and knowledgeable about the care of patients with substance abuse. For all people with disabilities, including adolescents, nurses must assess actual or potential substance abuse. Fifty percent of spinal cord injuries are related to substance abuse, and approximately 50% of all patients with traumatic brain injury were intoxicated at the time of injury (U.S. Department of Health and Human Services [HHS], 2010).

Substance abuse is a critical issue in rehabilitation, especially for people with disabilities who are attempting to gain employment via vocational rehabilitation. The rates of substance abuse, including alcohol abuse, in people with disabilities are two to four times as high as in the general population, and this increased abuse is associated with numerous risks that may have an adverse impact. These risks include medication and health problems, societal enabling (i.e., acceptance and tolerance of substance abuse by key social and cultural groups), a lack of identification of potential problems, and a lack of accessible and appropriate prevention and treatment services. Treatment for alcoholism and drug dependencies includes thorough physical and psychosocial evaluations; detoxification; counseling; medical treatment; psychological assistance for patients and families; treatment of any coexisting psychiatric illness; and referral to community resources for social, legal, spiritual, or vocational assistance. The length of treatment and the rehabilitation process depends on the patient's needs. Self-help groups are also encouraged, although attendance at meetings of such groups (e.g., Alcoholics Anonymous, Narcotics Anonymous) poses various challenges for people who have neurologic disorders, are permanent wheelchair users, or must adapt to encounters with nondisabled attendees who may not understand disability.

Assessment of Functional Ability

Comprehensive assessment of functional capacity is the basis for developing a rehabilitation program. Functional capacity is a person's ability to perform activities of daily living and instrumental activities of daily living. **Activities of daily living (ADLs)** are those self-care activities that the patient must accomplish each day to meet personal needs; they include personal hygiene/bathing, dressing/grooming, feeding, and toileting. Many patients cannot perform such activities easily. **Instrumental activities of daily living (IADLs)** include those complex skills needed for independent living, including meal preparation, grocery shopping, household management, finances, and transportation.

The nurse observes the patient performing specific activities (e.g., eating, dressing) and notes the degree of independence; the time taken; the patient's mobility, coordination, and endurance; and the amount of assistance required. The nurse also carefully assesses joint motion, muscle strength, cardiovascular reserve, and neurologic function, because functional ability depends on these factors as well. Observations are recorded on a functional assessment tool. These tools provide a way to standardize assessment parameters and include a scale or score against which improvements may be measured. They also clearly communicate the patient's level of functioning to all members of the rehabilitation team. Rehabilitation staff members use these tools to provide an initial assessment of the patient's abilities and to monitor the patient's progress in achieving independence.

One of the most frequently used tools to assess the patient's level of independence is the Functional Independence Measure (FIM™) (Keith, Granger, Hamilton, et al., 1987). The FIM™ is a minimum data set, measuring 18 self-care items including eating, bathing, grooming, dressing upper body, dressing lower body, toileting, bladder management, and bowel management. The FIM™ addresses transfers and the ability to ambulate and climb stairs and also includes communication and social cognition items. Scoring is based on a seven-point scale, with items used to assess the patient's level of independence. The Alpha FIM™, a short

version of the FIM™, is used frequently within 72 hours of admission in acute care settings to measure functional independence and the amount of assistance the patient needs to perform ADLs.

Although there are many disease-specific tools used to assess the patient's functional ability, some frequently used generic measures include the following:

- The PULSES profile (Granger, Albrecht, & Hamilton, 1979) is used to assess physical condition (e.g., health/illness status), upper extremity functions (e.g., eating, bathing), lower extremity functions (e.g., transfer, ambulation), sensory function (e.g., vision, hearing, speech), bowel and bladder function (i.e., control of bowel or bladder), and situational factors (e.g., social and financial support). Each of these areas is rated on a scale from one (independent) to four (greatest dependency).
- The Barthel Index (Mahoney & Barthel, 1965) is used to measure the patient's level of independence in ADLs, continence, toileting, transfers, and ambulation (or wheelchair mobility). This scale does not address communicative or cognitive abilities.
- The Patient Evaluation Conference System (PECS) (Harvey, Hollis, & Jellinek, 1981), which contains 15 categories, is a comprehensive assessment scale that includes such areas as medications, pain, nutrition, use of assistive devices, psychological status, vocation, and recreation.

A detailed functional evaluation of secondary conditions related to the patient's disability, such as muscle atrophy and deconditioning, skin integrity, bowel and bladder control, and sexual function, together with residual strengths unaffected by disease or disability, is necessary. In addition, the nurse assesses the patient's physical, mental, emotional, spiritual, social, and economic status, as well as cultural and familial environment. These elements may provide a context to the functional findings and influence the rehabilitation plan. For example, the patient's perception of what it means to have a disability and the implications that this might have on familial and social roles can influence the rehabilitation process.

NURSING PROCESS

The Patient With Self-Care Deficits in Activities of Daily Living

An ADL program is started as soon as the rehabilitation process begins, because the ability to perform ADLs is frequently the key to independence, return to the home, and reentry into the community.

Assessment

The nurse must observe and assess the patient's ability to perform ADLs to determine the level of independence in self-care and the need for nursing intervention. Chart 10-2 depicts indications of potential problems in function or movement. For example, bathing requires obtaining bath water and items used for bathing (e.g., soap, washcloth), washing, and drying the body after bathing. Dressing requires getting clothes from the closet, putting on and taking off clothing, and

ASSESSMENT
Assessing Potential Problems in Function or Movement

Be alert for the following behaviors, which may indicate problems in function or movement:

- Holding onto a handrail to pull the body while going up stairs
- Holding onto a bedside rail or bedcovers to pull to a sitting position in bed
- Leaning to one side and using both hands on the handrail while going down the stairs or a ramp
- Holding onto furniture or doorways and watching the feet while walking in the house
- Lifting a leg (or arm) by using the other leg (or arm) as support or by lifting with the pants leg (or sleeve)
- Tilting the head to reach the back or side of the hair while grooming
- Pushing up, rocking forward and back, and/or leaning the body over for momentum ("nose over toes") when rising to stand from a chair
- Leaning over from the waist without bending the knees and then placing one hand on the thigh, as if it were a prop, and pushing against the thigh to assist in moving to the upright position
- Turning to reach for an object and then using the other arm or an object to support the reaching arm at the elbow or wrist
- Positioning a chair before sitting down by using the front or back of the knees and then using the back of the knees to guide sitting down; using the torso and hips to lean against a table or chair
- Reaching and leaning with the body rather than with an arm
- Walking with a lean to one side, a limp, a waddle, or other variation of a gait
- Scanning (i.e., observing or being aware of surroundings) ineffectively while eating or grooming
- Rolling or scooting the body, sliding forward in a seat, or other maneuvers to move off a bed or out of a chair

Adapted from Hoeman, S. P. (2008). *Rehabilitation nursing: Prevention, intervention, and outcomes* (4th ed.). St. Louis: Mosby.

fastening the clothing. Self-feeding requires using utensils to bring food to the mouth and chewing and swallowing the food. Toileting includes removing clothing to use the toilet, cleansing oneself, and readjusting clothing. Grooming activities include combing hair, brushing one's teeth, shaving or applying makeup, and handwashing. Patients who can sit up and raise their hands to their head can begin self-care activities. Assistive devices are often essential in achieving some level of independence in ADLs.

The nurse should also be aware of the patient's medical conditions or other health problems, the effect that they have on the ability to perform ADLs, and the family's involvement in the patient's ADLs. This information is valuable in setting goals and developing the plan of care to maximize self-care.

Nursing Diagnosis

Based on the assessment data, major nursing diagnoses may include the following:

- Self-care deficit: bathing, dressing, feeding, toileting

Planning and Goals

The major goals include performing the following activities independently or with assistance, using adaptive or assistive devices as appropriate: bathing/hygiene, dressing/grooming, feeding, and toileting. Another goal is patient expression of

satisfaction with the extent of independence achieved in self-care activities.

Nursing Interventions

Repetition, practice, and demonstrations help patients achieve maximum independence in personal care activities. The nurse's role is to provide an optimal learning environment that minimizes distractions. The nurse can identify the patient's optimal time to work on activities, encourage concentration, identify endurance issues that may affect safety, and provide cues and reminders to patients with specific disabilities (e.g., hemiparesis or hemineglect) (Hoeman, 2008). Patients with impaired mobility, sensation, strength, or dexterity may need to use assistive devices to accomplish self-care.

Fostering Self-Care Abilities

A patient's approach to self-care may be affected by altered or impaired mobility and influenced by family or cultural expectations. The inability to perform self-care as carried out previously may lead to ineffective coping behaviors such as social isolation, dependency on caregivers, or depression. The nurse must motivate the patient to learn and accept responsibility for self-care. It helps to encourage an "I'd rather do it myself" attitude. The nurse must also help the patient identify the safe limits of independent activity; knowing when to ask for assistance is particularly important.

The nurse educates, guides, and supports the patient who is learning or relearning how to perform self-care activities while maintaining a focus on patient strengths and optimal level of function. Consistency in instructions and assistance given by health care providers, including rehabilitation therapists (e.g., physiotherapists, occupational therapists, recreation therapists, speech language pathologists, and physicians) facilitates the learning process. Recording the patient's performance provides data for evaluating progress and may be used as a source for motivation and morale building. Guidelines for educating patients and families about ADLs are presented in Chart 10-3.

Often, performing a simple maneuver requires the patient with a disability to concentrate intensely and exert considerable effort; therefore, self-care techniques need to be adapted to accommodate the individual patient's lifestyle. Because a self-care activity usually can be accomplished in several ways, common sense and a little ingenuity may promote increased independence. For example, a person who cannot quite reach his or her head may be able to do so by leaning forward. Encouraging the patient to participate in a support group may also help the patient discover creative solutions to self-care problems.

Preexisting cultural norms may influence the degree of self-care the patient is willing to consider. Cultural and ethnic beliefs about hygiene can vary among individuals and families. The nurse must recognize these beliefs, work through any issues with the patient and family, and communicate pertinent findings to the rehabilitation team.

Recommending Adaptive and Assistive Devices

If the patient has difficulty performing an ADL, an adaptive or assistive device (self-help device) may be useful. Such devices may be obtained commercially or can be constructed by the nurse, occupational therapist, patient, or family. The devices may include built-up handles on toothbrushes or razors; long,

Chart 10-3 — Educating Patients About Activities of Daily Living

1. Define the goal of the activity with the patient. Be realistic. Set short-term goals that can be accomplished in the near future.
2. Identify several approaches to accomplish the task (e.g., there are several ways to put on a given garment).
3. Select the approach most likely to succeed.
4. Specify the approach on the patient's plan of care and the patient's level of accomplishment on the progress notes.
5. Identify the motions necessary to accomplish the activity (e.g., to pick up a glass, extend arm with hand open; place open hand next to glass; flex fingers around glass; move arm and hand holding glass vertically; flex arm toward body).
6. Focus on gross functional movements initially, and gradually include activities that use finer motions (e.g., buttoning clothes, eating with a fork).
7. Encourage the patient to perform the activity up to maximal capacity within the limitations of the disability.
8. Monitor the patient's tolerance.
9. Minimize frustration and fatigue.
10. Support the patient by giving appropriate praise for effort put forth and for acts accomplished.
11. Assist the patient to perform and practice the activity in real-life situations and in a safe environment.

curved handles on mirrors or shoe horns; suction cups to hold items in place; shower chairs; raised toilet seats; and universal cuffs to grip self-care items. Some of these are shown in Figure 10-1. To assist premenopausal women with managing menstruation, clothing adaptations (e.g., Velcro crotch flaps for ease of access), mirrors, self-sticking sanitary pads, packaged wipes, and loose underwear may be used.

⚑ Quality and Safety Nursing Alert

To avoid injury or bleeding, people who take anticoagulant medication should be encouraged to use an electric razor. Women may wish to consider depilatory creams or electrolysis.

A wide selection of computerized devices is available, or devices can be designed to help individual patients with severe disabilities to function more independently. The Able-Data project (see Resources list at the end of this chapter) offers a computerized listing of commercially available aids and equipment for patients with disabilities.

The nurse should be alert to "gadgets" coming on the market and evaluate their potential usefulness. The nurse must exercise professional judgment and caution in recommending devices,

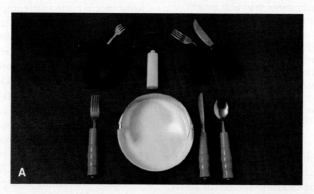

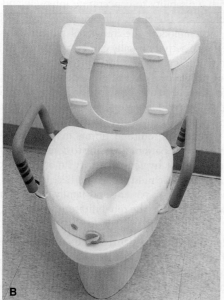

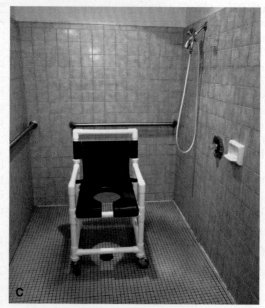

FIGURE 10-1 • Adaptive and assistive devices. **A.** Feeding tools. **B.** Raised toilet seat. **C.** Shower chair.

because in the past, unscrupulous vendors have marketed unnecessary, overly expensive, or useless items to patients.

Helping Patients Accept Limitations

If the patient has a severe disability, independent self-care may be an unrealistic goal. In this situation, the nurse educates the patient how to take charge by directing his or her care. The patient may require a personal attendant to perform ADLs. Family members may not be appropriate for providing bathing/hygiene, dressing/grooming, feeding, and toileting assistance, and spouses may have difficulty providing bowel and bladder care for patients and maintaining the role of sexual partners. If a personal caregiver is necessary, the patient and family members must learn how to manage an employee effectively. The nurse helps the patient accept self-care dependency. Independence in other areas, such as social interaction, should be emphasized to promote a positive self-concept.

Evaluation

Expected patient outcomes may include:

1. Demonstrates independent self-care in bathing/hygiene or with assistance, using adaptive devices as appropriate
   a. Bathes self at maximal level of independence
   b. Uses adaptive and assistive devices effectively
   c. Reports satisfaction with level of independence in bathing/hygiene
2. Demonstrates independent self-care in dressing/grooming or with assistance, using adaptive devices as appropriate
   a. Dresses/grooms self at maximal level of independence
   b. Uses adaptive devices effectively
   c. Reports satisfaction with level of independence in dressing/grooming
   d. Demonstrates increased interest in appearance
3. Demonstrates independent self-care in feeding or with assistance, using adaptive and assistive devices as appropriate
   a. Feeds self at maximal level of independence
   b. Uses adaptive and assistive devices effectively
   c. Demonstrates increased interest in eating
   d. Maintains adequate nutritional intake
4. Demonstrates independent self-care in toileting or with assistance, using adaptive and assistive devices as appropriate
   a. Toilets self at maximal level of independence
   b. Uses adaptive and assistive devices effectively
   c. Indicates positive feelings regarding level of toileting independence
   d. Experiences adequate frequency of bowel and bladder elimination
   e. Does not experience incontinence, constipation, urinary tract infection, or other complications

NURSING PROCESS

The Patient With Impaired Physical Mobility

Problems commonly associated with immobility include weakened muscles, joint contracture, and deformity. Each joint of the body has a normal range of motion; if the range is limited, the functions of the joint and the muscles that move

the joint are impaired, and painful deformities may develop. The nurse must identify patients at risk for such complications. The nurse needs to assess, plan, and intervene to prevent complications of immobility.

Another problem frequently seen in rehabilitation nursing is an altered ambulatory/mobility pattern. Patients with disabilities may be either temporarily or permanently unable to walk independently and unaided. The nurse assesses the mobility of the patient and designs care that promotes independent mobility within the prescribed therapeutic limits. If a patient cannot exercise and move his or her joints through their full range of motion, contractures may develop. A contracture is a shortening of the muscle and tendon that leads to deformity and limits joint mobility. When the contracted joint is moved, the patient experiences pain; in addition, more energy is required to move when joints are contracted.

Assessment

Mobility may be restricted owing to pain, paralysis, loss of muscle strength, systemic disease, an immobilizing device (e.g., cast, brace), or prescribed limits to promote healing. Assessment of mobility includes positioning, ability to move, muscle strength and tone, joint function, and the prescribed mobility limits. The nurse must collaborate with physical therapists or other team members to assess mobility.

During position change, transfer, and ambulation activities, the nurse assesses the patient's abilities, the extent of disability, and residual capacity for physiologic adaptation. The nurse observes for orthostatic hypotension, pallor, diaphoresis, nausea, tachycardia, and fatigue.

In addition, the nurse assesses the patient's ability to use various assistive devices that promote mobility. If the patient cannot ambulate without assistance, the nurse assesses the patient's ability to balance, transfer, and use assistive devices (e.g., crutches, walker). Crutch walking requires high energy expenditure and produces considerable cardiovascular stress; therefore, people with reduced exercise capacity, decreased arm strength, and problems with balance because of aging or multiple diseases may be unable to use them. A walker is more stable and may be a better choice for such patients. If the patient uses an orthosis, the nurse monitors the patient for effective use and potential problems associated with its use.

Nursing Diagnosis

Based on the assessment data, major nursing diagnoses may include the following:

- Impaired physical mobility
- Activity intolerance
- Risk for injury
- Risk for disuse syndrome
- Impaired walking
- Impaired wheelchair mobility
- Impaired bed mobility

Planning and Goals

Major goals may include absence of contracture and deformity, maintenance of muscle strength and joint mobility, independent mobility, increased activity tolerance, and prevention of further disability.

Nursing Interventions

Positioning to Prevent Musculoskeletal Complications

Deformities and contractures can often be prevented by proper positioning. Maintaining correct body alignment when the patient is in bed is essential regardless of the position selected. During each patient contact, the nurse evaluates the patient's position and assists the patient to achieve and maintain proper positioning and alignment. The most common positions that patients assume in bed are supine (dorsal), side-lying (lateral), and prone. The nurse helps the patient assume these positions and uses pillows to support the body in correct alignment. At times, a splint (e.g., wrist or hand splint) may be made by the occupational therapist to support a joint and prevent deformity. The nurse must ensure proper use of the splint and provide skin care.

Preventing External Rotation of the Hip. The patient who is in bed for an extended period of time may develop external rotation deformity of the hip because the ball-and-socket joint of the hip tends to rotate outward when the patient lies on his or her back. A trochanter roll (i.e., a flannel sheet or bath towel folded in thirds lengthwise and rolled toward the patient or a commercially manufactured roll) extending from the crest of the ilium to the midthigh prevents this deformity; with correct placement, it serves as a mechanical wedge under the projection of the greater trochanter.

 Concept Mastery Alert

Abduction moves the body part away from the body; adduction moves the body part toward the body. External rotation occurs as the leg moves outward. To prevent external rotation deformity, the patient's hip should *not* be abducted or moved away from the body.

Preventing Footdrop. Footdrop is a deformity in which the foot is plantar flexed (the ankle bends in the direction of the sole of the foot). If the condition continues without correction, the patient will not be able to hold the foot in a normal position and will be able to walk only on his or her toes, without touching the ground with the heel of the foot. The deformity is caused by contracture of both the gastrocnemius and soleus muscles. Damage to the peroneal nerve or loss of flexibility of the Achilles tendon may also result in footdrop. To prevent this disabling deformity, the patient is positioned to sit at a 90-degree angle in a wheelchair with his or her feet on the footrests or flat on the floor.

When the patient is supine in bed, padded splints or protective boots are used to keep the patient's feet at right angles to the legs. Frequent skin inspection of the feet must also be performed to determine whether positioning devices have created any unwanted pressure areas.

The patient is encouraged to perform the following ankle exercises several times each hour: dorsiflexion and plantar flexion of the feet, flexion and extension (curl and stretch) of the toes, and eversion and inversion of the feet at the ankles. The nurse provides frequent passive range-of-motion exercises if the patient cannot perform active exercises.

 Quality and Safety Nursing Alert

Prolonged bed rest, lack of exercise, incorrect positioning in bed, and the weight of bedding that forces the toes into plantar flexion must be avoided to prevent footdrop. Patients should be encouraged to wear shoes for support and protection to prevent footdrop.

Maintaining Muscle Strength and Joint Mobility

Optimal function depends on the strength of the muscles and joint motion, and active participation in ADLs promotes maintenance of muscle strength and joint mobility. Range-of-motion exercises and specific therapeutic exercises may be included in the nursing plan of care.

Performing Range-of-Motion Exercises. Range of motion involves moving a joint through its full range in all appropriate planes (Chart 10-4). To maintain or increase the motion of a joint, range-of-motion exercises are initiated as soon as the patient's condition permits. The exercises are planned for individual patients to accommodate the wide variation in the degrees of motion that people of varying body builds and age groups can attain.

Range-of-motion exercises may be active (performed by the patient under the supervision of the nurse), assisted (with the nurse helping if the patient cannot do the exercise independently), or passive (performed by the nurse). Unless otherwise prescribed, a joint should be moved through its range of motion three times, at least twice a day. The joint to be exercised is supported, the bones above the joint are stabilized, and the body part distal to the joint is moved through the range of motion of the joint. For example, the humerus must be stabilized while the radius and ulna are moved through their range of motion at the elbow joint.

Chart 10-4 **Range-of-Motion Terminology**

Abduction: movement away from the midline of the body
Adduction: movement toward the midline of the body
Flexion: bending of a joint so that the angle of the joint diminishes
Extension: the return movement from flexion; the joint angle is increased
Rotation: turning or movement of a part around its axis
   Internal: turning inward, toward the center
   External: turning outward, away from the center
Dorsiflexion: movement that flexes or bends the hand back toward the body or the foot toward the leg
Palmar flexion: movement that flexes or bends the hand in the direction of the palm
Plantar flexion: movement that flexes or bends the foot in the direction of the sole
Pronation: rotation of the forearm so that the palm of the hand is down
Supination: rotation of the forearm so that the palm of the hand is up
Opposition: touching the thumb to each fingertip on same hand
Inversion: movement that turns the sole of the foot inward
Eversion: movement that turns the sole of the foot outward

A joint should not be moved beyond its free range of motion; the joint is moved to the point of resistance and stopped at the point of pain. If muscle spasms are present, the joint is moved slowly to the point of resistance. Gentle, steady pressure is then applied until the muscle relaxes, and the motion is continued to the joint's final point of resistance.

To perform assisted or passive range-of-motion exercises, the patient must be in a comfortable supine position with the arms at the sides and the knees extended. Good body posture is maintained during the exercises. The nurse also uses good body mechanics during the exercise session.

Performing Therapeutic Exercises. Therapeutic exercises are prescribed by the primary provider and performed with the assistance and guidance of the physical therapist or nurse. The patient should have a clear understanding of the goal of the prescribed exercise. Written instructions about the frequency, duration, and number of repetitions, as well as simple line drawings of the exercise, help to ensure adherence to the exercise program. Return demonstration of the exercises also helps the patient and family to follow the instructions correctly.

When performed correctly, exercise assists in maintaining and building muscle strength, maintaining joint function, preventing deformity, stimulating circulation, developing endurance, and promoting relaxation. Exercise is also valuable in helping to restore motivation and the well-being of the patient. Weight-bearing exercises may slow the bone loss that occurs with disability. There are five types of exercise: passive, active-assistive, active, resistive, and isometric. The description, purpose, and action of each of these exercises are summarized in Table 10-1.

Promoting Independent Mobility

When the patient's condition stabilizes, his or her physical condition permits, and the patient is able to stand, the patient is assisted to sit up on the side of the bed and then to stand. Tolerance of this activity is assessed. Orthostatic (postural) hypotension may develop when the patient assumes a vertical position. Because of inadequate vasomotor reflexes, blood pools in the splanchnic (visceral or intestinal) area and in the legs, resulting in inadequate cerebral circulation. If indicators of orthostatic hypotension (e.g., drop in blood pressure, pallor, diaphoresis, nausea, tachycardia, dizziness) are present, the activity is stopped, and the patient is assisted to a supine position in bed.

Some disabling conditions, such as spinal cord injury, acute brain injury, and other conditions that require extended periods in the recumbent position, prevent the patient from assuming an upright position at the bedside. Several strategies can be used to help the patient assume a 90-degree sitting position. A reclining wheelchair with elevating leg rests allows a slow and controlled progression from a supine position to a 90-degree sitting position. A tilt table (a board that can be tilted in 10-degree increments from a horizontal to a vertical position) may also be used. The tilt table promotes vasomotor adjustment to positional changes and helps patients with limited standing balance and limited weight-bearing activities avoid the decalcification of bones and low bone mass associated with disuse syndrome and lack of weight-bearing exercise. Physical therapists may use a tilt table for patients who have not been upright owing to illness or disability. Gradual elevation of the head of the bed may help. When getting patients with spinal cord injury out of bed, it is important to gradually raise the head of the bed to a 90-degree angle; this may take approximately 10 to 15 minutes.

TABLE 10-1	**Therapeutic Exercises**		
	Description	**Purposes**	**Action**
Passive	An exercise carried out by the therapist or the nurse without assistance from the patient	To retain as much joint range of motion as possible; to maintain circulation	Stabilize the proximal joint and support the distal part; move the joint smoothly, slowly, and gently through its full range of motion; avoid producing pain.
Active-assistive	An exercise carried out by the patient with the assistance of the therapist or the nurse	To encourage normal muscle function	Support the distal part, and encourage the patient to take the joint actively through its range of motion; give no more assistance than is necessary to accomplish the action; short periods of activity should be followed by adequate rest periods.
Active	An exercise accomplished by the patient without assistance; activities include turning from side to side and from back to abdomen and moving up and down in bed	To increase muscle strength	When possible, active exercise should be performed against gravity; the joint is moved through full range of motion without assistance; make sure that the patient does not substitute another joint movement for the one intended.
Resistive	An active exercise carried out by the patient working against resistance produced by either manual or mechanical means	To provide resistance to increase muscle power	The patient moves the joint through its range of motion while the therapist resists slightly at first and then with progressively increasing resistance; sandbags and weights can be used and are applied at the distal point of the involved joint; the movements should be performed smoothly.
Isometric or Muscle Setting	Alternately contracting and relaxing a muscle while keeping the part in a fixed position; this exercise is performed by the patient	To maintain strength when a joint is immobilized	Contract or tighten the muscle as much as possible without moving the joint, hold for several seconds, then let go and relax; breathe deeply.

Graduated compression stockings are used to prevent venous stasis. For some patients, a compression garment (leotard) or snug-fitting abdominal binder and elastic compression bandaging of the legs are needed to prevent venous stasis and orthostatic hypotension. When the patient is standing, the feet are protected with a pair of properly fitted shoes. Extended periods of standing are avoided because of venous pooling and pressure on the soles of the feet. The nurse monitors the patient's blood pressure and pulse and observes for signs and symptoms of orthostatic hypotension and cerebral insufficiency (e.g., the patient reports feeling faint and weak), which suggest intolerance of the upright position. If the patient does not tolerate the upright position, the nurse should return the patient to the reclining position and elevate his or her legs.

Assisting Patients With Transfer. A transfer is movement of the patient from one place to another (e.g., bed to chair, chair to commode, wheelchair to tub). As soon as the patient is permitted out of bed, transfer activities are started. The nurse assesses the patient's ability to participate actively in the transfer and determines, in conjunction with occupational therapists or physical therapists, the adaptive equipment required to promote independence and safety. A lightweight wheelchair with brake extensions, removable and detachable armrests, and leg rests minimizes structural obstacles during the transfer. Tub seats or benches make transfers in and out of the tub easier and safer. Raised, padded commode seats may also be warranted for patients who must avoid flexing the hips greater than 90 degrees when transferring to a toilet. It is important that the nurse educate the patient about hip precautions (e.g., no adduction past the midline, no flexion greater than 90 degrees, and no internal rotation); abduction pillows can be used to keep the hip in correct alignment if precautions are warranted.

It is important that the patient maintains muscle strength and, if possible, performs push-up exercises to strengthen the arm and shoulder extensor muscles. The push-up exercises require the patient to sit upright in bed; a book is placed under each of the patient's hands to provide a hard surface, and the patient is instructed to push down on the book, raising the body. The nurse should encourage the patient to raise and move the body in different directions by means of these push-up exercises.

The nurse or physical therapist instructs the patient how to transfer. There are several methods of transferring from the bed to the wheelchair when the patient cannot stand, and the technique chosen should take into account the patient's abilities and disabilities (Fig. 10-2). It is helpful to demonstrate the technique to the patient. If the physical therapist is involved in teaching the patient to transfer, the nurse and physical therapist must collaborate so that consistent instructions are given to the patient. During transfer, the nurse assists and coaches the patient. For example, with a weight-bearing transfer from bed to chair, the patient stands up, pivots until his back is opposite the new seat, and sits down. If the patient's muscles are not strong enough to overcome the resistance of body weight, a polished lightweight board (transfer board, sliding board) may be used to bridge the gap between the bed and the chair. The patient slides across on the board with or without assistance from a caregiver. This

board may also be used to transfer the patient from the chair to the toilet or bathtub bench. It is important to avoid the effects of shear on the patient's skin while sliding across the board. The nurse should make sure that the patient's fingers do not curl around the edge of the board during the transfer, because the patient's body weight can crush the fingers as he or she moves across the board.

Safety is a primary concern during a transfer, and the following guidelines are recommended:

- Wheelchairs and beds must be locked before transfer begins.
- Detachable arm- and footrests are removed to make getting in and out of the chair easier.
- One end of the transfer board is placed under the buttocks and the other end on the surface to which the transfer is being made (e.g., the chair).
- The patient is instructed to lean forward, push up with his or her hands, and then slide across the board to the other surface.

Nurses frequently assist weak and incapacitated patients out of bed. The nurse supports and gently assists the patient during position changes, protecting the patient from injury. The nurse avoids pulling on a weak or paralyzed upper extremity to prevent dislocation of the shoulder. The patient is assisted to move toward the stronger side.

In the home setting, getting in and out of bed and performing chair, toilet, and tub transfers are difficult for patients with weak muscles and loss of hip, knee, and ankle motion. A rope attached to the headboard of the bed enables a patient to move toward the center of the bed, and the use of a rope attached to the footboard facilitates getting in and out of bed. The height of a chair can be raised with cushions on the seat or with hollowed-out blocks placed under the chair legs. Grab bars can be attached to the wall near the toilet and tub to provide leverage and stability.

Preparing for Ambulation. Regaining the ability to walk is a prime morale builder. However, to be prepared for ambulation—whether with a brace, walker, cane, or crutches—the patient must strengthen the muscles required. Therefore, exercise is the foundation of preparation. The nurse and physical therapist instruct and supervise the patient in these exercises.

For ambulation, the quadriceps muscles, which stabilize the knee joint, and the gluteal muscles are strengthened. To perform quadriceps-setting exercises, the patient contracts the quadriceps muscle by attempting to push the popliteal area against the mattress and at the same time raising the heel. The patient maintains the muscle contraction for a count of five and relaxes for a count of five. The exercise is repeated 10 to 15 times hourly. Exercising the quadriceps muscles prevents flexion contractures of the knee. In gluteal setting, the patient contracts or "pinches" the buttocks together for a count of five, relaxes for a count of five; the exercise is repeated 10 to 15 times hourly.

If assistive devices (i.e., walker, cane, crutches) will be used, the muscles of the upper extremities are exercised and strengthened. Push-up exercises are especially useful. While in a sitting position, the patient raises the body by pushing the hands against the chair seat or mattress. The patient should be encouraged to do push-up exercises while in a prone position as well. Pull-up exercises done on a trapeze while lifting the

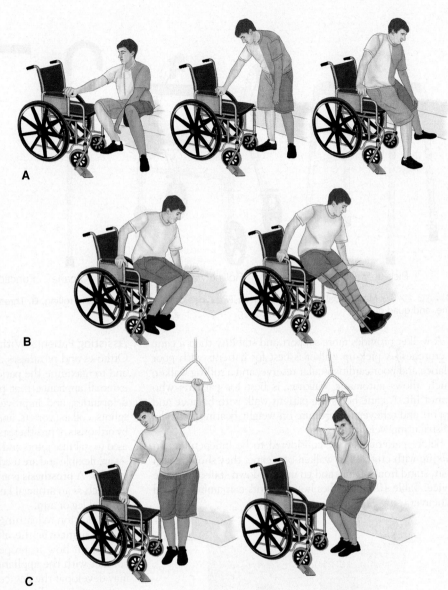

FIGURE 10-2 • Methods of patient transfer from the bed to a wheelchair. The wheelchair is in a locked position. Colored areas indicate non–weight-bearing body parts. **A.** Weight-bearing transfer from bed to chair. The patient stands up, pivots until his back is opposite the new seat, and sits down. **B.** (*Left*) Non–weight-bearing transfer from chair to bed. (*Right*) With legs braced. **C.** (*Left*) Non–weight-bearing transfer, combined method. (*Right*) Non–weight-bearing transfer, pull-up method. One of the wheelchair arms is removed to make getting in and out of the chair easier.

body are also effective for conditioning. The patient is taught to raise the arms above the head and then lower them in a slow, rhythmic manner while holding weights. Gradually, the weight is increased. The hands are strengthened by squeezing a rubber ball.

Typically, the physical therapist designs exercises to help the patient develop sitting and standing balance, stability, and coordination needed for ambulation. After sitting and standing balance is achieved, the patient is able to use parallel bars. Under the supervision of the physical therapist, the patient practices shifting weight from side to side, lifting one leg while supporting weight on the other, and then walking between the parallel bars.

A patient who is ready to begin ambulation must be fitted with the appropriate assistive device, instructed about the prescribed weight-bearing limits (e.g., non–weight-bearing, partial weight-bearing ambulation), and taught how to use the device safely. Figure 10-3 illustrates some of the more common assistive devices used in rehabilitation settings.

The nurse continually assesses the patient for stability and adherence to weight-bearing precautions and protects the patient from falling. The nurse provides contact guarding by holding on to a gait belt that the patient wears around the waist. The patient should wear sturdy, well-fitting shoes and be advised of the dangers of wet or highly polished floors and throw rugs. The patient should also learn how to ambulate on inclines, uneven surfaces, and stairs.

Ambulating With an Assistive Device: Crutches, a Walker, or a Cane

Crutches are for partial weight-bearing or non–weight-bearing ambulation. Good balance, adequate cardiovascular reserve, strong upper extremities, and erect posture are essential for crutch walking. Ambulating a functional distance (at least the length of a room or house) or maneuvering stairs on crutches requires significant arm strength, because the arms must bear the patient's weight (Fig. 10-4). The nurse or physical therapist determines which gait is best (Chart 10-5).

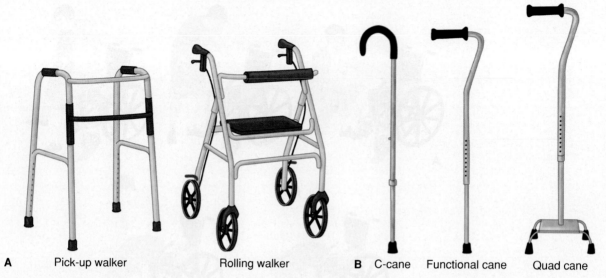

A   Pick-up walker   Rolling walker   B   C-cane   Functional cane   Quad cane

FIGURE 10-3 • Mechanical aids to walking. **A.** Two types of walkers: pick-up and rolling. **B.** Three types of canes: C-cane, functional cane, and quad cane.

A walker provides more support and stability than a cane or crutches. A pick-up walker is best for patients with poor balance and poor cardiovascular reserve, and a rolling walker, which allows automatic walking, is best for patients who cannot lift. A cane helps the patient walk with balance and support and relieves the pressure on weight-bearing joints by redistributing weight.

Before patients can be considered to be independent in walking with crutches, a walker, or a cane, they should learn to sit, stand from sitting, and go up and down stairs using the device. Table 10-2 describes how patients can ambulate and maneuver using each of the three devices.

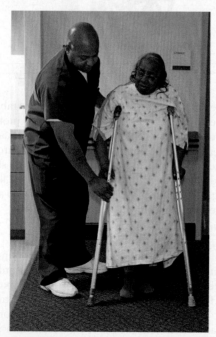

FIGURE 10-4 • For a person walking with crutches, the tripod stance, with crutches out to the sides and in front of the toes, increases stability.

Assisting Patients With an Orthosis or Prosthesis

Orthoses and prostheses are designed to facilitate mobilization and to maximize the patient's quality of life. An **orthosis** is an external appliance that provides support, prevents or corrects deformities, and improves function. Orthoses include braces, splints, collars, corsets, and supports that are designed and fitted by orthotists or prosthetists. Static orthoses (no moving parts) are used to stabilize joints and prevent contractures. Dynamic orthoses are flexible and are used to improve function by assisting weak muscles. A **prosthesis** is an artificial body part that may be internal, such as an artificial knee or hip joint, or external, such as an artificial leg or arm.

In addition to learning how to apply and remove the orthosis and maneuver the affected body part correctly, patients must learn how to properly care for the skin that comes in contact with the appliance. Skin problems or pressure ulcers may develop if the device is applied too tightly or too loosely, or if it is adjusted improperly. The nurse instructs the patient to clean and inspect the skin daily, to make sure the brace fits snugly without being too tight, to check that the padding distributes pressure evenly, and to wear a cotton garment without seams between the orthosis and the skin.

If the patient has had an amputation, the nurse promotes tissue healing, uses compression dressings to promote residual limb shaping, and minimizes contracture formation. A permanent prosthetic limb cannot be fitted until the tissue has healed completely and the residual limb shape is stable and free from edema. The nurse also helps the patient cope with the emotional issues surrounding loss of a limb and encourages acceptance of the prosthesis. The prosthetist, nurse, and primary provider collaborate to provide instructions related to skin care and care of the prosthesis.

Evaluation

Expected patient outcomes may include:
1. Demonstrates improved physical mobility
   a. Maintains muscle strength and joint mobility
   b. Does not develop contractures
   c. Participates in exercise program

(text continues on page 167)

Chart 10-5 Crutch Gaits

Shaded areas are weight bearing. Arrow indicates advance of foot or crutch. (Read chart from bottom, starting with beginning stance.)

4-POINT GAIT	2-POINT GAIT	3-POINT GAIT	SWING-TO	SWING-THROUGH
• Partial weight bearing both feet • Maximal support provided • Requires constant shift of weight	• Partial weight bearing both feet • Provides less support • Faster than a 4-point gait	• Non–weight bearing • Requires good balance • Requires arm strength • Faster gait • Can use with walker	• Weight bearing both feet • Provides stability • Requires arm strength • Can use with walker	• Weight bearing • Requires arm strength • Requires coordination/ balance • Most advanced gait
4. Advance right foot	4. Advance right foot and left crutch	4. Advance right foot	4. Lift both feet/swing forward/land feet next to crutches	4. Lift both feet/swing forward/land feet in front of crutches
3. Advance left crutch	3. Advance left foot and right crutch	3. Advance left foot and both crutches	3. Advance both crutches	3. Advance both crutches
2. Advance left foot	2. Advance right foot and left crutch	2. Advance right foot	2. Lift both feet/swing forward/land feet next to crutches	2. Lift both feet/swing forward/land feet in front of crutches
1. Advance right crutch	1. Advance left foot and right crutch	1. Advance left foot and both crutches	1. Advance both crutches	1. Advance both crutches
Beginning stance	Beginning stance	Beginning stance	Beginning stance	Beginning stance

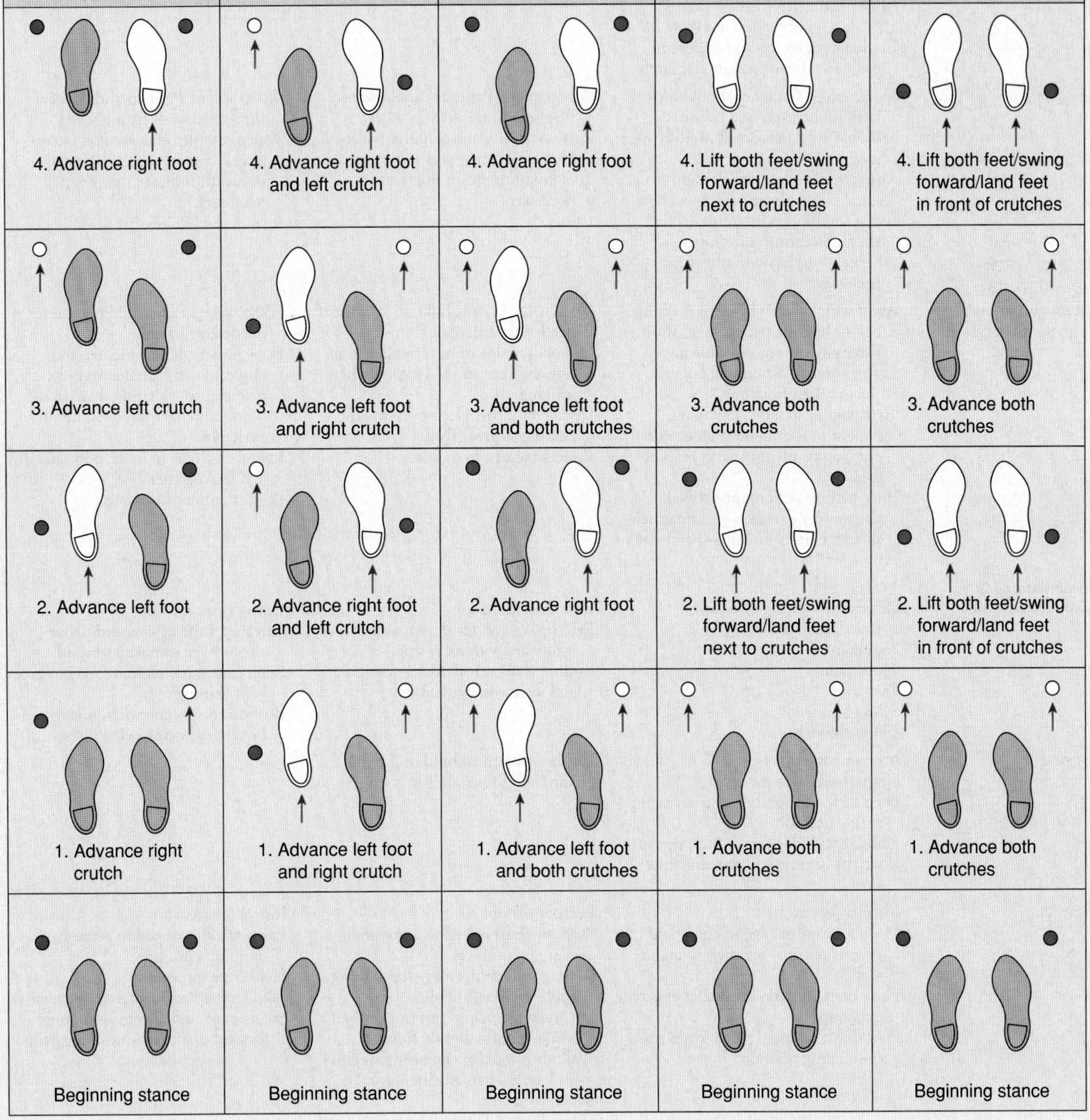

TABLE 10-2	Nursing Actions Involved in Using Assistive Devices		
	Crutches	**Walker**	**Cane**
Patient Preparation			
Adjusting device to fit patient	Measure patient standing or lying down: If standing, set crutch length approximately 5 cm (2 inches) below axilla. If lying down, measure from anterior fold of axilla to sole of the foot and add 5 cm. If using patient's height, subtract 40 cm (16 inches) to obtain crutch height. Adjust hand grip to allow 20 to 30 degrees of flexion at elbow. Use foam rubber pad on underarm piece to relieve pressure of crutch.	Adjust height to individual patient. Patient's arms should be in 20 to 30 degrees of flexion at elbows when hands are resting on hand grips.	With patient flexing elbow at 30-degree angle, hold handle of cane level with greater trochanter and place tip of cane 15 cm (6 inches) lateral to base of 5th toe. Fit cane with gently flaring tip that has flexible, concentric rings to provide stability, absorb shock, and enable greater speed and less fatigue with walking.
Assessment	Assess safety. Crutches should have large rubber tips, and patients should wear firm-soled, well-fitting shoes. Assess balance by asking patient to stand on unaffected leg by a chair. Assess stability and stamina (tolerance). Sweating and shortness of breath indicate that rest is necessary.	Assess safety. Patients should wear firm-soled, well-fitting shoes. Assess stability and stamina (tolerance). Sweating and shortness of breath indicate that rest is necessary.	Assess safety. Patients should wear firm-soled, well-fitting shoes. Assess stability and stamina (tolerance). Sweating and shortness of breath indicate that rest is necessary.
Interventions and patient education	Assist with balance by using a transfer belt or holding patient near waist. Have patient practice shifting weight and maintaining balance. Protect patient from falls. To maximize stability, encourage patient to use tripod stance, with crutches to the front and sides of toes. Have patient perform prescribed preparatory exercises to strengthen shoulder girdle and upper extremity muscles.*	Walk with patient, holding at waist if needed for balance. Instruct patient to never pull self up using walker and to look up when walking. Discuss full, partial, or non–weight bearing as prescribed. Protect patient from falls.	Walk with patient, holding at waist if needed for balance. Have patient hold cane in hand opposite to affected extremity, if possible, to widen the base of support and reduce stress on involved extremity. Instruct patient to move opposite arm and leg together. Protect patient from falls.
Ambulation			
Gait/action used	Determine which gait is best (see Chart 10-5)** Four-point Three-point Two-point Swing-to Swing-through	Instruct patient to: Pick-up walker: lift device and move it forward with each step. Rolling walker: roll device forward and walk automatically.	Instruct patient to: Advance cane at same time that affected leg is moved forward. Keep cane fairly close to body to prevent leaning. Bear down on cane when unaffected extremity begins swing phase.
Sitting	Instruct patient to: Grasp hand piece for control. Bend forward slightly while assuming sitting position. Place affected leg forward to prevent weight bearing and flexion while sitting.	Instruct patient to hold walker on hand grips for stability.	
Standing	Instruct patient to: Move forward to edge of chair, and keep unaffected leg slightly under seat. Place both crutches on side of affected extremity. Push down on hand piece while rising to standing position.	Instruct patient to: Push off chair or bed to come to a standing position. Rolling walker: if walker has a brake, apply it before standing. Lift walker, placing it in front of self while leaning slightly forward. Walk into walker, supporting weight on hands when advancing. Balance on feet. Lift walker and place it in front of self again.	Instruct patient to: Push off chair or bed to come to a standing position. Hold cane for stability. Step forward on unaffected extremity. Swing cane and affected extremity forward in a normal walking gait.

	Crutches	Walker	Cane
Going down stairs	Instruct patient to: Walk forward as far as possible. Advance crutches to lower step; advance affected leg, then unaffected leg.	Continue pattern.	Instruct patient to: Step down on unaffected extremity. Place the cane and then affected extremity on down step.
Going up stairs	Instruct patient to: Advance unaffected leg first up next step. Advance crutches and affected extremity. Unaffected leg goes up first and comes down first.	n/a	Instruct patient to: Step up on unaffected extremity. Place cane and affected extremity up on step.

n/a, not applicable.

*For patients who cannot support their weight through the wrist and hand because of arthritis or fracture, platform crutches that support the forearm and allow the weight to be borne through the elbow are available. If weight is borne on the axilla, the pressure of the crutch can damage the brachial plexus nerves, producing "crutch paralysis".

**Teach patients two gaits so that they can change from one to another to avoid fatigue. In addition, a faster gait can be used when walking an uninterrupted distance, and a slower gait can be used for short distances or in crowded places.

2. Transfers safely
   a. Demonstrates assisted transfers
   b. Performs independent transfers
3. Ambulates with maximum independence
   a. Uses ambulatory aid safely
   b. Adheres to weight-bearing prescription
   c. Requests assistance as needed
4. Demonstrates increased activity tolerance
   a. Does not experience episodes of orthostatic hypotension
   b. Reports absence of fatigue with ambulatory efforts
   c. Gradually increases distance and speed of ambulation

NURSING PROCESS

The Patient With Impaired Skin Integrity

Pressure ulcers are localized areas of necrotic soft tissue that occur when pressure applied to the skin over time is greater than normal capillary closure pressure, which is about 32 mm Hg. Critically ill patients have a lower capillary closure pressure and a greater risk of pressure ulcers. Patients who are prone to pressure ulcers include those confined to bed for long periods, those with motor or sensory dysfunction, and those who experience muscular atrophy and reduction of padding between the overlying skin and the underlying bone (Lyder & Ayello, 2008).

The Healthcare Cost and Utilization Project (HCUP) reported that 503,300 hospitalizations annually in the United States are complicated by pressure ulcers (Russo, Steiner, & Spector, 2008); this represents a nearly 80% increase over a 10-year period. The average length of stay for hospitalizations related to pressure ulcers is 13.4 days, with an average treatment cost of nearly $20,000 for each affected patient. All possible efforts to prevent skin breakdown must be made because the treatment of pressure ulcers is costly in terms of health care dollars and quality of life for patients at risk.

The initial sign of pressure is erythema (redness of the skin) caused by reactive hyperemia, which normally resolves in less than 1 hour. Unrelieved pressure results in tissue ischemia or anoxia. The cutaneous tissues become broken or destroyed, leading to progressive destruction and necrosis of underlying soft tissue, and the resulting pressure ulcer is painful and slow to heal.

Assessment

Nursing assessment involves identifying and evaluating risk for development of pressure ulcers as well as assessment of the skin.

Assessment of Risk Factors

Immobility, impaired sensory perception or cognition, decreased tissue perfusion, decreased nutritional status, friction and shear forces, increased moisture, and age-related skin changes all contribute to the development of pressure ulcers. Chart 10-6 lists risk factors for pressure ulcers. Scales such as the Braden scale (Table 10-3) or Norton scale (Norton, McLaren, & Exon-Smith, 1962) may be used to facilitate systematic assessment and quantification of a patient's risk for pressure ulcer, although the nurse should recognize that the reliability of these scales is not well established for all patient populations.

Specific nursing actions related to assessing risk include:
- Evaluate level of mobility.
- Note safety and assistive devices (e.g., restraints, splints).
- Assess neurovascular status.
- Evaluate circulatory status (e.g., peripheral pulses, edema).

Chart 10-6

RISK FACTORS
Pressure Ulcers

- Prolonged pressure on tissue
- Immobility, compromised mobility
- Loss of protective reflexes, sensory deficit/loss
- Poor skin perfusion, edema
- Malnutrition, hypoproteinemia, anemia, vitamin deficiency
- Friction, shearing forces, trauma
- Incontinence of urine or feces
- Altered skin moisture: excessively dry, excessively moist
- Advanced age, debilitation
- Equipment: casts, traction, restraints

TABLE 10-3 Braden Scale for Predicting Pressure Ulcer Risk

Patient's Name _____ Evaluator's Name _____

					Date of Assessment			
Sensory Perception Ability to respond meaningfully to pressure-related discomfort	**1. Completely Limited** Unresponsive (does not moan, flinch, or grasp) to painful stimuli, due to diminished level of consciousness or sedation OR limited ability to feel pain over most of body.	**2. Very Limited** Responds only to painful stimuli. Cannot communicate discomfort except by moaning or restlessness OR has a sensory impairment that limits the ability to feel pain or discomfort over 1/2 of body.	**3. Slightly Limited** Responds to verbal commands, but cannot always communicate discomfort or the need to be turned. OR has some sensory impairment that limits ability to feel pain or discomfort in 1 or 2 extremities.	**4. No Impairment** Responds to verbal commands. Has no sensory deficit that would limit ability to feel or voice pain or discomfort.				
Moisture Degree to which skin is exposed to moisture	**1. Constantly Moist** Skin is kept moist almost constantly by perspiration, urine, etc. Dampness is detected every time patient is moved or turned.	**2. Very Moist** Skin is often, but not always, moist. Linen must be changed at least once a shift.	**3. Occasionally Moist** Skin is occasionally moist, requiring an extra linen change approximately once a day.	**4. Rarely Moist** Skin is usually dry, linen only requires changing at routine intervals.				
Activity Degree of physical activity	**1. Bedfast** Confined to bed.	**2. Chairfast** Ability to walk severely limited or nonexistent. Cannot bear own weight and/or must be assisted into chair or wheelchair.	**3. Walks Occasionally** Walks occasionally during day, but for very short distances, with or without assistance. Spends majority of each shift in bed or chair.	**4. Walks Frequently** Walks outside room at least twice a day and inside room at least once every two hours during waking hours.				
Mobility Ability to change and control body position	**1. Completely Immobile** Does not make even slight changes in body or extremity position without assistance.	**2. Very Limited** Makes occasional slight changes in body or extremity position but unable to make frequent or significant changes independently.	**3. Slightly Limited** Makes frequent though slight changes in body or extremity position independently.	**4. No Limitation** Makes major and frequent changes in position without assistance.				
Nutrition Usual food intake pattern	**1. Very Poor** Never eats a complete meal. Rarely eats more than a 1/3 of any food offered. Eats 2 servings or less of protein (meat or dairy products) per day. Takes fluids poorly. Does not take a liquid dietary supplement OR is NPO and/or maintained on clear liquids or IVs for more than 5 days.	**2. Probably Inadequate** Rarely eats a complete meal and generally eats only about 1/2 of any food offered. Protein intake includes only 3 servings of meat or dairy products per day. Occasionally will take a dietary supplement OR receives less than optimum amount of liquid diet or tube feeding.	**3. Adequate** Eats half of most meals. Eats a total of 4 servings of protein (meat, dairy products) per day. Occasionally will refuse a meal, but will usually take a supplement when offered OR is on a tube feeding or TPN regimen, which probably meets most of nutritional needs.	**4. Excellent** Eats most of every meal. Never refuses a meal. Usually eats a total of 4 or more servings of meat and dairy products. Occasionally eats between meals. Does not require supplementation.				
Friction and Shear	**1. Problem** Requires moderate to maximum assistance in moving. Complete lifting without sliding against sheets is impossible. Frequently slides down in bed or chair, requiring frequent repositioning with maximum assistance. Spasticity, contractures, or agitation leads to almost constant friction.	**2. Potential Problem** Moves feebly or requires minimum assistance. During a move, skin probably slides to some extent against sheets, chair, restraints, or other devices. Maintains relatively good position in chair or bed most of the time but occasionally slides down.	**3. No Apparent Problem** Moves in bed and in chair independently and has sufficient muscle strength to lift up completely during move. Maintains good position in bed or chair.					
					Total Score			

NPO, nothing by mouth; TPN, total parenteral nutrition.

- Note present health problems.
- Evaluate nutritional and hydration status.
- Review the results of the patient's laboratory studies, including hematocrit, hemoglobin, electrolytes, albumin, transferrin, and creatinine.
- Determine presence of incontinence.
- Review current medications.

▶ Quality and Safety Nursing Alert

Pressure ulcers are associated with increased costs of treatment and length of hospital stay as well as diminished quality of life for patients. It is imperative that nurses perform a skin assessment on every patient admitted to a hospital, inpatient rehabilitation facility, or skilled nursing facility.

Immobility. When a person is immobile and inactive, pressure is exerted on the skin and subcutaneous tissue by objects on which the person rests, such as a mattress, chair seat, or cast. The development of pressure ulcers is directly related to the duration of immobility: If pressure continues long enough, small vessel thrombosis and tissue necrosis occur and a pressure ulcer results. Weight-bearing bony prominences are most susceptible to pressure ulcer development because they are covered only by skin and small amounts of subcutaneous tissue. Susceptible areas include the sacrum and coccygeal areas, ischial tuberosities (especially in people who sit for prolonged periods), greater trochanter, heel, knee, malleolus, medial condyle of the tibia, fibular head, scapula, and elbow (Fig. 10-5).

Impaired Sensory Perception or Cognition. Patients with sensory loss, impaired level of consciousness, or paralysis may not be aware of the discomfort associated with prolonged pressure on the skin and therefore may not change their positions to relieve the pressure. This prolonged pressure impedes blood flow, reducing nourishment of the skin and underlying tissues. A pressure ulcer may develop in a short period of time.

Decreased Tissue Perfusion. Any condition that reduces the circulation and nourishment of the skin and subcutaneous tissue (altered peripheral tissue perfusion) increases the risk of pressure ulcer development. Patients with diabetes have compromised microcirculation. Similarly, patients with edema have impaired circulation and poor nourishment of the skin tissue. Patients who are obese have large amounts of poorly vascularized adipose tissue, which is susceptible to breakdown.

Decreased Nutritional Status. Nutritional deficiencies, anemias, and metabolic disorders also contribute to development of pressure ulcers. Anemia, regardless of its cause, decreases the blood's oxygen-carrying ability and predisposes the patient to pressure ulcers. Poor nutritional status can prolong the inflammatory phase of pressure ulcer healing and can reduce the quality and strength of wound healing (Agency for Healthcare Research and Quality [AHRQ], 2012; Doley, 2010). Serum albumin and prealbumin levels are sensitive indicators of protein deficiency. Serum albumin levels of less than 3 g per dL are associated with hypoalbuminemic tissue edema and increased risk of pressure ulcers. Prealbumin levels are more sensitive indicators of protein status than albumin

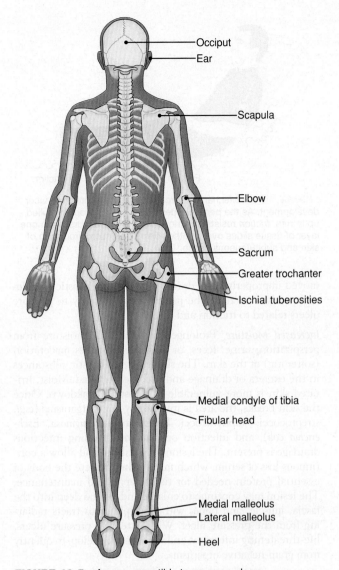

FIGURE 10-5 • Areas susceptible to pressure ulcers.

Occiput
Ear
Scapula
Elbow
Sacrum
Greater trochanter
Ischial tuberosities
Medial condyle of tibia
Fibular head
Medial malleolus
Lateral malleolus
Heel

levels, but they are more costly to assess. The nurse should assess the patient's prealbumin and albumin values and electrolyte panel.

Friction and Shear. Mechanical forces also contribute to the development of pressure ulcers. Friction is the force of rubbing two surfaces against one another and is often caused by pulling a patient over a bed sheet (commonly known as sheet burn) or from a poorly fitted prosthetic device. Shear is the result of gravity pushing down on the patient's body and the resistance between the patient and the chair or bed (European Pressure Ulcer Advisory Panel, 2012). When shear occurs, tissue layers slide over one another, blood vessels stretch and twist, and the microcirculation of the skin and subcutaneous tissue is disrupted. Evidence of deep tissue damage may be slow to develop and may present through the development of a sinus tract, which is an area of destroyed tissue that extends from the edge of a wound. The sacrum and heels are most susceptible to the effects of shear. Pressure ulcers from friction and shear occur when the patient slides down in bed (Fig. 10-6) or when the patient is positioned or

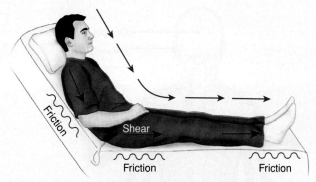

FIGURE 10-6 • Mechanical forces contribute to pressure ulcer development. As the person slides down or is improperly pulled up in bed, *friction* resists this movement. *Shear* occurs when one layer of tissue slides over another, disrupting microcirculation of skin and subcutaneous tissue.

moved improperly (e.g., dragged up in bed). Spastic muscles and paralysis increase the patient's vulnerability to pressure ulcers related to friction and shear.

Increased Moisture. Prolonged contact with moisture from perspiration, urine, feces, or drainage produces maceration (softening) of the skin. The skin reacts to caustic substances in the excreta or drainage and becomes irritated. Moist, irritated skin is more vulnerable to pressure breakdown. Once the skin breaks, the area is invaded by microorganisms (e.g., streptococci, staphylococci, *Pseudomonas aeruginosa, Escherichia coli*), and infection occurs. Foul-smelling infectious drainage is present. The lesion may enlarge and allow a continuous loss of serum, which may further deplete the body of essential protein needed for tissue repair and maintenance. The lesion may continue to enlarge and extend deep into the fascia, muscle, and bone, with multiple sinus tracts radiating from the pressure ulcer. With extensive pressure ulcers, life-threatening infections and sepsis may develop, frequently from gram-negative organisms.

Gerontologic Considerations. In older adults, the normal aging process leads to diminished epidermal thickness, dermal collagen, and tissue elasticity. The skin is drier as a result of diminished sebaceous and sweat gland activity. Cardiovascular changes result in decreased tissue perfusion. Muscles atrophy and bone structures become prominent. Diminished sensory perception and reduced ability to reposition oneself contribute to prolonged pressure on the skin. Therefore, older adults are more susceptible to pressure ulcers, which cause pain, suffering, and reduced quality of life.

Assessment of Skin and Existing Ulcers

In addition to assessing risk, nursing actions to assess skin include:

- Assess total skin condition at least twice a day.
- Inspect each pressure site for erythema.
- Assess areas of erythema for blanching response.
- Palpate the skin for increased warmth.
- Inspect for dry skin, moist skin, and breaks in skin.
- Note drainage and odor.

If a pressure ulcer is seen, the nurse documents its size and location and uses a grading system to describe severity and provides a description of the site (Chart 10-7). The appearance of purulent drainage or foul odor suggests an infection.

With an extensive pressure ulcer, deep pockets of infection are often present. Drying and crusting of exudate may be present. Infection of a pressure ulcer may advance to osteomyelitis, pyarthrosis (pus formation within a joint cavity), sepsis, and septic shock.

Nursing Diagnosis

Based on the assessment data, nursing diagnoses may include the following:

- Risk for impaired skin integrity
- Impaired skin integrity related to immobility, decreased sensory perception, decreased tissue perfusion, decreased nutritional status, friction and shear forces, excessive moisture, or advanced age

Planning and Goals

The major goals may include relief of pressure, improved mobility, improved sensory perception, improved tissue perfusion, improved nutritional status, minimized friction and shear forces, dry surfaces in contact with skin, and healing of pressure ulcer, if present.

Nursing Interventions

Relieving Pressure

Frequent changes of position are needed to relieve and redistribute the pressure on the patient's skin and to promote blood flow to the skin and subcutaneous tissues. This can be accomplished by instructing the patient to change position or by turning and repositioning the patient. The patient's family members should be educated about how to position and turn the patient at home to prevent pressure ulcers. Shifting weight allows the blood to flow into the ischemic areas and helps tissues recover from the effects of pressure.

For patients who spend long periods in a wheelchair, pressure can be relieved by:

- *Push-ups:* The patient pushes down on armrests and raises buttocks off the seat of the chair (Fig. 10-7).
- *One half push-up:* The patient repeats the push-up on the right side and then the left, pushing up on one side by pushing down on the armrest.
- *Moving side to side:* The patient moves from one side to the other while sitting in the chair.
- *Shifting:* The patient bends forward with the head down between the knees (if able) and constantly shifts in the chair.

Positioning the Patient

The degree of ability to move independently—the comfort, fatigue, loss of sensation, overall physical and mental status, and specific disorder—influences plans for changing position. Patients should be positioned laterally, prone, and dorsally in sequence unless a position is not tolerated or is contraindicated. Generally, those who experience discomfort after 30 to 60 minutes of lying prone need to be repositioned. The recumbent position is preferred to the semi-Fowler's position because of increased supporting body surface area in this position.

Patients able to shift their weight every 15 to 20 minutes and move independently may change total position every 2 to 4 hours. Indications for routine repositioning every 2 hours or more frequently include loss of sensation, paralysis, coma, and edema.

Chart 10-7 Stages in the Development of Pressure Ulcers

Suspected Deep Tissue Injury

- There may be a purple or maroon localized area of discolored intact skin or blood-filled blister.
- The area may be preceded in appearance by tissue that is painful, firm, mushy, boggy, and warmer or cooler as compared to adjacent tissue.
- Evolution may include a thin blister over a dark wound bed.
- The wound may further evolve and become covered by thin eschar.
- Evolution may be rapid, exposing additional layers of tissue even with optimal treatment.

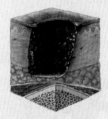

Stage I

- Intact skin
- Nonblanchable redness of a localized area, usually over a bony prominence
- Darkly pigmented skin may not have visible blanching.
- Color may differ from surrounding area.
- Area may be painful, firm, soft, and warmer or cooler as compared to adjacent tissue.

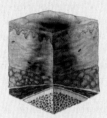

Stage II

- Partial thickness loss of dermis, presenting as a shallow open ulcer with red-pink wound bed without slough
- May present as an intact or open/ruptured serum-filled blister
- May present as a shiny or dry shallow ulcer without slough or bruising; bruising indicates suspected deep tissue injury
- Does not include skin tears, tape burns, perineal dermatitis, maceration, or excoriation

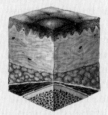

Stage III

- Full-thickness tissue loss
- Subcutaneous fat may be visible; however, bone, tendon, or muscle is not exposed.

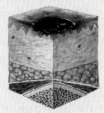

- Slough may be present but does not obscure the depth of tissue loss.
- May include undermining and tunneling
- Depth of a stage III pressure ulcer varies by anatomic location. The bridge of the nose, ear, occiput, and malleolus do not have subcutaneous tissue; stage III ulcers can be shallow in these areas. Areas of significant adiposity can develop extremely deep stage III pressure ulcers.

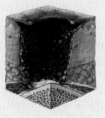

Stage IV

- Ulcer presents with full-thickness tissue loss with exposed bone, tendon, or muscle.
- Slough or eschar may be present on some parts of the wound.
- Often includes undermining and tunneling
- Depth of a stage IV pressure ulcer varies by anatomic location. The bridge of the nose, ear, occiput, and malleolus do not have subcutaneous tissue; stage IV ulcers can be shallow in these areas. Stage IV ulcers can extend into muscle and/or supporting structures (e.g., fascia, tendon, or joint capsule); osteomyelitis is possible. Exposed bone/tendon is visible or directly palable.

Unstageable

- Full-thickness tissue loss in which the base of the ulcer is covered by slough (yellow, tan, gray, green, or brown) and/or eschar (tan, brown, or black) in the wound bed
- Until enough slough and/or eschar is removed to expose the base of the wound, the true depth, and therefore stage, cannot be determined.
- Stable (dry, adherent, intact without erythema or fluctuance) eschar on the heels serves as "the body's natural (biological) cover" and should not be removed.

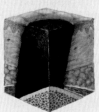

Adapted from Peirce, B., Mackey, D., & McNichol, L. (2009). *Wound Ostomy Continence Nurses Society guidance on OASIS-C integumentary items.* Available at: www.nursingcenter.com/pdf.asp?AID=1239554. Illustrations used with permission of the National Pressure Ulcer Advisory Panel. © NPUAP.

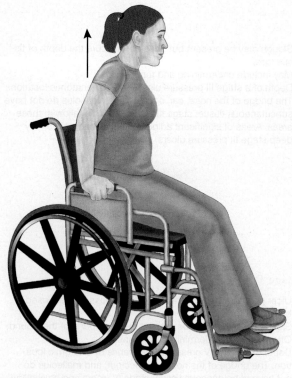

FIGURE 10-7 • Wheelchair push-up to prevent ischial pressure ulcers. These push-ups should become an automatic routine (every 15 minutes) for the person with paraplegia. The person should stay up and out of contact with the seat for several seconds. The wheels are kept in the locked position during the exercise.

In addition to regular turning, small shifts of body weight, such as repositioning of an ankle, elbow, or shoulder, are necessary. The skin is inspected at each position change and assessed for temperature elevation. If redness or heat is noted or if the patient complains of discomfort, pressure on the area must be relieved.

Another way to relieve pressure over bony prominences is the bridging technique, accomplished through the correct positioning of pillows. Just as a bridge is supported on pillars to allow traffic to move underneath, the body can be supported by pillows to allow for space between bony prominences and the mattress. A pillow or commercial heel protector may be used to support the heels off the bed when the patient is supine. Placing pillows superior and inferior to the sacrum relieves sacral pressure. Supporting the patient in a 30-degree side-lying position avoids pressure on the trochanter. In older adult patients, frequent small shifts of body weight may be effective. Placing a small rolled towel or sheepskin under a shoulder or hip allows a return of blood flow to the skin in the area on which the patient is sitting or lying. The towel or sheepskin is moved around the patient's pressure points in a clockwise fashion. A turning schedule can help the family keep track of the patient's turns.

Using Pressure-Relieving Devices

At times, special equipment and beds may be needed to help relieve the pressure on the skin. This is particularly important for patients who cannot get out of bed and who are at high risk for pressure ulcer development. These devices are designed to provide support for specific body areas or to distribute pressure evenly.

A patient who sits in a wheelchair for prolonged periods should have wheelchair cushions fitted and adjusted on an individualized basis, using pressure measurement techniques as a guide to selection and fitting. The aim is to redistribute pressure away from areas at risk for ulcers; however, no cushion can eliminate excessive pressure completely. The patient should be reminded to shift weight frequently and to rise for a few seconds every 15 minutes while sitting in a chair.

Static support devices (e.g., high-density foam, air, or liquid mattress overlays) distribute pressure evenly by bringing more of the patient's body surface into contact with the supporting surface. Gel-type flotation pads and air-fluidized beds reduce pressure. The weight of a body floating on a fluid system is evenly distributed over the entire supporting surface. Therefore, as the body sinks into the fluid, additional surface becomes available for weight bearing, body weight per unit area is decreased, and there is less pressure on the body parts.

Soft, moisture-absorbing padding is also useful because the softness and resilience of padding provide for more even distribution of pressure and the dissipation and absorption of moisture, along with freedom from wrinkles and friction. Bony prominences may be protected by gel pads, sheepskin padding, or soft foam rubber beneath the sacrum, the trochanters, heels, elbows, scapulae, and back of the head when there is pressure on these sites.

Specialized beds are designed to prevent pressure on the skin. Air-fluidized beds allow the patient to float. Dynamic support surfaces, such as low air-loss pockets, alternately inflate and deflate sections to change support pressure for very high risk patients who are critically ill and debilitated and cannot be repositioned to relieve pressure. Oscillating or kinetic beds change pressure by means of rocking movements of the bed that redistribute the patient's weight and stimulate circulation. These beds may be used with patients who have injuries attributed to multiple trauma. Specialized beds, which are more expensive than mattress overlays, are no more effective at preventing pressure ulcers than the overlays; there is insufficient evidence to support the choice of one specific bed surface over another (Stechmiller, Cowan, Whitney, et al., 2008).

Improving Mobility

The patient is encouraged to remain active and is ambulated whenever possible. When sitting, the patient is reminded to change positions frequently to redistribute weight. Active and passive exercises increase muscular, skin, and vascular tone. For patients at risk for pressure ulcers, turning and exercise schedules are essential, and repositioning must occur around the clock.

Improving Sensory Perception

The nurse helps the patient recognize and compensate for altered sensory perception. Depending on the origin of the alteration (e.g., decreased level of consciousness, spinal cord lesion), specific interventions are selected. Strategies to improve cognition and sensory perception may include stimulating the patient to increase awareness of self in the environment, encouraging the patient to participate in self-care, or supporting the patient's efforts toward active compensation for loss of sensation (e.g., a patient with paraplegia lifting up from the sitting position every 15 minutes). A patient with quadriplegia should be weight shifted every 30 minutes while sitting in a wheelchair. When decreased sensory perception exists, the patient and caregivers are taught to inspect potential pressure areas visually every morning and evening, using a mirror if necessary, for evidence of pressure ulcer development.

Improving Tissue Perfusion

Activity, exercise, and repositioning improve tissue perfusion. Massage of erythematous areas is avoided because damage to the capillaries and deep tissue may occur (Fonder, Lazarus, Cowan, et al., 2008).

> ◄ *Quality and Safety Nursing Alert*
>
> The nurse should avoid massaging reddened areas because this may increase the damage to already traumatized skin and tissue.

In patients who have evidence of compromised peripheral circulation (e.g., edema), positioning and elevation of the edematous body part to promote venous return and diminish congestion improve tissue perfusion. In addition, the nurse or family must be alert to environmental factors (e.g., wrinkles in sheets, pressure of tubes) that may contribute to pressure on the skin and diminished circulation and remove the source of pressure.

Improving Nutritional Status

The patient's nutritional status must be adequate and a positive nitrogen balance must be maintained because pressure ulcers develop more quickly and are more resistant to treatment in patients with nutritional disorders. A high-protein diet with protein supplements may be helpful. Iron preparations may be necessary to raise the hemoglobin concentration so that tissue oxygen levels can be maintained within acceptable limits. Ascorbic acid (vitamin C) is necessary for tissue healing. Other nutrients associated with healthy skin include vitamin A, B vitamins, zinc, and sulfur. With adequate nutrition and hydration, the skin can remain healthy, and damaged tissues can be repaired (Table 10-4).

To assess the patient's nutritional status in response to therapeutic strategies, the nurse monitors the patient's hemoglobin, prealbumin level, and body weight weekly. Nutritional assessment is described in further detail in Chapter 5.

Reducing Friction and Shear

Raising the head of the bed by even a few centimeters increases the shearing force over the sacral area; therefore, the semireclining position is avoided in patients at risk. Proper positioning with adequate support is also important when the patient is sitting in a chair.

> ◄ *Quality and Safety Nursing Alert*
>
> To avoid shearing forces when repositioning patients, the nurse must lift and avoid dragging patients across a surface. Lift devices should be used to prevent occupational injuries.

Minimizing Irritating Moisture

Continuous moisture on the skin must be prevented by meticulous hygiene measures. It is important to pay special attention to skin folds, including areas under the breasts, arms, and groin, and between the toes. Perspiration, urine, stool, and drainage must be removed from the skin promptly. The soiled skin should be washed immediately with mild soap and water and blotted dry with a soft towel. The skin may be lubricated with a bland lotion to keep it soft and pliable. Drying agents and powders are avoided. Topical barrier ointments (e.g., petroleum jelly) may be helpful in protecting the skin of patients who are incontinent.

Absorbent pads that wick moisture away from the body should be used to absorb drainage. Patients who are incontinent need to be checked regularly and have their wet incontinence pads and linens changed promptly. Their skin needs to be cleansed and dried promptly.

Promoting Pressure Ulcer Healing

Regardless of the stage of the pressure ulcer, the pressure on the area must be eliminated because the ulcer will not heal until all pressure is removed. The patient must not lie or sit on the pressure ulcer, even for a few minutes. Individualized

TABLE 10-4	Nutritional Requirements to Promote Healing of Pressure Ulcers	
Nutrient	**Rationale**	**Recommended Amount**
Protein	Tissue repair	1.25–1.50 g/kg/d
Calories	Spare protein Restore normal weight	30–35 calories/kg/d
Water	Maintain homeostasis	1 mL/calorie fed or 30 mL/kg/d
Multivitamin	Promote collagen formation	1 daily
Vitamin C	Promote collagen synthesis Support integrity of capillary wall	500–1,000 mg daily
Zinc sulfate	Cofactor for collagen formation and protein synthesis Normal lymphocyte and phagocyte response	220 mg daily
Vitamin A	Stimulate epithelial cells Stimulate immune response *Caution:* An excess can cause an extreme inflammatory response that could impair healing.	

Adapted from Agency for Healthcare Research and Quality. (2009). *AHRQ news and numbers: Pressure ulcers increasing among hospital patients.* Available at: www.ahrq.gov/legacy/research/jan09/0109RA22.htm; Doley, J. (2010). Nutrition management of pressure ulcers. *Nutrition in Clinical Practice, 25*(1), 50–60.

positioning and turning schedules must be written in the plan of nursing care and followed meticulously.

In addition, inadequate nutritional status and fluid and electrolyte abnormalities must be corrected to promote healing. Wounds from which body fluids and protein drain place the patient in a catabolic state and predispose to hypoproteinemia and serious secondary infections. Protein deficiency must be corrected to promote the healing of the pressure ulcer. Carbohydrates are necessary to "spare" the protein and to provide an energy source. Vitamin C and trace elements, especially zinc, are necessary for collagen formation and wound healing. (Refer to Chart 10-7 for descriptions of stages of pressure ulcers.)

Deep Tissue Injury. These tissue injuries may evolve rapidly, and immediate pressure relief to the affected area is indicated. Therefore, the nurse must be vigilant in assessing for these types of injuries (European Pressure Ulcer Advisory Panel & National Pressure Ulcer Advisory Panel, 2009).

Stage I Pressure Ulcers. To permit healing of stage I pressure ulcers, the pressure is removed to allow increased tissue perfusion, nutritional and fluid and electrolyte balance are maintained, friction and shear are reduced, and moisture to the skin is avoided (European Pressure Ulcer Advisory Panel & National Pressure Ulcer Advisory Panel, 2009).

Stage II Pressure Ulcers. In addition to measures listed for stage I pressure ulcers, a moist environment, in which migration of epidermal cells over the ulcer surface occurs more rapidly, should be provided to aid wound healing. The ulcer is gently cleansed with sterile saline solution. The use of a heat lamp to dry the open wound is avoided, as is the use of antiseptic solutions that damage healthy tissues and delay wound healing. Semipermeable occlusive dressings, hydrocolloid wafers, or wet saline dressings are helpful in providing a moist environment for healing and in minimizing the loss of fluids and proteins from the body (European Pressure Ulcer Advisory Panel & National Pressure Ulcer Advisory Panel, 2009).

Stage III Pressure Ulcers. Stage III pressure ulcers are characterized by extensive tissue damage, including **slough** (i.e., soft, moist avascular tissue), tunneling (i.e., formation of a sinus tract), and **undermining** (i.e., extensive tunneling under wound edge), to name a few. Given the extensive damage to tissue and necrosis that characterize stage III pressure ulcers, they must be cleaned (débrided) to create an area that will heal, in addition to the measures listed for stage I pressure ulcers. Necrotic, devitalized tissue favors bacterial growth, delays granulation, and inhibits healing. Wound cleaning and dressing are uncomfortable; therefore, the nurse must prepare the patient for the procedure by explaining what will occur and administering prescribed analgesia (European Pressure Ulcer Advisory Panel & National Pressure Ulcer Advisory Panel, 2009).

Stage IV Pressure Ulcers. Surgical interventions are required for these extensive pressure ulcers (European Pressure Ulcer Advisory Panel & National Pressure Ulcer Advisory Panel, 2009). (See the following Other Treatment Methods section.)

Other Treatment Methods

Débridement may be accomplished by wet-to-damp dressing changes, mechanical flushing of necrotic and infective exudate, application of prescribed enzyme preparations that dissolve necrotic tissue, or surgical dissection. If eschar (dry scab) covers the ulcer, it is removed surgically to ensure the wound is clean and vitalized. Exudate may be absorbed by dressings or special hydrophilic powders, beads, or gels. Cultures of infected pressure ulcers are obtained to guide the selection of antibiotic therapy.

After the pressure ulcer is clean, a topical treatment is prescribed to promote granulation. New granulation tissue must be protected from reinfection, drying, and damage, and care should be taken to prevent pressure and further trauma to the area. Dressings, solutions, and ointments applied to the ulcer should not disrupt the healing process. For chronic, noninfected ulcers that are healing by secondary intention (healing of an open wound from the base upward by laying down new tissue), vacuum-assisted closure (VAC) or hyperbaric oxygen treatment may be used. VAC involves the use of a negative-pressure sponge dressing in the wound to increase blood flow, increasing formation of granulation tissue and nutrient uptake and decreasing bacterial load. Hyperbaric oxygen therapy involves either the application of topical oxygen at increased pressure directly to the wound or placing the patient into a hyperbaric oxygen chamber. Both methods of hyperbaric oxygen therapy promote wound healing by stimulating new vascular growth and aiding in the preservation of damaged tissue (Goldman, 2009).

Multiple agents and protocols are used to treat pressure ulcers; however, consistency is an important key to success. Objective evaluation of the pressure ulcer (e.g., measurement of the size and depth of the pressure ulcer, inspection for granulation tissue) for response to the treatment protocol must be made every 4 to 6 days. Taking photographs at weekly intervals is a reliable strategy for monitoring the healing process, which may take weeks to months.

Surgical intervention is necessary when the ulcer is extensive, when complications (e.g., fistula) exist, and when the ulcer does not respond to treatment. Surgical procedures include débridement, incision and drainage, bone resection, and skin grafting. Osteomyelitis is a common complication of wounds of stage IV depth. (See Chapter 42 for more information on osteomyelitis.)

Preventing Recurrence

It may take more than a year for healing tissue to regain the strength of pre-injury skin; thus, care must be taken to prevent recurrence of pressure ulcers. However, recurrence of pressure ulcers should be anticipated; therefore, active, preventive intervention and frequent continuing assessments are essential. For example, between 36% and 50% of all persons with spinal cord injury who have had a pressure ulcer develop another one within the first year after initial healing (Vaishampayan, Clark, Carlson, et al., 2011). Recurrence rates in general range from 21% to 79%, regardless of treatment (Gelis, Dupeyron, Legros, et al., 2009). The patient's tolerance for sitting or lying on the healed pressure area is increased gradually by increasing the time that pressure is allowed on the area in 5- to 15-minute increments. The patient is instructed to increase mobility and to follow a regimen of turning, weight shifting, and repositioning. The patient education plan includes strategies to reduce the risk of pressure ulcers and methods to detect, inspect, and minimize pressure areas. Early recognition and intervention are keys to long-term management of potential impaired skin integrity. Research findings suggest that individualized education and structured monthly contacts may help to reduce the frequency of pressure ulcers or to delay their recurrence after surgical repair of an ulcer (Rintala, Garber, Friedman, et al., 2008).

Evaluation

Expected patient outcomes may include:

1. Maintains intact skin
   a. Exhibits no areas of nonblanchable erythema at bony prominences
   b. Avoids massage of bony prominences
   c. Exhibits no breaks in skin
2. Limits pressure on bony prominences
   a. Changes position every 1 to 2 hours
   b. Uses bridging techniques to reduce pressure
   c. Uses special equipment as appropriate
   d. Raises self from seat of wheelchair every 15 minutes
3. Increases mobility
   a. Performs range-of-motion exercises
   b. Adheres to turning schedule
   c. Advances sitting time as tolerated
4. Has improved sensory and cognitive ability
   a. Demonstrates improved level of consciousness
   b. Remembers to inspect potential pressure ulcer areas every morning and evening
5. Demonstrates improved tissue perfusion
   a. Exercises to increase circulation
   b. Elevates body parts susceptible to edema
6. Attains and maintains adequate nutritional status
   a. Verbalizes the importance of protein and vitamin C in diet
   b. Eats diet high in protein and vitamin C
   c. Exhibits acceptable levels of hemoglobin, electrolyte, prealbumin, transferrin, and creatinine
7. Avoids friction and shear
   a. Avoids semireclining position
   b. Uses heel protectors when appropriate
   c. Lifts body instead of sliding across surfaces
8. Maintains clean, dry skin
   a. Avoids prolonged contact with wet or soiled surfaces
   b. Keeps skin clean and dry
   c. Uses lotion to keep skin lubricated

NURSING PROCESS

The Patient With Altered Elimination Patterns

Urinary incontinence and bowel incontinence or constipation and impaction are problems that often occur in patients with disabilities. Incontinence curtails the person's independence, causing embarrassment and isolation. Incontinence occurs in as much as 15% of the community-based older adult population, and nearly 50% of nursing home residents have bowel or bladder incontinence or both (Abrams, Cardozo, Khoury, et al., 2011). For patients with disabilities who experience constipation, complete and predictable evacuation of the bowel is the goal. If a bowel routine is not established, the patient may experience abdominal distention; small, frequent oozing of stool; or impaction.

Assessment

Urinary incontinence may result from multiple causes, including urinary tract infection, detrusor instability, bladder outlet obstruction or incompetence, neurologic impairment, bladder spasm or contracture, and inability to reach the toilet in time. Urinary incontinence can be classified as urge, reflex, stress, functional, or total:

- *Urge incontinence* occurs when involuntary elimination of urine is associated with a strong perceived need to void.
- *Reflex (neurogenic) incontinence* is associated with a spinal cord lesion that interrupts cerebral control, resulting in no sensory awareness of the need to void.
- *Stress incontinence* is associated with weakened perineal muscles that permit leakage of urine when intra-abdominal pressure is increased (e.g., with coughing or sneezing).
- *Functional incontinence* occurs in patients with intact urinary physiology who experience mobility impairment, environmental barriers, or cognitive problems and cannot reach and use the toilet before soiling themselves.
- *Total incontinence* occurs in patients who cannot control excreta because of physiologic or psychological impairment. Management of the excreta is an essential focus of nursing care.

The health history is used to explore bladder and bowel function, symptoms associated with dysfunction, physiologic risk factors for elimination problems, perception of micturition (urination, or voiding) and defecation cues, and functional toileting abilities. Previous and current fluid intake and voiding patterns may be helpful in designing the plan of nursing care. A record of times of voiding and amounts voided is kept for at least 48 hours. In addition, episodes of incontinence and associated activity (e.g., coughing, sneezing, lifting), fluid intake time and amount, and medications are recorded. This record is analyzed and used to determine patterns and relationships of incontinence to other activities and factors.

The ability to get to the bathroom, manipulate clothing, and use the toilet are important functional factors that may be related to incontinence. Related cognitive functioning (perception of need to void, verbalization of need to void, and ability to learn to control urination) must also be assessed. In addition, the nurse reviews the results of the diagnostic studies (e.g., urinalysis, urodynamic tests, postvoiding residual volumes).

Bowel incontinence and constipation may result from multiple causes, such as diminished or absent sphincter control, cognitive or perceptual impairment, neurogenic factors, diet, and immobility. The origin of the bowel problem must be determined. The nurse assesses the patient's normal bowel patterns, nutritional patterns, use of laxatives, gastrointestinal problems (e.g., colitis), bowel sounds, anal reflex and tone, and functional abilities. The character and frequency of bowel movements are recorded and analyzed.

Nursing Diagnosis

Based on the assessment data, major nursing diagnoses may include the following:

- Functional urinary incontinence

- Urge urinary incontinence
- Reflex urinary incontinence
- Stress urinary incontinence
- Impaired urinary elimination
- Urinary retention
- Constipation
- Bowel incontinence

Planning and Goals

The major goals may include control of urinary incontinence or urinary retention, control of bowel incontinence, and regular elimination patterns.

Nursing Interventions

Promoting Urinary Continence

After the nature of the urinary incontinence has been identified, a plan of nursing care is developed based on analysis of the assessment data. Various approaches to promote urinary continence have been developed (Registered Nurses' Association of Ontario [RNAO], 2011; Wagg, Duckett, McClurg, et al., 2011). Most approaches attempt to condition the body to control urination or to minimize the occurrence of unscheduled urination. Selection of the approach depends on the cause and type of the incontinence. For the program to be successful, participation by the patient and a desire to avoid incontinence episodes are crucial; an optimistic attitude with positive feedback for even slight gains is essential for success. Accurate recording of intake and output and of the patient's response to selected strategies is essential for evaluation.

At no time should the fluid intake be restricted to decrease the frequency of urination. Sufficient fluid intake (2,000 to 3,000 mL per day, according to patient needs) must be ensured. To optimize the likelihood of voiding as scheduled, measured amounts of fluids may be administered about 30 minutes before voiding attempts. In addition, most of the fluids should be consumed before evening to minimize the need to void frequently during the night.

> ◤ *Quality and Safety Nursing Alert*
>
> Carbonated soft drinks, milk shakes, alcohol, tomato juice, and citrus fruit juices are alkaline-producing drinks that promote bacterial growth in the urine. Patients should be encouraged to drink more acid-producing fluids (e.g., cranberry and cranapple juice) to reduce the chance of urinary tract infection. Water is a preferred fluid because it flushes the kidneys and bladder.

The goal of bladder training is to restore the bladder to normal function. Bladder training can be used with cognitively intact patients experiencing urge incontinence. A voiding and toileting schedule is developed based on analysis of the assessment data. The schedule specifies times for the patient to try to empty the bladder using a bedpan, toilet, or commode. Privacy should be provided during voiding efforts. The interval between voiding times in the early phase of the bladder training period is short (90 to 120 minutes). The patient is encouraged not to void until the specified voiding time. Voiding success and episodes of incontinence are recorded. As the patient's bladder capacity and control increase, the interval is lengthened.

Usually, there is a temporal relationship between drinking, eating, exercising, and voiding. Alert patients can participate in recording intake, activity, and voiding and can plan the schedule to achieve maximum continence. Barrier-free access to the toilet and modification of clothing can help patients with functional incontinence achieve self-care in toileting and continence.

Habit training is used to try to keep patients dry by strict adherence to a toileting schedule and may be successful with stress, urge, or functional incontinence. If the patient is confused, caregivers take the patient to the toilet according to the schedule before involuntary voiding occurs. Simple cuing and consistency promote success. Periods of continence and successful voiding are positively reinforced.

Biofeedback is a system through which patients learn to consciously contract urinary sphincters and control voiding cues. Cognitively intact patients who have stress or urge incontinence may gain bladder control through biofeedback.

Pelvic floor exercises (Kegel exercises) strengthen the pubococcygeus muscle. The patient is instructed to tighten the pelvic floor muscles for 4 seconds 10 times, and this is repeated 4 to 6 times a day. Stopping and starting the stream during urination is recommended to increase control. Daily practice is essential. These exercises are helpful for cognitively intact women who experience stress incontinence.

Suprapubic tapping or stroking of the inner thigh may produce voiding by stimulating the voiding reflex arc in patients with reflex incontinence. However, this method is not always effective, owing to a lack of detrusor sphincter muscle coordination. As the bladder reflexively contracts to expel urine, the bladder sphincter reflexively closes, producing a high residual urine volume and an increased incidence of urinary tract infection.

Intermittent self-catheterization is an appropriate alternative for managing reflex incontinence, urinary retention, and overflow incontinence attributed to an overdistended bladder. The nurse emphasizes regular emptying of the bladder rather than sterility. Patients with disabilities may reuse and clean catheters with bleach or hydrogen peroxide solutions or soap and water and may use a microwave oven to sterilize catheters. Aseptic intermittent catheterization technique is required in health care institutions because of the potential for bladder infection from resistant organisms. Intermittent self-catheterization may be difficult for patients with limited mobility, dexterity, or vision; however, family members can be taught the procedure.

Self-catheterization is also particularly pertinent for patients with spinal cord injury, because most of these patients do not have voluntary control of urination. Even those patients with spinal cord injuries who can voluntarily void should measure their residual urine (the amount of urine that remains in the bladder after voluntary or involuntary voiding) by self-catheterization.

Indwelling catheters are avoided if at all possible because of the high incidence of urinary tract infections associated with their use. Short-term use may be needed during treatment of severe skin breakdown due to continued incontinence. Patients with disabilities who cannot perform intermittent self-catheterization may elect to use suprapubic catheters for long-term bladder management. Suprapubic catheters are easier to maintain than indwelling catheters.

External catheters (condom catheters) and leg bags to collect spontaneous voidings are useful for male patients with reflex or total incontinence. The appropriate design and size must be chosen for maximal success, and the patient or caregiver must be taught how to apply the condom catheter and how to provide daily hygiene, including skin inspection. Instruction on emptying the leg bag must also be provided, and modifications can be made for patients with limited hand dexterity.

Incontinence pads (briefs) may be useful at times for patients with stress or total incontinence to protect clothing but should be avoided whenever possible. Incontinence pads only manage, rather than solve, the incontinence problem. In addition, they have a negative psychological effect on patients, because many people think of the pads as diapers. Every effort should be made to reduce the incidence of incontinence episodes through the other methods that have been described. When incontinence pads are used, they should wick moisture away from the body to minimize contact of moisture and excreta with the skin. Wet incontinence pads must be changed promptly, the skin cleansed, and a moisture barrier applied to protect the skin. It is important for the patient's self-esteem to avoid use of the term *diapers*.

Promoting Bowel Continence

The goals of a bowel training program are to develop regular bowel habits and to prevent uninhibited bowel elimination. Regular, complete emptying of the lower bowel results in bowel continence. A bowel training program takes advantage of the patient's natural reflexes. Regularity, timing, nutrition and fluids, exercise, and correct positioning promote predictable defecation (National Institute for Health and Clinical Excellence, 2010).

The nurse records defecation time, character of stool, nutritional intake, cognitive abilities, and functional self-care toileting abilities for 5 to 7 days. Analysis of this record is helpful when designing a bowel program for patients with fecal incontinence.

Consistency in implementing the plan is essential. A regular time for defecation is established, and attempts at evacuation should be made within 15 minutes of the designated time daily. Natural gastrocolic and duodenocolic reflexes occur about 30 minutes after a meal; therefore, after breakfast is one of the best times to plan for bowel evacuation. However, if the patient had a previously established habit pattern at a different time of day, it should be followed.

The anorectal reflex may be stimulated by a rectal suppository (e.g., glycerin) or by mechanical stimulation (e.g., digital stimulation with a lubricated gloved finger or anal dilator). Mechanical stimulation should be used only in patients with a disability who have no voluntary motor function and no sensation as a result of injuries above the sacral segments of the spinal cord, such as patients with quadriplegia, high paraplegia, or severe brain injuries. The technique is not effective in patients who do not have an intact sacral reflex arc (e.g., those with flaccid paralysis). Mechanical stimulation, suppository insertion, or both should be initiated about 30 minutes before the scheduled bowel elimination time, and the interval between stimulation and defecation is noted for subsequent modification of the bowel program. Once the bowel routine is well established, stimulation with a suppository may not be necessary.

The patient should assume the normal squatting position and be in a private bathroom for defecation if at all possible, although a padded commode chair or bedside toilet is an alternative. An elevated toilet seat is a simple modification that may make use of the toilet easier for the patient with a disability. Seating time is limited in patients who are at risk for skin breakdown. Bedpans should be avoided. A patient with a disability who cannot sit on a toilet should be positioned on the left side with legs flexed and the head of the bed elevated 30 to 45 degrees to increase intra-abdominal pressure. Protective padding is placed behind the buttocks. When possible, the patient is instructed to bear down and to contract the abdominal muscles. Massaging the abdomen from right to left facilitates movement of feces in the lower tract.

Preventing Constipation

The record of bowel elimination, character of stool, food and fluid intake, level of activity, bowel sounds, medications, and other assessment data are reviewed to develop the plan of care. Multiple approaches may be used to prevent constipation. The diet should include adequate intake of high-fiber foods (vegetables, fruits, bran) to prevent hard stools and to stimulate peristalsis. Daily fluid intake should be 2 to 3 L unless contraindicated. Drinking prune juice (120 mL) 30 minutes before a meal once daily is helpful in some cases when constipation is a problem. Physical activity and exercise are encouraged, as is self-care in toileting. Patients are encouraged to respond to the natural urge to defecate. Privacy during toileting is provided. Stool softeners, bulk-forming agents, mild stimulants, and suppositories may be prescribed to stimulate defecation and to prevent constipation.

Evaluation

Expected patient outcomes may include:
1. Demonstrates control of bowel and bladder function
   a. Experiences no episodes of incontinence
   b. Avoids constipation
   c. Achieves independence in toileting
   d. Expresses satisfaction with level of bowel and bladder control
2. Achieves urinary continence
   a. Uses therapeutic approach that is appropriate to type of incontinence
   b. Maintains adequate fluid intake
   c. Washes and dries skin after episodes of incontinence
3. Achieves bowel continence
   a. Participates in bowel program
   b. Verbalizes need for regular time for bowel evacuation
   c. Modifies diet to promote continence
   d. Uses bowel stimulants as prescribed and needed
4. Experiences relief of constipation
   a. Uses high-fiber diet, fluids, and exercise to promote defecation
   b. Responds to urge to defecate

Promoting Home and Community-Based Care

An important goal of rehabilitation is to assist the patient to return to the home environment after learning to manage the disability. A referral system maintains continuity of care when the patient is transferred to the home or to a long-term care facility. The plan for discharge is formulated when the patient is first admitted to the hospital, and discharge plans are made with the patient's functional potential in mind.

Educating Patients About Self-Care

Significant expenditures of time and resources are necessary to ensure that patients gain the skills and confidence to self-manage their health effectively after discharge from the hospital. Formal programs provide patients with effective strategies for interpreting and managing disease-specific issues and skills needed for problem solving, as well as building and maintaining self-awareness and self-efficacy. Self-care programs often use multifaceted approaches, including didactic teaching, group sessions, individual learning plans, and Web-based resources. When planning the approach to self-care, the nurse must consider the individual patient's knowledge, experience, social and cultural background, level of formal education, and psychological status. The preparation for self-care must also be spread out over the course of the recovery period, and it must be monitored and updated regularly as the patient masters aspects of self-care. Preparation for self-care is also highly relevant for informal caregivers of patients in rehabilitation.

Chart 10-8

HOME CARE CHECKLIST
Managing the Therapeutic Regimen at Home

At the completion of home care education, the patient or caregiver will be able to:	PATIENT	CAREGIVER
• State the impact of disability on physiologic functioning.	✔	✔
• State changes in lifestyle necessary to maintain health.	✔	✔
• State the name, dose, side effects, frequency, and schedule for all medications.	✔	✔
• State how to obtain medical supplies after discharge.	✔	✔
• Identify durable medical equipment needs, proper usage, and maintenance necessary for safe utilization: [ ] Wheelchair—manual/power [ ] Bedside toilet [ ] Cushion [ ] Crutches [ ] Grab bars [ ] Walker [ ] Sliding board [ ] Prosthesis [ ] Mechanical lift [ ] Orthosis [ ] Raised padded commode seat [ ] Specialty bed [ ] Padded commode wheelchair	✔	✔
• Demonstrate usage of adaptive equipment for activities of daily living: [ ] Long-handled sponge [ ] Rocker-knife, spork, weighted utensils [ ] Reacher [ ] Special closures for clothing [ ] Universal cuff [ ] Other [ ] Plate mat and guard	✔	✔
• Demonstrate mobility skills: [ ] Transfers: bed to chair; in and out of toilet and tub; in and out of car [ ] Negotiate ramps, curbs, stairs [ ] Assume sitting from supine position [ ] Turn side to side in bed [ ] Maneuver wheelchair; manage armrests and leg rests; lock brakes [ ] Ambulate safely using assistive devices [ ] Perform range-of-motion exercises [ ] Perform muscle-strengthening exercises	✔	✔
• Demonstrate skin care: [ ] Inspect bony prominences every morning and evening [ ] Identify stage I pressure ulcer and actions to take if present [ ] Change dressings for stage II to IV pressure ulcers [ ] State dietary requirements to promote healing of pressure ulcers [ ] Demonstrate pressure relief at prescribed intervals [ ] State sitting schedule and demonstrate weight lifts in wheelchair [ ] Demonstrate adherence to bed turning schedule, bed positioning, and the use of bridging techniques [ ] Apply and wear protective boots at prescribed times [ ] Demonstrate correct wheelchair sitting posture [ ] Demonstrate techniques to avoid friction and shear in bed [ ] Demonstrate proper hygiene to maintain skin integrity	✔	✔

Chart 10-8

HOME CARE CHECKLIST

Managing the Therapeutic Regimen at Home (continued)

At the completion of home care education, the patient or caregiver will be able to:	PATIENT	CAREGIVER
• Demonstrate bladder care: [ ] State schedule for voiding, toileting, and catheterization [ ] Identify relationship of fluid intake to voiding and catheterization schedule [ ] State how to perform pelvic floor exercises [ ] Demonstrate clean self-intermittent catheterization and care of catheterization equipment [ ] Demonstrate indwelling catheter care [ ] Demonstrate application of external condom catheter [ ] Demonstrate application, emptying, and cleaning of urinary drainage bag [ ] Demonstrate application of incontinence pads and performance of perineal hygiene [ ] State signs and symptoms of urinary tract infection	✔	✔

• Demonstrate bowel care:
[ ] State optimum dietary intake to promote evacuation
[ ] Identify schedule for optimum bowel evacuation
[ ] Demonstrate techniques to increase intra-abdominal pressure; Valsalva maneuver;
  abdominal massage; leaning forward
[ ] Demonstrate techniques to stimulate bowel movements: ingesting warm liquids; digital stimulation;
insertion of suppositories
[ ] Demonstrate optimum position for bowel evacuation: on toilet with knees higher than hips;
  left side in bed with knees flexed and head of bed elevated 30 to 45 degrees
[ ] Identify complications and corrective strategies for bowel retraining: constipation, impaction, diarrhea,
  hemorrhoids, rectal bleeding, anal tears
	✔	✔

• Identify community resources for peer and family support: [ ] Identify phone numbers of support groups for people with disabilities [ ] State meeting locations and times	✔	✔
• Demonstrate how to access transportation: [ ] Identify locations of wheelchair accessibility for public buses or trains [ ] Identify phone numbers for private wheelchair van [ ] Contact Division of Motor Vehicles for handicapped parking permit [ ] Contact Division of Motor Vehicles for driving test when appropriate [ ] Identify resources for adapting private vehicle with hand controls or wheelchair lift	✔	✔
• Identify vocational rehabilitation resources: [ ] State name and phone number of vocational rehabilitation counselor [ ] Identify educational opportunities that may lead to future employment	✔	✔
• Identify community resources for recreation: [ ] State local recreation centers that offer programs for people with disabilities [ ] Identify leisure activities that can be pursued in the community	✔	✔
• Identify the need for health promotion and screening activities	✔	✔

When a patient is discharged from acute care or a rehabilitation facility, informal caregivers, typically family members, often assume the care and support of the patient. Although the most obvious care tasks involve physical care (e.g., personal hygiene, dressing, meal preparation), other elements of the caregiving role include psychosocial support and a commitment to this supportive role. Thus, the nurse must assess the patient's support system (family, friends) well in advance of discharge. The positive attitudes of family and friends toward the patient, his or her disability, and the return home are important in making a successful transition to home. Not all families can carry out the arduous programs of exercise, physical therapy, and personal care that the patient may need. They may not have the resources or stability to care for family members with a severe disability. The physical, emotional, economic, and energy strains of a disabling condition may overwhelm even a stable family. Members of the reha-

bilitation team must not judge the family but rather should provide supportive interventions that help the family to attain its highest level of function.

The family members need to know as much as possible about the patient's condition and care so that they do not fear the patient's return home. The nurse develops methods to help the patient and family cope with problems that may arise. For example, the nurse may develop an ADL checklist individualized for the patient and family to ensure that the family is proficient in assisting the patient with certain tasks (Chart 10-8).

Continuing Care

A home care nurse may visit the patient in the hospital, interview the patient and the family, and review the ADL sheet to learn which activities the patient can perform. This helps to ensure that continuity of care is provided and that the patient does not regress yet maintains the independence gained while in the hospital or rehabilitation setting. The family may need to purchase, borrow, or improvise needed equipment, such as safety rails, a raised toilet seat or commode, or a tub bench. Ramps may need to be built or doorways widened to allow full access.

Family members are taught how to use equipment and are given a copy of the equipment manufacturer's instruction booklet, the names of resource people, lists of equipment-related supplies, and locations where they may be obtained. A written summary of the care plan is included in family education. The patient and family members are reminded about the importance of routine health screening and other health promotion strategies.

A network of support services and communication systems may be required to enhance opportunities for independent living. The nurse uses collaborative, administrative skills to coordinate these activities and pull together the network of care. The nurse also provides skilled care, initiates additional referrals when indicated, and serves as a patient advocate and counselor when obstacles are encountered. The nurse continues to reinforce prior patient education and helps the patient to set and achieve attainable goals. The degree to which the patient adapts to the home and community environment depends on the confidence and self-esteem developed during the rehabilitation process and on the acceptance, support, and reactions of family members, employers, and community members.

There is a growing trend toward independent living by people with severe disabilities, either alone or in groups that share resources. Preparation for independent living should include training in managing a household and working with personal care attendants as well as training in mobility. The goal is integration into the community—living and working in the community with accessible housing, employment, public buildings, transportation, and recreation.

State rehabilitation administration agencies provide services to assist people with disabilities in obtaining the help they need to engage in gainful employment. These services include diagnostic, medical, and mental health services. Counseling, training, placement, and follow-up services are available to help people with disabilities select and obtain jobs.

If the patient is transferred to a long-term care facility, the transition is planned to promote continued progress. Independence gained continues to be supported, and progress is fostered. Adjustment to the facility is promoted through communication. Family members are encouraged to visit, to be involved, and to take the patient home on weekends and holidays if possible.

Critical Thinking Exercises

1 [PQ] A 24-year-old woman was involved in a motor vehicle crash resulting in multiple traumatic injuries, including a complete transection of her spinal cord at T12. She had surgery to stabilize her spine. As a result of her spinal cord injury, she is incontinent and has lost all sensation and motor function in her legs. She is now admitted to the long-term acute care hospital unit. She expresses disappointment that she has not regained any function after her surgery, that she cannot walk anymore, and that she has to depend on a catheter to void her urine. She expresses embarrassment that sometimes she has stool and urine leakage. What challenges now confront the rehabilitation nursing staff in helping this patient establish goals and maintain motivation? What are your priority nursing diagnoses for this patient as you plan your care for her?

2 [ebp] Recently, several community-dwelling older adult patients fell in their homes, resulting in hospital admission, surgery, and subsequent rehabilitation on your unit. Although frail, these patients had all been independent in their IADLs prior to these falls. Getting some of these patients discharged back to their homes was a slow process, and others were eventually placed in long-term care facilities. As a nurse on the rehabilitation unit, you wonder if there is a benefit in initiating a program to prevent older community-dwelling patients from falls at home. Identify a specific question related to these patients in order to conduct a relevant and focused literature search. What key words would you use in this search, and what sources would be appropriate to search?

3 You are caring for a 65-year-old patient post stroke (cerebrovascular accident) who is experiencing difficulty adjusting to her physical deficits, thus limiting her participation in rehabilitation sessions. You wish to create the necessary "space" for this patient so that she may practice the tasks and activities requisite to successful rehabilitation, without her becoming unduly frustrated. How do you ensure that you incorporate this patient's central concerns, including her preferences and values, into clinical decisions around the rehabilitation services offered to her? Describe how you would provide emotional support to this woman for the losses that now confront her and her family.

Brunner Suite Resources
Explore these additional resources to enhance learning for this chapter:
• NCLEX-Style Questions and Other Resources on thePoint, http://thePoint.lww.com/Brunner13e
• Study Guide
• PrepU
• Clinical Handbook
• Handbook of Laboratory and Diagnostic Tests

References

*Asterisk indicates nursing research.
**Double asterisk indicates classic reference.

Books

Abrams, P., Cardozo, L., Khoury, A., et al. (2011). *Incontinence*. Paris, France: Health Publication Ltd.

European Pressure Ulcer Advisory Panel and National Pressure Ulcer Advisory Panel. (2009). *Treatment of pressure ulcers: Quick reference guide*. Washington DC: National Pressure Ulcer Advisory Panel.

Hoeman, S. (2008). *Rehabilitation nursing: Prevention, intervention, and outcomes* (4th ed.). St. Louis: Mosby.

Lyder, C. H., & Ayello, E. A. (2008). Pressure ulcers: A patient safety issue. In R. G. Hughes (Ed.): *Patient safety and quality: An evidence-based handbook for nurses*. AHRQ Publication No. 08-0043; Rockville, MD: Agency for Healthcare Research and Quality.

**Norton, D., McLaren, R., & Exton-Smith, A. N. (1962). *An investigation of geriatric nursing problems in hospital*. London: National Corporation for the Care of Old People.

Journals and Electronic Documents

Ackerman, P., Asindua, S., Blouin, M., et al. (2011). Rehabilitation: World Health Organization report on disability. Available at: www.who.int/disabilities/world_report/2011/report.pdf

Agency for Healthcare Research and Quality. (2009). *AHRQ news and numbers: Pressure ulcers increasing among hospital patients*. Available at: www.ahrq.gov/legacy/research/jan09/0109RA22.htm

Centers for Medicare and Medicaid Services, DMEPOS Accreditation Program. (2011). *Standards manual with survey preparation questions* (3rd ed.). Available at: www.carf.org/Accreditation/QualityStandards/OnlineStandards/

Doley, J. (2010). Nutrition management of pressure ulcers. *Nutrition in Clinical Practice, 25*(1), 50–60.

European Pressure Ulcer Advisory Panel. (2012). *Pressure ulcer prevention guidelines*. Available at: www.guideline.gov/content.aspx?id=12262

Fonder, M. A., Lazarus, G. S., Cowan, D. A., et al. (2008). Treating the chronic wound: A practical approach to the care of nonhealing wounds and wound care dressings. *Journal of the American Academy of Dermatology, 58*(2), 185–206.

Gelis, A., Dupeyron, A., Legros, P., et al. (2009). Pressure ulcer risk factors in persons with spinal cord injury, part 2: The chronic stage. *Spinal Cord, 47*(9), 651–661.

Goldman, R. J. (2009). Hyperbaric oxygen therapy for wound healing and limb salvage: A systematic review. *Physical Medicine and Rehabilitation, 1*(5), 471–489.

**Granger, C., Albrecht, G., & Hamilton, B. (1979). Outcomes of comprehensive medical rehabilitation: Measurement by PULSES profile and the Barthel Index. *Archives of Physical and Medical Rehabilitation, 60*(4), 145–154.

**Harvey, R. F., Hollis, M., & Jellinek, M. (1981). Functional performance assessment: A program approach. *Archives of Physical Medicine and Rehabilitation, 62*(9), 456–461.

**Keith, R. A., Granger, C. V., Hamilton, B. B, et al. (1987). The functional independence measure: A new tool for rehabilitation. *Advances in Clinical Rehabilitation, 1*, 6–18.

**Mahoney, F., & Barthel, D. (1965). Functional evaluation: The Barthel Index. *Maryland State Medical Journal, 14*, 61–65.

National Institute for Health and Clinical Excellence. (2010). *Faecal incontinence: The management of faecal incontinence in adults (bowel control guidelines)*. Available at: publications/nice/org/uk/faecal-incontinence-cg49

National Rehabilitation Information Center. (2011). Information sources on spinal cord injury (SCI). Available at: www.naric.com/?q=node/72

*Pryor, J., & O'Connell, B. (2009). Incongruence between nurses' and patients' understandings and expectations of rehabilitation. *Journal of Clinical Nursing, 18*(2), 1766–1774.

Registered Nurses' Association of Ontario. (2011). *Nursing best practice guideline: Shaping the future of nursing. Promoting continence using prompted voiding*. Available at: rnao.ca/bpg/guidelines/promoting-continence-using-prompted-voiding

Rintala, D. H., Garber, S. L., Friedman, J. D., et al. (2008). Preventing recurrent pressure ulcers in veterans with spinal cord injury: Impact of a structured education and follow-up intervention. *Archives of Physical and Medical Rehabilitation, 89*(8), 1429–1441.

Russo, C., Steiner, C., & Spector, W. (2008). *Hospitalizations related to pressure ulcers among adults 18 years and older, 2006*. HCUP Statistical Brief No. 64. Healthcare Cost and Utilization Project, Rockville, MD. Available at: www.hcup-us.ahrq.gov/reports/statbriefs/sb64.pdf

*Stechmiller, J., Cowan, L., Whitney, J., et al. (2008). Guidelines for the prevention of pressure ulcers. *Wound Repair and Regeneration, 16*(2), 151–168.

U.S. Department of Health and Human Services. (2010). *Office on Disability, Substance Abuse, and Disability fact sheet: A companion to chapter 26 of Healthy People 2010*. Available at: www.hhs.gov/od/about/fact_sheets/substanceabuse.html

Vaishampayan, A., Clark, F., Carlson, B., et al. (2011). Preventing pressure ulcers in people with spinal cord injury: Targeting risky life circumstances through community-based interventions. *Advances in Skin and Wound Care, 24*(6), 275–284.

Wagg, A., Duckett, J., McClurg, D., et al. (2011). To what extent are national guidelines for the management of urinary incontinence in women adhered to? Data from a national audit. *BJOG: An International Journal of Obstetrics and Gynaecology, 118*(13), 1592.

*Zampieron, A., Silla, A., & Marilisa, C. (2011). A retrospective study of nursing diagnoses, outcomes, and interventions for patients admitted to a cardiology rehabilitation unit. *International Journal of Nursing Terminologies and Classifications, 22*(4), 148–156.

Resources

AbleData, www.abledata.com

Agency for Healthcare Research and Quality (AHRQ), www.ahrq.gov

American Association of People with Disabilities (AAPD), www.aapd.com

American Society of Addiction Medicine (ASAM), www.asam.org

Assistive Technology Industry Association (ATIA), www.atia.org

Association of Rehabilitation Nurses (ARN), www.rehabnurse.org

Canine Companions for Independence, www.caninecompanions.org

Council for Disability Rights, www.disabilityrights.org

National Association on Alcohol, Drugs and Disability (NAADD), www.naadd.org

National Center for Health Statistics (NCHS), www.cdc.gov/nchs

National Center for the Dissemination of Disability Research (NCDDR), www.ncddr.org

National Council on Alcoholism and Drug Dependence, Inc. (NCADD), www.ncadd.org

National Council on Disability (NCD), www.ncd.gov

National Institute on Disability and Rehabilitation Research (NIDRR), www2.ed.gov/about/offices/list/osers/nidrr/index.html

National Rehabilitation Information Center (NARIC), www.naric.com

National Spinal Cord Injury Association (NSCIA), www.spinalcord.org

Sexuality Information and Education Council of the United States (SIECUS), www.siecus.org

Stroke Engine, McGill University general information, http://strokengine.ca

Substance Abuse Resources and Disability Issues (SARDI), www.med.wright.edu/citar/sardi

U.S. Census Bureau, www.census.gov

U.S. Department of Health and Human Services, www.hhs.gov

World Health Organization, health topics: rehabilitation, www.who.int/topics/rehabilitation/en/

Learning Objectives

On completion of this chapter, the learner will be able to:

1 Describe the demographic trends and the physiologic aspects of aging in older adults in the United States.
2 Describe the significance of preventive health care and health promotion for the older adult.
3 Compare and contrast the common physical and mental health problems of aging and their effects on the functioning of older people and their families.
4 Identify the role of the nurse in meeting the health care needs, including medication therapy, of the older patient.
5 Examine the concerns of older people and their families in the home and community, in the acute care setting, and in the long-term care facility.
6 Discuss the potential economic effect on health care of the large aging population in the United States.

Glossary

activities of daily living (ADLs): basic personal care activities; bathing, dressing, grooming, eating, toileting, and transferring

advance directive: a formal, legally endorsed document that provides instructions for care ("living will")

ageism: a bias that discriminates, stigmatizes, and disadvantages older people based solely on their chronologic age

comorbidity: having more than one illness at the same time (e.g., diabetes and congestive heart failure)

delirium: an acute, confused state that begins with disorientation and if not recognized and treated early can progress to changes in level of consciousness, irreversible brain damage, and sometimes death

dementia: broad term for a syndrome characterized by a general decline in higher brain functioning, such as reasoning, with a pattern of eventual decline in ability to perform even basic activities of daily living, such as toileting and eating

depression: the most common affective (mood) disorder of old age; results from changes in reuptake of the neurochemical serotonin in response to chronic illness and emotional stresses related to the physical and social changes associated with the aging process

durable power of attorney: a formal, legally endorsed document that identifies a proxy decision maker who can make decisions if the signer becomes incapacitated

elder abuse: the physical, emotional, or financial harm to an older person by one or more of the individual's children, caregivers, or others; includes neglect

geriatric syndromes: common conditions found in older adults that tend to be multifactorial and do not fall under discrete disease categories, such as falls, delirium, frailty, dizziness, and urinary incontinence

geriatrics: a field of practice that focuses on the physiology, pathology, diagnosis, and management of the disorders and diseases of older adults

gerontologic/geriatric nursing: the field of nursing that relates to the assessment, planning, implementation, and evaluation of older adults in all environments, including acute, intermediate, and skilled care as well as within the community

gerontology: the combined biologic, psychological, and sociologic study of older adults within their environment

instrumental activities of daily living (IADLs): activities that are essential for independent living, such as shopping, cooking, housework, using the telephone, managing medications and finances, and being able to travel by car or public transportation

orientation: a person's ability to recognize who and where he or she is in a time continuum; used to evaluate one's basic cognitive status

polypharmacy: the prescription, use, or administration of more medications than is clinically indicated

presbycusis: the decreased ability to hear high-pitched tones that naturally begins in midlife as a result of irreversible inner ear changes

presbyopia: the decrease in visual accommodation that occurs with advancing age

sundowning (sundown syndrome): increased confusion and/or agitation at night

urinary incontinence: the unplanned loss of urine

Aging, the normal process of time-related change, begins with birth and continues throughout life. Americans are living longer and healthier than any previous generation. As a result of the baby boomers turning 65 years of age beginning in 2011, older Americans are the most rapidly expanding segment of the population. Whenever nurses work with an adult population, they are likely to encounter older adult patients. This chapter presents demographics of aging, normal age-related changes, health problems associated with aging, and ways that nurses can address the health issues of older adults.

Overview of Aging

Demographics of Aging

The proportion of Americans 65 years of age and older has tripled in the past 100 years (4.1% in 1900 to 13% of the population in 2010) (Howden & Meyer, 2011). Life expectancy—the average number of years that a person can expect to live—varies by gender and race, with women living longer than men and white women having the longest life expectancy. Life expectancy has risen dramatically in the past 100 years. In 1900, average life expectancy was 47 years, and by 2009, that figure had increased to 78.2 years (Kochanek, Xu, Murphy, et al., 2011). As the older adult population increases, the number of people who live to a very old age is also dramatically increasing.

The older adult population is becoming more diverse, reflecting changing demographics in the United States. Although this population will increase in number for all racial and ethnic groups, the rate of growth is projected to be fastest in the Hispanic population, which is expected to increase from 6 million in 2004 to an estimated 17.5 million by 2050. Proportionally, there will be a significant decline in the percentage of the White non-Hispanic population. By 2050, it is estimated that the White non-Hispanic population will decrease to 59% of the older adult population; 20% will be Hispanic, 11% Black, and 8% Asian (Administration on Aging [AoA], 2010a).

Health Status of the Older Adult

Although many older adults enjoy good health, most have at least one chronic illness, and many have multiple health conditions. Chronic conditions, many of which are preventable or treatable, are the major cause of disability and pain among older adults (Fig. 11-1).

Most deaths in the United States occur in people 65 years of age and older; 48% of these are caused by heart disease and cancer (Kochanek et al., 2011). Owing to improvements in the prevention, early detection, and treatment of diseases, there has been a noticeable impact on the health of people in this age group. In the past 60 years, there has been a decline in overall deaths—specifically, deaths from heart disease. In addition, there has been a recent decline in deaths from cancer and cerebrovascular disease.

Preliminary analysis of data suggests that chronic lower respiratory diseases have risen to the third leading cause of death, and cerebrovascular disease is now the fourth leading cause of death among this population of adults (Kochanek et al., 2011). Deaths from Alzheimer's disease (AD) have risen more than 50% between 1999 and 2007 (Kochanek et al., 2011).

More than 70% of noninstitutionalized Americans aged 65 years and older rate their health as good, very good, or excellent (AoA, 2010b). Men and women report comparable levels of health; however, positive health reports decline with advancing age, and Blacks, Hispanics, and Latinos appear less likely to report good health than their White or Asian counterparts. Most Americans 75 years of age and older remain functionally independent regardless of how they perceive their health, and the proportion of older Americans reporting a limitation in activities declined from 49% in 2002 to 42% in 2007 (AoA, 2010b). These declines in limitations may reflect trends in health promotion and disease prevention activities, such as improved nutrition, decreased smoking, increased exercise, and early detection and treatment of risk factors such as hypertension and elevated serum cholesterol levels.

Many chronic conditions commonly found among older people can be managed, limited, and even prevented. Older people are more likely to maintain good health and functional

FIGURE 11-1 • Percentage of people 65 years and older who reported having selected chronic health conditions, by sex, 2009–2010. From Federal Interagency Forum on Aging-Related Statistics. (2012). *2010 older Americans: Key indicators of well-being.* Washington, DC: U.S. Government Printing Office. Available at www.agingstats.gov/agingstatsdotnet/Main_Site/Data/Data_2012.aspx

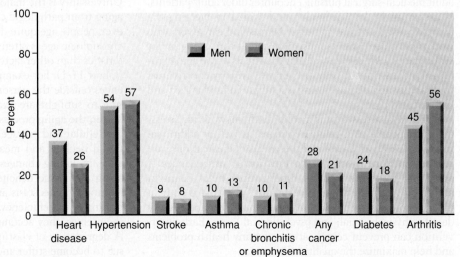

independence if encouraged to do so and if appropriate community-based support services are available (Miller, 2012). Nurses are challenged to promote positive lifelong health behaviors, because the impact of unhealthy behaviors and choices can result in chronic disease.

Nursing Care of the Older Adult

Gerontology, the scientific study of the aging process, is a multidisciplinary field that draws from the biologic, psychological, and sociologic sciences. **Geriatrics** is the practice (medical or nursing) that focuses on the physiology, pathology, diagnosis, and management of the disorders and diseases of older adults. Because aging is a normal process, care for older adults cannot be limited to one discipline but is best provided through a cooperative effort. An interdisciplinary approach to providing care combines expertise and resources to provide comprehensive geriatric assessment and intervention. Nurses collaborate with the team to obtain appropriate services for patients and provide a holistic approach to care.

Gerontologic/geriatric nursing is the field of nursing that specializes in the care of older adults. The Scope and Standards of Gerontological Nursing Practice were originally developed in 1969 by the American Nurses Association (ANA) and revised in 2010 (ANA, 2010). The nurse gerontologist can be either a specialist or a generalist providing comprehensive nursing care to older people by combining the basic nursing process with a specialized knowledge of aging. Gerontologic nursing is provided in acute care, skilled and assisted living, the community, and home settings. The goals of care include promoting and maintaining functional status as well as helping older adults identify and use their strengths to achieve optimal independence.

Nurses who are certified in geriatric nursing have specialized knowledge of the acute and chronic changes specific to older people. The use of advanced practice nurses who have been educated in geriatric nursing concepts has proved to be very effective when dealing with the complex care needs of an older patient. When best practices are used and current scientific knowledge applied to clinical problems, there is significantly less deterioration in the overall health of aging patients (ANA, 2010; Mauk, 2010).

In addition to specialists, nurses who work in all areas of adult medical-surgical nursing encounter older adult patients. Nurses must be knowledgeable and skilled in meeting the complex needs of these patients. Nurses and caregivers who work with older patients must understand that aging is not synonymous with disease and that the effects of the aging process alone are not the only or even the primary contributors to disability and disease. Aging is a highly individualized and multifaceted process.

Functional assessment is a common framework for assessing older people. Age-related changes, as well as additional risk factors such as disease and the effects of medications, can reduce function. Assessing the functional consequences of aging and proposing practical interventions helps maintain and improve the health of older adults. The goal is to help older people sustain maximum functional level and dignity despite physical, social, and psychological losses. Early intervention can prevent complications of many health problems and help maximize the quality of life.

Theories of Aging

Aging has been defined chronologically by the passing of time—subjectively, as in how a person feels, and functionally, as in changes in physical or mental capabilities. The many theories of aging attempt to provide a framework in which to understand aging from different perspectives (Meiner, 2011). Clinicians can use each theory to gain insight into different aspects of aging.

In addition to the biologic, developmental, and sociologic theories of aging, Miller (2012) developed the Functional Consequences Theory, which challenges nurses to consider the effects of normal age-related changes as well as the damage incurred through disease or environmental and behavioral risk factors when planning care. Miller suggests that nurses can alter the outcome for patients through nursing interventions that address the consequences of these changes. Age-related changes and risk factors may negatively interfere with patient outcomes and impair patient activity and quality of life. For example, normal age-related changes in vision may increase sensitivity to glare. Alterations in the environment that reduce glare may enhance patient comfort and safety. In contrast, the development of cataracts, which is not a normal age-related change, also may increase sensitivity to glare. The nurse must differentiate between normal, irreversible age-related changes and modifiable risk factors. Doing so helps the nurse design appropriate nursing interventions that have a positive impact on outcomes for older patients—most importantly, for their quality of life.

Age-Related Changes

The well-being of older people depends on physical, psychosocial, mental, social, economic, and environmental factors. A total assessment includes an evaluation of all major body systems, social and mental status, and the person's ability to function independently (Weber & Kelley, 2010).

Physical Aspects of Aging

Intrinsic aging (from within the person) refers to those changes caused by the normal aging process that are genetically programmed and essentially universal within a species. Universality is the major criterion used to distinguish normal aging from pathologic changes associated with illness. However, people age quite differently and at different rates; thus, chronologic age is often less predictive of obvious age characteristics than other factors, such as one's genetics and lifestyle (Chart 11-1). For example, extrinsic aging results from influences outside the person. Air pollution and excessive exposure to sunlight are examples of extrinsic factors that may hasten the aging process and can be eliminated or reduced.

Cellular and extracellular changes of old age cause functional decline and measurable changes in physical appearance, including changes in shape and body makeup. Cellular aging and tissue deficits also diminish the body's ability to maintain homeostasis and prevent organ systems from functioning at full efficiency. As cells become less able to replace themselves, they accumulate a pigment known as lipofuscin. A degradation of elastin and collagen causes connective tissue to become stiffer and less elastic. These changes result in

Chart 11-1

GENETICS IN NURSING PRACTICE
Genetics Concepts and the Older Adult

Studies of older adults suggest that they are largely unsure of the underlying scientific basis of genetics but are interested in learning more. In addition, although older adults may have information about genetics, that information is not always accurate. They typically defer to their provider's opinion about genetic testing and gene-based interventions. Older adults also have a positive attitude about the opportunities presented by genetic testing for clinical purposes and research. However, they need accurate information about the reasons for and the implications of such genetic testing.

Nursing Assessments

Family History Assessment

- Assess patient's understanding of the role of family history in health and disease.
- Assess and collect family history on both maternal and paternal sides of the family for three generations.

Patient Assessment

- Assess older adult patient's knowledge and understanding of genetics, genetic testing, and gene-based therapies.
- Assess older adult patient's health literacy needs.
- Cultural, social, and spiritual assessment—assess for individual and family perceptions and beliefs around topics related to genetics.
- Assess patient's communication capacities so that communication strategies about genetics are tailored to his or her needs and abilities.

Management Issues Specific to Genetics

- Inquire whether DNA mutation or other genetic testing has been performed on affected family members.
- Refer for further genetic counseling and evaluation as warranted so that family members can discuss inheritance, risk to other family members, and availability of genetic testing and gene-based interventions.
- Offer appropriate genetic information and resources that take into consideration older patient's literacy needs.
- Evaluate older patient's understanding before, during, and after the introduction of genetic information and services.
- Assess patient's understanding of genetic information.
- Take the time to explain the concepts of genetic testing clearly to older patients.
- Ensure that consent obtained for genetic testing is voluntary and informed.
- Provide support to families with a newly diagnosed genetic disorder.
- Participate in the management and coordination of care of older patients with genetic conditions and individuals predisposed to develop or pass on a genetic condition.

Genetics Resources

BiomedSearch.com: provides understanding of genetics among older adults, www.biomedsearch.com

U.S. Department of Health and Human Services: provides information about health literacy and older adults, www.health.gov/communication/literacy/olderadults/literacy.htm

See Chapter 8, Chart 8-6 for additional resources.

---

diminished capacity for organ function and increased vulnerability to disease and stress. Age-related changes in the hematopoietic system influence red blood cell production leading to increased rates of anemia (Bross, Soch, & Smith-Knuppel, 2010; Vanasse & Berliner, 2010).

Table 11-1 summarizes the signs and symptoms of age-related changes in the functioning of body systems. More in-depth information about age-related changes can be found in the chapters pertaining to each organ system. Specifics of diseases, medical and surgical management, and nursing interventions are also presented in the related chapters.

When assessing the physical aspects of aging, nurses should know that some research suggests that the ability to attend to internal physical symptoms declines with age, which may cause poor early symptom detection (Riegel, Dickson, Cameron, et al., 2010).

Cardiovascular System

Heart disease is the leading cause of death in older adults. Heart failure is the leading cause of hospitalization among Medicare recipients, and it is also a major cause of morbidity and mortality among the older adult population in the United States (Riegel et al., 2010). Age-related changes reduce the efficiency of the heart and contribute to decreased compliance of the heart muscle. These changes include myocardial hypertrophy, which changes left ventricular strength and function; fibrosis and stenosis of the valves; and decreased pacemaker cells. As a result, the heart valves become thicker and stiffer, and the heart muscle and arteries lose their elasticity, resulting in a reduced stroke volume. Calcium and fat deposits accumulate within arterial walls, and veins become increasingly stiff and tortuous, increasing arterial resistance; this increases the workload of the heart (Porth & Matfin, 2009).

It is difficult to differentiate between age- and disease-related changes in cardiovascular function because of the significant influence of behavioral factors on cardiovascular health. When cross-cultural studies are conducted, cardiovascular changes that in the past were thought to be age related do not consistently appear. For example, the higher blood pressure found in older adults in Western societies does not occur in less-developed societies and may be a result of different lifestyle behaviors rather than normal age-related changes (Miller, 2012). Under normal circumstances, the cardiovascular system can adapt to the normal age-related changes, and an older person is unaware of any significant decline in cardiovascular performance. However, when challenged, the cardiovascular system of an older person is less efficient under conditions of stress and exercise and when life-sustaining activities are needed.

Careful assessment of older people is necessary because they often present with different symptoms than those seen in younger patients. Older people are more likely to have dyspnea or neurologic symptoms associated with heart disease, and they may experience mental status changes or report vague symptoms such as fatigue, nausea, and syncope. Rather

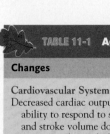

TABLE 11-1 Age-Related Changes in Body Systems and Health Promotion Strategies

Changes	Subjective and Objective Findings	Health Promotion Strategies
Cardiovascular System Decreased cardiac output; diminished ability to respond to stress; heart rate and stroke volume do not increase with maximum demand; slower heart recovery rate; increased blood pressure	Complaints of fatigue with increased activity Increased heart rate recovery time *Optimal blood pressure:* ≤120/80 mm Hg *Prehypertension:* >120–139/80–89 mm Hg *Hypertension:* ≥140/90 mm Hg	Exercise regularly; pace activities; avoid smoking; eat a low-fat, low-salt diet; participate in stress-reduction activities; check blood pressure regularly; adherence to medications; weight control (body mass index <25 kg/m²).
Respiratory System Increase in residual lung volume; decrease in muscle strength, endurance, and vital capacity; decreased gas exchange and diffusing capacity; decreased cough efficiency	Fatigue and breathlessness with sustained activity; decreased respiratory excursion and chest/lung expansion with less effective exhalation; difficulty coughing up secretions	Exercise regularly; avoid smoking; take adequate fluids to liquefy secretions; receive yearly influenza immunization and pneumonia vaccine at 65 years of age; avoid exposure to upper respiratory tract infections.
Integumentary System Decreased subcutaneous fat, interstitial fluid, muscle tone, glandular activity, and sensory receptors, resulting in decreased protection against trauma, sun exposure, and temperature extremes; diminished secretion of natural oils and perspiration; capillary fragility	Thin, wrinkled, and dry skin; complaints of injuries, bruises, and sunburn; complaints of intolerance to heat; prominent bone structure	Limit solar exposure to 10–15 minutes daily for vitamin D (use protective clothing and sunscreen); dress appropriately for temperature; maintain a safe indoor temperature; take shower rather than hot tub bath if possible; lubricate skin with lotions that contain petroleum or mineral oil.
Reproductive System *Female:* Vaginal narrowing and decreased elasticity; decreased vaginal secretions *Male:* Less firm testes and decreased sperm production *Male and female:* Slower sexual response	*Female:* Painful intercourse; vaginal bleeding following intercourse; vaginal itching and irritation; delayed orgasm *Male:* Delayed erection and achievement of orgasm	May require vaginal estrogen replacement; gynecology/urology follow-up; use a lubricant with sexual intercourse.
Musculoskeletal System Loss of bone density; loss of muscle strength and size; degenerated joint cartilage	Height loss; prone to fractures; kyphosis; back pain; loss of strength, flexibility, and endurance; joint pain	Exercise regularly; eat a high-calcium diet; limit phosphorus intake; take calcium and vitamin D supplements as prescribed.
Genitourinary System *Male:* Benign prostatic hyperplasia *Female:* Relaxed perineal muscles; detrusor instability (urge incontinence); urethral dysfunction (stress urinary incontinence)	Urinary retention; irritative voiding symptoms including frequency, feeling of incomplete bladder emptying, multiple nighttime voiding Urgency/frequency syndrome; decreased "warning time"; drops of urine lost with cough, laugh, position change	Limit drinking in evening (e.g., caffeinated beverages, alcohol); do not wait long periods between voiding; empty bladder all the way when passing urine. Wear easily manipulated clothing; drink adequate fluids; avoid bladder irritants (e.g., caffeinated beverages, alcohol, artificial sweeteners); perform pelvic floor muscle exercises, preferably learned via biofeedback; consider urologic workup.
Gastrointestinal System Decreased sense of thirst, smell, and taste; decreased salivation; difficulty swallowing food; delayed esophageal and gastric emptying; reduced gastrointestinal motility	Risk of dehydration, electrolyte imbalances, and poor nutritional intake; complaints of dry mouth; complaints of fullness, heartburn, and indigestion; constipation, flatulence, and abdominal discomfort	Use ice chips, mouthwash; brush, floss, and massage gums daily; receive regular dental care; eat small, frequent meals; sit up and avoid heavy activity after eating; limit antacids; eat a high-fiber, low-fat diet; limit laxatives; toilet regularly; drink adequate fluids.
Nervous System Reduced speed in nerve conduction; increased confusion with physical illness and loss of environmental cues; reduced cerebral circulation (becomes faint, loses balance)	Slower to respond and react; learning takes longer; becomes confused with hospital admission; faintness; frequent falls	Pace teaching; with hospitalization, encourage visitors; enhance sensory stimulation; with sudden confusion, look for cause; encourage slow rising from a resting position.
Special Senses *Vision:* Diminished ability to focus on close objects; inability to tolerate glare; difficulty adjusting to changes of light intensity; decreased ability to distinguish colors	Holds objects far away from face; complaints of glare; poor night vision; confuses colors	Wear eyeglasses and use sunglasses outdoors; avoid abrupt changes from dark to light; use adequate indoor lighting with area lights and nightlights; use large-print books; use magnifier for reading; avoid night driving; use contrasting colors for color coding; avoid glare of shiny surfaces and direct sunlight.
Hearing: Decreased ability to hear high-frequency sounds; tympanic membrane thinning and loss of resiliency	Gives inappropriate responses; asks people to repeat words; strains forward to hear	Recommend a hearing examination; reduce background noise; face person; enunciate clearly; speak with a low-pitched voice; use nonverbal cues.
Taste and smell: Decreased ability to taste and smell	Uses excessive sugar and salt	Encourage us Encourage use of lemon, spices, herbs; recommend smoking cessation.

than the typical substernal chest pain associated with myocardial ischemia, older patients may report burning or sharp pain or discomfort in an area of the upper body. Complicating the assessment is the fact that many older patients have more than one underlying disease. When a patient complains of symptoms related to digestion and breathing and upper extremity pain, cardiac disease must be considered. The absence of chest pain in an older patient is not a reliable indicator of the absence of heart disease. Researchers reported in one study that patients 73 years of age and older with heart failure had more difficulty detecting and interpreting shortness of breath compared to the patients younger than 73 years (Riegel et al., 2010).

Hypotension may be a concern. The risk of orthostatic and postprandial hypotension increases significantly after 75 years of age (Miller, 2012). A patient experiencing hypotension should be counseled to rise slowly (from a lying, to a sitting, to a standing position), avoid straining when having a bowel movement, and consider having five or six small meals each day, rather than three, to minimize the hypotension that can occur after a large meal. Extremes in temperature, including hot showers and whirlpool baths, should be avoided.

Respiratory System

The respiratory system seems to be able to compensate best for the functional changes of aging. In general, healthy, nonsmoking older adults show very little decline in respiratory function; however, there are substantial individual variations. The age-related changes that do occur are subtle and gradual, and healthy older adults are able to compensate for these changes. Diminished respiratory efficiency and reduced maximal inspiratory and expiratory force may occur as a result of calcification and weakening of the muscles of the chest wall. Lung mass decreases, and residual volume increases (Bickley, 2009).

Conditions of stress, such as illness, may increase the demand for oxygen and affect the overall function of other systems. Like cardiovascular diseases, respiratory diseases manifest more subtly in older adults than in younger adults and do not necessarily follow the typical pattern of cough, chills, and fever. Older adults may exhibit headache, weakness, lethargy, anorexia, dehydration, and mental status changes (Miller, 2012).

Smoking is the most significant risk factor for respiratory diseases. Therefore, a major focus of health promotion activities should be on smoking cessation and avoidance of environmental smoke. Activities that help older people maintain adequate respiratory function include regular exercise, appropriate fluid intake, pneumococcal vaccination, yearly influenza immunizations, and avoidance of people who are ill. Hospitalized older adults should be frequently reminded to cough and take deep breaths, particularly postoperatively, because their decreased lung capacity and decreased cough efficiency predispose them to atelectasis and respiratory infections.

Integumentary System

The functions of the skin include protection, temperature regulation, sensation, and excretion. Aging affects skin function and appearance. Epidermal proliferation decreases, and the dermis becomes thinner. Elastic fibers are reduced in number, and collagen becomes stiffer. Subcutaneous fat diminishes, particularly in the extremities, but gradually increases in other areas, such as the abdomen (men) and thighs (women), leading to an overall increase in body fat in older people (Tabloski, 2009). Decreased numbers of capillaries in the skin result in diminished blood supply. These changes cause a loss of resiliency, wrinkling, and sagging of the skin. The skin becomes drier and more susceptible to burns, injury, and infection. Hair pigmentation may change, and balding may occur; genetic factors strongly influence these changes. These changes in the integument reduce tolerance to temperature extremes and sun exposure.

Lifestyle practices are likely to have a large impact on skin changes. Strategies to promote healthy skin function include not smoking, avoiding exposure to the sun, using a sun protection factor (SPF) of 15 or higher, using emollient skin cream containing petrolatum or mineral oil, avoiding hot soaks in the bathtub, and maintaining optimal nutrition and hydration. Older adults should be encouraged to have any changes in the skin examined, because early detection and treatment of precancerous or cancerous lesions are essential for the best outcome.

Reproductive System

Contrary to the common misperception that older adults are asexual, older adults report maintaining a fairly stable and active sex life as long as there is a partner available (Hooyman & Kiyak, 2008). Sexual activity declines with the loss of a partner, primarily for women as a result of widowhood and for men as a result of poor heath, erectile dysfunction, medications, and emotional factors (Karraker, DeLamatar & Schwartz, 2011). However, although good health is a predictor of sexual activity, older adults with chronic illnesses may be able to have a sexually active life as well. Because of the many factors that influence the ability to be sexually active, nurses and the older person need to understand the physiologic, psychological, and social factors that affect reproductive and sexual functioning as aging progresses.

Ovarian production of estrogen and progesterone declines with menopause. Changes that occur in the female reproductive system include thinning of the vaginal wall, along with a shortening of the vagina and a loss of elasticity; decreased vaginal secretions, resulting in vaginal dryness, itching, and decreased acidity; involution (atrophy) of the uterus and ovaries; and decreased pubococcygeal muscle tone, resulting in a relaxed vagina and perineum. Without the use of water-soluble lubricants, these changes may contribute to vaginal bleeding and painful intercourse.

In older men, the testes become less firm but may continue to produce viable sperm up to 90 years of age. At about 50 years of age, production of testosterone begins to diminish (Tabloski, 2009). Decreased libido and erectile dysfunction may develop but are more likely to be associated with factors other than age-related changes. These risk factors include cardiovascular disease; neurologic disorders; diabetes; respiratory disease; pain; and medications such as vasodilators, antihypertensive agents, and tricyclic antidepressants.

In both older men and women, it may take longer to become sexually aroused, longer to complete intercourse, and longer before sexual arousal can occur again. Although a less intense response to sexual stimulation and a decline in sexual activity occurs with increasing age, sexual desire does not disappear. Many couples are unaware of the causes of decreased libido or erectile dysfunction and are often reluctant to discuss decreased sexual function. Many methods of improving the quality of sexual interactions exist, and assessment and communication require sensitivity and expert knowledge in the field of sexual dysfunction. If sexual dysfunction is present, referral to a gynecologist, urologist, or sex therapist may be warranted.

Genitourinary System

The genitourinary system continues to function adequately in older people, although kidney mass is decreased, primarily because of a loss of nephrons. However, the loss of nephrons does not typically become significant until about 90 years of age, and changes in kidney function vary widely; approximately one third of older people show no decrease in renal function (Tabloski, 2009). Changes in renal function may be attributable to a combination of aging and pathologic conditions such as hypertension. The changes most commonly seen include a decreased filtration rate, diminished tubular function with less efficiency in resorbing and concentrating the urine, and a slower restoration of acid–base balance in response to stress. In addition, older adults who take medications may experience serious consequences owing to decline in renal function because of impaired absorption, decreased ability to maintain fluid and electrolyte balance, and decreased ability to concentrate urine.

Certain genitourinary disorders are more common in older adults than in the general population. In the United States, almost 50% of women 80 years of age and older suffer from **urinary incontinence** (i.e., urine leakage or problems controlling urine flow). This condition should not be mistaken as a normal consequence of aging (Weber & Kelley, 2010). Costly and often embarrassing, it should be evaluated, because in many cases it is reversible or can be treated. (See Chapter 55 for further discussion of urinary incontinence.) Benign prostatic hyperplasia (enlarged prostate gland), a common finding in older men, causes a gradual increase in urine retention and overflow incontinence. Changes in the urinary tract increase the susceptibility to urinary tract infections. Adequate consumption of fluids is an important nursing intervention that reduces the risk of bladder infections and also helps decrease urinary incontinence.

Gastrointestinal System

Digestion of food is less influenced by age-related changes than by the risk of poor nutrition. Older people can adjust to the age-related changes but may have difficulty purchasing, preparing, and enjoying their meals. The sense of smell diminishes as a result of neurologic changes and environmental factors such as smoking, medications, and vitamin B_{12} deficiencies. The ability to recognize sweet, sour, bitter, or salty foods diminishes over time, altering satisfaction with food. Salivary flow does not decrease in healthy adults; however, approximately 30% of older people may experience a dry mouth as a result of medications and diseases (Miller, 2012). Difficulties with chewing and swallowing are generally associated with lack of teeth and disease.

Experts disagree on the extent of gastric changes that occur as a result of normal aging. However, gastric motility appears to slow modestly, which results in delayed emptying of stomach contents and early satiety (feeling of fullness). Diminished secretion of gastric acid and pepsin, seemingly the result of pathologic conditions rather than normal aging, reduces the absorption of iron, calcium, and vitamin B_{12}. Absorption of nutrients in the small intestine, particularly calcium and vitamin D, appears to diminish with age. Functions of the liver, gallbladder, and pancreas are generally maintained, although absorption and tolerance to fat may decrease. The incidence of gallstones and common bile duct stones increases progressively with advancing years.

Difficulty swallowing, or dysphagia, increases with age and is a major health care problem in older patients. Normal aging alters some aspects of the swallowing function. In addition, dysphagia is a frequent complication of stroke and a significant risk factor for development of aspiration pneumonia; it can be life threatening. Dysphagia is caused by interruption or dysfunction of neural pathways. It may also result from dysfunction of the striated and smooth muscles of the gastrointestinal tract in patients with Parkinson's disease. Aspiration of food or fluid is the most serious complication and can occur in the absence of coughing or choking.

Constipation is a common pathologic condition that affects as many as 74% of institutionalized and 50% of community-dwelling older adults (Rao & Go, 2010). Symptoms of mild constipation are abdominal discomfort and flatulence; more serious constipation leads to fecal impaction that contributes to diarrhea around the impaction, fecal incontinence, and obstruction. Predisposing factors for constipation include lack of dietary bulk, prolonged use of laxatives, some medications, inactivity, insufficient fluid intake, and excessive dietary fat. Ignoring the urge to defecate may also be a contributing factor.

Practices that promote gastrointestinal health include regular tooth brushing and flossing; receiving regular dental care; eating small, frequent meals; avoiding heavy activity after eating; eating a high-fiber, low-fat diet; drinking enough fluids; and avoiding the use of laxatives and antacids. Understanding that there is a direct correlation between loss of smell and taste perception and food intake helps caregivers intervene to maintain the nutritional health of older patients.

Nutritional Health

The social, psychological, and physiologic functions of eating influence the dietary habits of older people. Increasing age alters nutrient requirements; older adults require fewer calories and a more nutrient-rich, healthy diet in response to alterations in body mass and a more sedentary lifestyle. Recommendations include reducing fat intake while consuming sufficient protein, vitamins, minerals, and dietary fiber for health and prevention of disease. Decreased physical activity and a slower metabolic rate reduce the number of calories needed by older adults to maintain an ideal weight. As stated previously, age-related changes that alter pleasure in eating include a decrease in taste and smell. Older people are likely to maintain a taste for sweetness but require more sugar to achieve a sweet flavor. They also may lose the ability to differentiate sour, salty, and bitter tastes. Apathy, immobility, depression, loneliness, poverty, inadequate knowledge, and poor oral health also contribute to suboptimal nutrient intake. Budgetary constraints and

MyPlate for Older Adults

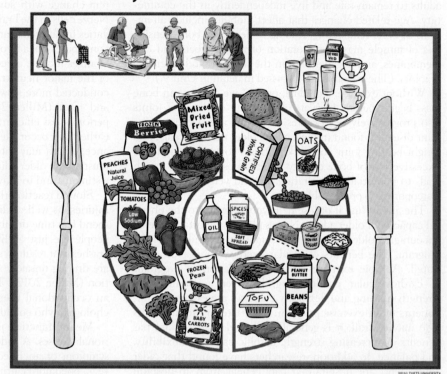

FIGURE 11-2 • MyPlate for older adults. Used with permission from the Jean Mayer USDA Human Nutrition Research Center on Aging (HNRCA) at Tufts University.

physical limitations may interfere with food shopping and meal preparation.

Health promotion for older adults is based on the individual's physiologic, pathologic, and psychosocial conditions. The goals of nutrition therapy are to maintain or restore maximal independent functioning and health and to maintain the sense of dignity and quality of life by imposing as few restrictions as possible. Dietary changes should be incorporated into the older adult's existing food pattern as much as possible (Dudek, 2010). Figure 11-2 lists modified dietary guidelines for older adults.

Women older than 50 years and men older than 70 years should have a daily calcium intake of 1,200 mg. To foster the absorption of calcium, adults should have 600 IU of vitamin D until 70 years of age and 800 IU after 70 years of age to maintain bone health (National Institutes of Health [NIH], 2011a, 2011b).

Undernutrition, which can lead to malnutrition, may be a problem for older adults and is an important quality-of-life issue. A recent unintentional weight loss may be a result of an illness or other factors, such as depression, that may have serious consequences and affect a person's ability to maintain health and fight illness (Dudek, 2010). Many people are unaware of dietary deficits. Nurses are in an ideal position to identify nutritional problems among their patients and to work within the patient's own framework of knowledge of his or her health status to improve health behaviors. (See Chapter 5 for more information on nutritional assessment.)

Sleep

Studies suggest that older adults have increased complaints about their sleep as they age, and as many as 57% complain of sleep disturbances such as periodic limb movements (45%) and restless leg syndrome (12%), insomnia (29%) obstructive sleep apnea (24%), and early morning awakening (19%) (Bloom, Ahmed, Alessi, et al., 2009). Consequently, they may feel less satisfied with their sleep. Older adults sleep an average of 7 hours each night, with more time spent in light sleep (Vance, Heaton, Eaves, et al., 2011). The lack of quality sleep at night may increase napping during the day. Older people are more likely to awaken because of factors such as noise, pain, or nocturia. The incidence of sleep apnea (a sleep disorder characterized by brief periods in which respirations are absent) increases with age. Having insomnia symptoms and a sleep-related disorder (snoring, choking, or pauses in breathing) is associated with significantly impaired daytime functioning and longer psychomotor reaction times compared with having either condition. (Sleep apnea is discussed in more detail in Chapter 22.)

The nurse often observes patients while they are sleeping and can identify problems. The nurse can provide health education on sleep hygiene behaviors such as avoiding use of the bed for activities other than sleeping (or sex), maintaining a consistent bedtime routine, avoiding or limiting daytime napping, and limiting alcohol intake to one drink a day. Additional suggestions include avoiding stimulants such as caffeine and nicotine after noon; curbing the amount of liquids in the evening to avoid nocturia; and engaging in regular physical activity, preferably in bright outside light (Vance et al., 2011).

Musculoskeletal System

Intact musculoskeletal and neurologic systems are essential for the maintenance of safe mobility, performance of **activities of daily living (ADLs)** (basic personal care activities), and **instrumental activities of daily living (IADLs)** (activities that are essential for independent living), thus allowing older adults to remain safe and live independently in the community. Age-related changes that affect mobility include alterations in bone remodeling, leading to decreased bone density, loss of muscle mass, deterioration of muscle fibers and cell membranes, and degeneration in the function and efficiency of joints. (These factors are discussed in detail in Unit 9.)

Without exercise, a gradual, progressive decrease in bone mass begins before 40 years of age. The cartilage of joints also progressively deteriorates in middle age. Degenerative joint disease is found in most adults older than 70 years, and weight-bearing joint and back pain is a common complaint. Excessive loss of bone density results in osteoporosis, which leads to potentially life-altering hip and vertebral fractures. Osteoporosis is preventable.

The axiom "use it or lose it" is very relevant to the physical capacity of older adults. Nurses play an important role by encouraging older people to participate in a regular exercise program. The benefits of regular exercise cannot be overstated. Aerobic exercises are the foundation of programs of cardiovascular conditioning; however, resistance and strength training and flexibility exercises are essential components of an exercise program. Even late in life, in adults who may be frail, it is generally believed that exercise has benefits of increasing strength, aerobic capacity, flexibility, and balance. In addition, researchers have found that older adults who are hospitalized can benefit from in-hospital physical activity (Chart 11-2).

Nervous System

Homeostasis is difficult to maintain with aging, but older people have a tremendous ability to adapt and function adequately, retaining their cognitive and intellectual abilities in the absence of pathologic changes. However, normal aging changes in the nervous system can affect all parts of the body.

The structure, chemistry, and function of the nervous system change with advanced age (Murphy & Hickey, 2010). Nerve cells in the brain decrease; the quantity of neuronal loss varies in different parts of the brain, but the overall decrease contributes to a progressive loss of brain mass. Chemical changes include a decrease in the synthesis and metabolism of the major neurotransmitters. Because nerve impulses are conducted more slowly, older people take longer to respond and react (Miller, 2012). The autonomic nervous system performs less efficiently, and postural hypotension, discussed earlier, may occur. Neurologic changes can affect gait and balance, which may interfere with mobility and safety. Nurses must advise older adults to allow a longer time to respond to a stimulus and to move more deliberately.

Slowed reaction time puts older people at risk for falls and injuries, as well as driving errors. Even though older adults spend less time driving compared with younger people, older people are just as likely to be involved in motor vehicle crashes that result in serious injury or death. Older adults who are driving unsafely should receive a driving fitness evaluation (Miller, 2012). The evaluation is often administered by an occupational therapist in conjunction with a neuropsychologist, who conducts more detailed cognitive testing.

Mental function may be threatened by physical or emotional stresses. A sudden onset of confusion may be the first symptom of an infection or change in physical condition (e.g., pneumonia, urinary tract infection, medication interactions, and dehydration).

Sensory System

People interact with the world through their senses. Losses associated with old age affect all sensory organs, and it can be devastating not to be able to see to read or watch television, hear conversation well enough to communicate, or discriminate taste well enough to enjoy food. Nearly half of older men and one third of older women report difficulty hearing

---

Chart 11-2

NURSING RESEARCH PROFILE

Low Mobility During Hospitalization

Zisberg, A., Shadmi, E., Sinoff, G., et al. (2011). Low mobility during hospitalization and functional decline in older adults. *Journal of the American Geriatric Society, 59*(2), 266–273.

Purpose

The main objective of this study was to examine the association of mobility levels of older hospitalized adults and functional outcomes.

Design

This prospective cohort study examined the effects of in-hospital mobility levels on the functional outcomes of 526 older adults who were hospitalized for nondisabling conditions. A baseline assessment of level of mobility and function was conducted using various scales that assessed activities of daily living (ADLs) and instrumental activities of daily living (IADLs). Hospital mobility levels were assessed through daily interviews with either the participants or their surrogate. Participants were asked about their ability to transfer as well as the frequency and distance of all mobility efforts of any type, including physical therapy. Upon discharge from the hospital and 1 month later, participants or

surrogates were interviewed about the participants' mobility and functional abilities.

Findings

Among the participants, 46% had declined in ADLs at discharge, and 49% had declined at follow-up 1 month later. There was a strong positive relationship between levels of in-hospital mobility and functional outcomes even among those who were identified as functionally stable and generally would be characterized as at low risk for decline. In the low-risk group, 44% were significantly affected by low mobility during hospitalization.

Nursing Implications

This study demonstrated the value of in-hospital mobilization for all older adults. Promoting mobility throughout the hospital stay is an important nursing intervention for all patients. Nurses can be proactive by encouraging hospital policies that promote in-hospital mobility, keeping patients out of bed and moving, recommending ongoing exercise to older patients, and identifying patients who are demonstrating a functional decline and referring them to moderate exercise programs geared toward older adults.

without a hearing aid. Most adults have a decrease in visual acuity beginning at the age of 50 years (Miller, 2012). An uncompensated sensory loss negatively affects the functional ability and quality of life of the older adult. However, assistive devices such as glasses and hearing aids can compensate for a sensory loss.

Sensory Loss Versus Sensory Deprivation

In contrast to sensory loss, sensory deprivation is the absence of stimuli in the environment or the inability to interpret existing stimuli (perhaps as a result of a sensory loss). Sensory deprivation can lead to boredom, confusion, irritability, disorientation, and anxiety. A decline in sensory input can mimic a decline in cognition that is in fact not present. Meaningful sensory stimulation provided to the older person is often helpful in correcting this problem. In some situations, one sense can substitute for another in observing and interpreting stimuli. Nurses can enhance sensory stimulation in the environment with colors, pictures, textures, tastes, smells, and sounds. The stimuli are most meaningful if they are appropriate for older people and the stimuli are changed often. Cognitively impaired people tend to respond well to touch and to familiar music.

Vision

As new cells form on the outside surface of the lens of the eye, the older central cells accumulate and become yellow, rigid, dense, and cloudy, leaving only the outer portion of the lens elastic enough to change shape (accommodate) and focus at near and far distances. As the lens becomes less flexible, the near point of focus gets farther away. This common condition—**presbyopia**—usually begins in the fifth decade of life and requires the person to wear reading glasses to magnify objects (Miller, 2012). In addition, the yellowing, cloudy lens causes light to scatter and sensitivity to glare. The ability to distinguish colors decreases, particularly blue from green. The pupil dilates slowly and less completely because of increased stiffness of the muscles of the iris, thus the older person takes more time to adjust when going to and from light and dark settings and needs brighter light for close vision. Pathologic visual conditions are not a part of normal aging; however, the incidence of eye disease (most commonly cataracts, glaucoma, diabetic retinopathy, and age-related macular degeneration) increases in older people.

Age-related macular degeneration is the primary cause of vision loss in older adults. Approximately 18% of people between 70 and 74 years of age and 47% of people 85 years or older have some signs of this disease (Miller, 2012). Macular degeneration does not affect peripheral vision, which means that it does not cause blindness. However, it affects central vision, color perception, and fine detail, greatly affecting common visual skills such as reading, driving, and seeing faces. Risk factors include sunlight exposure, cigarette smoking, and heredity. People with fair skin and blue eyes may be at increased risk. Sunglasses and hats with visors provide some protection, and stopping smoking is paramount in preventing the disease. Although there is no definitive treatment and no cure that restores vision, several treatment options are available, depending on factors such as the location of the abnormal blood vessels. Laser photocoagulation and photodynamic therapy are commonly used, and there are many promising ongoing clinical trials (Miller, 2012). The earlier this condition is diagnosed, the greater the chances of preserving sight. (See Chapter 63 for more information on altered vision.)

Hearing

Auditory changes begin to be noticed at about 40 years of age. Environmental factors, such as exposure to noise, medications, and infections, as well as genetics, may contribute to hearing loss as much as age-related changes. **Presbycusis** is a gradual sensorineural loss that progresses from the loss of the ability to hear high-frequency tones to a generalized loss of hearing. It is attributed to irreversible inner ear changes. Older people often cannot follow conversation because tones of high-frequency consonants (the sounds *f, s, th, ch, sh, b, t, p*) all sound alike. Hearing loss may cause older people to respond inappropriately, misunderstand conversation, and avoid social interaction. This behavior may be erroneously interpreted as confusion. Wax buildup or other correctable problems may also be responsible for hearing difficulties. A properly prescribed and fitted hearing aid may be useful in reducing some types of hearing deficits. (See Chapter 64 for discussion of alterations in hearing.)

Taste and Smell

The senses of taste and smell are reduced in older adults (Murphy & Hickey, 2010). Of the four basic tastes (sweet, sour, salty, and bitter), sweet tastes are particularly dulled in older people. Blunted taste may contribute to the preference for salty, highly seasoned foods, but herbs, onions, garlic, and lemon can be used as substitutes for salt to flavor food.

Changes in the sense of smell are related to cell loss in the nasal passages and in the olfactory bulb in the brain. Environmental factors such as long-term exposure to toxins (e.g., dust, pollen, and smoke) contribute to the cellular damage.

Psychosocial Aspects of Aging

Successful psychological aging is reflected in the ability of older people to adapt to physical, social, and emotional losses and to achieve life satisfaction. Because changes in life patterns are inevitable over a lifetime, older people need resiliency and coping skills when confronting stresses and change. A positive self-image enhances risk taking and participation in new, untested roles.

Although attitudes toward older people differ in ethnic subcultures, a subtle theme of **ageism**—prejudice or discrimination against older people—predominates in our society, and many myths surround aging. Ageism is based on stereotypes—simplified and often untrue beliefs that reinforce society's negative image of older people. Although older people make up an extremely heterogeneous and increasingly a racially and ethnically diverse group, these negative stereotypes are sometimes attributed to all older people.

Fear of aging and the inability of many to confront their own aging process may trigger ageist beliefs. Retirement and perceived nonproductivity are also responsible for negative feelings, because a younger working person may falsely see older people as not contributing to society, as draining economic resources, and may actually feel that they are in competition with children for resources. Concern about the large numbers of older persons leaving the workforce (baby boomers began to turn age 65 in 2011) is fueling this debate.

Negative images are so common in society that older adults themselves often believe and perpetuate them. An understanding of the aging process and respect for each person as an individual can dispel the myths of aging. Nurses can facilitate successful aging by recommending health promotion strategies such as anticipatory planning for retirement, including ensuring adequate income, developing routines not associated with work, and relying on other people and groups in addition to spouse to fill leisure time (Pender, Murdaugh, & Parsons, 2011).

Stress and Coping in the Older Adult

Coping patterns and the ability to adapt to stress develop over the course of a lifetime and remain consistent later in life. Experiencing success in younger adulthood helps a person develop a positive self-image that remains solid through old age. A person's abilities to adapt to change, make decisions, and respond predictably are also determined by past experiences. A flexible, well-functioning person will probably continue as such. However, losses may accumulate within a short period of time and become overwhelming. The older person often has fewer choices and diminished resources to deal with stressful events. Common stressors of old age include normal aging changes that impair physical function, activities, and appearance; disabilities from injury or chronic illness; social and environmental losses related to loss of income and decreased ability to perform previous roles and activities; and the deaths of significant others. Many older adults rely strongly on their spiritual beliefs for comfort during stressful times.

Living Arrangements

Many older people have more than adequate financial resources and good health even until very late in life; therefore, they have many housing options. More than 90% of older adults live in the community, with a relatively small percentage (4.1%) residing in nursing homes and a comparable percentage living in some type of senior housing. Eighty percent of those older than 65 years own their homes. Thirty percent of noninstitutionalized older people live alone, and widowed women predominate. Seventy-two percent of men older than 65 years are married compared with 42% of women in the same age group. Among those 85 years of age or older, about 55% of men are married compared with 15% of women. This difference in marital status is a result of several factors: Women have a longer life expectancy than men; women tend to marry older men; and women tend to remain widowed, whereas men often remarry (AoA, 2010b).

Older people tend to relocate in response to changes in their lives such as retirement or widowhood, a significant deterioration in health, or disability. The type of housing they choose depends on their reason for moving (Hooyman & Kiyak, 2008). With increasing disability and illness, older people may move to retirement facilities or assisted living communities that provide some support such as meals, transportation, and housekeeping but otherwise allow them to live somewhat independently. If they develop a serious illness or disability and can no longer live independently or semi-independently, they may need to move to a setting where additional support is available, such as a relative's home or a long-term care or assisted living facility near an adult child's home.

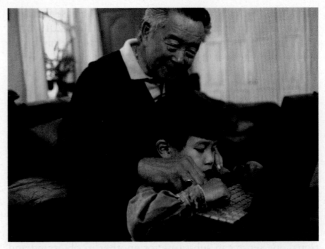

FIGURE 11-3 • Families are an important source of psychosocial and physical support for all people. Caring interaction among grandchildren, grandparents, and other family members typically contributes to the health of all.

Living at Home or With Family

Most older people want to remain in their own homes; in fact, they function best in their own environment. The family home and familiar community may have strong emotional significance for them, and this should not be ignored. However, with advanced age and increasing disability, adjustments to the environment may be required to allow older adults to remain in their own homes or apartments. Additional family support or more formal support may be necessary to compensate for declining function and mobility. There are many services and organizations to assist older adults to successfully "age in place" in their own homes or in assisted living facilities (Marchant & Williams, 2011; Wick & Zanni, 2009).

Sometimes older adults or couples move in with adult children. This can be a rewarding experience as the children, their parents, and the grandchildren interact and share household responsibilities (Fig. 11-3). It can also be stressful, depending on family dynamics. Adult children and their older parents may choose to pool their financial resources by moving into a house that has an attached "in-law suite." This arrangement provides security for the older adult and privacy for both families. Many older people and their adult children make housing decisions in times of crisis, such as during a serious illness or after the death of a spouse. Older people and their families often are unaware of the ramifications of shared housing and assuming care for an increasingly dependent person. Families can be helped by anticipatory guidance and long-term planning before a crisis occurs. Older adults should participate in decisions that affect them as much as possible.

Continuing Care Retirement Communities

Continuing care retirement communities (CCRCs) offer three levels of living arrangements and care that provide for aging in place (Meiner, 2011; Miller 2012). CCRCs consist of independent single-dwelling houses or apartments for people who can manage their day-to-day needs, assisted living apartments for those who need limited assistance with their daily living needs, and skilled nursing services when continuous nursing assistance is required. CCRCs usually contract for a large down payment before the resident moves into the community. This payment gives a person or couple the option of residing in the same community from the time of total independence through the need for assisted or skilled nursing care. Decisions about living arrangements and health care can be made before any decline in health status occurs. CCRCs also provide continuity at a time in an older adult's life when many other factors, such as health status, income, and availability of friends and family members, may be changing.

Assisted Living Facilities

Assisted living facilities are an option when an older person's physical or cognitive changes necessitate at least minimal supervision or assistance. Assisted living allows for a degree of independence while providing minimal nursing assistance with administration of medication, assistance with ADLs, or other chronic health care needs. Other services, such as laundry, cleaning, and meals, may also be included. Both assisted living and CCRCs are costly and primarily paid out-of-pocket (Meiner, 2011).

Long-Term Care Facilities

Many types of nursing homes, nursing facilities, or long-term care facilities offer continuous nursing care. Contrary to the myth of family abandonment and the fear of "ending up in a nursing home," the actual percentage of long-term nursing home residents has declined, from 5.4% in 1985 to 4.1% in 2009 (AoA, 2010b). However, the actual number of older people who reside in long-term care facilities has risen owing to the large increase in the aging population and the use of nursing homes for short-term rehabilitation.

Short-term nursing facility care is often reimbursed by Medicare if the patient is recovering from an acute illness such as a stroke, myocardial infarction, or cancer and requires skilled nursing care or therapy for recuperation. Usually, if an older adult suffers a major health event and is hospitalized and then goes to a nursing facility, Medicare covers the cost of the first 30 to 90 days in a skilled nursing facility if ongoing therapy is needed. The requirement for continued Medicare coverage during this time is documentation of persistent improvement in the condition that requires therapy, most often physical therapy, occupational therapy, respiratory therapy, and cognitive therapy. Some adults choose to have long-term care insurance as a means of paying, at least in part, for the cost of these services should they become necessary. For older people who are living in nursing homes and are medically stable, even though they may have multiple chronic and debilitating health issues, costs are primarily paid out-of-pocket by the patient. When a person's financial resources become exhausted as a result of prolonged nursing home care, the patient, the institution, or both may apply for Medicaid reimbursement. Family members are not responsible for nursing home costs.

An increasing number of skilled nursing facilities offer subacute care. This area of the facility offers a high level of nursing care that may either avoid the need for a resident to be transferred to a hospital from the nursing home or allow a hospitalized patient to be transferred back to the nursing facility sooner.

The Role of the Family

Planning for care and understanding the psychosocial issues confronting older people must be accomplished within the context of the family. If dependency needs occur, the spouse often assumes the role of primary caregiver. In the absence of a surviving spouse, an adult child may assume caregiver responsibilities and need help in providing or arranging for care and support.

Two common myths in American society are that adult children and their aged parents are socially alienated, and that adult children abandon their parents when health and other dependency problems arise. In reality, the family has been and continues to be an important source of support for older people; similarly, older family members provide a great deal of support to younger family members.

Although adult children are not financially responsible for their older parents, social attitudes and cultural values often dictate that adult children should provide services and assume the burden of care if their aged parents cannot care for themselves. Estimates indicate that 75% of the 4.5 million individuals with AD receive some of their care from informal caregivers (Elliott, Burgio, & DeCoster, 2010). Caregiving, which may continue for many years, can become a source of family stress and is a well-known risk for psychiatric and physical morbidity. Evidence-based interventions to reduce distress and enhance well-being in caregivers have been identified. Three broad types of effective programs include (1) psychoeducational skill building, (2) cognitive behavioral therapy, and (3) using a combination of at least two approaches such as education, family meetings, and skill building (Coon & Evans, 2009).

Cognitive Aspects of Aging

Cognition can be affected by many variables, including sensory impairment, physiologic health, environment, sleep, and psychosocial influences. Older adults may experience temporary changes in cognitive function when hospitalized or admitted to skilled nursing facilities, rehabilitation centers, or long-term care facilities. These changes are related to differences in the environment or in medical therapy or to alteration in role performance. A commonly used assessment tool is the Mini-Mental State Examination (MMSE) (Chart 11-3).

Good sleep hygiene can improve cognition, as can treatment of depression and anxiety (Vance et al., 2011). Several researchers are evaluating cognitive remediation (Vance, Keltner, McGuinness, et al., 2010) and memory enhancement programs for older adults (Marchant & Williams, 2011) as strategies to address cognitive decline. When intelligence test scores from people of all ages are compared, test scores for older adults show a progressive decline beginning in midlife. However, research has shown that environment and health have a considerable influence on scores, and that certain types of intelligence (e.g., spatial perceptions and retention of nonintellectual information) decline, whereas others (e.g., problem-solving ability based on past experiences, verbal comprehension, and mathematical ability) do not. Cardiovascular health, a stimulating environment, and high levels of education, occupational status, and income all appear to have a positive effect on intelligence scores in later life.

Chart 11-3 ASSESSMENT
Assessing Mental Status: Mini-Mental State Examination Sample Items

Orientation to Time

"What is the date?"

Registration

"Listen carefully. I am going to say three words. You say them back after I stop. Ready? Here they are . . . APPLE (pause), PENNY (pause), TABLE (pause). Now repeat those words back to me." [Repeat up to five times, but only score the first trial.]

Naming

"What is this?" [Point to a pencil.]

Reading

"Please read this and do what it says." [Show examinee the words on the stimulus form.] CLOSE YOUR EYES.

Reproduced by special permission of the Publisher, Psychological Assessment Resources, Inc., 16204 North Florida Avenue, Lutz, FL 33549, from the Mini Mental State Examination, by Marshall Folstein and Susan Folstein, Copyright 1975, 1998, 2001 by Mini Mental LLC, Inc. Published 2001 by Psychological Assessment Resources, Inc. Further reproduction is prohibited without permission of PAR, Inc. The MMSE can be purchased from PAR, Inc. by calling (813) 968-3003. Used with permission.

According to Hooyman and Kiyak (2008), significant age-related declines in intelligence, learning, and memory are not inevitable. These authors summarized the major studies on cognitive function in later years and provided the following overview. Many factors affect the ability of older people to learn and remember and to perform well in testing situations. Older adults who have higher levels of education, good sensory function, good nutrition, and jobs that require complex problem-solving skills continue to demonstrate intelligence, memory, and the capacity for learning. Part of the challenge in testing older adults is determining what is actually being tested (e.g., speed of response) and whether the test results are indicative of a normal age-related change, a sensory deficit, or poor health. However, age differences continue to emerge even with untimed tests and when the tests are controlled for variations in motor and sensory function. In general, fluid intelligence—the biologically determined intelligence used for flexibility in thinking and problem solving—declines. Crystallized intelligence—gained through education and lifelong experiences (e.g., verbal skills)—remains intact. These differences exemplify the classic aging pattern of intelligence. Despite these slight declines, many older people continue to learn and participate in varied educational experiences. Good health and motivation are important influences on learning (Chart 11-4).

Pharmacologic Aspects of Aging

Because an increasing number of chronic conditions affect older people, they use more medications than any other age group. Approximately 94% of adults between the ages of 65 and 74 years take medications of some type (Meiner, 2011). Although medications improve health and well-being by

Chart 11-4 Nursing Strategies for Promoting Cognitive Function

Nurses can support the processes by which older adults learn by using the following strategies:

- Supply mnemonics to enhance recall of related data.
- Encourage ongoing learning.
- Link new information with familiar information.
- Use visual, auditory, and other sensory cues.
- Encourage learners to wear prescription glasses and hearing aids.
- Provide glare-free lighting.
- Provide a quiet, nondistracting environment.
- Set short-term goals with input from the learner.
- Keep teaching periods short.
- Pace learning tasks according to the endurance of the learner.
- Encourage verbal participation by learners.
- Reinforce successful learning in a positive manner.

relieving pain and discomfort, treating chronic illnesses, and curing infectious processes, adverse drug reactions are common because of medication interactions, multiple medication effects, incorrect dosages, and the use of multiple medications.

Drug Interactions and Adverse Effects

Polypharmacy, or the prescription, use, or administration of more medications than is clinically indicated, is common in older adults (Meiner, 2011; Miller, 2012). The potential for drug–drug interactions increases with increased medication use and with multiple coexisting diseases (**comorbidity**) that affect the absorption, distribution, metabolism, and elimination of the medications. Such interactions are responsible for numerous emergency department and physician visits, which cost billions of dollars annually.

Any medication is capable of altering nutritional status, and the nutritional health of an older adult may already be compromised by a marginal diet or by chronic disease and its treatment. Medications can affect the appetite, cause nausea and vomiting, irritate the stomach, cause constipation or diarrhea, and decrease absorption of nutrients. In addition, these medications may alter electrolyte balance as well as carbohydrate and fat metabolism. For example, antacids may cause thiamine deficiency; laxatives diminish absorption; antibiotics and phenytoin (Dilantin) reduce utilization of folic acid; and phenothiazines, estrogens, and corticosteroids increase appetite and cause weight gain.

Combining multiple medications with alcohol, as well as with over-the-counter and herbal medications, further complicates gastrointestinal problems. For example, St. John's wort, a common herbal supplement effective for mild depression, decreases the anticoagulant effect of warfarin (Coumadin) and interacts with many other medications metabolized in the liver (Miller, 2012).

Altered Pharmacokinetics

Alterations in absorption, metabolism, distribution, and excretion occur as a result of normal aging and may also result from drug and food interactions (Meiner, 2011). Absorption may be affected by changes in gastric pH and a decrease in gastrointestinal motility. Drug distribution may be altered

TABLE 11-2 Altered Drug Responses in Older People

Age-Related Changes	Effect of Age-Related Change	Applicable Medications
Absorption		
Reduced gastric acid; increased pH (less acid)	Rate of drug absorption—possibly delayed	Vitamins
Reduced gastrointestinal motility; prolonged gastric emptying	Extent of drug absorption—not affected	Calcium
Distribution		
Decreased albumin sites	Serious alterations in drug binding to plasma proteins (the unbound drug gives the pharmacologic response); highly protein-bound medications have fewer binding sites, leading to increased effects and accelerated metabolism and excretion.	*Selected highly protein-binding medications:* Oral anticoagulants (warfarin) Oral hypoglycemic agents (sulfonylureas) Barbiturates Calcium channel blockers Furosemide (Lasix) Nonsteroidal anti-inflammatory drugs (NSAIDs) Sulfonamides Quinidine Phenytoin (Dilantin)
Reduced cardiac output	Decreased perfusion of many bodily organs	
Impaired peripheral blood flow	Decreased perfusion	
Increased percentage of body fat	Proportion of body fat increases with age, resulting in increased ability to store fat-soluble medications; this causes drug accumulation, prolonged storage, and delayed excretion.	*Selected fat-soluble medications:* Barbiturates Diazepam (Valium) Lidocaine Phenothiazines (antipsychotics) Ethanol Morphine
Decreased lean body mass	Decreased body volume allows higher peak levels of medications.	
Metabolism		
Decreased cardiac output and decreased perfusion of the liver	Decreased metabolism and delay of breakdown of medications, resulting in prolonged duration of action, accumulation, and drug toxicity	All medications metabolized by the liver
Excretion		
Decreased renal blood flow; loss of functioning nephrons; decreased renal efficiency	Decreased rates of elimination and increased duration of action; danger of accumulation and drug toxicity	*Selected medications with prolonged action:* Aminoglycoside antibiotics Cimetidine (Tagamet) Chlorpropamide (Diabinese) Digoxin Lithium Procainamide

as a result of decrease in body water and increase in body fat. Normal age-related changes and diseases that alter blood flow, liver and renal function, or cardiac output may affect distribution and metabolism (Table 11-2).

Nursing Implications

Prescription principles that have been identified as appropriate for older patients include starting with a low dose, going slowly, and keeping the medication regimen as simple as possible (Meiner, 2011; Miller, 2012). A comprehensive assessment that begins with a thorough medication history, including use of alcohol, recreational drugs, and over-the-counter and herbal medications, is essential. It is best to ask the patient or reliable informants to provide all medications for review. Assessing the patient's understanding of when and how to take each medication, as well as the purpose of each medication, allows the nurse to assess the patient's knowledge about and compliance with the medication regimen. The patient's beliefs and concerns about the medications should be identified, including beliefs on whether a given medication is helpful.

Nonadherence with medication regimens can lead to significant morbidity and mortality among older adults. The many contributing factors include the number of medications prescribed, the complexity of the regimen, difficulty opening containers, inadequate patient education, financial cost, and the disease or medication interfering with the patient's life (Meiner, 2011). Furthermore, visual and hearing problems may make it difficult to read or to hear directions.

Multifaceted interventions tailored to the individual patient are the most effective strategies in improving adherence (Messina & Escallier, 2011) (Chart 11-5).

Nursing Strategies for Improving Medication Management and Adherence

The following strategies can help patients manage their medications and improve adherence:

- Explain the purpose, adverse effects, and dosage of each medication.
- Provide the medication schedule in writing.
- Encourage the use of standard containers without safety lids (if there are no children in the household).
- Suggest the use of a multiple-day, multiple-dose medication dispenser to help the patient adhere to the medication schedule.
- Destroy or remove old, unused medications.
- Encourage the patient to inform the primary health care provider about the use of over-the-counter medications and herbal agents, alcohol, and recreational drugs.
- Encourage the patient to keep a list of all medications, including over-the-counter and herbal medications, in his or her purse or wallet to share with the primary care provider at each visit and in case of an emergency.
- Review the medication schedule periodically, and update it as necessary.
- Recommend using one supplier for prescriptions; pharmacies frequently track patients and are likely to notice a prescription problem such as duplication or contraindications in the medication regimen.
- If the patient's competence is doubtful, identify a reliable family member or friend who might monitor the patient for adherence.

Mental Health Problems in the Older Adult

Changes in cognitive ability, excessive forgetfulness, and mood swings are not a part of normal aging. These symptoms should not be dismissed as age-related changes; a thorough assessment may reveal a treatable, reversible physical or mental condition. Changes in mental status may be related to many factors, such as alterations in diet and fluid and electrolyte balance, fever, or low oxygen levels associated with many cardiovascular and pulmonary diseases. Cognitive changes may be reversible when the underlying condition is identified and treated. However, the susceptibility to depression, delirium, and incidence of dementia increases with age. Older adults are less likely than younger people to acknowledge or seek treatment for mental health symptoms. Therefore, health professionals must recognize, assess, refer, collaborate, treat, and support older adults who exhibit noticeable changes in intellect or affect.

Depression

Depression is the most common affective or mood disorder of old age. Nearly 15% of older Americans suffer from depression, and between 10% and 20% of older adults have bipolar disorder (Meiner, 2011).

Depression among older adults can follow a major precipitating event or loss and is often related to chronic illness or pain. It may also be secondary to a medication interaction or an undiagnosed physical condition. Signs of depression include feelings of sadness, fatigue, diminished memory and concentration, feelings of guilt or worthlessness, sleep disturbances, appetite disturbances with excessive weight loss or gain, restlessness, impaired attention span, and suicidal ideation. Mild depression with symptoms that do not meet the criteria for a major depression is common and reduces quality of life and function (Meiner, 2011; Naegle, 2011).

The risk of suicide is increased in older adults, with approximately 84% of suicides carried out by white men (Meiner, 2011). There is a need for routine assessment of patients for depression and risk for suicide. Geriatric depression may be confused with dementia. However, the cognitive impairment resulting from depression is owing to apathy rather than decline in brain function. When depression and medical illnesses coexist, as they often do, neglect of the depression can impede physical recovery. Assessing the patient's mental status, including depression, is vital and must not be overlooked. A commonly used assessment tool is the Geriatric Depression Scale (GDS) (Chart 11-6).

Depression does respond appropriately to treatment but is often not recognized and therefore is undertreated. Initial management involves evaluation of the patient's medication regimen and eliminating or changing any medications that contribute to depression. Furthermore, treatment of underlying medical conditions that may produce depressive symptoms may alleviate the depression. For mild depression, nonpharmacologic measures such as exercise, bright lighting, increasing interpersonal interactions, cognitive therapy, and reminiscence therapy are effective. However, for major depression, antidepressants and short-term psychotherapy, particularly in combination, are effective in older adults. Atypical antidepressants, such as bupropion (Wellbutrin), venlafaxine (Effexor), mirtazapine (Remeron), and nefazodone (Serzone), as well as selective serotonin reuptake inhibitors, such as paroxetine (Paxil), are effective (Karch, 2012; Kauffman, 2009). Tricyclic antidepressants can be useful for treating major depression in some patients. Electroconvulsive therapy is highly effective when antidepressant medications are not tolerated, not effective, or pose a significant medical risk (Miller, 2012).

Most antidepressant medications have anticholinergic, cardiac, and orthostatic adverse effects (Karch, 2012). They also interact with other medications and therefore should be used with care to avoid medication toxicity, hypotensive events, and falls. Good patient education is needed to make sure older adults understand that it may take 4 to 6 weeks for symptoms to diminish. During this period, nurses should offer support, encouragement, and strategies to maintain safety, such as changing positions slowly and maintaining adequate hydration (Miller, 2012).

Substance Abuse

Substance abuse caused by misuse of alcohol and drugs may be related to depression. Thirty-six percent of adults 65 years and older report that they are current drinkers; 2% of men and less than 1% of women meet the criteria for alcohol abuse (Miller, 2012). Moderate levels of alcohol consumption may be associated with positive health risks, such as lowering the risks for cardiovascular disease. Alcohol abuse, while rare, is especially dangerous in older people because of age-related changes in renal and liver function as well as the high risk of

Chart 11-6   Geriatric Depression Scale

Choose the best answer for how you felt this past week.

*1.	Are you basically satisfied with your life?	YES	NO
2.	Have you dropped many of your activities and interests?	YES	NO
3.	Do you feel that your life is empty?	YES	NO
4.	Do you often get bored?	YES	NO
*5.	Are you hopeful about the future?	YES	NO
6.	Are you bothered by thoughts you can't get out of your head?	YES	NO
*7.	Are you in good spirits most of the time?	YES	NO
8.	Are you afraid that something bad is going to happen to you?	YES	NO
*9.	Do you feel happy most of the time?	YES	NO
10.	Do you often feel helpless?	YES	NO
11.	Do you often get restless and fidgety?	YES	NO
12.	Do you prefer to stay at home, rather than going out and doing new things?	YES	NO
13.	Do you frequently worry about the future?	YES	NO
14.	Do you feel you have more problems with memory than most?	YES	NO
*15.	Do you think it is wonderful to be alive now?	YES	NO
16.	Do you often feel downhearted and blue?	YES	NO
17.	Do you feel pretty worthless the way you are now?	YES	NO
18.	Do you worry a lot about the past?	YES	NO
*19.	Do you find life very exciting?	YES	NO
20.	Is it hard for you to get started on new projects?	YES	NO
*21.	Do you feel full of energy?	YES	NO
22.	Do you feel that your situation is hopeless?	YES	NO
23.	Do you think that most people are better off than you are?	YES	NO
24.	Do you frequently get upset over little things?	YES	NO
25.	Do you frequently feel like crying?	YES	NO
26.	Do you have trouble concentrating?	YES	NO
*27.	Do you enjoy getting up in the morning?	YES	NO
28.	Do you prefer to avoid social gatherings?	YES	NO
*29.	Is it easy for you to make decisions?	YES	NO
*30.	Is your mind as clear as it used to be?	YES	NO

Score: _____ (*Number of "depressed" answers*)

Norms

Normal: 5 ± 4
Mildly depressed: 15 ± 6
Very depressed: 23 ± 5

*Appropriate (nondepressed) answers = yes; all others = no.
From Yesavage, J., Brink, T. L., Rose, T. L., et al. (1983). Development and validation of a geriatric screening scale: A preliminary report. *Journal of Psychiatric Research*, *17*(1), 37–49. Reprinted with permission from Pergamon Press Ltd., Headington Hill Hall, Oxford OX3 OBW, UK. Used with permission.

interactions with prescription medications and the resultant adverse effects. Alcohol and drug-related problems in older people often remain hidden because many older adults deny their habit when questioned. Assessing for drug and alcohol use with direct questions in a nonaccusatory manner should be part of the routine physical assessment (Meiner, 2011; Miller, 2012). (See Chapter 5 for more information and specific assessment tools.)

Delirium

Delirium, often called *acute confusional state*, begins with confusion and progresses to disorientation. It is a common and life-threatening complication for the hospitalized older adult and the most frequent complication of hospitalization, occurring in 7% to 61% of older people, with associated morbidity ranging from 6% to 18% in this group (Meiner, 2011). Patients may experience an altered level of consciousness, ranging from stupor (hypoalert–hypoactive) to excessive activity (hyperalert–hyperactive); alternatively, they may have a combination of these two types (mixed). Thinking is disorganized, and the attention span is short. Hallucinations, delusions, fear, anxiety, and paranoia may also be evident. Patients who tend to be hyperalert and hyperactive demand more attention from nurses and thus are easier to diagnose, whereas those who are hypoalert or hypoactive tend to be less problematic and pose diagnostic difficulties. Recognition of delirium can also be complicated in patients with the mixed disorders. Patients with the hypoalert–hypoactive type of delirium have higher mortality rates and even poorer outcomes of care because the delirium tends not to be recognized and treated (Meiner, 2011; Miller, 2012).

Attentive clinical assessment is essential because delirium is sometimes mistaken for dementia; Table 11-3 compares dementia and delirium. It helps to know an individual patient's usual mental status and whether the changes noted are long term, which probably represents dementia, or are abrupt in onset, which is more likely delirium.

Delirium occurs secondary to numerous causes, including physical illness, medication or alcohol toxicity, dehydration,

TABLE 11-3   Summary of Differences Between Dementia and Delirium

	Dementia		Delirium
	Alzheimer's Disease (AD)	**Vascular (Multi-Infarct) Dementia**	**Delirium**
Etiology	Early onset (familial, genetic [chromosomes 14, 19, 21]) Late-onset sporadic	Cardiovascular (CV) disease Cerebrovascular disease Hypertension	Drug toxicity and interactions; acute disease; trauma; chronic disease exacerbation Fluid and electrolyte disorders
Risk factors	Advanced age; genetics	Preexisting CV disease	Preexisting cognitive impairment
Occurrence	50%–60% of dementias	10%–20% of dementias	7%–61% among hospitalized people
Onset	Slow	Often abrupt Follows a stroke or transient ischemic attack	Rapid, acute onset A harbinger of acute medical illness
Age of onset	Early-onset AD: 30s–65 y Late onset AD: 65+ y Most commonly: 85+ y	Most commonly 50–70 y	Any age, although predominantly in older persons
Gender	Males and females equally	Predominantly males	Males and females equally
Course	Chronic, irreversible; progressive, regular, downhill	Chronic, irreversible Fluctuating, stepwise progression	Acute onset Hypoalert–hypoactive Hyperalert–hyperactive Mixed hypo–hyper
Duration	2–20 y	Variable; years	Lasts 1 d to 1 mo
Symptom progress	Onset insidious: *Early*—mild and subtle *Middle and late*—intensified Progression to death (infection or malnutrition)	Depends on location of infarct and success of treatment; death attributed to underlying CV disease	Symptoms are fully reversible with adequate treatment; can progress to chronicity or death if underlying condition is ignored.
Mood	Early depression (30%)	Labile: mood swings	Variable
Speech/language	Speech remains intact until late in disease: *Early*—mild anomia (cannot name objects); deficits progress until speech lacks meaning; echoes and repeats words and sounds; mutism *Early*—no motor deficits	May have speech deficit/aphasia depending on location of lesion	Fluctuating; often cannot concentrate long enough to speak May be somnolent
Physical signs	*Middle*—apraxia (70%) (cannot perform purposeful movement) *Late*—Dysarthria (impaired speech) *End stage*—loss of all voluntary activity; positive neurologic signs	According to location of lesion: focal neurologic signs, seizures Commonly exhibits motor deficits	Signs and symptoms of underlying disease
Orientation	Becomes lost in familiar places (topographic disorientation) Has difficulty drawing three-dimensional objects (visual and spatial disorientation) Disorientation to time, place, and person—with disease progression		May fluctuate between lucidity and complete disorientation to time, place, and person
Memory	Loss is an early sign of dementia; loss of recent memory is soon followed by progressive decline in recent and remote memory		Impaired recent and remote memory; may fluctuate between lucidity and confusion
Personality	Apathy, indifference, irritability: *Early disease*—social behavior intact; hides cognitive deficits *Advanced disease*—disengages from activity and relationships; suspicious; paranoid delusions caused by memory loss; aggressive; catastrophic reactions		Fluctuating; cannot focus attention to converse; alarmed by symptoms (when lucid); hallucinations; paranoid
Functional status, activities of daily living	Poor judgment in everyday activities; has progressive decline in ability to handle money, use telephone, use computer and other electronic devices, function in home and workplace		Impaired
Attention span	Distractible; short attention span		Highly impaired; cannot maintain or shift attention
Psychomotor activity	Wandering, hyperactivity, pacing, restlessness, agitation		Variable; alternates between high agitation, hyperactivity, restlessness, and lethargy
Sleep–wake cycle	Often impaired; wandering and agitation at nighttime		Takes brief naps throughout day and night

fecal impaction, malnutrition, infection, head trauma, lack of environmental cues, and sensory deprivation or overload. Older adults are particularly vulnerable to acute confusion because of their decreased biologic reserve and the large number of medications they may take. Nurses must recognize the implications of the acute symptoms of delirium and report them immediately. Because of the acute and unexpected onset of symptoms and the unknown underlying cause, delirium is a medical emergency. If the delirium goes unrecognized and the underlying cause is not treated, permanent, irreversible brain damage or death can follow.

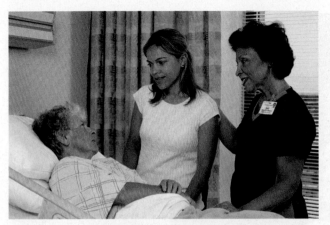

FIGURE 11-4 • Talking to family members may increase the comfort of patients with delirium.

The most effective approach is prevention. Strategies include providing therapeutic activities for cognitive impairment, ensuring early mobilization, controlling pain, minimizing the use of psychoactive drugs, preventing sleep deprivation, enhancing communication methods (particularly eye glasses and hearing aids) for vision and hearing impairment, maintaining oxygen levels and fluid and electrolyte balance, and preventing surgical complications (Meiner, 2011; Miller, 2012).

Once delirium occurs, treatment of the underlying cause is most important. Therapeutic interventions vary depending on the cause. Delirium increases the risk of falls; therefore, management of patient safety and behavioral problems is essential. Because medication interactions and toxicity are often implicated, nonessential medications should be discontinued. Nutritional and fluid intake should be supervised and monitored. The environment should be quiet and calm. To increase function and comfort, the nurse provides familiar environmental cues and encourages family members or friends to touch and talk to the patient (Fig. 11-4). Ongoing mental status assessments using prior mental cognitive status as a baseline are helpful in evaluating responses to treatment and upon admission to a hospital or extended care facility. If the underlying problem is adequately treated, the patient often returns to baseline within several days. Several resources specific to delirium are included in the Resources section at the end of the chapter.

Dementia

The cognitive, functional, and behavioral changes that characterize **dementia** eventually destroy a person's ability to function. The symptoms are usually subtle in onset and often progress slowly until they are obvious and devastating. The two most common types of dementia are AD and vascular or multi-infarct dementia (Meiner, 2011; Miller, 2012). Other non-Alzheimer dementias include Parkinson's disease, acquired immunodeficiency syndrome (AIDS)-related dementia, Pick's disease, and other types of frontotemporal dementia. It is important to identify reversible dementia, which occurs when pathologic conditions masquerade as dementia (Meiner, 2011).

Alzheimer's Disease

AD, the fifth leading cause of death for older adults, is a progressive, irreversible, degenerative neurologic disease that begins insidiously and is characterized by gradual losses of cognitive function and disturbances in behavior and affect. AD can occur in people as young as 40 years of age but is uncommon before 65 years of age. Although the prevalence of AD increases dramatically with increasing age, affecting as many as half of those 85 years and older, it is important to note that AD is not a normal part of aging. Without a cure or any preventive measures, it is estimated that 13.4 million Americans will have this disease by 2050 (Meiner, 2011).

There are numerous theories about the cause of age-related cognitive decline. Although the greatest risk factor for AD is increasing age, many environmental, dietary, and inflammatory factors also may determine whether a person suffers from this cognitive disease. AD is a complex brain disorder caused by a combination of various factors that may include genetics, neurotransmitter changes, vascular abnormalities, stress hormones, circadian changes, head trauma, and the presence of seizure disorders.

AD can be classified into two types: familial or early-onset AD and sporadic or late-onset AD (see Table 8-5). Familial AD is rare, accounting for less than 10% of all cases, and is frequently associated with genetic mutations. It occurs in middle-aged adults. If family members have at least one other relative with AD, then there is a familial component, which nonspecifically includes both environmental triggers and genetic determinants.

Pathophysiology

Specific neuropathologic and biochemical changes are found in patients with AD. These include neurofibrillary tangles (tangled masses of nonfunctioning neurons) and senile or neuritic plaques (deposits of amyloid protein, part of a larger protein called *amyloid precursor protein* in the brain) (Fig. 11-5). The neuronal damage occurs primarily in the cerebral cortex and results in decreased brain size. Similar changes are found in the normal brain tissue of older adults, although to a lesser extent. Cells that use the neurotransmitter acetylcholine are principally affected by AD. At the biochemical level, the enzyme active in producing acetylcholine, which is specifically involved in memory processing, is decreased.

Scientists have been studying complex neurodegenerative diseases such as AD and have focused on two key issues: whether a gene might influence a person's overall risk of developing the disease, and whether a gene might influence some particular aspect of a person's risk, such as the age at which the disease begins (age at onset). There are genetic differences in early- and late-onset forms of AD. Researchers are investigating what predisposes people to develop the plaques and neurofibrillary tangles that can be seen at autopsy in the brains of patients with AD. Understanding of the complex ways in which aging and genetic and nongenetic factors affect brain cells over time, eventually leading to AD, continues to increase. Researchers have discovered how amyloid plaques form and cause neuronal death, the possible relationship between various forms of *tau* protein and impaired function, the roles of inflammation and oxidative stress, and the contribution of brain infarctions to the disease (Meiner, 2011).

Clinical Manifestations

In the early stages of AD, forgetfulness and subtle memory loss occur. Patients may experience small difficulties in

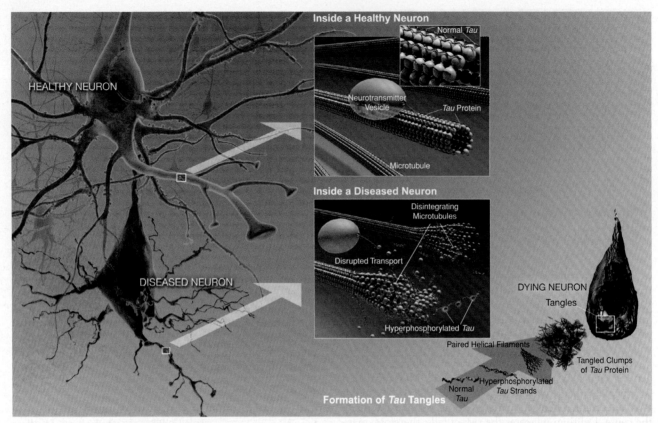

FIGURE 11-5 • Healthy and diseased neurons and formation of *tau* tangles. From National Institute on Aging, National Institutes of Health, Alzheimer's Disease Education and Referral Center. Available at: www.nia.nih.gov/alzheimers/scientific-images

work or social activities but have adequate cognitive function to compensate for the loss and continue to function independently. With further progression of AD, the deficits can no longer be concealed. Forgetfulness is manifested in many daily actions; patients may lose their ability to recognize familiar faces, places, and objects, and they may become lost in a familiar environment. They may repeat the same stories because they forget that they have already told them. Trying to reason with people with AD and using reality **orientation** only increase their anxiety without increasing function. Conversation becomes difficult, and word-finding difficulties occur. The ability to formulate concepts and think abstractly disappears—for example, a patient can interpret a proverb only in concrete terms. Patients are often unable to recognize the consequences of their actions and therefore exhibit impulsive behavior—for example, on a hot day, a patient may decide to wade in the city fountain fully clothed. Patients have difficulty with everyday activities, such as operating simple appliances and handling money.

Personality changes are also usually evident. Patients may become depressed, suspicious, paranoid, hostile, and even combative. Progression of the disease intensifies the symptoms: Speaking skills deteriorate to nonsense syllables, agitation and physical activity increase, and patients may wander at night. Eventually, assistance is needed for most ADLs, including eating and toileting, because dysphagia and incontinence develop. The terminal stage, in which patients are usually immobile and require total care, may last months or years. Occasionally, patients may recognize family members or caregivers. Death occurs as a result of complications such as pneumonia, malnutrition, or dehydration.

Assessment and Diagnostic Findings

A definitive diagnosis of AD can be made only at autopsy; however, an accurate clinical diagnosis can be made in approximately 90% of cases. The most important goal is to rule out other causes of dementia or reversible causes of confusion, such as other types of dementia, depression, delirium, alcohol or drug abuse, or inappropriate drug dosage or drug toxicity (Murphy & Hickey, 2010). AD is a diagnosis of exclusion, and a diagnosis of probable AD is made when the medical history, physical examination, and laboratory tests have excluded all known causes of other dementias.

The health history—including medical history, family history, social and cultural history, and medication history—and the physical examination, including functional and mental health status, are essential to the diagnosis of probable AD. Diagnostic tests, including complete blood count, chemistry profile, and vitamin B_{12} and thyroid hormone levels, as well as screening with electroencephalography, computed tomography (CT) scanning, magnetic resonance imaging (MRI), and examination of the cerebrospinal fluid may all refute or support a diagnosis of probable AD.

Depression can closely mimic early-stage AD and coexists in many patients. Therefore, assessing the patient for underlying depression is important. The GDS is a useful tool to assess for depression (see Chart 11-6).

Tools such as the MMSE (see Chart 11-3) are useful for assessing cognitive status and screening for AD. Both CT scanning and MRI of the brain are useful for excluding hematoma, brain tumor, stroke, normal-pressure hydrocephalus, and atrophy but are not reliable in making a definitive diagnosis of AD (Murphy & Hickey, 2010). Infections and physiologic disturbances, such as hypothyroidism, Parkinson's disease, and vitamin B_{12} deficiency, can cause cognitive impairment that may be misdiagnosed as AD. Biochemical abnormalities can be excluded through examination of the blood and cerebrospinal fluid.

Medical Management

In AD, the primary goal is to manage the cognitive and behavioral symptoms. Although there is no cure, several medications have been introduced to slow the progression of the disease (Meiner, 2011). The cholinesterase inhibitors (CEIs) donepezil hydrochloride (Aricept), rivastigmine tartrate (Exelon), and galantamine hydrobromide (Razadyne [formerly known as Reminyl]) enhance acetylcholine uptake in the brain, thus maintaining memory skills for a period of time; these and other medications are used for mild to moderate symptoms. Cognitive ability may improve within 6 to 12 months of therapy; however, cessation of the medications results in disease progression and cognitive decline. It is recommended that treatment continue at least through the moderate stage of the illness. Combination of a CEI with memantine (Namenda) may be useful for mild to moderate cognitive symptoms (Press & Alexander, 2011).

Behavioral problems such as agitation and psychosis can be managed by behavioral and psychosocial therapies. Associated depression and behavioral problems can also be treated pharmacologically if other interventions fail. Because symptoms change over time, all patients with AD should be reevaluated routinely, and the nurse should document and report both positive or negative responses to medications (Meiner, 2011; Miller, 2012).

Nursing Management

Nurses play an important role in the recognition of dementia, particularly in hospitalized older adults, by assessing for signs (e.g., repeating or asking the same thing over and over, getting lost) during the nursing admission assessment. Nursing interventions for dementia are aimed at promoting patient function and independence for as long as possible (Murphy & Hickey, 2010). Other important goals include promoting the patient's physical safety, promoting independence in self-care activities, reducing anxiety and agitation, improving communication, providing for socialization and intimacy, promoting adequate nutrition, promoting balanced activity and rest, and supporting and educating family caregivers. These nursing interventions apply to all patients with dementia, regardless of cause.

Supporting Cognitive Function. Because dementia of any type is degenerative and progressive, patients display a decline in cognitive function over time. In the early phase of dementia, minimal cuing and guidance may be all that are needed for the patient to function fairly independently for a number of years. However, as the patient's cognitive ability declines, family members must provide more and more assistance and supervision. A calm, predictable environment helps people with dementia interpret their surroundings and activities. Environmental stimuli are limited, and a regular routine is established. A quiet, pleasant manner of speaking, clear and simple explanations, and the use of memory aids and cues help minimize confusion and disorientation and give patients a sense of security. Prominently displayed clocks and calendars may enhance orientation to time. Color-coding the doorway may help patients who have difficulty locating their room. Active participation may help patients maintain cognitive, functional, and social interaction abilities for a longer period. Physical activity and communication have also been demonstrated to slow some of the cognitive decline of AD.

Promoting Physical Safety. A safe home and hospital environment allows the patient to move about as freely as possible and relieves the family of constant worry about safety. To prevent falls and other injuries, all obvious hazards are removed and hand rails are installed in the home. A hazard-free environment allows the patient maximum independence and a sense of autonomy. Adequate lighting, especially in halls, stairs, and bathrooms, is necessary. Nightlights are helpful, particularly if the patient has increased confusion at night (**sundowning**). Driving is prohibited, and smoking is allowed only with supervision. The patient may have a short attention span and be forgetful. Wandering behavior can often be reduced by gentle persuasion, distraction, or by placing the patient close to the nursing station. Restraints should be avoided because they increase agitation. Doors leading from the house must be secured. Outside the home, all activities must be supervised to protect the patient, and the patient should wear an identification bracelet or neck chain in case of separation from the caregiver.

Promoting Independence in Self-Care Activities. Pathophysiologic changes in the brain make it difficult for people with AD to maintain physical independence. Patients should be assisted to remain functionally independent for as long as possible. One way to do this is to simplify daily activities by organizing them into short, achievable steps so that the patient experiences a sense of accomplishment. Frequently, occupational therapists can suggest ways to simplify tasks or recommend adaptive equipment. Direct patient supervision is sometimes necessary; however, maintaining personal dignity and autonomy is important for people with AD, who should be encouraged to make choices when appropriate and to participate in self-care activities as much as possible.

Reducing Anxiety and Agitation. Despite profound cognitive losses, patients are sometimes aware of their diminishing abilities. Patients need constant emotional support that reinforces a positive self-image. When loss of skills occurs, goals are adjusted to fit the patient's declining ability.

The environment should be kept familiar and noise free. Excitement and confusion can be upsetting and may precipitate a combative, agitated state known as a catastrophic reaction (overreaction to excessive stimulation). The patient may respond by screaming, crying, or becoming abusive (physically or verbally); this may be the patient's only way of expressing an inability to cope with the environment. When this occurs, it is important to remain calm and unhurried. Forcing the patient to proceed with the activity only increases the agitation. It is better to postpone the activity until later, even to another day. Frequently, the patient quickly forgets what triggered the reaction. Measures such as moving to a familiar environment, listening to music, stroking, rocking, or distraction may quiet the patient. Structuring activity is also helpful. Becoming familiar with a particular patient's predicted responses to certain stressors helps caregivers avoid similar situations.

Patients with dementia who have progressed to the late stages of the disease often reside in nursing homes and are predominantly cared for by unlicensed assistive personnel. Dementia education for caregivers is essential to minimize patient agitation and can be effectively taught by geriatric advanced nurse practitioners.

Improving Communication. To promote the patient's interpretation of messages, the nurse should remain unhurried and reduce noises and distractions. Use of clear, easy-to-understand sentences to convey messages is essential because patients frequently forget the meaning of words or have difficulty organizing and expressing thoughts. In the earlier stages of dementia, lists and simple written instructions that serve as reminders may be helpful. In later stages, the patient may be able to point to an object or use nonverbal language to communicate. Tactile stimuli, such as hugs or hand pats, are usually interpreted as signs of affection, concern, and security.

Providing for Socialization and Intimacy Needs. Because socialization with friends can be comforting, visits, letters, and phone calls are encouraged. Visits should be brief and nonstressful; limiting visitors to one or two at a time helps reduce overstimulation. Recreation is important, and people with dementia are encouraged to participate in simple activities. Realistic goals for activities that provide satisfaction are appropriate. Hobbies and activities such as walking, exercising, and socializing can improve quality of life. The nonjudgmental friendliness of a pet may provide stimulation, comfort, and contentment. Care of plants or a pet can also be satisfying and an outlet for energy.

AD does not eliminate the need for intimacy. Patients and their spouses may continue to enjoy sexual activity. Spouses should be encouraged to talk about any sexual concerns, and sexual counseling may be necessary. Simple expressions of love, such as touching and holding, are often meaningful.

Promoting Adequate Nutrition. Mealtime can be a pleasant social occasion or a time of upset and distress, and it should be kept simple and calm, without confrontations. Patients prefer familiar foods that look appetizing and taste good. To avoid any "playing" with food, one dish is offered at a time. Food is cut into small pieces to prevent choking. Liquids may be easier to swallow if they are converted to gelatin. Hot food and beverages are served warm, and the temperature of the foods should be checked to prevent burns.

When lack of coordination interferes with self-feeding, adaptive equipment is helpful (Fig. 11-6). Some patients may do well eating with a spoon or with their fingers. If this is the case, an apron or a smock, rather than a bib, is used to protect clothing. As deficits progress, it may become necessary to feed the patient. Forgetfulness, disinterest, dental problems, lack of coordination, overstimulation, and choking all serve as barriers to good nutrition and hydration.

Promoting Balanced Activity and Rest. Many patients with dementia exhibit sleep disturbances, wandering, and

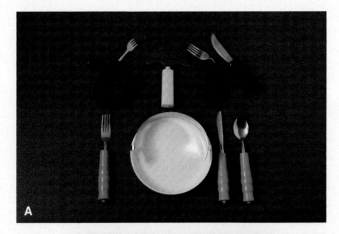

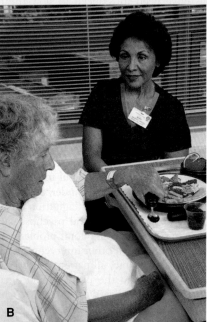

FIGURE 11-6 • A. Assistive feeding devices make it easy for patients to grasp and get food on utensils. B. Assistive feeding devices may be required for patients who are weak, fatigued, or paralyzed or have neuromuscular impairment.

behaviors that may be considered inappropriate. These behaviors are most likely to occur when there are unmet underlying physical or psychological needs. Caregivers must identify the needs of patients who are exhibiting these behaviors because further health decline may occur if the source of the problem is not corrected. Adequate sleep and physical exercise are essential. If sleep is interrupted or the patient cannot fall asleep, music, warm milk, or a back rub may help the patient relax. During the day, patients should be encouraged to participate in exercise because a regular pattern of activity and rest enhances nighttime sleep. Long periods of daytime sleeping are discouraged.

Supporting Home and Community-Based Care. The emotional burden on the families of patients with all types of dementia is enormous. The physical health of the patient is often very stable, and the mental degeneration is gradual. Family members may cling to the hope that the diagnosis is incorrect and that their relative will improve with greater effort. Family members are faced with numerous difficult decisions (e.g., when the patient should stop driving, when to assume responsibility for the patient's financial affairs). Aggression and hostility exhibited by the patient are often misunderstood by families or caregivers, who feel unappreciated, frustrated, and angry. Feelings of guilt, nervousness, and worry contribute to caregiver fatigue, depression, and family dysfunction.

Neglect or abuse of the patient can occur, and this has been documented in home situations as well as in institutions. If neglect or abuse of any kind—including physical, emotional, sexual, or financial abuse—is suspected, the local adult protective services agency must be notified. The responsibility of the nurse is to report the suspected abuse, not to prove it.

The Alzheimer's Association is a coalition of family members and professionals who share the goals of family support and service, education, research, and advocacy. Family support groups, respite (relief) care, and adult day care may be available through different community resources, such as the Area Agency on Aging, in which concerned volunteers are trained to provide structure to caregiver support groups. Respite care is a commonly provided service in which caregivers can get away from the home for short periods while someone else tends to the needs of the patient.

Vascular Dementia

Vascular dementia is associated with cerebrovascular disease in the form of multiple infarcts or strokes, a single larger infarct, or small vessel disease (Grand, Caspar, & MacDonald, 2011). Vascular dementia affects approximately 10% to 20% of people with dementia; the rate is higher in men than women, tends to have a more abrupt onset than AD, and is characterized by an uneven, stepwise downward decline in mental function. Multi-infarct dementia, the most common form of vascular dementia, has an unpredictable course and is characterized by variable impairment depending on the affected sites in the brain. The patient may present with a deficit in only one domain, such as word retrieval, whereas other cognitive abilities may be intact. Diagnosis may be even more difficult if a patient has vascular dementia as well as AD.

Because vascular dementia is associated with hypertension and cardiovascular disease, risk factors (e.g., hypercholesterolemia, history of smoking, diabetes) are similar. Prevention and management are also similar. Therefore, measures to decrease blood pressure and lower cholesterol levels may prevent future infarcts.

Geriatric Syndromes

Older people tend to acquire multiple problems and illnesses as they age. The decline of physical function leads to a loss of independence and increasing frailty as well as to susceptibility to both acute and chronic health problems, which generally result from several factors rather than from a single cause. When combined with a decrease in host resistance, these factors can lead to illness or injury. A number of problems commonly experienced by older adults are becoming recognized as **geriatric syndromes**. These conditions do not fit into discrete disease categories and require a multidisciplinary and comprehensive assessment to identify the underlying cause or causes. Examples include skin impairment, poor nutrition, falls or functional decline, incontinence, cognitive impairment, skin impairment, and sleep disturbances (Weber & Kelley, 2010). Although these conditions may develop slowly, the onset of symptoms is often acute. Furthermore, the presenting symptoms may appear in other body systems before becoming apparent in the affected system. For example, an older patient may present with confusion, and the underlying disease may be a urinary tract infection, dehydration, or a heart attack.

An additional term, *geriatric triad*, includes changes in cognitive status, falls, and incontinence (Meiner, 2011). This term is used to bring attention to these three conditions that need particular attention and the implementation of preventative measures during the hospitalization of older patients.

Impaired Mobility

The causes of decreased mobility are many and varied. Common causes include strokes, Parkinson's disease, diabetic neuropathy, cardiovascular compromise, osteoarthritis, osteoporosis, and sensory deficits. To avoid immobility, older people should be encouraged to stay as active as possible. During illness, bed rest should be kept to a minimum, even with hospitalized patients, because brief periods of bed rest quickly lead to deconditioning and, consequently, to a wide range of complications. When bed rest cannot be avoided, patients should perform active range-of-motion and strengthening exercises with the unaffected extremities, and nurses or family caregivers should perform passive range-of-motion exercises on the affected extremities (Meiner, 2011; Miller 2012). Frequent position changes help offset the hazards of immobility. Both the health care staff and the patient's family can assist in maintaining the current level of mobility. Nurse researchers have identified benefits from in-hospital physical activity for older patients (see Chart 11-2).

Dizziness

Older people frequently seek help for dizziness, which presents a particular challenge because there are numerous possible causes. For many, the problem is complicated by an inability to differentiate between true dizziness (a sensation of disorientation in relation to position) and vertigo (a spinning sensation). Other similar sensations include nearsyncope and disequilibrium. The causes for these sensations range in severity from minor (e.g., buildup of ear wax) to severe (e.g., dysfunction of the cerebral cortex, cerebellum, brain stem, proprioceptive receptors, or vestibular system). Even a minor reversible cause, such as ear wax impaction, can result in a loss of balance and a subsequent fall and injury. Because dizziness has many predisposing factors, nurses should seek to identify any potentially treatable factors related to the condition.

Falls and Falling

Injuries rank seventh as a cause of death for older people, and falls are the most common cause of nonfatal injuries and hospital admissions. In 2007, more than 18,000 older adults died from unintentional fall injuries (Centers for Disease Control and Prevention [CDC], 2010). The incidence of falls rises with increasing age. It tends to be highest in people who are 85 years and older, and outcomes are worst in these adults. Some causes of falls are treatable.

Although many falls by older adults do not result in injury, between 20% and 30% of older people who fall sustain moderate to serious injury. Overall, older women who fall sustain a greater degree of injury than do older men; however, men are more likely to die of a fall injury (CDC, 2010). Hip fracture is a common type of fracture that can occur as a result of a fall. Many older adults who fall and sustain a hip fracture are unable to regain their pre-fracture ability. Causes of falls are multifactorial. Both extrinsic factors such as changes in the environment or poor lighting and intrinsic factors such as physical illness, neurologic changes, or sensory impairment play a role. Mobility difficulties, medication effects, foot problems or unsafe footwear, postural hypotension, visual problems, and tripping hazards are common and treatable causes. Polypharmacy, medication interactions, and the use of alcohol precipitate falls by causing drowsiness, decreased coordination, and postural hypotension. Falls have physical dangers as well as serious psychological and social consequences. It is not uncommon for an older person who has experienced a fall to become fearful and lose self-confidence (Meiner, 2011; Miller, 2012).

Nurses can encourage older adults and their families to make lifestyle and environmental changes to prevent falls. Adequate lighting with minimal glare and shadow can be achieved through the use of small area lamps, indirect lighting, sheer curtains to diffuse direct sunlight, dull rather than shiny surfaces, and nightlights. Sharply contrasting colors can be used to mark the edges of stairs. Grab bars by the bathtub, shower, and toilet are useful. Loose clothing, improperly fitting shoes, scatter rugs, small objects, and pets create hazards and increase the risk of falls. Older adults function best in familiar settings when the arrangement of furniture and objects remains unchanged.

> ▶ **Quality and Safety Nursing Alert**
>
> In hospitalized and institutionalized older adults, physical restraints (lap belts; geriatric chairs; vest, waist, and jacket restraints) and chemical restraints (medications) precipitate many of the injuries they were meant to prevent. Because of the overwhelming negative consequences of restraint use, accrediting agencies of nursing homes and acute care facilities now maintain stringent guidelines concerning their use.

Urinary Incontinence

Urinary incontinence may be acute, occurring during an illness, or may develop chronically over a period of years. Older patients often do not report this very common problem unless specifically asked. Transient causes may be attributed to *d*elirium and *d*ehydration; *r*estricted mobility; *i*nflammation, *i*nfection, and *i*mpaction; and *p*harmaceuticals and *p*olyuria (the acronym *drip* may be used to remember them). Once identified, the causative factor can be eliminated.

Older patients with incontinence should be urged to seek help from appropriate health care providers because incon-

tinence can be both emotionally devastating and physically debilitating. Nurses who specialize in behavioral approaches to urinary incontinence management can help patients regain full continence or significantly improve the level of continence. Although medications such as anticholinergics may decrease some of the symptoms of urge incontinence (detrusor instability), the adverse effects of these medications (dry mouth, slowed gastrointestinal motility, and confusion) may make them inappropriate choices for older adults. Various surgical procedures are also used to manage urinary incontinence, particularly stress urinary incontinence.

Detrusor hyperactivity with impaired contractility is a type of urge incontinence that is seen predominantly in the older adult population. In this variation of urge incontinence, patients have no warning that they are about to urinate. They often void only a small volume of urine or none at all and then experience a large volume of incontinence after leaving the bathroom. The nursing staff should be familiar with this form of incontinence and should not show disapproval when it occurs. Many patients with dementia suffer from this type of incontinence, because both incontinence and dementia are a result of dysfunction in similar areas of the brain. Prompted, timed voiding can be of assistance in these patients, although clean intermittent catheterization may be necessary because of postvoid residual urine. (See Chapter 55 for information on management of urinary disorders.)

Increased Susceptibility to Infection

Infectious diseases present a significant threat of morbidity and mortality to older people, in part because of the blunted response of host defenses caused by a reduction in both cell-mediated and humoral immunity (see Chapters 35 and 36). Age-related loss of physiologic reserve and chronic illnesses also contribute to increased susceptibility. Pneumonia, urinary tract infections, tuberculosis (TB), gastrointestinal infections, and skin infections are some of the common infections in older people.

The effects of influenza and pneumococcal infections on older people are significant. Estimates by the CDC (2011a) reveal that 90% of seasonal flu–related deaths and more than 60% of seasonal flu–related hospitalizations occur in those 65 years and older, primarily because of age-related weakened immune response. More than half of the deaths occurred in adults who had not received the recommended vaccination against pneumococcal disease. There is a national goal to achieve an increase in coverage for pneumococcal polysaccharide vaccine among persons 65 years and older. By 2009, almost 67% of those in this age group reported receiving an influenza vaccination during the past 12 months, and 61% reported that they had ever received a pneumococcal vaccination (AoA, 2010b).

Influenza and pneumococcal vaccinations lower the risks of hospitalization and death in older people. The influenza vaccine, which is prepared yearly to adjust for the specific immunologic characteristics of the influenza viruses at that time, should be administered annually in autumn. The pneumococcal vaccine, which has 23 type-specific capsular polysaccharides, should be administered every 5 years. Both of these injections can be received at the same time in separate injection sites. Nurses should urge older people to be vaccinated. All health care providers working with older people or high-risk chronically ill people should also be immunized.

TB affects a significant number of older adults. Case rates for TB are highest among those who are 65 years or older, with the exception of people with human immunodeficiency virus (HIV) infection. Residents of long-term care facilities account for most TB cases in older adults. Much of the infection rate is attributed to reactivation of old infection. Pulmonary TB and extrapulmonary TB often have subtle, nonspecific symptoms, which is of particular concern in nursing facilities because an active case of TB places patients and staff at risk for infection.

CDC guidelines suggest that all patients newly admitted to nursing homes have a Mantoux (purified protein derivative [PPD]) test unless there is a history of TB or a previous positive response (CDC, 2011b). All patients whose tests are negative (a positive test is indicated by induration of more than 10 mm at 48 to 72 hours) should have a second test in 1 to 2 weeks. The first PPD serves to boost the suppressed immune response that may occur in older people. Chest x-rays and possibly sputum studies should be used to follow up on PPD-positive responders and converters. For positive converters, a course of preventive therapy for 6 to 9 months with isoniazid (INH) is effective in eliminating active disease. All patients who test negative should be periodically retested (see Chapter 23).

AIDS occurs across the age spectrum. It is increasingly recognized that AIDS does not spare the older segment of society, and many who are living with HIV/AIDS are aging. In the past, male homosexual contact and blood transfusions were the predominant modes of transmission among older patients. Transmission by contaminated blood is now rare, and the predominant mode of transmission in older people is through sexual contact (Meiner, 2011).

Atypical Responses

Many altered physical, emotional, and systemic reactions to disease are attributed to age-related changes in older people. Physical indicators of illness that are useful and reliable in young and middle-aged people cannot be relied on for the diagnosis of potential life-threatening problems in older adults. The response to pain in older people may be lessened because of reduced acuity of touch, alterations in neural pathways, and diminished processing of sensory data.

Older adults who are experiencing a myocardial infarction may not have chest pain. Hiatal hernia or upper gastrointestinal distress is often the cause of chest pain. Acute abdominal conditions may go unrecognized in older people because of atypical signs and absence of pain.

The baseline body temperature for older people is about 1°F lower than it is for younger people (Weber & Kelley, 2010). In the event of illness, the body temperature of an older person may not be high enough to qualify as a traditionally defined fever. A temperature of 37.8°C (100°F) in combination with systemic symptoms may signal infection. A temperature of 38.3°C (101°F) almost certainly indicates a serious infection that needs prompt attention. A blunted fever in the face of an infection often indicates a poor prognosis. Temperatures rarely exceed 39.5°C (103°F). Nurses must be alert to other subtle signs of infection, such as mental confusion, increased respirations, tachycardia, and a change in skin color.

Altered Emotional Impact

The emotional component of illness in older people may differ from that in younger people. Many older adults equate good health with the ability to perform their daily activities and believe that "you are as old as you feel." An illness that requires hospitalization or a change in lifestyle is an imminent threat to well-being. Older people admitted to the hospital are at high risk for disorientation, confusion, change in level of consciousness, and other symptoms of delirium, as well as anxiety and fear. In addition, economic concerns and fear of becoming a burden to families often lead to high anxiety in older people. Nurses must recognize the implications of fear, anxiety, and dependency in older patients. They should encourage autonomy, independent decision making, and early mobilization. A positive and confident demeanor in nurses and family members promotes a positive mental outlook in older patients.

Altered Systemic Response

In an older person, illness has far-reaching repercussions. The decline in organ function that occurs in every system of the aging body eventually depletes the body's ability to respond at full capacity. Illness places new demands on body systems that have little or no reserve to meet the crisis. Homeostasis is jeopardized. Older people may be unable to respond effectively to an acute illness or, if a chronic health condition is present, they may be unable to sustain appropriate responses over a long period. Furthermore, their ability to respond to definitive treatment is impaired. The altered responses of older adults reinforce the need for nurses to monitor all body system functions closely, being alert to signs of impending systemic complication.

Other Aspects of Health Care of the Older Adult

Elder Neglect and Abuse

Older adults who live in communities and institutions can be at risk for abuse and neglect. Because of different definitions and terminology and the pattern of underreporting, a clear picture of the incidence and prevalence of abuse among older adults is lacking. Furthermore, one of the major barriers to fully understanding **elder abuse** is that most professionals in all professions, including law enforcement, are not equipped to recognize and report this type of abuse. Both victims and perpetrators are reluctant to report the abuse, and clinicians are unaware of the frequency of the problems.

Neglect is the most common type of abuse. Other forms of abuse include physical, psychological or emotional, sexual, abandonment, and financial exploitation or abuse (Meiner, 2011). Contributing factors include a family history of violence, mental illness, and drug or alcohol abuse, as well as financial dependency on the older person. In addition, diminished cognitive and physical function or disruptive and abusive behavior on the part of the older person can lead to caregiver strain and emotional exhaustion. Older people with disabilities of all types are at increased risk for abuse from family members and paid caregivers.

Nurses should be alert to possible elder abuse and neglect. During the health history, the older adult should be asked about abuse during a private portion of the interview. Most states require that care providers, including nurses, report suspected abuse. Preventive action should be taken when caregiver strain is evident—before elder abuse occurs. Early detection and intervention may provide sufficient resources to the family or person at risk to ensure patient safety. Interdisciplinary team members, including the psychologist, social worker, or chaplain, can be enlisted to help the caregiver develop self-awareness, increased insight, and an understanding of the disease or aging process. Community resources such as caregiver support groups, respite services, and local offices of Area Agencies on Aging are useful for both the older adult and the caregiver.

Social Services

Many social programs exist for older Americans, including Medicare, Medicaid, the Older Americans Act, Supplemental Security Income (SSI), Social Security amendments, Section 202 housing, and Title XX social services legislation. These federal programs have increased health care options and financial support for older Americans. The Older Americans Act mandated creation of a federal aging network, resulting in the establishment of the Area Agencies on Aging, a national system of social services and networks providing many community services for older adults. Each state has an advisory network that is charged with overseeing statewide planning and advocacy for older adults throughout the state. Among the services provided by the Area Agencies on Aging are assessment of need, information and referral, case management, transportation, outreach, homemaker services, day care, nutritional education and congregate meals, legal services, respite care, senior centers, and part-time community work. The agencies target low-income, ethnic minority, rural-living, and frail older adults who are at risk for institutionalization; however, the assessment and information services are available to all older people (Hooyman & Kiyak, 2008). Similar services such as homemaker, home health aide, and chore services can be obtained at an hourly rate through these agencies or through local community nursing services if the family does not meet the low-income criteria. Informal sources of help, such as family, friends, mail carriers, church members, and neighbors, can all keep an informal watch on community-dwelling senior citizens.

Other community support services are available to help older people outside the home. Senior centers have social and health promotion activities, and some provide a nutritious noontime meal. Adult day care facilities offer daily supervision and social opportunities for older people who cannot be left alone. Adult day care services, although expensive, provide respite and enable family members to carry on daily activities while the older person is at the day care center.

Health Care Costs of Aging

Health care is a major expenditure for older adults, especially for those with chronic illness and limited financial resources.

Older adults, who make up about 13% of the population, consume more than 30% of health care costs, particularly in the last year of life (Hooyman & Kiyak, 2008).

The two major programs that finance health in the United States are Medicare and Medicaid, both of which are overseen by the Centers for Medicaid and Medicare Services (CMS). Both programs cover acute care needs such as inpatient hospitalization, physician care, outpatient care, home health services, and skilled nursing care in a nursing facility. Medicare is federally funded, whereas Medicaid is administered by states; therefore, eligibility and reimbursements for Medicaid services vary from state to state. For older adults with limited incomes, even with the support of Medicare or Medicaid, paying out-of-pocket expenses can be a hardship. Out-of-pocket health care expenses represent 28% of the income of poor and near-poor older people (AoA, 2010a, 2010b). Despite the recent additional Medicare prescription benefit plan, out-of-pocket expenditures and prescription costs can be burdensome. As more and more people in the United States become eligible for publicly funded health programs, there are serious concerns about whether sufficient health services will be available.

Home Health Care

The use of home care services and skilled nursing home care increases with age. Because of the rapidly growing older adult population and the availability of Medicare funding for acute care, home health care in the United States has rapidly expanded. (See Chapter 2 for more information on home health care.)

Hospice Services

Hospice is a program of supportive and palliative services for terminally ill patients and their families that includes physical, psychological, social, and spiritual care. In most cases, patients are not expected to live longer than 6 months. The goal of hospice is to improve the quality of life by focusing on symptom management, pain control, and emotional support (Meiner, 2011). Under Medicare and Medicaid, medical and nursing services are provided to keep patients as pain free and comfortable as possible. Hospice services may be incorporated into the care of residents in long-term care facilities and include care for end-stage dementia and other chronic diseases such as end-stage heart failure. (For an in-depth discussion of hospice care, see Chapter 16.)

Aging With a Disability

As the life expectancy of people with all types of physical, cognitive, and mental disabilities has increased, individuals must deal with the normal changes associated with aging in addition to their preexisting disabilities. There are still large gaps in our understanding of the interaction between disabilities and aging, including how this interaction varies depending on the type and degree of disability and other factors such as socioeconomics and gender. For adults without disabilities, the changes associated with aging may be minor inconveniences. For adults with disorders such as polio, multiple sclerosis, and cerebral palsy, aging may lead to greater disability. In addition, many people with disabilities are greatly concerned and fearful about what will happen to them as they age and whether assistance will be available when they need care.

It has been proposed that nurses view people with disabilities as capable, responsible individuals who are able to function effectively despite having a disability. Both the interface and the biopsychosocial models of disability can serve as a basis for the role of nurses as advocates for removal of barriers to health care (Sharts-Hopko, Smeltzer, Ott, et al. 2010; Smeltzer, 2007). The use of such models would also encourage public policies that support full participation of all citizens through greater availability of personal assistants and affordable and accessible transportation. (See Chapter 10 for discussion of other disability models.)

Today, children born with intellectual and physical disabilities and those who acquire them early in life are also living into middle and older age. Often, their care has been provided by the family, primarily by the parents. As parents age and can no longer provide the needed care, they seek additional help with the care or long-term care alternatives for their children. However, few services are available at present to support a smooth transition between caregiving by parents and then by others. Research and public policy must focus on supports and interventions that allow people with disabilities who are aging to increase or maintain function within their personal environment as well as in the outside community. Important questions include who will provide the care and how will it be financed. The National Institute on Aging has identified aging with a disability as a focus and is striving to provide streamlined information and access to those with a disability and their family caregivers.

Ethical and Legal Issues Affecting the Older Adult

Nurses play an important role in supporting and informing patients and families when making treatment decisions. This nursing role becomes even more important in the care of aging patients who are facing life-altering and possibly end-of-life decisions. Loss of rights, victimization, and other serious problems might occur if a patient has not made plans for personal and property management in the event of disability or death. As advocates, nurses should encourage end-of-life discussions and educate older people to prepare advance directives before incapacitation (Meiner, 2011; Miller, 2012).

An **advance directive** is a formal, legally endorsed document that provides instructions for care (living will) or names a proxy decision maker (**durable power of attorney**). It is to be implemented if the signer becomes incapacitated. This written document must be signed by the person and by two witnesses, and a copy should be given to the physician and placed in the medical record. The person must understand that the advance directive is not meant to be used only when certain (or all) types of medical treatment are withheld; rather, it allows for a detailed description of all health care preferences, including full use of all available medical interventions. The health care proxy may have the authority to interpret the patient's wishes on the basis of medical circumstances and is not restricted to the decisions or situations stated in the living will, such as whether life-sustaining treatment can be withdrawn or withheld.

When such serious decisions are made, possibilities exist for significant conflict of values among patients, family members, health care providers, and the legal representative. Autonomy and self-determination are Western concepts, and people from different cultures may view advance directives as a method for denial of care. Older people from some cultures may be unwilling to consider the future, or they may wish to protect relatives and not want them to be informed about a serious illness. Nurses can facilitate the decision-making process by being sensitive to the complexity of patients' values and respecting their decisions. Directives must be focused on the wishes of the patient, not those of the family or the designated proxy.

If no advance arrangement has been made and the older person appears unable to make decisions, the court may be petitioned for a competency hearing. If the court rules that an older adult is incompetent, the judge appoints a guardian—a third party who is given powers by the court to assume responsibility for making financial or personal decisions for that person.

People with communication difficulties or mild dementia may be viewed as incapable of self-determination. Most people with mild dementia have sufficient cognitive capability to make some, but perhaps not all, decisions. For example, a patient may be able to identify a proxy decision maker yet be unable to select specific treatment options. People with mild dementia may be competent to understand the nature and significance of such decisions.

In 1990, the Patient Self-Determination Act (PSDA), a federal law, was enacted to require patient education about advance directives at the time of hospital admission, as well as documentation of this education. Nursing homes are also mandated to enhance residents' autonomy by increasing their involvement in health care decision making. A growing body of research indicates that nursing homes implement the PSDA more vigorously than hospitals. However, in both settings, the documentation and placement of advance directives in the medical record and the education of patients about advance directives vary considerably. Periodically, it is important to ensure that the directives reflect the current wishes of the patient and that all providers have a copy so that they are aware of the patient's wishes.

Critical Thinking Exercises

1 **ebp** Your health history and physical examination of an older male patient alerts you to the possibility of substance abuse. Explain how you would address this. What is the evidence base for available assessments to assist in a more comprehensive evaluation of substance abuse in an older adult patient? Identify the criteria used to evaluate the strength of the evidence for this practice.

2 You are conducting an admission assessment on a 68-year-old woman admitted for a planned hip replacement. Her husband reports that she has become confused in the past 3 days. What assessment parameters and tools would you use to differentiate among the possibilities of infection, other physical conditions, dementia, and Alzheimer's disease? What information should you provide to the patient's husband? What actions and interventions are indicated?

---

3 [pq] Identify the priorities, approach, and techniques you would use to perform a comprehensive home assessment on an 88-year-old patient who has a paid caregiver. How would your priorities, approach, and techniques differ if the patient is disoriented? If the patient has a visual impairment or is hard of hearing? If the patient is from a culture with very different values from your own?

Brunner Suite Resources
Explore these additional resources to enhance learning for this chapter:
 • NCLEX-Style Questions and Other Resources
on thePoint, http://thePoint.lww.com/Brunner13e
• Study Guide
• PrepU
• Clinical Handbook
• Handbook of Laboratory and Diagnostic Tests

References

*Asterisk indicates nursing research.
**Double asterisk indicates classic reference.

Books

American Nurses Association. (2010). *Gerontological nursing: Scope and standards of practice.* Silver Spring, MD: Author.

Bickley, L. S. (2009). *Bates' guide to physical examination and history taking* (10th ed.). Philadelphia: Lippincott Williams & Wilkins.

Dudek, S. G. (2010). *Nutrition essentials for nursing practice* (6th ed.). Philadelphia: Lippincott Williams & Wilkins.

Hooyman, N. R., & Kiyak, H. A. (2008). *Social gerontology: A multidisciplinary perspective* (8th ed.). Boston: Allyn & Bacon.

Karch, A. M. (2012). *2012 Lippincott's nursing drug guide.* Philadelphia: Lippincott Williams & Wilkins.

Mauk, K. L. (2010). *Gerontological nursing: Competencies for care.* Sudbury, MA: Jones & Bartlett.

Meiner, S. E. (2011). *Gerontologic nursing* (4th ed.). St Louis: Mosby-Elsevier.

Miller, C. A. (2012). *Nursing for wellness in older adults* (6th ed.). Philadelphia: Lippincott Williams & Wilkins.

Murphy, K. P., & Hickey, J. V. (2010). Geriatric issues. In M. K. Bader & L. Littlejohns (Eds.). *AANN core curriculum for neuroscience nurses* (5th ed.). Glenview, IL: American Association of Neuroscience Nurses.

Pender, N. J., Murdaugh, C. L., & Parsons, M. A. (Eds.). (2011). *Health promotion in nursing practice* (6th ed.). Upper Saddle River, NJ: Prentice Hall Health.

Porth, C. M., & Matfin, G. (2009). *Pathophysiology: Concepts of altered health states* (8th ed.). Philadelphia: Lippincott Williams & Wilkins.

Tabloski, P. A. (2009). *Gerontological nursing: The essential guide to clinical practice* (2nd ed.). Upper Saddle River, NJ: Prentice Hall Health.

Weber, J., & Kelley, J. (2010). *Health assessment in nursing* (4th ed.). Philadelphia: Lippincott Williams & Wilkins.

Journals and Electronic Documents

Administration on Aging. (2010a). *A profile of older Americans: 2010.* Available at: www.aoa.gov/aoaroot/aging_statistics/Profile/2010/docs/2010profile.pdf

Administration on Aging. (2010b). *Older Americans 2010: Key indicators of well-being.* Available at: www.agingstats.gov/agingstatsdotnet/Main_Site/Data/2010_Documents/Docs/OA_2010.pdf

Bloom, H. G., Ahmed, I., Alessi, C. A., et al. (2009). Evidence-based recommendations for the assessment and management of sleep disorders in older persons. *Journal of the American Geriatric Society, 57*(5), 761–789.

Bross, M., Soch, K., & Smith-Knuppel, T. (2010). Anemia in older persons. *American Family Physician, 82*(5), 480–487.

Centers for Disease Control and Prevention. (2010). *Falls among older adults: An overview.* Available at: www.cdc.gov/homeandrecreationalsafety/falls/adultfalls.html

Centers for Disease Control and Prevention. (2011a). *Pneumococcal disease.* Available at: www.cdc.gov/vaccines/pubs/pinkbook/downloads/pneumo.pdf

Centers for Disease Control and Prevention. (2011b). *Enhancing use of clinical preventive services among older adults.* Available at: www.cdc.gov/aging and www.aarp.org/healthpros

Coon, D. W., & Evans, G. (2009). Empirically based treatments for caregiver distress: What works and where do we go from here? *Geriatric Nursing, 30*(6), 426–435.

Elliott, A. F., Burgio, L. D., & DeCoster, J. (2010). Enhancing caregiver health: Findings from the resources for enhancing the Alzheimer's caregiver health II intervention. *Journal of the American Geriatric Society, 58*(1), 30–37.

Grand, J. H., Caspar, S., & MacDonald, S. W. (2011). Clinical features and multidisciplinary approaches to dementia care. *Journal of Multidisciplinary Healthcare, 4,* 125–147.

Howden, L. M., & Meyer, J. A. (2011). *Age and sex composition: 2010.* 2010 Census Briefs No. C2010BR-03. Available at: www.census.gov/prod/cen2010/briefs/c2010br-03.pdf

Karraker, A., DeLamater, J., & Schwartz, C. R. (2011). Sexual frequency decline from midlife to later life. *Journals of Gerontology. Series B, Psychological Sciences and Social Sciences, 66B*(4), 502–512.

Kauffman, J. M. (2009). Selective serotonin reuptake inhibitor (SSRI) drugs: More risks than benefits? *Journal of American Physicians & Surgeons, 14*(1), 7–12.

Kochanek, K. D., Xu, J., Murphy, S. L., et al. (2011). Deaths: Preliminary data for 2009. *National Vital Statistics Report, 59*(4):1–54. Available at: www.cdc.gov/nchs/data/nvsr/nvsr59/nvsr59_04.pdf

Marchant, J. A., & Williams, K. N. (2011). Memory matters in assisted living. *Rehabilitation Nursing, 36*(2), 83–88.

Messina, B A., & Escallier, L. A. (2011). Take the 'hyper' out of pharmacotherapy. *Nursing, 2011*(7), 51–53.

Naegle, M. A. (2011). Detecting and screening for depression in older adults. *American Nurse Today, 6*(11), 18–20.

National Institutes of Health. (2011a). *Dietary supplement fact sheet: Calcium.* Available at: ods.od.nih.gov/factsheets/calcium

National Institutes of Health. (2011b). *Dietary supplement fact sheet: Vitamin D.* Available at: ods.od.nih.gov/factsheets/VitaminD-HealthProfessional

Press, D., & Alexander, M. (2011) *Cholinesterase inhibitors in the treatment of dementia.* UpToDate. Available at: http://www.uptodate.com/contents/cholinesterase-inhibitors-in-the-treatment-of-dementia

Rao, S. S., & Go, J. T. (2010). Update on the management of constipation in the elderly: New treatment options. *Clinical Interventions in Aging, 9*(5), 163–171.

*Riegel, B., Dickson, V. V., Cameron, J., et al. (2010). Symptom recognition in elders with heart failure. *Journal of Nursing Scholarship, 42*(1), 92–100.

*Sharts-Hopko, N. C., Smeltzer, S., Ott, B. B., et al. (2010). Healthcare experiences of women with visual impairment. *Clinical Nurse Specialist, 24*(3), 149–153.

*Smeltzer, S. C. (2007). Improving the health and wellness of persons with disabilities. A call to action too important for nursing to ignore. *Nursing Outlook, 55*(4), 189–193.

Vance, D. E., Heaton, K., Eaves, Y., et al. (2011). Sleep and cognition on everyday functioning in older adults: Implications for nursing practice and research. *Journal of Neuroscience Nursing, 43*(5), 261–271.

Vance, D. E., Keltner, N. L., McGuinness, T., et al. (2010). The future of cognitive remediation training in older adults. *Journal of Neuroscience Nursing, 42*(5), 255–266.

Vanasse, G. J., & Berliner, N. (2010). Anemia in the elderly: An emerging problem for the 21st century. *Hematology, 2010,* 271–275.

Wick, J. Y., & Zanni, G. R. (2009). Aging in place: Multiple options, multiple choices. *Consultant Pharmacist, 24*(11), 804–806, 808, 811–812.

**Yesavage, J., Brink, T. L., Rose, T. L., et al. (1983). Development and validation of a geriatric screening scale: A preliminary report. *Journal of Psychiatric Research, 17*(1), 37–49.

*Zisberg, A., Shadmi, E., Sinoff, G., et al. (2011). Low mobility during hospitalization and functional decline in older adults. *Journal of the American Geriatric Society, 59*(2), 266–273.

Resources

Administration on Aging (AoA), www.aoa.gov
Alzheimer's Association, www.alz.org
American Association for Geriatric Psychiatry (AAGP), www.aagponline.org
American Association of Retired Persons (AARP), www.aarp.org
American Federation for Aging Research (AFAR), www.afar.org
American Geriatrics Society (AGS), www.americangeriatrics.org
Association for Gerontology in Higher Education (AGHE), www.aghe.org

Children of Aging Parents (CAPS), www.caps4caregivers.org
Family Caregiver Alliance (FCA), www.caregiver.org
Gerontological Society of America (GSA), www.geron.org
Hartford Institute for Geriatric Nursing, www.consultgerirn.org
Hospital Elder Life Program (HELP), www.hospitalelderlifeprogram.org
LeadingAge (formerly American Association of Homes and Services for the Aging), www.leadingage.org
MedicAlert + Alzheimer's Association Safe Return (program for locating lost patients), www.alz.org/care/dementia-medic-alert-safe-return.asp
National Caucus and Center on Black Aged (NCBA), www.ncba-aged.org
National Council on Aging (NCOA), www.ncoa.org
National Gerontological Nursing Association (NGNA), www.ngna.org
National Institute on Aging (NIA), Alzheimer's Disease Education and Referral (ADEAR) Center, www.nia.nih.gov/Alzheimers

Unit
3

Concepts and Challenges in Patient Management

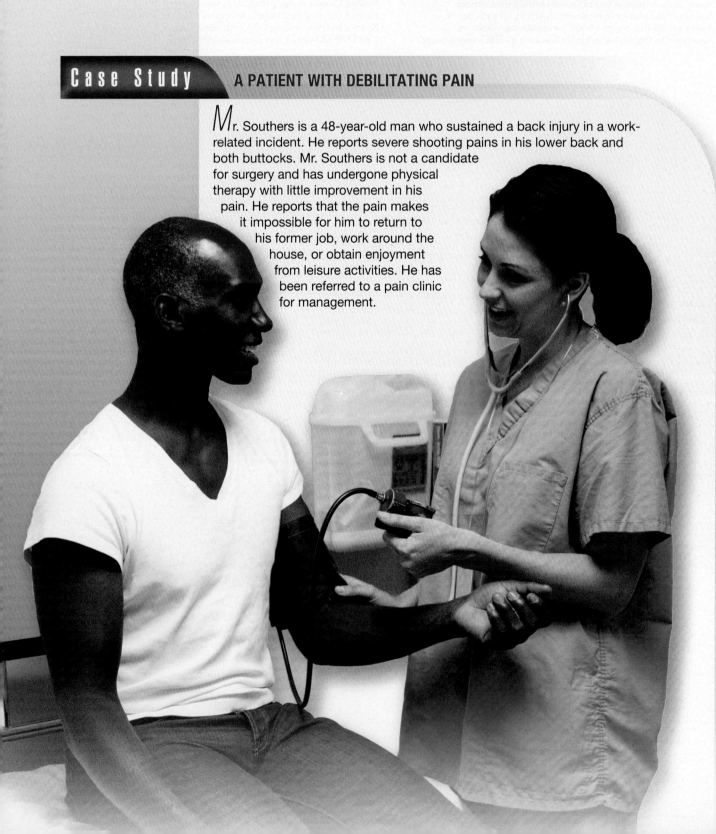

Case Study   A PATIENT WITH DEBILITATING PAIN

Mr. Southers is a 48-year-old man who sustained a back injury in a work-related incident. He reports severe shooting pains in his lower back and both buttocks. Mr. Southers is not a candidate for surgery and has undergone physical therapy with little improvement in his pain. He reports that the pain makes it impossible for him to return to his former job, work around the house, or obtain enjoyment from leisure activities. He has been referred to a pain clinic for management.

QSEN Competency Focus: *Patient-Centered Care*

The complexities inherent in today's health care system challenge nurses to demonstrate integration of specific interdisciplinary core competencies. These competencies are aimed at ensuring the delivery of safe, quality patient care (Institute of Medicine, 2003). The concepts from the Quality and Safety Education for Nurses (QSEN) Institute (2012) provide a framework for the knowledge, skills, and attitudes (KSAs) required for nurses to demonstrate competency in these key areas, which include *patient-centered care, interdisciplinary teamwork and collaboration, evidence-based practice, quality improvement, safety,* and *informatics*.

Patient-Centered Care Definition: Recognize the patient or designee as the source of control and full partner in providing compassionate and coordinated care based on respect for patient's preferences, values, and needs.

SELECTED PRE-LICENSURE KSAs	APPLICATION AND REFLECTION
Knowledge	
Demonstrate comprehensive understanding of the concepts of pain and suffering, including physiologic models of pain and comfort.	Describe the interplay between Mr. Southers's injury and the pathophysiologic mechanisms that may explain the pain he is experiencing.
Skills	
Assess presence and extent of pain and suffering. Elicit expectations of patient and family for relief of pain, discomfort, or suffering. Initiate effective treatments to relieve pain and suffering in light of patient values, preferences, and expressed needs.	How would you assess and measure Mr. Southers's pain? When and how would you reassess his pain? How would you determine his expectations for relief of pain? Describe how you would assess his values, preferences, and needs and then incorporate these into an individualized nursing plan of care with interventions and expected outcomes targeted at providing relief of his pain.
Attitudes	
Recognize personally held values and beliefs about the management of pain or suffering. Appreciate the role of the nurse in relief of all types and sources of pain or suffering.	Back-related injuries are a frequent cause of workers' compensation–related claims. Reflect on your attitude toward Mr. Southers and patients with work-related back pain that prevents them from working. Do you believe Mr. Southers's report of pain? Might your attitude toward him or patients like him have an effect on the nursing care that you provide?

Cronenwett, L., Sherwood, G., Barnsteiner, J., et al. (2007). Quality and safety education for nurses. *Nursing Outlook, 55*(3), 122–131.
Institute of Medicine. (2003). *Health professions education: A bridge to quality*. Washington, DC: National Academies Press.
QSEN Institute (2012). *Competencies: Prelicensure KSAs*. Available at: qsen.org/competencies/pre-licensure-ksas

Read More About This Case

More information about this case study and the relationships between nursing diagnoses, interventions, and expected outcomes is available online. Visit thePoint for Applying Concepts From NANDA-I, NIC, and NOC.

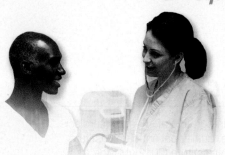

12

Pain Management

On completion of this chapter, the learner will be able to:

1 Identify the fundamental concepts of pain.
2 Distinguish between the types of pain.
3 Describe the four processes of nociception.
4 Explain underlying mechanisms of neuropathic pain.
5 Identify methods to perform a pain assessment.
6 List the first-line analgesic agents from the three groups of analgesic agents.

7 Identify the effects of select analgesic agents on older adults.
8 Identify practical nonpharmacologic methods that can be used in the clinical setting in patients with pain.
9 Use the nursing process as a framework for the care of patients with pain.

Glossary

addiction: a chronic neurologic and biologic disease defined by pain specialists and characterized by behaviors that include one or more of the following: impaired control over drug use, compulsive use, continued use despite harm, and craving to use the opioid for effects other than pain relief

adjuvant analgesic agent: a drug that has a primary indication other than pain (e.g., anticonvulsant, antidepressant, sodium channel blocker, or muscle relaxant) but is an analgesic agent for some painful conditions; sometimes referred to as co-analgesic

agonist-antagonist: a type of opioid (e.g., nalbuphine [Nubain] and butorphanol [Stadol]) that binds to the kappa opioid receptor site acting as an agonist (capable of producing analgesia) and simultaneously to the mu opioid receptor site acting as an antagonist (reversing mu agonist effects)

allodynia: pain due to a stimulus that does not normally provoke pain, such as touch; typically experienced in the skin around areas affected by nerve injury and commonly seen with many neuropathic pain syndromes

antagonist: drug that competes with agonists for opioid receptor binding sites; can displace agonists, thereby inhibiting their action

breakthrough pain (BTP): a transitory increase in pain that occurs on a background of otherwise controlled persistent pain

ceiling effect: an analgesic dose above which further dose increments produce no change in effect

central sensitization: a key central mechanism of neuropathic pain; the abnormal hyperexcitability of central neurons in the spinal cord, which results from complex changes induced by the incoming afferent barrages of nociceptors

comfort-function goal: the pain rating identified by the individual patient above which the patient experiences interference with function and quality of life (e.g., activities the patient needs or wishes to perform)

efficacy: the extent to which a drug or another treatment "works" and can produce the effect in question—analgesia in this context

half-life: the time it takes for the plasma concentration (amount of drug in the body) to be reduced by 50% (After starting a drug, or increasing its dose, four to five half-lives are required to approach a steady-state level in the blood, irrespective of the dose, dosing interval, or route of administration; after four to five half-lives, a drug that has been discontinued generally is considered to be mostly eliminated from the body.)

hydrophilic: readily absorbed in aqueous solution

intraspinal: "within the spine"; refers to the spaces or potential spaces surrounding the spinal cord into which medications can be administered

lipophilic: readily absorbed in fatty tissues

metabolite: the product of biochemical reactions during drug metabolism

mu agonist: any opioid that binds to the mu opioid receptor subtype and produces analgesic effects (e.g., morphine); used interchangeably with the terms *full agonist, pure agonist,* and *morphinelike drug*

neuropathic (pathophysiologic) pain: pain sustained by injury or dysfunction of the peripheral or central nervous systems and distinctly different from nociceptive (physiologic) pain

neuroplasticity: the ability of the peripheral and central nervous systems to change both structure and function as a result of noxious stimuli

nociceptive (physiologic) pain: pain that is sustained by ongoing activation of the sensory system that conducts the perception of noxious stimuli; implies the existence of damage to somatic or visceral tissues sufficient to activate the nociceptive system

nociceptor: a type of primary afferent neuron that has the ability to respond to a noxious stimulus or to a stimulus that would be noxious if prolonged

nonopioid: refers to analgesic agents that include acetaminophen (Tylenol) and nonsteroidal anti-inflammatory drugs (NSAIDs); term is used instead of "nonnarcotic"

NSAID: an acronym for nonsteroidal anti-inflammatory drug (pronounced "en said"); also referred to as aspirinlike drugs

opioid: refers to codeine, morphine, and other natural, semisynthetic, and synthetic drugs that relieve pain by binding to multiple types of opioid receptors; term is preferred to "narcotic"

opioid dose-sparing effect: occurs when a nonopioid or adjuvant is added to an opioid, allowing the opioid dose to be lowered without diminishing analgesic effects

opioid-induced hyperalgesia (OIH): a phenomenon in which exposure to an opioid induces increased sensitivity, or a lowered threshold, to the neural activity conducting pain perception; it is the "flip side" of tolerance

opioid naïve: denotes a person who has not recently taken enough opioid on a regular enough basis to become tolerant to the opioid's effects

opioid tolerant: denotes a person who has taken opioids long enough at doses high enough to develop tolerance to many of the opioid's effects, including analgesia and sedation

peripheral sensitization: a key peripheral mechanism of neuropathic pain that occurs when there are changes in the number and location of ion channels; in particular, sodium channels abnormally accumulate in injured nociceptors, producing a lower nerve depolarization threshold, ectopic discharges, and an increase in the response to stimuli

physical dependence: the body's normal response to administration of an opioid for 2 or more weeks; withdrawal symptoms may occur if an opioid is abruptly stopped or an antagonist is administered

placebo: any medication or procedure, including surgery, that produces an effect in a patient because of its implicit or explicit intent and not because of its specific physical or chemical properties

preemptive analgesic agents: pre-injury pain treatments (e.g., preoperative epidural analgesia and preincision local anesthetic infiltration) to prevent the establishment of peripheral and central sensitization of pain

refractory: nonresponsive or resistant to therapeutic interventions such as analgesic agents

self-report: the ability of an individual to give a report—in this case, of pain, especially intensity; the most essential component of pain assessment

titration: upward or downward adjustment of the amount (dose) of an analgesic agent

tolerance: a process characterized by decreasing effects of a drug at its previous dose, or the need for a higher dose of drug to maintain an effect

---

Nurses play a key role in the management of pain as experts in assessment, drug administration, and patient education. They are uniquely positioned to assume this role as the only members of the health care team that are at the patient's bedside 24 hours a day, 7 days a week. These characteristics have led to their distinction as the patient's primary pain manager (Pasero, Eksterowicz, & McCaffery, 2009).

Fundamental Concepts

Understanding the definition, effects, and types of pain lays the foundation for proper pain assessment and management.

Definition of Pain

The American Pain Society (APS) (2008) defines pain as "an unpleasant sensory and emotional experience associated with actual or potential tissue damage, or described in terms of such damage" (p. 1). This definition describes pain as a complex phenomenon that can impact a person's psychosocial, emotional, and physical functioning. The clinical definition of pain reinforces that pain is a highly personal and subjective experience: "Pain is whatever the experiencing person says it is, existing whenever he says it does" (McCaffery, 1968, p. 8). All accepted guidelines consider the patient's report to be the most reliable indicator of pain and the most essential component of pain assessment (APS, 2008; McCaffery, Herr, & Pasero, 2011).

Effects of Pain

Pain affects individuals of every age, sex, race, and socioeconomic class (American Geriatrics Society, 2009; Johannes, Le, Zhou, et al., 2010; Walco, Dworkin, Krane, et al., 2010). It is the primary reason people seek health care and one of the most common conditions that nurses treat (International Association for the Study of Pain, 2011). Unrelieved pain has the potential to affect every system in the body and cause numerous harmful effects, some of which may last a person's lifetime (Table 12-1). Despite many advances in the understanding of the underlying mechanisms of pain and the availability of improved analgesic agents and technology, as well as nonpharmacologic pain management methods, all types of pain continue to be undertreated (Portenoy, 2011; Turk, Wilson, & Cahana, 2011; Wu & Raja, 2011).

Types and Categories of Pain

There are many ways to categorize pain, and clear distinctions are not always possible. Pain often is described as being acute or chronic (persistent) (Pasero & Portenoy, 2011). Acute pain differs from chronic pain primarily in its duration. For example, tissue damage as a result of surgery, trauma, or burns produces acute pain, which is expected to have a relatively short duration and resolve with normal healing. Chronic pain is subcategorized as being of cancer or noncancer origin and can be time limited (e.g., may resolve within months) or persist throughout the course of a person's life. Examples of noncancer pain include peripheral neuropathy from diabetes, back or neck pain after injury, and osteoarthritis pain from joint degeneration. Some conditions can produce both acute and chronic pain. For example, some patients with cancer have continuous chronic pain and also experience acute exacerbations of pain periodically—called **breakthrough pain (BTP)**—or endure

TABLE 12-1	**Harmful Effects of Unrelieved Pain**
Domains Affected	**Specific Responses to Pain**
Endocrine	↑ Adrenocorticotrophic hormone (ACTH), ↑ cortisol, ↑ antidiuretic hormone (ADH), ↑ epinephrine, ↑ norepinephrine, ↑ growth hormone (GH), ↑ catecholamines, ↑ renin, ↑ angiotensin II, ↑ aldosterone, ↑ glucagon, ↑ interleukin-1; ↓ insulin, ↓ testosterone
Metabolic	Gluconeogenesis, hepatic glycogenolysis, hyperglycemia, glucose intolerance, insulin resistance, muscle protein catabolism, ↑ lipolysis
Cardiovascular	↑ Heart rate, ↑ cardiac workload, ↑ peripheral vascular resistance, ↑ systemic vascular resistance, hypertension, ↑ coronary vascular resistance, ↑ myocardial oxygen consumption, hypercoagulation, deep vein thrombosis
Respiratory	↓ Flows and volumes, atelectasis, shunting, hypoxemia, ↓ cough, sputum retention, infection
Genitourinary	↓ Urinary output, urinary retention, fluid overload, hypokalemia
Gastrointestinal	↓ Gastric and bowel motility
Musculoskeletal	Muscle spasm, impaired muscle function, fatigue, immobility
Cognitive	Reduction in cognitive function, mental confusion
Immune	Depression of immune response
Developmental	↑ Behavioral and physiologic responses to pain, altered temperaments, higher somatization; possible altered development of the pain system, ↑ vulnerability to stress disorders, addictive behavior, and anxiety states
Future pain	Debilitating chronic pain syndromes: postmastectomy pain, postthoracotomy pain, phantom pain, postherpetic neuralgia
Quality of life	Sleeplessness, anxiety, fear, hopelessness, ↑ thoughts of suicide

Copyright 1999, Pasero C., McCaffery M. Used with permission. Pasero, C., & McCaffery, M. (2011). *Pain assessment and pharmacologic management.* St. Louis: Mosby-Elsevier.

acute pain from repetitive painful procedures during cancer treatment (McCaffery et al., 2011).

Pain is better classified by its inferred pathology as being either nociceptive pain or neuropathic pain (Table 12-2). **Nociceptive (physiologic) pain** refers to the normal functioning of physiologic systems that leads to the perception of noxious stimuli (tissue injury) as being painful (Pasero & Portenoy, 2011). This is why nociception is described as "normal" pain transmission. **Neuropathic (pathophysiologic) pain** is pathologic and results from abnormal processing of sensory input by the nervous system as a result of damage to the peripheral or central nervous system or both (Pasero & Portenoy, 2011).

Patients may have a combination of nociceptive and neuropathic pain. For example, a patient may have nociceptive pain as a result of tumor growth and also report radiating sharp and shooting neuropathic pain if the tumor is pressing against a nerve plexus. Sickle cell pain is usually a combination of nociceptive pain from the clumping of sickled cells and resulting perfusion deficits, and neuropathic pain from nerve ischemia.

Nociceptive Pain

Nociception includes four specific processes: transduction, transmission, perception, and modulation. Figure 12-1 illustrates these processes, and following is an overview of each.

Transduction

Transduction refers to the processes by which noxious stimuli, such as a surgical incision or burn, activate primary afferent neurons called **nociceptors**, which are located throughout the body in the skin, subcutaneous tissue, and visceral (organ) and somatic (musculoskeletal) structures (Pasero & Portenoy, 2011). These neurons have the ability to respond selectively to noxious stimuli generated as a result of tissue damage from mechanical (e.g., incision, tumor growth), thermal (e.g., burn, frostbite), chemical (e.g., toxins, chemotherapy), and infectious sources. Noxious stimuli cause the release of a number of excitatory compounds (e.g., serotonin, bradykinin, histamine, substance P, and prostaglandins), which move pain along the pain pathway (Pasero & Portenoy, 2011) (see Fig. 12-1A).

Prostaglandins are lipid compounds that initiate inflammatory responses that increase tissue swelling and pain at the site of injury (Vadivelu, Whitney, & Sinatra, 2009). They form when the enzyme phospholipase breaks down phospholipids into arachidonic acid. In turn, the enzyme cyclo-oxygenase (COX) acts on the arachidonic acid to produce prostaglandins (Fig. 12-2). COX-1 and COX-2 are isoenzymes of COX and play an important role in producing the effects of the **nonopioid** analgesic agents, which include the nonsteroidal anti-inflammatory drugs (**NSAIDs**) and acetaminophen. NSAIDs produce pain relief primarily by blocking the formation of prostaglandins in the periphery (Pasero, Portenoy, & McCaffery 2011). The nonselective NSAIDs, such as ibuprofen (Motrin, Advil), naproxen (Naprosyn), diclofenac (Voltaren), and ketorolac (Toradol), inhibit both COX-1 and COX-2, and the COX-2 selective NSAIDs, such as celecoxib (Celebrex), inhibit only COX-2. As Figure 12-2 illustrates, both types of NSAIDs produce anti-inflammation and pain relief through the inhibition of COX-2. Acetaminophen is known to be a COX inhibitor that has minimal peripheral effect, is not anti-inflammatory, and can both relieve pain and reduce fever by preventing the formation of prostaglandins in the central nervous system (CNS) (Pasero & Portenoy, 2011).

Other analgesic agents work at the site of transduction by affecting the flux of ions. For example, sodium channels are closed and inactive at rest but undergo changes in response to nerve membrane depolarization. Transient channel opening leads to an influx of sodium that results in nerve conduction (Dib-Hajj, Black, & Waxman, 2009). Local anesthetics reduce nerve conduction by blocking sodium channels. Anticonvulsants also produce pain relief by reducing the flux of other ions, such as calcium and potassium (Pasero & Portenoy, 2011).

Transmission

Transmission is the second process involved in nociception. Effective transduction generates an action potential that is transmitted along the A-delta (δ) and C fibers (Pasero & Portenoy, 2011). A-δ fibers are lightly myelinated and faster conducting than the unmyelinated C fibers (see Fig. 12-1B).

TABLE 12-2 Classification of Pain by Inferred Pathology

	Nociceptive Pain	Neuropathic Pain	Mixed Pain
Physiologic Processes	Normal processing of stimuli that damages tissues or has the potential to do so if prolonged; can be somatic or visceral	Abnormal processing of sensory input by the peripheral or central nervous system or both	Components of both nociceptive and neuropathic pain; poorly defined
Categories and Examples	*Somatic Pain* Arises from bone joint, muscle, skin, or connective tissue. It is usually described as aching or throbbing in quality and is well localized. *Examples:* Surgical, trauma; wound and burn pain; cancer pain (tumor growth) and pain associated with bony metastases; labor pain (cervical changes and uterine contractions); osteoarthritis and rheumatoid arthritis pain; osteoporosis pain; pain of Ehlers-Danlos syndrome; ankylosing spondylitis *Visceral Pain* Arises from visceral organs, such as the GI tract and pancreas. This may be subdivided: • Tumor involvement of the organ capsule that causes aching and fairly well-localized pain • Obstruction of hollow viscus, which causes intermittent cramping and poorly localized pain *Examples:* Organ-involved cancer pain; ulcerative colitis; irritable bowel syndrome; Crohn's disease; pancreatitis	*Centrally Generated Pain* *Deafferentation pain:* Injury to either the peripheral or central nervous system; burning pain below the level of a spinal cord lesion reflects injury to the central nervous system. *Examples:* Phantom pain as a result of peripheral nerve damage; post stroke pain; pain following spinal cord injury *Sympathetically maintained pain:* Associated with dysregulation of the autonomic nervous system *Example:* Complex regional pain syndrome *Peripherally Generated Pain* *Painful polyneuropathies:* Pain is felt along the distribution of many peripheral nerves. *Examples:* Diabetic neuropathy; postherpetic neuralgia; alcohol-nutritional neuropathy; some types of neck, shoulder, and back pain; pain of Guillain-Barré syndrome *Painful mononeuropathies:* Usually associated with a known peripheral nerve injury; pain is felt at least partly along the distribution of the damaged nerve. *Examples:* Nerve root compression, nerve entrapment; trigeminal neuralgia; some types of neck, shoulder, and back pain	No identified categories *Examples:* Fibromyalgia; some types of neck, shoulder, and back pain; some headaches; pain associated with HIV; some myofascial pain; pain associated with Lyme disease
Pharmacologic Treatment	Most responsive to nonopioids, opioids, and local anesthetics	Adjuvant analgesic agents, such as antidepressants, anticonvulsants, and local anesthetics, but there is wide variability in terms of efficacy and adverse-effect profiles.	Adjuvant analgesic agents, such as antidepressants, anticonvulsants, and local anesthetics, but there is wide variability in terms of efficacy and adverse-effect profiles.

HIV, human immunodeficiency virus; GI, gastrointestinal.
Copyright 1999, Pasero C., McCaffery M. Used with permission. Pasero, C., & McCaffery, M. (2011). *Pain assessment and pharmacologic management.* St. Louis: Mosby.

The endings of A-δ fibers detect thermal and mechanical injury, allow relatively quick localization of pain, and are responsible for a rapid reflex withdrawal from the painful stimulus. Unmyelinated C fibers are slow impulse conductors and respond to mechanical, thermal, and chemical stimuli. They produce poorly localized and often aching or burning pain. A-beta (β) fibers are the largest of the fibers and respond to touch, movement, and vibration but do not normally transmit pain (Pasero & Portenoy, 2011).

Noxious information passes through the dorsal root ganglia and synapses in the dorsal horn of the spinal cord (see Fig. 12-1B). An action potential is generated, and the impulse ascends up to the spinal cord and transmits the information to the brain, where pain is perceived. Extensive modulation occurs in the dorsal horn via complex neurochemical mechanisms (see Fig. 12-1B inset). The primary A-δ fibers and C fibers release various transmitters including glutamate, neurokinins, and substance P. Glutamate is a key neurotransmitter because it binds to the N-methyl-D-aspartate (NMDA) receptor and promotes pain transmission. The drug ketamine, an NMDA receptor **antagonist**, produces analgesia by preventing glutamate from binding to the NMDA receptor sites. Endogenous and exogenous (therapeutically administered) **opioids** bind to opioid receptor sites in the dorsal horn to block substance P and thereby produce analgesia (Pasero & Portenoy, 2011). The opioid methadone (Dolophine) binds to opioid receptor sites and has NMDA antagonist properties (Pasero, Quinn, Portenoy, et al., 2011).

Perception

The third process involved in nociception is perception. Perception is the result of the neural activity associated with transmission of noxious stimuli (Pasero & Portenoy, 2011). It requires activation of higher brain structures for the occurrence of awareness, emotions, and drives associated with pain (see Fig. 12-1C). The physiology of perception of pain continues to be studied but can be targeted by mind–body therapies, such as distraction and imagery, which are based on the belief that brain processes can strongly influence pain perception (Bruckenthal, 2010).

Modulation

Modulation of the information generated in response to noxious stimuli occurs at every level from the periphery to the cortex and involves many different neurochemicals (Pasero & Portenoy, 2011) (see Fig. 12-1D). For example, serotonin and norepinephrine are inhibitory neurotransmitters that are released in the spinal cord and brain stem by

NOCICEPTION

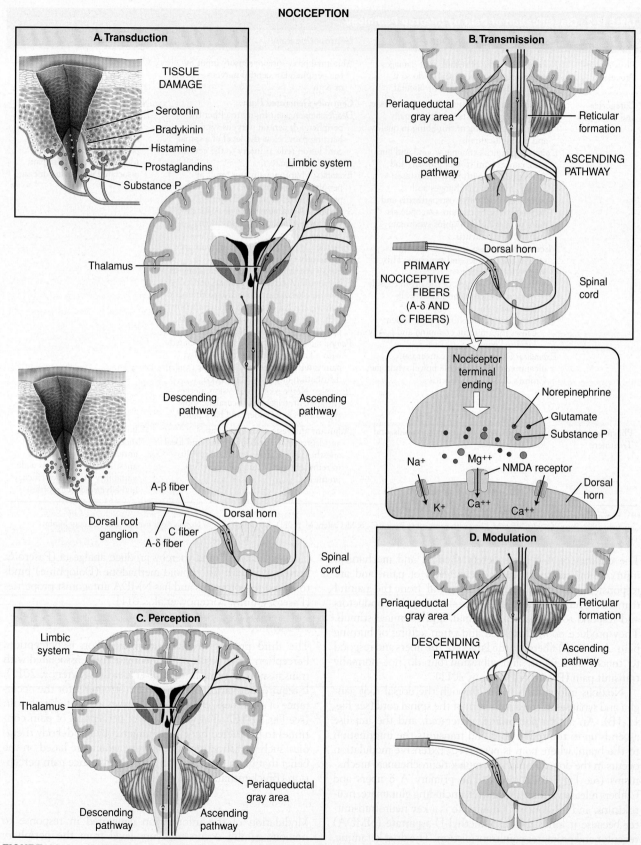

FIGURE 12-1 • Nociception. **A.** Transduction. **B.** Transmission. **C.** Perception. **D.** Modulation. Redrawn from Pasero C., & McCaffery M. (2011). *Pain assessment and pharmacologic management* (p. 5). St. Louis: Mosby-Elsevier. Copyright 2011, Pasero C., McCaffery M. Used with permission.

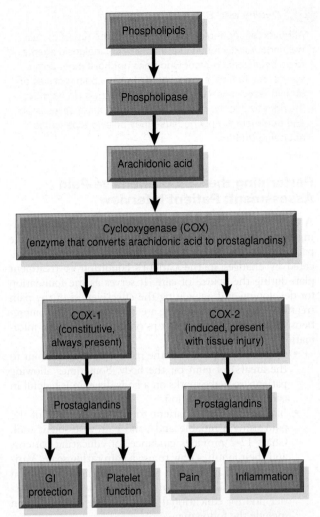

FIGURE 12-2 • Enzyme pathway: COX-1 and COX-2. Redrawn from Pasero, C., & McCaffery, M. (2011). *Pain assessment and pharmacologic management* (p. 6). St. Louis: Mosby-Elsevier. Copyright 2004, Pasero C., McCaffery M. Used with permission.

the descending (efferent) fibers of the modulatory system. Some antidepressants provide pain relief by blocking the body's reuptake (resorption) of serotonin and norepinephrine, extending their availability to fight pain. Endogenous opioids are located throughout the peripheral and central nervous systems, and like exogenous opioids, they bind to opioid receptors in the descending system and inhibit pain transmission. Dual-mechanism analgesic agents, such as tramadol (Ultram) and tapentadol (Nucynta), bind to opioid receptor sites and block the reuptake of serotonin and/or norepinephrine (Pasero, Quinn et al., 2011).

Neuropathic Pain

Neuropathic pain is sustained by mechanisms that are driven by damage to, or dysfunction of, the peripheral or central nervous system and is the result of abnormal processing of stimuli (Pasero & Portenoy, 2011) (Fig. 12-3). Unlike nociceptive pain, neuropathic pain may occur in the absence of tissue damage and inflammation, even when acute neuropathic pain serves no useful purpose. Extensive research is ongoing to better define the peripheral and central mechanisms that initiate and maintain neuropathic pain.

Peripheral Mechanisms

At any point from the periphery to the CNS, the potential exists for the development of neuropathic pain. Hyperexcitable nerve endings in the periphery can become damaged, leading to abnormal reorganization of the nervous system called **neuroplasticity**, an underlying mechanism of some neuropathic pain states (Pasero & Portenoy, 2011). Changes in the number and location of ion channels can occur. For example, sodium channels abnormally accumulate in injured nociceptors, which can lower the threshold for nerve depolarization and increase response to stimuli, setting off ectopic nerve discharges (Argoff, Albrecht, Irving, et al., 2009). These and many other processes lead to a phenomenon called **peripheral sensitization**, which is thought to contribute to the maintenance of neuropathic

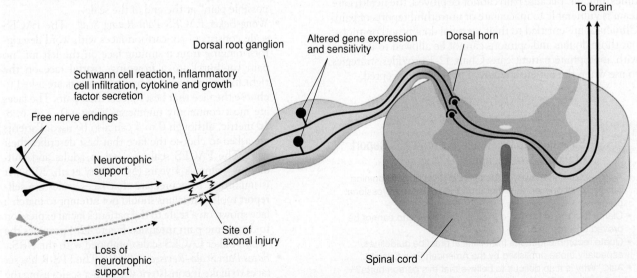

FIGURE 12-3 • Neuropathic pain. Nociceptive injury or inflammation may result in an altered physiologic response within the nociceptive system. These changes cause release of inflammatory cytokines that may alter gene expression and sensitivity in nociceptive fibers. In turn, these alter nociceptive activity, causing neuropathic pain. Used with permission from Golan, D. E., Tashjian, A. H., & Armstrong, E. J. (2008). *Principles of pharmacology: The pathophysiologic basis of drug therapy* (2nd ed.). Baltimore: Wolters Kluwer Health | Lippincott Williams & Wilkins.

pain. Topical local anesthetics, such as lidocaine patch 5% (Lidoderm), produce effects in the tissues right under the site of application by "dampening" neuropathic pain mechanisms in the peripheral nervous system (Pasero, Polomano, Portenoy, et al., 2011).

Central Mechanisms

Central mechanisms also play a role in the establishment of neuropathic pain. **Central sensitization** is defined as abnormal hyperexcitability of central neurons in the spinal cord, which results from complex changes induced by incoming afferent barrages of nociceptors (Pasero & Portenoy, 2011). Extensive release and binding of excitatory neurotransmitters, such as glutamate, activate the NMDA receptor and cause an increase in intracellular calcium levels into the neuron, resulting in pain. Similar to what happens in the peripheral nervous system, an increase in the influx of sodium is thought to lower the threshold for nerve activation, increase response to stimuli, and enlarge the receptive field served by the affected neuron.

As in the peripheral nervous system, anatomic changes can occur in the CNS. For example, injury to a nerve route can lead to reorganization in the dorsal horn of the spinal cord. Nerve fibers can invade other locations and create abnormal sensations in the area of the body served by the injured nerve. **Allodynia**, or pain from a normally nonnoxious stimulus (e.g., touch), is one such type of abnormal sensation and a common feature of neuropathic pain. In patients with allodynia, the mere weight of clothing or bed sheets on the skin can be excruciatingly painful (Pasero & Portenoy, 2011).

Pain Assessment

The highly subjective nature of pain causes challenges in assessment and management; however, the patient's **self-report** is the undisputed standard for assessing the existence and intensity of pain (APS, 2008; McCaffery et al., 2011). Accepting and acting on the patient's report of pain are sometimes difficult. Because pain cannot be proved, the health care team is vulnerable to inaccurate or untruthful reports of pain. Clinicians are entitled to their personal doubts and opinions, but those doubts and opinions cannot be allowed to interfere with appropriate patient care. Chart 12-1 provides strategies to use when the patient's report of pain is not accepted.

Chart 12-1	Strategies to Use When the Patient's Report of Pain Is Not Accepted

- Acknowledge that everyone is entitled to a personal opinion, but personal opinion does not form the basis for professional practice.
- Clarify that the sensation of pain is subjective and cannot be proved or disproved.
- Quote recommendations from clinical practice guidelines, especially those published by the American Pain Society.
- Ask, "Why is it so difficult to believe that this person hurts?"

Copyright 2011, Pasero C., McCaffery M. Used with permission from Pasero, C., & McCaffery, M. (2011). *Pain assessment and pharmacologic management*. St. Louis: Mosby.

> **Quality and Safety Nursing Alert**
>
> Although accepting and responding to the report of pain will undoubtedly result in administering analgesic agents to an occasional patient who does not have pain, doing so ensures that everyone who does have pain receives attentive responses. Health care professionals do not have the right to deprive any patient of appropriate assessment and treatment simply because they believe a patient is not being truthful.

Performing the Comprehensive Pain Assessment: Patient Interview

A comprehensive pain assessment should be conducted during the admission assessment or initial interview with the patient, with each new report of pain, and whenever indicated by changes in the patient's condition or treatment plan during the course of care. It serves as the foundation for developing and evaluating the effectiveness of the pain treatment plan. The following are components of a comprehensive pain assessment and tips on how to elicit the information from the patient:

- *Location(s) of pain:* Ask the patient to state or point to the area(s) of pain on the body. Sometimes allowing patients to make marks on a body diagram is helpful in gaining this information.
- *Intensity:* Ask the patient to rate the severity of the pain using a reliable and valid pain assessment tool. Chart 12-2 provides guidance for educating patients and their families how to use a pain rating scale. Various scales translated in several languages have been evaluated and made available for use in clinical practice and for educational practice. The most common include the following:
- *Numeric Rating Scale (NRS):* The NRS is most often presented as a horizontal 0-to-10 point scale, with word anchors of "no pain" at one end of the scale, "moderate pain" in the middle of the scale, and "worst possible pain" at the end of the scale.
- *Wong-Baker FACES Pain Rating Scale:* The FACES scale consists of six cartoon faces with word descriptors, ranging from a smiling face on the left for "no pain (or hurt)" to a frowning, tearful face on the right for "worst pain (or hurt)." Patients are asked to choose the face that best reflects their pain. The faces are most commonly numbered using a 0, 2, 4, 6, 8, 10 metric, although 0 to 5 can also be used. Patients are asked to choose the face that best describes their pain. The FACES scale is used in adults and children as young as 3 years (McCaffery et al., 2011). It is important to appreciate that faces scales are self-report tools; clinicians should not attempt to match a face shown on a scale to the patient's facial expression to determine pain intensity. Figure 12-4 provides the Wong-Baker FACES scale combined with the NRS.
- *Faces Pain Scale–Revised (FPS-R):* The FPS-R has six faces to make it consistent with other scales using the 0 to 10 metric. The faces range from a neutral facial expression to one of intense pain and are numbered 0, 2, 4, 6, 8, and 10. As with the Wong-Baker FACES

Chart
12-2

PATIENT EDUCATION

Educating Patients and Their Families How to Use a Pain Rating Scale*

Step 1. Show the pain rating scale to the patient and family and explain its primary purpose.

Example: "This is a pain rating scale that many of our patients use to help us understand their pain and to set goals for pain relief. We will ask you regularly about pain, but any time you have pain you must let us know. We do not always know when you hurt."

Step 2. Explain the parts of the pain rating scale. If the patient does not like it or understand it, switch to another scale (e.g., vertical presentation, VDS, or faces).

Example: "On this pain rating scale, 0 means no pain and 10 means the worst possible pain. The middle of the scale, around 5, means moderate pain. A 2 or 3 would be mild pain, but 7 or higher means severe pain."

Step 3. Discuss pain as a broad concept that is not restricted to a severe and intolerable sensation.

Example: "Pain refers to any kind of discomfort anywhere in your body. Pain also means aching and hurting. Pain can include pulling, tightness, burning, knifelike feelings, and other unpleasant sensations."

Step 4. Verify that the patient understands the broad concept of pain. Ask the patient to mention two examples of pain he or she has experienced. If the patient is already in pain that requires treatment, use the present situation as the example.

Example: "I want to be sure that I have explained this clearly, so would you give me two examples of pain you have had recently?" If the patient's examples include various parts of the body and various pain characteristics, that indicates that he or she understands pain as a fairly broad concept. An example of what a patient might say is "I have a mild, sort of throbbing headache now, and yesterday my back was aching."

Step 5. Ask the patient to practice using the pain rating scale with the present pain or select one of the examples mentioned.

Example: "Using the scale, what is your pain right now? What is it at its worst?" OR "Using the pain rating scale and one of your examples of pain, what is that pain usually? What is it at its worst?"

Step 6. Set goals for comfort and function/recovery/quality of life. Ask patients what pain rating would be acceptable or satisfactory, considering the activities required for recovery or for maintaining a satisfactory quality of life.

Example for a surgical patient: "I have explained the importance of coughing and deep breathing to prevent pneumonia and other complications. Now we need to determine the pain rating that will not interfere with this so that you may recover quickly."

Example for patient with chronic pain or terminal illness: "What do you want to do that pain keeps you from doing? What pain rating would allow you to do this?"

VDS, verbal descriptor scale.

*When a patient is obviously in pain or not focused enough to learn to use a pain rating scale, pain treatment should proceed without pain ratings. Education can be undertaken when pain is reduced to a level that facilitates understanding how to use a pain scale.

scale, patients are asked to choose the face that best reflects their pain. Faces scales have been shown to be reliable and valid measures in children as young as 3 years of age; however, the ability to optimally quantify pain (identify a number) is not acquired until approximately 8 years of age (Spagrud, Piira, & Von Baeyer, 2003). Some research shows that the FPS-R is preferred by both cognitively intact and impaired older and minority populations (Li, Liu, & Herr, 2007; Ware, Epps, Herr, et al., 2006).

- *Verbal descriptor scale (VDS):* A VDS uses different words or phrases to describe the intensity of pain, such as "no pain, mild pain, moderate pain, severe pain, very severe pain, and worst possible pain."

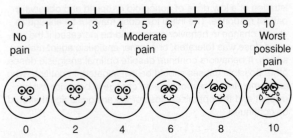

FIGURE 12-4 • Example of how the Numerical Rating Scale (NRS) can be combined with the Wong-Baker FACES Pain Rating Scale. From Hockenberry, M. J., & Wilson, D. (2009). *Wong's essentials of pediatric nursing* (8th ed.). St. Louis: Mosby. Used with permission. Copyright Mosby.

The patient is asked to select the phrase that best describes pain intensity.

- *Visual Analog Scale (VAS):* The VAS is a horizontal (sometimes vertical) 10-cm line with word anchors at the extremes, such as "no pain" on one end and "pain as bad as it could be" or "worst possible pain" on the other end. Patients are asked to make a mark on the line to indicate intensity of pain, and the length of the mark from "no pain" is measured and recorded in centimeters or millimeters. Although often used in research, the VAS is impractical for use in daily clinical practice and rarely used in that setting.

- *Quality:* Ask the patient to describe how the pain feels. Descriptors such as "sharp," "shooting," or "burning" may help identify the presence of neuropathic pain.

- *Onset and duration:* Ask the patient when the pain started and whether it is constant or intermittent.

- *Aggravating and relieving factors:* Ask the patient what makes the pain worse and what makes it better.

- *Effect of pain on function and quality of life:* The effect of pain on the ability to perform recovery activities should be regularly evaluated in the patient with acute pain. It is particularly important to ask patients with persistent pain about how pain has affected their lives, what could they do before the pain began that they can no longer do, or what they would like to do but cannot do because of the pain.

- *Comfort-function (pain intensity) goal:* For patients with acute pain, identify short-term functional goals and reinforce to the patient that good pain control will more likely lead to successful achievement of the goals. For example, surgical patients are told that they will be expected to ambulate or participate in physical therapy postoperatively. Patients with chronic pain can be asked to identify their unique functional or quality-of-life goals, such as being able to work or walk the dog. Patients are then asked to identify (using a pain intensity scale) a level of pain that will allow accomplishment of the functional goals with reasonable ease. A realistic goal for most patients is a rating of "2" or "3"; pain intensity that is consistently above the goal warrants further evaluation and consideration of an intervention and possible adjustment of the treatment plan (McCaffery et al., 2011).

- *Other information:* The patient's culture, past pain experiences, and pertinent medical history such as comorbidities, laboratory tests, and diagnostic studies are considered when establishing a treatment plan.

Patients who are unable to report their pain are at higher risk for undertreated pain than those who can report (McCaffery et al., 2011). In the adult population, this includes patients who are cognitively impaired, critically ill (intubated, unresponsive), comatose, or imminently dying.

Patients who are receiving neuromuscular blocking agents or are sedated from anesthesia and other drugs given during surgery are also among this at-risk population.

The Hierarchy of Pain Measures is recommended as a framework for assessing pain in nonverbal patients (McCaffery et al., 2011). The key components of the hierarchy require the nurse to (1) attempt to obtain self-report, (2) consider underlying pathology or conditions and procedures that might be painful (e.g., surgery), (3) observe behaviors, (4) evaluate physiologic indicators, and (5) conduct an analgesic trial. Chart 12-3 provides detailed information on each component of the Hierarchy of Pain Measures.

Reassessing Pain

Following initiation of the pain management plan, pain is reassessed and documented on a regular basis to evaluate the effectiveness of treatment. At a minimum, pain should be reassessed with each new report of pain and before and after the administration of analgesic agents (McCaffery et al., 2011). The frequency of reassessment depends on the stability of the patient's pain and is guided by institutional policy. For example, in the postanesthesia care unit (PACU),

---

Chart 12-3 **Hierarchy of Pain Measures**

1. Attempt to obtain the patient's self-report, the single most reliable indicator of pain. Do not assume a patient cannot provide a report of pain; many cognitively impaired patients are able to use a self-report tool if simple actions are taken.
   - Try using standard pain assessment tools (see text).
   - Increase the size of the font and other features of the scale.
   - Present the tool in vertical format (rather than the frequently used horizontal).
   - Try using alternative words, such as "ache," "hurt," and "sore," when discussing pain.
   - Ensure eyeglasses and hearing aids are functioning.
   - Ask about pain in the present.
   - Repeat instructions and questions more than once.
   - Allow ample time to respond.
   - Remember that head nodding and eye blinking or squeezing the eyes tightly can also be used to signal presence of pain and sometimes used to rate intensity.
   - Ask awake and oriented intubated patients to point to a number on the numerical scale if they are able.
   - Repeat instructions and show the scale each time pain is assessed.

2. Consider the patient's condition or exposure to a procedure that is thought to be painful. If appropriate, assume pain is present and document as such when approved by institution policy and procedure. As an example, pain should be assumed to be present in an unresponsive, mechanically ventilated, critically ill trauma patient.

3. Observe behavioral signs, e.g., facial expressions, crying, restlessness, and changes in activity. A pain behavior in one patient may not be in another. Try to identify pain behaviors that are unique to the patient ("pain signature"). There are many behavioral pain assessment tools available that will yield a pain behavior score and may help to determine if pain is present. However, it is important to remember that a behavioral score is not the same as a pain intensity score. Behavioral tools are used to help identify the presence of pain, but the pain intensity is unknown if the patient is unable to provide it.
   - A surrogate who knows the patient well (e.g., parent, spouse, or caregiver) may be able to provide information about underlying painful pathology or behaviors that may indicate pain.

4. Evaluate physiologic indicators with the understanding that they are the *least* sensitive indicators of pain and may signal the existence of conditions other than pain or a lack of it (e.g., hypovolemia, blood loss) (Arbour & Gelinas, 2010; Gelinas & Arbour, 2009). Patients quickly adapt physiologically despite pain and may have normal or below normal vital signs in the presence of severe pain. The overriding principle is that the absence of an elevated blood pressure or heart rate does not mean the absence of pain.

5. Conduct an analgesic trial to confirm the presence of pain and to establish a basis for developing a treatment plan if pain is thought to be present. An analgesic trial involves the administration of a low dose of nonopioid or opioid and observing patient response. The initial low dose may not be enough to elicit a change in behavior and should be increased if the previous dose was tolerated, or another analgesic agent may be added. If behaviors continue despite optimal analgesic doses, other possible causes should be investigated. In patients who are completely unresponsive, no change in behavior will be evident and the optimized dose of the analgesic agent should be continued.

From Arbour, C., & Gelinas, C. (2010). Are vital signs valid indicators for the assessment of pain in postoperative cardiac surgery ICU adults? *Intensive Critical Care Nursing*, 26(2), 83–90; Gelinas, C., & Arbour, C. (2009). Behavioral and physiologic indicators during a nociceptive procedure in conscious and unconscious mechanically ventilated patients: Similar or different? *Journal of Critical Care*, 24(4), 7–17; Pasero, C. (2009). Challenges in pain assessment. *Journal of PeriAnesthesia Nursing*, 24(1), 50–54; Pasero, C., & McCaffery, M. (2011). *Pain assessment and pharmacologic management.* St. Louis: Mosby-Elsevier.

reassessment may be necessary as often as every 10 minutes when pain is unstable during opioid **titration** but may be done every 4 to 8 hours in patients with satisfactory and stable pain 24 hours after surgery.

Pain Management

Achieving optimal pain relief is best viewed on a continuum, with the primary objective being to provide both effective and safe analgesia (Pasero, Quinn et al., 2011). The quality of pain control should be addressed whenever patient care is passed on from one clinician to another, such as at change of shift and transfer from one clinical area to another. Optimal pain relief is the responsibility of *every* member of the health care team and begins with titration of the analgesic agent followed by continued prompt assessment and analgesic agent administration during the course of care to safely achieve pain intensities that allow patients to meet their functional goals with relative ease.

Although it may not always be possible to achieve a patient's pain intensity goal within the short time the patient is in an area like the PACU or emergency department (ED), this goal provides direction for ongoing analgesic care. Important information to provide during transfer report is the patient's **comfort-function goal**, how close the patient is to achieving it, what has been done thus far to achieve it (analgesic agents and doses), and how well the patient has tolerated administration of the analgesic agent (adverse effects) (Pasero, Quinn et al., 2011).

> ▶ *Quality and Safety Nursing Alert*
>
> Pain control is the responsibility of every member of the health care team and begins with systematic assessment and initial analgesic titration followed by reassessment and analgesic administration throughout the course of care to safely achieve a level of pain that allows patients to meet their functional goals with relative ease.

Pharmacologic Management of Pain: Multimodal Analgesia

Pain is a complex phenomenon involving multiple underlying mechanisms and as such, requires more than one analgesic agent to manage it safely and effectively (Pasero, Quinn et al., 2011). The recommended approach for the treatment of all types of pain in all age groups is called *multimodal analgesia* (Dworkin, O'Connor, Audette, et al., 2010; Portenoy, 2011; Pasero, Quinn, et al., 2011; Wu & Raja, 2011). A multimodal regimen combines drugs with different underlying mechanisms, which allows lower doses of each of the drugs in the treatment plan, reducing the potential for each to produce adverse effects. Further, multimodal analgesia can result in comparable or greater pain relief than can be achieved with any single analgesic agent (Pasero, Quinn et al., 2011).

Routes of Administration

The oral route is the preferred route of analgesic administration and should be used whenever feasible because it is generally the least expensive, best tolerated, and easiest to administer (Pasero, Quinn et al., 2011). When the oral route is not possible, such as in patients who cannot swallow or are NPO (nothing by mouth) or nauseated, other routes of administration are used. For example, patients with cancer pain who are unable to swallow may take analgesic agents by the transdermal, rectal, or subcutaneous route of administration.

In the immediate postoperative period, the intravenous (IV) route is the first-line route of administration for analgesic delivery, and patients are transitioned to the oral route as tolerated. (See Chapter 19 for the management of postoperative pain.)

The rectal route of analgesic administration is an alternative route when oral or IV analgesic agents are not an option (Pasero, Quinn et al., 2011). The rectum allows passive diffusion of medications and absorption into the systemic circulation. This route of administration can be less expensive and does not involve the skill and expertise required of the parenteral route of administration. Drawbacks are that drug absorption can be unreliable and depends on many factors including rectal tissue health and administrator technique. Some patients may be resistant to or fearful of rectal administration. The rectal route is contraindicated in patients who are neutropenic or thrombocytopenic because of potential rectal bleeding. Diarrhea, perianal abscess or fistula, and abdominoperineal resection are also relative contraindications (Pasero, Quinn et al., 2011).

The topical route of administration is used for both acute and chronic pain. For example, the nonopioid diclofenac is available in patch and gel formulations for application directly over painful areas. Local anesthetic creams, such as EMLA (eutectic mixture or emulsion of local anesthetics) and L.M.X.4 (lidocaine cream 4%), can be applied directly over the injection site prior to painful needle stick procedures, and the lidocaine patch 5% is often used for well-localized types of neuropathic pain, such as postherpetic neuralgia. It is important to distinguish between topical and transdermal drug delivery. Although both routes require the drug to cross the stratum corneum to produce analgesia, transdermal drug delivery requires absorption into the systemic circulation to achieve effects; topical agents produce effects in the tissues immediately under the site of application (referred to as targeted peripheral analgesia).

Some of the more invasive methods used to manage pain are accomplished via catheter techniques such as **intraspinal** analgesia, sometimes referred to as "neuraxial" analgesia. Delivery of analgesic agents by the intraspinal routes is accomplished by inserting a needle into the subarachnoid space (for intrathecal [spinal] analgesia) or the epidural space and injecting the analgesic agent, or threading a catheter through the needle and taping it in place temporarily for bolus dosing or continuous administration (Pasero, Quinn et al., 2011). Intrathecal catheters for acute pain management are used most often for providing anesthesia or a single bolus dose of an analgesic agent. Temporary epidural catheters for acute pain management are removed after 2 to 4 days. Epidural analgesia is administered by clinician-administered bolus, continuous infusion (basal rate), and patient-controlled epidural analgesia (PCEA). The most common opioids administered intraspinally are morphine, fentanyl, and hydromorphone (Dilaudid). These are usually combined with a local anesthetic, most often ropivacaine (Naropin) or bupivacaine (Marcaine), to improve analgesia and produce an **opioid dose-sparing effect** (Pasero, Quinn et al., 2011).

A relatively new pain management technique that involves the use of an indwelling catheter is the continuous peripheral nerve block (also called *perineural anesthesia*), whereby an initial local anesthetic block is established and followed by the placement of a catheter or catheters through which an infusion of local anesthetic, usually ropivacaine or bupivacaine, is infused continuously to the targeted site of innervation (Pasero, Polomano et al., 2011). The American Society for Pain Management Nursing (ASPMN) and others provide extensive guidelines for care of patients receiving analgesia via catheter (ASPMN, 2007a; Pasero, Polomano et al., 2011; Pasero, Quinn et al., 2011).

Dosing Regimen

Two basic principles of providing effective pain management are preventing pain and maintaining a pain intensity that allows the patient to accomplish functional or quality-of-life goals with relative ease (Pasero, Quinn et al., 2011). Accomplishment of these goals may require the mainstay analgesic agent to be administered on a scheduled around-the-clock (ATC) basis, rather than PRN (as needed) to maintain stable analgesic blood levels. ATC dosing regimens are designed to control pain for patients who report pain being present 12 hours or more during a 24-hour period. PRN dosing of analgesic agents is appropriate for intermittent pain, such as prior to painful procedures and for BTP (pain that "breaks through" the pain being managed by the mainstay analgesic agent), for which supplemental doses of analgesia are provided (Pasero, Quinn et al., 2011).

Patients with persistent pain in the hospital setting should be awakened to take their pain medication (see Sedation and Respiratory Depression section). Awakening postoperative patients with moderate to severe pain to take their pain medication is especially important during the first 24 to 48 hours after surgery to keep pain under control. Patients should be told that this helps to avoid waking up with severe pain and that if their pain is well controlled, they are likely to go back to sleep quickly. The patient can transition gradually to PRN dosing as pain resolves (Pasero, Quinn et al., 2011).

Patient-Controlled Analgesia

Patient-controlled analgesia (PCA) is an interactive method of pain management that allows patients to treat their pain by self-administering doses of analgesic agents. It is used to manage all types of pain by multiple routes of administration, including oral, IV, subcutaneous, epidural, and perineural (Pasero, Quinn et al., 2011). A PCA infusion device is programmed so that the patient can press a button (pendant) to self-administer a dose of an analgesic agent (PCA dose) at a set time interval (demand or lockout) as needed. Patients who use PCAs must be able to understand the relationships between pain, pushing the PCA button or taking the analgesic agent, and pain relief and must be cognitively and physically able to use any equipment that is utilized to administer the therapy.

The use of a basal rate (continuous infusion) is common when PCEA is used, and it is often added for patients who are **opioid tolerant** and sometimes for patients who are **opioid naïve** and receiving IV PCA to allow them to manage their pain and rest better. However, it is important to recognize that the patient has no control over the delivery of a continuous infusion. Therefore, extreme caution in using basal rates for acute pain management in opioid-naïve individuals is recommended (APS, 2008). Essential to the safe use of a basal rate with PCA is close monitoring by nurses of sedation and respiratory status and prompt decreases in opioid dose (e.g., discontinue basal rate) if increased sedation is detected (Pasero, Quinn et al., 2011).

The primary benefit of PCA is that it recognizes that only the patient can feel the pain and only the patient knows how much analgesic will relieve it. This reinforces that PCA is for patient use only and that unauthorized activation of the PCA button (PCA by proxy) should be discouraged.

 Quality and Safety Nursing Alert

Staff, family, and other visitors should be instructed to contact the nurse if they have concerns about pain control rather than pressing the PCA button for the patient.

For some patients who are candidates for PCA but unable to use the PCA equipment, the nurse or a capable family member may be authorized to manage the patient's pain using PCA equipment. This is referred to as Authorized Agent Controlled Analgesia; guidelines are available for the safe administration of this therapy (ASPMN, 2007b; Pasero, Quinn et al., 2011).

Analgesic Agents

Analgesic agents are categorized into three main groups: (1) nonopioid analgesic agents, which include acetaminophen and NSAIDs; (2) opioid analgesic agents, which include, among others, morphine, hydromorphone, fentanyl, and oxycodone; and (3) **adjuvant analgesic agents** (sometimes referred to as co-analgesic agents). The adjuvant analgesic agents comprise the largest group and include various agents with unique and widely differing mechanisms of action. Examples are local anesthetics and some anticonvulsants and antidepressants.

Nonopioid Analgesic Agents

Acetaminophen and NSAIDs comprise the group of nonopioid analgesic agents (refer to earlier discussion of the two categories of NSAIDs; see Fig. 12-2).

Indications and Administration. Nonopioids are flexible analgesic agents used for a wide variety of painful conditions. They are appropriate alone for mild to some moderate nociceptive pain (e.g., from surgery, trauma, or osteoarthritis) and are added to opioids, local anesthetics, and/or anticonvulsants as part of a multimodal analgesic regimen for more severe nociceptive pain (Pasero, Quinn et al., 2011). Acetaminophen and an NSAID may be given concomitantly, and there is no need for staggered doses. Unless contraindicated, all surgical patients should routinely be given acetaminophen and an NSAID in scheduled doses throughout the postoperative course, preferably initiated preoperatively (Pasero, Portenoy et al., 2011).

The nonopioids are often combined in a single tablet with opioids, such as oxycodone (Percocet) or hydrocodone (Vicodin, Lortab), and are very popular for the treatment of mild to moderate acute pain. They are the most common choice after invasive pain management therapies are discontinued and for pain treatment after hospital discharge and dental surgery when an opioid is prescribed. Many people with persistent pain also take a combination nonopioid-opioid analgesic agent; however, it is important to remember that these combination drugs are not appropriate for severe pain of any type because the maximum daily dose of the nonopioid limits the escalation of the opioid dose (Pasero, Quinn et al., 2011).

Acetaminophen is versatile in that it can be given by multiple routes of administration, including oral, rectal, and IV. Oral acetaminophen has a long history of safety in recommended doses in all age groups. It is increasingly added to multimodal treatment plans for postoperative pain (Pasero, Portenoy et al., 2011).

IV acetaminophen (Ofirmev) is approved for treatment of pain and fever and is given by a 15-minute infusion in single or repeated doses (Groudine & Fossum, 2011). It may be given alone for mild to moderate pain or in combination with opioid analgesic agents for more severe pain and has been shown to be well tolerated and to produce a significant opioid dose-sparing effect and superior pain relief compared with placebo (Macario & Royal, 2011) (see later discussion of placebos). Recommended dosing is 1,000 mg every 6 hours for a maximum of 4,000 mg in patients weighing more than 50 kg, and 15 mg/kg every 6 hours in patients weighing less than 50 kg. Repeated doses for up to 5 days have been shown to be safe and well tolerated (Candiotti, Bergese, Viscusi, et al., 2010; Uysal, Takmaz, Yaman, et al., 2011).

A benefit of the NSAID group is the availability of a wide variety of agents for administration via noninvasive routes. Ibuprofen, naproxen, and celecoxib are the most widely used oral NSAIDs in the United States. When rectal formulations are unavailable, an intact oral tablet may be administered rectally by inserting the tablet, or a crushed tablet in a gelatin capsule, into the rectum. Higher rectal than oral doses may be required to achieve similar analgesic effects (Pasero, Quinn et al., 2011). Diclofenac can be prescribed in patch and gel form for topical administration, and an intranasal patient-controlled formulation of ketorolac (Sprix) has been approved for treatment of postoperative pain.

IV formulations of ketorolac (Toradol) and ibuprofen (Caldolor) are available for acute pain treatment. Both have been shown to produce excellent analgesia alone for moderate nociceptive pain and significant opioid dose-sparing effects when administered as part of a multimodal analgesia plan for more severe nociceptive pain (Brown, Moodie, Bisley, et al., 2009; Chen, Ko, Wen, et al., 2009; Singla, Rock, & Pavliv, 2010).

Adverse Effects of Nonopioid Analgesic Agents. Acetaminophen is widely considered one of the safest and best tolerated analgesic agents (Candiotti et al., 2010; Pasero, Portenoy et al., 2011). Its most serious complication is hepatotoxicity (liver damage) as a result of overdose. In the healthy adult, a maximum daily dose below 4,000 mg is rarely associated with

liver toxicity (Groudine & Fossum, 2011). Nevertheless, one manufacturer of oral acetaminophen (Tylenol) voluntarily changed its dosing recommendations in 2011, calling for a maximum daily dose of 3,000 mg (Ortho-McNeil Pharmaceuticals, 2011). Acetaminophen does not increase bleeding time and has a low incidence of gastrointestinal (GI) adverse effects, making it the analgesic agent of choice in many individuals with comorbidities.

NSAIDs have considerably more adverse effects than acetaminophen, with gastric toxicity and ulceration being the most common (Pasero, Portenoy et al., 2011). The primary underlying mechanism of NSAID-induced gastric ulceration is the inhibition of COX-1, which leads to a reduction in GI-protective prostaglandins (see Fig. 12-2). This is a systemic (rather than local) effect and can occur regardless of the route of administration of the NSAID. Risk factors include advanced age (older than 60 years), presence of prior ulcer disease, and cardiovascular (CV) disease and other comorbidities (Pasero, Portenoy et al., 2011). The use of a COX-2 selective NSAID (e.g., celecoxib) if not contraindicated by CV risk or the least ulcerogenic nonselective NSAID (e.g., ibuprofen) plus a proton pump inhibitor is recommended in patients with elevated risk (AGS, 2009; Pasero, Portenoy et al., 2011). GI adverse effects are also related to the dose and duration of NSAID therapy; the higher the NSAID dose and the longer the duration of NSAID use, the higher the risk of GI toxicity. A principle of nonopioid analgesic use is to administer the lowest dose for the shortest time necessary (Pasero, Portenoy et al., 2011).

All NSAIDs carry a risk of CV adverse effects through prostaglandin inhibition, and the risk is increased with COX-2 inhibition, whether it is produced by a COX-2 selective NSAID (e.g., celecoxib) or by NSAIDs that are nonselective inhibitors of both COX-1 and COX-2 (e.g., ibuprofen, naproxen, and ketorolac) (Pasero, Portenoy et al., 2011). The U.S. Food and Drug Administration (FDA) cautions against the use of any NSAIDs following high-risk open heart surgery because of an elevated CV risk with NSAIDs in this population (U.S. FDA, 2007).

The COX isoenzymes play an important role in renal function through their effects on prostaglandin formation. Overall, adverse renal effects occur in approximately 1% to 5% of long-term NSAID users (Pasero, Quinn et al., 2011). NSAID-induced renal toxicity can occur but is relatively rare in otherwise healthy adults who are given NSAIDs for short-term pain management (e.g., in the perioperative period); however, individuals with acute or chronic volume depletion or hypotension rely on prostaglandin synthesis to maintain adequate renal blood flow, and NSAID inhibition of prostaglandin synthesis in such patients can cause acute renal failure. Attention to adequate hydration is essential when administering NSAIDs to prevent this complication (Pasero, Portenoy et al., 2011).

Most nonselective NSAIDs increase bleeding time though inhibition of COX-1. This is both drug- and dose related, so the lowest dose of nonopioids with minimal or no effect on bleeding time should be used in patients or procedures with high risk for bleeding. Options include acetaminophen, celecoxib, choline magnesium trisalicylate, salsalate (Disalcid), and nabumetone (Relafen) (Pasero, Portenoy et al., 2011).

Opioid Analgesic Agents

Although it is often used, the term *narcotic* is considered obsolete and inaccurate when discussing the use of opioids for pain management, in part because it is a term used loosely by law enforcement and the media to refer to various substances of potential abuse, which include opioids as well as cocaine and other illicit substances. Legally, controlled substances classified as narcotics include opioids, cocaine, and others. The preferred term is *opioid analgesics* when discussing these agents in the context of pain management; patients prefer the term *pain medications* or *pain medicine* (Pasero, Quinn et al., 2011).

Opioid analgesic agents are divided into two major groups: (1) **mu agonist** opioids (also called *morphinelike drugs*) and (2) **agonist-antagonist** opioids. The mu agonist opioids comprise the larger of the two groups and include morphine, hydromorphone, hydrocodone, fentanyl, oxycodone, and methadone, among others. The agonist-antagonist opioids include buprenorphine (Buprenex, Butrans), nalbuphine (Nubain), and butorphanol (Stadol).

Opioid analgesic agents exert their effects by interacting with opioid receptor sites located throughout the body, including in the peripheral tissues, GI system, and CNS; they are abundant in the dorsal horn of the spinal cord. There are three major classes of opioid receptor sites involved in analgesia: the mu, delta, and kappa. The pharmacologic differences in the various opioids are the result of their interaction with these opioid receptor types (Pasero, Quinn et al., 2011). When an opioid binds to the opioid receptor sites, it produces analgesia as well as unwanted effects, such as constipation, nausea, sedation, and respiratory depression.

The opioid analgesic agents that are designated as first line (e.g., morphine, hydromorphone, fentanyl, and oxycodone) belong to the mu opioid agonist class because they bind primarily to the mu-type opioid receptors. The agonist-antagonist opioids are designated as "mixed" because they bind to more than one opioid receptor site. They bind as agonists, producing analgesia, at the kappa opioid receptor sites, and as weak antagonists at the mu opioid receptor sites. Their propensity to antagonize the effects of mu opioid analgesic agents limits their usefulness in pain management (Pasero, Quinn et al., 2011). They should be avoided in patients receiving long-term mu opioid therapy because their use may trigger severe pain and opioid withdrawal syndrome characterized by rhinitis, abdominal cramping, nausea, agitation, and restlessness.

Antagonists (e.g., naloxone, naltrexone) are drugs that also bind to opioid receptors but produce no analgesia. If an antagonist is present, it competes with opioid molecules for binding sites on the opioid receptors and has the potential to block analgesia and other effects. They are used most often to reverse adverse effects, such as respiratory depression.

Administration. Safe and effective use of opioid analgesic agents requires the development of an individualized treatment plan based on a comprehensive pain assessment, which includes clarifying the goals of treatment and discussing options with the patient and family (Pasero, Quinn et al., 2011). Goals are periodically reevaluated and changes made depending on patient response and in some cases disease progression.

Many factors are considered when determining the appropriate opioid analgesic agent for the patient with pain. These include the unique characteristics of the various opioids and patient factors, such as pain intensity, age, coexisting disease, current drug regimen and potential drug interactions, prior treatment outcomes, and patient preference. In all cases, a multimodal approach that may rely on the selection of appropriate analgesic agents from the nonopioid, opioid, and adjuvant analgesic agent groups is recommended to manage all types of pain (Portenoy, 2011; Turk et al., 2011; Wu & Raja, 2011). Chart 12-4 lists the key considerations when developing an opioid pain treatment plan.

Titration of the opioid dose is usually required at the start and throughout the course of treatment when opioids are administered. Whereas patients with cancer pain most often are titrated upward over time for progressive pain, patients with acute pain, particularly postoperative pain, are eventually titrated downward as pain resolves (Pasero, Quinn et al., 2011). The dose and analgesic effect of mu agonist opioids have no **ceiling effect**, although the dose may be limited by adverse effects. The absolute dose administered is unimportant as long as a balance between pain relief and adverse effects is favorable. The goal of titration is to use the smallest dose that provides satisfactory pain relief with the fewest adverse effects. When an increase in the opioid dose is necessary and safe, this can be done by percentages. When a slight improvement in analgesia is needed, a 25% increase in the opioid dose may be sufficient and a 50% increase for moderate improvement; a 100% increase may be indicated for strong improvement, such as when treating severe pain (Pasero, Quinn et al., 2011). The time at which the dose can be increased is determined by the onset and peak effects of the opioid and its formulation. For example, the frequency of IV opioid doses during initial titration may be as often as every 5 to 15 minutes. In contrast, at least 24 hours should elapse before the dose of transdermal fentanyl is increased after the first patch application (Pasero, Quinn et al., 2011).

Equianalgesia. The term *equianalgesia* means approximately "equal analgesia." An equianalgesic chart provides a list of doses of analgesic agents, both oral and parenteral (IV, subcutaneous, and intramuscular), that are approximately equal to each other in ability to provide pain relief. Equianalgesic conversion of doses is used to help ensure that patients are not overdosed or underdosed when they are switched from one opioid or route of administration to another. It requires a series of calculations based on the daily dose of the current opioid to determine the equianalgesic dose of the opioid to which the patient is to be switched. Several excellent guidelines are available to assist in calculating equianalgesic doses (McPherson, 2010; Pasero, Quinn et al., 2011) (Table 12-3).

Formulation Terminology. The terms *short acting, immediate release,* and *normal release* have been used interchangeably to describe oral opioids that have an onset of action of approximately 30 minutes and a relatively short duration of 3 to 4 hours. The term *immediate release* is misleading because none of the oral analgesic agents have an immediate onset of analgesia; *short acting* is preferred. The terms *modified release, extended release, sustained release, controlled release,* and long acting are used to describe opioids that are formulated to release over a prolonged period of time. For the purposes of this chapter, the term *modified release* will be used when discussing these opioid formulations.

Chart 12-4 Use of Opioids

- Perform a comprehensive assessment that addresses pain, co-morbidities, and functional status.
- Develop an individualized treatment plan that includes specific goals related to pain intensity, activities (function/quality of life), and adverse effects (e.g., pain intensity rating of 3 on a 0 to 10 numerical rating scale to ambulate accompanied by minimal or no sedation).
- Use multimodal analgesia (e.g., add acetaminophen and NSAID; anticonvulsant in patients at risk for persistent postsurgical pain).
- Assess for presence preoperatively of underlying persistent pain in surgical patients and optimize its treatment.
- Consider **preemptive analgesic agents** before surgery, particularly for those at risk for severe postoperative pain or a persistent postsurgical pain syndrome.
- Provide analgesic agents prior to all painful procedures.
- Drug selection
  - Consider diagnosis, condition, or surgical procedure, current or expected pain intensity, age, presence of major organ dysfunction or failure, and presence of coexisting disease.
  - Consider pharmacologic issues (e.g., accumulation of metabolites and effects of concurrent drugs).
  - Consider prior treatment outcomes and patient preference.
  - Be aware of available routes of administration (oral, transdermal, rectal, intranasal, IV subcutaneous, perineural, intraspinal) and formulations (e.g., short acting, modified release).
  - Be aware of cost differences.
- Route of administration selection
  - Use least invasive route possible.
  - Consider convenience and patient's ability to adhere to the regimen.
  - Consider staff's (or patient's or caregiver's) ability to monitor and provide care required.
- Dosing and titration
  - Consider previous dosing requirement and relative analgesic potencies when initiating therapy.
  - Use equianalgesic dose chart (see Table 12-3) to determine starting dose with consideration of patient's current status

(e.g., sedation and respiratory status) and co-morbidities (e.g., medical frailty), and then titrate until adequate analgesia is achieved or dose-limiting adverse effects are encountered.
  - Use appropriate dosing schedule (e.g., around-the-clock for continuous pain; PRN for intermittent pain).
  - When dose is safe but additional analgesia is desired, titrate upward by 25% for slight increase, 50% for moderate increase, and 100% for considerable increase in analgesia.
  - Provide supplemental doses for breakthrough pain; consider PCA if appropriate.
- Treatment of adverse effects
  - Be aware of the prevalence and impact of opioid adverse effects.
  - Remember that most opioid adverse effects are dose dependent; always consider decreasing the opioid dose as a method of treating or eliminating an adverse effect; adding nonopioid analgesic agents for additive analgesia facilitates this approach.
  - Use a preventive approach in the management of constipation, including for patients receiving short-term opioid treatment.
  - Prevent respiratory depression by monitoring sedation levels and respiratory status frequently and decreasing the opioid dose as soon as increased sedation is detected.
- Monitoring
  - Continually and consistently evaluate the plan on the basis of the specific goals identified at the outset and assess pain intensity, adverse effects, and activity levels.
  - Make necessary modifications to treatment plan to maintain efficacy and safety.
- Tapering and cessation of treatment
  - If a decrease in dose or cessation of treatment is appropriate, do so in accordance with decreased pain intensity and after evaluation of functional outcomes.
  - Be aware of the potential for withdrawal syndrome (rhinitis, abdominal cramping, diarrhea, restlessness, agitation) and need for tapering schedule in patients who have been receiving opioid therapy for more than a few days.

NSAID, nonsteroidal anti-inflammatory drug; IV, intravenous; PRN, as needed; PCA, patient-controlled analgesia.
Copyright 2011, Pasero C., McCaffery M. Modified and used with permission. Pasero, C., & McCaffery, M. (2011). *Pain assessment and pharmacologic management.* St. Louis: Mosby-Elsevier.

Addiction, Physical Dependence, and Tolerance. The terms *physical dependence* and *tolerance* often are confused with addiction, thus clarification of definitions is important (Pasero, Quinn et al., 2011). More than a decade ago, the American Academy of Pain Medicine, the APS, and the American Society of Addiction Medicine (2001) proposed definitions that continue to be widely accepted today:

- **Physical dependence** is a normal response that occurs with repeated administration of the opioid for 2 or more weeks and cannot be equated with addictive disease. It is manifested by the occurrence of withdrawal symptoms when the opioid is suddenly stopped or rapidly reduced or an antagonist such as naloxone is given. Withdrawal symptoms may be suppressed by the natural, gradual reduction of the opioid as pain decreases or by gradual, systematic reduction, referred to as tapering.
- **Tolerance** is also a normal response that occurs with regular administration of an opioid and consists of a decrease in one or more effects of the opioid (e.g., decreased analgesia, sedation, or respiratory depression).

It cannot be equated with addictive disease. Tolerance to analgesia usually occurs in the first days to 2 weeks of opioid therapy but is uncommon after that. It may be treated with increases in dose. However, disease progression, not tolerance to analgesia, appears to be the reason for most dose escalations. Stable pain usually results in stable opioid doses. Thus, tolerance poses very few clinical problems. With the exception of constipation, tolerance to the opioid adverse effects develops with regular daily dosing of opioids over several days (Pasero, Quinn et al., 2011).

- Opioid **addiction**, or addictive disease, is a chronic neurologic and biologic disease. The development and characteristics of addiction are influenced by genetic, psychosocial, and environmental factors. No single cause of addiction, such as taking an opioid for pain relief, has been found. It is characterized by behaviors that include one or more of the following: impaired control over drug use, compulsive use, continued use despite harm, and craving to use the opioid for effects

TABLE 12-3 **Equianalgesic Dose Chart for Common mu Opioid Analgesic Agents**

- *Equianalgesic* means approximately the same pain relief.
- The equianalgesic chart is a guideline for selecting doses for opioid-naïve patients. Doses and intervals between doses are titrated according to individuals' responses.
- The equianalgesic chart is helpful when switching from one drug or route of administration to another.

Opioid	Oral	Parenteral	Comments
Morphine	30 mg	10 mg	Standard for comparison; first-line opioid via multiple routes of administration; once-daily and twice-daily oral formulations; clinically significant metabolites
Fentanyl	No formulation	100 mcg IV 100 mcg/h of transdermal fentanyl is approximately equal to 4 mg/h of IV morphine; 1 mcg/h of transdermal fentanyl is approximately equal to 2 mg/24 h of oral morphine	First-line opioid via IV, transdermal, and intraspinal routes; available in oral transmucosal and buccal formulations for breakthrough pain in opioid tolerant patients; no clinically relevant metabolites
Hydrocodone	30 mg (Not recommended)	No formulation	Available only in combination with acetaminophen (e.g., Vicodin, Lortab) and as such is appropriate only for mild to some moderate pain
Hydromorphone (Dilaudid)	7.5 mg	1.5 mg	First-line opioid via multiple routes of administration; once-daily oral formulation; clinically significant metabolites noted with long-term and high-dose infusion
Oxycodone	20 mg	No formulation in the United States	Short-acting and twice-daily oral formulations
Oxymorphone	10 mg	1 mg	Parenteral and short-acting and twice-daily oral formulations

IV, intravenous.

From Pasero, C., & McCaffery, M. (2011). *Pain assessment and pharmacologic management.* St. Louis: Mosby.

other than pain relief. This statement reinforces that taking opioids for pain relief is not addiction, no matter how long a person takes opioids or at what doses.

Pseudoaddiction is a mistaken diagnosis of addictive disease (Weissman & Haddox, 1989). When a patient's pain is not well controlled, the patient may begin to manifest symptoms suggestive of addictive disease. In an effort to obtain adequate pain relief, the patient may respond with demanding behavior, escalating demands for more or different medications, and repeated requests for opioids on time or before the prescribed interval between doses has elapsed. Pain relief typically eliminates these behaviors and is often accomplished by increasing opioid doses or decreasing intervals between doses (Pasero, Quinn et al., 2011).

The incidence of addiction as a result of taking an opioid for therapeutic reasons is thought to be quite rare (Jackson, 2009; Rowbotham, Serrano-Gomez, & Heffernan, 2009). An evidence-based review of the development of addiction *and* aberrant drug-related behaviors in patients with persistent noncancer pain being treated with opioids calculated the percentage of abuse or addiction to be 0.19% (Fishbain, Cole, Lewis, et al., 2008). This suggests that patients with no past or present history of abuse or addiction usually remain responsible medication users over time. Similarly, a registry study of 227 patients who were treated with modified-release oxycodone and followed for up to 3 years after participating in a clinical trial also showed a very low occurrence of problematic drug-related behavior—there were just six cases of misuse and no cases of new addiction (Portenoy, Farrar, Backonja, et al., 2007).

Opioid Naïve Versus Opioid Tolerant. Patients are often characterized as being either *opioid naïve* or *opioid tolerant.* Whereas an opioid-naïve individual has not recently taken enough opioid on a regular basis to become tolerant to the effects of an opioid, an opioid-tolerant individual has taken an opioid long enough at doses high enough to develop tolerance to many of the effects, including analgesia and sedation. There is no set time for the development of tolerance, and there is great individual variation with some not developing tolerance at all. By convention, most clinicians consider a patient who has taken opioids regularly for approximately 7 or more days to be opioid tolerant (Pasero, Quinn et al., 2011).

Opioid-Induced Hyperalgesia. Hyperalgesia means increased sensitivity to pain. **Opioid-induced hyperalgesia (OIH)** is a paradoxical situation in which increasing doses of opioid result in increasing sensitivity to pain (Compton, 2008). The incidence of clinically significant OIH has not been determined; however, it appears to be a rare but serious consequence of opioid administration (Chu, Angst, & Clark, 2008). At this time, it is not possible to predict who will develop OIH as a result of opioid exposure, and the mechanisms underlying OIH are largely unknown. In general, OIH is thought to be the result of changes in the central and peripheral nervous systems that produce increased transmission of nociceptive signals (Compton, 2008).

Some experts characterize OIH and analgesic tolerance as "opposite sides of the coin" (Pasero, Quinn et al., 2011). In tolerance, increasing doses of opioid are needed to provide the same level of pain relief because opioid exposure induces neurophysiologic changes that reverse analgesia; in OIH, opioid exposure induces neurophysiologic changes that produce pain or increase sensitivity to noxious input (Angst & Clark, 2006). In other words, tolerance may be inferred clinically when opioid treatment leads to decreased sensitivity to opioid analgesia over time (in the absence of another process that would explain this), whereas OIH may be inferred clinically when opioid treatment leads to increased pain or sensitivity to pain over time (DuPen, Shen, & Ersek, 2007). When OIH is suspected, a thorough differential assessment that rules out all other possible explanations is recommended (Pasero, Quinn et al., 2011).

Selected Opioid Analgesic Agents. Morphine is the standard against which all other opioid drugs are compared. It is the most widely used opioid worldwide, particularly for cancer pain, and its use is established by extensive research and clinical experience (Pasero, Quinn et al., 2011). It is available in a wide variety of short-acting and modified-release oral formulations and is given by multiple routes of administration. It was the first drug to be administered intraspinally and remains a first-line choice for long-term intraspinal analgesia. It is the only opioid uniquely formulated to produce analgesia for up to 48 hours following epidural administration for acute pain management (extended-release epidural morphine [Depo-Dur]). Morphine is a **hydrophilic** drug (readily absorbed in aqueous solution), which accounts for its slow onset and long duration of action when compared with other opioid analgesic agents (Table 12-4; see Table 12-3). It has two principal, clinically significant **metabolites:** morphine-3-glucuronide (M3G) and morphine-6-glucuronide (M6G). M6G may be responsible for some of the analgesic effect of morphine; accumulation of M3G can produce neurotoxicity, which necessitates switching the patient to a different opioid (Pasero, Quinn et al., 2011).

In contrast to morphine, fentanyl (Sublimaze) is a **lipophilic** (readily absorbed in fatty tissues) opioid, and as such has a fast onset and short duration of action (see Tables 12-3 and 12-4). These characteristics make it the most commonly used IV opioid when rapid analgesia is desired, such as for the treatment of severe, escalating acute pain, and for procedural pain when a short duration of action is desirable. The drug is a good choice for patients with end-organ failure because it has no clinically relevant metabolites. It also produces minimal hemodynamic adverse effects; thus, fentanyl is often preferred in patients who are hemodynamically unstable, such as the critically ill (Pasero, Quinn et al., 2011).

Its lipophilicity makes fentanyl ideal for drug delivery by transdermal patch (Duragesic) for long-term opioid administration and by the oral transmucosal (Actiq) and buccal (Fentora) routes for BTP treatment in patients who are opioid tolerant. Following application of the transdermal patch, a subcutaneous depot of fentanyl is established in the skin near the patch. After absorption from the depot into the systemic circulation, the drug distributes to fat and muscle. When the first patch is applied, 12 to 18 hours are required for clinically significant analgesia to be obtained; attention must be paid to providing adequate supplemental analgesia during that time. The patch is changed every 48 to 72 hours depending on patient response (Gallagher, Welz-Bosna, & Gammaitoni, 2007).

> ### Quality and Safety Nursing Alert
>
> The application of heat (heat packs, heating pads, or hot tubs or showers) directly over the patch can cause increased absorption of transdermal fentanyl, which can lead to life-threatening respiratory depression.

Hydromorphone (Dilaudid) is less hydrophilic than morphine but less lipophilic than fentanyl, which contributes to an onset and duration of action that is intermediate between morphine and fentanyl (see Tables 12-3 and 12-4). The drug is often used as an alternative to morphine, especially for acute pain because the two drugs produce similar analgesia and have comparable adverse effect profiles (Pasero, Quinn et al., 2011). It is a first- or second-choice opioid (after morphine) for postoperative pain management via IV PCA and is available in a once-daily modified-release oral formulation for chronic pain management. Accumulation of its neuroexcitatory metabolite hydromorphone-3-glucuronide (H3G) may occur with high-dose, long-term infusion therapy, which would necessitate a switch to another opioid (Pasero, Quinn et al., 2011).

Oxycodone is available in the United States for administration by the oral route only and is used to treat all types of pain. In combination with acetaminophen or ibuprofen, it is appropriate for mild to some moderate pain. Single-entity short-acting (OxyIR) and modified-release (OxyContin) oxycodone formulations are used most often for moderate to severe cancer pain and in some patients with moderate to severe noncancer pain (see Table 12-3). It has been used successfully as part of a multimodal treatment plan for postoperative pain as well (Pasero, Quinn et al., 2011).

Oxymorphone has been available for many years in parenteral formulation and more recently in short-acting (Opana IR) and modified-release (Opana ER) oral tablets for treatment of moderate to severe chronic pain (see Table 12-3). It must be taken on an empty stomach (1 hour before or 2 hours after a meal), and coingestion of alcohol at the time of dosing must be avoided, because food and alcohol can increase the serum concentration of the drug (Pasero, Quinn et al., 2011).

Hydrocodone is available only in combination with non-opioids (e.g., with acetaminophen in Vicodin or Lortab), which limits its use to the treatment of mild to some moderate pain (see Table 12-3). It is one of the most commonly prescribed analgesic agents in the United States; however, its prescription for treatment of persistent pain (except for breakthrough dosing) should be carefully evaluated because of its ceiling on **efficacy** and safety inherent in the nonopioid constituent (Pasero, Quinn et al., 2011).

Methadone (Dolophine) is a unique opioid analgesic agent that may have advantages over other opioids in carefully selected patients. In addition to being a mu opioid, it is

TABLE 12-4	Characteristics of Selected First-Line Opioid Analgesic Agents*		
Opioid	**Onset (minutes)**	**Peak (minutes)**	**Duration (hours)**
Morphine	30–60 (PO)	60–90 (PO)	3–6 (PO)
	5–10 (IV)	15–30 (IV)	3–4 (IV)
Fentanyl	5 (OT)	15 (OT)	2–5 (OT)
	3–5 (IV)	15–30 (IV)	2 (IV)
Hydromorphone	15–30 (PO)	30–90 (PO)	3–4 (PO)
	5 (IV)	10–20 (IV)	3–4 (IV)

PO, oral; IV, intravenous; OT, oral transmucosal.
*Characteristics do not apply to modified-release formulations.
From Pasero, C., & McCaffery, M. (2011). *Pain assessment and pharmacologic management.* St. Louis: Mosby-Elsevier.

an antagonist at the NMDA receptor site and thus has the potential to produce analgesic effects as a second- or third-line option for some neuropathic pain states (Dworkin et al., 2010). It is often used as an alternative when it is necessary to switch a patient to a new opioid because of inadequate analgesia or unacceptable adverse effects. The use of conventional equianalgesic dose conversion is not recommended when switching patients to and from methadone. Extensive guidelines on how to safely accomplish this are available elsewhere (Pasero, Quinn et al., 2011).

Methadone usually is administered orally but has also been given by virtually every other route of administration. Although it has no active metabolites, methadone has a very long and highly variable **half-life** (5 to 100-plus hours; average is 20 hours), which makes it a good choice for treatment of addictive disease but impacts clinical management during its titration for pain management; patients must be watched closely for excessive sedation, a sign of drug accumulation during this time period. (The drug is described as "long acting" because of its exceptionally long half-life.) Other limitations are its propensity to interact with a large number of medications and prolong the QTc interval on the electrocardiogram. Despite these characteristics, methadone can be an effective and safe drug when prescribed by practitioners who have an appreciation of the drug's characteristics and experience in its use (Pasero, Quinn et al., 2011).

Dual-Mechanism Analgesic Agents. The dual-mechanism analgesic agents tramadol (Ultram) and tapentadol (Nucynta) are relatively new to pain management. These drugs bind weakly to the mu opioid receptor site and block the reuptake (resorption) of the inhibitory neurotransmitters serotonin and/or norepinephrine at central synapses in the spinal cord and brain stem of the modulatory descending pain pathway (Pasero & Portenoy, 2011). This makes these neurotransmitters more available to fight pain. Dual-mechanism analgesic agents have been described as providing automatic "built-in" multimodal analgesia because a single tablet produces an effect on more than one analgesic action site (Pasero, 2011). The underlying mechanisms of tapentadol and tramadol differ in that tramadol blocks the reuptake of both serotonin and norepinephrine, but tapentadol blocks the reuptake of only norepinephrine. This is pertinent because norepinephrine is thought to play a more significant role than serotonin in the endogenous analgesia pathways (Veves, Backonja, & Malik, 2008). Serotonin may be the more powerful mediator of depression; low serotonin levels are associated with depression. This helps to explain why selective serotonin reuptake inhibitors (SSRIs), such as fluoxetine (Prozac) and paroxetine (Paxil), which block only serotonin, are effective for the treatment of depression but not pain (Pasero, Polomano et al., 2011).

Tramadol is used for both acute and chronic pain and is available in oral short-acting and modified-release (Ultram ER) formulations, including a short-acting tablet in combination with acetaminophen (Ultracet). It has been designated as a second-line analgesic agent for the treatment of neuropathic pain (Dworkin et al., 2010). The drug can lower seizure threshold and interact with other drugs that block the reuptake of serotonin, such as the SSRIs, although serotonin syndrome, characterized by agitation, diarrhea,

heart and blood pressure changes, and loss of coordination, appears to rarely be a problem in the clinical setting (Dworkin et al., 2010).

Tapentadol (NUCYNTA) is available in short-acting and modified-release oral formulations. The drug has been shown to produce dose-dependent analgesia comparable to oxycodone. Research suggests the drug can be given concomitantly with nonopioid analgesic agents commonly used in multimodal treatment plans for acute pain (Pasero, 2011). Major benefits are that it has no active metabolites and a significantly more favorable adverse effect profile (particularly GI) compared with opioid analgesic agents. These characteristics make tapentadol an attractive alternative to traditional oral opioid analgesic agents for many patients with pain.

Opioids to Avoid. Research suggests that codeine with acetaminophen (Tylenol #3) is less efficacious and associated with more adverse effects than NSAIDs, such as ibuprofen and naproxen, for acute pain (Mitchell, van Zanten, Inglis, et al., 2008; Nauta, Landsmeer, & Koren, 2009).

Meperidine (Demerol) has either been removed from or severely restricted on hospital formularies for the treatment of pain in an effort to improve patient safety (Pasero, Quinn et al., 2011). (It is accepted practice to use it in low doses [12.5 to 25 mg IV] to treat shivering associated with general anesthesia.) A major drawback to the use of meperidine is its active metabolite, normeperidine, which is a CNS stimulant and can cause delirium, irritability, tremors, myoclonus, and generalized seizures. Propoxyphene (Darvon) and propoxyphene plus acetaminophen (Darvocet) were prescribed for many years for mild to moderate pain but were withdrawn from the U.S. market in 2010.

Adverse Effects of Opioid Analgesic Agents. The most common adverse effects of opioid analgesic agents are constipation, nausea, vomiting, pruritus, and sedation (Pasero, Quinn et al., 2011). Respiratory depression is less common but the most feared of the opioid adverse effects (Pasero, 2009). In surgical patients, postoperative ileus can become a major complication as well. A common perception is that opioids cause hypotension; however, research findings from one study indicate that the opioid doses commonly used for pain management rarely cause this adverse effect (Ho & Gan, 2009).

Opioids can result in delayed gastric emptying, slowed bowel motility, and decreased peristalsis, all of which result in slow-moving, hard stool that is difficult to pass. Risk is elevated with opioid use, advanced age, and immobility; however, it is an almost universal opioid adverse effect (i.e., tolerance rarely develops). Constipation is a primary reason people stop taking their pain medication, which underscores the importance of taking a preventive approach and aggressive management if symptoms are detected. Prevention includes reminding patients to take a daily stool softener plus mild peristaltic stimulant, for as long as they are taking opioids (Pasero, Quinn et al., 2011).

Postoperative nausea and vomiting (PONV) are among the most unpleasant of the adverse effects associated with surgery, and it can have a negative impact on patient outcomes and increase the need for nursing intervention (Miaskowski,

2009). Guidelines recommend that all patients be evaluated for PONV risk, baseline risk factors be reduced if possible, multimodal analgesia be provided so that no opioid or the lowest effective opioid dose can be given, and prophylactic treatment (e.g., dexamethasone [Decadron] and a serotonin receptor antagonist such as ondansetron [Zofran] at the end of surgery) be given to patients with moderate risk (American Society of PeriAnesthesia Nurses, 2006). More aggressive interventions should be utilized in patients with high risk (Pasero, Quinn et al., 2011). (See Chapter 19 for further discussion of PONV.)

Pruritus is an adverse effect, not an allergic reaction, to opioids (Ho & Gan, 2009). Although antihistamines such as diphenhydramine (Benadryl) are commonly used, there is no strong evidence that they relieve opioid-induced pruritus (Grape & Schug, 2008). Patients may report being less bothered by itching after taking an antihistamine, although this is likely the result of sedating effects (Ho & Gan, 2009). Sedation can be problematic in those already at risk for excessive sedation, such as postoperative patients, because this can lead to life-threatening respiratory depression (Pasero, Quinn et al., 2011). A common clinical observation is that patients with postoperative opioid-induced pruritus usually have well-controlled pain. This may be because painful stimuli can inhibit itching, and inhibition of pain processing may enhance itching (Ho & Gan, 2009). This helps to explain why the single most effective, safest, and least expensive treatment for pruritus is opioid dose reduction. In fact, simply decreasing the opioid dose is sufficient to eliminate or make most of the adverse effects tolerable for most patients (Pasero, Quinn et al, 2011). Nonsedating analgesic agents can be added to facilitate this approach.

In addition to dose reduction strategies, most opioid pain treatment plans include orders for medications that can be used to treat adverse effects should they occur. Nonpharmacologic agents may also be effective, such as the application of a cool damp cloth over affected areas to help relieve the discomfort of pruritus.

As patients become opioid tolerant, tolerance to the opioid adverse effects (with the exception of constipation) develops. It is reassuring for patients receiving long-term opioid therapy to know that most of the adverse effects will subside with regular daily doses of opioids over several days.

Sedation and Respiratory Depression. Most patients experience sedation at the beginning of opioid therapy and whenever the opioid dose is increased significantly. If left untreated, excessive sedation can progress to clinically significant respiratory depression. Like other opioid adverse effects, sedation and respiratory depression are dose related. Prevention of clinically significant opioid-induced respiratory depression begins with administration of the lowest effective opioid dose, careful titration, and close nurse monitoring of sedation and respiratory status throughout therapy (Pasero, Quinn et al., 2011). In most cases (exceptions may apply at end of life), nurses should promptly reduce opioid doses or stop titration whenever advancing sedation is detected to prevent respiratory depression (Pasero, 2009; Pasero, Quinn et al., 2011). In some patients (e.g., those with obstructive sleep apnea, pulmonary dysfunction),

monitoring (i.e., capnography or pulse oximetry) is warranted (Jarzyna, Junquist, Pasero, et al., 2011).

> ▶ *Quality and Safety Nursing Alert*
>
> Opioid-induced respiratory depression is dose related and preceded by increasing sedation. Prevention of clinically significant opioid-induced respiratory depression begins with administration of the lowest effective opioid dose, careful titration, close nurse monitoring of sedation and respiratory status throughout therapy, and prompt dose reduction when advancing sedation is detected.

The observation that excessive sedation precedes opioid-induced respiratory depression indicates that systematic sedation assessment is an essential aspect of the care of patients receiving opioid therapy (Nisbet & Mooney-Cotter, 2009; Pasero, 2009) (Chart 12-5). Nursing assessment of sedation is convenient, inexpensive, and takes minimal time to perform. A simple, easy-to-understand sedation scale, developed for assessment of *unwanted* sedation and that includes what should be done at each level of sedation is widely recommended to enhance accuracy and consistency of assessment, monitor trends, and communicate effectively between members of the health care team (Jarzyna et al., 2011; Nisbet & Mooney-Cotter, 2009; Pasero, 2009; Pasero, Quinn et al., 2011). Chart 12-6 presents a widely used sedation scale.

Respiratory depression is assessed on the basis of what is normal for a particular individual and is usually described as clinically significant when there is a decrease in the rate, depth, and regularity of respirations from baseline, rather than just by a specific number of respirations per minute (Pasero, Quinn et al., 2011). There are many risk factors for opioid-induced respiratory depression, including older age (65 years or older), obesity, obstructive sleep apnea, and pre-existing pulmonary dysfunction or other comorbidities (Jarzyna et al., 2011). Risk is elevated during the first 24 hours following surgery and in patients who require a high dose of opioid in a short period of time (e.g., more than 10 mg of IV morphine or equivalent in the PACU).

A comprehensive respiratory assessment constitutes more than counting a patient's respiratory rate (Pasero, 2009). A proper assessment requires watching the rise and fall of the patient's chest to determine rate, depth, and regularity of respirations. Listening to the sound of the patient's respirations is critical as well—snoring indicates airway obstruction and must be attended to promptly with repositioning and, depending on severity, a request for respiratory therapy consultation and further evaluation (Pasero, 2009; Pasero, Quinn et al., 2011).

In most cases (exceptions may apply at end of life), the opioid antagonist naloxone is promptly administered IV to reverse clinically significant opioid-induced respiratory depression (Pasero, Quinn et al., 2011). The goal is to reverse only the sedation and respiratory depressant effects of the opioid. To this end, it should be diluted and titrated very slowly to prevent severe pain and other adverse effects, which can include hypertension, tachycardia, ventricular dysrhythmias, pulmonary edema, and cardiac arrest (APS, 2008) (see Chart 12-6, footnote 3, for correct technique). Sometimes more than one dose of naloxone is necessary,

NURSING RESEARCH PROFILE

Chart 12-5   Scales for Opioid-Induced Sedation: A Comparison of Opioid-Induced Sedation Scales Used in Nursing Practice

Nisbet, A. T., & Mooney-Cotter, F. (2009). Selected scales for reporting opioid-induced sedation. *Pain Management Nursing, 10*(3), 154–164.

Purpose

The observation that sedation precedes opioid-induced respiratory depression suggests that nurses play an important role in the prevention of life-threatening respiratory depression during opioid administration for pain management. The use of a simple and accurate sedation assessment scale facilitates communication among all members of the health care team. The ideal sedation scale would lead nurses to quickly and accurately make informed decisions that maximize patient safety during opioid administration. The purpose of this study was to compare the validity and reliability of three commonly used sedation scales (Inova Sedation Scale [ISS], Richmond Agitation Sedation Scale [RASS], and Pasero Opioid-Induced Sedation Scale [POSS]) and to determine if there were differences in the correct sedation scores and nursing actions chosen by nurses who used each of these scales and in-performance metrics used to gauge the usefulness of each of these scales.

Design

A sample of 96 nurses caring for adult patients on various medical and surgical units in an 830 bed suburban level I trauma center participated in the study. These nurse participants were invited to participate via poster announcements, staff and leadership meetings, and personal contact by the researchers. This study used a 25-question hospital intranet (online) questionnaire that asked nurse participants to read a hypothetical patient scenario and then choose the best response to score the patient's sedation using each scale, choose the appropriate next action, and rate each scale for ease of use, as well as information offered to assist in decision making and confidence in score and actions chosen.

Findings

A panel of 20 pain experts (10 from the study site and 10 from the American Society for Pain Management Nursing and American Pain Society) established content validity for the RASS and POSS; however, there was not enough discrimination between scale items to establish validity for the ISS. Acceptable reliability was demonstrated for the ISS ($\alpha = .803$), RASS ($\alpha = .770$), and POSS ($\alpha = .903$).

The use of the RASS was associated with more correct sedation scores and nursing actions chosen compared with the ISS, and the POSS was associated with more correct sedation scores and nursing actions than the RASS. The researchers inferred that use of the POSS would also result in significantly more correct scores compared with the ISS. Similarly, the nurses rated the RASS significantly higher than the ISS for ease of use, providing more helpful information to inform clinical decision making and greater confidence in sedation score obtained. In these same categories, the nurses rated the POSS significantly higher than the RASS. Again, the researchers inferred that the POSS would result in higher ratings than the ISS. The use of the POSS also resulted in the highest agreement among the experts and the study sample for correct responses and correct nursing actions.

Nursing Implications

The researchers concluded that both the POSS and the RASS are valid and reliable scales for assessment of unwanted sedation during opioid administration, but the POSS demonstrated the highest reliability. Furthermore, use of the POSS was associated with more correct sedation scores and nursing actions, was rated as the easiest to use, provided more useful information for making decisions, and resulted in greater confidence in selected sedation score and action. The POSS may be an ideal tool to screen for sedation among patients receiving opioids.

Chart 12-6   Pasero Opioid-Induced Sedation Scale (POSS) With Interventions

Each level of sedation is followed by the appropriate action in italics.

S = Sleep, easy to arouse
Acceptable; no action necessary; may increase opioid dose if needed

1 = Awake and alert
Acceptable; no action necessary; may increase opioid dose if needed

2 = Slightly drowsy, easily aroused
Acceptable; no action necessary; may increase opioid dose if needed

3 = Frequently drowsy, arousable, drifts off to sleep during conversation
Unacceptable; monitor respiratory status and sedation level closely until sedation level is stable at less than 3 and

respiratory status is satisfactory; decrease opioid dose 25% to 50%[1] or notify primary[2] or anesthesia provider for orders; consider administering a non-sedating, opioid-sparing nonopioid, such as acetaminophen or a NSAID, if not contraindicated; ask patient to take deep breaths every 15–30 minutes.

4 = Somnolent, minimal or no response to verbal and physical stimulation
Unacceptable; stop opioid; consider administering naloxone[3,4]; call Rapid Response Team (Code Blue); stay with patient, stimulate, and support respiration as indicated by patient status; notify primary[2] or anesthesia provider; monitor respiratory status and sedation level closely until sedation level is stable at less than 3 and respiratory status is satisfactory.

[1]Opioid analgesic agent prescriptions or a hospital protocol should include the expectation that a nurse will decrease the opioid dose if a patient is excessively sedated.

[2]For example, the physician, nurse practitioner, advanced practice nurse, or physician assistant responsible for the pain management prescription.

[3]For adults experiencing respiratory depression, mix 0.4 mg of naloxone and 10 mL of normal saline in syringe and administer this dilute solution very slowly (0.5 mL over 2 minutes) while observing the patient's response (titrate to effect).

[4]Hospital protocols should include the expectation that a nurse will administer naloxone to any patient suspected of having life-threatening opioid-induced sedation and respiratory depression.

Copyright 1994, Pasero C. Used with permission. Pasero, C., & McCaffery, M. (2011). *Pain assessment and pharmacologic management.* St. Louis: Mosby-Elsevier.

because naloxone has a shorter duration of action (1 hour in most patients) than most opioids.

Adjuvant Analgesic Agents

The adjuvant analgesic agents comprise the largest group of analgesic agents, which is diverse and offers many options. Drug selection and dosing is based on both experience and evidence-based guideline recommendations. There is considerable variability among individuals in their response to adjuvant analgesic agents, including to agents within the same class; often a "trial and error" strategy is used in the outpatient setting. Treatment in the outpatient setting is primarily for neuropathic pain and involves the use of low initial doses and gradual dose escalation to allow tolerance to the adverse effects. Patients must be forewarned in this setting that the onset of analgesia is likely to be delayed (Pasero, Polomano et al., 2011). Following is an overview of the most commonly used adjuvant analgesic agents.

Local Anesthetics. Local anesthetics have a long history of safe and effective use for all types of pain management. They are given by various routes of administration and are generally well tolerated by most individuals (Pasero, Polomano et al., 2011). Injectable and topical local anesthetics are commonly used for procedural pain treatment. Local anesthetics are added to opioid analgesic agents and other agents to be given intraspinally for the treatment of both acute and chronic pain. They are also infused for continuous peripheral nerve blocks, primarily after surgery.

The lidocaine patch 5% (Lidoderm) is placed directly over or adjacent to the painful area for absorption into the tissues directly below. The drug produces minimal systemic absorption and adverse effects. The patch is left in place for 12 hours then removed for 12 hours (12 hours on, 12 hours off regimen). This application process is repeated as needed for continuous analgesia. The drug is approved for the neuropathic pain syndrome postherpetic neuralgia; however, research suggests that it is effective and safe for a wide variety of acute and chronic pain conditions (Pasero, Polomano et al., 2011).

Allergy to local anesthetics is rare, and adverse effects are dose related. CNS signs of systemic toxicity include ringing in the ears, metallic taste, irritability, and seizures. Signs of cardiotoxicity include circumoral tingling and numbness, bradycardia, cardiac dysrhythmias, and CV collapse (Pasero, Polomano et al., 2011).

Anticonvulsants. The anticonvulsants gabapentin (Neurontin) and pregabalin (Lyrica) are first-line analgesic agents for neuropathic pain (Dworkin et al., 2010) and are increasingly being added to postoperative pain treatment plans to address the neuropathic component of surgical pain (Pasero, Polomano et al., 2011). Although further research is needed, their addition has been shown to improve analgesia, allow lower doses of other analgesic agents, and help prevent persistent neuropathic postsurgical pain syndromes, such as phantom limb, post thoracotomy, post hernia, and post mastectomy pain (Dauri, Faria, Gatti, et al., 2009). They are also effective in improving the acute pain associated with burn injuries as well as reducing the potential for subsequent neuropathic pain (Gray, Kirby, Smith, et al., 2011). Analgesic anticonvulsant therapy is initiated with low doses and titration according to patient response. Primary adverse effects of anticonvulsants

are sedation and dizziness, which are usually transient and most notable during the titration phase of treatment.

Antidepressants. Antidepressant adjuvant analgesic agents are divided into two major groups: the tricyclic antidepressants (TCAs) and the serotonin and norepinephrine reuptake inhibitors (SNRIs). Evidence-based guidelines recommend the TCAs desipramine (Norpramin) and nortriptyline (Aventyl, Pamelor) and the SNRIs duloxetine (Cymbalta) and venlafaxine (Effexor) as first-line options for neuropathic pain treatment (Dworkin et al., 2010). Their delayed onset of action makes them inappropriate for acute pain treatment. Analgesic antidepressant therapy is initiated with low doses and titration according to patient response.

Primary adverse effects of TCAs are dry mouth, sedation, dizziness, mental clouding, weight gain, and constipation (Pasero, Polomano et al., 2011). Orthostatic hypotension is a potentially serious TCA adverse effect. The most serious adverse effect is cardiotoxicity, and patients with significant heart disease are at high risk. SNRIs are thought to have a more favorable adverse effect profile and to be better tolerated than the TCAs (Pasero, Polomano et al., 2011). The most common SNRI adverse effects are nausea, headache, sedation, insomnia, weight gain, impaired memory, sweating, and tremors.

Ketamine. Ketamine (Ketalar) is a dissociative anesthetic with dose-dependent analgesic, sedative, and amnestic properties (Pasero, Polomano et al., 2011). As an NMDA antagonist, it blocks the binding of glutamate at the NMDA receptors and thus prevents the transmission of pain to the brain via the ascending pathway (Rakhman, Shmain, White, et al., 2011) (see Fig. 12-1B inset). At high doses, the drug can produce psychomimetic effects (e.g., hallucinations, dreamlike feelings); however, these are minimized when low doses are administered (Panzer, Moitra, & Sladen, 2009). A benefit of the drug is that it does not produce respiratory depression. Ketamine is given most often by the IV route but can also be given by the oral, rectal, intranasal, and subcutaneous routes. Epidural ketamine is not approved for use in the United States. Ketamine has been used for the treatment of persistent neuropathic pain, but its adverse effect profile makes it less favorable than other analgesic agents for long-term therapy. It is, however, increasingly used as a third-line analgesic agent for **refractory** acute pain (Pasero, Polomano et al., 2011).

 Gerontologic Considerations

Older adults are often sensitive to the effects of the adjuvant analgesic agents that produce sedation and other CNS effects, such as antidepressants and anticonvulsants. Therapy should be initiated with low doses, and titration should proceed slowly with systematic assessment of patient response.

Older adults are also at increased risk for NSAID-induced GI toxicity. Acetaminophen should be used for mild pain. It is recommended as first line for musculoskeletal pain (e.g., osteoarthritis) in older adults but is less effective than NSAIDs for chronic inflammatory pain (e.g., rheumatoid arthritis) (American Geriatrics Society, 2009). If an NSAID is needed for inflammatory pain, a COX-2 selective NSAID (if not contraindicated by an increased cardiovascular risk) or the least nonselective NSAID least likely to cause an ulcer is recommended. The addition of a proton pump inhibitor to NSAID therapy, or opioid analgesic agents rather than an

NSAID, is recommended for high risk patients. The American Geriatric Society has proposed that opioids are a safer choice than NSAIDs in many older adults because of the increased risk for NSAID-induced GI adverse effects in that population (American Geriatrics Society, 2009).

Age is considered an important factor to consider when selecting an opioid dose. The starting opioid dose should be reduced by 25% to 50% in adults older than 70 years because they are more sensitive to opioid adverse effects than younger adults; the amount of subsequent doses is based on patient response (American Geriatrics Society, 2009).

Use of Placebos

A **placebo** is defined as any medication or procedure, including surgery, that produces an effect in a patient because of its implicit or explicit intent and not because of its specific physical or chemical properties (McCaffery et al., 2011). A saline injection is one example of a placebo. Administration of a medication at a known subtherapeutic dose (e.g., 0.05 mg of morphine in an adult) is also considered a placebo.

Placebos are appropriately used as controls in research evaluating the effects of a new medication. The new drug is compared with the effects of a placebo and must show more favorable effects than placebos to warrant further investigation or marketing of the drug (McCaffery et al., 2011). When a person responds to a placebo in accordance with its intent, it is called a *positive placebo response* (ASPMN, 2010). Patients or volunteers who participate in placebo-controlled research must be able to give informed consent or have a guardian who can provide informed consent.

Occasionally, placebos may be used clinically in a deceitful manner and without informed consent. This is typically done when the clinician does not accept the patient's report of pain (see Chart 12-1). Pain relief resulting from a placebo is mistakenly believed to invalidate a patient's report of pain. This typically results in the patient being deprived of pain-relief measures, despite research showing that many patients who have obvious physical stimuli for pain (e.g., abdominal surgery) report pain relief after placebo administration (McCaffery et al., 2011). The reason for this is a mystery, but it is one of the many reasons that pain guidelines, position papers, nurse practice acts, and hospital policies nationwide agree that there are no individuals for whom and no condition for which placebos are the recommended treatment. The deceptive use of placebos has both ethical and legal implications, violates the nurse–patient relationship, and inevitably deprives patients of more appropriate methods of assessment or treatment (ASPMN, 2010; McCaffery et al., 2011).

Nonpharmacologic Methods of Pain Management

Most individuals use self-management strategies to deal with their health issues and promote well-being (Bruckenthal, 2010; National Center for Complementary and Alternative Medicine, 2010). One study suggested an association between adherence to pain self-management strategies and reduced pain, disability, and depressive symptoms in individuals with chronic pain (Nicholas, Asghari, Corbett, et al., 2011). The participants in this study used various techniques, including activity pacing, stretching exercises, goal setting, thought challenging (identifying unhelpful thoughts), and desensitization (observing pain in a calm manner rather than trying to escape it).

Nonpharmacologic interventions are categorized as being body-based (physical) modalities, mind–body (cognitive behavioral) methods, biologically based therapies, and energy therapies (Bruckenthal, 2010). Table 12-5 lists examples of interventions in the four categories of nonpharmacologic methods. Biologically based and energy therapies are used most often in the outpatient setting. For example, one study reported improvements in psychological functioning and reductions in pain and stress hormone (cortisol) levels in women with fibromyalgia who participated in a 75-minute yoga class twice weekly for 8 weeks (Curtis, Osadchuk, & Katz, 2011). The physical modalities are used most often in the inpatient setting because of their ease in implementation (McCaffery, 2002). Most of the physical modalities require a prescription in this setting.

Nonpharmacologic methods are usually effective alone for mild to some moderate-intensity pain, and they should complement, but not replace, pharmacologic therapies for more severe pain (McCaffery, 2002). The effectiveness of nonpharmacologic methods can be unpredictable, and although not all will relieve pain, they offer many benefits to patients with pain. For example, research suggests that nonpharmacologic methods can facilitate relaxation and reduce anxiety and stress (Allred, Byers, & Sole, 2010; Kwekkeboom, Cherwin, Lee, et al., 2010; McCaffery, 2002). Many patients find that the use of nonpharmacologic methods helps them cope better with their pain and feel greater control over the pain experience.

TABLE 12-5 **Nonpharmacologic Methods of Pain Management**		
Category	**Examples**	**Nursing Considerations**
Body-based (physical) modalities	Proper body alignment; application of heat and/or cold; massage; transcutaneous electrical nerve stimulation (TENS); acupuncture; physical therapy; and aqua therapy	Some of these methods require a prescription in the inpatient setting, as inappropriate use can cause harm (e.g., burns or frostbite from extreme temperatures and prolonged thermal application).
Mind–body (cognitive behavioral) methods	Relaxation breathing; listening, singing, or rhythmic tapping to music; imagery; humor; pet therapy; prayer; meditation; hypnosis	Prior to use, evaluate patient's cognitive ability to learn and perform necessary activities.
Biologically based therapies	Taking herbs, vitamins, and proteins	Evaluate use to identify potential adverse effects.
Energy therapies	Yoga, Reiki, and T'ai chi	Prior to use, evaluate patient's physical ability to perform necessary activities.

From Bruckenthal, P. (2010). Integrating nonpharmacologic and alternative strategies into a comprehensive management approach for older adults with pain. *Pain Management Nursing, 11*(2), S23–S31.

Chart 12-7 | Considerations in Selecting and Using Nonpharmacologic Methods

- Does the patient, family, and health care team understand the relationship between nonpharmacologic pain management and analgesics? Patients who have been taking analgesic agents may mistakenly assume that when clinicians suggest a nonpharmacologic method, the purpose is to reduce the use or dose of analgesic agents. All involved must understand that nonpharmacologic methods are used to complement—not replace—pharmacologic methods.
- Does the patient understand the limitations of nonpharmacologic methods? Nonpharmacologic methods are valuable as comfort measures; however, not all such measures relieve pain and should not be promoted as such.
- Is the patient interested in using a nondrug method, and have any been tried previously? If so, what happened? Is the patient using nondrug methods because of unfounded fears about analgesic agents? Willingness and interest are important for successful use of nonpharmacologic methods; however, patients may fear taking analgesic agents that clearly are indicated for their pain, such as nonsteroidal anti-inflammatory drugs (NSAIDs) for an inflammatory painful condition. Such fears should be explored and accurate information and appropriate treatment provided. Alternately, the reasons a patient refuses to use a nonpharmacologic method also should be explored, but the patient's right to refuse must be respected.

- What are the patient's preferences and coping styles? Encouraging patients to choose from a variety of techniques allows them to match the technique to their individual and cultural preferences. If none of the choices appeal to the patient, the patient's right to refuse use should be respected.
- Does the patient have the physical and cognitive abilities necessary for using the nonpharmacologic method? Does the patient have sufficient energy to learn and perform any tasks involved? For example, physical and mental fatigue can interfere with the use of distraction and relaxation imagery techniques. Does the patient want to dedicate the necessary time required for the nonpharmacologic method? For example, those who do not find a 20-minute self-sustained relaxation technique appealing may be more suited for passive application of cold or heat.
- Do others (e.g., family, friends) want to be involved in helping the patient? Is the method a potential vehicle for improving relationships between the patient and others? For example, a method that patients cannot do for themselves, such as massage, may be a burden to some caregivers in the home, whereas others may welcome that opportunity to be physically close to a loved one.
- Are support materials and patient education resources available? Whenever possible, verbal, written, and in some cases video education should be provided.

From McCaffery, M. (2002). What is the role of nondrug methods in the nursing care of patients with acute pain? (Guest Editorial). *Pain Management Nursing, 3*, 77–80; and McCaffery, M., & Pasero, C. (1999). *Pain: Clinical manual*. St. Louis: Mosby.

There are several nonpharmacologic methods that can be used in the clinical setting to provide comfort and pain relief for all types of pain; however, time is often limited in this setting for implementation of these methods (McCaffery, 2002). Nurses play an important role in providing them and instructing patients about their use (Gatlin & Schulmeister, 2007). Many of the methods are relatively easy for nurses to incorporate into daily clinical practice and may be used individually or in combination with other nonpharmacologic therapies. Chart 12-7 provides points for nurses to consider prior to using nonpharmacologic methods.

Nursing Implications of Pain Management

The provision of optimal pain management requires a collaborative approach between patients with pain, their families, and members of the health care team. Everyone involved must share common goals, a common knowledge base, and a common language with regard to the analgesics and nonpharmacologic methods used to manage pain. Whether nurses provide care in the home, hospital, or any other setting, they are in a unique position to coordinate a comprehensive, evidence-based approach to meet the needs of people with pain. Chart 12-8 provides a plan of nursing care for the patient with pain.

PLAN OF NURSING CARE
Care of the Patient With Pain

NURSING DIAGNOSIS: Pain
GOAL: Achievement and maintenance of patient's comfort-function goal

Nursing Intervention	Rationale	Expected Outcomes
1. Perform and document a comprehensive pain assessment.	1. The comprehensive pain assessment is the foundation of the pain treatment plan; documentation ensures communication between team members.	• If able, provides information about the pain • Expresses understanding of the link between function and pain control and establishes a realistic comfort-function goal • Reports a pain intensity that allows participation in important functional activities
a. Use a reliable and valid tool to determine pain intensity.	a. The use of valid and reliable tools helps ensure accuracy and consistency in assessment.	

(continues on page 234)

PLAN OF NURSING CARE

Chart 12-8

Care of the Patient With Pain (continued)

Nursing Intervention	Rationale	Expected Outcomes
b. Accept the patient's report of pain.	**b.** Accepting the patient's report of pain is the undisputed standard of pain assessment.	• If not able to report pain, demonstrates behaviors that indicate pain relief and participation in important functional activities
c. Assist the patient in establishing a comfort-function goal.	**c.** The comfort-function goal links function to pain control and provides direction for necessary adjustments in the treatment plan to maximize function.	• Expresses satisfaction with the use of nonpharmacologic methods
d. Apply the Hierarchy of Pain Measures in patients who are unable to report their pain.	**d.** The use of the Hierarchy of Pain Measures provides a process to ensure pain treatment in the patient who cannot report pain.	• Tolerates pharmacologic and nonpharmacologic interventions without adverse effects
2. Administer analgesic agents as prescribed.	**2.** Pharmacologic interventions are the cornerstone of pain management.	• Demonstrates an understanding of the treatment plan and goals of care
3. Offer and educate patient how to use appropriate nonpharmacologic interventions.	**3.** Nonpharmacologic methods are used to supplement pharmacologic interventions.	
4. Reassess for degree of pain relief and presence of adverse effects at peak effect time of intervention.	**4.** Reassessment permits evaluation of both the effectiveness and safety of interventions.	
5. Obtain additional prescriptions as needed.	**5.** Prescriptions for additional analgesic agents or adjustment in dose are often needed to maximize pain control.	
6. Prevent and treat adverse effects.	**6.** Adverse effects are prevented whenever possible and promptly treated to reduce patient discomfort and prevent harm.	
7. Educate patient and family about the effects of analgesic agents and the goals of care; explain how adverse effects will be prevented and treated; address fears of addiction.	**7.** An understanding of the treatment plan and goals of care educates patients and their families how to partner with the health care team to optimize pain control.	

Critical Thinking Exercises

1 **ebp** A 52-year-old woman is admitted to the gynecologic surgery unit following a total abdominal hysterectomy. She is receiving a continuous epidural infusion of hydromorphone and the local anesthetic ropivacaine for pain control. Her comfort-function goal is 3 on the 0-to-10 numerical rating scale to deep breathe and cough. Her pain assessment reveals a current pain intensity of 1, and she is satisfied with her comfort level. She is alert, and assessment of her respiratory status reveals no abnormalities; however, she reports significant discomfort from facial pruritus and intermittently scratches her face. Identify the evidence base for a nonpharmacologic action that could be taken to help relieve this patient's discomfort from the pruritus. Identify the criteria used to evaluate the strength of the evidence for this practice.

2 A 48-year-old man is admitted to the medical unit with renal calculi. He passed two calculi in the ED and was given 75 mcg of IV fentanyl and 1,000 mg of IV acetaminophen for analgesia. His comfort-function goal is 2 on the 0 to 10 numerical rating scale. He reports a pain intensity rating of 1 related to the acute pain; however, he describes a history of neck pain since an automobile acci-

dent 5 years ago. He rates the neck pain as 6 and describes it as continuous and burning. His prescribed analgesic agents include acetaminophen 1,000 mg IV every 6 hours and morphine 3 mg IV every hour PRN. Explain the deficiencies in this patient's analgesic agent prescriptions and what could be done to address his pain in a more comprehensive manner. What nonpharmacologic methods might be helpful?

3 **pcg** A 78-year-old woman is admitted to the orthopedic unit after repair of a right hip fracture. Her comfort-function goal is "mild pain" on the verbal descriptor scale to rest adequately. She received a total of 1 mg of hydromorphone in IV boluses in the PACU followed by initiation of IV PCA hydromorphone with a prescription that provides a basal rate of 0.1 mg per hour and allows the patient to self-administer 0.2 mg every 8 minutes as needed. She reports "moderate pain" and moans when transferred from the stretcher to the bed. She has an adequate respiratory status but is excessively sedated and unable to respond to a question without falling asleep in the middle of a sentence. Identify the first action to take for this patient. Who would you consult to implement this action? Describe other actions that could be taken to provide safer pain control for this patient.

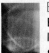

Brunner Suite Resources

Explore these additional resources to enhance learning for this chapter:

- NCLEX-Style Questions and Other Resources on thePoint, http://thePoint.lww.com/Brunner13e
- Study Guide
- PrepU
- Clinical Handbook
- Handbook of Laboratory and Diagnostic Tests

References

*Asterisk indicates nursing research.
**Double asterisk indicates classic reference.

Books

American Pain Society. (2008). *Principles of analgesic use in the treatment of acute and cancer pain* (6th ed.). Glenview, IL: Author.

Grape, S., & Schug, S. A. (2008). Epidural and spinal analgesia. In P. E. Macintyre, S. M. Walker, & D. J. Rowbotham (Eds.). *Clinical pain management. Acute pain* (2nd ed.; pp. 255–270). London: Hodder Arnold.

Ho, K. T., & Gan, T. J. (2009). Opioid-related adverse effects and treatment options. In: R. S. Sinatra, O. A. de Leon-Casasola, B. Ginsberg, & E. R. Viscusi (Eds.). *Acute pain management* (pp. 406–415). New York: Cambridge University Press.

Jackson, K. C. (2009). Opioid pharmacology. In H. S. Smith (Ed.): *Current therapy in pain* (pp. 78–84). Philadelphia: Saunders Elsevier.

**McCaffery, M. (1968). *Nursing practice theories related to cognition, bodily pain, and man-environment interactions.* Los Angeles: University of California, Los Angeles.

McCaffery, M., Herr, K., & Pasero, C. (2011). Assessment. In C. Pasero & M. McCaffery (Eds.). *Pain assessment and pharmacologic management* (pp. 13–176). St. Louis: Mosby-Elsevier.

**McCaffery, M., & Pasero, C. (1999). *Pain: Clinical manual.* St. Louis: Mosby.

McPherson, M. L. (2010). *Demystifying opioid conversion calculations. A guide to effective dosing.* Bethesda, MD: American Society of Health-System Pharmacists.

Pasero, C., Eksterowicz, N., & McCaffery, M. (2009). The nurse's perspective on acute pain management. In R. S. Sinatra, A. O. de Leon-Casasola, B. Ginsberg, & E. R. Viscusi (Eds.). *Acute pain management* (pp. 597–606). New York: Cambridge University Press.

Pasero, C., Polomano, R. C., Portenoy, R. K., et al. (2011). Adjuvant analgesics. In C. Pasero & M. McCaffery (Eds.). *Pain assessment and pharmacologic management* (pp. 623–818). St. Louis: Mosby-Elsevier.

Pasero, C., & Portenoy, R. K. (2011). Neurophysiology of pain and analgesia and the pathophysiology of neuropathic pain. In C. Pasero & M. McCaffery (Eds.). *Pain assessment and pharmacologic management* (pp. 1–12). St. Louis: Mosby-Elsevier.

Pasero, C., Portenoy, R. K., & McCaffery, M. (2011). Nonopioid analgesics. In C. Pasero & M. McCaffery (Eds.). *Pain assessment and pharmacologic management* (pp. 177–276). St. Louis: Mosby-Elsevier.

Pasero, C., Quinn, T. E., Portenoy, R. K., et al. (2011). Opioid analgesics. In C. Pasero & M. McCaffery (Eds.). *Pain assessment and pharmacologic management* (pp. 277–622). St. Louis: Mosby-Elsevier.

Rowbotham, D. J., Serrano-Gomez, A., & Heffernan, A. (2009). Clinical pharmacology: Opioids. In: P. E. Macintyre, S. M. Walker, & D. J. Rowbotham (Eds.). *Clinical pain management. Acute pain* (2nd ed.; pp. 53–67). London: Hodder Arnold.

Vadivelu, N., Whitney, C. J., & Sinatra, R. S. (2009). Pain pathways and acute pain processing. In R. S. Sinatra, A. O. de Leon-Casasola, B. Ginsberg, & E. R. Viscusi, E. R. (Eds.). *Acute pain management* (pp. 3–20). New York: Cambridge University Press.

Journals and Electronic Documents

*Allred, K. D., Byers, J., & Sole, M. L. (2010). The effect of music on postoperative pain and anxiety. *Pain Management Nursing, 11*(1), 15–25.

American Geriatrics Society. (2009). Pharmacological management of persistent pain in older persons. *Journal of the American Geriatrics Society, 57*(6), 1331–1346.

American Society for Pain Management Nursing. (2007a). *Registered nurse management and monitoring of analgesia by catheter techniques: Position statement.* Available at: www.aspmn.org/Organization/documents/Registered-NurseManagementandMonitoringofAnalgesiaByCatheterTechniquesPMN-version.pdf

American Society for Pain Management Nursing. (2007b). *Authorized and unauthorized ("PCA by proxy") dosing of analgesic infusion pumps: Position statement with clinical practice recommendations.* Available at: aspmn.org/Organization/documents/PMNVersionPCA.pdf

American Society for Pain Management Nursing. (2010). *Position statement: Use of placebos in pain management.* Available at: www.aspmn.org/Organization/documents/Placebo_Position_FINAL.pdf

**American Society of Addiction Medicine. (2001). *Definitions related to the use of opioids for the treatment of pain.* Available at: www.painmed.org/Workarea/DownloadAsset.aspx?id=3204

*American Society of PeriAnesthesia Nurses. (2006). ASPAN's evidence-based clinical practice guideline for the prevention and/or management of PONV/PDNV. *Journal of PeriAnesthesia Nursing, 21*(4), 230–250.

**Angst, M. S., & Clark, D. (2006). Opioid-induced hyperalgesia. *Anesthesiology, 104*(3), 570–587.

*Arbour, C., & Gelinas, C. (2010). Are vital signs valid indicators for the assessment of pain in postoperative cardiac surgery ICU adults? *Intensive Critical Care Nursing, 26*(2), 83–90.

Argoff, C. E., Albrecht, P., Irving, G., et al. (2009). Multimodal analgesia for chronic pain: Rationale and future directions. *Pain Medicine, 10*(Suppl 2), S53–S66.

Brown, C., Moodie, J., Bisley, E., et al. (2009). Intranasal ketorolac for postoperative pain: A phase 3, double-blind, randomized study. *Pain Medicine, 10*(6), 1106–1114.

*Bruckenthal, P. (2010). Integrating nonpharmacologic and alternative strategies into a comprehensive management approach for older adults with pain. *Pain Management Nursing, 11*(2), S23–S31.

Candiotti, K. A., Bergese, S. D., Viscusi, E. R., et al. (2010). Safety of multiple-dose intravenous acetaminophen in adult inpatients. *Pain Medicine, 11*(12), 1841–1848.

Chen, J. Y., Ko, T. L., Wen, Y. R., et al. (2009). Opioid-sparing effects of ketorolac and its correlation with the recovery of postoperative bowel function in colorectal surgery patients. A prospective randomized double-blinded study. *Clinical Journal of Pain, 25*(6), 485–489.

Chu, L. F., Angst, M. S., & Clark, D. (2008). Opioid-induced hyperalgesia in humans: Molecular mechanisms and clinical considerations. *Clinical Journal of Pain, 24*(6), 479–496.

*Compton, P. (2008). *The OIH paradox: Can opioids make pain worse?* Pain Treatment Topics. Available at: pain-topics.org/pdf/Compton-OIH-Paradox.pdf

Curtis, K., Osadchuk, A., & Katz, J. (2011). An eight-week yoga intervention is associated with improvements in pain, psychological functioning and mindfulness, and changes in cortisol levels in women with fibromyalgia. *Journal of Pain Research, 2011*(4), 189–201.

Dauri, M., Faria, S., Gatti, A., et al. (2009). Gabapentin and pregabalin for the acute post-operative pain management. A systematic-narrative review of the recent clinical evidences. *Current Drug Targets, 10*(8), 716–733.

Dib-Jajj, S. D., Black, J. A., & Waxman, S. G. (2009). Voltage-gated sodium channels: Targets for pain. *Pain Medicine, 10*(7), 1260–1269.

*DuPen, A., Shen, D., & Ersek, M. (2007). Mechanisms of opioid-induced tolerance and hyperalgesia. *Pain Management Nursing, 8*(3), 113–121.

Dworkin, R. H., O'Connor, A. B., Audette, J. B., et al. (2010). Recommendations for pharmacological management of neuropathic pain. *Mayo Clinic Proceedings, 85*(3 Suppl), S3–S14.

Fishbain, D. A., Cole, B., Lewis, J., et al. (2008). What percentage of chronic nonmalignant pain patients exposed to chronic opioid analgesic therapy develop abuse/addiction and/or aberrant drug-related behaviors? A structured evidence-based review. *Pain Medicine, 9*(4), 444–459.

Gallagher, R. M., Welz-Bosna, M., & Gammaitoni, A. (2007). Assessment of dosing frequency of sustained-release opioid preparations in patients with chronic nonmalignant pain. *Pain Medicine, 8*(1), 71–74.

*Gatlin, C. G., & Schulmeister, L. (2007). When medication is not enough: Nonpharmacologic management of pain. *Clinical Journal of Oncology Nursing, 11*(5), 699–704.

*Gelinas, C., & Arbour, C. (2009). Behavioral and physiologic indicators during a nociceptive procedure in conscious and unconscious mechanically ventilated patients: Similar or different? *Journal of Critical Care, 24*(4), 7–17.

Gray, P., Kirby, J., Smith, M. T., et al. (2011). Pregabalin in severe burn injury pain: A double-blind, randomised placebo-controlled trial. *Pain, 152*(6), 1279–1288.

Groudine, S., & Fossum, S. (2011). Use of intravenous acetaminophen in the treatment of postoperative pain. *Journal of PeriAnesthesia Nursing, 26*(2), 74–80.

International Association for the Study of Pain. (2011). *Global year against acute pain.* Available at: www.iasp-pain.org/Content/NavigationMenu/GlobalYearAgainstPain/GlobalYearAgainstAcutePain/default.htm

*Jarzyna, D., Junquist, C., Pasero, C., et al. (2011). American Society for Pain Management evidence-based guideline on monitoring for opioid-induced sedation and respiratory depression. *Pain Management Nursing, 12*(3), 118–145.

Johannes, C. B., Le, T. K., Zhou, X., et al. (2010). The prevalence of chronic pain in United States adults: Results of an Internet-based survey. *Journal of Pain, 11*(11), 1230–1239.

*Kwekkeboom, K. L., Cherwin, C. H., Lee, J. W., et al. (2010). Mind-body treatments for the pain-fatigue-sleep disturbance symptom cluster in persons with cancer. *Journal of Pain and Symptom Management, 39*(1), 126–138.

*Li, L., Liu, X., & Herr, K. (2007). Postoperative pain intensity assessment: A comparison of four scales in Chinese adult. *Pain Medicine, 8*(3), 223–234.

Macario, A., & Royal, M. A. (2011). A literature review of randomized clinical trials of intravenous acetaminophen (paracetamol) for acute postoperative pain. *Pain Practice, 11*(3), 209–296.

**McCaffery, M. (2002). What is the role of nondrug methods in the nursing care of patients with acute pain? (Guest Editorial). *Pain Management Nursing, 3*(3), 77–80.

*Miaskowski, C. (2009). A review of the incidence, causes, consequences, and management of gastrointestinal effects associated with postoperative opioid administration. *Journal of PeriAnesthesia Nursing, 24*(4), 222–228.

Mitchell, A., van Zanten, S. V., Inglis, K., et al. (2008). A randomized controlled trial comparing acetaminophen plus ibuprofen versus acetaminophen plus codeine plus caffeine after outpatient general surgery. *Journal of the American College of Surgeons, 206*(3), 472–479.

National Center for Complementary and Alternative Medicine. (2010). *What is complementary and alternative medicine?* Available at: nccam.nih.gov/health/whatiscam/

Nauta, M., Landsmeer, M. L., & Koren, G. (2009). Codeine-acetaminophen versus nonsteroidal anti-inflammatory drugs in the treatment of post-abdominal surgery pain: A systematic review of randomized trials. *American Journal of Surgery, 198*(2), 256–261.

Nicholas, M. K., Asghari, A., Corbett, M., et al. (2011). Is adherence to pain self-management strategies associated with improved pain, depression and disability in those with disabling chronic pain? *European Journal of Pain, 16*(1), 93–104.

*Nisbet, A. T., & Mooney-Cotter, F. (2009). Selected scales for reporting opioid-induced sedation. *Pain Management Nursing, 10*(3), 154–164.

Ortho-McNeil Pharmaceuticals. (2011). *New initiatives to help encourage appropriate use of acetaminophen.* Available at: www.tylenol.com/page2.jhtml?id=tylenol/news/newdosing.inc

Panzer, O., Moitra, V., & Sladen, R. N. (2009). Pharmacology of sedative-analgesic agents: Dexmedetomidine, remifentanil, ketamine, volatile anesthetics and the role of peripheral mu antagonists. *Critical Care Clinics, 25*(3), 451–469.

*Pasero, C. (2009). Assessment of sedation during opioid administration for pain management. *Journal of PeriAnesthesia Nursing, 24*(3), 186–190.

*Pasero, C. (2011). Tapentadol for multimodal pain management. *Journal of PeriAnesthesia Nursing, 26*(5), 343–346.

Portenoy, R. K. (2011). Treatment of cancer pain. *Lancet, 377*(9784), 2236–2247.

*Portenoy, R. K., Farrar, J. T., Backonja, M. M., et al. (2007). Long-term use of controlled-release oxycodone for noncancer pain: Results of a 3-year registry study. *Clinical Journal of Pain, 23*(4), 287–299.

Rakhman, E., Shmain, D, White, I., et al. (2011). Repeated and escalating preoperative subanesthetic doses of ketamine for postoperative pain control in patients undergoing tumor resection: A randomized, placebo-controlled, double-blind trial. *Clinical Therapeutics, 33*(7), 863–873.

Singla, N., Rock, A., & Pavliv, L. (2010). A multi-center, randomized, double-blind placebo-controlled trial of intravenous-ibuprofen (IV-ibuprofen) for treatment of pain in post-operative orthopedic adult patients. *Pain Medicine, 11*(8), 1284–1292.

*Spagrud, L. J., Piira, T., & Von Baeyer, C. L. (2003). Children's self-report of pain intensity. The faces pain scale—revised. *American Journal of Nursing, 103*(12), 62–64.

Turk, D. C., Wilson, H. D., & Cahana, A. (2011). Treatment of chronic noncancer pain. *Lancet, 377*(9784), 2226–2235.

U.S. Food and Drug Administration. (2007). *Medication guide for non-steroidal anti-inflammatory drugs (NSAIDs).* Available at: www.fda.gov/downloads/Drugs/DrugSafety/ucm089165.pdf

Uysal, H. Y., Takmaz, S. A., Yaman, F., et al. (2011). The efficacy of intravenous paracetamol versus tramadol for postoperative analgesia after adenotonsillectomy in children. *Journal of Clinical Anesthesia, 23*(1), 53–57.

Veves, A., Backonja, M., & Malik, R. A. (2008). Painful diabetic neuropathy: Epidemiology, natural history, early diagnosis, and treatment options. *Pain Medicine, 9*(6), 660–674.

Walco, G. A., Dworkin, R. H., Krane, E. J., et al. (2010). Neuropathic pain in children: Special considerations. *Mayo Clinic Proceedings, 85*(3 Suppl), S33–S41.

*Ware, L., Epps, D. E., Herr, K., et al. (2006). Evaluation of the Revised Faces Pain Scale, Verbal Descriptor Scale, Numeric Rating Scale, and Iowa Pain Thermometer in older minority adults. *Pain Management Nursing, 71*(3), 117–125.

**Weissman, D. E., & Haddox, J. D. (1989). Opioid pseudoaddiction—an iatrogenic syndrome. *Pain, 36*(3), 363–366.

Wu, C. L., & Raja, S. N. (2011). Treatment of acute postoperative pain. *Lancet, 377*(9784), 2215–2225.

Resources

American Academy of Pain Management, aapainmanage.org

American Academy of Pain Medicine (AAPM), painmed.org

American Chronic Pain Association, theacpa.org

American Pain Foundation (APF), painfoundation.org

American Pain Society, ampainsoc.org

American Society for Pain Management Nursing (ASPMN), aspmn.org

City of Hope Pain and Palliative Care Resource Center, www.cityofhope.org/education/health-professional-education/nursing-education/pain-resource-nurse-training/Pages/default.aspx

National Center for Complementary and Alternative Medicine (NCCAM), nccam.nih.gov/

Pain and Policies Studies Group, www.painpolicy.wisc.edu

Pain Treatment Topics, pain-topics.org

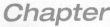

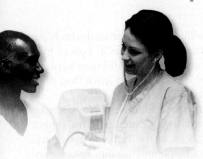

Fluid and Electrolytes: Balance and Disturbance

Learning Objectives

On completion of this chapter, the learner will be able to:

1. Differentiate between osmosis, diffusion, filtration, and active transport.
2. Describe the role of the kidneys, lungs, and endocrine glands in regulating the body's fluid composition and volume.
3. Identify the effects of aging on fluid and electrolyte regulation.
4. Plan effective care of patients with the following imbalances: fluid volume deficit and fluid volume excess, sodium deficit (hyponatremia) and sodium excess (hypernatremia), and potassium deficit (hypokalemia) and potassium excess (hyperkalemia).
5. Describe the cause, clinical manifestations, management, and nursing interventions for the following imbalances: calcium deficit (hypocalcemia) and calcium excess (hypercalcemia), magnesium deficit (hypomagnesemia) and magnesium excess (hypermagnesemia), phosphorus deficit (hypophosphatemia) and phosphorus excess (hyperphosphatemia), and chloride deficit (hypochloremia) and chloride excess (hyperchloremia).
6. Explain the roles of the lungs, kidneys, and chemical buffers in maintaining acid–base balance.
7. Compare metabolic acidosis and alkalosis with regard to causes, clinical manifestations, diagnosis, and management.
8. Compare respiratory acidosis and alkalosis with regard to causes, clinical manifestations, diagnosis, and management.
9. Interpret arterial blood gas measurements.
10. Identify a safe and effective procedure of venipuncture.
11. Describe measures used for preventing complications of intravenous therapy.

Glossary

acidosis: an acid–base imbalance characterized by an increase in H$^+$ concentration (decreased blood pH) (A low arterial pH due to reduced bicarbonate concentration is called *metabolic acidosis*; a low arterial pH due to increased PCO$_2$ is called *respiratory acidosis*.)

ascites: a type of edema in which fluid accumulates in the peritoneal cavity

active transport: physiologic pump that moves fluid from an area of lower concentration to one of higher concentration; active transport requires adenosine triphosphate for energy

alkalosis: an acid–base imbalance characterized by a reduction in H$^+$ concentration (increased blood pH) (A high arterial pH with increased bicarbonate concentration is called *metabolic alkalosis*; a high arterial pH due to reduced PCO$_2$ is called *respiratory alkalosis*.)

diffusion: the process by which solutes move from an area of higher concentration to one of lower concentration; does not require expenditure of energy

homeostasis: maintenance of a constant internal equilibrium in a biologic system that involves positive and negative feedback mechanisms

hydrostatic pressure: the pressure created by the weight of fluid against the wall that contains it. In the body, hydrostatic pressure in blood vessels results from the

weight of fluid itself and the force resulting from cardiac contraction.

hypertonic solution: a solution with an osmolality higher than that of serum

hypotonic solution: a solution with an osmolality lower than that of serum

isotonic solution: a solution with the same osmolality as serum and other body fluids

osmolality: the number of milliosmoles (the standard unit of osmotic pressure) per kilogram of solvent; expressed as milliosmoles per kilogram (mOsm/kg) (The term *osmolality* is used more often than *osmolarity* to evaluate serum and urine.)

osmolarity: the number of milliosmoles (the standard unit of osmotic pressure) per liter of solution; expressed as milliosmoles per liter (mOsm/L); describes the concentration of solutes or dissolved particles

osmosis: the process by which fluid moves across a semipermeable membrane from an area of low solute concentration to an area of high solute concentration; the process continues until the solute concentrations are equal on both sides of the membrane

tonicity: fluid tension or the effect that osmotic pressure of a solution with impermeable solutes exerts on cell size because of water movement across the cell membrane

Fluid and electrolyte balance is a dynamic process that is crucial for life and **homeostasis**. Potential and actual disorders of fluid and electrolyte balance occur in every setting, with every disorder, and with a variety of changes that affect healthy people (e.g., increased fluid and sodium loss with strenuous exercise and high environmental temperature, inadequate intake of fluid and electrolytes) as well as those who are ill.

Fundamental Concepts

Nurses need to understand the physiology of fluid and electrolyte balance and acid–base balance to anticipate, identify, and respond to possible imbalances. Nurses also must use effective education and communication skills to help prevent and treat various fluid and electrolyte disturbances.

Amount and Composition of Body Fluids

Approximately 60% of a typical adult's weight consists of fluid (water and electrolytes). Factors that influence the amount of body fluid are age, gender, and body fat. In general, younger people have a higher percentage of body fluid than older people, and men have proportionately more body fluid than women. People who are obese have less fluid than those who are thin, because fat cells contain little water. The skeleton also has low water content. Muscle, skin, and blood contain the highest amounts of water (Porth, 2011).

Body fluid is located in two fluid compartments: the intracellular space (fluid in the cells) and the extracellular space (fluid outside the cells). Approximately two thirds of body fluid is in the intracellular fluid (ICF) compartment and is located primarily in the skeletal muscle mass. Approximately one third is in the extracellular fluid (ECF) compartment.

The ECF compartment is further divided into the intravascular, interstitial, and transcellular fluid spaces:

- The intravascular space (the fluid within the blood vessels) contains plasma, the effective circulating volume. Approximately 3 L of the average 6 L of blood volume in adults is made up of plasma. The remaining 3 L is made up of erythrocytes, leukocytes, and thrombocytes.
- The interstitial space contains the fluid that surrounds the cell and totals about 11 to 12 L in an adult. Lymph is an interstitial fluid.
- The transcellular space is the smallest division of the ECF compartment and contains approximately 1 L. Examples of transcellular fluids include cerebrospinal, pericardial, synovial, intraocular, and pleural fluids, sweat, and digestive secretions.

Circulatory and neurologic symptoms, physical examination findings, and laboratory test results can be used to identify the compartment from which fluid is lost (McPhee, Papadakis, & Rabow, 2012).

As the next section describes, the ECF transports electrolytes; it also carries other substances, such as enzymes and hormones.

Body fluid normally moves between the two major compartments or spaces in an effort to maintain equilibrium between the spaces. Loss of fluid from the body can disrupt this equilibrium. Sometimes fluid is not lost from the body but is unavailable for use by either the ICF or ECF. Loss of ECF into a space that does not contribute to equilibrium between the ICF and the ECF is referred to as a third-space fluid shift, or third spacing (McPhee et al., 2012).

Early evidence of a third-space fluid shift is a decrease in urine output despite adequate fluid intake. Urine output decreases because fluid shifts out of the intravascular space; the kidneys then receive less blood and attempt to compensate by decreasing urine output. Other signs and symptoms of third spacing that indicate an intravascular fluid volume deficit (FVD) include increased heart rate, decreased blood pressure, decreased central venous pressure, edema, increased body weight, and imbalances in fluid intake and output (I&O). Third-space shifts occur in patients who have hypocalcemia, decreased iron intake, severe liver diseases, alcoholism, hypothyroidism, malabsorption, immobility, burns, and cancer (Guyton & Hall, 2011).

Electrolytes

Electrolytes in body fluids are active chemicals (cations that carry positive charges and anions that carry negative charges). The major cations in body fluid are sodium, potassium, calcium, magnesium, and hydrogen ions. The major anions are chloride, bicarbonate, phosphate, sulfate, and proteinate ions.

These chemicals unite in varying combinations. Therefore, electrolyte concentration in the body is expressed in terms of milliequivalents (mEq) per liter, a measure of chemical activity, rather than in terms of milligrams (mg), a unit of weight. More specifically, a milliequivalent is defined as being equivalent to the electrochemical activity of 1 mg of hydrogen. In a solution, cations and anions are equal in milliequivalents per liter.

Electrolyte concentrations in the ICF differ from those in the ECF, as reflected in Table 13-1. Because special techniques are required to measure electrolyte concentrations in the ICF, it is customary to measure the electrolytes in the most accessible portion of the ECF—namely, the plasma.

Sodium ions, which are positively charged, far outnumber the other cations in the ECF. Because sodium concentration affects the overall concentration of the ECF, sodium is important in regulating the volume of body fluid. Retention of sodium is associated with fluid retention, and excessive loss of sodium is usually associated with decreased volume of body fluid.

As shown in Table 13-1, the major electrolytes in the ICF are potassium and phosphate. The ECF has a low concentration of potassium and can tolerate only small changes in potassium concentrations. Therefore, release of large stores of intracellular potassium, typically caused by trauma to the cells and tissues, can be extremely dangerous.

The body expends a great deal of energy maintaining the high extracellular concentration of sodium and the high intracellular concentration of potassium. It does so by means of cell membrane pumps that exchange sodium and potassium ions. Normal movement of fluids through the capillary wall into the tissues depends on **hydrostatic pressure** (the pressure exerted by the fluid on the walls of the blood vessel) at both the arterial and the venous ends

TABLE 13-1	Approximate Major Electrolyte Content in Body Fluids	
Electrolytes		**mEq/L**
Extracellular Fluid (Plasma)		
Cations		
Sodium (Na$^+$)		142
Potassium (K$^+$)		5
Calcium (Ca^{++})		5
Magnesium (Mg^{++})		2
Total cations		154
Anions		
Chloride (Cl$^-$)		103
Bicarbonate (HCO$_3^-$)		26
Phosphate (HPO$_4^-$)		2
Sulfate (SO$_4^-$)		1
Organic acids		5
Proteinate		17
Total anions		154
Intracellular Fluid		
Cations		
Potassium (K$^+$)		150
Magnesium (Mg^{++})		40
Sodium (Na$^+$)		10
Total cations		200
Anions		
Phosphates and sulfates		150
Bicarbonate (HCO$_3^-$)		10
Proteinate		40
Total anions		200

of the vessel and the osmotic pressure exerted by the protein of plasma. The direction of fluid movement depends on the differences in these two opposing forces (hydrostatic vs. osmotic pressure).

Regulation of Body Fluid Compartments

Osmosis and Osmolality

When two different solutions are separated by a membrane that is impermeable to the dissolved substances, fluid shifts through the membrane from the region of low solute concentration to the region of high solute concentration until the solutions are of equal concentration. This diffusion of water caused by a fluid concentration gradient is known as **osmosis** (Fig. 13-1A). The magnitude of this force depends on the number of particles dissolved in the solutions, not on their weights. The number of dissolved particles contained in a unit of fluid determines the osmolality of a solution, which influences the movement of fluid between the fluid compartments. **Tonicity** is the ability of all solutes to cause an osmotic driving force that promotes water movement from one compartment to another. The control of tonicity determines the normal state of cellular hydration and cell size. Sodium, mannitol, glucose, and sorbitol are effective osmoles (capable of affecting water movement). Three other terms are associated with osmosis— *osmotic pressure, oncotic pressure,* and *osmotic diuresis*:

- Osmotic pressure is the amount of hydrostatic pressure needed to stop the flow of water by osmosis. It is primarily determined by the concentration of solutes.
- Oncotic pressure is the osmotic pressure exerted by proteins (e.g., albumin).

- Osmotic diuresis is the increase in urine output caused by the excretion of substances such as glucose, mannitol, or contrast agents in the urine.

Diffusion

Diffusion is the natural tendency of a substance to move from an area of higher concentration to one of lower concentration (see Fig. 13-1B). It occurs through the random movement of ions and molecules (Porth, 2011). Examples of diffusion are the exchange of oxygen and carbon dioxide (CO_2) between the pulmonary capillaries and alveoli and the tendency of sodium to move from the ECF compartment, where the sodium concentration is high, to the ICF, where its concentration is low.

Filtration

Hydrostatic pressure in the capillaries tends to filter fluid out of the intravascular compartment into the interstitial fluid. Movement of water and solutes occurs from an area of high hydrostatic pressure to an area of low hydrostatic pressure. The kidneys filter approximately 180 L of plasma per day. Another example of filtration is the passage of water and electrolytes from the arterial capillary bed to the interstitial fluid; in this instance, the hydrostatic pressure results from the pumping action of the heart.

Sodium–Potassium Pump

The sodium concentration is greater in the ECF than in the ICF; because of this, sodium tends to enter the cell by diffusion. This tendency is offset by the sodium–potassium pump that is maintained by the cell membrane and actively moves sodium from the cell into the ECF. Conversely, the high intracellular potassium concentration is maintained by pumping potassium into the cell. By definition, **active transport** implies that energy must be expended for the movement to occur against a concentration gradient.

Concept Mastery Alert

Filtration is a type of passive transport that results from hydrostatic pressure. Nurses must be careful to avoid confusing this pressure with energy expenditure during active transport of sodium out of the cell by the sodium–potassium pump. Visit thePoint to view a Fluid and Electrolytes Tutorial to review filtration and other fundamental concepts.

Systemic Routes of Gains and Losses

Water and electrolytes are gained in various ways. Healthy people gain fluids by drinking and eating, and their daily average I&O of water are approximately equal (Table 13-2).

Kidneys

The usual daily urine volume in the adult is 1 to 2 L (Porth, 2011). A general rule is that the output is approximately 1 mL of urine per kilogram of body weight per hour (1 mL/kg/h) in all age groups.

Skin

Sensible perspiration refers to visible water and electrolyte loss through the skin (sweating). The chief solutes in sweat

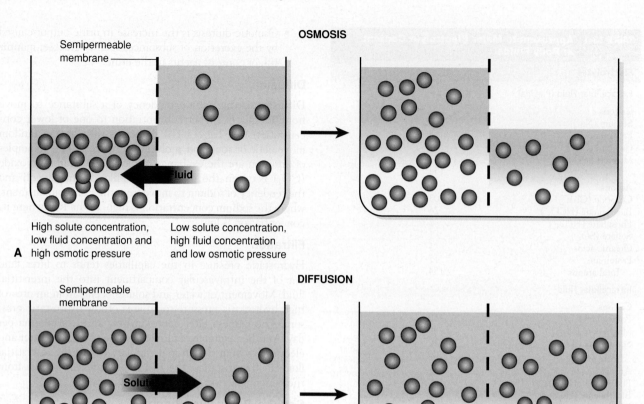

FIGURE 13-1 • A. Osmosis: movement of fluid from an area of lower solute concentration to an area of higher solute concentration with eventual equalization of the solute concentrations. **B.** Diffusion: movement of solutes from an area of greater concentration to an area of lesser concentration, leading ultimately to equalization of the solute concentrations.

are sodium, chloride, and potassium. Actual sweat losses can vary from 0 to 1,000 mL or more every hour, depending on factors such as the environmental temperature. Continuous water loss by evaporation (approximately 500 mL/day) occurs through the skin as insensible perspiration, a nonvisible form of water loss (Porth, 2011). Fever greatly increases insensible water loss through the lungs and the skin, as does the loss of the natural skin barrier (e.g., through major burns).

Lungs

The lungs normally eliminate water vapor (insensible loss) at a rate of approximately 300 mL every day (Porth, 2011). The

loss is much greater with increased respiratory rate or depth, or in a dry climate.

Gastrointestinal Tract

The usual loss through the gastrointestinal (GI) tract is 100 to 200 mL daily, even though approximately 8 L of fluid circulates through the GI system every 24 hours. Because the bulk of fluid is normally reabsorbed in the small intestine, diarrhea and fistulas cause large losses.

> ⚑ *Quality and Safety Nursing Alert*
>
> When fluid balance is critical, all routes of systemic gain and loss must be recorded and all volumes compared. Organs of fluid loss include the kidneys, skin, lungs, and GI tract.

Laboratory Tests for Evaluating Fluid Status

Osmolality is the concentration of fluid that affects the movement of water between fluid compartments by osmosis. Osmolality measures the solute concentration per kilogram in blood and urine. It is also a measure of a solution's ability to create osmotic pressure and affect the movement of water. Serum osmolality primarily reflects the concentration

TABLE 13-2	Sources of Body Water Gains and Losses in the Adult		
Intake (mL)		**Output (mL)**	
Oral Intake		Urine	1,500
As water	1,000	Stool	200
In food	1,300	Insensible	
Water of oxidation	200	Lungs	300
		Skin	500
Total gain*	2,500	Total loss*	2,500

*Approximate volumes.
From Porth, C. M. (2011). *Essentials of pathophysiology* (3rd ed.). Philadelphia: Lippincott Williams & Wilkins.

TABLE 13-3 Factors Affecting Serum and Urine Osmolality

Fluid	Factors Increasing Osmolality	Factors Decreasing Osmolality
Serum (270–300 mOsm/kg water)	• Severe dehydration • Free water loss • Diabetes insipidus • Hypernatremia • Hyperglycemia • Stroke or head injury • Renal tubular necrosis • Consumption of methanol or ethylene glycol (antifreeze) • High ion gap metabolic acidosis • Mannitol therapy • Advanced liver disease • Alcoholism • Burns	• Fluid volume excess • Syndrome of inappropriate antidiuretic hormone (SIADH) • Acute renal failure • Diuretic use • Adrenal insufficiency • Hyponatremia • Overhydration • Paraneoplastic syndrome associated with lung cancer
Urine (200–800 mOsm/kg water)	• Fluid volume deficit • SIADH • Congestive heart failure • Acidosis • Prerenal failure	• Fluid volume excess • Diabetes insipidus • Hyponatremia • Aldosteronism • Pyelonephritis • Acute tubular necrosis

of sodium, although blood urea nitrogen (BUN) and glucose also play a major role in determining serum osmolality. Urine osmolality is determined by urea, creatinine, and uric acid. When measured with serum osmolality, urine osmolality is the most reliable indicator of urine concentration. Osmolality is reported as milliosmoles per kilogram of water (mOsm/kg) (Guyton & Hall, 2011).

In healthy adults, normal serum osmolality is 270 to 300 mOsm/kg (Crawford & Harris, 2011c). Sodium predominates in ECF osmolality and holds water in this compartment. Factors that increase and decrease serum and urine osmolality are identified in Table 13-3. Serum osmolality may be measured directly through laboratory tests or estimated at the bedside by doubling the serum sodium level or by using the following formula:

$$Na^+ \times 2 = \frac{Glucose}{18} + \frac{BUN}{3}$$

$$= \text{Approximate value of serum osmolality}$$

Osmolarity, another term that describes the concentration of solutions, is measured in milliosmoles per liter (mOsm/L). However, the term osmolality is used more often in clinical practice. The value of osmolarity is usually within 10 mOsm of the value of osmolality.

Urine specific gravity measures the kidneys' ability to excrete or conserve water. The specific gravity of urine is compared to the weight of distilled water, which has a specific gravity of 1.000. The normal range of urine specific gravity is 1.010 to 1.025. Urine specific gravity can be measured at the bedside by placing a calibrated hydrometer or urinometer in a cylinder of approximately 20 mL of urine. Specific gravity can also be assessed with a refractometer or dipstick with a reagent for this purpose. Specific gravity varies inversely with urine volume; normally, the larger the volume of urine, the lower the specific gravity is. Specific gravity is a less reliable indicator of concentration than urine osmolality; increased glucose or protein in urine can cause a falsely elevated specific gravity. Factors that increase or decrease urine osmolality are the same as those for urine specific gravity.

BUN is made up of urea, which is an end product of the metabolism of protein (from both muscle and dietary intake) by the liver. Amino acid breakdown produces large amounts of ammonia molecules, which are absorbed into the bloodstream. Ammonia molecules are converted to urea and excreted in the urine. The normal BUN is 10 to 20 mg/dL (3.6 to 7.2 mmol/L). The BUN level varies with urine output. Factors that increase BUN include decreased renal function, GI bleeding, dehydration, increased protein intake, fever, and sepsis. Those that decrease BUN include end-stage liver disease, a low-protein diet, starvation, and any condition that results in expanded fluid volume (e.g., pregnancy).

Creatinine is the end product of muscle metabolism. It is a better indicator of renal function than BUN because it does not vary with protein intake and metabolic state. The normal serum creatinine is approximately 0.7 to 1.4 mg/dL (62 to 124 mmol/L); however, its concentration depends on lean body mass and varies from person to person. Serum creatinine levels increase when renal function decreases.

Hematocrit measures the volume percentage of red blood cells (erythrocytes) in whole blood and normally ranges from 42% to 52% for males and 35% to 47% for females. Conditions that increase the hematocrit value are dehydration and polycythemia, and those that decrease hematocrit are overhydration and anemia.

Urine sodium values change with sodium intake and the status of fluid volume: As sodium intake increases, excretion increases; as the circulating fluid volume decreases, sodium is conserved. Normal urine sodium levels range from 75 to 200 mEq/24 hours (75 to 200 mmol/24 hours). A random specimen usually contains more than 40 mEq/L of sodium. Urine sodium levels are used to assess volume status and are useful in the diagnosis of hyponatremia and acute renal failure.

Homeostatic Mechanisms

The body is equipped with remarkable homeostatic mechanisms to keep the composition and volume of body fluid within narrow limits of normal. Organs involved in homeostasis include the kidneys, heart, lungs, pituitary gland, adrenal glands, and parathyroid glands (Porth, 2011).

Kidney Functions

Vital to the regulation of fluid and electrolyte balance, the kidneys normally filter 180 L of plasma every day in the adult and excrete 1 to 2 L of urine. They act both autonomously and in response to bloodborne messengers, such as aldosterone and antidiuretic hormone (ADH) (Porth, 2011). Major functions of the kidneys in maintaining normal fluid balance include the following:

- Regulation of ECF volume and osmolality by selective retention and excretion of body fluids
- Regulation of normal electrolyte levels in the ECF by selective electrolyte retention and excretion
- Regulation of pH of the ECF by retention of hydrogen ions
- Excretion of metabolic wastes and toxic substances (Guyton & Hall, 2011)

Given these functions, failure of the kidneys results in multiple fluid and electrolyte abnormalities.

Heart and Blood Vessel Functions

The pumping action of the heart circulates blood through the kidneys under sufficient pressure to allow for urine formation. Failure of this pumping action interferes with renal perfusion and thus with water and electrolyte regulation.

Lung Functions

The lungs are also vital in maintaining homeostasis. Through exhalation, the lungs remove approximately 300 mL of water daily in the normal adult (Porth, 2011). Abnormal conditions, such as hyperpnea (abnormally deep respiration) or continuous coughing, increase this loss; mechanical ventilation with excessive moisture decreases it. The lungs also play a major role in maintaining acid–base balance.

Pituitary Functions

The hypothalamus manufactures ADH, which is stored in the posterior pituitary gland and released as needed to conserve water. Functions of ADH include maintaining the osmotic pressure of the cells by controlling the retention or excretion of water by the kidneys and by regulating blood volume (Fig. 13-2).

Adrenal Functions

Aldosterone, a mineralocorticoid secreted by the zona glomerulosa (outer zone) of the adrenal cortex, has a profound effect on fluid balance. Increased secretion of aldosterone causes sodium retention (and thus water retention) and potassium loss. Conversely, decreased secretion of aldosterone causes sodium and water loss and potassium retention.

Cortisol, another adrenocortical hormone, has less mineralocorticoid action. However, when secreted in large quantities (or administered as corticosteroid therapy), it can also produce sodium and fluid retention.

Parathyroid Functions

The parathyroid glands, embedded in the thyroid gland, regulate calcium and phosphate balance by means of parathyroid hormone (PTH). PTH influences bone reabsorption, calcium absorption from the intestines, and calcium reabsorption from the renal tubules.

Other Mechanisms

Changes in the volume of the interstitial compartment within the ECF can occur without affecting body function. However, the vascular compartment cannot tolerate change as readily and must be carefully maintained to ensure that tissues receive adequate nutrients.

Baroreceptors

The baroreceptors are located in the left atrium and the carotid and aortic arches. These receptors respond to changes in the circulating blood volume and regulate sympathetic and parasympathetic neural activity as well as endocrine activities.

As arterial pressure decreases, baroreceptors transmit fewer impulses from the carotid and the aortic arches to the vasomotor center. A decrease in impulses stimulates the sympathetic nervous system and inhibits the parasympathetic nervous system. The outcome is an increase in cardiac rate, conduction, and contractility and an increase in circulating blood volume. Sympathetic stimulation constricts renal arterioles; this increases the release of aldosterone, decreases glomerular filtration, and increases sodium and water reabsorption (Guyton & Hall, 2011).

Renin–Angiotensin–Aldosterone System

Renin is an enzyme that converts angiotensinogen, a substance formed by the liver, into angiotensin I (Porth, 2011). Renin is released by the juxtaglomerular cells of the kidneys in response to decreased renal perfusion. Angiotensin-converting enzyme (ACE) converts angiotensin I to angiotensin II. Angiotensin II, with its vasoconstrictor properties, increases arterial perfusion pressure and stimulates thirst. As the sympathetic nervous system is stimulated, aldosterone is released in response to an increased release of renin. Aldosterone is a volume regulator and is also released as serum potassium increases, serum sodium decreases, or adrenocorticotropic hormone (ACTH) increases.

Antidiuretic Hormone and Thirst

Antidiuretic hormone (ADH) and the thirst mechanism have important roles in maintaining sodium concentration and oral intake of fluids. Oral intake is controlled by the thirst center located in the hypothalamus (Porth, 2011). As serum concentration or osmolality increases or blood volume decreases, neurons in the hypothalamus are stimulated by intracellular dehydration; thirst then occurs, and the person increases his or her intake of oral fluids. Water excretion is controlled by ADH, aldosterone, and baroreceptors, as mentioned previously. The presence or absence of ADH is the most significant factor in determining whether the urine that is excreted is concentrated or dilute.

Osmoreceptors

Located on the surface of the hypothalamus, osmoreceptors sense changes in sodium concentration. As osmotic pressure increases, the neurons become dehydrated and quickly release impulses to the posterior pituitary, which increases the release of ADH, which then travels in the blood to the kidneys, where it alters permeability to water, causing

Physiology ⋮⋱⋮ Pathophysiology

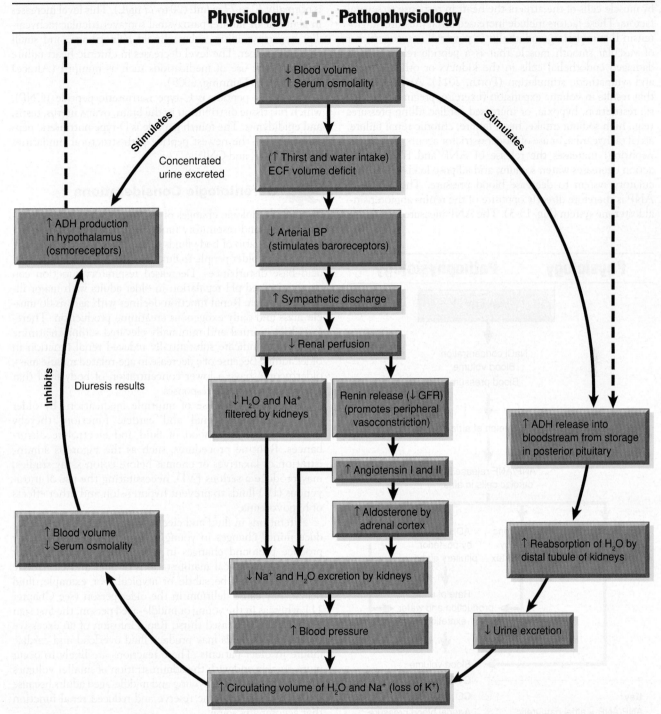

FIGURE 13-2 • Fluid regulation cycle. ADH, antidiuretic hormone; BP, blood pressure; ECF, extracellular fluid; GFR, glomerular filtration rate.

increased reabsorption of water and decreased urine output. The retained water dilutes the ECF and returns its concentration to normal. Restoration of normal osmotic pressure provides feedback to the osmoreceptors to inhibit further ADH release (Fig. 13-2).

Natriuretic Peptides

Natriuretic peptide hormones affect fluid volume and cardiovascular function through the excretion of sodium (natriure-

sis), direct vasodilation, and the opposition of the rennin–angiotensin–aldosterone system. Four peptides have been identified. The first is atrial natriuretic peptide (ANP) produced by the atrial myocardium with tissue distribution in the cardiac atria and ventricles. The second is brain natriuretic peptide (BNP) produced by the ventricular myocardium with tissue distribution in the brain and cardiac ventricles. ANP, also called *atrial natriuretic factor, atrial natriuretic hormone,* or *atriopeptin,* is a peptide that is synthesized, stored, and released by muscle cells of the atria of the heart in response to several factors. These factors include increased atrial pressure, angiotensin II stimulation, endothelin (a powerful vasoconstrictor of vascular smooth muscle that is a peptide released from damaged endothelial cells in the kidneys or other tissues), and sympathetic stimulation (Porth, 2011). Any condition that results in volume expansion (exercise, pregnancy), calorie restriction, hypoxia, or increased cardiac filling pressures (e.g., high sodium intake, heart failure, chronic renal failure, atrial tachycardia, or use of vasoconstrictor agents such as epinephrine) increases the release of ANP and BNP. ANP's action decreases water, sodium, and adipose loads on the circulatory system to decrease blood pressure. The action of ANP is therefore directly opposite of the renin–angiotensin–aldosterone system (Fig. 13-3). The ANP measured in plasma is normally 20 to 77 pg/mL (20 to 77 ng/L). This level increases in acute heart failure, paroxysmal supraventricular tachycardia, hyperthyroidism, subarachnoid hemorrhage, and small cell lung cancer. The level decreases in chronic heart failure and with the use of medications such as ramipril (Altace) (Fischbach & Dunning, 2009).

The third peptide is C-type natriuretic peptide (CNP), which has tissue distribution in the brain, ovary, uterus, testis, and epididymis. The fourth peptide is D-type natriuretic peptide (DNP)—the newest peptide with structural similarities to ANP, BNP, and CNP.

Gerontologic Considerations

Normal physiologic changes of aging, including reduced cardiac, renal, and respiratory function and reserve and alterations in the ratio of body fluids to muscle mass, may alter the responses of older people to fluid and electrolyte changes and acid–base disturbances. Decreased respiratory function can cause impaired pH regulation in older adults with major illness or trauma. Renal function declines with age, as do muscle mass and daily exogenous creatinine production. Therefore, high-normal and minimally elevated serum creatinine values may indicate substantially reduced renal function in older adults. Because of a decrease in age-related muscle mass, older people have a lower concentration of body fluid that may alter physiologic responses.

In addition, the use of multiple medications by older adults can affect renal and cardiac function, thereby increasing the likelihood of fluid and electrolyte disturbances. Routine procedures, such as the vigorous administration of laxatives or enemas before colon x-ray studies, may produce a serious FVD, necessitating the use of intravenous (IV) fluids to prevent hypotension and other effects of hypovolemia.

Alterations in fluid and electrolyte balance that may produce minor changes in young and middle-aged adults may produce profound changes in older adults. In many older patients, the clinical manifestations of fluid and electrolyte disturbances may be subtle or atypical. For example, fluid deficit may cause delirium in the older person (see Chapter 11), whereas in the young or middle-aged person, the first sign commonly is increased thirst. Rapid infusion of an excessive volume of IV fluids may produce fluid overload and cardiac failure in older patients. These reactions are likely to occur more quickly and with the administration of smaller volumes of fluid than in healthy young and middle-aged adults because of the decreased cardiac reserve and reduced renal function that accompany aging.

Dehydration is the rapid loss of more than 3% of body weight owing to the loss of either water or sodium (Collins & Claros, 2011). Dehydration in older adults is common because of decreased kidney mass, decreased glomerular filtration rate, decreased renal blood flow, decreased ability to concentrate urine, inability to conserve sodium, decreased excretion of potassium, and a decrease of total body water.

Loss of subcutaneous supporting tissue and resultant thinning of the skin occurs with aging; the dermis is dehydrated and loses strength and elasticity. These skin changes affect placement of peripheral IV catheters in older adults (Infusion Nurses Society [INS], 2011).

Physiology · · · Pathophysiology

ANP/ANF

↓

↑NaCl concentration
↑Blood volume
↑Blood pressure

↓

↑Stretch of atria

↓

↑ANP/ANF release from cardiac cells in atria

Suppression of RA system, thus ↓angiotensin II | ↓Aldosterone release by adrenal cortex | ↓ADH release by posterior pituitary gland | ↑GFR

↑Na⁺ excretion → ↑Na+ excretion

↑Rate of urine production and water excretion

↓

↓Blood volume
↓CVP
↓CO
↓Arterial blood pressure
↓Preload
↓HR

Key:
ANP/ANF = atrial natriuretic peptide/atrial natriuretic factor
CO = Cardiac output
CVP = Central venous pressure
GFR = Glomerular filtration rate
HR = Heart rate
RA = Renin–angiotensin

FIGURE 13-3 • Role of atrial natriuretic peptide in maintenance of fluid balance.

FLUID VOLUME DISTURBANCES

Hypovolemia

FVD, or hypovolemia, occurs when loss of ECF volume exceeds the intake of fluid. It occurs when water and electrolytes are lost in the same proportion as they exist in normal body fluids, thus the ratio of serum electrolytes to water remains the same. FVD should not be confused with dehydration, which refers to loss of water alone, with increased serum sodium levels. FVD may occur alone or in combination with other imbalances. Unless other imbalances are present concurrently, serum electrolyte concentrations remain essentially unchanged.

Pathophysiology

FVD results from loss of body fluids and occurs more rapidly when coupled with decreased fluid intake. FVD can also develop with a prolonged period of inadequate intake. Causes of FVD include abnormal fluid losses, such as those resulting from vomiting, diarrhea, GI suctioning, and sweating; decreased intake, as in nausea or lack of access to fluids; and third-space fluid shifts, or the movement of fluid from the vascular system to other body spaces (e.g., with edema formation in burns, ascites with liver dysfunction). Additional causes include diabetes insipidus (a decreased ability to concentrate urine owing to a defect in the kidney tubules that interferes with water reabsorption), adrenal insufficiency, osmotic diuresis, hemorrhage, and coma.

Clinical Manifestations

FVD can develop rapidly, and its severity depends on the degree of fluid loss. Clinical signs and symptoms and laboratory findings are presented in Table 13-4.

Assessment and Diagnostic Findings

Laboratory data useful in evaluating fluid volume status include BUN and its relation to serum creatinine concentration. A volume-depleted patient has a BUN elevated out of proportion to the serum creatinine (ratio greater than 20:1). The BUN can be elevated because of dehydration or decreased renal perfusion and function. The presence and cause of hypovolemia may be determined through the health history and physical examination. In addition, the hematocrit level is greater than normal because there is a decreased plasma volume (Chernecky & Berger, 2008).

Serum electrolyte changes may also exist. Potassium and sodium levels can be reduced (hypokalemia, hyponatremia) or elevated (hyperkalemia, hypernatremia).

- Hypokalemia occurs with GI and renal losses.
- Hyperkalemia occurs with adrenal insufficiency.
- Hyponatremia occurs with increased thirst and ADH release.
- Hypernatremia results from increased insensible losses and diabetes insipidus.

Urine specific gravity is increased in relation to the kidneys' attempt to conserve water and is decreased with diabetes insipidus. Aldosterone is secreted when fluid volume is low causing reabsorption of sodium and chloride, resulting in decreased urinary sodium and chloride. Urine osmolality can be greater than 450 mOsm/kg because the kidneys try to compensate by conserving water. Normal values for laboratory data are listed in Appendix A on thePoint.

 ## Gerontologic Considerations

Increased sensitivity to fluid and electrolyte changes in older patients requires careful assessment of I&O of fluids from all sources, assessment of changes in daily weight, careful monitoring of side effects and interactions of medications, and prompt reporting and management of disturbances. It is normally useful to monitor skin turgor serially to detect subtle changes. However, assessment of skin turgor is not as valid in older adults because the skin has lost some of its elasticity; therefore, other assessment measures (e.g., slowness in filling of veins of the hands and feet) become more useful in detecting FVD (Weber & Kelley, 2010).

The nurse also performs a functional assessment of the older patient's ability to determine fluid and food needs and to obtain adequate intake in addition to assessments discussed earlier in this chapter. For example, is the patient cognitively intact, able to ambulate and to use both arms and hands to reach fluids and foods, and able to swallow? Results of this assessment have a direct bearing on how the patient will be able to meet his or her own need for fluids and foods (Collins & Claros, 2011). During an older patient's hospital stay, the nurse provides fluids if the patient is unable to carry out self-care activities.

The nurse should also recognize that some older patients deliberately restrict their fluid intake to avoid embarrassing episodes of incontinence. In this situation, the nurse identifies interventions to deal with the incontinence, such as encouraging the patient to wear protective clothing or devices, to carry a urinal in the car, or to pace fluid intake to allow access to toilet facilities during the day. Older people without cardiovascular or renal dysfunction should be reminded to drink adequate fluids, particularly in very warm or humid weather.

Medical Management

When planning the correction of fluid loss for the patient with FVD, the primary provider considers the patient's maintenance requirements and other factors (e.g., fever) that can influence fluid needs. If the deficit is not severe, the oral route is preferred, provided the patient can drink. However, if fluid losses are acute or severe, the IV route is required. Isotonic electrolyte solutions (e.g., lactated Ringer's solution, 0.9% sodium chloride) are frequently the first-line choice to treat the hypotensive patient with FVD because they expand plasma volume (Crawford & Harris, 2011c). As soon as the patient becomes normotensive, a hypotonic electrolyte solution (e.g., 0.45% sodium chloride) is often used to provide both electrolytes and water for renal excretion of metabolic wastes. These and additional fluids are listed in Table 13-5.

Accurate and frequent assessments of I&O, weight, vital signs, central venous pressure, level of consciousness, breath sounds, and skin color should be performed to determine when therapy should be slowed to avoid volume overload.

TABLE 13-4 Major Fluid and Electrolyte Imbalances		
Imbalance	**Contributing Factors**	**Signs/Symptoms and Laboratory Findings**
Fluid volume deficit (hypovolemia)	Loss of water and electrolytes, as in vomiting, diarrhea, fistulas, fever, excess sweating, burns, blood loss, gastrointestinal suction, and third-space fluid shifts; and decreased intake, as in anorexia, nausea, and inability to gain access to fluid. Diabetes insipidus and uncontrolled diabetes both contribute to a depletion of extracellular fluid volume.	Acute weight loss, ↓ skin turgor, oliguria, concentrated urine, capillary filling time prolonged, low CVP, ↓ BP, flattened neck veins, dizziness, weakness, thirst and confusion, ↑ pulse, muscle cramps, sunken eyes, nausea, increased temperature; cool, clammy, pale skin *Labs indicate:* ↑ hemoglobin and hematocrit, ↑ serum and urine osmolality and specific gravity, ↓ urine sodium, ↑ BUN and creatinine, ↑ urine specific gravity and osmolality
Fluid volume excess (hypervolemia)	Compromised regulatory mechanisms, such as renal failure, heart failure, and cirrhosis; overzealous administration of sodium-containing fluids; and fluid shifts (i.e., treatment of burns). Prolonged corticosteroid therapy, severe stress, and hyperaldosteronism augment fluid volume excess.	Acute weight gain, peripheral edema and ascites, distended jugular veins, crackles, elevated CVP, shortness of breath, ↑ BP, bounding pulse and cough, ↑ respiratory rate, ↑ urine output *Labs indicate:* ↓ hemoglobin and hematocrit, ↓ serum and urine osmolality, ↓ urine sodium and specific gravity
Sodium deficit (hyponatremia) Serum sodium <135 mEq/L	Loss of sodium, as in use of diuretics, loss of GI fluids, renal disease, and adrenal insufficiency. Gain of water, as in excessive administration of D₅W and water supplements for patients receiving hypotonic tube feedings; disease states associated with SIADH such as head trauma and oat-cell lung tumor; medications associated with water retention (oxytocin and certain tranquilizers); and psychogenic polydipsia. Hyperglycemia and heart failure cause a loss of sodium.	Anorexia, nausea and vomiting, headache, lethargy, dizziness, confusion, muscle cramps and weakness, muscular twitching, seizures, papilledema, dry skin, ↑ pulse, ↓ BP, weight gain, edema *Labs indicate:* ↓ serum and urine sodium, ↓ urine specific gravity and osmolality
Sodium excess (hypernatremia) Serum sodium >145 mEq/L	Water deprivation in patients unable to drink at will, hypertonic tube feedings without adequate water supplements, diabetes insipidus, heatstroke, hyperventilation, watery diarrhea, burns, and diaphoresis. Excess corticosteroid, sodium bicarbonate, and sodium chloride administration, and saltwater near-drowning victims.	Thirst, elevated body temperature, swollen dry tongue and sticky mucous membranes, hallucinations, lethargy, restlessness, irritability, simple partial or tonic–clonic seizures, pulmonary edema, hyperreflexia, twitching, nausea, vomiting, anorexia, ↑ pulse, and ↑ BP *Labs indicate:* ↑ serum sodium, ↓ urine sodium, ↑ urine specific gravity and osmolality, ↓ CVP
Potassium deficit (hypokalemia) Serum potassium <3.5 mEq/L	Diarrhea, vomiting, gastric suction, corticosteroid administration, hyperaldosteronism, carbenicillin, amphotericin B, bulimia, osmotic diuresis, alkalosis, starvation, diuretics, and digoxin toxicity	Fatigue, anorexia, nausea and vomiting, muscle weakness, polyuria, decreased bowel motility, ventricular asystole or fibrillation, paresthesias, leg cramps, ↓ BP, ileus, abdominal distention, hypoactive reflexes. *ECG:* flattened T waves, prominent U waves, ST depression, prolonged PR interval
Potassium excess (hyperkalemia) Serum potassium >5.0 mEq/L	Pseudohyperkalemia, oliguric renal failure, use of potassium-conserving diuretics in patients with renal insufficiency, metabolic acidosis, Addison's disease, crush injury, burns, stored bank blood transfusions, rapid IV administration of potassium, and certain medications such as ACE inhibitors, NSAIDs, cyclosporine	Muscle weakness, tachycardia → bradycardia, dysrhythmias, flaccid paralysis, paresthesias, intestinal colic, cramps, abdominal distention, irritability, anxiety. *ECG:* tall tented T waves, prolonged PR interval and QRS duration, absent P waves, ST depression
Calcium deficit (hypocalcemia) Serum calcium <8.5 mg/dL	Hypoparathyroidism (may follow thyroid surgery or radical neck dissection), malabsorption, pancreatitis, alkalosis, vitamin D deficiency, massive subcutaneous infection, generalized peritonitis, massive transfusion of citrated blood, chronic diarrhea, decreased parathyroid hormone, diuretic phase of renal failure, ↑ PO₄, fistulas, burns, alcoholism	Numbness, tingling of fingers, toes, and circumoral region; positive Trousseau's sign and Chvostek's sign; seizures, carpopedal spasms, hyperactive deep tendon reflexes, irritability, bronchospasm, anxiety, impaired clotting time, ↓ prothrombin, diarrhea, ↓ BP. *ECG:* prolonged QT interval and lengthened ST *Labs indicate:* ↓ Mg⁺⁺
Calcium excess (hypercalcemia) Serum calcium >10.5 mg/dL	Hyperparathyroidism, malignant neoplastic disease, prolonged immobilization, overuse of calcium supplements, vitamin D excess, oliguric phase of renal failure, acidosis, corticosteroid therapy, thiazide diuretic use, increased parathyroid hormone, and digoxin toxicity	Muscular weakness, constipation, anorexia, nausea and vomiting, polyuria and polydipsia, dehydration, hypoactive deep tendon reflexes, lethargy, deep bone pain, pathologic fractures, flank pain, calcium stones, hypertension. *ECG:* shortened ST segment and QT interval, bradycardia, heart blocks
Magnesium deficit (hypomagnesemia) Serum magnesium <1.8 mg/dL	Chronic alcoholism, hyperparathyroidism, hyperaldosteronism, diuretic phase of renal failure, malabsorptive disorders, diabetic ketoacidosis, refeeding after starvation, parenteral nutrition, chronic laxative use, diarrhea, acute myocardial infarction, heart failure, decreased serum K⁺ and Ca⁺⁺ and certain pharmacologic agents (such as gentamicin, cisplatin, and cyclosporine)	Neuromuscular irritability, positive Trousseau's sign and Chvostek's sign, insomnia, mood changes, anorexia, vomiting, increased tendon reflexes, and ↑ BP. *ECG:* PVCs, flat or inverted T waves, depressed ST segment, prolonged PR interval, and widened QRS
Magnesium excess (hypermagnesemia) Serum magnesium >2.7 mg/dL	Oliguric phase of renal failure (particularly when magnesium-containing medications are administered), adrenal insufficiency, excessive IV magnesium administration, diabetic ketoacidosis, and hypothyroidism	Flushing, hypotension, muscle weakness, drowsiness, hypoactive reflexes, depressed respirations, cardiac arrest and coma, diaphoresis. *ECG:* tachycardia → bradycardia, prolonged PR interval and QRS, peaked T waves

Imbalance	Contributing Factors	Signs/Symptoms and Laboratory Findings
Phosphorus deficit (hypophosphatemia) Serum phosphorus <2.5 mg/dL	Refeeding after starvation, alcohol withdrawal, diabetic ketoacidosis, respiratory and metabolic alkalosis, ↓ magnesium, ↓ potassium, hyperparathyroidism, vomiting, diarrhea, hyperventilation, vitamin D deficiency associated with malabsorptive disorders, burns, acid–base disorders, parenteral nutrition, and diuretic and antacid use	Paresthesias, muscle weakness, bone pain and tenderness, chest pain, confusion, cardiomyopathy, respiratory failure, seizures, tissue hypoxia, and increased susceptibility to infection, nystagmus
Phosphorus excess (hyperphosphatemia) Serum phosphorus >4.5 mg/dL	Acute and chronic renal failure, excessive intake of phosphorus, vitamin D excess, respiratory and metabolic acidosis, hypoparathyroidism, volume depletion, leukemia/lymphoma treated with cytotoxic agents, increased tissue breakdown, rhabdomyolysis	Tetany, tachycardia, anorexia, nausea and vomiting, muscle weakness, signs and symptoms of hypocalcemia; hyperactive reflexes; soft tissue calcifications in lungs, heart, kidneys, and cornea
Chloride deficit (hypochloremia) Serum chloride <96 mEq/L	Addison's disease, reduced chloride intake or absorption, untreated diabetic ketoacidosis, chronic respiratory acidosis, excessive sweating, vomiting, gastric suction, diarrhea, sodium and potassium deficiency, metabolic alkalosis; loop, osmotic, or thiazide diuretic use; overuse of bicarbonate, rapid removal of ascitic fluid with a high sodium content, IV fluids that lack chloride (dextrose and water), draining fistulas and ileostomies, heart failure, cystic fibrosis	Agitation, irritability, tremors, muscle cramps, hyperactive deep tendon reflexes, hypertonicity, tetany, slow shallow respirations, seizures, dysrhythmias, coma *Labs indicate:* ↓ serum chloride, ↓ serum sodium, ↑ pH, ↑ serum bicarbonate, ↑ total carbon dioxide content, ↓ urine chloride level, ↓ serum potassium
Chloride excess (hyperchloremia) Serum chloride >108 mEq/L	Excessive sodium chloride infusions with water loss, head injury (sodium retention), hypernatremia, renal failure, corticosteroid use, dehydration, severe diarrhea (loss of bicarbonate), respiratory alkalosis, administration of diuretics, overdose of salicylates, Kayexalate, acetazolamide, phenylbutazone and ammonium chloride use, hyperparathyroidism, metabolic acidosis	Tachypnea, lethargy, weakness, deep rapid respirations, decline in cognitive status, ↓ cardiac output, dyspnea, tachycardia, pitting edema, dysrhythmias, coma *Labs indicate:* ↑ serum chloride, ↑ serum potassium and sodium, ↓ serum pH, ↓ serum bicarbonate, normal anion gap, ↑ urinary chloride level

↑, increased; ↓, decreased; →, followed by; CVP, central venous pressure; BP, blood pressure; BUN, blood urea nitrogen; GI, gastrointestinal; D₅W, dextrose 5% in water; SIADH, syndrome of inappropriate secretion of antidiuretic hormone; ECG, electrocardiogram; IV, intravenous; ACE, angiotensin-converting enzyme; NSAIDs, nonsteroidal anti-inflammatory drugs; PVCs, premature ventricular contractions.

The rate of fluid administration is based on the severity of loss and the patient's hemodynamic response to volume replacement (Porth, 2011).

If the patient with severe FVD is not excreting enough urine and is therefore oliguric, the primary provider needs to determine whether the depressed renal function is caused by reduced renal blood flow secondary to FVD (prerenal azotemia) or, more seriously, by acute tubular necrosis from prolonged FVD. The test used in this situation is referred to as a fluid challenge test. During a fluid challenge test, volumes of fluid are administered at specific rates and intervals while the patient's hemodynamic response to this treatment is monitored (i.e., vital signs, breath sounds, orientation status, central venous pressure, urine output).

An example of a typical fluid challenge test involves administering 100 to 200 mL of normal saline solution over 15 minutes. The goal is to provide fluids rapidly enough to attain adequate tissue perfusion without compromising the cardiovascular system. The response by a patient with FVD but normal renal function is increased urine output and an increase in blood pressure and central venous pressure.

Shock can occur when the volume of fluid lost exceeds 25% of the intravascular volume or when fluid loss is rapid. (Shock and its causes and treatment are discussed in detail in Chapter 14.)

Nursing Management

To assess for FVD, the nurse monitors and measures fluid I&O at least every 8 hours, and sometimes hourly. As FVD develops, body fluid losses exceed fluid intake through excessive urination (polyuria), diarrhea, vomiting, or other mechanisms. Once FVD has developed, the kidneys attempt to conserve body fluids, leading to a urine output of less than 1 mL/kg/h in an adult. Urine in this instance is concentrated and represents a healthy renal response. Daily body weights are monitored; an acute loss of 0.5 kg (1 lb) represents a fluid loss of approximately 500 mL (1L of fluid weighs approximately 1 kg, or 2.2 lb) (Crawford & Harris, 2011c).

Vital signs are closely monitored. The nurse observes for a weak, rapid pulse and orthostatic hypotension (i.e., a decrease in systolic pressure exceeding 20 mm Hg when the patient moves from a lying to a sitting position) (Weber & Kelley, 2010). A decrease in body temperature often accompanies FVD, unless there is a concurrent infection.

Skin and tongue turgor are monitored on a regular basis. In a healthy person, pinched skin immediately returns to its normal position when released (Weber & Kelley, 2010). This elastic property, referred to as turgor, is partially dependent on interstitial fluid volume. In a person with FVD, the skin flattens more slowly after the pinch is released. In a person with severe FVD, the skin may remain elevated for many seconds. Tissue turgor is best measured by pinching the skin over the sternum, inner aspects of the thighs, or forehead. Tongue turgor is not affected by age (see previous Gerontologic Considerations), and evaluating this may be more valid than evaluating skin turgor. In a normal person, the tongue has one longitudinal furrow. In the person with FVD, there are additional longitudinal furrows and the tongue is smaller because of fluid loss. The degree of oral mucous membrane moisture is also assessed; a dry mouth may indicate either FVD or mouth breathing.

TABLE 13-5   Selected Water and Electrolyte Solutions

Solution	Comments
Isotonic Solutions	
0.9% NaCl (isotonic, also called *normal saline* [NS]) Na⁺ 154 mEq/L Cl⁻ 154 mEq/L (308 mOsm/L) Also available with varying concentrations of dextrose (a 5% dextrose concentration is commonly used)	• An isotonic solution that expands the extracellular fluid (ECF) volume; used in hypovolemic states, resuscitative efforts, shock, diabetic ketoacidosis, metabolic alkalosis, hypercalcemia, mild Na⁺ deficit • Supplies an excess of Na⁺ and Cl⁻; can cause fluid volume excess and hyperchloremic acidosis if used in excessive volumes, particularly in patients with compromised renal function, heart failure, or edema • Not desirable as a routine maintenance solution, as it provides only Na⁺ and Cl⁻ (and these are provided in excessive amounts) • When mixed with 5% dextrose, the resulting solution becomes hypertonic in relation to plasma and, in addition to the previously described electrolytes, provides 170 cal/L • Only solution that may be administered with blood products • Tonicity similar to plasma
Lactated Ringer's Solution Na⁺ 130 mEq/L K⁺ 4 mEq/L Ca⁺⁺ 3 mEq/L Cl⁻ 109 mEq/L Lactate (metabolized to bicarbonate) 28 mEq/L (274 mOsm/L) Also available with varying concentrations of dextrose (the most common is 5% dextrose)	• An isotonic solution that contains multiple electrolytes in roughly the same concentration as found in plasma (note that solution is lacking in Mg⁺⁺); provides 9 cal/L • Used in the treatment of hypovolemia, burns, fluid lost as bile or diarrhea, and for acute blood loss replacement • Lactate is rapidly metabolized into HCO₃⁻ in the body. Lactated Ringer's solution should not be used in lactic acidosis because the ability to convert lactate into HCO₃⁻ is impaired in this disorder. • Not to be given with a pH >7.5 because bicarbonate is formed as lactate breaks down, causing alkalosis • Should not be used in renal failure because it contains potassium and can cause hyperkalemia • Tonicity similar to plasma
5% dextrose in water (D₅W) No electrolytes 50 g of dextrose	• An isotonic solution that supplies 170 cal/L and free water to aid in renal excretion of solutes • Used in treatment of hypernatremia, fluid loss, and dehydration • Should not be used in excessive volumes in the early postoperative period (when antidiuretic hormone secretion is increased due to stress reaction) • Should not be used solely in treatment of fluid volume deficit because it dilutes plasma electrolyte concentrations • Contraindicated in head injury because it may cause increased intracranial pressure • Should not be used for fluid resuscitation because it can cause hyperglycemia • Should be used with caution in patients with renal or cardiac disease because of risk of fluid overload • Electrolyte-free solutions may cause peripheral circulatory collapse, anuria in patients with sodium deficiency, and increased body fluid loss. • Converts to hypotonic solution as dextrose is metabolized by body. Over time, D₅W without NaCl can cause water intoxication (intracellular fluid volume excess [FVE]) because the solution is hypotonic. • Fluid therapy for an extended period of time without electrolytes may result in hypokalemia.
Hypotonic Solutions	
0.45% NaCl (half-strength saline) Na⁺ 77 mEq/L Cl⁻ 77 mEq/L (154 mOsm/L) Also available with varying concentrations of dextrose (the most common is a 5% concentration)	• Provides Na⁺, Cl⁻, and free water • Free water is desirable to aid the kidneys in elimination of solute. • Lacking in electrolytes other than Na⁺ and Cl⁻ • When mixed with 5% dextrose, the solution becomes slightly hypertonic to plasma and in addition to the previously described electrolytes provides 170 cal/L. • Used to treat hypertonic dehydration, Na⁺ and Cl⁻ depletion, and gastric fluid loss • Not indicated for third-space fluid shifts or increased intracranial pressure • Administer cautiously, because it can cause fluid shifts from vascular system into cells, resulting in cardiovascular collapse and increased intracranial pressure
Hypertonic Solutions	
3% NaCl (hypertonic saline) Na⁺ 513 mEq/L Cl⁻ 513 mEq/L (1,026 mOsm/L)	• Used to increase ECF volume, decrease cellular swelling • Highly hypertonic solution used only in critical situations to treat hyponatremia • Must be administered slowly and cautiously, because it can cause intravascular volume overload and pulmonary edema • Supplies no calories • Assists in removing intracellular fluid excess
5% NaCL (hypertonic solution) Na⁺ 855 mEq/L Cl⁻ 855 mEq/L (1,710 mOsm/L)	• Highly hypertonic solution used to treat symptomatic hyponatremia • Administer slowly and cautiously because it can cause intravascular volume overload and pulmonary edema. • Supplies no calories
Colloid Solutions Dextran in NS or D₅W Available in low-molecular-weight (Dextran 40) and high-molecular-weight (Dextran 70) forms	• Colloid solution used as volume/plasma expander for intravascular part of ECF • Affects clotting by coating platelets and decreasing ability to clot • Remains in circulatory system up to 24 h • Used to treat hypovolemia in early shock to increase pulse pressure, cardiac output, and arterial blood pressure • Improves microcirculation by decreasing red blood cell aggregation • Contraindicated in hemorrhage, thrombocytopenia, renal disease, and severe dehydration • Not a substitute for blood or blood products

Urine concentration is monitored by measuring the urine specific gravity. In a volume-depleted patient, the urine specific gravity should be greater than 1.020, indicating healthy renal conservation of fluid.

Mental function is eventually affected, resulting in delirium in severe FVD as a result of decreasing cerebral perfusion. Decreased peripheral perfusion can result in cold extremities. In patients with relatively normal cardiopulmonary function, a low central venous pressure is indicative of hypovolemia. Patients with acute cardiopulmonary decompensation require more extensive hemodynamic monitoring of pressures in both sides of the heart to determine if hypovolemia exists.

Preventing Hypovolemia

To prevent FVD, the nurse identifies patients at risk and takes measures to minimize fluid losses. For example, if the patient has diarrhea, measures should be implemented to control diarrhea and replacement fluids administered. This includes administering antidiarrheal medications and small volumes of oral fluids at frequent intervals.

Correcting Hypovolemia

When possible, oral fluids are administered to help correct FVD, with consideration given to the patient's likes and dislikes. The type of fluid the patient has lost is also considered, and fluids most likely to replace the lost electrolytes are appropriate. If the patient is reluctant to drink because of oral discomfort, the nurse assists with frequent mouth care and provides nonirritating fluids. The patient may be offered small volumes of oral rehydration solutions (e.g., Rehydralyte, Elete, Cytomax). These solutions provide fluid, glucose, and electrolytes in concentrations that are easily absorbed. If nausea is present, an antiemetic may be needed before oral fluid replacement can be tolerated.

If the deficit cannot be corrected by oral fluids, therapy may need to be initiated by an alternative route (enteral or parenteral) until adequate circulating blood volume and renal perfusion are achieved. Isotonic fluids are prescribed to increase ECF volume (Crawford & Harris, 2011c).

Hypervolemia

Fluid volume excess (FVE), or hypervolemia, refers to an isotonic expansion of the ECF caused by the abnormal retention of water and sodium in approximately the same proportions in which they normally exist in the ECF. It is most often secondary to an increase in the total body sodium content, which, in turn, leads to an increase in total body water. Because there is isotonic retention of body substances, the serum sodium concentration remains essentially normal.

Pathophysiology

FVE may be related to simple fluid overload or diminished function of the homeostatic mechanisms responsible for regulating fluid balance. Contributing factors can include heart failure, renal failure, and cirrhosis of the liver. Another contributing factor is consumption of excessive amounts of table or other sodium salts. Excessive administration of sodium-containing fluids in a patient with impaired regulatory mechanisms may predispose him or her to a serious FVE as well.

Clinical Manifestations

Clinical manifestations of FVE result from expansion of the ECF and may include edema, distended neck veins, and crackles (abnormal lung sounds). Further discussion of clinical signs and symptoms and laboratory findings can be found in Table 13-4.

Assessment and Diagnostic Findings

Laboratory data useful in diagnosing FVE include BUN and hematocrit levels. In FVE, both of these values may be decreased because of plasma dilution, low protein intake, and anemia. In chronic renal failure, both serum osmolality and the sodium level are decreased owing to excessive retention of water. The urine sodium level is increased if the kidneys are attempting to excrete excess volume. A chest x-ray may reveal pulmonary congestion. Hypervolemia occurs when aldosterone is chronically stimulated (i.e., cirrhosis, heart failure, and nephrotic syndrome). Therefore, the urine sodium level does not increase in these conditions.

Medical Management

Management of FVE is directed at the causes, and if related to excessive administration of sodium-containing fluids, discontinuing the infusion may be all that is needed. Symptomatic treatment consists of administering diuretics and restricting fluids and sodium.

Pharmacologic Therapy

Diuretics are prescribed when dietary restriction of sodium alone is insufficient to reduce edema by inhibiting the reabsorption of sodium and water by the kidneys. The choice of diuretic is based on the severity of the hypervolemic state, the degree of impairment of renal function, and the potency of the diuretic. Thiazide diuretics block sodium reabsorption in the distal tubule, where only 5% to 10% of filtered sodium is reabsorbed. Loop diuretics, such as furosemide (Lasix), bumetanide (Bumex), or torsemide (Demadex), can cause a greater loss of both sodium and water because they block sodium reabsorption in the ascending limb of Henle's loop, where 20% to 30% of filtered sodium is normally reabsorbed. Generally, thiazide diuretics, such as hydrochlorothiazide (HydroDIURIL) or chlorthalidone (Thalitone), are prescribed for mild to moderate hypervolemia and loop diuretics for severe hypervolemia (Karch, 2012).

Electrolyte imbalances may result from the effect of the diuretic. Hypokalemia can occur with all diuretics except those that work in the last distal tubule of the nephrons. Potassium supplements can be prescribed to avoid this complication. Hyperkalemia can occur with diuretics that work in the distal tubule (e.g., spironolactone [Aldactone], a potassium-sparing diuretic), especially in patients with decreased renal function. Hyponatremia occurs with diuresis owing to increased release of ADH secondary to reduction in circulating volume. Decreased magnesium levels occur with administration of loop and thiazide diuretics due to decreased reabsorption and increased excretion of magnesium by the kidney.

Azotemia (increased nitrogen levels in the blood) can occur with FVE when urea and creatinine are not excreted owing to decreased perfusion by the kidneys and decreased excretion of wastes. High uric acid levels (hyperuricemia) can also occur from increased reabsorption and decreased excretion of uric acid by the kidneys.

Dialysis

If renal function is so severely impaired that pharmacologic agents cannot act efficiently, other modalities are considered to remove sodium and fluid from the body. Hemodialysis or peritoneal dialysis may be used to remove nitrogenous wastes and control potassium and acid–base balance, and to remove sodium and fluid. Continuous renal replacement therapy may also be required. (See Chapter 54 for a discussion of these treatment modalities.)

Nutritional Therapy

Treatment of FVE usually involves dietary restriction of sodium. An average daily diet not restricted in sodium contains 6 to 15 g of salt, whereas low-sodium diets can range from a mild restriction to as little as 250 mg of sodium per day, depending on the patient's needs. A mild sodium-restricted diet allows only light salting of food (about half the usual amount) in cooking and at the table, and no addition of salt to commercially prepared foods that are already seasoned. Foods high in sodium must be avoided. It is the sodium salt (sodium chloride) rather than sodium itself that contributes to edema. Therefore, patients are instructed to read food labels carefully to determine salt content.

Because about half of ingested sodium is in the form of seasoning, seasoning substitutes can play a major role in decreasing sodium intake. Lemon juice, onions, and garlic are excellent substitute flavorings, although some patients prefer salt substitutes. Most salt substitutes contain potassium and must therefore be used cautiously by patients taking potassium-sparing diuretics (e.g., spironolactone, triamterene [Dyrenium], amiloride [Midamor]). They should not be used at all in conditions associated with potassium retention, such as advanced renal disease. Salt substitutes containing ammonium chloride can be harmful to patients with liver damage.

In some communities, drinking water may contain too much sodium for a sodium-restricted diet. Depending on its source, water may contain as little as 1 mg or more than 1,500 mg of sodium per quart. Patients may need to use distilled water if the local water supply is very high in sodium. Bottled water can have a sodium content that ranges from 0 to 1,200 mg/L; therefore, if sodium is restricted, the label must be carefully examined for sodium content before purchasing and drinking bottled water. Also, patients on sodium-restricted diets should be cautioned to avoid water softeners that add sodium to water in exchange for other ions, such as calcium. Protein intake may be increased in patients who are malnourished or who have low serum protein levels in an effort to increase capillary oncotic pressure and pull fluid out of the tissues into vessels for excretion by the kidneys.

Nursing Management

To assess for FVE, the nurse measures I&O at regular intervals to identify excessive fluid retention. The patient is weighed daily, and rapid weight gain is noted. An acute weight gain of 1 kg (2.2 lb) is equivalent to a gain of approximately 1 L of fluid. Breath sounds are assessed at regular intervals in at-risk patients, particularly if parenteral fluids are being administered. The nurse monitors the degree of edema in the most dependent parts of the body, such as the feet and ankles in ambulatory patients and the sacral region in patients confined to bed (Crawford & Harris, 2011c). Pitting edema is assessed by pressing a finger into the affected part, creating a pit or indentation that is evaluated on a scale of 1+ (minimal) to 4+ (severe). Peripheral edema is monitored by measuring the circumference of the extremity with a tape marked in millimeters (Weber & Kelley, 2010).

Preventing Hypervolemia

Specific interventions vary with the underlying condition and the degree of FVE. However, most patients require sodium-restricted diets in some form, and adherence to the prescribed diet is encouraged. Patients are instructed to avoid over-the-counter (OTC) medications without first checking with a health care provider, because these substances may contain sodium. If fluid retention persists despite adherence to a prescribed diet, hidden sources of sodium, such as the water supply or use of water softeners, should be considered.

Detecting and Controlling Hypervolemia

It is important to detect FVE before the condition becomes severe. Interventions include promoting rest, restricting sodium intake, monitoring parenteral fluid therapy, and administering appropriate medications.

Regular rest periods may be beneficial, because bed rest favors diuresis of fluid. The mechanism is related to diminished venous pooling and the subsequent increase in effective circulating blood volume and renal perfusion. Sodium and fluid restriction should be instituted as indicated. Because most patients with FVE require diuretics, the patient's response to these agents is monitored. The rate of parenteral fluids and the patient's response to these fluids are also closely monitored (Crawford & Harris, 2011c). If dyspnea or orthopnea is present, the patient is placed in a semi-Fowler's position to promote lung expansion. The patient is turned and repositioned at regular intervals because edematous tissue is more prone to skin breakdown than normal tissue. Because conditions predisposing to FVE are likely to be chronic, patients are taught to monitor their response to therapy by documenting fluid I&O and body weight changes. The importance of adhering to the treatment regimen is emphasized.

Educating Patients About Edema

Because edema is a common manifestation of FVE, patients need to recognize its symptoms and understand its importance. The nurse gives special attention to edema when instructing the patient with FVE. Edema can occur as a result of increased capillary fluid pressure, decreased capillary oncotic pressure, or increased interstitial oncotic pressure, causing expansion of the interstitial fluid compartment (Guyton & Hall, 2011). Edema can be localized (e.g., in the ankle, as in rheumatoid arthritis) or generalized (as in cardiac and renal failure). Severe generalized edema is called *anasarca*.

Edema occurs when there is a change in the capillary membrane, increasing the formation of interstitial fluid or decreasing the removal of interstitial fluid. Sodium retention is a frequent cause of the increased ECF volume. Burns and infection are examples of conditions associated with increased interstitial fluid volume. Obstruction to lymphatic outflow, a plasma albumin level less than 1.5 to 2 g/dL, or a decrease in plasma oncotic pressure contributes to increased interstitial fluid volume. The kidneys retain sodium and water when there is decreased ECF volume as a result of decreased cardiac output from heart failure. A thorough medication history is necessary to identify any medications that could cause edema, such as nonsteroidal anti-inflammatory drugs (NSAIDs), estrogens, corticosteroids, and antihypertensive agents.

Ascites is a type of edema in which fluid accumulates in the peritoneal cavity; it results from nephrotic syndrome, cirrhosis, and some malignant tumors. The patient commonly reports shortness of breath and a sense of pressure because of pressure on the diaphragm.

The goal of treatment is to preserve or restore the circulating intravascular fluid volume. Thus, in addition to treating the cause of the edema, other treatments may include diuretic therapy, restriction of fluids and sodium, elevation of the extremities, application of anti-embolism stockings, paracentesis, dialysis, and continuous renal replacement therapy in cases of renal failure or life-threatening fluid volume overload (see Chapter 54).

ELECTROLYTE IMBALANCES

Disturbances in electrolyte balances are common in clinical practice and may need to be corrected based on history, physical examination findings, and laboratory values (with comparison to previous values) (see Table 13-4).

Sodium Imbalances

Sodium (Na^+) is the most abundant electrolyte in the ECF; its concentration ranges from 135 to 145 mEq/L (135 to 145 mmol/L), and it is the primary determinant of ECF volume and osmolality (Crawford & Harris, 2011b). Sodium has a major role in controlling water distribution throughout the body, because it does not easily cross the cell wall membrane and because of its abundance and high concentration in the body. Sodium is regulated by ADH, thirst, and the renin–angiotensin–aldosterone system. A loss or gain of sodium is usually accompanied by a loss or gain of water. Sodium also functions in establishing the electrochemical state necessary for muscle contraction and the transmission of nerve impulses (Fischbach & Dunning, 2009).

The syndrome of inappropriate secretion of antidiuretic hormone (SIADH) may be associated with sodium imbalance. When there is a decrease in the circulating plasma osmolality, blood volume, or blood pressure, arginine vasopressin (AVP) is released from the posterior pituitary. Oversecretion of AVP can cause SIADH. Patients at risk are older adults, those with acquired immunodeficiency syndrome

(AIDS), those on mechanical ventilation, and people taking selective serotonin reuptake inhibitors (SSRIs).

Sodium imbalance can develop under simple or complex circumstances. The two most common sodium imbalances are sodium deficit and sodium excess.

■ Sodium Deficit (Hyponatremia)

Hyponatremia refers to a serum sodium level that is less than 135 mEq/L (135 mmol/L) (Fischbach & Dunning, 2009). Plasma sodium concentration represents the ratio of total body sodium to total body water. A decrease in this ratio can occur because of a low total body sodium with a lesser reduction in total body water, a normal total body sodium content with excess total body water, or an excess of total body sodium with an even greater excess of total body water. A hyponatremic state can be superimposed on an existing FVD or FVE.

Pathophysiology

Hyponatremia primarily occurs due to an imbalance of water rather than sodium. The urine sodium value assists in differentiating renal from nonrenal causes of hyponatremia. Low urine sodium occurs as the kidney retains sodium to compensate for nonrenal fluid loss (i.e., vomiting, diarrhea, sweating). High urine sodium concentration is associated with renal salt wasting (i.e., diuretic use). In dilutional hyponatremia, the ECF volume is increased without any edema.

A deficiency of aldosterone, as occurs in adrenal insufficiency, also predisposes to sodium deficiency. In addition, the use of certain medications, such as anticonvulsants (i.e., carbamazepine [Tegretol], oxcarbazepine (Trileptal), levetiracetam [Keppra]), SSRIs (fluoxetine [Prozac], sertraline [Zoloft], paroxetine [Paxil]), or desmopressin acetate (DDAVP) increases the risk of hyponatremia (Karch, 2012).

SIADH is seen in hyponatremia as well as hypernatremia. The physiologic disturbances include excessive ADH activity, with water retention and dilutional hyponatremia, and inappropriate urinary excretion of sodium in the presence of hyponatremia. SIADH can be the result of either sustained secretion of ADH by the hypothalamus or production of an ADH-like substance from a tumor (aberrant ADH production). Conditions affecting the central nervous system are associated with SIADH. (SIADH is discussed in more detail in Chapter 52.)

Clinical Manifestations

Clinical manifestations of hyponatremia depend on the cause, magnitude, and speed with which the deficit occurs. Poor skin turgor, dry mucosa, headache, decreased saliva production, orthostatic fall in blood pressure, nausea, vomiting, and abdominal cramping occur. Neurologic changes, including altered mental status, status epilepticus, and coma, are probably related to the cellular swelling and cerebral edema associated with hyponatremia. As the extracellular sodium level decreases, the cellular fluid becomes relatively more concentrated and pulls water into the cells (Fig. 13-4). In general, patients with an acute decrease in serum sodium levels have more cerebral edema and higher mortality rates than do those with more slowly developing hyponatremia. Acute decreases in sodium, developing in less than 48 hours, may be associated with brain

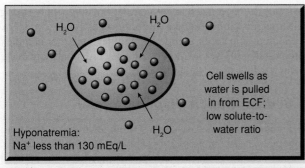

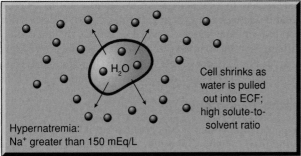

FIGURE 13-4 • Effect of extracellular sodium level on cell size.

herniation and compression of midbrain structures. Chronic decreases in sodium, developing over 48 hours or more, can occur in status epilepticus and other neurologic conditions.

Features of hyponatremia associated with sodium loss and water gain include anorexia, muscle cramps, and a feeling of exhaustion. The severity of symptoms increases with the degree of hyponatremia and the speed with which it develops. When the serum sodium level decreases to less than 115 mEq/L (115 mmol/L), signs of increasing intracranial pressure, such as lethargy, confusion, muscle twitching, focal weakness, hemiparesis, papilledema, seizures, and death, may occur.

Assessment and Diagnostic Findings

Assessment includes the history and physical examination, including a focused neurologic examination; evaluation of signs and symptoms as well as laboratory test results; identification of current IV fluids, if applicable; and a review of all medications the patient is taking. Regardless of the cause of hyponatremia, the serum sodium level is less than 135 mEq/L; in SIADH, it may be lower than 100 mEq/L (100 mmol/L). Serum osmolality is also decreased, except in azotemia with the accumulation of toxins. When hyponatremia is due primarily to sodium loss, the urinary sodium content is less than 20 mEq/L (20 mmol/L), suggesting increased proximal reabsorption of sodium secondary to ECF volume depletion, and the specific gravity is low (1.002 to 1.004). However, when hyponatremia is due to SIADH, the urinary sodium content is greater than 20 mEq/L, and the urine specific gravity is usually greater than 1.012. Although the patient with SIADH retains water abnormally and therefore gains body weight, there is no peripheral edema; instead, fluid accumulates inside the cells. This phenomenon sometimes manifests as pitting edema.

Medical Management

The key to treating hyponatremia is an assessment that focuses on the clinical symptoms of the patient and signs of

hyponatremia (including laboratory values). As a general rule, treating the underlying the condition is essential.

Sodium Replacement

The most common treatment for hyponatremia is careful administration of sodium by mouth, nasogastric tube, or a parenteral route. For patients who can eat and drink, sodium is easily replaced, because sodium is consumed abundantly in a normal diet. For those who cannot consume sodium, lactated Ringer's solution or isotonic saline (0.9% sodium chloride) solution may be prescribed. Serum sodium must not be increased by more than 12 mEq/L in 24 hours to avoid neurologic damage due to demyelination. This condition may occur when the serum sodium concentration is overcorrected (exceeding 140 mEq/L) too rapidly or in the presence of hypoxia or anoxia. It may produce lesions that show symmetric myelin destruction affecting all fiber tracts that can present with altered cognition and decreased alertness, ataxia, paraparesis, dysarthria, horizontal gaze paralysis, pseudobulbar palsy, and coma (Yee & Rabinstein, 2010; Lai, Tan, Lin, et al., 2011). The usual daily sodium requirement in adults is approximately 100 mEq, provided there are not excessive losses. Selected water and electrolyte solutions are described in Table 13-5.

In SIADH, the administration of hypertonic saline solution alone cannot change the plasma sodium concentration. Excess sodium would be excreted rapidly in highly concentrated urine. With the addition of the diuretic furosemide (Lasix), urine is not concentrated and isotonic urine is excreted to effect a change in water balance. In patients with SIADH, in whom water restriction is difficult, lithium (Eskalith) or demeclocycline (Declomycin) can antagonize the osmotic effect of ADH on the medullary collecting tubule.

Water Restriction

In patients with normal or excess fluid volume, hyponatremia is usually treated effectively by restricting fluid. However, if neurologic symptoms are severe (e.g., seizures, delirium, coma), or in patients with traumatic brain injury, it may be necessary to administer small volumes of a hypertonic sodium solution with the goal of alleviating cerebral edema (see Chapter 66). Incorrect use of these fluids is extremely dangerous, because 1 L of 3% sodium chloride solution contains 513 mEq of sodium and 1 L of 5% sodium chloride solution contains 855 mEq of sodium. The recommendation for hypertonic saline administration in patients with craniocerebral trauma is 3% saline between 0.10 to 1.0 mL/kg of body weight per hour (March, Criddle, Madden et al., 2010).

> ◢ **Quality and Safety Nursing Alert**
>
> Highly hypertonic sodium solutions (2% to 23% sodium chloride) should be administered slowly and the patient monitored closely, because only small volumes are needed to elevate the serum sodium concentration from a dangerously low level.

Pharmacologic Therapy

AVP receptor antagonists are new pharmacologic agents that treat hyponatremia by stimulating free water excretion. IV conivaptan hydrochloride (Vaprisol) use is limited to the treatment of hospitalized patients. It may be a useful therapy for those patients with moderate to severe symptomatic hyponatremia but is contraindicated in patients with seizures, delirium, or coma, which warrant the use of hypertonic saline. Tolvaptan (Samsca) is an oral medication indicated for clinically significant hypervolemic and euvolemic hyponatremia that must be initiated and monitored in the hospital setting (Crawford & Harris, 2011b; Karch, 2012).

Nursing Management

The nurse needs to identify and monitor patients at risk for hyponatremia. The nurse monitors fluid I&O as well as daily body weight.

Hyponatremia is a frequently overlooked cause of confusion in older patients, who are at increased risk because of decreased renal function and subsequent inability to excrete excess fluids. Administration of prescribed and OTC medications that cause sodium loss or water retention are predisposing factors. A diminished sense of thirst or loss of access to food or fluids may also contribute to the problem.

Detecting and Controlling Hyponatremia

Early detection and treatment are necessary to prevent serious consequences. For patients at risk, the nurse closely monitors fluid I&O as well as daily body weight. It is also necessary to monitor laboratory values (i.e., sodium) and be alert for GI manifestations such as anorexia, nausea, vomiting, and abdominal cramping. The nurse must be alert for central nervous system changes, such as lethargy, confusion, muscle twitching, and seizures. Neurologic signs are associated with very low sodium levels that have fallen rapidly because of fluid overloading. Serum sodium is monitored very closely in patients who are at risk for hyponatremia; when indicated, urine sodium and specific gravity are also monitored.

For a patient with abnormal losses of sodium who can consume a general diet, the nurse encourages foods and fluids with high sodium content to control hyponatremia. For example, broth made with one beef cube contains approximately 900 mg of sodium; 8 oz of tomato juice contains approximately 700 mg of sodium. The nurse also needs to be familiar with the sodium content of parenteral fluids (see Table 13-5).

If the primary problem is water retention, it is safer to restrict fluid intake than to administer sodium. In normovolemia or hypervolemia, administration of sodium predisposes a patient to fluid volume overload. In severe hyponatremia, the aim of therapy is to elevate the serum sodium level only enough to alleviate neurologic signs and symptoms. It is generally recommended that the serum sodium concentration be increased to no greater than 125 mEq/L (125 mmol/L) with a hypertonic saline solution.

> ### ▶ Quality and Safety Nursing Alert
>
> When administering fluids to patients with cardiovascular disease, the nurse assesses for signs of circulatory overload (e.g., cough, dyspnea, puffy eyelids, dependent edema, weight gain in 24 hours). The lungs are auscultated for crackles.

For the patient taking lithium, the nurse observes for lithium toxicity, particularly when sodium is lost. In such instances, supplemental salt and fluid are administered. Because diuretics promote sodium loss, the patient taking lithium is instructed not to use diuretics without close medical supervision. For all patients on lithium therapy, normal salt and oral fluid intake (2.5 L/day) should be encouraged (Karch, 2012).

Excess water supplements are avoided in patients receiving isotonic or hypotonic enteral feedings, particularly if abnormal sodium loss occurs or water is being abnormally retained (as in SIADH). Actual fluid needs are determined by evaluating fluid I&O, urine specific gravity, and serum sodium levels.

■ Sodium Excess (Hypernatremia)

Hypernatremia is a serum sodium level higher than 145 mEq/L (145 mmol/L) (Crawford & Harris, 2011b). It can be caused by a gain of sodium in excess of water or by a loss of water in excess of sodium. It can occur in patients with normal fluid volume or in those with FVD or FVE. With a water loss, the patient loses more water than sodium; as a result, the serum sodium concentration increases and the increased concentration pulls fluid out of the cell. This is both an extracellular and an intracellular FVD. In sodium excess, the patient ingests or retains more sodium than water.

Pathophysiology

A common cause of hypernatremia is fluid deprivation in unconscious patients who cannot perceive, respond to, or communicate their thirst (Porth, 2011). Most often affected are very old, very young, and cognitively impaired patients. Administration of hypertonic enteral feedings without adequate water supplements leads to hypernatremia, as does watery diarrhea and greatly increased insensible water loss (e.g., hyperventilation, burns). In addition, diabetes insipidus can lead to hypernatremia if the patient does not experience or cannot respond to thirst, or if fluids are excessively restricted.

Less common causes of hypernatremia are heat stroke, near drowning in seawater (which contains a sodium concentration of approximately 500 mEq/L), and malfunction of hemodialysis or peritoneal dialysis systems. IV administration of hypertonic saline or excessive use of sodium bicarbonate also causes hypernatremia. Exertional dysnatremia can occur in marathon runners and can result in life-threatening encephalopathy. Hypernatremia and exercise-associated hyponatremia may manifest similarly with confusion and disorientation. On-site testing can differentiate hyponatremia from hypernatremia, assist in the assessment of the severity of the dysnatremia, and guide appropriate therapy (Siegel, d'Hemecourt, Adner, et al., 2009).

Clinical Manifestations

The clinical manifestations of hypernatremia are owing to increased plasma osmolality caused by an increase in plasma sodium concentration (Crawford & Harris, 2011b). Water moves out of the cell into the ECF, resulting in cellular dehydration and a more concentrated ECF (see Fig. 13-4). Clinical signs and symptoms as well as laboratory findings can be found in Table 13-4. Dehydration (resulting in hypernatremia) is often overlooked as the cause of mental status and behavioral changes in older patients (Collins & Claros,

2011). Body temperature may increase mildly, but it returns to normal after the hypernatremia is corrected.

A primary characteristic of hypernatremia is thirst. Thirst is such a strong defender of serum sodium levels in healthy people that hypernatremia never occurs unless the person is unconscious or does not have access to water. However, those who are ill and older adults may have an impaired thirst mechanism.

Assessment and Diagnostic Findings

In hypernatremia, the serum sodium level exceeds 145 mEq/L (145 mmol/L) and the serum osmolality exceeds 300 mOsm/kg (300 mmol/L). The urine specific gravity and urine osmolality are increased as the kidneys attempt to conserve water (provided the water loss is from a route other than the kidneys). Patients with nephrogenic or central diabetes insipidus have hypernatremia and produce a dilute urine with a urine osmolality less than 250 mOsm/kg.

Medical Management

Treatment of hypernatremia consists of a gradual lowering of the serum sodium level by the infusion of a hypotonic electrolyte solution (e.g., 0.3% sodium chloride) or an isotonic nonsaline solution (e.g., dextrose 5% in water [D₅W]). D₅W is indicated when water needs to be replaced without sodium. Clinicians consider a hypotonic sodium solution to be safer than D₅W because it allows a gradual reduction in the serum sodium level, thereby decreasing the risk of cerebral edema. It is the solution of choice in severe hyperglycemia with hypernatremia. A rapid reduction in the serum sodium level temporarily decreases the plasma osmolality below that of the fluid in the brain tissue, causing dangerous cerebral edema. Diuretics also may be prescribed to treat the sodium gain.

There is no consensus about the exact rate at which serum sodium levels should be reduced. As a general rule, the serum sodium level is reduced at a rate no faster than 0.5 to 1 mEq/L/h to allow sufficient time for readjustment through diffusion across fluid compartments. Desmopressin acetate (DDAVP), a synthetic ADH, may be prescribed to treat diabetes insipidus if it is the cause of hypernatremia (Porth, 2011).

Nursing Management

As in hyponatremia, fluid losses and gains are carefully monitored in patients who are at risk for hypernatremia. The nurse should assess for abnormal losses of water or low water intake and for large gains of sodium, as might occur with ingestion of OTC medications that have a high sodium content (e.g., Alka-Seltzer). In addition, the nurse obtains a medication history, because some prescription medications have a high sodium content. The nurse also notes the patient's thirst or elevated body temperature and evaluates it in relation to other clinical signs and symptoms. The nurse monitors for changes in behavior, such as restlessness, disorientation, and lethargy.

Preventing Hypernatremia

The nurse attempts to prevent hypernatremia by providing oral fluids at regular intervals, particularly in debilitated patients who are unable to perceive or respond to thirst. If fluid intake remains inadequate or the patient is unconscious, the nurse consults with the physician to plan an alternative route for intake, either by enteral feedings or by the parenteral route. If enteral feedings are used, sufficient water should be administered to keep the serum sodium and BUN within normal limits. As a rule, the higher the osmolality of the enteral feeding, the greater is the need for water supplementation. Herbal medications, including goldenrod, can also increase serum sodium levels (Karch, 2012).

For patients with diabetes insipidus, adequate water intake must be ensured. If the patient is alert and has an intact thirst mechanism, merely providing access to water may be sufficient. If the patient has a decreased level of consciousness or other disability interfering with adequate fluid intake, parenteral fluid replacement may be prescribed. This therapy can be anticipated in patients with neurologic disorders, particularly in the early postoperative period.

Correcting Hypernatremia

When parenteral fluids are necessary for managing hypernatremia, the nurse monitors the patient's response to the fluids by reviewing serial serum sodium levels and by observing for changes in neurologic signs (Crawford & Harris, 2011b). With a gradual decrease in the serum sodium level, the neurologic signs should improve. Toorapid reduction in the serum sodium level renders the plasma temporarily hypo-osmotic to the fluid in the brain tissue, causing movement of fluid into brain cells and dangerous cerebral edema.

Potassium Imbalances

Potassium (K⁺) is the major intracellular electrolyte; in fact, 98% of the body's potassium is inside the cells. The remaining 2% is in the ECF and is important in neuromuscular function. Potassium influences both skeletal and cardiac muscle activity. For example, alterations in its concentration change myocardial irritability and rhythm. Under the influence of the sodium–potassium pump, potassium is constantly moving in and out of cells. The normal serum potassium concentration ranges from 3.5 to 5 mEq/L (3.5 to 5 mmol/L), and even minor variations are significant (Crawford & Harris, 2011b). Potassium imbalances are commonly associated with various diseases, injuries, medications (e.g., NSAIDs and angiotensin-converting enzyme [ACE] inhibitors), and acid–base imbalances (McPhee et al., 2012).

To maintain potassium balance, the renal system must function, because 80% of the potassium excreted daily leaves the body by way of the kidneys; the other 20% is lost through the bowel and in sweat. The kidneys regulate potassium balance by adjusting the amount of potassium that is excreted in the urine. As serum potassium levels increase, so does the potassium level in the renal tubular cell. A concentration gradient occurs, favoring the movement of potassium into the renal tubule and excretion of potassium in the urine. Aldosterone also increases the excretion of potassium by the kidney. Because the kidneys do not conserve potassium as well as they conserve sodium, potassium may still be lost in urine in the presence of a potassium deficit.

■ *Potassium Deficit (Hypokalemia)*

Hypokalemia (serum potassium level below 3.5 mEq/L [3.5 mmol/L]) usually indicates a deficit in total potassium stores. However, it may occur in patients with normal potassium stores: When **alkalosis** is present, a temporary shift of serum potassium into the cells occurs (see later discussion).

Pathophysiology

Potassium-losing diuretics, such as the thiazides and loop diuretics, can induce hypokalemia (Karch, 2012). Other medications that can lead to hypokalemia include corticosteroids, sodium penicillin, carbenicillin, and amphotericin B. GI loss of potassium is another common cause of potassium depletion. Vomiting and gastric suction frequently lead to hypokalemia, partly because potassium is actually lost when gastric fluid is lost and because potassium is lost through the kidneys in response to metabolic alkalosis. Because relatively large amounts of potassium are contained in intestinal fluids, potassium deficit occurs frequently with diarrhea, which may contain as much potassium as 30 mEq/L. Potassium deficit also occurs from prolonged intestinal suctioning, recent ileostomy, and villous adenoma (a tumor of the intestinal tract characterized by excretion of potassium-rich mucus).

Alterations in acid–base balance have a significant effect on potassium distribution due to shifts of hydrogen and potassium ions between the cells and the ECF. Respiratory or metabolic alkalosis promotes the transcellular shift of potassium and can have a variable and unpredictable effect on serum potassium. For example, hydrogen ions move out of the cells in alkalotic states to help correct the high pH, and potassium ions move in to maintain an electrically neutral state (see later discussion of acid–base balance).

Hyperaldosteronism increases renal potassium wasting and can lead to severe potassium depletion. Primary hyperaldosteronism is seen in patients with adrenal adenomas. Secondary hyperaldosteronism occurs in patients with cirrhosis, nephrotic syndrome, heart failure, or malignant hypertension.

Because insulin promotes the entry of potassium into skeletal muscle and hepatic cells, patients with persistent insulin hypersecretion may experience hypokalemia, which is often the case in patients receiving high-carbohydrate parenteral nutrition.

Patients who do not eat a normal diet for a prolonged period are at risk for hypokalemia. This may occur in debilitated older people and in patients with alcoholism or anorexia nervosa. In addition to poor intake, people with bulimia frequently suffer increased potassium loss through self-induced vomiting, misuse of laxatives, diuretics, and enemas. Magnesium depletion causes renal potassium loss and must be corrected first; otherwise, urine loss of potassium will continue.

Clinical Manifestations

Potassium deficiency can result in widespread derangements in physiologic function. Severe hypokalemia can cause death through cardiac or respiratory arrest. Clinical signs develop when the potassium level decreases to less than 3 mEq/L (3 mmol/L) (Crawford & Harris, 2011b). Clinical signs and symptoms and laboratory findings can be found in Table 13-4. If prolonged, hypokalemia can lead to an inability of the kidneys

to concentrate urine, causing dilute urine (resulting in polyuria, nocturia) and excessive thirst. Potassium depletion suppresses the release of insulin and results in glucose intolerance.

Assessment and Diagnostic Findings

In hypokalemia, the serum potassium concentration is less than the lower limit of normal. Electrocardiographic (ECG) changes can include flat T waves or inverted T waves or both, suggesting ischemia, and depressed ST segments (Fig. 13-5). An elevated U wave is specific to hypokalemia (Crawford &

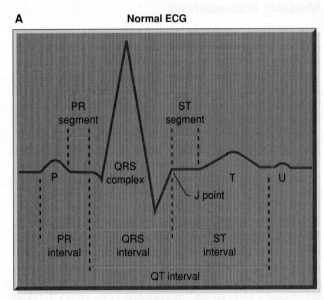

A **Normal ECG**

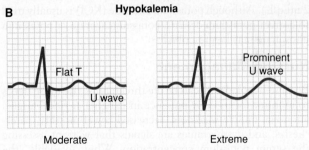

B **Hypokalemia**

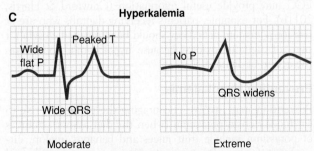

C **Hyperkalemia**

FIGURE 13-5 • Effect of potassium on the electrocardiogram (ECG). **A.** Normal tracing. **B.** Hypokalemia: serum potassium level below normal. *Left:* Flattening of the T wave and the appearance of a U wave. *Right:* Further flattening with prominent U wave. **C.** Hyperkalemia: serum potassium level above normal. *Left:* Moderate elevation with wide, flat P wave; wide QRS complex; and peaked T wave. *Right:* ECG changes seen with extreme potassium elevation: widening of QRS complex and absence of P wave.

Harris, 2011b). Hypokalemia increases sensitivity to digitalis, predisposing the patient to digitalis toxicity at lower digitalis levels. Metabolic alkalosis is commonly associated with hypokalemia. This is discussed further in the section on acid–base disturbances in this chapter.

The source of the potassium loss is usually evident from a careful history. However, if the cause of the loss is unclear, a 24-hour urinary potassium excretion test can be performed to distinguish between renal and extrarenal loss. Urinary potassium excretion exceeding 20 mEq/day with hypokalemia suggests that renal potassium loss is the cause.

Medical Management

If hypokalemia cannot be prevented by conventional measures such as increased intake in the daily diet or by oral potassium supplements for deficiencies, then it is treated cautiously with IV replacement therapy (Crawford & Harris, 2011b). Potassium loss must be corrected daily; administration of 40 to 80 mEq/day of potassium is adequate in the adult if there are no abnormal losses of potassium.

For patients who are at risk for hypokalemia, a diet containing sufficient potassium should be provided. Dietary intake of potassium in the average adult is 50 to 100 mEq/day. Foods high in potassium include most fruits and vegetables, legumes, whole grains, milk, and meat (Dudek, 2010).

When dietary intake is inadequate for any reason, oral or IV potassium supplements may be prescribed (Crawford & Harris, 2011b). Many salt substitutes contain 50 to 60 mEq of potassium per teaspoon and may be sufficient to prevent hypokalemia. If oral administration of potassium is not feasible, the IV route is indicated. The IV route is mandatory for patients with severe hypokalemia (e.g., serum level of 2 mEq/L). Although potassium chloride (KCl) is usually used to correct potassium deficits, potassium acetate or potassium phosphate may be prescribed.

Nursing Management

Because hypokalemia can be life threatening, the nurse needs to monitor for its early presence in patients at risk. Fatigue, anorexia, muscle weakness, decreased bowel motility, paresthesias, and dysrhythmias are signals that warrant assessing the serum potassium concentration. When available, the ECG may provide useful information (Crawford & Harris, 2011b). For example, patients receiving digitalis who are at risk for potassium deficiency should be monitored closely for signs of digitalis toxicity, because hypokalemia potentiates the action of digitalis.

Preventing Hypokalemia

Prevention may involve encouraging the patient at risk to eat foods rich in potassium (when the diet allows). Sources of potassium include fruit juices and bananas, melon, citrus fruits, fresh and frozen vegetables, lean meats, milk, and whole grains (Crawford & Harris, 2011b). If the hypokalemia is caused by abuse of laxatives or diuretics, patient education may help alleviate the problem. Part of the health history and assessment should be directed at identifying problems that are amenable to prevention through education. Careful monitoring of fluid I&O is necessary, because 40 mEq of potassium is lost for every liter of urine output. The ECG is monitored

for changes, and arterial blood gas values are checked for elevated bicarbonate and pH levels.

Correcting Hypokalemia

The oral route is ideal to treat mild to moderate hypokalemia because oral potassium supplements are absorbed well. Care should be exercised when administering potassium, particularly in older adults, who have lower lean body mass and total body potassium levels and therefore lower potassium requirements. In addition, because of the physiologic loss of renal function with advancing years, potassium may be retained more readily in older than in younger people.

 Quality and Safety Nursing Alert

Oral potassium supplements can produce small bowel lesions; therefore, the patient must be assessed for and cautioned about abdominal distention, pain, or GI bleeding.

Administering Intravenous Potassium

Potassium should be administered only after adequate urine output has been established. A decrease in urine volume to less than 20 mL per hour for 2 consecutive hours is an indication to stop the potassium infusion until the situation is evaluated. Potassium is primarily excreted by the kidneys; when oliguria occurs, potassium administration can cause the serum potassium concentration to rise dangerously.

 Quality and Safety Nursing Alert

Potassium is *never* administered by IV push or intramuscularly to avoid replacing potassium too quickly. IV potassium must be administered using an infusion pump.

Each health care facility has its own policy for the administration of potassium, which must be consulted. Administration of IV potassium is done with extreme caution using an infusion pump with the patient monitored by continuous ECG (Crawford & Harris, 2011b). Caution must be used when selecting a premixed solution of IV fluid containing KCl, as the concentrations range from 10 to 40 mEq/100 mL. Renal function should be monitored through BUN and creatinine levels and urine output if the patient is receiving potassium replacement. During replacement therapy, the patient is monitored for signs of worsening hypokalemia as well as hyperkalemia.

■ Potassium Excess (Hyperkalemia)

Hyperkalemia (serum potassium level greater than 5 mEq/L [5 mmol/L]) seldom occurs in patients with normal renal function (Crawford & Harris, 2011b). In older adults, there is an increased risk of hyperkalemia due to decreases in renin and aldosterone as well as an increased number of comorbid cardiac conditions (Domino, 2011). Like hypokalemia, hyperkalemia is often caused by iatrogenic (treatment-induced) causes. Although hyperkalemia is less common than hypokalemia, it is usually more dangerous because cardiac arrest is more frequently associated with high serum potassium levels.

Pathophysiology

Major causes of hyperkalemia are decreased renal excretion of potassium, rapid administration of potassium, and movement of potassium from the ICF compartment to the ECF compartment. Hyperkalemia is commonly seen in patients with untreated renal failure, particularly those in whom potassium levels increase as a result of infection or excessive intake of potassium in food or medications. Patients with hypoaldosteronism or Addison's disease are at risk for hyperkalemia because deficient adrenal hormones lead to sodium loss and potassium retention.

Medications have been identified as a probable contributing factor in more than 60% of hyperkalemic episodes. Medications commonly implicated are KCl, heparin, ACE inhibitors, NSAIDs, beta-blockers, cyclosporine (Neoral), tacrolimus (Prograf), and potassium-sparing diuretics (Karch, 2012). Potassium regulation is compromised in acute and chronic renal failure, with a glomerular filtration rate less than 10% to 20% of normal.

Improper use of potassium supplements predisposes all patients to hyperkalemia, especially if salt substitutes are used. Not all patients receiving potassium-losing diuretics require potassium supplements, and patients receiving potassium-conserving diuretics should not receive supplements.

> ◤ *Quality and Safety Nursing Alert*
>
> Potassium supplements are extremely dangerous for patients who have impaired renal function and thus decreased ability to excrete potassium. Even more dangerous is the IV administration of potassium to such patients, because serum levels can rise very quickly. Aged (stored) blood should not be administered to patients with impaired renal function, because the serum potassium concentration of stored blood increases due to red blood cell deterioration. It is possible to exceed the renal tolerance of any patient with rapid IV potassium administration, as well as when large amounts of oral potassium supplements are ingested.

In **acidosis**, potassium moves out of the cells and into the ECF. This occurs as hydrogen ions enter the cells to buffer the pH of the ECF (see later discussion). An elevated ECF potassium level should be anticipated when extensive tissue trauma has occurred, as in burns, crushing injuries, or severe infections. Similarly, it can occur with lysis of malignant cells after chemotherapy (i.e., tumor lysis syndrome).

Pseudohyperkalemia (a false hyperkalemia) has several causes, including the improper collection or transport of a blood sample, a traumatic venipuncture, and use of a tight tourniquet around an exercising extremity while drawing a blood sample, producing hemolysis of the sample before analysis (Crawford & Harris, 2011b). Other causes include marked leukocytosis (white blood cell count exceeding 200,000/mm^3) and thrombocytosis (platelet count exceeding 1 million/mm^3); drawing blood above a site where potassium is infusing; and familial pseudohyperkalemia, in which potassium leaks out of the red blood cells while the blood is awaiting analysis. Lack of awareness of these causes of pseudohyperkalemia can lead to aggressive treatment of a non-

existent hyperkalemia, resulting in serious lowering of serum potassium levels. Therefore, measurements of grossly elevated levels in the absence of clinical manifestations (e.g., normal ECG) should be verified by retesting.

Clinical Manifestations

Clinical signs and symptoms and laboratory findings can be found in Table 13-4. The most important consequence of hyperkalemia is its effect on the myocardium. Cardiac effects of elevated serum potassium are usually not significant when the level is less than 7 mEq/L (7 mmol/L); however, they are almost always present when the level is 8 mEq/L (8 mmol/L) or greater. As the plasma potassium level rises, disturbances in cardiac conduction occur. The earliest changes, often occurring at a serum potassium level greater than 6 mEq/L (6 mmol/L), are peaked, narrow T waves; ST-segment depression; and a shortened QT interval. If the serum potassium level continues to increase, the PR interval becomes prolonged and is followed by disappearance of the P waves. Finally, there is decomposition and widening of the QRS complex (see Fig. 13-5). Ventricular dysrhythmias and cardiac arrest may occur (Porth, 2011).

Assessment and Diagnostic Findings

Serum potassium levels and ECG changes are crucial to the diagnosis of hyperkalemia, as discussed previously. Arterial blood gas analysis may reveal both a metabolic and respiratory acidosis. Correcting the acidosis helps correct the hyperkalemia.

Medical Management

An ECG should be obtained immediately to detect changes. Shortened repolarization and peaked T waves are seen initially. To verify results, a repeat serum potassium level should be obtained from a vein without an IV infusing a potassium-containing solution.

In nonacute situations, restriction of dietary potassium and potassium-containing medications may correct the imbalance. For example, eliminating the use of potassium-containing salt substitutes in a patient who is taking a potassium-conserving diuretic may be all that is needed to deal with mild hyperkalemia.

Administration, either orally or by retention enema, of cation exchange resins (e.g., sodium polystyrene sulfonate [Kayexalate]) may be necessary (Crawford & Harris, 2011b). Cation exchange resins cannot be used if the patient has a paralytic ileus, because intestinal perforation can occur. Kayexalate binds with other cations in the GI tract and contributes to the development of hypomagnesemia and hypocalcemia; it may also cause sodium retention and fluid overload and should be used with caution in patients with heart failure.

Emergency Pharmacologic Therapy

If serum potassium levels are dangerously elevated, it may be necessary to administer IV calcium gluconate (Crawford & Harris, 2011b). Within minutes after administration, calcium antagonizes the action of hyperkalemia on the heart but does not reduce the serum potassium concentration. Calcium chloride and calcium gluconate are not interchangeable; calcium gluconate contains 4.5 mEq of calcium, and calcium chloride contains 13.6 mEq of calcium. Therefore, caution is required.

Monitoring the blood pressure is essential to detect hypotension, which may result from the rapid IV administration of calcium gluconate. The ECG should be continuously monitored during administration; the appearance of bradycardia is an indication to stop the infusion. The myocardial protective effects of calcium last about 30 minutes. Extra caution is required if the patient has been "digitalized" (i.e., has received accelerated dosages of a digitalis-based cardiac glycoside to reach a desired serum digitalis level rapidly); parenteral administration of calcium sensitizes the heart to digitalis and may precipitate digitalis toxicity.

IV administration of sodium bicarbonate may be necessary in severe metabolic acidosis to alkalinize the plasma, shift potassium into the cells, and furnish sodium to antagonize the cardiac effects of potassium (Crawford & Harris, 2011b). Effects of this therapy begin within 30 to 60 minutes and may persist for hours; however, they are temporary.

Circulatory overload and hypernatremia can occur when large amounts of hypertonic sodium bicarbonate are given. Bicarbonate therapy should be guided by the bicarbonate concentration or calculated base deficit obtained from blood gas analysis or laboratory measurement (Neumar, Otto, Link, et al., 2010).

IV administration of regular insulin and a hypertonic dextrose solution causes a temporary shift of potassium into the cells. Glucose and insulin therapy has an onset of action within 30 minutes and lasts for several hours. Loop diuretics, such as furosemide (Lasix), increase excretion of water by inhibiting sodium, potassium, and chloride reabsorption in the ascending loop of Henle and distal renal tubule.

Beta-2 agonists, such as albuterol (Proventil, Ventolin), are highly effective in decreasing potassium; however, their use remains controversial because they can cause tachycardia and chest discomfort (Porth, 2011). Beta-2 agonists move potassium into the cells and may be used in the absence of ischemic cardiac disease. Their use is a stopgap measure that only temporarily protects the patient from hyperkalemia. If the hyperkalemic condition is not transient, actual removal of potassium from the body is required through cation exchange resins, peritoneal dialysis, hemodialysis, or other forms of renal replacement therapy.

Nursing Management

Patients at risk for potassium excess (e.g., those with renal failure) need to be identified and closely monitored for signs of hyperkalemia. The nurse monitors I&O and observes for signs of muscle weakness and dysrhythmias. When measuring vital signs, an apical pulse should be taken (Crawford & Harris, 2011b). The presence of paresthesias and GI symptoms such as nausea and intestinal colic are noted. Serum potassium levels, as well as BUN, creatinine, glucose, and arterial blood gas values, are monitored for patients at risk for developing hyperkalemia.

Preventing Hyperkalemia

Measures are taken to prevent hyperkalemia in patients at risk, when possible, by encouraging the patient to adhere to the prescribed potassium restriction. Potassium-rich foods to be avoided include many fruits and vegetables, legumes, whole-grain breads, lean meat, milk, eggs, coffee, tea, and cocoa (Dudek, 2010). Conversely, foods with minimal potassium content include butter, margarine, cranberry juice or sauce, ginger ale, gumdrops or jellybeans, hard candy, root beer, sugar, and honey. Labels of cola beverages must be checked carefully because some are high in potassium and some are not.

Correcting Hyperkalemia

It is possible to exceed the tolerance for potassium if administered rapidly by the IV route. Therefore, care is taken to administer and monitor potassium solutions closely. Particular attention is paid to the solution's concentration and rate of administration. IV administration is via an infusion pump (Crawford & Harris, 2011b).

The nurse must caution patients to use salt substitutes sparingly if they are taking other supplementary forms of potassium or potassium-conserving diuretics. In addition, potassium-conserving diuretics such as spironolactone (Aldactone), triamterene (Dyrenium), and amiloride (Midamor), potassium supplements, and salt substitutes should not be administered to patients with renal dysfunction.

Calcium Imbalances

More than 99% of the body's calcium (Ca^{++}) is located in the skeletal system; it is a major component of bones and teeth. About 1% of skeletal calcium is rapidly exchangeable with blood calcium, and the rest is more stable and only slowly exchanged. The small amount of calcium located outside the bone circulates in the serum, partly bound to protein and partly ionized. Calcium plays a major role in transmitting nerve impulses and helps regulate muscle contraction and relaxation, including cardiac muscle. Calcium is instrumental in activating enzymes that stimulate many essential chemical reactions in the body, and it also plays a role in blood coagulation. Because many factors affect calcium regulation, both hypocalcemia and hypercalcemia are relatively common disturbances.

The normal total serum calcium level is 8.6 to 10.2 mg/dL (2.2 to 2.6 mmol/L). Calcium exists in plasma in three forms: ionized, bound, and complexed. Approximately 50% of the serum calcium exists in a physiologically active ionized form that is important for neuromuscular activity and blood coagulation; this is the only physiologically and clinically significant form. The normal ionized serum calcium level is 4.5 to 5.1 mg/dL (1.1 to 1.3 mmol/L). Less than half of the plasma calcium is bound to serum proteins, primarily albumin. The remainder is combined with nonprotein anions: phosphate, citrate, and carbonate.

Calcium is absorbed from foods in the presence of normal gastric acidity and vitamin D. It is excreted primarily in the feces, with the remainder excreted in the urine. The serum calcium level is controlled by parathyroid hormone (PTH) and calcitonin. As ionized serum calcium decreases, the parathyroid glands secrete PTH. This, in turn, increases calcium absorption from the GI tract, increases calcium reabsorption from the renal tubule, and releases calcium from the bone. The increase in calcium ion concentration suppresses PTH secretion. When calcium increases excessively, the thyroid gland secretes calcitonin, which inhibits calcium reabsorption from bone and decreases the serum calcium concentration.

■ Calcium Deficit (Hypocalcemia)

Hypocalcemia (serum calcium value lower than 8.6 mg/dL [2.15 mmol/L]) occurs in a variety of clinical situations. A patient may have a total body calcium deficit (as in osteoporosis) but a normal serum calcium level. Older people and those with disabilities, who spend an increased amount of time in bed, have an increased risk of hypocalcemia, because bed rest increases bone resorption.

Pathophysiology

Several factors can cause hypocalcemia, including primary hypoparathyroidism and surgical hypoparathyroidism. The latter is far more common. Not only is hypocalcemia associated with thyroid and parathyroid surgery, but it can also occur after radical neck dissection and is most likely in the first 24 to 48 hours after surgery. Transient hypocalcemia can occur with massive administration of citrated blood (i.e., massive hemorrhage and shock), because citrate can combine with ionized calcium and temporarily remove it from the circulation.

Inflammation of the pancreas causes the breakdown of proteins and lipids. It is thought that calcium ions combine with the fatty acids released by lipolysis, forming soaps. As a result of this process, hypocalcemia occurs and is common in pancreatitis. Hypocalcemia may be related to excessive secretion of glucagon from the inflamed pancreas, which results in increased secretion of calcitonin.

Hypocalcemia is common in patients with renal failure, because these patients frequently have elevated serum phosphate levels. Hyperphosphatemia usually causes a reciprocal drop in the serum calcium level. Other causes of hypocalcemia include inadequate vitamin D consumption, magnesium deficiency, medullary thyroid carcinoma, low serum albumin levels, alkalosis, and alcohol abuse. Medications predisposing to hypocalcemia include aluminum-containing antacids, aminoglycosides, caffeine, cisplatin, corticosteroids, mithramycin, phosphates, isoniazid, and loop diuretics.

Clinical Manifestations

Tetany, the most characteristic manifestation of hypocalcemia and hypomagnesemia, refers to the entire symptom complex induced by increased neural excitability. Clinical signs and symptoms are caused by spontaneous discharges of both sensory and motor fibers in peripheral nerves and are outlined in Table 13-4.

Chvostek's sign (Fig. 13-6A) consists of twitching of muscles enervated by the facial nerve when the region that is about 2 cm anterior to the earlobe, just below the zygomatic arch, is tapped (Porth, 2011). Trousseau's sign (Fig. 13-6B) can be elicited by inflating a blood pressure cuff on the upper arm to about 20 mm Hg above systolic pressure; within 2 to 5 minutes, carpal spasm (an adducted thumb, flexed wrist and metacarpophalangeal joints, extended interphalangeal joints with fingers together) will occur as ischemia of the ulnar nerve develops (Porth, 2011).

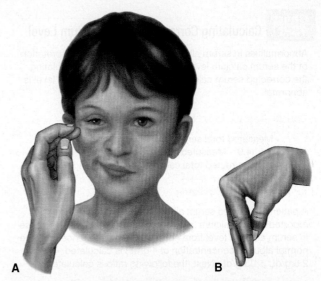

FIGURE 13-6 • **A.** Chvostek's sign: a contraction of the facial muscles elicited in response to light tap over the facial nerve in front of the ear. **B.** Trousseau's sign: a carpopedal spasm induced by inflating a blood pressure cuff above systolic blood pressure. Adapted from Bullock, B. A., & Henze, R. J. (2000). *Focus on pathophysiology* (p. 173). Philadelphia: Lippincott Williams & Wilkins.

Seizures may occur because hypocalcemia increases irritability of the central nervous system as well as the peripheral nerves. Other changes associated with hypocalcemia include mental changes such as depression, impaired memory, confusion, delirium, and hallucinations. A prolonged QT interval is seen on the ECG due to prolongation of the ST segment, and torsades de pointes, a type of ventricular tachycardia, may occur. Respiratory effects with decreasing calcium include dyspnea and laryngospasm. Signs and symptoms of chronic hypocalcemia include hyperactive bowel sounds, dry and brittle hair and nails, and abnormal clotting.

Osteoporosis is associated with prolonged low intake of calcium and represents a total body calcium deficit, even though serum calcium levels are usually normal. This disorder occurs in millions of Americans and is most common in postmenopausal women. It is characterized by loss of bone mass, which causes bones to become porous and brittle and therefore susceptible to fracture. (See Chapter 40 for further discussion of osteoporosis.)

Assessment and Diagnostic Findings

When evaluating serum calcium levels, the serum albumin level and the arterial pH must also be considered. Because abnormalities in serum albumin levels may affect interpretation of the serum calcium level, it may be necessary to calculate the corrected serum calcium if the serum albumin level is abnormal. For every decrease in serum albumin of 1 g/dL below 4 g/dL, the total serum calcium level is underestimated by approximately 0.8 mg/dL. Chart 13-1 displays a quick method that nurses can use to calculate the corrected serum calcium level.

Clinicians often discount a low serum calcium level in the presence of a similarly low serum albumin level. The ionized calcium level is usually normal in patients with reduced total serum calcium levels and concomitant

> ## Chart 13-1 Calculating Corrected Serum Calcium Level
>
> Abnormalities in serum albumin levels may affect interpretation of the serum calcium level. Below is a method for calculating the corrected serum calcium level if the serum albumin level is abnormal.
>
> ### Quick Calculation Method
>
> Measured total serum Ca^{++} level (mg/dL) + 0.8
> × (4.0 – Measured albumin level [g/dL])
> = (Corrected total calcium concentration (mg/dL)
>
> ### Example Calculation
>
> A patient's reported serum albumin level is 2.5 g/dL; the reported serum calcium level is 10.5 mg/dL. First, the decrease in serum albumin level from normal (i.e., the difference from the normal albumin concentration of 4 g/dL) is calculated: 4 g/dL – 2.5 g/dL = 1.5 g/dL. Next, the following ratio is calculated:
>
> 0.8 mg/dL : 1 g/dL = X mg/dL : 1.5 mg/dL
> X = 0.8 × 1.5 mg/dL
> X = 1.2 mg/dL calcium
>
> Finally, 1.2 mg/dL is added to 10.5 mg/dL (the reported serum calcium level) to obtain the corrected total serum calcium level: 1.2 mg/dL + 10.5 mg/dL = 11.7 mg/dL.

hypoalbuminemia. When the arterial pH increases (alkalosis), more calcium becomes bound to protein. As a result, the ionized portion decreases. Symptoms of hypocalcemia may occur with alkalosis. Acidosis (low pH) has the opposite effect—that is, less calcium is bound to protein and therefore more exists in the ionized form. However, relatively small changes in serum calcium levels occur in these acid–base abnormalities.

Ideally, the ionized level of calcium should be measured in the laboratory. However, in many laboratories, only the total calcium level is reported; therefore, the concentration of the ionized fraction must be estimated by simultaneous measurement of the serum albumin level. PTH levels are decreased in hypoparathyroidism. Magnesium and phosphorus levels need to be assessed to identify possible causes of decreased calcium.

Medical Management

Emergency Pharmacologic Therapy

Acute symptomatic hypocalcemia is life threatening and requires prompt treatment with IV administration of a calcium salt. Parenteral calcium salts include calcium gluconate and calcium chloride (Karch, 2012). Although calcium chloride produces a significantly higher ionized calcium level than calcium gluconate does, it is not used as often because it is more irritating and can cause sloughing of tissue if it infiltrates. IV administration of calcium is particularly dangerous in patients receiving digitalis-derived medications, because calcium ions exert an effect similar to that of digitalis and can cause digitalis toxicity, with adverse cardiac effects. The IV site must be observed often for any evidence of infiltration because of the risk of extravasation and resultant cellulitis or necrosis. A 0.9% sodium chloride solution should not be used with calcium because it increases renal calcium loss.

Solutions containing phosphates or bicarbonate should not be used with calcium because they cause precipitation when calcium is added. The nurse must clarify with the physician and pharmacist which calcium salt to administer, because calcium gluconate yields 4.5 mEq of calcium and calcium chloride provides 13.6 mEq of calcium. Calcium replacement can cause postural hypotension; therefore, the patient is kept in bed during IV infusion, and blood pressure is monitored.

 Quality and Safety Nursing Alert

Too-rapid IV administration of calcium can cause cardiac arrest, preceded by bradycardia. Therefore, calcium should be diluted in D_5W and administered as a slow IV bolus or a slow IV infusion using an infusion pump.

Nutritional Therapy

Vitamin D therapy may be instituted to increase calcium absorption from the GI tract; otherwise, the amount of calcium absorbed may not satisfy the body's calcium requirement. In addition, aluminum hydroxide, calcium acetate, or calcium carbonate antacids may be prescribed to decrease elevated phosphorus levels before treating hypocalcemia in the patient with chronic renal failure. Increasing the dietary intake of calcium to at least 1,000 to 1,500 mg/day in the adult is recommended. Calcium-containing foods include milk products; green, leafy vegetables; canned salmon; sardines; and fresh oysters. Hypomagnesemia can also cause tetany; if the tetany responds to IV calcium, then a low magnesium level is considered as a possible cause in chronic renal failure.

Nursing Management

It is important to assess for hypocalcemia in at-risk patients. Seizure precautions are initiated if hypocalcemia is severe. The status of the airway is closely monitored, because laryngeal stridor can occur. Safety precautions are taken, as indicated, if confusion is present.

The nurse must educate the patient with hypocalcemia about foods that are rich in calcium. The nurse must also advise the patient to consider calcium supplements if sufficient calcium is not consumed in the diet. Such supplements should be taken in divided doses with meals. Alcohol and caffeine in high doses inhibit calcium absorption, and moderate cigarette smoking increases urinary calcium excretion. The patient is also cautioned to avoid the overuse of laxatives and antacids that contain phosphorus, because their use decreases calcium absorption.

■ Calcium Excess (Hypercalcemia)

Hypercalcemia (serum calcium value greater than 10.2 mg/dL [2.6 mmol/L]) is a dangerous imbalance when severe; in fact, hypercalcemic crisis has a mortality rate as high as 50% if not treated promptly.

Pathophysiology

The most common causes of hypercalcemia are malignancies and hyperparathyroidism (Fischbach & Dunning, 2009).

Malignant tumors can produce hypercalcemia by various mechanisms. The excessive PTH secretion associated with hyperparathyroidism causes increased release of calcium from the bones and increased intestinal and renal absorption of calcium. Calcifications of soft tissue occur when the calcium–phosphorus product (serum calcium × serum phosphorus) exceeds 70 mg/dL.

Bone mineral is lost during immobilization, and sometimes this causes elevation of total (and especially ionized) calcium in the bloodstream. However, symptomatic hypercalcemia from immobilization is rare; when it does occur, it is limited to people with high calcium turnover rates (e.g., adolescents during a growth spurt). Most cases of hypercalcemia secondary to immobility occur after severe or multiple fractures or spinal cord injury.

Thiazide diuretics can cause a slight elevation in serum calcium levels because they potentiate the action of PTH on the kidneys, reducing urinary calcium excretion. Vitamin A and D intoxication, as well as chronic lithium use and theophylline toxicity, can cause calcium excess. Calcium levels are inversely related to phosphorus levels.

Hypercalcemia reduces neuromuscular excitability because it suppresses activity at the myoneural junction. Decreased tone in smooth and striated muscle may cause symptoms such as muscle weakness, incoordination, anorexia, and constipation. Cardiac standstill can occur when the serum calcium level is about 18 mg/dL (4.5 mmol/L). Calcium enhances the inotropic effect of digitalis; therefore, hypercalcemia aggravates digitalis toxicity.

Clinical Manifestations

Clinical signs and symptoms and laboratory findings can be found in Table 13-4. The symptoms of hypercalcemia are proportional to the degree of elevation of the serum calcium level. The more severe symptoms tend to appear when the serum calcium level is approximately 16 mg/dL (4 mmol/L) or higher. However, some patients become profoundly disturbed with serum calcium levels of only 12 mg/dL (3 mmol/L). These symptoms resolve as serum calcium levels return to normal after treatment.

Hypercalcemic crisis refers to an acute rise in the serum calcium level to 17 mg/dL (4.3 mmol/L) or higher. Severe thirst and polyuria are often present. Other findings may include muscle weakness, intractable nausea, abdominal cramps, severe constipation, diarrhea, peptic ulcer symptoms, and bone pain. Lethargy, confusion, and coma may also occur. This condition is dangerous and may result in cardiac arrest. Emergency treatment with calcitonin is indicated (see later discussion under Pharmacologic Therapy).

Assessment and Diagnostic Findings

The serum calcium level is greater than 10.2 mg/dL (2.6 mmol/L). Cardiovascular changes may include a variety of dysrhythmias (e.g., heart blocks) and shortening of the QT interval and ST segment. The PR interval is sometimes prolonged. The double-antibody PTH test may be used to differentiate between primary hyperparathyroidism and malignancy as a cause of hypercalcemia: PTH levels are increased in primary or secondary hyperparathyroidism and suppressed in malignancy. X-rays may reveal bone changes if the patient has hypercalcemia secondary to a malignancy, bone cavitations, or urinary calculi. The Sulkowitch urine test analyzes the amount of calcium in the urine; in hypercalcemia, dense precipitation is observed due to hypercalciuria.

Medical Management

Therapeutic aims include decreasing the serum calcium level and reversing the process causing the hypercalcemia. Treating the underlying cause (e.g., chemotherapy for a malignancy, partial parathyroidectomy for hyperparathyroidism) is essential.

Pharmacologic Therapy

Measures include administering fluids to dilute serum calcium and promote its excretion by the kidneys, mobilizing the patient, and restricting dietary calcium intake. IV administration of 0.9% sodium chloride solution temporarily dilutes the serum calcium level and increases urinary calcium excretion by inhibiting tubular reabsorption of calcium. Administering IV phosphate can cause a reciprocal drop in serum calcium. Furosemide (Lasix) is often used in conjunction with administration of a saline solution; in addition to causing diuresis, furosemide increases calcium excretion. Although often overlooked, fluids and medications that contain calcium and dietary sources of calcium should be halted.

Calcitonin can be used to lower the serum calcium level and is particularly useful for patients with heart disease or renal failure who cannot tolerate large sodium loads. Calcitonin reduces bone resorption, increases the deposition of calcium and phosphorus in the bones, and increases urinary excretion of calcium and phosphorus (Karch, 2012). Although several forms are available, calcitonin derived from salmon is commonly used. Skin testing for allergy to salmon calcitonin is necessary before the hormone is administered. Systemic allergic reactions are possible because this hormone is a protein; resistance to the medication may develop later because of antibody formation. Calcitonin is administered by intramuscular injection rather than subcutaneously, because patients with hypercalcemia have poor perfusion of subcutaneous tissue.

For patients with cancer, treatment is directed at controlling the condition by surgery, chemotherapy, or radiation therapy. Corticosteroids may be used to decrease bone turnover and tubular reabsorption for patients with sarcoidosis, myelomas, lymphomas, and leukemias; patients with solid tumors are less responsive. Some bisphosphonates (e.g., etidronate disodium [Didronel], pamidronate disodium [Aredia], and ibandronate sodium [Boniva]) inhibit osteoclast activity. IV forms can cause fever, transient leukopenia, eye inflammation, nephrotic syndrome, and jaw osteonecrosis (Karch, 2012). Mithramycin, a cytotoxic antibiotic, inhibits bone resorption and thus lowers the serum calcium level. This agent must be used cautiously because it has significant side effects, including thrombocytopenia, nephrotoxicity, rebound hypercalcemia when discontinued, and hepatotoxicity. Inorganic phosphate salts can be administered orally or by nasogastric tube (in the form of Phospho-Soda or Neutra-Phos), rectally (as retention enemas), or IV. IV phosphate therapy is used with extreme caution in the treatment of hypercalcemia, because it can cause severe calcification in various tissues, hypotension, tetany, and acute renal failure.

Nursing Management

The nurse must monitor for hypercalcemia in at-risk patients. Interventions such as increasing patient mobility and encouraging fluids can help prevent hypercalcemia, or at least minimize its severity. Hospitalized patients at risk should be encouraged to ambulate as soon as possible. Those who are outpatients and receive home care are educated about the importance of frequent ambulation.

When encouraging oral fluids, the nurse considers the patient's likes and dislikes. Fluids containing sodium should be administered unless contraindicated, because sodium assists with calcium excretion. Patients are encouraged to drink 2.8 ro 3.8 L (3 to 4 quarts) of fluid daily. Adequate fiber in the diet is encouraged to offset the tendency for constipation. Safety precautions are implemented, as necessary, when altered mental status is present. The patient and family are informed that these mental changes are reversible with treatment. Increased calcium increases the effects of digitalis; therefore, the patient is assessed for signs and symptoms of digitalis toxicity. Because ECG changes (premature ventricular contractions, paroxysmal atrial tachycardia, and heart block) can occur, the cardiac rate and rhythm are monitored for any abnormalities.

Magnesium Imbalances

Magnesium (Mg^{++}) is an abundant intracellular cation. It acts as an activator for many intracellular enzyme systems and plays a role in both carbohydrate and protein metabolism. The normal serum magnesium level is 1.3 to 2.3 mg/dL (0.62 to 0.95 mmol/L). Approximately one third of serum magnesium is bound to protein; the remaining two thirds exists as free cations—the active component (Mg^{++}). Magnesium balance is important in neuromuscular function. Because magnesium acts directly on the myoneural junction, variations in the serum level affect neuromuscular irritability and contractility. For example, an excess of magnesium diminishes the excitability of the muscle cells, whereas a deficit increases neuromuscular irritability and contractility. Magnesium produces its sedative effect at the neuromuscular junction, probably by inhibiting the release of the neurotransmitter acetylcholine. It also increases the stimulus threshold in nerve fibers.

Magnesium also affects the cardiovascular system, acting peripherally to produce vasodilation and decreased peripheral resistance. Approximately one third of magnesium in the ECF is bound to protein (mostly albumin), and the other two thirds are free or ionized (Crawford & Harris, 2011a).

■ Magnesium Deficit (Hypomagnesemia)

Hypomagnesemia refers to a below-normal serum magnesium concentration (1.3 mg/dL [0.62 mmol/L]) and is frequently associated with hypokalemia and hypocalcemia. Magnesium is similar to calcium in two aspects: (1) it is the ionized fraction of magnesium that is primarily involved in neuromuscular activity and other physiologic processes, and (2) magnesium levels should be evaluated in combination with albumin levels. Because about 30% of magnesium is protein bound, principally to albumin, a decreased serum albumin level can reduce the measured total magnesium concentration; however, it does not reduce the ionized plasma magnesium concentration (Crawford & Harris, 2011a).

Pathophysiology

An important route of magnesium loss is the GI tract; such loss can occur with nasogastric suction, diarrhea, or fistulas. Because fluid from the lower GI tract has a higher concentration of magnesium (10 to 14 mEq/L) than fluid from the upper tract (1 to 2 mEq/L), losses from diarrhea and intestinal fistulas are more likely to induce magnesium deficit than are those from gastric suction. Although magnesium losses are relatively small in nasogastric suction, hypomagnesemia occurs if losses are prolonged and magnesium is not replaced through IV infusion. Because the distal small bowel is the major site of magnesium absorption, any disruption in small bowel function (e.g., intestinal resection or inflammatory bowel disease) can lead to hypomagnesemia. Hypomagnesemia is a common yet often overlooked imbalance in acutely and critically ill patients. It may occur with withdrawal from alcohol and administration of tube feedings or parenteral nutrition.

Chronic alcohol abuse is a major cause of symptomatic hypomagnesemia in the United States (Crawford & Harris, 2011a). The serum magnesium level should be measured at least every 2 or 3 days in patients undergoing withdrawal from alcohol. The level may be normal on admission but may decrease as a result of metabolic changes, such as the intracellular shift of magnesium associated with IV glucose administration.

During nutritional replacement, the major cellular electrolytes move from the serum to newly synthesized cells. Therefore, if the enteral or parenteral feeding formula is deficient in magnesium content, serious hypomagnesemia will occur. Because of this, serum magnesium levels should be measured at regular intervals in patients who are receiving parenteral or enteral feedings, especially those who have undergone a period of starvation. Other causes of hypomagnesemia include the administration of aminoglycosides, cyclosporine, cisplatin, diuretics, digitalis, and amphotericin, as well as the rapid administration of citrated blood, especially to patients with renal or hepatic disease. Magnesium deficiency often occurs in diabetic ketoacidosis, secondary to increased renal excretion during osmotic diuresis and shifting of magnesium into the cells with insulin therapy. Other causes include administration of certain medications and citrated blood (Crawford & Harris, 2011a).

Clinical Manifestations

Clinical signs and symptoms and laboratory findings can be found in Table 13-4. Some clinical manifestations of hypomagnesemia are due directly to the low serum magnesium level; others are due to secondary changes in potassium and calcium metabolism. Symptoms do not usually occur until the serum magnesium level has dropped to less than 1 mEq/L (0.5 mmol/L). Chvostek's and Trousseau's signs (see earlier discussion) occur, in part, because of accompanying hypocalcemia (Crawford & Harris, 2011a).

Hypomagnesemia may be accompanied by marked alterations in psychological status. Apathy, depressed mood, apprehension, and extreme agitation have been noted, as well as ataxia, dizziness, insomnia, and confusion. At times, delirium, auditory or visual hallucinations, and frank psychoses may occur.

Magnesium deficiency can disturb the ECG by prolonging the QRS, depressing the ST segment, and predisposing to cardiac dysrhythmias, such as premature ventricular contractions, supraventricular tachycardia, torsades de pointes (a form of ventricular tachycardia), and ventricular fibrillation. Increased susceptibility to digitalis toxicity is associated with low serum magnesium levels. This is important, because patients receiving digoxin are also likely to be receiving diuretic therapy, predisposing them to renal loss of magnesium. Hypercalcemia and hypokalemia may be refractory to correction until the magnesium level is corrected.

Assessment and Diagnostic Findings

On laboratory analysis, the serum magnesium level is less than 1.3 mg/dL (0.62 mmol/L). Urine magnesium may help identify the cause of magnesium depletion, and levels are measured after a loading dose of magnesium sulfate is administered. Additional diagnostic techniques (nuclear magnetic resonance spectroscopy and the ion-selective electrode) are sensitive and direct means of measuring ionized serum magnesium levels.

Medical Management

Mild magnesium deficiency can be corrected by diet alone. Principal dietary sources of magnesium include green leafy vegetables, nuts, seeds, legumes, whole grains, seafood, peanut butter, and cocoa.

If necessary, magnesium salts can be administered orally in an oxide or gluconate form to replace continuous losses but can produce diarrhea. Patients receiving parenteral nutrition require magnesium in the IV solution to prevent hypomagnesemia. Overt symptoms of hypomagnesemia are treated with parenteral administration of magnesium. A bolus dose of magnesium sulfate given too rapidly can produce alterations in cardiac conduction leading to heart block or asystole. Vital signs must be assessed frequently during magnesium administration to detect changes in cardiac rate or rhythm, hypotension, and respiratory distress. Monitoring urine output is essential before, during, and after magnesium administration; the physician is notified if urine volume decreases to less than 100 mL over 4 hours. Calcium gluconate must be readily available to treat hypocalcemic tetany or hypermagnesemia.

Quality and Safety Nursing Alert

IV magnesium sulfate must be administered by an infusion pump and at a rate not to exceed 150 mg/min, or 67 mEq over 8 hours.

Nursing Management

The nurse should be aware of patients at risk for hypomagnesemia and observe them for its signs and symptoms. Patients receiving digitalis are monitored closely, because a deficit of magnesium can predispose them to digitalis toxicity. If hypomagnesemia is severe, seizure precautions are implemented. Other safety precautions are instituted, as indicated, if confusion is observed. Because difficulty in swallowing (dysphagia) may occur in those with magnesium depletion, these patients should be screened for dysphagia.

Patient education plays a major role in treating magnesium deficit. The patient is educated about sources of magnesium-rich foods, including green vegetables, nuts, legumes, bananas, and oranges (Crawford & Harris, 2011a).

■ Magnesium Excess (Hypermagnesemia)

Hypermagnesemia (serum magnesium level higher than 2.3 mg/dL [0.95 mmol/L]) is a rare electrolyte abnormality, because the kidneys efficiently excrete magnesium. A serum magnesium level can appear falsely elevated if blood specimens are allowed to hemolyze or are drawn from an extremity with a tourniquet that was applied too tightly.

Pathophysiology

By far, the most common cause of hypermagnesemia is renal failure (Crawford & Harris, 2011a). In fact, most patients with advanced renal failure have at least a slight elevation in serum magnesium levels. This condition is aggravated when such patients receive magnesium to control seizures.

Hypermagnesemia can occur in patients with untreated diabetic ketoacidosis when catabolism causes the release of cellular magnesium that cannot be excreted because of profound fluid volume depletion and resulting oliguria. A surplus of magnesium can also result from excessive magnesium administered to treat hypertension of pregnancy or to treat hypomagnesemia. Increased serum magnesium levels can also occur in adrenocortical insufficiency, Addison's disease, or hypothermia. Excessive use of magnesium-based antacids (e.g., Maalox, Riopan, Mylanta) or laxatives (Milk of Magnesia) and medications that decrease GI motility, including opioids and anticholinergics, can also increase serum magnesium levels. Decreased elimination of magnesium or its increased absorption due to intestinal hypomotility from any cause can contribute to hypermagnesemia. Lithium intoxication can also cause an increase in serum magnesium levels. Extensive soft tissue injury or necrosis as with trauma, shock, sepsis, cardiac arrest, or severe burns can also result in hypermagnesemia.

Clinical Manifestations

Acute elevation of the serum magnesium level depresses the central nervous system as well as the peripheral neuromuscular junction. Clinical signs and symptoms and laboratory findings can be found in Table 13-4. The respiratory center is depressed when serum magnesium levels exceed 10 mEq/L (5 mmol/L). Coma, atrioventricular heart block, and cardiac arrest can occur when the serum magnesium level is greatly elevated and not treated. High levels of magnesium also result in platelet clumping and delayed thrombin formation (Chernecky & Berger, 2008).

Assessment and Diagnostic Findings

On laboratory analysis, the serum magnesium level is greater than 2.3 mg/dL (0.95 mmol/L). Increased potassium and calcium are present concurrently. As creatinine clearance decreases to less than 3.0 mL/min, the serum magnesium levels increase. ECG findings may include a prolonged PR interval, tall T waves, a widened QRS, and a prolonged QT interval, as well as an atrioventricular block.

Medical Management

Hypermagnesemia can be prevented by avoiding the administration of magnesium to patients with renal failure and by carefully monitoring seriously ill patients who are receiving magnesium salts. In patients with severe hypermagnesemia, all parenteral and oral magnesium salts are discontinued. In emergencies, such as respiratory depression or defective cardiac conduction, ventilatory support and IV calcium gluconate are indicated. In addition, hemodialysis with a magnesium-free dialysate can reduce the serum magnesium to a safe level within hours. Administration of loop diuretics (e.g., furosemide) and sodium chloride or lactated Ringer's IV solution enhances magnesium excretion in patients with adequate renal function. IV calcium gluconate antagonizes the cardiovascular and neuromuscular effects of magnesium.

Nursing Management

Patients at risk for hypermagnesemia are identified and assessed. If hypermagnesemia is suspected, the nurse monitors the vital signs, noting hypotension and shallow respirations. The nurse also observes for decreased deep tendon reflexes (DTRs) and changes in the level of consciousness. Medications that contain magnesium are not administered to patients with renal failure or compromised renal function, and patients with renal failure are cautioned to check with their health care providers before taking OTC medications. Caution is essential when preparing and administering magnesium-containing fluids parenterally, because available parenteral magnesium solutions (e.g., 2-mL ampules, 50-mL vials) differ in concentration.

Phosphorus Imbalances

Phosphorus (HPO_4^-) is a critical constituent of all body tissues. It is essential to the function of muscle and red blood cells; the formation of adenosine triphosphate (ATP) and of 2,3-diphosphoglycerate, which facilitates release of oxygen from hemoglobin; and the maintenance of acid–base balance, as well as the nervous system and the intermediary metabolism of carbohydrate, protein, and fat. It provides structural support to bones and teeth. Phosphorus is the primary anion of the ICF. About 85% of phosphorus is located in bones and teeth, 14% in soft tissue, and less than 1% in the ECF. The normal serum phosphorus level is 2.5 to 4.5 mg/dL (0.8 to 1.45 mmol/L) in adults. PTH assists in phosphate homeostasis by varying phosphate reabsorption in the proximal tubule of the kidney, and it allows the shift of phosphate from bone to plasma.

▪ *Phosphorus Deficit (Hypophosphatemia)*

Hypophosphatemia is indicated by a value below 2.5 mg/dL (0.8 mmol/L). Although it often indicates phosphorus deficiency, hypophosphatemia may occur under a variety of circumstances in which total body phosphorus stores are normal. Conversely, phosphorus deficiency is an abnormally low content of phosphorus in lean tissues that may exist in the absence of hypophosphatemia. It can be caused by an intracellular shift of potassium from serum into cells, by increased urinary excretion of potassium, or by decreased intestinal absorption of potassium.

Pathophysiology

Hypophosphatemia may occur during the administration of calories to patients with severe protein–calorie malnutrition. It is most likely to result from overzealous intake or administration of simple carbohydrates. This syndrome can be induced in any person with severe protein–calorie malnutrition (e.g., patients with anorexia nervosa or alcoholism, older debilitated patients who are unable to eat).

Marked hypophosphatemia may develop in malnourished patients who receive parenteral nutrition if the phosphorus loss is not corrected. Other causes of hypophosphatemia include heat stroke, prolonged intense hyperventilation, alcohol withdrawal, poor dietary intake, diabetic ketoacidosis, respiratory alkalosis, hepatic encephalopathy, and major thermal burns. Low magnesium levels, low potassium levels, and hyperparathyroidism related to increased urinary losses of phosphorus contribute to hypophosphatemia. Loss of phosphorus through the kidneys also occurs with acute volume expansion, osmotic diuresis, the use of carbonic anhydrase inhibitors (acetazolamide [Diamox]), and some malignancies. Respiratory alkalosis can cause a decrease in phosphorus because of an intracellular shift of phosphorus.

Excess phosphorus binding by antacids may decrease the phosphorus available from the diet to an amount lower than required to maintain serum phosphorus balance. The degree of hypophosphatemia depends on the amount of phosphorus in the diet compared to the dose of antacid. Hypophosphatemia can occur with chronic diarrhea, Crohn's disease, vit.D deficiency, anorexia, alcoholism, malabsorption. Vitamin D regulates intestinal ion absorption; therefore, a deficiency of vitamin D may cause decreased calcium and phosphorus levels, which may lead to osteomalacia (softened, brittle bones).

Clinical Manifestations

Most of the signs and symptoms of phosphorus deficiency result from a deficiency of ATP, 2,3-diphosphoglycerate, or both. ATP deficiency impairs cellular energy resources; diphosphoglycerate deficiency impairs oxygen delivery to tissues, resulting in a wide range of neurologic manifestations. Clinical signs and symptoms and laboratory findings can be found in Table 13-4. Hypoxia leads to an increase in respiratory rate and respiratory alkalosis, causing phosphorus to move into the cells and potentiating hypophosphatemia. In laboratory animals, hypophosphatemia is associated with depression of the chemotactic, phagocytic, and bacterial activity of granulocytes.

Muscle damage may develop as the ATP level in the muscle tissue declines. Clinical manifestations are muscle weakness, which may be subtle or profound and may affect any muscle group; muscle pain; and at times acute rhabdomyolysis (breakdown of skeletal muscle). Weakness of respiratory muscles may greatly impair ventilation. Hypophosphatemia also may predispose a person to insulin resistance and thus hyperglycemia. Chronic loss of phosphorus can cause bruising and bleeding from platelet dysfunction.

Assessment and Diagnostic Findings

On laboratory analysis, the serum phosphorus level is less than 2.5 mg/dL (0.80 mmol/L). When reviewing laboratory results, the nurse should keep in mind that glucose or insulin administration causes a slight decrease in the serum phosphorus level. PTH levels are increased in hyperparathyroidism. Serum magnesium may decrease due to increased urinary excretion of magnesium. Alkaline phosphatase is increased with osteoblastic activity. X-rays may show skeletal changes of osteomalacia or rickets.

Medical Management

Prevention of hypophosphatemia is the goal. In patients at risk for hypophosphatemia, serum phosphate levels should be closely monitored and correction initiated before deficits become severe. Adequate amounts of phosphorus should be added to parenteral solutions, and attention should be paid to the phosphorus levels in enteral feeding solutions.

Severe hypophosphatemia is dangerous and requires prompt attention. Aggressive IV phosphorus correction is usually limited to the patient whose serum phosphorus levels decrease to less than 1 mg/dL (0.3 mmol/L) and whose GI tract is not functioning. Possible effects of IV administration of phosphorus include tetany from hypocalcemia and calcifications in tissues (blood vessels, heart, lung, kidney, eyes) from hyperphosphatemia. IV preparations of phosphorus are available as sodium or potassium phosphate. The rate of phosphorus administration should not exceed 10 mEq per hour, and the site should be carefully monitored because tissue sloughing and necrosis can occur with infiltration. In less acute situations, oral phosphorus replacement is usually adequate.

Nursing Management

The nurse identifies patients at risk for hypophosphatemia and monitors them. Because malnourished patients receiving parenteral nutrition are at risk when calories are introduced too aggressively, preventive measures involve gradually introducing the solution to avoid rapid shifts of phosphorus into the cells.

For patients with documented hypophosphatemia, careful attention is given to preventing infection, because hypophosphatemia may alter the granulocytes. In patients requiring correction of phosphorus losses, the nurse frequently monitors serum phosphorus levels and documents and reports early signs of hypophosphatemia (apprehension, confusion, change in level of consciousness). If the patient experiences mild hypophosphatemia, foods such as milk and milk products, organ meats, nuts, fish, poultry, and whole grains should be encouraged. With moderate hypophosphatemia, supplements such as Neutra-Phos capsules, K-Phos, and Fleet's Phospho-Soda may be prescribed.

■ *Phosphorus Excess (Hyperphosphatemia)*

Hyperphosphatemia is a serum phosphorus level that exceeds 4.5 mg/dL (1.45 mmol/L).

Pathophysiology

Various conditions can lead to hyperphosphatemia; however, the most common is renal failure (Fischbach & Dunning, 2009). Other causes include increased intake, decreased output, or a shift from the intracellular to extracellular space. Conditions such as excessive vitamin D intake, administration of total parenteral nutrition, chemotherapy for neoplastic disease, hypoparathyroidism, metabolic or respiratory acidosis, diabetic ketoacidosis, acute hemolysis, high phosphate intake, profound muscle necrosis, and increased phosphorus absorption may also lead to this phosphorus imbalance. The primary complication of increased phosphorus is metastatic calcification (soft tissue, joints, and arteries), which occurs when the calcium–magnesium product (calcium × magnesium) exceeds 70 mg/dL.

Clinical Manifestations

Clinical signs and symptoms and laboratory findings can be found in Table 13-4. Most symptoms result from decreased calcium levels and soft tissue calcifications. The most important short-term consequence is tetany. Because of the reciprocal relationship between phosphorus and calcium, a high serum phosphorus level tends to cause a low serum calcium concentration.

The major long-term consequence is soft tissue calcification, which occurs mainly in patients with a reduced glomerular filtration rate. High serum levels of inorganic phosphorus promote precipitation of calcium phosphate in nonosseous sites, decreasing urine output, impairing vision, and producing palpitations.

Assessment and Diagnostic Findings

On laboratory analysis, the serum phosphorus level exceeds 4.5 mg/dL (1.5 mmol/L). The serum calcium level is useful also for diagnosing the primary disorder and assessing the effects of treatments. X-rays may show skeletal changes with abnormal bone development. PTH levels are decreased in hypoparathyroidism. BUN and creatinine levels are used to assess renal function.

Medical Management

When possible, treatment is directed at the underlying disorder. For example, hyperphosphatemia may be related to volume depletion or respiratory or metabolic acidosis. In renal failure, elevated PTH production contributes to a high phosphorus level and bone disease. Measures to decrease the serum phosphate level and bind phosphorus in the GI tract of these patients include vitamin D preparations, such as calcitriol, which is available in both oral (Rocaltrol) and parenteral (Calcijex, paricalcitol [Zemplar]) forms. IV administration of calcitriol does not increase the serum calcium unless its dose is excessive, thus permitting more aggressive treatment of hyperphosphatemia with calcium-binding antacids (calcium carbonate or calcium citrate). Administration of Amphojel with meals is effective but can cause bone and central nervous system toxicity with long-term use. Restriction of dietary phosphate, forced diuresis with a loop diuretic, volume replacement with saline, and dialysis may also lower phosphorus. Surgery may be indicated for removal of large calcium and phosphorus deposits.

Nursing Management

The nurse monitors patients at risk for hyperphosphatemia. If a low-phosphorus diet is prescribed, the patient is instructed to avoid phosphorus-rich foods such as hard cheeses, cream, nuts, meats, whole-grain cereals, dried fruits, dried vegetables, kidneys, sardines, sweetbreads, and foods made with milk. When appropriate, the nurse instructs the patient to avoid phosphate-containing laxatives and enemas. The nurse also educates the patient about recognizing the signs of impending hypocalcemia and monitoring for changes in urine output.

Chloride Imbalances

Chloride (Cl⁻), the major anion of the ECF, is found more in interstitial and lymph fluid compartments than in blood. Chloride is also contained in gastric and pancreatic juices, sweat, bile, and saliva. Sodium and chloride make up the largest electrolyte composition of the ECF and assist in determining osmotic pressure. Chloride is produced in the stomach, where it combines with hydrogen to form hydrochloric acid. Chloride control depends on the intake of chloride and the excretion and reabsorption of its ions in the kidneys. A small amount of chloride is lost in the feces.

The normal serum chloride level is 97 to 107 mEq/L (97 to 107 mmol/L). Inside the cell, the chloride level is 4 mEq/L. The serum level of chloride reflects a change in dilution or concentration of the ECF and does so in direct proportion to the sodium concentration. Serum osmolality parallels chloride levels as well. Aldosterone secretion increases sodium reabsorption, thereby increasing chloride reabsorption. The choroid plexus, which secretes cerebrospinal fluid in the brain, depends on sodium and chloride to attract water to form the fluid portion of the cerebrospinal fluid. Bicarbonate has an inverse relationship with chloride. As chloride moves from plasma into the red blood cells (called the *chloride shift*), bicarbonate moves back into the plasma. Hydrogen ions are formed, which then help release oxygen from hemoglobin. When the level of one of these three electrolytes (sodium, bicarbonate, or chloride) is disturbed, the other two are also affected. Chloride assists in maintaining acid–base balance and works as a buffer in the exchange of oxygen and CO_2 in red blood cells (Fischbach & Dunning, 2009). Chloride is primarily obtained from the diet as table salt.

■ Chloride Deficit (Hypochloremia)

Hypochloremia is a serum chloride level below 97 mEq/L (97 mmol/L).

Pathophysiology

Hypochloremia can occur with GI tube drainage, gastric suctioning, gastric surgery, and severe vomiting and diarrhea. Administration of chloride-deficient IV solutions, low sodium intake, decreased serum sodium levels, metabolic alkalosis,

massive blood transfusions, diuretic therapy, burns, and fever may cause hypochloremia. Administration of aldosterone, ACTH, corticosteroids, bicarbonate, or laxatives decreases serum chloride levels as well. As chloride decreases (usually because of volume depletion), sodium and bicarbonate ions are retained by the kidney to balance the loss. Bicarbonate accumulates in the ECF, which raises the pH and leads to hypochloremic metabolic alkalosis.

Clinical Manifestations

The signs and symptoms of hypochloremia are outlined in Table 13-4. The signs and symptoms of hyponatremia, hypokalemia, and metabolic alkalosis may also be present. Metabolic alkalosis is a disorder that results in a high pH and a high serum bicarbonate level as a result of excess alkali intake or loss of hydrogen ions. With compensation, the partial pressure of carbon dioxide in arterial blood ($PaCO_2$) increases to 50 mm Hg. Hyperexcitability of muscles, tetany, hyperactive DTRs, weakness, twitching, and muscle cramps may result. Hypokalemia can cause hypochloremia, resulting in cardiac dysrhythmias. In addition, because low chloride levels parallel low sodium levels, a water excess may occur. Hyponatremia can cause seizures and coma.

Assessment and Diagnostic Findings

In addition to the chloride level, sodium and potassium levels are also evaluated, because these electrolytes are lost along with chloride. Arterial blood gas analysis identifies the acid–base imbalance, which is usually metabolic alkalosis. The urine chloride level, which is also measured, decreases in hypochloremia.

Medical Management

Treatment involves correcting the cause of hypochloremia and the contributing electrolyte and acid–base imbalances. Normal saline (0.9% sodium chloride) or half-strength saline (0.45% sodium chloride) solution is administered by IV to replace the chloride. If the patient is receiving a diuretic (loop, osmotic, or thiazide), it may be discontinued or another diuretic prescribed.

Ammonium chloride, an acidifying agent, may be prescribed to treat metabolic alkalosis; the dosage depends on the patient's weight and serum chloride level. This agent is metabolized by the liver, and its effects last for about 3 days. Its use should be avoided in patients with impaired liver or renal function.

Nursing Management

The nurse monitors the patient's I&O, arterial blood gas values, and serum electrolyte levels. Changes in the patient's level of consciousness and muscle strength and movement are reported to the physician promptly. Vital signs are monitored, and respiratory assessment is carried out frequently. The nurse provides and educates the patient about foods with high chloride content, which include tomato juice, bananas, dates, eggs, cheese, milk, salty broth, canned vegetables, and processed meats. A person who drinks free water (water without electrolytes) or bottled water and excretes large amounts of chloride needs instruction to avoid drinking this kind of water.

■ *Chloride Excess (Hyperchloremia)*

Hyperchloremia exists when the serum level of chloride exceeds 107 mEq/L (107 mmol/L). Hypernatremia, bicarbonate loss, and metabolic acidosis can occur with high chloride levels.

Pathophysiology

High serum chloride levels are almost exclusively a result of iatrogenically induced hyperchloremic metabolic acidosis, stemming from excessive administration of chloride relative to sodium, most commonly as 0.9% normal saline solution, 0.45% normal saline solution, or lactated Ringer's solution. This condition can also be caused by the loss of bicarbonate ions via the kidney or the GI tract with a corresponding increase in chloride ions. Chloride ions in the form of acidifying salts accumulate, and acidosis occurs with a decrease in bicarbonate ions. Head trauma, increased perspiration, excess adrenocortical hormone production, and decreased glomerular filtration can lead to a high serum chloride level.

Clinical Manifestations

The signs and symptoms of hyperchloremia are the same as those of metabolic acidosis: hypervolemia and hypernatremia. Tachypnea, weakness, lethargy, deep and rapid respirations, diminished cognitive ability, and hypertension occur. If untreated, hyperchloremia can lead to a decrease in cardiac output, dysrhythmias, and coma. A high chloride level is accompanied by a high sodium level and fluid retention.

Assessment and Diagnostic Findings

The serum chloride level is 108 mEq/L (108 mmol/L) or greater, the serum sodium level is greater than 145 mEq/L (145 mmol/L), the serum pH is less than 7.35, and the serum bicarbonate level is less than 22 mEq/L (22 mmol/L). Urine chloride excretion increases.

Medical Management

Correcting the underlying cause of hyperchloremia and restoring electrolyte, fluid, and acid–base balance are essential. Hypotonic IV solutions may be administered to restore balance. Lactated Ringer's solution may be prescribed to convert lactate to bicarbonate in the liver, which increases the bicarbonate level and corrects the acidosis. IV sodium bicarbonate may be administered to increase bicarbonate levels, which leads to the renal excretion of chloride ions because bicarbonate and chloride compete for combination with sodium. Diuretics may be administered to eliminate chloride as well. Sodium, chloride, and fluids are restricted.

Nursing Management

Monitoring vital signs, arterial blood gas values, and I&O is important to assess the patient's status and the effectiveness of treatment. Assessment findings related to respiratory, neurologic, and cardiac systems are documented, and changes are discussed with the physician. The nurse educates the patient about the diet that should be followed to manage hyperchloremia and maintain adequate hydration.

 ACID–BASE DISTURBANCES

Acid–base disturbances are commonly encountered in clinical practice, especially in critical care units. Identification of the specific acid–base imbalance is important in ascertaining the underlying cause of the disorder and determining appropriate treatment.

Plasma pH is an indicator of hydrogen ion (H$^+$) concentration and measures the acidity or alkalinity of the blood (Pruitt, 2010). Homeostatic mechanisms keep pH within a normal range (7.35 to 7.45) (Fischbach & Dunning, 2009; Fournier, 2009). These mechanisms consist of buffer systems, the kidneys, and the lungs. The H$^+$ concentration is extremely important: The greater the concentration, the more acidic the solution and the lower the pH. The lower the H$^+$ concentration, the more alkaline the solution and the higher the pH. The pH range compatible with life (6.8 to 7.8) represents a 10-fold difference in H$^+$ concentration in plasma.

Buffer systems prevent major changes in the pH of body fluids by removing or releasing H$^+$; they can act quickly to prevent excessive changes in H$^+$ concentration. Hydrogen ions are buffered by both intracellular and extracellular buffers. The body's major extracellular buffer system is the bicarbonate–carbonic acid buffer system, which is assessed when arterial blood gases are measured. Normally, there are 20 parts of bicarbonate (HCO$_3^-$) to one part of carbonic acid (H$_2$CO$_3$). If this ratio is altered, the pH will change. It is the ratio of HCO$_3^-$ to H$_2$CO$_3$ that is important in maintaining pH, not absolute values. CO$_2$ is a potential acid; when dissolved in water, it becomes carbonic acid (CO$_2$ + H$_2$O = H$_2$CO$_3$). Therefore, when CO$_2$ is increased, the carbonic acid content is also increased, and vice versa. If either bicarbonate or carbonic acid is increased or decreased so that the 20:1 ratio is no longer maintained, acid–base imbalance results.

Less important buffer systems in the ECF include the inorganic phosphates and the plasma proteins. Intracellular buffers include proteins, organic and inorganic phosphates, and, in red blood cells, hemoglobin.

The kidneys regulate the bicarbonate level in the ECF; they can regenerate bicarbonate ions as well as reabsorb them from the renal tubular cells. In respiratory acidosis and most cases of metabolic acidosis, the kidneys excrete hydrogen ions and conserve bicarbonate ions to help restore balance. In respiratory and metabolic alkalosis, the kidneys retain hydrogen ions and excrete bicarbonate ions to help restore balance. The kidneys obviously cannot compensate for the metabolic acidosis created by renal failure. Renal compensation for imbalances is relatively slow (a matter of hours or days).

The lungs, under the control of the medulla, control the CO$_2$ and thus the carbonic acid content of the ECF. They do so by adjusting ventilation in response to the amount of CO$_2$ in the blood. A rise in the partial pressure of CO$_2$ in arterial blood (PaCO$_2$) is a powerful stimulant to respiration. Of course, the partial pressure of oxygen in arterial blood (PaO$_2$) also influences respiration. However, its effect is not as marked as that produced by the PaCO$_2$.

In metabolic acidosis, the respiratory rate increases, causing greater elimination of CO$_2$ (to reduce the acid load). In metabolic alkalosis, the respiratory rate decreases, causing CO$_2$ to be retained (to increase the acid load) (Fournier, 2009).

Acute and Chronic Metabolic Acidosis (Base Bicarbonate Deficit)

Metabolic acidosis is a common clinical disturbance characterized by a low pH (increased H^+ concentration) and a low plasma bicarbonate concentration. It can be produced by a gain of hydrogen ion or a loss of bicarbonate (Fournier, 2009). It can be divided clinically into two forms, according to the values of the serum anion gap: high anion gap acidosis and normal anion gap acidosis (Porth, 2009). The sum of all negatively charged electrolytes (anions) equals the sum of all positively charged electrolytes (cations), with several anions that are not routinely measured leading to an anion gap. The anion gap reflects normally unmeasured anions (phosphates, sulfates, and proteins) in plasma that increase the anion gap by replacing bicarbonate. Measuring the anion gap is essential in analyzing acid–base disorders. The anion gap can be calculated by either of the following equations:

$$\text{Anion gap} = Na^+ + K^+ - (Cl^- + HCO_3^-)$$
$$\text{Anion gap} = Na^+ - (Cl^- + HCO_3^-)$$

Potassium is often omitted from the equation because of its low level in the plasma; therefore, the second equation is used more often than the first.

The normal value for an anion gap is 8 to 12 mEq/L (8 to 12 mmol/L) without potassium in the equation. If potassium is included in the equation, the normal value for the anion gap is 12 to 16 mEq/L (12 to 16 mmol/L). The unmeasured anions in the serum normally account for less than 16 mEq/L of the anion production. A person diagnosed with metabolic acidosis is determined to have normal anion gap metabolic acidosis if the anion gap is within this normal range. An anion gap greater than 16 mEq (16 mmol/L) suggests excessive accumulation of unmeasured anions and would indicate high anion gap metabolic acidosis as the type. An anion gap occurs because not all electrolytes are measured. More anions are left unmeasured than cations. A low or negative anion gap may be attributed to hypoproteinemia. Disorders that cause a decreased or negative anion gap are less common compared to those related to an increased or high anion gap.

Pathophysiology

Normal anion gap acidosis results from the direct loss of bicarbonate, as in diarrhea, lower intestinal fistulas, ureterostomies, and the use of diuretics; early renal insufficiency; excessive administration of chloride; and the administration of parenteral nutrition without bicarbonate or bicarbonate-producing solutes (e.g., lactate). Normal anion gap acidosis is also referred to as hyperchloremic acidosis.

High anion gap acidosis results from excessive accumulation of fixed acid. If increased to 30 mEq/L (30 mmol/L) or more, then a high anion gap metabolic acidosis is present regardless of the values of pH and HCO_3^-. High anion gap occurs in ketoacidosis, lactic acidosis, the late phase of salicylate poisoning, uremia, methanol or ethylene glycol toxicity, and ketoacidosis with starvation. The hydrogen is buffered by HCO_3^-, causing the bicarbonate concentration to fall. In all of these instances, abnormally high levels of anions flood the system, increasing the anion gap above normal limits.

 Concept Mastery Alert

Metabolic acidosis is characterized by a low pH and low plasma bicarbonate concentration. Nurses need to remember that the anion gap is calculated primarily to identify the cause (pathology) of metabolic acidosis (Porth, 2011):

	Reduced or Negative Anion Gap	Normal Anion Gap	High Anion Gap
Anion Gap Without Potassium	<8	8–12 mEq/L	>12
Anion Gap With Potassium	<12	12–16 mEq/L	>16
Clinical Significance	Hypoproteinemia	Normal anion gap metabolic acidosis	High anion gap metabolic acidosis

Clinical Manifestations

Signs and symptoms of metabolic acidosis vary with the severity of the acidosis but include headache, confusion, drowsiness, increased respiratory rate and depth, nausea, and vomiting (Fournier, 2009; Jones, 2010). Peripheral vasodilation and decreased cardiac output occur when the pH drops to less than 7. Additional physical assessment findings include decreased blood pressure, cold and clammy skin, dysrhythmias, and shock. Chronic metabolic acidosis is usually seen with chronic renal failure.

Assessment and Diagnostic Findings

Arterial blood gas measurements are valuable in diagnosing metabolic acidosis (Fischbach & Dunning, 2009; Fournier, 2009). Expected blood gas changes include a low bicarbonate level (less than 22 mEq/L) and a low pH (less than 7.35). The cardinal feature of metabolic acidosis is a decrease in the serum bicarbonate level. Hyperkalemia may accompany metabolic acidosis as a result of the shift of potassium out of the cells. Later, as the acidosis is corrected, potassium moves back into the cells and hypokalemia may occur. Hyperventilation decreases the CO_2 level as a compensatory action. Calculation of the anion gap is helpful in determining the cause of metabolic acidosis. An ECG detects dysrhythmias caused by the increased potassium.

Medical Management

Treatment is directed at correcting the metabolic imbalance (Fischbach & Dunning, 2009; Fournier, 2009). If the problem results from excessive intake of chloride, treatment is aimed at eliminating the source of the chloride. When necessary, bicarbonate is administered; however, the administration of sodium bicarbonate during cardiac arrest can result in paradoxical intracellular acidosis. Hyperkalemia may occur with acidosis and hypokalemia with reversal of the acidosis and subsequent movement of potassium back into the cells.

Therefore, the serum potassium level is monitored closely, and hypokalemia is corrected as acidosis is reversed.

In chronic metabolic acidosis, low serum calcium levels are treated before the chronic metabolic acidosis is treated to avoid tetany resulting from an increase in pH and a decrease in ionized calcium. Alkalizing agents may be administered. Treatment modalities may also include hemodialysis or peritoneal dialysis.

Acute and Chronic Metabolic Alkalosis (Base Bicarbonate Excess)

Metabolic alkalosis is a clinical disturbance characterized by a high pH (decreased H⁺ concentration) and a high plasma bicarbonate concentration. It can be produced by a gain of bicarbonate or a loss of H⁺ (Porth, 2011).

Pathophysiology

A common cause of metabolic alkalosis is vomiting or gastric suction with loss of hydrogen and chloride ions. The disorder also occurs in pyloric stenosis, in which only gastric fluid is lost. Gastric fluid has an acid pH (usually 1 to 3), and loss of this highly acidic fluid increases the alkalinity of body fluids. Other situations predisposing to metabolic alkalosis include those associated with loss of potassium, such as diuretic therapy that promotes excretion of potassium (e.g., thiazides, furosemide), and ACTH secretion (as in hyperaldosteronism and Cushing syndrome).

Hypokalemia produces alkalosis in two ways: (1) the kidneys conserve potassium, and therefore H⁺ excretion increases, and (2) cellular potassium moves out of the cells into the ECF in an attempt to maintain near-normal serum levels (as potassium ions leave the cells, hydrogen ions must enter to maintain electroneutrality). Excessive alkali ingestion from antacids containing bicarbonate or from the use of sodium bicarbonate during cardiopulmonary resuscitation can also cause metabolic alkalosis.

Chronic metabolic alkalosis can occur with long-term diuretic therapy (thiazides or furosemide), villous adenoma, external drainage of gastric fluids, significant potassium depletion, cystic fibrosis, and the chronic ingestion of milk and calcium carbonate.

Clinical Manifestations

Alkalosis is primarily manifested by symptoms related to decreased calcium ionization, such as tingling of the fingers and toes, dizziness, and hypertonic muscles. The ionized fraction of serum calcium decreases in alkalosis as more calcium combines with serum proteins. Because it is the ionized fraction of calcium that influences neuromuscular activity, symptoms of hypocalcemia are often the predominant symptoms of alkalosis. Respirations are depressed as a compensatory action by the lungs. Atrial tachycardia may occur. As the pH increases and hypokalemia develops, ventricular disturbances may occur. Decreased motility and paralytic ileus may also be evident.

Symptoms of chronic metabolic alkalosis are the same as for acute metabolic alkalosis, and as potassium decreases, frequent premature ventricular contractions or U waves are seen on the ECG.

Assessment and Diagnostic Findings

Evaluation of arterial blood gases reveals a pH greater than 7.45 and a serum bicarbonate concentration greater than 26 mEq/L (Fischbach & Dunning, 2009; Fournier, 2009). The PaCO₂ increases as the lungs attempt to compensate for the excess bicarbonate by retaining CO₂. This hypoventilation is more pronounced in semiconscious, unconscious, or debilitated patients than in alert patients. The former may develop marked hypoxemia as a result of hypoventilation. Hypokalemia may accompany metabolic alkalosis.

Urine chloride levels may help identify the cause of metabolic alkalosis if the patient's history provides inadequate information (Fischbach & Dunning, 2009). Metabolic alkalosis is the setting in which urine chloride concentration may be a more accurate estimate of fluid volume than the urine sodium concentration. Urine chloride concentrations help to differentiate between vomiting, diuretic therapy, and excessive adrenocorticosteroid secretion as the cause of the metabolic alkalosis. In patients with vomiting or cystic fibrosis, those receiving nutritional repletion, and those receiving diuretic therapy, hypovolemia and hypochloremia produce urine chloride concentrations lower than 25 mEq/L. Signs of hypovolemia are not present, and the urine chloride concentration exceeds 40 mEq/L in patients with mineralocorticoid excess or alkali loading; these patients usually have expanded fluid volume. The urine chloride concentration should be less than 15 mEq/L when decreased chloride levels and hypovolemia occur.

Medical Management

Treatment of both acute and chronic metabolic alkalosis is aimed at correcting the underlying acid–base disorder (Fischbach & Dunning, 2009; Fournier, 2009). Because of volume depletion from GI loss, the patient's fluid I&O must be monitored carefully.

Sufficient chloride must be available for the kidney to absorb sodium with chloride (allowing the excretion of excess bicarbonate). Treatment includes restoring normal fluid volume by administering sodium chloride fluids (because continued volume depletion perpetuates the alkalosis). In patients with hypokalemia, potassium is administered as KCl to replace both K⁺ and Cl⁻ losses. H₂ receptor antagonists, such as cimetidine (Tagamet), reduce the production of gastric hydrogen cloride (HCl), thereby decreasing the metabolic alkalosis associated with gastric suction. Carbonic anhydrase inhibitors are useful in treating metabolic alkalosis in patients who cannot tolerate rapid volume expansion (e.g., patients with heart failure).

Acute and Chronic Respiratory Acidosis (Carbonic Acid Excess)

Respiratory acidosis is a clinical disorder in which the pH is less than 7.35 and the PaCO₂ is greater than 42 mm Hg and a compensatory increase in the plasma HCO₃ occurs. It may be either acute or chronic.

Pathophysiology

Respiratory acidosis is always owing to inadequate excretion of CO_2 with inadequate ventilation, resulting in elevated plasma CO_2 concentrations and, consequently, increased levels of carbonic acid. In addition to an elevated $PaCO_2$, hypoventilation usually causes a decrease in PaO_2. Acute respiratory acidosis occurs in emergency situations, such as acute pulmonary edema, aspiration of a foreign object, atelectasis, pneumothorax, overdose of sedatives, sleep apnea, morbid obesity, administration of oxygen to a patient with chronic hypercapnia (excessive CO_2 in the blood), severe pneumonia, and acute respiratory distress syndrome. Respiratory acidosis can also occur in diseases that impair respiratory muscles, such as muscular dystrophy, multiple sclerosis, myasthenia gravis, and Guillain-Barré syndrome. Mechanical ventilation may be associated with hypercapnia if the rate of ventilation is inadequate and CO_2 retained.

Clinical Manifestations

Clinical signs in acute and chronic respiratory acidosis vary. Sudden hypercapnia (elevated $PaCO_2$) can cause increased pulse and respiratory rate, increased blood pressure, mental cloudiness or confusion, and a feeling of fullness in the head, or a decrease in the level of consciousness. An elevated $PaCO_2$, greater than 60 mm Hg, causes cerebrovascular vasodilation and increased cerebral blood flow. Ventricular fibrillation may be the first sign of respiratory acidosis in anesthetized patients.

If respiratory acidosis is severe, intracranial pressure may increase, resulting in papilledema and dilated conjunctival blood vessels. Hyperkalemia may result as the hydrogen concentration overwhelms the compensatory mechanisms and H^+ moves into cells, causing a shift of potassium out of the cell.

Chronic respiratory acidosis occurs with pulmonary diseases such as chronic emphysema and bronchitis, obstructive sleep apnea, and obesity. As long as the $PaCO_2$ does not exceed the body's ability to compensate, the patient will be asymptomatic. However, if the $PaCO_2$ increases rapidly, cerebral vasodilation will increase the intracranial pressure, and cyanosis and tachypnea will develop. Patients with chronic obstructive pulmonary disease (COPD) who gradually accumulate CO_2 over a prolonged period (days to months) may not develop symptoms of hypercapnia because compensatory renal changes have had time to occur.

> ### Quality and Safety Nursing Alert
>
> If the $PaCO_2$ is chronically greater than 50 mm Hg, the respiratory center becomes relatively insensitive to CO_2 as a respiratory stimulant, leaving hypoxemia as the major drive for respiration. Oxygen administration may remove the stimulus of hypoxemia, and the patient develops "carbon dioxide narcosis" unless the situation is quickly reversed. Therefore, oxygen is administered only with extreme caution.

Assessment and Diagnostic Findings

Arterial blood gas analysis reveals a pH less than 7.35, a $PaCO_2$ greater than 42 mm Hg, and a variation in the bicarbonate level, depending on the duration of the acute respiratory acidosis. When compensation (renal retention of bicarbonate) has fully occurred, the arterial pH is within the lower limits of normal. Depending on the cause of respiratory acidosis, other diagnostic measures include monitoring of serum electrolyte levels, chest x-ray for determining any respiratory disease, and a drug screen if an overdose is suspected. An ECG to identify any cardiac involvement as a result of COPD may be indicated as well.

Medical Management

Treatment is directed at improving ventilation; exact measures vary with the cause of inadequate ventilation (Fournier, 2009). Pharmacologic agents are used as indicated. For example, bronchodilators help reduce bronchial spasm, antibiotics are used for respiratory infections, and thrombolytics or anticoagulants are used for pulmonary emboli (see Chapter 21).

Pulmonary hygiene measures are initiated, when necessary, to clear the respiratory tract of mucus and purulent drainage. Adequate hydration (2 to 3 L/day) is indicated to keep the mucous membranes moist and thereby facilitate the removal of secretions. Supplemental oxygen is administered as necessary.

Mechanical ventilation, used appropriately, may improve pulmonary ventilation (Fournier, 2009). Inappropriate mechanical ventilation (e.g., increased dead space, insufficient rate or volume settings, high fraction of inspired oxygen [FiO_2] with excessive CO_2 production) may cause such rapid excretion of CO_2 that the kidneys are unable to eliminate excess bicarbonate quickly enough to prevent alkalosis and seizures. For this reason, the elevated $PaCO_2$ must be decreased slowly. Placing the patient in a semi-Fowler's position facilitates expansion of the chest wall.

Treatment of chronic respiratory acidosis is the same as for acute respiratory acidosis.

Acute and Chronic Respiratory Alkalosis (Carbonic Acid Deficit)

Respiratory alkalosis is a clinical condition in which the arterial pH is greater than 7.45 and the $PaCO_2$ is less than 38 mm Hg. As with respiratory acidosis, acute and chronic conditions can occur.

Pathophysiology

Respiratory alkalosis is always caused by hyperventilation, which causes excessive "blowing off" of CO_2 and, hence, a decrease in the plasma carbonic acid concentration. Causes include extreme anxiety, hypoxemia, early phase of salicylate intoxication, gram-negative bacteremia, and inappropriate ventilator settings.

Chronic respiratory alkalosis results from chronic hypocapnia, and decreased serum bicarbonate levels are the consequence. Chronic hepatic insufficiency and cerebral tumors are predisposing factors.

Clinical Manifestations

Clinical signs consist of lightheadedness due to vasoconstriction and decreased cerebral blood flow, inability to concentrate, numbness and tingling from decreased calcium ionization, tinnitus, and sometimes loss of consciousness. Cardiac

TABLE 13-6 Acid–Base Disorders and Compensation		
Disorder	Initial Event	Compensation
Respiratory acidosis	↓ pH, ↑ or normal HCO_3^-, ↑ $PaCO_2$	↑ Renal acid excretion (↑ $PaCO_2$) and ↑ serum HCO_3^- >26 mEq/L
Respiratory alkalosis	↑ pH, ↓ or normal HCO_3^-, ↓ $PaCO_2$	↓ Renal acid excretion (↓ $PaCO_2$) and ↓ serum HCO_3^- <21 mEq/L
Metabolic acidosis	↓ pH, ↓ HCO_3^-, ↓ or normal $PaCO_2$	Hyperventilation with resulting ↓ $PaCO_2$ (>45 mm Hg) ↓ HCO_3
Metabolic alkalosis	↑ pH, ↑ HCO_3^-, ↑ or normal $PaCO_2$	Hypoventilation with resulting ↑ $PaCO_2$ (<35 mm Hg) ↑ HCO_3

effects of respiratory alkalosis include tachycardia and ventricular and atrial dysrhythmias (Fournier, 2009).

Assessment and Diagnostic Findings

Analysis of arterial blood gases assists in the diagnosis of respiratory alkalosis (Pruitt, 2010). In the acute state, the pH is elevated above normal as a result of a low $PaCO_2$ and a normal bicarbonate level. (The kidneys cannot alter the bicarbonate level quickly.) In the compensated state, the kidneys have had sufficient time to lower the bicarbonate level to a near-normal level. Evaluation of serum electrolytes is indicated to identify any decrease in potassium, as hydrogen is pulled out of the cells in exchange for potassium; decreased calcium, as severe alkalosis inhibits calcium ionization, resulting in carpopedal spasms and tetany; or decreased phosphate due to alkalosis, causing an increased uptake of phosphate by the cells. A toxicology screen should be performed to rule out salicylate intoxication.

Patients with chronic respiratory alkalosis are usually asymptomatic, and the diagnostic evaluation and plan of care are the same as for acute respiratory alkalosis.

Medical Management

Treatment depends on the underlying cause of respiratory alkalosis. If the cause is anxiety, the patient is instructed to breathe more slowly to allow CO_2 to accumulate or to breathe into a closed system (such as a paper bag). An anti-anxiety agent may be required to relieve hyperventilation in very anxious patients. Treatment of other causes of respiratory alkalosis is directed at correcting the underlying problem.

Mixed Acid–Base Disorders

Patients can simultaneously experience two or more independent acid–base disorders. A normal pH in the presence of changes in the $PaCO_2$ and plasma HCO_3^- concentration immediately suggests a mixed disorder. An example of a mixed disorder is the simultaneous occurrence of metabolic acidosis and respiratory acidosis during respiratory and cardiac arrest. The only mixed disorder that cannot occur is a mixed respiratory acidosis and alkalosis, because it is impossible to have alveolar hypoventilation and hyperventilation at the same time.

Compensation

Generally, the pulmonary and renal systems compensate for each other to return the pH to normal. In a single acid–base disorder, the system not causing the problem tries to compensate by returning the ratio of bicarbonate to carbonic acid to the normal 20:1. The lungs compensate for metabolic disturbances by changing CO_2 excretion. The kidneys compensate

for respiratory disturbances by altering bicarbonate retention and H^+ secretion.

In respiratory acidosis, excess hydrogen is excreted in the urine in exchange for bicarbonate ions. In respiratory alkalosis, the renal excretion of bicarbonate increases, and hydrogen ions are retained. In metabolic acidosis, the compensatory mechanisms increase the ventilation rate and the renal retention of bicarbonate. In metabolic alkalosis, the respiratory system compensates by decreasing ventilation to conserve CO_2 and increase the $PaCO_2$. Because the lungs respond to acid–base disorders within minutes, compensation for metabolic imbalances occurs faster than compensation for respiratory imbalances. Table 13-6 summarizes compensation effects.

Blood Gas Analysis

Blood gas analysis is often used to identify the specific acid–base disturbance and the degree of compensation that has occurred (Fischbach & Dunning, 2009; Fournier, 2009). The analysis is usually based on an arterial blood sample; however, if an arterial sample cannot be obtained, a mixed venous sample may be used. Results of arterial blood gas analysis provide information about alveolar ventilation, oxygenation, and acid–base balance. It is necessary to evaluate the concentrations of serum electrolytes (sodium, potassium, and chloride) and CO_2 along with arterial blood gas data, because they are often the first sign of an acid–base disorder. The health history, physical examination, previous blood gas results, and serum electrolytes should always be part of the assessment used to determine the cause of the acid–base disorder (Porth, 2011). Responding to isolated sets of blood gas results without these data can lead to serious errors in interpretation. Treatment of the underlying condition usually corrects most acid–base disorders. Table 13-7 compares normal ranges of venous and arterial blood gas values. See also Chart 13-2.

TABLE 13-7 Normal Values for Arterial and Mixed Venous Bloods		
Parameter	Arterial Blood	Mixed Venous Blood
pH	7.35–7.45	7.32–7.42
PCO_2	35–45 mm Hg	38–52 mm Hg
PO_2*	>80 mm Hg	24–48 mm Hg
HCO_3^-	22–26 mEq/L	19–25 mEq/L
Base excess/deficit	±2 mEq/L	±5 mEq/L
Oxygen saturation (SaO_2%)	>94%	65%–75%

*At altitudes of 3,000 feet and higher; age dependent.
Adapted from Fischbach, F., & Dunning, M. B. (2009). *A manual of laboratory and diagnostic tests* (8th ed.). Philadelphia: Lippincott Williams & Wilkins.

ASSESSMENT

Assessing for Arterial Blood Gases

Chart 13-2

The following steps are recommended to evaluate arterial blood gas values. They are based on the assumption that the average values are:

pH = 7.4
$PaCO_2$ = 40 mm Hg
HCO_3^- = 24 mEq/L

1. *First, note the pH.* It can be high, low, or normal, as follows:

    pH >7.4 (alkalosis)

    pH <7.4 (acidosis)

    pH = 7.4 (normal)

    A normal pH may indicate perfectly normal blood gases, *or* it may indicate a *compensated* imbalance. A compensated imbalance is one in which the body has been able to correct the pH by either respiratory or metabolic changes (depending on the primary problem). For example, a patient with primary metabolic acidosis starts out with a low bicarbonate level but a normal CO_2 level. Soon afterward, the lungs try to compensate for the imbalance by exhaling large amounts of CO_2 (hyperventilation). As another example, a patient with primary respiratory acidosis starts out with a high CO_2 level; soon afterward, the kidneys attempt to compensate by retaining bicarbonate. If the compensatory mechanism is able to restore the bicarbonate-to-carbonic acid ratio back to 20:1, full compensation (and thus normal pH) will be achieved.

2. The next step is to determine the primary cause of the disturbance. This is done by evaluating the $PaCO_2$ and HCO_3^- in relation to the pH.

    Example: pH >7.4 (alkalosis)

    a. If the $PaCO_2$ is <40 mm Hg, the primary disturbance is respiratory alkalosis. (This situation occurs when a patient hyperventilates and "blows off" too much CO_2. Recall that CO_2 dissolved in water becomes carbonic acid, the acid side of the "carbonic acid–bicarbonate buffer system.")

    b. If the HCO_3^- is >24 mEq/L, the primary disturbance is metabolic alkalosis. (This situation occurs when the body gains too much bicarbonate, an alkaline substance. Bicarbonate is the basic or alkaline side of the "carbonic acid–bicarbonate buffer system.")

    Example: pH <7.4 (acidosis)

    a. If the $PaCO_2$ is >40 mm Hg, the primary disturbance is respiratory acidosis. (This situation occurs when a patient

hypoventilates and thus retains too much CO_2, an acidic substance.)

    b. If the HCO_3^- is <24 mEq/L, the primary disturbance is metabolic acidosis. (This situation occurs when the body's bicarbonate level drops, either because of direct bicarbonate loss or because of gains of acids such as lactic acid or ketones.)

3. The next step involves determining if compensation has begun. This is done by looking at the value other than the primary disorder. If it is moving in the same direction as the primary value, compensation is under way. Consider the following gases:

	pH	$PaCO_2$	HCO_3^-
(1)	7.2	60 mm Hg	24 mEq/L
(2)	7.4	60 mm Hg	37 mEq/L

    The first set (1) indicates acute respiratory acidosis without compensation (the $PaCO_2$ is high, the HCO_3^- is normal). The second set (2) indicates chronic respiratory acidosis. Note that compensation has taken place—that is, the HCO_3^- has elevated to an appropriate level to balance the high $PaCO_2$ and produce a normal pH.

4. Two distinct acid–base disturbances may occur simultaneously. These can be identified when the pH does not explain one of the changes. When the $PaCO_2$ is ↑ and the HCO_3 is ↓, respiratory acidosis and metabolic acidosis coexist. When the $PaCO_2$ is ↓ and the HCO_3 is ↑, respiratory alkalosis and metabolic alkalosis coexist.

    Example: Metabolic and respiratory acidosis

a.	pH	7.2	Decreased acid
b.	$PaCO_2$	52	Increased acid
c.	HCO_3	13	Decreased acid

5. If metabolic acidosis exists, then calculate the anion gap (AG) to determine the cause of the metabolic acidosis (AG vs. non-AG):

$$AG = Na - (CL + HCO3)$$

Normal AG = 10–14 mmol/L

6. Evaluate the patient to determine if the clinical signs and symptoms are compatible with the acid–base analysis.

Adapted from Pruitt, B. (2010). Interpreting ABGs: An inside look at your patient's status. *Nursing, 40*(7), 31–35.

PARENTERAL FLUID THERAPY

When no other route of administration is available, fluids are administered by IV in hospitals, outpatient diagnostic and surgical settings, clinics, and homes to replace fluids, administer medications, and provide nutrients.

Purpose

The choice of an IV solution depends on the purpose of its administration (INS, 2011). Generally, IV fluids are administered to achieve one or more of the following goals:

- To provide water, electrolytes, and nutrients to meet daily requirements
- To replace water and correct electrolyte deficits
- To administer medications and blood products

IV solutions contain dextrose or electrolytes mixed in various proportions with water. Pure, electrolyte-free water can never be administered by IV because it rapidly enters red blood cells and causes them to rupture.

Types of Intravenous Solutions

Solutions are often categorized as **isotonic**, **hypotonic**, or **hypertonic**, according to whether their total osmolality is the same as, less than, or greater than that of blood, respectively (see earlier discussion of osmolality). Electrolyte solutions are considered isotonic if the total electrolyte content (anions + cations) is between 250 and 375 mEq/L, hypotonic if the total electrolyte content is less than 250 mEq/L, and hypertonic if the total electrolyte content is greater than 375 mEq/L (Crawford & Harris, 2011c). The nurse must also consider a solution's osmolality, keeping in mind that the osmolality of plasma is approximately 300 mOsm/L (300 mmol/L). For example, a 10% dextrose solution has an osmolality of approximately 505 mOsm/L.

Isotonic Fluids

Fluids that are classified as isotonic have a total osmolality close to that of the ECF and do not cause red blood cells to shrink or swell. The composition of these fluids may or may not approximate that of the ECF. Isotonic fluids expand the ECF volume. One liter of isotonic fluid expands the ECF by 1 L; however, it expands the plasma by only 0.25 L because it is a crystalloid fluid and diffuses quickly into the ECF compartment. For the same reason, 3 L of isotonic fluid is needed to replace 1 L of blood loss. Because these fluids expand the intravascular space, patients with hypertension and heart failure should be carefully monitored for signs of fluid overload.

D₅W

A solution of D₅W is unique in that it may be both isotonic and hypotonic (Crawford & Harris, 2011c). Once administered, the glucose is rapidly metabolized, and this initially isotonic solution (same osmolality as serum) then disperses as a hypotonic fluid—one third extracellular and two thirds intracellular. It is essential to consider this action of D₅W, especially if the patient is at risk for increased intracranial pressure. During fluid resuscitation, this solution should not be used because hyperglycemia can result. Therefore, D₅W is used mainly to supply water and to correct an increased serum osmolality. About 1 L of D₅W provides fewer than 170 kcal and is a minor source of the body's daily caloric requirements (Crawford & Harris, 2011c).

Normal Saline Solution

Normal saline (0.9% sodium chloride) solution contains water, salt, and chloride (Crawford & Harris, 2011c). Because the osmolality is entirely contributed by electrolytes, the solution remains within the ECF. For this reason, normal saline solution is often used to correct an extracellular volume deficit but is not identical to ECF. It is used with administration of blood transfusions and to replace large sodium losses, such as in burn injuries. It is not used for heart failure, pulmonary edema, renal impairment, or sodium retention. Normal saline does not supply calories.

Other Isotonic Solutions

Several other solutions contain ions in addition to sodium and chloride and are somewhat similar to the ECF in composition. Lactated Ringer's solution contains potassium and calcium in addition to sodium chloride. It is used to correct dehydration and sodium depletion and replace GI losses. Lactated Ringer's solution contains bicarbonate precursors as well. These solutions are marketed, with slight variations, under various trade names.

Hypotonic Fluids

One purpose of hypotonic solutions is to replace cellular fluid, because it is hypotonic compared with plasma. Another is to provide free water for excretion of body wastes. At times, hypotonic sodium solutions are used to treat hypernatremia and other hyperosmolar conditions. Half-strength saline

(0.45% sodium chloride) solution is frequently used (Crawford & Harris, 2011c). Multiple-electrolyte solutions are also available. Excessive infusions of hypotonic solutions can lead to intravascular fluid depletion, decreased blood pressure, cellular edema, and cell damage. These solutions exert less osmotic pressure than the ECF.

Hypertonic Fluids

When normal saline solution or lactated Ringer's solution contains 5% dextrose, the total osmolality exceeds that of the ECF. However, the dextrose is quickly metabolized, and only the isotonic solution remains. Therefore, any effect on the intracellular compartment is temporary. Similarly, with hypotonic multiple-electrolyte solutions containing 5% dextrose, once the dextrose is metabolized, these solutions disperse as hypotonic fluids. Higher concentrations of dextrose, such as 50% dextrose in water, are strongly hypertonic and must be administered into central veins so that they can be diluted by rapid blood flow.

> ▶ *Quality and Safety Nursing Alert*
>
> The nurse must know that solutions with higher concentrations of dextrose, such as 50% dextrose in water, are strongly hypertonic and must be administered into central veins so that they can be diluted by rapid blood flow.

Saline solutions are also available in osmolar concentrations greater than that of the ECF. These solutions draw water from the ICF to the ECF and cause cells to shrink. If administered rapidly or in large quantity, they may cause an extracellular volume excess and precipitate circulatory overload and dehydration. As a result, these solutions must be administered cautiously and usually only when the serum osmolality has decreased to dangerously low levels. Hypertonic solutions exert an osmotic pressure greater than that of the ECF.

Other Intravenous Therapies

When the patient is unable to tolerate food, nutritional requirements are often met using the IV route. Solutions may include high concentrations of glucose (such as 50% dextrose in water), protein, or fat to meet nutritional requirements (see Chapter 45). The IV route may also be used to administer colloids, plasma expanders, and blood products. Examples of blood products include whole blood, packed red blood cells, albumin, and cryoprecipitate (these are discussed in more detail in Chapter 33).

Many medications are also delivered by the IV route, either by continuous infusion or intermittent bolus directly into the vein. Because IV medications enter the circulation rapidly, administration by this route is potentially hazardous. All medications can produce adverse reactions; however, medications administered by the IV route can cause these reactions within seconds to minutes after administration, because the medications are delivered directly into the bloodstream. Administration rates and recommended dilutions for individual medications are available in specialized texts pertaining to IV medications and in manufacturers' package inserts; these should be consulted to ensure safe IV administration of medications.

Nursing Management of the Patient Receiving Intravenous Therapy

In many settings, the ability to perform venipuncture to gain access to the venous system for administering fluids and medication is an expected nursing skill (Chart 13-3). This responsibility includes selecting the appropriate venipuncture site and type of cannula and being proficient in the technique of vein entry. The nurse should demonstrate competency in and knowledge of catheter placement according to the Nurse Practice Act applicable in his or her state and should follow the rules and regulations, organizational policies and procedures, and practice guidelines of that state's board of nursing (Alexander, Corrigan, Gorski, et al., 2010).

Infusion therapy is initiated by a primary provider who prescribes the type and amount of solution, additives (if any), and rate of flow. When administering parenteral fluids, the nurse monitors the patient's response to the fluids, considering the fluid volume, the fluid content, and the patient's clinical status.

Preparing to Administer Intravenous Therapy

Before performing venipuncture, the nurse carries out hand hygiene, applies gloves, and informs the patient about the procedure. The nurse selects the most appropriate insertion site and type of cannula for a particular patient.

Choosing an Intravenous Site

Many sites can be used for IV therapy, but ease of access and potential hazards vary. Veins of the extremities are designated as peripheral locations and are ordinarily the main sites used by nurses. Because they are relatively safe and easy to enter, arm veins are most commonly used (Fig. 13-7). The metacarpal, cephalic, basilic, and median veins and their branches are recommended sites because of their size and ease of access (O'Grady, Alexander, Burns, et al., 2011). Leg veins should rarely, if ever, be used because of the high risk of thromboembolism. Additional sites to avoid include veins distal to a previous IV infiltration or phlebitic area; sclerosed or thrombosed veins; an arm with an arteriovenous shunt or fistula; and an arm affected by edema, infection, blood clot, deformity, severe scarring, or skin breakdown. The arm on the side of a mastectomy is avoided because of impaired lymphatic flow.

Central veins commonly used by physicians include the subclavian and internal jugular veins. It is possible to gain access to (or cannulate) these larger vessels even when peripheral sites have collapsed, and they allow for the administration of hyperosmolar solutions. However, the potential hazards are much greater and include inadvertent entry into an artery or the pleural space.

Ideally, both arms and hands are carefully inspected before a specific venipuncture site that does not interfere with mobility is chosen. For this reason, the antecubital

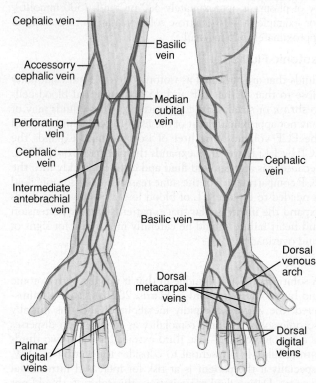

FIGURE 13-7 • Site selection for peripheral cannulation of veins: anterior (palmar) veins at left, posterior (dorsal) veins at right. Adapted from Agur, A. M. R., Lee, M. J., & Boileau Grant, M. J. (1999). *Grant's atlas of anatomy* (10th ed.). Philadelphia: Lippincott Williams & Wilkins.

fossa is avoided, except as a last resort. The most distal site of the arm or hand is generally used first so that subsequent IV access sites can be moved progressively upward. The following factors should be considered when selecting a site for venipuncture (INS, 2011):

- Condition of the vein
- Type of fluid or medication to be infused
- Duration of therapy
- Patient's age, size, and activity level
- Whether the patient is right- or left-handed
- Patient's medical history and current health status
- Setting in which the therapy will take place

After applying a tourniquet, the nurse palpates and inspects the vein. The vein should feel firm, elastic, engorged, and round—not hard, flat, or bumpy. Because arteries lie close to veins in the antecubital fossa, the vessel should be palpated for arterial pulsation (even with a tourniquet on), and cannulation of pulsating vessels should be avoided. General guidelines for selecting a cannula include the following:

- *Length:* 0.75 to 1.25 inches long
- *Diameter:* Narrow diameter of the cannula to occupy minimal space within the vein
- *Gauge:*
  - 20 to 22 gauge for most IV fluids; a larger gauge for caustic or viscous solutions
  - 14 to 18 gauge for blood administration and for trauma patients and those undergoing surgery
  - 22 to 24 gauge for older patients

Chart 13-3

GUIDELINES

Guidelines for Starting a Peripheral Intravenous Infusion

Equipment (as Needed)

- Single-use tourniquet
- Single use scissors or clippers for hair removal
- IV solution, tubing, connector, and catheter
- Chlorhexidine gluconate, povidone–iodine, or alcohol swabs
- Nonlatex gloves
- Transparent dressing, bandage, or sterile gauze
- Padded, appropriate-length arm board

- Tape
- Topical analgesics
- Preservative-free 0.9% NaCL flush solution
  Padded, appropriate-length arm board or finger splint
- Electronic infusion pump

Implementation

Nursing Action	Rationale
1. Verify prescription for IV therapy, check solution label, and identify patient. Check for allergies (i.e., latex, iodine).	1. Serious errors can be avoided by careful checking. Checking for allergies reduces risk of allergic reaction.
2. Explain procedure to patient.	2. Knowledge increases patient comfort and cooperation.
3. Perform hand hygiene, and put on disposable nonlatex gloves.	3. Asepsis is essential to prevent infection. The use of nonlatex gloves prevents exposure of nurse to patient's blood and of patient and nurse to latex.
4. Apply a tourniquet 4 to 6 inches above the site, and identify a suitable vein.	4. This will distend the veins and allow them to be visualized. A new tourniquet should be used for each patient to prevent the transmission of microorganisms. A blood pressure cuff may be used for older patients to avoid rupture of the veins.
5. Choose site. Use distal veins of hands and arms first.	5. Careful site selection will increase likelihood of successful venipuncture and preservation of vein. Using distal sites first preserves sites proximal to the previously cannulated site for subsequent venipunctures. Veins of feet and lower extremity should be avoided due to risk of thrombophlebitis. (In consultation with the physician, the saphenous vein of the ankle or dorsum of the foot may occasionally be used.)
6. Choose IV cannula or catheter and inspect carefully.	6. Length and gauge of cannula should be appropriate for both site and purpose of infusion. The shortest gauge and length needed to deliver prescribed therapy should be used. Inspect the needle or cannula to make sure there are no imperfections.
7. Prepare equipment by connecting infusion bag and tubing, run solution through tubing to displace air, and cover end of tubing.	7. This prevents delay; equipment must be ready to connect immediately after successful venipuncture to prevent clotting.
8. Raise bed to comfortable working height and position for patient; adjust lighting. Position patient's arm below heart level to encourage capillary filling. Place protective pad on bed under patient's arm.	8. Proper positioning will increase likelihood of success and provide comfort for patient.
9. Depending on agency policy and procedure, lidocaine 1% (without epinephrine) 0.1 to 0.2 mL may be injected locally to the IV site or a transdermal analgesic cream (EMLA) may be applied to the site prior to IV placement. Alternatively, topical application of lidocaine (Numby Stuff) or an intradermal injection of bacteriostatic 0.9% sodium chloride may be used to produce a local anesthetic effect.	9. This reduces pain locally from procedure and decreases anxiety about pain.
10. Palpate for a pulse distal to the tourniquet. Ask patient to open and close fist several times, or position patient's arm in a dependent position to distend a vein. Warm packs can be applied for 10 to 20 minutes prior to venipuncture to promote vasodilation.	10. The tourniquet should never be tight enough to occlude arterial flow. If a radial pulse cannot be palpated distal to the tourniquet, it is too tight. A clenched fist encourages the vein to become round and turgid. Positioning the arm below the level of the patient's heart promotes capillary filling.
11. Prepare site by scrubbing with chlorhexidine gluconate or povidone–iodine swabs for 2 to 3 minutes in circular motion, moving outward from injection site. Allow to dry. a. If the site selected is excessively hairy, clip hair. (Check agency's policy and procedure about this practice.) b. Isopropyl alcohol 70% is an alternative solution that may be used.	11. Strict asepsis and careful site preparation are essential to prevent infection. a. Hair removal should be performed with scissors or electric clippers. Hair should not be shaved with a razor because of the potential for microabrasions, which increase the risk of infection. Depilatories should not be used due to the potential for dermal allergic reactions and/or irritation.

(continues on page 276)

Chart 13-3

Guidelines for Starting a Peripheral Intravenous Infusion (continued)

Nursing Action	Rationale
12. With the hand not holding the venous access device, steady patient's arm and use finger or thumb to pull skin taut over vessel.	12. Applying traction to the vein helps to stabilize it.
13. Holding needle bevel up and at 5- to 25-degree angle, depending on the depth of the vein, pierce skin to reach but not penetrate vein. Use bevel-down technique for small veins to prevent extravasation.	13. One-step method of catheter insertion directly into vein with immediate thrust through the skin is excellent for large veins but may cause a hematoma if used in small veins.
14. Decrease angle of needle further until nearly parallel with skin, then enter vein either directly above or from the side in one quick motion.	14. Two-stage procedure decreases chance of thrusting needle through posterior wall of vein as skin is entered. No attempt should be made to reinsert the stylet because of risk of severing or puncturing the catheter.
15. If backflow of blood is visible, straighten angle and advance needle. Additional steps for catheter inserted over needle: a. Advance needle 0.6 cm (1/4 to 1/2 inch) after successful venipuncture. b. Hold needle hub, and slide catheter over the needle into the vein. Never reinsert needle into a plastic catheter or pull the catheter back into the needle. c. Remove needle while pressing lightly on the skin over the catheter tip; hold catheter hub in place. d. Never reinsert a stylet back into a catheter. e. Never reuse the same catheter.	15. Backflow may not occur if vein is small; this position decreases chance of puncturing posterior wall of vein. a. Advancing the needle slightly makes certain the plastic catheter has entered the vein. b. Reinsertion of the needle or pulling the catheter back can sever the catheter, causing catheter embolism. c. Slight pressure prevents bleeding before tubing is attached. d. The stylet can shear off a piece of the plastic if reinserted. e. Reusing the same catheter can cause infection.
16. Release tourniquet and attach infusion tubing; open clamp enough to allow drip.	16. Releasing the tourniquet restores blood flow and avoids potential ischemic damage to the area distal to the IV insertion site.
17. Cover the insertion site with a transparent dressing, bandage, or sterile gauze according to hospital policy and procedure. Tape in place with nonallergenic tape but do not encircle extremity. Tape a small loop of IV tubing onto dressing.	17. Transparent dressings allow assessment of the insertion site for phlebitis, infiltration, and infection without removing the dressing. Tape applied around extremity can act as a tourniquet and impede blood flow and infusion of fluid. The loop decreases the chance of inadvertent cannula removal if the tubing is pulled.
18. Label with type and length of cannula, date, time, and initials.	18. Labeling facilitates assessment and safe discontinuation.
19. A padded, appropriate-length arm board may be applied to an area of flexion (neurovascular checks should be performed frequently).	19. This secures cannula placement and allows correct flow rate (neurovascular checks assess nerve, muscle, and vascular function to be sure function is not affected by immobilization).
20. Calculate infusion rate and regulate flow of infusion. For hourly IV rate, use the following formula: gtt/mL of infusion set/60 (minutes in an hour) × Total hourly vol = gtt/min	20. Infusion must be regulated carefully to prevent overinfusion or underinfusion. Calculation of the IV rate is essential for the safe delivery of fluids. Safe administration requires knowledge of the volume of fluid to be infused, total infusion time, and calibration of the administration set (found on the IV tubing package; 10, 12, 15, or 60 drops to deliver 1 mL of fluid).
21. Document date and time therapy initiated; type and amount of solution; additives and dosages; flow rate; gauge, length, and type of vascular access device; catheter insertion site; type of dressing applied; patient response to procedure; patient education and name and title of the health care provider who inserted the catheter.	21. Documentation is essential to promote continuity of care.
22. Discard needles, stylets, or guidewires into a puncture-resistant needle container that meets OSHA guidelines. Remove gloves and perform hand hygiene.	22. Proper disposal of sharps decreases risk of needlesticks.

Adapted from Alexander, M., Corrigan, A., Gorski, L., et al. (Eds.). (2010). *Infusion nursing: An evidence-based approach* (3rd ed.). St. Louis: Saunders Elsevier.

Hand veins are easiest to cannulate. Cannula tips should not rest in a flexion area (e.g., the antecubital fossa), because this could inhibit the IV flow (Phillips, 2010).

Selecting Venipuncture Devices

Equipment used to gain access to the vasculature includes cannulas, needleless IV delivery systems, and peripherally inserted central catheter (PICC) or midline catheter vascular access devices.

Cannulas

Most peripheral access devices are cannulas. They have an obturator inside a tube that is later removed. *Catheter* and *cannula* are terms that are used interchangeably. The main types of cannula devices available are those referred to as winged infusion sets (butterfly) with a steel needle or as over-the-needle catheters with wings, indwelling plastic cannulas that are inserted over a steel needle, and indwelling plastic cannulas that are inserted through a steel needle.

Scalp vein or butterfly needles are short steel needles with plastic wing handles. These are easy to insert, but because they are small and nonpliable, infiltration occurs easily. The use of these needles should be limited to obtaining blood specimens or administering bolus injections or infusions lasting only a few hours, because they increase the risk of vein injury and infiltration. Insertion of an over-the-needle catheter requires the additional step of advancing the catheter into the vein after venipuncture. Because these devices are less likely to cause infiltration, they are frequently preferred over winged infusion sets.

Plastic cannulas inserted through a hollow needle are usually called *intracatheters*. They are available in long lengths and are well suited for placement in central locations. Because insertion requires threading the cannula through the vein for a relatively long distance, these can be difficult to insert. The most commonly used infusion device is the over-the-needle catheter. A hollow metal stylet is preinserted into the catheter and extends through the distal tip of the catheter to allow puncture of the vessel, in an effort to guide the catheter as the venipuncture is performed. The vein is punctured and a flashback of blood appears in the closed chamber behind the catheter hub. The catheter is threaded through the stylet into the vein and the stylet is then removed.

To select the ideal product for use, the nurse must consider the patient's age and condition, the setting, and the prescribed therapy (INS, 2011). All devices should be radiopaque to determine catheter location by x-ray, if necessary. All catheters increase the risk of thrombus formation to varying degrees. Biocompatibility, another characteristic of a catheter, ensures that inflammation and irritation do not occur. Catheters may be made of steel polytetrafluoroethylene (Teflon), polyurethane, silicone, and Vialon. Teflon is less thrombogenic and less inflammatory than polyurethane or polyvinyl chloride (PVC), and Vialon is a newer material that is nonhemolytic and free of plasticizers (Phillips, 2010).

Needleless Intravenous Delivery Systems

In an effort to decrease needlestick injuries and exposure to bloodborne pathogens, the federal government has legislated and agencies have implemented needleless IV delivery systems. These systems have built-in protection against needlestick injuries and provide a safe means of using and disposing of an IV administration set (which consists of tubing, an area for inserting the tubing into the container of IV fluid, and an adapter for connecting the tubing to the needle). Numerous companies produce needleless components. IV line connectors allow the simultaneous infusion of IV medications and other intermittent medications (known as a piggyback delivery) without the use of needles; this method is being used more frequently, moving away from use of the traditional stylet. An example is a self-sheathing stylet that is recessed into a rigid chamber at the hub of the catheter when its insertion is complete. Other designs have placed the stylet at the end of a flexible wire to avoid needlesticks.

Many types of these devices are on the market. Each institution must evaluate products to determine its own needs based on Occupational Safety and Health Administration (OSHA) guidelines and the institution's policies and procedures.

Peripherally Inserted Central Catheter or Midline Catheter Access Lines

Patients who need moderate- to long-term parenteral therapy often receive a PICC or a midline catheter. These catheters are also used for patients with limited peripheral access (e.g., patients who are obese or emaciated, IV/injection drug users) who require IV antibiotics, blood, and parenteral nutrition. For these devices to be used, the veins must be pliable (not sclerosed or hardened) and not subject to repeated puncture. If these veins are damaged, then central venous access via the subclavian or internal jugular vein, or surgical placement of an implanted port or a vascular access device, must be considered as an alternative (Alexander et al., 2010). Table 13-8 compares PICC and midline catheters. Both PICC and midline catheters have the advantages of reducing cost, avoiding repeated venipunctures, and decreasing the incidence of catheter-related infections when compared with centrally placed catheters.

The principles for inserting these lines are much the same as those for inserting peripheral catheters; however, their insertion should be undertaken only by practitioners who have received training in inserting these IV lines.

The physician prescribes the line and the solution to be infused. Insertion of either catheter requires sterile technique. The size of the catheter lumen chosen is based on the type of solution, the patient's body size, and the vein to be used. The patient's consent is obtained before use of these catheters. Use of the dominant arm is recommended as the site for inserting the cannula to ensure adequate arm movement, which encourages blood flow and reduces the risk of dependent edema.

Educating the Patient

Except in emergency situations, the patient should be prepared in advance for an IV infusion. The venipuncture, the expected length of infusion, and activity restrictions are explained. If the patient requires alternative formats (e.g., interpreter, large-print written materials) to understand the procedure, they should be provided. Then the patient should have an opportunity to ask questions and express concerns. For example, some patients believe that they will die if small bubbles in the tubing enter their veins. After acknowledging this fear, the nurse can explain that usually only relatively large volumes of air administered rapidly are dangerous.

Preparing the Intravenous Site

Before preparing the skin, the nurse should ask the patient if he or she is allergic to latex or iodine—products commonly used in preparing the skin for IV therapy. Excessive hair at the selected site may be removed by clipping to increase the visibility of the veins and to facilitate insertion of the cannula and adherence of dressings to the IV insertion site. Because infection can be a major complication of IV therapy, the IV device, the fluid, the container, and the tubing must be sterile. The nurse must perform hand hygiene and put on gloves (O'Grady et al., 2011). Gloves (nonsterile, disposable) must be worn during the venipuncture procedure because of the likelihood of coming into contact with bloodborne pathogens. The insertion site is prepared according to institutional policy (INS, 2011).

TABLE 13-8	**Comparison of Peripherally Inserted Central and Midline Catheters**	
	PICC	**Midline Catheter**
Indications	Parenteral nutrition; IV fluid replacement; administration of chemotherapy agents, analgesics, and antibiotics; removal of blood specimens; administration of blood products	Parenteral nutrition; IV fluid replacement; administration of analgesics and antibiotics (no solution or medications with a pH <5 or >9 or osmolality >600 mOsm/L); removal of blood specimens
Features	Single- and multi-lumen catheters available (16 to 23 gauge) 50 to 60 cm in length; sizes range from 2 to 7 Fr	Single- and double-lumen catheters available (16 to 24 gauge) 7.5 to 20 cm in length; catheter can increase two gauges in size as it softens
Material	Radiopaque, polymer (polyurethane), silastic materials; flexible. May be impregnated with antimicrobials to decrease infection.	Silicone, polyurethane, and their derivatives; available impregnated with heparin to ↓ thrombogenicity (radiopaque or clear, with radiopaque strip) or antibiotics to ↓ infection.
Insertion sites	Venipuncture performed in the antecubital fossa, above or below it into the basilic, cephalic, median cubital to brachial veins	Venipuncture performed 1-1/2 inches above or below antecubital fossa through brachial, cephalic, or basilic vein. Basilic vein preferred due to vein diameter.
Catheter placement	Tip of catheter lies in lower third of superior vena cava. Catheter is placed via median basilic, brachial, median cubital, or median cephalic vein at antecubital fossa.	Catheter lies between antecubital area and head of clavicle (tip in axilla region). Tip terminates in the proximal portion of extremity below axilla and proximal to central veins and is advanced 3 to 10 inches.
Insertion method	Sedation and NPO not required. Through-the-needle technique, with or without a guidewire, breakaway needle with introducer or cannula with introducer (peel-away sheath). (A PICC can also be used as midline catheter.) Insertion can be accomplished at bedside using sterile technique. Right arm placement is a more direct route to vena cava. Arm to be used should be positioned in abduction to 90-degree angle. Consent is required. Ultrasound-guided placement can allow access to difficult veins at bedside or in x-ray department with fluoroscopy. Catheter may stay in place for up to 12 months or as long as required without complications. Do not use scissors to change the length of the catheter as irregular surfaces occur. Follow only the manufacturers' guidelines for altering the length of the catheter.	No separate guidewire or introducer needed. Stiff catheter is passed using catheter advancement tab. Ultrasound guidance can be used for placement to observe real-time anatomy and select vessels. Insertion can be accomplished at bedside using sterile technique. Arm to be used should be positioned in abduction to 45-degree angle. Consent is required. The catheter should never be reused. Catheter may stay in place for 1 to 4 weeks. Do not use scissors to change the length of the catheter, as irregular surfaces occur. Follow only the manufacturers' guidelines for altering the length of the catheter.
Potential complications	Malposition, pneumothorax, hemothorax, hydrothorax, dysrhythmias, nerve or tendon damage, respiratory distress, catheter embolism, thrombophlebitis, or catheter occlusion. Compared with centrally placed catheters, venipuncture in antecubital space reduces risk of insertion complications.	Thrombosis, phlebitis, air embolism, infection, vascular perforation, bleeding, catheter transection, occlusion
Contraindications	Dermatitis, cellulitis, lymphedema, compromised anatomy, burns, high fluid volume infusions, rapid bolus injections, hemodialysis, and venous thrombosis. No clamping of this catheter or splinting of arm permitted. No blood pressure or tourniquets to be used on extremity where PICC is inserted.	Dermatitis, cellulitis, burns, high fluid volume infusions, rapid bolus injection, hemodialysis, and venous thrombosis. No blood pressure or tourniquet to be used on extremity where catheter is placed. Patient should avoid heavy lifting with arm that has catheter.
Catheter maintenance	Sterile, transparent, semipermeable dressing is used to cover site. Types and changes are according to agency protocol, training, and competency requirements. Catheter is secured with stabilization device.	Sterile, transparent, semipermeable dressing is used to cover site. Types and changes are according to agency protocol, training, and competency requirements. Catheter must be anchored securely to prevent its dislodgment and can be secured with stabilization device.
Postplacement	Chest x-ray needed to confirm placement of catheter tip prior to initiation of ordered infusion.	Chest x-ray to assess placement may be obtained if unable to flush catheter, if no free-flow blood return, if difficulty with catheter advancement, if guidewire is difficult to remove or bent on removal, or catheter migration is suspected.
Assessment	Daily measurement of arm circumference (4 inches above insertion site) and length of exposed catheter	Daily measurement of arm circumference (4 inches above insertion site) and length of exposed catheter
Removal	Catheter should be removed when no longer indicated for use, if contaminated, or if complications occur. Arm is abducted during removal. Patient should be in dorsal recumbent position with head of bed flat and should perform Valsalva maneuver while catheter is withdrawn. Pressure is applied on removal with sterile dressing and antiseptic ointment to site. Dressing is changed every 24 to 48 hours until epithelialization occurs.	Catheter should be removed when no longer indicated for use, if contaminated, or if complications occur. Arm is abducted during removal. Pull gently from insertion site no more than 1/4 to 1/2 inch at a time to prevent vasospasm. Pressure is applied on removal with a sterile dressing and antiseptic ointment to site. Dressing is changed every 24 to 48 hours until epithelialization occurs.

PICC, peripherally inserted central catheter; IV, intravenous; ↓, decrease; NPO, nothing by mouth.

Performing Venipuncture

Guidelines and a suggested sequence for venipuncture are presented in Chart 13-3. For veins that are very small or particularly fragile, modifications in the technique may be necessary. Alternative methods can be found in journal articles or in specialized textbooks on IV therapy. Institutional policies and procedures determine whether nurses must be certified to perform venipuncture. A nurse certified in IV therapy or an IV team can be consulted to assist with initiating IV therapy. To avoid multiple unsuccessful attempts, causing unnecessary trauma to the patient and limiting future vascular access, no more than two attempts at cannulation by any one nurse should be made (Alexander et al., 2010).

Maintaining Therapy

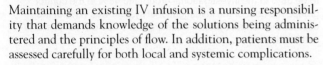

Maintaining an existing IV infusion is a nursing responsibility that demands knowledge of the solutions being administered and the principles of flow. In addition, patients must be assessed carefully for both local and systemic complications.

Factors Affecting Flow

The flow of an IV infusion is governed by the same principles that govern fluid movement in general:

- Flow is directly proportional to the height of the liquid column. Raising the height of the infusion container may improve a sluggish flow.
- Flow is directly proportional to the diameter of the tubing. The clamp on IV tubing regulates the flow by changing the tubing diameter. In addition, the flow is faster through large-gauge rather than small-gauge cannulas.
- Flow is inversely proportional to the length of the tubing. Adding extension tubing to an IV line decreases the flow.
- Flow is inversely proportional to the viscosity of a fluid. Viscous IV solutions, such as blood, require a larger cannula than do water or saline solutions.

Monitoring Flow

Because so many factors influence an IV set to gravity flow, a solution does not necessarily continue to run at the speed originally set. Therefore, the nurse monitors IV infusions frequently to make sure that the fluid is flowing at the intended rate. The IV container should be marked or a time tape used to indicate at a glance whether the correct amount has infused. The flow rate is calculated when the solution is originally started and then monitored at least hourly. To calculate the flow rate, the nurse determines the number of drops delivered per milliliter; this varies with equipment and is usually printed on the administration set packaging. The following formula can be used to calculate the drop rate:

$$\text{gtt/mL of infusion set}/60 \text{ (minutes in 1 hour)}$$
$$\times \text{ total hourly volume} = \text{gtt/min}$$

Flushing of a vascular device is performed to ensure patency and to prevent the mixing of incompatible medications or solutions. This procedure should be carried out at established intervals, according to hospital policy and procedure, especially for intermittently used catheters. Preservative-free 0.9% sodium chloride for flushing should be used (Alexander et al., 2010). The volume of the flush solution should be at least twice the internal volume capacity of the catheter. The catheter should be clamped before the syringe is completely empty and withdrawn to prevent reflux of blood into the lumen, which could cause catheter clotting.

A variety of electronic infusion devices (EIDs) are available to assist in IV fluid delivery. These EIDs allow more accurate administration of fluids and medications than is possible with routine gravity-flow setups. The choice of EID varies according to the age and condition of the patient, the setting, and the prescribed therapy (INS, 2011).

All EIDs calculate the volume delivered by measuring the volume in a reservoir that is part of the set and is calibrated in milliliters per hour (mL/h). A controller is a device that relies on gravity for infusion; the volume is calibrated in drops (gtt) per minute. A controller uses a drop sensor to monitor the flow, which decreases the possibility of rapidly infusing large amounts of fluids. Factors essential for the safe use of pumps include alarms to signify the presence of air in the IV line or an occlusion. The manufacturer's directions must be read carefully before using an EID, because there are many variations in models. The use of an EID does not eliminate the need for the nurse to monitor the infusion and the patient frequently. The nurse must be knowledgeable about EIDs and competent regarding their use.

Discontinuing an Infusion

IV therapy should be discontinued as prescribed by an appropriate health care provider or on assessment by the nurse that contamination, phlebitis, or infiltration has occurred. The removal of an IV catheter is associated with two possible dangers: bleeding and catheter embolism. To prevent excessive bleeding, a dry, sterile pressure dressing should be held over the site as the catheter is removed. Firm pressure is applied until bleeding stops.

If a plastic IV catheter is severed, the loose fragment can travel to the right ventricle and block blood flow. To detect this complication when the catheter is removed, the nurse compares the expected length of the catheter with its actual length. Plastic catheters should be withdrawn carefully and their length measured to detect if a fragment has broken off in the vein. Both of these actions must be documented in the patient's medical record.

Great care must be exercised when using scissors around the dressing site. The use of sterile, disposable scissors in the presence of vascular and nonvascular access devices should be limited to suture removal and during the procedure of catheter repair. Scissors are not to be used for removing dressings, tape, or stabilization devices due to the potential of severing the catheter or administration set and patient injury (Alexander et al., 2010). If the catheter clearly has been severed, the nurse can attempt to occlude the vein above the site by applying a tourniquet to prevent the catheter from entering the central circulation (until surgical removal is possible). The physician must be notified immediately. It is better to prevent a potentially fatal problem than to deal with it after it has occurred. Catheter embolism can be prevented easily by following simple rules:

- Avoid using scissors near the catheter.
- Avoid withdrawing the catheter through the insertion needle.
- Follow the manufacturer's guidelines carefully (e.g., cover the needle point with the bevel shield to prevent severing the catheter).

NURSING RESEARCH PROFILE

Peripheral Intravenous Catheter Stabilization

Chart 13-4

Bausone-Gazda, D., Lefaiver, C., & Walters, S. (2010). A randomized controlled trial to compare the complications of 2 peripheral intravenous catheter-stabilization systems. *Journal of Infusion Nursing, 33*(6), 371–384.

Purpose

Almost every patient in the hospital has a peripheral IV catheter inserted, and complications can occur. Inadequate stabilization of the catheter can lead to phlebitis, leakage at the site, pain, dislodgement, and infection. Restarting an IV (materials and time), treatment of complications, and additional days spent in the hospital are costly. This study compared the complications of two peripheral catheter stabilization systems and the costs of the two systems.

Design

The design utilized a prospective, randomized controlled trial to compare two catheter stabilization systems. The subjects included 302 medical-surgical patients: 150 participants (50%) were allocated to the investigational group, and 152 participants were assigned to the control group. The venous access device (VAD) team nurses enrolled the participants and collected the data. Participants were at least 18 years of age and were inpatients who required a peripheral IV for 96 hours (4 days). For stabilization, a StatLock device was used in the control group, and a specially designed Tegaderm dressing was used in the investigational group. Catheter stabilization and patency, performance of the stabilization device, and any complications were evaluated every 24 hours by the VAD nurses.

Findings

No significant differences between study groups were found for gender, age, or medical diagnoses. Approximately 70% of patients needed the IV for both hydration and medication administration. Complications rates in the investigational group were reported to be no worse than those in the control group. The stabilization-related complication rates of up to 72 hours were estimated to be 32% in the investigational group and 43% in the control group; complication rates for 96 hours were estimated to be 38% in the investigational group and 48% in the control group. The cost of the investigational system was 75% of the cost for the control system—a savings of $1.91 per peripheral IV catheter insertion.

Nursing Implications

Nurses preferred the ease of using the investigational catheter system for both application and removal (56% compared with 36% for the control group; $p \leq .001$). It was concluded that the custom designed Tegaderm dressing was an attractive alternative to the traditional IV stabilization practices used in this hospital, as it provided cost savings and similar performance in preventing complications.

Managing Systemic Complications

IV therapy predisposes the patient to numerous hazards, including both local (see Chart 13-4) and systemic complications. Systemic complications occur less frequently but are usually more serious than local complications. They include circulatory overload, air embolism, febrile reaction, and infection.

Fluid Overload

Overloading the circulatory system with excessive IV fluids causes increased blood pressure and central venous pressure. Signs and symptoms of fluid overload include moist crackles on auscultation of the lungs, cough, restlessness, distended neck veins, edema, weight gain, dyspnea, and rapid, shallow respirations. Possible causes include rapid infusion of an IV solution or hepatic, cardiac, or renal disease. The risk of fluid overload and subsequent pulmonary edema is especially increased in older patients with cardiac disease; this is referred to as circulatory overload. Its treatment includes decreasing the IV rate, monitoring vital signs frequently, assessing breath sounds, and placing the patient in a high Fowler's position. The physician is contacted immediately. This complication can be avoided by using an infusion pump and by carefully monitoring all infusions. Complications of circulatory overload include heart failure and pulmonary edema.

Air Embolism

The risk of air embolism is rare but ever-present. It is most often associated with cannulation of central veins and directly related to the size of the embolus and the rate of entry. Air entering into central veins gets to the right ventricle, where it lodges against the pulmonary valve and blocks the flow of blood from the ventricle into the pulmonary arteries. Manifestations of air embolism include palpitations, dyspnea, continued coughing, jugular venous distension, wheezing, and cyanosis; hypotension; weak, rapid pulse; altered mental status; and chest, shoulder, and low back pain. Treatment calls for immediately clamping the cannula and replacing a leaking or open infusion system, placing the patient on the left side in the Trendelenburg position, assessing vital signs and breath sounds, and administering oxygen. Air embolism can be prevented by using locking adapters on all lines, filling all tubing completely with solution, and using an air detection alarm on an IV infusion pump. Complications of air embolism include shock and death. The amount of air necessary to induce death in humans is not known; however, the rate of entry is probably as important as the actual volume of air.

Infection

Pyogenic substances in either the infusion solution or the IV administration set can cause bloodstream infections. Signs and symptoms include an abrupt temperature elevation shortly after the infusion is started, backache, headache, increased pulse and respiratory rate, nausea and vomiting, diarrhea, chills and shaking, and general malaise. Additional symptoms include erythema, edema, and induration or drainage at the insertion site. In severe sepsis, vascular collapse and septic shock may occur. (See Chapter 14 for a discussion of septic shock.)

Infection ranges in severity from local involvement of the insertion site to systemic dissemination of organisms through the bloodstream, as in sepsis. Measures to prevent infection are essential at the time the IV line is inserted and throughout the entire infusion. Prevention includes the following:

- Performing careful hand hygiene before every contact with any part of the infusion system or the patient
- Examining the IV containers for cracks, leaks, or cloudiness, which may indicate a contaminated solution
- Using strict aseptic technique
- Firmly anchoring the IV cannula to prevent to-and-fro motion (e.g., a catheter stabilization device will help). Sutureless securement devices avoid disruption around the catheter entry site and may decrease the degree of bacterial contamination.
- Inspecting the IV site daily and replacing a soiled or wet dressing with a dry sterile dressing (antimicrobial agents that should be used for site care include 2% tincture of iodine, 10% povidone–iodine, alcohol, or chlorhexidine gluconate, used alone or in combination)
- Disinfecting injection/access ports with antimicrobial solution before and after each use
- Removing the IV cannula at the first sign of local inflammation, contamination, or complication
- Replacing the peripheral IV cannula according to agency policy and procedure
- Replacing the IV cannula inserted during emergency conditions (with questionable asepsis) as soon as possible
- Using a 0.2-μm air-eliminating and bacteria/particulate retentive filter with non–lipid-containing solutions that require filtration. The filter can be added to the proximal or distal end of the administration set. If added to the proximal end between the fluid container and the tubing spike, the filter ensures sterility and particulate removal from the infusate container and prevents inadvertent infusion of air. If added to the distal end of the administration set, it filters air particles and contaminants introduced from add-on devices, secondary administration sets, or interruptions to the primary system. Filters should be located as close to the catheter insertion site as possible and changed to coincide with administration set changes (Alexander et al., 2010).
- Replacing the solution bag and administration set in accordance with agency policy and procedure (Rickard, Vannapraseuth, McGrail, et al., 2009)
- Infusing or discarding medication or solution within 24 hours of its addition to an administration set
- Changing primary and secondary continuous administration sets according to agency policy and procedure, or immediately if contamination is suspected
- Using administration sets with a twist-lock design

Managing Local Complications

Local complications of IV therapy include infiltration and extravasation, phlebitis, thrombophlebitis, hematoma, and clotting of the needle.

Infiltration and Extravasation

Infiltration is the unintentional administration of a non-vesicant solution or medication into surrounding tissue. This can occur when the IV cannula dislodges or perforates the wall of the vein. Infiltration is characterized by edema around the insertion site, leakage of IV fluid from the insertion site, discomfort and coolness in the area of infiltration, and a significant decrease in the flow rate. When the solution is particularly irritating, sloughing of tissue may result. Close monitoring of the insertion site is necessary to detect infiltration before it becomes severe.

Infiltration is usually easily recognized if the insertion area is larger than the same site of the opposite extremity but is not always so obvious. A common misconception is that a backflow of blood into the tubing proves that the catheter is properly placed within the vein. However, if the catheter tip has pierced the wall of the vessel, IV fluid will seep into tissues and flow into the vein. Although blood return occurs, infiltration may have occurred as well. A more reliable means of confirming infiltration is to apply a tourniquet above (or proximal to) the infusion site and tighten it enough to restrict venous flow. If the infusion continues to drip despite the venous obstruction, infiltration is present.

As soon as the nurse detects infiltration, the infusion should be stopped, the IV catheter discontinued, and a sterile dressing applied to the site after careful inspection to determine the extent of infiltration. The infiltration of any amount of blood product, irritant, or vesicant is considered the most severe.

The IV infusion should be started in a new site or proximal to the infiltration site if the same extremity must be used again. A warm compress may be applied to the site if small volumes of noncaustic solutions have infiltrated over a long period, or if the solution was isotonic with a normal pH; the affected extremity should be elevated to promote the absorption of fluid. If the infiltration is recent and the solution was hypertonic or had an increased pH, a cold compress may be applied to the area. Infiltration can be detected and treated early by inspecting the site every hour for redness, pain, edema, blood return, coolness at the site, and IV fluid leaking from the IV site. Using the appropriate size and type of cannula for the vein prevents this complication. The use of EIDs does not cause an infiltration or extravasation; however, these devices will exacerbate the problem until the infusion is turned off. The Infusion Nursing Standards of Practice state that a standardized infiltration scale should be used to document the infiltration (Alexander et al., 2010) (Chart 13-5).

Extravasation is similar to infiltration, with an inadvertent administration of vesicant or irritant solution or medication into the surrounding tissue. Medications such as vasopressors, potassium and calcium preparations, and chemotherapeutic agents can cause pain, burning, and redness at the site. Blistering, inflammation, and necrosis of tissues can occur. Older patients, comatose or anesthetized patients, patients with diabetes, and patients with peripheral vascular or cardiovascular disease are at greater risk for extravasation; other risk factors include high pressure infusion pumps, palpable cording of vein, and fluid leakage from the insertion site (Phillips, 2010). The extent of tissue damage is determined by the concentration of the medication, the quantity that extravasated, the location of the infusion site, the tissue response, and the duration of the process of extravasation.

When extravasation occurs, the infusion must be stopped and the provider notified promptly. The agency's protocol

ASSESSMENT
Chart 13-5 Assessing for Infiltration

Grade	Clinical Criteria
0	No clinical symptoms
1	Skin blanched, edema less than 1 inch in any direction, cool to touch, with or without pain
2	Skin blanched, edema 1 to 6 inches in any direction, cool to touch, with or without pain
3	Skin blanched, translucent, gross edema greater than 6 inches in any direction, cool to touch, mild to moderate pain, possible numbness
4	Skin blanched, translucent, skin tight, leaking, skin discolored, bruised, swollen, gross edema greater than 6 inches in any direction, deep pitting tissue edema, circulatory impairment, moderate to severe pain, infiltration of any amount of blood products, irritant, or vesicant

Adapted from Alexander, M., Corrigan, A., Gorski, L., et al. (Eds.). (2010). *Infusion nursing: An evidence-based approach* (3rd ed.). St. Louis: Saunders Elsevier; and Infusion Nurses Society. (2011). *Infusion nursing standards of practice.* Norwood, MA: Author.

to treat extravasation is initiated; the protocol may specify specific treatments, including antidotes specific to the medication that extravasated, and may indicate whether the IV line should remain in place or be removed before treatment. The protocol often specifies infiltration of the infusion site with an antidote prescribed after assessment by the provider, removal of the cannula, and application of warm compresses to sites of extravasation from alkaloids or cold compresses to sites of extravasation from alkylating and antibiotic vesicants. The affected extremity should not be used for further cannula placement. Thorough neurovascular assessments of the affected extremity must be performed frequently.

Reviewing the institution's IV policy and procedures and incompatibility charts and checking with the pharmacist before administering any IV medication, whether peripherally or centrally, are recommended to determine incompatibilities and vesicant potential to prevent extravasation. Careful, frequent monitoring of the IV site, avoiding insertion of IV devices in areas of flexion, securing the IV line, and using the smallest catheter possible that accommodates the vein help minimize the incidence and severity of this complication. In addition, when vesicant medication is administered by IV push, it should be given through a side port of an infusing IV solution to dilute the medication and decrease the severity of tissue damage if extravasation occurs. Extravasation is rated as grade 4 on the infiltration scale. Complications of an extravasation may include blister formation, skin sloughing and tissue necrosis, functional or sensory loss in the injured area, and disfigurement or loss of limb (Alexander et al., 2010).

Phlebitis

Phlebitis, or inflammation of a vein, can be categorized as chemical, mechanical, or bacterial; however, two or more of these types of irritation often occur simultaneously. Chemical phlebitis can be caused by an irritating medication or solution (increased pH or high osmolality of a solution), rapid infusion

rates, and medication incompatibilities. Mechanical phlebitis results from long periods of cannulation, catheters in flexed areas, catheter gauges larger than the vein lumen, and poorly secured catheters. Bacterial phlebitis can develop from poor hand hygiene, lack of aseptic technique, failure to check all equipment before use, and failure to recognize early signs and symptoms of phlebitis. Other factors include poor venipuncture technique, catheter in place for a prolonged period, and failure to adequately secure the catheter. Phlebitis is characterized by a reddened, warm area around the insertion site or along the path of the vein, pain or tenderness at the site or along the vein, and swelling. The incidence of phlebitis increases with the length of time the IV line is in place, the composition of the fluid or medication infused (especially its pH and tonicity), catheter material, emergency insertions, the size and site of the cannula inserted, ineffective filtration, inadequate anchoring of the line, and the introduction of microorganisms at the time of insertion. The INS has identified specific standards for assessing phlebitis (Alexander et al., 2010; INS, 2011); these appear in Chart 13-6. Phlebitis is graded according to the most severe presenting indication.

Treatment consists of discontinuing the IV line and restarting it in another site, and applying a warm, moist compress to the affected site (O'Grady et al., 2011). Phlebitis can be prevented by using aseptic technique during insertion, using the appropriate-size cannula or needle for the vein, considering the composition of fluids and medications when selecting a site, observing the site hourly for any complications, anchoring the cannula or needle well, and changing the IV site according to agency policy and procedures.

Thrombophlebitis

Thrombophlebitis refers to the presence of a clot plus inflammation in the vein. It is evidenced by localized pain, redness, warmth, and swelling around the insertion site or along the path of the vein, immobility of the extremity because of discomfort and swelling, sluggish flow rate, fever, malaise, and leukocytosis.

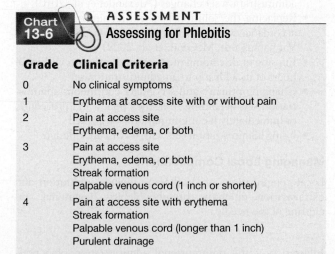

ASSESSMENT
Chart 13-6 Assessing for Phlebitis

Grade	Clinical Criteria
0	No clinical symptoms
1	Erythema at access site with or without pain
2	Pain at access site Erythema, edema, or both
3	Pain at access site Erythema, edema, or both Streak formation Palpable venous cord (1 inch or shorter)
4	Pain at access site with erythema Streak formation Palpable venous cord (longer than 1 inch) Purulent drainage

Adapted from Alexander, M., Corrigan, A., Gorski, L., et al. (Eds.). (2010). *Infusion nursing: An evidence-based approach* (3rd ed.). St. Louis: Saunders Elsevier; and Infusion Nurses Society. (2011). *Infusion nursing standards of practice.* Norwood, MA: Author.

Treatment includes discontinuing the IV infusion; applying a cold compress first to decrease the flow of blood and increase platelet aggregation, followed by a warm compress; elevating the extremity; and restarting the line in the opposite extremity. If the patient has signs and symptoms of thrombophlebitis, the IV line should not be flushed (although flushing may be indicated in the absence of phlebitis to ensure cannula patency and to prevent mixing of incompatible medications and solutions). The catheter should be cultured after the skin around the catheter is cleaned with alcohol. If purulent drainage exists, the site is cultured before the skin is cleaned.

Thrombophlebitis can be prevented by avoiding trauma to the vein at the time the IV line is inserted, observing the site every hour, and checking medication additives for compatibility.

Hematoma

Hematoma results when blood leaks into tissues surrounding the IV insertion site. Leakage can result if the opposite vein wall is perforated during venipuncture, the needle slips out of the vein, a cannula is too large for the vessel, or insufficient pressure is applied to the site after removal of the needle or cannula. The signs of a hematoma include ecchymosis, immediate swelling at the site, and leakage of blood at the insertion site.

Treatment includes removing the needle or cannula and applying light pressure with a sterile, dry dressing; applying ice for 24 hours to the site to avoid extension of the hematoma; elevating the extremity to maximize venous return, if tolerated; assessing the extremity for any circulatory, neurologic, or motor dysfunction; and restarting the line in the other extremity if indicated. A hematoma can be prevented by carefully inserting the needle and by using diligent care with patients who have a bleeding disorder, are taking anticoagulant medication, or have advanced liver disease.

Clotting and Obstruction

Blood clots may form in the IV line as a result of kinked IV tubing, a very slow infusion rate, an empty IV bag, or failure to flush the IV line after intermittent medication or solution administrations. The signs are decreased flow rate and blood backflow into the IV tubing.

If blood clots in the IV line, the infusion must be discontinued and restarted in another site with a new cannula and administration set. The tubing should not be irrigated or milked. Neither the infusion rate nor the solution container should be raised, and the clot should not be aspirated from the tubing. Clotting of the needle or cannula may be prevented by not allowing the IV solution bag to run dry, taping the tubing to prevent kinking and maintain patency, maintaining an adequate flow rate, and flushing the line after intermittent medication or other solution administration. In some cases, a specially trained nurse or physician may inject a thrombolytic agent into the catheter to clear an occlusion resulting from fibrin or clotted blood.

Promoting Home and Community-Based Care

Educating Patients About Self-Care

At times, IV therapy must be administered in the home setting, in which case much of the daily management rests with the patient and family. Education becomes essential to ensure that the patient and family can manage the IV fluid and infu-sion correctly and avoid complications. Written instructions as well as demonstration and return demonstration help reinforce the key points for all of these functions.

Continuing Care

Home infusion therapies cover a wide range of treatments, including antibiotic, analgesic, and antineoplastic medications; blood or blood component therapy; and parenteral nutrition. When direct nursing care is necessary, arrangements are made to have an infusion nurse visit the home and administer the IV therapy as prescribed. In addition to implementing and monitoring the IV therapy, the nurse carries out a comprehensive assessment of the patient's condition and continues to educate the patient and family about the skills involved in overseeing the IV therapy setup. Any dietary changes that may be necessary because of fluid or electrolyte imbalances are explained or reinforced during such sessions.

Periodic laboratory testing may be necessary to assess the effects of IV therapy and the patient's progress. Blood specimens may be obtained by a laboratory near the patient's home, or a home visit may be arranged to obtain blood specimens for analysis.

The nurse collaborates with the case manager in assessing the patient, family, and home environment; developing a plan of care in accordance with the patient's treatment plan and level of ability; and arranging for appropriate referral and follow-up if necessary. Any necessary equipment may be provided by the agency or purchased by the patient, depending on the terms of the home care arrangements. Appropriate documentation is necessary to assist in obtaining third-party payment for the service provided.

Critical Thinking Exercises

1 A 38-year-old woman is admitted to the emergency department following a motor vehicle crash. She is hypotensive and her pulse rate is 110 bpm. Her laboratory test results are as follows: pH 7.32; sodium 151 mEq/L; glucose 120 mg/dL; $PaCO_2$ 28 mm Hg; potassium 5.5 mEq/L; creatinine 1.4 mg/dL; HCO_3^- 14 mEq/L; chloride 95 mEq/L; BUN 30 mg/dL. What assessment parameters would you use to further evaluate this patient? What actions and interventions are indicated? Which electrolyte results should be followed? What IV fluids would you anticipate being prescribed? Give the rationale for their use.

2 A 54-year-old woman who has a history of COPD presents with a productive cough for the past 3 months and shortness of breath with little exertion. Her blood pressure is 130/90 mm Hg and pulse rate 126 bpm. Arterial blood gas results are as follows: pH 7.29; $PaCO_2$ 72 mm Hg; HCO_3^- 34 mEq/L; PaO_2 50 mm Hg. How do you interpret the patient's blood gas values? What treatment would you anticipate? Outline the nursing plan of care to address the patient's fluid and electrolyte or acid–base disorders. Give the rationale for the nursing interventions for this patient.

3 **ebp** An 85-year-old man is brought to the hospital with a decreased fluid intake for the past 4 days and weakness. He is unable to tolerate oral fluids, so IV fluids are prescribed. What is the evidence for selecting a site for IV placement and selecting a stabilization device for this patient? What criteria would you use to assess the strength of the evidence? What is the evidence for when to change the IV site?

4 **pq** Identify the priorities, approach, and techniques you would use to provide nursing care to a patient in respiratory alkalosis. How would your priorities, approach, and techniques differ if the patient is in respiratory acidosis? If the patient is in metabolic acidosis? If the patient is in metabolic alkalosis?

Brunner Suite Resources

Explore these additional resources to enhance learning for this chapter:
- NCLEX-Style Questions and Other Resources on thePoint, http://thePoint.lww.com/Brunner13e
- Study Guide
- PrepU
- Clinical Handbook
- Handbook of Laboratory and Diagnostic Tests

References

*Asterisk indicates nursing research.

Books

Alexander, M., Corrigan, A., Gorski, L., et al. (Eds.). (2010). *Infusion nursing: An evidence based approach* (3rd ed.). St. Louis: Saunders Elsevier.

Chernecky, C. C., & Berger, B. J. (2008). *Laboratory tests and diagnostic procedures* (5th ed.). Philadelphia: Saunders Elsevier.

Domino, F. (2011). *The 5-minute clinical consult*. Philadelphia: Lippincott Williams & Wilkins.

Dudek, S. G. (2010). *Nutrition essentials for nursing practice* (6th ed.). Philadelphia: Lippincott Williams & Wilkins.

Fischbach, F., & Dunning, M. B. (2009). *A manual of laboratory and diagnostic tests* (8th ed.). Philadelphia: Lippincott Williams & Wilkins.

Guyton, A. C., & Hall, J. E. (2011). *Textbook of medical physiology* (12th ed.). St. Louis: Elsevier Saunders.

Infusion Nurses Society. (2011). *Infusion nursing standards of practice*. Norwood, MA: Author.

Karch, A. M. (2012). *Lippincott's nursing drug guide*. Philadelphia: Lippincott Williams & Wilkins.

March, K., Criddle, L. M., Madden, L. K. et al. (2010). *Craniocerebral trauma*. In M. K. Bader, & L. R. Littlejohns (Eds.). *AANN core curriculum for neuroscience nursing* (5th ed.). Glenview, IL: American Association of Neuroscience Nursing.

McPhee, S. J., Papadakis, M., & Rabow M. (2012). *Current medical diagnosis and treatment* (51st ed.). New York: McGraw-Hill Medical.

Phillips, L. D. (2010). *Manual of IV therapeutics: Evidence-based practice for infusion therapy* (5th ed.). Philadelphia: F. A. Davis.

Porth, C. M. (2011). *Essentials of pathophysiology* (3rd ed.). Philadelphia: Lippincott Williams & Wilkins.

Weber, J., & Kelley, J. (2010). *Health assessment in nursing* (4th ed.). Philadelphia: Lippincott Williams & Wilkins.

Journals and Electronic Documents

*Bausone-Gazda, D., Lefaiver, C., & Walters S. (2010). A randomized controlled trial to compare the complications of 2 peripheral intravenous catheter stabilization systems. *Journal of Infusion Nursing, 33*(6), 371–384.

Collins, M., & Claros, E. (2011). Recognizing the face of dehydration. *Nursing, 41*(8), 26–31.

Crawford, A., & Harris, H. (2011a). Balancing act: Hypomagnesemia and hypermagnesemia. *Nursing, 41*(10), 52–55.

Crawford, A., & Harris, H. (2011b). Balancing act: Sodium (NA+) and potassium (K+). *Nursing, 41*(7), 44–50.

Crawford, A., & Harris, H. (2011c). I.V. fluids: What nurses need to know. *Nursing, 41*(5), 30–38.

Fournier, M. (2009). Perfecting your acid-base balancing act: How to detect and correct acid-base disorders. *American Nurse Today, 4*(1), 17–22.

Jones, M. B. (2010). Basic interpretation of metabolic acidosis. *Critical Care Nurse, 30*(5), 63–69.

Lai, C. C., Tan, C. K., Lin, S. H., et al. (2011). Central pontine myelinolysis. *Canadian Medical Association Journal, 183*(9), E605.

Neumar, R. W., Otto, C. W., Link, M. S., et al. (2010). Adult advanced cardiovascular life support: 2010 American Heart Association guidelines for cardiopulmonary resuscitation and emergency cardiovascular care. *Circulation, 122*, S729–S767.

O'Grady, N. P., Alexander, M., Burns, L., et al. (2011). *Guidelines for the prevention of intravascular catheter-related infections, 2011*. Centers for Disease Control and Prevention. Available at: www.cdc.gov/hicpac/pdf/guidelines/bsi-guidelines-2011.pdf

Pruitt, B. (2010). Interpreting ABGs: An inside look at your patient's status. *Nursing, 40*(7), 31–35.

*Rickard, C. M., Vannapraseuth, B., McGrail, M. R., et al. (2009). The relationship between intravenous infusate colonization and fluid container hang time. *Journal of Clinical Nursing, 18*(21), 3022–3028.

Siegel, A. J., d'Hemecourt, P., Adner, M. M., et al. (2009). Exertional dysnatremia in collapsed marathon runners: A critical role for point-of-care testing to guide appropriate therapy. *American Journal of Clinical Pathology, 132*(3), 336–340.

Yee, A. H., & Rabinstein A. A. (2010). Neurologic presentations of acid-base imbalance, electrolyte abnormalities and endocrine emergencies. *Neurologic Clinics, 28*(1), 1–16.

Resources

Infusion Nurses Society (INS), www.ins1.org
Safe Needles Save Lives—It's the Law, www.nursingworld.org/safeneedles
Stop Sticks Campaign, www.cdc.gov/niosh/stopsticks

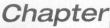

Chapter

14

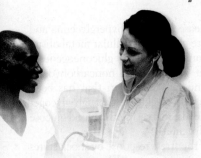

Shock and Multiple Organ Dysfunction Syndrome

Glossary

anaphylactic shock: circulatory shock state resulting from a severe allergic reaction producing an overwhelming systemic vasodilation and relative hypovolemia

biochemical mediators: messenger substances that may be released by a cell to create an action at that site or may be carried by the bloodstream to a distant site before being activated; also called *cytokines* or *inflammatory mediators*

cardiogenic shock: shock state resulting from impairment or failure of the myocardium

circulatory shock: shock state resulting from displacement of intravascular volume creating a relative hypovolemia and inadequate delivery of oxygen to the cells; also called *distributive shock*

colloids: intravenous solutions that contain molecules that are too large to pass through capillary membranes

crystalloids: intravenous electrolyte solutions that move freely between the intravascular compartment and interstitial spaces

hypovolemic shock: shock state resulting from decreased intravascular volume due to fluid loss

multiple organ dysfunction syndrome: presence of altered function of two or more organs in an acutely ill patient such that interventions are necessary to support continued organ function

neurogenic shock: shock state resulting from loss of sympathetic tone causing relative hypovolemia

septic shock: circulatory shock state resulting from overwhelming infection causing relative hypovolemia

shock: physiologic state in which there is inadequate blood flow to tissues and cells of the body

systemic inflammatory response syndrome (SIRS): overwhelming inflammatory response in the absence of infection causing relative hypovolemia and decreased tissue perfusion

Shock is a life-threatening condition that results from inadequate tissue perfusion. Many conditions may cause shock; irrespective of the cause, tissue hypoperfusion prevents adequate oxygen delivery to cells, leading to cell dysfunction and death. The progression of shock is neither linear nor predictable, and shock states, especially septic shock, comprise a current area of aggressive clinical research. Nurses caring for patients with shock and those at risk for shock must understand the underlying mechanisms of the various shock states (i.e., hypovolemic, cardiogenic, neurogenic, anaphylactic, and septic) and recognize the subtle as well as more obvious signs of each of these states. Rapid assessment with early recognition and response to shock states is essential to the patient's recovery.

Overview of Shock

Shock can best be defined as a clinical syndrome that results from inadequate tissue perfusion creating an imbalance between the delivery of and requirement for oxygen and nutrients that support cellular function (Maier, 2011). Adequate blood flow to the tissues and cells requires an effective cardiac pump, adequate vasculature or circulatory system, and sufficient blood volume. If one of these components is impaired, perfusion to the tissues is threatened or compromised. Without treatment, inadequate blood flow to the cells results in poor delivery of oxygen and nutrients, cellular hypoxia, and cell death that progresses to organ dysfunction and eventually death.

Shock affects all body systems. It may develop rapidly or slowly, depending on the underlying cause. During shock, the body struggles to survive, calling on all its homeostatic mechanisms to restore blood flow. Any insult to the body can create a cascade of events resulting in poor tissue perfusion. Therefore, almost any patient with any disease state may be at risk for developing shock. Conventionally, the primary underlying pathophysiologic process and underlying disorder are used to classify the shock state (e.g., hypovolemic shock, cardiogenic shock, and circulatory shock [i.e., neurogenic, anaphylactic, septic] [all discussed later in the chapter]).

Regardless of the initial cause of shock, certain physiologic responses are common to all types of shock. These physiologic responses include hypoperfusion of tissues, hypermetabolism, and activation of the inflammatory response. The body responds to shock states by activating the sympathetic nervous system and mounting a hypermetabolic and inflammatory response. Failure of compensatory mechanisms to effectively restore physiologic balance is the final pathway of all shock states and results in end-organ dysfunction and death (Dellinger, Levy, Rhodes, et al. 2013; Funk, Sebat, & Kumar, 2009; Maier, 2011).

Nursing care of patients with shock requires ongoing systematic assessment. Many of the interventions required in caring for patients with shock call for close collaboration with other members of the health care team and rapid implementation of prescribed therapies. Nurses are in key positions to identify early signs of shock and anticipate rapid therapy.

Normal Cellular Function

Energy metabolism occurs within the cell, where nutrients are chemically broken down and stored in the form of adenosine triphosphate (ATP). Cells use this stored energy to perform necessary functions, such as active transport, muscle contraction, and biochemical synthesis, as well as specialized cellular functions, such as the conduction of electrical impulses. ATP can be synthesized aerobically (in the presence of oxygen) or anaerobically (in the absence of oxygen). Aerobic metabolism yields far greater amounts of ATP per mole of glucose than does anaerobic metabolism; therefore, it is a more efficient and effective means of producing energy. In addition, anaerobic metabolism results in the accumulation of the toxic end product lactic acid, which must be removed from the cell and transported to the liver for conversion into glucose and glycogen.

Pathophysiology

Cellular Changes

In shock, the cells lack an adequate blood supply and are deprived of oxygen and nutrients; therefore, they must produce energy through anaerobic metabolism. This results in low energy yields from nutrients and an acidotic intracellular environment. Because of these changes, normal cell function ceases (Fig. 14-1). The cell swells and the cell membrane becomes more permeable, allowing electrolytes and fluids to seep out of and into the cell. The sodium–potassium pump becomes impaired; cell structures, primarily the mitochondria, are damaged; and death of the cell results.

Glucose is the primary substrate required for the production of cellular energy in the form of ATP. In stress states, catecholamines, cortisol, glucagons, and inflammatory cytokines and mediators are released, causing hyperglycemia and insulin resistance to mobilize glucose for cellular metabolism. Activation of these substances promotes gluconeogenesis, which is the formation of glucose from noncarbohydrate sources such as proteins and fats. Glycogen that has been stored in the liver is converted to glucose through glycogenolysis to meet metabolic needs, increasing the blood glucose concentration (i.e., hyperglycemia).

Continued activation of the stress response by shock states causes a depletion of glycogen stores, resulting in increased proteolysis and eventual organ failure (Strehlow, 2010). The body's inability to have enough nutrients and oxygen for normal cellular metabolism causes a buildup of metabolic end products in the cells and interstitial spaces. The clotting cascade, also associated with the inflammatory process, becomes activated, which compounds this pathologic cycle. With significant cell injury or death caused by shock, the clotting cascade is overproductive, resulting in small clots lodging in microcirculation, further hampering cellular perfusion (Wilmot, 2010). This up-regulation of the clotting cascade further compromises microcirculation of tissues, exacerbating cellular hypoperfusion (Strehlow, 2010). Cellular metabolism is impaired, and a self-perpetuating negative situation (i.e., a positive feedback loop) is initiated.

Vascular Responses

Local regulatory mechanisms, referred to as autoregulation, stimulate vasodilation or vasoconstriction in response to **biochemical mediators** (i.e., cytokines) released by the cell, communicating the need for oxygen and nutrients (Wilmot, 2010). A biochemical mediator is a substance released by a cell or immune cells such as macrophages; the substance triggers an action at a cell site or travels in the bloodstream to a distant site, where it triggers action. Researchers are learning more every day about the physiologic actions of more than 170 known cytokines (Pierrakos & Vincent, 2010).

Blood Pressure Regulation

Three major components of the circulatory system—blood volume, the cardiac pump, and the vasculature—must respond effectively to complex neural, chemical, and hormonal feedback systems to maintain an adequate blood pressure (BP) and perfuse body tissues. BP is regulated through a complex interaction of neural, chemical, and hormonal feedback systems affecting both cardiac output and peripheral resistance. This relationship is expressed in the following equation:

$$\text{Mean arterial BP} = \text{Cardiac output} \times \text{Peripheral resistance}$$

Cardiac output is a product of the stroke volume (the amount of blood ejected from the left ventricle during systole) and heart rate. Peripheral resistance is primarily determined by the diameter of the arterioles.

Tissue perfusion and organ perfusion depend on mean arterial pressure (MAP), or the average pressure at which blood moves through the vasculature. MAP must exceed 65 mm Hg for cells to receive the oxygen and nutrients needed to metabolize energy in amounts sufficient to sustain life (Dellinger et al., 2013; Tuggle, 2010). True MAP can be calculated only by complex methods.

BP is regulated by baroreceptors (pressure receptors) located in the carotid sinus and aortic arch. These pressure

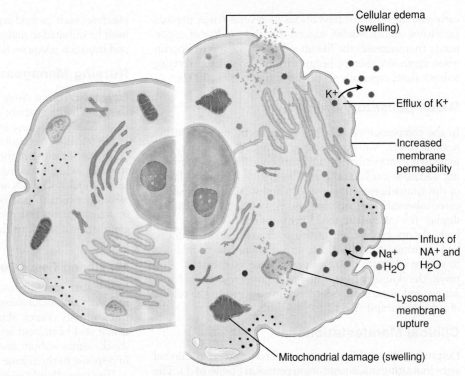

FIGURE 14-1 • Cellular effects of shock. The cell swells and the cell membrane becomes more permeable; fluids and electrolytes seep from and into the cell. Mitochondria and lysosomes are damaged, and the cell dies.

Normal Cell   Effects of shock

receptors are responsible for monitoring the circulatory volume and regulating neural and endocrine activities (see Chapter 31 for further description). When BP drops, catecholamines (epinephrine and norepinephrine) are released from the adrenal medulla. These increase heart rate and cause vasoconstriction, thus restoring BP. Chemoreceptors, also located in the aortic arch and carotid arteries, regulate BP and respiratory rate using much the same mechanism in response to changes in oxygen and carbon dioxide (CO_2) concentrations in the blood. These primary regulatory mechanisms can respond to changes in BP on a moment-to-moment basis.

The kidneys regulate BP by releasing renin, an enzyme needed for the eventual conversion of angiotensin I to angiotensin II, a potent vasoconstrictor. This stimulation of the renin–angiotensin mechanism and the resulting vasoconstriction indirectly lead to the release of aldosterone from the adrenal cortex, which promotes the retention of sodium and water (i.e., hypernatremia). Hypernatremia then stimulates the release of antidiuretic hormone (ADH) by the pituitary gland. ADH causes the kidneys to retain water further in an effort to raise blood volume and BP. These secondary regulatory mechanisms may take hours or days to respond to changes in BP. The relationship between the initiation of shock and the responsiveness of primary and secondary regulatory mechanisms that compensate for deficits in blood volume, the pumping effectiveness of the heart, or vascular tone, which may result because of the shock state is noted in Figure 14-2.

Stages of Shock

Shock progresses along a continuum and can be identified as early or late, depending on the signs and symptoms and the

overall severity of organ dysfunction. A convenient way to understand the physiologic responses and subsequent clinical signs and symptoms of shock is to divide the continuum into separate stages: compensatory (stage 1), progressive (stage 2), and irreversible (stage 3). The earlier that interventions are initiated along this continuum, the greater the patient's chance of survival. Current research is focusing on assessing patients at greatest risk for shock and implementing

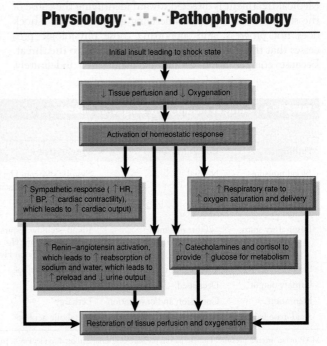

FIGURE 14-2 • Compensatory mechanisms in shock.

early and aggressive interventions to reverse tissue hypoxia (Strehlow, 2010). Studies suggest that the window of opportunity that increases the likelihood of patient survival occurs when aggressive therapy begins within 6 hours of identifying a shock state, especially septic shock (Funk et al., 2009).

■ Compensatory Stage

In the compensatory stage of shock, the BP remains within normal limits. Vasoconstriction, increased heart rate, and increased contractility of the heart contribute to maintaining adequate cardiac output. This results from stimulation of the sympathetic nervous system and subsequent release of catecholamines (epinephrine and norepinephrine). Patients display the often-described "fight-or-flight" response. The body shunts blood from organs such as the skin, kidneys, and gastrointestinal (GI) tract to the brain, heart, and lungs to ensure adequate blood supply to these vital organs. As a result, the skin may be cool and pale, bowel sounds are hypoactive, and urine output decreases in response to the release of aldosterone and ADH.

Clinical Manifestations

Despite a normal BP, the patient shows numerous clinical signs indicating inadequate organ perfusion (Table 14-1). The result of inadequate perfusion is anaerobic metabolism and a buildup of lactic acid, producing metabolic acidosis. The respiratory rate increases in response to the need to increase oxygen to the cells and in compensation for metabolic acidosis. This rapid respiratory rate facilitates removal of excess CO_2 but raises the blood pH and often causes a compensatory respiratory alkalosis. The patient may experience change in affect, express feeling anxious, or be confused. If treatment begins in this stage of shock, the prognosis for the patient is better than in later stages.

Medical Management

Medical treatment is directed toward identifying the cause of the shock, correcting the underlying disorder so that shock does not progress, and supporting those physiologic processes that thus far have responded successfully to the threat. Because compensation cannot be maintained indefinitely,

measures such as fluid replacement and medication therapy must be initiated to maintain an adequate BP and reestablish and maintain adequate tissue perfusion (Maier, 2011).

Nursing Management

Early intervention along the continuum of shock is the key to improving the patient's prognosis (Jones, Brown, Trzeciak, et al., 2008). The nurse must systematically assess the patient at risk for shock, recognizing subtle clinical signs of the compensatory stage before the patient's BP drops. Early interventions include identifying the cause of shock, administering intravenous (IV) fluids and oxygen, and obtaining necessary laboratory tests to rule out and treat metabolic imbalances or infection. Special considerations related to recognizing early signs of shock in the older adult patient are discussed in Chart 14-1.

Monitoring Tissue Perfusion

In assessing tissue perfusion, the nurse observes for changes in level of consciousness, vital signs (including pulse pressure), urinary output, skin, and laboratory values (e.g., base deficit and lactic acid levels). In the compensatory stage of shock, serum sodium and blood glucose levels are elevated in response to the release of aldosterone and catecholamines.

The nurse should monitor the patient's hemodynamic status and promptly report deviations to the primary provider, assist in identifying and treating the underlying disorder by continuous in-depth assessment of the patient, administer prescribed fluids and medications, and promote patient safety. Vital signs are key indicators of hemodynamic status, and BP is an indirect measure of tissue hypoxia. The nurse should report a systolic BP lower than 90 mm Hg or a drop in systolic BP of 40 mm Hg from baseline or a MAP less than 65 mm Hg (Dellinger et al., 2013; Funk et al., 2009; Powers & Burchell, 2010).

Pulse pressure correlates well with stroke volume. Pulse pressure is calculated by subtracting the diastolic measurement from the systolic measurement; the difference is the pulse pressure. Normally, the pulse pressure is 30 to 40 mm Hg. Narrowing or decreased pulse pressure is an earlier indicator of shock than a drop in systolic BP (Strehlow, 2010). Decreased or narrowing pulse pressure, an early indication

---

TABLE 14-1 Clinical Findings in Stages of Shock

| Finding | Stage | | |
	Compensatory	Progressive	Irreversible
Blood pressure	Normal	Systolic <90 mm Hg; MAP <65 mm Hg Requires fluids resuscitation to support blood pressure	Requires mechanical or pharmacologic support
Heart rate	>100 bpm	>150 bpm	Erratic or asystole
Respiratory status	>20 breaths/min PaCO$_2$ <32 mm Hg	Rapid, shallow respirations; crackles PaO$_2$ <80 mm Hg PaCO$_2$ >45 mm Hg	Requires intubation and mechanical ventilation and oxygenation
Skin	Cold, clammy	Mottled, petechiae	Jaundice
Urinary output	Decreased	<0.5 mL/kg/h	Anuric, requires dialysis
Mentation	Confusion and/or agitation	Lethargy	Unconscious
Acid–base balance	Respiratory alkalosis	Metabolic acidosis	Profound acidosis

MAP, mean arterial pressure; PaCO$_2$, partial pressure of arterial carbon dioxide; PaO$_2$, partial pressure of arterial oxygen.

Chart 14-1   Recognizing Shock in Older Patients

The physiologic changes associated with aging, coupled with pathologic and chronic disease states, place older people at increased risk for developing a state of shock and possibly multiple organ dysfunction syndrome. Older adults can recover from shock if it is detected and treated early with aggressive and supportive therapies. Nurses play an essential role in assessing and interpreting subtle changes in older patients' responses to illness.

- Medications such as beta-blocking agents (metoprolol [Lopressor]) used to treat hypertension may mask tachycardia, a primary compensatory mechanism to increase cardiac output, during hypovolemic states.
- The aging immune system may not mount a truly febrile response (temperature greater than 38°C [100.4°F]); however, a lack of a febrile response (temperature less than 37°C [98.6°F]) or an increasing trend in body temperature should be addressed. The patient may also report increased fatigue and malaise in the absence of a febrile response.
- The heart does not function well in hypoxemic states, and the aging heart may respond to decreased myocardial oxygenation with dysrhythmias that may be misinterpreted as a normal part of the aging process.
- There is a progressive decline in respiratory muscle strength, maximal ventilation, and response to hypoxia. Older patients have a decreased respiratory reserve and decompensate more quickly.
- Changes in mentation may be inappropriately misinterpreted as dementia. Older people with a sudden change in mentation should be aggressively assessed for acute delirium and treated for the presence of infection and organ hypoperfusion.

of decreased stroke volume, is illustrated in the following example:

$$\text{Systolic BP} - \text{Diastolic BP} = \text{Pulse pressure}$$

Normal pulse pressure:

$$120 \text{ mm Hg} - 80 \text{ mm Hg} = 40 \text{ mm Hg}$$

Narrowing of pulse pressure:

$$90 \text{ mm Hg} - 70 \text{ mm Hg} = 20 \text{ mm Hg}$$

Elevation of the diastolic BP with release of catecholamines and attempts to increase venous return through vasoconstriction is an early compensatory mechanism in response to decreased stroke volume, BP, and overall cardiac output.

 Quality and Safety Nursing Alert

By the time BP drops, damage has already been occurring at the cellular and tissue levels. Therefore, the patient at risk for shock must be assessed and monitored closely before the BP falls.

Continuous central venous oximetry ($Sc\bar{v}O_2$) monitoring may be used to evaluate mixed venous blood oxygen saturation and severity of tissue hypoperfusion states. A central catheter is introduced into the superior vena cava (SVC), and a sensor on the catheter measures the oxygen saturation of the blood in the SVC as blood returns to the heart and pulmonary system for re-oxygenation. A normal $Sc\bar{v}O_2$ value

is 70% (Ramos & Azevedo, 2010). Body tissues use approximately 25% of the oxygen delivered to them during normal metabolism. During stressful events, such as shock, more oxygen is consumed and the $Sc\bar{v}O_2$ saturation is lower, indicating that the tissues are consuming more oxygen.

Interventions focus on decreasing tissue oxygen requirements and increasing perfusion to deliver more oxygen to the tissues. For instance, sedating agents may be administered to lower metabolic demands, or the patient's pain may be treated with IV opioid agents to decrease metabolic demands for oxygen. Supplemental oxygen and mechanical ventilation may be required to increase the delivery of oxygen in the blood. Administration of IV fluids and medications supports BP and cardiac output, and the transfusion of packed red blood cells enhances oxygen transport. Monitoring tissue oxygen consumption with $Sc\bar{v}O_2$ is a minimally invasive measure to more accurately assess tissue oxygenation in the compensatory stage of shock before changes in vital signs detect altered tissue perfusion (Dellinger et al., 2013; Ramos & Azevedo, 2010).

Newer technologies allow clinicians to detect changes in tissue perfusion before changes in classic signs (BP, heart rate, and urine output) indicative of hypoperfusion occur. Sublingual capnometry, a noninvasive technology, provides information about the degree of hypoperfusion based on the sublingual partial pressure of CO_2 (Strehlow, 2010). A probe is placed under the patient's tongue, and CO_2 levels are derived from the blood flow found in the mucosal bed. During shock, an elevated CO_2 indicates poor tissue perfusion. Near-infrared spectroscopy (StO_2), a continuous noninvasive technology, uses light transmission to measure skeletal muscle oxygenation as an indicator of shock. The StO_2 probe is applied to the thenar muscle that is located on the palm of the hand near the thumb, and it measures the oxygen saturation of tissue by determining the amount of infrared light absorption. Low values of tissue oxygenation (e.g., less than 80%) indicate severity of shock; the lower the value, the more severe the tissue hypoxia.

Although treatments are prescribed and initiated by the physician, the nurse usually implements them, operates and troubleshoots equipment used in treatment, monitors the patient's status during treatment, and evaluates the immediate effects of treatment. In addition, the nurse assesses the response of the patient and family to the crisis and its treatment.

Reducing Anxiety

Patients and their families often become anxious and apprehensive when they face a major threat to health and well-being and are the focus of attention of many health care providers. Providing brief explanations about the diagnostic and treatment procedures, supporting the patient during these procedures, and providing information about their outcomes are usually effective in reducing stress and anxiety and thus promoting the patient's physical and mental well-being. Speaking in a calm, reassuring voice and using gentle touch also help ease the patient's concerns. These actions may provide comfort for critically ill, frightened patients (Bradley, Lensky, & Brassel, 2011). Research suggests that family members have certain needs during a health-related crisis, including the need for honest, consistent, and thorough communication with health care providers; physical and emotional closeness to the patient; sensing that health care providers care about their patients; seeing the patient frequently; and knowing exactly what has been done for the patient (Bradley et al., 2011).

The nurse should advocate that family members be present during procedures and while patient care is provided. The presence of family provides a necessary connection and support for the patient during a time of crisis.

Promoting Safety

The nurse must be vigilant for potential threats to the patient's safety, because a high anxiety level and altered mental status impair judgment. In this stage of shock, patients who were previously cooperative and followed instructions may now disrupt IV lines and catheters and complicate their condition. Therefore, close monitoring, frequent reorientation, hourly rounding, and implementing interventions to prevent falls (e.g., bed alarms) are essential.

■ Progressive Stage

In the second stage of shock, the mechanisms that regulate BP can no longer compensate, and the MAP falls below normal limits. Patients are clinically hypotensive; this is defined as a systolic BP of less than 90 mm Hg or a decrease in systolic BP of 40 mm Hg from baseline. The patient shows signs of declining mental status (Dellinger et al., 2013; VonRueden, Bolton, & Vary, 2009).

Pathophysiology

Although all organ systems suffer from hypoperfusion at this stage, several events perpetuate the shock syndrome. First, the overworked heart becomes dysfunctional, the body's inability to meet increased oxygen requirements produces ischemia, and biochemical mediators cause myocardial depression (Dellinger et al., 2013; VonRueden et al., 2009). This leads to failure of the cardiac pump, even if the underlying cause of the shock is not of cardiac origin. Second, the autoregulatory function of the microcirculation fails in response to the numerous biochemical mediators released by the cells, resulting in increased capillary permeability, with areas of arteriolar and venous constriction further compromising cellular perfusion (VonRueden et al., 2009). At this stage, the prognosis worsens. The relaxation of precapillary sphincters causes fluid to leak from the capillaries, creating interstitial edema and decreased return to the heart. In addition, the inflammatory response to injury is activated, and proinflammatory and anti-inflammatory mediators are released, which activate the coagulation system in an effort to reestablish homeostasis (Wilmot, 2010). The body mobilizes energy stores and increases oxygen consumption to meet the increased metabolic needs of the underperfused tissues and cells.

Even if the underlying cause of the shock is reversed, the sequence of compensatory responses to the decrease in tissue perfusion perpetuates the shock state, and a vicious cycle ensues. The cellular reactions that occur during the progressive stage of shock are an active area of clinical research. It is believed that the body's response to shock or lack of response in this stage of shock may be the primary factor determining the patient's survival.

Clinical Manifestations

Chances of survival depend on the patient's general health before the shock state as well as the amount of time it takes to restore tissue perfusion. As shock progresses, organ systems decompensate (see Table 14-1).

Respiratory Effects

The lungs, which become compromised early in shock, are affected at this stage. Subsequent decompensation of the lungs increases the likelihood that mechanical ventilation will be needed. Respirations are rapid and shallow. Crackles are heard over the lung fields. Decreased pulmonary blood flow causes arterial oxygen levels to decrease and CO_2 levels to increase. Hypoxemia and biochemical mediators cause an intense inflammatory response and pulmonary vasoconstriction, perpetuating pulmonary capillary hypoperfusion and hypoxemia. The hypoperfused alveoli stop producing surfactant and subsequently collapse. Pulmonary capillaries begin to leak, causing pulmonary edema, diffusion abnormalities (shunting), and additional alveolar collapse. This condition is called *acute lung injury* (ALI); as ALI continues, interstitial inflammation and fibrosis are common consequences, leading to acute respiratory distress syndrome (ARDS) (Girard, Kess, Fuchs, et al., 2008). Further explanation of ALI and ARDS, as well as their nursing management, can be found in Chapter 23.

Cardiovascular Effects

A lack of adequate blood supply leads to dysrhythmias and ischemia. The heart rate is rapid, sometimes exceeding 150 bpm. The patient may complain of chest pain and even suffer a myocardial infarction (MI). Levels of cardiac enzymes and biomarkers (e.g., myocardial creatine kinase [CK-MB] and cardiac troponin I [cTn-I]) increase. In addition, myocardial depression and ventricular dilation may further impair the heart's ability to pump enough blood to the tissues to meet oxygen requirements.

Neurologic Effects

As blood flow to the brain becomes impaired, mental status deteriorates. Changes in mental status occur with decreased cerebral perfusion and hypoxia. Initially, the patient may exhibit subtle changes in behavior or agitation and confusion. Subsequently, lethargy increases, and the patient begins to lose consciousness.

Renal Effects

When the MAP falls below 65 mm Hg (Martin, 2010), the glomerular filtration rate of the kidneys cannot be maintained, and drastic changes in renal function occur. Acute kidney injury (AKI) is characterized by an increase in blood urea nitrogen (BUN) and serum creatinine levels, fluid and electrolyte shifts, acid–base imbalances, and a loss of the renal-hormonal regulation of BP. Urinary output usually decreases to less than 0.5 mL/kg per hour (or less than 30 mL per hour) but may vary depending on the phase of AKI. (See Chapter 54 for further information about AKI.)

Hepatic Effects

Decreased blood flow to the liver impairs the ability of liver cells to perform metabolic and phagocytic functions.

Consequently, the patient is less able to metabolize medications and metabolic waste products, such as ammonia and lactic acid. Metabolic activities of the liver, including gluconeogenesis and glycogenolysis, are impaired. The patient becomes more susceptible to infection as the liver fails to filter bacteria from the blood. Liver enzymes (aspartate aminotransferase [AST], alanine aminotransferase [ALT], lactate dehydrogenase [LDH]), and bilirubin levels are elevated, and the patient develops jaundice.

Gastrointestinal Effects

GI ischemia can cause stress ulcers in the stomach, putting the patient at risk for GI bleeding. In the small intestine, the mucosa can become necrotic and slough off, causing bloody diarrhea. Beyond the local effects of impaired perfusion, GI ischemia leads to bacterial toxin translocation, in which bacterial toxins enter the bloodstream through the lymphatic system. In addition to causing infection, bacterial toxins can cause cardiac depression, vasodilation, increased capillary permeability, and an intense inflammatory response with activation of additional biochemical mediators. The net result is interference with healthy cellular functioning and the ability to metabolize nutrients (VonRueden et al., 2009).

Hematologic Effects

The combination of hypotension, sluggish blood flow, metabolic acidosis, coagulation system imbalance, and generalized hypoxemia can interfere with normal hemostatic mechanisms. In shock states, the inflammatory cytokines activate the clotting cascade, causing deposition of microthrombi in multiple areas of the body and consumption of clotting factors. The alterations of the hematologic system, including imbalance of the clotting cascade, are linked to the overactivation of the inflammatory response of injury (VonRueden et al., 2009). Disseminated intravascular coagulation (DIC) may occur either as a cause or as a complication of shock. In this condition, widespread clotting and bleeding occur simultaneously. Bruises (ecchymoses) and bleeding (petechiae) may appear in the skin. Coagulation times (e.g., prothrombin time [PT], activated partial thromboplastin time [aPTT]) are prolonged. Clotting factors and platelets are consumed and require replacement therapy to achieve hemostasis. (Further discussion of DIC appears in Chapter 33.)

 ## Medical Management

Specific medical management in the progressive stage of shock depends on the type of shock, its underlying cause, and the degree of decompensation in the organ systems. Medical management specific to each type of shock is discussed later in this chapter. Although medical management in the progressive stage differs by type of shock, some medical interventions are common to all types. These include the use of appropriate IV fluids and medications to restore tissue perfusion by the following methods:

- Supporting the respiratory system
- Optimizing intravascular volume
- Supporting the pumping action of the heart
- Improving the competence of the vascular system

Other aspects of management may include early enteral nutritional support, targeted hyperglycemic control with IV insulin and use of antacids, histamine-2 (H_2) blockers, or antipeptic medications to reduce the risk of GI ulceration and bleeding.

Tight glycemic control (serum glucose of 80 to 100 mg/dL) is no longer recommended, as hypoglycemic events associated with regulating tight control in critically ill patients have been found to result in adverse patient outcomes (Griesdale, DeSouza, VanDam, et al., 2009). Current evidence suggests that maintaining serum glucose between 140 and 180 mg/dL with aggressive insulin therapy and close monitoring is indicated in the management of the critically ill patient (Kavanagh & McCowen, 2010)

 Quality and Safety Nursing Alert

Glycemic control is linked to outcomes in the patient in shock. Although tight glycemic control is no longer indicated, evidence shows that maintaining serum glucose between 140 and 180 mg/dL is linked to best outcomes.

 ## Nursing Management

Nursing care of patients in the progressive stage of shock requires expertise in assessing and understanding shock and the significance of changes in assessment data. Early interventions are essential to the survival of patients; therefore, suspecting that a patient may be in shock and reporting subtle changes in assessment are imperative. Patients in the progressive stage of shock are cared for in the intensive care setting to facilitate close monitoring (hemodynamic monitoring, electrocardiographic [ECG] monitoring, arterial blood gases, serum electrolyte levels, physical and mental status changes); rapid and frequent administration of various prescribed medications and fluids; and possibly interventions with supportive technologies, such as mechanical ventilation, dialysis (e.g., continuous renal replacement therapy), and intra-aortic balloon pump.

Working closely with other members of the health care team, the nurse carefully documents treatments, medications, and fluids that are administered, recording the time, dosage or volume, and patient response. In addition, the nurse coordinates both the scheduling of diagnostic procedures that may be carried out at the bedside and the flow of health care personnel involved in care of patients.

Preventing Complications

The nurse helps reduce the risk of related complications and monitors the patient for early signs of complications. Monitoring includes evaluating blood levels of medications, observing invasive vascular lines for signs of infection, and checking neurovascular status if arterial lines are inserted, especially in the lower extremities. Simultaneously, the nurse promotes the patient's safety and comfort by ensuring that all procedures, including invasive procedures and arterial and venous punctures, are carried out using correct aseptic techniques and that venous and arterial puncture and infusion sites are maintained with the goal of preventing infection. Nursing interventions that reduce the incidence of ventilator-associated pneumonia (VAP) must also be implemented. These include frequent oral care, aseptic suction technique, turning, and elevating the head of the bed at least 30 degrees to prevent aspiration (Dellinger et al, 2013; Zilberberg &

Shorr, 2011). See Chart 21-13 for an overview of the evidence-based ("bundled") interventions aimed at preventing VAP. Positioning and repositioning of the patient to promote comfort and maintain skin integrity are essential.

Promoting Rest and Comfort

Efforts are made to minimize the cardiac workload by reducing the patient's physical activity and treating pain and anxiety. Because promoting patient rest and comfort is a priority, the nurse performs essential nursing activities in blocks of time, allowing the patient to have periods of uninterrupted rest. To conserve the patient's energy, the nurse should protect the patient from temperature extremes (e.g., excessive warmth or cold, and shivering), which can increase the metabolic rate and oxygen consumption and thus the cardiac workload.

Supporting Family Members

Because patients in shock receive intense attention by the health care team, families may be overwhelmed and frightened. Family members may be reluctant to ask questions or seek information for fear that they will be in the way or will interfere with the attention given to the patient. The nurse should make sure that the family is comfortably situated and kept informed about the patient's status. Often, families need advice from the health care team to get some rest; family members are more likely to take this advice if they feel that the patient is being well cared for and that they will be notified of any significant changes in the patient's status. A visit from the hospital chaplain may be comforting and provides some attention to the family while the nurse concentrates on the patient. Ensuring patient- and family-centered care is central to the delivery of high-quality care. This helps meet the emotional well-being of the patient and family as well as the physiologic needs of the patient (Bradley et al., 2011).

■ *Irreversible Stage*

The irreversible (or refractory) stage of shock represents the point along the shock continuum at which organ damage is so severe that the patient does not respond to treatment and cannot survive. Despite treatment, BP remains low. Renal and liver dysfunction, compounded by the release of necrotic tissue toxins, creates an overwhelming metabolic acidosis. Anaerobic metabolism contributes to a worsening lactic acidosis. Reserves of ATP are almost totally depleted, and mechanisms for storing new supplies of energy have been destroyed. Respiratory system dysfunction prevents adequate oxygenation and ventilation despite mechanical ventilatory support, and the cardiovascular system is ineffective in maintaining an adequate MAP for perfusion. Multiple organ dysfunction progressing to complete organ failure has occurred, and death is imminent. Multiple organ dysfunction can occur as a progression along the shock continuum or as a syndrome unto itself and is described in more detail later in this chapter.

Concept Mastery Alert

The irreversible stage of shock is aptly named because it correlates with significantly severe organ damage and dysfunction. Critical body functions are affected, leading to profound acidosis, unconsciousness, and the need for support of vital functions.

Medical Management

Medical management during the irreversible stage of shock is usually the same as for the progressive stage. Although the patient may have progressed to the irreversible stage, the judgment that the shock is irreversible can be made only retrospectively on the basis of the patient's failure to respond to treatment. Strategies that may be experimental (e.g., investigational medications, such as antibiotic agents and immunomodulation therapy) may be tried to reduce or reverse the severity of shock.

Nursing Management

As in the progressive stage of shock, the nurse focuses on carrying out prescribed treatments, monitoring the patient, preventing complications, protecting the patient from injury, and providing comfort. Offering brief explanations to the patient about what is happening is essential even if there is no certainty that the patient hears or understands what is being said. Simple comfort measures, including reassuring touches, should continue to be provided despite the patient's nonresponsiveness to verbal stimuli (Bradley et al., 2011).

As it becomes obvious that the patient is unlikely to survive, the family must be informed about the prognosis and likely outcome. Opportunities should be provided—throughout the patient's care—for the family to see, touch, and talk to the patient. Close family friends or spiritual advisors may be of comfort to the family members in dealing with the inevitable death of their loved one. Whenever possible and appropriate, the patient's family should be approached regarding any living wills, advance directives, or other written or verbal wishes the patient may have shared in the event that he or she became unable to participate in end-of-life decisions. In some cases, ethics committees may assist families and health care teams in making difficult decisions.

During this stage of shock, the family may misinterpret the actions of the health care team. They have been told that nothing has been effective in reversing the shock and that the patient's survival is very unlikely, yet they find physicians and nurses continuing to work feverishly on the patient. Distraught, grieving families may interpret this as a chance for recovery when none exists, and family members may become angry when the patient dies. Conferences with all members of the health care team and the family promote better understanding by the family of the patient's prognosis and the purpose for management measures. Engaging palliative care specialists can be beneficial in developing a plan of care that maximizes comfort and effective symptom management as well as assisting the family with difficult decisions (Hudson, Payne, & Dip, 2011). During these conferences, it is essential to explain that the equipment and treatments being provided are intended for patient comfort and do not suggest that the patient will recover. Family members should be encouraged to express their views of life-support measures (Hudson et al., 2011).

General Management Strategies in Shock

As described previously and in the discussion of types of shock to follow, management in all types and all phases of shock includes the following:

- Support of the respiratory system with supplemental oxygen and/or mechanical ventilation to provide optimal oxygenation (see Chapter 21)
- Fluid replacement to restore intravascular volume
- Vasoactive medications to restore vasomotor tone and improve cardiac function
- Nutritional support to address the metabolic requirements that are often dramatically increased in shock

Therapies described in this section require collaboration among all members of the health care team.

Fluid Replacement

Fluid replacement, also referred to as fluid resuscitation, is administered in all types of shock. The type of fluids administered and the speed of delivery vary; however, fluids are administered to improve cardiac and tissue oxygenation, which in part depends on flow. The fluids administered may include **crystalloids** (electrolyte solutions that move freely between intravascular compartment and interstitial spaces), **colloids** (large-molecule IV solutions), and blood components (packed red blood cells, fresh frozen plasma, and platelets).

Crystalloid and Colloid Solutions

In emergencies, the "best" fluid is often the fluid that is readily available. Fluid resuscitation should be initiated early in shock to maximize intravascular volume. There is no consensus regarding whether crystalloids or colloids should be used; however, with crystalloids, more fluid is necessary to restore intravascular volume (Perel & Roberts, 2011).

Isotonic crystalloid solutions are often selected because they contain the same concentration of electrolytes as the extracellular fluid and therefore can be given without altering the concentrations of electrolytes in the plasma. IV crystalloids commonly used for resuscitation in hypovolemic shock include 0.9% sodium chloride solution (normal saline) and lactated Ringer's solution (Boswell & Scalea, 2009). Ringer's lactate is an electrolyte solution containing the lactate ion, which should not be confused with lactic acid. The lactate ion is converted to bicarbonate, which helps buffer the overall acidosis that occurs in shock. A disadvantage of using isotonic crystalloid solutions is that some of the volume administered is lost to the interstitial compartment and some remains in the intravascular compartment. This occurs as a consequence of cellular permeability that occurs during shock. Diffusion of crystalloids into the interstitial space means that more fluid must be administered than the amount lost (Perel & Roberts, 2011).

Care must be taken when rapidly administering isotonic crystalloids to avoid both underresuscitating and overresuscitating the patient in shock. Insufficient fluid replacement is associated with a higher incidence of morbidity and mortality from lack of tissue perfusion, whereas excessive fluid administration can cause systemic and pulmonary edema that progresses to ARDS (see Chapter 23), abdominal hypertension and abdominal compartment syndrome (ACS), and multiple organ dysfunction syndrome (MODS) (see later discussion).

ACS is a serious complication that may occur when large volumes of fluid are administered. It may also occur after trauma, abdominal surgery, severe pancreatitis, or sepsis (Paula, 2011). In ACS, fluid leaks into the intra-abdominal cavity, increasing pressure that is displaced onto surround-

ing vessels and organs. Venous return, preload, and cardiac output are compromised. The pressure also elevates the diaphragm, making it difficult to breathe effectively. The renal and GI systems also begin to show signs of dysfunction (e.g., decreased urine output, absent bowel sounds, intolerance of tube feeding). Abdominal compartment pressure can be measured. Normally, it is 0 to 5 mm Hg, and a pressure of 12 mm Hg is considered to be indicative of intra-abdominal hypertension (Paula, 2011). If ACS is present, interventions that usually include surgical decompression are necessary to relieve the pressure.

 Concept Mastery Alert

Elevated pressure in an enclosed area puts pressure on surrounding structures. Thus, when the pressure in the abdomen increases, the diaphragm rises, placing additional pressure in the chest and compromising the patient's airway and breathing.

Depending on the cause of the hypovolemia, a hypertonic crystalloid solution, often 3% sodium chloride, may be administered in hypovolemic shock. These solutions exert a large osmotic force that pulls fluid from the intracellular space to the extracellular space to achieve a fluid balance (Coimbra, 2011). This osmotic effect results in fewer fluids being administered to restore intravascular volume. Complications associated with use of hypertonic solutions include excessive serum osmolality, which can cause rapid fluid shifts, overwhelming the heart and leading to hypernatremia. Continued research is needed as to the benefits of hypertonic saline infusion in the treatment of shock (Coimbra, 2011).

Generally, IV colloidal solutions are similar to plasma proteins, in that they contain molecules that are too large to pass through capillary membranes. Colloids expand intravascular volume by exerting oncotic pressure, thereby pulling fluid into the intravascular space. Colloidal solutions have the same effect as hypertonic solutions in increasing intravascular volume, but less volume of fluid is required than with crystalloids. In addition, colloids have a longer duration of action than crystalloids, because the molecules remain within the intravascular compartment longer.

Typically, if colloids are used to treat tissue hypoperfusion, albumin is the agent prescribed. Albumin is a plasma protein; an albumin solution is prepared from human plasma and is heated during production to reduce its potential to transmit disease. The disadvantage of albumin is its high cost compared to crystalloid solutions.

 Quality and Safety Nursing Alert

With all colloidal solutions, side effects include the rare occurrence of anaphylactic reactions. Nurses must monitor patients closely.

Complications of Fluid Administration

Close monitoring of the patient during fluid replacement is necessary to identify side effects and complications. The most common and serious side effects of fluid replacement are cardiovascular overload and pulmonary edema. The patient receiving fluid replacement must be monitored frequently for adequate urinary output, changes in mental status, skin perfusion, and changes in vital signs. Lung sounds are auscultated frequently to detect signs of fluid accumulation. Adventitious lung sounds, such as crackles, may indicate pulmonary edema.

▶ Quality and Safety Nursing Alert

When administering large volumes of crystalloid solutions, the nurse must monitor the lungs for adventitious sounds and signs and symptoms of interstitial edema (e.g., ACS).

Often, a central venous pressure (CVP) line is inserted (typically into the subclavian or jugular vein) and is advanced until the tip of the catheter rests near the junction of the SVC and right atrium. The CVP is used to measure right atrial pressure. In addition to physical assessment, the CVP value assists in monitoring the patient's response to fluid replacement. A normal CVP is 4 to 12 mm Hg or cm H_2O. Several readings are obtained to determine a range, and fluid replacement is continued to achieve a CVP between 8 to 12 mm Hg (Dellinger et al., 2013). Interpreting blood volume based on CVP readings has been recently challenged in the literature; therefore, CVP readings should be used in conjunction with other assessment variables to assess blood volume (Marik, Baram, & Vahid, 2008). With newer technologies, CVP catheters can be placed that allow the monitoring of intravascular pressures and venous oxygen levels. Assessment of venous oxygenation (venous oxygen saturation ([$S\bar{v}O_2$], or $Sc\bar{v}O_2$ with a CVP line) is helpful in evaluating the adequacy of intravascular volume (Rivers, McIntyre, Morro, et al., 2005; Strehlow, 2010). Hemodynamic monitoring with arterial and pulmonary artery lines may be implemented to allow close monitoring of the patient's perfusion and cardiac status as well as response to therapy. Advances in noninvasive or minimally invasive technology (e.g., esophageal Doppler, pulse contour cardiac output devices) provide additional hemodynamic monitoring options (Peyton & Chong, 2010). (For additional information about hemodynamic monitoring, see Chapter 25.)

Placement of central lines for fluid administration and monitoring requires collaborative practice between the provider and nurse to ensure that all measures to prevent central line–associated bloodstream infection (CLABSI) are implemented. Several interventions aimed at preventing CLABSI should be implemented collaboratively while the central line is being placed as well as during ongoing nursing management of the central line itself. Chart 14-2 describes the evidence-based ("bundled") interventions that have been found to reduce CLABSI.

Vasoactive Medication Therapy

Vasoactive medications are administered in all forms of shock to improve the patient's hemodynamic stability when fluid therapy alone cannot maintain adequate MAP. Specific medications are selected to correct the particular hemodynamic alteration that is impeding cardiac output. These medications help increase the strength of myocardial contractility, regulate the heart rate, reduce myocardial resistance, and initiate vasoconstriction.

Vasoactive medications are selected for their action on receptors of the sympathetic nervous system. These receptors are known as alpha-adrenergic and beta-adrenergic receptors. Beta-adrenergic receptors are further classified as beta-1 and beta-2 adrenergic receptors. When alpha-adrenergic receptors are stimulated, blood vessels constrict in the cardiorespiratory and GI systems, skin, and kidneys. When beta-1 adrenergic receptors are stimulated, heart rate and myocardial contraction increase. When beta-2 adrenergic receptors are stimulated, vasodilation occurs in the heart and skeletal muscles, and the bronchioles relax. The medications used in treating shock consist of various combinations of vasoactive medications to maximize tissue perfusion by stimulating or blocking the alpha- and beta-adrenergic receptors.

When vasoactive medications are administered, vital signs must be monitored frequently (at least every 15 minutes until stable, or more often if indicated). Vasoactive medications should be administered through a central venous line, because infiltration and extravasation of some vasoactive medications can cause tissue necrosis and sloughing.

Individual medication dosages are usually titrated by the nurse, who adjusts drip rates based on the prescribed dose and target outcome parameter (e.g., BP, heart rate) and the patient's response. Dosages are changed to maintain the MAP at a physiologic level that ensures adequate tissue perfusion (usually greater than 65 mm Hg).

▶ Quality and Safety Nursing Alert

Vasoactive medications should never be stopped abruptly, because this could cause severe hemodynamic instability, perpetuating the shock state.

Dosages of vasoactive medications must be tapered. When vasoactive medications are no longer needed or are necessary to a lesser extent, the infusion should be weaned with frequent monitoring of BP (every 15 minutes). Table 14-2 presents some of the commonly prescribed vasoactive medications used in the treatment of shock. Occasionally, the patient does not respond as expected to vasoactive medications. A current topic of active research is evaluation of patients' adrenal function. Recent studies suggest that critically ill patients should be evaluated for corticosteroid insufficiency (also referred to as relative adrenal insufficiency or critical illness–related corticosteroid insufficiency) and, if this condition is present, corticosteroid replacement (e.g., hydrocortisone) should be considered (Cohen & Venkatesh, 2010; Dellinger et al., 2013).

Nutritional Support

Nutritional support is an important aspect of care for patients with shock. Increased metabolic rates during shock increase energy requirements and therefore caloric requirements. Patients in shock may require more than 3,000 calories daily. The release of catecholamines early in the shock continuum causes depletion of glycogen stores in about 8 to 10 hours. Nutritional energy requirements are then met by breaking down lean body mass. In this catabolic process, skeletal muscle mass is broken down even when the patient has large stores of fat or adipose tissue. Loss of skeletal muscle greatly prolongs the patient's recovery time.

Chart 14-2   Collaborative Practice Interventions to Prevent Central Venous Line–Associated Bloodstream Infections

Current best practices can include the implementation of specific evidence-based bundle interventions that when used together (i.e., as a "bundle") improve patient outcomes. This chart outlines specific parameters for the central venous line bundled collaborative interventions that have been found to reduce central venous line–associated bloodstream infections (CLABSI).

What are the five key elements of the central venous line bundle?

- Hand hygiene
- Maximal barrier precautions (see later discussion)
- Chlorhexidine skin antisepsis
- Optimal catheter site selection with avoidance of using the femoral vein for central venous access in adult patients
- Daily review of line necessity, with prompt removal of unnecessary lines

When should hand hygiene be performed in the care of a patient with a central venous line?

- All clinicians who provide care to the patient should adhere to good hand hygiene practices, particularly:
  - Before and after palpating the catheter insertion site
  - With all dressing changes to the intravascular catheter access site
  - When hands are visibly soiled or contamination of hands is suspected
  - Before donning and after removing gloves

What changes can be made to improve hand hygiene?

- Implement a central venous line procedure checklist that requires that clinicians perform hand hygiene as an essential step in care.
- Post signage stating the importance of hand hygiene.
- Have soap and alcohol-based hand sanitizers prominently placed to facilitate hand hygiene practices.

What are maximal barrier precautions?

- These are implemented during central venous line insertion:
  - For the primary provider, this means strict compliance with wearing a cap, mask, sterile gown, and sterile gloves. The cap should cover all hair, and the mask should cover the nose and mouth tightly. The nurse should also wear a cap and mask.
  - For the patient, this means covering the patient from head to toe with a sterile drape, with a small opening for the site of insertion. If a full-size drape is not available, two drapes may be applied to cover the patient or the operating room may be consulted to determine how to procure full-size sterile drapes, because these are routinely used in surgical settings.

- Nurses should be empowered to enforce use of a central line checklist to be sure all processes related to central line placement are properly executed for every line placed.

Which antiseptic should be used to prepare the patient's skin for central venous line insertion?

- Chlorhexidine skin antisepsis has been proven to provide better skin antisepsis than other antiseptic agents, such as povidone–iodine solutions.
- Chlorhexidine 2% in 70% isopropyl alcohol should be applied using a back-and-forth friction scrub for at least 30 seconds; this should not be wiped or blotted dry.
- The antiseptic solution should be allowed time to dry completely before the insertion site is punctured/accessed (approximately 2 minutes).

What nursing interventions are essential to reduce the risk of infection?

- Maintaining sterile technique when changing the central venous line dressing
- Always performing hand hygiene before manipulating or accessing the line ports
- Wearing clean gloves prior to accessing the line port
- Performing a 15- to 30-second "hub scrub" using chlorhexidine or alcohol and friction in a twisting motion on the access hub (reduces biofilm on the hub that may contain pathogens)

When should central venous lines be discontinued?

- Assessment for removal of central venous lines should be included as part of the nurse's daily goal sheets.
- The time and date of central venous line placement should be recorded and evaluated by staff to aid in decision making.
- The need for the central venous line access should be reviewed as part of multidisciplinary rounds.
- During these rounds, the "line day" should be stated to remind everyone how long the central venous line has been in place (e.g., "Today is line day 6").
- An appropriate timeframe for regular review of the necessity for a central venous line should be identified, such as weekly, when central venous lines are placed for long-term use (e.g., chemotherapy, extended antibiotic administration).

Quality improvement processes that trend CLABSI rates and the compliance with CLABSI bundle prevention strategies have been found to effectively engage the multidisciplinary team in achieving goals to reduce infections related to central venous lines.

Adapted from Institute for Healthcare Improvement. (2012a). *How-to guide: Prevent central line-associated bloodstream infection.* Available at: www.ihi.org/knowledge/Pages/Tools/HowtoGuidePreventCentralLineAssociatedBloodstreamInfection.aspx; and Kaler, W. (2007). Successful disinfection of needleless mechanical access ports: A matter of time and friction. *Journal of the Association of Vascular Access, 12*(4), 203–205.

Parenteral or enteral nutritional support should be initiated as soon as possible. Enteral nutrition is preferred, promoting GI function through direct exposure to nutrients and limiting infectious complications associated with parenteral feeding (Blackhead, Boullata, Brantley, et al., 2009). Implementation of an evidence-based enteral feeding protocol that is tolerant of increased gastric residual volumes ensures the delivery of adequate nutrition to critically ill patients (Makic, VonRueden, Rauen, et al., 2011). Gastric residual volume does not predict a patient's risk of aspiration (Blackhead et al., 2009). (See Chapter 45 for further discussion of monitoring gastric residual volumes.)

Stress ulcers occur frequently in acutely ill patients because of the compromised blood supply to the GI tract. Therefore, antacids, H$_2$ blockers (e.g., famotidine [Pepcid],

ranitidine [Zantac]), and proton pump inhibitors (e.g., lansoprazole [Prevacid], esomeprazole magnesium [Nexium]) are prescribed to prevent ulcer formation by inhibiting gastric acid secretion or increasing gastric pH.

Hypovolemic Shock

Hypovolemic shock, the most common type of shock, is characterized by decreased intravascular volume. Body fluid is contained in the intracellular and extracellular compartments. Intracellular fluid accounts for about two thirds of the total body water. The extracellular body fluid is found in one of two compartments: intravascular (inside blood vessels) or interstitial (surrounding tissues). The volume of interstitial

TABLE 14-2	Vasoactive Agents Used in Treating Shock	
Medication	Desired Action in Shock	Disadvantages
Inotropic Agents		
Dobutamine (Dobutrex) Dopamine (Intropin) Epinephrine (Adrenalin) Milrinone (Primacor)	Improve contractility, increase stroke volume, increase cardiac output	Increase oxygen demand of the heart
Vasodilators		
Nitroglycerin (Tridil) Nitroprusside (Nipride)	Reduce preload and afterload, reduce oxygen demand of heart	Cause hypotension
Vasopressor Agents		
Norepinephrine (Levophed) Dopamine (Intropin) Phenylephrine (Neo-Synephrine) Vasopressin (Pitressin)	Increase blood pressure by vasoconstriction	Increase afterload, thereby increasing cardiac workload; compromise perfusion to skin, kidneys, lungs, gastrointestinal tract

fluid is about three to four times that of intravascular fluid. Hypovolemic shock occurs when there is a reduction in intravascular volume by 15% to 30%, which represents a loss of 750 to 1,500 mL of blood in a 70-kg (154-lb) person (American College of Surgeons, 2008).

Pathophysiology

Hypovolemic shock can be caused by external fluid losses, as in traumatic blood loss, or by internal fluid shifts, as in severe dehydration, severe edema, or ascites (Chart 14-3). Intravascular volume can be reduced both by fluid loss and by fluid shifting between the intravascular and interstitial compartments.

The sequence of events in hypovolemic shock begins with a decrease in the intravascular volume. This results in decreased venous return of blood to the heart and subsequent decreased ventricular filling. Decreased ventricular filling results in decreased stroke volume (amount of blood ejected from the heart) and decreased cardiac output. When cardiac output drops, BP drops and tissues cannot be adequately perfused (Fig. 14-3).

 ## Medical Management

Major goals in the treatment of hypovolemic shock are to restore intravascular volume to reverse the sequence of events leading to inadequate tissue perfusion, to redistribute fluid volume, and to correct the underlying cause of the fluid loss as quickly as possible. Depending on the severity of shock and the patient's condition, often all three goals are addressed simultaneously.

Chart 14-3   RISK FACTORS
Hypovolemic Shock

External: Fluid Losses
- Trauma
- Surgery
- Vomiting
- Diarrhea
- Diuresis
- Diabetes insipidus

Internal: Fluid Shifts
- Hemorrhage
- Burns
- Ascites
- Peritonitis
- Dehydration

Treatment of the Underlying Cause

If the patient is hemorrhaging, efforts are made to stop the bleeding. This may involve applying pressure to the bleeding site or surgical interventions to stop internal bleeding. If the cause of the hypovolemia is diarrhea or vomiting, medications to treat diarrhea and vomiting are administered while efforts are made to identify and treat the cause. In older adult patients, dehydration may be the cause of hypovolemic shock.

Fluid and Blood Replacement

Beyond reversing the primary cause of the decreased intravascular volume, fluid replacement is of primary concern. At least two large-gauge IV lines are inserted to establish access for fluid administration. If an IV catheter cannot be quickly inserted, an intraosseous catheter may be used

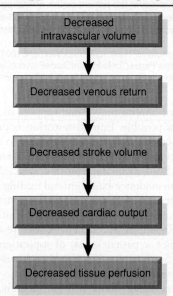

Physiology → Pathophysiology

Decreased intravascular volume → Decreased venous return → Decreased stroke volume → Decreased cardiac output → Decreased tissue perfusion

FIGURE 14-3 • Pathophysiologic sequence of events in hypovolemic shock.

TABLE 14-3	**Fluid Replacement in Shock***	
Fluids	**Advantages**	**Disadvantages**
Crystalloids		
0.9% sodium chloride (normal saline solution)	Widely available, inexpensive	Requires large volume of infusion; can cause hypernatremia, pulmonary edema, abdominal compartment syndrome
Lactated Ringer's	Lactate ion that helps buffer metabolic acidosis	Requires large volume of infusion; can cause metabolic acidosis, pulmonary edema, abdominal compartment syndrome
Hypertonic saline (3%)	Small volume needed to restore intravascular volume	Danger of hypernatremia and cardiovascular compromise from rapid fluid shifts
Colloids		
Albumin (5%, 25%)	Rapidly expands plasma volume	Expensive; requires human donors; limited supply; can cause heart failure

*Deliver a minimum of 20 mL/kg of crystalloid (or colloid equivalent).

for access in the sternum, legs, arms, or pelvis to facilitate rapid fluid replacement (Day, 2011). Multiple IV lines allow simultaneous administration of fluid, medications, and blood component therapy if required. Because the goal of the fluid replacement is to restore intravascular volume, it is necessary to administer fluids that will remain in the intravascular compartment to avoid fluid shifts from the intravascular compartment into the intracellular compartment. Table 14-3 summarizes the fluids commonly used in the treatment of shock.

As discussed earlier, crystalloid solutions such as lactated Ringer's solution or 0.9% sodium chloride solution are commonly used to treat hypovolemic shock, as large amounts of fluid must be administered to restore intravascular volume. If hypovolemia is primarily due to blood loss, the American College of Surgeons (2008) recommends administration of 3 mL of crystalloid solution for each milliliter of estimated blood loss. This is referred to as the 3:1 rule. Colloid solutions (e.g., albumin) may also be used. Hetastarch and dextran solutions are not indicated for fluid administration because these agents interfere with platelet aggregation.

Blood products, which are also colloids, may need to be administered, particularly if the cause of the hypovolemic shock is hemorrhage. The decision to give blood is based on the patient's lack of response to crystalloid resuscitation, the volume of blood lost, the need for hemoglobin to assist with oxygen transport, and the necessity to correct the patient's coagulopathy. It should be noted that research indicates that patients who receive massive blood transfusions to achieve near-normal hemoglobin levels tend to have poorer outcomes than those with low hemoglobin levels (e.g., less than 7 g/dL) (Santry & Alam, 2010).

Packed red blood cells are administered to replenish the patient's oxygen-carrying capacity in conjunction with other fluids that will expand volume. The need for transfusions is based on the patient's oxygenation needs, which are determined by vital signs, blood gas values, and clinical appearance rather than an arbitrary laboratory value. An area of active research is the development of synthetic forms of blood (i.e., compounds capable of carrying oxygen in the same way that blood does) as potential alternatives to blood component therapy.

Redistribution of Fluid

In addition to administering fluids to restore intravascular volume, positioning the patient properly assists fluid redistribution. A modified Trendelenburg position (Fig. 14-4) is

recommended in hypovolemic shock. Elevation of the legs promotes the return of venous blood. A full Trendelenburg position makes breathing difficult and does not increase BP or cardiac output (Bridges & Jarquin-Valdivia, 2005; Makic et al., 2011).

Pharmacologic Therapy

If fluid administration fails to reverse hypovolemic shock, then vasoactive medications that prevent cardiac failure are given. Medications are also administered to reverse the cause of the dehydration. For example, insulin is administered if dehydration is secondary to hyperglycemia, desmopressin (DDAVP) is administered for diabetes insipidus, antidiarrheal agents for diarrhea, and antiemetic medications for vomiting.

Nursing Management

Primary prevention of shock is an essential focus of nursing care. Hypovolemic shock can be prevented in some instances by closely monitoring patients who are at risk for fluid deficits and assisting with fluid replacement before intravascular volume is depleted. In other circumstances, nursing care focuses on assisting with treatment targeted at the cause of the shock and restoring intravascular volume.

General nursing measures include ensuring safe administration of prescribed fluids and medications and documenting their administration and effects. Another important nursing role is monitoring for complications and side effects of treatment and reporting them promptly.

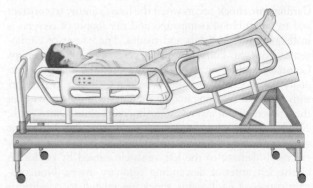

FIGURE 14-4 • Proper positioning (modified Trendelenburg) for the patient who shows signs of shock. The lower extremities are elevated to an angle of about 20 degrees; the knees are straight, the trunk is horizontal, and the head is slightly elevated.

Administering Blood and Fluids Safely

Administering blood transfusions safely is a vital nursing role. In emergency situations, it is important to acquire blood specimens quickly, to obtain a baseline complete blood count, and to type and cross-match the blood in anticipation of blood transfusions. A patient who receives a transfusion of blood products must be monitored closely for adverse effects (see Chapter 33).

Fluid replacement complications can occur, especially when large volumes are administered rapidly. Therefore, the nurse monitors the patient closely for cardiovascular overload, signs of difficulty breathing, and pulmonary edema. The risk of these complications is increased in older adults and in patients with preexisting cardiac disease. ACS is also a possible complication of excessive fluid resuscitation and may initially present with respiratory symptoms (difficulty breathing) and decreased urine output (Paula, 2011). Hemodynamic pressure, vital signs, arterial blood gases, serum lactate levels, hemoglobin and hematocrit levels, bladder pressure monitoring, and fluid intake and output (I&O) are among the parameters monitored. Temperature should also be monitored closely to ensure that rapid fluid resuscitation does not cause hypothermia. IV fluids may need to be warmed when large volumes are administered. Physical assessment focuses on observing the jugular veins for distention and monitoring jugular venous pressure. Jugular venous pressure is low in hypovolemic shock; it increases with effective treatment and is significantly increased with fluid overload and heart failure. The nurse must monitor cardiac and respiratory status closely and report changes in BP, pulse pressure, CVP, heart rate and rhythm, and lung sounds to the primary provider.

Implementing Other Measures

Oxygen is administered to increase the amount of oxygen carried by available hemoglobin in the blood. A patient who is confused may feel apprehensive with an oxygen mask or cannula in place, and frequent explanations about the need for the mask may reduce some of the patient's fear and anxiety. Simultaneously, the nurse must direct efforts to the safety and comfort of the patient.

Cardiogenic Shock

Cardiogenic shock occurs when the heart's ability to contract and to pump blood is impaired and the supply of oxygen is inadequate for the heart and tissues. The causes of cardiogenic shock are known as either coronary or noncoronary. Coronary cardiogenic shock is more common than noncoronary cardiogenic shock and is seen most often in patients with acute MI resulting in damage to a significant portion of the left ventricular myocardium (Buerke, Lemm, Dietz, et al., 2011). Patients who experience an anterior wall MI are at greatest risk for cardiogenic shock because of the potentially extensive damage to the left ventricle caused by occlusion of the left anterior descending coronary artery. Noncoronary causes of cardiogenic shock are related to conditions that stress the myocardium (e.g., severe hypoxemia, acidosis, hypoglycemia, hypocalcemia, tension pneumothorax) as well as conditions that result in ineffective myocardial function

(e.g., cardiomyopathies, valvular damage, cardiac tamponade, dysrhythmias).

Pathophysiology

In cardiogenic shock, cardiac output, which is a function of both stroke volume and heart rate, is compromised. When stroke volume and heart rate decrease or become erratic, BP falls and tissue perfusion is reduced. Blood supply for tissues and organs and for the heart muscle itself is inadequate, resulting in impaired tissue perfusion. Because impaired tissue perfusion weakens the heart and impairs its ability to pump, the ventricle does not fully eject its volume of blood during systole. As a result, fluid accumulates in the lungs. This sequence of events can occur rapidly or over a period of days (Fig. 14-5).

Clinical Manifestations

Patients in cardiogenic shock may experience the pain of angina, develop dysrhythmias, complain of fatigue, express feelings of doom, and show signs of hemodynamic instability.

 Medical Management

The goals of medical management in cardiogenic shock are to limit further myocardial damage and preserve the healthy myocardium and to improve cardiac function by increasing cardiac contractility, decreasing ventricular afterload, or both (Buerke et al., 2011). In general, these goals are achieved by increasing oxygen supply to the heart muscle while reducing oxygen demands.

Correction of Underlying Causes

As with all forms of shock, the underlying cause of cardiogenic shock must be corrected. It is necessary first to treat the oxygenation needs of the heart muscle to ensure its continued ability to pump blood to other organs. In the case of coronary cardiogenic shock, the patient may require thrombolytic/fibrinolytic therapy, a percutaneous coronary intervention (PCI),

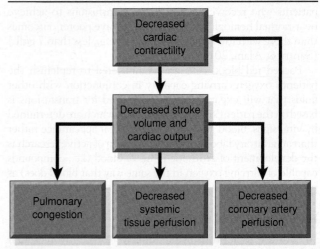

FIGURE 14-5 • Pathophysiologic sequence of events in cardiogenic shock.

coronary artery bypass graft (CABG) surgery, intra-aortic balloon pump therapy, or some combination of these treatments. In the case of noncoronary cardiogenic shock, interventions focus on correcting the underlying cause, such as replacement of a faulty cardiac valve, correction of a dysrhythmia, correction of acidosis and electrolyte disturbances, or treatment of a tension pneumothorax. If the cause of the cardiogenic shock was related to a cardiac arrest, once the patient is successfully resuscitated, targeted temperature management, also called *therapeutic hypothermia*, may be initiated to actively lower the body temperature to a targeted core temperature (e.g., 32°C [89.6°F] to 34°C [93.2°F]) to preserve neurologic function (Neumer, Barnhart, Berg, et al., 2011; Nunnally, Jaeschke, Bellingan, et al., 2011). (See Chapter 27 for more information regarding MI.)

Initiation of First-Line Treatment

Oxygenation

In the early stages of shock, supplemental oxygen is administered by nasal cannula at a rate of 2 to 6 L/min to achieve an oxygen saturation exceeding 90%. Monitoring of arterial blood gas values, pulse oximetry values, and ventilatory effort helps determine whether the patient requires a more aggressive method of oxygen delivery (including mechanical ventilation).

Pain Control

If a patient experiences chest pain, IV morphine is administered for pain relief. In addition to relieving pain, morphine dilates the blood vessels. This reduces the workload of the heart by both decreasing the cardiac filling pressure (preload) and reducing the pressure against which the heart muscle has to eject blood (afterload). Morphine also decreases the patient's anxiety.

Hemodynamic Monitoring

Hemodynamic monitoring is initiated to assess the patient's response to treatment. In many institutions, this is performed in the intensive care unit (ICU), where an arterial line can be inserted. The arterial line enables accurate and continuous monitoring of BP and provides a port from which to obtain frequent arterial blood samples without having to perform repeated arterial punctures. A multilumen pulmonary artery catheter may be inserted to allow measurement of the pulmonary artery pressures, myocardial filling pressures, cardiac output, and pulmonary and systemic resistance. (For more information, see Chapter 25.)

Laboratory Marker Monitoring

Laboratory markers for ventricular dysfunction (e.g., B-type natriuretic peptide [BNP]) and cardiac enzyme levels and biomarkers (CK-MB and cTn-I) are measured, and serial 12-lead ECGs are obtained to assess the degree of myocardial damage. Continuous ECG and ST segment monitoring is also used to closely monitor the patient for ischemic changes. An active area of research in the treatment of cardiogenic shock includes monitoring proinflammatory cytokine markers such as C-reactive protein (CRP) and procalcitonin levels (Shpektor, 2010).

Fluid Therapy

Appropriate fluid administration is also necessary in the treatment of cardiogenic shock. Administration of fluids must be monitored closely to detect signs of fluid overload. Incremental IV fluid boluses are cautiously administered to determine optimal filling pressures for improving cardiac output.

 Quality and Safety Nursing Alert

A fluid bolus should never be given rapidly, because rapid fluid administration in patients with cardiac failure may result in acute pulmonary edema.

Pharmacologic Therapy

Vasoactive medication therapy consists of multiple pharmacologic strategies to restore and maintain adequate cardiac output. In coronary cardiogenic shock, the aims of vasoactive medication therapy are improved cardiac contractility, decreased preload and afterload, and stabilized heart rate and rhythm.

Because improving contractility and decreasing cardiac workload are opposing pharmacologic actions, two types of medications may be administered in combination: inotropic agents and vasodilators. Inotropic medications increase cardiac output by mimicking the action of the sympathetic nervous system, activating myocardial receptors to increase myocardial contractility (inotropic action) or increasing the heart rate (chronotropic action). These agents may also enhance vascular tone, increasing preload. Vasodilators are used primarily to decrease afterload, reducing the workload of the heart and oxygen demand. Vasodilators also decrease preload. Medications commonly combined to treat cardiogenic shock include dobutamine, nitroglycerin, and dopamine (see Table 14-2).

Dobutamine. Dobutamine produces inotropic effects by stimulating myocardial beta-receptors, increasing the strength of myocardial activity and improving cardiac output. Myocardial alpha-adrenergic receptors are also stimulated, resulting in decreased pulmonary and systemic vascular resistance (decreased afterload) (Hollenberg, 2011).

Nitroglycerin. IV nitroglycerin in low doses acts as a venous vasodilator and therefore reduces preload. At higher doses, nitroglycerin causes arterial vasodilation and therefore reduces afterload as well. These actions, in combination with dobutamine, increase cardiac output while minimizing cardiac workload. In addition, vasodilation enhances blood flow to the myocardium, improving oxygen delivery to the weakened heart muscle (Buerke et al., 2011).

Dopamine. Dopamine is a sympathomimetic agent that has varying vasoactive effects depending on the dosage. It may be used with dobutamine and nitroglycerin to improve tissue perfusion. Doses of 2 to 8 μg/kg/min improve contractility (inotropic action), slightly increase the heart rate (chronotropic action), and may increase cardiac output. Doses that are higher than 8 μg/kg/min predominantly cause vasoconstriction, which increases afterload and thus increases cardiac workload. Because this effect is undesirable in patients with cardiogenic shock, dopamine doses must be carefully titrated.

Low-dose dopamine (i.e., 0.5 to 3 μg/kg/min) neither improves renal flow, changes the need for renal support, nor reduces mortality (Makic, Rauen, & Bridges, 2009) Thus, low-dose dopamine is no longer recommended. However, some patients respond to lower dosages of dopamine for its inotropic effects (Hollenberg, 2011).

In severe metabolic acidosis, which occurs in the later stages of shock, the effectiveness of dopamine is diminished. To maximize the effectiveness of any vasoactive agent, metabolic acidosis must first be corrected (Dellinger et al., 2013).

Other Vasoactive Medications. Additional vasoactive agents that may be used in managing cardiogenic shock include norepinephrine, epinephrine, milrinone, vasopressin, and phenylephrine. Each of these medications stimulates different receptors of the sympathetic nervous system. A combination of these medications may be prescribed, depending on the patient's response to treatment. All vasoactive medications have adverse effects, making specific medications more useful than others at different stages of shock. Diuretics such as furosemide may be administered to reduce the workload of the heart by reducing fluid accumulation (see Table 14-2).

Antiarrhythmic Medications. Multiple factors, such as hypoxemia, electrolyte imbalances, and acid–base imbalances, contribute to serious cardiac dysrhythmias in all patients with shock. In addition, as a compensatory response to decreased cardiac output and BP, the heart rate increases beyond normal limits. This impedes cardiac output further by shortening diastole and thereby decreasing the time for ventricular filling. Consequently, antiarrhythmic medications are required to stabilize the heart rate. General principles regarding the administration of vasoactive medications are discussed later in this chapter. (For a full discussion of cardiac dysrhythmias as well as commonly prescribed medications, see Chapter 26.)

Mechanical Assistive Devices

If cardiac output does not improve despite supplemental oxygen, vasoactive medications, and fluid boluses, mechanical assistive devices are used temporarily to improve the heart's ability to pump. Intra-aortic balloon counterpulsation is one means of providing temporary circulatory assistance (see Chapter 29). Other means of mechanical assistance include left and right ventricular assist devices and total temporary artificial hearts (see Chapters 28 and 29.) Another short-term means of providing cardiac or pulmonary support to the patient in cardiogenic shock is through an extracorporeal device similar to the cardiopulmonary bypass (CPB) system used in open-heart surgery (see Chapter 27). CPB is used only in emergency situations until definitive treatment, such as heart transplantation, can be initiated.

 Nursing Management

Preventing Cardiogenic Shock

Identifying at-risk patients early, promoting adequate oxygenation of the heart muscle, and decreasing cardiac workload can prevent cardiogenic shock. This can be accomplished by conserving the patient's energy, promptly relieving angina, and administering supplemental oxygen. Often, however, cardiogenic shock cannot be prevented. In such instances, nursing management includes working with other members of the health care team to prevent shock from progressing and to restore adequate cardiac function and tissue perfusion.

Monitoring Hemodynamic Status

A major role of the nurse is monitoring the patient's hemodynamic and cardiac status. Arterial lines and ECG monitoring equipment must be well maintained and functioning properly. The nurse anticipates the medications, IV fluids, and equipment that might be used and is ready to assist in implementing these measures. Changes in hemodynamic, cardiac, and pulmonary status and laboratory values are documented and reported promptly. In addition, adventitious breath sounds, changes in cardiac rhythm, and other abnormal physical assessment findings are reported immediately.

Administering Medications and Intravenous Fluids

The nurse plays a critical role in the safe and accurate administration of IV fluids and medications. Fluid overload and pulmonary edema are risks because of ineffective cardiac function and accumulation of blood and fluid in the pulmonary tissues. The nurse documents medications and treatments that are administered as well as the patient's response to treatment.

The nurse must be knowledgeable about the desired effects as well as the side effects of medications. For example, the nurse monitors the patient for decreased BP after administering morphine or nitroglycerin. Arterial and venous puncture sites must be observed for bleeding, and pressure must be applied at the sites if bleeding occurs. IV infusions must be observed closely because tissue necrosis and sloughing may occur if vasopressor medications infiltrate the tissues. The nurse must also monitor urine output, BUN, and serum creatinine levels to detect decreased renal function secondary to the effects of cardiogenic shock or its treatment.

Maintaining Intra-aortic Balloon Counterpulsation

The nurse plays a critical role in caring for the patient receiving intra-aortic balloon counterpulsation (see Chapter 29). The nurse makes ongoing timing adjustments of the balloon pump to maximize its effectiveness by synchronizing it with the cardiac cycle. The patient is at risk of circulatory compromise to the leg on the side where the catheter for the balloon has been inserted; therefore, the nurse must check the neurovascular status of the lower extremities frequently.

Enhancing Safety and Comfort

The nurse must take an active role in safeguarding the patient, enhancing comfort, and reducing anxiety. This includes administering medication to relieve chest pain, preventing infection at the multiple arterial and venous line insertion sites, protecting the skin, and monitoring respiratory and renal function. Proper positioning of the patient promotes effective breathing without decreasing BP and may also increase patient comfort while reducing anxiety.

Brief explanations about procedures that are being performed and the use of comforting touch often provide reassurance to the patient and family. The family is usually anxious and benefits from opportunities to see and talk to the patient. Explanations of treatments and the patient's responses are often comforting to family members.

Circulatory Shock

Circulatory shock, also called *distributive shock*, occurs when intravascular volume pools in peripheral blood vessels. This abnormal displacement of intravascular volume causes a relative hypovolemia because not enough blood returns to the heart, which leads to inadequate tissue perfusion. The ability of the blood vessels to constrict helps return the blood to the heart. The vascular tone is determined both by central regulatory mechanisms, as in BP regulation, and by local regulatory mechanisms, as in tissue demands for oxygen and nutrients. Therefore, circulatory shock can be caused either by a loss of sympathetic tone or by release of biochemical mediators from cells that causes vasodilation.

The varied mechanisms leading to the initial vasodilation in circulatory shock provide the basis for the further subclassification of shock into three types: septic shock, neurogenic shock, and anaphylactic shock. These subtypes of circulatory shock cause variations in the pathophysiologic chain of events and are explained here separately. In all types of circulatory shock, massive arterial and venous dilation promotes peripheral pooling of blood. Arterial dilation reduces systemic vascular resistance. Initially, cardiac output can be high, both from the reduction in afterload (systemic vascular resistance) and from the heart muscle's increased effort to maintain perfusion despite the incompetent vasculature. Pooling of blood in the periphery results in decreased venous return. Decreased venous return results in decreased stroke volume and decreased cardiac output. Decreased cardiac output, in turn, causes decreased BP and ultimately decreased tissue perfusion. Figure 14-6 presents the pathophysiologic sequence of events in circulatory shock.

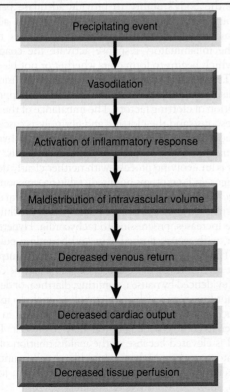

Physiology ········ Pathophysiology

Precipitating event

↓

Vasodilation

↓

Activation of inflammatory response

↓

Maldistribution of intravascular volume

↓

Decreased venous return

↓

Decreased cardiac output

↓

Decreased tissue perfusion

FIGURE 14-6 • Pathophysiologic sequence of events in circulatory shock.

■ *Septic Shock*

Septic shock, the most common type of circulatory shock, is caused by widespread infection or sepsis. Sepsis occurs in stages that may progress from uncomplicated sepsis, to severe sepsis, to septic shock (Chart 14-4). Despite the increased sophistication of antibiotic therapy, the incidence of septic shock has continued to rise. It is the leading cause of death in noncoronary ICU patients. More than 18 million cases of severe sepsis occur each year, resulting in approximately 1,400 deaths worldwide every day. The number of severe sepsis cases in the United States is anticipated to grow at a rate of 1.5% per year, from the current annual incidence of 3.0 cases per 1,000 of the U.S. population, or approximately 1 million cases per year by 2020 (Surviving Sepsis Campaign, 2011). Finding and aggressively treating the source of infection and quickly restoring tissue perfusion are important interventions that may positively influence the clinical outcome.

Health care–associated infections (infections not incubating at the time of admission to the health care setting) in critically ill patients that may progress to septic shock most frequently originate in the bloodstream (bacteremia), lungs (pneumonia), and urinary tract (urosepsis). Other infections include intra-abdominal infections and wound infections. Of increasing concern are bacteremias associated with intravascular catheters and indwelling urinary catheters (Institute for Healthcare Improvement [IHI], 2012a).

Additional risk factors that contribute to the growing incidence of septic shock are the increased use of invasive procedures and indwelling medical devices, the increased number of antibiotic-resistant microorganisms, and the increasingly older population (Funk et al., 2009). Older adult patients are at particular risk for sepsis because of decreased physiologic reserves and an aging immune system (Tiruvoipati, Ong, Gangopadhyay, et al., 2010). Other patients at risk are those undergoing surgical and other invasive procedures, especially patients who have emergency surgery or multiple surgeries (Fried, Weissman & Sprung, 2011); those with malnutrition or immunosuppression; and those with chronic illness such as diabetes, hepatitis, chronic renal failure, and immunodeficiency disorders (Gustot, 2011).

The incidence of septic shock can be reduced by using strict infection control practices, beginning with thorough hand-hygiene techniques (Fried et al., 2011). Other interventions

---

Chart 14-5 Definitions to Promote Recognition and Earlier Treatment of Patients With Sepsis

- **Bacteremia:** the presence of bacteria in the blood
- **Infection:** the presence of microorganisms that trigger an inflammatory response
- **Hypotension:** a systolic blood pressure <90 mm Hg or a drop in systolic blood pressure of >40 mm Hg from the patient's baseline blood pressure
- **Systemic inflammatory response syndrome (SIRS):** a syndrome resulting from a *severe clinical insult* that initiates an overwhelming inflammatory response by the body; clinical signs and symptoms may include:
  - Temperature >38°C (>100.4°F) or <36°C (<96.8°F)
  - Heart rate >90 bpm
  - Respiratory rate >20 breaths/min or partial pressure of arterial carbon dioxide ($PaCO_2$) <32 mm Hg
  - White blood cell (WBC) count >12,000 cells/mm^3, <4,000 cells/mm^3, or >10% immature WBC (bands)
- **Sepsis:** a systemic response to *infection;* manifested by two or more of the SIRS criteria as a consequence of documented or presumed infection
- **Severe sepsis:** the presence of signs and symptoms of sepsis associated with organ dysfunction, hypotension, and/or hypoperfusion; clinical signs and symptoms include those of sepsis as well as:

- Lactic acidosis
- Oliguria
- Altered level of consciousness
- Thrombocytopenia and coagulation disorders
- Altered hepatic function
- **Septic shock:** shock associated with sepsis; characterized by symptoms of sepsis plus hypotension and hypoperfusion despite adequate fluid volume replacement
- **Multiple organ dysfunction syndrome (MODS):** the presence of altered function of more than one organ in an acutely ill patient requiring intervention and support of the organs to achieve physiologic functioning required for homeostasis; clinical signs and symptoms may be:
  - *Cardiovascular:* hypotension and hypoperfusion
  - *Respiratory:* hypoxemia, hypercarbia, adventitious breath sounds
  - *Renal:* increased creatinine, decreased urine output
  - *Hematologic:* thrombocytopenia, coagulation abnormalities
  - *Metabolic:* lactic acidemia, metabolic acidosis
  - *Neurologic:* altered level of consciousness
  - *Hepatic:* elevated liver function tests, hyperbilirubinemia

Adapted from Levy, M. M., Fink, M. P., Marshall, J. C., et al. (2003). 2001 SCCM/ESICM/ACCP/ATS/SIS International Sepsis Definitions Conference. *Critical Care Medicine, 31*(4), 1250–1256; and Dellinger, R. P., Levy, M. M., Rhodes, A., et al. (2013). Surviving Sepsis Campaign: International guidelines for management of severe sepsis and septic shock: 2012. *Critical Care Medicine, 41*(2), 580–637.

---

include implementing programs to prevent central line infection; ensuring early removal of invasive devices that are no longer necessary (e.g., indwelling urinary catheters); implementing prevention programs to prevent VAP; early débriding of wounds to remove necrotic tissue; carrying out standard precautions and adhering to infection prevention/control practices, including the use of meticulous aseptic technique; and properly cleaning equipment and the patient environment.

A significant body of research has been conducted in the past two decades that is aimed at reducing the morbidity and mortality caused by septic shock and at clarifying the understanding of sepsis and related disorders (Chart 14-5). In 1991, 2003, 2008, and again in 2012, critical care experts and infectious disease experts systematically reevaluated the body of research and provided evidence-based recommendations for the acute management of patients with sepsis and septic shock (Dellinger et al., 2013; Surviving Sepsis Campaign, 2013). Developing and implementing protocols that focus on prevention and early detection and management of patients with sepsis have reduced the mortality of hospitalized patients (Westphal, Koenig, Filho, et al., 2011).

Pathophysiology

Gram-negative bacteria traditionally have been the most commonly implicated microorganisms in septic shock. However, there is an increased incidence of gram-positive bacterial infections, viral infections, and fungal infections that can also cause sepsis (Funk et al., 2009). Although a site of infection is identified in most cases, up to 30% of patients with severe sepsis may never have an identifiable site of infection (Surviving Sepsis Campaign, 2011).

When microorganisms invade body tissues, patients exhibit an immune response. This immune response provokes the activation of biochemical cytokines and mediators associated with an inflammatory response and produces a complex cascade of physiologic events that leads to poor tissue perfusion. Increased capillary permeability results in fluid seeping from the capillaries. Capillary instability and vasodilation interrupt the body's ability to provide adequate perfusion, oxygen, and nutrients to the tissues and cells. In addition, proinflammatory and anti-inflammatory cytokines released during the inflammatory response activate the coagulation system, which begins to form clots whether or not bleeding is present. This results not only in microvascular occlusions that further disrupt cellular perfusion but also in an inappropriate consumption of clotting factors. The imbalance of the inflammatory response and the clotting and fibrinolysis cascades are considered critical elements of the devastating physiologic progression that occurs in patients with severe sepsis.

Sepsis is an evolving process, with neither clearly definable clinical signs and symptoms nor predictable progression. In the early stage of septic shock, BP may remain within normal limits, or the patient may be hypotensive but responsive to fluids. The heart rate increases, progressing to tachycardia. Hyperthermia and fever, with warm, flushed skin and bounding pulses, are present. The respiratory rate is elevated. Urinary output may remain at normal levels or decrease. GI status may be compromised, as evidenced by nausea, vomiting, diarrhea, or decreased gastric motility. Signs of hypermetabolism include increased serum glucose and insulin resistance. Subtle changes in mental status, such as confusion or agitation, may be present. The lactate level is elevated because of the maldistribution of blood. Inflammatory markers such as white blood cell counts, CRP and procalcitonin levels are also elevated (Heyland, Johnson, Reynolds, et al., 2011; Powers & Burchell, 2010).

As sepsis progresses, tissues become less perfused and acidotic, compensation begins to fail, and the patient begins to

Chart 14-6 Early Identification and Management of Patients With Sepsis and Severe Sepsis

Questions to Ask

Does the patient meet criteria for systemic inflammatory response syndrome (SIRS) (see Chart 14-5)?

Does the patient have signs or symptoms of infection?
- Positive blood cultures
- Currently receiving antibiotic or antifungal therapy
- Examination or chest x-ray suggestive of pneumonia
- Suspected infected wound, abdomen, urine, or other source of infection

Does the patient have signs of acute organ dysfunction?
- *Cardiovascular:* systolic blood pressure (BP) <90 mm Hg or mean arterial pressure (MAP) <65 mm Hg, or drop in systolic BP >40 mm Hg from baseline BP:
  - Is hypotension responsive to fluid resuscitation, or is vasopressor support needed?
  - Is the serum lactate >4 mmol/L?
- *Respiratory:* respiratory rate >20 breaths/min or partial pressure of arterial carbon dioxide ($PaCO_2$) <32 mm Hg:
  - Is increasing oxygen and/or mechanical ventilator support needed?
- *Renal:* urine output <0.5 mL/kg/h
- *Hematologic:* laboratory analysis and signs and symptoms of coagulopathies
- *Metabolic:* insulin resistance, metabolic acidosis, and/or serum lactate >4 mmol/L
- *Hepatic:* elevated liver function tests and/or hyperbilirubinemia
- *Central nervous system:* changes in level of consciousness ranging from agitation to coma

Early Management (Sepsis Bundle)

- Initiate aggressive fluid resuscitation in patients with hypotension or elevated serum lactate (>4 mmol/L):

- Fluid resuscitate using crystalloids at 30 mL/kg (or colloid equivalent)
- Fluid challenges of 1,000 mL of crystalloids or 300 to 500 mL of colloids over 30 min may be required to treat tissue hypoperfusion
- Administer fluids to achieve a target central venous pressure of 8 to 12 mm Hg, MAP >65 mm Hg, urine output >0.5 mL/kg/h, and a central venous oxygen saturation ($Sc\overline{v}O_2$) >70%.
- Vasopressor agents are used if fluid resuscitation does not restore an effective BP and cardiac output:
  - Norepinephrine centrally administered is the initial vasopressor of choice.
  - Epinephrine, phenylephrine, or vasopressin should not be administered as the initial vasopressor in septic shock.
- Obtain blood, sputum, urine, and wound cultures, and administer broad spectrum antibiotics:
  - Cultures should be obtained prior to antibiotic administration.
  - Antibiotic administration should occur within 3 hours of admission to the emergency department or within 1 hour of inpatient admission.
- Support the respiratory system with supplemental oxygen and mechanical ventilation.
- Transfuse with packed red blood cells when hemoglobin is <7 g/dL to achieve a target hemoglobin of 7 to 9 g/dL in adults.
- Provide adequate IV sedation and analgesia; avoid the use of neuromuscular blockade agents when possible.
- Control serum glucose <180 mg/dL with IV insulin therapy.
- Implement interventions and medications to prevent deep vein thrombosis and stress ulcer prophylaxis.
- Consider IV hydrocortisone therapy if the patient is not responding to fluid resuscitation and vasopressor therapy.
- Discuss advance care planning with patients and families.

Adapted from Dellinger, R. P., Levy, M. M., Rhodes, A., et al. (2013). Surviving Sepsis Campaign: International guidelines for management of severe sepsis and septic shock: 2012. *Critical Care Medicine, 41*(2), 580–637; and Surviving Sepsis Campaign. (2011). Available at: www.survivingsepsis.org.

show signs of organ dysfunction. The cardiovascular system also begins to fail, the BP does not respond to fluid resuscitation and vasoactive agents, and signs of end-organ damage are evident (e.g., AKI, pulmonary dysfunction, hepatic dysfunction). As sepsis progresses to septic shock, the BP drops and the skin becomes cool, pale, and mottled. Temperature may be normal or below normal. Heart and respiratory rates remain rapid. Urine production ceases, and multiple organ dysfunction progressing to death occurs.

Systemic inflammatory response syndrome (SIRS) presents like sepsis clinically and is part of the initial continuum of sepsis. The physiologic presentation of SIRS is similar to sepsis, except there is no identifiable source of infection (Dellinger et al., 2013). SIRS stimulates an overwhelming inflammatory immunologic and hormonal response seen in septic patients and may progress to sepsis. Therefore, despite an absence of infection, antibiotic agents may still be administered because of the possibility of unrecognized infection. Additional therapies directed to support patients with SIRS are similar to those for sepsis. If the inflammatory process progresses, septic shock may develop.

 Medical Management

Current treatment of sepsis and septic shock involves identification and elimination of the cause of infection. Current

goals are to identify and treat patients in early sepsis within 6 hours to optimize patient outcome (Surviving Sepsis Campaign, 2011). Several evidence-based screening tools can be used to help identify patients for severe sepsis. Chart 14-6 provides key elements of assessment and interventions that, when used together, may help identify patients with sepsis and guide early interventions in the treatment of severe sepsis and septic shock (IHI, 2012b; Surviving Sepsis Campaign, 2011).

Rapid identification of the infectious source is a critical element in managing sepsis. Specimens of blood, sputum, urine, wound drainage, and tips of invasive catheters are collected for culture using aseptic technique. IV lines are removed and reinserted at alternate sites. If possible, urinary catheters are removed or changed. Any abscesses are drained, and necrotic areas are débrided. All cultures should be obtained prior to antibiotic administration. Current guidelines suggest that antibiotics should be initiated within the first hour of treatment of a patient with sepsis (Surviving Sepsis Campaign, 2011).

Research efforts are focusing on better identification and early aggressive treatment of patients with sepsis, rapid and effective restoration of tissue perfusion, evaluation and treatment of the patient's immune response, and treatment of dysregulation of the coagulation system that occurs with severe sepsis (Funk et al., 2009).

Fluid Replacement Therapy

Fluid replacement must be instituted to correct tissue hypoperfusion that results from the incompetent vasculature and the inflammatory response. Reestablishing tissue perfusion through aggressive fluid resuscitation is key to the management of severe sepsis and septic shock (Dellinger et al., 2013; Nee & Rivers, 2011). Fluid challenges of 1,000 mL of crystalloids or 300 to 500 mL of colloids over 30 minutes may be required to aggressively treat sepsis-induced tissue hypoperfusion. In addition to monitoring BP, CVP, and urine output, serum lactate levels are monitored to assess effectiveness of fluid resuscitation. See Chart 14-6 for a list of the treatment endpoints of fluid resuscitation.

Pharmacologic Therapy

If the infecting organism is unknown, broad-spectrum antibiotic agents are started until culture and sensitivity reports are received (Dellinger et al., 2013; IHI, 2012b), at which time the antibiotic agents may be changed to agents that are more specific to the infecting organism and less toxic to the patient.

The 2008 guidelines for management of severe sepsis and septic shock recommend the administration of recombinant human activated protein C (rhAPC; drotrecogin alfa [Xigris]) to patients with end-organ dysfunction and high risk of death (Dellinger et al., 2013). However, ongoing research has found that the medication did not positively impact the outcome of patients with severe sepsis, and it is no longer available for patient use (Eli Lilly and Company, 2011).

If fluid therapy alone does not effectively improve tissue perfusion, vasopressor agents, specifically norepinephrine or dopamine, may be initiated to achieve a MAP of 65 mmHg or higher. Inotropic agents may also be administered to provide pharmacologic support to the myocardium. Packed red blood cells may be ordered to support oxygen delivery and transport to the tissues. Neuromuscular blockade agents and sedation agents may be required to reduce metabolic demands and provide comfort to the patient. Deep vein thrombosis (DVT) prophylaxis with low-dose unfractionated heparin or low-molecular-weight heparin, in combination with mechanical prophylaxis (e.g., sequential compression devices [SCDs]) should be initiated, as well as medications for stress ulcer prophylaxis (e.g., H$_2$ blocking agents, proton pump inhibitors).

Nutritional Therapy

Aggressive nutritional supplementation should be initiated within 24 to 48 hours of ICU admission to address the hypermetabolic state present with septic shock (Aikten, Williams, Harvey, et al., 2011). Malnutrition further impairs the patient's resistance to infection. Enteral feedings are preferred to the parenteral route because of the increased risk of iatrogenic infection associated with IV catheters; however, enteral feedings may not be possible if decreased perfusion to the GI tract reduces peristalsis and impairs absorption.

Nursing Management

Nurses caring for patients in any setting must keep in mind the risks of sepsis and the high mortality rate associated with sepsis, severe sepsis, and septic shock. All invasive procedures must be carried out with aseptic technique after careful hand hygiene. In addition, IV lines, arterial and venous puncture sites, surgical incisions, traumatic wounds, and urinary catheters must be monitored for signs of infection. Nursing interventions to prevent infection, specifically VAP, as well as actions to prevent pressure ulcers need to be implemented in the care of all patients. Nurses should identify patients who are at particular risk for sepsis and septic shock (i.e., older adults and immunosuppressed patients and those with extensive trauma, burns, or diabetes), keeping in mind that these high-risk patients may not develop typical or classic signs of infection and sepsis. For example, confusion may be the first sign of infection and sepsis in older adult patients.

When caring for a patient with septic shock, the nurse collaborates with other members of the health care team to identify the site and source of sepsis and the specific organisms involved. The nurse often obtains appropriate specimens for culture and sensitivity. Chart 14-7 highlights nursing considerations believed to be instrumental in preventing and treating severe sepsis.

Elevated body temperature (hyperthermia) is common with sepsis and raises the patient's metabolic rate and oxygen consumption. Fever is one of the body's natural mechanisms for fighting infections. Therefore, elevated temperatures may not be treated unless they reach dangerous levels (more than 40°C [104°F]) or unless the patient is uncomfortable. Efforts may be made to reduce the temperature by administering acetaminophen or applying a hypothermia blanket. During these therapies, the nurse monitors the patient closely for shivering, which increases oxygen consumption. Efforts to increase comfort are important if the patient experiences fever, chills, or shivering.

The nurse administers prescribed IV fluids and medications, including antibiotic agents and vasoactive medications, to restore vascular volume. Because of decreased perfusion, serum concentrations of antibiotic agents that are normally cleared by the kidneys and liver may increase and produce toxic effects. Therefore, the nurse monitors blood levels (peak and trough levels of antibiotic agents, procalcitonin, CRP, BUN, creatinine, white blood cell count, hemoglobin, hematocrit, platelet levels, coagulation studies) and reports changes to the primary provider. As with other types of shock, the nurse monitors the patient's hemodynamic status, fluid I&O, and nutritional status. Daily weights and close monitoring of serum albumin and prealbumin levels help determine the patient's protein requirements.

◼ Neurogenic Shock

In **neurogenic shock**, vasodilation occurs as a result of a loss of balance between parasympathetic and sympathetic stimulation. Sympathetic stimulation causes vascular smooth muscle to constrict, and parasympathetic stimulation causes vascular smooth muscle to relax or dilate. The patient experiences a predominant parasympathetic stimulation that causes vasodilation lasting for an extended period, leading to a relative hypovolemic state. However, blood volume is adequate, because the vasculature is dilated; the blood volume is displaced, producing a hypotensive (low BP) state. The overriding parasympathetic stimulation that occurs with neurogenic

NURSING RESEARCH PROFILE

Chart 14-7

Best Nursing Practices That Prevent and Treat Sepsis and Severe Sepsis

Aitken, L. M., Williams, G., Harvey, M., et al. (2011). Nursing considerations to complement the Surviving Sepsis Campaign guidelines. *Critical Care Medicine, 39*(7), 1800–1818.

Purpose

The Surviving Sepsis Campaign (SSC) guidelines provide a systematic and evidence-based review of best practices targeted at reducing sepsis-related morbidity and mortality throughout the globe. However, these practices do not specify implications for nursing care crucial to meeting these aims. Therefore, the purpose of this initiative was to provide evidence-based recommendations for best nursing practices that might supplement or augment the SSC guidelines.

Design

This study utilized a modified Delphi method that sampled focus-group teams of internationally recognized critical care nursing experts. It was conducted under the supervision of the World Federation of Critical Care Nurses. Sampled experts systematically reviewed the literature and utilized the GRADE system (i.e., Grades of Recommendation, Assessment, Development, and Evaluation) to rate the strength and quality of the evidence for various nursing practices and did not support a recommendation until full consensus was reached.

Findings

Sixty-three best nursing practice recommendations were made that were classified under the categories of infection prevention, infection management, severe sepsis and septic shock initial resuscitation, and severe sepsis and septic shock hemodynamic

support, as well as other supportive nursing care. Recommended infection prevention practices included implementing multifaceted best practice education initiatives, promoting cultures of safety, continuously surveying for nosocomial infections, promoting good hand hygiene, and utilizing practices aimed at preventing respiratory infections, catheter-related bloodstream infections, surgical site infections, and urinary tract infections. Infection management practices that were endorsed included promoting infection source control (i.e., removing suspected sources of infection such as IV and other catheters) and ensuring pathogen transmission precautions (e.g., implementing contact, droplet, and airborne precautions as needed). It was recommended that nurses participate in the initial resuscitation of patients diagnosed with severe sepsis or septic shock by using early warning systems and screening tools, seeking interdisciplinary medical assistance, initiating rapid response systems, and ensuring the provision of adequate resources, including adequate nursing staffing. With these same patients, it was recommended that nurses provide hemodynamic support by improving tissue oxygenation and improving macrocirculation. Other best nursing practices that were endorsed pertained to nutritional support, eye care, and pressure ulcer prevention and management.

Nursing Implications

This review summarizes the best and most current evidence of nursing practices aimed at preventing and treating severe sepsis and septic shock. Whereas endorsed best practices aimed at managing patients with severe sepsis and septic shock are targeted primarily at critical care nurses, the best practices aimed at preventing and managing infections have implications for nursing practice in any setting or any specialty.

---

shock causes a drastic decrease in the patient's systemic vascular resistance and bradycardia. Inadequate BP results in the insufficient perfusion of tissues and cells that is common to all shock states.

Neurogenic shock can be caused by spinal cord injury, spinal anesthesia, or other nervous system damage (see Chart 14-4). It may also result from the depressant action of medications or from lack of glucose (e.g., insulin reaction). Neurogenic shock may have a prolonged course (spinal cord injury) or a short one (syncope or fainting). Normally, during states of stress, the sympathetic stimulation causes the BP and heart rate to increase. In neurogenic shock, the sympathetic system is not able to respond to body stressors. Therefore, the clinical characteristics of neurogenic shock are signs of parasympathetic stimulation. It is characterized by dry, warm skin rather than the cool, moist skin seen in hypovolemic shock. Another characteristic is hypotension with bradycardia, rather than the tachycardia that characterizes other forms of shock.

 Medical Management

Treatment of neurogenic shock involves restoring sympathetic tone, either through the stabilization of a spinal cord injury or, in the instance of spinal anesthesia, by positioning the patient properly. Specific treatment depends on the cause of the shock. (Further discussion of management of patients with a spinal cord injury is presented in Chapter 68.)

Nursing Management

It is important to elevate and maintain the head of the bed at least 30 degrees to prevent neurogenic shock when a patient receives spinal or epidural anesthesia. Elevation of the head helps prevent the spread of the anesthetic agent up the spinal cord. In suspected spinal cord injury, neurogenic shock may be prevented by carefully immobilizing the patient to prevent further damage to the spinal cord (Bader & Littlejohns, 2010).

Nursing interventions are directed toward supporting cardiovascular and neurologic function until the usually transient episode of neurogenic shock resolves. Patients with neurogenic shock have a higher risk for venous thromboembolism (VTE) formation because of increased pooling of blood from vascular dilation; this risk is greater in patients with neurogenic shock related to spinal cord injury (Christie, Thibault-Halman, Casha, 2009; Raslan, Fields, Bhardwaj, 2010). Therefore, the nurse must check the patient daily for any lower-extremity pain, redness, tenderness, and warmth. If the patient complains of pain and objective assessment of the calf is suspicious, the patient should be evaluated for DVT. Passive range of motion of the immobile extremities helps promote circulation. Early interventions to prevent VTE include the application of pneumatic compression devices often combined with antithrombotic agents (e.g., low-molecular-weight heparin).

A patient who has experienced a spinal cord injury may not report pain caused by internal injuries. Therefore, in the immediate postinjury period, the nurse must monitor the patient closely for signs of internal bleeding that could lead to hypovolemic shock.

■ Anaphylactic Shock

Anaphylactic shock is caused by a severe allergic reaction when patients who have already produced antibodies to a foreign substance (antigen) develop a systemic antigen–antibody reaction; specifically, an immunoglobulin E (IgE)-mediated response (see Chart 14-4). This antigen–antibody reaction provokes mast cells to release potent vasoactive substances, such as histamine or bradykinin, and activates inflammatory cytokines, causing widespread vasodilation and capillary permeability. The most common triggers are foods (especially peanuts), medications, and insects (Lee & Vadas, 2011). Anaphylaxis has three defining characteristics (Lee & Vadas, 2011):

- Acute onset of symptoms
- Presence of two or more symptoms that include respiratory compromise, reduced BP, GI distress, and skin or mucosal tissue irritation
- Cardiovascular compromise from minutes to hours after exposure to the antigen

Signs and symptoms of anaphylaxis may present within 5 to 30 minutes of exposure to the antigen; however, occasionally some reactions may not develop for several hours (Khan & Kemp, 2011). The patient may complain of headache, lightheadedness, nausea, vomiting, acute abdominal pain or discomfort, pruritus, and feeling of impending doom. Assessment may reveal diffuse erythema and generalized flushing, difficulty breathing (laryngeal edema), bronchospasm, cardiac dysrhythmias, and hypotension. Characteristics of severe anaphylaxis usually include rapid onset of hypotension, neurologic compromise, respiratory distress, and cardiac arrest (Khan & Kemp, 2011). Anaphylactoid reactions present similarly to anaphylaxis but are not mediated by IgE responses. Anaphylaxis and anaphylactoid reactions are often clinically indistinguishable (Lee & Vadas, 2011).

 Medical Management

Treatment of anaphylactic shock requires removing the causative antigen (e.g., discontinuing an antibiotic agent), administering medications that restore vascular tone, and providing emergency support of basic life functions. Fluid management is critical, as massive fluid shifts can occur within minutes due to increased vascular permeability (Lee & Vadas, 2011). Intramuscular epinephrine is administered for its vasoconstrictive action. Diphenhydramine (Benadryl) is administered IV to reverse the effects of histamine, thereby reducing capillary permeability. Nebulized medications, such as albuterol (Proventil), may be given to reverse histamine-induced bronchospasm.

If cardiac arrest and respiratory arrest are imminent or have occurred, cardiopulmonary resuscitation (CPR) is performed. Endotracheal intubation may be necessary to establish an airway. IV lines are inserted to provide access for administering fluids and medications. (See Chapter 38 for further discussion of anaphylaxis and specific chemical mediators.)

 Nursing Management

The nurse has an important role in prevention and early recognition of anaphylactic shock. The nurse must assess all patients for allergies or previous reactions to antigens (e.g., medications, blood products, foods, contrast agents, latex) and communicate the existence of these allergies or reactions to others. In addition, the nurse assesses the patient's understanding of previous reactions and steps taken by the patient and family to prevent further exposure to antigens. When new allergies are identified, the nurse advises the patient to wear or carry identification that names the specific allergen or antigen.

When administering any new medication, the nurse observes all patients for allergic reactions. This is especially important with antibiotics, beta-blockers, angiotensin inhibitors (angiotensin-converting enzyme [ACE] inhibitors, angiotensin receptor blockers [ARBs]), aspirin (ASA), and nonsteroidal anti-inflammatory drugs (NSAIDs) (Lee & Vadas, 2011). Previous adverse drug reactions increase the risk that the patient will develop a reaction to a new medication. If the patient reports an allergy to a medication, the nurse must be aware of the risks involved in the administration of similar medications.

At hospital and outpatient diagnostic testing sites, the nurse must identify patients who are at risk for anaphylactic reactions to contrast agents (radiopaque, dyelike substances that may contain iodine) used for diagnostic tests. Patients with a known allergy to iodine or fish and those who have had previous allergic reactions to contrast agents are at high risk. This information must be communicated to the staff at the diagnostic testing site, including x-ray personnel. The nurse must be knowledgeable about the clinical signs of anaphylaxis, must take immediate action if signs and symptoms occur, and must be prepared to begin CPR if cardiorespiratory arrest occurs.

Community health and home care nurses who administer medications, including antibiotic agents, in the patient's home or other settings, must be prepared to administer epinephrine intramuscularly in the event of an anaphylactic reaction.

After recovery from anaphylaxis, the patient and family require an explanation of the event. Furthermore, the nurse provides education about avoiding future exposure to antigens and administering emergency medications to treat anaphylaxis (see Chapter 38).

Multiple Organ Dysfunction Syndrome

Multiple organ dysfunction syndrome (MODS) is altered organ function in acutely ill patients that requires medical intervention to support continued organ function. It is another phase in the progression of shock states. The actual incidence of MODS is difficult to determine, because it develops with acute illnesses that compromise tissue perfusion. Dysfunction of one organ system is associated with 20% mortality, and if more than four organs fail, the mortality may reach 65% (Gustot, 2011).

Pathophysiology

MODS may be a complication of any form of shock, but it is most commonly seen in patients with severe sepsis and is a result of inadequate tissue perfusion. The precise mechanism by which MODS occurs remains unknown. However, MODS frequently occurs toward the end of the continuum of septic shock when tissue perfusion cannot be effectively restored. It is not possible to predict which patients who experience shock will develop MODS, partly because much of the organ damage occurs at the cellular level and therefore cannot be directly observed or measured.

The clinical presentation of MODS is insidious; tissues become hypoperfused at both a microcellular and macrocellular level, eventually causing organ dysfunction that requires mechanical and pharmacologic intervention to support organ function. Organ failure usually begins in the lungs, and cardiovascular instability as well as failure of the hepatic, GI, renal, immunologic, and central nervous systems follow (VonRueden et al., 2009).

Clinical Manifestations

While it is not possible to predict MODS, clinical severity assessment tools may be used to anticipate patient risk of organ dysfunction and mortality. These clinical assessment tools include APACHE (Acute Physiology and Chronic Health Evaluation); SAPS (Simplified Acute Physiology Score); PIRO (Predisposing factors, the Infection, the host Response, and Organ dysfunction); and SOFA (Sequential Organ Failure Assessment) score (Gustot, 2011).

In MODS, the sequence of organ dysfunction varies depending on the patient's primary illness and comorbidities prior to experiencing shock. Advanced age, malnutrition, and coexisting disease appear to increase the risk of MODS in acutely ill patients. For simplicity of presentation, the classic pattern is described. Typically, the lungs are the first organs to show signs of dysfunction. The patient experiences progressive dyspnea and respiratory failure that is manifested as ALI or ARDS, requiring intubation and mechanical ventilation (see Chapters 23 and 25). The patient usually remains hemodynamically stable but may require increasing amounts of IV fluids and vasoactive agents to support BP and cardiac output. Signs of a hypermetabolic state, characterized by hyperglycemia (elevated blood glucose level), hyperlactic acidemia (excess lactic acid in the blood), and increased BUN, are present. The metabolic rate may be 1.5 to 2 times the basal metabolic rate. At this time, there is a severe loss of skeletal muscle mass (autocatabolism) to meet the high energy demands of the body.

After approximately 7 to 10 days, signs of hepatic dysfunction (e.g., elevated bilirubin and liver function tests) and renal dysfunction (e.g., elevated creatinine and anuria) are evident. As the lack of tissue perfusion continues, the hematologic system becomes dysfunctional, with worsening immunocompromise, increasing the risk of bleeding. The cardiovascular system becomes unstable and unresponsive to vasoactive agents, and the patient's neurologic response progresses to a state of unresponsiveness or coma.

The goal of all shock states is to reverse the tissue hypoperfusion and hypoxia. If effective tissue perfusion is restored before organs become dysfunctional, the patient's condition stabilizes. Along the septic shock continuum, the onset of organ dysfunction is an ominous prognostic sign; the more organs that fail, the worse the outcome.

 ## Medical Management

Prevention remains the top priority in managing MODS. Older adult patients are at increased risk for MODS because of the lack of physiologic reserve and the natural degenerative process, especially immune compromise (Rubulotta, Marshall, Ramsay, et al., 2009). Early detection and documentation of initial signs of infection are essential in managing MODS in older adult patients. Subtle changes in mentation and a gradual rise in temperature are early warning signs. Other patients at risk for MODS are those with chronic illness, malnutrition, immunosuppression, or surgical or traumatic wounds.

If preventive measures fail, treatment measures to reverse MODS are aimed at (1) controlling the initiating event, (2) promoting adequate organ perfusion, (3) providing nutritional support, and (4) maximizing patient comfort.

 ## Nursing Management

The general plan of nursing care for patients with MODS is the same as that for patients with septic shock. Primary nursing interventions are aimed at supporting the patient and monitoring organ perfusion until primary organ insults are halted. Providing information and support to family members is a critical role of the nurse. The health care team must address end-of-life decisions to ensure that supportive therapies are congruent with the patient's wishes (see Chapter 16).

Promoting Communication

Nurses should encourage frequent and open communication about treatment modalities and options to ensure that the patient's wishes regarding medical management are met. Patients who survive MODS must be informed about the goals of rehabilitation and expectations for progress toward these goals, because massive loss of skeletal muscle mass makes rehabilitation a long, slow process. A strong nurse–patient relationship built on effective communication provides needed encouragement during this phase of recovery.

Promoting Home and Community-Based Care

Educating Patients About Self-Care

Patients who experience and survive shock may have been unable to get out of bed for an extended period of time and are likely to have a slow, prolonged recovery. The patient and family are educated about strategies to prevent further episodes of shock by identifying the factors implicated in the initial episode. In addition, the patient and family require education about assessments needed to identify the complications that may occur after the patient is discharged from the hospital. Depending on the type of shock and its management, the patient or family may require education about treatment modalities such as emergency administration of medications, IV therapy, parenteral or enteral nutrition, skin care, exercise, and ambulation. The patient and family are also educated about the need for gradual increases in ambulation and other activity. The need for adequate nutrition is another crucial aspect of education.

Continuing Care

Because of the physical toll associated with recovery from shock, patients may be cared for in a long-term care facility or rehabilitation setting after hospital discharge. Alternatively, a referral may be made for home care. The home care nurse assesses the patient's physical status and monitors recovery. The nurse also assesses the adequacy of treatments that are continued at home and the ability of the patient and family to cope with these treatments. The patient is likely to require close medical supervision until complete recovery occurs. The home care nurse reinforces the importance of continuing medical care and helps the patient and family identify and mobilize community resources.

Critical Thinking Exercises

1 **pq** A patient preparing to have a valve replacement is prescribed a prophylactic dose of IV cefazolin preoperatively. The patient's chart states that he has no known drug allergies. Five minutes after the medication is administered, the patient complains of anxiety, shortness of breath, and chest discomfort. He is flushed and visibly uncomfortable. What are your nursing priorities in providing care to this patient? What assessment data do you need to obtain to determine if this patient is experiencing shock? Based on the history associated with the patient presentation, what type of shock do you anticipate the patient may be experiencing and why? What nursing interventions and medical treatments would you anticipate?

2 **ebp** A community-dwelling older woman is admitted to the hospital with a hip fracture after falling at home. She is now 72 hours post hip fracture repair. Initial shift assessment reveals the patient to be confused and somewhat combative in behavior. You know that changes in mental status may be an early sign of sepsis in older adults. How would you assess this patient for the possibility of sepsis? What risk factors place an older patient at higher risk for sepsis? What risk factors does this patient have that placed her at increased risk for sepsis? How would you ensure the accuracy of vital signs and interpretation of vital signs in the older patient experiencing sepsis? What is the evidence base for these risk factors? How would the management of the older adult patient differ from that of a younger patient?

3 A 34-year-old patient underwent left knee replacement surgery. He had regional anesthesia for the surgery and currently has a patent epidural catheter for pain management. What types of shock are possible in this patient? What therapy directed at prevention or treatment of shock would you anticipate? Describe the rationale for the therapies that you have identified. How would you use the patient's history and symptom presentation to help you identify shock states? Describe likely symptoms and the underlying pathophysiology of the shock state.

4 A 57-year-old construction worker presents to the emergency department complaining of generalized fatigue

and left-sided chest and arm pain. What clinical condition do you believe the patient may be experiencing? What type of shock may progress from his suspected clinical condition? If cardiogenic shock is suspected, what nursing interventions do you anticipate initiating in the care of this patient? What vasopressor and inotropic agents may need to be started? What risk factors can be identified for this patient related to his presenting condition and subsequent shock state?

Brunner Suite Resources

Explore these additional resources to enhance learning for this chapter:
- NCLEX-Style Questions and Other Resources on **thePoint**, http://thePoint.lww.com/Brunner13e
- Study Guide
- PrepU
- Clinical Handbook
- Handbook of Laboratory and Diagnostic Tests

References

*Asterisk indicates nursing research.
**Double asterisk indicates classic reference.

Books

American College of Surgeons, Committee on Trauma. (2008). *Resources for optimal care of the injured patient 2008.* Chicago: American College of Surgeons.

Bader, M. K., & Littlejohns, L. R. (2010). *AANN core curriculum for neuroscience nursing* (5th ed.). Chicago: AANN Publishers.

Boswell, S., & Scalea, T. M. (2009). Initial management of traumatic shock. In K. McQuillan, M. B. Flynn Makic, & E. Whalen (Eds.). *Trauma nursing from resuscitation through rehabilitation* (4th ed.). Philadelphia: Elsevier.

Maier, R. V. (2011). Approach to the patient with shock. In A. S. Fauci, E. Braunwald, D. L. Kasper, et al. (Eds.). *Harrison's principles of internal medicine* (18th ed.). New York: McGraw-Hill Medical.

VonRueden, K. T., Bolton, P. J., & Vary T. C. (2009). Shock and multiple organ dysfunction syndrome. In K. McQuillan, M. B. Flynn Makic, & E. Whalen (Eds.). *Trauma nursing from resuscitation through rehabilitation* (4th ed.). Philadelphia: Elsevier.

Journals and Electronic Documents

*Aitken, L. M., Williams, G., Harvey, M., et al. (2011). Nursing considerations to complement the surviving sepsis campaign guidelines. *Critical Care Medicine, 39*(7), 1800–1818.

Blackhead, R., Boullata, J., Brantley S., et al. (2009). ASPEN Board of Directors, Enteral nutrition practice recommendations. *Journal of Parenteral and Enteral Nutrition, 33,* 165–167.

Bradley, C., Lensky, M., & Brassel, K. (2011). Implementation of a family presence during resuscitation protocol. *Journal of Palliative Care, 14*(1), 98–99.

**Bridges, N., & Jarquin-Valdivia, A. A. (2005). Use of the Trendelenburg position as the resuscitation position: To T or not to T? *American Journal of Critical Care, 14*(3), 364–367.

Buerke, M., Lemm, H., Dietz, S., et al. (2011). Pathophysiology, diagnosis, and treatment of infarction-related cardiogenic shock. *Herz, 36*(2), 73–83.

Christie, S., Thibault-Halman, G., & Casha, S. (2009). Acute pharmacological DVT prophylaxis after spinal cord injury. *Journal of Neurotrauma, 28*(8), 1509–1514.

Cohen, J., & Venkatesh, B. (2010). Relative adrenal insufficiency in the intensive care population: Background and critical appraisal of the evidence. *Anaesthesia and Intensive Care, 38*(3), 425–436.

Coimbra, R. (2011). 3% and 5% hypertonic saline. *Journal of Trauma, Infection, Injury and Critical Care, 70*(5S), S25–S26.

Day, M. (2011). Intraosseous devices for intravascular access in adult trauma patients. *Critical Care Nurse, 31*(2), 76–89.

**Dellinger, R. P., Levy, M. M., Rhodes, A., et al., (2013). Surviving Sepsis Campaign: International guidelines for management of severe sepsis and septic shock: 2012. *Critical Care Medicine, 41*(2), 580–637.

Eli Lilly and Company. (October 25, 2011). *Lilly announces withdrawal of Xigris® following recent clinical trial results.* Available at: newsroom.lilly.com/releasedetail.cfm?releaseid=617602

Fried, E., Weissman, C., & Sprung, C. (2011). Postoperative sepsis. *Current Opinion in Critical Care, 17*(4), 396–401.

Funk, D., Sebat, F., & Kumar, A. (2009). A systems approach to the early recognition and rapid administration of best practice therapy in sepsis and septic shock. *Current Opinion in Critical Care, 15*(4), 301–307.

Girard, T. D., Kess, J. P., Fuchs, B. D., et al. (2008). Efficacy and safety of a paired sedation and ventilator weaning protocol for mechanically ventilated patients in intensive care. *Lancet, 371*(1), 126–134.

Griesdale, D. E., DeSouza, R. J., VanDam, R. M., et al. (2009). Intensive insulin therapy and mortality among critically ill patients: A meta-analysis including NICE-Sugar study data. *Canadian Medical Association Journal, 180*(8), 821–827.

Gustot, T. (2011). Multiple organ failure in sepsis: Prognosis and role of systemic inflammatory response. *Current Opinion in Critical Care, 17*(2), 153–159.

Heyland, D. K., Johnson, A. P., Reynolds, S. C., et al. (2011). Procalcitonin for reduced antibiotic exposure in the critical care setting: A systematic review and an economic evaluation. *Critical Care Medicine, 39*(7), 1792–1798.

Hollenberg, S. M. (2011). Vasoactive drugs in circulatory shock. *American Journal of Respiratory and Critical Care, 183*(7), 847–855.

Hudson, P., Payne, S., & Dip, N, H. (2011). Family care givers and palliative care: Current status and agenda for the future. *Journal of Palliative Medicine, 14*(7), 864–869.

Institute for Healthcare Improvement. (2012a). *How-to guide: Prevent central line–associated bloodstream infection.* Available at: www.ihi.org/knowledge/Pages/Tools/HowtoGuidePreventCentralLineAssociatedBloodstreamInfection.aspx

Institute for Healthcare Improvement. (2012b). *Implement the sepsis resuscitation bundle.* Available at: www.ihi.org/knowledge/Pages/Changes/ImplementtheSepsisResuscitationBundle.aspx

Jones, A. E., Brown, M. D., Trzeciak, S., et al. (2008). The effect of a quantitative resuscitation strategy on mortality in patients with sepsis: A meta-analysis. *Critical Care Medicine, 36*(10), 2734–2739.

**Kaler, W. (2007). Successful disinfection of needleless mechanical access ports: A matter of time and friction. *Journal of the Association of Vascular Access, 12*(4), 203–205.

Kavanagh, B. P., & McCowen, K. C. (2010). Glycemic control in the ICU. *New England Journal of Medicine, 363,* 2540–2546.

Khan, B. Q., & Kemp, S. F. (2011). Pathophysiology of anaphylaxis. *Current Opinion in Allergy and Clinical Immunology, 11*(4), 319–325.

Lee, J. K., & Vadas, P. (2011). Anaphylaxis: Mechanisms and management. *Clinical and Experimental Allergy, 41*(7), 923–938.

Makic, M. B. F., Rauen, C. A., & Bridges, E. (2009). Evidence-based practice habits: Transforming research into bedside practice. *Critical Care Nurse, 29*(2), 46–59.

Makic, M. B. F., VonRueden, K. T., Rauen, C. A., et al. (2011). Evidence-based practice habits: Putting more sacred cows out to pasture. *Critical Care Nurse, 31*(2), 38–62.

**Marik, P. E., Baram, M., & Vahid, B. (2008). Does central venous pressure predict fluid responsiveness? A systematic review of the literature and the tale of seven mares. *Chest, 134*(1), 172–178.

Martin, R. K. (2010). Acute kidney injury: Advances in definition, pathophysiology, and diagnosis. *AACN Advanced Critical Care, 21*(4), 350–356.

Nee, P. A., & Rivers, E. P. (2011). The end of the line for the Surviving Sepsis Campaign but not for early goal-directed therapy. *Emergency Medicine Journal, 28*(1), 3–5.

Neumer, R. W., Barnhart, J. M., Berg, R. A., et al. (2011). Implementation strategies for improving survival after out-of-hospital cardiac arrest in the United States. *Circulation, 123*(24), 2898–2911.

Nunnally, M. E., Jaeschke, R. N., Bellingan, G. J., et al. (2011). Target temperature management in critical care: A report and recommendations from five professional societies. *Critical Care Medicine, 39*(5), 1113–1125.

Paula, R. (August 26, 2011). Abdominal compartment syndrome. *Medscape.* Available at: emedicine.medscape.com/article/829008-overview

Perel, P., & Roberts, I. (2011). Colloids versus crystalloids for fluid resuscitation in critically ill patients (Review). *Cochrane Database of Systematic Reviews,* (4), CD000567.

Peyton, P. J., & Chong, S. W. (2010). Minimally invasive measurement of cardiac output during surgery and critical care. *Anesthesiology, 113*(5), 1220–1235.

Pierrakos, C., & Vincent, J. L. (2010). Sepsis biomarkers: A review. *Critical Care, 14,* 1–18. Available at: ccforum.com/content/14/1/R15

Powers, K. A., & Burchell, P. L. (2010). Sepsis alert: Avoiding the shock. *Nursing, 40*(4), 35–38.

Ramos, F. J., & Azevedo, L. C. P. (2010). Hemodynamic and perfusion end points for volemic resuscitation in sepsis. *Shock, 34*(1), 43–39.

Raslan, A. M., Fields, J. D., & Bhardwaj, A. (2010). Prophylaxis for venous thromboembolism in neurocritical care: A critical appraisal. *Neurocritical Care, 12*(2), 297–309.

**Rivers, E. P., McIntyre, L., Morro, D. C., et al. (2005). Early and innovative interventions for severe sepsis and septic shock: Taking advantage of a window of opportunity. *Canadian Medical Association Journal, 173*(9), 1054–1065.

Rubulotta, F., Marshall, J. C., Ramsay, G., et al. (2009). Predisposition, insult, infection, response, and organ dysfunction: A new model for staging severe sepsis. *Critical Care Medicine, 37*(4), 1329–1335.

Santry, H. P., & Alam, H. B. (2010). Fluid resuscitation: Past, present, and the future. *Shock, 33*(3), 229–241.

Shpektor, A. (2010). Cardiogenic shock: The role of inflammation. *Acute Cardiac Care, 12*(4), 115–118.

Strehlow, M. C. (2010). Early identification of shock in critically ill patients. *Emergency Medicine Clinics of North America, 28*(1), 57–66.

Surviving Sepsis Campaign. (2011). Available at: www.survivingsepsis.org

Tiruvoipati, R., Ong, K., Gangopadhyay, H., et al. (2010). Hypothermia predicts mortality in critically ill elderly patients with sepsis. *BioMed Central Geriatrics, 10,* 70. Available at: www.biomedcentral.com/1471-2318/10/70

Tuggle, D. (2010). Hypotension and shock: The truth about blood pressure. *Nursing, 40*(10), 1–5.

Westphal, G. A., Koenig, A., Filho, M. C., et al. (2011). Reduced mortality after the implementation of a protocol for the early detection of severe sepsis. *Journal of Critical Care, 26*(1), 76–81.

Wilmot, L. A. (2010). Shock: Early recognition and management. *Journal of Emergency Nursing, 36*(2), 134–139.

Zilberberg, M. D., & Shorr, A. F. (2011). Ventilator-associated pneumonia as a model for approaching cost effectiveness for infection prevention in the ICU. *Current Opinion in Critical Care, 24*(4), 385–389.**

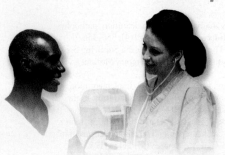

Oncology: Nursing Management in Cancer Care

On completion of this chapter, the learner will be able to:

1 Compare the function and behavior of normal and cancer cells.
2 Differentiate between benign and malignant tumors.
3 Identify agents and factors that have been found to be carcinogenic.
4 Describe the role of nurses in health education and prevention in decreasing the incidence of cancer.
5 Differentiate among the goals of cancer care: prevention, diagnosis, cure, control, and palliation.
6 Describe the roles of surgery, radiation therapy, chemotherapy, hematopoietic stem cell transplantation, hyperthermia, targeted therapy, and symptom management in treating cancer.
7 Use the nursing process as a framework for the care of patients with cancer.
8 Identify potential complications for the patient with cancer and discuss associated nursing care.
9 Identify assessment parameters and nursing management of patients with oncologic emergencies.

alopecia: hair loss
anaplasia: pattern of growth in which cells lack normal characteristics and differ in shape and organization with respect to their cells of origin; usually, anaplastic cells are malignant
angiogenesis: growth of new blood vessels that allows cancer cells to grow
apoptosis: programmed cell death
benign: not cancerous; benign tumors may grow but are unable to spread to other organs or body parts
biologic response modifier (BRM) therapy: the use of agents or treatment methods that can alter the immunologic relationship between the tumor and the host to provide a therapeutic benefit
biopsy: a diagnostic procedure in which a small sample of tissue is removed and examined microscopically to detect malignant cells
brachytherapy: delivery of radiation therapy through internal implants
cancer: a disease process whereby cells proliferate abnormally, ignoring growth-regulating signals in the environment surrounding the cells
carcinogenesis: process of transforming normal cells into malignant cells
carcinogens: chemicals, physical factors, and other agents that cause cancer
chemotherapy: the use of medications to kill tumor cells by interfering with cellular functions and reproduction
control: containment of the growth of cancer cells
cure: prolonged survival and disappearance of all evidence of disease so that the patient has the same life expectancy as anyone else in his or her age group
cytokines: substances produced primarily by cells of the immune system to enhance production and functioning of components of the immune system

extravasation: leakage of medication from the veins into the subcutaneous tissues
grading: identification of the type of tissue from which the tumor originated and the degree to which the tumor cells retain the functional and structural characteristics of the tissue of origin
graft-versus-host disease (GVHD): an immune response initiated by T lymphocytes of donor tissue against the recipient's tissues (skin, gastrointestinal tract, liver); an undesirable response
graft-versus-tumor effect: the donor cell response against the malignancy; a desirable response
malignant: having cells or processes that are characteristic of cancer
metastasis: spread of cancer cells from the primary tumor to distant sites
mucositis: inflammation of the lining of the gastrointestinal tract often associated with cancer therapies
myelosuppression: suppression of the blood cell–producing function of the bone marrow
nadir: lowest point of white blood cell depression after therapy that has toxic effects on the bone marrow
neoplasia: uncontrolled cell growth that follows no physiologic demand
neutropenia: abnormally low absolute neutrophil count
oncology: field or study of cancer
palliation: relief of symptoms and promotion of comfort and quality of life
radiation therapy: the use of ionizing radiation to kill malignant cells
staging: process of determining the extent of disease, including tumor size and spread or metastasis to distant sites
stomatitis: inflammation of the oral tissues, often associated with some chemotherapeutic agents and radiation therapy to the head and neck region

targeted therapies: cancer treatments that seek to minimize the negative effects on healthy tissues by disrupting specific cancer cell functions, such as malignant transformation, communication pathways, processes for growth and metastasis, and genetic coding

thrombocytopenia: decrease in the number of circulating platelets; associated with the potential for bleeding

tumor-specific antigen (TSA): protein on the membrane of cancer cells that distinguishes the malignant cell from a benign cell of the same tissue type

vesicant: substance that can cause tissue necrosis and damage

xerostomia: dry oral cavity resulting from decreased function of salivary glands

Cancer is not a single disease with a single cause; rather, it is a group of distinct diseases with different causes, manifestations, treatments, and prognoses. Because cancer can involve any organ system and treatment approaches have the potential for multisystem effects, cancer nursing practice overlaps numerous nursing specialties. Cancer nursing practice covers all age groups and is carried out in various settings, including acute care institutions, outpatient centers, rehabilitation facilities, the home, and long-term care facilities. The scope, responsibilities, and goals of cancer nursing, also called **oncology** nursing, are as diverse and complex as those of any nursing specialty. Cancer nursing practice addresses the care of patients throughout the cancer trajectory from prevention through end-of-life care (Fig. 15-1).

Despite significant advances in the understanding of cancer, including causes, prevention, early detection, diagnostic tools, prognostic indicators, treatment, and symptom management, many people still associate cancer with pain and death. Nurses need to identify their own perception of cancer and set realistic goals to meet the challenges inherent in caring for patients with cancer. In addition, nurses caring for patients with cancer must be prepared to support patients and families through a wide range of physical, emotional, social, cultural, financial, and spiritual challenges.

Epidemiology of Cancer

In 2011, more than 1.5 million Americans were diagnosed with cancer affecting various locations within the body. Cancer is second only to cardiovascular disease as a cause of death in the United States. Although the number of cancer deaths has decreased, more than 570,000 Americans were expected to die of a malignant process in 2011. The leading causes of cancer death in the United States in order of frequency and location are lung, prostate, and colorectal cancer in men and

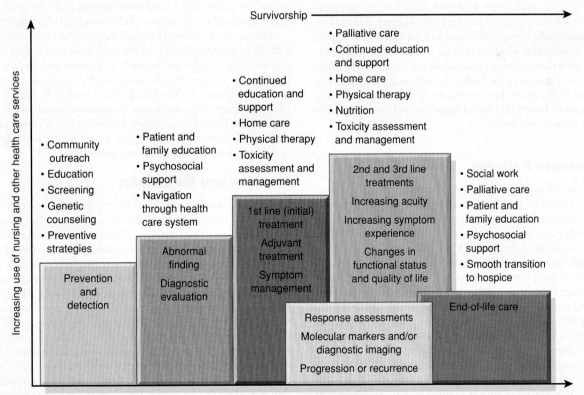

FIGURE 15-1 • Cancer care trajectory. The cancer care trajectory reflects the phases and care required during the continuum of the cancer experience from prevention and early detection through end-of-life care. Specialized nursing care is provided throughout the entire trajectory.

lung, breast, and colorectal cancer in women (Siegel, Ward, Brawley, et al., 2011). Most cancer occurs in people older than 65 years. Overall, the incidence of cancer is higher in men than in women and higher in industrialized nations.

Although the overall rate of cancer deaths has declined, cancer death rates in African American men remain substantially higher than those among Caucasian men and twice those of Hispanic men. Despite progress in screening, diagnosis, and treatment, progress has not benefited all segments of the population equally; cancer death rates for individuals with the least education are more than twice those of the most educated. The elimination of educational and racial disparities could potentially have avoided about 37% of the premature cancer deaths in 2007 among individuals 25 to 64 years of age (Siegel et al., 2011).

Disparities in treatment, morbidity, and mortality are related to patient, physician, and system factors that exist, interact, and affect each other within the health care system and the patient's community (Korber, Padula, Gray, et al., 2011). Factors include attitudes, knowledge, cultural beliefs, socioeconomic issues, level of education, insurance coverage, lifestyle choices such as the use of tobacco, misconceptions, communication skills, and other epidemiologic factors.

Pathophysiology of the Malignant Process

Cancer is a disease process that begins when a cell is transformed by genetic mutations of the cellular DNA. Genetic mutations may result from inherited and/or acquired mutations that lead to abnormal cell behavior (Eggert, 2011). The initial genetically altered cell forms a clone and begins to proliferate abnormally, evading normal intracellular and extracellular growth-regulating processes or signals as well as other defense mechanisms of the body. The cells acquire a variety of capabilities that allow them to invade surrounding tissues and gain access to lymph and blood vessels, which carry the cells to other areas of the body.

Proliferative Patterns

During the lifespan, various body tissues normally undergo periods of rapid or proliferative growth that must be distinguished from malignant growth activity. Several patterns of cell growth exist: hyperplasia, metaplasia, dysplasia, anaplasia, and neoplasia (see Chapter 6). Cancerous cells, described as **malignant** neoplasms, demonstrate uncontrolled cell growth that follows no physiologic demand (**neoplasia**). Although both **benign** (noncancerous) and malignant growths are classified and named by tissue of origin, the *International Classification of Diseases for Oncology* (Fitz, Percy, Jack, et al., 2011) is used by scientists and clinicians around the world as the nomenclature for malignant disease (Table 15-1).

Benign and malignant cells differ in many cellular growth characteristics, including the method and rate of growth, ability to metastasize or spread, general effects, destruction of tissue, and ability to cause death. These differences are summarized in Table 15-2. The degree of **anaplasia** (a pattern of growth in which cells lack normal characteristics and differ in shape and organization with respect to their cells of origin) is associated with increased malignant potential.

Characteristics of Malignant Cells

Despite individual differences, cancer cells share some common behavioral capabilities that foster uncontrolled growth, survival, and the ability to invade adjacent tissues and/or spread to other body sites. These capabilities include uncontrolled proliferation, evasion of growth suppression signals, replicative immortality, invasion and metastasis, resistance to cell death, uncontrolled **angiogenesis** (growth of new blood vessels that allows cancer cells to grow), reprogrammed cell metabolism, and evasion of the immune system (Hanahan & Weinberg, 2011).

Malignant cell membranes have been found to contain proteins called **tumor-specific antigens (TSAs)** (e.g., carcinoembryonic antigen [CEA] and prostate-specific antigen [PSA]), which develop over time as the cells become differentiated (mature). These proteins distinguish malignant cells from benign cells of the same tissue type. Many of the TSAs that have been identified have aided in assessing the extent of disease in a person and in tracking the course of illness during treatment or relapse. Malignant cellular membranes also contain less fibronectin, a cellular cement, making them less cohesive and less likely to adhere to adjacent cells readily.

Typically, nuclei of cancer cells are large and irregularly shaped (pleomorphism). Nucleoli—structures within the nucleus that house ribonucleic acid (RNA)—are larger and more numerous in malignant cells, perhaps because of increased RNA synthesis. Chromosomal abnormalities (translocations, deletions, additions) and fragility of chromosomes are commonly found when cancer cells are analyzed. (See Chapter 8 for discussion of chromosomal abnormalities.)

Mitosis (cell division) occurs more rapidly in malignant cells than in normal cells. As the cells grow and divide, more glucose and oxygen are needed. If glucose and oxygen are unavailable, malignant cells use anaerobic metabolic channels for cell proliferation (Vander Heiden, Cantley, & Thompson, 2009). Cancer cells utilize an increased amount of glucose even in the presence of oxygen, known as the Warburg effect (Vander Heiden et al., 2009). This increase in glucose uptake is the basis for positron emission tomography (PET).

Invasion and Metastasis

Malignant diseases have the ability to spread or transfer cancerous cells from one organ or body part to another by invasion and metastasis. Invasion, which refers to the growth of the primary tumor into the surrounding host tissues, occurs in several ways. Mechanical pressure exerted by rapidly proliferating neoplasms may force fingerlike projections of tumor cells into surrounding tissue and interstitial spaces. Malignant cells are less adherent and may break off from the primary tumor and invade adjacent structures. Malignant cells are thought to possess or produce specific destructive enzymes (proteinases), such as collagenases (specific to collagen), plasminogen activators (specific to plasma), and lysosomal hydrolyses. These enzymes are thought to destroy surrounding tissue, including the structural tissues of the vascular basement membrane, facilitating invasion of malignant cells into blood and lymphatic vessels. The mechanical pressure of a rapidly growing tumor may enhance this process.

TABLE 15-1 Classification of Cancer by Tissue of Origin

Classification	Tissue of Origin	Characteristics	Term	Examples
Carcinoma	Epithelial	Account for 80%–90% of all cancers		
	• Glandular epithelium	Organs or glands capable of secretion	Adenocarcinoma	Adenocarcinoma of the breast, lung, prostate
	• Squamous epithelium	Covers or lines all external and internal body surfaces	Squamous cell carcinoma	Squamous cell cancer of the skin, lung, esophagus
Sarcoma	Connective or Supportive			
	• Bone	Most common form of cancer of the bone	Osteosarcoma	Osteosarcoma of the femur, humerus
	• Cartilage	Rare, arises from within bones	Chondrosarcoma	Chondrosarcoma of the femur, pelvis
	• Adipose	Arises from deep soft tissue	Liposarcoma	Liposarcoma of the retroperitoneum, thigh
	• Smooth muscle	Very rare	Leiomyosarcoma	Leiomyosarcoma of the uterus, intestines, stomach
	• Skeletal muscle	Most common in young children	Rhabdosarcoma	Rhabdosarcoma of the head and neck, limbs
	• Fibrous tissue	Often involves long or flat bones	Fibrosarcoma	Fibrosarcoma of the femur, tibia, mandible
	• Membranes lining body cavities	Most often related to asbestos exposure	Mesothelial sarcoma or mesothelioma	Mesothelioma of the pleura or peritoneum
	• Blood vessels	With liver involvement may be related to occupational exposure to vinyl chloride monomer	Angiosarcoma	Angiosarcoma of the liver, heart
Myeloma	Plasma cells	Produced by B-cell lymphocytes; plasma cells produce antibodies	Not applicable (N/A)	N/A
Lymphoma	Lymphocytes	Two main classifications; may involve lymph nodes and/or body organs	Non-Hodgkin lymphoma	B-cell lymphoma, T-cell lymphoma
			Hodgkin lymphoma	N/A
Leukemia	Hematopoietic cells in the bone marrow	May involve various cell lines produced in the bone marrow		
	• White blood cells (WBCs)	N/A	Myelogenous	Acute myelogenous leukemia
	• Lymphocytes	N/A	Lymphocytic	Acute lymphocytic leukemia
	• Red blood cells (RBCs)	Involves overproduction of RBCs and is associated with increased levels of WBCs and platelets; also risk of additional bone marrow disease	Erythremia	Polycythemia vera

Adapted from Fitz, A., Percy, C., Jack, A. et al. (2011). *International classification of disease for oncology.* World Health Organization: Geneva.

TABLE 15-2 Characteristics of Benign and Malignant Tumors

Characteristics	Benign	Malignant
Cell	Well-differentiated cells resemble normal cells of the tissue from which the tumor originated.	Cells are undifferentiated and may bear little resemblance to the normal cells of the tissue from which they arose.
Mode of growth	Tumor grows by expansion and does not infiltrate the surrounding tissues; usually encapsulated.	Grows at the periphery and overcomes contact inhibition to invade and infiltrate surrounding tissues
Rate of growth	Rate of growth is usually slow.	Rate of growth is variable and depends on level of differentiation; the more anaplastic the tumor, the faster its growth.
Metastasis	Does not spread by metastasis	Gains access to the blood and lymphatic channels and metastasizes to other areas of the body
General effects	Is usually a localized phenomenon that does not cause generalized effects unless its location interferes with vital functions	Often causes generalized effects, such as anemia, weakness, systemic inflammation, weight loss, and CACS
Tissue destruction	Does not usually cause tissue damage unless its location interferes with blood flow	Often causes extensive tissue damage as the tumor outgrows its blood supply or encroaches on blood flow to the area; may also produce substances that cause cell damage
Ability to cause death	Does not usually cause death unless its location interferes with vital functions	Usually causes death unless growth can be controlled

CACS, cancer-related anorexia-cachexia syndrome.
Adapted from Porth, C. M., & Matfin, G. (2009). *Pathophysiology: Concepts of altered health states* (8th ed.). Philadelphia: Lippincott Williams & Wilkins.

Metastasis is the dissemination or spread of malignant cells from the primary tumor to distant sites by direct spread of tumor cells to body cavities or through lymphatic and blood circulation. Tumors growing in or penetrating body cavities may shed cells or emboli that travel within the body cavity and seed the surfaces of other organs. This occurs in ovarian cancer when malignant cells enter the peritoneal cavity and seed the peritoneal cavity or surfaces of abdominal organs such as the liver or pancreas. Patterns of metastasis can be partially explained by circulatory patterns and by the affinity for certain malignant cells to bind to molecules in specific body tissues. Patterns of metastasis associated with various types of cancer are often referred to as the natural history of the disease.

Lymphatic and Hematogenous Spread

Lymph and blood are key mechanisms by which cancer cells spread. Lymphatic spread (the transport of tumor cells through the lymphatic circulation) is the most common mechanism of metastasis. Tumor emboli enter the lymph channels by way of the interstitial fluid, which communicates with lymphatic fluid. Malignant cells also may penetrate lymphatic vessels by invasion. After entering the lymphatic circulation, malignant cells either lodge in the lymph nodes or pass between the lymphatic and venous circulations. Tumors arising in areas of the body with rapid and extensive lymphatic circulation are at high risk for metastasis through lymphatic channels. Breast tumors frequently metastasize in this manner through axillary, clavicular, and thoracic lymph channels.

Hematogenous spread—the dissemination of malignant cells via the bloodstream—is directly related to the vascularity of the tumor. Few malignant cells can survive the turbulence of arterial circulation, insufficient oxygenation, or destruction by the body's immune system. In addition, the structure of most arteries and arterioles is far too secure to permit malignant invasion. Those malignant cells that do survive are able to attach to endothelium and attract fibrin, platelets, and clotting factors to seal themselves from immune system surveillance. The endothelium retracts, allowing the malignant cells to enter the basement membrane and secrete proteolytic enzymes. These enzymes degrade the extracellular matrix, allowing implantation.

Angiogenesis

Angiogenesis is the growth of new blood vessels from the host tissue stimulated by the release of growth factors such as vascular endothelial growth factor (VEGF). Rapid formation of new blood vessels helps malignant cells obtain the necessary nutrients and oxygen. However, the vessels formed in this deregulated process are morphologically abnormal and function inefficiently. It is also through this vascular network that tumor emboli can enter the systemic circulation and travel to distant sites. Large tumor emboli that become trapped in the microcirculation of distant sites may further metastasize to other sites. Therapies that target VEGF or its receptors are being used to treat many cancers effectively (see the Targeted Therapies section).

Carcinogenesis

Molecular Process

Malignant transformation, or **carcinogenesis**, is thought to be at least a three-step cellular process, involving initiation,

promotion, and progression. Agents that initiate or promote cellular transformation are referred to as carcinogens. During *initiation*, **carcinogens** (substances that can cause cancer), such as chemicals, physical factors, and biologic agents, cause mutations in the cellular deoxyribonucleic acid (DNA). Normally, these alterations are reversed by DNA repair mechanisms or the changes initiate programmed cellular death (**apoptosis**) or cell senescence. Occasionally, cells escape these protective mechanisms, and permanent cellular mutations occur. These mutations usually are not significant to cells until the second step of carcinogenesis.

During *promotion*, repeated exposure to promoting agents (co-carcinogens) causes proliferation and expansion of initiated cells with increased expression or manifestations of abnormal genetic information, even after long latency periods. Latency periods for the promotion of cellular mutations vary with the type of agent, the dosage of the promoter, and the innate characteristics and genetic stability of the target cell. The promotion phase generally leads to the formation of a preneoplastic or benign lesion.

During *progression*, the altered cells exhibit increasingly malignant behavior. These cells acquire the ability to stimulate angiogenesis, to invade adjacent tissues, and to metastasize.

Cellular oncogenes are responsible for vital cell functions, including proliferation and differentiation. Cellular proto-oncogenes, such as those for the epidermal growth factor receptor (EGFR), transcription factors such as c-Myc, or cell signaling proteins such as *Kirsten ras* (*KRAS*), act as "on switches" for cellular growth. Amplification of proto-oncogenes or overexpression of growth factors, such as epidermal growth factor (EGF), can lead to uncontrolled cell proliferation. Mutations that increase the activity of oncogenes also deregulate cell proliferation. Genetic alterations in the gene for *KRAS* have been associated with some types of colon, pancreatic, and lung cancer (Bokemeyer, Bondarenko, Makhson, et al., 2009; Suda, Tomizawa, & Mitsudomi, 2010). Just as proto-oncogenes "turn on" cellular growth, cancer suppressor genes "turn off," or regulate, unneeded cellular proliferation. When suppressor genes are mutated or silenced, thus losing their regulatory capabilities, malignant cell reproduction continues uncontrolled. The *p53* (*TP53*) gene, a tumor suppressor gene, is implicated in as many as 50% of all noninherited human cancers (Soussi, 2011). This gene determines whether cells will live or die (via apoptosis) after DNA damage. Alterations in *TP53* may decrease apoptotic signals, thus giving rise to a survival advantage for mutant cell populations. Mutant *TP53* is associated with a poor prognosis and may be associated with determining response to treatment. Once this genetic expression occurs in cells, the cells begin to produce mutant cell populations that are different from their original cellular ancestors.

Etiology

Factors implicated or known to induce carcinogenesis include viruses and bacteria, physical agents, chemicals, genetic or familial factors, diet, and hormones. Additional research is needed for a better understanding of the relationships between etiologic factors and cancer.

Viruses and Bacteria

It is estimated that about 20% of all cancers worldwide are linked to viral and bacterial infections (De Flora & Bonanni,

2011). Viruses are associated with cancer in one of two ways. After infecting individuals, DNA viruses insert a part of their own DNA near the infected cell genes causing cell division. The newly formed cells that now carry viral DNA lack normal controls on growth. Examples of these viruses that are known to cause cancer include human papillomavirus (HPV) (cervical and head and neck cancers), hepatitis B virus (HBV) (liver cancer), and Epstein-Barr virus (EBV) (Burkitt lymphoma and nasopharyngeal cancer) (Callaway, 2011; Faridi, Zahra, Khan, et al., 2011). Other viruses carry a gene that causes the infected cell to degrade tumor suppressor proteins or overexpress proto-oncogenes, which, in turn, induces uncontrolled cell proliferation.

There is little evidence to support the link of most bacteria to cancer, although chronic inflammatory reactions to bacteria and the production of carcinogenic metabolites are possible mechanisms that continue to be investigated. *Helicobacter pylori* is one bacterium identified as a cause of cancer in humans (Fontham, Thun, Ward, et al., 2009). *H. pylori* has been associated with an increased incidence of gastric malignancy related to chronic superficial gastritis, with resultant atrophic and metaplastic changes to the gastric mucosa.

Physical Agents

Physical factors associated with carcinogenesis include exposure to sunlight or radiation, chronic irritation or inflammation, and tobacco use.

Excessive exposure to the ultraviolet rays of the sun, especially in fair-skinned people, increases the risk of skin cancers. Factors such as clothing styles (sleeveless shirts or shorts), the use of sunscreens, occupation, recreational habits, and environmental variables, including humidity, altitude, and latitude, all play a role in the amount of exposure to ultraviolet light.

Exposure to ionizing radiation can occur with repeated diagnostic x-ray procedures or with radiation therapy used to treat disease. Improved x-ray equipment minimizes the risk of extensive radiation exposure. Radiation therapy used in cancer treatment and exposure to radioactive materials at nuclear weapon manufacturing sites or nuclear power plants in the past have been associated with a higher incidence of leukemias, multiple myeloma, and cancers of the lung, bone, breast, thyroid, and other tissues. Background radiation from the natural decay processes that produce radon has also been associated with lung cancer. Ventilation is advised in homes with high levels of trapped radon to allow the gas to disperse into the atmosphere.

Chemical Agents

Many cancers are thought to be related to environmental factors (American Cancer Society [ACS], 2011b; Eggert, 2011). Most hazardous chemicals produce their toxic effects by altering DNA structure in body sites distant from chemical exposure.

Tobacco smoke, thought to be the single most lethal chemical carcinogen, accounts for at least 30% of cancer deaths in humans (Fontham et al., 2009). Smoking is strongly associated with cancers of the lung, head and neck, esophagus, stomach, pancreas, cervix, kidney, and bladder and with acute myeloblastic leukemia. More than 4,000 individual chemicals have been identified in tobacco and tobacco smoke, including more than 60 chemicals that are known carcinogens. Tobacco may also act synergistically with other substances, such as alcohol, asbestos, radiation, and viruses, to promote cancer development. Chewing tobacco is associated with cancers of the oral cavity, which primarily occur in men younger than 40 years (ACS, 2011b). Passive smoke (i.e., secondhand smoke) has been linked to lung cancer; nonsmokers who live with a smoker have about a 20% to 30% greater risk of developing lung cancer (ACS, 2012). There is also evidence suggesting that passive smoke may be linked with childhood leukemia and cancers of the larynx, pharynx, brain, bladder, rectum, stomach, and breast (ACS, 2009).

Many chemical substances found in the workplace are carcinogens or cocarcinogens. In the United States, carcinogens are classified by two federal agencies: the National Toxicology Program of the Department of Health and Human Services (HHS) and the Environmental Protection Agency's (EPA) Integrated Risk Information System (IRIS). The Centers for Disease Control and Prevention (CDC) established the National Institute for Occupational Safety and Health (NIOSH) to provide occupational exposure limits and guidelines for protection of the workforce as regulated by the Occupational Safety and Health Act of 1970. The extensive list of suspected chemical substances continues to grow and includes aromatic amines and aniline dyes; pesticides and formaldehydes; arsenic, soot, and tars; asbestos; benzene; betel nut and lime; cadmium; chromium compounds; nickel and zinc ores; wood dust; beryllium compounds; and polyvinyl chloride.

Genetics and Familial Factors

Almost every cancer type has been shown to run in families. This may be owing to genetics, shared environments, cultural or lifestyle factors, or chance alone. Genetic factors play a role in cancer cell development. Abnormal chromosomal patterns and cancer have been associated with extra chromosomes, too few chromosomes, or translocated chromosomes. Specific cancers with underlying genetic abnormalities include Burkitt lymphoma, chronic myelogenous leukemia, meningiomas, acute leukemia, retinoblastomas, Wilms tumor, and skin cancers, including malignant melanoma. Additionally, there are syndromes that represent a cluster of cancers that are identified by a specific genetic alteration that is inherited across generations of a family. In these families, the associated genetic mutation is found in all cells and represents an inherited susceptibility to cancer for all family members who carry the mutation.

Approximately 5% to 10% of cancers in adults display a pattern of cancers suggestive of a familial predisposition (MacDonald, 2011). The hallmarks of families with a hereditary cancer syndrome include cancer in two or more first-degree or second-degree relatives, early onset of cancer in family members younger than 50 years, the same type of cancer in several family members, individual family members with more than one type of cancer, and a rare cancer in one or more family members (Aiello-Laws, 2011). There is also evidence of an autosomal dominant inheritance pattern of cancers affecting several generations of a family.

There have been considerable advances in the recognition of inherited cancer susceptibility syndromes and in the ability to isolate and identify the inherited genetic

Chart 15-1 Genetics Concepts and Cancer

Cancer is a genetic disease. Every phase of carcinogenesis is affected by multiple gene mutations. Some of these mutations are inherited (present in germ-line cells); however, most (90%) are somatic mutations that are acquired mutations in specific cells. Examples of cancers influenced by genetics include:

- Cowden syndrome
- Familial adenomatous polyposis
- Familial melanoma syndrome
- Hereditary breast and ovarian cancer
- Hereditary nonpolyposis colon cancer
- Neurofibromatosis type 1
- Retinoblastoma

Nursing Assessments

Family History Assessment

- Obtain information about both maternal and paternal sides of family for three generations.
- Obtain cancer history for at least three generations.
- Look for clustering of cancers that occur at young ages, multiple primary cancers in one individual, cancer in paired organs, and two or more close relatives with the same type of cancer suggestive of hereditary cancer syndromes.

Patient Assessment

- Physical findings that may predispose the patient to cancer, such as multiple colon polyps, suggestive of a polyposis syndrome
- Skin findings, such as atypical moles, that may be related to familial melanoma syndrome

- Multiple *café-au-lait* spots, axillary freckling, and two or more neurofibromas associated with neurofibromatosis type 1
- Facial trichilemmomas, mucosal papillomatosis, multinodular thyroid goiter or thyroid adenomas, macrocephaly, fibrocystic breasts, and other fibromas or lipomas related to Cowden syndrome

Management Issues Specific to Genetics

- Assess patient's understanding of genetics factors related to his or her cancer.
- Refer for cancer risk assessment when a hereditary cancer syndrome is suspected so that patient and family can discuss inheritance risk with other family members and availability of genetic testing.
- Offer appropriate genetics information and resources.
- Assess patient's understanding of genetics information.
- Provide support to patients and families with known genetic test results for hereditary cancer syndromes.
- Participate in the management and coordination of risk reduction measures for those with known gene mutations.

Genetics Resources

American Cancer Society: offers general information about cancer and support resources for families, www.cancer.org
National Cancer Institute: a listing of cancers with clinical summaries and treatment reviews, information on genetic risks for cancer, listing of cancer centers providing genetic cancer risk assessment services, www.cancernet.nci.nih.gov
See also Chapter 8, Chart 8-6 for additional resources.

mutations responsible for cancer. These advances have enabled the appropriate identification of families at risk for certain syndromes. Examples include hereditary breast and ovarian cancer syndrome (*BRCA1* and *BRCA2*) and multiple endocrine neoplasia syndrome (*MEN1* and *MEN2*) (Chart 15-1). Other cancers associated with familial inheritance syndromes include nephroblastomas, pheochromocytomas, and colorectal, stomach, thyroid, renal, prostate, and lung cancers (Weitzel, Blazer, MacDonald, et al., 2011).

Dietary Factors

Dietary factors are also linked to environmental cancers. Dietary substances can be proactive (protective), carcinogenic, or cocarcinogenic. The risk of cancer increases with long-term ingestion of carcinogens or cocarcinogens or chronic absence of protective substances in the diet.

Dietary substances that appear to increase the risk of cancer include fats, alcohol, salt-cured or smoked meats, nitrate- and nitrite-containing foods, and red and processed meats. Alcohol increases the risk of cancers of the mouth, pharynx, larynx, esophagus, liver, colon, rectum, and breast. Alcohol intake should be limited to no more than two drinks per day for men and one drink per day for women. Greater consumption of vegetables and fruits is associated with a decreased risk of lung, esophageal, stomach, and colorectal cancers (ACS, 2011a).

Poor diet and obesity have been identified as contributing factors to the development of cancers of the breast (in postmenopausal women), colon, endometrium, esophagus,

and kidney. Obesity is also associated with increased risk for cancers of the pancreas, gallbladder, thyroid, ovary, and cervix, and for multiple myeloma, Hodgkin lymphoma, and an aggressive form of prostate cancer (Kagawa-Singer, Dadia, Yu, et al., 2010). Recent epidemiologic studies have suggested an association between diabetes and cancer development. Although a scientific basis has yet to be identified, diabetes and cancer share common risk factors and incidence patterns (Giovannucci, Harlan, Archer, et al., 2010).

Nutritional guidelines for cancer prevention can be found in Chart 15-2. A healthy weight needs to be achieved and maintained. A healthy diet is plant based with at least 2-1/2 cups of fruits and vegetables each day (ACS, 2012; Dudek, 2010).

Hormonal Agents

Tumor growth may be promoted by disturbances in hormonal balance, either by the body's own (endogenous) hormone production or by administration of exogenous hormones. Cancers of the breast, prostate, and uterus are thought to depend on endogenous hormonal levels for growth. Diethylstilbestrol (DES) has long been recognized as a cause of vaginal carcinomas. Oral contraceptives and prolonged estrogen therapy are associated with an increased incidence of hepatocellular, endometrial, and breast cancers but decrease the risk of ovarian cancer. The combination of estrogen and progesterone appears safer than estrogen alone in decreasing the risk of endometrial cancers; however, studies support discontinuing hormonal therapy containing both estrogen and progestin because of the increased risk of breast cancer, coronary artery disease, stroke, and blood clots (ACS, 2010).

Hormonal changes related to the female reproductive cycle are also associated with cancer incidence. Early onset of menses before age 12 and delayed onset of menopause after age 55, nulliparity (never giving birth), and delayed childbirth after age 30 are all associated with an increased risk of breast cancer. Increased numbers of pregnancies are associated with a decreased incidence of breast, endometrial, and ovarian cancers.

Role of the Immune System

In humans, malignant cells are capable of developing on a regular basis. However, through surveillance, cells of the immune system can detect the development of transformed cells and destroy them before cell growth becomes uncontrolled. When the immune system fails to identify and stop the growth of transformed cells, cancer develops.

Patients who are immunocompromised have an increased incidence of cancer. Renal transplant recipients who receive immunosuppressive therapy to prevent rejection of the transplanted organ have an increased incidence of lymphoma, Kaposi's sarcoma, and cancers of the skin and cervix (Chandraker, Milford, & Sayegh, 2012). Patients with immunodeficiency diseases, such as acquired immunodeficiency syndrome (AIDS), have an increased incidence of Kaposi's sarcoma, non-Hodgkin's lymphoma, and cervical carcinoma. In addition, there is also an increase in the incidence of various non–AIDS-defining malignancies, including Hodgkin lymphoma; multiple myeloma; leukemia; melanoma; and cervical, brain,

testicular, oral, lung, gastric, liver, renal, and anal cancers (Fauci & Lane, 2012). Patients who were previously treated with alkylating chemotherapy agents, allogeneic hematopoietic stem cell transplantation (HSCT) involving total-body irradiation, and certain types of chest radiation are at increased risk for secondary primary cancers related to treatment-associated immunosuppression (Sharp, Kinahan, & Didwania, 2010). Autoimmune diseases, such as rheumatoid arthritis and Sjögren syndrome, are associated with increased development of cancer. Finally, age-related changes, such as declining organ function, increased incidence of chronic diseases, and diminished immunocompetence, may contribute to an increased incidence of cancer in older people.

Normal Immune Responses

Through the process of surveillance, an intact immune system usually has the ability to recognize and combat cancer cells through multiple, interacting cells and actions of the innate, humoral, and cellular components of the immune system. Tumor-associated antigens (TAAs; also called *tumor cell antigens*) are found on the membranes of many cancer cells. TAAs are processed by antigen-presenting cells (APCs) (e.g., macrophages and dentritic cells [very specialized cells of the immune system] that present antigens to both T- and B lymphocytes) and are presented to T lymphocytes that recognize the antigen-bearing cells as foreign. Multiple TAAs have been identified—some are found in many types of cancer, some exist in the normal tissues of origin as well as the cancer cells, some exist in both normal and cancer cells but are overexpressed (exist in higher concentrations) in cancer cells, and others are very specific to a limited number of cancer types (Flechner, Finke, & Fairchild, 2011).

In response to recognizing TAAs as foreign, T-cell lymphocytes release several cytokines that elicit various immune system actions, including (1) proliferation of cytotoxic (cell-killing) T lymphocytes capable of direct destruction of cancer cells, (2) induction of cancer cell apoptosis, and (3) recruitment of additional immune system cells (B-cell lymphocytes that produce antibodies, natural killer cells, and macrophages) that contribute to the destruction and degradation of cancer cells.

Immune System Evasion

Several theories postulate how malignant cells can survive and proliferate, evading the elaborate immune system defense mechanisms. If the body fails to recognize the TAAs on cancer cells or the function of the APCs is impaired, the immune response is not stimulated. Some cancer cells have been found to have altered cell membranes that interfere with APC binding and presentation to T lymphocytes. Tumors can also express molecules that induce T-lymphocyte anergy or tolerance such as PD-1 ligand. These molecules bind to PD-1 proteins on T lymphocytes and either block killing of the tumor or induce cell death in the lymphocyte. In addition, cancer cells have been found to release cytokines that inhibit APCs as well as other cells of the immune system. When tumors do not possess TAAs that label them as foreign, the immune response is not alerted. This allows the tumor to grow too large to be managed by normal immune mechanisms.

Through genetic mutations, the immunogenicity (immunologic appearance) of cancer cells can be altered, allowing the cells to evade immune cell recognition. Tumor antigens may combine with the antibodies produced by the immune system and hide or disguise themselves from normal immune defense mechanisms. The tumor antigen–antibody complexes that evade recognition lead to a false message to decrease further production of antibodies as well as other immune system components.

Overexpression (abnormally high concentrations) of host suppressor T lymphocytes induced through the release of cytokines by malignant cells are thought to play a role in uncontrolled cancer cell growth (Hanahan & Weinberg, 2011). Suppressor T lymphocytes normally assist in regulating lymphocyte production and diminishing immune responses (i.e., antibody production) when they are no longer required. Low levels of antibodies and high levels of suppressor cells have been found in patients with multiple myeloma, which is a cancer associated with hypogammaglobulinemia (low amounts of serum antibodies). Alternatively, there is evidence that proliferation of helper T lymphocytes, responsible for "turning on" immune responses, is impaired by cytokines produced by cancer cells (Hanahan & Weinberg, 2011). Without proliferation of helper T lymphocytes, the immune system response is limited and the cancer cells continue to proliferate uncontrolled. Understanding the role of the immune system and identification of the ways in which cancer evades the body's natural defenses provides the foundation for therapeutic approaches that seek to support and enhance the immune system's role in combating cancer (see Chapter 35).

Detection and Prevention of Cancer

The primary, secondary, and tertiary prevention of cancer has become increasingly important for addressing cancer burden. All individuals are encouraged to comply with detection efforts suggested by the ACS (Table 15-3).

Primary Prevention

Primary prevention is concerned with reducing the risks of disease through health promotion and risk reduction strategies. It is estimated that almost 75% of all cancers in the United States are related to environmental and lifestyle factors (ACS, 2011b). By acquiring the knowledge and skills necessary to educate the community about cancer risks, nurses in all settings play a key role in cancer prevention. One way to reduce the risk of cancer is to help individuals avoid known carcinogens. Another strategy involves encouraging individuals to make dietary and lifestyle changes (smoking cessation, decreased caloric and alcohol intake, increased physical activity) that studies show influence the risk for cancer (McCullough, Patel, Kushi, et al., 2011). Nurses use their education and counseling skills to provide patient education and support public education campaigns through organizations, such as the ACS, that guide individuals and families in taking steps to reduce cancer risks through health promotion behaviors (see Chart 15-2).

Clinical trials that explore the use of medications for reducing the incidence of certain types of cancer are numerous. For example, large-scale breast cancer prevention studies supported by the National Cancer Institute (NCI) indicated that chemoprevention with the medications tamoxifen (Nolvadex) or raloxifene (Evista) can reduce the incidence of breast cancer by 50% in women at high risk for breast cancer (Vogel, Costantino, Wickerham, et al., 2010). Daily aspirin has been reported to reduce colorectal cancers. Currently, the NCI (2011) lists more than 100 ongoing clinical trials exploring cancer prevention strategies.

Secondary Prevention

Secondary prevention involves screening and early detection activities that seek to identify early stage cancer in individuals who lack signs and symptoms suggestive of cancer. The goal is to decrease cancer morbidity and mortality associated with advanced stages of cancer and complex treatment approaches. Many organizations conduct cancer screening events that focus on cancers with the highest incidence rates or those that have improved survival rates if diagnosed early, such as breast or prostate cancer. These events offer education and appropriate assessments such as mammograms, digital rectal examinations, and PSA blood tests for minimal or no cost. Many screening and detection programs target people who do not regularly practice health-promoting behaviors or lack access to health care due to health insurance issues, financial or transportation limitations, competing priorities, or lack of knowledge. Nurses continue to develop evidence-based approaches for community-based screening and detection programs that reflect the cultural beliefs of the target population (Conde, Landier, Ishida, et al., 2011; Gwede, William, Thomas, et al., 2010; Meade, Menard, Thervil, et al., 2009; Northington, Martin, Walker, et al., 2011).

TABLE 15-3	American Cancer Society Screening Guidelines for the Early Detection of Cancer in Average-Risk Asymptomatic People		
Cancer Site	**Population**	**Test or Procedure**	**Frequency**
Breast	Women, age 20+	Breast self-examination (BSE)	Beginning in their early 20s, women should be told about the benefits and limitations of BSE. The importance of prompt reporting of any new breast symptoms to a health professional should be emphasized. Women who choose to do BSE should receive instruction and have their technique reviewed on the occasion of a periodic health examination. It is acceptable for women to choose not to do BSE or to do BSE irregularly.
		Clinical breast examination (CBE)	For women in their 20s and 30s, it is recommended that CBE be part of a periodic health examination, preferably at least every 3 years. Asymptomatic women age 40 years and over should continue to receive a CBE as part of a periodic health examination, preferably annually.
		Mammography	Begin annual mammography at age 40.*
Colorectal[†]	Men and women, age 50+	*Tests that find polyps and cancer:* Flexible sigmoidoscopy,[‡] or	Every 5 years, starting at age 50
		Colonoscopy, or	Every 10 years, starting at age 50
		Double-contrast barium enema (DCBE),[‡] or	Every 5 years, starting at age 50
		CT colonography (virtual colonoscopy)[‡]	Every 5 years, starting at age 50
		Tests that mainly find cancer: Fecal occult blood test (FOBT) with at least 50% test sensitivity for cancer, or fecal immunochemical test (FIT) with at least 50% test sensitivity for cancer[‡ §] or	Annual, starting at age 50
		Stool DNA test (sDNA)[‡]	Interval uncertain, starting at age 50
Prostate	Men, age 50+	Prostate-specific antigen (PSA) test with or without digital rectal exam (DRE)	Asymptomatic men who have at least a 10-year life expectancy should have an opportunity to make an informed decision with their health care provider about screening for prostate cancer after receiving information about the uncertainties, risks, and potential benefits associated with screening. Prostate cancer screening should not occur without an informed decision-making process.[¶]
Cervix	Women, age 21–29	Pap test	Cytology alone every 3 years (liquid or conventional). Recommend AGAINST annual cytology.
	Women, age 30–65	Co-testing with human papillomavirus (HPV) test and Pap test	HPV + cytology "co-testing" every 5 years (preferred) or every 3 years with cytology alone (acceptable). Recommend AGAINST more frequent screening.
	Women, age >65		Discontinue after age 65 if 3 negative cytology tests or 2 negative HPV tests in past 10 years with most recent test in past 5 years.
Endometrial	Women, at menopause	At the time of menopause, women at average risk should be informed about risks and symptoms of endometrial cancer and strongly encouraged to report any unexpected bleeding or spotting to their physicians.	N/A
Cancer-related checkup	Men and women, age 20+	On the occasion of a periodic health examination, the cancer-related checkup should include examination for cancers of the thyroid, testicles, ovaries, lymph nodes, oral cavity, and skin, as well as health counseling about tobacco, sun exposure, diet and nutrition, risk factors, sexual practices, and environmental and occupational exposures.	N/A

*Beginning at age 40, annual CBE should be performed prior to mammography.
[†]Individuals with a personal or family history of colorectal cancer or adenomas, inflammatory bowel disease, or high-risk genetic syndromes should continue to follow the most recent recommendations for individuals at increased or high risk.
[‡]Colonoscopy should be done if test results are positive.
[§]For FOBT or FIT used as a screening test, the take-home multiple sample method should be used. A FOBT or FIT done during a DRE in the doctor's office is not adequate for screening.
[¶]Information should be provided to men about the benefits and limitations of testing so that an informed decision can be made with the clinician's assistance.
Reprinted with permission from American Cancer Society. *Cancer Prevention & Early Detection Facts and Figures 2012.* Atlanta: American Cancer Society, Inc.

The evolving understanding of the role of genetics in cancer cell development has contributed to prevention and screening efforts. Many centers offer cancer risk evaluation programs that provide interdisciplinary in-depth assessment, screening, education, and counseling as well as follow-up monitoring for people who are found to be at high risk for cancer (Aiello-Laws, 2011). Several professional organizations provide guidelines outlining standards for the practice of cancer risk assessment, counseling, education, and genetic testing (Weitzel et al., 2011).

Tertiary Prevention

Improved screening, diagnosis, and treatment approaches have led to an estimated 13.7 million cancer survivors in the United States (Mariotto, Yabroff, Shao, et al., 2011). Tertiary prevention efforts focus on monitoring for and preventing recurrence of the primary cancer as well as screening for development of second malignancies in cancer survivors. Survivors are assessed for the development of second malignancies such as lymphoma and leukemia, which have been associated with certain chemotherapy agents and the use of radiation therapy

(ACS, 2011d). Survivors may also develop second malignancies not related to treatment but genetic mutations related to inherited cancer syndromes, environmental exposures, and lifestyle factors.

Diagnosis of Cancer

A cancer diagnosis is based on assessment of physiologic and functional changes and results of the diagnostic evaluation. Patients with suspected cancer undergo extensive testing to (1) determine the presence and extent of cancer, (2) identify possible spread (metastasis) of disease or invasion of other body tissues, (3) evaluate the function of involved and uninvolved body systems and organs, and (4) obtain tissue and cells for analysis, including evaluation of tumor stage and grade. The diagnostic evaluation includes a review of systems; physical examination; imaging studies; laboratory tests of blood, urine, and other body fluids; procedures; and pathology analysis. Knowledge of suspicious symptoms and the behavior of particular types of cancer assists in determining relevant diagnostic tests (Table 15-4).

TABLE 15-4   Diagnostic Tests Used to Detect Cancer

Test	Description	Examples of Diagnostic Uses
Tumor marker identification	Analysis of substances found in tumor tissue, blood, or other body fluids that are indicative of cancer cells or specific characteristics of cancer cells. These substances may also be found in some normal body tissues.	Breast, colon, lung, ovarian, testicular, prostate cancers
Genetic tumor markers	Analysis for the presence of mutations (alterations) in genes found in tumors or body tissues. Assists in diagnosis, selection of treatment, prediction of response to therapy, and risk of progression or recurrence.	Breast, lung, kidney, ovarian, brain cancers; leukemia, and lymphoma. Many uses of genetic profiling are considered investigational.
Mammography	Use of x-ray images of the breast	Breast cancer
Magnetic resonance imaging (MRI)	Use of magnetic fields and radiofrequency signals to create sectioned images of various body structures	Neurologic, pelvic, abdominal, thoracic, breast cancers
Computed tomography (CT) scan	Use of narrow-beam x-ray to scan successive layers of tissue for a cross-sectional view	Neurologic, pelvic, skeletal, abdominal, thoracic cancers
Fluoroscopy	Use of x-rays that identify contrasts in body tissue densities; may involve the use of contrast agents	Skeletal, lung, gastrointestinal cancers
Ultrasonography (ultrasound)	High-frequency sound waves echoing off body tissues are converted electronically into images; used to assess tissues deep within the body.	Abdominal and pelvic cancers
Endoscopy	Direct visualization of a body cavity or passageway by insertion of an endoscope into a body cavity or opening; allows tissue biopsy, fluid aspiration, and excision of small tumors. Used for diagnostic and therapeutic purposes.	Bronchial, gastrointestinal cancers
Nuclear medicine imaging	Uses IV injection or ingestion of radioisotope substances followed by imaging of tissues that have concentrated the radioisotopes	Bone, liver, kidney, spleen, brain, thyroid cancers
Positron emission tomography (PET)	Through the use of a tracer, provides black and white or color-coded images of the biologic activity of a particular area, rather than its structure. Used in detection of cancer or its response to treatment.	Lung, colon, liver, pancreatic, head and neck cancers; Hodgkin and non-Hodgkin lymphoma and melanoma
PET fusion	Use of a PET scanner and a CT scanner in one machine to provide an image combining anatomic detail, spatial resolution, and functional metabolic abnormalities	See PET.
Radioimmunoconjugates	Monoclonal antibodies are labeled with a radioisotope and injected IV into the patient; the antibodies that aggregate at the tumor site are visualized with scanners.	Colorectal, breast, ovarian, head and neck cancers; lymphoma and melanoma
Vascular imaging	Use of contrast agents that are injected into veins or arteries and monitored by fluoroscopy, CT, or MRI imaging in order to assess tumor vasculature. Used to assess tumor vascularity prior to surgical procedures. Use in assessing the efficacy of antiangiogenesis (preventing new blood vessel formation) drugs is largely investigational.	Liver and brain cancers

Patients undergoing extensive testing may be fearful of the procedures and anxious about possible test results. Nurses help relieve the patient's fear and anxiety by explaining the tests to be performed, the sensations likely to be experienced, and the patient's role in the test procedures. The nurse encourages the patient and family to voice their fears about the test results, supports the patient and family throughout the test period, and reinforces and clarifies information conveyed by the physician. The nurse also encourages the patient and family to communicate and share their concerns and to discuss their questions and concerns with one another.

Tumor Staging and Grading

A complete diagnostic evaluation includes identifying the stage and grade of the tumor. This is accomplished prior to treatment to provide baseline data for evaluating outcomes of therapy and to maintain a systematic and consistent approach to ongoing diagnosis and treatment. Treatment options and prognosis are based on tumor stage and grade.

Staging provides a common language used by health care providers and scientists to accurately communicate about cancer in and across clinical settings and in research. These systems also provide a convenient shorthand notation that condenses lengthy descriptions into manageable terms for comparisons of treatments and prognoses.

Staging determines the size of the tumor, the existence of local invasion, lymph node involvement, and distant metastasis. Several systems exist for classifying the anatomic extent of disease. The tumor, nodes, and metastasis (TNM) system (Chart 15-3) is one system used to describe many solid tumors (Edge, Byrd, Compton, et al., 2010).

Chart 15-3 TNM Classification System

T The extent of the primary tumor
N The absence or presence and extent of regional lymph node metastasis
M The absence or presence of distant metastasis

The use of numerical subsets of the TNM components indicates the progressive extent of the malignant disease.

Primary Tumor (T)

Tx Primary tumor cannot be assessed
T0 No evidence of primary tumor
Tis Carcinoma in situ
T1, T2, T3, T4 Increasing size and/or local extent of the primary tumor

Regional Lymph Nodes (N)

Nx Regional lymph nodes cannot be assessed
N0 No regional lymph node metastasis
N1, N2, N3 Increasing involvement of regional lymph nodes

Distant Metastasis (M)

Mx Distant metastasis cannot be assessed
M0 No distant metastasis
M1 Distant metastasis

Adapted from Edge, S. B., Byrd, D. R., Compton, C. C., et al. (Eds.). (2010). *AJCC cancer staging manual* (7th ed.). New York: Springer.

Grading is the pathologic classification of tumor cells. Grading systems seek to define the type of tissue from which the tumor originated and the degree to which the tumor cells retain the functional and histologic characteristics of the tissue of origin (differentiation). Samples of cells used to establish the tumor grade may be obtained from tissue scrapings, body fluids, secretions, washings, biopsy, or surgical excision. This information helps providers predict the behavior and prognosis of various tumors. The grade corresponds with a numeric value ranging from I to IV. Grade I tumors, also known as well-differentiated tumors, closely resemble the tissue of origin in structure and function. Tumors that do not clearly resemble the tissue of origin in structure or function are described as poorly differentiated or undifferentiated and are assigned grade IV. These tumors tend to be more aggressive, less responsive to treatment, and associated with a poorer prognosis as compared to well-differentiated, grade I tumors. Various staging and grading systems are used to characterize cancers.

Anatomic Stage Group

Once the diagnosis, clinical stage, and histologic grade have been determined, the anatomic stage group, designated by I through IV (representing increasing severity of disease), is assigned to facilitate communication, treatment decisions, and estimation of prognosis. The anatomic stage group is also useful for comparing clinical outcomes.

Management of Cancer

Treatment options offered to patients with cancer are based on treatment goals for each specific type, stage, and grade of cancer. The range of possible treatment goals includes complete eradication of malignant disease (**cure**), prolonged survival and containment of cancer cell growth (**control**), or relief of symptoms associated with the disease and improvement of quality of life (**palliation**). Treatment approaches are not initiated until the diagnosis of cancer has been confirmed and staging and grading has been completed

The health care team and the patient and family must have a clear understanding of the treatment options and goals. Open communication and support are vital as those involved periodically reassess treatment plans and goals when complications of therapy develop or disease progresses.

Multiple modalities are commonly used in cancer treatment. Various approaches, including surgery, radiation therapy, chemotherapy, HSCT, hyperthermia, and targeted therapy, may be used together or at different times throughout treatment. Understanding the principles of each and how they interrelate is important in understanding the rationale and goals of treatment.

■ Surgery

Surgical removal of the entire cancer remains the ideal and most frequently used treatment method. However, the specific surgical approach may vary for several reasons. Diagnostic surgery is the definitive method for obtaining tissue to identify the cellular characteristics that influence all treatment decisions. Surgery may be the primary method of treatment, or it may be prophylactic, palliative, or reconstructive.

Diagnostic Surgery

Diagnostic surgery, or **biopsy**, is performed to obtain a tissue sample for histologic analysis of cells suspected to be malignant. In most instances, the biopsy is taken from the actual tumor; however, in some situations, it is necessary to biopsy lymph nodes near the suspicious tumor. Many cancers can metastasize from the primary site to other areas of the body through the lymphatic circulation. Knowing whether adjacent lymph nodes contain tumor cells helps health care providers plan the best therapeutic approach to combat tumor cells that have gone beyond the primary tumor site. The use of injectable dyes and nuclear medicine imaging can help identify the sentinel lymph node or the initial lymph node to which the primary tumor and surrounding tissue drains. Sentinel lymph node biopsy (SLNB), also known as sentinel lymph node mapping, is a minimally invasive surgical approach that in many instances has replaced more invasive lymph node dissections (lymphadenectomy) and the associated complications such as lymphedema and delayed healing. SLNB has been widely adopted for regional lymph node staging in selected cases of melanoma and breast cancer (National Comprehensive Cancer Network [NCCN], 2011a).

Biopsy Types

The three most common biopsy methods are the excisional, incisional, and needle methods (Drake & Lynes, 2010). The biopsy type is determined by the size and location of the tumor, the type of treatment anticipated if the cancer diagnosis is confirmed, and the need for surgery and general anesthesia. The biopsy method that allows for the least invasive approach while permitting the most representative tissue sample is chosen. Occasionally, diagnostic imaging techniques are used to assist in locating the suspicious lesion and to facilitate accurate tissue sampling. The patient and family are provided the opportunity and time to discuss the options before definitive plans are made.

Excisional biopsy is most frequently used for small, easily accessible tumors of the skin, breast, and upper or lower gastrointestinal and upper respiratory tracts. In many cases, the surgeon can remove the entire tumor as well as the surrounding marginal tissues. The removal of normal tissue beyond the tumor area decreases the possibility that residual microscopic malignant cells may lead to a recurrence of the tumor. This approach not only provides the pathologist with the entire tissue specimen for determination of stage and grade but also decreases the chance of seeding tumor cells (disseminating cancer cells throughout surrounding tissues).

Incisional biopsy is performed if the tumor mass is too large to be removed. In this case, a wedge of tissue from the tumor is removed for analysis. The cells of the tissue wedge must be representative of the tumor mass so that the pathologist can provide an accurate diagnosis. If the specimen does not contain representative tissue and cells, negative biopsy results do not guarantee the absence of cancer.

Excisional and incisional approaches are often performed through endoscopy. However, a surgical procedure may be required to determine the anatomic extent or stage of the tumor. For example, a diagnostic or staging laparotomy (the surgical opening of the abdomen to assess malignant abdominal disease) may be necessary to assess malignancies such as gastric or colon cancer.

Needle biopsy is performed to sample suspicious masses that are easily and safely accessible, such as some masses in the breasts, thyroid, lung, liver, and kidney. Needle biopsies are most often performed on an outpatient basis. They are fast, relatively inexpensive, easy to perform, and usually require only local anesthesia. In general, the patient experiences slight and temporary physical discomfort. In addition, the surrounding tissues are minimally disturbed, thus decreasing the likelihood of seeding cancer cells. Fine-needle aspiration (FNA) biopsy involves aspirating cells rather than intact tissue through a needle guided into a suspected diseased area. This type of specimen can only be analyzed by cytologic examination. Often, x-ray, computed tomography (CT) scanning, ultrasonography, or magnetic resonance imaging (MRI) is used to help locate the suspicious area and guide placement of the needle. FNA does not always yield enough material to permit accurate diagnosis, necessitating additional biopsy procedures. A core needle biopsy uses a specially designed needle to obtain a small core of tissue that permits histologic analysis. Most often, this specimen is sufficient to permit accurate diagnosis.

Surgery as Primary Treatment

When surgery is the primary approach in treating cancer, the goal is to remove the entire tumor or as much as is feasible (a procedure sometimes called *debulking*) as well as any involved surrounding tissue, including regional lymph nodes.

Two common surgical approaches used for treating primary tumors are local and wide excisions. Local excision, often performed on an outpatient basis, is warranted when the mass is small. It includes removal of the mass and a small margin of normal tissue that is easily accessible. Wide or radical excisions (en bloc dissections) include removal of the primary tumor, lymph nodes, adjacent involved structures, and surrounding tissues that may be at high risk for tumor spread. This surgical method can result in disfigurement and altered functioning, necessitating rehabilitation and/or reconstructive procedures. However, wide excisions are considered if the tumor can be removed completely and the chances of cure or control are good.

Minimally invasive surgical techniques are increasingly replacing traditional surgery associated with large incisions for a variety of cancers. The advantages of minimally invasive approaches include minimization of surgical trauma, decreased blood loss, decreased incidence of wound infection and other complications associated with surgery, decreased surgical time and requirement for anesthesia, decreased postoperative pain and limited mobility, and shorter periods of recovery.

Video-assisted endoscopic surgery, an example of minimally invasive surgery, uses an endoscope with intense lighting and an attached multichip mini-camera that is inserted into the body through a small incision. The surgical instruments are inserted into the surgical field through one or two additional small incisions, each about 3 cm in length. The camera transmits the image of the involved area to a monitor so the surgeon can manipulate the instruments to perform the necessary procedure. Such surgery is used for many thoracic and abdominal procedures. The use of robotics during

TABLE 15-5 **Selected Techniques Used for Localized Destruction of Tumor Tissue**

Type of Procedure	Description	Examples of Use
Chemosurgery	Use of chemicals or chemotherapy applied directly to tissue to cause destruction	Intraperitoneal chemotherapy for ovarian cancer involving the abdomen and peritoneum
Cryoablation	Use of liquid nitrogen or a very cold probe to freeze tissue and cause cell destruction	Cervical, prostate, and rectal cancers
Electrosurgery	Use of an electric current to destroy tumor cells	Basal and squamous cell skin cancers
Laser surgery	Use of light and energy aimed at an exact tissue location and depth to vaporize cancer cells (also referred to as photocoagulation or photoablation)	Dyspnea associated with endobronchial obstructions
Photodynamic therapy	IV administration of a light-sensitizing agent (hematoporphyrin derivative [HPD]) that is taken up by cancer cells, followed by exposure to laser light within 24–48 hours; causes cancer cell death	Palliative treatment of dysphagia associated with esophageal and dyspnea associated with endobronchial obstructions
Radiofrequency ablation (RFA)	Uses localized application of thermal energy that destroys cancer cells through heat: temperatures exceed 50°C (122°F)	Nonresectable liver tumors, pain control with bone metastasis

laparoscopic procedures permits the removal of tumors with more precision and dexterity than could be accomplished by laparoscopic surgery alone (Castiglia, Drummond, & Purden 2011). Laparoscopic robotic assisted surgery has been used for prostate and gynecologic cancers. Transoral robotic assisted surgery is being used in some centers for certain types of oral and laryngeal cancers (Scarpa, 2011).

Salvage surgery is an additional treatment option that uses an extensive surgical approach to treat the local recurrence of cancer after the use of a less extensive primary approach. Mastectomy to treat recurrent breast cancer after primary lumpectomy and radiation is an example of salvage surgery.

In addition to surgery that uses surgical blades or scalpels to excise the mass and surrounding tissues, several other types of techniques are available. Table 15-5 provides examples of these techniques.

A multidisciplinary approach to patient care is essential for the patient undergoing cancer-related surgery. The effects of surgery on the patient's body image, self-esteem, and functional abilities are addressed. If necessary, a plan for postoperative rehabilitation is made before the surgery is performed. The growth and dissemination of cancer cells may have produced distant micrometastases by the time the patient seeks treatment. Therefore, attempting to remove wide margins of tissue in the hope of "getting all the cancer" may not be feasible. This reality substantiates the need for a coordinated multidisciplinary approach to cancer therapy.

Once the surgery has been completed, one or more additional (or adjuvant) modalities may be chosen to increase the likelihood of eradicating the remaining cancer cells. However, some cancers that are treated surgically in the very early stages (e.g., skin and testicular cancers) are considered to be curable without additional therapies.

Prophylactic Surgery

Prophylactic surgery involves removing nonvital tissues or organs that are at increased risk of developing cancer. The following factors are considered when discussing possible prophylactic surgery:

- Family history and genetic predisposition
- Presence or absence of signs and symptoms

- Potential risks and benefits
- Ability to detect cancer at an early stage
- Alternative options for managing increased risk
- The patient's acceptance of the postoperative outcome

Colectomy, mastectomy, and oophorectomy are examples of prophylactic surgeries. Identification of genetic markers indicative of a predisposition to develop some types of cancer plays a role in decisions concerning prophylactic surgeries. However, what is adequate justification for prophylactic surgery remains controversial. For example, several factors are considered when deciding to proceed with a prophylactic mastectomy, including a strong family history of breast cancer; positive *BRCA1* or *BRCA2* findings; an abnormal physical finding on breast examination, such as progressive nodularity and cystic disease; a proven history of breast cancer in the opposite breast; abnormal mammography findings; abnormal biopsy results; and individual factors that may influence the patient's decision-making process (McQuirter, Castiglia, Loiselle, et al., 2010). Prophylactic surgery is discussed with patients and families along with other approaches for managing increased risk of cancer development. Preoperative education and counseling, as well as long-term follow-up, are provided.

Palliative Surgery

When surgical cure is not possible, the goals of surgical interventions are to relieve symptoms, make the patient as comfortable as possible, and promote quality of life as defined by the patient and family. Palliative surgery and other interventions are performed in an attempt to relieve complications of cancer, such as ulceration, obstruction, hemorrhage, pain, and malignant effusions (Table 15-6). Honest and informative communication with the patient and family about the goal of surgery is essential to avoid false hope and disappointment.

Reconstructive Surgery

Reconstructive surgery may follow curative or radical surgery in an attempt to improve function or obtain a more desirable cosmetic effect. It may be performed in one operation or in stages. The surgeon who will perform the surgery discusses possible reconstructive surgical options with the patient

TABLE 15-6 **Types of Palliative Surgery and Interventions**

Procedure	Indications
Abdominal shunt placement	Ascites
Biliary stent placement	Biliary obstruction
Bone stabilization	Displaced bone fracture related to metastatic disease
Colostomy or ileostomy	Bowel obstruction
Cordotomy	Pain
Epidural catheter placement (for administering epidural analgesics)	Pain
Excision of solitary metastatic lesion	Metastatic lung, liver, or brain lesion
Gastrostomy, jejunostomy tube placement	Upper gastrointestinal tract obstruction
Hormone manipulation (removal of ovaries, testes, adrenals, pituitary)	Tumors that depend on hormones for growth
Nerve block	Pain
Percutaneous enteral gastrostomy (PEG) tube placement	Enteral nutrition
Pericardial drainage tube placement	Pericardial effusion
Peritoneal drainage tube placement	Ascites
Pleural drainage tube placement	Pleural effusion
Ureteral stent placement	Ureteral obstruction
Venous access device placement (for administering parenteral analgesics)	Pain

Adapted from Drake, D., & Lynes, B. (2010). Surgery. In J. Eggert (Ed.). *Cancer basics*. Pittsburgh: Oncology Nursing Society; and Walker, S. J., & Bryden, G. (2010). Managing pleural effusions: Nursing care of patients with a Tenckhoff catheter. *Clinical Journal of Oncology Nursing, 14*(1), 59–64.

before the primary surgery is performed. Reconstructive surgery may be indicated for breast, head and neck, and skin cancers.

The nurse assesses the patient's needs and the impact that altered functioning and body image may have on quality of life. Nurses provide patients and families with opportunities to discuss these issues. The individual needs of the patient undergoing reconstructive surgery and their families must be accurately recognized and addressed.

Nursing Management

Patients undergoing surgery for cancer require general perioperative nursing care, as described in Unit 4 of this text. Surgical care is individualized according to age, organ impairment, specific deficits, comorbities, cultural implications (Baldwin, 2010), and altered immunity, as all can increase the risk of postoperative complications. Combining other treatment methods, such as radiation and chemotherapy, with surgery also contributes to postoperative complications, such as infection, impaired wound healing, altered pulmonary or renal function, and the development of venous thromboembolism (VTE). The nurse completes a thorough preoperative assessment for factors that may affect the patient undergoing the surgical procedure.

Preoperatively, the nurse provides the patient and family with verbal and written information about the surgical procedure as well as other interventions that may take place intraoperatively (i.e., radiation implants). Instructions concerning

prophylactic antibiotic requirements, diet, and bowel preparation are also provided.

Patients who are undergoing surgery for the diagnosis or treatment of cancer may be anxious about the surgical procedure, possible findings, postoperative limitations, changes in normal body functions, and prognosis. The patient and family require time and assistance to process the possible changes and outcomes resulting from the surgery (Chart 15-4).

The nurse serves as the patient advocate and liaison and encourages the patient and family to take an active role in decision making when possible. If the patient or family asks about the results of diagnostic testing and surgical procedures, the nurse's response is guided by the information that was conveyed previously. The nurse may be asked to explain and clarify information for patients and families that was provided initially but was not grasped because of anxiety and overwhelming feelings. It is important that the nurse, as well as other members of the health care team, provide information that is consistent from one clinician to another.

Postoperatively, the nurse assesses patient responses to surgery and monitors the patient for possible complications, such as infection, bleeding, thrombophlebitis, wound dehiscence, fluid and electrolyte imbalance, and organ dysfunction. The nurse also provides for the patient's comfort. Postoperative education addresses wound care, pain management, activity, nutrition, and medication information.

Plans for discharge, follow-up, home care, and subsequent treatment are initiated as early as possible to ensure continuity of care from hospital to home or from a cancer referral center to the patient's local hospital and health care provider. Patients and families are encouraged to use community resources such as the ACS for support and information (see the Resources section at the end of this chapter).

■ Radiation Therapy

Approximately 60% of patients with cancer receive **radiation therapy** at some point during treatment (Gosselin, 2010). Radiation may be used to cure cancer, as in thyroid carcinomas, localized cancers of the head and neck, and cancers of the cervix. Radiation therapy may also be used to control cancer when a tumor cannot be removed surgically or when local nodal metastasis is present. Neoadjuvant (prior to local definitive treatment) radiation therapy, with or without chemotherapy, is used to reduce tumor size in order to facilitate surgical resection. Radiation therapy may be administered prophylactically to prevent spread of the primary cancer to a distant area (e.g., irradiating the brain to prevent leukemic infiltration or metastatic lung cancer). Palliative radiation therapy is used to relieve the symptoms of metastatic disease, especially when the cancer has spread to the brain, bone, or soft tissue, or to treat oncologic emergencies, such as superior vena cava syndrome, bronchial airway obstruction, or spinal cord compression.

Two types of ionizing radiation—electromagnetic radiation (x-rays and gamma rays) and particulate radiation (electrons, beta particles, protons, neutrons, and alpha particles)—can be used to kill cells. The most lethal damage is the direct alteration of the DNA molecule within the cells of both malignant and normal tissue. Ionizing radiation can directly break the strands of the DNA helix, leading to cell

Chart 15-4

NURSING RESEARCH PROFILE

Coping and Recovery Following Breast Cancer Surgery

Greenslade, M., V., Elliott, B., & Mandville-Anstey, S. A. (2010). Same-day breast cancer surgery: A qualitative study of women's lived experiences. *Oncology Nursing Forum, 37*(2), E92–E97.

Purpose

The purpose of this research was to understand the experiences of women having same-day breast cancer surgery and to make recommendations to facilitate changes that enhance quality of care and patient outcomes. There is little nursing research to inform clinicians about factors that make women good candidates for same-day surgery or nursing interventions that foster optimal patient outcomes.

Design

The methodology of this study involved in-depth interviews about 8 weeks after surgery and comparative analysis to identify themes and a connecting essential thread. A purposive sample of 13 women who had undergone same-day breast cancer surgery was obtained from outpatient departments of two city hospitals on the east coast of Canada. Participants, who all lived with family members, ranged in age from 32 to 74 years, with a mean age of 53 years. Nine participants (69%) came from an urban area, whereas four (31%) were from rural areas. Data were collected during audiotaped, unstructured interviews including open-ended questions used to stimulate discussion. Data that were transcribed verbatim were examined individually and collaboratively by the researchers in order to identify themes and

to develop a description of the experience of having same-day breast surgery.

Findings

The findings illustrated four interrelated themes that had an impact on women's coping: preparation, timing, supports, and community health nursing intervention. The themes were of tremendous importance for effective coping and recovery, both of which were independent of the type (lumpectomy vs. mastectomy) or complexity of surgery performed. In general, the women who reported a positive experience with same-day breast cancer surgery also reported having (1) adequate preparation through preoperative education about surgery, discharge, and recovery; (2) appropriate timing of and time devoted to preadmission education; (3) availability of strong support systems through family and/or friends; and (4) availability of community health nursing services including weekends and holidays when needed due to the timing of surgical procedures.

Nursing Implications

The researchers note that for women with breast cancer, the length of time has decreased from initial presentation to surgical intervention. Women are challenged to cope with a cancer diagnosis and to absorb an overwhelming amount of information in a relatively short period of time. The researchers suggest that future research should explore optimal methods and timing of preoperative education.

---

death. It can also indirectly damage DNA through the formation of free radicals. If the DNA cannot be repaired, the cell may die immediately or may initiate apoptosis, a genetically programmed normal process of cell death (Kelvin, 2010). Cells are most vulnerable to the disruptive effects of radiation during DNA synthesis and mitosis (early S, G_2, and M phases of the cell cycle; Fig. 15-2). Therefore, those body tissues that undergo frequent cell division are most sensitive to radiation therapy. These tissues include bone marrow, lymphatic tissue, epithelium of the gastrointestinal tract, hair cells, and gonads. Slower-growing tissues and tissues at rest (e.g., muscle, cartilage, and connective tissues) are relatively radioresistant (less sensitive to the effects of radiation). However, it is important to remember that radiation therapy is localized treatment, and only the tissues that are within the treatment field are affected.

A radiosensitive tumor is one that can be destroyed by a dose of radiation that still allows for cell repair and regeneration in the normal tissue. Tumors that are well oxygenated also appear to be more sensitive to radiation. In theory, therefore, radiation therapy may be enhanced if more oxygen can be delivered to tumors. In addition, if the radiation is delivered when most tumor cells are cycling through the cell cycle, the number of cancer cells destroyed (cell kill) is maximal. Radiation sensitivity is enhanced in tumors that are smaller in size and that contain cells that are rapidly dividing (highly proliferative) and poorly differentiated (no longer resembling the tissue of origin).

Certain chemicals, including chemotherapy agents, act as radiosensitizers and facilitate the effects of radiation therapy

on hypoxic (oxygen-poor) tumors. Combinations of chemotherapy and radiation therapy are typically used to take advantage of the radiosensitizing effects of chemotherapy and achieve improved tumor response and patient survival. Combined modality therapy can, however, result in increased toxicities.

Radiation Dosage

The radiation dosage depends on the sensitivity of the target tissues to radiation, the size of the tumor, tissue tolerance of the surrounding normal tissues, and critical structures adjacent to the tumor target. The lethal tumor dose is defined as the dose that will eradicate 95% of the tumor yet preserve normal tissue. In external-beam radiation therapy (EBRT), the total radiation dose is delivered over several weeks in daily doses called *fractions*. This allows healthy tissue to repair and achieves greater cell kill by exposing more cells to the radiation as they begin active cell division. Repeated radiation treatments over time (fractionated doses) also allow for the periphery of the tumor to be reoxygenated repeatedly, because tumors shrink from the outside inward. This increases the radiosensitivity of the tumor, thereby increasing tumor cell death (Kelvin, 2010).

Administration of Radiation

Radiation therapy can be administered in various ways depending on the source of radiation used, the location of the tumor, and the type of cancer targeted. The primary applications include teletherapy (external-beam radiation),

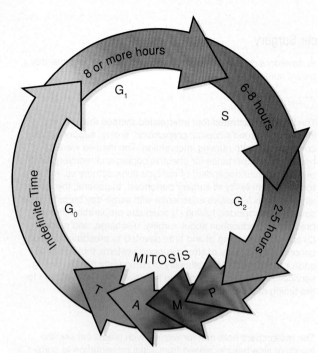

FIGURE 15-2 • Phases of the cell cycle extend over the interval between the midpoint of mitosis and the subsequent endpoint in mitosis in a daughter cell. G_1 is the postmitotic phase during which ribonucleic acid (RNA) and protein syntheses are increased and cell growth occurs. G_0 is the resting, or dormant, phase of the cell cycle. In the S phase, nucleic acids are synthesized and chromosomes are replicated in preparation for cell mitosis. During G_2, RNA and protein synthesis occur as in G_1. P, prophase; M, metaphase; A, anaphase; T, telophase. Redrawn from Porth, C. M., & Matfin, G. (2009). *Pathophysiology: Concepts of altered health states* (8th ed.). Philadelphia: Lippincott Williams & Wilkins.

brachytherapy (internal radiation), systemic (radioisotopes), and contact or surface molds.

External Radiation

EBRT is the most commonly used form of radiation therapy. The energy utilized in EBRT is either generated from a linear accelerator or from a unit that generates energy directly from a core source of radioactive material such as a GammaKnife™ unit. Through computerized software programs, both approaches are able to shape an invisible beam of highly charged electrons to penetrate the body and target the tumor with pinpoint accuracy.

Advances in computer technology allow multiple imaging modalities (CT, MRI, and PET scans) to be used to provide three-dimensional images of the tumor, neighboring tissues at risk for microscopic spread, and surrounding normal tissues or organs at risk for radiation-induced toxicity. These images, referred to as volumetric images, allow the radiation oncologist to plan for multiple radiation beams directed from different angles and different planes so that the beams conform precisely around the tumor (referred to as conformal radiation). The dose of radiation that reaches the surrounding normal tissues is reduced, leading to much less toxicity than in older forms of radiation therapy (Mallick & Waldron, 2009). Treatment enhancements in EBRT include the ability to control different intensity or energy levels of radiation beams at different angles directed at the tumor, a process

known as intensity-modulated radiation therapy (IMRT), which enables higher doses to be delivered to the tumor while sparing the important healthy structures surrounding the tumor (Khan, 2010). IMRT can be administered as standard daily fractions or as "hyperfractionated" twice-daily fractions, which shortens the duration of the patient's treatment schedule. Image-guided radiation therapy (IGRT) uses continuous monitoring of the tumor with ultrasound, x-ray, or CT scans during the treatment to allow for automatic adjustment of the beams as the tumor changes shape or position in an effort to spare the healthy surrounding tissue and reduce side effects. Additional treatment enhancements include respiratory gating, where the treatment delivery is actually synchronized with the patient's respiratory cycle, enabling the beam to be adjusted as the tumor or organ moves (Mallick & Waldron, 2009). These treatment advancements improve tumor destruction while reducing acute and long-term toxicities.

Gamma rays generated from the spontaneous decay of naturally occurring solid source of radioactivity, such as cobalt-60, is one of the oldest forms of EBRT. With the advent of modern linear accelerators, the use of solid radioactive elements are confined primarily to the GammaKnife™ stereotactic radiosurgery unit, which is used as a one-time, high-dose delivery of EBRT for treatment of both benign and malignant intracranial lesions.

Stereotactic body radiotherapy (SBRT) is another form of EBRT that uses higher doses of radiation to penetrate very deeply into the body to control deep-seated tumors that cannot be treated by other approaches such as surgery. SBRT is delivered with considerably higher treatment fraction doses over a short span of time, usually 1 to 5 treatment days, in contrast to daily treatments for 5 days per week for 6 to 8 weeks for conventional EBRT. Specialized linear accelerators with the capability of robotically moving around the patient are used to deliver SBRT, such as the CyberKnife™, Trilogy™, and TomoTherapy™ delivery systems, which are now more commonly available in community hospital settings.

Proton therapy is another very different approach to EBRT. Proton therapy utilizes high linear energy transfer (LET) in the form of charged protons generated by a large magnetic unit called a *cyclotron*. The advantage of proton therapy is that it is capable of delivering its high-energy dose to a deep-seated tumor, with decreased doses of radiation to the tissues in front of the tumor while virtually no energy exits through the patient's healthy tissue behind the tumor (Kelvin, 2010). Proton therapy permits treatment of deep tumors in close proximity to critical structures such as the heart or major blood vessels. Because of high costs and the limited number of proton units in the United States, most treatment has been investigational in the areas of localized prostate cancer, inoperable early-stage lung cancer, uveal melanoma, and head and neck tumors.

Internal Radiation

Internal radiation implantation, or brachytherapy, delivers the dose of radiation to a localized area. The specific radioisotope for implantation is selected on the basis of its half-life, which is the time it takes for half of its radioactivity to decay. Internal radiation can be implanted by means of needles or rods, seeds, beads, ribbons, or catheters placed into body cavities (vagina, abdomen, pleura) or interstitial compartments (breast, prostate). Patients may have many fears or concerns about internal radiation, and the nurse explains the various approaches and safety precautions that will be used to protect the patient, family, and health care staff.

Brachytherapy may be delivered as a temporary or a permanent implant. Temporary applications may be delivered as high-dose radiation (HDR) for short periods of time or low-dose radiation (LDR) for a more extended period of time. The primary advantage of HDR sources of brachytherapy is that treatment time is shorter, there is reduced exposure to personnel, and the procedure can typically be performed on an outpatient basis over several days. HDR brachytherapy can be used for intraluminal, surface, interstitial, and intracavitary lesions.

Intraluminal brachytherapy involves the insertion of catheters or hollow tubes into the lumens of organs so that the radioisotope can be delivered as close to the tumor bed as possible. Obstructive lesions in the bronchus, esophagus, or bile duct can be treated with this approach. Contact or surface application is used for treatment of tumors of the eye, such as retinoblastoma in children or ocular melanoma in adults.

Interstitial implants, used in treating such malignancies as prostate, pancreatic, or breast cancer, may be temporary or permanent, depending on the site and radioisotope used. Based on the dose to be delivered (LDR or HDR), the implants may consist of seeds, needles, wires, strands, or small catheters positioned to provide a local radiation source. Prostate HDR therapy is one form of interstitial brachytherapy, in which radioactive strands or wires are placed, while the patient is under anesthesia, into hollow catheters that have been inserted in the perineum close to the prostate gland (Waring & Gosselin, 2010).

Intracavitary radioisotopes are used to treat gynecologic cancers. In these malignancies, the radioisotopes are inserted into specially positioned applicators within the vagina. The applicator placement is verified by x-ray. Treatment can be achieved with either HDR or LDR brachytherapy sources, depending on the extent of disease. LDR therapy requires hospitalization because the patient is treated over several days.

Systemic radiotherapy (radiopharmaceutical therapy) involves the intravenous (IV) administration of a therapeutic radioactive isotope targeted to a specific tumor. Radioactive iodine (I-131) is a widely used form of systemic brachytherapy that is the primary treatment for thyroid cancer. Strontium 89 is utilized for bone metastases, samarium 153 is used for metastatic bone lesions, and phosphorus 32 is used for treatment of malignant ascites associated with ovarian cancer. Radioisotopes are also used as radioimmunotherapy for the treatment of refractory non-Hodgkin lymphoma. (See Chapter 34 for more information on lymphoma.)

Toxicity

Toxicities associated with radiation therapy are most often localized in the region being irradiated. Toxicity may be increased if concomitant chemotherapy is administered. Acute or early toxicities that most often begin within 2 weeks of the initiation of treatment occur when normal cells within the treatment area are damaged and cellular death exceeds cellular regeneration. Body tissues most affected are those that normally proliferate rapidly, such as the skin, the epithelial lining of the gastrointestinal tract, and the bone marrow.

Altered skin integrity is common and can include **alopecia** (hair loss) associated with whole brain radiation. Other skin reactions, referred to as radiation dermatitis, are identified and graded by severity along a continuum ranging from erythema and dry desquamation (flaking of skin), to moist desquamation (dermis exposed, skin oozing serous fluid), and, potentially, ulceration. Up to 95% of patients who receive radiation will experience some degree of radiation dermatitis (Feight, Baney, Bruce, et al., 2011). Severe radiation dermatitis may necessitate treatment interruption, delays, or cessation of therapy. Reepithelialization occurs after treatments have been completed (McQuestion, 2011). Hyperpigmentation, a less severe radiation-associated skin reaction, may develop about 2 to 4 weeks after the initiation of treatment.

 Concept Mastery Alert

Alopecia is mainly a side effect of some chemotherapy drugs. Radiation only results in alopecia when targeted at the whole brain; radiation of other parts of the body does not lead to hair loss.

Alterations in oral mucosa secondary to radiation therapy in the head and neck region include **stomatitis** (inflammation of the oral tissues), decreased salivation and **xerostomia** (dryness of the mouth), and change in or loss of taste. Depending on the targeted region, any portion of the gastrointestinal mucosa may be involved, causing **mucositis** (inflammation of the lining of the gastrointestinal tract). For example, patients receiving thoracic irradiation for lung cancer may experience acute esophageal irritation–associated chest pain and dysphagia. Anorexia, nausea, vomiting, and diarrhea may occur if the stomach or colon is in the radiation field. Symptoms subside and gastrointestinal reepithelialization occurs after treatments have been completed. Bone marrow cells proliferate rapidly, and if sites containing bone marrow (e.g., the iliac crest or sternum) are included in the radiation field, anemia, leukopenia (decreased white blood cells [WBCs]), and **thrombocytopenia** (a decrease in platelets) may result. The patient is then at increased risk for infection and bleeding until blood cell counts return to normal. Research to develop cytoprotective agents that can protect normal tissue from radiation damage continues. The only approved cytoprotectant is amifostine (Ethyol), which is occasionally utilized in patients with head and neck cancers to reduce acute and chronic xerostomia while preserving antitumor efficacy of the necessary radiation doses (Mettler, Brenner, Coleman, et al., 2011).

Systemic side effects are commonly experienced by patients receiving radiation therapy. These include fatigue, malaise, and anorexia that may be secondary to substances released when tumor cells are destroyed. Early effects tend to be temporary and most often subside within 6 months of the cessation of treatment.

Late effects (approximately 6 months to years after treatment) of radiation therapy may occur in body tissues that were in the field of radiation. These effects are chronic, usually a result of permanent damage to tissues, loss of elasticity, and changes secondary to a decreased vascular supply. Severe late effects include fibrosis, atrophy, ulceration, and necrosis and may affect the lungs, heart, central nervous system, and bladder. With advances in treatment planning and the accuracy of treatment delivery, the occurrence of late toxicities has diminished. However, late or chronic symptoms, such as dysphagia, incontinence, cognitive impairment, and sexual dysfunction, may persist for several years with implications for survivors' overall health and quality of life (Howlett, Koetters, Edrington, et al., 2010; Mallick & Waldron, 2009).

Nursing Management

Nursing care of the hospitalized patient receiving LDR focuses on effective safe delivery of the therapy and prevention of complications. The patient is maintained on bed rest in a specially prepared private room typically for 72 hours and log-rolled to prevent displacement of any intracavitary delivery device. An indwelling urinary catheter is inserted to ensure that the bladder remains empty. Low-residue diets and antidiarrheal agents are provided to prevent bowel movements during therapy, which could displace the radioisotopes. Visitors and personnel must limit their time and proximity to the patient due to the risk of radiation exposure. HDR intracavitary brachytherapy is typically delivered as an outpatient procedure in the radiation therapy department over several days.

The area of the body being irradiated partially guides the focus of nursing assessments. For the patient receiving EBRT, regardless of the targeted area, the nurse assesses the patient's skin regularly throughout the course of treatment and for the first several weeks after completion of therapy. In addition, nutritional status and general feelings of well-being are assessed throughout the course of treatment. Evidence-based treatment protocols for nursing management of the toxicities associated with radiation therapy are used. If systemic symptoms, such as weakness and fatigue, occur, the nurse explains that these symptoms are a result of the treatment and do not represent deterioration or progression of the disease.

Protecting Caregivers

When the patient has a radioactive implant in place, the nurse and other health care providers need to protect themselves, as well as the patient, from the effects of radiation. Patients receiving internal radiation emit radiation while the implant is in place; therefore, contact with the health care team is guided by principles of time, distance, and shielding to minimize exposure of personnel to radiation. Specific instructions are provided by the radiation safety officer from the radiology department and specify the maximum time that can be spent safely in the patient's room, the shielding equipment to be used, and special precautions and actions to be taken if the implant is dislodged (Kelvin, 2010). Safety precautions used in caring for a patient receiving brachytherapy include assigning the patient to a private room, posting appropriate notices about radiation safety precautions, having staff members wear dosimeter badges, making sure that pregnant staff members are not assigned to the patient's care, prohibiting visits by children or pregnant visitors, limiting visits from others to 30 minutes daily, and seeing that visitors maintain a 6-foot distance from the radiation source.

Patients with seed implants typically are able to return home; radiation exposure to others is minimal. Information about any precautions, if needed, is provided to the patient and family members to ensure safety. Depending on the dose and energy emitted by a systemic radionuclide, patients may or may not require special precautions or hospitalization (Kelvin, 2010). The nurse should explain the rationale for these precautions to keep the patient from feeling unduly isolated.

■ Chemotherapy

Chemotherapy involves the use of antineoplastic drugs in an attempt to destroy cancer cells by interfering with cellular functions, including replication and DNA repair (Levine, 2010). Chemotherapy is used primarily to treat systemic disease rather than localized lesions that are amenable to surgery or radiation. Chemotherapy may be combined with surgery, radiation therapy, or both to reduce tumor size preoperatively (neoadjuvant), to destroy any remaining tumor cells postoperatively (adjuvant), or to treat some forms of leukemia or lymphoma (primary). The goals of chemotherapy (cure, control, or palliation) must be realistic because they will determine the medications that are used and the aggressiveness of the treatment plan.

Cell Kill and the Cell Cycle

Each time a tumor is exposed to chemotherapy, a percentage of the tumor cells (20% to 99%, depending on dosage and agent) are destroyed. Repeated doses of chemotherapy are necessary over a prolonged period to achieve regression of the tumor. Eradication of 100% of the tumor is almost impossible; the goal of treatment is eradication of enough of the tumor so that the remaining malignant cells can be destroyed by the body's immune system (Levine, 2010).

Actively proliferating cells within a tumor are the most sensitive to chemotherapy (the ratio of dividing cells to resting cells is referred to as the growth fraction). Nondividing cells capable of future proliferation are the least sensitive to antineoplastic medications and consequently are potentially dangerous. However, the nondividing cells must be destroyed to eradicate the disease. Repeated cycles of chemotherapy or sequencing of multiple chemotherapeutic agents are used to achieve more tumor cell destruction by destroying the nondividing cells as they begin active cell division.

Reproduction of both healthy and malignant cells follows the cell cycle pattern (see Fig. 15-2). The cell cycle time is the time required for one cell to divide and reproduce two identical daughter cells. The cell cycle of any cell has four distinct phases, each with a vital underlying function:

1. G_1 phase—RNA and protein synthesis occur
2. S phase—DNA synthesis occurs
3. G_2 phase—premitotic phase; DNA synthesis is complete, mitotic spindle forms
4. Mitosis—cell division occurs

The G_0 phase, the resting or dormant phase of cells, can occur after mitosis and during the G_1 phase. Within the G_0 phase are those dangerous cells that are not actively dividing but have the potential for replicating. Protocols (standardized regimens) for administration of certain chemotherapeutic agents (as well as some other forms of therapy) are developed and coordinated with an understanding of the cell cycle (Levine, 2010).

Classification of Chemotherapeutic Agents

Chemotherapeutic agents may be classified by their mechanism of action in relation to the cell cycle. Agents that exert their maximal effect during specific phases of the cell cycle are termed *cell cycle–specific agents*. These agents destroy cells that are actively reproducing by means of the cell cycle; most affect cells in the S phase by interfering with DNA and RNA synthesis. Other agents, such as the vinca or plant alkaloids, are specific to the M phase, where they halt mitotic spindle formation. Chemotherapeutic agents that act independently of the cell cycle phases are termed *cell cycle–nonspecific agents*. These agents usually have a prolonged effect on cells, leading to cellular damage or death. Many treatment plans combine cell cycle–specific and cell cycle–nonspecific agents to increase the number of vulnerable tumor cells killed during a treatment period (Levine, 2010).

Chemotherapeutic agents are also classified by chemical group, each with a different mechanism of action. These include the alkylating agents, nitrosoureas, antimetabolites, antitumor antibiotics, topoisomerase inhibitors, plant alkaloids (also referred to as mitotic inhibitors), hormonal agents, and miscellaneous agents. The classification, mechanism of action, cell cycle specificity, and common side effects of selected antineoplastic agents are listed in Table 15-7.

Chemotherapeutic agents from multiple categories may be used together to maximize cell destruction. Combination chemotherapy relies on agents with varying mechanisms, potential synergistic actions, and differing toxicities. The use of combination therapy also helps prevent the development of drug-resistant cells.

Adjunct Chemotherapeutic Agents

In certain regimens, additional medications are administered with chemotherapy agents to enhance activity or protect normal cells from injury. For example, leucovorin (Wellcovorin) is often given with fluorouracil (5-FU) to treat colorectal cancer. Leucovorin, a compound similar to folic acid, helps fluorouracil bind with an enzyme inside of cancer cells and enhances the ability of fluorouracil to remain in the intracellular environment. Leucovorin also rescues normal cells from the toxic effects of high doses of methotrexate (Trexall).

When given at certain doses for the treatment of some forms of leukemia or lymphoma, methotrexate causes a folic acid deficiency in cells, resulting in cell death. Significant toxicity, including severe bone marrow suppression, mucositis, diarrhea and liver, and lung and kidney damage, can occur. Leucovorin helps to prevent or lessen these toxicities.

Administration of Chemotherapeutic Agents

Chemotherapy may be administered in the hospital, outpatient center, or home setting by multiple routes. The route of administration depends on the type of agent; the required dose; and the type, location, and extent of malignant disease being treated. Standards for the safe administration of chemotherapy have been developed by the Oncology Nursing Society (ONS) and the American Society of Clinical Oncology (ASCO) (Jacobson, Polovich, McNiff, et al., 2009). Patient education is essential to maximize safety when chemotherapy is administered in the home (Chart 15-5).

Dosage

The dosage of chemotherapeutic agents is based primarily on the patient's total body surface area, weight, previous response to chemotherapy or radiation therapy, and function of major organ systems. Dosages are determined to maximize cell kill while minimizing impact on healthy tissues and subsequent toxicities. The therapeutic effect may be compromised if modified and inadequate dosing is required due to toxicities. Modification of dosage is often required if critical laboratory values or the patient's symptoms indicate unacceptable or dangerous toxicities. Chemotherapy treatment regimens include standard-dose therapy, dose-dense regimens, and myeloablative regimens for HSCT. For certain chemotherapeutic agents, there is a maximum lifetime dose limit that must be adhered to because of the danger of long-term irreversible organ complications (e.g., because of the risk of cardiomyopathy, doxorubicin [Adriamycin] has a cumulative lifetime dose limit of 550 mg/m^2).

Extravasation

Chemotherapy agents are additionally classified by their potential to damage tissue if they inadvertently leak from

Chart 15-5	HOME CARE CHECKLIST Chemotherapy Administration		
At the completion of home care education, the patient or caregiver will be able to:		**PATIENT**	**CAREGIVER**
• Demonstrate how to administer the chemotherapy agent in the home.		✔	✔
• Describe safe storage and handling of oral chemotherapy/targeted agents in the home.		✔	✔
• Demonstrate safe disposal of needles, syringes, IV supplies, or unused chemotherapy medications.		✔	✔
• List possible side effects of chemotherapeutic agents and suggested management approaches.		✔	✔
• List complications of medications necessitating a call to the nurse or primary provider.		✔	✔
• List complications of medications necessitating a visit to the emergency department.		✔	✔
• Locate list of names and telephone numbers of resource personnel involved in care (i.e., home care nurse, infusion services, IV vendor, equipment company).		✔	✔
• Explain treatment plan and importance of upcoming visits to the primary provider.		✔	✔

TABLE 15-7 Select Antineoplastic Agents

Drug Class and Examples	Mechanism of Action	Cell Cycle Specificity	Common Side Effects
Alkylating Agents			
Busulfan (Busulfex, Myleran), carboplatin (Paraplatin), chlorambucil (Leukeran), cisplatin (Platinol-AQ), cyclophosphamide (Cytoxan), dacarbazine (DTIC-Dome), altretamine (Hexalen), ifosfamide (Ifex), melphalan (Alkeran), nitrogen mustard (Mustargen), oxaliplatin (Eloxatin), thiotepa (Thioplex)	Bond with DNA, RNA and protein molecules leading to impaired DNA replication, RNA transcription, and cell functioning; all resulting in cell death	Cell cycle–nonspecific	Bone marrow suppression, nausea, vomiting, cystitis (cyclophosphamide, ifosfamide), stomatitis, alopecia, gonadal suppression, renal toxicity (cisplatin), and development of secondary malignancies
Nitrosoureas			
Carmustine (BCNU [BiCNU, Gliadel]), lomustine or CCNU (CeeNU), semustine (methyl-CCNU [MeCCNU]), streptozocin (Zanosar)	Similar to alkylating agents; cross the blood–brain barrier	Cell cycle–nonspecific	Delayed and cumulative myelosuppression, especially thrombocytopenia; nausea, vomiting, pulmonary, hepatic and renal damage
Topoisomerase I Inhibitors			
Irinotecan (Camptosar) Topotecan (Hycamtin) **Topoisomerase II Inhibitors** Etoposide (Etopophos, VePesid) Teniposide (Vumon, VM-26)	Induce breaks in the DNA strand by binding to enzyme topoisomerase, preventing cells from dividing	Cell cycle–specific (S phase)	Bone marrow suppression, diarrhea, nausea, vomiting, flulike symptoms (topotecan), rash (etoposide), hepatotoxicity (teniposide)
Antimetabolites			
5-Azacytidine (Vidaza), capecitabine (Xeloda), cytarabine (DepoCyt, Tarabine) edatrexate fludarabine (Fludara), 5-fluorouracil (5-FU), gemcitabine (Gemzar), hydroxyurea (Droxia, Hydrea), cladribine (Leustatin), 6-mercaptopurine (Purinethol), methotrexate (Trexall, Rheumatrex), pentostatin (Nipent), 6-thioguanine (Tabloid)	Interferes with the biosynthesis of metabolites or nucleic acids necessary for RNA and DNA synthesis; inhibits DNA replication and repair	Cell cycle–specific (S phase)	Nausea, vomiting, diarrhea, bone marrow suppression, stomatitis, renal toxicity (methotrexate), hepatotoxicity (6-thioguanine), hand-foot syndrome (capecitibine)
Antitumor Antibiotics			
Bleomycin (BLM, Blenoxane), dactinomycin (Cosmegen), daunorubicin (DaunoXome), doxorubicin (Adriamycin), epirubicin, idarubicin (Idamycin), mitomycin (Mutamycin), mitoxantrone (Novantrone), plicamycin (Mithracin)	Interfere with DNA synthesis by binding DNA; prevent RNA synthesis	Cell cycle–nonspecific	Bone marrow suppression, nausea, vomiting, alopecia, anorexia, cardiac toxicity (daunorubicin, doxorubicin), red urine (doxorubicin, idarubicin, epirubicin), pulmonary fibrosis (bleomycin)
Mitotic Spindle Inhibitors			
Plant alkaloids: vinblastine (Velban), vincristine (VCR [Oncovin]), vinorelbine (Navelbine)	Arrest metaphase by inhibiting mitotic tubular formation (spindle); inhibit DNA and protein synthesis	Cell cycle–specific (M phase)	Bone marrow suppression (mild with VCR), peripheral neuropathies, nausea and vomiting
Taxanes: paclitaxel (Taxol), docetaxel (Taxotere)	Arrest metaphase by inhibiting tubulin depolymerization	Cell cycle–specific (M phase)	Hypersensitivity reactions, bone marrow suppression, alopecia, peripheral neuropathies, mucositis
Epothilones: ixabepilone (Ixempra)	Alters microtubules and inhibits mitosis	Cell cycle–specific (M phase)	Peripheral neuropathies, bone marrow suppression, hypersensitivity reactions, hepatic impairment
Hormonal Agents			
Androgens and antiandrogens, estrogens and antiestrogens, progestins and antiprogestins, aromatase inhibitors, luteinizing hormone–releasing hormone analogues, steroids	Bind to hormone receptor sites that alter cellular growth; block binding of estrogens to receptor sites (antiestrogens); inhibit RNA synthesis; suppress cytochrome P450 system	Cell cycle–nonspecific	Hypercalcemia, jaundice, increased appetite, masculinization, feminization, sodium and fluid retention, nausea, vomiting, hot flashes, vaginal estrogen dryness
Miscellaneous Agents			
Asparaginase (Elspar), procarbazine (Matulane)	Inhibits protein, DNA, and RNA synthesis	Varies	Anorexia, nausea, vomiting, bone marrow suppression, hepatotoxicity, hypersensitivity reaction, pancreatitis
Arsenic trioxide (Trisenox)	Causes fragmentation of DNA resulting in cell death; in acute promyelocytic leukemia, it corrects protein changes and changes malignant cells into normal white blood cells.		Nausea, vomiting, electrolyte imbalances, fever, headache, cough, dyspnea, electrocardiogram abnormalities

Adapted from Levine, A. (2010). Chemotherapy. In J. Eggert (Ed.). *Cancer basics*. Pittsburgh: Oncology Nursing Society; and Polovich, M., Whitford, J., & Olsen, M. (Eds.). (2009). *Chemotherapy and biotherapy guidelines and recommendations for practice* (3rd ed.). Pittsburgh: Oncology Nursing Society.

a vein into surrounding tissue (**extravasation**). The consequences of extravasation range from mild discomfort to severe tissue destruction, depending on whether the agent is classified as a nonvesicant, irritant, or vesicant. The pH of irritant agents (<5 or >9) induce inflammatory reactions but usually cause no permanent tissue damage (Schulmeister, 2009, 2011).

Vesicants are those agents that, if deposited into the subcutaneous or surrounding tissues (extravasation), cause tissue damage and possibly necrosis of tendons, muscles, nerves, and blood vessels. Although the mechanism of vesicant actions vary with each drug, some agents bind to cell DNA and cause cell death that progresses to involve neighboring cells, whereas other agents are metabolized into cells and cause a localized, painful reaction that usually improves over time (Schulmeister, 2010). Sloughing and ulceration of the tissue may progress to tissue necrosis that is so severe that skin grafting becomes necessary. The full extent of tissue damage may take several weeks to become apparent. Examples of commonly used agents classified as vesicants include cisplatin (Platinol-AQ), dactinomycin (Cosmegen), daunorubicin (DaunoXome), doxorubicin, nitrogen mustard (Mustargen), mitomycin (Mutamycin), paclitaxel (Taxol), vinblastine (Velban), vincristine (Oncovin), vindesine (Eldisine), and vinorelbine (Navelbine). The ASCO and the ONS chemotherapy administration safety standards require the availability of defined extravasation management procedures including antidote order sets and accessibility of antidotes in all settings where vesicant chemotherapy is administered (Jacobson et al., 2009).

To ensure patient safety, chemotherapy is administered only by those who have the knowledge and established competencies for vesicant and extravasation management (Schulmeister, 2010). Prevention of extravasation is essential. Vesicant chemotherapy should never be administered in peripheral veins involving the hand or wrist. Peripheral administration is permitted for short-duration infusions only, and placement of the venipuncture site should be on the forearm area using a soft, plastic catheter. For any frequent or prolonged administration of antineoplastic vesicants, right atrial silastic catheters, implanted venous access devices, or peripherally inserted central catheters (PICCs) should be inserted to promote safety during medication administration and reduce problems with access to the circulatory system (Figs. 15-3 and 15-4). Indwelling or subcutaneous catheters require vigilance.

Hypersensitivity Reactions

Although hypersensitivity reactions (HSRs) can occur with any medication, many chemotherapy agents pose much higher risks and have been associated with life-threatening outcomes.

Although most reactions coincide with chemotherapy or targeted therapy administration and are successfully treated with resolution of symptoms (uniphasic reactions), some reactions can recur between 1 and 72 hours after the original episode (biphasic reactions) (Viale & Yamamoto, 2010). Protracted reactions may last for 24 hours or longer, requiring hospitalization and continued medical treatment and observation. Delayed HSRs in the form of mild to severe signs and symptoms may occur after several uneventful courses

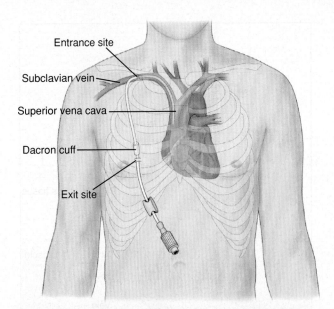

FIGURE 15-3 • Right atrial catheter. The right atrial catheter is inserted into the subclavian vein and advanced until its tip lies in the superior vena cava just above the right atrium. The proximal end is then tunneled from the entry site through the subcutaneous tissue of the chest wall and brought out through an exit site on the chest. The Dacron cuff anchors the catheter in place and serves as a barrier to infection.

of therapy. Although patients may react to the first infusion of a chemotherapy agent, repeated exposure increases the likelihood of a reaction along with other predisposing risk factors such as preexisting allergic reactions to food, blood products, and other medications, concurrent autoimmune disease or asthma, older age, preexisting cardiac or pulmonary dysfunction, higher than standard drug doses, concomitant T-lymphocyte counts in excess of 25,000/mm^3, concomitant beta-adrenergic blocker therapy, and female gender (Vogel, 2010).

The usual chemotherapy HSR is categorized as a type I immediate, immunoglobulin E (IgE [antibody])-mediated reaction; an allergic reaction. Examples of agents that may cause an allergic, IgE-mediated response include carboplatin, oxaliplatin (Eloxatin), and L-asparaginase. However, some HSRs, such as anaphylactoid reactions, are non–IgE-mediated (nonallergic) and a result of cytokine release. When the chemotherapy agent or targeted agent binds with malignant cells, cytokines are released and recruit cells of the immune system to help destroy the cancer cells. When the cancer cells are destroyed, multiple cytokines are released into the circulation (cytokine-release syndrome), causing the clinical signs and symptoms of a HSR (Viale & Yamamoto, 2010; Vogel, 2010). Examples of agents associated with a non–IgE-mediated response include paclitaxel (Taxol) and docetaxel (Taxotere), rituximab, and cetuximab. Regardless of the underlying pathophysiology, both allergic and anaphylactoid HSRs are characterized by very similar and potentially progressive signs and symptoms involving multiple body systems. Signs and symptoms of HSRs commonly occur within 15 to 30 minutes of the initiation of IV administration (Epting, 2010).

When signs and symptoms of HSR occur, the medication should be discontinued immediately and emergency procedures initiated. Many institutions have developed

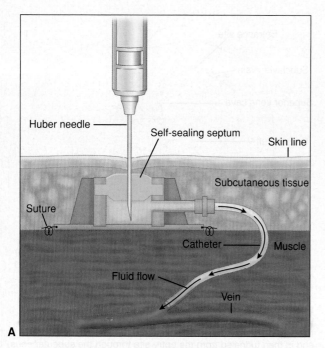

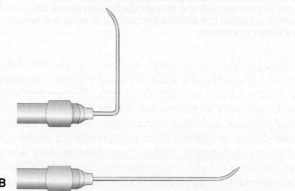

FIGURE 15-4 • Implanted vascular access device. **A.** A schematic diagram of an implanted vascular access device used for administration of medications, fluids, blood products, and nutrition. The self-sealing septum permits repeated puncture by Huber needles without damage or leakage. **B.** Two Huber needles used to enter the implanted vascular port. The 90-degree needle is used for top-entry ports for continuous infusions.

specific protocols for responding to HSRs, including standing orders for administration of emergency medications (Epting, 2010). (Chapter 38 presents further discussion of allergic reactions.)

For some chemotherapeutic agents, especially if they are essential in the treatment plan, desensitization procedures may be possible, and the patient is retreated with the agent at reduced dosages or slower infusion rates. Premedication regimens including corticosteroids, histamine-1 and histamine-2 antagonists, and antipyretics are routinely preadministered for certain chemotherapy agents to prevent or minimize potential reactions.

Doxorubicin or daunorubicin (DaunoXome) can create localized allergic reactions referred to as a *flare reaction.* Patients typically experience a hot, flushed sensation with urticaria and pruritis. The nurse confirms that the reaction is indeed a flare and not an extravasation. The infusion can be

temporarily discontinued and restarted at a slower infusion rate after consultation with the physician and IV administration of hydrocortisone (Solu-Cortef, Hydrocortone).

Toxicity

Toxicity associated with chemotherapy can be acute or chronic. Cells with rapid growth rates (e.g., epithelium, bone marrow, hair follicles, sperm) are very susceptible to damage, and the effects may manifest in virtually any body system.

Gastrointestinal System

Nausea and vomiting are the most common side effects of chemotherapy, which may persist for 24 to 48 hours with delayed nausea and vomiting up to 1 week after administration. The experience of chemotherapy-induced nausea and vomiting (CINV) tends to be underestimated and undertreated (Nevidjon & Chaudhary, 2010). CINV may affect quality of life, nutrition, fluid and electrolyte status, functional ability, and compliance with treatment. It has financial considerations due to the high cost of medical care for CINV that is not adequately controlled (Prechtel-Dunphy & Walker, 2010). In addition, comorbidities, the underlying malignancy, other treatment approaches, other medications, and symptoms (i.e., pain) may contribute to nausea and vomiting.

Several mechanisms are responsible for the occurrence of nausea and vomiting, including activation of multiple receptors found in the vomiting center of the medulla, the chemoreceptor trigger zone, the gastrointestinal tract, the pharynx, and the cerebral cortex. Activation of neurotransmitter receptors in these areas is thought to induce CINV. Stimulation may originate through peripheral, autonomic, vestibular, or cognitive pathways. The primary neuroreceptors known to be implicated in CINV are 5-hydroxytryptamine (5-HT or serotonin) and dopamine receptors (NCCN, 2011c).

The approach for managing CINV is based on knowledge of the probability of emesis of the chemotherapy agents used. There are four classification levels of emesis: minimal, low, moderate, and high risk (Grunberg, Warr, Gralla, et al., 2011). Algorithms used to prevent and treat CINV are based on national guidelines that consider this classification of chemotherapy agents (Prechtel-Dunphy & Walker, 2010). Medications that decrease nausea and vomiting include serotonin receptor blockers such as ondansetron (Zofran), granisetron (Kytril), dolasetron (Anzemet), and palonosetron (Aloxi); dopaminergic receptor blockers such as metoclopramide (Reglan) and prochlorperazine (Compazine); and neurokinin 1 receptor antagonists such as aprepitant (Emend) (Karch, 2012).

Corticosteroids, phenothiazines, sedatives, and histamines are helpful, especially when used in combination with serotonin blockers to provide improved antiemetic protection (Cotter, 2009; NCCN, 2011c). Due to delayed nausea and vomiting, some antiemetic medications are administered for the first week at home after chemotherapy. Nonpharmacologic approaches such as relaxation techniques, imagery, and acupressure (Prechtel-Dunphy & Walker, 2010) can also help decrease stimuli contributing to symptoms. Small, frequent meals, bland foods, and comfort foods may reduce the frequency or severity of symptoms.

Stomatitis is commonly associated with some chemotherapy agents because of the rapid turnover of epithelium that lines the oral cavity. The entire gastrointestinal tract is susceptible to mucositis (inflammation of the mucosal lining) with diarrhea. Antimetabolites and antitumor antibiotics are the major culprits in mucositis and other gastrointestinal symptoms, which can be severe in some patients.

Hematopoietic System

Many chemotherapy agents cause some degree of **myelosuppression** (depression of bone marrow function), resulting in decreased WBCs (leukopenia), granulocytes (neutropenia), red blood cells (RBCs) (anemia), and platelets (thrombocytopenia) and increased risk of infection and bleeding. Depression of these cells is the usual reason for limiting the dose of the chemotherapy. Myelosuppression is predictable; for most agents, patients usually reach the point at which blood counts are lowest 7 to 14 days after chemotherapy has been administered. During these 2 weeks, nurses anticipate associated toxicities, especially a fever associated with neutrophil count less than 1,500 cells/mm³. Frequent monitoring of blood cell counts is essential, and patients are educated about strategies to protect against infection, injury, and blood loss, particularly while counts are low (Saria, 2011).

Other agents—colony-stimulating factors (granulocyte colony-stimulating factor [G-CSF] and granulocyte-macrophage colony-stimulating factor [GM-CSF])—can be administered after chemotherapy to stimulate the bone marrow to produce WBCs, especially neutrophils, at an accelerated rate, thus decreasing the duration of neutropenia. G-CSF and GM-CSF decrease the episodes of infection and the need for antibiotics and allow for more timely treatment cycles of chemotherapy with less need to reduce the dosage (Quirion, 2009). Erythropoietin (EPO) stimulates RBC production, thus decreasing the symptoms of treatment-induced chronic anemia and reducing the need for blood transfusions. Interleukin 11 (IL-11) (oprelvekin [Neumega]) stimulates the production of megakaryocytes (precursors to platelets) and can be used to prevent and treat severe thrombocytopenia but has had limited use because of toxicities such as HSR; capillary leak syndrome; pulmonary edema; atrial dysrhythmias; and nausea, vomiting, and diarrhea (Polovich, Whitford, & Olsen, 2009).

Renal System

Some chemotherapy agents can damage the kidneys because they impair water secretion, leading to syndrome of inappropriate secretion of antidiuretic hormone (SIADH), decrease renal perfusion, precipitate end products after cell lysis, and cause interstitial nephritis (Polovich et al., 2009). Cisplatin (Platinol), methotrexate, and mitomycin (Mutamycin) are particularly toxic to the kidneys. Rapid tumor cell lysis after chemotherapy results in increased urinary excretion of uric acid, which can cause renal damage. In addition, intracellular contents are released into the circulation, resulting in hyperkalemia, hyperphosphatemia, and hypocalcemia and obstructive nephropathy. (See later discussion of tumor lysis syndrome.)

Monitoring laboratory values of blood urea nitrogen (BUN), serum creatinine, creatinine clearance, and serum electrolytes is essential. Adequate hydration, diuresis, alkalinization of the urine to prevent formation of uric acid crystals, and administration of allopurinol (Zyloprim) may be used to prevent renal toxicity. Amifostine has demonstrated an ability to minimize renal toxicities associated with cisplatin, cyclophosphamide (Cytoxan), and ifosfamide (Ifex) therapy.

Hemorrhagic cystitis is a bladder toxicity that can result from cyclophosphamide and ifosfamide therapy. Hematuria can range from microscopic to frank bleeding with symptoms ranging from transient irritation during urination, dysuria, and suprapubic pain to life-threatening hemorrhage. Protection of the bladder focuses on aggressive IV hydration, frequent voiding, and diuresis. Mesna (Mesnex) is a cytoprotectant agent that binds with the toxic metabolites of cyclophosphamide or ifosfamide in the kidneys to prevent hemorrhagic cystitis (Harris, 2010).

Cardiopulmonary System

Several agents are associated with cardiac toxicity. Anthracyclines (e.g., daunorubicin, doxorubicin) are known to cause irreversible cumulative cardiac toxicities, especially when total dosage reaches 600 mg/m² and 550 mg/m², respectively. If these agents are administered in the presence of thoracic radiation therapy or other agents with cardiotoxicity potential, their cumulative dose limit is reduced to 450 mg/m². Patients at increased risk for the development of cardiopulmonary toxicities include those older than 65 years, those with a history of preexisting cardiopulmonary disease, tobacco use, renal or hepatic dysfunction, and longer survival time (Camp-Sorrell, 2010). Dexrazoxane (Zinecard) has been utilized as a cardioprotectant when doxorubicin is needed in individuals who have already received a cumulative dose of 300 mg/m² and continuation of therapy is deemed beneficial. Patients with known cardiac disease (e.g., heart failure) are treated with lower doses or agents not known to be associated with cardiac toxicity. Cardiac ejection fraction (volume of blood ejected from the heart with each beat) and other signs of heart failure must be monitored closely.

Bleomycin (Blenoxane), carmustine (BCNU), and busulfan (Busulfex, Myleran), among other agents, have cumulative toxic effects on lung function, resulting in pulmonary fibrosis. Therefore, patients are monitored closely for changes in pulmonary function, including pulmonary function test results. Total cumulative doses of bleomycin should not exceed 400 U, and carmustine should not exceed 1,400 mg. Patients with known pulmonary disease are treated with alternative agents not known to cause pulmonary toxicity (Camp-Sorrell, 2010).

Capillary leak syndrome with resultant pulmonary edema is an effect of cytarabine (DepoCyt, Tarabine, Ara-C), mitomycin C, cyclophosphamide, and carmustine. Subtle onset of dyspnea and cough may progress rapidly to acute respiratory distress and subsequent respiratory failure. Patients who are at significant risk for capillary leak syndrome are monitored closely.

Reproductive System

Testicular and ovarian function can be affected by chemotherapeutic agents, resulting in possible sterility (Lee, 2011). Women may develop problems with ovulation or early menopause, whereas men may develop temporary or permanent azoospermia (absence of spermatozoa). Because treatment may damage reproductive cells, banking of sperm is often recommended for men before treatment is initiated. Options available for women prior to initiation of chemotherapy include freezing (cryopreservation) of oocytes, embryos, or ovarian tissue (Shear, 2010). Patients and their partners are informed about potential changes in reproductive function resulting from chemotherapy. In addition, many chemotherapy agents are known or thought to be teratogenic. Therefore, patients are advised to use reliable methods of birth control while receiving chemotherapy and not to assume that sterility has resulted.

Neurologic System

Chemotherapy-induced neurotoxicity, a potentially dose-limiting toxicity, can affect the central nervous system, peripheral nervous system, and/or the cranial nerves. Neurotoxicity characterized by metabolic encephalopathy can occur with ifosfamide, high-dose methotrexate, and cytarabine. With repeated doses, the taxanes and plant alkaloids, especially vincristine, can cause cumulative peripheral nervous system damage with sensory alterations in the feet and hands. These sensations can be described as tingling, pricking, or numbness of the extremities; burning or freezing pain; sharp, stabbing, or electric shock–like pain; and extreme sensitivity to touch. If unreported by patients or undetected, progressive motor axon damage can lead to loss of deep tendon reflexes, with muscle weakness, loss of balance and coordination, and paralytic ileus.

Severe peripheral neuropathies may lead to diminished quality of life and functional abilities and result in dose reductions, a change in chemotherapy regimen, or early cessation of treatment, all of which compromise the success of cancer therapy (Tofthagen, 2010). Although often reversible, these side effects may take many months to resolve or persist indefinitely. Along with the usual paresthesias of the hands and feet, oxaliplatin has a unique and frightening neurotoxicity presentation that is often precipitated by exposure to cold and is characterized by pharyngolaryngeal dysesthesia consisting of lip paresthesia, discomfort or tightness in the back of the throat, inability to breathe, and jaw pain.

> ### ▶ *Quality and Safety Nursing Alert*
>
> Patients receiving oxaliplatin must be instructed to avoid drinking cold fluids or going outside with hands and feet exposed to cold temperatures to avoid exacerbation of these symptoms. Cisplatin may cause peripheral neuropathies and hearing loss due to damage to the acoustic nerve.

Cognitive Impairment

Many patients with cancer experience difficulty with remembering dates, multitasking, managing numbers and finances, organization, face or object recognition, inability to follow directions, feeling easily distracted, and motor and behavioral changes. Although not completely understood, these are viewed as symptoms of cognitive impairment, defined as a decline in the information-handling processes of attention and concentration, executive function, information processing speed, language, visual–spatial skill, psychomotor ability, learning, and memory (Jansen, 2010). Commonly referred to

by patients as "chemo brain," cognitive impairment has been associated with both cancer and cancer treatments including surgery, radiation, chemotherapy, and targeted agents (Evens & Eschiti, 2009). The symptoms may be subtle or profound with potential negative effects on functional abilities, employment, independence, quality of life, and psychosocial status. Comorbidities, age, medications, pain, impaired nutrition, anemia, fatigue, fluid and electrolyte disturbances, organ dysfunction, infection, and hormonal imbalances are factors that may contribute to the experience of cognitive impairment and make it difficult to fully understand. Proposed underlying mechanisms of cognitive impairment in patients with cancer currently being explored include direct neurotoxic effects, oxidative stress, hormonal changes, immune dysregulation, cytokine release, clotting, and genetic predisposition (Von Ah, Jansen, Hutchinson, et al., 2011).

Fatigue

Fatigue, a subjective and distressing side effect for most patients that greatly affects quality of life, can last for months after treatment. The health care team works together to identify effective pharmacologic and nonpharmacologic approaches for fatigue management (Wanchai, Armer, & Stewart, 2011).

Nursing Management

Nurses play an important role in assessing and managing many of the problems experienced by patients receiving chemotherapy. Chemotherapy agents affect both normal and malignant cells; therefore, their effects are often widespread, affecting many body systems.

Laboratory and physical assessments of metabolic indices and the hematologic, hepatic, renal, cardiovascular, neurologic, and pulmonary systems are critical in evaluating the body's response to chemotherapy. These assessments are performed prior to, during, and after a course of chemotherapy to determine optimal treatment options, evaluate the patient's response, and monitor toxicity.

Assessing Fluid and Electrolyte Status

Anorexia, nausea, vomiting, altered taste, mucositis, and diarrhea put patients at risk for nutritional and fluid and electrolyte disturbances. Therefore, it is important for the nurse to assess the patient's nutritional and fluid and electrolyte status on an ongoing basis and to identify creative ways to encourage an adequate fluid and dietary intake.

Assessing Cognitive Status

The topic of cognitive impairment has been frequently overlooked in patient education about cancer and cancer treatments. Patients should be reassessed routinely for the development of cognitive impairment, just as they are for other side effects. Prior to the initiation of treatment, patients and families should be informed about the possibility of cognitive impairment.

Modifying Risks for Infection and Bleeding

Suppression of the bone marrow and immune system is expected and frequently serves as a guide in determining appropriate chemotherapy dosage but increases the risk of anemia, infection, and bleeding disorders. Nursing assessment and care address factors that would further increase the patient's risk. The nurse's role in decreasing the risk of infection and bleeding is discussed further in the Nursing Care of Patients With Cancer section (see Chart 15-7).

Administering Chemotherapy

Nurses must be aware of chemotherapy and other agents most associated with HSRs, strategies for prevention, signs and symptoms characteristic of HSRs, and the appropriate early and time-sensitive interventions for preventing progression to anaphylaxis. Nurses provide patient and family education that emphasizes two key points: the importance of adhering to prescribed self-administered premedication before presenting to the infusion center, and recognizing and reporting the signs and symptoms to the nurse once the infusion has started. Patients and families are also educated about signs and symptoms that may occur at home following discharge from the infusion area that may warrant medication administration or immediate transport to the emergency department for further assessment and treatment.

The local effects of the chemotherapeutic agent are also of concern. The patient is observed closely during administration of the agent because of the risk and consequences of extravasation, particularly of vesicant agents. Prevention of extravasation is essential and relies on vigilant nursing care. Selection of peripheral veins, skilled venipuncture, and careful administration of medications are essential. Peripheral administration is limited to short duration (less than 1 hour; IV push or bolus) infusions using only a soft, plastic catheter placed in the forearm area. Continuous-infusion vesicants whose administration takes longer than 1 hour or are administered frequently are given only via a central line, such as a right atrial silastic catheter, implanted venous access device, or PICC. These long-term venous access devices promote safety during medication administration and reduce problems with repeated access to the circulatory system (see Figs. 15-3 and 15-4). Indwelling or subcutaneous venous access devices require consistent nursing care. Complications include infection and thrombosis (Levine, 2010).

Indications of extravasation during administration of vesicant agents include the following:

- Absence of blood return from the IV catheter
- Resistance to flow of IV fluid
- Burning or pain, swelling, or redness at the site

> ▶ *Quality and Safety Nursing Alert*
>
> If extravasation is suspected, the medication administration is stopped immediately, and depending on the drug, the nurse may attempt to aspirate any remaining drug from the extravasation site.

An extravasation kit should be readily available with emergency equipment and antidote medications, as well as a quick reference for how to properly manage an extravasation of the specific vesicant agent used (although evidence-based data regarding effective antidotes is limited). Application of heat or cold is very dependent on the drug administered; nurses should refer to their organization's policy and procedures. Recommendations and guidelines for managing vesicant extravasation, which vary with each agent, have been issued by individual medication manufacturers, pharmacies, and the ONS (Schulmeister, 2011).

Difficulties or problems with administration of chemotherapeutic agents are brought to the attention of the primary provider promptly so that corrective measures can be taken to minimize local tissue damage. (See previous discussion of extravasation.)

The nurse evaluates the patient receiving neurotoxic chemotherapy, communicates findings with the medical oncologist, provides education to patients and families, and makes appropriate referrals for complete neurologic evaluation and occupational or rehabilitative therapies (Tofthagen McAllister, & McMillan, 2011).

Preventing Nausea and Vomiting

Nurses are integral to the prevention and management of CINV. They collaborate with other members of the oncology care team to identify factors contributing to the experience of CINV and select effective antiemetic regimens that maximize currently available therapies. Nurses provide education for patients and families regarding antiemetic regimens and care for delayed CINV that may continue at home after the chemotherapy infusion has completed (Rogers & Blackburn, 2010).

Managing Cognitive Changes

Although several approaches have been explored, no evidence-based guidelines for the prevention, treatment, or management of cognitive impairment have been established. Examples of nonpharmacologic approaches that nurses recommend to patients include exercise, natural restorative environmental intervention (walking in nature or gardening), and cognitive training programs. Nurses should assist patients to address factors such as fluid and electrolyte imbalances, nutrition deficits, fatigue, pain, and infection to minimize their contribution to cognitive impairment.

Managing Fatigue

Fatigue is a common side effect of chemotherapy. Nurses assist patients to explore the role that the underlying disease processes, combined treatments, other symptoms and psychosocial status play in the patient's experience of fatigue (Scott, Lasch, Barsevick, et al., 2011). In addition, nurses work with the patient and other team members to identify effective approaches for fatigue management (Wanchai et al., 2011).

Protecting Caregivers

Nurses involved in handling chemotherapeutic agents may be exposed to low doses of the agents by direct contact, inhalation, or ingestion. Studies suggest that nurses and others preparing chemotherapy agents or handling linens and other materials that are contaminated with body fluids of patients receiving chemotherapy have been unknowingly exposed (Nixon & Schulmeister, 2009). Skin and eye irritation, nausea, vomiting, nasal mucosal ulcerations, infertility, low-birth-weight babies, congenital anomalies, spontaneous abortions, and mutagenic substances in urine have been reported in nurses preparing and handling chemotherapy agents (Levine, 2010). Although long-term studies of nurses who handle chemotherapy agents have not been conducted, it is known that these agents are associated with

Safety in Handling Chemotherapy for Health Care Providers

- When preparing (compounding, reconstituting) chemotherapy for administration, use the following safety equipment to prevent exposure through inhalation, direct contact, and ingestion:
  - Class II or III biological safety cabinet (BSC)
  - Closed system transfer devices
  - Puncture and leak-proof containers, IV bags
  - Needleless systems (i.e., IV tubing and syringes)
- If BSC is not available when preparing chemotherapy for administration, use the following safety equipment to minimize exposure:
  - Surgical N-95 respirator to provide respiratory and splash protection
  - Eye and face protection (both face shield and goggles) working at or above eye level or cleaning a spill
- When preparing or administering chemotherapy or handling linens and other materials contaminated with chemotherapy or blood and body fluids of patients receiving chemotherapy, wear the following for personal protection:
  - Double layer of powder-free gloves specifically designated for chemotherapy handling (the inner glove is worn under the gown cuff and the outer glove is worn over the cuff)
  - Long sleeve, disposable gowns (without seams or closures that can allow drugs to pass through) made of polyethylene-coated polypropylene or other laminate materials
- Linens contaminated with chemotherapy or blood and body fluids of patients receiving chemotherapy should be placed in the following:
  - Closed-system, puncture- and leak-proof containers labeled "hazardous: chemotherapy contaminated linens"

- Above referenced container maintained in the infusion center soiled utility room for outpatient settings
- Above referenced container maintained in the patient room and/or soiled utility room for inpatient settings
- Chemotherapy preparation equipment (i.e., syringes, tubing, empty vials, etc.), gowns, and gloves should be disposed of in:
  - Closed-system, puncture- and leak-proof containers labeled "hazardous: chemotherapy contaminated waste"
- Wash hands with soap and water after removing gloves used to prepare or administer chemotherapy or clean contaminated linens and other materials.
- "Spill kits" with the appropriate gowns, gloves, disposable absorbent materials for cleansing large areas, and hazard sign should be kept in all areas where chemotherapy is prepared and administered.
- Implement a quality improvement program addressing safe chemotherapy handling that includes the following:
  - Standard operating policies and procedures for:
    - Chemotherapy handling, preparation, and disposal
    - Handling and disposal of chemotherapy spills
    - Handling and disposal of blood and body fluids and contaminated materials of patients receiving chemotherapy
  - Conduct competency-based education, training, and performance evaluations regarding chemotherapy safety procedures at orientation and at subsequent regular intervals.
  - Medical monitoring program to identify indicators of exposure
  - Root cause analysis for all chemotherapy spills and exposure incidents

Adapted from National Institute for Occupational Safety and Health. (2010). *Personal protective equipment for health care workers who work with hazardous drugs.* Available at: www.cdc.gov/niosh/docs/wp-solutions/2009-106/pdfs/2009-106.pdf

secondary formation of cancers and chromosome abnormalities. The Occupational and Safety Health Administration (OSHA), the ONS, hospitals, and other health care agencies have developed specific precautions for health care providers involved in the preparation and administration of chemotherapy and for handling materials exposed to body fluids of those who have received these hazardous agents (Chart 15-6) (National Institute for Occupational Safety and Health [NIOSH], 2010). Nurses must be familiar with their institutional policies and procedures regarding personal protective equipment, handling and disposal of chemotherapy agents and supplies, and management of accidental spills or exposures. Emergency spill kits should be readily available in any treatment area where chemotherapy is prepared or administered. Precautions must also be taken when handling any bodily fluids or excreta from the patient, as many agents are excreted unaltered in urine and feces. Nurses in all treatment settings have a responsibility to educate patients, families, caregivers, assistive personnel, and housekeepers concerning precautions.

■ Hematopoietic Stem Cell Transplantation

HSCT has been used to treat several malignant and nonmalignant diseases for many years. The use of HSCT for solid tumors is limited to clinical trials (Devine, Tierney, Schmit-Pokorny, et al., 2010). However, the use of HSCT in the treatment of certain adult hematologic malignancies (i.e., malignant myeloma, acute leukemias, and non-Hodgkin lymphoma) is considered the standard of care (Devine et al., 2010; Harris, 2010).

The process of obtaining hematopoietic stem cells (HSCs) has evolved over the years. Historically, HSCs were obtained in the operating room by harvesting large amounts of bone marrow tissue from a donor under general anesthesia. However, peripheral blood stem cell collection using the process of apheresis has gained widespread use. The cells collected are specially processed and ultimately reinfused into the patient. This method of collecting HSCs is a safe and a more cost-effective means of collection than the process of harvesting of marrow (Devine et al., 2010). Stem cells can also be collected from umbilical cord blood harvested from the placenta of newborns at birth.

Types of Hematopoietic Stem Cell Transplantation

Types of HSCT are based on the source of donor cells and the treatment (conditioning) regimen used to prepare the patient for stem cell infusion and eradicate malignant cells. These include:

- *Allogeneic HSCT* (AlloHSCT): From a donor other than the patient (may be a related donor such as a family member or a matched unrelated donor from the National Bone Marrow Registry or Cord Blood Registry)
- *Autologous*: From the patient
- *Syngeneic*: From an identical twin

- *Myeloablative:* Consists of giving patients high-dose chemotherapy and, occasionally, total-body irradiation
- *Nonmyeloablative:* Also called *mini-transplants;* does not completely destroy bone marrow cells

AlloHSCTs are used primarily for diseases of the bone marrow and are dependent on the availability of a human leukocyte antigen–matched donor, which greatly limits the number of possible transplants. An advantage of AlloHSCT is that the transplanted cells should not be immunologically tolerant of a patient's malignancy and should cause a lethal **graft-versus-tumor effect** in which the donor cells recognize the malignant cells and act to eliminate them.

AlloHSCT may involve either myeloablative (high-dose) or nonmyeloablative (mini-transplant) chemotherapy. In ablative AlloHSCT, the recipient receives high doses of chemotherapy and possibly total-body irradiation to completely eradicate (ablate) the bone marrow and any malignant cells and help prevent rejection of the donor stem cells. The collected HSCs that are infused IV into the recipients travel to sites in the body where they produce bone marrow and establish themselves through the process of engraftment. Once engraftment is complete (2 to 4 weeks, sometimes longer), the new bone marrow becomes functional and begins producing RBCs, WBCs, and platelets. In nonablative AlloHSCT, the chemotherapy doses are lower and are aimed at destroying malignant cells (without completely eradicating the bone marrow), thus suppressing the recipient's immune system to allow engraftment of donor stem cells. The lower doses of chemotherapy, associated with less organ toxicity and infection, can be used for older patients or those with underlying organ dysfunction for whom high-dose chemotherapy would be prohibitive. After engraftment, it is hoped that the donor cells will create a graft-versus-tumor effect (Devine et al., 2010; Harris, 2010). Before engraftment, patients are at high risk for infection, sepsis, and bleeding. Side effects of the high-dose chemotherapy and total-body irradiation can be acute and chronic. Acute side effects include alopecia, hemorrhagic cystitis, nausea, vomiting, diarrhea, encephalopathy, pulmonary edema, acute renal failure, fluid and electrolyte imbalances, and severe mucositis (Rimkus, 2009). Chronic side effects include sterility; pulmonary, cardiac, renal, neurologic, and hepatic dysfunction; osteoporosis; avascular bone necrosis; diabetes; and secondary malignancy (Harris & Eilers, 2009).

During the first 30 days after the conditioning regimen, AlloHSCT patients are at risk for developing hepatic sinusoidal obstructive syndrome (HSOS) (previously referred to as veno-oclusive disease) related to chemotherapy-induced inflammation of the sinusoidal epithelium. Inflammation causes embolization of RBCs, resulting in destruction, fibrosis, and occlusion of the sinusoids (Rimkus, 2009). Signs and symptoms of HSOS may include weight gain, hepatomegaly, increased bilirubin, and ascites. Although various approaches have been used to treat HSOS, evidence-based strategies have not emerged. The use of peripheral stem cells, specific chemotherapy dosing, and nonmyeloablative regimens have been associated with a decreased incidence (Harris, 2010).

Graft-versus-host disease (GVHD), a major cause of morbidity and mortality in 30% to 50% of the allogeneic transplant population, occurs when the donor lymphocytes initiate an immune response against the recipient's tissues (skin, gastrointestinal tract, liver) during the beginning of engraftment (Harris, 2010). The donor cells view the recipient's tissues as foreign or immunologically different from what they recognize as "self" in the donor. To prevent GVHD, patients receive immunosuppressant drugs, such as cyclosporine (Sandimmune), methotrexate, tacrolimus (Prograf), or mycophenolate mofetil (MMF). GVHD may be acute or chronic. Clinical manifestations of acute GVHD include diffuse rash progressing to blistering and desquamation similar to second-degree burns; mucosal inflammation of the eyes and the entire gastrointestinal tract with subsequent diarrhea that may exceed 2 L per day; and biliary stasis with abdominal pain, hepatomegaly, and elevated liver enzymes progressing to obstructive jaundice. The first 100 days or so after AlloHSCT are crucial for patients; the immune system and blood-making capacity (hematopoiesis) must recover sufficiently to prevent infection and hemorrhage. Most acute side effects, such as nausea, vomiting, and mucositis, resolve during this period of time. However, there are some complications that may occur, such as encephalopathy, hemolytic uremia syndrome, hemolytic anemia, and thrombotic thrombocytopenia purpura (Rimkus, 2009).

Autologous HSCT (AuHSCT) is considered for patients with disease of the bone marrow who do not have a suitable donor for AlloHSCT or for patients who have healthy bone marrow but require bone marrow–ablative doses of chemotherapy to cure an aggressive malignancy. The most common malignancies treated with AuHSCT include lymphoma and multiple myeloma. However, the use of AuHSCT has gained increasing acceptance in treating neuroblastoma, Ewing's sarcoma, and germ cell tumors (Devine et al., 2010). Stem cells are collected from the patient and preserved for reinfusion; if necessary, they are treated to kill any malignant cells within the marrow, called *purging.* The patient is then treated with ablative chemotherapy and, possibly, total-body irradiation to eradicate any remaining tumor. Stem cells are then reinfused. Until engraftment occurs in the bone marrow sites of the body, there is a high risk of infection, sepsis, and bleeding. Acute and chronic toxicities from chemotherapy and radiation therapy may be severe. The risk of HSOS is also present after autologous transplantation. No immunosuppressant medications are necessary after AuHSCT, because the patient does not receive foreign tissue. A disadvantage of AuHSCT is the risk that tumor cells may remain in the bone marrow despite high-dose chemotherapy (conditioning regimens).

Syngeneic transplants result in less incidence of GVHD and graft rejection; however, there is also less graft-versus-tumor effect to fight the malignancy. Syngeneic transplant is associated with transmission of genetic defects (Harris, 2010). For this reason, even when an identical twin is available for marrow donation, another matched sibling or even an unrelated donor may be the most suitable donor to combat an aggressive malignancy.

Nursing Management

Nursing care of patients undergoing HSCT is complex and demands a high level of skill. The success of HSCT is greatly influenced by nursing care throughout the transplantation process.

Implementing Care Before Treatment

All patients must undergo extensive pretransplantation evaluations to assess the current clinical status of the disease. Nutritional assessments, extensive physical examinations, organ function tests, and psychological evaluations are conducted. Blood work includes assessing past infectious antigen exposure (e.g., hepatitis virus, cytomegalovirus, herpes simplex virus, human immunodeficiency virus, and syphilis). The patient's social support systems, financial, and insurance resources are also evaluated. Informed consent and patient education about the procedure and care before and after HSCT are vital.

Providing Care During Treatment

Skilled nursing care is required during the treatment phase of HSCT when high-dose chemotherapy (conditioning regimen) and total-body irradiation are administered. The acute toxicities of nausea, diarrhea, mucositis, and hemorrhagic cystitis require close monitoring and symptom management by the nurse.

Nursing management during stem cell infusion consists of monitoring the patient's vital signs and blood oxygen saturation; assessing for adverse effects such as fever, chills, shortness of breath, chest pain, cutaneous reactions, nausea, vomiting, hypotension or hypertension, tachycardia, anxiety, and taste changes; and providing strategies for symptom control, ongoing support, and patient education. During stem cell infusion, patients may experience adverse reactions to the cryoprotectant dimethylsulfoxide (DMSO) used to preserve the harvested stem cells. These reactions may include nausea, vomiting, chills, dyspnea, cardiac dysrhythmias, and hypotension progressing to cardiac or respiratory arrest. Less common toxicities include neurologic and renal impairment (Rimkus, 2009).

> ### ▶ *Quality and Safety Nursing Alert*
>
> **Until engraftment of the new marrow occurs, the patient is at high risk for death from sepsis and bleeding.**

A cluster of symptoms referred to as engraftment syndrome may occur during the neutrophil recovery phase in both allogeneic and autologous transplants. Clinical features of this syndrome vary widely but may include noninfectious fever associated with skin rash, weight gain, diarrhea, and pulmonary infiltrates, with improvement noted after the initiation of corticosteroid therapy rather than antibiotic therapy (Harris, 2010). Until engraftment is well established, the patient requires support with blood products and hemopoietic growth factors.

Potential infections may be bacterial, viral, fungal, or protozoan in origin. During the first 30 days following transplant, the patient is most at risk for developing reactivations of viral infections including herpes simplex, EBV, cytomegalovirus, and varicella zoster. Mucosal denudement poses a risk for *Candida* (yeast) infection locally and systemically. Pulmonary toxicities offer the opportunity for fungal infections such as *Aspergillus*. Renal complications arise from the nephrotoxic

chemotherapy agents used in the conditioning regimen or those used to treat infection (amphotericin B, aminoglycosides). Tumor lysis syndrome and acute tubular necrosis are also risks after HSCT. Nursing assessment for signs of these complications is essential for early identification and treatment. GVHD requires skillful nursing assessment to detect early effects on the skin, liver, and gastrointestinal tract. HSOS resulting from the conditioning regimens used can result in fluid retention, jaundice, abdominal pain, ascites, tender and enlarged liver, and encephalopathy. Pulmonary complications, such as pulmonary edema, interstitial pneumonia, and other pneumonias, often complicate recovery.

Providing Care After Treatment

Caring for Recipients

Ongoing nursing assessment during follow-up visits is essential to detect late effects of therapy after HSCT, which may occur 100 days or more after the procedure. Late effects include infections (e.g., varicella-zoster infection), restrictive pulmonary abnormalities, and recurrent pneumonias. Sterility often results due to total-body irradiation and/or chemotherapy as components of the ablative regimen. Chronic GVHD involves the skin, liver, intestine, esophagus, eyes, lungs, joints, and vaginal mucosa. Cataracts may also develop after total-body irradiation.

The potential psychological impact of HSCT has been described as unique and unlike other experiences (Cooke, Gemmill, Kravits, et al., 2009). Psychosocial assessments by nursing staff must be ongoing and a priority. In addition to the multiple physical and psychological stressors affecting patients at each phase of the transplantation experience, the nature of the treatment and patient experience can place extreme emotional, social, financial, and physical demands on family, friends, and donors. Nurses assess the family and other caregivers' needs and provide education, support, and information about resources.

Caring for Donors

Like HSCT recipients, donors also require nursing care. They may experience mood alterations, decreased self-esteem, and guilt from feelings of failure if the transplantation fails. Family members must be educated and supported to reduce anxiety and promote coping during this difficult time. In addition, they must also be assisted to maintain realistic expectations of themselves as well as of the patient.

■ *Hyperthermia*

The use of hyperthermia (thermal therapy), which is the generation of temperatures greater than physiologic fever range (greater than 41.5°C [106.7°F]), has been used for many years to destroy cancerous tumors. Hyperthermia is most effective when combined with radiation therapy, chemotherapy, or biologic therapy. Hyperthermia and radiation therapy are thought to work well together because hypoxic tumor cells and cells in the S phase of the cell cycle are more sensitive to heat than radiation, and the addition of heat damages tumor cells so that they cannot repair themselves after radiation therapy. Hyperthermia preferentially damages tumor blood vessels, partly because these vessels are of inadequate size to dissipate the heat generated by hyperthermia.

Hyperthermia is thought to alter cellular membrane permeability when used with chemotherapy, allowing for an increased uptake of the chemotherapeutic agent. Hyperthermia may enhance the function of immune system cells, such as macrophages and T cells, to assist in combating malignant cells. Resistance to hyperthermia may develop during the treatment because cells adapt to repeated thermal insult. Research into the effectiveness of hyperthermia is ongoing (Gosselin, 2010).

Heat can be produced by using radio waves, ultrasound, microwaves, magnetic waves, hot-water baths, or even hot-wax immersions. Hyperthermia may be local or regional, or it may include the whole body. Local or regional hyperthermia may be delivered into a tumor, on the skin, into a body orifice, or by regional perfusion (i.e., an extremity affected by melanoma). Heated intraperitoneal chemotherapy has been used (in combination with surgery) to treat metastasis to the peritoneum for both colon and ovarian cancers (Chua, Yan, Saxena, et al., 2009). Side effects of hyperthermia treatments include burns, fatigue, hypotension, peripheral neuropathies, thrombophlebitis, nausea, vomiting, diarrhea, and electrolyte imbalances. Cardiovascular stress may develop in patients receiving hyperthermia to a large area or whole body due to changes in pulse and blood pressure.

Nursing Management

Although hyperthermia has been used for years, patients and their families may be unfamiliar with this cancer treatment. Consequently, they need explanations about the procedure, its goals, and its effects. The nurse assesses the patient for adverse effects and acts to reduce their occurrence and severity. Local skin care at the site of the implanted probes is necessary.

◼ Targeted Therapies

Normal cell growth is regulated by well-defined communication pathways between the environment surrounding the cell and the internal cell environment, the nucleus, and the intracellular cytoplasm. The cell membrane contains important protein receptors that respond to signals transmitted from the external cell environment and transmit that signal to the internal cell environment using enzymatic pathways called *signal transduction pathways*. Although normal cells have transduction pathways, scientific advances have led to the recognition that cancer, at the cellular level, is characterized by deregulated cell signaling transduction pathways (both intra- and extracellular pathways), and receptors and proteins that play an important role in tumor initiation, growth, and spread (Goetsch, 2009). This improved understanding of cancer cell behavior has allowed scientists to develop molecular-based therapies, called **targeted therapies**. These specifically target (like a lock and key mechanism) receptors, proteins, signal transduction pathways, and other processes to prevent the continued growth of cancer cells. Targeted therapies seek to work against cancer cell capabilities such as malignant transformation, uncontrolled reproduction, growth and metastasis, blocking apoptosis, and altered genetic coding. Examples of targeted therapies include biologic response modifiers (BRMs), monoclonal antibodies (MoAbs), several types of growth factors and cytokines, and gene therapy (Eggert, 2011; Goetsch, 2009).

Biologic Response Modifiers

Biologic response modifier (BRM) therapy involves the use of naturally occurring or recombinant (reproduced through genetic engineering) agents or treatment methods that can alter the immunologic relationship between the tumor and the patient with cancer (host) to provide a therapeutic benefit. Although the mechanisms of action vary with each type of BRM, the goal is to destroy or stop the malignant growth. The basis of BRM treatment lies in the restoration, modification, stimulation, or augmentation of the body's natural immune defenses against cancer (Polovich et al., 2009).

Nonspecific Biologic Response Modifiers

Early investigations of the stimulation of the immune system involved nonspecific agents such as bacille Calmette-Guérin (BCG) and *Corynebacterium parvum*. When injected into the patient, these agents serve as antigens that stimulate an immune response. The hope is that the stimulated immune system will then eradicate malignant cells. Extensive animal and human investigations with BCG have shown promising results, especially in treating localized malignant melanoma. In addition, BCG bladder instillation is a standard form of treatment for localized bladder cancer (Polovich et al, 2009). However, the use of nonspecific agents in advanced cancer remains limited, and research is ongoing to identify other uses and agents.

Monoclonal Antibodies

MoAbs, another type of BRM, have become available through technologic advances, enabling investigators to grow and produce targeted antibodies for specific malignant cells. Theoretically, this type of specificity allows MoAbs to destroy the cancer cells and spare normal cells. The specificity of MoAbs is dependent on identifying key antigen proteins on the surface of tumors that are not present on normal tissues. When the MoAb attaches to the cell surface antigen, an important signal transduction pathway for communication between the malignant cells and the extracellular environment is blocked. The results may include an inability to initiate apoptosis, reproduce, or invade surrounding tissues. There are several categories of TAAs, including oncofetal antigens such as CEA, a prominent tumor marker identified in colon cancer; growth factors such as EGFs and VEGFs; and oncogenes such as *C-erb* or *Bcr-Abl* (Cook & Figg, 2010).

The production of MoAbs involves injecting tumor cells that act as antigens into mice. B-cell lymphocytes in the spleen of the mouse produce immunoglobulin (antibodies) made in response to the injected antigens. Antibody-producing B cells are combined with a cancer cell that has the ability to grow indefinitely in culture medium and continue producing more antibodies.

The combination of spleen cells and the cancer cells is referred to as a hybridoma. From hybridomas that continue to grow in the culture medium, the desired antibodies are harvested, purified, and prepared for diagnostic or therapeutic use (Fig. 15-5). Advances in genetic engineering have led to the production of MoAbs with combinations of mouse and human components (*chimeric MoAbs*) or all-human components (*human MoAbs*). MoAbs made with human genes have

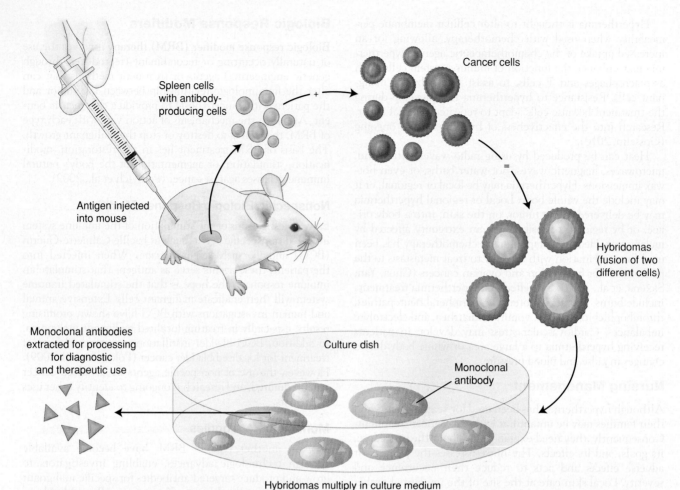

FIGURE 15-5 • Antibody-producing spleen cells are fused with cancer cells. This process produces cells called *hybridomas*. These cells, which can grow indefinitely in a culture medium, produce antibodies that are harvested, purified, and prepared for diagnostic or treatment purposes.

greater immunologic properties and are less likely to cause allergic reactions (Polovich et al., 2009).

Several MoAbs have been approved for treatment in cancer using various extracellular (on the cell membrane) and intracellular targets. Trastuzumab (Herceptin) has the ability to target the HER2 protein, an error of gene overexpression found in some breast cancers. Currently, clinical trials are exploring the use of trastuzumab in other cancers (gastric, colon, bladder, uterine, cervical, head and neck, and esophageal cancers) that have also demonstrated overexpression of the HER2 protein (Goetsch, 2009). Rituxumab (Rituxin) is a MoAb that binds specifically with the CD20 antigen expressed by non-Hodgkin lymphoma and B-cell chronic lymphocytic leukemia (Polovich et al., 2009). Ipilimumab (Yervoy) is used in the treatment of advanced malignant melanoma. In the process of specifically targeting cytotoxic T-lymphocyte antigen-4 (CTLA-4), this MoAb prevents inactivation of T-cell lymphocytes so that the body's normal T-cell–mediated antitumor immune response can destroy melanoma cells (Ledezma, Binder, & Hamid, 2011; Roman, 2011).

Some MoAbs are used alone, whereas others are used in combination with agents that facilitate their antitumor actions. Ibritumomab tiuxetan (Zevalin), a MoAb conjugated with a radioactive isotope, is used in the treatment of certain types of lymphoma (Lapka & Franson, 2010). MoAbs are also used as aids in diagnostic evaluation of both primary and metastatic tumors through radiologic imaging and laboratory techniques. For example, the process of immunohistochemistry uses a MoAb tagged with a stain that binds with the protein of interest, providing a visual stain for the presence or absence of the protein (Goetsch, 2009). This type of test is used to identify the presence of estrogen and progesterone receptors on breast cancer cells to see if the cells will be responsive to hormonal agents. Immunohistochemistry testing is also used to detect several proteins associated with hereditary nonpolyposis colon cancer (Goetsch, 2009). MoAbs are used to assist in the diagnosis of ovarian, colorectal, breast, and prostate cancers and some types of leukemia and lymphoma. MoAbs are also used in purging residual tumor cells from peripheral stem cell collections for patients who are undergoing HSCT after high-dose cytotoxic therapy. Researchers continue to explore the development and use of MoAbs, either alone or in combination with other substances such as radioactive materials, chemotherapy agents, toxins, hormones, or other BRMs.

Cytokines

Cytokines, substances produced primarily by cells of the immune system to enhance or suppress the production and functioning of components of the immune system, are used to treat cancer or the adverse effects of some cancer treatments. Cytokines are grouped into families, such as interferons (IFNs), interleukins (ILs), colony-stimulating factors, and tumor necrosis factor. Colony-stimulating factors were described earlier in this chapter for their supportive role in myelosuppressive treatment modalities. (Refer to Chapter 35 for more detailed discussion of the immune system.)

Interferons

IFNs are cytokines with antiviral, antitumor, and immunomodulatory (inhibition or stimulation of the immune system) properties (Lapka & Franson, 2010). Multiple antitumor effects of IFNs include antiangiogenesis, direct destruction of tumor cells, inhibition of growth factors, and disruption of the cell cycle. IFN-α is used in treatment of hairy-cell leukemia, Kaposi's sarcoma, chronic myelogenous leukemia, high-grade non-Hodgkin lymphoma, renal cell cancer, cutaneous T-cell lymphoma, and melanoma. IFN is administered by subcutaneous, intramuscular, IV, and intracavitary routes. Efforts are under way to establish the effectiveness of IFN in combination with other treatment regimens for treatment of various malignancies.

Interleukins

ILs are a subgroup of cytokines known as lymphokines and monokines produced by lymphocytes and monocytes, respectively. Various ILs that have been identified act by signaling and coordinating other cells of the immune system and thus require an intact immune system to achieve their therapeutic effects. IL-2 is an approved treatment option for renal cell cancer and metastatic melanoma in adults. IL-2 stimulates the production and activation of several different types of lymphocytes, enhances the production of other types of cytokines, and affects both humoral and cell-mediated immunity. Side effects of ILs range from mild to severe, including flulike symptoms, fatigue, migranes, and anorexia. More serious toxicities include severe diarrhea, capillary leak syndrome, pulmonary edema, profound hypotension, oliguria, HSRs, cardiac dysrhythmias, and altered mental status. When given in elevated doses or combined with other cytokines, administration of IL-2 requires hospitalization and monitoring due to the potential for life-threatening toxicities (Polovich et al., 2009).

Clinical trials are ongoing that explore the role of ILs in treatment of other cancers. Some early-stage clinical trials are assessing their effects when combined with chemotherapy and as growth factors for treatment of myelosuppression after the use of some forms of chemotherapy.

Tyrosine Kinase Inhibitors

Tyrosine kinases (TKs) are enzymes that, when activated, set in motion signaling pathways that regulate cell proliferation and various other processes that characterize cancer cell behavior (Goetsch, 2009). The genetic mutations found in malignant cells may cause TK activation despite, or in the absence of, the normal signals that should control TK activity. Alternatively, genetic mutations may lead to abnormally high levels of TK activation or prevent the usual signals that deactivate TK. Angiogenesis (the formation of tumor-associated blood vessels or circulation), the ability to invade surrounding cells and tissues, the ability to travel to distant body sites (metastasis), and malignant cell resistance to chemotherapy are all examples of processes and cancer cell characteristics that are related to TK activation. Several types of targeted therapies have been approved for use or are being evaluated in clinical trials because of their role in targeting TK overactivity (Bauer & Romvari, 2009; Goetsch, 2009; Lapka & Franson, 2010). Examples of TK targets include EGFRs, VEGF, and Bcr-Abl TK. A broader classification of drugs that target TK are also referred to as tyrosine kinase inhibitors (TKIs).

Epidermal Growth Factor Receptor Antagonists

EGFRs are proteins found on normal cells (expressed) but found in abundance (overexpressed) in many types of cancer, such as colon, rectal, and head and neck cancers. Activation of EGFRs in cancer cells can influence malignant cell growth, survival, and the ability to metastasize to other areas of the body. Targeted therapies, known as EGFR antagonists, act by blocking the pathway for EGFR activation and result in inhibiting cell growth and local invasion and metastasis (Goetsch, 2009). At least two approved EGFR antagonists are also MoAbs.

Vascular Endothelial Growth Factor Inhibitors

The process of new blood vessel formation—angiogenesis—is needed by tumors to provide blood supply for growth and metastasis. Angiogenesis is activated by VEGF when this growth factor attaches to endothelial cell receptors. Targeted agents that inhibit angiogenesis by blocking the endothelial receptors or directly targeting VEGF block the formation of new blood vessels and limit the supply of nutrients to tumor cells; contributing to cell death and prevention of local invasion and metastasis.

Bcr-Abl Tyrosine Kinase Inhibitors

In chronic myelogenous leukemia, there often is a gene mutation that causes abnormal activity of the TK Bcr-Abl (Bauer & Romvari, 2009; Galinsky & Buchanan, 2009). This mutation is occasionally associated with gastrointestinal stromal cell tumors and acute lymphocytic leukemia (Goetsch, 2009). Bcr-Abl TKIs act by opposing the gene mutation and inhibiting cell proliferation. Ultimately, this inhibition leads to cancer cell apoptosis. Continuing research will explore the identification of Bcr-Abl in association with other types of cancer and the effect of TKIs that specifically target receptors for this enzyme.

In addition to clinical trials exploring TK targeted therapies, there are trials seeking to identify other targets and agents. Poly (ADP-ribose) polymerases (PARPs) are a group of enzymes that play a role in DNA repair. If DNA repair mechanisms are negatively altered, it is posited that cancer cells will not be able to survive. Currently, research is exploring the role of PARP inhibitors in the treatment of cancers associated with BRCA1 and BRCA2 mutations such as breast, ovarian, prostate, and pancreatic cancers (Yap, Sandhu, Carden, et al., 2011).

Cancer Vaccines

Cancer vaccines mobilize the body's immune response to recognize and destroy cancer cells (Lapka & Franson, 2010). Cancer vaccines contain either portions of cancer cells alone or portions of cells in combination with other substances (adjuvants) that can augment or boost immune responses. *Autologous* vaccines are made from the patient's own cancer cells, which are obtained from tumor tissue during diagnostic biopsy or surgery. The cancer cells are killed and prepared for injection back into the patient. *Allogeneic* vaccines are made from cancer cells that are obtained from other people who have a specific type of cancer. These cancer cells are grown in a laboratory and eventually killed and prepared for injection.

Prophylactic vaccines prevent disease. Quadrivalent HPV recombinant vaccine (Gardasil) protects against HPV types 6, 11, 16, and 18 associated with common genital warts (type 6 and 11) and development of cervical cancer (types 16 and 18). It is administered over a series of three doses to females age 9 to 26 years to prevent HPV-associated cervical cancer (Merck & Co. Inc., 2011). Cervarix is another vaccine approved to combat two strains of HPV. Recombivax HB (Merck) and Engerix-B (GlaxoSmithKline) are U.S. Food and Drug Administration (FDA) approved vaccines against hepatitis B infection, which is associated with the development of hepatocellular cancer.

Therapeutic vaccines kill existing cancer cells and provide long-lasting immunity against further cancer development. In 2010, the FDA approved the first therapeutic cancer vaccine, Sipuleucel-T (Provenge, Dendreon Corp.), for use in men with metastatic prostate cancer that is no longer responding to hormone therapy. Sipuleucel-T is customized to each patient. Patients first undergo apheresis to isolate cells; the cells are then processed, resulting in a vaccine with hundreds of millions of "activated" cells loaded with an antigen commonly found on most prostate cancer cells. The resultant individualized vaccine is then administered IV to the patient, stimulating the patient's immune system to neutralize tumor cells that express the antigen. Patients receive three treatments over the course of 4 to 6 weeks, with each round requiring the same process (Phillips, 2010). This vaccine does not cure cancer but is associated with improved patient survival.

Challenges to the therapeutic activity of cancer vaccines include the size of the tumor burden, the mechanisms that allow tumor cells to avoid recognition as "nonself" by the immune system, and immune tolerance as the result of previous exposure to the tumor antigens. Multiple clinical trials are being conducted to develop therapeutic vaccines for cancers of the prostate, breast, kidney, and lung, as well as for melanoma, myeloma, and lymphoma (Lapka & Franson, 2010).

Gene Therapy

Gene therapy includes approaches that correct genetic defects, manipulate genes to induce tumor cell destruction, or assist the body's immune defenses in the hope of preventing or combating disease. One of the challenges confronting cancer gene therapy is the multiple somatic mutations involved in the development of cancer, making it difficult to identify the most effective gene therapy approach.

Considerable advances have been made in the identification of effective tumor cell targets and evaluation of the most appropriate vectors. Vectors serve as a vehicle or carrier to transport a gene into the target cell. With improved understanding of cell surface proteins and signaling pathways, many clinical trials are under way.

At this time, there are no FDA-approved gene therapies for cancer. Three approaches have been used in the development of gene therapies, with adenoviruses showing the most promise in each:

- *Tumor-directed therapy* is the introduction of a therapeutic gene (suicide gene) into tumor cells in an attempt to destroy them. This approach is challenging because it is difficult to identify the gene that would cause optimal tumor destruction, and patients with widespread disease would require multiple injections to treat every site of disease.
- *Active immunotherapy* is the administration of genes that will invoke the antitumor responses of the immune system.
- *Adoptive immunotherapy* is the administration of genetically altered lymphocytes that are programmed to cause tumor destruction.

Nursing Management

Patients receiving targeted therapies have many of the same needs as patients undergoing other cancer treatments. However, manipulation and stimulation of the immune system create unique challenges. Consequently, the nurse must assess the need for education, support, and additional resources for both the patient and family and assist in planning and evaluating patient care.

Monitoring Therapeutic and Adverse Effects

The nurse must become familiar with each agent administered and its potential effects. Adverse effects such as fever, myalgia, nausea, and vomiting, as seen with IFN therapy, may not be life threatening. Other adverse effects (e.g., capillary leak syndrome, pulmonary edema, hypotension) that may become life threatening can occur with BRM approaches such as high-dose IL-2 therapy. MoAbs are associated with both common and unique adverse effects. Although mild to moderate infusion reactions are more commonly associated with chimeric MoAbs, severe HSRs have been seen with MoAb infusions. Nurses must be aware of the adverse effects of BRMs and recognize the signs and symptoms of serious reactions to emergently institute appropriate interventions and supportive care. Nurses monitor patients for the impact of adverse effects on performance status and quality of life so that appropriate measures can be implemented to improve patient outcomes.

Nurses also need to be familiar with common and unique adverse effects associated with TKIs. Dermatologic toxicities, the most common side effects associated with EGFR inhibitors, may lead to poor patient adherence to treatment, interruptions, or discontinuation of therapy, especially for the oral agents that are self-administered by the patient at home (Given, Spoelstra, & Grant, 2011). Toxicities include dose-limiting papulopustular rashes, pruritis, purulent nail changes, nail fissures, and skin flaking. Patients may also develop corneal dryness and abrasions, eyelid changes, photosensitivity, alopecia, or hirsutism (Boucher, Olson, & Piperdi, 2011). Nurses use evidence-based practices for managing toxicities, promoting comfort, and improving patients' quality of life in hope of maximizing adherence to treatment and avoidance of treatment delays or discontinuation (Schneider, Hess, & Gosselin, 2011).

Promoting Home and Community-Based Care

The nurse educates patients about self-care and assists in providing for continuing care. Some targeted therapies can be administered subcutaneously by the patient or family members at home. As needed, the home care nurse educates the patient and family how to administer these agents and monitors the use of appropriate technique as well as safe disposal of sharps and contaminated materials. The nurse also provides instructions about side effects and helps the patient and family identify strategies to manage many of the common side effects of BRM therapy, such as fatigue, anorexia, and flulike symptoms.

The use of oral medications to treat cancer has risen greatly in the past several years, especially with advances in targeted therapies, many of which are given by mouth. It has been estimated that almost half of the new antineoplastic drugs in development are oral agents (Given et al., 2011). This shifts the responsibility for delivery of treatment to patients and families in the home setting (Given et al., 2011) and increases the need for home care referral. Regardless of the setting, nurses play an important role in identifying factors affecting adherence to oral antineoplastic agents and in developing strategies to address adherence barriers (Table 15-8).

The nurse collaborates with physicians, social workers, third-party payers, and pharmaceutical companies to help the patient obtain reimbursement or support for the cost of oral targeted therapies and other required medications. The nurse also reminds the patient about the importance of keeping follow-up appointments with the physician and assesses the patient's need for symptom management related to the underlying diseases and/or adverse effects of treatment. Home care nurses maintain communication with the physician regarding patient adherence and tolerance of treatment so that changes in care can be implemented in a timely fashion.

■ *Complementary and Alternative Medicine*

For many patients and clinicians, the challenge of managing symptoms related to cancer and its treatments is in finding the balance between achieving a reasonable quality of life while undergoing potentially toxic and lifesaving modalities. It is estimated that about 4 in 10 adults in the United States use some type of complementary or alternative medicine, with the rate being higher among patients with serious illnesses such as cancer (Bell, 2010).

The National Center for Complementary and Alternative Medicine (NCCAM) (2011) defines *complementary and alternative medicine* (CAM) as diverse medical and health care systems, practices, and products that are not presently considered to be part of conventional medicine. NCCAM defines *complementary medicine* as therapies used in conjunction with conventional medicine, whereas *alternative medicine* is therapies used instead of conventional medicine. More recently, the term *integrative* or *integrated medicine* has been used, which refers to a combination of conventional medicine and CAM with evidence of effectiveness and safety (NCCAM, 2011). Patients use CAM to manage symptoms related to cancer and associated treatments (Fouladbakhsh & Stommel, 2010).

Patients do not routinely communicate CAM practices to their health care providers because they were never asked about its use; they withhold the information, fearing that their physicians would not approve, or they feel that the use of CAM will not affect the conventional treatment they are receiving (Carroll-Johnson, 2010).

Although many CAM modalities can be a source of comfort and emotional support for patients, assessment of CAM use is important for patient safety. Patients often perceive vitamins and dietary supplements as harmless, natural products that have no side effects or potential toxicities. However, in patients receiving chemotherapy, the use of herbs or botanicals may interfere with drug metabolism, decrease or increase desired effects, or contain elements of uncertain pharmacologic capacities (ACS, 2009). Deep tissue massage and other manipulative therapies are contraindicated in patients with open wounds, radiation dermatitis, thrombocytopenia, VTE, and coagulation disorders, and in those taking anticoagulants (Running & Turnbeaugh, 2011).

Using a nonjudgmental approach, nurses include the assessment of CAM practices as part of the overall patient assessment. Cultural sensitivity and assessment of the patient's motivation in using CAM is essential for understanding patient needs (Bell, 2010). In addition, nurses reflect a willingness to assist patients to identify safe and acceptable CAM practices according to patient needs and desires. This requires that nurses develop familiarity and knowledge related to CAM, strength of supporting evidence, and credible sources of information to facilitate patient education and decision making.

Patients have access to frequently unreliable claims of "miracle cures" that range from plant remedies to metabolic therapy using special diets, supplements, or "detoxification" regimens involving unconventional enemas and colonic cleansing procedures. The ACS established a clearinghouse along with NCCAM to investigate and identify potentially dangerous and harmful unproven therapies. Information about unproven methods (unconventional treatments) can be obtained on the ACS Web site (ACS, 2011c).

Nursing Care of Patients With Cancer

The outlook for patients with cancer has greatly improved because of scientific and technologic advances. However, as a result of the underlying disease or various treatment modalities, patients with cancer may experience a variety of secondary problems such as reduced WBC counts, infection, bleeding, skin and nutritional problems, pain, fatigue, and psychological stress. Chart 15-7 provides a nursing care plan for patients with cancer.

TABLE 15-8 Strategies for Promoting Adherence to Oral Antineoplastic Agents

Assess for factors that may interfere with adherence to oral antineoplastic agents; develop plan of care that addresses specific assessment findings.

Barriers to Adherence	Strategies for Promoting Adherence
Sociodemographic Factors • Limited financial resources • Competing priorities for financial resources • Joblessness • Limited or no insurance • Racial or ethnic disparities • Lower level of education • Poor health literacy • Illiteracy • Non–English speaking • Lack of transportation • Lack of or limited social support • Rural residence	• Refer to financial counseling through health care facility, local nonprofit health/oncology support/advocacy, or other nonprofit community advocacy organizations. • Refer to social worker for referrals as described above and/or for disability applications through employer or Social Security Administration, Medicaid, or Medicare applications. • Explore patient assistance programs for costs of health care, copays, medications, household costs, transportation services (costs or availability), and home care available through nonprofit organizations, oncology support/advocacy or other nonprofit community advocacy organizations, religious institutions, philanthropic organizations, pharmaceutical industry–sponsored programs, health care institution–specific programs; assist with financial documentation and application procedures as needed. • Explore assistance programs for other priorities competing for financial resources (i.e., for utility costs, gas, child care, food). • Assist patient to identify family, friends or other available supports to assist with activities of daily living, household responsibilities, errands, shopping, meals, transportation or other responsibilities; assist with delegation of needs and schedules of availability if needed. • Assess preferred method of learning (i.e., verbal, visual, written materials); tailor instructional materials to patient needs, including language. • Include family, significant other, and friends in education whenever feasible. • Use return demonstration of behaviors and devices used to support adherence. • Provide contact information that spans 24 hours for questions or problems. • Contact patient by phone or other means (e-mail) to assess for concerns in between follow-up visits to physician. • Encourage patient to use adherence reminders such as pill boxes, medication calendars, checklists, medication diaries, alarms on cell phone or other devices/timers; explore availability of programmed telephone reminder services, text messages from family member, friend, or other caregiver; review diary at each visit. • Instruct patient to bring pill bottles to each follow-up visit; perform pill counts to monitor adherence. • Send postcard reminder to patient weekly (or less often) or 1 week prior to due date for medication refill. • Refer to home care for continued education, and follow up on adherence. • Identify local pharmacies that supply oral cancer therapies. Instruct patients to contact nurse if the pharmacy cannot fill the prescription within 24 hours. • Remind patients to anticipate need for adequate supply of medications prior to travel or vacation.
Age • Older adults; especially those >75 years	• Ensure that written education materials and instructions are written in black using at least 14-point sans serif font such as Arial or Calibri. • Use illustrated education materials. • Review and revise adherence strategies if patient status declines or changes. • Explore availability of alarmed medication box.
Beliefs • Oral medications less effective or important than IV treatments • Fatalism about disease outcomes	• Provide education regarding oral versus IV medications. • Discuss goals of care and ongoing assessment of response to treatment.
Comorbidities • Preexisting chronic disease • Vision or hearing impairments	• Communicate with primary care and other providers involved in care of patient regarding current cancer disease status and treatment; collaborate with other providers for ongoing management of nononcology issues or exacerbation of issues that may impact cancer treatment adherence. • Collaborate with appropriate resources to assist with special needs and assistive devices for vision or hearing impairments.
Polypharmacy • Multiple medications for comorbidities and/or cancer treatment and symptom management	• Review all medications prescribed by oncology physicians and other providers involved in care of patient for preexisting chronic disease. • Assess patient use of over-the-counter medications and other agents. • Consult with pharmacist to identify medications and other agents that may be contraindicated or that may interfere with antineoplastic regimen. • Collaborate with all providers prescribing medications in order to simplify and/or reduce number of required medications if possible. • Provide patient, family, or other caregiver education regarding specific instructions when multiple medications are required. • Provide written checklist for patient to utilize daily to check off each medication when taken. • Do not give patients prescriptions that allow for refills; prescriptions should be for a finite period of time that concludes with next scheduled visit.
Psychiatric, Psychological, or Cognitive Concerns • Psychiatric disease • Depression • Cognitive impairments • Anxiety	• Avoid initial education regarding oral medications at same time of first physician visit; have patient and other learners return for another appointment to see nurse for education, and follow up with subsequent visit if deemed to be at high risk for adherence challenges. • Discuss with physician the necessity for referral to psychiatrist to evaluate need for psychotropic medications. • Refer patient for professional mental health counseling as needed. • Identify additional supports for care and education as discussed earlier.

Barriers to Adherence	Strategies for Promoting Adherence
Disease Factors • Symptoms such as pain, nausea, fatigue, skin rashes, etc. • Impaired mobility	• Proactively assess and manage symptoms related to underlying disease and/or treatments. • Provide patient, family, or other caregivers education about expected side effects and management strategies. • Instruct patient to premedicate with antiemetic as prescribed 30 minutes prior to taking oral antineoplastic agent if needed for nausea and/or vomiting. • Identify additional supports for care as discussed earlier. • Assess need for referral to home physical and/or occupational therapy to address impaired mobility and need for assistive devices.
Communication Issues • Patient–Clinician • Clinician—clinician	• Establish rapport and allow patients, families, and other caregivers time and opportunity to ask questions. • Do not assume adherence to oral antineoplastic agents; assess potential barriers consistently throughout course of treatment at each follow-up visit. • Communicate with primary provider regarding current cancer disease status, treatment and information regarding antineoplastic agents, such as drug–drug interactions, expected toxicities, and toxicities requiring prompt intervention.

Adapted from Streeter, S. B., Schwartzberg, L., Husain, N., et al. (2011). Patient and plan characteristics affecting abandonment of oral oncolytic prescriptions. *Journal of Oncology Practice*, 7(3S), 46S–51S; Given, B. A., Spoelstra, S. L., & Grant, M. (2011). The challenges of oral agents as antineoplastic treatments. *Seminars in Oncology Nursing*, 27(2), 93–103; and Mathews, M., & Park, A. D. (2009). Identifying patients in financial need: Cancer care providers' perceptions of barriers. *Clinical Journal of Oncology Nursing*, 13(5), 501–505.

Maintaining Tissue Integrity

Some of the most frequently encountered disturbances of tissue integrity include stomatitis, skin and tissue reactions to radiation therapy, cutaneous toxicities associated with targeted therapy, alopecia, and metastatic skin lesions.

Stomatitis

Mucositis, a common side effect of radiation and some types of chemotherapy, refers to an inflammatory process involving the mucous membranes of the oral cavity and the gastrointestinal tract. Stomatitis, a form of mucositis, is an inflammatory process of the mouth including the mucosa and tissues surrounding the teeth (Eilers & Million, 2011). Stomatitis is characterized by changes in sensation, mild redness (erythema), and edema or, if severe, by painful ulcerations, bleeding, and secondary infection. Stomatitis commonly develops 5 to 14 days after patients receive certain chemotherapeutic agents, such as doxorubicin and 5-fluorouracil, and BRMs, such as IL-2 and IFN. Stomatitis affects up to 100% of patients undergoing high-dose chemotherapy with HSCT, 80% of patients with malignancies of the head and neck receiving radiotherapy, and up to 40% of patients receiving standard-dose chemotherapy. Oropharyngeal mucositis may be worse in patients with head and neck cancers who receive combined modality therapy of both radiation and chemotherapy (Kurtin, 2009).

Stomatitis and mucositis are attributed to a cascade of molecular processes and submucosal endothelial cell destruction that begin almost immediately after the initiation of radiation and certain types of chemotherapy prior to the development of signs and symptoms. Mucositis develops as a consequence of a sequence of related and interacting biologic events, culminating in injury and apoptosis of basal epithelial cells, which results in the loss of epithelial renewal, atrophy, and ulceration. Gram-positive and gram-negative organisms can invade the ulcerated tissue and result in infection.

Risk factors and comorbidities associated with stomatitis include poor oral hygiene, general debilitation, existing dental disease, prior irradiation to the head and neck region, impaired salivary gland function, the use of other medications that dry mucous membranes, myelosuppression (bone marrow depression), advanced age, tobacco use, previous stomatoxic chemotherapy, diminished renal function, and impaired nutritional status (Eilers & Million, 2011).

Because chemotherapy-associated neutropenia is better managed now, patients may receive higher doses of chemotherapy than in the past. However, stomatitis is now more prevalent and frequently causes treatment delays and dose reductions that may ultimately contribute to poor treatment outcomes (Eilers & Million, 2011). Severe oral pain can significantly affect swallowing, nutritional intake, speech, quality of life, coping abilities, and willingness to adhere to treatment regimens. Severe mucositis may lead to more frequent health care visits, hospitalizations, and increased health care costs (Eilers & Million, 2011).

Nursing assessment begins with understanding the patient's usual practices for oral hygiene and identification of individuals at risk for stomatitis. The patient is also assessed for dehydration, infection, pain, and nutritional impairment resulting from stomatitis and mucositis.

Optimal evidence-based prevention and treatment approaches for stomatitis remain severely limited but continue to be studied across disciplines (Eilers & Million, 2011). Most clinicians agree that maintenance of good oral hygiene, including brushing, flossing, rinsing, and dental care, is necessary to minimize the risk of oral complications associated with cancer therapies.

Palifermin (Kepivance), an IV administered synthetic form of human keratinocyte growth factor, is beneficial in the prevention of oral mucositis in patients with hematologic malignancies who are preparing for HSCT, as well as head and neck cancer treated with chemotherapy and radiation (Eilers & Million, 2011; Le, Kim, Schneider, et al., 2011). Palifermin promotes epithelial cell repair and accelerated replacement of cells in the mouth and gastrointestinal tract. Careful timing of administration and monitoring are essential for maximum effectiveness and to detect adverse effects.

Radiation-Associated Skin Impairment

Although advances in radiation therapy have resulted in decreased incidence and severity of skin impairments, patients

(text continues on page 356)

Chart 15-7

PLAN OF NURSING CARE

The Patient With Cancer

NURSING DIAGNOSIS: Risk for infection related to inadequate defenses related to myelosuppression secondary to radiation or antineoplastic agents

GOAL: Prevention of infection

Nursing Interventions	Rationale	Expected Outcomes
1. Assess patient for evidence of infection. a. Check vital signs every 4 hours. b. Monitor white blood cell (WBC) count and differential each day. c. Inspect all sites that may serve as entry ports for pathogens (IV sites, wounds, skin folds, bony prominences, perineum, and oral cavity).	1. Signs and symptoms of infection may be diminished in the immunocompromised host. Prompt recognition of infection and subsequent initiation of therapy will reduce morbidity and mortality associated with infection.	• Demonstrates normal temperature and vital signs • Exhibits absence of signs of inflammation: local edema, erythema, pain, and warmth • Exhibits normal breath sounds on auscultation
2. Report fever (≥38.3°C [101°F] or ≥38°C [100.4°F] for >1 hour) (see Table 15-10), chills, diaphoresis, swelling, heat, pain, erythema, exudate on any body surfaces. Also report change in respiratory or mental status, urinary frequency or burning, malaise, myalgias, arthralgias, rash, or diarrhea.	2. Early detection of infection facilitates early intervention.	• Takes deep breaths and coughs every 2 hours to prevent respiratory dysfunction and infection. • Exhibits absence of pathogens on cultures • Avoids contact with others with infections • Avoids crowds
3. Obtain cultures and sensitivities as indicated before initiation of antimicrobial treatment (wound exudate, sputum, urine, stool, blood).	3. Tests identify the organism and indicate the most appropriate antimicrobial therapy. The use of inappropriate antibiotics enhances proliferation of additional flora and encourages growth of antibiotic-resistant organisms.	• All personnel carry out hand hygiene after each voiding and bowel movement. • Excoriation and trauma of skin are avoided. • Trauma to mucous membranes is avoided (avoidance of rectal thermometers, suppositories, vaginal tampons, perianal trauma).

4. Initiate measures to minimize infection.
 a. Discuss with patient and family:
  (1) Placing patient in private room if absolute WBC count <1,000/mm³.
  (2) Importance of patient avoiding contact with people who have known or recent infection or recent vaccination.
 b. Instruct all personnel in careful hand hygiene before and after entering room.
 c. Avoid rectal or vaginal procedures (rectal temperatures, examinations, suppositories; vaginal tampons).
	4. Exposure to infection is reduced.
	 a. Preventing contact with pathogens helps prevent infection.
	
	 b. Hands are significant source of contamination.
	
	 c. Incidence of rectal and perianal abscesses and subsequent systemic infection is high. Manipulation may cause disruption of membrane integrity and enhance progression of infection.
		• Uses evidence-based procedures and techniques if participating in management of invasive lines or catheters
		• Uses electric razor
		• Is free of skin breakdown and stasis of secretions
		• Adheres to dietary and environmental precautions
		• Exhibits no signs of sepsis or septic shock
		• Exhibits normal vital signs, cardiac output, and arterial pressures when monitored
		• Demonstrates ability to administer colony-stimulating factor
		• Has bowel movements at regular intervals without constipation or straining

d. Use stool softeners to prevent constipation and straining. e. Assist patient in practice of meticulous personal hygiene. f. Instruct patient to use electric razor. g. Encourage patient to ambulate in room unless contraindicated. h. Provide patient and family education on food hygiene and safe food handling.	d. Minimizes trauma to tissues e. Prevents skin irritation f. Minimizes skin trauma g. Minimizes chance of skin breakdown and stasis of pulmonary secretions h. No evidence supports dietary restrictions of avoiding raw or fresh fruit and vegetables for patients who are neutropenic (Tarr & Allen, 2009). General precautions regarding food handling and storage are recommended.	• Patient hygiene is maintained. • Absence of IV catheter–related infection • Absence of skin abcesses • Absence of urinary catheter–related infection
i. Each day, change water pitcher, denture cleaning fluids, and respiratory equipment containing water.	i. Stagnant water is a source of infection.	

**Chart
15-7**

PLAN OF NURSING CARE

The Patient With Cancer (continued)

Nursing Intervention	Rationale	Expected Outcomes
5. Assess IV sites every day for evidence of infection.	5. Nosocomial staphylococcal septicemia is closely associated with IV catheters.	
a. Change peripheral short-term IV sites every other day.	a. Incidence of infection is increased when catheter is in place >72 hours.	
b. Cleanse skin with povidone–iodine before arterial puncture or venipuncture.	b. Povidone–iodine is effective against many gram-positive and gram-negative pathogens.	
c. Change central venous catheter dressings every 48 hours.	c. Allows observation of site and removes source of contamination	
d. Change all solutions and infusion sets every 72–96 hours.	d. Once introduced into the system, microorganisms are capable of growing in infusion sets despite replacement of container and high flow rates.	
e. Follow Infusion Nursing Society guidelines for care of peripheral and central venous access devices.	e. Infusion Nursing Society collaborates with other nursing subspecialties in determining guidelines for IV access care.	
6. Avoid intramuscular injections.	6. Reduces risk for skin abscesses.	
7. Avoid insertion of urinary catheters; if catheters are necessary, use aseptic technique.	7. Rates of infection greatly increase after urinary catheterization.	
8. Educate patient or family member to administer granulocyte (or granulocyte-macrophage) colony-stimulating factor when prescribed.	8. Granulocyte colony-stimulating factor decreases the duration of neutropenia and the potential for infection.	
9. Advise patient to avoid exposure to animal excreta; discuss dental procedures with primary provider; avoid vaginal douche; and avoid vaginal or rectal manipulation during sexual contact during period of neutropenia.	9. Minimizes exposure to potential sources of infection and disruption of skin integrity	

NURSING DIAGNOSIS: Risk for impaired skin integrity: erythematous and wet desquamation reactions to radiation therapy
GOAL: Maintenance of skin integrity

Nursing Intervention	Rationale	Expected Outcomes
1. In erythematous areas:	1. Care to the affected areas must focus on preventing further skin irritation, drying, and damage.	• Avoids use of soaps, powders, and other cosmetics on site of radiation therapy • States rationale for special care of skin • Exhibits minimal change in skin • Avoids trauma to affected skin region (avoids shaving, constricting and irritating clothing, extremes of temperature, and the use of adhesive tape) • Reports change in skin promptly • Demonstrates proper care of blistered or open areas • Exhibits absence of infection of blistered and opened areas. • Wound is free of development of eschar.
a. Avoid the use of soaps, cosmetics, perfumes, powders, lotions, and ointments; non–aluminum-based deodorant may be used on intact skin (McQuestion, 2011).	a. These substances may cause pain and additional skin irritation and damage.	
b. Use only lukewarm water to bathe the area.	b. Avoiding water of extreme temperatures and soap minimizes additional skin damage, irritation, and pain.	
c. Avoid rubbing or scratching the area.	c. Rubbing and or scratching will lead to additional skin irritation, damage, and increased risk of infection.	
d. Avoid shaving the area with a straight-edged razor.	d. The use of razors may lead to additional irritation and disruption of skin integrity and increased risk of infection.	
e. Avoid applying hot-water bottles, heating pads, ice, and adhesive tape to the area.	e. Avoiding extreme temperatures minimizes additional skin damage, irritation, burns, and pain.	
f. Avoid exposing the area to sunlight or cold weather.	f. Sun exposure or extreme cold weather may lead to additional skin damage and pain.	
g. Avoid tight clothing in the area. Use cotton clothing.	g. Allows air circulation to affected area	
h. Apply vitamin A and D ointment to the area.	h. May aid healing; however, evidence that supports its use is lacking.	

(continues on page 348)

Chart 15-7

PLAN OF NURSING CARE

The Patient With Cancer (continued)

Nursing Intervention	Rationale	Expected Outcomes
i. Apply calendula cream or hyaluronic acid to decrease the incidence of moist desquamation.	**i.** Limited data supports the use of calendula cream to decrease the incidence of moist desquamation, and some formulations of hyaluronic acid may be effective (McQuestion, 2011).	
2. If wet desquamation occurs:	**2.** Open weeping areas are susceptible to bacterial infection. Care must be taken to prevent introduction of pathogens.	
a. Do not disrupt any blisters that have formed.	**a.** Disruption of skin blisters disrupts skin integrity and may lead to increased risk of infection.	
b. Avoid frequent washing of the area.	**b.** Frequent washing may lead to increased irritation and skin damage, with increased risk of infection.	
c. Report any blistering.	**c.** Blistering of skin represents progression of skin damage.	
d. Use *prescribed* creams or ointments.	**d.** Anecdotally believed to decrease irritation and inflammation of the area and promote healing; although a variety of products are used in many settings, there are few randomized controlled trials with evidence to support one product or intervention over another (McQuestion, 2011).	
e. If area weeps, apply a nonadhesive absorbent dressing.	**e.** Easier to remove and associated with less pain and trauma when drainage dries and adheres to dressing.	
f. If the area is without drainage, the use of moisture and vapor-permeable dressings, such as hydrocolloids and hydrogels on noninfected areas, have been used in many settings.	**f.** May promote healing; however, randomized controlled clinical trial support is lacking in the setting of moist desquamation. Hydrocolloid dressings have demonstrated promotion of comfort (McQuestion, 2011).	
g. Consult with wound-ostomy-continence nurse (WOCN) and primary provider if eschar forms.	**g.** Eschar must be removed to promote healing and prevent infection. WOCNs have expertise in the care of wounds.	

NURSING DIAGNOSIS: Impaired oral mucous membrane: stomatitis
GOAL: Maintenance of intact oral mucous membranes

Nursing Intervention	Rationale	Expected Outcomes
1. Assess oral cavity daily using the same assessment criteria or rating scale (Caplinger, Royse, & Martens, 2010).	**1.** Provides baseline for later evaluation; maintains consistency in assessment findings	• States rationale for frequent oral assessment and hygiene
2. Identify individuals at increased risk for stomatitis and related complications.	**2.** Patient and treatment variables are associated with incidence and severity of stomatitis as well as related complications such as delayed healing and infection (Eilers & Million, 2011).	• Factors associated with incidence, severity, and complications are identified prior to initiation of cancer treatment • Oral mucosal assessment is conducted at baseline and on an ongoing basis.
3. Instruct patient to report oral burning, pain, areas of redness, open lesions on oropharyngeal mucosa and lips, pain associated with swallowing, or decreased tolerance to temperature extremes of food.	**3.** Identification of initial stages of stomatitis will facilitate prompt interventions, including modification of treatment as prescribed by primary provider.	• Oral hygiene practices are initiated prior to development of stomatitis. • Identifies signs and symptoms of stomatitis to report to nurse or primary provider • Participates in recommended oral hygiene regimen • Avoids mouthwashes with alcohol
4. Encourage and assist as needed in oral hygiene.	**4.** Patients who are having discomfort or pain, or other symptoms related to the disease and treatment, may require encouragement and assistance in performing oral hygiene. Oral hygiene is maintained to prevent complications of stomatitis, such as infection (Eilers & Million, 2011).	• Brushes teeth and mouth with soft toothbrush • Uses lubricant to keep lips soft and nonirritated • Avoids hard-to-chew, spicy, hot foods or other irritating foods • Maintains adequate hydration

**Chart
15-7**

PLAN OF NURSING CARE
The Patient With Cancer (continued)

Nursing Intervention	Rationale	Expected Outcomes
Preventive 1. Advise patient to avoid irritants such as commercial mouthwashes, alcoholic beverages, and tobacco. 2. Brush with soft toothbrush using nonabrasive toothpaste for 90 seconds after meals and at bedtime; allow toothbrush to air dry before storing; floss at least once daily or as advised by the clinician; patients who have not previously flossed regularly should not initiate flossing during stomatoxic treatment; rinse mouth four times a day with a bland rinse (normal saline, sodium bicarbonate, or saline and sodium bicarbonate); avoid irritating foods (acidic, hot, rough, and spicy); use water-based moisturizers to protect lips. 3. Maintain adequate hydration. 4. Provide written instruction and education to patients on above items (Harris & Eilers, 2009).	1. Alcohol content of mouthwashes and tobacco smoke will dry oral tissues and potentiate breakdown. 2. Limits trauma and removes debris. Patients who have not previously flossed regularly do initiate flossing during stomatoxic treatment due to potential for injury to the oral mucosa and increased susceptibility to infection. 3. Maintenance of hydration prevents mucosal drying and breakdown. 4. Written information reinforces patient education and provides the patient and family with a source.	• Exhibits clean, intact oral mucosa • Exhibits no ulcerations or infections of oral cavity • Exhibits no evidence of bleeding • Reports absent or decreased oral pain • Reports no difficulty swallowing • Exhibits healing (reepithelialization) of oral mucosa within 5–7 days (mild stomatitis)
Mild stomatitis (generalized erythema, limited ulcerations, small white patches: *Candida*) 1. Use bland mouth rinses every 1–4 hours. 2. Use soft toothbrush or toothette. 3. Remove dentures except for meals; be certain that dentures fit well. 4. Apply water-soluble lip lubricant. 5. Avoid foods that are spicy or hard to chew and those with extremes of temperature.	1. Assists in removing debris, thick secretions, and bacteria 2. Minimizes trauma 3. Minimizes friction and discomfort 4. Promotes comfort 5. Prevents local trauma	• Exhibits healing of oral tissues within 10–14 days (severe stomatitis) • Exhibits no bleeding or oral ulceration • Consumes adequate fluid and food • Exhibits absence of dehydration and weight loss • Exhibits no evidence of infection
Severe stomatitis (confluent ulcerations with bleeding and white patches covering >25% of oral mucosa) 1. Obtain tissue samples for culture and sensitivity tests of areas of infection. 2. Assess ability to chew and swallow; assess gag reflex. 3. Use bland oral rinses (may combine in solution saline, anti-*Candida* agent, such as Mycostatin, and topical anesthetic agent [described later]) as prescribed, or place patient on side and irrigate mouth; have suction available. 4. Remove dentures. 5. Use toothette or gauze soaked with solution for cleansing. 6. Use water-soluble lip lubricant. 7. Provide liquid or pureed diet. 8. Monitor for dehydration.	1. Assists in identifying need for antimicrobial therapy 2. Patient may be in danger of aspiration. 3. Facilitates cleansing and provides for safety and comfort 4. Prevents trauma from ill-fitting dentures 5. Limits trauma and promotes comfort 6. Promotes comfort and minimizes loss of skin integrity 7. Ensures intake of easily digestible foods without chewing 8. Decreased oral intake and ulcerations potentiate fluid deficits.	

(continues on page 350)

Chart 15-7

PLAN OF NURSING CARE

The Patient With Cancer (continued)

Nursing Intervention	Rationale	Expected Outcomes

9. Minimize discomfort.
  a. Consult primary provider for use of topical anesthetic, such as dyclonine and diphenhydramine, or viscous lidocaine.
  b. Administer systemic analgesics as prescribed.
 	
  c. Perform mouth care as described.
	a. Alleviates pain and increases sense of well-being; promotes participation in oral hygiene and nutritional intake
	
	b. Adequate management of pain related to severe stomatitis can facilitate improved quality of life, participation in other aspects of activities of daily living, oral intake, and verbal communication.
	c. Promotes removal of debris, healing, and comfort	

NURSING DIAGNOSIS: Impaired tissue integrity: alopecia
GOAL: Maintenance of tissue integrity; coping with hair loss

Nursing Intervention	Rationale	Expected Outcomes

1. Discuss potential hair loss and regrowth with patient and family; advise that hair loss may occur on body parts other than the head.
2. Explore potential impact of hair loss on self-image, interpersonal relationships, and sexuality.
3. Prevent or minimize hair loss through the following:
  a. Use scalp hypothermia and scalp tourniquets, if appropriate.
 	
  b. Cut long hair before treatment.
 	
  c. Use mild shampoo and conditioner, gently pat dry, and avoid excessive shampooing.
  d. Avoid electric curlers, curling irons, dryers, clips, barrettes, hair sprays, hair dyes, and permanent waves.
  e. Avoid excessive combing or brushing; use wide-toothed comb.
4. Prevent trauma to scalp.
  a. Lubricate scalp with vitamin A and D ointment to decrease itching.
  b. Have patient use sunscreen or wear hat when in the sun.
5. Suggest ways to assist in coping with hair loss.
  a. Purchase wig or hairpiece before hair loss.
 	
  b. If hair loss has occurred, take photograph to wig shop to assist in selection.
  c. Begin to wear wig before hair loss.
 	
  d. Contact the American Cancer Society for donated wigs or a store that specializes in this product.
  e. Wear hat, scarf, or turban.
6. Encourage patient to wear own clothes and retain social contacts.
7. Explain that hair growth usually begins again once therapy is completed.
	1. Provides information so patient and family can begin to prepare cognitively and emotionally for loss
	
	2. Facilitates coping and maintenance of interpersonal relationships
	
	3. Retains hair as long as possible.
	
	  a. Decreases hair follicle uptake of chemotherapy (not used for patients with leukemia or lymphoma because tumor cells may be present in blood vessels or scalp tissue)
	  b–e. Minimizes hair loss due to the weight and manipulation of hair
	
	4. Preserves tissue integrity
	  a. Assists in maintaining skin integrity
	
	  b. Prevents ultraviolet light exposure
	
	5. Minimizes change in appearance
	
	  a. Wig that closely resembles hair color and style is more easily selected if hair loss has not begun.
	  b. Facilitates adjustment
	
	  c. Enables patient to be prepared for loss and facilitates adjustment
	  d. Provides options to patient and assists with financial burden if necessary
	  e. Conceals loss and protects scalp
	6. Assists in maintaining personal identity
	
	7. Reassures patient that hair loss is usually temporary
		• Identifies alopecia as potential side effect of treatment
		• Identifies positive and negative feelings and threats to self-image
		• Verbalizes meaning that hair and possible hair loss have for him or her
		• States rationale for modifications in hair care and treatment
		• Uses mild shampoo and conditioner, and shampoos hair only when necessary
		• Avoids hair dryer, curlers, sprays, and other stresses on hair and scalp
		• Wears hat or scarf over hair when exposed to sun
		• Takes steps to deal with possible hair loss before it occurs; purchases wig or hairpiece if desired
		• Maintains hygiene and grooming
		• Interacts and socializes with others
		• States that hair loss and the use of wig or head covering are temporary

PLAN OF NURSING CARE

Chart
15-7

The Patient With Cancer (continued)

NURSING DIAGNOSIS: Imbalanced nutrition: less than body requirements, related to nausea and vomiting
GOAL: Patient experiences less nausea and vomiting associated with chemotherapy; weight loss is minimized

Nursing Intervention	Rationale	Expected Outcomes
1. Assess the patient's previous experiences and expectations of nausea and vomiting, including causes and interventions used. 2. Adjust diet before and after drug administration according to patient preference and tolerance. 3. Prevent unpleasant sights, odors, and sounds in the environment. 4. Use distraction, music therapy, biofeedback, self-hypnosis, relaxation techniques, and guided imagery before, during, and after chemotherapy. 5. Administer prescribed antiemetics, sedatives, and corticosteroids before chemotherapy and afterward as needed. 6. Ensure adequate fluid hydration before, during, and after drug administration; assess intake and output. 7. Encourage frequent oral hygiene. 8. Provide pain-relief measures, if necessary. 9. Consult with dietician as needed. 10. Assess and address other contributing factors to nausea and vomiting, such as other symptoms, constipation, gastrointestinal irritation, electrolyte imbalance, radiation therapy, medications, and central nervous system metastasis.	1. Identifies patient concerns, misinformation, and potential strategies for intervention; also gives patient sense of empowerment and control 2. Each patient responds differently to food after chemotherapy. A diet containing foods that relieve or prevent nausea or vomiting is most helpful. 3. Unpleasant sensations can stimulate the nausea and vomiting center. 4. Decreases anxiety, which can contribute to nausea and vomiting. Psychological conditioning may also be decreased. 5. Administration of antiemetic regimen before onset of nausea and vomiting limits the adverse experience and facilitates control. Combination drug therapy reduces nausea and vomiting through various triggering mechanisms. 6. Adequate fluid volume dilutes drug levels, decreasing stimulation of vomiting receptors. 7. Reduces unpleasant taste sensations 8. Increased comfort increases physical tolerance of symptoms. 9. Interdisciplinary collaboration is essential in addressing complex patient needs. 10. Multiple factors may contribute to nausea and vomiting.	• Identifies previous triggers of nausea and vomiting • Exhibits decreased apprehension and anxiety • Identifies previously used successful interventions for nausea and vomiting • Reports decrease in nausea • Reports decrease in incidence of vomiting • Consumes adequate fluid and food when nausea subsides • Demonstrates use of distraction, relaxation, and imagery when indicated • Exhibits normal skin turgor and moist mucous membranes • Reports no additional weight loss

NURSING DIAGNOSIS: Imbalanced nutrition: less than body requirements, related to anorexia, cachexia, or malabsorption
GOAL: Maintenance of nutritional status and of weight within 10% of pretreatment weight

Nursing Intervention	Rationale	Expected Outcomes
1. Assess and address factors that interfere with oral intake or are associated with increased risk of decreased nutritional status.	1. Multiple patient or treatment-related factors are associated with increased risk of impaired nutritional intake, such as radiation to the head, neck, and thorax; stomatoxic or emetogenic chemotherapy; prior oral, head, and neck surgery; mucositis; impaired swallowing or dysphagia; poor dentition; cough or shortness of breath (Granda-Cameron, DeMille, Lynch, et al., 2010).	• Factors associated with increased risk for impaired nutritional intake are identified. • Factors associated with increased risk of impaired nutritional intake are identified and addressed, whenever possible, through interdisciplinary collaboration. • Patient and family identify minimal nutritional requirements • Maintains or increases weight and body cell mass as per goals identified by nutritionist • Reports decreasing anorexia and increased interest in eating • Demonstrates normal skin turgor • Identifies rationale for dietary modifications; patient and family verbalize strategies to minimize nutritional deficits

(continues on page 352)

Chart 15-7

PLAN OF NURSING CARE
The Patient With Cancer (continued)

Nursing Intervention	Rationale	Expected Outcomes
2. Initiate appropriate referrals for interdisciplinary collaboration to manage factors that interfere with oral intake.	2. Other disciplines may be more appropriate for assessment and management of issues such as swallowing impairments (speech therapy), fatigue and decreased physical ability (physical and occupational therapy), nutritional assessment and determination of patient needs (nutritionist), cough and shortness of breath (respiratory therapy), poor dentition (dental medicine), depression/anxiety (social worker, psychologist, or psychiatrist).	• Participates in calorie counts and diet histories • Uses relaxation techniques and guided imagery before meals • Exhibits laboratory and clinical findings indicative of adequate nutritional intake: normal serum levels of protein, albumin, transferrin, iron, blood urea nitrogen (BUN), creatinine, vitamin D, electrolytes, hemoglobin, hematocrit, and lymphocytes; normal urinary creatinine levels • Consumes diet containing required nutrients • Carries out oral hygiene before meals • Reports decreased pain and/or other symptoms; symptoms do not interfere with oral intake • Reports decreasing episodes of nausea and vomiting • Participates in increasing levels of activity as measured by assessment of performance status • States rationale for use of tube feedings or parenteral nutrition • Demonstrates ability to manage enteral feedings or parenteral nutrition, if prescribed • Maintains body position and alignment needed to facilitate chewing and swallowing
3. Educate patient to avoid unpleasant sights, odors, and sounds in the environment during mealtime.	3. Anorexia can be stimulated or increased with noxious stimuli.	
4. Suggest foods that are preferred and well tolerated by the patient, preferably high-calorie and high-protein foods. Respect ethnic and cultural food preferences.	4. Foods preferred, well tolerated, and high in calories and protein maintain nutritional status during periods of increased metabolic demand.	
5. Encourage adequate fluid intake, but limit fluids at mealtime.	5. Fluids are necessary to eliminate wastes and prevent dehydration. Increased fluids with meals can lead to early satiety.	
6. Suggest smaller, more frequent meals.	6. Smaller, more frequent meals are better tolerated because early satiety is less likely to occur.	
7. Promote relaxed, quiet environment during mealtime with increased social interaction as desired.	7. A quiet environment promotes relaxation. Social interaction at mealtime may foster appetite, divert focus on food, and promote enjoyment of eating.	
8. If patient desires, serve wine at mealtime with foods.	8. Wine may stimulate appetite and add calories.	
9. Consider cold foods, if desired.	9. Cold, high-protein foods are often more tolerable and less odorous than hot foods.	
10. Encourage nutritional supplements and high-protein foods between meals.	10. Supplements and snacks add protein and calories to meet nutritional requirements.	
11. Encourage frequent oral hygiene, particularly prior to meals.	11. Oral hygiene may stimulate appetite and increase saliva production.	
12. Address pain and other symptom management needs.	12. Pain and other symptoms impair appetite and nutritional intake.	
13. Increase activity level as tolerated.	13. Increased activity promotes appetite.	
14. Decrease anxiety by encouraging verbalization of fears and concerns; use relaxation techniques and guided imagery at mealtime.	14. Relief of anxiety may increase appetite.	
15. Instruct patient and family about body alignment and proper positioning at mealtime.	15. Proper body position and alignment are necessary to aid chewing and swallowing.	
16. Collaborate with dietician to instruct patient and family regarding enteral tube feedings of commercial liquid diets, elemental diets, or blenderized foods as prescribed.	16. Tube feedings may be necessary in the severely debilitated patient who has a functioning gastrointestinal system but is unable to maintain adequate oral intake.	
17. Collaborate with dietician or nutrition support team to instruct patient and family regarding home parenteral nutrition with lipid supplements as prescribed.	17. Parenteral nutrition with supplemental fats supplies needed calories and proteins to meet nutritional demands, especially in the nonfunctional gastrointestinal system.	

Chart 15-7

PLAN OF NURSING CARE
The Patient With Cancer (continued)

Nursing Intervention	Rationale	Expected Outcomes
18. Administer appetite stimulants as prescribed by primary provider.	18. Although the mechanism is unclear, medications such as megestrol acetate (Megace) have been noted to improve appetite in patients with cancer and human immunodeficiency virus infection.	
19. Encourage family and friends not to nag or cajole patient about eating.	19. Pressuring patient to eat may cause conflict and unnecessary stress.	
20. Assess and address other contributing factors to nausea, vomiting, and anorexia such as electrolyte imbalance, radiation therapy, medications, and central nervous system metastasis.	20. Multiple factors contribute to anorexia and nausea.	

NURSING DIAGNOSIS: Fatigue
GOAL: Decreased fatigue level

Nursing Intervention	Rationale	Expected Outcomes
1. Assess patient and treatment factors that are associated with or increase fatigue.	1. Multiple factors are associated with or contribute to cancer-related fatigue. Although fatigue is common in patients receiving chemotherapy or radiation therapy, there are several factors that can be modified or addressed, such as dehydration, electrolye abnormalities, organ impairment, anemia, impaired nutrition, pain and other symptoms, depression, anxiety, impaired mobility, and shortness of breath.	• Factors contributing to fatigue are assessed and managed whenever possible. • Exhibits acceptable serum value levels for nutritional indices (See Imbalanced Nutrition) • Reports decreased pain and/or other symptoms • Consumes diet with recommended nutritional intake • Maintains adequate hydration • Reports decreasing levels of fatigue • Increases participation in activities gradually
2. Encourage rest periods during the day, especially before and after physical exertion.	2. During rest, energy is conserved and levels are replenished. Several shorter rest periods may be more beneficial than one longer rest period.	• Rests when fatigued • Reports restful sleep • Requests assistance with activities appropriately
3. At minimum, promote patient's normal sleep habits.	3. Sleep helps to restore energy levels. Prolonged napping during the day may interfere with sleep habits.	• Reports adequate energy to participate in activities important to him or her (e.g., visiting with family, hobbies)
4. Rearrange daily schedule and organize activities to conserve energy expenditure.	4. Reorganization of activities can reduce energy losses and stressors.	• Uses relaxation exercises and imagery to decrease anxiety and promote rest • Reports no breathlessness during activities
5. Encourage patient to ask for others' assistance with necessary chores, such as housework, child care, shopping, and cooking.	5. Conserves energy	• Reports improved ability to relax and rest • Exhibits improved mobility and decreased fatigue
6. Encourage reduced job workload, if necessary and possible, by reducing number of hours worked per week.	6. Reducing workload decreases physical and psychological stress and increases periods of rest and relaxation.	
7. Encourage adequate protein and calorie intake.	7. Protein and calorie depletion decreases activity tolerance.	
8. Encourage the use of relaxation techniques and guided imagery.	8. Promotion of relaxation and psychological rest decreases physical fatigue.	
9. Encourage participation in planned exercise programs as identified through collaboration with physical therapy.	9. Various approaches to exercise programs have demonstrated increases in endurance and stamina and lower fatigue (Wanchai, Armer, & Stewart, 2011).	
10. For collaborative management, administer blood products as prescribed.	10. Lowered hemoglobin and hematocrit predispose patient to fatigue due to decreased oxygen availability.	
11. Assess for fluid and electrolyte disturbances.	11. May contribute to altered nerve transmission and muscle function	
12. Collaborate with physical and occupational therapy to identify strategies to facilitate mobility.	12. Impaired mobility requires increased energy expenditure.	

(continues on page 354)

PLAN OF NURSING CARE

Chart 15-7

The Patient With Cancer (continued)

NURSING DIAGNOSIS: Chronic pain
GOAL: Relief of pain and discomfort

Nursing Intervention	Rationale	Expected Outcomes
1. Use pain scale to assess pain and discomfort characteristics: location, quality, frequency, duration, etc., at baseline and on an ongoing basis.	1. Provides baseline for assessing changes in pain level and evaluation of interventions	• Reports decreased level of pain and discomfort on pain scale
2. Assure patient that you know the pain is real and will assist him or her in reducing it.	2. Fear that pain will not be considered real increases anxiety and reduces pain tolerance.	• Reports less disruption in activity and quality of life from pain and discomfort
3. Assess other factors contributing to patient's pain: fear, fatigue, other symptoms, psychosocial distress, etc.	3. Provides data about factors that decrease patient's ability to tolerate pain and increase pain level	• Reports decrease in other symptoms and psychosocial distress
4. Provide education to patient and family regarding prescribed analgesic regimen and importance of analgesics (e.g., around the clock, long acting; analgesics for breakthrough pain episodes).	4. Analgesics tend to be more effective when administered early in pain cycle, around the clock at regular intervals, or when administered in long-acting forms; breaks the pain cycle; premedication with analgesics is used for activities that cause increased pain or breakthrough pain.	• Adheres to analgesic regimen as prescribed
		• Barriers to adequately addressing pain do not interfere with strategies for managing pain.
		• Takes an active role in administration of analgesia
5. Address myths or misconceptions and lack of knowledge about the use of opioid analgesics.	5. Barriers to adequate pain management involve patients' fear of side effects, fatalism about the possibility of achieving pain control, fear of distracting providers from treating the cancer, belief that pain is indicative of progressive disease, and fears about addiction. Professional health providers also have demonstrated limited knowledge about pain management, potential analgesic side effects, and management and risk of addiction (Paice & Ferrell, 2011).	• Identifies additional effective pain-relief strategies
		• Uses previously employed successful pain-relief strategies appropriately
		• Reports effective use of nonpharmacologic pain-relief strategies and decrease in pain
		• Reports that decreased level of pain permits participation in other activities and events and quality of life
6. Collaborate with patient, primary provider, and other health care team members when changes in pain management are necessary.	6. New methods of administering analgesia must be acceptable to patient, primary provider, and health care team to be effective; patient's participation decreases the sense of powerlessness.	
7. Encourage strategies of pain relief that patient has used successfully in previous pain experience.	7. Encourages success of pain-relief strategies accepted by patient and family.	
8. Offer nonpharmacologic strategies to relieve pain and discomfort: distraction, imagery, relaxation, cutaneous stimulation, etc.	8. Increases number of options and strategies available to patient that serve as adjuncts to pharmacologic interventions.	

NURSING DIAGNOSIS: Grieving related to loss; altered role functioning
GOAL: Appropriate progression through grieving process

Nursing Intervention	Rationale	Expected Outcomes
1. Encourage verbalization of fears, concerns, and questions regarding disease, treatment, and future implications.	1. An increased and accurate knowledge base decreases anxiety and dispels misconceptions.	The patient and family:
2. Explore previous successful coping strategies.	2. Provides frame of reference and examples of coping	• Progress through the phases of grief as evidenced by increased verbalization and expression of grief.
3. Encourage active participation of patient or family in care and treatment decisions.	3. Active participation maintains patient independence and control.	• Identify resources available to aid coping strategies during grieving.
		• Use resources and supports appropriately.
4. Visit family and friends to establish and maintain relationships and physical closeness.	4. Frequent contacts promote trust and security and reduce feelings of fear and isolation.	• Discuss the future openly with each other.
		• Discuss concerns and feelings openly with each other.
5. Encourage ventilation of negative feelings, including projected anger and hostility, within acceptable limits.	5. This allows for emotional expression without loss of self-esteem.	• Use nonverbal expressions of concern for each other.
		• Develop positive or adaptive coping mechanisms for processing of grief.

PLAN OF NURSING CARE

The Patient With Cancer (continued)

Nursing Intervention	Rationale	Expected Outcomes
6. Allow for periods of crying and expression of sadness.	6. These feelings are necessary for separation and detachment to occur.	
7. Involve spiritual advisor as desired by the patient and family.	7. This facilitates the grief process and spiritual care.	
8. Refer patient and family to professional counseling as indicated to alleviate pathologic or nonadaptive grieving.	8. Goal is to facilitate the grief process or adaptive methods of coping.	
9. Allow for progression through the grieving process at the individual pace of the patient and family.	9. Grief work is variable. Not every person uses every phase of the grief process, and the time spent in dealing with each phase varies with every person. To complete grief work, this variability must be allowed.	

NURSING DIAGNOSIS: Disturbed body image and situational low self-esteem related to changes in appearance, function, and roles
GOAL: Improved body image and self-esteem

Nursing Intervention	Rationale	Expected Outcomes
1. Assess patient's feelings about body image and level of self-esteem.	1. Provides baseline assessment for evaluating changes and assessing effectiveness of interventions	• Identifies concerns of importance • Takes active role in activities • Maintains participation in decision making
2. Identify potential threats to patient's self-esteem (e.g., altered appearance, decreased sexual function, hair loss, decreased energy, role changes). Validate concerns with patient.	2. Anticipates changes and permits patient to identify importance of these areas to him or her	• Verbalizes feelings and reactions to losses or threatened losses • Participates in self-care activities • Permits others to assist in care when he
3. Encourage continued participation in activities and decision making.	3. Encourages and permits continued control of events and self	or she is unable to be independent • Exhibits interest in appearance, main-
4. Encourage patient to verbalize concerns.	4. Identifying concerns is an important step in coping with them.	tains grooming, and uses aids (cosmetics, scarves, etc.) appropriately if desired
5. Individualize care for the patient.	5. Prevents or reduces depersonalization and emphasizes patient's self-worth	• Participates with others in conversations and social events and activities
6. Assist patient in self-care when fatigue, lethargy, nausea, vomiting, and other symptoms prevent independence.	6. Physical well-being improves self-esteem.	• Verbalizes concern about sexual partner and/or significant others • Explores alternative ways of expressing
7. Assist patient in selecting and using cosmetics, scarves, hair pieces, hats, and clothing that increase his or her sense of attractiveness.	7. Promotes positive body image	concern and affection • The patient and significant other are able to maintain level of intimacy and express affection and acceptance.
8. Encourage patient and partner to share concerns about altered sexuality and sexual function and to explore alternatives to their usual sexual expression.	8. Provides opportunity for expressing concern, intimacy, affection, and acceptance	
9. Refer to collaborating specialists as needed.	9. Interdisciplinary collaboration is essential in meeting patient needs.	

COLLABORATIVE PROBLEM: Potential complication: risk for bleeding problems
GOAL: Prevention of bleeding

Nursing Intervention	Rationale	Expected Outcomes
1. Assess for potential for bleeding: monitor platelet count.	1. Mild risk: 50,000–100,000/mm^3 (0.05–0.1 × 10^{12}/L); moderate risk: 20,000–50,000/mm^3 (0.02–0.05 × 10^{12}/L); severe risk: <20,000/mm^3 (0.02 × 10^{12}/L)	• Signs and symptoms of bleeding are identified. • Exhibits no blood in feces, urine, or emesis
2. Assess for bleeding.	2. Early detection promotes early intervention.	• Exhibits no bleeding of gums or injection/venipuncture sites • Exhibits no ecchymosis (bruising) or
a. Petechiae or ecchymosis (bruising)	a. Indicates injury to microcirculation and larger vessels	petechiae • Patient and family identify ways to prevent bleeding.
b. Decrease in hemoglobin or hematocrit	b–e. Indicates blood loss	• Uses recommended measures to reduce risk of bleeding (uses soft toothbrush,
c. Prolonged bleeding from invasive procedures, venipunctures, minor cuts or scratches		shaves with electric razor only)

(continues on page 356)

Chart 15-7

PLAN OF NURSING CARE

The Patient With Cancer (continued)

Nursing Intervention	Rationale	Expected Outcomes

d. Frank or occult blood in any body excretion, emesis, sputum
e. Bleeding from any body orifice
f. Altered mental status
3. Instruct patient and family about ways to minimize bleeding.
  a. Use soft toothbrush or toothette for mouth care.
  b. Avoid commercial mouthwashes.
 	
  c. Use electric razor for shaving.
  d. Use emery board for nail care.
  e. Avoid foods that are difficult to chew.
4. Initiate measures to minimize bleeding.
  a. Draw all blood for lab work with one daily venipuncture.
  b. Avoid taking temperature rectally or administering suppositories and enemas.
  c. Avoid intramuscular injections; use smallest needle possible.
  d. Apply direct pressure to injection and venipuncture sites for at least 5 minutes.
  e. Lubricate lips with water-based lubricant
  f. Avoid bladder catheterizations; use smallest catheter if catheterization is necessary.
  g. Maintain fluid intake of at least 3 L per 24 hours unless contraindicated.
  h. Use stool softeners or increase bulk in diet.
  i. Avoid medications that will interfere with clotting (e.g., aspirin).
  j. Recommend use of water-based lubricant before sexual intercourse.
5. When platelet count is <20,000/mm³, institute the following:
 	
  a. Bed rest with padded side rails
  b. Avoidance of strenuous activity
 	
  c. Platelet transfusions as prescribed; administer prescribed diphenhydramine hydrochloride (Benadryl) or hydrocortisone sodium succinate (Solu-Cortef) to prevent reaction to platelet transfusion.
  d. Supervise activity when out of bed.
  e. Caution against forceful nose blowing.
	f. Indicates neurologic involvement
	3. Patient can participate in self-protection.
	  a. Prevents trauma to oral tissues
	
	  b. Contain high alcohol content that will dry oral tissues
	  c. Prevents trauma to skin
	  d. Reduces risk of trauma to nailbeds
	  e. Prevents oral tissue trauma
	4. Preserves circulating blood volume
	  a. Minimizes trauma and blood loss
	
	  b. Prevents trauma to rectal mucosa
	
	  c. Prevents intramuscular bleeding
	
	  d. Minimizes blood loss
	
	  e. Prevents skin from drying
	
	  f. Prevents trauma to urethra
	
	  g. Hydration helps to prevent skin drying.
	  h. Prevents constipation and straining that may injure rectal tissue
	  i. Minimizes risk of bleeding
	
	  j. Prevents friction and tissue trauma
	
	5. Platelet count <20,000/mm³ (0.02 × 10¹²/L) is associated with increased risk of spontaneous bleeding.
	  a. Reduces risk of injury
	  b. Increases intracranial pressure and risk of cerebral hemorrhage
	  c. Allergic reactions to blood products are associated with antigen–antibody reaction that causes platelet destruction.
	
	  d. Reduces risk of falls
	  e. Prevents trauma to nasal mucosa and increased intracranial pressure
		• Exhibits normal vital signs
		• Reports that environmental hazards have been reduced or removed
		• Maintains hydration
		• Reports absence of constipation
		• Avoids substances interfering with clotting
		• Absence of tissue destruction
		• Exhibits normal mental status and absence of signs of intracranial bleeding
		• Avoids medications that interfere with clotting (e.g., aspirin)
		• Absence of epistaxis and cerebral bleeding

where the platelet count is noted as $<20,000/mm^3$ $(0.02 \times 10^{12}/L)$.

may still develop radiation dermatitis that may be associated with pain, irritation, pruritus, burning, and diminished quality of life. Nursing care for patients with radiation dermatitis includes maintenance of skin integrity, cleansing, promotion of comfort, pain reduction, prevention of additional trauma, prevention and management of infection, and promotion of a moist wound-healing environment (Gosselin, Schneider, Plambeck, et al., 2010; McQuestion, 2011). Although a variety of methods and products are used in clinical practice for patients with radiation-induced skin impairment, there is limited evidence to support their value. Patients with skin and tissue reactions to radiation therapy require careful skin care to prevent further skin irritation, drying, and damage, as discussed in the nursing care plan (see Chart 15-7, Risk for impaired skin integrity: erythematous and wet desquamation reactions to radiation therapy).

Alopecia

The temporary or permanent thinning or complete loss of hair is a potential adverse effect of whole brain radiation therapy and various chemotherapeutic agents. Alopecia usually begins 2 to 3 weeks after the initiation of treatment; regrowth most often begins within 8 weeks after the last treatment. Some patients who undergo radiation to the head may sustain permanent hair loss. Although health care providers may view hair loss as a minor issue, for many patients it is a major assault on body image, resulting in challenges to self-esteem, anger, and feelings of rejection and isolation. In some cases, patients' anticipation of hair loss may contribute to a sense of helplessness, reluctance, fear, and depression (Borsellino & Young, 2011). To patients and families, hair loss can serve as a constant reminder of the challenges cancer places on their coping abilities, interpersonal relationships, and sexuality.

Although few studies have addressed methods to minimize the impact of alopecia, nurses provide information about hair loss and support the patient and family in coping with changes in body image. Nurses help patients identify proactive choices that may empower them to improve responses to cancer and perceived lack of control (Borsellino & Young, 2011), as discussed in the nursing care plan (see Chart 15-7, Impaired tissue integrity: alopecia).

Malignant Skin Lesions

Skin lesions may occur with local extension or metastasis of the tumor into the epithelium and its surrounding lymph and blood vessels. Either locally invasive or metastatic cancer to the skin may result in redness (erythema), discolored nodules, or progression to wounds involving edema, exudates, and tissue necrosis. The most extensive lesions involve ulceration (referred to as fungating lesions) with an overgrowth of malodorous microorganisms. These lesions are a source of considerable pain, discomfort, and embarrassment. Although skin lesions occur in various malignancies, they are most commonly associated with breast cancer (Kalmykow & Walker, 2011).

Ulcerating skin lesions usually indicate advanced or disseminated disease that is unlikely to be eradicated but may be controlled or palliated through systemic treatment (chemotherapy and targeted therapy) or radiation therapy. Local care of these lesions is a nursing priority. Nurses carefully assess malignant skin lesions for the size, appearance, condition of surrounding tissue, odor, bleeding, drainage, and associated pain or other symptoms, including evidence of infection. The potential for serious complications such as hemorrhage, vessel compression/obstruction, or airway obstruction, especially in head and neck cancer, should be noted so that the caregiver can be instructed in palliative measures to maintain patient comfort.

Nursing care (see Chart 15-7) also includes wound cleansing, reduction of superficial bacteria, control of bleeding, odor reduction, protection from further skin trauma, and pain management (Kalmykow & Walker, 2011). The patient and family require emotional support, assistance, and guidance in providing wound care and addressing comfort measures at home.

Promoting Nutrition

Nutritional Problems

Most patients with cancer experience some weight loss during their illness. Anorexia, malabsorption, and cancer-related

---

Chart 15-8	**Potential Consequences of Impaired Nutrition in Patients With Cancer**

- Anemia
- Decreased survival
- Immune incompetence and increased incidence of infection
- Delayed tissue and wound healing
- Fatigue
- Diminished functional ability
- Decreased capacity to continue antineoplastic therapy
- Increased hospital admissions
- Increased length of hospital stay
- Impaired psychosocial functioning

anorexia-cachexia syndrome (CACS) are some common nutritional problems. Impaired nutritional status may contribute to both physical and psychosocial consequences (Chart 15-8). Nutritional concerns include decreased protein and caloric intake, metabolic or mechanical effects of the cancer, systemic disease, side effects of the treatment, or the patient's emotional status.

Anorexia

Among the many causes of anorexia in patients with cancer are alterations in taste, manifested by increased salty, sour, and metallic taste sensations, and altered responses to sweet and bitter flavors. Taste changes contribute to decreased appetite and nutritional intake and subsequently protein–calorie malnutrition. Taste alterations may result from mineral (e.g., zinc) deficiencies, increases in circulating amino acids and cellular metabolites, or the administration of chemotherapeutic agents. Patients undergoing radiation therapy to the head and neck may experience "mouth blindness," which is a severe impairment of taste.

Anorexia may occur because patients develop early satiety after eating only a small amount of food. This sense of fullness occurs secondary to a decrease in digestive enzymes, abnormalities in the metabolism of glucose and triglycerides, and prolonged stimulation of gastric volume receptors, which convey the feeling of being full. Psychological distress (e.g., fear, pain, depression, and isolation) throughout illness may also have a negative impact on appetite. Patients may develop an aversion to food because of nausea and vomiting associated with treatment.

Malabsorption

Some patients with cancer are unable to absorb nutrients from the gastrointestinal system as a result of tumor activity and/or cancer treatments. Malignancy can affect gastrointestinal activity in several ways (i.e., impaired enzyme production, interference with both protein and fat digestion) that can lead to increased gastrointestinal irritation, peptic ulcer disease, and fistula formation.

Chemotherapy and radiation associated with mucositis cause damage to mucosal cells of the bowel, resulting in impaired nutrient absorption. Abdominal irradiation has been associated with sclerosis of intestinal blood vessels and fibrotic changes in the gastrointestinal tissue, both impacting nutrient absorption. Surgical intervention may change peristaltic patterns, alter gastrointestinal secretions, and reduce the absorptive surfaces of gastrointestinal mucosa, all of which contribute to malabsorption.

Cancer-Related Anorexia-Cachexia Syndrome

CACS is a complex biologic process that results from a combination of increased energy expenditure and decreased intake (Walz, 2010). This syndrome can occur in both the curative and palliative stages of treatment and care (Gabison, Gibbs, Uziely, et al., 2010). Combined immunologic, neuroendocrine, and metabolic processes give rise to anorexia, unintentional weight loss, and increased metabolic demand with impaired metabolism of glucose and lipids. As this syndrome continues, altered metabolic processes and tumor responses lead to cytokine release, causing generalized systemic inflammation. The patient experiences continued weight loss and malnutrition characterized by loss of adipose tissue, visceral protein, and skeletal muscle mass. Patients with CACS complain of loss of appetite, early satiety, and fatigue. As many as 50% to 75% of all patients with cancer experience some degree of cachexia (Granda-Cameron, DeMille, Lynch, et al., 2010). Protein losses are associated with the development of anemia, peripheral edema, and progressive debilitation (Walz, 2010). Changes in eating habits, fatigue, impaired mobility, and progressive debilitation are associated with decreased quality of life, psychological distress, and anxiety for both patient and family as they respond to actual and perceived impending losses, fear, lack of control, and helplessness.

Nursing care is integral to an interdisciplinary approach that addresses the multiple factors contributing to impaired nutritional status in patients with cancer (see Chart 15-7).

General Nutrition Considerations

Assessment of the patient's nutritional status is conducted at diagnosis and monitored throughout the course of treatment and follow-up. Early identification of patients at risk for problems with intake, absorption, and cachexia, particularly during the early stages of disease, can facilitate timely implementation of specifically targeted interventions that attempt to improve quality of life, treatment outcomes, and survival (Gabison et al., 2010). Current weight, weight loss, diet and medication history, patterns of anorexia, nausea and vomiting, and situations and foods that aggravate or relieve symptoms are assessed and addressed.

The type of cancer, stage, and treatment approaches are considered so that proactive measures to support nutrition can be identified. For example, patients with head and neck cancers who are treated with radiation therapy, or some combination of surgery, radiation, and chemotherapy, are at high risk for inadequate oral intake and nutritional deficits. In many centers, these patients have a percutaneous endoscopic gastrostomy (PEG) tube placed for enteral nutrition prior to initiation of treatment and the onset of mucositis, weight loss, and other consequences of impaired oral intake (Hayward & Shea, 2009).

A speech consult may be helpful for patients with oropharyngeal or laryngeal tumors or surgical interventions that are anticipated to effect swallowing, secretion management, speech, or respiratory function.

Whenever possible, every effort is made to maintain adequate nutrition through the oral route. Prokinetic agents such as metoclopramide (Reglan) are used in some settings to increase gastric emptying in patients with early satiety

and delayed gastric emptying. Other pharmacologic interventions such as megestrol acetate (Megace) or corticosteroids may be used to improve appetite. Oral nutritional supplements are encouraged to meet nutritional needs and to improve weight gain and physical functioning. Supplements containing n-3 polyunsaturated fatty acids (omega-3), arginine, and nucleotides are suggested to decrease the inflammatory response and improve oxygen metabolism and intestinal function (Walz, 2010). If adequate nutrition cannot be maintained by oral intake, nutritional support via the enteral route may be necessary as discussed previously. When needed, the patient and family are taught to administer enteral nutrition in the home. Home care nurses assist with patient education and monitor the patient's symptoms and response to enteral nutrition.

If malabsorption is a problem, enzyme and vitamin replacement may be instituted. Additional strategies include changing the feeding schedule, using simple diets, and relieving diarrhea. If malabsorption is severe, or the cancer involves the upper gastrointestinal tract, parenteral nutrition may be necessary. However, patients receiving parenteral nutrition are at increased risk for complications including catheter-related and systemic infection. The use of parenteral nutrition in patients with advanced or end-stage cancer is seldom used and controversial (Walz, 2010). Parenteral nutrition can be administered in several ways: by a long-term venous access device such as a right atrial catheter, implanted venous port, or PICC (Fig. 15-6). The nurse educates the patient and family to care for the venous access device and to administer parenteral nutrition. Home care nurses provide education and assist with or supervise parenteral nutrition administration in the home.

Relieving Pain

More than half of patients with cancer experience pain throughout the cancer trajectory. Moderate to severe pain is reported by approximately 30% to 70% of patients with cancer during treatment and by as many as 90% of those with advanced disease (Edrington, Sun, Wong, et al., 2009). Although the pain may be acute, it is more frequently

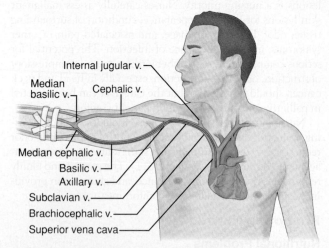

Internal jugular v.
Median basilic v.
Cephalic v.
Median cephalic v.
Basilic v.
Axillary v.
Subclavian v.
Brachiocephalic v.
Superior vena cava

FIGURE 15-6 • A peripherally inserted central catheter is advanced through the cephalic or basilic vein to the axillary, subclavian, or brachiocephalic vein or the superior vena cava.

TABLE 15-9	Examples of Sources of Cancer Pain	
Source	**Descriptions**	**Underlying Cancer**
Bone metastasis	Throbbing, aching	Breast, prostate, myeloma
Ischemia	Sharp, throbbing	Kaposi's sarcoma
Lymphatic or venous obstruction	Dull, aching, tightness	Lymphoma, breast, Kaposi's sarcoma
Nerve compression, infiltration	Burning, sharp, tingling	Breast, prostate, lymphoma
Organ obstruction	Dull, crampy, gnawing	Colon, gastric
Organ infiltration	Distention, crampy	Liver, pancreatic
Skin inflammation, ulceration, infection, necrosis	Burning, sharp	Breast, head and neck, Kaposi's sarcoma

characterized as chronic. (See Chapter 12 for more information on pain.) As in other situations involving pain, the experience of cancer pain is influenced by physical, psychosocial, cultural, and spiritual factors.

Cancer can cause pain in various ways (Table 15-9). Initially, pain is most often related to the underlying cancer process. Pain is also associated with various cancer treatments. Acute pain is linked with trauma from surgery. Occasionally, chronic pain syndromes, such as postsurgical neuropathies (pain related to nerve tissue injury), occur. Some chemotherapeutic agents cause tissue necrosis, peripheral neuropathies, and stomatitis—all potential sources of pain—whereas radiation therapy can cause pain secondary to skin, nervous tissue, or organ inflammation. Patients with cancer may have other sources of pain, such as arthritis or migraine headaches, that are unrelated to the underlying cancer or its treatment.

The nurse assesses the patient for the source and site of pain as well as those factors that influence the patient's perception and experience of pain, such as fear and apprehension, fatigue, anger, and social isolation. Pain assessment scales (see Chapter 12) are useful for assessing the patient's pain before and after pain-relieving interventions are instituted to assess the effectiveness of interventions. Other symptoms that contribute to the pain experience, such as nausea and fatigue, are assessed and addressed as well.

In today's society, most people expect pain to disappear or resolve quickly. Although it is often controllable, advanced cancer pain is commonly irreversible and not quickly resolved. For many patients, pain is often seen as a signal that cancer is advancing and that death is approaching. As patients anticipate pain and anxiety increases, pain perception heightens, producing fear and further pain. Thus, chronic cancer pain can lead to a cycle progressing from pain to anxiety to fear and back to pain, especially when the pain is not adequately managed. Inadequate pain management is most often the result of misconceptions and insufficient knowledge about pain assessment and management on the part of patients, families, and health care providers (Running & Turnbeaugh, 2011). Chapter 12 provides information concerning factors contributing to the pain experience, pain perception, and tolerance as well as pharmacologic and nonpharmacologic nursing interventions addressing pain. The nursing care plan (see Chart 15-7) also provides strategies for nursing assessment and management of chronic pain.

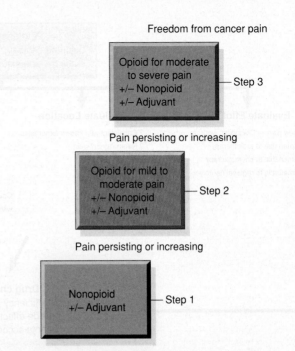

Freedom from cancer pain

Opioid for moderate to severe pain
+/– Nonopioid
+/– Adjuvant — Step 3

Pain persisting or increasing

Opioid for mild to moderate pain
+/– Nonopioid
+/– Adjuvant — Step 2

Pain persisting or increasing

Nonopioid
+/– Adjuvant — Step 1

FIGURE 15-7 • Adapted from the World Health Organization three-step ladder approach to relieving cancer pain. Various opioid (narcotic) and nonopioid medications may be combined with other medications to control pain.

The World Health Organization advocates a three-step approach to treat cancer pain (Fig. 15-7). Analgesics are administered based on the patient's reported level of pain. A cancer pain algorithm, developed as a set of analgesic guiding principles, is given in Figure 15-8.

Pharmacologic and nonpharmacologic approaches, even those that may be invasive, are considered in managing cancer-related pain regardless of the patient's status along the cancer trajectory. The nurse assists the patient and family to take an active role in managing pain. The nurse provides education and support to correct fears and misconceptions about opioid use. Inadequate pain management leads to a diminished quality of life characterized by distress, suffering, anxiety, fear, immobility, isolation, and depression.

Decreasing Fatigue

Fatigue is one of the most significant and frequent symptoms experienced by patients receiving cancer therapy. Patients report that fatigue persists and interferes with activities of daily living for months to years after the completion of treatment (NCCN, 2011d). Fatigue rarely exists in isolation; patients typically experience other symptoms concurrently, such as pain, dyspnea, anemia, sleep disturbances, or depression.

In assessing fatigue, the nurse distinguishes between *acute fatigue*, which occurs after an energy-demanding experience, and *cancer-related fatigue*, which is defined as "a distressing persistent, subjective sense of physical, emotional and/or cognitive tiredness or exhaustion related to cancer or cancer treatment that is not proportional to recent activity and interferes with usual functioning" (NCCN, 2011d). Acute fatigue serves a protective function, whereas cancer-related fatigue does not. The exact mechanisms of fatigue are not well understood and are most probably multifactorial in nature.

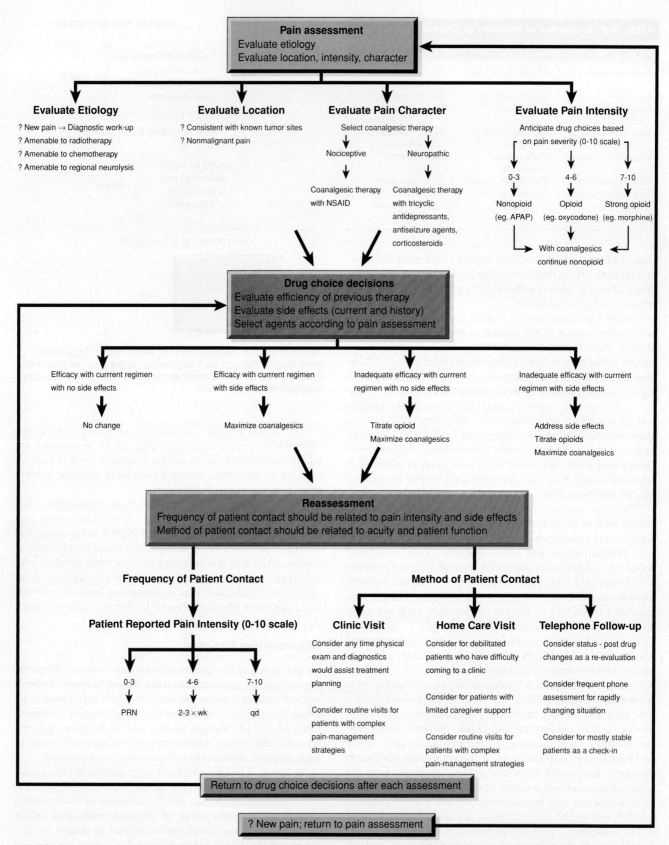

FIGURE 15-8 • The cancer pain algorithm (highest-level view) is a decision-tree model for pain treatment that was developed as an interpretation of the AHCPR Guideline for Cancer Pain, 1994. Redrawn with permission from DuPen, A. R., DuPen, S., Hansberry, J., et al. (2000). An educational implementation of a cancer pain algorithm for ambulatory care. *Pain Management Nursing, 1*(4), 118.

<table>
<tr><td>

Chart 15-9 **Sources of Fatigue in Patients With Cancer**

- Pain, pruritus
- Imbalanced nutrition related to nausea, vomiting, cancer-related anorexia-cachexia syndrome
- Electrolyte imbalance related to vomiting, diarrhea
- Ineffective protection related to neutropenia, thrombocytopenia, anemia
- Impaired tissue integrity related to stomatitis, mucositis
- Impaired physical mobility related to neurologic impairments, surgery, bone metastasis, pain, and analgesic use
- Uncertainty and deficient knowledge related to disease process, treatment
- Anxiety related to fear, diagnosis, role changes, uncertainty of future
- Ineffective breathing patterns related to cough, shortness of breath, and dyspnea
- Disturbed sleep pattern related to cancer therapies, anxiety, and pain

</td></tr>
</table>

Despite the commonly occurring experience of fatigue in patients with cancer, a reliable assessment tool has not been identified. The experience of fatigue is highly subjective, with patient descriptors varying greatly (Scott, Lasch, Barsevick, et al., 2011). The nurse assesses physiologic and psychological factors that can contribute to fatigue (Chart 15-9).

Wanchai and colleagues (2011) report a systematic review of nonpharmacologic interventions for fatigue that identifies various exercise options, cognitive therapy, and sleep therapy as effective interventions for fatigue as well as improved quality of life. Nurses assist patients with additional nonpharmacologic strategies to minimize fatigue or help the patient cope with existing fatigue as described in the nursing care plan (see Chart 15-7, Fatigue). Occasionally, pharmacologic interventions are utilized, including antidepressants for patients with depression, anxiolytics for those with anxiety, hypnotics for patients with sleep disturbances, and psychostimulants for some patients with advanced cancer or fatigue that does not respond to other interventions (NCCN, 2011d).

Improving Body Image and Self-Esteem

The nurse identifies potential threats to the patient's body image and assesses the patient's ability to cope with the many assaults to body image that may be experienced throughout the course of disease and treatment. Entry into the health care system is often accompanied by depersonalization. Threats to self-concept occur as the patient faces the realization of illness, disfigurement, possible disability, and death. To accommodate treatments or because of the disease, many patients with cancer are forced to alter their lifestyles. Priorities and values change when body image is threatened. Disfiguring surgery, hair loss, cachexia, skin changes, altered communication patterns, and sexual dysfunction can threaten the patient's self-esteem and body image.

A creative and positive approach is essential when caring for patients with altered body image. Nursing approaches for addressing issues related to body image and self-esteem are included in the nursing care plan (see Chart 15-7). The nurse serves as a listener and counselor to both the patient and family. Possible influences of the patient's culture and age are considered when discussing concerns and potential interventions.

The physiologic processes associated with cancer, potential short- and long-term effects of cancer treatments, and psychosocial, emotional, and spiritual responses to the entire experience may lead patients to confront a variety of sexuality-based issues. Patients with breast, gynecologic, or genitourinary cancers may be at even greater risk for sexual dysfunction (Kaplan & Pacelli, 2011). Although sexuality is an important component of overall health, multiple barriers contribute to nurses failing to include sexual assessment and discussion in their patient care. Julien and colleagues (2010) explored oncology nurses' attitudes and beliefs about patient sexual health assessment. They identified the following barriers: a misconception that patients do not expect nurses to discuss sexual concerns, feelings that patients rather than nurses should initiate these discussions, feelings of being inadequately prepared to discuss sexual concerns, a belief that these discussions should be deferred to the physician, working night shift, limited nursing experience, nurses younger than 40 years, lack of oncology certification, and working in an acute care inpatient setting.

Patients prefer that their health care providers take the lead in inquiring about their sexual health (Julien et al., 2010). In offering a holistic approach to the care of patients with cancer, nurses should initiate discussions about sexuality and assess sexual health, including factors that contribute to patient and partner (when appropriate) areas of concern. Physiologic, interpersonal, and psychological factors are addressed to help patients and their partners (when appropriate) achieve the outcomes of importance to them. When necessary, nurses assist patients to seek further specialized evaluation and intervention.

Assisting in the Grieving Process

A cancer diagnosis need not indicate a fatal outcome. Many forms of cancer are curable, and others may be controlled for long periods of time similar to the course of other chronic diseases. Despite the tremendous advances in cancer, many patients and their families still view cancer as a fatal disease that is inevitably accompanied by pain, suffering, debilitation, and emaciation. Grieving is a normal response to these fears and to actual or potential losses: loss of health, normal sensations, body image, social interaction, intimacy, independence, and usual social roles (Hottensen, 2010). Patients, families, and friends may grieve for the loss of quality time to spend with others, the loss of future and unfulfilled plans, and the loss of control over the patient's body and emotional reactions. Nurses continue to assess the patient and family for positive or maladaptive coping behaviors, interpersonal communication, and evidence of the need for additional psychosocial support or interventions such as referral for professional counseling.

If the patient enters the terminal phase of disease, the nurse may assess that the patient and family members are at different stages of grief. In such cases, the nurse assists the patient and family to acknowledge and cope with their reactions and feelings. The nurse also empowers the patient and family to explore preferences for issues related to end-of-life care, such as withdrawal of active disease treatment, desire for the use of life-support measures, and symptom management approaches. Oncology nurses respectfully support the patient's spiritual or religious views and facilitate contact with their preferred clergy member, if desired. In addition, nurses consider the patient's cultural beliefs and practices when addressing issues related to grief. After the death of a patient with cancer, home care and/or hospice nurses follow up with surviving family members for bereavement counseling to facilitate expression and coping with feelings of loss and grief. (See Chapter 16 for further discussion of end-of-life issues.)

Monitoring and Managing Potential Complications

Infection

For patients in all stages of cancer, the nurse assesses factors associated with the development of infection. Although infection-associated morbidity and mortality has greatly decreased, prevention and prompt treatment of infection is essential in patients with cancer. Often, more than one predisposing factor is present in patients with cancer. The nurse monitors laboratory studies to detect early changes in WBC counts. Common sites of infection, such as the pharynx, skin, perianal area, urinary, and respiratory tracts, are assessed on a regular basis. However, the typical signs of infection (swelling, redness, drainage, and pain) may not occur in myelosuppressed patients because of decreased circulating WBCs and a diminished local inflammatory response. Fever may be the only sign of infection (Johnson, 2010). The nurse monitors the patient for sepsis, particularly if invasive catheters or long-term IV catheters are in place.

WBC function is often impaired in patients with cancer. Among the five types of WBCs, (neutrophils [granulocytes], lymphocytes, monocytes, basophils, and eosinophils), neutrophils serve as the body's primary initial defense against invading organisms. Comprising 60% to 70% of the body's WBCs, neutrophils act by engulfing and destroying infective organisms through phagocytosis. Both the total WBC count and the concentration of neutrophils are important in determining the patient's ability to fight infection. A decrease in circulating WBCs is referred to as leukopenia. Granulocytopenia is a decrease in neutrophils.

A differential WBC count identifies the relative numbers of WBCs and permits tabulation of polymorphonuclear neutrophils (PMNs) or segmented neutrophils (mature neutrophils, reported as "polys," PMNs, or "segs") and immature forms of neutrophils (reported as bands, metamyelocytes, and "stabs"). The absolute neutrophil count (ANC) is calculated by the following formula:

$$ANC = (\text{Segmented neutrophils [\%]} + \text{bands [\%]}) \times \text{WBC count (cells/mm}^3)$$

$$Example: (25\% \text{ segs} + 25\% \text{ bands}) \times 6,000 \text{ WBC cells/mm}^3 = 3,000 \text{ ANC}$$

Neutropenia, an abnormally low ANC, is associated with an increased risk of infection. The risk of infection rises as the ANC decreases. As the ANC declines below 1,500 cells/mm^3, the risk of infection rises. An ANC less than 500 cells/mm^3 reflects a severe risk of infection (NCI, 2010). **Nadir** is the lowest ANC after myelosuppressive chemotherapy, targeted therapy, or radiation therapy that suppresses bone

marrow function. Severe neutropenia may necessitate delays in administration of myelosuppressive therapies or treatment dose adjustments, although the use of the hematopoietic growth factors (i.e., colony-stimulating factors; see previous discussion) has reduced the severity and duration of treatment-associated neutropenia as well as infection-related morbidity, mortality, and early death (Saria, 2011). The administration of these growth factors assists in maintaining treatment schedules, drug dosages, treatment effectiveness, and quality of life.

Febrile patients who are neutropenic are assessed for factors that increase the risk of infection and for sources of infection through cultures of blood, sputum, urine, stool, IV and urinary or other catheters, and wounds, if appropriate (Table 15-10). In addition, a chest x-ray is usually obtained to assess for pulmonary infection.

Defense against infection is compromised in many different ways. The integrity of the skin and mucous membranes is challenged by multiple invasive diagnostic procedures, by the adverse effects of all cancer treatment modalities, and by the detrimental effects of immobility. Impaired nutrition as a result of CACS, nausea, vomiting, diarrhea, and the underlying disease alters the body's ability to combat invading organisms. Medications such as antibiotics disturb the balance of normal flora, allowing the overgrowth of normal flora and pathogenic organisms. Other medications can also alter the immune response (see Chapter 35). Cancer itself may lead to defects in cellular and humoral immunity. Advanced cancer may cause obstruction of hollow viscera (e.g., intestines), blood, and lymphatic vessels, creating a favorable environment for proliferation of pathogenic organisms. In some patients, tumor cells infiltrate bone marrow and prevent normal production of WBCs.

Nurses are in a key position to assist in preventing and identifying symptoms of infection, as discussed in the nursing care plan (see Chart 15-7). Although multiple infection control practices are employed, there is limited evidence to support many of them (Saria, 2011). Evidence-based, clinical practice guidelines developed by the ONS, the Infusion Nurses Society (INS), the NCCN, and the ASCO are used to guide prevention and management of infection. Interventions to prevent infection and alternative patient education formats for infection-related instruction are high nursing research priorities.

Gram-positive bacteria (*Streptococcus*, enterococci, and *Staphylococcus* species) and gram-negative organisms (*Escherichia coli*, *Klebsiella pneumoniae*, *Enterobacter*, and *Pseudomonas aeruginosa*) are the most frequently isolated causes of infection. Fungal organisms, such as *Candida albicans*, also contribute to the incidence of serious infection. Viral infections in immunocompromised patients are caused most often by herpes simplex, respiratory syncytial, parainfluenza, and influenza A and B viruses.

Fever is an important sign of infection in patients with impaired immune defenses. Patients with neutropenic fever (see Table 15-10) are assessed for infection and reported promptly (NCCN, 2011b). Antibiotics may be prescribed after cultures of wound drainage, exudates, sputum, urine, stool, or blood are obtained. Careful consideration is given to the underlying malignancy, prior antineoplastic treatment, ANC, comorbidities, and other patient-related factors prior to the identification of the most appropriate antibiotic therapy. Evidence-based guidelines are available for prevention and treatment of

TABLE 15-10 Assessment of Neutropenic Fever in Patients With Cancer	
Fever Criteria	**Neutropenia Criteria**
• Any one-time temperature of 38.3°C (101°F) **or** • Any temperature of ≥38°C (100.4°F) or ≥1 h	• <500 neutrophils/mcL **or** • <1,000 neutrophils/mcL and predicted to decline to ≤500 neutrophils/mcL over the next 48 h

Assessment Targets for Neutropenic Fever Evaluation			
Infection Risk Factors	**Physical Assessment**	**Diagnostic Procedures**	**Microbiologic Cultures**
• Chronic comorbid illnesses • Underlying malignancy • Age ≥65 y • Limited mobility and/or debilitation • Medications (e.g., corticosteroids such as prednisone) • Antibiotic therapy or prophylaxis • Recent surgery for diagnosis or treatment • Chemotherapy received within 7–10 d • Recent radiation therapy • Prior documented infections • Impaired skin integrity • Invasive drainage or urinary catheters • Peripheral or central venous access devices • Exposures (travel, others with infection, blood administration, pets) • Diarrhea • Poor nutritional status • Recent lumbar puncture or indwelling Ommaya reservoir™ (long-term intraventricular catheter for administration of chemotherapy into CSF and ventricles)	• Skin, pressure points, wounds • Surgical or biopsy incision sites • IV access or reservoir sites • Drainage catheter sites • Tracheostomy site • Lungs and sinuses • Perivaginal and perirectal area • Alimentary canal, abdomen • Neurologic assessment • Vital signs	• Diagnostic imaging as appropriate to identify abscesses, fistulas, pneumonia, obstruction, etc. • Complete blood count/differential • Serum chemistries, liver function tests • Renal function tests • Pulse oximetry or arterial blood gases • Lumbar puncture for CSF analysis	• Blood (peripheral and central venous access if applicable) • Urine (especially with indwelling catheter) • Skin wounds, lesions, incision sites, catheter exit sites • Catheter tips when feasible • Drainage from catheters • Stool, diarrhea • Sputum • CSF

CSF, cerebrospinal fluid.
Adapted from National Comprehensive Cancer Network. (2011b). *Clinical practice guidelines: Prevention and treatment of cancer related infections (v2.2011)*. Available at: www.nccn.org/professionals/physician_gls/pdf/infections.pdf

cancer-related infections (NCCN, 2011b). Patients with neutropenia are treated with broad-spectrum antibiotics before the infecting organism is identified because of the increased risk of mortality associated with untreated infection. Broad-spectrum antibiotic therapy targets the most likely major pathogenic organisms. It is important for these medications to be administered and taken promptly as scheduled to achieve adequate blood levels. Once the offending organism is identified, more specific antimicrobial therapy is prescribed as appropriate. Nurses provide education for patients and families regarding prevention of infection, signs and symptoms to report, and the importance of adherence to prescribed antimicrobial therapy.

 Septic Shock

The nurse assesses the patient frequently for signs and symptoms of infection and inflammation throughout the trajectory of cancer care. Sepsis and septic shock are life-threatening complications that must be prevented or detected and treated promptly. Although all patients with cancer are at risk, patients who are neutropenic or who have hematologic malignancies are at the greatest risk. Patients with signs and symptoms of impending sepsis and septic shock require immediate hospitalization and aggressive treatment in the intensive care setting. (See Chapter 14 for discussion of sepsis and septic shock.)

Bleeding and Hemorrhage

Platelets are essential for normal blood clotting and coagulation (hemostasis). Thrombocytopenia, a decrease in the circulating platelet count, is the most common cause of bleeding in patients with cancer and is usually defined as a platelet count less than 100,000/mm³ (0.1 × 10¹²/L). The risk of bleeding increases when the platelet count decreases to between 20,000 and 50,000/mm³ (0.02 to 0.05 × 10¹²/L). A platelet count lower than 20,000/mm³ (0.02 × 10¹²/L) is associated with an increased risk for spontaneous bleeding; most patients with a platelet count in this range require platelet transfusion.

Thrombocytopenia often results from bone marrow depression after certain types of chemotherapy and radiation therapy and with tumor infiltration of the bone marrow. In some cases, platelet destruction is associated with an enlarged spleen (hypersplenism) and abnormal antibody function, which occur with leukemia and lymphoma. The nursing care plan addresses nursing assessment parameters and interventions for patients at risk for bleeding (see Chart 15-7).

 Quality and Safety Nursing Alert

Although laboratory test results confirm the diagnosis of thrombocytopenia, the patient who is developing thrombocytopenia may display early signs and symptoms. Thus, nurses need to observe keenly for petechiae and ecchymoses, which are early indicators of decreasing platelet levels. Early detection promotes early intervention.

In limited circumstances, the nurse may administer IL-11 to prevent severe thrombocytopenia and reduce the need for platelet transfusions after myelosuppressive chemotherapy in patients with nonmyeloid malignancies, as described previously. Additional medications may be prescribed to address bleeding due to disorders of coagulation. (Refer to

Chapter 33 for further discussion of assessment and treatment of thrombocytopenia and coagulopathies.)

Acutely ill, hospitalized patients are assessed and monitored on an ongoing basis for VTE. The risk of VTE needs to be evaluated and recommendations for prophylaxis followed according to the risk category (Kahn, Lim, Dunn, et al., 2012).

Promoting Home and Community-Based Care

Educating Patients About Self-Care

Most commonly, patients with cancer are diagnosed and treated in the outpatient setting. Nurses in outpatient settings often have the responsibility for patient education and for coordinating care in the home. The shift of care from acute care to the home or outpatient setting places a great deal of the responsibility for care on the patient and family; this requires instruction that enables them to function relatively independently in providing care. Education initially focuses on the most immediate care needs likely to be encountered at home.

Side effects of treatments and changes in the patient's status that should be reported are reviewed verbally and reinforced with written information. Strategies to deal with side effects of treatment or symptom management are discussed with the patient and family. Other learning needs are based on the priorities conveyed by the patient and family as well as on the complexity of care required in the home.

Technologic advances allow home administration of chemotherapy, enteral or parenteral nutrition, blood products, parenteral antibiotics, and analgesics, as well as management of symptoms and care of vascular access devices. Patients are assessed and monitored on an ongoing basis for VTE. The risk of VTE in outpatients with cancer (with no additional risk factors) is thought to be low, and the current recommendations do not include routine medical prophylaxis (Kahn et al., 2012). Although home care nurses provide care and support for patients receiving this type of care, patients and families need instruction and support to enable them to feel comfortable and proficient in managing these treatments at home. Follow-up visits and telephone calls from the home care nurse or the nurse in the ambulatory care setting assist in identifying problems and are often reassuring, increasing the patient's and family's comfort in dealing with complex and new aspects of care. Continued contact facilitates evaluation of the patient's progress and assessment of the ongoing needs of the patient and family.

Continuing Care

Referral for home care is often indicated for patients with cancer. The responsibilities of the home care nurse include assessing the home environment, suggesting modifications in the home or in care to help the patient and family address the patient's physical and safety needs, and assessing the psychological and emotional impact of the illness on the patient and family.

Assessing changes in the patient's physical status and reporting relevant changes helps to ensure that appropriate and timely modifications in therapy are made. The home care nurse also assesses the adequacy of pain management and the effectiveness of other strategies to prevent or manage the side effects of treatment modalities and disease progression.

It is necessary to assess the patient's and family's understanding of the treatment plan and management strategies and to reinforce previous education. The nurse facilitates coordination of patient care by maintaining close communication with all involved health care providers. The nurse may make referrals and coordinate available community resources (e.g., local office of the ACS, home aides, church groups, faith community nurses, support groups) to assist patients and caregivers.

 Gerontologic Considerations

More than 60% of all new cancers occur in people older than 65 years, and about 70% of all cancer deaths occur in people 65 years and older (Pal, Katheria, & Hurria, 2010). The rising number of individuals over age 65 with cancer has led to the emergence of geriatric oncology, a multidimensional and multidisciplinary approach to treating growing numbers of older adults with cancer.

Nurses working with older adults must understand the normal physiologic changes that occur with aging and the implications for the patient with cancer (Table 15-11). These

---

TABLE 15-11   Age-Related Changes and Their Effects on Patients With Cancer

Age-Related Changes	Implications
Impaired immune system	Use special precautions to avoid infection; monitor for atypical signs and symptoms of infection.
Altered drug absorption, distribution, metabolism, and elimination	Mandates careful calculation of chemotherapy and frequent assessment for drug response and side effects; dose adjustments may be necessary.
Increased prevalence of other chronic diseases	Monitor for effect of cancer or its treatment on patient's other chronic diseases; monitor patient's tolerance for cancer treatment; monitor for interactions with medications used to treat chronic diseases.
Diminished renal, respiratory, and cardiac reserve	Be proactive in prevention of decreased renal function, atelectasis, pneumonia, and cardiovascular compromise; monitor for side effects of cancer treatment.
Decreased skin and tissue integrity; reduction in body mass; delayed healing	Prevent pressure ulcers secondary to immobility; monitor skin and mucous membranes for changes related to radiation or chemotherapy; monitor nutritional status.
Decreased musculoskeletal strength	Prevent falls; assess support for performing activities of daily living in home setting; encourage safe use of assistive mobility devices.
Decreased neurosensory functioning: loss of vision, hearing, and distal extremity tactile senses	Provide instruction modified for patient's hearing and vision changes; provide instruction concerning safety and skin care for distal extremities; assess home for safety.
Altered social and economic resources	Assess for financial concerns, living conditions, and resources for support.
Potential changes in cognitive and emotional capacity	Provide education and support modified for patient's level of functioning and safety.

Emergency	Clinical Manifestations and Diagnostic Findings	Management
About 70% of compressions occur at the thoracic level, 20% in the lumbosacral level, and 10% in the cervical region (Kaplan, 2009). The prognosis depends on the severity and rapidity of onset.	• Neurologic dysfunction and related motor and sensory deficits (numbness, tingling, feelings of coldness in the affected area, inability to detect vibration, loss of positional sense) • Motor loss ranging from subtle weakness to flaccid paralysis • Bladder and/or bowel dysfunction depending on level of compression (above S2, overflow incontinence; from S3 to S5, flaccid sphincter tone and bowel incontinence). **Diagnostic** • Percussion tenderness at the level of compression • Abnormal reflexes • Sensory and motor abnormalities • MRI is preferred diagnostic tool; may also utilize spinal cord x-rays, bone scans, and CT scan. CT-guided myelogram is reserved for patients who are unable to undergo MRI (Kaplan, 2009).	• Vertebroplasty has been used to stabilize vertebrae when patients have pain without neurologic dysfunction; vertebroplasty involves percutaneous injection of polymethyl methacrylate (PMMA), a bone cement filler, into the vertebral body (Kaplan, 2009). • Chemotherapy as adjuvant to radiation therapy for patients with lymphoma or small cell lung cancer • *Note:* Despite treatment, patients with poor neurologic function before treatment are less likely to regain complete motor and sensory function; patients who develop complete paralysis usually do not regain all neurologic function (Kaplan, 2009). **Nursing** • Perform ongoing assessment of neurologic function to identify existing and progressing dysfunction. • Control pain with pharmacologic and nonpharmacologic measures. • Prevent complications of immobility resulting from pain and decreased function (e.g., skin breakdown, urinary stasis, thrombophlebitis, decreased clearance of pulmonary secretions). • Maintain muscle tone by assisting with range-of-motion exercises in collaboration with physical and occupational therapists; patients with unstable vertebral fractures do not initiate physical therapy until spine stabilization procedures have been completed. • Institute intermittent urinary catheterization and bowel training programs for patients with bladder or bowel dysfunction. • Provide encouragement and support to patient and family coping with pain and altered functioning, lifestyle, roles, and independence. • Institute appropriate referrals for home care and physical and occupational therapy.

Hypercalcemia
Hypercalcemia is a potentially life-threatening metabolic abnormality resulting when the calcium released from the bones is more than the kidneys can excrete or the bones can reabsorb.
• It may result from production of cytokines, hormonal substances, and growth factors by cancer cells, or by the body in response to substances produced by cancer cells; which lead to bone breakdown and calcium release.
• Most commonly seen in breast, lung, and renal cancers; myeloma; and some types of leukemia (Lewis et al., 2011)
	Clinical
	Fatigue, weakness, confusion, decreased level of responsiveness, hyporeflexia, nausea, vomiting, constipation, ileus, polyuria (excessive urination), polydipsia (excessive thirst), dehydration, and dysrhythmias
	Diagnostic
	Total serum calcium level >10.5 mg/dL (2.74 mmol/L)
	Ionized serum calcium >1.29 mmol/L
		Medical
		See Chapter 13. Nursing
		• Identify patients at risk for hypercalcemia and assess for signs and symptoms of hypercalcemia.
		• Educate patient and family; prevention and early detection can prevent fatality.
		• Educate at-risk patients to recognize and report signs and symptoms of hypercalcemia.
		• Provide patient and family education regarding:
		  • Need to consume 2–4 L of fluid daily unless contraindicated by existing renal or cardiac disease
		  • Use of dietary and pharmacologic interventions such as stool softeners and laxatives for constipation
		  • Maintenance of nutritional intake without restricting normal calcium intake
		  • Antiemetic therapy for nausea and vomiting
		  • Promotion of mobility and emphasis on importance in preventing demineralization and breakdown of bones
		  • Safety precautions for patients with impaired mental and mobility status

(continues on page 368)

TABLE 15-13 Oncologic Emergencies: Manifestations and Management (continued)

Emergency	Clinical Manifestations and Diagnostic Findings	Management
Tumor Lysis Syndrome (TLS) Potentially fatal complication that occurs spontaneously or more commonly following radiation, biotherapy, or chemotherapy-induced cell destruction of large or rapidly growing cancers such as leukemia, lymphoma, and small cell lung cancer. The release of tumor intracellular contents (nuclei acids, electrolytes, and debris) leads to rapidly induced electrolyte imbalances—hyperkalemia, hyperphosphatemia (leading to hypocalemia), and hyperuricemia—that can have life-threatening end-organ effects on the myocardium, kidneys, and central nervous system (Lewis et al., 2011).	**Clinical** Clinical manifestations depend on the extent of metabolic abnormalities. Clinical TLS is diagnosed when ≥1 of three conditions arise either 3 days prior to or 7 days after cytotoxic cancer therapy: acute renal failure (defined as a rise in creatinine to ≥1.5 times the upper limit of normal that is not attributable to medications), dysrhythmias (including sudden cardiac death), and seizures (Lewis et al., 2011). • *Neurologic:* Fatigue, weakness, memory loss, altered mental status, muscle cramps, tetany, paresthesias (numbness and tingling), seizures • *Cardiac:* Elevated blood pressure, shortened QT complexes, widened QRS waves, altered T waves, dysrhythmias, cardiac arrest • *GI:* Anorexia, nausea, vomiting, abdominal cramps, diarrhea, increased bowel sounds • *Renal:* Flank pain, oliguria, anuria, renal failure, acidic urine pH • *Other:* Gout, malaise, pruritis **Diagnostic** • Electrolyte imbalances identified by serum electrolyte measurement and urinalysis (see Chapter 13); electrocardiogram to detect cardiac dysrhythmias	**Medical** • To prevent renal failure and restore electrolyte balance, aggressive fluid hydration is initiated 24–48 hours before and after the initiation of cytotoxic therapy to increase urine volume and eliminate uric acid and electrolytes; urine is alkalinized by adding sodium bicarbonate to IV fluid to maintain a urine pH of 7–7.5; this prevents renal failure secondary to uric acid precipitation in the kidneys. • Diuresis with a loop diuretic or osmotic diuretic if urine output is not sufficient • Allopurinol (Zyloprim) therapy to inhibit the conversion of nucleic acids to uric acid; rasburicase (Elitek) may be used to convert already formed uric acid to allantoin, which is highly water soluble and eliminated in urine. • Administration of a cation-exchange resin, such as sodium polystyrene sulfonate (Kayexalate), to treat hyperkalemia by binding and eliminating potassium through the bowel • Administration of IV sodium bicarbonate, hypertonic dextrose, and regular insulin temporarily shifts potassium into cells and lowers serum potassium levels if rapid decrease in potassium is necessary. • Administration of phosphate-binding gels, such as aluminum hydroxide, to treat hyperphosphatemia by promoting phosphate excretion in the feces • Hemodialysis when patients are unresponsive to the standard approaches for managing uric acid and electrolyte abnormalities **Nursing** • Identify at-risk patients, including those in whom TLS may develop up to 1 week after therapy for hematologic malignancies and up to several weeks for solid tumors. • Institute essential preventive measures (e.g., fluid hydration, medications) as prescribed. • Assess patient for signs and symptoms of electrolyte imbalances. • Assess urine pH to confirm alkalization. • Monitor serum electrolyte and uric acid levels for evidence of fluid volume overload secondary to aggressive hydration. • Instruct patients to monitor for and report symptoms indicating electrolyte disturbances.

From Camp-Sorrell, D. (2010). Cardiac and pulmonary toxicity. In J. Eggert (Ed.). *Cancer basics.* Pittsburgh: Oncology Nursing Society; Kaplan, M. (2009). Back pain: Is it spinal cord compression? *Clinical Journal of Oncology Nursing, 13*(5), 592–595; and Lewis, M. A., Hendrickson, A. W., & Moynihan, T. J. (2011). Oncologic emergencies: Pathophysiology, presentation, diagnosis, and treatment. *CA: A Cancer Journal for Clinicians, 61*(5), 287–314.

prevention and appropriate management of pain. The use of long-acting analgesic agents at set intervals, rather than on an "as needed" basis, is recommended in addressing pain management. Working with the patient and family, as well as with other health care providers, to manage pain is essential to increase the patient's comfort and offer some sense of control. Other medications (e.g., sedatives, tranquilizers, muscle relaxants, antiemetics) are added to assist in palliating additional symptoms and promoting quality of life.

If the patient is a candidate for radiation therapy or surgical interventions to relieve pain or other symptoms, the potential benefits and risks of these procedures (e.g., percutaneous nerve block, cordotomy) are explained to the patient and family. Measures are taken to prevent complications that result from altered sensation, immobility, and changes in bowel and bladder function.

Weakness, altered mobility, fatigue, and inactivity typically increase with advanced cancer as a result of the disease, treatment, inadequate nutritional intake, or dyspnea. The nurse works with the patient and family to identify realistic goals and promote comfort. Measures include use of energy conservation methods to accomplish tasks and activities that the patient values most.

Efforts are made to provide the patient with as much control and independence as desired but with assurance that support and assistance are available when needed. In addition, health care teams work with the patient and family to ascertain and comply with the patient's wishes about treatment methods and care as the terminal phase of illness and death approach.

Hospice

The needs of patients with end-stage illness are best met by a comprehensive interdisciplinary specialty program that focuses on quality of life, palliation of symptoms, and provision of physical, psychosocial, and spiritual support for patients and families when cure and control of the disease are no longer possible. The concept of hospice best addresses these needs.

Because of the high costs associated with maintaining freestanding hospices, care is often delivered through coordination of specialty services provided by hospitals, home care programs, and the community. The view that hospice and palliative care services are necessary only in the last few days of life prevents timely referral, limits patient and family access to needed services, and diminishes satisfaction with care (Hill & Hacker, 2010). Patients should be referred to hospice services in a timely fashion so that complex patient and family needs can be addressed. (See Chapter 16 for detailed discussion of end-of-life care.)

Critical Thinking Exercises

1 **ebp** A patient assigned to your care is about to begin multimodality therapy with chemotherapy, surgery, and radiation for pharyngeal cancer. Based on your understanding of the site of disease and planned treatments, what evidence-based nursing interventions would you implement to minimize side effects? Would you anticipate that this patient will experience any nutritional concerns? Are there any preventive measures that should be considered to address nutritional needs? What is the evidence for the interventions that you identified? How strong is that evidence, and what criteria did you use to assess the strength of that evidence?

2 **pq** A 78-year-old patient with bone metastasis from an unknown primary cancer has been receiving an opioid through a continuous subcutaneous infusion of analgesia with an infusion pump to relieve severe pain. His wife tells you that both she and her husband fear that he will become addicted to the opioid; his adult children report that his pain remains severe and unrelieved. As a home care nurse, what assessments would be of highest priority to you during your initial visit to this patient? What would be your top three nursing interventions for the patient and his wife?

3 A 39-year-old woman has presented to the cancer center for treatment of breast cancer. In reviewing her family history, you note that her mother and aunt (the mother's sibling) (who are both deceased) had metastatic breast cancer. You also note that she has one twin sister and a daughter 18 years of age. What information is important in this family history and why? What type of referral would be appropriate for this woman and her family? How would you best advise this woman and her family regarding cancer risks and screening practices?

4 A 58-year-old patient with metastatic lung cancer returns to the clinic for follow-up care. He tells you that he has been unable to button his collar, his wedding ring is too tight to remove, and he becomes short of breath when reclining at night. Describe the underlying pathology that can lead to the signs and symptoms of superior vena cava syndrome. Identify your assessment parameters with this patient. What will you tell the patient about the likely procedures that he will need to diagnose superior vena cava syndrome? Describe the medical and nursing management strategies that will be used for this patient.

Brunner Suite Resources

Explore these additional resources to enhance learning for this chapter:
- NCLEX-Style Questions and Other Resources on **thePoint**, http://thePoint.lww.com/Brunner13e
- Study Guide
- PrepU
- Clinical Handbook
- Handbook of Laboratory and Diagnostic Tests

References

*Asterisk indicates nursing research.
**Double asterisk indicates classic reference.

Books

American Cancer Society. (2009). *Complete guide to complementary and alternative cancer therapies* (2nd ed.). Atlanta: Author.

Baldwin, C. M. (2010). Cultural differences in cancer care. In J. Eggert (Ed.). *Cancer basics*. Pittsburgh: Oncology Nursing Society.

Camp-Sorrell, D. (2010). Cardiac and pulmonary toxicity. In J. Eggert (Ed.). *Cancer basics*. Pittsburgh: Oncology Nursing Society.

Carroll-Johnson, R. M. (2010). Complementary and alternative medicine. In J. Eggert (Ed.). *Cancer basics*. Pittsburgh: Oncology Nursing Society.

Chandraker, A., Milford, E. L., & Sayegh, M. H. (2012). Transplantation in the treatment of renal failure. In D. L. Longo, A. S. Fauci, D. L. Kasper, et al. (Eds.). *Harrison's principles of internal medicine* (18th ed.). New York: McGraw-Hill Professional.

Drake, D., & Lynes, B. (2010). Surgery. In J. Eggert (Ed.). *Cancer basics*. Pittsburgh: Oncology Nursing Society.

Dudek, S. G. (2010). *Nutrition essentials for nursing practice* (6th ed.). Philadelphia: Lippincott Williams & Wilkins.

Edge, S. B., Byrd, D. R., Compton, C. C., et al. (Eds.). (2010). *AJCC cancer staging manual* (7th ed.). New York: Springer.

Epting, S. P. (2010). Hypersensitivity. In J. Eggert (Ed.). *Cancer basics*. Pittsburgh: Oncology Nursing Society.

Fauci, A., & Lane, C. (2012). Human immunodeficiency virus disease: AIDS and related disorders. In D. L. Longo, A. S. Fauci, D. L. Kasper, et al. (Eds.). *Harrison's principles of internal medicine* (18th ed.). New York: McGraw-Hill Professional.

Fitz, A., Percy, C., Jack, A. et al. (2011). *International classification of disease for oncology*. World Health Organization: Geneva.

Flechner, S. M., Finke, J. H., & Fairchild, R. L. (2011). Principles of immunology in urology. In A. J. Wein, L. R. Kavoussi, A. C. Novick, et al. (Eds.). *Campbell Walsh urology* (10th ed.). Philadelphia: Elsevier-Saunders.

Gosselin, T. K. (2010). Principles of radiation therapy. In C. Henke Yarbro, D. Wujcik, & B. H. Holmes (Eds.). *Cancer nursing: Principles and practice* (7th ed). Sudbury, MA: Jones & Bartlett.

Harris, D. J. (2010). Transplantation. In J. Eggert (Ed.). *Cancer basics*. Pittsburgh: Oncology Nursing Society.

Harris, D. J., & Eilers, J. G. (2009). Mucositis. In: L. H. Eaton & J. M. Tipton (Eds.). *Putting Evidence into practice—improving oncology patient outcomes*. Pittsburgh: Oncology Nursing Society.

**Hewitt, M., Greenfield, S., & Stovall, E. (Eds.). (2006). *From cancer patient to cancer survivor*. Washington, DC: Institute of Medicine and National Research Council, National Academies Press. (Components of survivorship care provided by the Institute of Medicine report on cancer survivorship.)

Jansen, C. (2010). Cognitive changes. In J. Eggert (Ed.). *Cancer basics*. Pittsburgh: Oncology Nursing Society.

Johnson, G. B. (2010). Hematologic issues. In J. Eggert (Ed.). *Cancer basics*. Pittsburgh: Oncology Nursing Society.

Karch, A.M. (2012). *Lippincott's 2012 drug guide*. Philadelphia: Lippincott Williams & Wilkins.

Kelvin, J. F. (2010). Radiation therapy. In J. Eggert (Ed.). *Cancer basics*. Pittsburgh: Oncology Nursing Society.

Khan, F. M. (2010). *Physics of radiation therapy* (4th ed.). Philadelphia: Lippincott Williams & Wilkins.

Lapka, D. V., & Franson, P. J. (2010). Biologics and targeted therapies. In J. Eggert (Ed.). *Cancer basics*. Pittsburgh: Oncology Nursing Society.

Levine, A. (2010). Chemotherapy. In J. Eggert (Ed.). *Cancer basics*. Pittsburgh: Oncology Nursing Society.

Polovich, M., Whitford, J., & Olsen, M. (Eds.). (2009). *Chemotherapy and biotherapy guidelines and recommendations for practice* (3rd ed.). Pittsburgh: Oncology Nursing Society.

Prechtel-Dunphy, E., & Walker, S. (2010). Gastrointestinal symptoms. In J. Eggert (Ed.). *Cancer basics*. Pittsburgh: Oncology Nursing Society.

Sharp, L. K., Kinahan, K. E., & Didwania, A. (2010). Care for the adult childhood cancer survivor. In J. Eggert (Ed.). *Cancer basics*. Pittsburgh: Oncology Nursing Society.

Journals and Electronic Documents

General Oncology

Devine, H., Tierney, K., Schmit-Pokorny, K., et al. (2010). Mobilization of hemopoietic stem cells for use in autologous transplantation. *Clinical Journal of Oncology Nursing, 14*(2), 212–222.

Hill, K. K., & Hacker, E. D. (2010). Helping patients with cancer prepare for hospice. *Clinical Journal of Oncology Nursing, 14*(2), 180–188.

Kahn, S. R., Lim, W., Dunn, A. S., et al. (2012). Prevention of VTE in non-surgical patients. *Chest, 14*(2), e195S–e226S.

*Korber, S. F., Padula, C., Gray, J., et al. (2011). A breast navigator program: Barriers, enhancers, and nursing interventions. *Oncology Nursing Forum, 38*(1), 44–50.

Mariotto, A. B., Yabroff, K. R., Shao, Y., et al. (2011). Projections of the cost of cancer care in the United States: 2010-2020. *Journal of the National Cancer Institute, 103*(2), 117–128.

National Comprehensive Cancer Network. (2011a). *Clinical practice guidelines: Breast*. Available at: www.nccn.org/professionals/physician_gls/PDF/infections.pdf

National Comprehensive Cancer Network. (2011b). *Clinical practice guidelines: Prevention and treatment of cancer related infections (v2.2011)*. Available at: www.nccn.org/professionals/physician_gls/pdf/infections.pdf

Pal, S. K., Katheria, V., & Hurria, A. (2010). Evaluating the older patient with cancer: Understanding frailty and the geriatric assessment. *CA: A Cancer Journal for Clinicians, 60*(2), 120–132.

Siegel, R., Ward, E., Brawley, O., et al. (2011). Cancer statistics, 2011: The impact of eliminating socioeconomic and racial disparities on premature cancer deaths. *CA: A Cancer Journal for Clinicians, 61*(4), 212–236.

Vander Heiden, M. G., Cantley, L. C., & Thompson, C. B. (2009). Understanding the Warberg effect: The metabolic requirements of cell proliferation. *Science, 324*(10), 1049–1033.

Biologic Response Modifier Therapy

Merck & Co. Inc. (2011). *Gardasil: Human papillomavirus quadrivalent (types 6, 11, 16, and 18) vaccine, recombinant*. Available at: www.gardasil.com/prescribe-gardasil/index.html

Phillips, C. (2010). FDA approves first therapeutic cancer vaccine. *NCI Cancer Bulletin, 7*(9). Available at: www.cancer.gov/ncicancerbulletin/050410/page2

Roman, R. A. (2011). Immunotherapy for advanced melanoma: The emerging role of therapeutic antibodies against CTLA-4 for metastatic melanoma. *Clinical Journal of Oncology Nursing, 15*(5), E58–E65.

Cancer Development

American Cancer Society. (2011d). *Second cancers caused by cancer treatment*. Available at: www.cancer.org/Cancer/CancerCauses/OtherCarcinogens/MedicalTreatments/second-cancers-caused-by-cancer-treatment

American Cancer Society. (2012). *Secondhand smoke*. Available at: www.cancer.org/cancer/cancercauses/tobaccocancer/secondhand-smoke

Bokemeyer C., Bondarenko I., Makhson A., et al. (2009). Fluorouracil, leucovorin, and oxaliplatin with and without cetuximab in the first-line treatment of metastatic colorectal cancer. *Journal of Clinical Oncology, 27*(5), 663–671.

Callaway, C. (2011). Rethinking the head and neck cancer population: The human papillomavirus association. *Clinical Journal of Oncology Nursing, 15*(2), 165–170.

De Flora, S., & Bonanni, P. (2011). The prevention of infection-associated cancers. *Carcinogenesis, 32*(6), 787–795.

Eggert, J. (2011). The biology of cancer: What do oncology nurses really need to know. *Seminars in Oncology Nursing, 27*(1), 3–12.

Faridi, R., Zahra A., Khan K., et al. (2011). Oncogenic potential of human papillomavirus (HPV) and its relation with cervical cancer. *Virology Journal, 8*(269), 2–8.

Fontham, E. T. H., Thun, M. J., Ward, E., et al. (2009). American Cancer Society perspectives on environmental factors and cancer. *CA: A Cancer Journal for Clinicians, 59*(6), 343–351.

Giovannucci, E., Harlan, D. M., Archer, M. C., et al. (2010). Diabetes and cancer: A consensus report. *CA: A Cancer Journal for Clinicians, 60*(4), 207–221.

Hanahan D., & Weinberg R. A. (2011). Hallmarks of cancer: The next generation. *Cell, 144*(5), 646–674.

Kagawa-Singer, M., Dadia, A. V., Yu, M. C., et al. (2010). Cancer, culture, and health disparities: Time to chart a new course? *CA: A Cancer Journal for Clinicians, 60*(1), 12–39.

Soussi, T. (2011). *The TP53 web site: Inactivating p53 pathway in cancer*. Available at: p53.free.fr/p53_info/p53_cancer.html

Suda K., Tomizawa K., & Mitsudomi T. (2010). Biological and clinical significance of KRAS mutations in lung cancer: An oncogenic driver that contrasts with EGFR mutation. *Cancer & Metastasis Reviews, 29*(1), 49–60.

Chemotherapy

Chua, T. C., Yan, T. D., Saxena, A., et al. (2009). Should the treatment of peritoneal carcinomatosis by cytoreductive surgery and hyperthermic intraperitoneal chemotherapy still be regarded as a highly morbid procedure? A systematic review of morbidity and mortality. *Annals of Surgery, 249*(6), 900–907.

Cooke, L., Gemmill, R., Kravits, K., et al. (2009). Psychological issues of stem cell transplant. *Seminars in Oncology Nursing, 25*(2), 139–150.

Jacobson, J. O., Polovich, M., McNiff, K. K., et al. (2009). American Society of Clinical Oncology/Oncology Nursing Society chemotherapy administration safety standards. *Oncology Nursing Forum, 36*(6), 651–658.

National Institute for Occupational Safety and Health. (2010). *Personal protective equipment for health care workers who work with hazardous drugs*. Available at: www.cdc.gov/niosh/docs/wp-solutions/2009-106/pdfs/2009-106.pdf

Nixon, S., & Schulmeister, L. (2009). Safe handling of hazardous drugs: Are you protected? *Clinical Journal of Oncology Nursing, 13*(4), 433–439.

Rimkus, C. (2009). Acute complications of stem cell transplant. *Seminars in Oncology Nursing, 25*(2), 129–138.

Schulmeister, L. (2011). Extravasation management: Clinical update. *Seminars in Oncology Nursing, 27*(1), 82–90.

Schulmeister, L. (2010). Preventing and managing vesicant chemotherapy extravasations. *Journal of Supportive Oncology, 8*(5), 212–215.

Schulmeister, L. (2009). Vesicant chemotherapy extravasation antidotes and treatments. *Clinical Journal of Oncology Nursing, 13*(4), 395–398.

Viale, P. H., & Yamamoto, D. S. (2010). Biphasic and delayed hypersensitivity reactions: Implications for oncology nursing. *Clinical Journal of Oncology Nursing, 14*(3), 347–356.

Vogel, W. H. (2010). Infusion reactions: Diagnosis, assessment and management. *Clinical Journal of Oncology Nursing, 14*(2), E10–E21.

Complementary and Alternative Medicine

American Cancer Society. (2011c). *Complementary and alternative methods for cancer management*. Available at: www.cancer.org/Treatment/TreatmentandSideEffects/ComplementaryandAlternativeMedicine/complementary-and-alternative-methods-for-cancer-management

Bell, R. M. (2010). A review of complementary and alternative medicine practices among cancer survivors. *Clinical Journal of Oncology Nursing, 14*(3), 365–370.

*Fouladbakhsh, J. M., & Stommel, M. (2010). Gender, symptom experience, and use of complementary and alternative medicine practices among cancer survivors in the U.S. cancer population. *Oncology Nursing Forum, 37*(1), E7–E15.

National Center for Complementary and Alternative Medicine. (2011). *What is complementary and alternative medicine?* Available at: nccam.nih.gov/health/whatiscam/

Running, A., & Turnbeaugh, E. (2011). Oncology pain and complementary therapy: A review of the literature. *Clinical Journal of Oncology Nursing, 15*(4), 374–379.

Complications

Evens, K., & Eschiti V. S. (2009). Cognitive effects of cancer treatment: "Chemo brain" explained. *Clinical Journal of Oncology Nursing, 13*(6), 661–666.

National Cancer Institute Cancer Therapy Evaluation Program. (2010). *Common terminology criteria for adverse events (version 4.0)*. Available at: safetyprofiler-ctep.nci.nih.gov/CTC/CTC.aspx

Quirion, E. (2009). Filgrastim and pegfilgrastim use in patients with neutropenia. *Clinical Journal of Oncology Nursing, 13*(5), 324–328.

Saria, M. (2011). Preventing and managing infections in neutropenic stem cell transplantation recipients: Evidence-based review. *Clinical Journal of Oncology Nursing, 15*(2), 133–139.

Tarr, S., & Allen, D. (2009). Evidence does not support the use of a neutropenic diet. *Clinical Journal of Oncology Nursing, 13*(6), 617–619.

Von Ah, D., Jansen, C., Hutchinson A., et al. (2011). Putting evidence into practice: Evidence-based interventions for cancer and cancer treatment-related cognitive impairment. *Clinical Journal of Oncology Nursing, 15*(6), 607–615.

Genetics

Aiello-Laws, L. (2011). Genetic cancer risk assessment. *Seminars in Oncology Nursing, 27*(1), 13–20.

MacDonald, D. J. (2011). Germline mutations in cancer susceptibility genes: An overview for nurses. *Seminars in Oncology Nursing, 27*(1), 21–33.

Weitzel, J. N., Blazer, K. R., Macdonald, D. J., et al. (2011). Genetics, genomics, and cancer risk assessment state of the art and future directions in the era of personalized medicine. *CA: A Cancer Journal for Clinicians, 61*(5), 327–359.

Prevention and Detection

American Cancer Society. (2011a). *ACS guidelines on nutrition and physical activity for cancer prevention*. Available at: http://www.cancer.org/healthy/eathealthygetactive/acsguidelinesonnutritionphysicalactivityforcancer-prevention/acs-guidelines-on-nutrition-and-physical-activity-for-cancer-prevention-intro

American Cancer Society. (2011b). *Cancer prevention and early detection facts and figures*. Atlanta, GA: Author. Available at: http://www.cancer.org/research/cancerfactsfigures/cancerpreventionearlydetectionfactsfigures/index

American Cancer Society. (2010). *Menopausal hormone therapy and cancer risk*. Available at: www.cancer.org/Cancer/CancerCauses/OtherCarcinogens/MedicalTreatments/menopausal-hormone-replacement-therapy-and-cancer-risk

*Conde, F. A., Landier, W., Ishida, D., et al. (2011). Barriers and facilitators of prostate cancer screening among Filipino men in Hawaii. *Oncology Nursing Forum, 38*(2), 227–233.

*Gwede, C. K., William, C. M., Thomas K. B., et al. (2010). Exploring disparities and variability in perceptions and self-reported colorectal cancer screening among three ethnic subgroups in U.S. blacks. *Oncology Nursing Forum, 37*(5), 581–591.

McCullough, M. L., Patel, A. V., Kushi, L. H., et al. (2011). Cancer, cardiovascular disease, and all-cause mortality following cancer prevention guidelines reduces risk of cancer. *Cancer Epidemiology, Biomarkers & Prevention, 20*(6), 1089–1097.

*Meade, C. D., Menard, J., Thervil, C., et al. (2009). Addressing cancer disparities through community engagement: Improving breast health among Haitian women. *Oncology Nursing Forum, 36*(6), 716–722.

National Cancer Institute. (2011). *Clinical trials search: Cancer prevention*. Available at: www.cancer.gov/clinicaltrials/search/results?protocolsearchid=9589346

*Northington, L., Martin, T., Walker, J. T., et al. (2011). Integrated community education model: Breast health awareness to impact late-stage breast cancer. *Clinical Journal of Oncology Nursing, 15*(4), 387–392.

Vogel, V. G., Costantino, J. P., Wickerham, D. L., et al. (2010). Update of the national surgical adjuvant breast and bowel project study of Tamoxifen and Raloxifene (STAR) P-2 Trial: Preventing breast cancer. *Cancer Prevention Research, 3*(6), 696–706.

Radiation Therapy

Feight, D., Baney, T., Bruce, S., et al. (2011). Putting evidence into practice: Evidence-based interventions for radiation dermatitis. *Clinical Journal of Oncology Nursing, 15*(5), 481–492.

*Gosselin, T. K., Schneider, S. M., Plambeck, M. A., et al. (2010). A prospective randomized, placebo-controlled skin care study in women diagnosed with breast cancer undergoing radiation therapy. *Oncology Nursing Forum, 37*(5), 619–626.

Mallick, I., & Waldron, J. N. (2009). Radiation therapy for head and neck cancers. *Seminars in Oncology Nursing, 25*(3), 193–202.

McQuestion, M. (2011). Evidence-based skin care management in radiation therapy: Clinical update. *Seminars in Oncology Nursing, 27*(2), E1–E17.

Mettler, F. A., Brenner, D., Coleman, C. N., et al. (2011). Can radiation risks to patients be reduced without reducing radiation exposure? The status of chemical radioprotectants. *American Journal of Roentgenology, 196*(3), 616–618.

Waring, J., & Gosselin, T. (2010). Developing a high-dose-rate prostate brachytherapy program. *Clinical Journal of Oncology Nursing, 14*(2), 199–205.

Sexuality

*Howlett, K., Koetters, T., Edrington, J., et al. (2010). Changes in sexual function on mood and quality of life in patients undergoing radiation therapy of prostate cancer. *Oncology Nursing Forum, 37*(1), E58–E66.

*Julien, J. O., Thom, B., & Kline, N. E. (2010). Identification of barriers to sexual health assessment in oncology nursing practice. *Oncology Nursing Forum, 37*(3), E186–E190.

Kaplan, M., & Pacelli, R. (2011). The sexuality discussion: Tools for the oncology nurse. *Clinical Journal of Oncology Nursing, 15*(1), 15–17.

Lee, J. J. (2011). Sexual dysfunction after hematopoietic stem cell transplantation. *Oncology Nursing Forum, 38*(4), 409–412.

Shear, A. (2010). Fertility preservation: An option for women with cancer? *Clinical Journal of Oncology Nursing, 14*(2), 240–242.

Survivorship

Griffith, K. A., Mcguire, D. B., & Russo, M. (2010). Meeting survivors' unmet needs: An integrated framework for survivor and palliative care. *Seminars of Oncology Nursing, 26*(4), 231–242.

Jacobs, L. A., Palmer, S. C., Schwartz, L. A., et al. (2009). Adult cancer survivorship: Evolution, research, and planning care. *CA: Cancer Journal for Clinicians, 59*(6), 391–410.

Haylock, P. J. (2010). Advanced cancer: Emergence of a new survivor population. *Seminars in Nursing, 26*(3), 144–150.

Symptom Management

Borsellino, M., & Young, M. M. (2011). Anticipatory coping: Taking control of hair loss. *Clinical Journal of Oncology Nursing, 15*(3), 311–315.

*Caplinger, J., Royse, M., & Martens, J. (2010). Implementation of an oral care protocol to promote early detection and management of stomatitis. *Clinical Journal of Oncology Nursing, 14*(6), 799–802.

*Cotter, J. (2009). Efficacy of crude marijuana and synthetic delta-9-tetrahydrocannabinol as treatment for chemotherapy-induced nausea and vomiting: A systematic literature review. *Oncology Nursing Forum, 36*(3), 345–352.

*Edrington, J., Sun, A., Wong, C., et al. (2009). Barriers to pain management in a community sample of Chinese American patients with cancer. *Journal of Pain and Symptom Management, 37*(4), 665–675.

Eilers, J., & Million, R. (2011). Clinical update: Prevention and management of oral mucositis in patients with cancer. *Seminars in Oncology Nursing, 27*(4), E1–E16.

*Gabison, R., Gibbs, M., Uziely, M., et al. (2010). The cachexia assessment scale: Development and psychometric properties. *Oncology Nursing Forum, 37*(5), 635–640.

Granda-Cameron, C., DeMille, D., Lynch, M. P., et al. (2010). An interdisciplinary approach to manage cancer cachexia. *Clinical Journal of Oncology Nursing, 14*(1), 72–80.

Grunberg, S. M., Warr, D., Gralla, D. J., et al. (2011). Evaluation of new antiemetic agents and definition of antineoplastic emetogenicity—state of the art. *Supportive Care in Cancer, 19*(1), S43–S47.

Hayward, M. C., & Shea, A. M. (2009). Nutritional needs of patients with malignancies of the head and neck. *Seminars in Oncology Nursing, 25*(3), 203–211.

Hottensen, D. (2010). Anticipatory grief in patients with cancer. *Clinical Journal of Oncology Nursing, 14*(1), 106–107.

Kalmykow, B., & Walker, S. (2011). Cutaneous metastases in breast cancer. *Clinical Journal of Oncology Nursing, 15*(1), 99–101.

Kurtin, S. E. (2009). Systemic therapies for squamous cell carcinoma of the head and neck. *Seminars in Oncology Nursing, 25*(3), 183–192.

Le, Q. T., Kim, H. E., Schneider, C. J., et al. (2011). Palifermin reduces severe mucositis in definitive chemoradiotherapy of locally advanced head and neck cancer: A randomized, placebo-controlled study. *Journal of Clinical Oncology, 29*(20), 2808–2814.

National Comprehensive Cancer Network. (2011c). *NCCN Clinical Practice Guidelines in Oncology™: Antiemesis (v. 1. 2012).* Available at: www.nccn. org/professionals/physician_gls/pdf/antiemesis.pdf

National Comprehensive Cancer Network. (2011d). *NCCN Clinical Practice Guidelines in Oncology™: Cancer-related fatigue (v. 1. 2011).* Available at: www.nccn.org/professionals/physician_gls/pdf/fatigue.pdf

Nevidjon, B., & Chaudhary R. (2010). Controlling emesis: Evolving challenges, novel strategies. *Journal of Supportive Oncology, 8*(4 Suppl. 2), 1–10.

Paice, J. A., & Ferrell, B. (2011). The management of cancer pain. *Cancer: A Journal for Clinicians, 61*(3), 157–182.

*Rogers, M. P., & Blackburn, L. (2010). Use of neurokinin-1 receptor antagonists in patients receiving moderately or highly emetogenic chemotherapy. *Clinical Journal of Oncology Nursing, 14*(4), 500–550.

*Scott, J. A., Lasch, K. E., Barsevick, A. M., et al. (2011). Patients' experiences with cancer-related fatigue: A review and synthesis of qualitative research. *Oncology Nursing Forum, 38*(3), E191–E203.

*Tofthagen, C. (2010). Patient perceptions associated with chemotherapy-induced peripheral neuropathy. *Clinical Journal of Oncology Nursing, 14*(3), E22–E28.

*Tofthagen, C., McAllister, R. D., & McMillan, S. C. (2011). Peripheral neuropathy in patients with colorectal cancer receiving oxaliplatin. *Clinical Journal of Oncology Nursing, 15*(2), 182–188.

Walz, D. A. (2010). Cancer-related anorexia-cachexia syndrome. *Clinical Journal of Oncology Nursing, 14*(3), 283–287.

*Wanchai, A., Armer, J. M., & Stewart, B. R. (2011). Nonpharmacologic supportive strategies to promote quality of life in patients experiencing cancer-related fatigue: A systematic review. *Clinical Journal of Oncology Nursing, 15*(2), 203–214.

Surgery

Castiglia, L. L., Drummond, N., & Purden, M. A. (2011). Development of a teaching tool for women with a gynecologic malignancy undergoing minimally invasive robotic-assisted surgery. *Clinical Journal of Oncology Nursing, 15*(4), 404–410.

*Greenslade, M., V., Elliott, B., & Mandville-Anstey, S. A. (2010). Same-day breast cancer surgery: A qualitative study of women's lived experiences. *Oncology Nursing Forum, 37*(2), E92–E97.

*McQuirter, M., Castiglia, L. L., Loiselle, C. G., et al. (2010). Decision-making process of women carrying a BRCA1 or BRCA2 mutation who have chosen prophylactic mastectomy. *Oncology Nursing Forum, 37*(3), 313–320.

Scarpa, R. (2011). Surgical management of head and neck carcinoma. *Seminars in Oncology Nursing, 25*(3), 172–182.

Targeted Therapies

Bauer, S., & Romvari, E. (2009). Treatment of chronic myeloid leukemia following imatinib resistance: A nursing guide to second-line treatment options. *Clinical Journal of Oncology Nursing, 13*(5), 523–534.

Boucher, J., Olson, L., & Piperdi, B. (2011). Preemptive management of dermatologic toxicities associated with epidermal growth factor receptor inhibitors. *Clinical Journal of Oncology Nursing, 15*(5), 501–508.

Cook, K. M., & Figg, W. D. (2010). Angiogenesis inhibitors: Current strategies and future prospects. *CA: A Cancer Journal for Clinicians, 60*(4), 223–243.

Galinsky, I., & Buchanan, S. (2009). Practical management of dasatinib for maximum patient benefit. *Clinical Journal of Oncology Nursing, 13*(3), 329–335.

Given, B. A., Spoelstra, S. L., & Grant, M. (2011). The challenges of oral agents as antineoplastic treatments. *Seminars in Oncology Nursing, 27*(2), 93–103.

Goetsch, C. M. (2009). Genetic tumor profiling and genetically targeted cancer therapy. *Seminars in Oncology Nursing, 27*(1), 34–44.

Ledezma, B., Binder, S., & Hamid, O. (2011). Atypical clinical response patterns to ipilimumab: Four case studies of advanced melanoma. *Clinical Journal of Oncology Nursing, 15*(4), 393–403.

Schneider, S. M., Hess, K., & Gosselin, T. (2011). Interventions to promote adherence with oral agents. *Seminars in Oncology Nursing, 27*(2), 133–141.

Yap, T. A., Sandhu, S. K., Carden, C. P., et al. (2011). Poly(ADP-ribose) polymerase (PARP) inhibitors: Exploiting a synthetic lethal strategy in the clinic. *CA: A Cancer Journal for Clinicians, 61*(1), 31–49.

Resources

American Cancer Society (ACS), www.cancer.org/

American Pain Society (APS), www.ampainsoc.org

American Society of Clinical Oncology (ASCO), www.asco.org

Centers for Disease Control and Prevention: Preventing Infections in Cancer Patients, www.cdc.gov/Features/PreventInfections/

Coalition of Cancer Cooperative Groups, www.cancertrialshelp.org/

Hospice and Palliative Nurses Association (HPNA), www.hpna.org

LIVESTRONG Survivorship Centers of Excellence, www.livestrong.org

National Cancer Institute (NCI), www.cancer.gov

National Center for Complementary and Alternative Medicine (NCCAM), nccam.nih.gov

National Coalition for Cancer Survivorship, www.canceradvocacy.org

National Comprehensive Cancer Network (NCCN), www.nccn.org

National Hospice and Palliative Care Organization, www.nhpco.org

OncoLink (cancer resources), www.oncolink.org

Oncology Nursing Society (ONS), www.ons.org

Quackwatch, www.quackwatch.org

The Wellness Community, www.twccaz.org

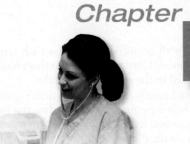

Chapter

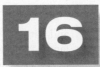

End-of-Life Care

Learning Objectives

On completion of this chapter, the learner will be able to:

1. Discuss the historical, legal, and sociocultural perspectives of palliative and end-of-life care in the United States.
2. Define palliative care.
3. Compare and contrast the settings where palliative care and end-of-life care are provided.
4. Describe the principles and components of hospice care.
5. Identify barriers to improving care at the end of life.
6. Reflect on personal experience with and attitudes toward death and dying.
7. Apply skills for communicating with terminally ill patients and their families.
8. Provide culturally and spiritually sensitive care to terminally ill patients and their families.
9. Implement nursing measures to manage physiologic responses to terminal illness.
10. Support actively dying patients and their families.
11. Identify components of uncomplicated grief and mourning, and implement nursing measures to support patients and families.

Glossary

assisted suicide: the use of pharmacologic agents to hasten the death of a terminally ill patient; illegal in most states

autonomy: self-determination; in the health care context, the right of the individual to make choices about the use and discontinuation of medical treatment

bereavement: period during which mourning for a loss takes place

euthanasia: Greek for "good death"; has evolved to mean the intentional killing by act or omission of a dependent human being for his or her alleged benefit

grief: personal feelings that accompany an anticipated or actual loss

hospice: a coordinated program of interdisciplinary care and services provided primarily in the home to terminally ill patients and their families

interdisciplinary collaboration: communication and cooperation among members of diverse health care disciplines jointly to plan, implement, and evaluate care

Medicare Hospice Benefit: a Medicare entitlement that provides for comprehensive, interdisciplinary palliative care and services for eligible beneficiaries who have a terminal illness and a life expectancy of less than 6 months

mourning: individual, family, group, and cultural expressions of grief and associated behaviors

palliative care: philosophy of and system for delivering care that expands on traditional medical care for serious, progressive illness to include a focus on quality of life, function, decision making, and opportunities for personal growth

palliative sedation: the use of pharmacologic agents, at the request of the terminally ill patient or the patient's legal proxy, to induce sedation, or near-sedation, when symptoms have not responded to other management measures; the purpose is not to hasten the patient's death but to relieve intractable symptoms

prognosis: the expected course of an illness and the chance for recovery

spirituality: personal belief systems that focus on a search for meaning and purpose in life, intangible elements that impart meaning and vitality to life, and a connectedness to a higher or transcendent dimension

terminal illness: progressive, irreversible illness that despite cure-focused medical treatment will result in the patient's death

Nurses can have a significant and lasting effect on the way in which patients live until they die, the manner in which the death occurs, and the enduring memories of that death for the families. Nursing has a long history of holistic, person- and family-centered care. Indeed, the definition of nursing highlights nursing's commitment to the diagnosis and treatment of *human responses to illness* (American Nurses Association [ANA], 2010a). There may be no setting or circumstance in which nursing care—that is, attention to human responses—is more important than in caring for seriously ill and dying patients.

Knowledge about palliative and end-of-life principles of care and patients' and families' unique responses to illness are essential to supporting their unique values and goals. Nurses have an opportunity to bring research, education, and practice together to change the culture of dying, bringing much-needed improvement to care that is relevant across practice settings, age groups, cultural backgrounds, and illnesses. The National Institute of Nursing Research (NINR) was designated in 1997 as the lead institute to coordinate research-related to end-of-life care within the National Institutes of

Health (NIH) and included end-of-life care in its strategic plan (NINR, 2012). In its 2011 summit, *The Science of Compassion: Future Directions in End-of-Life and Palliative Care,* national experts concluded that many barriers remain to fully appreciating and responding to patient and family needs during serious illness and at end of life (NINR, 2011). Nurses in all settings are likely to encounter end-of-life care. This chapter presents concepts about death and dying in the United States, settings for end-of-life care of the dying, and ways that nurses can address the health issues of terminally ill patients.

Nursing and End-of-Life Care

Death and Dying in America

The focus on care of the dying has been motivated by the aging of the population, the prevalence of and publicity surrounding life-threatening illnesses (e.g., cancer and acquired immunodeficiency syndrome [AIDS]), and the increasing likelihood of a prolonged period of chronic illness prior to death. Although there are more opportunities than ever before to allow peaceful death, the knowledge and technologies available to providers have made the process of dying anything but peaceful. Patients and clinicians may view death as what happens when medicine fails. This attitude has placed the issue of death and improvement of the dying process outside the focus of modern medicine and health care. Numerous initiatives aimed at improving end-of-life care have been launched in recent years, spurred by a widespread call for substantive change in the way Americans deal with death.

The National Consensus Project for Quality Palliative Care (NCP, 2009) identified the following eight key domains underlying a more comprehensive and humane approach to care of the dying. These include:

- *Structure and processes of care:* The timely plan of care is based on a comprehensive interdisciplinary assessment of the patient and family.
- *Physical aspects of care:* Pain, other symptoms, and side effects are managed based on the best available evidence, with attention to disease-specific pain and symptoms, which is skillfully and systematically applied.
- *Psychological and psychiatric aspects of care:* Psychological status is assessed and managed based on the best available evidence, which is skillfully and systematically applied. When necessary, psychiatric issues are addressed and treated.
- *Social aspects of care:* Comprehensive interdisciplinary assessment identifies the social needs of patients and their families, and a plan of care is developed to respond to these needs as effectively as possible.
- *Spiritual, religious, and existential aspects of care:* Spiritual and existential dimensions are assessed and responded to based on the best available evidence, which is skillfully and systematically applied.
- *Cultural aspects of care:* The palliative care program assesses and attempts to meet the needs of the patient, family, and community in a culturally sensitive manner.
- *Care of the imminently dying patient:* Signs and symptoms of impending death are recognized and communicated in developmentally appropriate language for children

and patients with cognitive disabilities with respect to family preferences. Care appropriate to this phase of illness is provided to the patient and family.
- *Ethical and legal aspects of care:* The patient's goals, preferences, and choices are respected within the limits of applicable state and federal law, within current accepted standards of medical care, and form the basis for the plan of care.

Major organizations, such as the National Hospice and Palliative Care Organization (NHPCO), National Quality Forum (NQF), and others have used the NCP clinical guidelines to structure quality palliative and end-of-life programs.

Technology and End-of-Life Care

In the 20th century, chronic, degenerative diseases replaced communicable diseases as the major causes of death. In the earlier part the 20th century, most deaths occurred at home and most families had direct experience with death, providing care to family members at the end of life and then mourning their losses. As the place of death shifted from home to hospitals, families became increasingly distanced from the death experience.

The application of technology to prolong life raises numerous ethical issues. One major question is: Because we *can* prolong life through increasingly sophisticated technology, does it necessarily follow that we *must* do so? In the later half of the 20th century, a "technologic imperative" practice pattern among health care professionals emerged, along with an expectation among patients and families that every available means to extend life must be tried. By the early 1970s, when hospice care was just beginning in this country, technology had become an expected companion of the critically and terminally ill.

In the 21st century, technologic intervention at the end of life continues to have profound implications, affecting how clinicians care for the dying, how family and friends participate in care, how patients and families understand and choose among end-of-life care options, how families prepare for **terminal illness** and death, and how they heal after the death of a loved one.

Sociocultural Context

Although each person experiences terminal illness uniquely, terminal illness is also shaped by the broader social and cultural contexts in which it occurs. The approach in the United States to serious illness has been described as "death denying"—that is, the health care system has been built on management of acute illness and the use of technology to cure (when possible) and to extend life. As a result, life-threatening illness, life-sustaining treatment decisions, dying, and death occur in a social environment in which illness is largely considered an enemy. Many common expressions reflect this dominant sociocultural view. For example, people talk about the "war" against cancer or "fighting" illness, and when patients choose not to pursue the most aggressive course of medical treatment available, many health care providers perceive this as "giving up." A care/cure dichotomy has emerged in which health care providers may view cure as the ultimate good and care as second best, a good only when cure is no longer possible. In such a model, alleviating suffering is not as valued as curing disease. Patients who cannot be cured feel distanced from the health care team, and when curative treatments have failed, they may feel that they too have failed. Patients and families may fear that any shift from curative goals to comfort-focused care will result in no care or lower-quality care, and that the clinicians on whom they have come to rely will abandon them if they withdraw from a focus on cure.

The statement in late-stage illness that exemplifies this care versus cure dichotomy is "nothing more can be done." This all-too-frequently used statement communicates the belief of many clinicians that there is nothing of value to offer patients beyond cure; however, in a care-focused perspective, there is always more that can be done. This expanded notion of healing implies that healing can take place throughout life. There are many opportunities for physical, spiritual, emotional, and social healing, even as body systems begin to fail at the end of life.

Clinicians' Attitudes Toward Death

Clinicians' attitudes toward the terminally ill and dying remain the greatest barrier to improving care at the end of life. Kübler-Ross illuminated the concerns of the seriously ill and dying in her seminal work, *On Death and Dying*, in 1969. At that time, it was common for patients to be kept uninformed about life-threatening diagnoses, particularly cancer, and for physicians and nurses to avoid open discussion of death and dying with their patients. Kübler-Ross's work revealed that, given open discussion, adequate time, and some help in working through the process, patients could reach a stage of acceptance in which they were neither angry nor depressed about their fate (see later discussion).

Clinicians' reluctance to discuss disease and death openly with patients stems from their own anxieties about death as well as misconceptions about what and how much patients want to know about their illnesses. In an early study of care of the dying in hospital settings, sociologists Glaser and Strauss (1965) discovered that health care professionals in hospital settings avoided direct communication about dying in hope that the patient would discover it on his or her own. They identified four "awareness contexts":

1. *Closed awareness:* The patient is unaware of his or her terminal state, whereas others are aware. Closed awareness may be characterized as a conspiracy between the family and health care professionals to guard the "secret," fearing that the patient may not be able to cope with full disclosure about his or her status, and the patient's acceptance of others' accounts of his or her "future biography" as long as the others give him or her no reason to be suspicious.

2. *Suspected awareness:* The patient suspects what others know and attempts to find out details about his or her condition. Suspected awareness may be triggered by inconsistencies in the family's and the clinician's communication and behavior, discrepancies between clinicians' accounts of the seriousness of the patient's illness, or a decline in the patient's condition or other environmental cues.

3. *Mutual pretense awareness:* The patient, the family, and the health care professionals are aware that the patient is dying, but all pretend otherwise.

4. *Open awareness:* The patient, the family, and the health care professionals are aware that the patient is dying and openly acknowledge that reality.

Glaser and Strauss (1965) also identified a pattern of clinician behavior in which those clinicians who feared or were uncomfortable discussing death developed and substituted "personal mythologies" for appraisals of what level of disclosure their patients actually wanted. For example, clinicians avoided direct communication with patients about the seriousness of their illness based on their beliefs that (1) patients already knew the truth or would ask if they wanted to know, or (2) patients would subsequently lose all hope, give up, or be psychologically harmed by disclosure.

Although Glaser and Strauss's findings were published decades ago, their observations remain valid today. The growth of palliative and hospice care programs has led to greater numbers of health care providers becoming comfortable with assessing patients' and families' information needs and disclosing honest information about the seriousness of illness (Ferrell & Coyle, 2010). However, in many settings, clinicians still avoid the topic of death in hope that patients will ask or find out on their own. Despite progress on many health care fronts, many who work with seriously ill and dying patients recognize a persistent conspiracy of silence about dying.

How to communicate truthfully with patients and encourage patient **autonomy** in a way that acknowledges where they are on the continuum of acceptance remains a challenge. Despite continued reluctance of health care providers to engage in open discussion about end-of-life issues, it has been confirmed that patients want information about their illness and end-of-life choices and that they are not harmed by open discussion about death (ANA, 2010b; Barclay, Momen, Case-Upton, et al., 2011). Timing of sensitive discussion takes experience, but speaking the truth can be a relief to patients and families, enhancing their autonomy by making way for truly informed consent as the basis for decision making.

Patient and Family Concerns

Patient and family denial about the seriousness of terminal illness also has been cited as a barrier to discussion about end-of-life treatment options. Yet research demonstrates that denial is a useful coping mechanism that enables the patient to gain temporary emotional distance from a situation that is too painful to contemplate fully (Benkel, Wijk, & Molander, 2010). Denial may become a barrier to care if patients or families refuse to acknowledge a diagnosis or refuse to hear about treatment options. Nurses must accept patients regardless of the degree to which they are in denial about their illness and work with other health care providers to present the same message.

Patient and family awareness of **prognosis** is a key factor in acceptance of and planning for death. Even patients and families who have received clear and honest information may not fully accept the situation. For patients who have been informed about terminal illness, their understanding of treatment goals and prognosis is dynamic and may sometimes require reinforcement.

Another concern is that patients' and their caregivers' understanding of treatment goals and prognosis can differ dramatically. In a study of patients receiving palliative radiation therapy for cancer metastases, researchers found that 25% of patients believed that their cancer was curable, and there was no change before and after therapy in belief that radiation therapy would cure the cancer and prolong their lives (Mitera, Zhang, Sahgal, et al., 2012). Such misunderstandings can complicate both delivery of effective care and informed consent for care.

Patients with noncancerous diagnoses such as heart failure, chronic obstructive pulmonary disease (COPD), renal failure, dementia, or neurodegenerative diseases such as amyotrophic lateral sclerosis, frequently do not receive adequate information and support to fully understand their prognosis, yet they often desire clear and honest information. For example, they may have troublesome symptoms and reduced quality of life paralleling or exceeding that of patients with cancer. Patients may want but are unlikely to receive clear information about disease progression, advance care planning, and prognosis. Similarly, in a qualitative study of preferences for prognosis communication among patients with end-stage heart failure, researchers found a strong preference for physician disclosure about treatment possibilities and probable outcomes (i.e., a balance of honest disclosure with hope) (Barclay et al., 2011). Clearly, further research is needed to examine the complex interactions between patients' misconceptions about advanced illness, their underlying psychological states, and barriers to clinicians' explanations of treatment expectations and prognosis.

Assisted Suicide

The assisted suicide debate has aimed a spotlight on the adequacy and quality of end-of-life care in the United States. **Assisted suicide** refers to providing another person the means to end his or her own life. Physician-assisted suicide involves the prescription by a physician of a lethal dose of medication for the purpose of ending someone's life (not to be confused with the ethically and legally supported practice of withholding or withdrawing medical treatment in accordance with the wishes of the terminally ill person).

Although assisted suicide is expressly prohibited under statutory or common law in the overwhelming majority of states, calls for legalized assisted suicide have highlighted inadequacies in the care of the dying. Public support for physician-assisted suicide has resulted in several state ballot initiatives. In 1994, Oregon voters approved the Oregon Death With Dignity Act, the first and—until 2008—only such legislative initiative to pass. This law provides for access to physician-assisted suicide by terminally ill patients under very controlled circumstances. After numerous challenges, the law was enacted in 1997. The number of Oregonians who have self-administered physician-prescribed lethal medication has remained small, totaling 596 persons who have died under the terms of the law since it was passed in 1997 (Oregon Public Health Division, 2011).

In November 2008, voters approved the Washington Death With Dignity Act. Modeled after the Oregon Death With Dignity law, the act contains the same safeguards and is administered through the Washington State Department of Health (Compassion and Choices of Washington, 2008). In 2009, Montana's Supreme Court ruled that physician aid in dying is not a crime, making this the third state to legalize assisted suicide. Numerous other states have considered

and rejected assisted suicide ballot initiatives. Gallup (2011) polls reflect a nearly even split among Americans with regard to the moral acceptability of assisted suicide, and it is likely that the issue will continue to be pursued in the courts and through ballot measures in other states.

Proponents of physician-assisted suicide argue that terminally ill people should have a legally sanctioned right to make independent decisions about the value of their lives and the timing and circumstances of their deaths, and its opponents argue for greater access to symptom management and psychosocial support for people approaching the end of life.

In its 2010 position statement on *Registered Nurses' Roles and Responsibilities in Providing Expert Care and Counseling at the End of Life*, the ANA acknowledges the complexity of the assisted suicide debate but clearly states that nursing participation in assisted suicide is a violation of the Code for Nurses. The ANA position statement further stresses the important role of the nurse in supporting effective symptom management, contributing to the creation of environments for care that honor the patient's and family's wishes, as well as identifying their concerns and fears (ANA, 2010b). Similarly, the Hospice and Palliative Nurses Association (HPNA) opposes the legalization of assisted suicide and affirms the value of comprehensive end-of-life care (HPNA, 2011). Although the Oncology Nursing Society (ONS, 2010) does not specifically oppose legalization of assisted suicide in its position statement, it too calls for quality palliative care and prompt discussion of requests to hasten death. The American Academy of Hospice and Palliative Medicine (AAHPM, 2007) has also recommended that clinicians carefully assess the fear and suffering that have led patients to request assisted suicide and to address these without hastening death (Chart 16-1).

Settings for End-of-Life Care

Palliative Care

Palliative care is an approach to care for the seriously ill that has long been a part of cancer care. More recently, it has been expanded to address the comprehensive symptom management, psychosocial care, and spiritual support needed to enhance the quality of life for patients with noncancerous diagnoses. Although hospice care is considered by many to be the gold standard for palliative care, the term *hospice* is generally associated with palliative care that is delivered at home or in special facilities to patients who are approaching the end of life (see later discussion). Palliative care and hospice care have been recognized as important bridges between cure-oriented treatment and the needs of terminally ill patients and their families for comprehensive care in the final years, months, or weeks of life (Fig. 16-1). Advocates for improved care for the dying have stated that acceptance, management, and understanding of death should become fully integrated concepts in mainstream health care.

Palliative care, which is conceptually broader than hospice care, is both an approach to care and a structured system for care delivery that aims to "prevent and relieve suffering and to support the best possible quality of life for patients and their families, regardless of the stage of the disease or the need for other therapies" (NCP, 2009, p. 6). Palliative

ETHICAL DILEMMA

Chart 16-1

What If a Patient Asks You to Help Him End His Life?

Case Scenario

You are a hospice nurse making a first home visit to a 52-year-old man with pancreatic cancer and metastasis to the liver. Prior to his illness, he was athletic and participated in triathlons. He now reports severe back and abdominal pain that is increasing and unrelieved by any of the pharmacologic and nonpharmacologic interventions that have been tried. In addition, he appears grossly jaundiced and cachectic. He is divorced and lives alone. His divorce was rancorous, and he does not enjoy a good relationship with his ex-wife but has reportedly enjoyed close, loving relationships with their twin daughters who are 12 years old. His ex-wife and daughters live in the same town. Until he was placed in hospice care, his daughters regularly spent weekends with him; however, he has not wanted them to visit him since that time and only speaks with them by phone. The patient tells you "I don't want my girls to see me like this" and then tells you "If you and your hospice won't help me end things on my own terms when I am good and ready, I will take one of my guns and do it myself."

Discussion

Assisted suicide remains a highly controversial topic—is it a matter of personal choice (i.e., does it preserve the autonomy of those who are dying), or does it constitute homicide by health care professionals who should "first do no harm" (i.e., nonmaleficence)? At this time, three states in the United States (Oregon, Washington, and Montana) legally permit physician-assisted suicide. However, the laws in these states include highly prescriptive criteria that must be present before a patient may be given a lethal prescription to end his or her own life. The professional role of the nurse is not clearly defined in these states as an accomplice to assisted suicide. However, the American Nurses Association (ANA, 1994) *Position Paper on Assisted Suicide* clearly stipulates that the nurse should not participate in assisted suicide.

Analysis

- How might you proceed with providing further consultation or follow-up with this patient? Would this follow-up be based upon whether or not he resided in a state where physician-assisted suicide is legal? Would his state of residence have any effect on your personal decision-making process?
- Further describe the ethical principles that are in conflict in this case and in other cases that surround requests for assisted suicide (see Chart 3-3). Which principle do you believe should have preeminence in deciding whether or not patients have the right to request assistance in suicide at the end of life?
- The ANA (1994) clearly notes that the nurse is not to participate in assisted suicide. Are there other discussion points or recommendations within the ANA (1994) *Position Paper on Assisted Suicide* that might be of help to you in providing competent professional nursing care to this patient?

Reference

American Nurses Association. (1994). *Position paper on assisted suicide*. Available at: www.nursingworld.org/MainMenu Categories/EthicsStandards/Ethics-Position-Statements/ prtetsuic14456.html

Resources

See Chapter 3, Chart 3-6 for ethics resources.

---

care emphasizes management of psychological, social, and spiritual problems in addition to control of pain and other physical symptoms. As the definition suggests, palliative care does not begin when cure-focused treatment ends but is most beneficial when it is provided along with disease-remitting treatments (World Health Organization, 2008). The goal of palliative care is to improve the patient's and family's quality of life, and many aspects of this type of comprehensive, comfort-focused approach to care are applicable earlier in the process of life-threatening disease and in conjunction with cure-focused treatment.

In palliative care, **interdisciplinary collaboration** is necessary to bring about the desired outcomes for patients and their families. Interdisciplinary collaboration, which is different from multidisciplinary practice, is based on communication and cooperation among the various disciplines, with each member of the team contributing to a single integrated care plan that addresses the needs of the patient and family. Multidisciplinary care refers to participation of clinicians with varied backgrounds and skill sets but without coordination and integration.

Palliative Care at the End of Life

The broadening of the concept of palliative care actually *followed* the development of hospice services in the United States. All hospice care is palliative care; however, not all palliative care is hospice care. The difference is that hospice care is an application of palliative care delivered at the end of life. Hospice care focuses on quality of life, and by necessity, it usually includes realistic emotional, social, spiritual, and financial preparation for death. After hospice care was recognized as a distinct program of services under Medicare in the early 1980s, organizations providing hospice care were able to receive Medicare reimbursement if they could demonstrate that the hospice program met the Medicare "conditions of participation," or regulations, for hospice providers.

Many chronic diseases do not have a predictable "end stage" that fits hospice eligibility criteria, and many patients

FIGURE 16-1 • The place of palliative care within the course of illness. From National Consensus Project for Quality Palliative Care. (2009). *Clinical practice guidelines for quality palliative care* (2nd ed., p. 6). Available at www. nationalconsensusproject.org

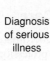
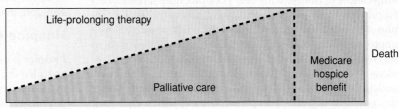

die after a long, slow, and often painful decline, without the benefit of the coordinated palliative care that is unique to hospice programs. The palliative approach to care could benefit many more patients if it were available across care settings and earlier in the disease process. Palliative care programs are now being developed in other settings for patients who are either not eligible for hospice or who do not choose to enroll in a formal hospice program. At this time, there is no dedicated reimbursement to providers for palliative care services when they are delivered outside the hospice setting, making the sustainability of such programs challenging.

Palliative Care in the Hospital Setting

Since the advent of diagnosis-related groups as the basis for prospective payment for hospital services in the 1980s, hospitals have had a financial incentive to transfer patients with terminal illnesses who are no longer in need of acute care to receive care in other settings, such as long-term care facilities and home. Despite the economic and human costs associated with death in the hospital setting, approximately 39% of all deaths among older adults occur in acute care settings (Kelley, Ettner, Wenger, et al., 2011). The landmark Study to Understand Prognoses and Preferences for Outcomes and Risks of Treatments (SUPPORT) documented troubling deficiencies in the care of the dying in hospital settings (SUPPORT Principal Investigators, 1995). Other studies have demonstrated that the health care system continues to be challenged when meeting seriously ill patients' needs for pain and symptom management and their families' needs for information and support. However, numerous guidelines have been issued in recent years in an effort to improve care for seriously ill and dying patients across settings. For example, in its 2000 to 2001 standards, the Joint Commission recognized pain as the "fifth vital sign" to ensure that pain is assessed routinely; in 2006, the NQF issued a consensus report on preferred practices for palliative and hospice care quality. The latter report builds on the NCP's eight domains of quality palliative and hospice care to develop 38 preferred practices to serve as a foundation for quality monitoring and reporting in health care organizations. In 2012, the NQF endorsed 12 new palliative and end-of-life quality measures that will guide quality improvement across settings where care is provided (NQF, 2006).

Many patients will continue to opt for hospital care or will by default find themselves in hospital settings at the end of life. Increasingly, hospitals are conducting system-wide assessments of end-of-life care practices and outcomes and are developing innovative models for delivering high-quality, person-centered care to patients approaching the end of life. A growing body of evidence supports the role of palliative care that is delivered *concurrently* with standard medical treatment. For example, in a study of referral to palliative care for patients newly diagnosed with metastatic non–small cell lung cancer (a disease with very poor prognosis), researchers found that those patients randomized to the palliative care plus standard oncology care arm of the trial not only showed improved quality of life and mood but also had longer median survival than those who received standard oncology care alone (Temel, Greer, Muzikansky, et al., 2010). This study underscores the value of palliative care and undercuts one of the principal objections to palliative care, which equates it with "giving up."

In 2011, the Joint Commission launched an advanced certification program for palliative care to recognize hospitals that provide exceptional patient and family-centered care. Hospitals cite considerable financial barriers to providing high-quality palliative care in acute care settings (Connor, 2007–2008). Public policy changes have been called for that would reimburse hospitals for care delivered via designated hospital-wide palliative care beds, clustered palliative care units, or palliative care consultation services in acute care settings. Resources are available for developing hospital–hospice partnerships to provide high-quality palliative care for hospitalized patients and for addressing the palliative care needs of other specialized populations, such as patients receiving such care in intensive care units (ICUs), pediatric patients, residents of long-term care facilities, and patients receiving care in community settings (Center to Advance Palliative Care, 2012).

Palliative Care in Long-Term Care Facilities

Experts estimate that the number of people who will need some form of long-term care in their lifetimes, whether in the community or in a residential care facility, will double by the year 2050 (Family Caregiver Alliance, 2012). As a result, the likely place of death for a growing number of Americans after age 65 years will be a long-term care facility. For those Americans younger than 65 years, the most common place for death remains the hospital (38%), although the proportion who die at home has increased steadily over the years. Similarly, for those older than 65 years, death at home has become more common (24%); however, the hospital (35%) and nursing home (28%) as the location of death still exceed the number of deaths at home, and although hospital death is decreasing, nursing home death is increasing (National Center for Health Statistics, 2010).

Residents of long-term care facilities typically have poor access to high-quality palliative care. Regulations that govern how care in these facilities is organized and reimbursed tend to emphasize restorative measures and serve as a disincentive to palliative care. Since 1989, home hospice programs have been permitted to enroll long-term care facility residents in hospice programs and to provide interdisciplinary services to residents who qualify for hospice care. Of the more than 939,000 Medicare beneficiaries who received hospice services in 2006, 31% resided in long-term care facilities (Office of the Inspector General [OIG], 2009). In 1997, the OIG, an oversight arm of the federal government, questioned whether hospice services in nursing homes are an unnecessary duplication of services already provided by long-term care facility staff. In 2008, the OIG reported on the appropriateness of payments for hospice care in nursing homes. Meanwhile, long-term care facilities are under increasing public pressure to improve care of the dying and are beginning to develop palliative care units or services; to contract with home hospice programs to provide hospice care in the facilities; and to educate staff, residents, and their families about pain and symptom management and end-of-life care.

Hospice Care

Hospice is a coordinated program of interdisciplinary services provided by professional caregivers and trained volunteers to patients with serious, progressive illnesses that are not responsive to cure. The root of the word *hospice* is *hospes*, meaning "host." According to Cicely Saunders, who founded the world-renowned St. Christopher's Hospice in London, the principles underlying hospice are as follows:

- Death must be accepted.
- The patient's total care is best managed by an interdisciplinary team whose members communicate regularly with one another.
- Pain and other symptoms of terminal illness must be managed.
- The patient and family should be viewed as a single unit of care.
- Home care of the dying is necessary.
- Bereavement care must be provided to family members.
- Research and education should be ongoing.

Hospice Care in the United States

Hospice in the United States is not a place, but a concept of care in which the end of life is viewed as a developmental stage. The hospice movement in the United States is based on the belief that meaningful living is achievable during terminal illness and that it is best supported in the home, free of technologic interventions to prolong physiologic dying. The concept of hospice care as an alternative to depersonalized death in institutions began in the early 1970s as a grassroots, volunteer-based, and spiritually centered movement. After the first hospice in the United States was founded in 1974 in Connecticut, the concept quickly spread and the number of hospice programs throughout the country increased dramatically. By 2010, there were more than 5,000 hospice programs in operation, serving an estimated 1.6 million patients (NHPCO, 2011).

Despite decades of existence in the United States, hospice remains an option for end-of-life care that has not been fully integrated into mainstream health care. Physicians are reluctant to refer patients to hospice, and patients are reluctant to accept this form of care. Reasons include the difficulties in making a terminal prognosis (especially for those patients with noncancerous diagnoses), the strong association of hospice with death, advances in "curative" treatment options in late-stage illness, and financial pressures on health care providers that may cause them to retain rather than refer hospice-eligible patients. As a result, many patients and families do not fully benefit from the comprehensive, interdisciplinary support offered by hospice programs; the median length of stay in a hospice program is just 21.3 days (NHPCO, 2011).

The goal of hospice is to enable the patient to remain at home, surrounded by the people and objects that have been important to him or her throughout life. The patient and family make up the unit of care. Hospice care does not seek to hasten death or encourage the prolongation of life through artificial means. Hospice care hinges on the competent patient's full or "open" awareness of dying; it embraces realism about death and helps patients and families understand the dying process so that they can live each moment as fully as possible. Approximately 20% of hospice programs have developed inpatient facilities or residences (NHPCO, 2011) where terminally ill patients without family support and those who desire inpatient care may receive hospice services.

Hospice Care Eligibility and Benefits

Since 1983, the **Medicare Hospice Benefit** has covered costs of hospice care for Medicare beneficiaries. State Medical Assistance (Medicaid) also provides coverage for hospice care, as do most commercial insurers. To receive Medicare payment for

| Chart 16-2 | Eligibility Criteria for Hospice Care |

General

- Serious, progressive illness
- Limited life expectancy
- Informed choice of palliative care over cure-focused treatment

Hospice Specific

- Presence of a family member or other caregiver continuously in the home when the patient is no longer able to safely care for himself or herself (some hospices have created special services within their programs for patients who live alone, although this varies widely)

Medicare and Medicaid Hospice Benefits

- Medicare Part A; Medical Assistance eligibility
- Waiver of traditional Medicare/Medicaid benefits for the terminal illness
- Life expectancy of ≤6 months
- Physician certification of terminal illness
- Care must be provided by a Medicare-certified hospice program

hospice services, programs are required to comply with rules known as "conditions of participation," which are enforced by the Centers for Medicare and Medicaid Services. In many aspects, Medicare standards have come to largely define hospice philosophy and services.

Eligibility criteria for hospice vary depending on the hospice program, but generally patients must have a progressive, irreversible illness and limited life expectancy and must opt for palliative care rather than cure-focused treatment. Chart 16-2 presents the eligibility criteria for hospice coverage under the Medicare Hospice Benefit. The patient who wishes to use his or her Medicare Hospice Benefit must be certified by a physician as terminally ill, with a life expectancy of 6 months or less if the disease follows its natural course. Thus, hospice has come to be defined as palliative care provided to terminally ill persons and their families in the last 6 months of the patient's life. Because of additional Medicare rules concerning a palliative focus for medical treatment under the Medicare Hospice Benefit, many patients delay enrollment in hospice programs until very close to the end of life.

Federal rules for hospices require that eligibility be reviewed periodically. Patients who live longer than 6 months under hospice care are *not* discharged, provided that their physician and the hospice medical director continue to certify that they are terminally ill with a life expectancy of 6 months or less (assuming that the disease continues its expected course). Once a patient meets eligibility criteria and elects to use the benefit, the Medicare-certified hospice program assumes responsibility for providing and paying for the care and treatment to palliate the terminal illness for which hospice care was elected. The Medicare-certified hospice is paid a predetermined dollar amount for each day of hospice care that each patient receives. Four levels of hospice care are covered under Medicare and Medicaid hospice benefits:

- *Routine home care:* All services provided are included in the daily rate to the hospice.

- *Inpatient respite care:* A 5-day inpatient stay, provided on an occasional basis to relieve the family caregivers.
- *Continuous care:* Continuous nursing care provided in the home for management of a medical crisis. Care reverts to the routine home care level after the crisis is resolved. (For example, seizure activity develops and a nurse is placed in the home continuously to monitor the patient and administer medications. After 72 hours, the seizure activity is under control, the family has been instructed how to care for the patient, and the continuous nursing care is discontinued.)
- *General inpatient care:* Inpatient stay for symptom management that cannot be provided in the home. This is not subject to the guidelines for a standard hospital inpatient stay.

Most hospice care is provided at the "routine home care" level and includes the services described in Chart 16-3. According to federal guidelines, hospices may provide no more than 20% of the aggregate annual patient-days at the inpatient level. Patients may "revoke" their hospice benefits at any time, resuming traditional coverage under Medicare or Medicaid for the terminal illness. Those who revoke their benefits may also reelect to use them at a later time.

Hospice Care Utilization

Hospice programs are reaching out to patients with very advanced illness and seeking ways to provide them with hospice services while they are completing courses of treatment that many programs previously defined as "life prolonging," such as disease-modifying therapies for dementia, enteral or parenteral nutritional support, and certain types of chemotherapy. The hospice industry has begun to refer to more flexible policies concerning disease-modifying medical treatment at the time of admission as "open access." The NHPCO acknowledges the concept of open access, stating that palliative care is "treatment that enhances comfort and improves the quality of an individual's life during the last phase of life. No specific therapy is excluded from consideration" (NHPCO, 2010, p. 1).

Hospice use has increased steadily since the inception of the Medicare Hospice Benefit. In 2009, approximately 42% of Medicare beneficiaries who died used hospice services compared to 23% in 2000 (Medicare Payment Advisory Commission [MedPAC], 2011). The most common primary hospice

diagnoses among Medicare patients are heart disease, general debility, dementia, and lung disease. Whereas most patients who enrolled in hospice in previous decades had cancer diagnoses, 64% of hospice enrollees in 2010 had noncancer diagnoses (NHPCO, 2011).

Although hospice utilization continues to increase, many patients who could benefit from hospice care do not receive it. Most terminally ill patients who are not enrolled in hospice die in hospitals and long-term care facilities.

Nursing Care of Terminally Ill Patients

Many patients suffer unnecessarily when they do not receive adequate attention for the symptoms accompanying serious illness. Careful evaluation of the patient should include not only the physical problems but also the psychosocial and spiritual dimensions of the patient's and family's experience of serious illness. This approach contributes to a more comprehensive understanding of how the patient's and family's life has been affected by illness and leads to nursing care that addresses their needs in every dimension.

Psychosocial and Regulatory Issues

Nurses are responsible for educating patients and their caregivers and for supporting them as they adapt to life with the illness. Nurses can assist patients and families with life review, values clarification, treatment decision making, and end-of-life goals. The only way to do this effectively is to try to appreciate and understand the illness from the patient's perspective.

Nurses should be both culturally aware and sensitive in their approaches to communication with patients and families about death. Attitudes toward open disclosure about terminal illness vary widely among different cultures, and direct communication with patients about such matters may be viewed as harmful (Long, 2011). To provide effective patient- and family-centered care at the end of life, nurses must be willing to set aside their own assumptions and attitudes so that they can discover what type and amount of disclosure is most meaningful to each patient and family within their unique belief systems (Table 16-1).

The social and legal evolution of advance directive documents represents some progress in people's willingness to both contemplate and communicate their wishes concerning the end of life (Chart 16-4). Now legally sanctioned in every state and federally sanctioned through the Patient Self-Determination Act of 1991, advance directives are written documents that allow competent people to document their preferences regarding the use or nonuse of medical treatment at the end of life, specify their preferred setting for care, and communicate other valuable insights into their values and beliefs. The addition of a proxy directive (the appointment and authorization of another person to make medical decisions on behalf of the person who created the advance directive when he or she can no longer speak for himself or herself) is an important addition to the living will or medical directive that specifies the signer's preferences. These documents are widely available from health care providers, community organizations, bookstores, and the Internet. However, their underuse reflects society's continued discomfort with openly

---

Chart 16-3

Home Hospice Services Covered Under the Medicare/Medicaid Hospice Benefit Routine Home Care Level

- Nursing care provided by or under the supervision of a registered nurse, available 24 hours a day
- Medical social services
- Physician's services
- Counseling services, including dietary counseling
- Home health aide/homemaker
- Physical/occupational/speech therapists
- Volunteers
- Bereavement follow-up (for up to 13 months after the death of the patient)
- Medical supplies for the palliation of the terminal illness
- Medical equipment for the palliation of the terminal illness
- Medications for the palliation of the terminal illness

TABLE 16-1 Overview of Religious and Cultural Beliefs and Views on Death and Dying

Religion	General Religious/Cultural Beliefs	Views About Death/Preparing for Death
Hinduism	• Each caste has a different view of death. • This life is a transition between the previous life and the next. • Bodies are cremated. During the first 10 days after death, relatives must create a new ethereal body. • "Good karma" leads to good rebirth or release, and "bad karma" leads to bad rebirth.	• Many older adults withdraw into their homes, where they prepare for death through prayer and meditation. • Family is very important; health care decisions may be made communally with senior family member as final authority. • A "good death" is timely, in the right place (on the ground at home), conscious and prepared, with the mind on God. All affairs should be in order. • A "bad death" is untimely, violent, and unprepared. The worst death is suicide.
Judaism	• Human beings are mortal, and their bodies belong to God. • Although the physician has the authority to determine the appropriate course of treatment, ultimately the patient has the right to choose, as long as the medical regimen follows Jewish law. • Disclosure is important. Most patients want to know the truth. • Jews are obligated to visit the sick.	• Traditional criteria for death are cessation of breathing and heartbeat. Conservative rabbis have accepted brain death as fulfilling these criteria. • Advance directives for health care are permissible. • Views on the use of artificial nutrition and hydration vary, depending on the particular sect/movement. • Most rabbis maintain that Jews may enroll in hospice.
Buddhism	• There is no central authority in the Buddhist religion. • Taboo and religious purity play little, if any, role, and religious law imposes no special requirements for medical treatment. • Treatment by someone of the same gender is preferable. • Cremation is the most common way of disposing of the dead. • Some Buddhists may be unwilling to take pain-relieving medications or strong sedatives. It is believed that an unclouded mind can lead to a better rebirth. • Buddhists believe that after death there is either rebirth or nirvana—the latter being enlightenment that frees the soul from the cycle of death and rebirth.	• Teachings emphasize the inevitability of death; therefore, Buddhists tend to be psychologically prepared to accept impending death with calmness and dignity. • Death occurs when a body is bereft of vitality, heat, and sentiency. Brain death is disputed as meeting the requirements for death. • It is often appropriate to decide that the patient is beyond medical help and to allow events to take their course. In these cases, it is justifiable to refuse or withdraw treatment in light of the overall prognosis. • Buddhism supports the use of hospice.
Islam	• Muslims believe in one God. • God revealed the message of God to Muhammad, the prophet, in the Qur'an (Koran), which states that Muslims should maintain a balanced diet and exercise. • Muslim patients may wish to engage in ritual prayer, practiced five times during the day. • Fasting during the month of Ramadan is a pillar of Islam. • Completion of the pilgrimage (hajj) to Mecca (money and health permitting), at least once, is also a pillar of Islam.	• Everyone will face death, and the way a person dies is of great individual importance. • Death cannot happen except by God's permission. However, it is recognized that diseases and trauma cause death. • There is a belief that God is the one who cures and physicians are a means to enact God's will. • Decisions are made within families, and disclosure of diagnosis and prognosis must be considered in this context. • Pain is a cleansing instrument of God. Pain can also be viewed as having an educational purpose (pain can compensate for sin). • The killing of a terminally ill person is an act of disobedience against God. However, pain relief or withholding or withdrawing of life support when there is no doubt that the person's disease is causing untreatable suffering is permissible as long as there is formal agreement among all parties concerned.
Traditional Christianity	• Christians believe in one God. • The belief in eternal salvation sets Christianity apart. • Beliefs vary. Some Christians hope to attain eternal salvation. • Even within family, religious views can differ. Some family members may not follow the religion at all.	• Intentionally bringing about death by either omission or commission is prohibited. • The appropriateness of analgesia and sedation to avoid terminal suffering and despair is acceptable, if it does not, by clouding consciousness, take away the final opportunity for repentance. • Christians are not obligated to postpone death; it is forbidden to try to save life at all costs. However, there could be a duty to use high-technology medicine to gain a last opportunity for repentance. • Impending death offers a final chance to become reconciled with those whom one has harmed and to ask God's forgiveness. • Liturgical (ceremonial) Christians generally regard last rites as integral to the relationship with God. Repentance can include confessing formally and receiving Communion and final anointing. This often involves particular ministers. • Christians who follow the religion at a cultural level are likely to have secular approaches to end-of-life decisions. • Advance directives allow patients to appoint decision makers and to provide instructions that ensure that their wishes are followed.

Information compiled from Firth, S. (2005). End of life: A Hindu view. *Lancet, 366*(9486), 682–686; Thrane, S. (2010). Hindu end of life. *Journal of Hospice and Palliative Nursing, 12*(6), 337–342; Dorff, E. N. (2005). End of life: Jewish perspectives. *Lancet, 366*(9488), 862–865; Engelhardt, H. T., & Smith Iltis, A. (2005). End of life: The traditional Christian view. *Lancet, 366*(9490), 1045–1049; Keown, D. (2005). End of life: The Buddhist view. *Lancet, 366*(9489), 952–955; Sachedina, A. (2005). End of life: The Islamic view. *Lancet, 366*(9487), 774–779; and Salman, K., & Zoucha, R. (2010). Considering faith within culture when caring for the terminally ill Muslim patient. *Journal of Hospice and Palliative Nursing, 12*(3), 156–163.

Chart 16-4 **Methods of Stating End-of-Life Preferences**

Advance directives: written documents that allow the individual of sound mind to document preferences regarding end-of-life care that should be followed when the signer is terminally ill and unable to verbally communicate his or her wishes. The documents are generally completed in advance of serious illness but may be completed after a diagnosis of serious illness if the signer is still of sound mind. The most common types are the durable power of attorney for health care and the living will.

Durable power of attorney for health care: a legal document through which the signer appoints and authorizes another individual to make medical decisions on his or her behalf when he or she is no longer able to speak for himself or herself. This is also known as a health care power of attorney or a proxy directive.

Living will: a type of advance directive in which the individual documents treatment preferences. It provides instructions for care in the event that the signer is terminally ill and not able to communicate his or her wishes directly and often is accompanied by a durable power of attorney for health care. This is also known as a medical directive or treatment directive.

Physician Orders for Life-Sustaining Treatment (POLST): a form that translates patient preferences expressed in advance directives to medical "orders" that are transferable across settings and readily available to all health care providers, including emergency medical personnel. The POLST form is a brightly colored form that specifies preferences related to cardiopulmonary resuscitation and use of IV medications or fluids, antibiotics, artificial nutrition, and other medical interventions. The form is signed by the patient or surrogate and the physician, advanced practice nurse, or physician assistant. The use of the POLST is subject to state laws and regulations. Numerous states have endorsed the POLST or a similar form.

Information about the advance care planning and state-specific advance directive documents and instructions is available at www.caringinfo.org. Information about the POLST is available at www.ohsu.edu/polst/

confronting the subject of death. Furthermore, the existence of a properly executed advance directive does not reduce the complexity of end-of-life decisions.

The Patient Self-Determination Act requires that health care entities receiving Medicare or Medicaid reimbursement must ask if patients have advance directives, provide information about advance directives, and incorporate advance directives into the medical record. However, advance directives should not be considered a substitute for ongoing communication among the health care provider, patient, and family as the end of life approaches.

 Concept Mastery Alert

A durable power of attorney for health care is different from a power of attorney. A *durable power of attorney* is an advance directive that authorizes another person to make medical decisions when the person is no longer able to do so. A *power of attorney* is a document that authorizes a designated individual to make decisions for another; however, these decisions are often related to financial and property issues.

Communication

Remarkable strides have been made in the ability to prolong life; however, attention to care for the dying lags behind. On one level, this should come as no surprise. Each of us will eventually face death, and most would agree that one's own demise is a subject that he or she would prefer not to contemplate. Confronting death in our patients uncovers our own deeply rooted fears.

To develop a level of comfort and expertise in communicating with seriously and terminally ill patients and their families, nurses must first consider their own experiences with and values concerning illness and death. Reflection, reading, and talking with family members, friends, and colleagues can help nurses examine beliefs about death and dying. Talking with people from different cultural and religious backgrounds can help nurses view personally held beliefs through a different lens and can increase their sensitivity to death-related beliefs and practices in other cultures. Discussion with nursing and non-nursing colleagues can also be useful; it may reveal the values shared by many health care professionals and may also identify diversity in the values of patients in their care. Values clarification and personal death awareness exercises can provide a starting point for self-discovery and discussion.

Skills for Communicating With the Seriously Ill

Nurses need to develop skill and comfort in assessing patients' and families' responses to serious illness and planning interventions that support their values and choices throughout the continuum of care (Back, Arnold, & Tulsky, 2009). Throughout the course of a serious illness, patients and their families encounter complicated treatment options and bad news about disease progression. They may have to make difficult decisions at the time of diagnosis, when disease-focused treatment fails, when the effectiveness of a particular intervention is being discussed, and when decisions about hospice care are presented. These critical points on the treatment continuum demand patience, empathy, and honesty from nurses. Discussing sensitive issues such as serious illness, hopes for survival, and fears associated with death is never easy. However, the art of therapeutic communication can be learned and, like other skills, must be practiced to gain expertise. Like other skills, communication should be practiced in a "safe" setting, such as a classroom or clinical skills laboratory with other students or clinicians.

Communication with each patient and family should be tailored to their particular level of understanding and values concerning disclosure. Before disclosing any health information about a patient to family members, nurses should follow their agency's policy for obtaining patient consent in accordance with Health Insurance Portability and Accountability Act (HIPAA) rules.

Nursing Interventions When Patients and Families Receive Bad News

Communicating about a life-threatening diagnosis or disease progression is best accomplished in any setting by the interdisciplinary team: A physician, nurse, social worker, and chaplain should be present whenever possible to provide information, facilitate discussion, and address

Chart 16-5 | COMFORT: A Framework for Communication in Palliative Care

Communication (C)

- Narrative clinical practice: Elicit and be fully present for the patient's and family's story.
- Verbal clarity: Use compassionate, nonambiguous language.
- Nonverbal immediacy: Use eye contact, body position, and self-awareness to show attentiveness.

Orientation (O)

- Support health literacy.
- Acknowledge vulnerability.
- Express cultural sensitivity.

Mindfulness (M)

- Stay in the moment: Avoid scripted responses.
- Avoid prejudgment: Do not have expectations that this patient and family will or should respond as others have in the past.
- Adapt to rapid changes: Be ready to shift to new topics and concerns that are revealed.

Family (F)

- Think of the family as a "second-order" patient: The family and the patient comprise the unit of care.
- Know that the family is a bridge to the patient: You must gain the family's trust to work effectively.

- Use family meetings (patient included) to clarify goals for treatment.

Openings (O)

- Address essential transitions in care or status.
- Seek a higher level of understanding of the disease process.
- Engage spiritual concerns.

Relating (R)

- Prioritize the turning point in illness.
- Understand that communication should be nonlinear: The patient and family may need to revisit topics multiple times and on multiple occasions.
- Know that the patient's and family's acceptance must drive communication.

Team (T)

- The interdisciplinary team includes members trained in various aspects of palliative care.
- Assure the patient and family that they will not be abandoned.
- Assure continuity of care across settings: Goals and plans should be clearly communicated to other providers.

Adapted with permission, Wittenberg-Lyles, E., Goldsmith, J., & Ragan, S. L. (2010). The COMFORT initiative: Palliative nursing and the centrality of communication. *Journal of Hospice and Palliative Nursing*, *12*(5), 282–292.

concerns. Most important, the presence of the team conveys caring and respect for the patient and family. If the patient wishes to have family present for the discussion, arrangements should be made to have the discussion at a time that is best for everyone. Creating the right setting is particularly important. A quiet area with a minimum of disturbances should be used. All clinicians present should turn off pagers, cell phones, and other communication devices for the duration of the meeting and should allow sufficient time for the patient and family to absorb and respond to the news. Finally, the space in which the meeting takes place should be conducive to seating all participants at eye level. It is difficult enough for the patient and family to be the recipients of bad news without having an array of clinicians standing uncomfortably over them at the foot of the patient's bed (Chart 16-5).

After the initial discussion of a life-threatening illness or progression of a disease, the patient and family will probably have many questions and may need to be reminded of factual information. Coping with news about a serious diagnosis or poor prognosis is an ongoing process. The nurse should be sensitive to these ongoing needs and may need to repeat previously provided information or simply be present while the patient and family react emotionally. The most important intervention the nurse can provide is listening empathetically. Seriously ill patients and their families need time and support to cope with the changes brought about by serious illness and the prospect of impending death. The nurse who is able to listen without judging and without trying to solve the patient's and family's problems provides an

invaluable intervention. Keys to effective listening include the following:

- Resist the impulse to fill the "empty space" in communication with talk.
- Allow the patient and family sufficient time to reflect and respond after asking a question.
- Prompt gently: "Do you need more time to think about this?"
- Avoid distractions (noise, interruptions).
- Avoid the impulse to give advice.
- Avoid canned responses: "I know just how you feel."
- Ask questions.
- Assess understanding—your own and the patient's—by restating, summarizing, and reviewing.

Responding With Sensitivity to Difficult Questions

Patients often direct questions or concerns to nurses before they have been able to fully discuss the details of their diagnosis and prognosis with their physicians or the entire health care team. Using open-ended questions allows the nurse to elicit the patient's and family's concerns, explore misconceptions and needs for information, and form the basis for collaboration with physicians and other team members.

For example, a seriously ill patient may ask the nurse, "Am I dying?" The nurse should avoid making unhelpful responses that dismiss the patient's real concerns or defer the issue to another care provider. Nursing assessment and intervention are always possible, even when a need for further discussion with a physician is clearly indicated. Whenever possible, discussions in response to a patient's concerns should occur when the patient expresses a need, although that may be the least convenient time for the nurse. Creating an uninterrupted space of just 5 minutes can do much to identify the source of the concern, allay anxieties, and plan for follow-up.

In response to the question "Am I dying?" the nurse could establish eye contact and follow with a statement acknowledging the patient's fears ("This must be very difficult for you") and an open-ended statement or question ("Tell me more about what is on your mind"). The nurse then needs to listen intently, ask additional questions for clarification, and provide reassurance only when it is realistic. In this example, the nurse might quickly ascertain that the patient's question emanates from a need for specific information—about diagnosis and prognosis from the physician, about the physiology of the dying process from the nurse, or perhaps about financial implications for the family from the social worker. The chaplain may also be called to talk with the patient about existential concerns.

As a member of the interdisciplinary team caring for the patient at the end of life, the nurse plays an important role in facilitating the team's understanding of the patient's values and preferences, family dynamics concerning decision making, and the patient's and family's response to treatment and changing health status. Many dilemmas in patient care at the end of life are related to poor communication between team members and the patient and family, as well as to failure of team members to communicate with one another effectively. Regardless of the care setting, the nurse can ensure a proactive approach to the psychosocial care of the patient and family. Periodic, structured assessments provide an opportunity for all parties to consider their priorities and plan for an uncertain future. The nurse can help the patient and family clarify their values and preferences concerning end-of-life care by using a structured approach. Sufficient time must be devoted to each step so that the patient and family have time to process new information, formulate questions, and consider their options. The nurse may need to plan several meetings to accomplish the steps described in Chart 16-5.

Providing Culturally Sensitive Care at the End of Life

Although death, grief, and mourning are universally accepted aspects of living, the values, expectations, and practices during serious illness as death approaches and after death are culturally bound and expressed. Health care providers may share similar values concerning end-of-life care and may find that they are inadequately prepared to assess for and implement care plans that support culturally diverse perspectives. Historical mistrust of the health care system and unequal access to even basic medical care may underlie the beliefs and attitudes among ethnically diverse populations (see Table 16-1). In addition, lack of education or knowledge about end-of-life care treatment options and language barriers influence decisions among many socioeconomically disadvantaged groups.

The nurse's role is to assess the values, preferences, and practices of every patient, regardless of ethnicity, socioeconomic status, or background. The nurse can share knowledge about a patient's and family's cultural beliefs and practices with the health care team and facilitate the adaptation of the care plan to accommodate these practices. For example, a nurse may find that a male patient prefers to have his eldest son make all of his care decisions. Institutional practices and laws governing informed consent are also rooted in the Western notion of autonomous decision making and informed consent. If a patient wishes to defer decisions to his son, the nurse can work with the team to negotiate informed consent, respecting the patient's right not to participate in decision making and honoring his family's cultural practice.

The nurse should assess and document the patient's and family's specific beliefs, preferences, and practices regarding end-of-life care, preparation for death, and after-death rituals. Chart 16-6 identifies topics that the nurse should cover and questions the nurse may use to elicit the information.

The nurse must use judgment and discretion about the timing and setting for eliciting this information. Some patients may wish to have a family member speak for them or may be unable to provide information because of advanced illness. The nurse should give the patient and family a context for the discussion, such as "It is very important to us to provide care that addresses your needs and the needs of your family. We want to honor and support your wishes, and want you to feel free to tell us how we are doing, and what we could do to better meet your needs. I'd like to ask you some questions; what you tell me will help me to understand and support what is most important to you at this time. You don't need to answer anything that makes you uncomfortable. Is it all right to ask some questions?" The assessment of end-of-life beliefs, preferences, and practices should be carried out in short segments over a period of time (e.g., across multiple days of an inpatient hospital stay or in conjunction with multiple patient visits to an outpatient setting or over several home care visits). The discomfort of novice nurses with asking questions and discussing this type of sensitive content can be reduced by prior practice in a classroom or clinical skills laboratory, observation of interviews conducted by experienced nurses, and partnering with experienced nurses during the first few assessments.

Goal Setting in Palliative Care at the End of Life

As treatment goals begin to shift in the direction of comfort care over aggressive disease-focused treatment, symptom relief and patient/family-defined quality of life assume greater prominence in treatment decision making. Throughout the course of the illness, and especially as the patient's functional status and symptoms indicate approaching death, the clinician should help the patient and family weigh the benefits of continued diagnostic testing and disease-focused medical treatment against the costs of those activities. The patient and family may be extremely reluctant to forego monitoring that has become routine throughout the illness (e.g., blood testing, x-rays) but that may contribute little to a primary focus on comfort. Likewise, health care providers may have difficulty discontinuing such diagnostic testing or medical treatment.

Specifically, the nurse should collaborate with other members of the interdisciplinary team to share assessment findings, develop a coordinated plan of care, and make decisions about

ASSESSMENT
Chart 16-6   Assessing End-of-Life Care Beliefs, Preferences, and Practices

Disclosure/truth telling: "Tell me how you/your family talk about very sensitive or serious matters."
- Content: "Are there any topics that you or your family are uncomfortable discussing?"
- Person responsible for disclosure: "Is there one person in the family who assumes responsibility for obtaining and sharing information?"
- Disclosure practices regarding children: "What kind of information may be shared with children in your family, and who is responsible for communicating with the children?"
- Sharing of information within the family or community group: "What kind/how much information should be shared with your immediate family? Your extended family? Others in the community (for example, members of a religious community)?"

Decision-making style: "How are decisions made in your family? Who would you like to be involved in decisions about your treatment or care?"
- Individual
- Family centered
- Family elder or patriarch/matriarch
- Deference to authority (such as the physician)

Symptom management: "How would you like us to help you to manage the physical effects of your illness?"
- Acceptability of medications used for symptom relief
- Beliefs regarding expression of pain and other symptoms
- Degree of symptom management desired

Life-sustaining treatment expectations: "Have you thought about what type of medical treatment you or your loved one would want as the end of life is nearing? Do you have

an advance directive (living will and/or durable power of attorney)?"
- Nutrition/hydration at the end of life
- Cardiopulmonary resuscitation
- Ventilator
- Dialysis
- Antibiotics
- Medications to treat infection

Desired location of dying: "Do you have a preference about being at home or in some other location when you die?"
- Desired role for family members in providing care: "Who do you want to be involved in caring for you at the end of life?"
- Gender-specific prohibitions: "Are you uncomfortable having either males or females provide your care or your loved one's personal care?"

Spiritual/religious practices and rituals: "Is there anything that we should know about your spiritual or religious beliefs about death? Are there any practices that you would like us to observe as death is nearing?"

Care of the body after the death: "Is there anything that we should know about how a body/your body should be treated after death?"

Expression of grief: "What types of losses have you and your family experienced? How do you and your family express grief?"

Funeral and burial practices: "Are there any rituals or practices associated with funerals or burial that are especially important to you?"

Mourning practices: "How have you and your family carried on after a loss in the past? Are particular behaviors or practices expected or required?"

---

diagnostic testing at the end of life (Fig. 16-2). In addition, the nurse should help the patient and family clarify their goals, expected outcomes, and values as they consider treatment options (Chart 16-7). The nurse should work with colleagues in other disciplines to ensure that the patient and family are referred for continuing psychosocial support, symptom management, and assistance with other care-related challenges (e.g., arrangements for home care or hospice support, referrals for financial assistance).

Spiritual Care

Attention to the spiritual component of the illness experienced by the patient and family is not new within the context of nursing care, yet many nurses lack the comfort or skills to assess and intervene in this dimension. **Spirituality** contains features of religiosity; however, the two concepts are not interchangeable (Puchalski, & Ferrell, 2010; Puchalski, Ferrell, Virani, et al., 2009). Spirituality includes domains such as how a person derives meaning and purpose from life, one's beliefs and faith, sources of hope, and attitudes toward death (Vachon, Fillion, & Achille, 2009). For most people, contemplating one's own death raises many issues, such as the meaning of existence, the purpose of suffering, and the existence of an afterlife. A survey on end-of-life issues conducted by the American Association of Retired Persons (AARP, 2009) revealed that although the greatest concerns among respondents were receiving honest answers from doctors

(74%) and understanding medical treatment options (64%), many also expressed spiritually themed concerns:
- Religious or spiritual comfort (37%)
- Giving to others (33%)
- Fulfilling personal goals (27%)

ASSESSMENT
Chart 16-7   Assessing the Patient and Family Perspective: Goal Setting in Palliative Care

- **Awareness of diagnosis, illness stage, and prognosis:** "Tell me your understanding of your illness right now."
- **Values:** "Tell me what is most important to you as you are thinking about the treatment options available to you/your loved one."
- **Preferences:** "You've said that being comfortable and pain free is most important to you right now. Where would you like to receive care (home, hospital, long-term care facility, doctor's office), and how can I help?"
- **Expected/desired outcomes:** "What are your hopes and expectations for this (diagnostic test [for example, CT scan] or treatment)?"
- **Benefits and burdens:** "Is there a point at which you would say that the testing or treatment is outweighed by the burdens it is causing you (for example, getting from home to the hospital, pain, nausea, fatigue, interference with other important activities)?"

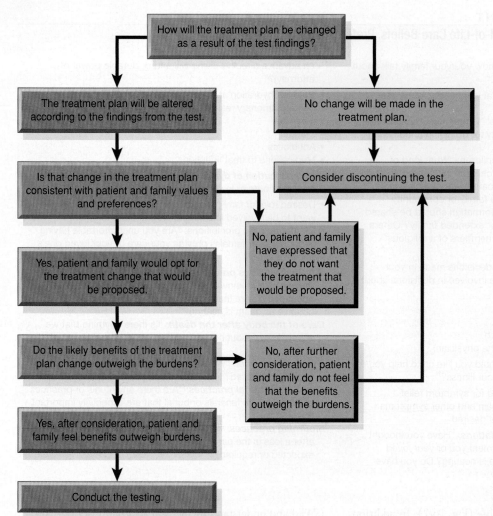

FIGURE 16-2 • An algorithm for decision making about diagnostic testing at the end of life.

The spiritual assessment is a key component of comprehensive nursing assessment for terminally ill patients and their families. Although the nursing assessment should include religious affiliation, spiritual assessment is conceptually much broader than religion and therefore is relevant regardless of a patient's expression of religious preference or affiliation. In addition to assessment of the role of religious faith and practices, important religious rituals, and connection to a religious community (see Table 16-1), the nurse should further explore:

- The harmony or discord between the patient's and the family's beliefs
- Other sources of meaning, hope, and comfort
- The presence or absence of a sense of peace of mind and purpose in life
- Spiritual or religious beliefs about illness, medical treatment, and care of the sick

A four-step spiritual assessment process using the acronym FICA involves asking the following questions (Borneman, Ferrell, & Puchalski, 2010):

- Faith and belief: Do you consider yourself to be a spiritual or religious person? What is your *faith* or belief? What gives your life meaning?
- Importance and Influence: What *importance* does faith have in your life? Have your beliefs influenced the way

you take care of yourself and your illness? What role do your beliefs play in regaining your health?
- Community: Are you a part of a spiritual or religious *community*? Is this of support to you and how? Is there a group of people you really love or who are important to you?
- Address in care: How would you like me to *address* these issues in your health care?

Hope

Clinicians and researchers have observed that although specific hopes may change over time, hope generally persists in some form across every stage of illness. In terminal illness, hope represents the patient's imagined future, forming the basis of a positive, accepting attitude and providing the patient's life with meaning, direction, and optimism. When hope is viewed in this way, it is not limited to cure of the disease; instead, it focuses on what is achievable in the time remaining. Many patients find hope in working on important relationships and creating legacies. Terminally ill patients can be extremely resilient, reconceptualizing hope repeatedly as they approach the end of life.

Numerous nurse researchers have studied the concept of hope, and they have related its presence to spirituality, quality of life, and transcendence. Hope is a multidimensional construct that provides comfort as a person endures life threats and personal challenges. The following are hope-fostering and hope-hindering activities among terminally ill hospice patients with various diagnoses:

- *Hope-fostering categories:* Love of family and friends, spirituality/faith, setting goals and maintaining independence, positive relationships with clinicians, humor, personal characteristics, and uplifting memories
- *Hope-hindering categories:* Abandonment and isolation, uncontrollable pain/discomfort, and devaluation of personhood

Nurses can support hope for the patient and family by using effective listening and communication skills, thus encouraging realistic hope that is specific to their needs for information, expectations for the future, and values and preferences concerning the end of life. Nurses must engage in self-reflection and identify their own biases and fears concerning illness, life, and death. As nurses becomes more skilled in working with seriously ill patients, they can become less determined to "fix" and more willing to listen; more comfortable with silence, grief, anger, and sadness; and more fully present with patients and their families.

Nursing interventions for enabling and supporting hope include the following:

- Listening attentively
- Encouraging sharing of feelings
- Providing accurate information
- Encouraging and supporting the patients' control over their circumstances, choices, and environment whenever possible
- Assisting patients to explore ways for finding meaning in their lives
- Encouraging realistic goals
- Facilitating effective communication within families
- Making referrals for psychosocial and spiritual counseling
- Assisting with the development of supports in the home or community when none exist

Managing Physiologic Responses to Terminal Illness

Patients approaching the end of life experience many of the same symptoms, regardless of their underlying disease processes. Symptoms in terminal illness may be caused by the disease, either directly (e.g., dyspnea owing to chronic obstructive lung disease) or indirectly (e.g., nausea and vomiting related to pressure in the gastric area), by the treatment for the disease, or by a coexisting disorder that is unrelated to the disease. Symptoms should be carefully and systematically assessed and managed. Questions that guide the assessment of symptoms are listed in Chart 16-8.

The patient's goals should guide symptom management. Medical interventions may be aimed at treating the underlying causes of the symptoms or reducing the impact of symptoms. For example, a medical intervention such as thoracentesis (an invasive procedure in which fluid is drained from the pleural space) may be performed to temporarily relieve dyspnea in a patient with pleural effusion secondary to lung cancer. Pharmacologic and nonpharmacologic methods of symptom management may be used in combination with

---

Chart 16-8

ASSESSMENT

Assessing Symptoms Associated With Terminal Illness

- How is this symptom affecting the patient's life?
- What is the meaning of the symptom to the patient? To the family?
- How does the symptom affect physical functioning, mobility, comfort, sleep, nutritional status, elimination, activity level, and relationships with others?
- What makes the symptom better?
- What makes it worse?
- Is it worse at any particular time of the day?
- What are the patient's expectations and goals for managing the symptom? The family's expectations?
- How is the patient coping with the symptom?
- What is the economic effect of the symptom and its management?

Adapted from Jacox, A., Carr, D. B., & Payne, R. (1994). *Management of cancer pain.* Rockville, MD: Agency for Health Care Policy and Research.

---

medical interventions to modify the physiologic causes of symptoms. In addition, pharmacologic management with low-dose oral morphine effectively relieves dyspnea (Kamal, McGuire, Wheeler, et al., 2012), and guided relaxation may reduce the anxiety associated with the sensation of breathlessness. As is true with pain, the principles of pharmacologic symptom management are the use of the smallest dose of the medication to achieve the desired effect, avoidance of polypharmacy, anticipation and management of adverse effects, and creation of a therapeutic regimen that is acceptable to the patient based on his or her goals for maximizing quality of life.

The patient's goals take precedence over the clinicians' goals. Although clinicians may believe that symptoms must be completely relieved whenever possible, the patient might choose instead to decrease symptoms to a tolerable level rather than to relieve them completely if the side effects of medications are unacceptable to him or her. This often allows the patient to have greater independence, mobility, and alertness and to devote attention to issues that he or she considers of higher priority and greater importance.

Anticipating and planning interventions for symptoms is a cornerstone of end-of-life care. Patients and family members cope more effectively with new symptoms and exacerbations of existing symptoms when they know what to expect and how to manage them. Hospice programs typically provide "emergency kits" containing ready-to-administer doses of various medications that are useful to treat symptoms in advanced illness. For example, a kit might contain small doses of oral morphine liquid for pain or shortness of breath, a benzodiazepine for restlessness, and an acetaminophen suppository for fever. Family members can be instructed to administer a prescribed dose from the emergency kit, often avoiding prolonged suffering for the patient as well as rehospitalization for symptom management.

Pain

In the final stages of illnesses such as cancer, AIDS, heart disease, COPD, and renal disease, pain and other symptoms are common. Pain results from the diseases as well as the modalities used to treat them. In a study of community-dwelling older adults, researchers found that the prevalence of pain was 46% in the last 4 months of life (Smith, Cenzer, Knight, et al., 2010). Chapter 12 presents the importance of pain assessment, assessment principles for pain that include identifying the effect of the pain on the patient's life, and the importance of believing the patient's report of the pain and its effect. Although the means to relieve pain have existed for many years, the continued, pervasive undertreatment of pain has been well documented. Poorly managed pain affects the psychological, emotional, social, and financial well-being of patients. Despite studies demonstrating the negative effects of inadequate pain management, practice has been slow to change (Institute of Medicine, 2011).

Patients who are receiving an established regimen of analgesics should continue to receive those medications as they approach the end of life. Inability to communicate pain should not be equated with the absence of pain. (See the Nursing Research Profile presented in Chart 16-9.) Although most pain can be managed effectively using the oral route, as the end of life nears, patients may be less able to swallow oral medications due to somnolence or nausea. Patients who have been receiving opioids should continue to receive equianalgesic doses via rectal or sublingual routes. Concentrated morphine solution can be effectively delivered by the sublingual route, because the small liquid volume is well tolerated even if swallowing is not possible. As long as the patient continues to receive opioids, a regimen to combat constipation must be implemented. If the patient cannot swallow laxatives or stool softeners, rectal suppositories or enemas may be necessary.

The nurse should educate the family about continuation of comfort measures as the patient approaches the end of life, how to administer analgesics via alternative routes, and how to assess for pain when the patient cannot verbally report pain intensity. Because the analgesics administered orally or rectally are short acting and typically scheduled as frequently as every 3 to 4 hours around the clock, there is always a strong possibility that a patient approaching the end of life will die in close proximity to the time of analgesic administration. If the patient is at home, family members administering analgesics should be prepared for this possibility. They need reassurance that they did not "cause" the death of the patient by administering a dose of analgesic medication.

Dyspnea

Dyspnea is an uncomfortable awareness of breathing that is common in patients approaching the end of life. A highly subjective symptom, dyspnea often is not associated with visible signs of distress, such as tachypnea, diaphoresis, or cyanosis. Patients with primary lung tumors, lung metastases, pleural effusion, restrictive lung disease, and advanced heart disease may experience significant dyspnea (Mahler, Selecky, Harrod, et al., 2010). Although the underlying cause of the dyspnea can be identified and treated in some cases, the burdens of additional diagnostic evaluation and treatment aimed at the physiologic problem may outweigh the benefits. The treatment of dyspnea varies depending on the patient's general physical condition and imminence of death. For example, a blood transfusion may provide temporary symptom relief for a patient with anemia earlier in the disease process; however, as the patient approaches the end of life, the benefits are typically short-lived or absent.

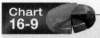

Chart 16-9

NURSING RESEARCH PROFILE
Assessing Pain in Nonresponsive Hospice Patients

McGuire, D. B., Reifsnyder, J., Soeken, K., et al. (2011). Assessing pain in non-responsive hospice patients: Development and preliminary testing of the Multidimensional Objective Pain Assessment Tool. *Journal of Palliative Medicine, 14*(3), 287–292.

Purpose

Pain is a subjective experience that is best assessed by way of patient self-report. For those patients who cannot self-report due to underlying medical conditions, disease progression, or other medical treatment, pain may not be assessed systematically or adequately. The purpose of this series of studies was to develop and refine an instrument to measure pain through observation and to evaluate the validity, reliability, and clinical utility of the Multidimensional Objective Pain Assessment Tool (MOPAT). Such research is needed so that accurate assessment and effective interventions can be developed for this group of patients.

Design

In a series of several small studies, researchers first engaged focus groups of hospice nurses to adapt an existing objective pain measure, tested the resulting measure (MOPAT) with a sample of cognitively impaired and alert/oriented hospice inpatients, and in subsequent studies evaluated the MOPAT's validity and reliability and nurses' perceptions of clinical utility.

Findings

Researchers found support for two subscales (behavioral and physiologic) and that the subscales yielded scores that changed significantly when used to assess pain before and after a pain-relieving intervention. This finding demonstrates that the instrument is sensitive to changes in pain. Nearly all hospice nurses rated the MOPAT as easy to use and feasible in daily practice.

Nursing Implications

Across all settings where health care is delivered, nurses assess and respond to pain. Pain is a subjective experience—that is, the patient is the expert concerning his or her own pain level and response to intervention. Pain has been recognized as the "fifth vital sign," and nurses are accustomed to eliciting pain intensity scores during their assessments. To date, there has been no instrument that nurses could use to systematically assess pain with populations of palliative care patients who cannot self-report. The risk to such patients is underappreciation and undertreatment of pain, leading to unnecessary suffering. This series of studies establishes the MOPAT as a valid, reliable, and feasible pain instrument that nurses can adopt to improve and standardize pain measurement—assuring that pain evaluations are consistent across nurses and across settings and that patients' responses to pain interventions are documented and used to guide practice.

Nursing Assessment

As with assessment of pain, reports of dyspnea by patients must be believed. As is true for physical pain, the meaning of dyspnea to an individual patient may increase his or her suffering. For example, the patient may interpret increasing dyspnea as a sign that death is approaching. For some patients, sensations of breathlessness may invoke frightening images of drowning or suffocation, and the resulting cycle of fear and anxiety may increase the sensation of breathlessness. Therefore, the nurse should conduct a careful assessment of the psychosocial and spiritual components of the dyspnea. Physical assessment parameters include symptom intensity, distress, and interference with activities; auscultation of lung sounds; assessment of fluid balance, including measurement of dependent edema (circumference of lower extremities) and abdominal girth; temperature; skin color; sputum quantity and character; and cough.

To determine the intensity of dyspnea and its interference with daily activities, the patient can be asked to report the severity of the dyspnea using a scale of 0 to 10, where 0 is no dyspnea and 10 is the worst imaginable dyspnea. The nurse should assess the patient's baseline rating before treatment and should elicit subsequent measurements taken during exacerbation of the symptom, periodically during treatment, and whenever the treatment plan changes; these parameters provide ongoing objective evidence for the efficacy of the treatment plan. In addition, physical assessment findings may assist in locating the source of the dyspnea and selecting nursing interventions to relieve the symptom. The components of the assessment change as the patient's condition changes. For example, when the patient who has been on daily weights can no longer get out of bed, the goal of comfort may outweigh the benefit of continued weights. Like other symptoms at the end of life, dyspnea can be managed effectively in the absence of assessment and diagnostic data (e.g., arterial blood gases) that are standard when a patient's illness or symptom is acute and considered reversible.

Concept Mastery Alert

Dyspnea is a subjective finding, as is pain. Therefore, a numeric rating scale similar to one that is used for assessing pain provides objective evidence of the severity of the patient's dyspnea.

Nursing Management

Nursing management of dyspnea at the end of life is directed toward administering medical treatment for the underlying pathology, monitoring the patient's response to treatment, helping the patient and family manage anxiety (which exacerbates dyspnea), altering the perception of the symptom, and conserving energy (Chart 16-10). Pharmacologic intervention is aimed at modifying lung physiology and improving performance as well as altering the perception of the symptom. Bronchodilators and corticosteroids are used to treat underlying obstructive pathology, thereby improving overall lung function. Low doses of opioids effectively relieve dyspnea, although the mechanism of relief is not entirely clear. Although dyspnea in terminal illness is typically not associated with diminished blood oxygen saturation, low-flow oxy-

---

Chart 16-10 Palliative Nursing Interventions for Dyspnea

Decrease Anxiety

- Administer prescribed anxiolytic medications as indicated for anxiety or panic associated with dyspnea.
- Assist with relaxation techniques, guided imagery.
- Provide patient with a means to call for assistance (call bell/light within reach in a hospital or long-term care facility; handheld bell or other device for home).

Treat Underlying Pathology

- Administer prescribed bronchodilators and corticosteroids (obstructive pathology).
- Administer blood products, erythropoietin as prescribed (typically not beneficial in advanced disease).
- Administer prescribed diuretics and monitor fluid balance.

Alter Perception of Breathlessness

- Administer prescribed oxygen therapy via nasal cannula, if tolerated; masks may not be well tolerated.
- Administer prescribed low-dose opioids via oral route (morphine sulfate is used most commonly).
- Provide air movement in the patient's environment with a portable fan.

Reduce Respiratory Demand

- Educate patient and family to implement energy conservation measures.
- Place needed equipment, supplies, and nourishment within reach.
- For home or hospice care, offer bedside commode, electric bed (with head that elevates).

---

gen often provides psychological comfort to both patients and families, particularly in the home setting.

As mentioned previously, dyspnea may be exacerbated by anxiety, and anxiety may trigger episodes of dyspnea, setting off a respiratory crisis in which the patient and family may panic. For patients receiving care at home, patient and family education should include anticipation and management of crisis situations and a clearly communicated emergency plan. The patient and family should be instructed about medication administration, condition changes that should be reported to the physician and nurse, and strategies for coping with diminished reserves and increasing symptomatology as the disease progresses. The patient and family require reassurance that the symptom can be effectively managed at home without the need for activation of the emergency medical services or hospitalization and that a nurse will be available at all times via telephone and to make a visit.

Nutrition and Hydration at the End of Life

Anorexia and cachexia are common in the seriously ill. The profound changes in the patient's appearance and a lack of interest in the socially important rituals of mealtime are particularly disturbing to families. The approach to the problem varies depending on the patient's stage of illness, level of disability associated with the illness, and desires. The anorexia–cachexia syndrome is characterized by disturbances in carbohydrate, protein, and fat metabolism; endocrine dysfunction;

and anemia. The syndrome results in severe asthenia (loss of energy).

Anorexia and cachexia differ from starvation (simple food deprivation) in several important ways. Appetite is lost early in the process, the body becomes catabolic in a dysfunctional way, and supplementation by gastric feeding (tube feeding) or parenteral nutrition in advanced disease does not replenish lean body mass that has been lost.

Anorexia

Although causes of anorexia may be controlled for a period of time, progressive anorexia is an expected and natural part of the dying process. Anorexia may be related to or exacerbated by situational variables (e.g., the ability to have meals with the family vs. eating alone in the "sick room"), progression of the disease, treatment for the disease, or psychological distress. The patient and family should be instructed in strategies to manage the variables associated with anorexia (Table 16-2).

Use of Pharmacologic Agents to Stimulate Appetite. Several pharmacologic agents are commonly used to stimulate appetite in patients with anorexia. These include dexamethasone (Decadron), megestrol acetate (Megace), and dronabinol (Marinol). Although these agents may result in temporary weight gain, their use is not associated with an increase in lean body mass in terminally ill patients. Therapy should be tapered or discontinued after 4 to 8 weeks if there is no response (Wrede-Seaman, 2008).

Dexamethasone initially increases appetite and may provide short-term weight gain in some patients. It should be considered for those patients whose life expectancy is less than 6 weeks because the beneficial effects may be limited to the first few weeks of therapy and side effects increase over time (Del Fabbro, Dalal, & Bruera, 2006). Therapy may need to be discontinued in patients with a longer life expectancy; after 3 to 4 weeks, corticosteroids interfere with the synthesis of muscle protein.

Megestrol acetate produces temporary weight gain of primarily fatty tissue, with little effect on protein balance. Because of the time required to see any effect from this agent, therapy should not be initiated if life expectancy is less than 30 days. With long-term use, megestrol acetate may have fewer side effects than dexamethasone (Del Fabbro et al., 2006).

Dronabinol is a psychoactive compound found in cannabis that may be helpful in reducing nausea and vomiting, appetite loss, pain, and anxiety, thereby improving food and fluid intake in some patients. However, in most patients, it is not as effective as other agents for appetite stimulation. Although dronabinol may have beneficial effects on appetite in patients with advanced cancer, it has not been shown

---

TABLE 16-2 Measures for Managing Anorexia

Nursing Interventions	Patient and Family Education Tips
Initiate measures to ensure adequate dietary intake without adding stress to the patient at mealtimes.	Reduce the focus on "balanced" meals; offer the same food as often as the patient desires it.
Assess the impact of medications (e.g., chemotherapy, antiretrovirals) or other therapies (radiation therapy, dialysis) that are being used to treat the underlying illness.	Increase the nutritional value of meals. For example, add dry milk powder to milk, and use this fortified milk to prepare cream soups, milkshakes, and gravies.
Administer and monitor effects of prescribed treatment for nausea, vomiting, and delayed gastric emptying.	
Encourage patient to eat when effects of medications have subsided.	Allow and encourage the patient to eat when hungry, regardless of usual mealtimes.
Assess and modify environment to eliminate unpleasant odors and other factors that cause nausea, vomiting, and anorexia.	Eliminate or reduce noxious cooking odors, pet odors, or other odors that may precipitate nausea, vomiting, or anorexia.
Remove items that may reduce appetite (soiled tissues, bedpans, emesis basins, clutter).	Keep patient's environment clean, uncluttered, and comfortable.
Assess and manage anxiety and depression to the extent possible.	Make mealtime a shared experience away from the "sick" room whenever possible.
	Reduce stress at mealtimes.
	Avoid confrontations about the amount of food consumed.
	Reduce or eliminate routine weighing of the patient.
Position to enhance gastric emptying.	Encourage patient to eat in a sitting position; elevate the head of the patient's bed.
	Plan meals (food selection and portion size) that the patient desires.
	Provide small frequent meals if they are easier for patient to eat.
Assess for constipation and/or intestinal obstruction.	Ensure that patient and family understand that prevention of constipation is essential, even when the patient's intake is minimal.
Prevent and manage constipation on an ongoing basis, even when the patient's intake is minimal.	Encourage adequate fluid intake, dietary fiber, and the use of a bowel program to prevent constipation.
Provide frequent mouth care, particularly following nourishment.	Assist the patient to rinse after every meal. Avoid mouthwashes that contain alcohol or glycerine, which dry mucous membranes.
Ensure that dentures fit properly.	Weight loss may cause dentures to loosen and cause irritation. Remove them to inspect the gums and to provide oral care.
Administer and monitor effects of topical and systemic treatment for oropharyngeal pain.	The patient's comfort may be enhanced if medications for pain relief given on an as-needed basis for breakthrough pain are administered before mealtimes.

to be more effective than megestrol. In addition, it possesses undesirable central nervous system side effects (Del Fabbro et al., 2006).

Cachexia

Cachexia refers to severe muscle wasting and weight loss associated with illness. Although anorexia may exacerbate cachexia, it is not the primary cause. Cachexia is associated with anabolic and catabolic changes in metabolism that relate to activity of neurohormones and proinflammatory cytokines, resulting in profound protein loss. These processes appear to be similar at the end stages of both cancer and some noncancerous illnesses, such as heart disease (Siddiqui, Pandya, Harvey, et al., 2006; Von Haehling, Doehner, & Anker, 2007). However, the pathophysiology of cachexia in terminal illness is not well understood. In terminal illness, the severity of tissue wasting is greater than would be expected from reduced food intake alone, and typically increasing appetite or food intake does not reverse cachexia.

At one time, it was believed that cancer patients with rapidly growing tumors developed cachexia because the tumor created an excessive nutritional demand and diverted nutrients from the rest of the body. Research links cytokines produced by the body in response to a tumor to a complex inflammatory-immune response present in patients whose tumors have metastasized, leading to anorexia, weight loss, and altered metabolism. An increase in cytokines occurs not only in cancer but also in AIDS and many other chronic diseases (Del Fabbro et al., 2006).

Artificial Nutrition and Hydration

Along with breathing, eating and drinking are essential to survival throughout life. Near the end of life, the body's nutritional needs change, and the desire for food and fluid may diminish. People may no longer be able to use, eliminate, or store nutrients and fluids adequately. Eating and sharing meals are important social activities in families and communities, and food preparation and enjoyment are linked to happy memories, strong emotions, and hope for survival. For patients with serious illness, food preparation and mealtimes often become battlegrounds in which well-meaning family members argue, plead, and cajole to encourage ill people to eat. Seriously ill patients often lose their appetites entirely, develop strong aversions to foods that they have enjoyed in the past, or crave a particular food to the exclusion of all other foods.

Although nutritional supplementation may be an important part of the treatment plan in early or chronic illness, unintended weight loss and dehydration are expected characteristics of progressive illness. As illness progresses, patients, families, and clinicians may believe that without artificial nutrition and hydration, terminally ill patients will "starve," causing profound suffering and hastened death. However, starvation should not be viewed as the failure to insert tubes for nutritional supplementation or hydration of terminally ill patients with irreversible progression of disease. Research has demonstrated that terminally ill patients with cancer who were hydrated did not have improved biochemical parameters and exhibited lower serum albumin levels, leading to fluid retention. The use of artificial nutrition and hydration (tube and intravenous [IV] fluids and feeding) carry consid-

erable risks and do not contribute to comfort at end of life (Casarett, Kapo, & Kaplan, 2005). Similarly, survival is not increased when terminally ill patients with advanced dementia receive enteral feeding, and no data support an association between tube feeding and improved quality of life in these patients (Mitchell, Black, Ersek, et al., 2012). Furthermore, in patients who are close to death, symptoms associated with dehydration such as dry mouth, confusion, and diminished alertness are common and typically do not respond to artificial nutrition. Dry mouth can generally be managed through nursing measures such as mouth care and environmental changes with medications to diminish confusion.

As the patient approaches the end of life, the family and health care providers should offer the patient what he or she prefers and can most easily tolerate. The nurse should instruct the family how to separate feeding from caring, demonstrating love, sharing, and caring by being with the loved one in other ways. Preoccupation with appetite, feeding, and weight loss diverts energy and time that the patient and family could use in other meaningful activities. In addition to those given in Table 16-2, the following are tips to promote nutrition for terminally ill patients:

- Offer small portions of favorite foods.
- Be aware that cool foods may be better tolerated than hot foods.
- Offer cheese, eggs, peanut butter, mild fish, chicken, or turkey. Meat (especially beef) may taste bitter and unpleasant.
- Add milk shakes, meal replacement drinks, or other liquid supplements.
- Place nutritious foods at the bedside (fruit juices, milk shakes in insulated drink containers with straws).
- Schedule meals when family members can be present to provide company and stimulation.
- Offer ice chips made from frozen fruit juices.
- Allow the patient to refuse foods and fluids.

Delirium

Many patients remain alert, arousable, and able to communicate until very close to death. Others sleep for long intervals and awaken only intermittently, with eventual somnolence until death. Delirium refers to concurrent disturbances in level of consciousness, psychomotor behavior, memory, thinking, attention, and sleep–wake cycle (Breibart & Alici, 2008). In some patients, a period of agitated delirium precedes death, sometimes causing families to be hopeful that suddenly active patients may be getting better. Confusion may be related to underlying, treatable conditions such as medication side effects or interactions, pain or discomfort, hypoxia or dyspnea, or a full bladder or impacted stool. In patients with cancer, confusion may be secondary to brain metastases. Delirium may also be related to metabolic changes, infection, and organ failure.

Patients with delirium may become hypoactive or hyperactive, restless, irritable, and fearful. Sleep deprivation and hallucinations may occur. If treatment of the underlying factors contributing to these symptoms brings no relief, a combination of pharmacologic intervention with neuroleptics or benzodiazepines may be effective in decreasing distressing symptoms. Haloperidol (Haldol) may reduce hallucinations and agitation. Benzodiazepines (e.g., lorazepam [Ativan]) can reduce anxiety but may contribute to worsening cognitive impairment if used alone.

Nursing interventions are aimed at identifying the underlying causes of delirium; acknowledging the family's distress over its occurrence; reassuring family members about what is normal; educating family members how to interact with and ensure safety for the patient with delirium; and monitoring the effects of medications used to treat severe agitation, paranoia, and fear. Confusion may mask the patient's unmet spiritual needs and fears about dying. Spiritual intervention, music therapy, gentle massage, and therapeutic touch may provide some relief. Reduction of environmental stimuli, avoidance of harsh lighting or very dim lighting (which may produce disturbing shadows), presence of familiar faces, and gentle reorientation and reassurance are also helpful.

Depression

Clinical depression should neither be accepted as an inevitable consequence of dying nor confused with sadness and anticipatory grieving, which are normal reactions to the losses associated with impending death. Emotional and spiritual support and control of disturbing physical symptoms are appropriate interventions for situational depression associated with terminal illness. Researchers have linked the psychological effects of cancer pain to suicidal thought and, less frequently, to carrying out a planned suicide (Robson, Scrutton, Wilkinson, et al., 2010). Patients and their families must be given space and time to experience sadness and to grieve; however, patients should not have to endure untreated depression at the end of their lives. An effective combined approach to clinical depression includes relief of physical symptoms, attention to emotional and spiritual distress, and pharmacologic intervention with psychostimulants, selective serotonin reuptake inhibitors, and tricyclic antidepressants (Lorenz, Lynn, Dy, et al., 2008).

Palliative Sedation at the End of Life

Effective control of symptoms can be achieved under most conditions; however, some patients may experience distressing, intractable symptoms. Although **palliative sedation** remains controversial, it is offered in some settings to patients who are close to death or who have symptoms that do not respond to conventional pharmacologic and nonpharmacologic approaches, resulting in unrelieved suffering. Palliative sedation is distinguished from **euthanasia** and physician-assisted suicide in that the intent of palliative sedation is to relieve symptoms, not to hasten death. Palliative sedation is most commonly used when the patient exhibits intractable pain, dyspnea, seizures, or delirium, and it is generally considered appropriate in only the most difficult situations. Before implementing palliative sedation, the health care team should assess for the presence of underlying and treatable causes of suffering, such as depression or spiritual distress. Finally, the patient and family should be fully informed about the use of this treatment and alternatives. Whereas proportionate palliative sedation uses the minimum drug necessary to relieve the symptom while preserving consciousness, palliative sedation induces unconsciousness, which is more controversial (Quill, Lo, Brock, et al., 2009).

Palliative sedation is accomplished through infusions of haloperidol, midazolam (or other benzodiazepine), phenobarbital, ketamine, and chlorpromazine (Thorazine) (McWilliams, Keeley, & Waterhouse, 2010) in doses adequate to eliminate signs of discomfort and, in some cases, induce sleep. For refractory symptoms, the anesthetic propofol (Diprivan) has been used successfully in some instances. Nurses act as collaborating members of the interdisciplinary health care team, providing emotional support to patients and families, facilitating clarification of values and preferences, and providing comfort-focused physical care. Once sedation has been induced, the nurse should continue to comfort the patient, monitor the physiologic effects of the sedation, support the family during the final hours or days of their loved one's life, and ensure communication within the health care team and between the team and family.

Nursing Care of Patients Who Are Close to Death

Providing care to patients who are close to death and being present at the time of death can be one of the most rewarding experiences a nurse can have. Patients and their families are understandably fearful of the unknown, and the approach of death may prompt new concerns or cause previous fears or issues to resurface. Family members who have always had difficulty communicating or who are part of families in which there are old resentments and hurts may experience heightened difficulty as their loved one nears death. However, the time at the end of life can also afford opportunities to resolve old hurts and learn new ways of being a family. Regardless of the setting, skilled practitioners can make dying patients comfortable, make space for their loved ones to remain present if they wish, and can give family members the opportunity to experience growth and healing. Likewise, patients and family members may be less apprehensive near the time of death if they know what to expect and how to respond.

Expected Physiologic Changes

As death approaches and organ systems begin to fail, observable, expected changes in the body take place. Nursing care measures aimed at patient comfort, such as pain medications (administered rectally or sublingually), turning, mouth care, eye care, positioning to facilitate draining of secretions, and measures to protect the skin from urine or feces (if the patient is incontinent), should be continued. The nurse should consult with the physician about discontinuing measures that no longer contribute to patient comfort, such as drawing blood, administering tube feedings, suctioning (in most cases), and invasive monitoring. The nurse should prepare the family for the normal, expected changes that accompany the period immediately preceding death. Although the exact time of death cannot be predicted, it is often possible to identify when the patient is very close to death. Hospice programs frequently provide written information for families so they know what to expect and what to do as death nears (Chart 16-11).

If family members have been prepared for the time of death, they are less likely to panic and are better able to be with their

Chart 16-11 Educating the Family: Signs of Approaching Death

The person shows less interest in eating and drinking. For many patients, refusal of food is an indication that they are ready to die. Fluid intake may be limited to that which will keep their mouths from feeling too dry.

- *What you can do:* Offer, but do not force, fluids and medication. Sometimes pain or other symptoms that have required medication in the past may no longer be present. For most patients, pain medications are still needed, and they can be provided by concentrated oral solutions placed under the tongue or by rectal suppository.

Urinary output may decrease in amount and frequency.

- *What you can do:* No response is needed unless the patient expresses a desire to urinate and cannot. Call the hospice nurse for advice if you are not sure.

As the body weakens, the patient will sleep more and begin to detach from the environment. He or she may refuse your attempts to provide comfort.

- *What you can do:* Allow your loved one to sleep. You may wish to sit with him or her, play soft music, or hold hands. Your loved one's withdrawal is normal and is not a rejection of your love.

Mental confusion may become apparent. This occurs because less oxygen is available to supply the brain. The patient may report strange dreams or visions.

- *What you can do:* As he or she awakens from sleep, remind him or her of the day and time, where he or she is, and who is present. This is best done in a casual, conversational way.

Vision and hearing may become somewhat impaired, and speech may be difficult to understand.

- *What you can do:* Speak clearly but no more loudly than necessary. Keep the room as light as the patient wishes, even at night. Carry on all conversations as if they can be heard, because hearing may be the last of the senses to cease functioning.
- Many patients are able to talk until minutes before death and are reassured by the exchange of a few words with a loved one.

Secretions may collect in the back of the throat and rattle or gurgle as the patient breathes though the mouth. He or she may try to cough, and his or her mouth may become dry and encrusted with secretions.

- *What you can do:* If the patient is trying to cough up secretions and is experiencing choking or vomiting, call the hospice nurse for assistance.
- Secretions may drain from the mouth if you place the patient on his or her side and provide support with pillows.

- Cleansing the mouth with moistened mouth swabs will help to relieve the dryness that occurs with mouth breathing.
- Offer water in small amounts to keep the mouth moist. A straw with one finger placed over the end can be used to transfer sips of water to the patient's mouth.

Breathing may become irregular with periods of no breathing (apnea). The patient may be working very hard to breathe and may make a moaning sound with each breath. As the time of death nears, the breathing remains irregular and may become more shallow and mechanical.

- *What you can do:* Raising the head of the bed may help the patient to breathe more easily. The moaning sound does not mean that the patient is in pain or other distress; it is the sound of air passing over very relaxed vocal cords.

As the oxygen supply to the brain decreases, the patient may become restless. It is not unusual to pull at the bed linens, to have visual hallucinations, or even to try to get out of bed at this point.

- *What you can do:* Reassure the patient in a calm voice that you are there. Prevent him or her from falling by trying to get out of bed. Soft music or a back rub may be soothing.

The patient may feel hot one moment and cold the next as the body loses its ability to control temperature. As circulation slows, the arms and legs may become cool and bluish. The underside of the body may darken. It may be difficult to feel a pulse at the wrist.

- *What you can do:* Provide and remove blankets as needed. Avoid using electric blankets, which may cause burns because the patient cannot tell you if he or she is too warm.
- Sponge the patient's head with a cool cloth if this provides comfort.

Loss of bladder and bowel control may occur around the time of death.

- *What you can do:* Protect the mattress with waterproof padding, and change the padding as needed to keep the patient comfortable.

As people approach death, many times they report seeing gardens, libraries, or family or friends who have died. They may ask you to pack their bags and find tickets or a passport. Sometimes they may become insistent and attempt to do these chores themselves. They may try getting out of bed (even if they have been confined to bed for a long time) so that they can "leave."

- *What you can do:* Reassure the patient that it is all right; he or she can "go" without getting out of bed. Stay close, share stories, and be present.

Used with permission from the Hospice of Philadelphia. Hospice and Palliative Nurses Association. (2011). *HPNA position statement: Legalization of assisted suicide*. Available at: www.hpna.org/DisplayPage.aspx?Title=Position%20Statements

loved one in a meaningful way. Noisy, gurgling breathing or moaning is generally most distressing to family members. In most cases, the sounds of breathing at the end of life are related to oropharyngeal relaxation and diminished awareness. Family members may have difficulty believing that the patient is not in pain or that the patient's breathing could not be improved by suctioning secretions. Patient positioning and family reassurance are the most helpful responses to these symptoms.

When death is imminent, patients may become increasingly somnolent and unable to clear sputum or oral secretions, which may lead to further impairment of breathing from pooled or dried and crusted secretions. The sound (terminal bubbling) and appearance of the secretions are often more distressing to family members than is the presence of

the secretions to the patient. Family distress over the changes in the patient's condition may be eased by supportive nursing care. Continuation of comfort-focused interventions and reassurance that the patient is not in any distress can do much to ease family concerns. Gentle mouth care with a moistened swab or very soft toothbrush helps maintain the integrity of the patient's mucous membranes. In addition, gentle oral suctioning, positioning to enhance drainage of secretions, and sublingual or transdermal administration of anticholinergic drugs (Table 16-3) reduce the production of secretions and provide comfort to the patient and support to the family. Deeper suctioning may cause significant discomfort to the dying patient and is rarely of any benefit because secretions reaccumulate rapidly.

TABLE 16-3	**Pharmacologic Management of Excess Oral/Respiratory Secretions When Death Is Imminent**
Medication	**Dose**
Atropine ophthalmic 1%	1 to 2 drops PO/SL every 4 to 6 hours ATC or PRN
Atropine solution for injection	0.4 mg to 0.6 mg IV/IM/SC every 4 to 6 hours ATC or PRN
Glycopyrrolate	1 mg to 2 mg PO every 8 hours ATC or PRN
Hyoscyamine regular release	0.125 mg to 0.25 mg PO/SL every 4 to 6 hours ATC or PRN
Hyoscyamine ER	0.375 mg PO every 12 hours
Scopolamine, transdermal patch (TRANSDERM SCOP®)	Apply 1 to 3 patches behind the ear every 3 days

PO, by mouth; SL, sublingually; ATC, around the clock; PRN, as needed; IV, intravenously; IM, intramuscularly; SC, subcutaneously; ER, extended-release.
Table reprinted with permission from excelleRx, Inc. (2010). *Hospice Pharmacia Medication Use Guidelines* (10th ed.). Philadelphia: Author.

The Death Vigil

Although each death is unique, it is often possible for experienced clinicians to assess that the patient is "actively" or imminently dying and to prepare the family in the final days or hours leading to death. As death nears, the patient may withdraw, sleep for longer intervals, or become somnolent. Death is generally preceded by a period of gradual diminishment of bodily functions, increased intervals between respirations, a weakened and irregular pulse, diminished blood pressure, and skin color changes or mottling. Family members should be encouraged to be with the patient, to speak and reassure the patient of their presence, to stroke or touch the patient, or to lie alongside the patient (even in the hospital or long-term care facility) if the family members are comfortable with this degree of closeness and can do so without causing discomfort to the patient.

The family may go to great lengths to ensure that their loved one will not die alone. However, despite the best intentions and efforts of the family and clinicians, the patient may die at a time when no one is present. In any setting, it is unrealistic for family members to be at the patient's bedside 24 hours a day. Experienced hospice clinicians have observed and reported that some patients appear to "wait" until family members are away from the bedside to die, perhaps to spare their loved ones the pain of being present at the time of death. Nurses can reassure family members throughout the death vigil by being present intermittently or continuously, modeling behaviors (such as touching and speaking to the patient), providing encouragement in relation to family caregiving, providing reassurance about normal physiologic changes, and encouraging family rest breaks. If a patient dies while family members are away from the bedside, they may express feelings of guilt and profound grief and may need emotional support.

After-Death Care

For patients who have received adequate management of symptoms and for families who have received adequate preparation and support, the actual time of death is commonly peaceful and occurs without struggle. Nurses may or may not be present at the time of a patient's death. In many states, nurses are authorized to make the pronouncement of death and sign the death certificate when death is expected. The determination of death is made through a physical examination that includes auscultation for the absence of breathing and heart sounds. Home care or hospice programs in which nurses make the time-of-death visit and pronounce death have policies and procedures to guide the nurse's actions during this visit. Immediately on cessation of vital functions, the body begins to change. It becomes dusky or bluish, waxen appearing, and cool; blood darkens and pools in dependent areas of the body (e.g., the back and sacrum if the body is in a supine position); and urine and stool may be evacuated.

Immediately after death, family members should be allowed and encouraged to spend time with the deceased. Normal responses of family members at the time of death vary widely and range from quiet expressions of grief to overt expressions that include wailing and prostration. The family's desire for privacy during their time with the deceased should be honored. Family members may wish to independently manage or assist with care of the body after death. In the home, after-death care of the body frequently includes culturally specific rituals such as bathing the body. Home care agencies and hospices vary in the policies surrounding removal of tubes. In the absence of specific guidance from the organization, the nurse should shut off infusions of any kind (IV or tube feeding) and leave IV access devices, feeding tubes, catheters, and wound dressings in place. When an expected death occurs in the home setting, the family generally will have received assistance with funeral arrangements in advance of the death. The funeral home has often been prearranged, and the funeral director will transport the body directly to the funeral home. In the hospital or long-term care facility, nurses follow the facility's procedure for preparation of the body and transportation to the facility's morgue. However, the needs of families to remain with the deceased, to wait until other family members arrive before the body is moved, and to perform after-death rituals should be honored.

Grief, Mourning, and Bereavement

A wide range of feelings and behaviors are normal, adaptive, and healthy reactions to the loss of a loved one. **Grief** refers to the personal feelings that accompany an anticipated or actual loss. **Mourning** refers to individual, family, group, and cultural expressions of grief and associated behaviors. **Bereavement** refers to the period of time during which mourning for a loss takes place. Both grief reactions and mourning behaviors change over time as people learn to live with the loss. Although the pain of the loss may be tempered by the passage of time, loss is an ongoing developmental process, and time does not heal the bereaved individual completely. That is, the bereaved do not get over a loss entirely, nor do they return to who they were before the loss. Rather, they develop a new sense of who they are and where they fit in a world that has changed dramatically and permanently.

Anticipatory Grief and Mourning

Denial, sadness, anger, fear, and anxiety are normal grief reactions in people with life-threatening illness and those close to

TABLE 16-4 Kübler-Ross's Five Stages of Grief

Stage	Nursing Implications
Denial: "This cannot be true." Feelings of isolation. May search for another health care professional who will give a more favorable opinion. May seek unproven therapies.	Denial can be an adaptive response, providing a buffer after bad news. It allows time to mobilize defenses but can be maladaptive when it prevents the patient or family from seeking help or when denial behaviors cause more pain or distress than the illness or interfere with everyday functions. Nurses should assess the patient's and family's coping style, information needs, and understanding of the illness and treatment to establish a basis for empathetic listening, education, and emotional support. Rather than confronting the patient with information that he or she is not ready to hear, the nurse can encourage him or her to share fears and concerns. Open-ended questions or statements such as "Tell me more about how you are coping with this new information about your illness" can provide a springboard for expression of concerns.
Anger: "Why me?" Feelings of rage, resentment or envy directed at God, health care professionals, family, others.	Anger can be very isolating, and loved ones or clinicians may withdraw. Nurses should allow the patient and family to express anger, treating them with understanding, respect, and knowledge that the root of the anger is grief over impending loss.
Bargaining: "I just want to see my grandchild's birth, then I'll be ready...." Patient and/or family plead for more time to reach an important goal. Promises are sometimes made with God.	Terminally ill patients are sometimes able to outlive prognoses and achieve some future goal. Nurses should be patient, allow expression of feelings, and support realistic and positive hope.
Depression: "I just don't know how my kids are going to get along after I'm gone." Sadness, grief, mourning for impending losses.	Normal and adaptive response. Clinical depression should be assessed and treated when present. Nurses should encourage the patient and family to fully express their sadness. Insincere reassurance or encouragement of unrealistic hopes should be avoided.
Acceptance: "I've lived a good life, and I have no regrets." Patient and/or family are neither angry nor depressed.	The patient may withdraw as his or her circle of interest diminishes. The family may feel rejected by the patient. Nurses need to support the family's expression of emotions and encourage them to continue to be present for the patient.

them. Kübler-Ross (1969) described five common emotional reactions to dying that are applicable to the experience of any loss (Table 16-4). Not every patient or family member experiences every stage; many patients never reach a stage of acceptance, and patients and families fluctuate on a sometimes daily basis in their emotional responses. Furthermore, although impending loss stresses the patient, people who are close to him or her, and the functioning of the family unit, awareness of dying also provides a unique opportunity for family members to reminisce, resolve relationships, plan for the future, and say goodbye.

Individual and family coping with the anticipation of death is complicated by the varied and conflicting trajectories that grief and mourning may assume in families. For example, the patient may be experiencing sadness while contemplating role changes that have been brought about by the illness, and the patient's spouse or partner may be expressing or suppressing feelings of anger about the current changes in role and impending loss of the relationship. Others in the family may be engaged in denial (e.g., "Dad will get better. He just needs to eat more"), fear ("Who will take care of us?" or "Will I get sick, too?"), or profound sadness and withdrawal. Although each of these behaviors is normal, tension may arise when one or more family members perceive that others are less caring, too emotional, or too detached.

The nurse should assess the characteristics of the family system and intervene in a manner that supports and enhances the cohesion of the family unit. Parameters for assessing the family facing life-threatening illness are identified in Chart 16-12. The nurse can suggest that family members talk about their feelings and understand them in the broader context of anticipatory grief and mourning. Acknowledging and expressing feelings, continuing to interact with the patient in meaningful ways, and planning for the time of death and bereavement are adaptive family behaviors. Professional support provided by grief counselors, whether in the community, at a local hospital, in the long-term care facility, or associated with a hospice program, can help both the patient and the family

Chart 16-12

ASSESSMENT

Assessing for Anticipatory Mourning in the Family Facing Life-Threatening Illness

Family Constellation

- Identify the members who constitute the patient's family. Who is important to the patient?
- Identify roles and relationships among the family members:
  - Who is the primary caregiver?
  - By what authority is this person the primary caregiver?

Cohesion and Boundaries

- How autonomous/interdependent are family members?
  - Degree of involvement with each other as individuals and as a family
  - Degree of bonding between family members
  - Degree of "teamwork" in the family
  - Degree of reliance on individual family members for specific tasks/roles
- How do family members differ in:
  - Personality?
  - Worldview?
  - Priorities?
- What are the implicit and explicit expectations or "rules" for behavior within the family?

Flexibility and Adaptability

- What is the family's ability to integrate new information?
- How does the family manage change?
- How able are the family members to assume new roles and responsibilities?

Communication

- What is the style of communication in the family, in terms of:
  - Openness?
  - Directness?
  - Clarity?
- What are the constraints on communication?
- What topics are avoided?

sort out and acknowledge feelings and make the end of life as meaningful as possible.

Grief and Mourning After Death

When a loved one dies, the family members enter a new phase of grief and mourning as they begin to accept the loss, feel the pain of permanent separation, and prepare to live a life without the deceased. Even if the loved one died after a long illness, preparatory grief experienced during the terminal illness does not preclude the grief and mourning that follow the death. With a death after a long or difficult illness, family members may experience conflicting feelings of relief that the loved one's suffering has ended, compounded by guilt and grief related to unresolved issues or the circumstances of death. Grief work may be especially difficult if a patient's death was painful, prolonged, accompanied by unwanted interventions, or unattended. Families who had no preparation or support during the period of imminent death may have a more difficult time finding a place for the painful memories.

Although some family members may experience prolonged or complicated mourning, most grief reactions fall within a "normal" range. The feelings are often profound; however, bereaved people eventually reconcile the loss and find a way to reengage with their lives. Grief and mourning are affected by several factors, including individual characteristics, coping skills, and experiences with illness and death; the nature of the relationship to the deceased; factors surrounding the illness and the death; family dynamics; social support; and cultural expectations and norms. Uncomplicated grief and mourning are characterized by emotional feelings of sadness, anger, guilt, and numbness; physical sensations such as hollowness in the stomach and tightness in the chest, weakness, and lack of energy; cognitions that include preoccupation with the loss and a sense of the deceased as still present; and behaviors such as crying, visiting places that are reminders of the deceased, social withdrawal, and restless overactivity (Zhang, El-Jawahri & Prigerson, 2006).

After-death rituals, including preparation of the body, funeral practices, and burial rituals, are socially and culturally significant ways in which family members begin to accept the reality and finality of death. Preplanning of funerals is becoming increasingly common, and hospice professionals in particular help the family make plans for death, often involving the patient, who may wish to play an active role. Preplanning of the funeral relieves the family of the burden of making decisions in the intensely emotional period after a death.

In general, the period of mourning is an adaptive response to loss during which mourners come to accept the loss as real and permanent, acknowledge and experience the painful emotions that accompany the loss, experience life without the deceased, overcome impediments to adjustment, and find a new way of living in a world without the loved one. Particularly immediately after the death, mourners begin to recognize the reality and permanence of the loss by talking about the deceased and telling and retelling the story of the illness and death. Societal norms in the United States are frequently at odds with the normal grieving processes of people; time excused from work obligations is typically measured in days, and mourners are often expected to get over the loss quickly and get on with life.

In reality, the work of grief and mourning takes time, and avoiding grief work after the death often leads to long-term adjustment difficulties. According to Rando (2000), mourning for a loss involves the "undoing" of psychosocial ties that bind mourners to the deceased, personal adaptation to the loss, and learning to live in the world without the deceased. Six key processes of mourning allow people to accommodate to the loss in a healthy way (Rando, 2000):

1. Recognition of the loss
2. Reaction to the separation, and experiencing and expressing the pain of the loss
3. Recollection and reexperiencing the deceased, the relationship, and the associated feelings
4. Relinquishing old attachments to the deceased
5. Readjustment to adapt to the new world without forgetting the old
6. Reinvestment

Although many people complete the work of mourning with the informal support of families and friends, many find that talking with others who have had a similar experience, such as in formal support groups, normalizes the feelings and experiences and provides a framework for learning new skills to cope with the loss and create a new life. Hospitals, hospices, religious organizations, and other community organizations often sponsor bereavement support groups. Groups for parents who have lost a child, children who have lost a parent, widows, widowers, and gay men and lesbians who have lost a life partner are some examples of specialized support groups available in many communities. Nursing interventions for those experiencing grief and mourning are identified in Chart 16-13.

Chart 16-13 **Nursing Interventions for Grief and Mourning**

Support the Expression of Feelings

- Encourage the telling of the story using open-ended statements or questions (e.g., "Tell me about your husband").
- Assist the mourner to find an outlet for his or her feelings: talking, attending a support group, keeping a journal, finding a safe outlet for angry feelings (writing letters that will not be mailed, physical activity).
- Assess emotional affect and reinforce the normalcy of feelings.
- Assess for guilt and regrets:
  - "Are you especially troubled by a certain memory or thought?"
  - "How do you manage those memories?"

Assess for the Presence of Social Support

- "Do you have someone to whom you can talk about your husband?"
- "May I help you find someone you can talk to?"

Assess Coping Skills

- "How are you managing day to day?"
- "Have you experienced other losses? How did you manage those?"
- "Are there things that you are having trouble doing?"
- "Do you have/need help with specific tasks?"

Assess for Signs of Complicated Grief and Mourning and Offer Professional Referral

Complicated Grief and Mourning

Complicated grief and mourning are characterized by prolonged feelings of sadness and feelings of general worthlessness or hopelessness that persist long after the death, prolonged symptoms that interfere with activities of daily living (anorexia, insomnia, fatigue, panic), or self-destructive behaviors such as alcohol or substance abuse and suicidal ideation or attempts. Complicated grief and mourning require professional assessment and can be treated with psychological interventions and, in some cases, with medications.

Coping With Death and Dying: Professional Caregiver Issues

Whether practicing in a trauma center, ICU or other acute care setting, home care, hospice, long-term care, or the many locations where patients and their families receive ambulatory services, nurses are closely involved with complex and emotionally laden issues surrounding loss of life. To be most effective and satisfied with the care they provide, nurses should attend to their own emotional responses to the losses witnessed every day. Well before exhibiting symptoms of stress or burnout, nurses should acknowledge the difficulty of coping with others' pain on a daily basis and establish healthy practices that guard against emotional exhaustion. In hospice settings, where death, grief, and loss are expected outcomes of patient care, interdisciplinary colleagues rely on one another for support, using meeting time to express frustration, sadness, anger, and other emotions; to learn coping skills from one another; and to speak about how they were affected by the lives of those patients who have died since the last meeting. In many settings, staff members organize or attend memorial services to support families and other caregivers, who find comfort in joining one another to remember and celebrate the lives of patients. Finally, healthy personal habits, including diet, exercise, stress reduction activities (e.g., dance, yoga, T'ai chi, meditation), and sleep, help guard against the detrimental effects of stress.

Critical Thinking Exercises

1 **ebp** You are the new unit manager on a hospice unit that is part of a long-term care facility. While reviewing documented nursing assessments, you note that pain intensity scores (0 to 10) are recorded for some residents, although for others, a mix of methods is used to evaluate pain. What is the evidence base for pain assessment in palliative care? Identify the criteria used to evaluate the strength of the evidence for this practice. How will you evaluate the implementation of a new tool or tools?

2 **pg** You are caring for a 68-year-old man with end-stage heart failure in a hospital-based palliative care unit. You observe that he has peripheral edema and cachexia. He reports dyspnea at rest, profound fatigue, and activity intolerance. He tells you that he would like to return home, but his wife becomes very anxious when he has pain or shortness of breath, causing him to become anxious as well. What priority assessments would you conduct? What specific information should you include first in a discussion with this man and his wife? What type of information and in what format would be appropriate for this man and his wife?

3 A 35-year-old married mother of two young children of Hispanic origin has been referred for hospice care. She has advanced breast cancer with metastases to the bone, liver, and lung. During your assessment visit, she tearfully states, "I don't know why I am still here. I want God to take me before I become a complete burden on my family." Discuss how you would carry out additional assessment and the recommendations that you might make based on findings from your assessment. Give examples of questions that you would ask to further assess the cultural and spiritual aspects of care. What types of services may be helpful for this woman and her family?

Brunner Suite Resources
Explore these additional resources to enhance learning for this chapter:
• NCLEX-Style Questions and Other Resources on **thePoint**, http://thePoint.lww.com/Brunner13e
• Study Guide
• PrepU
• Clinical Handbook
• Handbook of Laboratory and Diagnostic Tests

References

*Asterisk indicates nursing research.
**Double asterisk indicates classic reference.

Books

American Nurses Association. (2010a). *Nursing's social policy statement* (3rd ed.). Silver Spring, MD: Author.

Back, A., Arnold, A., & Tulsky, J. (2009). *Mastering communication with seriously ill patients: Balancing honesty with empathy and hope*. New York: Cambridge.

Ferrell, B. R., & Coyle, N. (Eds.). (2010). *Oxford textbook of palliative nursing* (3rd ed.). New York: Oxford.

**Glaser, B. G., & Strauss, A. (1965). *Awareness of dying*. Chicago: Aldine.

Hospice of Philadelphia. (2012). *Signs of approaching death*. Philadelphia: Author.

**Kübler-Ross, E. (1969). *On death and dying*. New York: Macmillan.

Puchalski, C. M., & Ferrell, B. R. (2010). *Making health care whole: Integrating spirituality into patient care*. West Conshohocken, PA: Templeton.

**Rando, T. A. (2000). Promoting healthy anticipatory mourning in intimates of the life-threatened or dying person. In T. A. Rando (Ed.): *Clinical dimensions of anticipatory mourning*. Champaign, IL: Research Press.

Wrede-Seaman, L. (2008). *Symptom management algorithms: A handbook for palliative care*. (2nd ed.). Yakima, WA: Intellicard.

Journals and Electronic Documents

American Academy of Hospice and Palliative Medicine. (2007). *Position statements: Physician-assisted death*. Available at: www.aahpm.org/positions/default/suicide.html

American Association of Retired Persons. (2009). *Caregiving and end of life issues: A survey of AARP members in Florida*. Available at: assets.aarp.org/rgcenter/il/fl_eol_08.pdf

**American Nurses Association. (2010b). *Position statement: Registered nurses' roles and responsibilities in providing expert care and counseling at the end of life*.

Available at: gm6.nursingworld.org/MainMenuCategories/EthicsStandards/Ethics-Position-Statements/etpain14426.pdf

Barclay, S., Momen, N., Case-Upton, S., et al. (2011). End-of-life care conversations with heart failure patients: A systematic literature review and narrative synthesis. *British Journal of General Practice*, e49–e62. Available at: cambridge.academia.edu/NatalieMomen/Papers/1295449/End-of-life_care_conversations_with_heart_failure_patients_a_systematic_literature_review_and_narrative_synthesis

*Benkel, I., Wijk, H., & Molander, U. (2010). Using coping strategies is not denial: Helping loved ones to adjust to living with a patent with a palliative diagnosis. *Journal of Hospice and Palliative Medicine*, 13(9), 1119–1123.

Borneman, T., Ferrell, B., & Puchalski, C. M. (2010). Evaluation of the FICA tool for spiritual assessment. *Journal of Pain and Symptom Management*, 40(2), 163–173.

Breibart, W., & Alici, Y. (2008). Agitation and delirium at the end of life. *Journal of the American Medical Association*, 300(24), 2898–2910.

**Casarett, D. J., Kapo, J., & Kaplan, A. (2005). Appropriate use of artificial nutrition and hydration—fundamental principles and recommendations. *New England Journal of Medicine*, 353(24), 2607–2612.

Center to Advance Palliative Care. (2012). *Palliative care and hospice care across the continuum*. Available at: www.capc.org/palliative-care-across-the-continuum/

Compassion and Choices of Washington. (2008). *Washington death with dignity act—Initiative 1000*. Available at: wei.sos.wa.gov/agency/osos/en/documents/i1000-text%20for%20web.pdf

Connor, S. R. (2007–2008). Development of hospice and palliative care in the United States. *Omega*, 56(1), 89–99.

Del Fabbro, E., Dalal, S., & Bruera, E. (2006). Symptom control in palliative care—part II: Cachexia/anorexia and fatigue. *Journal of Palliative Medicine*, 9(2), 409–421.

Family Caregiver Alliance. (2012). *Selected long-term care statistics*. Available at: www.caregiver.org/caregiver/jsp/content_node.jsp?nodeid=440

Gallup Poll. (2011). *Doctor-assisted suicide is moral issue dividing Americans most*. Available at: www.gallup.com/poll/147842/doctor-assisted-suicide-moral-issue-dividing-americans.aspx

Hospice and Palliative Nurses Association. (2011). *HPNA position statement: Legalization of assisted suicide*. Available at: www.hpna.org/DisplayPage.aspx?Title=Position%20Statements

Institute of Medicine. (2011). *Relieving pain in America: A blueprint for transforming prevention, care, education, and research*. Available at: www.iom.edu/~/media/Files/Report%20Files/2011/Relieving-Pain-in-America-A-Blueprint-for-Transforming-Prevention-Care-Education-Research/Pain%20Research%202011%20Report%20Brief.pdf

Joint Commission. (2011). *Facts about the advanced certification program for palliative care*. Available at: www.jointcommission.org/assets/1/18/Palliative_Care.pdf

Kamal, A. H., Maguire, J. M. ,Wheeler, J. L., et al. (2012). Dyspnea review for the palliative care professional: Treatment goals and therapeutic options. *Journal of Palliative Medicine*, 15(1), 106–114.

Kelley, A. S., Ettner, S. L., Wenger, N. S., et al. (2011). Determinants of death in the hospital among older adults. *Journal of the American Geriatric Society*, 59(12), 2321–2325.

Long, C. O. (2011). Ten best practices to enhance culturally competent communication in palliative care. *Journal of Pediatric Hematology/Oncology*, 33, S136–S139.

Lorenz, K., Lynn, J., Dy, S. M., et al. (2008). Evidence for improving palliative care at the end of life: A systematic review. *Annals of Internal Medicine*, 148(2), 147–159.

Mahler, D. A., Selecky, P. A., Harrod, C. G., et al. (2010). American College of Chest Physicians consensus statement on the management of dyspnea in patients with advanced lung or heart disease. *Chest*, 137(3), 674–691.

McWilliams, K., Keeley P. W., & Waterhouse, E. T. (2010). Propofol for palliative sedation in terminal care: A systematic review. *Journal of Palliative Medicine*, 13(1), 73–76.

Medicare Payment Advisory Commission. (2011). Hospice. In *Report to the Congress: Medicare payment policy*. Available at: medpac.gov/documents/Mar11_EntireReport.pdf

Mitchell, S. L., Black, B. S., Ersek, M., et al. (2012). Advanced dementia: State of the art and priorities for the next decade. *Annals of Internal Medicine*, 156(1), 45–51.

Mitera, G., Zhang, L., Sahgal, A., et al. (2012). A survey of expectations and understanding of palliative radiotherapy from patients with advanced cancer. *Clinical Oncology*, 24(2), 134–138.

National Center for Health Statistics. (2010). *Health, United States, 2010: With Special Feature on Death and Dying*. Hyattsville, MD.

National Consensus Project for Quality Palliative Care. (2009). *Clinical practice guidelines for quality palliative care* (2nd ed.). Available at: www.nationalconsensusproject.org

National Hospice and Palliative Care Organization. (2010). *Preamble and philosophy*. Available at: www.nhpco.org/i4a/pages/index.cfm?pageid=5308

National Hospice and Palliative Care Organization. (2011). *NHPCO facts and figures: Hospice care in America*. Alexandria VA: Author.

National Institute of Nursing Research. (2011). *The science of compassion: Future directions in end-of-life and palliative care*. Available at: www.ninr.nih.gov/researchandfunding/scienceofcompassion

National Institute of Nursing Research. (2012). *Areas of research emphasis*. Available at: www.ninr.nih.gov/aboutninr/budgetandlegislation/2012-senate-budgettestimony

National Quality Forum. (2006). *A national framework and preferred practices for palliative and hospice care quality: Executive summary*. Available at: www.rwjf.org/content/dam/farm/reports/reports/2006/rwjf13081

Office of the Inspector General. (2009). *Memorandum report: Medicare hospice care: Services provided to beneficiaries residing in nursing facilities*. Available at: www.oig.hhs.gov/oei/reports/oei-02-06-00223.pdf

Oncology Nursing Society. (2010). *Oncology Nursing Society position on nurses' responsibility to patients requesting assistance in hastening death*. Available at: www.ons.org/Publications/Positions/AssistedSuicide/

Oregon Public Health Division. (2011). *Oregon's Death with Dignity Act—2011*. Available at: public.health.oregon.gov/ProviderPartnerResources/EvaluationResearch/DeathwithDignityAct/Documents/year14.pdf

Puchalski, C., Ferrell, B. Virani, R., et al. (2009). Improving the quality of spiritual care as a dimension of palliative care: The report on the consensus conference. *Journal of Palliative Medicine*, 12(10), 885–904.

Quill, T. E., Lo, B., Brock, D. W., et al. (2009). Last-resort options for palliative sedation. *Annals of Internal Medicine*, 151(6), 421–424.

Robson, A., Scrutton, F., Wilkinson, L., et al. (2010). The risk of suicide in cancer patients: A review of the literature. *Psychooncology*, 19(12),1250–1258.

Siddiqui, R., Pandya, D., Harvey, K., et al. (2006). Nutrition modulation of cachexia/proteolysis. *Nutrition in Clinical Practice*, 21(2), 155–167.

Smith, A. K., Cenzer, I. S., Knight, S. J., et al. (2010). The epidemiology of pain during the last 2 years of life. *Annals of Internal Medicine*, 153(9), 563–569.

**SUPPORT Principal Investigators. (1995). A controlled trial to improve care for seriously ill hospitalized patients. *Journal of the American Medical Association*, 274(20), 1591–1598.

Temel, J. S., Greer, J. A., Muzikansky, A., et al. (2010). Early palliative care for patients with metastatic non-small-cell lung cancer. *New England Journal of Medicine*, 363(8), 733–742.

Vachon, M., Fillion, L., & Achille, M. (2009). A conceptual analysis of spirituality at the end of life. *Journal of Palliative Medicine*, 12(1), 53–59.

Von Haehling, S., Doehner, W., & Anker, S. D. (2007). Nutrition, metabolism, and the complex pathophysiology of cachexia in chronic heart failure. *Cardiovascular Research*, 73(2), 298–309.

World Health Organization. (2008). *Definition of palliative care*. Available at: www.who.int/cancer/palliative/definition/en/print.html

Zhang, B., El-Jawahri, A., & Prigerson, H. G. (2006). Update on bereavement research: Evidence-based guidelines for the diagnosis and treatment of complicated bereavement. *Journal of Palliative Medicine*, 9(5), 1188–1203.

Resources

American Academy of Hospice and Palliative Medicine (AAHPM), www.aahpm.org/

American Hospice Foundation, www.americanhospice.org/

Americans for Better Care of the Dying (ABCD), abcd-caring.org/

Association for Death Education and Counseling (ADEC), www.adec.org/

Caring Connections: a program of the National Hospice and Palliative Care Organization, www.caringinfo.org/i4a/pages/index.cfm?pageid=1

Center to Advance Palliative Care, www.capc.org/

Children's Hospice International, www.chionline.org/

Compassion and Choices, www.compassionandchoices.org/

End-of-Life Nursing Education Consortium (ELNEC), www.aacn.nche.edu/elnec

End of Life/Palliative Education Resource Center (EPERC), www.eperc.mcw.edu/

Epidemiology of Dying and End-of-Life Experience (EDELE), a resource for data on death and dying, www.edeledata.org/

Family Caregiver Alliance (FCA), www.caregiver.org/

Growth House, Inc., provides information and referral services for agencies working with death and dying issues, www.growthhouse.org/

Harvard Medical School Center for Palliative Care, Dana Farber Cancer Institute, www.hms.harvard.edu/pallcare/

Hospice and Palliative Nurses Association (HPNA), www.hpna.org

Hospice Association of America, National Association for Home Care, www.nahc.org/haa/

Hospice Education Institute, www.hospiceworld.org/

Hospice Foundation of America (HFA), www.hospicefoundation.org/

Hospice Net, provides information and support to patients and families facing life-threatening illnesses, www.hospicenet.org/

National Consensus Project for Quality Palliative Care (national guidelines), www.nationalconsensusproject.org

National Hospice and Palliative Care Organization (NHPCO), www.nhpco.org

National Palliative Care Research Center (NPCRC), Brookdale Department of Geriatrics and Adult Development, www.npcrc.org

National Prison Hospice Association, www.npha.org

Population-based Palliative Care Research Network (PoPCRN), www.ucdenver.edu/academics/colleges/medicalschool/departments/medicine/GIM/Popcrn/Pages/PopcrnHome.aspx

Promoting Excellence in End-of-Life Care, www.promotingexcellence.org/

StopPain.org, Department of Pain Medicine and Palliative Care at Beth Israel Medical Center, www.stoppain.org/

Supportive Care Coalition, www.supportivecarecoalition.org/

TIME: Toolkit of Instruments to Measure End-of-Life Care (Brown University) www.chcr.brown.edu/pcoc/toolkit.htm

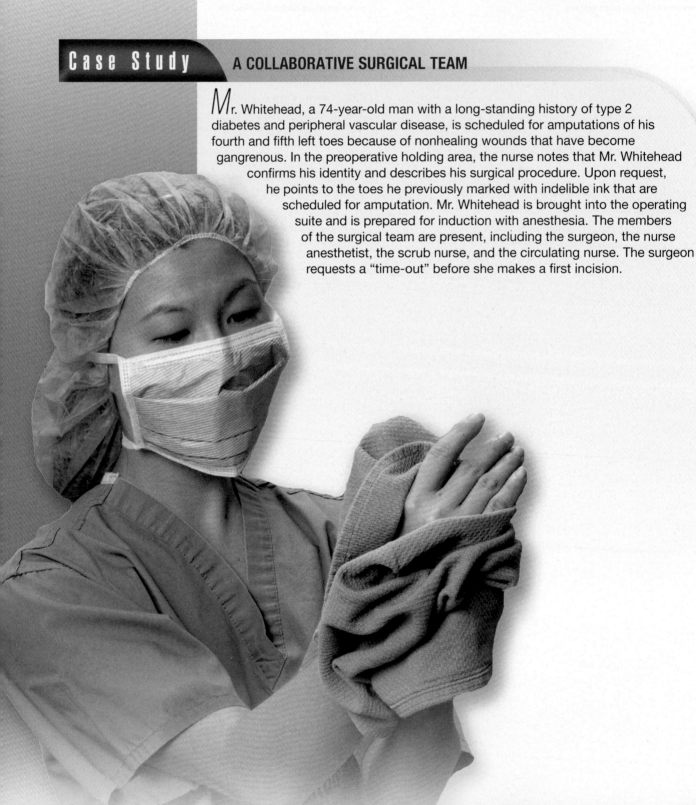

Unit 4

Perioperative Concepts and Nursing Management

Case Study A COLLABORATIVE SURGICAL TEAM

Mr. Whitehead, a 74-year-old man with a long-standing history of type 2 diabetes and peripheral vascular disease, is scheduled for amputations of his fourth and fifth left toes because of nonhealing wounds that have become gangrenous. In the preoperative holding area, the nurse notes that Mr. Whitehead confirms his identity and describes his surgical procedure. Upon request, he points to the toes he previously marked with indelible ink that are scheduled for amputation. Mr. Whitehead is brought into the operating suite and is prepared for induction with anesthesia. The members of the surgical team are present, including the surgeon, the nurse anesthetist, the scrub nurse, and the circulating nurse. The surgeon requests a "time-out" before she makes a first incision.

QSEN Competency Focus: *Teamwork and Collaboration*

The complexities inherent in today's health care system challenge nurses to demonstrate integration of specific interdisciplinary core competencies. These competencies are aimed at ensuring the delivery of safe, quality patient care (Institute of Medicine, 2003). The concepts from the Quality and Safety Education for Nurses (QSEN) Institute (2012) provide a framework for the knowledge, skills, and attitudes (KSAs) required for nurses to demonstrate competency in these key areas, which include *patient-centered care, interdisciplinary teamwork and collaboration, evidence-based practice, quality improvement, safety*, and *informatics*.

Teamwork and Collaboration Definition: Function effectively within nursing and interprofessional teams, fostering open communication, mutual respect, and shared decision making to achieve quality patient care.

RELEVANT PRE-LICENSURE KSAs	APPLICATION AND REFLECTION
Knowledge	
Examine strategies for improving systems to support team functioning.	Discuss what should happen during this pre-incisional time-out in the operating suite. What is the role of each member of the surgical team? Is any one of the members exempt from participating in this process?
Skills	
Participate in designing systems that support effective teamwork.	Give examples of checklists or other tools that may be used so that consistent processes are followed during time-outs.
Attitudes	
Value the influence of system solutions in achieving effective team functioning.	Think about times you performed a rote task over and over again, but, for some inexplicable reason, at one time made a mistake completing that task. If you were part of a team where each team member had been involved in and took responsibility for completing that task, and systematic processes were used to ensure task completion, might that mistake not have occurred? How can a team approach to job completion ensure best outcomes, generally speaking? Why is teamwork and collaboration of such great importance in ensuring best patient outcomes?

Cronenwett, L., Sherwood, G., Barnsteiner, J., et al. (2007). Quality and safety education for nurses. *Nursing Outlook, 55*(3), 122–131.
Institute of Medicine. (2003). *Health professions education: A bridge to quality.* Washington, DC: National Academies Press.
QSEN Institute. (2012). *Competencies: Pre-licensure KSAs.* Available at: qsen.org/competencies/pre-licensure-ksas

Read More About This Case

More information about this case study and the relationships between nursing diagnoses, interventions, and expected outcomes is available online. Visit thePoint for Applying Concepts From NANDA-I, NIC, and NOC.

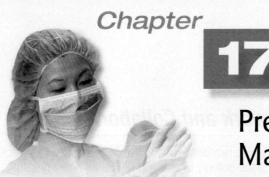

Preoperative Nursing Management

Learning Objectives

On completion of this chapter, the learner will be able to:

1 Define the three phases of perioperative patient care.
2 Describe a comprehensive preoperative assessment to identify surgical risk factors.
3 Describe the gerontologic considerations related to preoperative management.
4 Identify health factors that affect patients preoperatively.
5 Identify legal and ethical considerations related to obtaining informed consent for surgery.

6 Describe preoperative nursing measures that decrease the risk for infection and other postoperative complications.
7 Describe the immediate preoperative preparation of the patient.
8 Develop a preoperative education plan designed to promote the patient's recovery from anesthesia and surgery, thus preventing postoperative complications.

Glossary

ambulatory surgery: includes outpatient, same-day, or short-stay surgery that does not require an overnight hospital stay
bariatrics: having to do with patients who are obese
informed consent: the patient's autonomous decision about whether to undergo a surgical procedure, based on the nature of the condition, the treatment options, and the risks and benefits involved
intraoperative phase: period of time that begins with transfer of the patient to the operating room area and continues until the patient is admitted to the postanesthesia care unit
laparoscopy: visual examination of a body cavity or joint by means of an endoscope
minimally invasive surgery: surgical procedures that use specialized instruments inserted into the body

either through natural orifices or through small incisions
perioperative phase: period of time that constitutes the surgical experience; includes the preoperative, intraoperative, and postoperative phases of nursing care
postoperative phase: period of time that begins with the admission of the patient to the postanesthesia care unit and ends after follow-up evaluation in the clinical setting or home
preadmission testing: diagnostic testing performed before admission to the hospital
preoperative phase: period of time from when the decision for surgical intervention is made to when the patient is transferred to the operating room table

As techniques to perform surgery change with improved technology and expertise, surgery becomes less invasive and thereby less debilitating. The increased use of **minimally invasive surgery**—surgical procedures that use specialized instruments inserted into the body either through natural orifices or through small incisions—enables many surgeries to be performed on an outpatient basis. Surgery, however, remains a complex, stressful experience, whether elective or emergent. Even healthy patients having outpatient surgery may experience unanticipated complications during otherwise benign procedures.

Many patients enter the hospital 90 minutes prior to surgery and have necessary medical assessments and analyses preceding the surgical intervention. The surgical period is followed by a recovery period of a few hours in the postanesthesia care unit (PACU), then the patient returns home for recuperation the same day. For more invasive procedures, or when comorbidities exist, the patient may have laboratory

studies completed prior to admission, and may be required to be admitted to the hospital for a number of days postoperatively for physiotherapy, monitoring, and evaluation.

Traumatic and emergency surgery most often results in prolonged hospital stays. Patients who are acutely ill or undergoing major surgery and patients with concurrent medical disorders may require supportive supplementary care from other medical disciplines, which can be coordinated more easily within the hospital setting. The high acuity level of surgical inpatients and the greater complexity of procedures have placed greater demands on the practice of nursing in this setting (American Society of PeriAnesthesia Nurses [ASPAN], 2010). Although each setting (ambulatory, outpatient, or inpatient) offers its own unique advantages for the delivery of patient care, all patients require a comprehensive preoperative nursing assessment, patient education, and nursing interventions to prepare for surgery.

Perioperative Nursing

Communication, teamwork, and patient assessment are crucial to ensuring good patient outcomes in the perioperative setting. Professional perioperative and perianesthesia nursing standards encompass the domains of behavioral response, physiologic response, and patient safety and are used as guides toward development of nursing diagnoses, interventions, and plans. Perioperative nursing, which spans the entire surgical experience, consists of three phases that begin and end at particular points in the sequence of surgical experience events. The **preoperative phase** begins when the decision to proceed with surgical intervention is made and ends with the transfer of the patient onto the operating room (OR) bed. The **intraoperative phase** begins when the patient is transferred onto the OR bed and ends with admission to the PACU. Intraoperative nursing responsibilities involve acting as scrub nurse, circulating nurse, or registered nurse first assistant (see Chapter 18 for a description of these roles). The **postoperative phase** begins with the admission of the patient to the PACU and ends with a follow-up evaluation in the clinical setting or home (see Chapter 19).

Each **perioperative phase** includes the many diverse activities a nurse performs, using the nursing process, and based on the Standards of Practice of ASPAN (2010). Chart 17-1 presents nursing activities characteristic of the three perioperative phases of care. Each phase of the surgical experience is reviewed in more detail in this chapter and in the other chapters in this unit.

A conceptual model of patient care, published by the Association of PeriOperative Registered Nurses, formerly known as the Association of Operating Room Nurses (still abbreviated AORN), helps delineate the relationships between various components of nursing practice and patient outcomes. The Perioperative Nursing Data Set categorizes the practice of perioperative nursing practice into four domains: safety, physiologic responses, behavioral responses, and health care systems. The first three domains reflect phenomena of concern to perioperative nurses and are composed of nursing diagnoses, interventions, and outcomes. The fourth domain—the health care system—consists of structural data elements and focuses on clinical processes and outcomes. The model is used to depict the relationship of nursing process components to the achievement of optimal patient outcomes (Rothrock, 2010).

Technology and Anesthesia

Technological advancements continue to lead health care industry providers toward performing more complex procedures that are less invasive, and therefore cause less morbidity during the recovery phase of surgery (Becker, 2009). Innovative high-definition microsurgical and laser technology enable increasingly minute repairs of tissue resulting in accelerated tissue regeneration. Sophisticated bypass equipment and minimally invasive techniques have changed many cardiovascular surgeries into outpatient procedures (Massicotte, Chalaoui, Beaulieu, et al., 2009). The use of robots enables formerly debilitating orthopedic surgery to become minimally invasive procedures. The increased use of laparoscopic minimally invasive surgery promotes rapid healing and less morbidity in postoperative patients. Transplantation of multiple human organs occurs more frequently, along with the implantation of mechanical devices and the successful reattachment of body parts.

Enhanced anesthesia methodology complements advances in surgical technology. Modern methods of achieving airway patency, sophisticated monitoring devices, and new pharmacologic agents, such as short-acting anesthetics, have created a safer atmosphere in which to operate (Miller, Eriksson, Fleisher, et al., 2010). Effective antiemetics have reduced postoperative nausea and vomiting (Franck, Radtke, Apfel, et al., 2010). Improved postoperative pain management and shortened procedure and recovery times have improved the operative experience for surgical patients.

Surgical Classifications

The decision to perform surgery may be based on facilitating a diagnosis (a diagnostic procedure such as biopsy, exploratory laparotomy, or **laparoscopy**), a cure (e.g., excision of a tumor or an inflamed appendix), or repair (e.g., multiple wound repair). It may be reconstructive or cosmetic (such as mammoplasty or a facelift) or palliative (to relieve pain or correct a problem—as in debulking a tumor to permit comfort, or removal of a dysfunctional gallbladder). In addition, surgery might be rehabilitative (e.g., total joint replacement surgery to correct crippling pain or progression of degenerative osteoarthritis.) Surgery can also be classified based upon the degree of urgency involved: emergent, urgent, required, elective, and optional (Table 17-1).

Preadmission Testing

Concurrent with the increase in **ambulatory surgeries** (surgery that does not require an overnight hospital stay) have been changes in the delivery of and payment for health care. Incentives to reduce hospital stays and contain costs have resulted in diagnostic **preadmission testing** (PAT) and preoperative preparation prior to admission. Many facilities have a presurgical services department to facilitate PAT and to initiate the nursing assessment process, which focuses on admission data such as patient demographics, health history, and other information pertinent to the surgical procedure (i.e., appropriate consent forms, diagnostic and laboratory tests) (Rothrock, 2010). The increasing use of ambulatory, outpatient, or short-stay surgery means that patients leave the hospital sooner and recuperate quicker. These changes increase the need for patient education, discharge planning, preparation for self-care, and referral for home care and rehabilitation services (ASPAN, Schick, & Windle, 2010).

Special Considerations During the Perioperative Period

In an effort to reduce surgical complications, the Surgical Care Improvement Project (SCIP) was instituted as a national partnership of the Joint Commission and the Center for

Chart 17-1 Examples of Nursing Activities in the Perioperative Phases of Care

Preoperative Phase

Preadmission Testing (PAT)

1. Initiates initial preoperative assessment
2. Initiates education appropriate to patient's needs
3. Involves family in interview
4. Verifies completion of preoperative diagnostic testing
5. Verifies understanding of surgeon-specific preoperative orders (e.g., bowel preparation, preoperative shower)
6. Discusses and reviews advance directive document
7. Begins discharge planning by assessing patient's need for postoperative transportation and care

Admission to Surgical Center

1. Completes preoperative assessment
2. Assesses for risks for postoperative complications
3. Reports unexpected findings or any deviations from normal
4. Verifies that operative consent has been signed
5. Coordinates patient education and plan of care with nursing staff and other health team members
6. Reinforces previous education
7. Explains phases in perioperative period and expectations
8. Answers patient's and family's questions

In the Holding Area

1. Identifies patient
2. Assesses patient's status, baseline pain, and nutritional status
3. Reviews medical record
4. Verifies surgical site and that it has been marked per institutional policy
5. Establishes IV line
6. Administers medications if prescribed
7. Takes measures to ensure patient's comfort
8. Provides psychological support
9. Communicates patient's emotional status to other appropriate members of the health care team

Intraoperative Phase

Maintenance of Safety

1. Maintains aseptic, controlled environment
2. Effectively manages human resources, equipment, and supplies for individualized patient care
3. Transfers patient to operating room bed or table
4. Positions patient based on functional alignment and exposure of surgical site
5. Applies grounding device to patient
6. Ensures that the sponge, needle, and instrument counts are correct
7. Completes intraoperative documentation

Physiologic Monitoring

1. Calculates effects on patient of excessive fluid loss or gain
2. Distinguishes normal from abnormal cardiopulmonary data
3. Reports changes in patient's vital signs
4. Institutes measures to promote normothermia

Psychological Support (Before Induction and When Patient Is Conscious)

1. Provides emotional support to patient
2. Stands near or touches patient during procedures and induction
3. Continues to assess patient's emotional status

Postoperative Phase

Transfer of Patient to Postanesthesia Care Unit

1. Communicates intraoperative information:
   a. Identifies patient by name
   b. States type of surgery performed
   c. Identifies type and amounts of anesthetic and analgesic agents used
   d. Reports patient's vital signs and response to surgical procedure and anesthesia
   e. Describes intraoperative factors (e.g., insertion of drains or catheters, administration of blood, medications during surgery, or occurrence of unexpected events)
   f. Describes physical limitations
   g. Reports patient's preoperative level of consciousness
   h. Communicates necessary equipment needs
   i. Communicates presence of family or significant others

Postoperative Assessment Recovery Area

1. Determines patient's immediate response to surgical intervention
2. Monitors patient's vital signs and physiologic status
3. Assesses patient's pain level and administers appropriate pain-relief measures
4. Maintains patient's safety (airway, circulation, prevention of injury)
5. Administers medications, fluid, and blood component therapy, if prescribed
6. Provides oral fluids if prescribed for ambulatory surgery patient
7. Assesses patient's readiness for transfer to in-hospital unit or for discharge home based on institutional policy (e.g., Aldrete score, see Chapter 19)

Surgical Nursing Unit

1. Continues close monitoring of patient's physical and psychological response to surgical intervention
2. Assesses patient's pain level and administers appropriate pain-relief measures
3. Provides education to patient during immediate recovery period
4. Assists patient in recovery and preparation for discharge home
5. Determines patient's psychological status
6. Assists with discharge planning

Home or Clinic

1. Provides follow-up care during office or clinic visit or by telephone contact
2. Reinforces previous education and answers patient's and family's questions about surgery and follow-up care
3. Assesses patient's response to surgery and anesthesia and their effects on body image and function
4. Determines family's perception of surgery and its outcome

Medicare and Medicaid Services (CMS). The SCIP identifies performance measures aimed at preventing surgical complications, including venous thromboembolism (VTE) and surgical site infections (SSIs) (Joint Commission, 2011). In addition, if the surgical patient is currently using beta-blockers, particular attention is given to ensure timely administration of the beta-blocker and appropriate monitoring of vital signs. If the patient has not taken the usual dosage of this medication, the anesthesiologist and anesthetist must evaluate whether or not it should be administered prior to surgery or during the perioperative period. The nurse in the perioperative area needs to be alert for appropriate preoperative prescriptions

TABLE 17-1	Categories of Surgery Based on Urgency	
Classification	**Indications for Surgery**	**Examples**
I. Emergent—Patient requires immediate attention; disorder may be life threatening	Without delay	Severe bleeding Bladder or intestinal obstruction Fractured skull Gunshot or stab wounds Extensive burns
II. Urgent—Patient requires prompt attention	Within 24–30 h	Acute gallbladder infection Kidney or ureteral stones
III. Required—Patient needs to have surgery	Plan within a few weeks or months	Prostatic hyperplasia without bladder obstruction Thyroid disorders Cataracts
IV. Elective—Patient should have surgery	Failure to have surgery not catastrophic	Repair of scars Simple hernia Vaginal repair
V. Optional—Decision rests with patient	Personal preference	Cosmetic surgery

aimed at preventing VTE and SSI. If these are not present, they should be requested so that appropriate treatment begins before the start of surgery.

 ## Gerontologic Considerations

The hazards of surgery for older adults are proportional to the number and severity of coexisting morbidities and the nature and duration of the operative procedure. The underlying principle that guides the preoperative assessment, surgical care, and postoperative care is that older adult patients have less physiologic reserve (i.e., the ability of an organ to return to normal after a disturbance in its equilibrium) than younger patients (Johnson, Moorhead, Bulechek, et al., 2011). Respiratory and cardiac complications are the leading causes of postoperative morbidity and mortality in older adults (Tabloski, 2009). Cardiac reserves are lower, renal and hepatic functions are depressed, and gastrointestinal activity is likely to be reduced.

Dehydration, constipation, and malnutrition may occur postoperatively. Sensory limitations, such as impaired vision or hearing and reduced tactile sensitivity, frequently interact with the postoperative environment, so falls are more likely to occur (Meiner, 2011). Maintaining a safe environment for older adults requires alertness and planning. Arthritis is a common condition among older patients, and it affects mobility, creating difficulty turning from one side to the other or ambulating without discomfort. Protective measures include adequate foam padding for bony prominences and nerves, moving the patient slowly, protecting from prolonged pressure, and providing gentle massage and sequential compression devices to promote circulation and prevent VTE (Melnyk & Fineout-Overholt, 2010).

As the body ages, the ability to perspire decreases, leading to dry, itchy skin, which can become fragile and easily abraded. Precautions are taken when moving an older adult. Decreased subcutaneous fat makes older people more susceptible to temperature changes. A lightweight cotton blanket is an appropriate cover when an older patient is moved to and from the OR but never replaces asking patients if they feel sufficiently warm and attending to their desires.

Because the older patient may have greater perioperative risks, the following factors are critical: (1) skillful preoperative assessment and treatment (Tabloski, 2009), (2) proficient

anesthesia and surgical care, and (3) meticulous and competent postoperative and postanesthesia management. Nurses must educate patients about appropriate pain management and encourage pain communication to obtain greater postoperative pain relief. Older adults may need multiple explanations to understand and retain what is communicated (see Providing Patient Education section).

 ## Bariatric Patients

Bariatrics has to do with patients who are obese. Like age, obesity increases the risk and severity of complications associated with surgery. During surgery, fatty tissues are especially susceptible to infection. Wound infections are more common in the obese patient (Haupt & Reed, 2010). Obesity also increases technical and mechanical problems related to surgery, such as dehiscence (wound separation). It may be more challenging to provide care for the patient who is obese owing to the excessive weight and possible restrictions in movement. The estimation of about 25 additional miles of blood vessels needed for every 30 pounds of excess weight results in increased cardiac demand (Alvarex, Brodsky, Lemmens, et al., 2010). The patient tends to have shallow respirations when supine, increasing the risk of hypoventilation and postoperative pulmonary complications.

The acquired physical characteristics of short thick necks, large tongues, recessed chins, and redundant pharyngeal tissue, associated with increased oxygen demand and decreased pulmonary reserves, impedes intubation (Haupt & Reed, 2010). The anesthesiologist or anesthetist also assesses for obstructive sleep apnea, frequently diagnosed in bariatric patients and treated with continuous positive airway pressure (CPAP) preoperatively and postoperatively. The use of CPAP should continue throughout the patient's recovery when reclining or when sleeping (Alvarex et al., 2010). As the incidence of obesity continues to grow, nurses will be called on to be part of multidisciplinary teams that will develop and implement clinical plans for patients who are obese.

Patients With Disabilities

Special considerations for patients with mental or physical disabilities include the need for appropriate assistive devices, modifications in preoperative education, and additional assistance with and attention to positioning or transferring (De Lima, Borges, da Costa, et al., 2010). Assistive devices include hearing aids, eyeglasses, braces, prostheses, and other devices. People who are hearing impaired may need a sign interpreter or some alternative communication system perioperatively. If the patient relies on signing or speech (lip) reading and his or her eyeglasses or contact lenses are removed or the health care staff wears surgical masks, an alternative method of communication will be needed. These needs must be identified in the preoperative evaluation and clearly communicated to personnel. Specific strategies for accommodating the patient's needs must be identified in advance. Ensuring the security of assistive devices is important, because these devices are expensive and require time to replace if lost.

Most patients are directed to move from the stretcher to the OR bed prior to surgery and back again following the procedure. In addition to being unable to see or hear instructions, the patient with a disability may be unable to move without special devices or a great deal of assistance. The patient with a disability that affects body position (e.g., cerebral palsy, postpolio syndrome, and other neuromuscular disorders) may need special positioning during surgery to prevent pain and injury (Stannard & Krenzischek, 2012). Disabled patients may be unable to sense painful positioning if their extremities are incorrectly adjusted, or they may be unable to communicate their discomfort.

Patients with respiratory problems related to a disability (e.g., multiple sclerosis, muscular dystrophy) may experience difficulties unless the problems are made known to the anesthesiologist or anesthetist and adjustments are made (Spry, 2009). These factors need to be clearly identified in the preoperative period and communicated to the appropriate personnel.

Patients Undergoing Ambulatory Surgery

Ambulatory surgery includes outpatient, same-day, or short-stay surgery not requiring admission for an overnight hospital stay but may entail observation in a hospital setting for 23 hours or less. During the brief time the patient and family spend in the ambulatory setting, the nurse must quickly and comprehensively assess and anticipate the needs of the patient and at the same time begin planning for discharge and follow-up home care.

The nurse needs to be sure that the patient and family understand that the patient will first go to the preoperative holding area before going to the OR for the surgical procedure and then will spend some time in the PACU before being discharged home with the family member later that day. Other preoperative education content should also be verified and reinforced as needed (see later discussion). The nurse should ensure that any plans for follow-up home care or new assistive devices are in place if needed.

Patients Undergoing Emergency Surgery

Emergency surgeries are unplanned and occur with little time for preparation of the patient or the perioperative team. The unpredictable nature of trauma and emergency surgery poses unique challenges to the nurse throughout the perioperative period. It is important for the nurse to communicate with the patient and team members as calmly and effectively as possible in these situations. (See Chapter 18 for the duties of the members of the perioperative team.)

Factors that affect patients preparing to undergo surgery also apply to patients undergoing emergency surgery, although usually in a very condensed time frame. The only opportunity for preoperative assessment may take place at the same time as resuscitation in the emergency department. A quick visual survey of the patient is essential to identify all sites of injury if the emergency surgery is due to trauma (see Chapter 72 for more information). The patient, who may have undergone a traumatic experience, may need extra support and explanation of the surgery. For the unconscious patient, informed consent and essential information, such as pertinent past medical history and allergies, need to be obtained from a family member, if one is available.

Informed Consent

Informed consent is the patient's autonomous decision about whether to undergo a surgical procedure. Voluntary and written informed consent from the patient is necessary before nonemergent surgery can be performed to protect the patient from unsanctioned surgery and protect the surgeon from claims of an unauthorized operation or battery. Consent is a legal mandate, but it also helps the patient to prepare psychologically, because it helps to ensure that the patient understands the surgery to be performed (Rothrock, 2010).

The nurse may ask the patient to sign the consent form and witness the signature; however, it is the surgeon's responsibility to provide a clear and simple explanation of what the surgery will entail prior to the patient giving consent. The surgeon must also inform the patient of the benefits, alternatives, possible risks, complications, disfigurement, disability, and removal of body parts as well as what to expect in the early and late postoperative periods. The nurse clarifies the information provided, and if the patient requests additional information, the nurse notifies the physician. The nurse ascertains that the consent form has been signed before administering psychoactive premedication, because consent is not valid if it is obtained while the patient is under the influence of medications that can affect judgment and decision-making capacity.

> ► *Quality and Safety Nursing Alert*
>
> The signed consent form is placed in a prominent place on the patient's medical record and accompanies the patient to the OR.

Many ethical principles are integral to informed consent (Chart 17-2). Informed consent is necessary in the following circumstances:

- Invasive procedures, such as a surgical incision, a biopsy, a cystoscopy, or paracentesis
- Procedures requiring sedation and/or anesthesia (see Chapter 18 for a discussion of anesthesia)
- A nonsurgical procedure, such as an arteriography, that carries more than a slight risk to the patient
- Procedures involving radiation

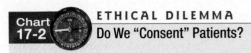

ETHICAL DILEMMA
Chart 17-2

Do We "Consent" Patients?

Case Scenario

You just completed the orientation program and assumed a new position as a staff nurse in an ambulatory surgery center. You finished obtaining informed consent from a patient scheduled for a minor procedure. As you walk past the charge nurse, you say, "I just consented Mrs. Owens." She sharply rebukes you, saying, "I would hope that you mean you obtained her informed consent."

Discussion

Although some clinicians claim that analyzing our choice of words is "hairsplitting" (i.e., nonconsequential), our choice of words, or semantics, do convey our point of view. For instance, when we refer to a patient among our peers as either a diagnosis (e.g., "the appendectomy") or by his or her assigned bed or room (e.g., "the patient in room 12"), we are not being respectful of our patients' identities. Not showing respect for personhood is tantamount to denying patient autonomy.

Analysis

- Describe the ethical principles that are in conflict in this case (see Chart 3-3). Which principle should have preeminence when you obtain informed consent from patients?
- Why is it not possible to say that you "consented a patient" and also assure that you obtained informed consent from a patient? How are these choices of terms at odds with each other? Do both choices of terms assure that patient autonomy is preserved?
- How would you respond to the charge nurse? Would you defend your choice of terms?

Resources

See Chapter 3, Chart 3-6 for ethics resources.

Chart 17-3

Valid Informed Consent

Voluntary Consent

Valid consent must be freely given, without coercion. Patient must be at least 18 years of age (unless an emancipated minor), a physician must obtain consent, and a professional staff member must witness patient's signature.

Incompetent Patient

Legal definition: individual who is *not* autonomous and cannot give or withhold consent (e.g., individuals who are cognitively impaired, mentally ill, or neurologically incapacitated).

Informed Subject

Informed consent should be in writing. It should contain the following:

- Explanation of procedure and its risks
- Description of benefits and alternatives
- An offer to answer questions about procedure
- Instructions that the patient may withdraw consent
- A statement informing the patient if the protocol differs from customary procedure

Patient Able to Comprehend

If the patient is non–English speaking, it is necessary to provide consent (written and verbal) in a language that is understandable to the client. A trained medical interpreter may be consulted. Alternative formats of communication (e.g., Braille, large print, sign interpreter) may be needed if the patient has a disability that affects vision or hearing. Questions must be answered to facilitate comprehension if material is confusing.

The patient personally signs the consent if of legal age and mentally capable. Permission is otherwise obtained from a surrogate, who most often is a responsible family member (preferably next of kin) or legal guardian. See Chart 17-3 for criteria for valid informed consent. State regulations and agency policy must be followed. In an emergency, it may be necessary for the surgeon to operate as a lifesaving measure without the patient's informed consent. However, every effort must be made to contact the patient's family. In such a situation, contact can be made by telephone, fax, or other electronic means and consent obtained.

If the patient has doubts and has not had the opportunity to investigate alternative treatments, a second opinion may be requested. No patient should be urged or coerced to give informed consent (Stell, 2009). Refusing to undergo a surgical procedure is a person's legal right and privilege. Such information must be documented and relayed to the surgeon so that other arrangements can be made. Additional explanations may be provided to the patient and family, or the surgery may be rescheduled. Consents for specific procedures such as sterilization, therapeutic abortion, disposal of severed body parts, organ donation, and blood product administration provide additional protection for the patient (Rothrock, 2010). States and regions may vary in their mandates.

Discussion with patients and their family members may be supplemented with audiovisual materials. Consent forms should be written in easily understandable words and concepts to facilitate the consent process and should use other strategies and resources as needed to help the patient understand the content (see Chart 17-3). Asking patients to describe in their own words the surgery they are about to have promotes nurses' understanding of patients' comprehension.

Preoperative Assessment

The goal in the preoperative period is for the patient to be as healthy as possible. Every attempt is made to assess for and address risk factors that may contribute to postoperative complications and delay recovery (Chart 17-4). A plan of action is designed so that potential complications are averted. Before any surgical treatment is initiated, a health history is obtained, a physical examination is performed during which vital signs are noted, and a database is established for future comparisons (Spry, 2009). During the physical examination, many factors that have the potential to affect the patient undergoing surgery are considered, such as joint mobility. Genetic considerations are also taken into account during assessment to prevent complications with anesthesia (Chart 17-5).

Asking the patient about use of prescription and over-the-counter (OTC) medications and herbal and other

RISK FACTORS
Chart 17-4 Surgical Complications

- Hypovolemia
- Dehydration or electrolyte imbalance
- Nutritional deficits
- Extremes of age (very young, very old)
- Extremes of weight (emaciation, obesity)
- Infection and sepsis
- Toxic conditions
- Immunologic abnormalities
- Pulmonary disease:
  - Obstructive disease
  - Restrictive disorder
  - Respiratory infection
- Renal or urinary tract disease:
  - Decreased renal function
  - Urinary tract infection
  - Obstruction
- Pregnancy:
  - Diminished maternal physiologic reserve
- Cardiovascular disease:
  - Coronary artery disease or previous myocardial infarction
  - Cardiac failure
  - Dysrhythmias
  - Hypertension
  - Prosthetic heart valve
  - Thromboembolism
  - Hemorrhagic disorders
  - Cerebrovascular disease
- Endocrine dysfunction:
  - Diabetes
  - Adrenal disorders
  - Thyroid malfunction
- Hepatic disease:
  - Cirrhosis
  - Hepatitis
- Preexisting mental or physical disability

supplements provides useful information. Activity level should be determined, including that involving regular aerobic exercise. Known allergies to drugs, foods, and latex could avert an anaphylactic response (Ewan, Dugué, Mirakian, et al., 2010). Patients may have early manifestations of a latex allergy and be unaware of this. If a patient states that he or she is allergic to kiwi, avocado, or banana, or cannot blow up balloons, there may be an association with an allergy to latex.

Latex, the milky fluid from the rubber tree, is found in many everyday products, and repeated exposure may cause some people to develop the allergy as an immune response to the protein (Australasian Society of Clinical Immunology and Allergy [ASCIA], 2011). Most hospital products today are latex free, especially in ORs; however, even the rubber stopper on a medication vial can trigger a deadly reaction following injection from that vial.

▶ Quality and Safety Nursing Alert

A latex allergy can manifest as a rash, asthma, or full anaphylactic shock.

Health care providers also should be alert for signs of abuse, which can occur at any age, in either sex, and in any socioeconomic, ethnic, and cultural group (Buscemi, 2011). Findings need to be reported accordingly (see Chapter 5 for further discussion of signs of abuse). Blood tests, x-rays, and other diagnostic tests are prescribed when indicated by information obtained from the history and physical examination.

Nutritional and Fluid Status

Optimal nutrition is an essential factor in promoting healing and resisting infection and other surgical complications. Assessment of a patient's nutritional status identifies factors that can affect the patient's surgical course, such as obesity,

GENETICS IN NURSING PRACTICE
Chart 17-5 Genetics Concepts and Perioperative Nursing

Nurses who are caring for patients undergoing surgery need to take various genetic considerations into account when assessing patients throughout the perioperative experience. For example, surgical outcomes may be altered by genetic conditions that may cause complications with anesthesia, including the following:

- Malignant hyperthermia
- Central core disease
- Duchenne muscular dystrophy
- Hyperkalemic periodic paralysis
- King-Denborough syndrome

Nursing Assessments

Family History Assessment

- Obtain a thorough assessment of personal and family history for three generations, inquiring about prior problems with surgery or anesthesia with specific attention to complications such as fever, rigidity, dark urine, and unexpected reactions.
- Inquire about any history of musculoskeletal complaints, history of heat intolerance, fevers of unknown origin, or unusual drug reactions.
- Assess for family history of any sudden or unexplained death, especially during participation in athletic events.

Patient Assessment

- Assess for subclinical muscle weakness.
- Assess for other physical features suggestive of an underlying genetic condition, such as contractures, kyphoscoliosis, and pterygium with progressive weakness.

Management Issues Specific to Genetics

- Inquire as to whether DNA mutation or other genetic testing has been performed on an affected family member.
- If indicated, refer for further genetic counseling and evaluation so that family members can discuss inheritance, risk to other family members, and availability of diagnostic/genetic testing.
- Offer appropriate genetics information and resources.
- Assess patient's understanding of genetics information.
- Provide support to families of patients with newly diagnosed malignant hyperthermia.
- Participate in management and coordination of care of patients with genetic conditions and individuals predisposed to develop or pass on a genetic condition.

Genetics Resources

See Chapter 8, Chart 8-6 for genetics resources.

TABLE 17-2 **Nutrients Important for Wound Healing**

Nutrient	Rationale for Increased Need	Possible Deficiency Outcome
Protein	To allow collagen deposition and wound healing to occur	Collagen deposition leading to impaired/delayed wound healing Decreased skin and wound strength Increased wound infection rates
Arginine (amino acid)	To provide necessary substrate for collagen synthesis and nitric oxide (crucial for wound healing) at wound site To increase wound strength and collagen deposition To stimulate T-cell response Associated with various essential reactions of intermediary metabolism	Impaired wound healing
Carbohydrates and fats	Primary source of energy in the body and consequently in the wound-healing process To meet the demand for increased essential fatty acids needed for cellular function after an injury To spare protein To restore normal weight	Signs and symptoms of protein deficiency due to the use of protein to meet energy requirements Extensive weight loss
Water	To replace fluid lost through vomiting, hemorrhage, exudates, fever, drainage, diuresis To maintain homeostasis	Signs, symptoms, and complications of dehydration, such as poor skin turgor, dry mucous membranes, oliguria, anuria, weight loss, increased pulse rate, decreased central venous pressure
Vitamin C	Important for capillary formation, tissue synthesis, and wound healing through collagen formation Needed for antibody formation	Impaired/delayed wound healing related to impaired collagen formation and increased capillary fragility and permeability Increased risk for infection related to decreased antibodies
Vitamin B complex	Indirect role in wound healing through their influence on host resistance	Decreased enzymes available for energy metabolism
Vitamin A	Increases inflammatory response in wounds, reduces anti-inflammatory effects of corticosteroids on wound healing	Impaired/delayed wound healing related to decreased collagen synthesis; impaired immune function Increased risk for infection
Vitamin K	Important for normal blood clotting Impaired intestinal synthesis associated with the use of antibiotics	Prolonged prothrombin time Hematomas contributing to impaired healing and predisposition to wound infections
Magnesium	Essential cofactor for many enzymes that are involved in the process of protein synthesis and wound repair	Impaired/delayed wound healing (impaired collagen production)
Copper	Required cofactor in the development of connective tissue	Impaired wound healing
Zinc	Involved in DNA synthesis, protein synthesis, cellular proliferation needed for wound healing Essential to immune function	Impaired immune response

Adapted from Dudek, S. G. (2010). *Nutrition essentials for nursing practice* (6th ed.). Philadelphia: Lippincott Williams & Wilkins; and Porth, C. M., & Matfin, G. (2009). *Pathophysiology: Concepts of altered health states* (8th ed.). Philadelphia: Lippincott Williams & Wilkins.

weight loss, malnutrition, deficiencies in specific nutrients, metabolic abnormalities, and the effects of medications on nutrition. Nutritional needs may be determined by measurement of body mass index and waist circumference. (See Chapter 5 for further discussion of nutritional assessment.)

Any nutritional deficiency should be corrected before surgery to provide adequate protein for tissue repair. The nutrients needed for wound healing are summarized in Table 17-2.

Dehydration, hypovolemia, and electrolyte imbalances can lead to significant problems in patients with comorbid medical conditions or in patients who are older. The severity of fluid and electrolyte imbalances is often difficult to determine. Mild volume deficits may be treated during surgery; however, additional time may be needed to correct pronounced fluid and electrolyte deficits to promote the best possible preoperative condition. The current shift to more minimally invasive abdominal surgical techniques has increased the need for bowel preparation. The depletion of fluids and electrolytes following bowel preparation can result in dehydration and chemical imbalances, even among healthy surgical patients. During surgery, dehydration and chemical imbalance is anticipated, planned for,

and addressed to maintain the patient in stable condition (Doran, 2010). The patient and family need to be informed of the need for fluid replacement following surgery.

Dentition

The condition of the mouth is an important health factor to assess. Dental caries, dentures, and partial plates are particularly significant to the anesthesiologist or anesthetist, because decayed teeth or dental prostheses may become dislodged during intubation and occlude the airway. This is especially important for older patients as well as those who may not have regular dental care. The condition of the mouth is also important because any bodily infection, even in the mouth, can be a source of postoperative infection.

Drug or Alcohol Use

Ingesting even moderate amounts of alcohol prior to surgery can weaken a patient's immune system and increase the likelihood of developing postoperative infections (Porth & Matfin, 2009). In addition, the use of illicit drugs and alcohol may impede the effectiveness of some medications. People who abuse drugs or alcohol frequently may deny or attempt to hide it. In such situations, the nurse who is obtaining the patient's health history needs to ask frank questions with patience, care, and a nonjudgmental attitude. (See Chapter 5 for an assessment of alcohol and drug use.)

Because acutely intoxicated people are susceptible to injury, surgery is postponed if possible. If emergency surgery is required, local, spinal, or regional block anesthesia is used for minor surgery (Faulk, Twite, Zuk, et al., 2010). Otherwise, to prevent vomiting and potential aspiration, a nasogastric tube is inserted before general anesthesia is administered.

The person with a history of chronic alcoholism often suffers from malnutrition and other systemic problems or metabolic imbalances that increase surgical risk. In patients who are alcohol dependent, alcohol withdrawal syndrome may be anticipated 2 to 4 days after the last drink and is associated with a significant mortality rate when it occurs postoperatively. This increase in mortality rate can be contributed to cardiac dysrhythmias, cardiomyopathy, and bleeding tendencies seen in long-term alcohol abuse (Riddle, Bush, Tittle, et al., 2010).

Respiratory Status

The patient is educated in breathing exercises and the use of an incentive spirometer, if indicated, to achieve optimal respiratory function prior to surgery. The potential compromise of ventilation during all phases of surgical treatment necessitates a proactive response to respiratory infections. Surgery is usually postponed for elective cases if the patient has a respiratory infection. Patients with underlying respiratory disease (e.g., asthma, chronic obstructive pulmonary disease) are assessed carefully for current threats to their pulmonary status. Patients also need to be assessed for comorbid conditions such as human immunodeficiency virus infection and Parkinson's disease, which may affect respiratory function (West, 2011).

Patients who smoke are urged to stop 4 to 8 weeks before surgery to significantly reduce pulmonary and wound healing complications. Preoperative smoking cessation interventions can be effective in changing smoking behavior and reducing the incidence of postoperative complications. Patients who smoke are more likely to experience poor wound healing, a higher incidence of SSI, and complications that include VTE and pneumonia (West, 2011).

Cardiovascular Status

Patient preparation for surgical intervention includes ensuring that the cardiovascular system can support the oxygen, fluid, and nutritional needs of the perioperative period. If the patient has uncontrolled hypertension, surgery may be postponed until the blood pressure is under control. At times, surgical treatment can be modified to meet the cardiac tolerance of the patient. For example, in a patient with obstruction of the descending colon and coronary artery disease, a temporary simple colostomy may be performed rather than a more extensive colon resection that would require a prolonged period of anesthesia.

Hepatic and Renal Function

The presurgical goal is optimal function of the liver and urinary systems so that medications, anesthetic agents, body wastes, and toxins are adequately metabolized and removed from the body. The liver, lungs, and kidneys are the routes for elimination of drugs and toxins.

The liver is important in the biotransformation of anesthetic compounds. Disorders of the liver may substantially affect how anesthetic agents are metabolized. Acute liver disease is associated with high surgical mortality; preoperative improvement in liver function is a goal. Careful assessment may include various liver function tests (see Chapter 49).

The kidneys are involved in excreting anesthetic medications and their metabolites; therefore, surgery is contraindicated if a patient has acute nephritis, acute renal insufficiency with oliguria or anuria, or other acute renal problems (see Chapter 54). Exceptions include surgeries performed as lifesaving measures, surgery to enable easier access for dialysis, or those necessary to improve urinary function (i.e., obstructive uropathy or hydronephrosis).

Endocrine Function

The patient with diabetes who is undergoing surgery is at risk for both hypoglycemia and hyperglycemia. Hypoglycemia may develop during anesthesia or postoperatively from inadequate carbohydrates or excessive administration of insulin. Hyperglycemia, which can increase the risk of surgical wound infection, may result from the stress of surgery, which can trigger increased levels of catecholamine. Other risks are acidosis and glucosuria. Although the surgical risk in the patient with controlled diabetes is no greater than in the patient without diabetes, strict glycemic control (80 to 110 mg/dL) leads to better outcomes (Alvarex et al., 2010). Frequent monitoring of blood glucose levels is important before, during, and after surgery. (See Chapter 51 for a discussion of the patient with diabetes.)

Patients who have received corticosteroids are at risk for adrenal insufficiency. The use of corticosteroids for any purpose during the preceding year must be reported to the anesthesiologist or anesthetist and surgeon. The patient is monitored for signs of adrenal insufficiency (see Chapter 52).

Patients with uncontrolled thyroid disorders are at risk for thyrotoxicosis (with hyperthyroid disorders) or respiratory failure (with hypothyroid disorders). The patient with an associated history of a thyroid disorder is assessed preoperatively (see Chapter 52).

Immune Function

An important function of the preoperative assessment is to determine the presence of allergies. It is especially important to identify and document any sensitivity to medications and past adverse reactions (ASCIA, 2011). The patient is asked to identify any substances that precipitated previous allergic reactions, including medications, blood transfusions, contrast agents, latex, and food products, and to describe the signs and symptoms produced by these substances. A sample latex allergy screening questionnaire is shown in Figure 17-1.

Immunosuppression is common with corticosteroid therapy, renal transplantation, radiation therapy, chemotherapy, and disorders affecting the immune system, such as acquired immunodeficiency syndrome and leukemia. The mildest symptoms or slightest temperature elevation must be investigated.

Latex Allergy Assessment

Ask the patient the following questions. Check "Yes" or "No" in the box.	YES	NO
1. Has a doctor ever told you that you are allergic to latex?		
2. Do you have on-the-job exposure to latex?		
3. Were you born with problems involving your spinal cord?		
4. Have you ever had allergies, asthma, hay fever, eczema, or problems with rashes?		
5. Have you ever had respiratory distress, rapid heart rate, or swelling?		
6. Have you ever had swelling, itching, hives, or other symptoms after contact with a balloon?		
7. Have you ever had swelling, itching, hives, or other symptoms after a dental examination or procedure?		
8. Have you ever had swelling, itching, hives, or other symptoms following a vaginal or rectal examination or after contact with a diaphragm or condom?		
9. Have you ever had swelling, itching, hives, or other symptoms during or within 1 hour after wearing rubber gloves?		
10. Have you ever had a rash on your hands that lasted longer than 1 week?		
11. Have you ever had swelling, itching, hives, runny nose, eye irritation, wheezing, or asthma after contact with any latex or rubber product?		
12. Have you ever had swelling, itching, hives, or other symptoms after being examined by someone wearing rubber or latex gloves?		
13. Are you allergic to bananas, avocados, kiwi, or chestnuts?		
14. Have you ever had an unexplained anaphylactic episode?		

Preop RN Signature: _____

Patient Name: _____

Procedure: _____

Scheduled Date / Time: _____

Surgeon: _____

FIGURE 17-1 • Example of a latex allergy assessment form. Courtesy of Inova Fair Oaks Hospital, Fairfax, VA.

Previous Medication Use

A medication history is obtained because of the possible interactions with medications that might be administered during surgery and the effects of any of these medications on the patient's perioperative course. Any medications the patient is using or has used in the past is documented, including OTC preparations and herbal agents, as well as the frequency with which they are used. Many medications have an effect on physiologic functions; interactions of such medications with anesthetic agents can cause serious problems, such as hypotension and circulatory collapse. Medications that cause particular concern are listed in Table 17-3.

Aspirin, a common OTC medication that inhibits platelet aggregation, should be prudently discontinued 7 to 10 days before surgery; otherwise, the patient may be at increased risk for bleeding (Rothrock, 2010). Any use of aspirin or other OTC medications is noted in the patient's medical record and conveyed to the anesthesiologist or anesthetist and surgeon. The anesthesiologist or anesthetist evaluates the potential effects of prior medication therapy, considering the length of time the patient has used the medication, the physical condition of the patient, and the nature of the proposed surgery (Miller et al., 2010).

> ### Quality and Safety Nursing Alert
>
> The possible adverse interactions of some medications require the nurse to assess and document the patient's use of prescription medications, OTC medications (especially aspirin), herbal agents, and the frequency with which medications are used. The nurse must clearly communicate this information to the anesthesiologist or anesthetist.

The use of medications is widespread among patients; approximately 40% of Americans report taking some form of these substances (Rowe & Baker, 2009). Commonly used herbal medications may include echinacea, garlic (*Allium sativum*), ginkgo biloba, ginseng, kava kava (*Piper methysticum*), St. John's wort (*Hypericum perforatum*), licorice extract (*Glycyrrhizic acid*), and valerian (*Valeriana officinalis*). Many patients fail to report the use of herbal medicines to health care providers; therefore, the nurse must ask surgical patients specifically about the use of these agents (Izzo & Ernst, 2009). It is recommended that patients anticipating surgery discontinue the use of herbal medicines at least 2 weeks before surgery, because many herbal agents can adversely affect surgical outcomes (Rowe & Baker, 2009).

Psychosocial Factors

The nurse anticipates that most patients have emotional reactions prior to surgery—obvious or veiled, normal or abnormal. Fear may be related to the unknown, lack of control, or of death and may be influenced by anesthesia, pain, complications, cancer, or prior surgical experience. Preoperative anxiety can be a preemptive response to a threat to the patient's role in life, a permanent incapacity or body integrity, increased responsibilities or burden on family members, or life itself. Less obvious concerns may occur because of previous experiences with the health care system and people the patient has known with the same condition. Psychological distress directly influences body functioning. Identification of anxiety by the health care team using supportive guidance at every juncture of the perioperative process helps to ease anxiety (Weber & Kelley, 2009).

People express fear in different ways. Some patients may ask repeated questions, regardless of information already shared with them. Others may withdraw, deliberately avoiding communication by reading, watching television, or talking about trivialities. Consequently, the nurse must be empathetic, listen well, and provide information that helps alleviate concerns.

TABLE 17-3   Examples of Medications With the Potential to Affect the Surgical Experience

Agent	Effect of Interaction With Anesthetics
Corticosteroids Prednisone (Deltasone)	Cardiovascular collapse can occur if discontinued suddenly. Therefore, a bolus of corticosteroid may be administered IV immediately before and after surgery.
Diuretics Hydrochlorothiazide (HydroDIURIL)	During anesthesia, may cause excessive respiratory depression resulting from an associated electrolyte imbalance
Phenothiazines Chlorpromazine (Thorazine)	May increase the hypotensive action of anesthetics
Tranquilizers Diazepam (Valium)	May cause anxiety, tension, and even seizures if withdrawn suddenly
Insulins	Interaction between anesthetics and insulin must be considered when a patient with diabetes is undergoing surgery. IV insulin may need to be administered to keep the blood glucose within the normal range.
Antibiotics Erythromycin (Ery-Tab)	When combined with a curariform muscle relaxant, nerve transmission is interrupted and apnea from respiratory paralysis may result.
Anticoagulants Warfarin (Coumadin)	Can increase the risk of bleeding during the intraoperative and postoperative periods; should be discontinued in anticipation of elective surgery. The surgeon will determine how long before the elective surgery the patient should stop taking an anticoagulant, depending on the type of planned procedure and the medical condition of the patient.
Antiseizure Medications	IV administration of medication may be needed to keep the patient seizure free in the intraoperative and postoperative periods.
Thyroid Hormone Levothyroxine sodium (Levothroid)	IV administration may be needed during the postoperative period to maintain thyroid levels.
Opioids Morphine sulfate (MS Contin)	Long-term use of opioids for chronic pain (≥6 mo) in the preoperative period may alter the patient's response to analgesic agents.

Adapted from Costantini, R., Affaitati, G., Fabrizio, A., et al. (2011). Controlling pain in the post-operative setting. *International Journal of Clinical Pharmacology & Therapeutics*, 49(2), 116–127.

An important outcome of the psychosocial assessment is the determination of the extent and role of the patient's support network. The value and reliability of available support systems are assessed. Other information, such as knowledge of the usual level of functioning and typical daily activities, may assist in the patient's care and recovery. Assessing the patient's readiness to learn and determining the best approach to maximize comprehension provides the basis for preoperative patient education. This is of particular importance in patients who are developmentally delayed and those who are cognitively impaired, where the approach to patient education and consent will include the legal guardian.

Spiritual and Cultural Beliefs

Spiritual beliefs play an important role in how people cope with fear and anxiety. Regardless of the patient's religious affiliation, spiritual beliefs can be as therapeutic as medication. Every attempt must be made to help the patient obtain the spiritual support that he or she requests. Therefore, the nurse must respect and support the beliefs of each patient. Some nurses may avoid the subject of a clergy visit lest the suggestion alarm the patient. Asking whether the patient's spiritual advisor knows about the impending surgery is a caring, nonthreatening approach.

Showing respect for a patient's cultural values and beliefs facilitates rapport and trust. Some areas of assessment include identifying the ethnic group to which the patient relates and the customs and beliefs the patient holds about illness and health care providers. Some ethnic groups are unaccustomed to expressing feelings openly with strangers (Engebretson, 2011). Nurses need to consider this pattern of communication when assessing pain. In some cultural groups, it is seen as impolite to make direct eye contact with others and doing so is seen as disrespectful (Buscemi, 2011). The nurse should know that this lack of eye contact is not avoidance nor does it reflect a lack of interest. Other ethnicities may view the top of the head as sacred; therefore, a nurse would not put the surgical cap on the patient but would ask the patient to don the cap.

Perhaps the most valuable skill at the nurse's disposal is listening carefully to the patient and observing body language, especially when obtaining the history. Invaluable information and insights may be gained through effective communication and interviewing skills. An unhurried, understanding, and caring nurse promotes confidence on the part of the patient.

Preoperative Nursing Interventions

A wide range of interventions are used to prepare the patient physically and psychologically and to maintain safety. Beginning with the nursing history and physical examination, listing of medications taken routinely, history of allergies, and surgical and anesthetic histories, the patient's overall health status and level of experience and understanding may be established.

Providing Patient Education

Nurses have long recognized the value of preoperative instruction (Rothrock, 2010). Each patient's education is individualized, with consideration for any unique concerns or learning needs. Multiple education strategies should be used (e.g., verbal, written, return demonstration), depending on the patient's needs and abilities.

Preoperative education is initiated as soon as possible, beginning in the physician's office, in the clinic, or at the time of PAT when diagnostic tests are performed. During PAT, the nurse or health care provider makes resources available related to patient education, such as written instructions (designed to be copied and given to patients), audiovisual resources, and telephone numbers, to ensure that education continues until the patient arrives for the surgical intervention. When possible, instruction is spaced over a period of time to allow the patient to assimilate information and ask questions as they arise.

Frequently, education sessions are combined with various preparation procedures to allow for an easy and timely flow of information. The nurse should guide the patient through the experience and allow ample time for questions. Education should go beyond descriptions of the procedure and should include explanations of the sensations the patient will experience. Telling the patient that preoperative medication will cause relaxation before the operation is not as effective as also noting that the medication will act quickly and may result in lightheadedness, dizziness, and drowsiness. Knowing what to expect will help the patient anticipate these reactions and attain a superior degree of relaxation. Overly detailed descriptions may increase anxiety in some patients; therefore, the nurse should be sensitive to this, by watching and listening, and provide less detail based on the individual patient's needs.

Concept Mastery Alert

Patient education serves to prepare the patient physically and emotionally for the surgery, with the ultimate goal of reducing the risk for complications and thus promoting an optimal recovery period. Legally, the surgeon is responsible for explaining simply and clearly what the surgery involves and what to expect in the early and late postoperative periods; the nurse often clarifies this information for the patient.

Deep Breathing, Coughing, and Incentive Spirometry

One goal of preoperative nursing care is to educate the patient how to promote optimal lung expansion and resulting blood oxygenation after anesthesia. The patient assumes a sitting position to enhance lung expansion. The nurse then demonstrates how to take a deep, slow breath and how to exhale slowly. After practicing deep breathing several times, the patient is instructed to breathe deeply, exhale through the mouth, take a short breath, and cough deeply in the lungs (Chart 17-6). The nurse or respiratory therapist also demonstrates how to use an incentive spirometer, a device that provides measurement and feedback related to breathing effectiveness (see Chapter 21). In addition to enhancing respiration, these exercises may help the patient relax. Research indicates that some patients benefit from intensive inspiratory muscle training in the preoperative period (West, 2011).

If a thoracic or abdominal incision is anticipated, the nurse demonstrates how to splint the incision to minimize pressure and control pain. The patient should put the palms of both hands together, interlacing the fingers snugly. Splinting or placing the hands across the incision site acts as an effective support when coughing. The patient is informed that medications are available to relieve pain and should be taken regularly for pain relief so that effective deep-breathing and coughing exercises can be performed comfortably. The goal in promoting coughing is to mobilize secretions so that they can be removed. Deep breathing before coughing stimulates the cough reflex. If the patient does not cough effectively, atelectasis (collapse of the alveoli), pneumonia, or other lung complications may occur.

Mobility and Active Body Movement

The goals of promoting mobility postoperatively are to improve circulation, prevent venous stasis, and promote optimal respiratory function. The patient should be taught that early and frequent ambulation postoperatively, as tolerated, will help prevent complications.

The nurse explains the rationale for frequent position changes after surgery and then shows the patient how to turn from side to side and how to assume the lateral position without causing pain or disrupting intravenous (IV) lines, drainage tubes, or other equipment. Any special position the patient needs to maintain after surgery (e.g., adduction or elevation of an extremity) is discussed, as is the importance of maintaining as much mobility as possible despite restrictions. Reviewing the process before surgery is helpful, because the patient may be too uncomfortable or drowsy after surgery to absorb new information.

Exercise of the extremities includes extension and flexion of the knee and hip joints (similar to bicycle riding while lying on the side) unless contraindicated by type of surgical procedure (e.g., hip replacement). The foot is rotated as though tracing the largest possible circle with the great toe (see Chart 17-6). The elbow and shoulder are also put through their range of motion. At first, the patient is assisted and reminded to perform these exercises. Later, the patient is encouraged to do them independently. Muscle tone is maintained so that ambulation will be easier. The nurse should remember to use proper body mechanics and to instruct the

Chart
17-6

PATIENT EDUCATION

Preoperative Instructions to Prevent Postoperative Complications

Diaphragmatic Breathing

Diaphragmatic breathing refers to a flattening of the dome of the diaphragm during inspiration, with resultant enlargement of the upper abdomen as air rushes in. During expiration, the abdominal muscles contract.

1. Practice in the same position you would assume in bed after surgery: a semi-Fowler's position, propped in bed with the back and shoulders well supported with pillows.
2. Feel the movement with your hands resting lightly on the front of the lower ribs and fingertips against the lower chest.

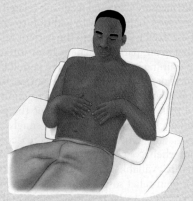

Diaphragmatic breathing

3. Breathe out gently and fully as the ribs sink down and inward toward midline.
4. Then take a deep breath through your nose and mouth, letting the abdomen rise as the lungs fill with air.
5. Hold this breath for a count of five.
6. Exhale and let out *all* the air through your nose and mouth.
7. Repeat this exercise 15 times with a short rest after each group of five.
8. Practice this twice a day preoperatively.

Coughing

1. Lean forward slightly from a sitting position in bed, interlace your fingers together, and place your hands across the incision site to act as a splint for support when coughing.

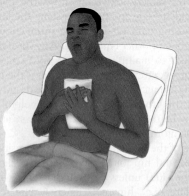

Splinting of chest when coughing

2. Breathe with the diaphragm as described under "Diaphragmatic Breathing."

3. With your mouth slightly open, breathe in fully.
4. "Hack" out sharply for three short breaths.
5. Then, keeping your mouth open, take in a quick deep breath and immediately give a strong cough once or twice. This helps clear secretions from your chest. It may cause some discomfort but will not harm your incision.

Leg Exercises

1. Lie in a semi-Fowler's position and perform the following simple exercises to improve circulation.
2. Bend your knee and raise your foot—hold it a few seconds, then extend the leg and lower it to the bed.

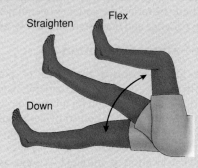

Leg exercises

3. Do this five times with one leg and then repeat with the other leg.
4. Then trace circles with the feet by bending them down, in toward each other, up, and then out.
5. Repeat these movements five times.

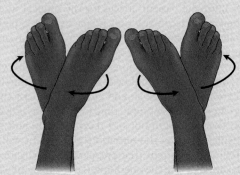

Foot exercises

Turning to the Side

1. Turn on your side with the uppermost leg flexed most and supported on a pillow.
2. Grasp the side rail as an aid to maneuver to the side.
3. Practice diaphragmatic breathing and coughing while on your side.

Getting Out of Bed

1. Turn on your side.
2. Push yourself up with one hand as you swing your legs out of bed.

Preoperative Pain Assessment and Education for Older Adults

The older person undergoing surgery may have a combination of chronic illnesses and health issues in addition to the specific one for which surgery is indicated. Older adults frequently do not report symptoms, perhaps because they fear a serious illness may be diagnosed or because they accept such symptoms as part of the aging process. Subtle clues alert the nurse to underlying problems. Some older patients believe that pain is inevitable with aging and is meant to be endured; therefore, nurses must educate the patient about the benefits of controlling pain. Older patients also report higher levels of preoperative anxiety; therefore, the nurse should be prepared to spend additional time, increase the amount of therapeutic touch utilized, and encourage family members to be present to decrease anxiety (Constantini, Affaitati, Fabrizio, et al., 2011).

patient to do the same. Whenever the patient is positioned, his or her body needs to be properly aligned.

Pain Management

A pain assessment should include differentiation between acute and chronic pain. A pain intensity scale should be introduced and explained to the patient to promote more effective postoperative pain management. (See Chapter 12 for examples of pain scales.) Preoperative patient education also needs to include the difference between acute and chronic pain so that the patient is prepared to differentiate acute postoperative pain from a chronic condition such as back pain. Preoperative pain assessment and education for the older patient may require additional attention (Chart 17-7).

Postoperatively, medications are administered to relieve pain and maintain comfort without suppressing respiratory function. The patient is instructed to take the medication as frequently as prescribed during the initial postoperative period for pain relief. Anticipated methods of administration of analgesic agents for inpatients include patient-controlled analgesia (PCA), epidural catheter bolus or infusion, or patient-controlled epidural analgesia (PCEA). (See Chapter 12 for discussion of PCA and PCEA.) A patient who is expected to go home will likely receive oral analgesic agents. These methods are discussed with the patient before surgery, and the patient's interest and willingness to use them are assessed.

Cognitive Coping Strategies

Cognitive strategies may be useful for relieving tension, overcoming anxiety, decreasing fear, and achieving relaxation. Examples of general strategies include:

- *Imagery:* The patient concentrates on a pleasant experience or restful scene.
- *Distraction:* The patient thinks of an enjoyable story or recites a favorite poem or song.
- *Optimistic self-recitation:* The patient recites optimistic thoughts ("I know all will go well").
- *Music:* The patient listens to soothing music (an easy-to-administer, inexpensive, noninvasive intervention).

Education for Patients Undergoing Ambulatory Surgery

Preoperative education for the same-day or ambulatory surgical patient comprises all previously discussed patient education

as well as collaborative planning with the patient and family for discharge and follow-up home care. The major difference in outpatient preoperative education is the environment.

Preoperative education content may be presented in a group class, in a media presentation, at PAT, or by telephone in conjunction with the preoperative interview. In addition to answering questions and describing what to expect, the nurse tells the patient when and where to report, what to bring (insurance card, list of medications and allergies), what to leave at home (jewelry, watch, medications, contact lenses), and what to wear (loose-fitting, comfortable clothes; flat shoes). The nurse in the surgeon's office may initiate education before the perioperative telephone contact.

During the final preoperative telephone call, education is completed or reinforced as needed, and last-minute instructions are given. The patient is reminded not to eat or drink for a specified period of time preoperatively.

Providing Psychosocial Interventions

Reducing Anxiety and Decreasing Fear

Perioperative nurses in the preoperative department have a limited amount of time to acquire information and establish trust. Nurses must introduce themselves, giving their title and a brief synopsis of their professional role and background. Each preoperative patient should be acknowledged as an individual, and each patient's needs and desires must be assessed. The patient should be thanked for choosing that particular hospital or surgical center. These methods facilitate establishing a positive nurse–patient relationship. Discussion of the surgical experience, its length, and explanation of what will happen may diminish the patient's anxiety.

During the preoperative assessment of psychological factors and spiritual and cultural beliefs, the nurse assists the patient to identify coping strategies that he or she has previously used to decrease fear. Discussions with the patient to help determine the source of fears can help with expression of concerns. The patient benefits from knowing when family and friends will be able to visit after surgery and that a spiritual advisor will be available if desired. The preoperative education and cognitive coping strategies addressed earlier help decrease preoperative anxiety in many patients (Moradipanah, Mohammadi, & Mohammadil, 2009). Knowing ahead of time about the possible need for a ventilator, drainage tubes, or other types of equipment helps decrease anxiety related to the postoperative period.

Respecting Cultural, Spiritual, and Religious Beliefs

Psychosocial interventions include identifying and showing respect for cultural, spiritual, and religious beliefs. In some cultures, for example, people are stoic in regard to pain, whereas in others they are more expressive. These responses should be recognized as normal for those patients and families and should be respected by perioperative personnel (Buscemi, 2011). If patients decline blood transfusions for religious reasons (Jehovah's Witnesses), this information needs to be clearly identified in the preoperative period, documented, and communicated to the appropriate personnel. Although minimally invasive surgery has significantly lowered blood loss, any surgical procedure has the potential for hemorrhage.

Chart 17-8

Summary of the 2012 National Patient Safety Goals

- Identify patients correctly.
- Improve staff communication.
- Use medicines safely.
- Prevent infection.
- Identify patient safety risks.
- Prevent mistakes in surgery.

Adapted from the Joint Commission. (2013). *2013 National Patient Safety Goals.* Available at: www.jointcommission.org/standards _information/npsgs.aspx

Maintaining Patient Safety

Protecting patients from injury is one of the major roles of the perioperative nurse. Adherence to AORN recommended practices and the Joint Commission's National Patient Safety Goals (Chart 17-8) are crucial (Rothrock, 2010). These apply to hospitals as well as to ambulatory surgery centers and office-based surgery facilities (Joint Commission, 2012). Researchers are investigating "near misses," or injuries that almost occur in the perioperative setting (Chart 17-9).

Managing Nutrition and Fluids

The major purpose of withholding food and fluid before surgery is to prevent aspiration. Until recently, fluid and food were restricted preoperatively overnight and often longer. The American Society of Anesthesiologists reviewed this practice and made new recommendations for people undergoing elective surgery who are otherwise healthy. Specific recommendations depend on the age of the patient and the type of food eaten. For example, adults may be advised to fast for 8 hours after eating fatty food and 4 hours after ingesting milk products. Healthy patients are allowed clear liquids up to 2 hours before an elective procedure (Crenshaw, 2011).

Preparing the Bowel

Enemas are not commonly prescribed preoperatively unless the patient is undergoing abdominal or pelvic surgery. In this case, a cleansing enema or laxative may be prescribed the evening before surgery and may be repeated the morning of surgery. The goals of this preparation are to allow satisfactory visualization of the surgical site and to prevent trauma to the intestine or contamination of the peritoneum by fecal material. Unless the condition of the patient presents some contraindication, the toilet or bedside commode, rather than the bedpan, is used for evacuating the enema if the patient is hospitalized during this time. In addition, antibiotics may be prescribed to reduce intestinal flora.

Preparing the Skin

The goal of preoperative skin preparation is to decrease bacteria without injuring the skin. If the surgery is not performed as an emergency, the patient may be instructed to use a soap containing a detergent-germicide to cleanse the skin area for several days before surgery to reduce the number of skin organisms; this preparation may be carried out at home.

Generally, hair is not removed preoperatively unless the hair at or around the incision site is likely to interfere with the operation. If hair must be removed, electric clippers are used for safe hair removal immediately before the operation (AORN, 2011). To ensure the correct site, the surgical site is typically marked by the patient and the surgeon prior to the procedure.

Immediate Preoperative Nursing Interventions

Immediately prior to the procedure, the patient changes into a hospital gown that is left untied and open in the back. The patient with long hair may braid it, remove hairpins, and cover the head completely with a disposable paper cap. The mouth is inspected, and dentures or plates are removed. If left in the mouth, these items could easily fall to the back of the throat during induction of anesthesia and cause respiratory obstruction.

Jewelry is not worn to the OR; wedding rings and jewelry or body piercings should be removed to prevent injury. If a patient objects to removing a ring, some institutions allow the ring to be securely fastened to the finger with tape. All

NURSING RESEARCH PROFILE

Chart 17-9

Causes of Near Misses

Cohoon, B. (2011). Causes of near misses: Perceptions of perioperative nurses. *AORN Journal, 93*(5), 551–565.

Purpose

Previous events indicate the potential for systemic problems, and the identification of near misses is an important method of predicting system failures. Events labeled near misses are injuries that almost always occur in the perioperative setting. The purpose of this study was to identify causes of near misses.

Design

At a health care system in the mid-Atlantic region of the United States, 377 possible participants from the perioperative setting completed up to four "near-miss" surveys from their personal experience in this descriptive mixed methods study. Power analysis indicated that a sample size of 100 surveys was necessary, with a minimum of 25 participants.

Findings

Six causal factors were identified (hospital characteristics, patient characteristics, workload, task, staffing, team), with inconsistent information and incorrect monitoring being the most common. Fifty-five nurses completed surveys, totaling 163 returned surveys. Tuesdays showed the highest number of near misses, with the operating room having 46%, postanesthesia care unit 16%, preoperative holding 35%, and 3% in other areas.

Nursing Implications

Examination of perioperative near-miss situations leads to an understanding of the causes and helps to define methods of avoiding errors in the future. The size of the study and the limitation of it having been conducted at only one hospital system limit the generalizability of the findings. Further research is needed to determine if causes of the near-miss experience are universal. If so, findings could lead to policy and procedure changes, which could lead to a safer perioperative environment.

articles of value, including assistive devices, dentures, glasses, and prosthetic devices, are given to family members or are labeled clearly with the patient's name and stored in a safe and secure place according to the institution's policy.

All patients (except those with urologic disorders) should void immediately before going to the OR. This is particularly important in promoting visibility of anatomy and continence during low abdominal surgery. Urinary catheterization is performed in the OR only as necessary.

Administering Preanesthetic Medication

The use of preanesthetic medication is minimal with ambulatory or outpatient surgery. If prescribed, it is usually administered in the preoperative holding area. If a preanesthetic medication is administered, the patient is kept in bed with the side rails raised, because the medication can cause lightheadedness or drowsiness. During this time, the nurse observes the patient for any untoward reaction to the medi-

cations. The immediate surroundings are kept quiet to promote relaxation, and some facilities use soft classical music (Moradipanah et al., 2009).

Often, surgery is delayed or schedules change, and it becomes impossible to request that a medication be given at a specific time. In these situations, the preoperative medication is prescribed "on call to OR." The nurse can have the medication ready to administer as soon as a call is received from the OR staff. It usually takes 15 to 20 minutes to prepare the patient for the OR. If the nurse gives the medication before attending to the other details of preoperative preparation, the patient will have at least partial benefit from the preoperative medication and will have a smoother anesthetic and operative course.

Maintaining the Preoperative Record

Preoperative checklists contain critical elements that must be checked and verified preoperatively (Rothrock, 2010). The nurse completes the preoperative checklist (Fig. 17-2). The

Preoperative Checklist

1. Patient's name: _____ Date: _____ Height: _____ Weight: _____
   Identification band present: _____
2. Informed consent signed: _____ Special permits signed: _____
3. Surgical site: _____ (Ex: Sterilization)
4. History & physical examination report present: _____ Date: _____
5. Laboratory records present: _____
   CBC: _____ Hgb: _____ Urinalysis: _____ Hct: _____

6. Item	Present	Removed
a. Natural teeth		
Dentures; upper, lower, partial		
Bridge, fixed; crown		
b. Contact lenses		
c. Other prostheses—type: _____		
d. Jewelry:		
Wedding band (taped/tied)		
Rings		
Earrings: pierced, clip-on		
Neck chains		
Any other body piercings		
e. Make-up		
Nail polish		
7. Clothing		
a. Clean patient gown		
b. Cap		
c. Sanitary pad, etc.		

8. Family instructed where to wait? _____
9. Valuables secured? _____
10. Blood available? _____ Ordered? _____ Where? _____
11. Preanesthetic medication given: _____
    Type: _____ Time: _____
12. Voided: _____ Amount: _____ Time: _____ Catheter: _____
    Mouth care given: _____
13. Vital signs: Temperature: _____ Pulse: _____ Resp: _____ Blood Pressure: _____
14. Special problems/precautions: (Allergies, deafness, etc.): _____
15. Area of skin preparation: _____
16. _____ Date: _____ Time: _____
    Signature: Nurse releasing patient

FIGURE 17-2 • Example of a preoperative checklist.

completed medical record (with the preoperative checklist and verification form) accompanies the patient to the OR with the surgical consent form attached, along with all laboratory reports and nurses' records. Any unusual last-minute observations that may have a bearing on anesthesia or surgery are noted prominently at the front of the medical record.

Transporting the Patient to the Presurgical Area

The patient is brought to the holding area or presurgical suite about 30 to 60 minutes before the anesthetic is to be given. The stretcher should be as comfortable as possible, with a sufficient number of blankets to prevent chilling in an air-conditioned room. A small head pillow is usually provided.

The patient is taken to the preoperative holding area, greeted by name, and positioned comfortably on the stretcher or bed. The surrounding area should be kept quiet if the preoperative medication is to have maximal effect. Unpleasant sounds or conversation should be avoided, because a sedated patient may misinterpret them.

Patient safety in the preoperative area is a priority. The use of a standard process or procedure to verify patient identification, the surgical procedure, and the surgical site is imperative to maximize patient safety (World Health Organization, 2008). This allows for prompt intervention if any discrepancies are identified.

Attending to Family Needs

Most hospitals and ambulatory surgery centers have a waiting room where family members and significant others can wait while the patient is undergoing surgery. This room may be equipped with comfortable chairs, televisions, telephones, and light refreshments. Volunteers may remain with the family, offer them coffee, and keep them informed of the patient's progress. After surgery, the surgeon may meet the family in the waiting room and discuss the outcome.

The family and significant others should never judge the seriousness of an operation by the length of time the patient is in the OR. A patient may be in the OR much longer than the actual operating time for several reasons:

- Patients are routinely transported well in advance of the actual operating time.
- The anesthesiologist or anesthetist often makes additional preparations that may take 30 to 60 minutes.
- The surgeon may take longer than expected with the preceding case, which delays the start of the next surgical procedure.

After surgery, the patient is taken to the PACU to ensure safe emergence from anesthesia. Family members and significant others waiting to see the patient after surgery should be informed that the patient may have certain equipment or devices (e.g., IV lines, indwelling urinary catheter, nasogastric tube, oxygen lines, monitoring equipment, blood transfusion lines) in place when he or she returns from surgery. When the patient returns to the room, the nurse provides explanations regarding the frequent postoperative observations that will be made. However, it is the responsibility of the surgeon, not the nurse, to relay the surgical findings and the prognosis, even when the findings are favorable.

Chart 17-10 **Expected Patient Outcomes in the Preoperative Phase of Care**

Relief of anxiety, evidenced when the patient:
- Discusses with the anesthesiologist, anesthetist, or nurse anesthetist concerns related to types of anesthesia and induction
- Verbalizes an understanding of the preanesthetic medication and general anesthesia
- Discusses last-minute concerns with the nurse or physician
- Discusses financial concerns with the social worker, when appropriate
- Requests visit with spiritual advisor, when appropriate
- Appears relaxed when visited by health care team members

Decreased fear, evidenced when the patient:
- Discusses fears with health care professionals or a spiritual advisor, or both
- Verbalizes an understanding of any expected bodily changes, including expected duration of bodily changes

Understanding of the surgical intervention, evidenced when the patient:
- Participates in preoperative preparation
- Demonstrates and describes exercises that he or she is expected to perform postoperatively
- Reviews information about postoperative care
- Accepts preanesthetic medication, if prescribed
- Remains in bed once premedicated
- Relaxes during transportation to the operating room or unit
- States rationale for use of side rails
- Discusses postoperative expectations

No evidence of preoperative complications

Expected Patient Outcomes

Expected patient outcomes in the preoperative phase of care are summarized in Chart 17-10.

Critical Thinking Exercises

1 **pq** During your preoperative assessment of your patient, a 68-year-old woman who is alert and oriented describes her surgery as "getting a new right knee." The OR schedule indicates that she is having a left knee arthroscopy. What are the priorities of the perioperative nurse? What further assessments are priorities? What nursing interventions are warranted?

2 **ebp** A morbidly obese 55-year-old man with a history of high blood pressure who takes insulin, antihypertensive medication, aspirin, and several herbal supplements daily is scheduled for laparoscopic gastric bypass surgery. What resources would you use to identify evidence-based practices for prevention of complications during the perioperative period? Identify the evidence, as well as the criteria used to evaluate the strength of the evidence, for the practices identified.

3 A patient is admitted to an outpatient surgery unit and claims an allergy to latex. What further assessment data are indicated to establish the extent of the latex allergy? How will you communicate this information to other team members? Describe how this patient's care will be affected in the perioperative area.

Brunner Suite Resources
Explore these additional resources to enhance
learning for this chapter:
• NCLEX-Style Questions and Other Resources
on thePoint, http://thePoint.lww.com/Brunner13e
• Study Guide
• PrepU
• Clinical Handbook
• Handbook of Laboratory and Diagnostic Tests

References

*Asterisk indicates nursing research.

Books

American Society of PeriAnesthesia Nurses. (2010). *2010–2012 perianesthesia nursing standards and practice recommendations.* Cherry Hill, NJ: Author.

Association of PeriOperative Registered Nurses. (2011). *Association of PeriOperative Registered Nurses (AORN) standards, recommended practice, and guidelines.* Denver: Author.

Alvarex, A., Brodsky, J. B., Lemmens, H. J., et al. (2010). *Morbid obesity: Peri-operative management* (2nd ed.). New York: Cambridge University Press.

ASPAN, Schick, L., & Windle, P. E. (2010). *PeriAnesthesia Nursing Core Curriculum: Preprocedure, phase I and phase II PACU nursing* (2nd ed.). St. Louis: Saunders.

Doran, D. (2010). *Nursing outcomes: State of the science* (2nd ed.). Sudbury, MA: Jones & Bartlett.

Haupt, M., & Reed, M. (2010). *Critical care considerations of the morbidly obese.* Philadelphia: Elsevier Saunders.

Johnson, M., Moorhead, S., Bulechek, G. et al. (2011). *NOC and NIC linkages to NANDA-I and clinical conditions: Supporting critical thinking and quality care* (3rd ed.). St. Louis: Mosby.

Meiner, S. E. (2011). *Gerontological nursing* (4th ed.). St. Louis: Elsevier Mosby.

Melnyk, B. M., & Fineout-Overholt, E. (2010). *Evidence-based practice in nursing and healthcare: A guide to best practices* (2nd ed.). Philadelphia: Lippincott Williams & Wilkins.

Miller, R. D., Eriksson, L. I., Fleisher, L. A., et al. (2010). *Miller's anesthesia* (7th ed.). New York: Elsevier/Churchill Livingstone.

Porth, C. M., & Matfin, G. (2009). *Pathophysiology: Concepts of altered health states* (8th ed.). Philadelphia: Lippincott Williams & Wilkins.

Rothrock, J. C. (2010). *Alexander's care of the patient in surgery* (14th ed.). St. Louis: Mosby.

Spry, C. (2009). *Essentials of perioperative nursing* (4th ed.). Sudbury, MA: Jones & Bartlett.

Stannard, D., & Krenzischek, D. A. (2012). *Perianesthesia nursing care: A bedside guide for safe recovery.* Sudbury, MA: Jones & Bartlett Learning.

Tabloski, P. A. (2009). *Gerontological nursing: The essential guide to clinical practice* (2nd ed.). Upper Saddle River, NJ: Prentice Hall.

Weber, J., & Kelley, J. H. (2009). *Health assessment in nursing* (4th ed.). Philadelphia: Lippincott Williams & Wilkins.

West, J. B. (2011). *Respiratory physiology: The essentials* (9th ed.). Baltimore: Lippincott Williams & Wilkins.

Journals and Electronic Documents

Australasian Society of Clinical Immunology and Allergy. (2011). *Latex allergy.* Available at: www.allergy.org.au

Becker, D. (2009). Preoperative medical evaluation: Part 1: General principles and cardiovascular considerations. *Anesthesia Progress, 56*(3), 92–102.

Buscemi, C. (2011). Acculturation: State of the science in nursing. *Journal of Cultural Diversity, 18*(2), 39–42.

*Cohoon, B. (2011). Causes of near misses: Perceptions of perioperative nurses. *AORN Journal, 93*(5), 551–565.

Costantini, R., Affaitati, G., Fabrizio, A., et al. (2011). Controlling pain in the post-operative setting. *International Journal of Clinical Pharmacology and Therapeutics, 49*(2), 116–127.

Crenshaw, J. T. (2011). Preoperative fasting: Will the evidence ever be put into practice? *American Journal of Nursing, 111*(10), 38–43.

De Lima, L., Borges, D., da Costa, S., et al. (2010). Classification of patients according to the degree of dependence on nursing care and illness severity in a post-anesthesia care unit. *Revista Latino-Americana De Enfermagem, 18*(5), 881–887.

*Dizer, B., Hatipoglu, S., Kaymakcioglu, N., et al. (2009). The effect of nurse-performed preoperative skin preparation on postoperative surgical site infections in abdominal surgery. *Journal of Clinical Nursing, 18*(5), 3325–3332.

Engebretson, J. (2011). Clinically applied medical ethnography: Relevance to cultural competence in patient care. *Nursing Clinics of North America, 46*(2), 145.

Ewan, P., Dugué, P., Mirakian, R., et al. (2010). BSACI guidelines for the investigation of suspected anaphylaxis during general anesthesia. *Clinical and Experimental Allergy: Journal of the British Society for Allergy and Clinical Immunology, 40*(1), 15–31.

Faulk, D., Twite, M., Zuk, J., et al. (2010). Hypnotic depth and the incidence of emergence agitation and negative postoperative behavioral changes. *Pediatric Anesthesia, 20*(1), 72–81.

Franck, M., Radtke, F., Apfel, C., et al. (2010). Documentation of postoperative nausea and vomiting in routine clinical practice. *Journal of International Medical Research, 38*(3), 1034–1041.

Izzo, A. A., & Ernst, E. (2009). Interactions between herbal medicines and prescribed drugs. *Drugs, 69*(13), 1777–1798.

Joint Commission. (2011). *Surgical Care Improvement Project.* Available at: www.jointcommission.org/surgical_care_improvement_project/

Joint Commission. (2013). *2013 National Patient Safety Goals.* Available at: www.jointcommission.org/standards_information/npsgs.aspx

*Kruzik, N. (2009). Benefits of preoperative education for adult elective surgery patients. *AORN Journal, 90*(3), 381–387.

Massicotte, L., Chalaoui, K., Beaulieu, D., et al. (2009). Comparison of spinal anesthesia with general anesthesia on morphine requirement after abdominal hysterectomy. *Acta Anaesthesiologica Scandinavica, 53*(5), 641–647.

Moradipanah, F., Mohammadi, E., & Mohammadil, A. (2009). Effect of music on anxiety, stress, and depression levels in patients undergoing coronary angiography. *Eastern Mediterranean Health Journal, 15*(3), 639–647.

National Patient Safety Goals. (2011). *Preventing health care associated infections due to multi-drug resistant organisms. Prevent central line associated blood stream infections.* Available at: www.centennialmedicalplaza.com/for_health_professionals/physicians/medical_staff_access/physicians_link/winter-2011/2011-national-patient-safety-goals.htm

Riddle, E., Bush, J., Tittle, M., et al. (2010). Alcohol withdrawal: Development of a standing order set. *Critical Care Nurse, 30*(3), 38–47.

Rowe, D. J., and Baker, A. C. (2009). Perioperative risks and benefits of herbal supplements in aesthetic surgery. *Aesthetic Surgery Journal, 29*(2), 150–157.

Stell, L. (2009). Clinical ethics and patient advocacy. *North Carolina Medical Journal, 70*(2), 131–135.

World Health Organization (WHO). (2008). New checklist to help make surgery safer. *WHO Bulletin, 86*(7), 496–576.

Resources

American Academy of Ambulatory Care Nursing (AACN), www.aaacn.org
American Association of Gynecologic Laparoscopy (AAGL), www.aagl.org
American Society for Metabolic and Bariatric Surgery (ASMBS), www.asbs.org
American Society of PeriAnesthesia Nurses (ASPAN), www.aspan.org
Association of PeriOperative Registered Nurses (AORN), www.aorn.org
Centers for Medicare and Medicaid Services (CMS), www.cms.hhs.gov
Joint Commission, www.jointcommission.org

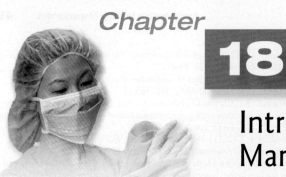

Chapter

18

Intraoperative Nursing Management

Glossary

anesthesia: a state of narcosis, analgesia, relaxation, and loss of reflexes

anesthesiologist: physician trained to deliver anesthesia and to monitor the patient's condition during surgery

anesthetic agent: the substance, such as a chemical or gas, used to induce anesthesia

anesthetist: health care professional, often a certified registered nurse anesthetist, who is trained to deliver anesthesia and to monitor the patient's condition during surgery

circulating nurse (or circulator): registered nurse who coordinates and documents patient care in the operating room

epidural anesthesia: state of narcosis, analgesia, relaxation, and loss of reflexes at and below the level where the spine is accessed, achieved by injecting an anesthetic agent into the epidural space of the spinal cord

general anesthesia: state of narcosis, analgesia, relaxation, and loss of reflexes produced by pharmacologic agents

laparoscope: a thin endoscope inserted through a small incision into a cavity or joint using fiber-optic technology to project live images of structures onto a video monitor; other small incisions allow additional instruments to be inserted to facilitate laparoscopic surgery

local anesthesia: injection of a solution containing the anesthetic agent into the tissues at the planned incision site, affecting only the local area

malignant hyperthermia: a rare life-threatening condition triggered by exposure to most anesthetic agents inducing a drastic and uncontrolled increase in skeletal muscle oxidative metabolism that can overwhelm the body's capacity to supply oxygen, remove carbon dioxide, and regulate body temperature, eventually leading to circulatory collapse and death if untreated; often inherited as an autosomal dominant disorder

moderate sedation: previously referred to as conscious sedation, involves the use of sedation to depress the level of consciousness without altering the patient's ability to maintain a patent airway and to respond to physical stimuli and verbal commands

monitored anesthesia care: moderate sedation administered by an anesthesiologist or anesthetist

regional anesthesia: an anesthetic agent is injected around nerves so that the area supplied by these nerves is anesthetized

registered nurse first assistant: a member of the operating room team whose responsibilities may include handling tissue, providing exposure at the operative field, suturing, and maintaining hemostasis

restricted zone: area in the operating room where scrub attire and surgical masks are required; includes operating room and sterile core areas

scrub role: registered nurse, licensed practical nurse, or surgical technologist who scrubs and dons sterile surgical attire, prepares instruments and supplies, and hands instruments to the surgeon during the procedure

semirestricted zone: area in the operating room where scrub attire is required; may include areas where surgical instruments are processed

spinal anesthesia: achieved when a local anesthetic agent is introduced into the subarachnoid space of the spinal cord

surgical asepsis: absence of microorganisms in the surgical environment to reduce the risk of infection

unrestricted zone: area in the operating room that interfaces with other departments; includes patient reception area and holding area

The intraoperative experience has undergone many changes and advances that make it safer and less disturbing to patients. Even with these advances, anesthesia and surgery still place the patient at risk for several complications or adverse events. Consciousness or full awareness, mobility, protective biologic functions, and personal control are totally or partially relinquished by the patient when entering the operating room (OR). Staff from the departments of anesthesia, nursing, and surgery work collaboratively to implement professional standards of care, to control iatrogenic and individual risks, to prevent complications, and to promote high-quality patient outcomes.

The Surgical Team

The surgical team consists of the patient, the anesthesiologist (physician) or anesthetist (e.g., certified registered nurse anesthetist [CRNA]), the surgeon, nurses, the surgical technicians, and the registered nurse first assistants (RFNAs) or certified surgical technologists (assistants). The anesthesiologist or anesthetist (often a CRNA) administers the **anesthetic agent** and monitors the patient's physical status throughout the surgery. The surgeon, nurses, and assistants scrub and perform the surgery. The person in the scrub role, either a nurse or a surgical technician, provides sterile instruments and supplies to the surgeon during the procedure by anticipating the surgical needs as the surgical case progresses. The circulating nurse coordinates the care of the patient in the OR. Care provided by the circulating nurse includes planning for and assisting with patient positioning, preparing the patient's skin for surgery, managing surgical specimens, anticipating the needs of the surgical team, and documenting intraoperative events. Collaboration of the core surgical team using evidence-based practices tailored to the specific case results in optimum patient care and improved outcomes (Chart 18-1).

The Patient

As the patient enters the OR, he or she may feel either relaxed and prepared or fearful and highly stressed. These feelings depend to a large extent on the amount and timing of preoperative sedation, preoperative education, and the individual patient. Fears about loss of control, the unknown, pain, death, changes in body structure, appearance, or function, and disruption of lifestyle all contribute to anxiety. These fears can increase the amount of anesthetic medication needed, the level of postoperative pain, and overall recovery time. (See Chapter 6 for more information on stress.)

The patient is also subject to several risks. Infection, failure of the surgery to relieve symptoms or correct a deformity, temporary or permanent complications related to the procedure or the anesthetic agent, and death are uncommon but potential outcomes of the surgical experience (Chart 18-2). In addition to fears and risks, the patient undergoing sedation and anesthesia temporarily loses both cognitive function and biologic self-protective mechanisms. Loss of the sense of pain, reflexes, and the ability to communicate subjects the intraoperative patient to possible injury. The OR nurse is the patient's advocate while surgery proceeds.

 Gerontologic Considerations

Approximately one third of surgical patients are 65 years of age or older as the baby boomer population enters the geriatric years (Barash, Cullen & Stoelting, 2009). Older adult patients are at higher risk for complications from anesthesia and surgery compared to younger adult patients due to several factors (Rothrock, 2010). There is a progressive loss of skeletal muscle mass in conjunction with an increase in adipose tissue (Tabloski, 2009). Comorbidities, advanced systemic disease, and increased susceptibility to illness, even in the healthiest geriatric patient, can complicate perioperative management. Age alone confers enough surgical risk that it is a clinical predictor of cardiovascular complications (Meiner, 2011).

 NURSING RESEARCH PROFILE

The Structure of Operating Room Staffing

Anderson, C., & Talsma, A. (2011). Characterizing the structure of operating room staffing using social network analysis. *Nursing Research, 60*(6), 378–385.

Purpose

Staffing characteristics of the operating room (OR) team is an essential component of safe patient care; however, there is very little research focused on this area. The purpose of this study was to determine how the OR staffing of two surgical specialties (general and neurosurgical) compared in terms of social network variables.

Design

Staffing data from all general and neurosurgical procedures that occurred in one hospital were analyzed with Social Network Analysis methods. Variables in this type of analysis include centrality, team coreness (how often the team worked together), and the core/periphery network structure. Additional techniques included multidimensional scaling, correlation, and descriptive statistics.

Findings

Both general and the neurosurgical services had the characteristic of the core/periphery network structure. Team coreness was associated with the length of the case ($p < .001$). The start time of the procedure predicted the team coreness measure, with cases beginning later in the day less likely to be staffed with a high-core team ($p < .001$). Registered nurses (RNs) constituted the majority of core team members in both groups.

Nursing Implications

The results of this study suggest that many OR procedures are staffed with personnel who are peripherally associated with the specialty. RNs, as core team members, are in a position to take the lead in communicating standards and process variations to noncore team members. The effect of late-starting cases staffed with lower coreness teams should be investigated further, as this may be an essential component of providing safe patient care.

Chart 18-2 **Potential Adverse Effects of Surgery and Anesthesia**

Anesthesia and surgery disrupt all major body systems. Although most patients can compensate for surgical trauma and the effects of anesthesia, all patients are at risk during the operative procedure. These risks include the following:

- Allergic reactions
- Anesthesia awareness
- Cardiac dysrhythmia from electrolyte imbalance or adverse effect of anesthetic agents
- Myocardial depression, bradycardia, and circulatory collapse
- Central nervous system agitation, seizures, and respiratory arrest
- Oversedation or undersedation
- Agitation or disorientation, especially in older adult patients
- Hypoxemia or hypercarbia from hypoventilation and inadequate respiratory support during anesthesia
- Laryngeal trauma, oral trauma, and broken teeth from difficult intubation
- Hypothermia from cool operating room temperatures, exposure of body cavities, and impaired thermoregulation secondary to anesthetic agents
- Hypotension from blood loss or adverse effect of anesthesia
- Infection
- Thrombosis from compression of blood vessels or stasis
- Malignant hyperthermia secondary to adverse effect of anesthesia
- Nerve damage and skin breakdown from prolonged or inappropriate positioning
- Electrical shock or burns
- Laser burns
- Drug toxicity, faulty equipment, and other types of human error

Biologic variations of particular importance include age-related cardiovascular and pulmonary changes. The aging heart and blood vessels have decreased ability to respond to stress. Reduced cardiac output and limited cardiac reserve make the older adult vulnerable to changes in circulating volume and blood oxygen levels (Becker, 2009). Excessive or rapid administration of intravenous (IV) solutions can cause pulmonary edema. A sudden or prolonged decline in blood pressure may lead to cerebral ischemia, thrombosis, embolism, infarction, and anoxia. Reduced gas exchange can result in cerebral hypoxia.

Lower doses of anesthetic agents are required in older adults due to decreased tissue elasticity (lung and cardiovascular systems) and reduced lean tissue mass. Older patients often experience an increase in the duration of clinical effects of medications. With decreased plasma proteins, more of the anesthetic agent remains free or unbound, and the result is more potent action (Barash et al., 2009).

In addition, body tissues of the older adult are made up predominantly of water, and those tissues with a rich blood supply, such as skeletal muscle, liver, and kidneys, shrink as the body ages. Reduced liver size decreases the rate at which the liver can inactivate many anesthetic agents, and decreased kidney function slows the elimination of waste products and anesthetic agents. Other factors that affect the older surgical patient in the intraoperative period include the following:

- Impaired ability to increase metabolic rate and impaired thermoregulatory mechanisms increase susceptibility to hypothermia.

- Bone loss (25% in women, 12% in men) necessitates careful manipulation and positioning during surgery.
- Reduced ability to adjust rapidly to emotional and physical stress influences surgical outcomes and requires meticulous observation of vital functions.

All of these factors lead to a higher likelihood of perioperative mortality and morbidity in older adult patients (Barash et al., 2009). (Further discussion of age-related physiologic changes can be found in Chapter 11.)

Nursing Care

Throughout surgery, nursing responsibilities include providing for the safety and well-being of the patient, coordinating the OR personnel, and performing scrub and circulating activities. Because the patient's emotional state remains a concern, the intraoperative nursing staff provides the patient with information and reassurance, continuing the care initiated by preoperative nurses. The nurse supports coping strategies and reinforces the patient's ability to influence outcomes by encouraging active participation in the plan of care, incorporating cultural, ethnic, and religious considerations as appropriate. The establishment of an environment of trust and relaxation through visualization techniques is another method of patient reassurance that can be used as the patient is anesthetically induced.

As patient advocates, intraoperative nurses monitor factors that have the potential to cause injury, such as patient position, equipment malfunction, and environmental hazards, and protect the patient's dignity and interests while the patient is under anesthesia. Additional responsibilities include maintaining surgical standards of care and identifying and minimizing risks and complications.

Cultural Diversity

Cultural, ethnic, and religious diversity are important considerations for all health care professionals. Nurses in the perioperative area should be aware of medications that may be prohibited by certain groups (e.g., Muslims and those of the Jewish faith cannot use porcine-based products [heparin (porcine or bovine)], Buddhists may choose not to use bovine products). In certain cultures, the head is a sacred area, and staff should allow patients to apply their own surgical cap in this case. When English is the second language of the patient having surgery under local anesthesia, certified medical translators can be provided to maintain understanding and comprehension by the patient (Miller, 2009). Translator phones are also available at most hospitals. Family members may have the ability to translate but should not be used as medical translators, as they may wish to save the patient anxiety and not provide an accurate translation, resulting in the patient not receiving complete information.

The Circulating Nurse

The **circulating nurse (or circulator)**, a qualified registered nurse, works in collaboration with surgeons, anesthesia providers, and other health care providers to plan the best course of action for each patient (Rothrock, 2010). In this leadership role, the circulating nurse manages the OR and protects the patient's safety and health by monitoring the activities of the surgical team, checking the OR conditions, and continually assessing the patient for signs of injury and implementing appropriate interventions. A foremost responsibility includes verifying consent; if not obtained, surgery may not commence. The team is coordinated by the circulating nurse, who ensures cleanliness, proper temperature, humidity, appropriate lighting, safe function of equipment, and the availability of supplies and materials.

The circulating nurse monitors aseptic practices to avoid breaks in technique while coordinating the movement of related personnel (medical, x-ray, and laboratory), as well as implementing fire safety precautions. The circulating nurse also monitors the patient and documents specific activities throughout the operation to ensure the patient's safety and well-being.

In addition, the circulating nurse is responsible for ensuring that the second verification of the surgical procedure and site takes place and is documented (Fig. 18-1). In some institutions, this is referred to as a time out, surgical pause, or universal protocol that takes place among the surgical team prior to induction of anesthesia with a briefing about anticipated problems, potential complications, allergies, and comorbidities. Every member of the surgical team verifies the patient's name, procedure, and surgical site using objective documentation and data before beginning the surgery (World Health Organization, 2008). Identifying patients correctly is a 2012 National Patient Safety Goal (see Chart 17-8 in Chapter 17).

Research suggests that the use of a surgical safety checklist reduces morbidity and mortality (Haynes, Weiser, Berry, et al., 2009). A team debriefing session that is led by the circulating nurse should be initiated following the completion of surgery to identify potential problems with the postsurgical care of the patient and areas for improvement (Robinson, Paull, Mazzia, et al., 2010).

Quality and Safety Nursing Alert

It is imperative that the correct patient identity, surgical procedure, and surgical site be verified prior to surgery. The surgical site should be marked by the patient and physician prior to coming to the OR suite during the consent process.

The Scrub Role

The registered nurse, licensed practical nurse, or surgical technologist (or assistant) performs the activities of the **scrub role,** including performing a surgical hand scrub; setting up the sterile tables; preparing sutures, ligatures, and special equipment (e.g., a **laparoscope,** which is a thin endoscope inserted through a small incision into a cavity or joint using fiber-optic technology to project live images of structures onto a video

World Health Organization	**SURGICAL SAFETY CHECKLIST** (First Edition)	
Before induction of anaesthesia ▶▶▶▶▶	Before skin incision ▶▶▶▶▶▶▶▶▶▶	Before patient leaves operating room
SIGN IN	**TIME OUT**	**SIGN OUT**
☐ PATIENT HAS CONFIRMED • IDENTITY • SITE • PROCEDURE • CONSENT	☐ CONFIRM ALL TEAM MEMBERS HAVE INTRODUCED THEMSELVES BY NAME AND ROLE	NURSE VERBALLY CONFIRMS WITH THE TEAM: ☐ THE NAME OF THE PROCEDURE RECORDED
☐ SITE MARKED/NOT APPLICABLE	☐ SURGEON, ANAESTHESIA PROFESSIONAL AND NURSE VERBALLY CONFIRM • PATIENT • SITE • PROCEDURE	☐ THAT INSTRUMENT, SPONGE AND NEEDLE COUNTS ARE CORRECT (OR NOT APPLICABLE)
☐ ANAESTHESIA SAFETY CHECK COMPLETED		
☐ PULSE OXIMETER ON PATIENT AND FUNCTIONING	**ANTICIPATED CRITICAL EVENTS**	☐ HOW THE SPECIMEN IS LABELLED (INCLUDING PATIENT NAME)
DOES PATIENT HAVE A: KNOWN ALLERGY?	☐ SURGEON REVIEWS: WHAT ARE THE CRITICAL OR UNEXPECTED STEPS, OPERATIVE DURATION, ANTICIPATED BLOOD LOSS?	☐ WHETHER THERE ARE ANY EQUIPMENT PROBLEMS TO BE ADDRESSED
☐ NO ☐ YES	☐ ANAESTHESIA TEAM REVIEWS: ARE THERE ANY PATIENT-SPECIFIC CONCERNS?	☐ SURGEON, ANAESTHESIA PROFESSIONAL AND NURSE REVIEW THE KEY CONCERNS FOR RECOVERY AND MANAGEMENT OF THIS PATIENT
DIFFICULT AIRWAY/ASPIRATION RISK? ☐ NO ☐ YES, AND EQUIPMENT/ASSISTANCE AVAILABLE	☐ NURSING TEAM REVIEWS: HAS STERILITY (INCLUDING INDICATOR RESULTS) BEEN CONFIRMED? ARE THERE EQUIPMENT ISSUES OR ANY CONCERNS?	
RISK OF >500ML BLOOD LOSS (7ML/KG IN CHILDREN)? ☐ NO ☐ YES, AND ADEQUATE INTRAVENOUS ACCESS AND FLUIDS PLANNED	HAS ANTIBIOTIC PROPHYLAXIS BEEN GIVEN WITHIN THE LAST 60 MINUTES? ☐ YES ☐ NOT APPLICABLE	
	IS ESSENTIAL IMAGING DISPLAYED? ☐ YES ☐ NOT APPLICABLE	

THIS CHECKLIST IS NOT INTENDED TO BE COMPREHENSIVE. ADDITIONS AND MODIFICATIONS TO FIT LOCAL PRACTICE ARE ENCOURAGED.

FIGURE 18-1 • Surgical safety checklist. Used with permission from World Health Organization. (2008). New checklist to help make surgery safer. *WHO Bulletin, 86* (7), 496–576. Available at: www.who.int/patientsafety/safesurgery/tools_resources/SSSL_Checklist_finalJun08.pdf

monitor); and assisting the surgeon and the surgical assistants during the procedure by anticipating the instruments and supplies that will be required, such as sponges, drains, and other equipment. As the surgical incision is closed, the scrub person and the circulating nurse count all needles, sponges, and instruments to be sure they are accounted for and not retained as a foreign body in the patient (Association of PeriOperative Registered Nurses [AORN], 2011; Rothrock, 2010). Standards call for all sponges used in surgery to be visible on x-ray and for sponge counts to take place at the beginning of surgery and twice at the end (when wound closure begins and again as the skin is being closed). Tissue specimens obtained during surgery are labeled by the person in the scrub role and sent to the laboratory by the circulating nurse.

The Surgeon

The surgeon performs the surgical procedure, heads the surgical team, and is a licensed physician (MD or DO), oral surgeon (DDS or DMD), or podiatrist (DPM) who is specially trained and qualified. Qualifications and training must adhere to Joint Commission standards, hospital standards, and local and state admitting practices and procedures (Rothrock, 2010).

The Registered Nurse First Assistant

The **registered nurse first assistant** is another member of the OR team. Although the scope of practice of the RNFA depends on each state's nurse practice act, the RNFA practices under the direct supervision of the surgeon. RNFA responsibilities may include handling tissue, providing exposure at the operative field, suturing, and maintaining hemostasis (Rothrock, 2010). The role requires a thorough understanding of anatomy and physiology, tissue handling, and the principles of surgical asepsis. The RNFA must be aware of the objectives of the surgery, must have the knowledge and ability to anticipate needs and to work as a skilled member of a team, and must be able to handle any emergency situation in the OR.

The Anesthesiologist and Anesthetist

An **anesthesiologist** is a physician specifically trained in the art and science of anesthesiology. An **anesthetist** is also a qualified and specifically trained health care professional who administers anesthetic medications. Most anesthetists are nurses who have graduated from an accredited nurse anesthesia master's program and have passed examinations sponsored by the American Association of Nurse Anesthetists to become a CRNA. The anesthesiologist or anesthetist assesses the patient before surgery, selects the anesthesia, administers it, intubates the patient if necessary, manages any technical problems related to the administration of the anesthetic agent, and supervises the patient's condition throughout the surgical procedure. Before the patient enters the OR, often at preadmission testing, the anesthesiologist or anesthetist visits the patient to perform an assessment, supply information, and answer questions. The type of anesthetic agent to be administered, previous reactions to anesthetic medications, and known anatomic abnormalities that would make airway management difficult are among the topics discussed.

The anesthesiologist or anesthetist uses the American Society of Anesthesiologists (ASA) Physical Status Classification System to determine the patient's status. A patient who is classified as P2, P3, or P4 has a systemic disease that may or may not be related to the cause of surgery. If a patient with a classification of P1, P2, P3, P4, or P5 requires emergency surgery, an E is added to the physical status designation (e.g., P1E, P2E). P6 refers to a patient who is brain dead and is undergoing surgery as an organ donor. The abbreviations ASA1 through ASA6 are often used interchangeably with P1 to P6 to designate physical status (Rothrock, 2010).

When the patient arrives in the OR, the anesthesiologist or anesthetist reassesses the patient's physical condition immediately prior to initiating anesthesia. The anesthetic agent is administered, and the patient's airway is maintained through an intranasal intubation (if the surgeon is using an oral approach to surgery), intubation with an endotracheal tube (ETT), or a laryngeal mask airway (LMA). During surgery, the anesthesiologist or anesthetist monitors the patient's blood pressure, pulse, and respirations, as well as the electrocardiogram (ECG), blood oxygen saturation level, tidal volume, blood gas levels, blood pH, alveolar gas concentrations, and body temperature. Monitoring by electroencephalography (EEG) is sometimes required. Levels of anesthetic medications in the body can also be determined; a mass spectrometer can provide instant readouts of critical concentration levels on display terminals. This information is used to assess the patient's ability to breathe unassisted or the need for mechanical assistance if ventilation is poor and the patient is not breathing well independently.

The Surgical Environment

The surgical environment is known for its stark appearance and cool temperature. The surgical suite is behind double doors, and access is limited to authorized, appropriately clad personnel. External precautions include adherence to principles of surgical asepsis; strict control of the OR environment is required, including traffic pattern restrictions. Policies governing this environment address such issues as the health of the staff; the cleanliness of the rooms; the sterility of equipment and surfaces; processes for scrubbing, gowning, and gloving; and OR attire.

To provide the best possible conditions for surgery, the OR is situated in a location that is central to all supporting services (e.g., pathology, x-ray, and laboratory). The OR has special air filtration devices to screen out contaminating particles, dust, and pollutants.

Many National Patient Safety Goals pertain to the perioperative areas (see Chart 17-8 in Chapter 17); however, the one with the most direct relevance to the OR is to identify patient safety risks. A unique risk is the risk of fire in the OR due to three factors: a source of fuel, an oxygen source, and a mechanism to ignite a fire (AORN, 2011). All surgical services personnel must familiarize themselves with the department fire emergency response plan and be competent in the use and safeguards of all combustible materials and equipment in the surgical environment (Rothrock, 2010). Surgical drapes provide an opportunity for oxygen to concentrate; a stray spark could more easily ignite a fire. This occurs most commonly in ambulatory surgery settings (Joint Commission, 2013). To further improve safety, electrical hazards, emergency exit clearances, and storage of equipment and anesthetic gases are monitored periodically by official agencies, such as the respective state Department of Health and the Joint Commission.

To help decrease microbes, the surgical area is divided into three zones: the **unrestricted zone**, where street clothes are allowed; the **semirestricted zone**, where attire consists of scrub clothes and caps; and the **restricted zone**, where scrub clothes, shoe covers, caps, and masks are worn. The surgeons and other surgical team members wear additional sterile clothing and protective devices during surgery.

The AORN recommends specific practices for personnel wearing surgical attire to promote a high level of cleanliness in a particular practice setting (AORN, 2011). OR attire includes close-fitting cotton dresses, pantsuits, jumpsuits, gowns, and jackets. Knitted cuffs on sleeves prevent organisms from shedding and being released into the immediate surroundings. Shirts and waist drawstrings should be tucked inside the pants to prevent accidental contact with sterile areas and to contain skin shedding. Wet or soiled garments should be changed.

Masks are worn at all times in the restricted zone of the OR. High-filtration masks decrease the risk of postoperative wound infection by containing and filtering microorganisms from the oropharynx and nasopharynx. Masks should fit tightly; should cover the nose and mouth completely; and should not interfere with breathing, speech, or vision. Masks must be adjusted to prevent venting from the sides. Disposable masks have a filtration efficiency exceeding 95%. Masks are changed between patients and should not be worn outside the surgical department. The mask must be either on or off; it must not be allowed to hang around the neck.

Headgear should completely cover the hair (head and neckline, including beard) so that hair, bobby pins, clips, and particles of dandruff or dust do not fall on the sterile field.

Shoes designated for use inside the OR (not worn home) should be comfortable and supportive. Shoe covers are used when spills or splashes are anticipated. If worn, the covers should be changed whenever they become wet, torn, or soiled (Rothrock, 2010).

Barriers such as scrub attire and masks do not entirely protect the patient from microorganisms. Upper respiratory tract infections, sore throats, and skin infections in staff and patients are sources of pathogens and must be reported.

Because artificial fingernails harbor microorganisms and can cause nosocomial infections, a ban on artificial nails by OR personnel is supported by the Centers for Disease Control and Prevention (CDC), AORN, and the Association for Professionals in Infection Control and Epidemiology (APIC). Research provides support for policies prohibiting artificial nails for health care workers (AORN, 2011). Short, natural fingernails are encouraged.

Principles of Surgical Asepsis

Surgical asepsis prevents the contamination of surgical wounds. The patient's natural skin flora or a previously existing infection may cause postoperative wound infection.

Rigorous adherence to the principles of surgical asepsis by OR personnel is basic to preventing surgical site infections.

All surgical supplies, instruments, needles, sutures, dressings, gloves, covers, and solutions that may come in contact with the surgical wound or exposed tissues must be sterilized before use (Rothrock, 2010). Traditionally, the surgeon, surgical assistants, and nurses prepared themselves by scrubbing their hands and arms with antiseptic soap and water; however, this practice is being challenged by research investigating the optimal length of time to scrub and the best preparation to use. In some institutions, various alcohol-based products or scrubless soaps are used to prepare for surgery (Rothrock, 2010) but are only effective when no gross contaminants are present.

Surgical team members wear long-sleeved, sterile gowns and gloves. Head and hair are covered with a cap, and a mask is worn over the nose and mouth to minimize the possibility that bacteria from the upper respiratory tract will enter the wound. During surgery, only personnel who have scrubbed, gloved, and gowned touch sterilized objects. Non-scrubbed personnel refrain from touching or contaminating anything sterile.

An area of the patient's skin larger than that requiring exposure during the surgery is meticulously cleansed, and an antiseptic solution is applied (Rothrock, 2010). If hair needs to be removed, this is done immediately before the procedure with clippers (not shaved) to minimize the risk of infection (AORN, 2011). The remainder of the patient's body is covered with sterile drapes.

Environmental Controls

In addition to the protocols described previously, surgical asepsis requires meticulous cleaning and maintenance of the OR environment. Floors and horizontal surfaces are cleaned between cases with detergent, soap, and water or a detergent-germicide. Sterilized equipment is inspected regularly to ensure optimal operation and performance.

All equipment that comes into direct contact with the patient must be sterile. Sterilized linens, drapes, and solutions are used. Instruments are cleaned and sterilized in a unit near the OR. Individually wrapped sterile items are used when additional individual items are needed.

Airborne bacteria are a concern. To decrease the amount of bacteria in the air, standard OR ventilation provides 15 air exchanges per hour, at least three of which are fresh air (Rothrock, 2010). A room temperature of 20°C to 24°C (68°F to 73°F), humidity between 30% and 60%, and positive pressure relative to adjacent areas are maintained. Staff members shed skin scales, resulting in about 1,000 bacteria-carrying particles (or colony-forming units [CFUs]) per cubic foot per minute. With the standard air exchanges, air counts of bacteria are reduced to 50 to 150 CFUs per cubic foot per minute. Systems with high-efficiency particulate air (HEPA) filters are needed to remove particles larger than 0.3 μm (Rothrock, 2010). Unnecessary personnel and physical movement may be restricted to minimize bacteria in the air and achieve an OR infection rate no greater than 3% to 5% in clean, infection-prone surgery.

Some ORs have laminar airflow units. These units provide 400 to 500 air exchanges per hour (Rothrock, 2010). When used appropriately, laminar airflow units result in fewer than 10 CFUs per cubic foot per minute during surgery. The goal for a laminar airflow–equipped OR is an infection rate of less than 1%. An OR equipped with a laminar airflow unit is frequently used for total joint replacement or organ transplant surgery.

Even using all precautions, wound contamination may inadvertently occur, resulting in a nosocomial infection and a prolonged hospitalization. Constant surveillance and conscientious technique in carrying out aseptic practices are necessary to reduce the risk of contamination and infection.

Basic Guidelines for Maintaining Surgical Asepsis

All practitioners involved in the intraoperative phase have a responsibility to provide and maintain a safe environment. Adherence to aseptic practice is part of this responsibility. The basic principles of aseptic technique follow:

- All materials in contact with the surgical wound or used within the sterile field must be sterile. Sterile surfaces or articles may touch other sterile surfaces or articles and remain sterile; contact with unsterile objects at any point renders a sterile area contaminated.
- Gowns of the surgical team are considered sterile in front from the chest to the level of the sterile field. The sleeves are also considered sterile from 2 inches above the elbow to the stockinette cuff.
- Sterile drapes are used to create a sterile field (Fig. 18-2). Only the top surface of a draped table is considered sterile. During draping of a table or patient, the sterile drape is held well above the surface to be covered and is positioned from front to back.
- Items are dispensed to a sterile field by methods that preserve the sterility of the items and the integrity of the sterile field. After a sterile package is opened, the edges are considered unsterile. Sterile supplies, including solutions, are delivered to a sterile field or handed to a scrubbed person in such a way that the sterility of the object or fluid remains intact.
- The movements of the surgical team are from sterile to sterile areas and from unsterile to unsterile areas. Scrubbed people and sterile items contact only sterile areas; circulating nurses and unsterile items contact only unsterile areas.

- Movement around a sterile field must not cause contamination of the field. Sterile areas must be kept in view during movement around the area. At least a 1-foot distance from the sterile field must be maintained to prevent inadvertent contamination.
- Whenever a sterile barrier is breached, the area must be considered contaminated. A tear or puncture of the drape permitting access to an unsterile surface underneath renders the area unsterile. Such a drape must be replaced.
- Every sterile field is constantly monitored and maintained. Items of doubtful sterility are considered unsterile. Sterile fields are prepared as close as possible to the time of use.
- The routine administration of hyperoxia (high levels of oxygen) is *not* recommended to reduce surgical site infections.

Health Hazards Associated With the Surgical Environment

Faulty equipment, improper use of equipment, exposure to toxic substances, surgical plume (smoke generated by electrosurgical cautery), as well as infectious waste, cuts, needlestick injuries, and lasers are some of the associated hazards in the surgical environment (Rothrock, 2010). Internal monitoring of the OR includes the analysis of surface swipe samples and air samples for infectious and toxic agents. In addition, policies and procedures for minimizing exposure to body fluids and reducing the dangers associated with lasers and radiation are identified in AORN standards (AORN, 2011).

Regardless of the size or location of an incision, unintentional retention of an object (e.g., sponge, instrument) can occur. A retained object can cause wound infection or disruption, an abscess can form, and fistulas may develop between organs (Rothrock, 2010).

Laser Risks

The AORN has recommended practices for laser safety (Rothrock, 2010). When lasers are in use, warning signs must be clearly posted to alert personnel. Safety precautions are implemented to reduce the possibility of exposing the eyes and skin to laser beams, to prevent inhalation of the laser plume (smoke and particulate matter), and to protect the patient and personnel from fire and electrical hazards (Zahiri, Stromberg, Skupsky, et al., 2011). Several types of lasers are available for clinical use; perioperative personnel should be familiar with the unique features, specific operation, and safety measures for each type of laser used in the practice setting and wear appropriate laser goggles for the type of laser beam in use. Registered nurses trained and certified in laser safety maintain the established standards in the OR.

Smoke evacuators are used in some procedures to remove the laser plume from the operative field. In recent years, this technology has been extended to all surgical cases to protect the surgical team from the potential hazards associated with the generalized smoke plume generated by standard electrocautery units.

Exposure to Blood and Body Fluids

OR attire has changed dramatically since the advent of acquired immunodeficiency syndrome. Double-gloving is

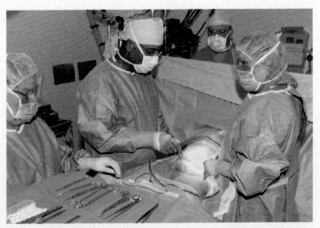

FIGURE 18-2 • Proper draping exposes only the surgical site, which decreases the risk of infection.

routine in trauma and other types of surgery where sharp bone fragments are present. In addition to the routine scrub suit and double gloves, some surgical personnel wear rubber boots, a waterproof apron, and sleeve protectors. Goggles, or a wraparound face shield, are worn to protect against splashing when the surgical wound is irrigated or when bone drilling is performed. In hospitals where numerous total joint procedures are performed, a complete bubble mask may be used. This mask provides full-barrier protection from bone fragments and splashes. Ventilation is accomplished through an accompanying hood with a separate air filtration system.

The Surgical Experience

During the surgical procedure, the patient will need sedation, anesthesia, or some combination of these.

Types of Anesthesia and Sedation

Research estimates anesthesia-related death rates in the United States to be less than 1 per 10,000 surgeries (Barash et al., 2009). For the patient, the anesthesia experience consists of having an IV line inserted, if it was not inserted earlier; receiving a sedating agent prior to induction with an anesthetic agent; losing consciousness; being intubated, if indicated; and then receiving a combination of anesthetic agents. Typically, the experience is a smooth one, and the patient has no recall of the events. The main types of anesthesia are general anesthesia (inhalation, IV), regional anesthesia (epidural, spinal, and local conduction blocks), moderate sedation (monitored anesthesia care [MAC]), and local anesthesia.

General Anesthesia

Anesthesia is a state of narcosis (severe central nervous system depression produced by pharmacologic agents), analgesia, relaxation, and reflex loss. Patients under **general anesthesia** are not arousable, not even to painful stimuli. They lose the ability to maintain ventilatory function and require assistance in maintaining a patent airway. Cardiovascular function may be impaired as well.

The Joint Commission has issued an alert regarding the phenomenon of patients being partially awake while under general anesthesia (referred to as anesthesia awareness). Patients at greatest risk of anesthesia awareness are cardiac, obstetric, and major trauma patients. The entire surgical team must be aware of this phenomenon and help prevent or manage it (Joint Commission, 2011a).

General anesthesia consists of four stages, each associated with specific clinical manifestations (Rothrock, 2010). Understanding of these stages is necessary for nurses because of the emotional support that the patient might need as anesthesia progresses.

- *Stage I: beginning anesthesia.* As the patient breathes in the anesthetic mixture, warmth, dizziness, and a feeling of detachment may be experienced. The patient may have a ringing, roaring, or buzzing in the ears and, although still conscious, may sense an inability to move the extremities easily. During this stage, noises are exaggerated; even low voices or minor sounds seem loud and unreal. For this reason, unnecessary noises and motions are avoided when anesthesia begins.

- *Stage II: excitement.* The excitement stage, characterized variously by struggling, shouting, talking, singing, laughing, or crying, is often avoided if IV anesthetic agents are administered smoothly and quickly. The pupils dilate, but they contract if exposed to light; the pulse rate is rapid, and respirations may be irregular. Because of the possibility of uncontrolled movements of the patient during this stage, the anesthesiologist or anesthetist must always be assisted by someone ready to help restrain the patient or to apply cricoid pressure in the case of vomiting to prevent aspiration. Manipulation increases circulation to the operative site and thereby increases the potential for bleeding.

- *Stage III: surgical anesthesia.* Surgical anesthesia is reached by administration of anesthetic vapor or gas and supported by IV agents as necessary. The patient is unconscious and lies quietly on the table. The pupils are small but contract when exposed to light. Respirations are regular, the pulse rate and volume are normal, and the skin is pink or slightly flushed. With proper administration of the anesthetic agent, this stage may be maintained for hours in one of several planes, ranging from light (1) to deep (4), depending on the depth of anesthesia needed.

- *Stage IV: medullary depression.* This stage is reached if too much anesthesia has been administered. Respirations become shallow, the pulse is weak and thready, and the pupils become widely dilated and no longer contract when exposed to light. Cyanosis develops and, without prompt intervention, death rapidly follows. If this stage develops, the anesthetic agent is discontinued immediately and respiratory and circulatory support is initiated to prevent death. Stimulants, although rarely used, may be administered; narcotic antagonists can be used if the overdose is due to opioids.

When opioid agents (narcotics) and neuromuscular blockers (relaxants) are administered, several of the stages are absent. During smooth administration of an anesthetic agent, there is no sharp division between stages I, II, and III, and there is no stage IV. The patient passes gradually from one stage to another, and it is through close observation of the signs exhibited by the patient that an anesthesiologist or anesthetist controls the situation. The responses of the pupils, the blood pressure, and the respiratory and cardiac rates are among the most reliable guides to the patient's condition.

Anesthetic agents used in general anesthesia are inhaled or administered IV. Anesthetic medications produce anesthesia because they are delivered to the brain at a high partial pressure that enables them to cross the blood–brain barrier. Relatively large amounts of anesthetic medication must be administered during induction and the early maintenance phases because the anesthetic agent is recirculated and deposited in body tissues. As these sites become saturated, smaller amounts of the anesthetic agent are required to maintain anesthesia because equilibrium or near-equilibrium has been achieved between brain, blood, and other tissues. When possible, the anesthesia induction (initiation) begins with IV anesthesia and is then maintained at the desired stage by inhalation methods, achieving a smooth transition and eliminating the obvious stages of anesthesia.

TABLE 18-1 Inhalation Anesthetic Agents

Agent	Administration	Advantages	Disadvantages	Implications/Considerations
Volatile Liquids				
Halothane (Fluothane)	Inhalation; special vaporizer	Not explosive or flammable Induction rapid and smooth Useful in almost every type of surgery Low incidence of postoperative nausea and vomiting	Requires skillful administration to prevent overdose May cause liver damage May produce hypotension Requires special vaporizer for administration	In addition to observation of pulse and respiration postoperatively, blood pressure must be monitored frequently.
Enflurane (Ethrane)	Inhalation	Rapid induction and recovery Potent analgesic agent Not explosive or flammable	Respiratory depression may develop rapidly, along with electrocardiogram abnormalities. Not compatible with epinephrine	Observe for possible respiratory depression. Administration with epinephrine may cause ventricular fibrillation.
Isoflurane (Forane)	Inhalation	Rapid induction and recovery Muscle relaxants are markedly potentiated.	A profound respiratory depressant	Monitor respirations closely and support when necessary.
Sevoflurane* (Ultane)	Inhalation	Rapid induction and excretion; minimal side effects	Coughing and laryngospasm; trigger for malignant hyperthermia	Monitor for malignant hyperthermia.
Desflurane (Suprane)	Inhalation	Rapid induction and emergence; rare organ toxicity	Respiratory irritation; trigger for malignant hyperthermia	Monitor for malignant hyperthermia and dysrhythmias.
Gases				
Nitrous oxide (N_2O)	Inhalation (semiclosed method)	Induction and recovery rapid Nonflammable Useful with oxygen for short procedures Useful with other agents for all types of surgery	Poor relaxant Weak anesthetic May produce hypoxia	Most useful in conjunction with other agents with longer action. Monitor for chest pain, hypertension, and stroke.
Oxygen (O_2)	Inhalation	Can increase O_2 available to tissues	High concentrations are hazardous.	Increased fire risk when used with lasers

*Currently most popular choice.

Any condition that diminishes peripheral blood flow, such as vasoconstriction or shock, may reduce the amount of anesthetic medication required. Conversely, when peripheral blood flow is unusually high, as in a muscularly active or apprehensive patient, induction is slower, and greater quantities of anesthetic agents are required because the brain receives a smaller quantity of anesthetic agent.

Inhalation

Inhaled anesthetic agents include volatile liquid agents and gases. Volatile liquid anesthetic agents produce anesthesia when their vapors are inhaled. Some commonly used inhalation agents are included in Table 18-1. All are administered in combination with oxygen and usually nitrous oxide as well.

Gas anesthetic agents are administered by inhalation and are always combined with oxygen. Nitrous oxide is the most commonly used gas anesthetic agent. When inhaled, the anesthetic agents enter the blood through the pulmonary capillaries and act on cerebral centers to produce loss of consciousness and sensation. When anesthetic administration is discontinued, the vapor or gas is eliminated through the lungs.

The vapor from inhalation anesthetic agents can be administered to the patient by several methods. The inhalation anesthetic agent may be administered through an LMA—a flexible tube with an inflatable silicone ring and cuff that can

be inserted into the larynx (Fig. 18-3A). The endotracheal technique for administering anesthetic medications consists of introducing a soft rubber or plastic ETT into the trachea, usually by means of a laryngoscope. The ETT may be inserted through either the nose (see Fig. 18-3B) or mouth (see Fig. 18-3C). When in place, the tube seals off the lungs from the esophagus so that if the patient vomits, stomach contents do not enter the lungs.

Intravenous Administration

General anesthesia can also be produced by the IV administration of various substances, such as barbiturates, benzodiazepines, nonbarbiturate hypnotics, dissociative agents, and opioid agents (Schifilliti, Grasso, Conti, et al., 2010). Table 18-2 lists commonly used IV anesthetic and analgesic agents, including IV medications used as muscle relaxants in the intraoperative period. These medications may be administered to induce or maintain anesthesia. Although they are often used in combination with inhalation anesthetic agents, they may be used alone. They may also be used to produce moderate sedation, as discussed later in this chapter.

An advantage of IV anesthesia is that the onset of anesthesia is pleasant; there is none of the buzzing, roaring, or dizziness known to follow administration of an inhalation anesthetic agent. The duration of action is brief, and the patient awakens with little nausea or vomiting.

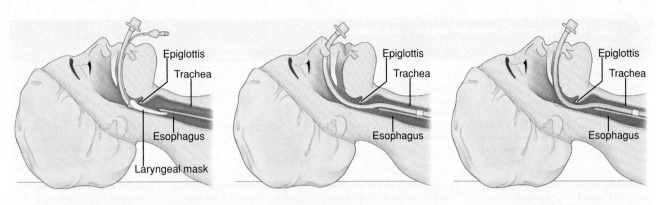

A. Laryngeal Mask Airway (LMA)   B. Intranasal intubation   C. Oral intubation

FIGURE 18-3 • Anesthetic delivery methods. **A.** Laryngeal mask airway (LMA). **B.** Nasal endotracheal catheter used when oral access will be required by the surgeon (in position with cuff inflated). **C.** Oral endotracheal intubation (tube is in position with cuff inflated).

The IV anesthetic agents are nonexplosive, require little equipment, and are easy to administer. The low incidence of postoperative nausea and vomiting makes the method useful in eye surgery, because in this setting vomiting would increase intraocular pressure and endanger vision in the operated eye. IV anesthesia is useful for short procedures but is used less often for the longer procedures of abdominal surgery. It is not indicated for children who have small veins or for those who require intubation because of their susceptibility to respiratory obstruction. The combination of IV and inhaled anesthetic agents produce an effective and smooth experience for the patient, with a controlled emergence following surgery.

IV neuromuscular blockers (muscle relaxants) block the transmission of nerve impulses at the neuromuscular junction of skeletal muscles. Muscle relaxants are used to relax muscles in abdominal and thoracic surgery, relax eye muscles in certain types of eye surgery, facilitate endotracheal intubation, treat laryngospasm, and assist in mechanical ventilation.

Regional Anesthesia

In **regional anesthesia**, an anesthetic agent is injected around nerves so that the region supplied by these nerves is anesthetized. The effect depends on the type of nerve involved. Motor fibers are the largest fibers and have the thickest myelin sheath. Sympathetic fibers are the smallest and have a minimal covering. Sensory fibers are intermediate. A local anesthetic agent blocks motor nerves least readily and sympathetic nerves most readily. An anesthetic agent is not considered metabolized until all three systems (motor, sensory, and autonomic) are no longer affected.

The patient receiving regional anesthesia is awake and aware of his or her surroundings unless medications are given to produce mild sedation or to relieve anxiety. The health care team must avoid careless conversation, unnecessary noise, and unpleasant odors; these may be noticed by the patient in the OR and may contribute to a negative response to the surgical experience. A quiet environment is therapeutic. The diagnosis must not be stated aloud if the patient is not to know it at this time.

Epidural Anesthesia

Epidural anesthesia is achieved by injecting a local anesthetic agent into the epidural space that surrounds the dura mater of the spinal cord (Fig. 18-4). The administered medication diffuses across the layers of the spinal cord to provide anesthesia and pain relief (Miller, Eriksson, Fleisher, et al., 2010). In contrast, spinal anesthesia involves injection through the dura mater into the subarachnoid space surrounding the spinal cord. Epidural anesthesia blocks sensory, motor, and autonomic functions; it differs from spinal anesthesia by the site of the injection and the amount of anesthetic agent used. Epidural doses are much higher because the epidural anesthetic agent does not make direct contact with the spinal cord or nerve roots (McKay, Lett, Chilibeck, et al., 2009).

An advantage of epidural anesthesia is the absence of headache that can result from spinal anesthesia. A disadvantage is the greater technical challenge of introducing the anesthetic agent into the epidural space rather than the subarachnoid space. If inadvertent puncture of the dura occurs during epidural anesthesia and the anesthetic agent travels toward the head, high spinal anesthesia can result; this can produce severe hypotension and respiratory depression and arrest. Treatment of these complications includes airway support, IV fluids, and the use of vasopressors.

Spinal Anesthesia

Spinal anesthesia is an extensive conduction nerve block that is produced when a local anesthetic agent is introduced into the subarachnoid space at the lumbar level, usually between L4 and L5 (see Fig. 18-4). It produces anesthesia of the lower extremities, perineum, and lower abdomen. For the lumbar puncture procedure, the patient usually lies on the side in a knee–chest position. Sterile technique is used as a spinal puncture is made and the medication is injected through the needle. As soon as the injection has been made, the patient is positioned on his or her back. If a relatively high level of block is sought, the head and shoulders are lowered.

The spread of the anesthetic agent and the level of anesthesia depend on the amount of agent injected, the speed with which it is injected, the positioning of the patient after the injection, and the specific gravity of the agent. If the specific gravity is greater than that of cerebrospinal fluid (CSF), the agent moves to the dependent position of the subarachnoid space. If the specific gravity is less than that of CSF, the anesthetic agent moves away from the dependent position.

TABLE 18-2 **Commonly Used Intravenous Medications**

Medication	Common Usage	Advantages	Disadvantages	Comments
Opioid Analgesic Agents				
Alfentanil (Alfenta)	Surgical analgesia in ambulatory patients	Ultra-short-acting (5–10 min) analgesic agent; duration of action 0.5 h; bolus or infusion	—	Potency: 750 µg; half-life 1.6 h
Fentanyl (Sublimaze)	Surgical analgesia; epidural infusion for postoperative analgesia; add to SAB	Good cardiovascular stability; duration of action 0.5 h	May cause muscle or chest wall rigidity	Most commonly used opioid; potency: 100 µg = 10 mg morphine sulfate; elimination half-life 3.6 h
Morphine sulfate (MS-Contin)	Preoperative pain; premedication; postoperative pain	Inexpensive; duration of action 4–5 h; euphoria; good cardiovascular stability	Nausea and vomiting; histamine release; postural ↓ BP and ↓ SVR	Epidural and intrathecal administration for postoperative pain; elimination half-life 3 h
Remifentanil (Ultiva)	IV infusion for surgical analgesia; small boluses for brief, intense pain	Easily titrated; very short duration; good cardiovascular stability. Ultiva is rapidly metabolized by hydrolysis of the propanoic acid–methyl ester linkage by nonspecific blood and tissue esterases.	New; expensive; requires mixing; may cause muscle rigidity	Potency: 25 µg = 10 mg morphine sulfate; 20–30 times potency of alfentanil; elimination half-life 3–10 min
Sufentanil (Sufenta)	Surgical analgesia	Duration of action 0.5 h; prolonged analgesia exceptionally potent (5–10 times more than fentanyl); provides good stability in cardiovascular surgery	Prolonged respiratory depression	Potency: 15 µg = 10 mg morphine sulfate; elimination half-life 2.7 h
Depolarizing Muscle Relaxants				
Succinylcholine	Relax skeletal muscles for surgery and orthopedic manipulations; short procedures; intubation	Short duration; rapid onset	No known effect on consciousness, pain threshold, or cerebration; fasciculations, postoperative myalgias, dysrhythmias; raises serum K⁺ in tissue trauma, muscular disease, paralysis, burns; histamine release is slight; requires refrigeration	Prolonged muscle relaxation with serum cholinesterase deficiency and some antibiotics; may trigger malignant hyperthermia
Nondepolarizing Muscle Relaxants—Intermediate Onset and Duration				
Atracurium besylate (Tracrium)	Intubation; maintenance of skeletal muscle relaxation	No significant cardiovascular or cumulative effects; good with renal failure	Requires refrigeration; slight histamine release; pregnancy risk category C; do not mix with lactated Ringer's solution or alkaline solutions such as barbiturates	Rapid IV bolus; use cautiously with geriatric and debilitated patients
Cisatracurium besylate (Nimbex)	Intubation; maintenance of skeletal muscle relaxation	Similar to atracurium	No histamine release	Similar to atracurium
Mivacurium (Mivacron)	Intubation; maintenance of skeletal muscle relaxation	Short acting; rapid metabolism by plasma cholinesterase; used as bolus or infusion	Expensive in longer cases	Competes with acetylcholine for receptor sites at the motor end plate, blocking neuromuscular transmission; new; rarely need to reverse; prolonged effect with plasma cholinesterase deficiency
Rocuronium (Zemuron)	Intubation; maintenance of relaxation	Rapid onset (dose dependent); elimination via kidney and liver	No known effect on consciousness, pain threshold, or cerebration; vagolytic; may ↑ HR	Duration similar to atracurium and vecuronium
Vecuronium (Norcuron)	Intubation; maintenance of relaxation	No significant cardiovascular or cumulative effects; no histamine release	Requires mixing	Mostly eliminated in bile, some in urine

Medication	Common Usage	Advantages	Disadvantages	Comments
Nondepolarizing Muscle Relaxants—Longer Onset and Duration				
d-Tubocurarine	Adjunct to anesthesia; maintenance of relaxation	—	No known effect on consciousness, pain threshold, or cerebration; might cause histamine release and transient ganglionic blockade	Mostly used for pretreatment with succinylcholine
Metocurine (Metubine)	Maintenance of relaxation	Good cardiovascular stability	Slight histamine release	Most commonly used opioid; potency: 100 μg = 10 mg morphine sulfate; elimination half-life 3.6 h
Pancuronium (Pavulon)	Maintenance of relaxation	—	May cause ↑ HR and ↑ BP	Used intrathecally and epidurally for postoperative pain; elimination half-life 3 h
Intravenous Anesthetic Agents				
Diazepam (Valium, Dizac)	Amnesia; hypnotic; relieves anxiety; preoperative	Good sedation	Long acting	Residual effects for 20–90 h; increased effect with alcohol
Etomidate (Amidate)	Induction of general anesthesia; indicated to supplement low-potency anesthetic agents	Short-acting hypnotic; good cardiovascular stability; fast, smooth induction and recovery	May cause brief period of apnea; pain with injection and myotonic movements	—
Ketamine (Ketalar)	Induction; occasional maintenance (IV or IM)	Short acting; profound analgesia; patient maintains airway; good in small children and burn patients	Large doses may cause hallucinations and respiratory depression; chest wall rigidity; laryngeal spasm	Need darkened, quiet room for recovery; often used in trauma cases
Midazolam (Versed)	Hypnotic; anxiolytic; sedation; often used as adjunct to induction	Excellent amnesia; water soluble (no pain with IV injection); short acting	Slower induction than thiopental	Often used for amnesia with insertion of invasive monitors or regional anesthesia; depresses all levels of CNS, including limbic and reticular formation, probably through increased action of GABA, which is major inhibitory neurotransmitter in brain
Propofol (Diprivan)	Induction and maintenance; sedation with regional anesthesia or MAC	Rapid onset; awakening in 4–8 min; produces sedation/hypnosis rapidly (within 40 s) and smoothly with minimal excitation; decreases intraocular pressure and systemic vascular resistance; rarely is associated with malignant hyperthermia and histamine release	May cause pain when injected; suppresses cardiac output and respiratory drive	Short elimination half-life (34–64 min)
Methohexital sodium (Brevital)	Induction; methohexital slows the activity of brain and nervous system	Ultra-short-acting barbiturate	May cause hiccups	Can be given rectally
Thiopental sodium (Pentothal)	Induction; stops seizures	—	May cause laryngospasm; can be given rectally	Large doses may cause apnea and cardiovascular depression

SAB, subarachnoid block; BP, blood pressure; SVR, stroke volume ratio; IV, intravenous; K⁺, potassium; HR, heart rate; IM, intramuscular; CNS, central nervous system; GABA, gamma-aminobutyric acid; MAC, monitored anesthesia care.

The anesthesiologist or anesthetist controls the administration of the agent. Table 18-3 presents types of regional anesthesia agents.

A few minutes after induction of a spinal anesthetic agent, anesthesia and paralysis affect the toes and perineum and then gradually the legs and abdomen. If the anesthetic agent reaches the upper thoracic and cervical spinal cord in high concentrations, a temporary partial or complete respiratory paralysis results (Massicotte, Chalaoui, Beaulieu, et al., 2009).

Paralysis of the respiratory muscles is managed by mechanical ventilation until the effects of the anesthetic agent on the cranial and thoracic nerves have worn off.

Nausea, vomiting, and pain may occur during surgery when spinal anesthesia is used. As a rule, these reactions result from manipulation of structures within the abdominal cavity. Adequate hydration and the IV administration of appropriate medications may prevent such reactions (Miller et al., 2010).

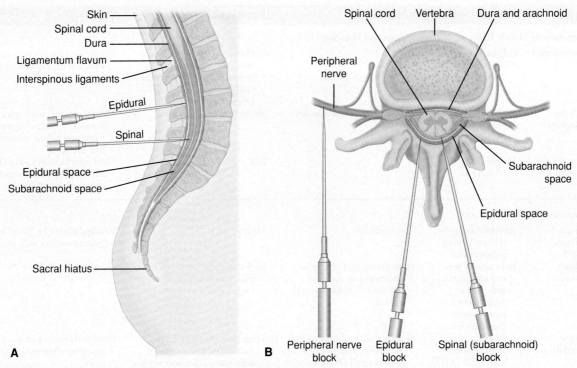

FIGURE 18-4 • **A.** Injection sites for spinal and epidural anesthesia. **B.** Cross-section of injection sites for peripheral nerve, epidural, and spinal blocks.

Headache may be an aftereffect of spinal anesthesia. Several factors are related to the incidence of headache: the size of the spinal needle used, the leakage of fluid from the subarachnoid space through the puncture site, and the patient's hydration status. Measures that increase cerebrospinal pressure are helpful in relieving headache. These include maintaining a quiet environment, keeping the patient lying flat, and keeping the patient well hydrated.

In continuous spinal anesthesia, the tip of a plastic catheter remains in the subarachnoid space during the surgical procedure so that more anesthetic medication may be injected as needed. This technique allows greater control of the dosage;

however, there is greater potential for postanesthetic headache because of the large-gauge needle used.

Local Conduction Blocks

Examples of common local conduction blocks include:
- Brachial plexus block, which produces anesthesia of the arm
- Paravertebral anesthesia, which produces anesthesia of the nerves supplying the chest, abdominal wall, and extremities
- Transsacral (caudal) block, which produces anesthesia of the perineum and, occasionally, the lower abdomen

TABLE 18-3 Selected Regional and Local Anesthetic Agents

Agent	Administration	Advantages	Disadvantages	Implications/Considerations
Lidocaine (Xylocaine)	Epidural, spinal, peripheral IV anesthesia, and local infiltration	Rapid. Longer duration of action (compared with procaine). Free of local irritative effect	Occasional	Useful topically for cystoscopy. Observe for untoward reactions—drowsiness, depressed respiration, seizures
Bupivacaine (Marcaine, Sensorcaine)	Epidural, spinal, peripheral IV anesthesia, and local infiltration	Duration is 2–3 times longer than lidocaine	Use cautiously in patients with known drug allergies or sensitivities.	A period of analgesia persists after return of sensation; therefore, need for strong analgesic agents is reduced. Greater potency and longer action than lidocaine
Tetracaine (Pontocaine)	Topical, infiltration, and nerve block	Long acting, produces good relaxation	Occasional allergic reaction	>10 times as potent as procaine (Novocaine)
Procaine (Novocaine)	Local infiltration	—	Occasional allergic reaction	Commonly used in oral or dental surgery

Moderate Sedation

Moderate sedation, previously referred to as conscious sedation, is a form of anesthesia that involves the IV administration of sedatives or analgesic medications to reduce patient anxiety and control pain during diagnostic or therapeutic procedures. It is being used increasingly for specific short-term surgical procedures in hospitals and ambulatory care centers (Rothrock, 2010). The goal is to depress a patient's level of consciousness to a moderate level to enable surgical, diagnostic, or therapeutic procedures to be performed while ensuring the patient's comfort during and cooperation with the procedures. With moderate sedation, the patient is able to maintain a patent airway, retain protective airway reflexes, and respond to verbal and physical stimuli.

Moderate sedation can be administered by an anesthesiologist, anesthetist, or other specially trained and credentialed physician or nurse. The patient receiving moderate sedation is never left alone and is closely monitored by a physician or nurse who is knowledgeable and skilled in detecting dysrhythmias, administering oxygen, and performing resuscitation. The continual assessment of the patient's vital signs, level of consciousness, and cardiac and respiratory function is an essential component of moderate sedation. Pulse oximetry, an ECG monitor, and frequent measurement of vital signs are used to monitor the patient. Regulations for the use and administration of moderate sedation differ from state to state, and its administration is addressed by standards issued by the Joint Commission and by institutional policies and nursing specialty organizations, including the American Society of PeriAnesthesia Nurses (ASPAN, 2010).

Monitored Anesthesia Care

Monitored anesthesia care, also referred to as monitored sedation, is moderate sedation administered by an anesthesiologist or anesthetist who must be prepared and qualified to convert to general anesthesia if necessary. The skills of an anesthesiologist or anesthetist may be necessary to manage the effects of a level of deeper sedation to return the patient to the appropriate level of sedation (Barash et al., 2009). MAC may be used for healthy patients undergoing relatively minor surgical procedures and for some critically ill patients who may be unable to tolerate anesthesia without extensive invasive monitoring and pharmacologic support (Rothrock, 2010).

Local Anesthesia

Local anesthesia is the injection of a solution containing the anesthetic agent into the tissues at the planned incision site. Often it is combined with a local regional block by injecting around the nerves immediately supplying the area. Advantages of local anesthesia are as follows:

- It is simple, economical, and nonexplosive.
- Equipment needed is minimal.
- Postoperative recovery is brief.
- Undesirable effects of general anesthesia are avoided.
- It is ideal for short and minor surgical procedures.

Local anesthesia is often administered in combination with epinephrine. Epinephrine constricts blood vessels, which prevents rapid absorption of the anesthetic agent and thus prolongs its local action and prevents seizures. Agents that can be used as local anesthetic agents are listed in Table 18-3; some of the same agents used in regional anesthesia are used as local anesthetic agents.

Local anesthesia is the preferred anesthetic method in any surgical procedure. However, contraindications include high preoperative levels of anxiety, because surgery with local anesthesia may increase anxiety. For some surgical procedures, local anesthesia is impractical because of the number of injections and the amount of anesthetic medication that would be required (e.g., breast reconstruction) and might result in toxic doses.

The skin is prepared as for any surgical procedure, and a small-gauge needle is used to inject a modest amount of the anesthetic medication into the skin layers. This produces blanching or a wheal. Additional anesthetic medication is then injected into the skin until an area the length of the proposed incision is anesthetized. A larger, longer needle then is used to infiltrate deeper tissues with the anesthetic agent. The action of the agent is almost immediate, so surgery may begin shortly after the injection is complete. The anesthetic may be mixed with a fast-acting analgesic of short duration to circumvent the burning felt when the longer-acting anesthetics are injected.

Potential Intraoperative Complications

The surgical patient is subject to several risks. Potential intraoperative complications include anesthesia awareness, nausea and vomiting, anaphylaxis, hypoxia, hypothermia, and malignant hyperthermia. The Surgical Care Improvement Project (SCIP) set a national goal of a 25% reduction in surgical complications by 2010. Targeted areas include surgical site infections as well as cardiac, respiratory, and venous thromboembolic complications (Joint Commission, 2011b).

■ Anesthesia Awareness

Publicity has increased patient's concerns about intraoperative awareness. It is important to discuss awareness with patients preoperatively so they realize that only general anesthesia is meant to create a state of oblivion. All other forms of anesthesia will eliminate pain, but sensation of pushing and pulling tissues may still be recognized and they may hear conversations among the operative team. In many cases, they may be able to respond to questions and involve themselves in the discussion. This is normal and is not what is referred to as anesthesia awareness.

Unintended intraoperative awareness refers to a patient becoming cognizant of surgical interventions while under general anesthesia and then recalling the incident. Neuromuscular blocks, sometimes required for surgical muscle relaxation, intensify the fear of the patient experiencing awareness because they are then unable to communicate during the episode. The frequency of anesthesia awareness may be as high as 0.1% to 0.2% of general anesthesia patients, equivalent to about 30,000 cases per year in the United States (Orser, 2008).

Indications of the occurrence of anesthesia awareness include an increase in the blood pressure, rapid heart rate, and patient movement. However, hemodynamic changes can be masked by paralytic medication, beta-blockers, and calcium channel blockers, thus the awareness may remain undetected. Premedication with amnesic agents and avoidance of muscle paralytics except when essential help to preclude the occurrence (Orser, 2008).

Nausea and Vomiting

Nausea and vomiting, or regurgitation, may affect patients during the intraoperative period. If gagging occurs, the patient is turned to the side, the head of the table is lowered, and a basin is provided to collect the vomitus. Suction is used to remove saliva and vomited gastric contents. The advent of new anesthetic agents has reduced the incidence; however, there is no single way to prevent nausea and vomiting. An interdisciplinary approach involving the surgeon, anesthesiologist or anesthetist, and nurse is best (Miller et al., 2010).

In some cases, the anesthesiologist or anesthetist administers antiemetics preoperatively or intraoperatively to counteract possible aspiration. If the patient aspirates vomitus, an asthmalike attack with severe bronchial spasms and wheezing is triggered. Pneumonitis and pulmonary edema can subsequently develop, leading to extreme hypoxia. Increasing medical attention is being paid to silent regurgitation of gastric contents (not related to preoperative fasting times), which occurs more frequently than previously realized. The volume and acidity of the aspirate determine the extent of damage to the lungs. Patients may be given citric acid and sodium citrate (Bicitra), a clear, nonparticulate antacid to increase gastric fluid pH or a histamine-2 (H_2) receptor antagonist such as cimetidine (Tagamet), ranitidine (Zantac), or famotidine (Pepcid) to decrease gastric acid production (Rothrock, 2010).

Anaphylaxis

Any time the patient comes into contact with a foreign substance, there is potential for an anaphylactic reaction. Because medications are the most common cause of anaphylaxis, intraoperative nurses must be aware of the type and method of anesthesia used as well as the specific agents (Erbe, 2011). An anaphylactic reaction can occur in response to many medications, latex, or other substances. The reaction may be immediate or delayed. Anaphylaxis is a life-threatening acute allergic reaction (Ewan, Dugué, Mirakian, et al., 2010).

Latex allergy—the sensitivity to natural rubber latex products—has become more prevalent, creating the need for alert responsiveness among health care professionals. The allergy exhibits with urticaria, asthma, rhinoconjunctivitis, and anaphylaxis (Australasian Society of Clinical Immunology and Allergy [ASCIA], 2011). If patients state that they have allergies to latex, even if they are wearing latex in their clothing, treatment must be latex free. In the OR, many products are latex free with the notable exception of softer latex catheters. Surgical cases should use latex-free gloves in anticipation of a possible allergy, and if no allergy is present, then personnel can switch to other gloves after the case starts if desired.

Fibrin sealants are used in various surgical procedures, and cyanoacrylate tissue adhesives are used to close wounds

without the use of sutures. These sealants have been implicated in allergic reactions and anaphylaxis (Rothrock, 2010). Although these reactions are rare, the nurse must be alert to the possibility and observe the patient for changes in vital signs and symptoms of anaphylaxis when these products are used. (Chapters 14 and 38 provide more details about the signs, symptoms, and treatment of anaphylaxis and anaphylactic shock.)

Hypoxia and Other Respiratory Complications

Inadequate ventilation, occlusion of the airway, inadvertent intubation of the esophagus, and hypoxia are significant potential complications associated with general anesthesia. Many factors can contribute to inadequate ventilation. Respiratory depression caused by anesthetic agents, aspiration of respiratory tract secretions or vomitus, and the patient's position on the operating table can compromise the exchange of gases. Anatomic variation can make the trachea difficult to visualize and result in insertion of the artificial airway into the esophagus rather than into the trachea. In addition to these dangers, asphyxia caused by foreign bodies in the mouth, spasm of the vocal cords, relaxation of the tongue, or aspiration of vomitus, saliva, or blood can occur. Brain damage from hypoxia occurs within minutes; therefore, vigilant monitoring of the patient's oxygenation status is a primary function of the anesthesiologist or anesthetist and the circulating nurse. Peripheral perfusion is checked frequently, and pulse oximetry values are monitored continuously.

Hypothermia

During anesthesia, the patient's temperature may fall. Glucose metabolism is reduced, and as a result, metabolic acidosis may develop. This condition is called *hypothermia* and is indicated by a core body temperature that is lower than normal (36.6°C [98°F] or less). Inadvertent hypothermia may occur as a result of a low temperature in the OR, infusion of cold fluids, inhalation of cold gases, open body wounds or cavities, decreased muscle activity, advanced age, or the pharmaceutical agents used (e.g., vasodilators, phenothiazines, general anesthetic medications). Hypothermia can depress neuronal activity and decrease cellular oxygen requirements below the minimum levels normally required for continued cell viability. As a result, it is used to protect function during some surgical procedures (e.g., carotid endarterectomy, cardiopulmonary bypass) (Barash et al., 2009).

Unintentional hypothermia needs to be avoided. If it occurs, it must be minimized or reversed. If hypothermia is intentional, the goal is safe return to normal body temperature. Environmental temperature in the OR can temporarily be set at 25°C to 26.6°C (78°F to 80°F). IV and irrigating fluids are warmed to 37°C (98.6°F). Wet gowns and drapes are removed promptly and replaced with dry materials, because wet materials promote heat loss. Warm air blankets and thermal blankets can also be used on the areas not exposed for surgery, and minimizing the area of the patient that is exposed will help maintain core temperature. Whatever methods are used to rewarm the patient, warming must be accomplished gradually, not rapidly. Conscientious monitoring of core temperature, urinary output, ECG, blood pressure, arterial blood gas levels, and serum electrolyte levels is required.

Malignant Hyperthermia

Malignant hyperthermia is a rare often inherited muscle disorder that is chemically induced by anesthetic agents (Rothrock, 2012). Malignant hyperthermia can be triggered by myopathies, emotional stress, heatstroke, neuroleptic malignant syndrome, strenuous exercise exertion, and trauma. It occurs in 1 in 50,000 to 100,000 adults. Mortality from malignant hyperthermia had been reported to be as high as 70%; however, with prompt recognition and rapid treatment, it has fallen to less than 10% (Hopkins & Ellis, 2011). Susceptible people include those with strong and bulky muscles, a history of muscle cramps or muscle weakness and unexplained temperature elevation, and an unexplained death of a family member during surgery that was accompanied by a febrile response (Hopkins & Ellis, 2011).

Pathophysiology

During anesthesia, potent agents such as inhalation anesthetic agents (halothane, enflurane) and muscle relaxants (succinylcholine) may trigger the symptoms of malignant hyperthermia (Rothrock, 2010). Stress and some medications, such as sympathomimetics (epinephrine), theophylline, aminophylline, anticholinergics (atropine), and cardiac glycosides (digitalis), can induce or intensify such a reaction.

The pathophysiology of malignant hyperthermia is related to a hypermetabolic condition that involves altered mechanisms of calcium function in skeletal muscle cells. This disruption of calcium causes clinical symptoms of hypermetabolism, which in turn increases muscle contraction (rigidity) and causes hyperthermia and subsequent damage to the central nervous system.

Clinical Manifestations

The initial symptoms of malignant hyperthermia are related to cardiovascular and musculoskeletal activity. Tachycardia (heart rate greater than 150 bpm) is often the earliest sign. Sympathetic nervous stimulation also leads to ventricular dysrhythmia, hypotension, decreased cardiac output, oliguria, and, later, cardiac arrest. With the abnormal transport of calcium, rigidity or tetanuslike movements occur, often in the jaw. Generalized muscle rigidity is one of the earliest signs. The rise in temperature is actually a late sign that develops rapidly; body temperature can increase 1°C to 2°C (2°F to 4°F) every 5 minutes, and core body temperature can exceed 42°C (107°F) (Hopkins & Ellis, 2011; Rothrock, 2010).

Medical Management

Recognizing symptoms early and discontinuing anesthesia promptly are imperative. Goals of treatment are to decrease metabolism, reverse metabolic and respiratory acidosis, correct dysrhythmias, decrease body temperature, provide oxygen and nutrition to tissues, and correct electrolyte imbalance. The Malignant Hyperthermia Association of the United States (MHAUS) publishes a treatment protocol that should be posted in the OR and be readily available on a malignant hyperthermia cart (MHAUS, 2011).

Anesthesia and surgery should be postponed. However, if end-tidal carbon dioxide (CO_2) monitoring and dantrolene sodium (Dantrium) are available and the anesthesiologist is experienced in managing malignant hyperthermia, the surgery may continue using a different anesthetic agent (Barash et al., 2009). Although malignant hyperthermia usually manifests about 10 to 20 minutes after induction of anesthesia, it can also occur during the first 24 hours after surgery.

Nursing Management

Although malignant hyperthermia is uncommon, the nurse must identify patients at risk, recognize the signs and symptoms, have the appropriate medication and equipment available, and be knowledgeable about the protocol to follow. Preparation may be lifesaving for the patient.

NURSING PROCESS

The Patient During Surgery

Intraoperative nurses focus on nursing diagnoses, interventions, and outcomes that surgical patients and their families experience. Additional priorities include collaborative problems and expected goals.

Assessment

Nursing assessment of the intraoperative patient involves obtaining data from the patient and the patient's medical record to identify factors that can affect care. These serve as guidelines for an individualized plan of patient care. The intraoperative nurse uses the focused preoperative nursing assessment documented on the patient record. This includes assessment of physiologic status (e.g., health–illness level, level of consciousness), psychosocial status (e.g., anxiety level, verbal communication problems, coping mechanisms), physical status (e.g., surgical site, skin condition, and effectiveness of preparation; mobility of joints), and ethical concerns.

Diagnosis

Nursing Diagnoses

Based on the assessment data, major nursing diagnoses may include the following:

- Anxiety related to surgical or environmental concerns
- Risk of latex allergy response due to possible exposure to latex in OR environment
- Risk for perioperative positioning injury related to positioning in the OR
- Risk for injury related to anesthesia and surgical procedure
- Disturbed sensory perception (global) related to general anesthesia or sedation

Collaborative Problems/Potential Complications

Based on the assessment data, potential complications may include the following:

- Anesthesia awareness
- Nausea and vomiting
- Anaphylaxis
- Hypoxia
- Unintentional hypothermia
- Malignant hyperthermia
- Infection

Planning and Goals

The major goals for care of the patient during surgery include reduced anxiety, absence of latex exposure, absence of positioning injuries, freedom from injury, maintenance of the patient's dignity, and absence of complications.

Nursing Interventions

Reducing Anxiety

The OR environment can seem cold, stark, and frightening to the patient, who may be feeling isolated and apprehensive. Introducing yourself, addressing the patient by name warmly and frequently, verifying details, providing explanations, and encouraging and answering questions provide a sense of professionalism and friendliness that can help the patient feel safe and secure. When discussing what the patient can expect in surgery, the nurse uses basic communication skills, such as touch and eye contact, to reduce anxiety. Attention to physical comfort (warm blankets, padding, and position changes) helps the patient feel more comfortable. Telling the patient who else will be present in the OR, how long the procedure is expected to take, and other details helps the patient prepare for the experience and gain a sense of control.

Reducing Latex Exposure

Patients with latex allergies require early identification and communication to all personnel about the presence of the allergy according to standards of care for patients with latex allergy (AORN, 2011; ASCIA, 2011). In most ORs, there are few latex items currently in use, but because there still remain some instances of latex use, maintenance of latex allergy precautions throughout the perioperative period must be observed. For safety, manufacturers and hospital materials managers need to take responsibility for identifying the latex content in items used by patients and health care personnel. (See Chapters 17 and 38 for assessment for latex allergy.)

> ### ▶ Quality and Safety Nursing Alert
>
> It is the responsibility of all nurses, and particularly perianesthesia and perioperative nurses, to be aware of latex allergies, necessary precautions, and products that are latex free. Hospital staff are also at risk for development of a latex allergy secondary to repeated exposure to latex products.

Preventing Perioperative Positioning Injury

The patient's position on the operating table depends on the surgical procedure to be performed as well as the patient's physical condition (Fig. 18-5). The potential for transient discomfort or permanent injury is present because many surgical positions are awkward. Hyperextending joints, compressing arteries, or pressing on nerves and bony prominences usually results in discomfort simply because the position must be sustained for a long period of time (Rothrock, 2010). Factors to consider include the following:

- The patient should be in as comfortable a position as possible, whether conscious or unconscious.
- The operative field must be adequately exposed.
- An awkward position, undue pressure on a body part, or the use of stirrups or traction should not obstruct the vascular supply.

- Respiration should not be impeded by pressure of arms on the chest or by a gown that constricts the neck or chest.
- Nerves must be protected from undue pressure. Improper positioning of the arms, hands, legs, or feet can cause serious injury or paralysis. Shoulder braces must be well padded to prevent irreparable nerve injury, especially when the Trendelenburg position is necessary.
- Precautions for patient safety must be observed, particularly with older adults, patients who are thin or obese, and those with a physical deformity.
- The patient may need light restraint before induction in case of excitement.

The usual position for surgery, called the *dorsal recumbent position*, is flat on the back. Both arms are positioned at the side of the table: one with the hand placed palm down and the other carefully positioned on an armboard to facilitate IV infusion of fluids, blood, or medications. This position is used for most abdominal surgeries, except for surgery of the gallbladder or pelvis (see Fig. 18-5A).

The Trendelenburg position usually is used for surgery on the lower abdomen and pelvis to obtain good exposure by displacing the intestines into the upper abdomen. In this position, the head and body are lowered. The patient is supported in position by padded shoulder braces (see Fig. 18-5B), bean bags, and foam padding. Reverse Trendelenburg position provides the space to operate on the upper abdomen by shifting the intestines into the pelvis. A padded footboard and other supportive cushioning preserve a safe environment for the patient.

The lithotomy position is used for nearly all perineal, rectal, and vaginal surgical procedures (see Fig. 18-5C). The patient is positioned on the back with the legs and thighs flexed. The position is maintained by placing the feet in stirrups.

The Sims or lateral position is used for renal surgery. The patient is placed on the nonoperative side with an air pillow 12.5 to 15 cm (5 to 6 inches) thick under the loin, or on a table with a kidney or back lift (see Fig. 18-5D).

Protecting the Patient From Injury

Various activities are used to address the diverse patient safety issues that arise in the OR. The nurse protects the patient from injury by providing a safe environment. Verifying information, checking the medical record for completeness, and maintaining surgical asepsis and an optimal environment are critical nursing responsibilities. Verification that all required documentation is completed is an important function of the intraoperative nurse. A surgical checklist is used prior to induction of anesthesia, before the skin incision is made, and before the patient leaves the OR (see Fig. 18-1). It is important to review the patient's record for the following:

- Correct informed surgical consent, with patient's signature
- Completed records for health history and physical examination
- Results of diagnostic studies
- Allergies (including latex)

In addition to checking that all necessary patient data are complete, the perioperative nurse obtains the necessary equipment specific to the procedure. The need for nonroutine medications, blood components, instruments, and other

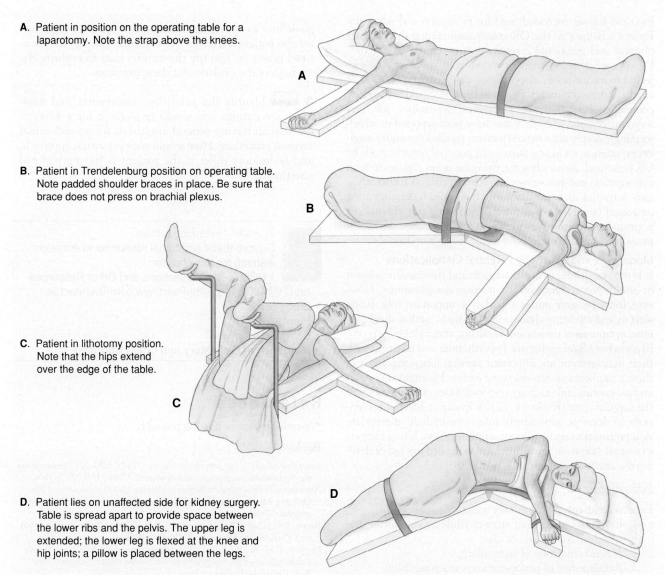

A. Patient in position on the operating table for a laparotomy. Note the strap above the knees.

B. Patient in Trendelenburg position on operating table. Note padded shoulder braces in place. Be sure that brace does not press on brachial plexus.

C. Patient in lithotomy position. Note that the hips extend over the edge of the table.

D. Patient lies on unaffected side for kidney surgery. Table is spread apart to provide space between the lower ribs and the pelvis. The upper leg is extended; the lower leg is flexed at the knee and hip joints; a pillow is placed between the legs.

FIGURE 18-5 • Patient positions on the operating table. Captions call attention to safety and comfort features. All surgical patients wear caps to cover the hair completely.

equipment and supplies is assessed, and the readiness of the room, completeness of physical setup, and completeness of instrument, suture, and dressing setups are determined. Any aspects of the OR environment that may negatively affect the patient are identified. These include physical features, such as room temperature and humidity; electrical hazards; potential contaminants (dust, blood, and discharge on floor or surfaces; uncovered hair; nonsterile attire of personnel; jewelry worn by personnel; chipped or artificial fingernails); and unnecessary traffic. The circulating nurse also sets up and maintains suction equipment in working order, sets up invasive monitoring equipment, assists with insertion of vascular access and monitoring devices (arterial, Swan-Ganz, central venous pressure, IV lines), and initiates appropriate physical comfort measures for the patient.

Preventing physical injury includes using safety straps and side rails and not leaving the sedated patient unattended. Transferring the patient from the stretcher to the OR table requires safe transferring practices. Other safety measures include properly positioning a grounding pad under the patient to prevent electrical burns and shock, removing excess antiseptic solution from the patient's skin, and promptly and completely draping exposed areas after the sterile field has been created to decrease the risk of hypothermia.

Nursing measures to prevent injury from excessive blood loss include blood conservation using equipment such as a cell saver (a device for recirculating the patient's own blood cells) and administration of blood products (Rothrock, 2010). Few patients undergoing an elective procedure require blood transfusion, but those undergoing high-risk procedures (such as orthopedic or cardiac surgeries) may require an intraoperative transfusion. The circulating nurse anticipates this need, checks that blood has been cross-matched and held in reserve, and is prepared to administer blood.

Serving as Patient Advocate

The patient undergoing general anesthesia or moderate sedation experiences temporary sensory or perceptual alteration or loss, and has an increased need for protection and advocacy. Patient advocacy in the OR entails maintaining the patient's physical and emotional comfort, privacy, rights, and dignity. Patients, whether conscious or unconscious, should not be subjected to excess noise, inappropriate conversation, or, most of all, derogatory comments. Banter in the OR should not include comments about the patient's physical appearance, job, personal history, and so forth. Cases have been reported in which seemingly deeply anesthetized patients recalled the entire surgical experience, including disparaging personal remarks made by OR personnel. As an advocate, the nurse never engages in such conversation and discourages others from doing so. Other advocacy activities include minimizing the clinical, dehumanizing aspects of being a surgical patient by making sure the patient is treated as a person, respecting cultural and spiritual values, providing physical privacy, and maintaining confidentiality.

Monitoring and Managing Potential Complications

It is the responsibility of the surgeon and the anesthesiologist or anesthetist to monitor and manage complications. However, intraoperative nurses also play an important role. Being alert to and reporting changes in vital signs, cardiac dysrhythmias, symptoms of nausea and vomiting, anaphylaxis, hypoxia, hypothermia, and malignant hyperthermia and assisting with their management are important nursing functions. Each of these complications was discussed earlier. Maintaining asepsis and preventing infection are responsibilities of all members of the surgical team (Rothrock, 2010). Evidence-based interventions to decrease surgical site infections include appropriate skin preparation and antibiotic administration. Using clippers to remove hair from the surgical site as needed instead of shaving the site is recommended (AORN, 2011).

Evaluation

Expected patient outcomes may include:

1. Exhibits low level of anxiety while awake during the intraoperative phase of care
2. Has no symptoms of latex allergy
3. Remains free of perioperative positioning injury
4. Experiences no unexpected threats to safety
5. Has dignity preserved throughout OR experience
6. Is free of complications (e.g., nausea and vomiting, anaphylaxis, hypoxia, hypothermia, malignant hyperthermia, or deep vein thrombosis) or experiences successful management of adverse effects of surgery and anesthesia should they occur

Critical Thinking Exercises

1 A 75-year-old patient with hypertension and decreased hearing is scheduled for hip replacement surgery. Generate a list of possible nursing diagnoses for this patient during the intraoperative period. Identify the nursing interventions that would be most appropriate for each of the possible nursing diagnoses and evaluation criteria for these interventions.

2 **ebp** A patient is undergoing a lengthy cardiac surgery. What resources would you use to identify the current

guidelines for avoiding intraoperative positioning injury for the patient? What is the evidence base for the identified practices? Identify the criteria used to evaluate the strength of the evidence for these practices.

3 **pq** Identify the priorities, assessments, and nursing interventions you would implement for a 45-year-old woman having general anesthesia for an abdominal surgical procedure. How would your priorities, approach, and techniques differ if the patient is having regional anesthesia?

 Brunner Suite Resources

Explore these additional resources to enhance learning for this chapter:
- NCLEX-Style Questions and Other Resources on **thePoint**, http://thePoint.lww.com/Brunner13e
- Study Guide
- PrepU
- Clinical Handbook
- Handbook of Laboratory and Diagnostic Tests

References

*Asterisk indicates nursing research.

Books

American Society of PeriAnesthesia Nurses. (2010). *2010–2012 perianesthesia nursing standards and practice recommendations.* Cherry Hill, NJ: Author.

Association of PeriOperative Registered Nurses. (2011). *Association of Peri-Operative Registered Nurses (AORN) standards, recommended practice, and guidelines.* Denver: Author.

Barash, P. G., Cullen, B. F., & Stoelting, R. K. (2009). *Clinical anesthesia* (6th ed.). Philadelphia: Lippincott Williams & Wilkins.

Hopkins, P. M., & Ellis, F. R. (2011). *Hyperthermic and hypermetabolic disorders: Exertional heat-stroke, malignant hyperthermia and related syndromes.* New York: Cambridge University Press.

Meiner, S. E. (2011). *Gerontologic nursing* (4th ed.). St. Louis: Elsevier Mosby.

Miller, C. A. (2009). *Nursing for wellness in older adults* (5th ed.). Philadelphia: Lippincott Williams & Wilkins.

Miller, R. D., Eriksson, L. I., Fleisher, L. A., et al. (2010). *Miller's anesthesia* (7th ed.). Philadelphia: Elsevier.

Rothrock, J. C. (Ed.). (2010). *Alexander's care of the patient in surgery* (14th ed.). St. Louis: Mosby.

Tabloski, P. A. (2009). *Gerontological nursing: The essential guide to clinical practice* (2nd ed.). Upper Saddle River, NJ: Prentice Hall Health.

Journals and Electronic Documents

*Anderson, C., & Talsma, A. (2011). Characterizing the structure of operating room staffing using social network analysis. *Nursing Research*, 60(6), 378–385.

Australasian Society of Clinical Immunology and Allergy. (2011). *Latex allergy.* Available at: www.allergy.org.au/

Becker, D. (2009). Preoperative medical evaluation: Part 1: General principles and cardiovascular considerations. *Anesthesia Progress*, 56(3), 92–102.

Erbe, B. (2011). Safe medication administration in the operating room. *Tar Heel Nurse*, 73(1), 10–13.

Ewan, P., Dugué, P., Mirakian, R., et al. (2010). BSACI guidelines for the investigation of suspected anaphylaxis during general anaesthesia. *Clinical and Experimental Allergy: Journal of the British Society for Allergy and Clinical Immunology*, 40(1), 15–31.

Haynes, A. B., Weiser, T. G., Berry, W. R., et al. (2009). A surgical safety checklist to reduce morbidity and mortality in a global population. *New England Journal of Medicine*, 360(5), 491–499.

Joint Commission. (2011a). *Sentinel alert: Patient alert under anesthesia.* Available at: www.jointcommission.org/sentinel_event_alert_issue_32_preventing_and_managing_the_impact_of_anesthesia_awareness/

Joint Commission. (2011b). *Surgical Care Improvement Project.* Available at: www.jointcommission.org/surgical_care_improvement_project

Joint Commission. (2013). *2013 National Patient Safety Goals.* Available at: www.jointcommission.org/standards_information/npsgs.aspx

Malignant Hyperthermia Association of the United States. (2011). *What is MH?* Available at: www.mhaus.org/index.cfm/fuseaction/OnlineBrochures.Display/BrochurePK/8AABF3FB-13B0-430F-BE20FB32516B02D6.cfm

Massicotte, L., Chalaoui, K., Beaulieu, D., et al. (2009). Comparison of spinal anesthesia with general anesthesia on morphine requirement after abdominal hysterectomy. *Acta Anaesthesiologica Scandinavia, 53*(5), 641–647.

McKay, W., Lett, B., Chilibeck, P., et al. (2009). Effects of spinal anesthesia on resting metabolic rate and quadriceps mechanomyography. *European Journal of Applied Physiology, 106*(4), 583–588.

Orser, B. A. (2008). Depth-of-anesthesia monitor and the frequency of intraoperative awareness. *New England Journal of Medicine, 358,* 1189–1191.

Robinson, L., Paull, D., Mazzia, L., et al. (2010). The role of the operating room nurse manager in the successful implementation of preoperative briefings and postoperative debriefings in the VA Medical Team Training Program. *Journal of Perianesthesia Nursing, 25*(5), 302–306.

Schifilliti, D., Grasso, G., Conti, A., et al. (2010). Anaesthetic-related neuroprotection: Intravenous or inhalational agents? *CNS Drugs, 24*(11), 893–907.

World Health Organization. (2008). New checklist to help make surgery safer. *WHO Bulletin, 86*(7), 496–576.

Zahiri, H., Stromberg, J., Skupsky, H., et al. (2011). Prevention of 3 "never events" in the operating room: Fires, gossypiboma, and wrong-site surgery. *Surgical Innovation, 18*(1), 55–60.

Resources

American Latex Allergy Association (ALAA), www.latexallergyresources.org

American Society of Anesthesiologists (ASA), www.asahq.org

American Society of PeriAnesthesia Nurses (ASPAN), www.aspan.org

Association of PeriOperative Registered Nurses, www.aorn.org

Centers for Disease Control and Prevention, Injury and Violence Prevention and Control, www.cdc.gov/injury

Joint Commission, www.jointcommission.org

Malignant Hyperthermia Association of the United States (MHAUS), www.mhaus.org

National SCIP Partnership, www.leapfroggroup.org/news/leapfrog_news/144968

World Health Organization (WHO), www.who.int/en/

Postoperative Nursing Management

Learning Objectives

On completion of this chapter, the learner will be able to:

1 Describe the responsibilities of the postanesthesia care nurse in the prevention of immediate postoperative complications.
2 Compare postoperative care of the ambulatory surgery patient with that of the hospitalized surgery patient.
3 Identify common postoperative problems and their management.

4 Describe the gerontologic considerations related to postoperative management.
5 Describe variables that affect wound healing.
6 Demonstrate postoperative dressing techniques.
7 Identify assessment parameters appropriate for the early detection of postoperative complications.

Glossary

dehiscence: partial or complete separation of wound edges

evisceration: protrusion of organs through the surgical incision

first-intention healing: method of healing in which wound edges are surgically approximated and integumentary continuity is restored without granulation

phase I PACU: area designated for care of surgical patients immediately after surgery and for patients whose condition warrants close monitoring

phase II PACU: area designated for care of surgical patients who have been transferred from a phase I PACU because their condition no longer requires the close monitoring provided in a phase I PACU

phase III PACU: setting in which the patient is cared for in the immediate postoperative period and then prepared for discharge from the facility

postanesthesia care unit (PACU): area where postoperative patients are monitored as they recover from anesthesia; formerly referred to as the recovery room or postanesthesia recovery room

second-intention healing: method of healing in which wound edges are not surgically approximated and integumentary continuity is restored by the process known as granulation

third-intention healing: method of healing in which surgical approximation of wound edges is delayed and integumentary continuity is restored by opposing areas of granulation

The postoperative period extends from the time the patient leaves the operating room (OR) until the last follow-up visit with the surgeon. This may be as short as a day or two or as long as several months. During the postoperative period, nursing care focuses on reestablishing the patient's physiologic equilibrium, alleviating pain, preventing complications, and educating the patient about self-care (Stannard & Krenzischek, 2012). Careful assessment and immediate intervention assist the patient in returning to optimal function quickly, safely, and as comfortably as possible. Ongoing care in the community through home care, clinic visits, office visits, or telephone follow-up facilitates an uncomplicated recovery.

Care of the Patient in the Postanesthesia Care Unit

The **postanesthesia care unit (PACU)**, formerly referred to as the recovery room or postanesthesia recovery room, is located adjacent to the OR suite. Patients still under anesthesia or recovering from anesthesia are placed in this unit for easy access to experienced, highly skilled nurses, anesthesiologists or anesthetists, surgeons, advanced hemodynamic and pulmonary monitoring and support, special equipment, and medications.

Phases of Postanesthesia Care

In some hospitals and ambulatory surgical centers, postanesthesia care is divided into three phases (Rothrock, 2010). In the **phase I PACU**, used during the immediate recovery phase, intensive nursing care is provided. In the **phase II PACU**, the patient is prepared for self-care or care in the hospital or an extended care setting. In **phase III PACU**, the patient is prepared for discharge. Recliners rather than stretchers or beds are standard in many phase III units, which may also be referred to as step-down, sit-up, or progressive care units. In many hospitals, phase II and phase III units are combined. Patients may remain in a PACU for as long as 4 to

6 hours, depending on the type of surgery and any preexisting conditions. In facilities without separate phase I, II, and III units, the patient remains in the PACU and may be discharged home directly from this unit.

Admitting the Patient to the Postanesthesia Care Unit

Transferring the postoperative patient from the OR to the PACU is the responsibility of the anesthesiologist or anesthetist and any other licensed member of the OR team. During transport from the OR to the PACU, the anesthesia provider remains at the head of the stretcher (to maintain the airway), and a surgical team member remains at the opposite end. Transporting the patient involves special consideration of the incision site, potential vascular changes, and exposure. The surgical incision is considered every time the postoperative patient is moved; many wounds are closed under considerable tension, and every effort is made to prevent further strain on the incision. The patient is positioned so that he or she is not lying on and obstructing drains or drainage tubes. Orthostatic hypotension may occur when a patient is moved too quickly from one position to another (e.g., from a lithotomy position to a horizontal position or from a lateral to a supine position), so the patient must be moved slowly and carefully. As soon as the patient is placed on the stretcher or bed, the soiled gown is removed and replaced with a dry gown. The patient is covered with lightweight blankets and warmed. Only three side rails may be raised to prevent falls because in many states raising all side rails constitutes restraint.

The nurse who admits the patient to the PACU reviews essential information with the anesthesiologist or anesthetist (Chart 19-1) and the circulating nurse. Oxygen is applied, monitoring equipment is attached, and an immediate physiologic assessment is conducted.

Nursing Management in the Postanesthesia Care Unit

The nursing management objectives for the patient in the PACU are to provide care until the patient has recovered from the effects of anesthesia (e.g., until resumption of motor and sensory functions), is oriented, has stable vital signs, and shows no evidence of hemorrhage or other complications (Spry, 2009).

Assessing the Patient

Frequent, skilled assessments of the patient's airway, respiratory function, cardiovascular function, skin color, level of consciousness, and ability to respond to commands are the cornerstones of nursing care in the PACU (Weber & Kelley, 2010). The nurse performs and documents a baseline assessment, then checks the surgical site for drainage or hemorrhage and makes sure that all drainage tubes and monitoring lines are connected and functioning. The nurse checks any intravenous (IV) fluids or medications currently infusing and verifies dosage and rate (ASPAN, Schick, & Windle, 2010).

After the initial assessment, vital signs are monitored and the patient's general physical status is assessed and documented at least every 15 minutes (Miller, Eriksson, Fleisher, et al., 2010). The nurse must be aware of any pertinent information from the patient's history that may be significant (e.g., patient is deaf or hard of hearing, has a history of seizures, has diabetes, or is allergic to certain medications or to latex). Administration of the patient's postoperative analgesic requirements is a top priority to provide pain relief before it becomes severe and facilitate early ambulation (Miller et al., 2010).

Maintaining a Patent Airway

The primary objective in the immediate postoperative period is to maintain ventilation and thus prevent hypoxemia (reduced oxygen in the blood) and hypercapnia (excess carbon dioxide in the blood). Both can occur if the airway is obstructed and ventilation is reduced (hypoventilation). Besides administering supplemental oxygen (as prescribed), the nurse assesses respiratory rate and depth, ease of respirations, oxygen saturation, and breath sounds.

Patients who have experienced prolonged anesthesia usually are unconscious, with all muscles relaxed. This relaxation extends to the muscles of the pharynx. When the patient lies on his or her back, the lower jaw and the tongue fall backward and the air passages become obstructed (Fig. 19-1A). This is called *hypopharyngeal obstruction*. Signs of occlusion include choking; noisy and irregular respirations; decreased oxygen saturation scores; and, within minutes, a blue, dusky color (cyanosis) of the skin. Because movement of the thorax and the diaphragm does not necessarily indicate that the patient is breathing, the nurse needs to place the palm of the hand at the patient's nose and mouth to feel the exhaled breath.

 Quality and Safety Nursing Alert

> The treatment of hypopharyngeal obstruction involves tilting the head back and pushing forward on the angle of the lower jaw, as if to push the lower teeth in front of the upper teeth (see Fig. 19-1B,C). This maneuver pulls the tongue forward and opens the air passages.

The anesthesiologist or anesthetist may leave a hard rubber or plastic airway in the patient's mouth to maintain a patent

---

Chart 19-1

Anesthesia Provider-to-Nurse Report and Nurse-to-Nurse Report: Information to Convey

Patient name, gender, age
Allergies
Surgical procedure
Length of time in the operating room
Anesthetic agents and reversal agents used
Estimated blood loss/fluid loss
Fluid/blood replacement
Last set of vital signs and any problems during the procedure
Complications encountered (anesthetic or surgical)
Medical comorbidities (e.g., diabetes, hypertension)
Considerations for immediate postoperative period (pain management, reversals, ventilator settings)
Language barrier
Location of patient's family

Ideally, the anesthesia provider should not leave the patient until the nurse is satisfied with the patient's airway and immediate condition.

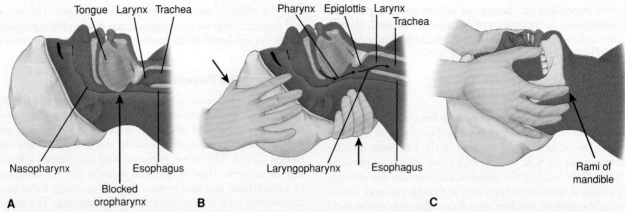

FIGURE 19-1 • A. A hypopharyngeal obstruction occurs when neck flexion permits the chin to drop toward the chest; obstruction almost always occurs when the head is in the midposition. **B.** Tilting the head back to stretch the anterior neck structure lifts the base of the tongue off the posterior pharyngeal wall. The direction of the *arrows* indicates the pressure of the hands. **C.** Opening the mouth is necessary to correct a valvelike obstruction of the nasal passage during expiration, which occurs in about 30% of unconscious patients. Open the patient's mouth (separate lips and teeth) and move the lower jaw forward so that the lower teeth are in front of the upper teeth. To regain backward tilt of the neck, lift with both hands at the ascending rami of the mandible.

airway (Fig. 19-2). Such a device should not be removed until signs such as gagging indicate that reflex action is returning. Alternatively, the patient may enter the PACU with an endotracheal tube still in place and may require continued mechanical ventilation. The nurse assists in initiating the use of the ventilator as well as the weaning and extubation processes. Some patients, particularly those who have had extensive or lengthy surgical procedures, may be transferred from the OR directly to the intensive care unit (ICU) or from the PACU to the ICU while still intubated and receiving mechanical ventilation. In most facilities, the patient is awakened and extubated in the OR (except in cases of trauma or a critically ill patient) and arrives in the PACU breathing without support.

If the teeth are clenched, the mouth may be opened manually but cautiously with a padded tongue depressor. The head

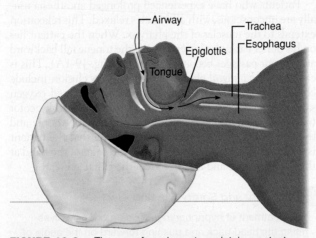

FIGURE 19-2 • The use of an airway to maintain a patent airway after anesthesia. The airway passes over the base of the tongue and permits air to pass into the pharynx in the region of the epiglottis. Patients often leave the operating room with an airway in place. The airway should remain in place until the patient recovers sufficiently to breathe normally. As the patient regains consciousness, the airway usually causes irritation and should be removed.

of the bed is elevated 15 to 30 degrees unless contraindicated, and the patient is closely monitored to maintain the airway as well as to minimize the risk of aspiration. If vomiting occurs, the patient is turned to the side to prevent aspiration and the vomitus is collected in the emesis basin. Mucus or vomitus obstructing the pharynx or the trachea is suctioned with a pharyngeal suction tip or a nasal catheter introduced into the nasopharynx or oropharynx to a distance of 15 to 20 cm (6 to 8 inches). Caution is necessary in suctioning the throat of a patient who has had a tonsillectomy or other oral or laryngeal surgery because of the risk of bleeding and discomfort.

Maintaining Cardiovascular Stability

To monitor cardiovascular stability, the nurse assesses the patient's mental status; vital signs; cardiac rhythm; skin temperature, color, and moisture; and urine output. Central venous pressure, pulmonary artery pressure, and arterial lines are monitored, if in place. The nurse also assesses the patency of all IV lines. The primary cardiovascular complications seen in the PACU include hypotension and shock, hemorrhage, hypertension, and dysrhythmias.

Hypotension and Shock

Hypotension can result from blood loss, hypoventilation, position changes, pooling of blood in the extremities, or side effects of medications and anesthetics. The most common cause is loss of circulating volume through blood and plasma loss. If the amount of blood loss exceeds 500 mL (especially if the loss is rapid), replacement is usually indicated.

> **⚑ Quality and Safety Nursing Alert**
>
> A systolic blood pressure of less than 90 mm Hg is usually considered immediately reportable. However, the patient's preoperative or baseline blood pressure is used to make informed postoperative comparisons. A previously stable blood pressure that shows a downward trend of 5 mm Hg at each 15-minute reading should also be reported.

Shock, which is one of the most serious postoperative complications, can result from hypovolemia and decreased intravascular volume. The types of shock are classified as hypovolemic, cardiogenic, neurogenic, anaphylactic, and septic (Ewan, Dugué, Mirakian, et al., 2010). The classic signs of hypovolemic shock (the most common type of shock) are pallor; cool, moist skin; rapid breathing; cyanosis of the lips, gums, and tongue; rapid, weak, thready pulse; narrowing pulse pressure; low blood pressure; and concentrated urine. (See Chapter 14 for a detailed discussion of shock.)

Hypovolemic shock can be avoided largely by the timely administration of IV fluids, blood, blood products, and medications that elevate blood pressure. The primary intervention for hypovolemic shock is volume replacement, with an infusion of lactated Ringer's solution, 0.9% sodium chloride solution, colloids, or blood component therapy (see Table 14-3 in Chapter 14). Oxygen is administered by nasal cannula, facemask, or mechanical ventilation. If fluid administration fails to reverse hypovolemic shock, then various cardiac, vasodilator, and corticosteroid medications may be prescribed to improve cardiac function and reduce peripheral vascular resistance.

The PACU bed provides easy access to the patient; is easily movable; can readily be positioned to facilitate the use of measures to counteract shock; and has features that facilitate care, such as IV poles, side rails, and wheel brakes. The patient is placed flat with the legs elevated. Respiratory rate, pulse rate, blood pressure, blood oxygen concentration, urinary output, level of consciousness, central venous pressure, pulmonary artery pressure, pulmonary artery wedge pressure, and cardiac output are monitored to provide information on the patient's respiratory and cardiovascular status. Vital signs are monitored continuously until the patient's condition has stabilized.

Other factors can contribute to hemodynamic instability, such as body temperature and pain. The PACU nurse implements measures to manage these factors. The nurse keeps the patient warm (while avoiding overheating to prevent cutaneous vessels from dilating and depriving vital organs of blood), avoids exposure, and maintains normothermia (to prevent vasodilation). Pain control measures are implemented, as discussed later in this chapter.

Hemorrhage

Hemorrhage is an uncommon yet serious complication of surgery that can result in hypovolemic shock and death. It can present insidiously or emergently at any time in the immediate postoperative period or up to several days after surgery (Table 19-1). The patient presents with hypotension; rapid, thready pulse; disorientation; restlessness; oliguria; and cold, pale skin. The early phase of shock will manifest in feelings of apprehension, decreased cardiac output, and vascular resistance. Breathing becomes labored, and "air hunger" will be exhibited; the patient will feel cold (hypothermia) and may experience tinnitus. If shock symptoms are left untreated, the patient will continually grow weaker but can remain conscious until near death (Miller et al., 2010; Rothrock, 2010).

Transfusing blood or blood products and determining the cause of hemorrhage are the initial therapeutic measures. The surgical site and incision should always be inspected for bleeding. If bleeding is evident, a sterile gauze pad and a pressure dressing are applied, and the site of the bleeding is elevated to heart level if possible. The patient is placed in the shock position (flat on back; legs elevated at a 20-degree angle; knees kept straight). If hemorrhage is suspected but cannot be visualized, the patient may be taken back to the OR for emergency exploration of the surgical site.

If hemorrhage is suspected, the nurse should be aware of any special considerations related to blood loss replacement. Certain patients may decline blood transfusions for religious or cultural reasons and may identify this request on their advance directives or living will.

Hypertension and Dysrhythmias

Hypertension is common in the immediate postoperative period secondary to sympathetic nervous system stimulation from pain, hypoxia, or bladder distention. Dysrhythmias are associated with electrolyte imbalance, altered respiratory function, pain, hypothermia, stress, and anesthetic agents. Both hypertension and dysrhythmias are managed by treating the underlying causes.

Relieving Pain and Anxiety

The PACU nurse monitors the patient's physiologic status, manages pain, and provides psychological support in an effort to relieve the patient's fears and concerns. The nurse checks the medical record for special needs and concerns of the patient. Opioid analgesic medications are administered mostly by IV in the PACU (Rothrock, 2010). IV opioids provide immediate pain relief and are short acting, thus minimizing the potential for drug interactions or prolonged respiratory depression while anesthetics are still active in the patient's system (West, 2011). When the patient's condition permits, a close member of the family may visit in the PACU to decrease the family's anxiety and make the patient feel more secure.

Controlling Nausea and Vomiting

Nausea and vomiting are common issues in the PACU. The nurse should intervene at the patient's first report of nausea to control the problem rather than wait for it to progress to vomiting.

TABLE 19-1 Classifications of Hemorrhage

Classification	Defining Characteristic
Time Frame	
Primary	Hemorrhage occurs at the time of surgery.
Intermediary	Hemorrhage occurs during the first few hours after surgery when the rise of blood pressure to its normal level dislodges insecure clots from untied vessels.
Secondary	Hemorrhage may occur some time after surgery if a suture slips because a blood vessel was not securely tied, became infected, or was eroded by a drainage tube.
Type of Vessel	
Capillary	Hemorrhage is characterized by a slow, general ooze.
Venous	Darkly colored blood flows quickly.
Arterial	Blood is bright red and appears in spurts with each heartbeat.
Visibility	
Evident	Hemorrhage is on the surface and can be seen.
Concealed	Hemorrhage is in a body cavity and cannot be seen.

TABLE 19-2 Medications Used to Control Postoperative Nausea and Vomiting

Drug Classes	Name	Nursing Implications
GI stimulant	Metoclopramide (Reglan)	Acts by stimulating gastric emptying and increasing GI transit time. Administration recommended at end of procedure. Available in oral, IM, and IV forms.
Phenothiazine antiemetic	Prochlorperazine (Compazine)	Indicated for control of severe nausea and vomiting. Available in oral, SR, rectal, IM, and IV forms.
Phenothiazine antiemetic antimotion sickness	Promethazine (Phenergan)	Recommended every 4–6 h for nausea and vomiting associated with anesthesia and surgery. Available in oral, IM, and IV forms.
Antimotion sickness	Dimenhydrinate (Dramamine)	Indicated for prevention of nausea, vomiting, or vertigo of motion sickness. Available in oral, IM, and IV forms.
Antiemetic	Hydroxyzine (Vistaril, Atarax)	Control of nausea and vomiting and as adjunct to analgesia preoperatively and postoperatively to allow decreased opioid dosage. Available in oral and IM forms.
Antiemetic antimotion sickness	Scopolamine (Transderm Scop)	Used to prevent and control of nausea and vomiting associated with motion sickness and recovery from surgery. Available in oral, transdermal SC, and IM forms.
Antiemetic	Ondansetron (Zofran)	Prevention of postoperative nausea and vomiting. Available in oral, IM, and IV forms. With few side effects, frequently the drug of choice

GI, gastrointestinal; IM, intramuscular; IV, intravenous; SR, sustained release; SC, subcutaneous.
Adapted from Karch, A. M. (2012). *2012 Lippincott's nursing drug guide*. Philadelphia: Lippincott Williams & Wilkins.

◣ Quality and Safety Nursing Alert

At the slightest indication of nausea, the patient is turned completely to one side to promote mouth drainage and prevent aspiration of vomitus, which can cause asphyxiation and death.

Many medications are available to control postoperative nausea and vomiting (PONV) without oversedating the patient; they are commonly administered during surgery as well as in the PACU. Table 19-2 contains some medications prescribed to control PONV (Constantini, Affaitati, Fabrizio, et al., 2011; Franck, Radtke, Apfel, et al., 2010).

The risk of PONV ranges from 30% in the general surgical population but increases to 80% with certain risk factors. These risks include general anesthesia, female gender, nonsmoker, history of PONV, and history of motion sickness (Franck et al., 2010). Surgical risks are increased with PONV due to an increase in intra-abdominal pressure, elevated central venous pressure, the potential for aspiration, increased heart rate, and systemic blood pressure, which increase the risk of myocardial ischemia and dysrhythmias. Postoperative pain is increased as well (Miller et al., 2010). Ongoing research is investigating the most efficacious combination of medications for patients with different risk profiles (Franck et al., 2010; Haupt & Reed, 2010; Rowe & Baker, 2009).

🌿 Gerontologic Considerations

The older patient, like all patients, is transferred from the OR table to the bed or stretcher slowly and gently. The effects of this action on blood pressure and ventilation are monitored. Special attention is given to keeping the patient warm, because older patients are more susceptible to hypothermia. The patient's position is changed frequently to stimulate respirations as well as promote circulation and comfort.

Immediate postoperative care for the older patient is the same as for any surgical patient; however, additional support is given if cardiovascular, pulmonary, or renal function is impaired. With careful monitoring, it is possible to detect cardiopulmonary deficits before signs and symptoms are apparent. Changes associated with the aging process, the prevalence of chronic diseases, alteration in fluid and nutrition status, and the increased use of medications result in the need for postoperative vigilance and slower recovery from anesthesia due to the prolonged time to eliminate sedatives and anesthetic agents (Tabloski, 2009).

Postoperative confusion and delirium may occur in up to half of all older patients. Acute confusion may be caused by pain, altered pharmacokinetics of analgesic agents, hypotension, fever, hypoglycemia, fluid loss, fecal impaction, urinary retention, or anemia (De Lima, Borges, da Costa, et al., 2010; Liukas, Kuusniemi, Aantaa, et al. 2011; Meiner, 2011). Providing adequate hydration, reorienting to the environment, and reassessing the doses of sedative, anesthetic, and analgesic agents may reduce the risk of confusion. Hypoxia can present as confusion and restlessness, as can blood loss and electrolyte imbalances. Exclusion of all other causes of confusion must precede the assumption that confusion is related to age, circumstances, and medications.

Determining Readiness for Postanesthesia Care Unit Discharge

A patient remains in the PACU until fully recovered from the anesthetic agent. Indicators of recovery include stable blood pressure, adequate respiratory function, and adequate oxygen saturation level compared with baseline.

Many hospitals use a scoring system (e.g., Aldrete score) to determine the patient's general condition and readiness for transfer from the PACU (Aldrete & Wright, 1992). Throughout the recovery period, the patient's physical signs are observed and evaluated by means of a scoring system based on a set of objective criteria. This evaluation guide allows an objective assessment of the patient's condition in the PACU (Fig. 19-3). The patient is assessed at regular intervals, and a total score is calculated and recorded on the assessment record. The Aldrete score is usually between 8 and 10 before discharge from the PACU. Patients with a

Post Anesthesia Care Unit
MODIFIED ALDRETE SCORE

Patient: _____   Final score: _____

Room: _____   Surgeon: _____

Date: _____   PACU nurse: _____

Area of Assessment	Point Score	Upon Admission	After			
			15 min	30 min	45 min	60 min
Activity						
(Able to move spontaneously or on command)						
• Ability to move all extremities	2					
• Ability to move 2 extremities	1					
• Unable to control any extremity	0					
Respiration						
• Ability to breathe deeply and cough	2					
• Limited respiratory effort (dyspnea or splinting)	1					
• No spontaneous effort	0					
Circulation						
• BP 20% of preanesthetic level	2					
• BP 20% –49% of preanesthetic level	1					
• BP 50% of preanesthetic level	0					
Consciousness						
• Fully awake	2					
• Arousable on calling	1					
• Not responding	0					
O_2 Saturation						
• Able to maintain O_2 sat >92% on room air	2					
• Needs O_2 inhalation to maintain O_2 sat >90%	1					
• O_2 sat <90% even with O_2 supplement	0					
Totals:						

Required for discharge from Post Anesthesia Care Unit: 7–8 points

Time of release   Signature of nurse

FIGURE 19-3 • Postanesthesia care unit record; modified Aldrete score. O_2 sat, oxygen saturation; BP, blood pressure. Adapted from Aldrete, A., & Wright, A. (1992). Revised Aldrete score for discharge. *Anesthesiology News, 18*(1), 17.

score of less than 7 must remain in the PACU until their condition improves or until they are transferred to an intensive care area, depending on their preoperative baseline score (Rothrock, 2010).

The patient is discharged from the phase I PACU by the anesthesiologist or anesthetist to the critical care unit, the medical-surgical unit, the phase II PACU, or home with a responsible adult. In some hospitals and ambulatory care centers,

patients are discharged to a phase III PACU, where they are prepared for discharge.

Preparing the Postoperative Patient for Direct Discharge

Ambulatory surgical centers frequently only have a stepdown PACU similar to a phase II PACU. Patient seen in this type of unit are usually healthy, and the plan is to discharge them directly to home. Prior to discharge, the patient will require verbal and written instructions and information about follow-up care.

Promoting Home and Community-Based Care

To ensure patient safety and recovery, expert patient education and discharge planning are necessary when a patient undergoes same-day or ambulatory surgery (Kruzik, 2009). Because anesthetics cloud memory for concurrent events, verbal and written instructions should be given to both the patient and the adult who will be accompanying the patient home. Alternative formats (e.g., large print, Braille) of instructions or the use of a sign language interpreter may be required to ensure patient and family understanding. A translator may be required if the patient and family members do not understand English.

Discharge Preparation

The patient and caregiver (e.g., family member or friend) are informed about expected outcomes and immediate postoperative changes anticipated (Doran, 2010; Kruzik, 2009). Chart 19-2 identifies important educational points; before discharging the patient, the nurse provides written instructions covering each of those points. Prescriptions are given to the patient. The nursing unit or surgeon's telephone number is provided, and the patient and caregiver are encouraged to call with questions and to schedule follow-up appointments.

Although recovery time varies depending on the type and extent of surgery and the patient's overall condition, instructions usually advise limited activity for 24 to 48 hours. During this time, the patient should not drive a vehicle, drink alcoholic beverages, or perform tasks that require energy or skill. Fluids may be consumed as desired and smaller than normal amounts may be eaten at mealtime. Patients are cautioned not to make important decisions at this time because the medications, anesthesia, and surgery may affect their decision-making ability.

Continuing Care

Although most patients who undergo ambulatory surgery recover quickly and without complications, some patients require referral for home care. These may be older or frail patients, those who live alone, and patients with other health care problems or disabilities that might interfere with self-care or resumption of usual activities. The home care nurse assesses the patient's physical status (e.g., respiratory and cardiovascular status, adequacy of pain management, the surgical incision, surgical complications) and the patient's and family's ability to adhere to the recommendations given at the time of discharge. Previous education is reinforced as needed. The home care nurse may change surgical dressings, monitor the patency of a drainage system, or administer medications. The patient and family are reminded about the importance of keeping follow-up appointments with the surgeon. Follow-up phone calls from the nurse or surgeon are also used to assess the patient's progress and to answer any questions.

Care of the Hospitalized Postoperative Patient

Most surgeries are now performed in ambulatory care centers, and surgical patients who require hospital stays include trauma patients, acutely ill patients, patients undergoing major surgery, patients who require emergency surgery, and patients with a concurrent medical disorder. Seriously ill patients and those who have undergone major cardiovascular, pulmonary, or neurologic surgery may be admitted to specialized ICUs for close monitoring and advanced interventions and support. The care required by these patients in the immediate postoperative period is discussed in specific chapters of this book. Patients admitted to the clinical unit for postoperative care have multiple needs and stay for a short period of time. Postoperative care for those surgical patients returning to the general medical-surgical unit is discussed later in this chapter.

Receiving the Patient in the Clinical Unit

The patient's room is readied by assembling the necessary equipment and supplies: IV pole, drainage receptacle holder,

---

Chart 19-2 🏠 **HOME CARE CHECKLIST**
Discharge After Surgery

At the completion of home care education, the patient or caregiver will be able to:	PATIENT	CAREGIVER
• Name the procedure that was performed and identify any permanent changes in anatomic structure or function.	✓	✓
• Describe ongoing postoperative therapeutic regimen, including medications, diet, activities to perform (e.g., walking and breathing exercises) and to avoid (e.g., driving a car, contact sports), adjuvant therapies, dressing changes and wound care, and any other treatments.	✓	✓
• Describe signs and symptoms of complications.	✓	✓
• State time and date of follow-up appointments.	✓	✓
• Identify interventions and strategies to use in adapting to any permanent changes in structure or function.	✓	✓
• Relate how to reach health care provider with questions or complications.	✓	✓
• State understanding of community resources and referrals (if any).	✓	✓
• Describe pertinent health promotion activities (e.g., weight reduction, smoking cessation, stress management).	✓	✓

Chart 19-3

GUIDELINES

Immediate Postoperative Nursing Interventions

Nursing Interventions	Rationale
1. Assess breathing and administer supplemental oxygen, if prescribed.	1. Assessment provides a baseline and helps identify signs and symptoms of respiratory distress early.
2. Monitor vital signs and note skin warmth, moisture, and color.	2. A careful baseline assessment helps identify signs and symptoms of shock early.
3. Assess the surgical site and wound drainage systems. Connect all drainage tubes to gravity or suction as indicated and monitor closed drainage systems.	3. Assessment provides a baseline and helps identify signs and symptoms of hemorrhage early.
4. Assess level of consciousness, orientation, and ability to move extremities.	4. These parameters provide a baseline and help identify signs and symptoms of neurologic complications.
5. Assess pain level, pain characteristics (location, quality), and timing, type, and route of administration of last dose of analgesic.	5. Assessment provides a baseline of current pain level and assesses effectiveness of pain management strategies.
6. Administer analgesic medications as prescribed and assess their effectiveness in relieving pain.	6. Administration of analgesic agents helps decrease pain.
7. Place the call light, emesis basin, ice chips (if allowed), and bedpan or urinal within reach.	7. Attending to these needs provides for comfort and safety.
8. Position the patient to enhance comfort, safety, and lung expansion.	8. This promotes safety and reduces risk of postoperative complications.
9. Assess IV sites for patency and infusions for correct rate and solution.	9. Assessing IV sites and infusions helps detect phlebitis and prevents errors in rate and solution type.
10. Assess urine output in closed drainage system or use bladder scanner to detect distention.	10. Assessment provides a baseline and helps identify signs of urinary retention.
11. Reinforce the need to begin deep breathing and leg exercises.	11. These activities help prevent complications.
12. Provide information to the patient and family.	12. Patient education helps decrease the patient's and family's anxiety.

suction equipment, oxygen, emesis basin, tissues, disposable pads, blankets, and postoperative documentation forms. When the call comes to the unit about the patient's transfer from the PACU, the need for any additional items is communicated. The PACU nurse reports relevant data about the patient to the receiving nurse (see Chart 19-1).

Usually, the surgeon speaks to the family after surgery and relates the general condition of the patient. The receiving nurse reviews the postoperative orders, admits the patient to the unit, performs an initial assessment, and attends to the patient's immediate needs (Chart 19-3).

Nursing Management After Surgery

During the first 24 hours after surgery, nursing care of the hospitalized patient on the general medical-surgical unit involves continuing to help the patient recover from the effects of anesthesia, frequently assessing the patient's physiologic status, monitoring for complications, managing pain, and implementing measures designed to achieve the long-range goals of independence with self-care, successful management of the therapeutic regimen, discharge to home, and full recovery (Ackley & Ladwig, 2010). In the initial hours after admission to the clinical unit, adequate ventilation, hemodynamic stability, incisional pain, surgical site integrity, nausea and vomiting, neurologic status, and spontaneous voiding are primary concerns. The pulse rate, blood pressure, and respiration rate are recorded at least every 15 minutes for the first hour and every 30 minutes for the next 2 hours. Thereafter, they are measured less frequently if they remain stable. The temperature is monitored every 4 hours for the first 24 hours (American Society of PeriAnesthesia Nurses [ASPAN], 2010).

Patients usually begin to return to their usual state of health several hours after surgery or after awaking the next morning. Although pain may still be intense, many patients feel more alert, less nauseous, and less anxious. They have begun their breathing and leg exercises as appropriate for the type of surgery, and many will have dangled their legs over the edge of the bed, stood, and ambulated a few feet or been assisted out of bed to the chair at least once. Many will have tolerated a light meal and had IV fluids discontinued. The focus of care shifts from intense physiologic management and symptomatic relief of the adverse effects of anesthesia to regaining independence with self-care and preparing for discharge.

NURSING PROCESS

The Hospitalized Patient Recovering From Surgery

Nursing care of the hospitalized patient recovering from surgery takes place in a compressed time frame, with much of the healing and recovery occurring after the patient is discharged to home or to a rehabilitation center.

Assessment

Assessment of the hospitalized postoperative patient includes monitoring vital signs and completing a review of systems upon the patient's arrival to the clinical unit (see Chart 19-3) and at regular intervals thereafter.

Respiratory status is important because pulmonary complications are among the most frequent and serious problems encountered by the surgical patient. The nurse monitors for airway patency and any signs of laryngeal edema. The quality of respirations, including depth, rate, and sound, are assessed regularly. Chest auscultation verifies that breath sounds are normal (or abnormal) bilaterally, and the findings are documented as a baseline for later comparisons. Often, because of the effects of analgesic and anesthetic medications, respirations are slow. Shallow and rapid respirations may be caused by pain, constricting dressings, gastric dilation, abdominal distention, or obesity. Noisy breathing may be due to obstruction by secretions or the tongue. Another possible complication is flash pulmonary edema that occurs when protein and fluid accumulate in the alveoli unrelated to elevated pulmonary artery occlusive pressure. Signs and symptoms include agitation; tachypnea; tachycardia; decreased pulse oximetry readings; frothy, pink sputum; and crackles on auscultation.

The nurse assesses the patient's pain level using a verbal or visual analogue scale and assesses the characteristics of the pain. The patient's appearance, pulse, respirations, blood pressure, skin color (adequate or cyanotic), and skin temperature (cold and clammy, warm and moist, or warm and dry) are clues to cardiovascular function. When the patient arrives in the clinical unit, the surgical site is assessed for bleeding, type and integrity of dressings, and drains.

The nurse also assesses the patient's mental status and level of consciousness, speech, and orientation and compares them with the preoperative baseline. Although a change in mental status or postoperative restlessness may be related to anxiety, pain, or medications, it may also be a symptom of oxygen deficit or hemorrhage. These serious causes must be investigated and excluded before other causes are pursued.

General discomfort that results from laying in one position on the operating table, the handling of tissues by the surgical team, the body's reaction to anesthesia, and anxiety are also common causes of restlessness. These discomforts may be relieved by administering the prescribed analgesic medication, changing the patient's position frequently, and assessing and alleviating the cause of anxiety. If tight, drainage-soaked bandages are causing discomfort, reinforcing or changing the dressing completely as prescribed by the physician may make the patient more comfortable. The bladder is assessed for distention (usually with a bladder scanner) because urinary retention can also cause restlessness (Palese, Buchini, Deroma, et al., 2010).

Diagnosis

Nursing Diagnoses

Based on the assessment data, major nursing diagnoses may include the following:

- Risk for ineffective airway clearance related to depressed respiratory function, pain, and bed rest
- Acute pain related to surgical incision
- Decreased cardiac output related to shock or hemorrhage
- Risk for activity intolerance related to generalized weakness secondary to surgery
- Impaired skin integrity related to surgical incision and drains
- Ineffective thermoregulation related to surgical environment and anesthetic agents

- Risk for imbalanced nutrition, less than body requirements related to decreased intake and increased need for nutrients secondary to surgery
- Risk for constipation related to effects of medications, surgery, dietary change, and immobility
- Risk for urinary retention related to anesthetic agents
- Risk for injury related to surgical procedure/positioning or anesthetic agents
- Anxiety related to surgical procedure
- Risk for ineffective therapeutic regimen management related to wound care, dietary restrictions, activity recommendations, medications, follow-up care, or signs and symptoms of complications

Collaborative Problems or Potential Complications

Based on the assessment data, potential complications may include the following:

- Pulmonary infection/hypoxia
- Deep vein thrombosis (DVT)
- Hematoma or hemorrhage
- Infection
- Pulmonary embolism (PE)
- Wound dehiscence or evisceration

Planning and Goals

The major goals for the patient include optimal respiratory function, relief of pain, optimal cardiovascular function, increased activity tolerance, unimpaired wound healing, maintenance of body temperature, and maintenance of nutritional balance. Further goals include resumption of usual pattern of bowel and bladder elimination, identification of any perioperative positioning injury, acquisition of sufficient knowledge to manage self-care after discharge, and absence of complications.

Nursing Interventions

Preventing Respiratory Complications

Respiratory depressive effects of opioid medications, decreased lung expansion secondary to pain, and decreased mobility combine to put the patient at risk for respiratory complications, particularly atelectasis (alveolar collapse; incomplete expansion of the lung), pneumonia, and hypoxemia (Overdyk & Guerra, 2011; Rothrock, 2010). Atelectasis remains a risk for the patient who is not moving well or ambulating or who is not performing deep-breathing and coughing exercises or using an incentive spirometer. Signs and symptoms include decreased breath sounds over the affected area, crackles, and cough. Pneumonia is characterized by chills and fever, tachycardia, and tachypnea. Cough may or may not be present and may or may not be productive. Hypostatic pulmonary congestion, caused by a weakened cardiovascular system that permits stagnation of secretions at lung bases, may develop; this condition occurs most frequently in older patients who are not mobilized effectively (Tabloski, 2009). The symptoms are often vague, with perhaps a slight elevation of temperature, pulse, and respiratory rate as well as a cough. Physical examination reveals dullness and crackles at the base of the lungs. If the condition progresses, the outcome may be fatal.

The types of hypoxemia that can affect postoperative patients are subacute and episodic. Subacute hypoxemia is a constant low level of oxygen saturation when breathing appears normal. Episodic hypoxemia develops suddenly, and the patient may be at risk for cerebral dysfunction, myocardial ischemia, and cardiac arrest. Risk for hypoxemia is increased in patients who have undergone major surgery (particularly abdominal), are obese, or have preexisting pulmonary problems. Hypoxemia is detected by pulse oximetry, which measures blood oxygen saturation. Factors that may affect the accuracy of pulse oximetry readings include cold extremities, tremors, atrial fibrillation, acrylic nails, and black or blue nail polish (these colors interfere with the functioning of the pulse oximeter; other colors do not).

Preventive measures and timely recognition of signs and symptoms help avert pulmonary complications. Crackles indicate static pulmonary secretions that need to be mobilized by coughing and deep-breathing exercises. When a mucus plug obstructs one of the bronchi entirely, the pulmonary tissue beyond the plug collapses, resulting in atelectasis.

To clear secretions and prevent pneumonia, the nurse encourages the patient to turn frequently, take deep breaths, cough, and use the incentive spirometer at least every 2 hours. These pulmonary exercises should begin as soon as the patient arrives on the clinical unit and continue until the patient is discharged. Even if he or she is not fully awake from anesthesia, the patient can be asked to take several deep breaths. This helps expel residual anesthetic agents, mobilize secretions, and prevent atelectasis. Careful splinting of abdominal or thoracic incision sites helps the patient overcome the fear that the exertion of coughing might open the incision (see Chapter 17, Chart 17-6). Analgesic agents are administered to permit more effective coughing, and oxygen is administered as prescribed to prevent or relieve hypoxia. To encourage lung expansion, the patient is encouraged to yawn or take sustained maximal inspirations to create a negative intrathoracic pressure of −40 mm Hg and expand lung volume to total capacity. Chest physical therapy may be prescribed if indicated. (See Chapter 21.)

Coughing is contraindicated in patients who have head injuries or who have undergone intracranial surgery (because of the risk for increasing intracranial pressure), as well as in patients who have undergone eye surgery (because of the risk for increasing intraocular pressure) or plastic surgery (because of the risk for increasing tension on delicate tissues).

Early ambulation increases metabolism and pulmonary aeration and, in general, improves all body functions. The patient is encouraged to be out of bed as soon as possible (i.e., on the day of surgery or no later than the first postoperative day). This practice is especially valuable in preventing pulmonary complications in older patients.

Relieving Pain

Most patients experience some pain after a surgical procedure. Complete absence of pain in the area of the surgical incision may not occur for a few weeks, depending on the site and nature of the surgery, but the intensity of postoperative pain gradually subsides on subsequent days. About one third of patients report severe pain, one third moderate pain, and one third little or no pain. This does not mean that the patients in the last group have no pain; rather, they appear to activate psychodynamic mechanisms that impair the registering of pain (nociceptive transmission). (See Chapter 12 for a more detailed discussion of pain.)

Many factors (motivational, affective, cognitive, emotional, and cultural) influence the pain experience (Buscemi, 2011). The degree and severity of postoperative pain and the patient's tolerance for pain depend on the incision site, the nature of the surgical procedure, the extent of surgical trauma, the type of anesthesia, and the route of administration. The preoperative preparation received by the patient (including information about what to expect, reassurance, psychological support, and educating specific communication techniques related to pain) is a significant factor in decreasing anxiety, apprehension, the amount of postoperative pain, and PONV (Miller et al., 2010).

Intense pain stimulates the stress response, which adversely affects the cardiac and immune systems. When pain impulses are transmitted, both muscle tension and local vasoconstriction increase, further stimulating pain receptors. This increases myocardial demand and oxygen consumption. The hypothalamic stress response also results in an increase in blood viscosity and platelet aggregation, increasing the risk of thrombosis and PE.

Often, the physician has prescribed different medications or dosages to cover various levels of pain. The nurse discusses these options with the patient to determine the best medication. The nurse assesses the effectiveness of the medication periodically, beginning 30 minutes after administration, or sooner if the medication is being delivered by patient-controlled analgesia (PCA).

Opioid Analgesic Medications. Opioid analgesic agents are commonly prescribed for pain and immediate postoperative restlessness. A preventive approach, rather than an "as needed" (PRN) approach, is more effective in relieving pain. With a preventive approach, the medication is administered at prescribed intervals rather than when the pain becomes severe or unbearable. Many patients (and some health care providers) are overly concerned about the risk of drug addiction in the postoperative patient. However, this risk is negligible with the use of opioid medications for short-term pain control (Faulk, Twite, Zuk, et al., 2010).

Patient-Controlled Analgesia. The nurse's goal is pain prevention rather than sporadic pain control. Patients recover more quickly when adequate pain relief measures are used, and PCA permits patients to administer their own pain medication when needed. Most patients are candidates for PCA. The two requirements for PCA are an understanding of the need to self-dose and the physical ability to self-dose. The amount of medication delivered by the IV or epidural route and the time span during which the opioid medication is released are controlled by the PCA device. PCA promotes patient participation in care, eliminates delayed administration of analgesic medications, maintains a therapeutic drug level, and enables the patient to move, turn, cough, and take deep breaths with less pain, thus reducing postoperative pulmonary complications (Rothrock, 2010).

Epidural Infusions and Intrapleural Anesthesia. Patients undergoing many types of procedures and surgeries benefit from the use of epidural infusion of opioids (McKay, Lett, Chilibeck, et al., 2009). Epidural infusions are used with caution in chest procedures because the analgesic may ascend along the spinal cord and affect respiration. Intrapleural anesthesia involves the administration of local anesthetic by a catheter between the parietal and visceral pleura. It provides sensory anesthesia without affecting motor function to the intercostal muscles. This anesthesia allows more effective coughing and deep breathing in conditions such as cholecystectomy, renal surgery, and rib fractures, in which pain in the thoracic region would interfere with these exercises.

A local opioid or a combination anesthetic (opioid plus local anesthetic agent) is used in the epidural infusion.

Other Pain Relief Measures. For pain that is difficult to control, a subcutaneous pain management system may be used. In this system, a nylon catheter is inserted at the site of the affected area. The catheter is attached to a pump that delivers a continuous amount of local anesthetic at a specific amount determined and prescribed by the physician (Fig. 19-4).

Nonpharmacologic pain relief measures, such as guided imagery, music, and application of heat or cold (if prescribed), have been successful in decreasing pain (Rothrock, 2010). Changing the patient's position, using distraction, applying cool washcloths to the face, and providing back massage may be useful in relieving general discomfort temporarily, promoting relaxation, and rendering medication more effective when it is administered.

Promoting Cardiac Output

If signs and symptoms of shock or hemorrhage occur, treatment and nursing care are implemented as described in the discussion of care in the PACU and in Chapter 14.

Although most patients do not hemorrhage or go into shock, changes in circulating volume, the stress of surgery, and the effects of medications and preoperative preparations all affect cardiovascular function. IV fluid replacement may be prescribed for up to 24 hours after surgery or until the patient is stable and tolerating oral fluids. Close monitoring is indicated to detect and correct conditions such as fluid volume deficit, altered tissue perfusion, and decreased cardiac output, all of which can increase the patient's discomfort, place him or her at risk of complications, and prolong the hospital stay. Some patients are at risk for fluid volume excess secondary to existing cardiovascular or renal disease, advanced age, and other factors (Meiner, 2011; Porth & Matfin, 2009). Consequently, fluid replacement must be carefully managed, and intake and output records must be accurate.

Nursing management includes assessing the patency of the IV lines and ensuring that the correct fluids are administered at the prescribed rate. Intake and output, including emesis and output from wound drainage systems, are recorded separately and totaled to determine fluid balance. If the patient has an indwelling urinary catheter, hourly outputs are monitored and rates of less than 30 mL per hour are reported; if the patient is voiding, an output of less than 240 mL per 8-hour shift is reported. Electrolyte levels and hemoglobin and hematocrit levels are monitored. Decreased hemoglobin and hematocrit levels can indicate blood loss or dilution of circulating volume by IV fluids. If dilution is contributing to the decreased levels, the hemoglobin and hematocrit will rise as the stress response abates and fluids are mobilized and excreted.

Venous stasis from dehydration, immobility, and pressure on leg veins during surgery put the patient at risk for venous thromboembolism. Leg exercises and frequent position changes are initiated early in the postoperative period to stimulate circulation. Patients should avoid positions that compromise venous return, such as raising the bed's knee gatch, placing a pillow under the knees, sitting for long periods, and dangling the legs with pressure at the back of the knees. Venous return is promoted by anti-embolism stockings and early ambulation.

Encouraging Activity

Early ambulation has a significant effect on recovery and the prevention of complications (e.g., atelectasis, hypostatic pneumonia, gastrointestinal [GI] discomfort, circulatory problems) (Rothrock, 2010). Postoperative activity orders are checked before the patient is assisted to get out of bed, in many instances, on the evening following surgery. Sitting up at the edge of the bed for a few minutes may be all that the patient who has undergone a major surgical procedure can tolerate at first.

Ambulation reduces postoperative abdominal distention by increasing GI tract and abdominal wall tone and stimulating peristalsis. Early ambulation prevents stasis of blood, and thromboembolic events occur less frequently. Pain is often decreased when early ambulation is possible, and the hospital stay is shorter and less costly.

Despite the advantages of early ambulation, patients may be reluctant to get out of bed on the evening of surgery. Reminding them of the importance of early mobility in preventing complications may help patients overcome their fears. When a patient gets out of bed for the first time, orthostatic hypotension, also called *postural hypotension*, is a concern. Orthostatic hypotension is an abnormal drop in blood pressure that occurs as the patient changes from a supine to a standing position. It is common after surgery

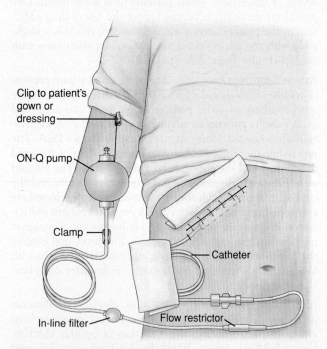

FIGURE 19-4 • Subcutaneous pain management system consists of a pump, filter, and catheter that delivers a specific amount of prescribed local anesthetic at the rate determined by the physician. Redrawn with permission from I-Flow Corporation, Lake Forest, CA.

Clip to patient's gown or dressing

ON-Q pump

Clamp

In-line filter

Catheter

Flow restrictor

because of changes in circulating blood volume and bed rest. Signs and symptoms include a decrease of 20 mm Hg in systolic blood pressure or 10 mm Hg in diastolic blood pressure, weakness, dizziness, and fainting (Weber & Kelley, 2010). Older adults are at increased risk for orthostatic hypotension secondary to age-related changes in vascular tone. To detect orthostatic hypotension, the nurse assesses the patient's blood pressure first in the supine position, after the patient sits up, again after the patient stands, and 2 to 3 minutes later. Gradual position change gives the circulatory system time to adjust. If the patient becomes dizzy, he or she is returned to the supine position, and ambulation is delayed for several hours.

To assist the postoperative patient in getting out of bed for the first time after surgery, the nurse:

1. Helps the patient move gradually from the lying position to the sitting position by raising the head of the bed and encourages the patient to splint the incision when applicable.
2. Positions the patient completely upright (sitting) and turned so that both legs are hanging over the edge of the bed.
3. Helps the patient stand beside the bed.

After becoming accustomed to the upright position, the patient may start to walk. The nurse should be at the patient's side to give physical support and encouragement. Care must be taken not to tire the patient; the extent of the first few periods of ambulation varies with the type of surgical procedure and the patient's physical condition and age.

Whether or not the patient can ambulate early in the postoperative period, bed exercises are encouraged to improve circulation. Bed exercises consist of the following:

- Arm exercises (full range of motion, with specific attention to abduction and external rotation of the shoulder)
- Hand and finger exercises
- Foot exercises to prevent DVT, footdrop, and toe deformities and to aid in maintaining good circulation
- Leg flexion and leg-lifting exercises to prepare the patient for ambulation
- Abdominal and gluteal contraction exercises

Hampered by pain, dressings, IV lines, or drains, many patients cannot engage in activity without assistance. Helping the patient increase his or her activity level on the first postoperative day is important to prevent complications related to prolonged inactivity. One way to increase the patient's activity is to have the patient perform as much routine hygiene care as possible. Setting up the patient to bathe with a bedside wash basin or, if possible, assisting the patient to the bathroom to sit in a chair at the sink not only gets the patient moving but helps restore a sense of self-control and prepares the patient for discharge.

For a safe discharge to home, patients need to be able to ambulate a functional distance (e.g., length of the house or apartment), get in and out of bed unassisted, and be independent with toileting. Patients can be asked to perform as much as they can and then to call for assistance. The patient and the nurse can collaborate on a schedule for progressive activity that includes ambulating in the room and hallway and sitting out of bed in a chair. Assessing the patient's vital signs before, during, and after a scheduled activity helps the nurse and patient determine the rate of progression. By providing physical support, the nurse maintains the patient's safety; by communicating a positive attitude about the patient's ability to perform the activity, the nurse promotes the patient's confidence. The nurse encourages the patient to continue to perform bed exercises, wear pneumatic compression or prescribed anti-embolism stockings when in bed, and rest as needed. If the patient has had orthopedic surgery of the lower extremities or will require a mobility aid (i.e., walker, crutches) at home, a physical therapist may be involved the first time the patient gets out of bed to educate him or her to ambulate safely or to use the mobility aid correctly.

Caring for Wounds

Wound Healing. Wounds heal by different mechanisms, depending on the condition of the wound. Surgical wound healing may occur in three ways, by **first-intention, second-intention**, and **third-intention wound healing** (Rothrock, 2010) (Chart 19-4). With shorter hospital stays, much of the healing takes place at home, and both the hospital and home care nurse should be informed about the principles of wound healing (Alvarex, Brodsky, Lemmens, et al., 2010).

Ongoing assessment of the surgical site involves inspection for approximation of wound edges, integrity of sutures or staples, redness, discoloration, warmth, swelling, unusual tenderness, or drainage. The area around the wound should also be inspected for a reaction to tape or trauma from tight bandages. As a wound heals, many factors, such as adequate nutrition, cleanliness, rest, and position, determine how quickly healing occurs. These factors are influenced by nursing interventions. Specific nursing assessments and interventions that address these factors and help promote wound healing are presented in Table 19-3.

Caring for Surgical Drains. Nursing interventions to promote wound healing also include management of surgical drains. Drains are tubes that exit the peri-incisional area, either into a portable wound suction device (closed) or into the dressings (open). The principle involved is to allow the escape of fluids that could otherwise serve as a culture medium for bacteria. In portable wound suction, the use of gentle, constant suction enhances drainage of these fluids and collapses the skin flaps against the underlying tissue, thus removing "dead space." Types of wound drains include the Penrose, Hemovac, and Jackson-Pratt drains (Fig. 19-5). Output (drainage) from wound systems is recorded. The amount of bloody drainage on the surgical dressing is assessed frequently. Spots of drainage on the dressings are outlined with a pen, and the date and time of the outline are recorded on the dressing so that increased drainage can be easily seen. A certain amount of bloody drainage in a wound drainage system or on the dressing is expected, but excessive amounts should be reported to the surgeon. Increasing amounts of fresh blood on the dressing should be reported immediately. Some wounds are irrigated heavily before closure in the OR, and open drains exiting the wound may be embedded in the dressings. These wounds may drain large amounts of blood-tinged fluid that saturate the dressing. The dressing can be reinforced with sterile gauze bandages; the time at which they were reinforced should be documented. If drainage continues, the surgeon should be notified so that the dressing can be changed. Multiple similar drains are numbered or otherwise labeled (e.g., left lower quadrant, left upper

Chart 19-4 Wound-Healing Mechanisms

First-Intention Healing

Wounds made aseptically with a minimum of tissue destruction that are properly closed heal with little tissue reaction by first intention (primary union). When wounds heal by first-intention healing, granulation tissue is not visible and scar formation is minimal. Postoperatively, many of these wounds are covered with a dry sterile dressing. If a cyanoacrylate tissue adhesive (LiquiBand) has been used to close the incision without sutures, a dressing is contraindicated.

Second-Intention Healing

Second-intention healing (granulation) occurs in infected wounds (abscess) or in wounds in which the edges have not been approximated. When an abscess is incised, it collapses partly, but the dead and dying cells forming its walls are still being released into the cavity. For this reason, a drainage tube or gauze packing is inserted into the abscess pocket to allow drainage to escape easily. Gradually, the necrotic material disintegrates and escapes, and the abscess cavity fills with a red, soft, sensitive tissue that bleeds easily. This tissue is composed of minute, thin-walled capillaries and buds that later form connective tissue. These buds, called *granulations*, enlarge until they fill the area left by the destroyed tissue. The cells surrounding the capillaries change their round shape to become long, thin, and intertwined to form a scar (cicatrix). Healing is complete when skin cells (epithelium) grow over these granulations. This method of repair is referred to as healing by granulation, and it takes place whenever pus is formed or when loss of tissue has occurred for any reason. When the postoperative wound is to be allowed to heal by secondary intention, it is usually packed with saline-moistened sterile dressings and covered with a dry sterile dressing.

Third-Intention Healing

Third-intention healing (secondary suture) is used for deep wounds that either have not been sutured early or break down and are resutured later, thus bringing together two opposing granulation surfaces. This results in a deeper and wider scar.

These wounds are also packed postoperatively with moist gauze and covered with a dry sterile dressing.

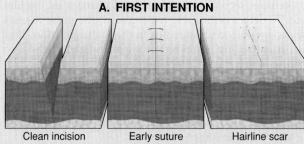

A. FIRST INTENTION

Clean incision   Early suture   Hairline scar

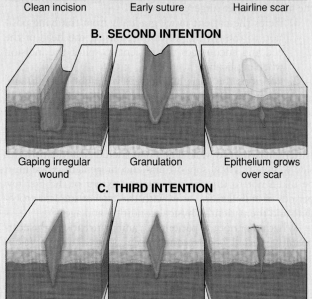

B. SECOND INTENTION

Gaping irregular wound   Granulation   Epithelium grows over scar

C. THIRD INTENTION

Wound   Increased granulation   Late suturing with wide scar

---

quadrant) so that output measurements can be reliably and consistently recorded.

Changing the Dressing. Although the first postoperative dressing is usually changed by a member of the surgical team, subsequent dressing changes in the immediate postoperative period are usually performed by the nurse. A dressing is applied to a wound for one or more of the following reasons: (1) to provide a proper environment for wound healing; (2) to absorb drainage; (3) to splint or immobilize the wound; (4) to protect the wound and new epithelial tissue from mechanical injury; (5) to protect the wound from bacterial contamination and from soiling by feces, vomitus, and urine; (6) to promote hemostasis, as in a pressure dressing; and (7) to provide mental and physical comfort for the patient.

The patient is told that the dressing is to be changed and that changing the dressing is a simple procedure associated with little discomfort. The dressing change is performed at a suitable time (e.g., not at mealtimes or when visitors are present). Privacy is provided, and the patient is not unduly exposed. The nurse should avoid referring to the incision as a

scar because the term may have negative connotations for the patient. Assurance is given that the incision will shrink as it heals and that the redness will fade.

The nurse performs hand hygiene before and after the dressing change and wears disposable gloves (sterile or clean as needed) for the dressing change itself. Most dressing changes following surgery are sterile. In accordance with standard precautions, dressings are never touched by ungloved hands because of the danger of transmitting pathogenic organisms. The tape or adhesive portion of the dressing is removed by pulling it parallel with the skin surface and in the direction of hair growth rather than at right angles. Alcohol wipes or nonirritating solvents aid in removing adhesive painlessly and quickly. The soiled dressing is removed and deposited in a container designated for disposal of biomedical waste.

Gloves are changed, and a new dressing is applied. If the patient is sensitive to adhesive tape, the dressing may be held in place with hypoallergenic tape. Many tapes are porous to prevent skin maceration. Some wounds become edematous after having been dressed, causing considerable

TABLE 19-3 Factors Affecting Wound Healing

Factors	Rationale	Nursing Interventions
Age of patient	The older the patient, the less resilient the tissues.	Handle all tissues gently.
Handling of tissues	Rough handling causes injury and delayed healing.	Handle tissues carefully and evenly.
Hemorrhage	Accumulation of blood creates dead spaces as well as dead cells that must be removed. The area becomes a growth medium for organisms.	Monitor vital signs. Observe incision site for evidence of bleeding and infection.
Hypovolemia	Insufficient blood volume leads to vasoconstriction and reduced oxygen and nutrients available for wound healing.	Monitor for volume deficit (circulatory impairment). Correct by fluid replacement as prescribed.
Local Factors		
Edema	Reduces blood supply by exerting increased interstitial pressure on vessels.	Elevate part; apply cool compresses.
Inadequate dressing technique:		
Too small	Permits bacterial invasion and contamination.	Follow guidelines for proper dressing technique.
Too tight	Reduces blood supply carrying nutrients and oxygen.	
Nutritional deficits	Protein–calorie depletion may occur.	Correct deficits; this may require parenteral nutritional therapy.
	Insulin secretion may be inhibited, causing blood glucose to rise.	Monitor blood glucose levels.
		Administer vitamin supplements as prescribed.
Foreign bodies	Foreign bodies retard healing.	Keep wounds free of dressing threads and talcum powder from gloves.
Oxygen deficit (tissue oxygenation insufficient)	Insufficient oxygen may be due to inadequate lung and cardiovascular function as well as localized vasoconstriction.	Encourage deep breathing, turning, and controlled coughing.
Drainage accumulation	Accumulated secretions hamper healing process.	Monitor closed drainage systems for proper functioning.
		Institute measures to remove accumulated secretions.
Medications		
Corticosteroids	May mask presence of infection by impairing normal inflammatory response	Be aware of action and effect of medications patient is receiving.
Anticoagulants	May cause hemorrhage	
Broad-spectrum and specific antibiotics	Effective if administered immediately before surgery for specific pathology or bacterial contamination. If administered after wound is closed, ineffective because of intravascular coagulation.	
Patient overactivity	Prevents approximation of wound edges. Resting favors healing.	Use measures to keep wound edges approximated: taping, bandaging, splints.
		Encourage rest.
Systemic Disorders		
Hemorrhagic shock	These depress cell functions that directly affect wound healing.	Be familiar with the nature of the specific disorder.
Acidosis		Administer prescribed treatment. Cultures may be indicated to determine appropriate antibiotic.
Hypoxia		
Renal failure		
Hepatic disease		
Sepsis		
Immunosuppressed state	Patient is more vulnerable to bacterial and viral invasion; defense mechanisms are impaired.	Provide maximum protection to prevent infection. Restrict visitors with colds; institute mandatory hand hygiene by all staff.
Wound Stressors		
Vomiting	Produce tension on wounds, particularly of the torso.	Encourage frequent turning and ambulation, and administer antiemetic medications as prescribed.
Valsalva maneuver		Assist patient in splinting incision.
Heavy coughing		
Straining		

tension on the tape. If the tape is not flexible, the stretching bandage will also cause a shear injury to the skin. This can result in denuded areas or large blisters and should be avoided. An elastic adhesive bandage (Elastoplast, 3M Microfoam) may be used to hold dressings in place over mobile areas, such as the neck or the extremities, or where pressure is required.

While changing the dressing, the nurse has an opportunity to educate the patient in how to care for the incision and change the dressings at home. The nurse observes for indicators of the patient's readiness to learn, such as looking at the incision, expressing interest, or assisting in the dressing change. Information on self-care activities and possible signs of infection is summarized in Chart 19-5.

Maintaining Normal Body Temperature

The patient is still at risk for malignant hyperthermia and hypothermia in the postoperative period. Efforts are made to identify malignant hyperthermia and to treat it early and promptly (Rothrock, 2010). (See the discussion of malignant hyperthermia in Chapter 18.)

Patients who have received anesthesia are susceptible to chills and drafts. Hypothermia management, begun in the intraoperative period, extends into the postoperative period to prevent significant nitrogen loss and catabolism (Schifilliti, Grasso, Conti, et al., 2010). Low body temperature is reported to the physician. The room is maintained at a comfortable temperature, and blankets are provided to prevent chilling. Treatment includes oxygen administration,

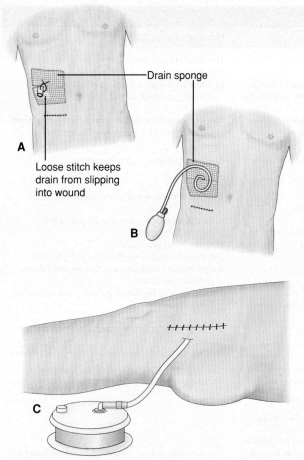

Drain sponge

A

Loose stitch keeps drain from slipping into wound

B

C

FIGURE 19-5 • Types of surgical drains: **A.** Penrose. **B.** Jackson-Pratt. **C.** Hemovac.

adequate hydration, and proper nutrition. The patient is also monitored for cardiac dysrhythmias. The risk of hypothermia is greater in older adults and in patients who were in the cool OR environment for a prolonged period.

Managing Gastrointestinal Function and Resuming Nutrition

Discomfort of the GI tract (nausea, vomiting, and hiccups) and resumption of oral intake are issues for both the patient and the nurse. See the earlier discussion of nausea and vomiting in the PACU.

If risk of vomiting is high due to the nature of surgery, a nasogastric tube is inserted preoperatively and remains in place throughout the surgery and the immediate postoperative period. A nasogastric tube also may be inserted before surgery if postoperative distention is anticipated. In addition, a nasogastric tube may be inserted if a patient who has food in the stomach requires emergency surgery.

Hiccups, produced by intermittent spasms of the diaphragm secondary to irritation of the phrenic nerve, can occur after surgery. The irritation may be direct, such as from stimulation of the nerve by a distended stomach, subdiaphragmatic abscess, or abdominal distention; indirect, such as from toxemia or uremia that stimulates the nerve; or reflexive, such as from irritation from a drainage tube or obstruction of the intestines. These occurrences usually are mild, transitory attacks that cease spontaneously. If hiccups persist, they may produce considerable distress and serious effects such as vomiting, exhaustion, and wound dehiscence. The physician may prescribe phenothiazine medications (e.g., chlorpromazine [Thorazine]) for intractable hiccups (Miller et al., 2010).

Chart 19-5

PATIENT EDUCATION
Wound Care Instructions

Until Sutures are Removed

1. Keep the wound dry and clean.
   - If there is no dressing, ask your nurse or physician if you can bathe or shower.
   - If a dressing or splint is in place, do not remove it unless it is wet or soiled.
   - If wet or soiled, change dressing yourself if you have been taught to do so; otherwise, call your nurse or physician for guidance.
   - If you have been taught, instruction might be as follows:
     - Cleanse area *gently* with sterile normal saline once or twice daily.
     - Cover with a sterile Telfa pad or gauze square large enough to cover wound.
     - Apply hypoallergenic tape (Dermicel or paper). Adhesive is not recommended because it is difficult to remove without possible injury to the incisional site.
2. Immediately report any of these signs of infection:
   - Redness, marked swelling exceeding ½ inch (2.5 cm) from incision site; tenderness; or increased warmth around wound
   - Red streaks in skin near wound
   - Pus or discharge, foul odor
   - Chills or temperature higher than 37.7°C (100°F)
3. If soreness or pain causes discomfort, apply a dry cool pack (containing ice or cold water) or take prescribed

acetaminophen tablets (2) every 4–6 hours. Avoid using aspirin without direction or instruction because bleeding can occur with its use.

4. Swelling after surgery is common. To help reduce swelling, elevate the affected part to the level of the heart.
   - Hand or arm:
     - Sleep—elevate arm on pillow at side
     - Sitting—place arm on pillow on adjacent table
     - Standing—rest affected hand on opposite shoulder; support elbow with unaffected hand
   - Leg or foot:
     - Sitting—place a pillow on a facing chair; provide support underneath the knee
     - Lying—place a pillow under affected leg

After Sutures are Removed

Although the wound appears to be healed when sutures are removed, it is still tender and will continue to heal and strengthen for several weeks.

1. Follow recommendations of physician or nurse regarding extent of activity.
2. Keep suture line clean; do not rub vigorously; pat dry. Wound edges may look red and may be slightly raised. This is normal.
3. If the site continues to be red, thick, and painful to pressure after 8 weeks, consult the health care provider. (This may be due to excessive collagen formation and should be checked.)

> ► *Quality and Safety Nursing Alert*
>
> Any condition that is persistent or considered intractable, such as hiccups, should be reported to the primary provider so that appropriate measures can be implemented.

Once nausea and vomiting have subsided and the patient is fully awake and alert, the sooner he or she can tolerate a usual diet, and the more quickly normal GI function will resume. Taking food by mouth stimulates digestive juices and promotes gastric function and intestinal peristalsis. The return to normal dietary intake should proceed at a pace set by the patient. The nature of the surgery and the type of anesthesia directly affect the rate at which normal gastric activity resumes. Liquids are typically the first substances desired and tolerated by the patient after surgery. Water, juice, and tea may be given in increasing amounts. Cool fluids are tolerated more easily than those that are ice cold or hot. Soft foods (gelatin, custard, milk, and creamed soups) are added gradually after clear fluids have been tolerated. As soon as the patient tolerates soft foods well, solid food may be given.

Assessment and management of GI function are important after surgery because the GI tract is subject to uncomfortable or potentially life-threatening complications. Any postoperative patient may suffer from distention. Postoperative distention of the abdomen results from the accumulation of gas in the intestinal tract. Manipulation of the abdominal organs during surgery may produce a loss of normal peristalsis for 24 to 48 hours, depending on the type and extent of surgery. Even though nothing is given by mouth, swallowed air and GI tract secretions enter the stomach and intestines; if not propelled by peristalsis, they collect in the intestines, producing distention and causing the patient to complain of fullness or pain in the abdomen. Most often, the gas collects in the colon. Abdominal distention is further increased by immobility, anesthetic agents, and the use of opioid medications.

After major abdominal surgery, distention may be avoided by having the patient turn frequently, exercise, and ambulate as early as possible. This also alleviates distention produced by swallowing air, which is common in anxious patients. A nasogastric tube inserted before surgery may remain in place until full peristaltic activity (indicated by the passage of flatus) has resumed. The nurse detects bowel sounds by listening to the abdomen with a stethoscope. Bowel sounds are documented so that diet progression can occur.

Paralytic ileus and intestinal obstruction are potential postoperative complications that occur more frequently in patients undergoing intestinal or abdominal surgery. (Refer to Chapter 48 for discussion of treatment.)

Promoting Bowel Function

Constipation is common after surgery and can be minor or a serious complication. Decreased mobility, decreased oral intake, and opioid analgesic medications contribute to difficulty having a bowel movement. In addition, irritation and trauma to the bowel during surgery may inhibit intestinal movement for several days. The combined effect of early ambulation, improved dietary intake, and a stool softener (if prescribed) promotes bowel elimination. Until the patient reports return of bowel function, the nurse should assess the abdomen for distention and the presence and frequency of bowel sounds. If the abdomen is not distended and bowel sounds are present, and if the patient does not have a bowel movement by the second or third postoperative day, the physician should be notified and a laxative or other test or intervention may be ordered as needed.

Managing Voiding

Urinary retention after surgery can occur for various reasons. Anesthetics, anticholinergic agents, and opioids interfere with the perception of bladder fullness and the urge to void and inhibit the ability to initiate voiding and completely empty the bladder. Abdominal, pelvic, and hip surgery may increase the likelihood of retention secondary to pain. In addition, some patients find it difficult to use the bedpan or urinal in the recumbent position.

Bladder distention and the urge to void should be assessed at the time of the patient's arrival on the unit and frequently thereafter. The patient is expected to void within 8 hours after surgery (this includes time spent in the PACU). If the patient has an urge to void and cannot, or if the bladder is distended and no urge is felt or the patient cannot void, catheterization is not delayed solely on the basis of the 8-hour time frame. All methods to encourage the patient to void should be tried (e.g., letting water run, applying heat to the perineum). The bedpan should be warm; a cold bedpan causes discomfort and automatic tightening of muscles (including the urethral sphincter). If the patient cannot void on a bedpan, it may be possible to use a commode or a toilet (if there is one in the PACU) rather than resorting to catheterization. Male patients are often permitted to sit up or stand beside the bed to use the urinal; however, safeguards should be taken to prevent the patient from falling or fainting due to loss of coordination from medications or orthostatic hypotension. If the patient cannot void in the specified time frame, the patient is catheterized and the catheter is removed after the bladder has emptied. Straight intermittent catheterization is preferred over indwelling catheterization because the risk of infection is increased with an indwelling catheter.

Even if the patient voids, the bladder may not necessarily be empty. The nurse notes the amount of urine voided and palpates the suprapubic area for distention or tenderness. A portable ultrasound device may also be used to assess residual volume. Intermittent catheterization may be prescribed every 4 to 6 hours until the patient can void spontaneously and the postvoid residual is less than 100 mL.

Maintaining a Safe Environment

During the immediate postoperative period, the patient recovering from anesthesia should have three side rails up, and the bed should be in the low position. The nurse assesses the patient's level of consciousness and orientation and determines whether the patient can resume wearing assistive devices as needed (e.g., eyeglasses or hearing aid). Impaired vision, inability to hear postoperative instructions, or inability to communicate verbally places the patient at risk for injury. All objects the patient may need should be within reach, especially the call light. Any immediate postoperative orders concerning special positioning, equipment, or interventions should be implemented as soon as possible. The patient is instructed to ask for assistance with any activity. Although restraints are occasionally necessary for the disoriented patient, they should be avoided if at all possible.

Agency policy on the use of restraints must be consulted and followed.

Any surgical procedure has the potential for injury due to disrupted neurovascular integrity resulting from prolonged awkward positioning in the OR, manipulation of tissues, inadvertent severing of nerves or blood vessels, or tight bandages. Any orthopedic or neurologic surgery or surgery involving the extremities carries a risk of peripheral nerve damage. Vascular surgeries, such as replacement of sections of diseased peripheral arteries or insertion of an arteriovenous graft, put the patient at risk for thrombus formation at the surgical site and subsequent ischemia of tissues distal to the thrombus. Assessment includes having the patient move the hand or foot distal to the surgical site through a full range of motion, assessing all surfaces for intact sensation, and assessing peripheral pulses (Rothrock, 2010).

Providing Emotional Support to the Patient and Family

Although patients and families are undoubtedly relieved that surgery is over, stress and anxiety levels may remain high in the immediate postoperative period (Chart 19-6). Many factors contribute to this stress and anxiety, including pain, being in an unfamiliar environment, inability to control one's circumstances or care for oneself, fear of the long-term effects of surgery, fear of complications, fatigue, spiritual distress, altered role responsibilities, ineffective coping, and altered body image, and all are potential reactions to the surgical experience. The nurse helps the patient and family work through their stress and anxieties by providing reassurance and information and by spending time listening to and addressing their concerns. The nurse describes hospital routines and what to expect in the time until discharge and explains the purpose of nursing assessments and interventions. Informing patients when they will be able to drink fluids or eat, when they will be getting out of bed, and when

TABLE 19-4 Potential Postoperative Complications

Body System/Type	Complications
Respiratory	Atelectasis, pneumonia, pulmonary embolism, aspiration
Cardiovascular	Shock, thrombophlebitis
Neurologic	Delirium, stroke
Skin/wound	Breakdown, infection, dehiscence, evisceration, delayed healing, hemorrhage, hematoma
Gastrointestinal	Constipation, paralytic ileus, bowel obstruction
Urinary	Acute urine retention, urinary tract infection
Functional	Weakness, fatigue, functional decline
Thromboembolic	Deep vein thrombosis, pulmonary embolism

tubes and drains will be removed helps them gain a sense of control and participation in recovery and engages them in the plan of care. Acknowledging family members' concerns and accepting and encouraging their participation in the patient's care assists them in feeling that they are helping their loved one. The nurse can modify the environment to enhance rest and relaxation by providing privacy, reducing noise, adjusting lighting, providing enough seating for family members, and encouraging a supportive atmosphere.

Managing Potential Complications

The postoperative patient is at risk for complications as outlined next and listed in Table 19-4.

Venous Thromboembolism. Serious potential venous thromboembolism complications of surgery include DVT and PE (Rothrock, 2010).

Prophylactic treatment is common for patients at risk for DVT and PE. Low-molecular-weight or low-dose heparin and low-dose warfarin (Coumadin) are other anticoagulants that may be used (Karch, 2012). External pneumatic compression and anti-embolism stockings can be used alone or in

---

Chart 19-6

NURSING RESEARCH PROFILE

Perioperative Pain, Psychological Distress, and Immune Function in Men Undergoing Prostatectomy

Yermal, S. J., Witek-Janusek, L., Peterson, J., et al. (2010). Perioperative pain, psychological distress, and immune function in men undergoing prostatectomy for cancer of the prostate. *Biological Research for Nursing, 11*(4), 351–362.

Purpose

The frequent occurrence of prostate cancer and the recommended treatment by prostatectomy cause pain, psychological distress, and altered immune function during the perioperative period. The purpose of this study was to assess the influence of psychological stress and pain perception on the immune parameters in men during the perioperative prostatectomy experience.

Design

A repeated measure comparative group design was used to study 42 men at baseline, 1 and 2 days postoperatively and at 4–6 weeks postoperatively. The men were compared to 20 cancer-free controls.

Findings

Patient evaluation pre- and postoperatively found intensified levels of anxiety, tension, and melancholy perceived by the

subjects with lowered vitality following surgery, and increased pain levels for as long as 6 weeks after the surgery. On the first postoperative day, natural killer cell activity (NKCA) was decreased as compared to the noncancer participant (control) group; however, no difference was apparent in the circulation of immune cells. By the second day, circulation of NKCA was comparable to the cancer-free group with no significant correlation between psychological influence and the change in NKCA levels, implying that the postoperative effect was owing to the stress of surgery.

Nursing Implications

This study suggests that psychological support and patient education that occurs from the time of the discovery of cancer through the progression of treatment can be used to decrease stress and anxiety. Suppression of immune function may place men at risk during a critical postoperative period when opportunistic tumor seeding can occur. More study is needed to identify supportive interventions.

combination with low-dose heparin. The stress response that is initiated by surgery inhibits the fibrinolytic system, resulting in blood hypercoagulability. Dehydration, low cardiac output, blood pooling in the extremities, and bed rest add to the risk of thrombosis formation. Although all postoperative patients are at some risk, factors such as a history of thrombosis, malignancy, trauma, obesity, indwelling venous catheters, and hormone use (e.g., estrogen) increase the risk. The first symptom of DVT may be a pain or cramp in the calf. Initial pain and tenderness may be followed by a painful swelling of the entire leg, often accompanied by fever, chills, and diaphoresis (Joint Commission, 2013).

The benefits of early ambulation and leg exercises in preventing DVT cannot be overemphasized, and these activities are recommended for all patients, regardless of their risk. It is important to avoid the use of blanket rolls, pillow rolls, or any form of elevation that can constrict vessels under the knees. Even prolonged "dangling" (having the patient sit on the edge of the bed with legs hanging over the side) can be dangerous and is not recommended in susceptible patients because pressure under the knees can impede circulation. Adequate hydration is also encouraged; the patient can be offered juices and water throughout the day to avoid dehydration. (Refer to Chapter 30 for a discussion of DVT and to Chapter 23 for discussion of PE.)

Hematoma. At times, concealed bleeding occurs beneath the skin at the surgical site. This hemorrhage usually stops spontaneously but results in clot (hematoma) formation within the wound. If the clot is small, it will be absorbed and need not be treated. If the clot is large, the wound usually bulges somewhat, and healing will be delayed unless the clot is removed. After several sutures are removed by the physician, the clot is evacuated and the wound is packed lightly with gauze. Healing occurs usually by granulation, or a secondary closure may be performed.

Infection (Wound Sepsis). The creation of a surgical wound disrupts the integrity of the skin, bypassing the body's primary defense and protection against infection. Exposure of deep body tissues to pathogens in the environment places the patient at risk for infection of the surgical site, and a potentially life-threatening complication such as infection increases length of hospital stay, costs of care, and risk of further complications. It is estimated that 14% to 16% of all health care–associated infections are surgical-site infections and that 77% of surgical patients who die succumb to sepsis associated with infections (Rothrock, 2010).

Multiple factors, including the type of wound, place the patient at risk for infection. Surgical wounds are classified according to the degree of contamination. Table 19-5 defines the terms used to describe surgical wounds and gives the expected rate of wound infection per category. Patient-related factors include age, nutritional status, diabetes, smoking, obesity, remote infections, endogenous mucosal microorganisms, altered immune response, length of preoperative stay, and severity of illness (Rothrock, 2010). Factors related to the surgical procedure include the method of preoperative skin preparation, surgical attire of the team, method of sterile draping, duration of surgery, antimicrobial prophylaxis, aseptic technique, factors related to surgical technique, drains or foreign material, OR ventilation, length of procedure, and exogenous microorganisms. Other risk factors for wound sepsis include wound contamination, foreign body, faulty suturing technique, devitalized tissue, hematoma, debilitation, dehydration, malnutrition, anemia, obesity, shock, duration of surgical procedure, and associated disorders (e.g., diabetes) (Alvarex et al., 2010). Efforts to prevent wound infection are directed at reducing risks. (Preoperative and intraoperative risks and interventions are discussed in Chapters 17 and 18.) Postoperative care of the wound centers on assessing the wound, preventing contamination and infection before wound edges have sealed, and enhancing healing.

Wound infection may not be evident until at least postoperative day 5. Most patients are discharged before that time, and more than half of wound infections are diagnosed after discharge, highlighting the importance of patient education regarding wound care (Kruzik, 2009). Signs and symptoms of wound infection include increased pulse rate and temperature; an elevated white blood cell

TABLE 19-5	Wound Classification and Associated Surgical Site Infection Risk	
Surgical Category	**Determinants of Category**	**Expected Risk of Postsurgical Infection (%)**
Clean	Nontraumatic site Uninfected site No inflammation No break in aseptic technique No entry into respiratory, alimentary, genitourinary, or oropharyngeal tracts	1–3
Clean contaminated	Entry into respiratory, alimentary, genitourinary, or oropharyngeal tracts without unusual contamination Appendectomy Minor break in aseptic technique Mechanical drainage	3–7
Contaminated	Open, newly experienced traumatic wounds Gross spillage from gastrointestinal tract Major break in aseptic technique Entry into genitourinary or biliary tract when urine or bile is infected	7–16
Dirty	Traumatic wound with delayed repair, devitalized tissue, foreign bodies, or fecal contamination Acute inflammation and purulent drainage encountered during procedure	16–29

count; wound swelling, warmth, tenderness, or discharge; and incisional pain. Local signs may be absent if the infection is deep. *Staphylococcus aureus* accounts for many postoperative wound infections. Other infections may result from *Escherichia coli*, *Proteus vulgaris*, *Aerobacter aerogenes*, *Pseudomonas aeruginosa*, and other organisms. Although they are rare, beta-hemolytic streptococcal or clostridial infections can be rapid and deadly and need strict infection control practices to prevent the spread of infection to others. Intensive medical and nursing care is essential if the patient is to survive.

When a wound infection is diagnosed in a surgical incision, the surgeon may remove one or more sutures or staples and, using aseptic precautions, separate the wound edges with a pair of blunt scissors or a hemostat. Once the incision is opened, a drain is inserted. If the infection is deep, an incision and drainage procedure may be necessary. Antimicrobial therapy and a wound care regimen are also initiated.

Wound Dehiscence and Evisceration. Wound **dehiscence** (disruption of surgical incision or wound) and **evisceration** (protrusion of wound contents) are serious surgical complications (Fig. 19-6). Dehiscence and evisceration are especially serious when they involve abdominal incisions or wounds. These complications result from sutures giving way, from infection, or, more frequently, from marked distention or strenuous cough. They may also occur because of increasing age, anemia, poor nutritional status, obesity, malignancy, diabetes, the use of steroids, and other factors in patients undergoing abdominal surgery (Haupt & Reed, 2010; Meiner, 2011).

When the wound edges separate slowly, the intestines may protrude gradually or not at all, and the earliest sign may be a gush of bloody (serosanguineous) peritoneal fluid from the wound. When a wound ruptures suddenly, coils of intestine may push out of the abdomen. The patient may report that "something gave way." The evisceration causes pain and may be associated with vomiting.

> ### Quality and Safety Nursing Alert
>
> If disruption of a wound occurs, the patient is placed in the low Fowler's position and instructed to lie quietly. These actions minimize protrusion of body tissues. The protruding coils of intestine are covered with sterile dressings moistened with sterile saline solution, and the surgeon is notified at once.

An abdominal binder can provide support and guard against dehiscence and often is used along with the primary dressing, especially in patients with weak or pendulous abdominal walls or when rupture of a wound has occurred.

Gerontologic Considerations. Older patients recover more slowly, have longer hospital stays, and are at greater risk for development of postoperative complications. Delirium, pneumonia, decline in functional ability, exacerbation of comorbid conditions, pressure ulcers, decreased oral intake, GI disturbance, and falls are all threats to recovery in the older adult (Tabloski, 2009; Tolson, Morley, Rolland, et al., 2011). Expert nursing care can help the older adult avoid these complications or minimize their effects (Rothrock, 2010).

Postoperative delirium, characterized by confusion, perceptual and cognitive deficits, altered attention levels, disturbed sleep patterns, and impaired psychomotor skills, is a significant problem for older adults (Meiner, 2011). Causes of delirium are multifactorial (Chart 19-7). Skilled and frequent assessment of mental status and of all physiologic factors influencing mental status helps the nurse plan for care because delirium may be the initial or only indicator of infection, fluid

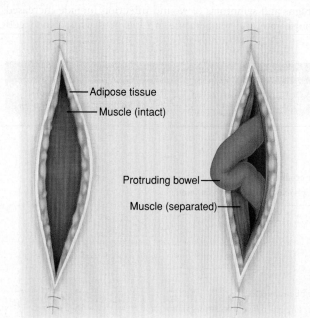

FIGURE 19-6 • **A.** Wound dehiscence. **B.** Wound evisceration.

Labels in figure: Adipose tissue · Muscle (intact) · Protruding bowel · Muscle (separated) · **A** · **B**

Chart 19-7 **Causes of Postoperative Delirium**

- Acid–base disturbances
- Age >80 years
- Fluid and electrolyte imbalance
- Dehydration
- History of dementialike symptoms
- Hypoxia
- Hypercarbia
- Infection (urinary tract, wound, respiratory)
- Medications (anticholinergics, benzodiazepines, central nervous system depressants)
- Unrelieved pain
- Blood loss
- Decreased cardiac output
- Cerebral hypoxia
- Heart failure
- Acute myocardial infarction
- Hypothermia or hyperthermia
- Unfamiliar surroundings and sensory deprivation
- Emergent surgery
- Alcohol withdrawal
- Urinary retention
- Fecal impaction
- Polypharmacy
- Presence of multiple diseases
- Sensory impairments
- High stress or anxiety levels

and electrolyte imbalance, or deterioration of respiratory or hemodynamic status in the older adult patient. Factors that determine whether a patient is at risk for delirium include age, history of alcohol abuse, preoperative cognitive function, physical function, serum chemistries, and type of surgery.

Recognizing postoperative delirium and identifying and treating its underlying cause are the goals of care. Postoperative delirium is sometimes mistaken for preexisting dementia or is attributed to age. In addition to monitoring and managing identifiable causes, the nurse implements supportive interventions. Keeping the patient in a well-lit room and in close proximity to staff can reduce sensory deprivation. At the same time, distracting and unfamiliar noises should be minimized. Because pain can contribute to postoperative delirium, adequate pain control without oversedation is essential (Rothrock, 2010).

The patient is reoriented as often as necessary, and staff should introduce themselves each time they come in contact with the patient. Engaging the patient in conversation and care activities and placing a clock and calendar nearby may improve cognitive function. Physical activity should not be neglected while the patient is confused because physical deterioration can worsen delirium and place the patient at increased risk for other complications. Restraints should be avoided because they can worsen confusion. A staff member is asked to stay with the patient instead. Medications may be administered during episodes of acute confusion but should be discontinued as soon as possible to avoid side effects.

Other problems confronting the older postoperative patient, such as pneumonia, altered bowel function, DVT, weakness, and functional decline, often can be prevented by early and progressive ambulation. Prolonged sitting positions are avoided at they promote venous stasis in the lower extremities. A physical therapy referral may be indicated to promote safe, regular exercise for the older adult.

Urinary incontinence can be prevented by providing easy access to the call bell and the commode and by prompting voiding. Early ambulation and familiarity with the room help the patient become self-sufficient sooner.

Optimal nutritional status is important for wound healing, return of normal bowel function, and fluid and electrolyte balance. The nurse and patient can consult with the dietitian to plan appealing, high-protein meals that provide sufficient fiber, calories, and vitamins. Nutritional supplements, such as Ensure™ or Sustacal™, may be recommended. Multivitamins, iron, and vitamin C supplements may be prescribed to aid in tissue healing, formation of new red blood cells, and overall nutritional status (Dudek, 2010).

In addition to monitoring and managing physiologic recovery of the older adult, the nurse identifies and addresses psychosocial needs. The older adult may require much encouragement and support to resume activities, and the pace may be slow. Sensory deficits may require frequent repetition of instructions, and decreased physiologic reserve may necessitate frequent rest periods. The older adult may require extensive discharge planning to coordinate both professional and family care providers, and the nurse, social worker, or nurse case manager may institute the plan for continuing care.

Promoting Home and Community-Based Care
Patient Self-Care. Patients have always required detailed discharge instructions to become proficient in special self-care needs after surgery; however, shorter hospital stays have increased the amount of information needed while reducing the amount of time in which to provide it. Although needs are specific to individual patients and the procedures they have undergone, general patient education needs prior to discharge have been identified (see Chart 19-2).

Continuing Care. Community-based services are frequently necessary after surgery. Older patients, patients who live alone, patients without family support, and patients with preexisting chronic illness or disabilities are often in greatest need. Planning for discharge involves arranging for necessary services early in the acute care hospitalization for wound care, drain management, catheter care, infusion therapy, and physical or occupational therapy. The home care nurse coordinates these activities and services.

During home care visits, the nurse assesses the patient for postoperative complications by assessment of the surgical incision, respiratory and cardiovascular status, adequacy of pain management, fluid and nutritional status, and the patient's progress in returning to preoperative status. The nurse evaluates the patient's and family's ability to manage dressing changes and drainage systems and other devices and to administer prescribed medications. The nurse may change dressings or catheters if needed. The nurse identifies any additional services that are needed and assists the patient and family to arrange for them. Previous education is reinforced, and the patient is reminded to keep follow-up appointments (Kruzik, 2009). The patient and family are instructed about signs and symptoms to be reported to the surgeon. In addition, the nurse provides information about how to obtain needed supplies and suggests resources or support groups.

Evaluation

Expected patient outcomes may include the following:

1. Maintains optimal respiratory function
   a. Performs deep-breathing exercises
   b. Displays clear breath sounds
   c. Uses incentive spirometer as prescribed
   d. Splints incisional site when coughing to reduce pain
2. Indicates that pain is decreased in intensity
3. Increases activity as prescribed
   a. Alternates periods of rest and activity
   b. Progressively increases ambulation
   c. Resumes normal activities within prescribed time frame
   d. Performs activities related to self-care
4. Wound heals without complication
5. Maintains body temperature within normal limits
6. Resumes oral intake
   a. Reports absence of nausea and vomiting
   b. Eats at least 75% of usual diet
   c. Is free of abdominal distress and gas pains
   d. Exhibits normal bowel sounds
7. Reports resumption of usual bowel elimination pattern
8. Resumes usual voiding pattern
9. Is free of injury
10. Exhibits decreased anxiety
11. Acquires knowledge and skills necessary to manage therapeutic regimen
12. Experiences no complications

Critical Thinking Exercises

1 `ebp` A 76-year-old man is admitted to the PACU following an arthroplasty of his right hip. He is complaining of pain and difficulty taking a deep breath. Develop an evidence-based plan of care for this patient that addresses priorities from admission to the unit until discharge. What resources would you use to identify the current safe practice guidelines for this older patient? Identify the criteria used to evaluate the strength of the evidence for these practices.

2 `pg` A 36-year-old man who is obese and has a history of diabetes is admitted to the phase II PACU following a laparoscopic procedure and is scheduled to be discharged home. Identify what information is essential to obtain during report from the OR. What are your first three priorities for immediate care of this patient in the PACU? Identify the discharge instructions that the patient will need.

3 A 25-year-old patient who is a smoker is admitted to the postoperative nursing unit after abdominal surgery. Identify the initial assessments that need to be performed. Develop a nursing plan of care for this patient that addresses care from admission to the unit until discharge to home. How will you modify the plan if the patient needs wound care after discharge?

Brunner Suite Resources

Explore these additional resources to enhance learning for this chapter:
• NCLEX-Style Questions and Other Resources on thePoint, http://thePoint.lww.com/Brunner13e
• Study Guide
• PrepU
• Clinical Handbook
• Handbook of Laboratory and Diagnostic Tests

References

*Asterisk indicates nursing research.
**Double asterisk indicates classic reference.

Books

Ackley, B. J., & Ladwig, G. B. (2010). *Nursing diagnosis handbook: An evidence-based guide to planning care* (9th ed.). St. Louis: Mosby.

Alvarex, A., Brodsky, J. B., Lemmens, H. J. M., et al. (2010). *Morbid obesity: Peri-operative management* (2nd ed.). New York: Cambridge University Press.

American Society of PeriAnesthesia Nurses. (2010). *2010–2012 perianesthesia nursing standards and practice recommendations*. Cherry Hill, NJ: Author.

ASPAN, Schick, L., Windle, P. E. (2010). *PeriAnesthesia nursing core curriculum: Preprocedure, Phase I and Phase II PACU nursing* (2nd ed.). St. Louis: Saunders.

Doran, D. (2010). *Nursing outcomes: State of the science* (2nd ed.). Sudbury, MA: Jones & Bartlett.

Dudek, S. G. (2010). *Nutrition essentials for nursing practice* (6th ed.). Philadelphia: Lippincott Williams & Wilkins.

Haupt, M., & Reed, M. (2010). *Critical care considerations of the morbidly obese*. Philadelphia: Elsevier Saunders.

Karch, A. M. (2012). *2012 Lippincott's nursing drug guide*. Philadelphia: Lippincott Williams & Wilkins.

Meiner, S. E. (2011). *Gerontologic nursing* (4th ed.). St. Louis: Elsevier Mosby.

Miller, R. D., Eriksson, L. I., Fleisher, L. A., et al. (2010). *Miller's anesthesia* (7th ed.). New York: Elsevier/Churchill Livingstone.

Porth, C. M., & Matfin, G. (2009). *Pathophysiology: Concepts of altered health states* (8th ed.). Philadelphia: Lippincott Williams & Wilkins.

Rothrock, J. C. (2010). *Alexander's care of the patient in surgery* (14th ed.). St. Louis: Mosby.

Spry, C. (2009). *Essentials of perioperative nursing* (4th ed.). Sudbury, MA: Jones & Bartlett.

Stannard, D., & Krenzischek, D. A. (2012). *Perianesthesia nursing care: A bedside guide*. Sudbury, MA: Jones & Bartlett.

Tabloski, P. A. (2009). *Gerontological nursing: The essential guide to clinical practice* (2nd ed.). Upper Saddle River, NJ: Prentice Hall Health.

Weber, J., & Kelley, J. H. (2010). *Health assessment in nursing* (4th ed.). Philadelphia: Lippincott Williams & Wilkins.

West, J. B. (2011). *Respiratory physiology: The essentials* (9th ed.). Baltimore: Lippincott Williams & Wilkins.

Journals and Electronic Documents

**Aldrete, A., & Wright, A. (1992). Revised Aldrete score for discharge. *Anesthesiology News*, 18(1), 17.

Buscemi, C. (2011). Acculturation: State of the science in nursing. *Journal of Cultural Diversity*, 18(2), 39–42.

Constantini, R., Affaitati, G., Fabrizio, A., et al. (2011). Controlling pain in the post-operative setting. *International Journal of Clinical Pharmacology and Therapeutics*, 49(2), 116–127.

De Lima, L., Borges, D., da Costa, S., et al. (2010). Classification of patients according to the degree of dependence on nursing care and illness severity in a post-anesthesia care unit. *Revista Latino-Americana De Enfermagem*, 18(5), 881–887.

Ewan, P., Dugué, P., Mirakian, R., et al. (2010). BSACI guidelines for the investigation of suspected anaphylaxis during general anesthesia. *Clinical and Experimental Allergy: Journal of the British Society for Allergy and Clinical Immunology*, 40(1), 15–31.

Faulk, D., Twite, M., Zuk, J., et al. (2010). Hypnotic depth and the incidence of emergence agitation and negative postoperative behavioral changes. *Paediatric Anaesthesia*, 20(1), 72–81.

Franck, M., Radtke, F., Apfel, C., et al. (2010). Documentation of post-operative nausea and vomiting in routine clinical practice. *Journal of International Medical Research*, 38(3), 1034–1041.

Joint Commission. (2013). *2013 National patient safety goals*. Available at: www.jointcommission.org/standards_information/npsgs.aspx

*Kruzik, N. (2009). Benefits of preoperative education for adult elective surgery patients. *AORN Journal*, 90(3), 381–387.

Liukas, A., Kuusniemi, K., Aantaa, R., et al. (2011). Elimination of intravenous oxycodone in the elderly. A pharmacokinetic study in postoperative orthopedic patients of different age groups. *Drugs & Aging*, 28(1), 41–50.

McKay, W., Lett, B., Chilibeck, P., et al. (2009). Effects of spinal anesthesia on resting metabolic rate and quadriceps mechanomyography. *European Journal of Applied Physiology*, 106(4), 583–588.

Overdyk, F. J., & Guerra, J. J. (2011). Improving outcomes in med-surg patients with opioid-induced respiratory depression. *American Nurse Today*, 6(11), 26–31.

*Palese, A., Buchini, S., Deroma, L., et al. (2010). The effectiveness of the ultrasound bladder scanner in reducing urinary tract infections: A meta-analysis. *Journal of Clinical Nursing*, 19(1), 2970–2979.

Rowe, D. J., & Baker, A. C. (2009). Perioperative risks and benefits of herbal supplements in aesthetic surgery. *Aesthetic Surgery Journal*, 29(2), 150–157.

Schifilliti, D., Grasso, G., Conti, A., et al. (2010). Anesthetic-related neuroprotection: Intravenous or inhalational agents. *CNS Drugs*, 24(11), 893–907.

Tolson, D., Morley, J., Rolland, Y., et al. (2011). Advancing nursing home practice: The International Association of Geriatrics and Gerontology recommendations. *Geriatric Nursing*, 32(3), 195–197.

*Yermal, S. J., Witek-Janusek, L., Peterson, J., et al. (2010). Perioperative pain, psychological distress, and immune function in men undergoing prostatectomy for cancer of the prostate. *Biological Research for Nursing*, 11(4), 351–362.

Resources

American Academy of Ambulatory Care Nursing (AAACN), www.aaacn.org
American Society of PeriAnesthesia Nurses (ASPAN), www.aspan.org
Association of PeriOperative Registered Nurses (AORN), www.aorn.org
Centers for Disease Control and Prevention (CDC), Surgical Site Infection Guideline, www.cdc.gov/ncidod/dhqp/gl_surgicalsite.html
Malignant Hyperthermia Association of the United States (MHAUS), www.mhaus.org

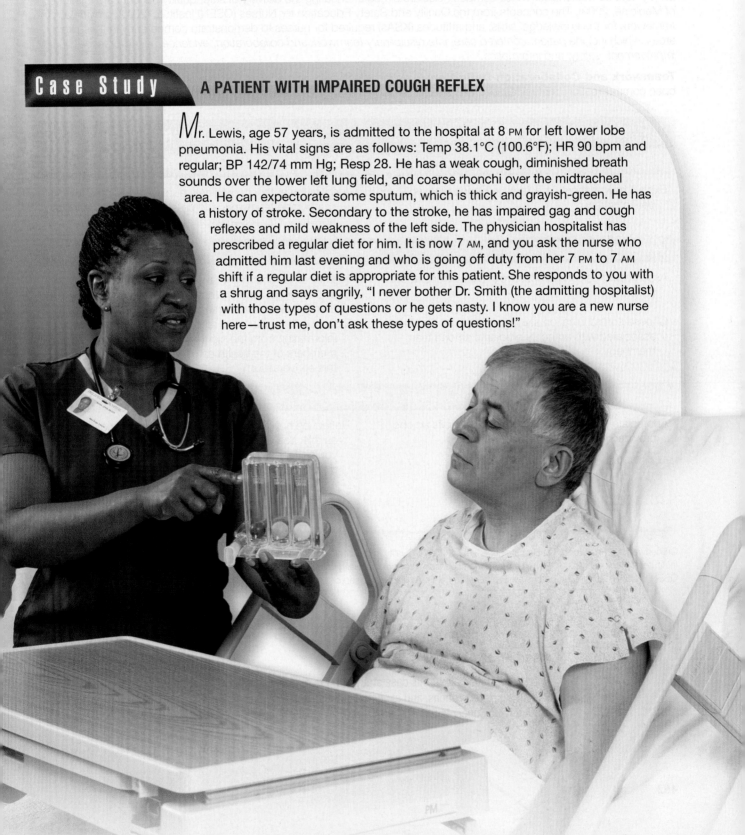

Unit 5

Gas Exchange and Respiratory Function

Case Study

A PATIENT WITH IMPAIRED COUGH REFLEX

Mr. Lewis, age 57 years, is admitted to the hospital at 8 PM for left lower lobe pneumonia. His vital signs are as follows: Temp 38.1°C (100.6°F); HR 90 bpm and regular; BP 142/74 mm Hg; Resp 28. He has a weak cough, diminished breath sounds over the lower left lung field, and coarse rhonchi over the midtracheal area. He can expectorate some sputum, which is thick and grayish-green. He has a history of stroke. Secondary to the stroke, he has impaired gag and cough reflexes and mild weakness of the left side. The physician hospitalist has prescribed a regular diet for him. It is now 7 AM, and you ask the nurse who admitted him last evening and who is going off duty from her 7 PM to 7 AM shift if a regular diet is appropriate for this patient. She responds to you with a shrug and says angrily, "I never bother Dr. Smith (the admitting hospitalist) with those types of questions or he gets nasty. I know you are a new nurse here—trust me, don't ask these types of questions!"

QSEN Competency Focus: *Teamwork and Collaboration*

The complexities inherent in today's health care system challenge nurses to demonstrate integration of specific interdisciplinary core competencies. These competencies are aimed at ensuring the delivery of safe, quality patient care (Institute of Medicine, 2003). The concepts from the Quality and Safety Education for Nurses (QSEN) Institute (2012) provide a framework for the knowledge, skills, and attitudes (KSAs) required for nurses to demonstrate competency in these key areas, which include *patient-centered care, interdisciplinary teamwork and collaboration, evidence-based practice, quality improvement, safety,* and *informatics*.

Teamwork and Collaboration Definition: Function effectively within nursing and interprofessional teams, fostering open communication, mutual respect, and shared decision making to achieve quality patient care.

RELEVANT PRE-LICENSURE KSAs	APPLICATION AND REFLECTION
Knowledge	
Explain how authority gradients influence teamwork and patient safety.	Identify the authority gradients at play in this case that discourage teamwork and collaboration, and describe how they may adversely affect Mr. Lewis's safety.
Skills	
Assert own position/perspective in discussions about patient care. Choose communication styles that diminish the risks associated with authority gradients among team members.	Identify steps you might take to determine the right type of diet for Mr. Lewis. Whom might you consult other than the night-shift nurse or Dr. Smith? Describe how you might respond to or seek further information from the night-shift nurse. Are there other members of the health care team you could bring into this conversation?
Attitudes	
Appreciate the risks associated with handoffs among providers and across transitions in care.	Reflect on how you might act or react in a situation such as this. You are the "junior" nurse on this team. Would you be fearful to seek clarification about Mr. Lewis's dietary needs? Would you feel comfortable seeking further clarification from the more seasoned night-shift nurse or from Dr. Smith? How might fear place Mr. Lewis at greater risk?

Cronenwett, L., Sherwood, G., Barnsteiner, J., et al. (2007). Quality and safety education for nurses. *Nursing Outlook, 55*(3), 122–131.
Institute of Medicine. (2003). *Health professions education: A bridge to quality.* Washington, DC: National Academies Press.
QSEN Institute (2012). *Competencies: Prelicensure KSAs.* Available at: qsen.org/competencies/pre-licensure-ksas

Read More About This Case

More information about this case study and the relationships between nursing diagnoses, interventions, and expected outcomes is available online. Visit thePoint for Applying Concepts From NANDA-I, NIC, and NOC.

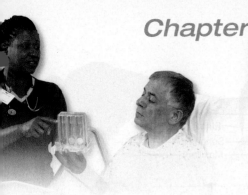

Assessment of Respiratory Function

On completion of this chapter, the learner will be able to:

1 Describe the structures and functions of the upper and lower respiratory tracts.
2 Describe ventilation, diffusion, perfusion, and ventilation–perfusion imbalances.
3 Explain proper techniques utilized to perform a comprehensive respiratory assessment.
4 Discriminate between normal and abnormal assessment findings identified by inspection, palpation, percussion, and auscultation of the respiratory system.
5 Recognize and evaluate the major symptoms of respiratory dysfunction by applying concepts from the patient's health history and physical assessment findings.
6 Identify the diagnostic tests and related nursing implications used to evaluate respiratory function.

apnea: temporary cessation of breathing

bronchophony: abnormal increase in clarity of transmitted voice sounds heard when auscultating the lungs

bronchoscopy: direct examination of the larynx, trachea, and bronchi using an endoscope

cilia: short hairs that provide a constant whipping motion that serves to propel mucus and foreign substances away from the lung toward the larynx

compliance: measure of the force required to expand or inflate the lungs

crackles: soft, high-pitched, discontinuous popping sounds during inspiration caused by delayed reopening of the airways

dyspnea: subjective experience that describes difficulty breathing; shortness of breath

egophony: abnormal change in tone of voice that is heard when auscultating the lungs

fremitus: vibrations of speech felt as tremors of the chest wall during palpation

hemoptysis: expectoration of blood from the respiratory tract

hypoxemia: decrease in arterial oxygen tension in the blood

hypoxia: decrease in oxygen supply to the tissues and cells

obstructive sleep apnea: temporary absence of breathing during sleep secondary to transient upper airway obstruction

orthopnea: inability to breathe easily except in an upright position

oxygen saturation: percentage of hemoglobin that is bound to oxygen

physiologic dead space: portion of the tracheobronchial tree that does not participate in gas exchange

pulmonary diffusion: exchange of gas molecules (oxygen and carbon dioxide) from areas of high concentration to areas of low concentration

pulmonary perfusion: blood flow through the pulmonary vasculature

respiration: gas exchange between atmospheric air and the blood and between the blood and cells of the body

rhonchi: low-pitched wheezing or snoring sound associated with partial airway obstruction, heard on chest auscultation

stridor: harsh high-pitched sound heard on inspiration, usually without need of a stethoscope, secondary to upper airway obstruction

tachypnea: abnormally rapid respirations

tidal volume: volume of air inspired and expired with each breath during normal breathing

ventilation: movement of air in and out of the airways

wheezes: continuous musical sounds associated with airway narrowing or partial obstruction

whispered pectoriloquy: whispered sounds heard loudly and clearly upon thoracic auscultation

Disorders of the respiratory system are common and are encountered by nurses in every setting, from the community to the intensive care unit. Expert assessment skills must be developed and used to provide the best care for patients with acute and chronic respiratory problems. Alterations in respiratory status are increasingly identified as one of the most sensitive predictors of clinical deterioration in hospitalized patients (Massey & Meredith, 2010). To differentiate between normal and abnormal assessment findings and recognize subtle changes that may negatively impact patient outcomes, nurses require an understanding of respiratory function and the significance of abnormal diagnostic test results.

Anatomic and Physiologic Overview

The respiratory system is composed of the upper and lower respiratory tracts. Together, the two tracts are responsible for

ventilation (movement of air in and out of the airways). The upper respiratory tract, known as the upper airway, warms and filters inspired air so that the lower respiratory tract (the lungs) can accomplish gas exchange or diffusion. Gas exchange involves delivering oxygen to the tissues through the bloodstream and expelling waste gases, such as carbon dioxide, during expiration. The respiratory system depends on the cardiovascular system for perfusion, or blood flow through the pulmonary system (Porth, 2011).

Anatomy of the Respiratory System

Upper Respiratory Tract

Upper airway structures consist of the nose; paranasal sinuses; pharynx, tonsils, and adenoids; larynx; and trachea.

Nose

The nose serves as a passageway for air to pass to and from the lungs. It filters impurities and humidifies and warms the air as it is inhaled. The nose is composed of an external and an internal portion. The external portion protrudes from the face and is supported by the nasal bones and cartilage. The anterior nares (nostrils) are the external openings of the nasal cavities.

The internal portion of the nose is a hollow cavity separated into the right and left nasal cavities by a narrow vertical divider, the septum. Each nasal cavity is divided into three passageways by the projection of the turbinates from the lateral walls. The turbinate bones are also called *conchae* (the name suggested by their shell-like appearance). Because of their curves, these bones increase the mucous membrane surface of the nasal passages and slightly obstruct the air flowing through them (Fig. 20-1).

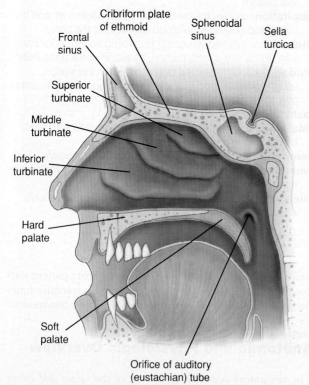

FIGURE 20-1 • Cross-section of nasal cavity.

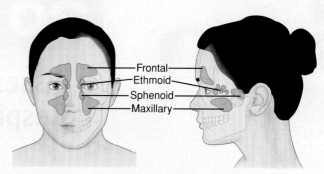

FIGURE 20-2 • The paranasal sinuses.

Air entering the nostrils is deflected upward to the roof of the nose, and it follows a circuitous route before it reaches the nasopharynx. It comes into contact with a large surface of moist, warm, highly vascular, ciliated mucous membrane (called *nasal mucosa*) that traps practically all of the dust and organisms in the inhaled air. The air is moistened, warmed to body temperature, and brought into contact with sensitive nerves. Some of these nerves detect odors; others provoke sneezing to expel irritating dust. Mucus, secreted continuously by goblet cells, covers the surface of the nasal mucosa and is moved back to the nasopharynx by the action of the **cilia** (fine hairs).

Paranasal Sinuses

The paranasal sinuses include four pairs of bony cavities that are lined with nasal mucosa and ciliated pseudostratified columnar epithelium. These air spaces are connected by a series of ducts that drain into the nasal cavity. The sinuses are named by their location: frontal, ethmoid, sphenoid, and maxillary (Fig. 20-2). A prominent function of the sinuses is to serve as a resonating chamber in speech. The sinuses are a common site of infection.

Pharynx, Tonsils, and Adenoids

The pharynx, or throat, is a tubelike structure that connects the nasal and oral cavities to the larynx. It is divided into three regions: nasal, oral, and laryngeal. The nasopharynx is located posterior to the nose and above the soft palate. The oropharynx houses the faucial, or palatine, tonsils. The laryngopharynx extends from the hyoid bone to the cricoid cartilage. The epiglottis forms the entrance to the larynx.

The adenoids, or pharyngeal tonsils, are located in the roof of the nasopharynx. The tonsils, the adenoids, and other lymphoid tissue encircle the throat. These structures are important links in the chain of lymph nodes guarding the body from invasion by organisms entering the nose and the throat. The pharynx functions as a passageway for the respiratory and digestive tracts.

Larynx

The larynx, or voice box, is a cartilaginous epithelium-lined organ that connects the pharynx and the trachea and consists of the following:

- *Epiglottis:* a valve flap of cartilage that covers the opening to the larynx during swallowing
- *Glottis:* the opening between the vocal cords in the larynx
- *Thyroid cartilage:* the largest of the cartilage structures; part of it forms the Adam's apple

- *Cricoid cartilage:* the only complete cartilaginous ring in the larynx (located below the thyroid cartilage)
- *Arytenoid cartilages:* used in vocal cord movement with the thyroid cartilage
- *Vocal cords:* ligaments controlled by muscular movements that produce sounds; located in the lumen of the larynx

Although the major function of the larynx is vocalization, it also protects the lower airway from foreign substances and facilitates coughing; it is therefore sometimes referred to as the "watchdog of the lungs" (Porth, 2011).

Trachea

The trachea, or windpipe, is composed of smooth muscle with C-shaped rings of cartilage at regular intervals. The cartilaginous rings are incomplete on the posterior surface and give firmness to the wall of the trachea, preventing it from collapsing. The trachea serves as the passage between the larynx and the right and left main stem bronchi, which enter the lungs through an opening called the *hilus.*

Lower Respiratory Tract

The lower respiratory tract consists of the lungs, which contain the bronchial and alveolar structures needed for gas exchange.

Lungs

The lungs are paired elastic structures enclosed in the thoracic cage, which is an airtight chamber with distensible walls

(Fig. 20-3). Each lung is divided into lobes. The right lung has upper, middle, and lower lobes, whereas the left lung consists of upper and lower lobes (Fig. 20-4). Each lobe is further subdivided into two to five segments separated by fissures, which are extensions of the pleura.

Pleura. The lungs and wall of the thoracic cavity are lined with a serous membrane called the *pleura.* The visceral pleura covers the lungs; the parietal pleura lines the thoracic cavity, lateral wall of the mediastinum diaphragm and inner aspects of the ribs. The visceral and parietal pleura and the small amount of pleural fluid between these two membranes serve to lubricate the thorax and lungs and permit smooth motion of the lungs within the thoracic cavity during inspiration and expiration.

Mediastinum. The mediastinum is in the middle of the thorax, between the pleural sacs that contain the two lungs. It extends from the sternum to the vertebral column and contains all of the thoracic tissue outside the lungs (heart, thymus, the aorta and vena cava, and esophagus).

Bronchi and Bronchioles. There are several divisions of the bronchi within each lobe of the lung. First are the lobar bronchi (3 in the right lung and 2 in the left lung). Lobar bronchi divide into segmental bronchi (10 on the right and 8 on the left); these structures facilitate effective postural drainage in the patient. Segmental bronchi then divide into subsegmental bronchi. These bronchi are surrounded by connective tissue that contains arteries, lymphatics, and nerves.

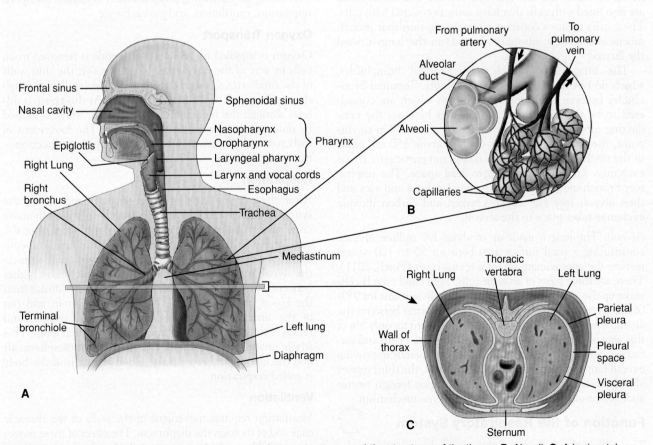

FIGURE 20-3 • The respiratory system. **A.** Upper respiratory structures and the structures of the thorax. **B.** Alveoli. **C.** A horizontal cross-section of the lungs.

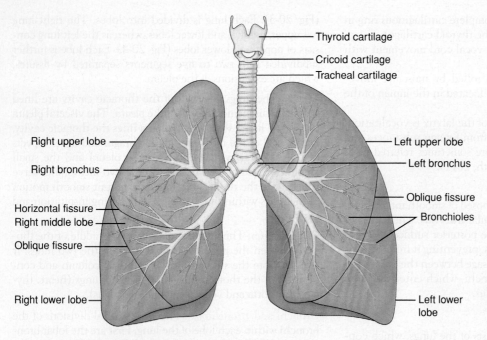

Thyroid cartilage
Cricoid cartilage
Tracheal cartilage

Right upper lobe
Right bronchus

Left upper lobe
Left bronchus

Horizontal fissure
Right middle lobe
Oblique fissure

Oblique fissure
Bronchioles

Right lower lobe

Left lower lobe

FIGURE 20-4 • Anterior view of the lungs. The lungs consist of five lobes. The right lung has three lobes (upper, middle, lower); the left has two (upper and lower). The lobes are further subdivided by fissures. The bronchial tree, another lung structure, inflates with air to fill the lobes.

The subsegmental bronchi then branch into bronchioles, which have no cartilage in their walls. Their patency depends entirely on the elastic recoil of the surrounding smooth muscle and on the alveolar pressure. The bronchioles contain submucosal glands, which produce mucus that covers the inside lining of the airways. The bronchi and bronchioles are also lined with cells that have surfaces covered with cilia. These cilia create a constant whipping motion that propels mucus and foreign substances away from the lungs toward the larynx.

The bronchioles branch into terminal bronchioles, which do not have mucous glands or cilia. Terminal bronchioles become respiratory bronchioles, which are considered to be the transitional passageways between the conducting airways and the gas exchange airways. Up to this point, the conducting airways contain about 150 mL of air in the tracheobronchial tree that does not participate in gas exchange, known as **physiologic dead space**. The respiratory bronchioles then lead into alveolar ducts and sacs and then alveoli (see Fig. 20-3). Oxygen and carbon dioxide exchange takes place in the alveoli.

Alveoli. The lung is made up of about 300 million alveoli, constituting a total surface area between 50 to 100 square meters, the approximate size of a tennis court (Porth, 2011). There are three types of alveolar cells. Type I and type II cells make up the alveolar epithelium. Type I cells account for 95% of the alveolar surface area and serve as a barrier between the air and the alveolar surface; type II cells account for only 5% of this area but are responsible for producing type I cells and surfactant. Surfactant reduces surface tension, thereby improving overall lung function. Alveolar macrophages, the third type of alveolar cells, are phagocytic cells that ingest foreign matter and, as a result, provide an important defense mechanism.

Function of the Respiratory System

The cells of the body derive the energy they need from the oxidation of carbohydrates, fats, and proteins. This process requires oxygen. Vital tissues, like the brain and heart, cannot survive long without a continuous supply of oxygen. As a result of oxidation, carbon dioxide is produced and must be removed from the cells to prevent the buildup of acid waste products. The respiratory system performs this function by facilitating life-sustaining processes such as oxygen transport, respiration, ventilation, and gas exchange.

Oxygen Transport

Oxygen is supplied to, and carbon dioxide is removed from, cells by way of the circulating blood through the thin walls of the capillaries. Oxygen diffuses from the capillary through the capillary wall to the interstitial fluid. At this point, it diffuses through the membrane of tissue cells, where it is used by mitochondria for cellular respiration. The movement of carbon dioxide occurs by diffusion in the opposite direction—from cell to blood.

Respiration

After these tissue capillary exchanges, blood enters the systemic venous circulation and travels to the pulmonary circulation. The oxygen concentration in blood within the capillaries of the lungs is lower than in the lungs' alveoli. Because of this concentration gradient, oxygen diffuses from the alveoli to the blood. Carbon dioxide, which has a higher concentration in the blood than in the alveoli, diffuses from the blood into the alveoli. Movement of air in and out of the airways continually replenishes the oxygen and removes the carbon dioxide from the airways and lungs. This whole process of gas exchange between the atmospheric air and the blood and between the blood and cells of the body is called **respiration**.

Ventilation

Ventilation requires movement of the walls of the thoracic cage and of its floor, the diaphragm. The effect of these movements is alternately to increase and decrease the capacity of the chest. When the capacity of the chest is increased, air enters through the trachea (inspiration) and moves into the bronchi, bronchioles, and alveoli, and inflates the lungs. When the chest wall and diaphragm return to their previous positions (expiration), the lungs recoil and force the air out through the bronchi and trachea. Inspiration occurs during the first third of the respiratory cycle; expiration occurs during the latter two thirds. The inspiratory phase of respiration normally requires energy; the expiratory phase is normally passive, requiring very little energy. Physical factors that govern airflow in and out of the lungs are collectively referred to as the mechanics of ventilation and include air pressure variances, resistance to airflow, and lung compliance.

Air Pressure Variances

Air flows from a region of higher pressure to a region of lower pressure. During inspiration, movements of the diaphragm and intercostal muscles enlarge the thoracic cavity and thereby lower the pressure inside the thorax to a level below that of atmospheric pressure. As a result, air is drawn through the trachea and bronchi into the alveoli. During expiration, the diaphragm relaxes and the lungs recoil, resulting in a decrease in the size of the thoracic cavity. The alveolar pressure then exceeds atmospheric pressure, and air flows from the lungs into the atmosphere.

Airway Resistance

Resistance is determined by the radius, or size of the airway through which the air is flowing, as well as by lung volumes and airflow velocity. Any process that changes the bronchial diameter or width affects airway resistance and alters the rate of airflow for a given pressure gradient during respiration (Chart 20-1). With increased resistance, greater-than-normal respiratory effort is required to achieve normal levels of ventilation.

Compliance

Compliance is the elasticity and expandability of the lungs and thoracic structures. Compliance allows the lung volume to increase when the difference in pressure between the atmosphere and thoracic cavity (pressure gradient) causes air to flow in. Factors that determine lung compliance are the surface tension of the alveoli, the connective tissue and water content of the lungs, and the compliance of the thoracic cavity.

Compliance is determined by examining the volume–pressure relationship in the lungs and the thorax. Compliance is normal (1 L/cm H_2O) if the lungs and thorax easily stretch and distend when pressure is applied. Increased compliance occurs if the lungs have lost their elastic recoil and become overdistended (e.g., in emphysema). Decreased compliance occurs if the lungs and thorax are "stiff." Conditions associated with decreased compliance include morbid obesity, pneumothorax, hemothorax, pleural effusion, pulmonary edema, atelectasis, pulmonary fibrosis, and acute respiratory distress syndrome (ARDS). Lungs with decreased compliance require greater-than-normal energy expenditure by the patient to achieve normal levels of ventilation.

Lung Volumes and Capacities

Lung function, which reflects the mechanics of ventilation, is viewed in terms of lung volumes and lung capacities. Lung volumes are categorized as tidal volume, inspiratory reserve volume, expiratory reserve volume, and residual volume. Lung capacity is evaluated in terms of vital capacity, inspiratory capacity, functional residual capacity, and total lung capacity. These terms are explained in Table 20-1.

Pulmonary Diffusion and Perfusion

Pulmonary diffusion is the process by which oxygen and carbon dioxide are exchanged from areas of high concentration to areas of low concentration at the air–blood interface. The alveolar–capillary membrane is ideal for diffusion because of its thinness and large surface area. In the normal healthy adult, oxygen and carbon dioxide travel across the alveolar–capillary membrane without difficulty as a result of differences in gas concentrations in the alveoli and capillaries.

Pulmonary perfusion is the actual blood flow through the pulmonary vasculature. The blood is pumped into the lungs by the right ventricle through the pulmonary artery. The pulmonary artery divides into the right and left branches to supply both lungs. Normally about 2% of the blood pumped by the right ventricle does not perfuse the alveolar capillaries. This shunted blood drains into the left side of the heart without participating in alveolar gas exchange. Bronchial arteries extending from the thoracic aorta also support perfusion but do not participate in gas exchange, further diluting oxygenated blood exiting through the pulmonary vein (Porth, 2011).

The pulmonary circulation is considered a low-pressure system because the systolic blood pressure in the pulmonary artery is 20 to 30 mm Hg and the diastolic pressure is 5 to 15 mm Hg. Because of these low pressures, the pulmonary vasculature normally can vary its capacity to accommodate the blood flow it receives. However, when a person is in an upright position, the pulmonary artery pressure is not great enough to supply blood to the apex of the lung against the force of gravity. Thus, when a person is upright, the lung may be considered to be divided into three sections: an upper part with poor blood supply, a lower part with maximal blood supply, and a section between the two with an intermediate supply of blood. When a person who is laying down turns to one side, more blood passes to the dependent lung.

Perfusion is also influenced by alveolar pressure. The pulmonary capillaries are sandwiched between adjacent alveoli. If the alveolar pressure is sufficiently high, the capillaries are squeezed. Depending on the pressure, some capillaries completely collapse, whereas others narrow.

Pulmonary artery pressure, gravity, and alveolar pressure determine the patterns of perfusion. In lung disease, these factors vary, and the perfusion of the lung may become abnormal.

Chart 20-1 **Causes of Increased Airway Resistance**

Common phenomena that may alter bronchial diameter, which affects airway resistance, include the following:

- Contraction of bronchial smooth muscle—as in asthma
- Thickening of bronchial mucosa—as in chronic bronchitis
- Obstruction of the airway—by mucus, a tumor, or a foreign body
- Loss of lung elasticity—as in emphysema, which is characterized by connective tissue encircling the airways, thereby keeping them open during both inspiration and expiration

TABLE 20-1 Lung Volumes and Lung Capacities

Term	Symbol	Description	Normal Value*	Significance
Lung Volumes				
Tidal volume	VT or TV	The volume of air inhaled and exhaled with each breath	500 mL or 5–10 mL/kg	The tidal volume may not vary, even with severe disease.
Inspiratory reserve volume	IRV	The maximum volume of air that can be inhaled after a normal inhalation	3,000 mL	
Expiratory reserve volume	ERV	The maximum volume of air that can be exhaled forcibly after a normal exhalation	1,100 mL	Expiratory reserve volume is decreased with restrictive conditions, such as obesity, ascites, pregnancy.
Residual volume	RV	The volume of air remaining in the lungs after a maximum exhalation	1,200 mL	Residual volume may be increased with obstructive disease.
Lung Capacities				
Vital capacity	VC	The maximum volume of air exhaled from the point of maximum inspiration: VC = TV + IRV + ERV	4,600 mL	A decrease in vital capacity may be found in neuromuscular disease, generalized fatigue, atelectasis, pulmonary edema, COPD, and obesity.
Inspiratory capacity	IC	The maximum volume of air inhaled after normal expiration: IC = TV + IRV	3,500 mL	A decrease in inspiratory capacity may indicate restrictive disease. It may also be decreased in obesity.
Functional residual capacity	FRC	The volume of air remaining in the lungs after a normal expiration: FRC = ERV + RV	2,300 mL	Functional residual capacity may be increased with COPD and decreased in ARDS and obesity.
Total lung capacity	TLC	The volume of air in the lungs after a maximum inspiration TLC = TV + IRV + ERV + RV	5,800 mL	Total lung capacity may be decreased with restrictive disease such as atelectasis and pneumonia and increased in COPD.

*Values for healthy men; women are 20% to 25% less.
ARDS, acute respiratory distress syndrome; COPD, chronic obstructive pulmonary disease.

Ventilation and Perfusion Balance and Imbalance

Adequate gas exchange depends on an adequate ventilation–perfusion ($\dot{V}/\dot{Q}$) ratio. In different areas of the lung, the ($\dot{V}/\dot{Q}$) ratio varies. Airway blockages, local changes in compliance, and gravity may alter ventilation. Alterations in perfusion may occur with a change in the pulmonary artery pressure, alveolar pressure, or gravity. Airway blockages, local changes in compliance, and gravity may alter ventilation.

($\dot{V}/\dot{Q}$) imbalance occurs as a result of inadequate ventilation, inadequate perfusion, or both. There are four possible ($\dot{V}/\dot{Q}$) states in the lung: normal ($\dot{V}/\dot{Q}$) ratio, low ($\dot{V}/\dot{Q}$) ratio (shunt), high ($\dot{V}/\dot{Q}$) ratio (dead space), and absence of ventilation and perfusion (silent unit) (Chart 20-2). ($\dot{V}/\dot{Q}$) imbalance causes shunting of blood, resulting in **hypoxia** (low level of cellular oxygen). Shunting appears to be the main cause of hypoxia after thoracic or abdominal surgery and most types of respiratory failure. Severe hypoxia results when the amount of shunting exceeds 20%. Supplemental oxygen may eliminate hypoxia, depending on the type of ($\dot{V}/\dot{Q}$) imbalance.

Gas Exchange

Partial Pressure of Gases

The air we breathe is a gaseous mixture consisting mainly of nitrogen (78.6%) and oxygen (20.8%), with traces of carbon dioxide (0.04%), water vapor (0.05%), helium, and argon. The atmospheric pressure at sea level is about 760 mm Hg. Partial pressure is the pressure exerted by each type of gas in a mixture of gases. The partial pressure of a gas is proportional to the concentration of that gas in the mixture. The total pressure exerted by the gaseous mixture, whether in the atmosphere or in the lungs, is equal to the sum of the partial pressures.

Based on these facts, the partial pressures of nitrogen and oxygen can be calculated. The partial pressure of nitrogen in the atmosphere at sea level is 78.6% of 760, or 597 mm Hg; that of oxygen is 20.8% of 760, or 158 mm Hg. Chart 20-3 identifies and defines terms and abbreviations related to partial pressure of gases.

Once the air enters the trachea, it becomes fully saturated with water vapor, which displaces some of the other gases. Water vapor exerts a pressure of 47 mm Hg when it fully saturates a mixture of gases at the body temperature of 37°C (98.6°F). Nitrogen and oxygen are responsible for almost all of the remaining 713 mm Hg pressure. Once this mixture enters the alveoli, it is further diluted by carbon dioxide. In the alveoli, the water vapor continues to exert a pressure of 47 mm Hg. The remaining 713 mm Hg pressure is now exerted as follows: nitrogen, 569 mm Hg (74.9%); oxygen, 104 mm Hg (13.6%); and carbon dioxide, 40 mm Hg (5.3%) (Porth, 2011).

When a gas is exposed to a liquid, the gas dissolves in the liquid until equilibrium is reached. The dissolved gas also exerts a partial pressure. At equilibrium, the partial pressure of the gas in the liquid is the same as the partial pressure of the gas in the gaseous mixture. Oxygenation of venous blood in the lung illustrates this point. In the lung, venous blood and alveolar oxygen are separated by a very thin alveolar membrane. Oxygen diffuses across this membrane to dissolve in the blood until the partial pressure of oxygen in the blood is the same as that in the alveoli (104 mm Hg). However, because carbon dioxide is a by-product of oxidation in the cells, venous blood contains carbon dioxide at a higher partial pressure than that in the alveolar gas. In the lung, carbon dioxide diffuses out of venous blood into the alveolar gas. At equilibrium, the partial pressure of carbon dioxide in the blood and in alveolar gas is the same (40 mm Hg). The changes in partial pressure are shown in Figure 20-5.

Chart 20-2   Ventilation–Perfusion Ratios

Normal Ratio (A)

In the healthy lung, a given amount of blood passes an alveolus and is matched with an equal amount of gas **(A).** The ratio is 1:1 (ventilation matches perfusion).

Low Ventilation–Perfusion Ratio: Shunts (B)

Low ventilation–perfusion states may be called *shunt-producing disorders.* When perfusion exceeds ventilation, a shunt exists **(B).** Blood bypasses the alveoli without gas exchange occurring. This is seen with obstruction of the distal airways, such as with pneumonia, atelectasis, tumor, or a mucus plug.

High Ventilation–Perfusion Ratio: Dead Space (C)

When ventilation exceeds perfusion, dead space results **(C).** The alveoli do not have an adequate blood supply for gas exchange to occur. This is characteristic of a variety of disorders, including pulmonary emboli, pulmonary infarction, and cardiogenic shock.

Silent Unit (D)

In the absence of both ventilation and perfusion or with limited ventilation and perfusion, a condition known as a silent unit occurs **(D).** This is seen with pneumothorax and severe acute respiratory distress syndrome.

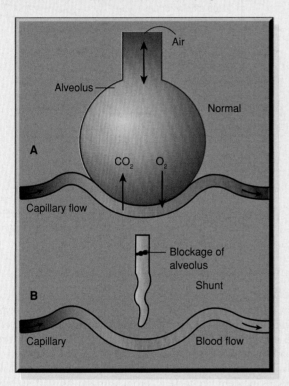

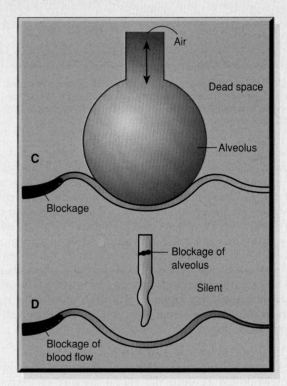

Effects of Pressure on Oxygen Transport

Oxygen and carbon dioxide are transported simultaneously, either dissolved in blood or combined with hemoglobin in red blood cells. Each 100 mL of normal arterial blood carries 0.3 mL of oxygen physically dissolved in the plasma and 20 mL of oxygen in combination with hemoglobin. Large amounts of oxygen can be transported in the blood because oxygen combines easily with hemoglobin to form oxyhemoglobin:

$$O_2 + Hgb \leftrightarrow HgbO_2$$

The volume of oxygen physically dissolved in the plasma is measured by the partial pressure of oxygen in the arteries (PaO_2). The higher the PaO_2, the greater the amount of oxygen dissolved. For example, at a PaO_2 of 10 mm Hg, 0.03 mL of oxygen is dissolved in 100 mL of plasma. At PaO_2 of 20 mm Hg, twice this amount is dissolved in plasma, and at PaO_2 of 100 mm Hg, 10 times this amount is dissolved. Therefore, the amount of dissolved oxygen is directly proportional to the partial pressure, regardless of how high the oxygen pressure becomes.

The amount of oxygen that combines with hemoglobin depends on both the amount of hemoglobin in the blood and on PaO_2, although only up to a PaO_2 of about 150 mm Hg.

Chart 20-3   Partial Pressure Abbreviations

P = pressure
PO_2 = partial pressure of oxygen
PCO_2 = partial pressure of carbon dioxide
PAO_2 = partial pressure of alveolar oxygen
$PACO_2$ = partial pressure of alveolar carbon dioxide
PaO_2 = partial pressure of arterial oxygen
$PaCO_2$ = partial pressure of arterial carbon dioxide
$Pv\text{–}O_2$ = partial pressure of venous oxygen
$Pv\text{–}CO_2$ = partial pressure of venous carbon dioxide
P_{50} = partial pressure of oxygen when the hemoglobin is 50% saturated

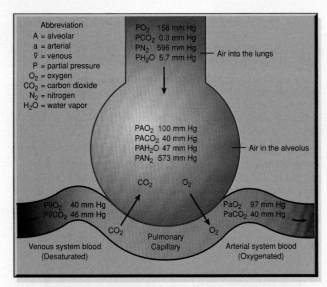

FIGURE 20-5 • Changes occur in the partial pressure of gases during respiration. These values vary as a result of the exchange of oxygen and carbon dioxide and the changes that occur in their partial pressures as venous blood flows through the lungs.

This is measured as O_2 saturation (SaO_2), the percentage of the O_2 that could be carried if all the hemoglobin held the maximum possible amount of O_2. When the PaO_2 is 150 mm Hg, hemoglobin is 100% saturated and does not combine with any additional oxygen. When hemoglobin is 100% saturated, 1 g of hemoglobin combines with 1.34 mL of oxygen. Therefore, in a person with 14 g/dL of hemoglobin, each 100 mL of blood contains about 19 mL of oxygen associated with hemoglobin. If the PaO_2 is less than 150 mm Hg, the percentage of hemoglobin saturated with oxygen decreases. For example, at a PaO_2 of 100 mm Hg (normal value), saturation is 97%; at a PaO_2 of 40 mm Hg, saturation is 70%.

Oxyhemoglobin Dissociation Curve

The oxyhemoglobin dissociation curve (Chart 20-4) shows the relationship between the partial pressure of oxygen (PaO_2) and the percentage of saturation of oxygen (SaO_2). The percentage of saturation can be affected by carbon dioxide, hydrogen ion concentration, temperature, and 2,3-diphosphoglycerate. An increase in these factors shifts the curve to the right, thus less oxygen is picked up in the lungs, but more oxygen is released to the tissues, if PaO_2 is unchanged. A decrease in these factors causes the curve to shift to the left, making the bond between oxygen and hemoglobin stronger. If the PaO_2 is still unchanged, more oxygen is picked up in the lungs, but less oxygen is given up to the tissues. The unusual shape of the oxyhemoglobin dissociation curve is a distinct advantage to the patient for two reasons:

1. If the PaO_2 decreases from 100 to 80 mm Hg as a result of lung disease or heart disease, the hemoglobin of the arterial blood remains almost maximally saturated (94%), and the tissues do not suffer from hypoxia.
2. When the arterial blood passes into tissue capillaries and is exposed to the tissue tension of oxygen (about 40 mm Hg), hemoglobin gives up large quantities of oxygen for use by the tissues.

Chart 20-4 Oxyhemoglobin Dissociation Curve

The oxyhemoglobin dissociation curve is marked to show three oxygen levels:

1. Normal levels—PaO_2 >70 mm Hg
2. Relatively safe levels—PaO_2 45–70 mm Hg
3. Dangerous levels—PaO_2 <40 mm Hg

The normal (middle) curve (N) shows that 75% saturation occurs at a PaO_2 of 40 mm Hg. If the curve shifts to the right (R), the same saturation (75%) occurs at the higher PaO_2 of 57 mm Hg. If the curve shifts to the left (L), 75% saturation occurs at a PaO_2 of 25 mm Hg.

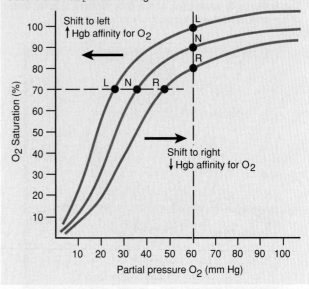

With a normal value for PaO_2 (80 to 100 mm Hg) and SaO_2 (95% to 98%), there is a 15% margin of excess oxygen available to the tissues. With a normal hemoglobin level of 15 mg/dL and a PaO_2 level of 40 mm Hg (SaO_2 75%), there is adequate oxygen available for the tissues but no reserve for physiologic stresses that increase tissue oxygen demand. If a serious incident occurs (e.g., bronchospasm, aspiration, hypotension, or cardiac dysrhythmias) that reduces the intake of oxygen from the lungs, tissue hypoxia results.

An important consideration in the transport of oxygen is cardiac output, which determines the amount of oxygen delivered to the body and affects lung and tissue perfusion. If the cardiac output is normal (5 L/min), the amount of oxygen delivered to the body per minute is normal. Under normal conditions, only 250 mL of oxygen is used per minute, which is approximately 25% of available oxygen. The rest of the oxygen returns to the right side of the heart, and the PaO_2 of venous blood drops from 80 to 100 mm Hg to about 40 mm Hg. If cardiac output falls, however, the amount of oxygen delivered to the tissues also falls and may be inadequate to meet the body's needs.

Carbon Dioxide Transport

At the same time that oxygen diffuses from the blood into the tissues, carbon dioxide diffuses from tissue cells to blood and is transported to the lungs for excretion. The amount of carbon dioxide in transit is one of the major determinants of the acid–base balance of the body. Normally, only 6% of the venous carbon dioxide is removed in the lungs, and enough remains in the arterial blood to exert a pressure of 40 mm Hg. Most of the carbon dioxide (90%) is carried by red blood cells; the small portion (5%) that remains dissolved in the plasma (partial pressure of carbon dioxide [PCO_2]) is the critical factor that determines carbon dioxide movement in or out of the blood.

Although the many processes involved in respiratory gas transport seem to occur in intermittent stages, the changes are rapid, simultaneous, and continuous.

Neurologic Control of Ventilation

Resting respiration is the result of cyclic excitation of the respiratory muscles by the phrenic nerve. The rhythm of breathing is controlled by respiratory centers in the brain. The inspiratory and expiratory centers in the medulla oblongata and pons control the rate and depth of ventilation to meet the body's metabolic demands.

The apneustic center in the lower pons stimulates the inspiratory medullary center to promote deep, prolonged inspirations. The pneumotaxic center in the upper pons is thought to control the pattern of respirations.

Several groups of receptor sites assist in the brain's control of respiratory function. The central chemoreceptors, located in the medulla, respond to chemical changes in the cerebrospinal fluid, which result from chemical changes in the blood. These receptors respond to an increase or decrease in the pH and convey a message to the lungs to change the depth and then the rate of ventilation to correct the imbalance. The peripheral chemoreceptors are located in the aortic arch and the carotid arteries and respond first to changes in PaO_2, then to partial pressure of carbon dioxide ($PaCO_2$) and pH.

Mechanoreceptors in the lung include stretch, irritant, and juxtacapillary receptors and respond to changes in resistance by altering breathing patterns to support optimal lung function. For example, the Hering-Breuer reflex is activated by stretch receptors in the alveoli. When the lungs are distended, inspiration is inhibited; as a result, the lungs do not become overdistended.

Proprioceptors in the muscles and chest wall respond to body movements, causing an increase in ventilation. Thus, range-of-motion exercises in an immobile patient stimulate breathing. Finally, baroreceptors, also located in the aortic and carotid bodies, respond to an increase or decrease in arterial blood pressure and cause reflex hypoventilation or hyperventilation.

 Gerontologic Considerations

A gradual decline in respiratory function begins in early to middle adulthood and affects the structure and function of the respiratory system. The vital capacity of the lungs and strength of the respiratory muscles peak between 20 and 25 years of age and decrease thereafter. With aging (40 years and older), changes occur in the alveoli that reduce the surface area available for the exchange of oxygen and carbon dioxide. At approximately 50 years of age, the alveoli begin to lose elasticity. A decrease in vital capacity occurs with loss of chest wall mobility, which restricts the tidal flow of air. The amount of respiratory dead space increases with age. These changes result in a decreased diffusion capacity for oxygen with increasing age, producing lower oxygen levels in the arterial circulation. Older adults have a decreased ability to rapidly move air in and out of the lungs.

Gerontologic changes in the respiratory system are summarized in Table 20-2. Despite these changes, in the absence

TABLE 20-2	**Age-Related Changes in the Respiratory System**		
	Structural Changes	**Functional Changes**	**History and Physical Findings**
Defense Mechanisms (Respiratory and Nonrespiratory)	↓ Number of cilia and ↓ mucus ↓ Cough and gag reflex Loss of surface area of the capillary membrane Lack of a uniform or consistent ventilation and/or blood flow	↓ Protection against foreign particles ↓ Protection against aspiration ↓ Antibody response to antigens ↓ Response to hypoxia and hypercapnia (chemoreceptors)	↓ Cough reflex and mucus ↑ Infection rate History of respiratory infections, chronic obstructive pulmonary disease (COPD), pneumonia. Risk factors: smoking, environmental exposure, exposure to tuberculosis (TB)
Lung	↓ Size of airway ↑ Diameter of alveolar ducts ↑ Collagen of alveolar walls ↑ Thickness of alveolar membranes ↓ Elasticity of alveolar sacs	↑ Airway resistance ↑ Pulmonary compliance ↓ Expiratory flow rate ↓ Oxygen diffusion capacity ↑ Dead space Premature closure of airways ↑ Air trapping ↓ Expiratory flow rates Ventilation–perfusion mismatch ↓ Exercise capacity ↑ Anteroposterior (AP) diameter	Unchanged total lung capacity (TLC) ↑ Residual volume (RV) ↓ Inspiratory reserve volume (IRV) ↓ Expiratory reserve volume (ERV) ↓ Forced vital capacity (FVC) and vital capacity (VC) ↑ Functional residual capacity (FRC) ↓ PaO_2 ↑ CO_2
Chest Wall and Muscles	Calcification of intercostal cartilages Arthritis of costovertebral joints ↓ Continuity of diaphragm Osteoporotic changes ↓ Muscle mass Muscle atrophy	↑ Rigidity and stiffness of thoracic cage ↓ Respiratory muscle strength ↑ Work of breathing ↓ Capacity for exercise ↓ Peripheral chemosensitivity ↑ Risk for inspiratory muscle fatigue	Kyphosis, barrel chest Skeletal changes ↑ AP diameter Shortness of breath ↑ Abdominal and diaphragmatic breathing ↓ Maximum expiratory flow rates

of chronic pulmonary disease, older adults are able to carry out activities of daily living, but they may have decreased tolerance for, and require additional rest after, prolonged or vigorous activity.

Assessment

Health History

The health history initially focuses on the patient's presenting problem and associated symptoms, with close attention to how all aspects of the patient's life, including activities of daily living and quality of life, are impacted. In conducting the history, the nurse should explore the onset, location, duration, character, aggravating and alleviating factors, radiation (if relevant), and timing of the presenting problem and associated symptoms.

Common Symptoms

The major signs and symptoms of respiratory disease are dyspnea, cough, sputum production, chest pain, wheezing, and hemoptysis. The nurse also assesses the impact of signs and symptoms on the patient's ability to perform activities of daily living and to participate in usual work and family activities.

Dyspnea

Dyspnea (subjective feeling of difficult or labored breathing, breathlessness, shortness of breath) is a multidimensional symptom common to many pulmonary and cardiac disorders, particularly when there is decreased lung compliance or increased airway resistance. Dyspnea may also be associated with allergic reactions, anemia, neurologic or neuromuscular disorders, trauma, and advanced disease. It is common at the end of life. Dyspnea can also occur after exercise in people without disease (Porth, 2011). Because dyspnea can occur with other conditions, these disorders also need to be considered when obtaining the patient's health history (Bickley, 2009; Porth, 2011).

In general, acute diseases of the lungs produce a more severe grade of dyspnea than do chronic diseases. Sudden dyspnea in a healthy person may indicate pneumothorax (air in the pleural cavity), acute respiratory obstruction, allergic reaction, or myocardial infarction. In immobilized patients, sudden dyspnea may denote pulmonary embolism. Dyspnea and **tachypnea** (abnormally rapid respirations) accompanied by progressive **hypoxemia** (low blood oxygen level) in a person who has recently experienced lung trauma, shock, cardiopulmonary bypass, or multiple blood transfusions may signal ARDS. **Orthopnea** (inability to breathe easily except in an upright position) may be found in patients with heart disease and occasionally in patients with chronic obstructive pulmonary disease (COPD); dyspnea with an expiratory wheeze occurs with COPD. Noisy breathing may result from a narrowing of the airway or localized obstruction of a major bronchus by a tumor or foreign body. The high-pitched sound heard (usually on inspiration) when someone is breathing through a partially blocked upper airway is called **stridor**. The circumstance that produces the dyspnea must be determined. Therefore, it is important to ask the patient the following questions:

- How much exertion triggers shortness of breath? Does it occur with exercise? Climbing stairs? At rest?

- Is the shortness of breath related to other symptoms? Is a cough present?
- Was the onset of shortness of breath sudden or gradual?
- At what time of day or night does the shortness of breath occur?
- Is the shortness of breath worse when lying flat?
- How severe is the shortness of breath? On a scale of 1 to 10, if 1 is not at all breathless and 10 is very breathless, how hard is it to breathe?

It is especially important to assess the patient's rating of the intensity of breathlessness, the effort required to breathe, and the psychological impact of dyspnea on the patient, because patients experiencing dyspnea frequently experience fear and anxiety (Ferrell & Coyle, 2010). Visual analogue or health-related quality-of-life scales that include dyspnea as a component can be used to assess the severity of dyspnea and its impact on the patient's life (Cox, 2010; Ferrell & Coyle, 2010; Wrede-Seaman, 2009). Patients use a variety of terms and phrases to describe breathlessness, and the nurse needs to clarify what terms are most familiar to the patient and what these terms mean.

Cough

Cough is a reflex that protects the lungs from the accumulation of secretions or the inhalation of foreign bodies. Its presence or absence can be a diagnostic clue because some disorders cause coughing and others suppress it. The cough reflex may be impaired by weakness or paralysis of the respiratory muscles, prolonged inactivity, the presence of a nasogastric tube, or depressed function of the brain's medullary centers (e.g., anesthesia, brain disorders).

Cough results from irritation or inflammation of the mucous membranes anywhere in the respiratory tract and is associated with multiple pulmonary disorders. Mucus, pus, blood, or an airborne irritant, such as smoke or a gas, may stimulate the cough reflex. Common causes of cough include asthma, gastrointestinal reflux disease, infection, aspiration, and side effects of medications, such as angiotensin-converting enzyme (ACE) inhibitors (Wrede-Seaman, 2009).

To help determine the cause of the cough, the nurse inquires about the onset and time of coughing. Coughing at night may indicate the onset of left-sided heart failure or bronchial asthma. A cough in the morning with sputum production may indicate bronchitis. A cough that worsens when the patient is supine suggests postnasal drip (rhinosinusitis). Coughing after food intake may indicate aspiration of material into the tracheobronchial tree. A cough of recent onset is usually from an acute infection.

The nurse assesses the character of the cough and associated symptoms. A dry, irritative cough is characteristic of an upper respiratory tract infection of viral origin, or it may be a side effect of ACE inhibitor therapy. An irritative, high-pitched cough can be caused by laryngotracheitis. A brassy cough is the result of a tracheal lesion, and a severe or changing cough may indicate bronchogenic carcinoma. Pleuritic chest pain that accompanies coughing may indicate pleural or chest wall (musculoskeletal) involvement. Violent coughing causes bronchial spasm, obstruction, and further irritation of the bronchi and may result in syncope (fainting).

A persistent cough may affect a patient's quality of life and may produce embarrassment, exhaustion, inability to sleep, and pain. Therefore, the nurse should explore a chronic cough's effect on the patient and the patient's view about the cough's significance and effect on his or her life.

Sputum Production

Sputum production is the reaction of the lungs to any constantly recurring irritant and often results from persistent coughing. It may also be associated with a nasal discharge. The nature of the sputum is often indicative of its cause. A profuse amount of purulent sputum (thick and yellow, green, or rust colored) or a change in color of the sputum is a common sign of a bacterial infection. Thin, mucoid sputum frequently results from viral bronchitis. A gradual increase of sputum over time may occur with chronic bronchitis or bronchiectasis. Pink-tinged mucoid sputum suggests a lung tumor. Profuse, frothy, pink material, often welling up into the throat, may indicate pulmonary edema. Foul-smelling sputum and bad breath point to the presence of a lung abscess, bronchiectasis, or an infection caused by fusospirochetal or other anaerobic organisms.

Chest Pain

Chest pain or discomfort may be associated with pulmonary, cardiac, gastrointestinal, or musculoskeletal disease or anxiety. Chest pain associated with pulmonary conditions may be sharp, stabbing, and intermittent, or it may be dull, aching, and persistent. The pain usually is felt on the side where the pathologic process is located, although it may be referred elsewhere—for example, to the neck, back, or abdomen.

Chest pain may occur with pneumonia, pulmonary infarction, or pleurisy, or as a late symptom of bronchogenic carcinoma. In carcinoma, the pain may be dull and persistent because the cancer has invaded the chest wall, mediastinum, or spine.

Lung disease does not always cause thoracic pain because the lungs and the visceral pleura lack sensory nerves and are insensitive to pain stimuli. However, the parietal pleura have a rich supply of sensory nerves that are stimulated by inflammation and stretching of the membrane. Pleuritic pain from irritation of the parietal pleura is sharp and seems to "catch" on inspiration; patients often describe it as being "like the stabbing of a knife." Patients are more comfortable when they lay on the affected side because this splints the chest wall, limits expansion and contraction of the lung, and reduces the friction between the injured or diseased pleurae on that side. Pain associated with cough may be reduced manually by splinting the rib cage.

The nurse assesses the quality, intensity, and radiation of pain and identifies and explores precipitating factors and their relationship to the patient's position. In addition, the nurse must assess the relationship of pain to the inspiratory and expiratory phases of respiration. (See Chapter 12 for further discussion on assessment of pain.)

Wheezing

Wheezing is a high-pitched, musical sound heard mainly on expiration (asthma) or inspiration (bronchitis). It is often the major finding in a patient with bronchoconstriction or airway narrowing. **Rhonchi** are low-pitched continuous sounds heard over the lungs in partial airway obstruction. Depending on their location and severity, these sounds may be heard with or without a stethoscope.

Hemoptysis

Hemoptysis is the expectoration of blood from the respiratory tract. It can present as small to moderate blood-stained sputum to a large hemorrhage and always warrants further investigation. The onset of hemoptysis is usually sudden, and it may be intermittent or continuous. The most common causes are:

- Pulmonary infection
- Carcinoma of the lung
- Abnormalities of the heart or blood vessels
- Pulmonary artery or vein abnormalities
- Pulmonary embolus and infarction

The nurse must determine the source of the bleeding, as the term *hemoptysis* is reserved for blood coming from the respiratory tract. Sources of bleeding include the gums, nasopharynx, lungs, or stomach. The nurse may be the only witness to the episode, and when documenting the bleeding episode, the following points should be considered:

- Bloody sputum from the nose or the nasopharynx is usually preceded by considerable sniffing, with blood possibly appearing in the nose.
- Blood from the lung is usually bright red, frothy, and mixed with sputum. Initial symptoms include a tickling sensation in the throat, a salty taste, a burning or bubbling sensation in the chest, and perhaps chest pain, in which case the patient tends to splint the bleeding side. This blood has an alkaline pH (greater than 7).
- Blood from the stomach is vomited rather than expectorated, may be mixed with food, and is usually much darker and often referred to as "coffee ground emesis." This blood has an acid pH (less than 7).

Past Health, Social, and Family History

In addition to the presenting problem and associated symptoms, the history should also focus on the patient's health, personal, and social history, as well as the family health history. Specific questions are asked about childhood illnesses, immunizations (including the most recent influenza and pneumonia vaccinations), medical conditions, injuries, hospitalizations, surgeries, allergies, and current medications (including over-the-counter medications and herbal remedies). Personal and social history addresses issues such as diet, exercise, sleep, recreational habits, and religion. Psychosocial factors that may affect the patient are also explored (Chart 20-5).

The nurse assesses for risk factors and genetic factors that may contribute to the patient's lung condition (Charts 20-6 and 20-7). Many lung disorders are related to or exacerbated by tobacco smoke; therefore, smoking history (including exposure to secondhand smoke) is also obtained. Smoking history is usually expressed in pack-years, which is the number of packs of cigarettes smoked per day times the number of years the patient has smoked. It is important to find out if the patient is still smoking or when the patient quit smoking. Finally, socioeconomic differences rooted in race and ethnicity may predispose certain groups to greater burdens related to lung disease and should also be considered (Chart 20-8).

If the patient is experiencing severe dyspnea, the nurse may need to modify the questions asked and the timing of the

ASSESSMENT
Chart 20-5 Assessing Psychosocial Factors Related to Respiratory Function and Disease

- What strategies does the patient use to cope with the signs, symptoms, and challenges associated with pulmonary disease?
- What effect has the pulmonary disease had on the patient's quality of life, goals, role within the family, and occupation?
- What changes has the pulmonary disease had on the patient's family and relationships with family members?
- Does the patient exhibit depression, anxiety, anger, hostility, dependency, withdrawal, isolation, avoidance, noncompliance, acceptance, or denial?
- What support systems does the patient use to cope with the illness?
- Are resources (relatives, friends, or community groups) available? Do the patient and family use them effectively?

RISK FACTORS
Chart 20-6 Respiratory Disease

- Smoking (the single most important contributor to lung disease)
- Exposure to secondhand smoke
- Personal or family history of lung disease
- Genetic makeup
- Exposure to allergens and environmental pollutants
- Exposure to certain recreational and occupational hazards
- Vitamin D deficiency
- Obesity
- Excessive exposure to acetaminophen prenatally and in the first 2 years of life

Adapted from Rubin, B. K., Dhand, R., Ruppel, G. L., et al. (2011). Respiratory care year in review 2010: Part 1. Asthma, COPD, pulmonary function testing, ventilator-associated pneumonia. *Respiratory Care, 56*(4), 488–502.

GENETICS IN NURSING PRACTICE
Chart 20-7 Respiratory Disorders

Various conditions that affect gas exchange and respiratory function are influenced by genetics factors, including:

- Asthma
- Chronic obstructive pulmonary disease
- Cystic fibrosis
- Alpha-1 antitrypsin deficiency

Nursing Assessments

Family History Assessment

- Assess family history for three generations for family members with histories of respiratory impairment.
- Assess family history for individuals with early-onset chronic pulmonary disease and family history of hepatic disease in infants (clinical symptoms of alpha-1 antitrypsin deficiency).
- Inquire about family history of cystic fibrosis, an autosomal recessive inherited respiratory disorder.

Patient Assessment

- Assess for symptoms such as changes in respiratory status associated with asthma (e.g., wheezing, hyperresponsiveness, mucosal edema, and mucus production).
- Assess for multisystem effects characteristic of cystic fibrosis (e.g., productive cough, wheezing, obstructive airways disease,

gastrointestinal problems including pancreatic insufficiency, clubbing of the fingers).

Management Issues Specific to Genetics

- Inquire whether DNA mutation or other genetic testing has been performed on affected family members.
- Refer for further genetics counseling and evaluation so that family members can discuss inheritance, risk to other family members, and availability of genetic testing and gene-based interventions.
- Offer appropriate genetics information and resources.
- Assess patient's understanding of genetics information.
- Provide support to families with newly diagnosed genetic-related respiratory disorders.
- Participate in management and coordination of care of patients with genetic conditions, as well as individuals predisposed to develop or pass on a genetic condition.

Genetics Resources

American Lung Association, www.lungusa.org
Cystic Fibrosis Foundation, www.cff.org
See also Chapter 8, Chart 8-6 for additional genetics resources.

Chart 20-8 Disparities in Pulmonary Health Related to Socioeconomics, Race, and Ethnicity: A Snapshot

- More African Americans and Hispanics live in areas with greater levels of air pollution and traffic and have higher prevalence rates of asthma compared to Caucasians.
- African Americans and Hispanics are less likely to receive influenza and pneumonia vaccinations when compared to Caucasians.
- Hispanics are more likely to work in occupations that expose them to greater levels of hazardous respiratory toxins.
- American Indians and Alaskan Natives have mortality rates from H1N1 influenza four times greater than the rate among all other groups, most likely related to higher rates of poverty, delays in accessing care, and chronic illness.

Adapted from American Lung Association. (2010). *State of lung disease in diverse communities 2010.* Available at: www.lungusa.org/assets/documents/publications/lung-disease-data/solddc_2010.pdf

health history to avoid increasing the patient's breathlessness and anxiety. Once the history is complete, the nurse conducts a comprehensive assessment. Data obtained from both the history and assessment guide the development of a nursing care plan and patient education.

Physical Assessment of the Respiratory System

General Appearance

The patient's general appearance may give clues to respiratory status. In particular, the nurse inspects for clubbing of the fingers and notes skin color.

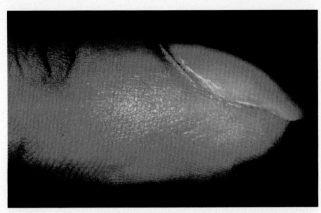

FIGURE 20-6 • Clubbed finger. In clubbing, the distal phalanx of each finger is rounded and bulbous. The nail plate is more convex, and the angle between the plate and the proximal nail fold increases to 180 degrees or more. The proximal nail fold, when palpated, feels spongy or floating. Among the many causes are chronic hypoxia and lung cancer.

Clubbing of the Fingers

Clubbing of the fingers is a change in the normal nail bed. It appears as sponginess of the nail bed and loss of the nail bed angle (Fig. 20-6). It is a sign of lung disease that is found in patients with chronic hypoxic conditions, chronic lung infections, or malignancies of the lung (Bickley, 2009). Approximately 75% patients who exhibit clubbing have an underlying pulmonary disease (Massey & Meredith, 2010).

Cyanosis

Cyanosis, a bluish coloring of the skin, is a very late indicator of hypoxia. The presence or absence of cyanosis is determined by the amount of unoxygenated hemoglobin in the blood. Cyanosis appears when there is at least 5 g/dL of unoxygenated hemoglobin. A patient with a hemoglobin level of 15 g/dL does not demonstrate cyanosis until 5 g/dL of that hemoglobin becomes unoxygenated, reducing the effective circulating hemoglobin to two thirds of the normal level.

A patient with anemia rarely manifests cyanosis, and a patient with polycythemia may appear cyanotic even if adequately oxygenated. Therefore, cyanosis is *not* a reliable sign of hypoxia.

Assessment of cyanosis is affected by room lighting, the patient's skin color, and the distance of the blood vessels from the surface of the skin. In the presence of a pulmonary condition, central cyanosis is assessed by observing the color of the tongue and lips. This indicates a decrease in oxygen tension in the blood. Peripheral cyanosis results from decreased blood flow to the body's periphery (fingers, toes, or earlobes), as in vasoconstriction from exposure to cold, and does not necessarily indicate a central systemic problem.

Upper Respiratory Structures

For a routine examination of the upper airway, only a simple light source, such as a penlight, is necessary. A more thorough examination requires the use of a nasal speculum.

Nose and Sinuses

The nurse inspects the external nose for lesions, asymmetry, or inflammation and then asks the patient to tilt the head backward. Gently pushing the tip of the nose upward, the nurse examines the internal structures of the nose, inspecting the mucosa for color, swelling, exudate, or bleeding. The nasal mucosa is normally redder than the oral mucosa. It may appear swollen and hyperemic if the patient has a common cold; however, in allergic rhinitis, the mucosa appears pale and swollen.

Next, the nurse inspects the septum for deviation, perforation, or bleeding. Most people have a slight degree of septal deviation, but actual displacement of the cartilage into either the right or left side of the nose may produce nasal obstruction. Such deviation usually causes no symptoms.

While the head is still tilted back, the nurse inspects the inferior and middle turbinates. In chronic rhinitis, nasal polyps may develop between the inferior and middle turbinates; they are distinguished by their gray appearance. Unlike the turbinates, they are gelatinous and freely movable.

Next, the nurse may palpate the frontal and maxillary sinuses for tenderness (Fig. 20-7). Using the thumbs, the nurse applies gentle pressure in an upward fashion at the supraorbital ridges (frontal sinuses) and in the cheek area adjacent to the nose (maxillary sinuses). Tenderness in either area suggests inflammation. The frontal and maxillary sinuses can be inspected by transillumination (passing a strong light through a bony area, such as the sinuses, to inspect the cavity; Fig. 20-8). If the light fails to penetrate, the cavity likely contains fluid or pus.

Mouth and Pharynx

After the nasal inspection, the nurse assesses the mouth and pharynx, instructing the patient to open the mouth wide and take a deep breath. Usually this flattens the posterior tongue and briefly allows a full view of the anterior and posterior pillars, tonsils, uvula, and posterior pharynx (see Fig. 46-2 in Chapter 46). The nurse inspects these structures for color, symmetry, and evidence of exudate, ulceration, or enlargement. If a tongue blade is needed to depress the tongue to visualize the pharynx, it is pressed firmly beyond the midpoint of the tongue to avoid a gagging response.

Trachea

Next, the position and mobility of the trachea are noted by direct palpation. This is performed by placing the thumb and

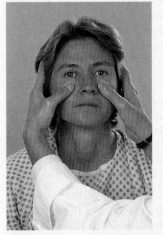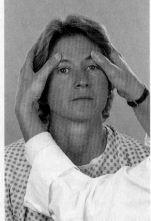

FIGURE 20-7 • Technique for palpating the frontal sinuses at left and the maxillary sinuses at right.

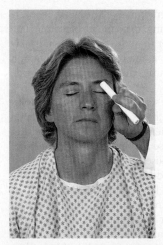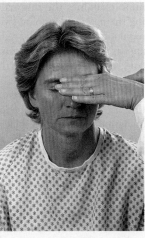

FIGURE 20-8 • At left, the nurse positions the light source for transillumination of the frontal sinus. At right, the nurse shields the patient's brow and shines the light. In normal conditions (a darkened room), the light should shine through the tissues and appear as a reddish glow (above the nurse's hand) over the sinus.

index finger of one hand on either side of the trachea just above the sternal notch. The trachea is highly sensitive, and palpating too firmly may trigger a coughing or gagging response. The trachea is normally in the midline as it enters the thoracic inlet behind the sternum; however, it may be deviated by masses in the neck or mediastinum. Pulmonary disorders such as a pneumothorax or pleural effusion may also displace the trachea.

Lower Respiratory Structures and Breathing

Assessment of the lower respiratory structures includes inspection, palpation, percussion, and auscultation of the thorax. The patient should be positioned as necessary prior to the assessment.

Positioning

To assess the posterior thorax and lungs, the patient should be in a sitting position with arms crossed in front of the chest and hands placed on the opposite shoulders (Bickley, 2009). This position separates the scapulae widely and exposes more lung area for assessment. If the patient is unable to sit, with the patient supine, the nurse should roll the patient from side to side to complete the posterior exam. To assess the anterior thorax and lungs, the patient should be either supine or sitting. The supine position allows easier displacement of the patient's breast tissue, improving the nurse's ability to perform the chest exam.

Thoracic Inspection

Inspection of the thorax provides information about the respiratory system, the musculoskeletal structure, and the patient's nutritional status. The nurse observes the skin over the thorax for color and turgor and for evidence of loss of subcutaneous tissue. It is important to note asymmetry, if present. In recording or reporting the findings, anatomic landmarks are used as points of reference (Chart 20-9).

Chest Configuration. Normally, the ratio of the anteroposterior diameter to the lateral diameter is 1:2. However, there are four main deformities of the chest associated with respiratory disease that alter this relationship: barrel chest, funnel

chest (pectus excavatum), pigeon chest (pectus carinatum), and kyphoscoliosis.

Barrel Chest. Barrel chest occurs as a result of overinflation of the lungs, which increases the anteroposterior diameter of the thorax. It occurs with aging and is a hallmark sign of emphysema and COPD. In a patient with emphysema, the ribs are more widely spaced and the intercostal spaces tend to bulge on expiration. The appearance of the patient with advanced emphysema is thus quite characteristic, allowing the nurse to detect its presence easily, even from a distance.

Funnel Chest (Pectus Excavatum). Funnel chest occurs when there is a depression in the lower portion of the sternum. This may compress the heart and great vessels, resulting in murmurs. Funnel chest may occur with rickets or Marfan's syndrome.

Pigeon Chest (Pectus Carinatum). A pigeon chest occurs as a result of the anterior displacement of the sternum, which also increases the anteroposterior diameter. This may occur with rickets, Marfan syndrome, or severe kyphoscoliosis.

Kyphoscoliosis. Kyphoscoliosis is characterized by elevation of the scapula and a corresponding S-shaped spine. This deformity limits lung expansion within the thorax. It may occur with osteoporosis and other skeletal disorders that affect the thorax.

Breathing Patterns and Respiratory Rates. Observing the rate and depth of respiration is a simple but important aspect of assessment. The normal adult who is resting comfortably takes 14 to 20 breaths per minute (Bickley, 2009; Massey & Meredith, 2010). Except for occasional sighs, respirations are quiet and regular in depth and rhythm. This normal pattern is described as eupnea. Certain patterns of respiration are characteristic of specific disease states. Respiratory rhythms and their deviation from normal are important observations that the nurse reports and documents. The rate and depth of various patterns of respiration are presented in Table 20-3.

 Concept Mastery Alert

There are subtle differences between Cheyne-Stokes and Biot's respiration patterns. Between regularly cycled periods of apnea, Cheyne-Stokes respirations demonstrate a regular pattern with the rate and depth of breathing increasing and then decreasing. In Biot's respiration, irregularly cycled periods of apnea are interspersed with cycles of normal rate and depth.

Temporary pauses of breathing, or **apnea**, may be noted. When apneas occur repeatedly during sleep, secondary to transient upper airway blockage, the condition is called **obstructive sleep apnea**. In thin people, it is quite normal to note a slight retraction of the intercostal spaces during quiet breathing. Bulging of the intercostal spaces during expiration implies obstruction of expiratory airflow, as in emphysema. Marked retraction on inspiration, particularly if asymmetric, implies blockage of a branch of the respiratory tree. Asymmetric bulging of the intercostal spaces, on either side of the thorax, is created by an increase in pressure within the hemithorax. This may be a result of air trapped under pressure within the pleural cavity, where it is not normally present

Chart 20-9 | **Locating Thoracic Landmarks**

With respect to the thorax, location is defined both horizontally and vertically. With respect to the lungs, location is defined by lobe.

Horizontal Reference Points

Horizontally, thoracic locations are identified according to their proximity to the rib or the intercostal space under the examiner's fingers. On the anterior surface, identification of a specific rib is facilitated by first locating the angle of Louis. This is where the manubrium joins the body of the sternum in the midline. The second rib joins the sternum at this prominent landmark.

Other ribs may be identified by counting down from the second rib. The intercostal spaces are referred to in terms of the rib immediately above the intercostal space; for example, the fifth intercostal space is directly below the fifth rib.

Locating ribs on the posterior surface of the thorax is more difficult. The first step is to identify the spinous process. This is accomplished by finding the seventh cervical vertebra (*vertebra prominens*), which is the most prominent spinous process. When the neck is slightly flexed, the seventh cervical spinous process stands out. Other vertebrae are then identified by counting downward.

Vertical Reference Points

Several imaginary lines are used as vertical referents or landmarks to identify the location of thoracic findings. The *midsternal line* passes through the center of the sternum. The *midclavicular line* is an imaginary line that descends from the middle of the

clavicle. The *point of maximal impulse* of the heart normally lies along this line on the left thorax.

When the arm is abducted from the body at 90 degrees, imaginary vertical lines may be drawn from the anterior axillary fold, from the middle of the axilla, and from the posterior axillary fold. These lines are called, respectively, the *anterior axillary line,* the *midaxillary line,* and the *posterior axillary line.* A line drawn vertically through the superior and inferior poles of the scapula is called the *scapular line,* and a line drawn down the center of the vertebral column is called the *vertebral line.* Using these landmarks, for example, the examiner communicates findings by referring to an area of dullness extending from the vertebral to the scapular line between the seventh and tenth ribs on the right.

Lobes of the Lungs

The lobes of the lung may be mapped on the surface of the chest wall in the following manner. The line between the upper and lower lobes on the left begins at the fourth thoracic spinous process posteriorly, proceeds around to cross the fifth rib in the midaxillary line, and meets the sixth rib at the sternum. This line on the right divides the right middle lobe from the right lower lobe. The line dividing the right upper lobe from the middle lobe is an incomplete one that begins at the fifth rib in the midaxillary line, where it intersects the line between the upper and lower lobes and traverses horizontally to the sternum. Thus, the upper lobes are dominant on the anterior surface of the thorax, and the lower lobes are dominant on the posterior surface. There is no presentation of the right middle lobe on the posterior surface of the chest.

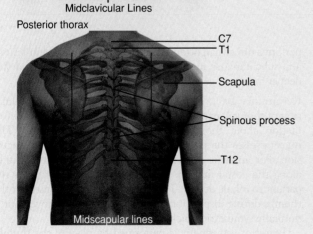

Anterior thorax — Clavicle, Suprasternal notch, First rib, First intercostal space, Angle of Louis, Manubrium, Xyphoid process, Costal angle, Costal margin, Midclavicular Lines

Posterior thorax — C7, T1, Scapula, Spinous process, T12, Midscapular lines

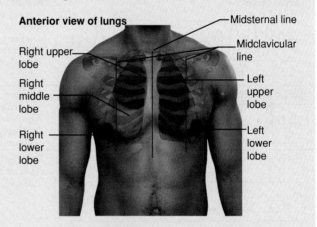

Anterior view of lungs — Midsternal line, Midclavicular line, Right upper lobe, Right middle lobe, Right lower lobe, Left upper lobe, Left lower lobe

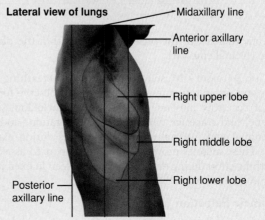

Lateral view of lungs — Midaxillary line, Anterior axillary line, Right upper lobe, Right middle lobe, Right lower lobe, Posterior axillary line

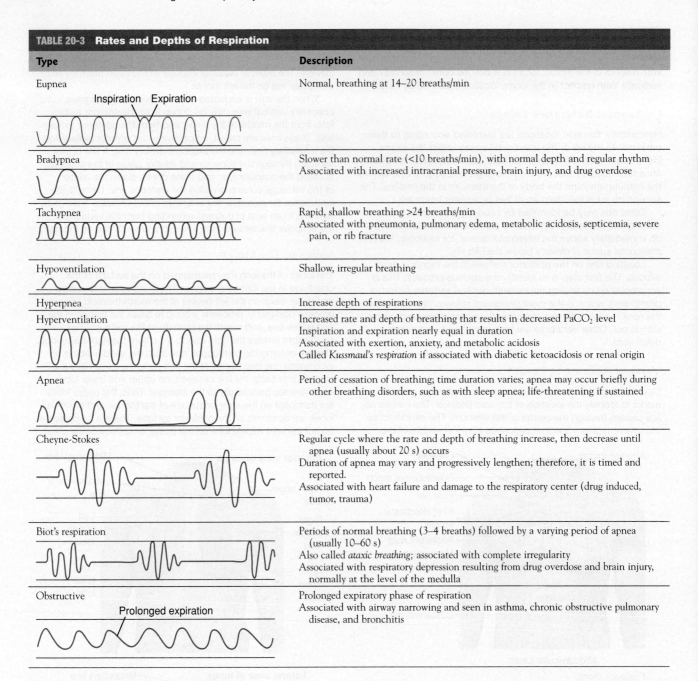

TABLE 20-3 **Rates and Depths of Respiration**

Type	Description
Eupnea	Normal, breathing at 14–20 breaths/min
Bradypnea	Slower than normal rate (<10 breaths/min), with normal depth and regular rhythm Associated with increased intracranial pressure, brain injury, and drug overdose
Tachypnea	Rapid, shallow breathing >24 breaths/min Associated with pneumonia, pulmonary edema, metabolic acidosis, septicemia, severe pain, or rib fracture
Hypoventilation	Shallow, irregular breathing
Hyperpnea	Increase depth of respirations
Hyperventilation	Increased rate and depth of breathing that results in decreased $PaCO_2$ level Inspiration and expiration nearly equal in duration Associated with exertion, anxiety, and metabolic acidosis Called *Kussmaul's respiration* if associated with diabetic ketoacidosis or renal origin
Apnea	Period of cessation of breathing; time duration varies; apnea may occur briefly during other breathing disorders, such as with sleep apnea; life-threatening if sustained
Cheyne-Stokes	Regular cycle where the rate and depth of breathing increase, then decrease until apnea (usually about 20 s) occurs Duration of apnea may vary and progressively lengthen; therefore, it is timed and reported. Associated with heart failure and damage to the respiratory center (drug induced, tumor, trauma)
Biot's respiration	Periods of normal breathing (3–4 breaths) followed by a varying period of apnea (usually 10–60 s) Also called *ataxic breathing*; associated with complete irregularity Associated with respiratory depression resulting from drug overdose and brain injury, normally at the level of the medulla
Obstructive	Prolonged expiratory phase of respiration Associated with airway narrowing and seen in asthma, chronic obstructive pulmonary disease, and bronchitis

(pneumothorax), or the pressure of fluid within the pleural space (pleural effusion).

Use of Accessory Muscles. In addition to breathing patterns and respiratory rates, the nurse should observe for the use of accessory muscles, such as the sternocleidomastoid, scalene, and trapezius muscles during inspiration, and the abdominal and internal intercostal muscles during expiration. These muscles provide additional support to assist the breathing effort during times of exertion as seen in exercise or certain disease states (Bickley, 2009).

Thoracic Palpation

The nurse palpates the thorax for tenderness, masses, lesions, respiratory excursion, and vocal fremitus. If the patient has reported an area of pain or if lesions are apparent, the nurse performs direct palpation with the fingertips (for skin lesions and subcutaneous masses) or with the ball of the hand (for deeper masses or generalized flank or rib discomfort).

Respiratory Excursion. Respiratory excursion is an estimation of thoracic expansion and may disclose significant information about thoracic movement during breathing. The nurse assesses the patient for range and symmetry of excursion. For anterior assessment, the nurse places the thumbs along the costal margin of the chest wall and instructs the patient to inhale deeply. The nurse observes movement of the thumbs during inspiration and expiration. This movement is normally symmetric (Bickley, 2009).

Posterior assessment is performed by placing the thumbs adjacent to the spinal column at the level of the 10th rib (Fig. 20-9). The hands lightly grasp the lateral rib cage. Sliding the

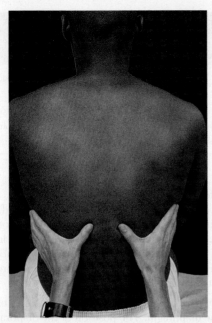

FIGURE 20-9 • Method for assessing posterior respiratory excursion. Place both hands posteriorly at the level of T9 or T10. Slide hands medially to pinch a small amount of skin between your thumbs. Observe for symmetry as the patient exhales fully following a deep inspiration.

thumbs medially about 2.5 cm (1 inch) raises a small skin fold between the thumbs. The patient is instructed to take a full inspiration and to exhale fully. The nurse observes for normal flattening of the skin fold and feels the symmetric movement of the thorax.

Decreased chest excursion may be caused by chronic fibrotic disease. Asymmetric excursion may be due to splinting secondary to pleurisy, fractured ribs, trauma, or unilateral bronchial obstruction.

Tactile Fremitus. Tactile **fremitus** describes vibrations of the chest wall that result from speech detected on palpation. Normally, sounds generated by the larynx travel distally along the bronchial tree to set the chest wall in resonant motion. This is most pronounced with consonant sounds.

Normal fremitus varies based on numerous factors. It is influenced by the thickness of the chest wall, especially muscle, and the subcutaneous tissue associated with obesity. It is also influenced by pitch; lower-pitched sounds travel better through the normal lung and produce greater vibration of the chest wall. Therefore, fremitus is more pronounced in men than in women because of the deeper male voice. Normally, fremitus is most pronounced where the large bronchi are closest to the chest wall, is more prominent on the right side, and is least palpable over the lower lung fields (Bickley, 2009).

The patient is asked to repeat "ninety-nine" or "one, two, three," or "eee, eee, eee," as the nurse's hands move down the patient's thorax. The vibrations are detected with the palmar surfaces of the fingers and hands, or the ulnar aspect of the extended hands, on the thorax. The hand or hands are moved in sequence down the thorax. Corresponding areas of the thorax are compared (Fig. 20-10). Bony areas are not assessed.

Air does not conduct sound well; however, a solid substance such as tissue does, provided that it has elasticity and is not compressed. Therefore, an increase in solid tissue per unit volume of lung enhances fremitus, and an increase in air per unit volume of lung impedes sound. Patients with emphysema exhibit almost no tactile fremitus. A patient with consolidation of a lobe of the lung from pneumonia has increased tactile fremitus over that lobe. Air in the pleural space does not conduct sound (Bickley, 2009).

Thoracic Percussion

Percussion produces audible and tactile vibration and allows the nurse to determine whether underlying tissues are filled

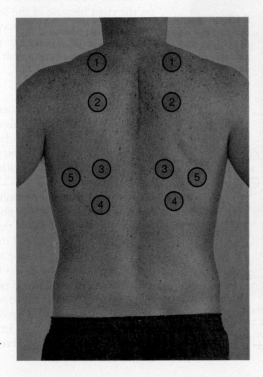 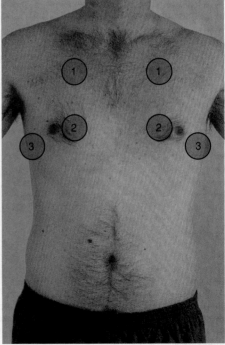

FIGURE 20-10 • Palpation sequence for tactile fremitus: posterior thorax (*left*) and anterior thorax (*right*).

TABLE 20-4	**Characteristics of Percussion Sounds**				
Sound	**Relative Intensity**	**Relative Pitch**	**Relative Duration**	**Location Example**	**Examples**
Flatness	Soft	High	Short	Thigh	Large pleural effusion
Dullness	Medium	Medium	Medium	Liver	Lobar pneumonia
Resonance	Loud	Low	Long	Normal lung	Simple chronic bronchitis
Hyperresonance	Very loud	Lower	Longer	None normally	Emphysema, pneumothorax
Tympany	Loud	High*	Medium	Gastric air bubble or puffed-out cheek	Large pneumothorax

*Distinguished mainly by its musical timbre.

with air, fluid, or solid material. Healthy lung tissue is resonant. Dullness over the lung occurs when air-filled lung tissue is replaced by fluid or solid tissue. Table 20-4 reviews percussion sounds and their characteristics. Percussion is also used to estimate the size and location of certain structures within the thorax (e.g., diaphragm, heart, liver).

Percussion usually begins with the posterior thorax. The nurse percusses across each shoulder top, locating the 5-cm width of resonance overlying the lung apices (Fig. 20-11). Then the nurse proceeds down the posterior thorax, percussing symmetric areas at intervals of 5 to 6 cm (2 to 2.5 inches). To perform percussion, the middle finger of the nondominant hand is firmly placed against the area of the chest wall to be percussed. The distal interphalangeal joint of this finger is struck with the tip of the middle finger of the dominant hand. This finger is partially flexed and percussion occurs in a smooth, dartlike fashion. Bony structures (scapulae or ribs) are not percussed.

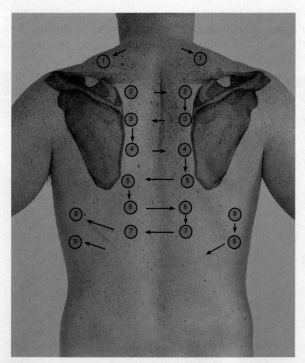

FIGURE 20-11 • Percussion of the posterior thorax. With the patient in a sitting position, symmetric areas of the lungs are percussed at 5-cm intervals. This progression starts at the apex of each lung and concludes with percussion of each lateral chest wall.

To perform percussion over the anterior chest, the nurse begins in the supraclavicular area and proceeds downward, from one intercostal space to the next. Dullness noted to the left of the sternum between the third and fifth intercostal spaces is a normal finding, because that is the location of the heart. Similarly, there is a normal span of liver dullness below the lung at the right costal margin (Bickley, 2009).

Diaphragmatic Excursion. The normal resonance of the lung stops at the diaphragm. The position of the diaphragm is different during inspiration and expiration.

To assess the position and motion of the diaphragm, the nurse instructs the patient to take a deep breath and hold it while the maximal descent of the diaphragm is percussed. The point at which the percussion note at the midscapular line changes from resonance to dullness is marked with a pen. The patient is then instructed to exhale fully and hold it while the nurse again percusses downward to the dullness of the diaphragm. This point is also marked. The distance between the two markings indicates the range of motion of the diaphragm.

Maximal excursion of the diaphragm may be as much as 8 to 10 cm (3 to 4 inches) in healthy, tall young men, but for most people it is usually 5 to 7 cm (2 to 2.75 inches). Normally, the diaphragm is about 2 cm (0.75 inches) higher on the right because of the location of the liver. Decreased diaphragmatic excursion may occur with pleural effusion. Atelectasis, diaphragmatic paralysis, or pregnancy may account for a diaphragm that is positioned high in the thorax (Bickley, 2009).

Thoracic Auscultation

Assessment concludes with auscultation of the anterior, posterior, and lateral thorax. Auscultation helps the nurse assess the flow of air through the bronchial tree and evaluate the presence of fluid or solid obstruction in the lung. The nurse auscultates for normal breath sounds, adventitious sounds, and voice sounds.

The nurse places the diaphragm of the stethoscope firmly against the bare skin of the chest wall as the patient breathes slowly and deeply through the mouth. Corresponding areas of the chest are auscultated in a systematic fashion from the apices to the bases and along midaxillary lines. The sequence of auscultation is similar to that used for percussion. The nurse may need to listen to two full inspirations and expirations at each anatomic location for valid interpretation of the sound heard. Repeated deep breaths may result in symptoms of hyperventilation (e.g., lightheadedness); this is avoided by having the patient rest and breathe normally periodically during the examination.

TABLE 20-5   Breath Sounds

	Duration of Sounds	Intensity of Expiratory Sound	Pitch of Expiratory Sound	Locations Where Heard Normally
Vesicular*	Inspiratory sounds last longer than expiratory ones.	Soft	Relatively low	Entire lung field except over the upper sternum and between the scapulae
Bronchovesicular	Inspiratory and expiratory sounds are about equal.	Intermediate	Intermediate	Often in the 1st and 2nd interspaces anteriorly and between the scapulae (over the main bronchus)
Bronchial	Expiratory sounds last longer than inspiratory ones.	Loud	Relatively high	Over the manubrium, if heard at all
Tracheal	Inspiratory and expiratory sounds are about equal.	Very loud	Relatively high	Over the trachea in the neck

*The thickness of the bars indicates intensity of breath sounds: The steeper their incline, the higher the pitch of the sounds.

Breath Sounds. Normal breath sounds are distinguished by their location over a specific area of the lung and are identified as vesicular, bronchovesicular, and bronchial (tubular) breath sounds (Table 20-5).

The location, quality, and intensity of breath sounds are determined during auscultation. When airflow is decreased by bronchial obstruction (atelectasis) or when fluid (pleural effusion) or tissue (obesity) separates the air passages from the stethoscope, breath sounds are diminished or absent. For example, the breath sounds of the patient with emphysema are faint or often completely inaudible. When they are heard, the expiratory phase is prolonged. In the patient who is obese, breath sounds may be inaudible. Bronchial and bronchovesicular sounds that are audible anywhere except over the main bronchus in the lungs signify pathology, usually indicating consolidation in the lung (e.g., pneumonia, heart failure). This finding requires further evaluation.

Adventitious Sounds. An abnormal condition that affects the bronchial tree and alveoli may produce adventitious (additional) sounds. Some adventitious sounds are divided into two categories: discrete, discontinuous sounds (**crackles**) and continuous musical sounds (**wheezes**) (Table 20-6). The duration of the sound is the important distinction to make in identifying the sound as discontinuous or continuous. Friction rubs may be either discontinuous or continuous.

Voice Sounds. The sound heard through the stethoscope as the patient speaks is known as vocal resonance. The nurse should assess voice sounds when abnormal breath sounds are auscultated. The vibrations produced in the larynx are transmitted to the chest wall as they pass through the bronchi and alveolar tissue. Voice sounds are evaluated by having the patient repeat "ninety-nine" or "eee" while the nurse listens with the stethoscope in corresponding areas of the chest from the apices to the bases. With normal physiology, the sounds are faint and indistinct. Pathology that increases lung density, such as pneumonia and pulmonary edema, alters this normal physiologic response and may result in the following sounds:

- **Bronchophony** describes vocal resonance that is more intense and clearer than normal.

- **Egophony** describes voice sounds that are distorted. It is best appreciated by having the patient repeat the letter E. The distortion produced by consolidation transforms the sound into a clearly heard A rather than E.
- **Whispered pectoriloquy** describes the ability to clearly and distinctly hear whispered sounds that should not normally be heard.

Whenever an abnormality is detected on exam, it should be evident using more than one assessment method. A change in tactile fremitus is more subtle and can be missed, but bronchophony can be noted loudly and clearly.

Interpreting Findings

The physical findings for the most common respiratory diseases are summarized in Table 20-7.

Assessment of Respiratory Function in the Acutely or Critically Ill Patient

Assessment of respiratory status is essential for the well-being of the patient who is acutely or critically ill. Often, such a patient is intubated and receiving mechanical ventilation. In addition to expertise in physical assessment, the nurse should be skilled in monitoring techniques and knowledgeable about possible ventilator-induced lung injury. The nurse reviews the patient's health history and performs a detailed assessment as described previously. The nurse analyzes these findings while considering laboratory and diagnostic results. After checking the ventilator settings to make sure that they are set as prescribed and that alarms are always in the "on" position, the nurse must assess for patient–ventilator synchrony and for agitation, restlessness, and other signs of respiratory distress (nasal flaring, excessive use of intercostals and accessory muscles, uncoordinated movement of the chest and abdomen, and a report by the patient of shortness of breath). The nurse must note changes in the patient's vital signs and evidence of hemodynamic instability and report them to the physician, because they may indicate that the mechanical ventilation is ineffective or that the patient's status has deteriorated. The patient's position must be assessed to ensure that the head of the bed is elevated to prevent aspiration, especially if the patient is receiving enteral feedings.

TABLE 20-6 Abnormal (Adventitious) Breath Sounds

Breath Sound	Description	Etiology
Crackles		
Crackles in general	Soft, high-pitched, discontinuous popping sounds that occur during inspiration (while usually heard on inspiration, they may also be heard on expiration); may or may not be cleared by coughing	Secondary to fluid in the airways or alveoli or to delayed opening of collapsed alveoli Associated with heart failure and pulmonary fibrosis
Coarse crackles	Discontinuous popping sounds heard in early inspiration; harsh, moist sound originating in the large bronchi	Associated with obstructive pulmonary disease
Fine crackles	Discontinuous popping sounds heard in late inspiration; sounds like hair rubbing together; originates in the alveoli	Associated with interstitial pneumonia, restrictive pulmonary disease (e.g., fibrosis); fine crackles in early inspiration are associated with bronchitis or pneumonia
Wheezes		
Wheezes in general	Usually heard on expiration but may be heard on inspiration depending on the cause	Associated with bronchial wall oscillation and changes in airway diameter Associated with chronic bronchitis or bronchiectasis
Sonorous wheezes (rhonchi)	Deep, low-pitched rumbling sounds heard primarily during expiration; caused by air moving through narrowed tracheo-bronchial passages	Associated with secretions or tumor
Sibilant wheezes	Continuous, musical, high-pitched, whistlelike sounds heard during inspiration and expiration caused by air passing through narrowed or partially obstructed airways; may clear with coughing	Associated with bronchospasm, asthma, and buildup of secretions
Friction Rubs		
Pleural friction rub	Harsh, crackling sound, like two pieces of leather being rubbed together (sound imitated by rubbing thumb and finger together near the ear) Heard during inspiration alone or during both inspiration and expiration May subside when patient holds breath; coughing will not clear sound Best heard over the lower lateral anterior surface of the thorax Sound can be enhanced by applying pressure to the chest wall with the diaphragm of the stethoscope.	Secondary to inflammation and loss of lubricating pleural fluid

In addition, the patient's mental status should be assessed and compared to previous status. Lethargy and somnolence may be signs of increasing carbon dioxide levels and should not be considered insignificant, even if the patient is receiving sedation or analgesic agents.

Chest auscultation, percussion, and palpation are essential and routine parts of the evaluation of the critically ill patient with or without mechanical ventilation. A recumbent patient must be turned to assess all lung fields. Dependent areas must be assessed for normal breath sounds and adventitious sounds. Failure to examine the dependent areas of the lungs can result in missing the findings associated with disorders such as atelectasis or pleural effusion. Percussion is performed to assess for pleural effusion; if pleural effusion is present, the affected lung fields are dull to percussion and breath sounds are absent. Upon auscultation, a pleural friction rub may also be present.

Tests of the patient's respiratory status are easily performed at the bedside by measuring the respiratory rate, tidal volume, minute ventilation, vital capacity, inspiratory force, and compliance. These tests are particularly important for patients who are at risk for pulmonary complications, including those who have undergone chest or abdominal surgery, have had

TABLE 20-7 Assessment Findings in Common Respiratory Disorders

Disorder	Tactile Fremitus	Percussion	Auscultation
Consolidation (e.g., pneumonia)	Increased	Dull	Bronchial breath sounds, crackles, bronchophony, egophony, whispered pectoriloquy
Bronchitis	Normal	Resonant	Normal to decreased breath sounds; possible scattered coarse crackles, rhonchi, or wheezes
Emphysema	Decreased	Hyperresonant	Absent or decreased breath sounds; possible crackles, wheezes, or rhonchi
Asthma	Decreased	Resonant to hyperresonant	Wheezes, occasional crackles
Pulmonary edema	Normal	Resonant	Crackles at lung bases, possibly wheezes
Pleural effusion	Decreased to absent but may be increased over large effusion	Dull to flat	Decreased to absent breath sounds, bronchial breath sounds sometimes heard atop of large effusion, possible pleural rub
Pneumothorax	Decreased to absent	Hyperresonant	Absent breath sounds, possible pleural rub
Atelectasis	Absent	Dull	Decreased to absent breath sounds; may be increased in right upper lobe atelectasis

prolonged anesthesia, or have preexisting pulmonary disease, and those who are older or obese. These tests are also used routinely for mechanically ventilated patients. Although some of these tests are performed by respiratory therapists or technicians, it is useful for nurses to understand the significance of results of these tests.

The patient whose chest expansion is limited by external restrictions such as obesity or abdominal distention and who cannot breathe deeply because of postoperative pain or sedation will inhale and exhale a low volume of air (referred to as low tidal volumes). Prolonged hypoventilation at low tidal volumes can produce alveolar collapse (atelectasis). Consequently, when the forced residual capacity decreases, compliance is reduced, and the patient must breathe faster to maintain the same degree of tissue oxygenation. These events can be exaggerated in patients who have preexisting pulmonary diseases; in older adult patients whose airways are less compliant because the small airways may collapse during expiration; or in patients who are obese, who have relatively low tidal volumes even when healthy. (More details of the assessment of the patient with lung disease are described in subsequent chapters in this unit and in Chapter 13.)

> ◢ *Quality and Safety Nursing Alert*
>
> The nurse should not rely only on visual inspection of the rate and depth of a patient's respiratory excursions to determine the adequacy of ventilation. Respiratory excursions may appear normal or exaggerated due to an increased work of breathing, but the patient may actually be moving only enough air to ventilate the dead space. If there is any question regarding adequacy of ventilation, the nurse should use auscultation or pulse oximetry (or both) for additional assessment of respiratory status.

Tidal Volume

The volume of each breath is referred to as the **tidal volume** (see Table 20-1 to review lung capacities and volumes). A spirometer is an instrument that can be used at the bedside to measure volumes. If the patient is breathing through an endotracheal tube or tracheostomy, the spirometer is directly attached to it and the exhaled volume is obtained from the reading on the gauge. In other patients, the spirometer is attached to a facemask or a mouthpiece positioned so that it is airtight, and the exhaled volume is measured.

The tidal volume may vary from breath to breath. To ensure that the measurement is reliable, it is important to measure the volumes of several breaths and to note the range of tidal volumes, together with the average tidal volume.

Minute Ventilation

Because respiratory rates and tidal volumes vary widely from breath to breath, these data alone are unreliable indicators of adequate ventilation. However, the tidal volume multiplied by the respiratory rate provides what is called *minute ventilation* or *minute volume*, the volume of air exchanged per minute. This value is useful in detecting respiratory failure. In practice, the minute volume is not calculated but is measured

> **Chart**
> **20-10** ⚠ **RISK FACTORS**
> ## Hypoventilation
>
> - Limited neurologic impulses transmitted from the brain to the respiratory muscles, as in spinal cord trauma, cerebrovascular accidents, tumors, myasthenia gravis, Guillain-Barré syndrome, polio, and drug overdose
> - Depressed respiratory centers in the medulla, as with anesthesia, sedation, and drug overdose
> - Limited thoracic movement (kyphoscoliosis), limited lung movement (pleural effusion, pneumothorax), or reduced functional lung tissue (chronic pulmonary diseases, severe pulmonary edema)

directly using a spirometer. In a patient receiving mechanical ventilation, minute volume is often monitored by the ventilator and can be viewed on the monitoring screen.

Minute ventilation may be decreased by a variety of conditions that result in hypoventilation. When the minute ventilation falls, alveolar ventilation in the lungs also decreases, and the $PaCO_2$ increases. Risk factors for hypoventilation are listed in Chart 20-10.

Vital Capacity

Vital capacity is measured by having the patient take in a maximal breath and exhale fully through a spirometer. The normal value depends on the patient's age, gender, body build, and weight.

> ◢ *Quality and Safety Nursing Alert*
>
> Most patients can generate a vital capacity twice the volume they normally breathe in and out (tidal volume). If the vital capacity is less than 10 mL/kg, the patient will be unable to sustain spontaneous ventilation and will require respiratory assistance.

When the vital capacity is exhaled at a maximal flow rate, the forced vital capacity (FVC) is measured. Most patients can exhale at least 80% of their vital capacity in 1 second (forced expiratory volume in 1 second, or FEV_1) and almost all of it in 3 seconds (FEV_3). A reduction in FEV_1 suggests abnormal pulmonary airflow. If the patient's FEV_1 and FVC are proportionately reduced, maximal lung expansion is restricted in some way. If the reduction in FEV_1 greatly exceeds the reduction in FVC (FEV_1/FVC less than 85%), the patient may have some degree of airway obstruction.

Inspiratory Force

Inspiratory force evaluates the effort the patient is making during inspiration. It does not require patient cooperation and therefore is a useful measurement in the patient who is unconscious. The equipment needed for this measurement includes a manometer that measures negative pressure and adapters that are connected to an anesthesia mask or a cuffed endotracheal tube. The manometer is attached, and the airway is completely occluded for 10 to 20 seconds while the inspiratory efforts of the patient are registered on the manometer. The normal inspiratory pressure is about 100 cm H_2O. If the negative pressure registered after 15 seconds of occluding the airway is less than about 25 cm H_2O, mechanical ventilation is usually required because the patient lacks sufficient muscle strength for deep breathing or effective coughing.

Diagnostic Evaluation

A wide range of diagnostic studies may be performed in patients with respiratory conditions. The nurse should educate the patient on the purpose of the studies, what to expect, and any possible side effects related to these examinations prior to testing. The nurse should note trends in results because they provide information about disease progression as well as the patient's response to therapy.

Pulmonary Function Tests

Pulmonary function tests (PFTs) are routinely used in patients with chronic respiratory disorders to aid diagnosis. They are performed to assess respiratory function and to determine the extent of dysfunction, response to therapy, and as screening tests in potentially hazardous industries, such as coal mining and those that involve exposure to asbestos and other noxious irritants. PFTs are also used prior to surgery to screen patients who are scheduled for thoracic and upper abdominal surgical procedures, patients who are obese, and symptomatic patients with a history suggesting high risk. Such tests include measurements of lung volumes, ventilatory function, and the mechanics of breathing, diffusion, and gas exchange.

PFTs generally are performed by a technician using a spirometer that has a volume-collecting device attached to a recorder that demonstrates volume and time simultaneously. Several tests are carried out because no single measurement provides a complete picture of pulmonary function. The most frequently used PFTs are described in Table 20-8. Technology is available that allows for more complex assessment of pulmonary function. Methods include exercise tidal flow–volume loops, negative expiratory pressure, nitric oxide, forced oscillation, and diffusing capacity for helium or carbon monoxide. These assessment methods allow for detailed evaluation of expiratory flow limitations and airway inflammation.

PFT results are interpreted on the basis of the degree of deviation from normal, taking into consideration the patient's height, weight, age, gender, and ethnicity. Because there is a wide range of normal values, PFTs may not detect early localized changes. The patient with respiratory symptoms usually undergoes a complete diagnostic evaluation, even if the results of PFTs are "normal." Patients with respiratory disorders may be taught how to measure their peak flow rate (which reflects maximal expiratory flow) at home using a spirometer. This allows them to monitor the progress of therapy, to alter medications and other interventions as needed based on caregiver guidelines, and to notify the health care provider if there is inadequate response to their own interventions. (Instructions for home care education are described in Chapter 24, which discusses asthma.)

Arterial Blood Gas Studies

Arterial blood gas (ABG) studies aid in assessing the ability of the lungs to provide adequate oxygen and remove carbon dioxide, which reflects ventilation, and the ability of the kidneys to reabsorb or excrete bicarbonate ions to maintain normal body pH, which reflects metabolic states. ABG levels are obtained through an arterial puncture at the radial, brachial, or femoral artery or through an indwelling arterial catheter. Pain (related to nerve injury or noxious stimulation), infection, and hemorrhage are potential complications that may be associated with obtaining ABGs (Chulay & Burns, 2010; Potter & Perry, 2010). (See Chapter 13 for discussion of ABG analysis.)

Pulse Oximetry

Pulse oximetry, or SpO_2, is a noninvasive method of continuously monitoring the **oxygen saturation** of hemoglobin (SaO_2). Although pulse oximetry does not replace ABG measurement, it is an effective tool to monitor for subtle or sudden changes in SaO_2 and can easily be used in the home and various health care settings.

A probe or sensor is attached to the fingertip (Fig. 20-12), forehead, earlobe, or bridge of the nose. The sensor detects

TABLE 20-8	Pulmonary Function Tests			
Term Used	**Symbol**	**Description**	**Remarks**	
Forced vital capacity	FVC	Vital capacity performed with a maximally forced expiratory effort	Forced vital capacity is often reduced in chronic obstructive pulmonary disease because of air trapping.	
Forced expiratory volume (qualified by subscript indicating the time interval in seconds)	FEV_t (usually FEV_1)	Volume of air exhaled in the specified time during the performance of forced vital capacity; FEV_1 is volume exhaled in 1 s	A valuable clue to the severity of the expiratory airway obstruction	
Ratio of timed forced expiratory volume to forced vital capacity	$FEV_t/FVC\%$, usually $FEV_1/FVC\%$	FEV_t expressed as a percentage of the forced vital capacity	Another way of expressing the presence or absence of airway obstruction	
Forced expiratory flow	$FEF_{200–1200}$	Mean forced expiratory flow between 200 and 1,200 mL of the FVC	An indicator of large airway obstruction	
Forced midexpiratory flow	$FEF_{25–75\%}$	Mean forced expiratory flow during the middle half of the FVC	Slowed in small airway obstruction	
Forced end expiratory flow	$FEF_{75–85\%}$	Mean forced expiratory flow during the terminal portion of the FVC	Slowed in obstruction of smallest airways	
Maximal voluntary ventilation	MVV	Volume of air expired in a specified period (12 s) during repetitive maximal effort	An important factor in exercise tolerance	

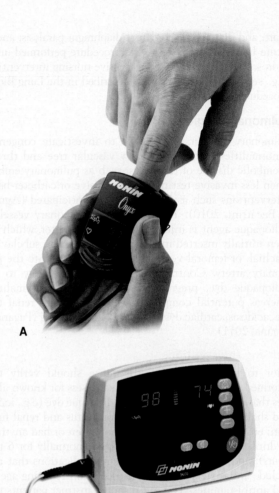

A

B

FIGURE 20-12 • Measuring blood oxygenation with pulse oximetry reduces the need for invasive procedures, such as drawing blood for analysis of oxygen levels. **A.** Self-contained digital fingertip pulse oximeter, which incorporates the sensor and the display into one unit. **B.** Tabletop model with sensor attached. Memory permits tracking heart rate and oxygen saturation over time.

changes in oxygen saturation levels by monitoring light signals generated by the oximeter and reflected by blood pulsing through the tissue at the probe. Normal SpO_2 values are 95% to 100%. Values less than 90% indicate that the tissues are not receiving enough oxygen, in which case further evaluation is needed. SpO_2 values are unreliable in cardiac arrest, shock, and other states of low perfusion (e.g., sepsis, peripheral vascular disease, hypothermia), and when vasoconstrictor medications have been used (Higginson & Jones, 2009). Additional causes of inaccurate pulse oximetry results include anemia, abnormal hemoglobin, high carbon monoxide level, the use of dyes (e.g., methylene blue), or if the patient has dark skin or is wearing nail polish. Bright light, particularly sunlight, fluorescent and xenon lights, and patient movement (including shivering) also affect accuracy. SpO_2 values cannot reliably detect hypoventilation when supplemental oxygen is in use (Higginson & Jones, 2009).

Cultures

Throat, nasal, and nasopharyngeal cultures can identify pathogens responsible for respiratory infections, such as pharyngitis. Throat cultures are performed in adults with severe or ongoing sore throats accompanied by fever and lymph node enlargement and are most useful in detecting streptococcal infection. Rapid strep tests are now available that can provide results within 15 minutes, often replacing the need for throat cultures. Other sources of infection, such as *Staphylococcus aureus* or *Influenza,* are detected via nasal or nasopharyngeal cultures. Ideally, all cultures should be obtained prior to the initiation of antibiotic therapy. Results usually take between 48 and 72 hours, with preliminary reports available usually within 24 hours. Cultures may be repeated to assess a patient's response to therapy (Pagana & Pagana, 2011).

Sputum Studies

Sputum is obtained for analysis to identify pathogenic organisms and to determine whether malignant cells are present. Periodic sputum examinations may be necessary for patients receiving antibiotics, corticosteroids, and immunosuppressive medications for prolonged periods because these agents are associated with opportunistic infections.

Sputum samples ideally are obtained early in the morning before the patient has had anything to eat or drink. The patient is instructed to clear the nose and throat and rinse the mouth to decrease contamination of the sputum, and not to simply spit saliva into the container. Rather, after taking a few deep breaths, the patient coughs deeply and expectorates sputum from the lungs into a sterile container.

If the patient cannot expel an adequate sputum sample following the above techniques, coughing can be induced by administering an aerosolized hypertonic solution via a nebulizer. Other methods of collecting sputum specimens include endotracheal or transtracheal aspiration or bronchoscopic removal. The nurse should label the specimen and send it to the laboratory as soon as possible to avoid contamination. (See Chapter 23 for procedures to obtain a sputum culture for tuberculosis.)

Imaging Studies

Imaging studies, including x-rays, computed tomography (CT), magnetic resonance imaging (MRI), and radioisotope or nuclear scans may be part of any diagnostic workup, ranging from a determination of the extent of infection in sinusitis to tumor growth in cancer.

Chest X-Ray

Normal pulmonary tissue is radiolucent because it consists mostly of air and gases; therefore, densities produced by fluid, tumors, foreign bodies, and other pathologic conditions can be detected by x-ray examination. In the absence of symptoms, a chest x-ray may reveal an extensive pathologic process in the lungs. The routine chest x-ray consists of two views: the posteroanterior projection and the lateral projection. Chest x-rays are usually taken after full inspiration because the lungs are best visualized when they are well aerated. In addition, the diaphragm is at its lowest level and the largest expanse of lung is visible. Patients therefore need to be able to take a deep breath and hold it without discomfort. Chest x-rays are contraindicated in pregnant women.

Computed Tomography

A CT scan is an imaging method in which the lungs are scanned in successive layers by a narrow-beam x-ray. The images produced provide a cross-sectional view of the chest. Whereas a chest x-ray shows major contrasts between body densities such as bone, soft tissue, and air, a CT scan can distinguish fine tissue density. A CT scan may be used to define pulmonary nodules and small tumors adjacent to pleural surfaces that are not visible on routine chest x-rays and to demonstrate mediastinal abnormalities and hilar adenopathy, which are difficult to visualize with other techniques. Contrast agents are useful when evaluating the mediastinum and its contents, particularly its vasculature. Advancements in CT scanning technology, referred to as multidetection, spiral, or helical CT, enable the chest to be scanned quickly while generating an extensive number of images that can generate a three-dimensional analysis; these newer methods have taken the place of more invasive testing (Pagana & Pagana, 2011). CT scans are now used routinely in place of pulmonary angiograms to diagnose pulmonary emboli (Agnelli & Becattini, 2010). Contraindications include allergy to dye, pregnancy, claustrophobia, and morbid obesity, whereas potential complications include acute renal failure and acidosis secondary to contrast (Pagana & Pagana, 2011).

Magnetic Resonance Imaging

MRI is similar to a CT scan except that magnetic fields and radiofrequency signals are used instead of radiation. MRI is able to better distinguish between normal and abnormal tissue when compared to CT and therefore yields a much more detailed diagnostic image. MRI is used to characterize pulmonary nodules; to help stage bronchogenic carcinoma (assessment of chest wall invasion); and to evaluate inflammatory activity in interstitial lung disease, acute pulmonary embolism, and chronic thrombolytic pulmonary hypertension. Patients scheduled for MRI should be instructed to remove all metal items such as hearing aids, hair clips, and medication patches with metallic foil components (e.g., nicotine patches). Contraindications for MRI include morbid obesity, claustrophobia, confusion and agitation, and having implanted metal or metal support devices that are considered unsafe (Pagana & Pagana, 2011). Various labels and icons are used to indicate if a medical device is safe or unsafe for use during MRI. Recent improvements in technology have contributed to the design of certain medical devices, such as infusion pumps and ventilators, deemed safe for the MRI room. The nurse should consult with specially trained MRI personnel to clarify the safety of various devices (Shellock & Spinazzi, 2008). Contrast agents used during MRI may potentially lead to the complication of acute renal failure (Pagana & Pagana, 2011; Shellock & Spinazzi, 2008).

Fluoroscopic Studies

Fluoroscopy, which allows live x-ray images to be generated via a camera to a video screen, is used to assist with invasive procedures, such as a chest needle biopsy or transbronchial biopsy, that are performed to identify lesions. It also may be used to study the movement of the chest wall, mediastinum, heart, and diaphragm; to detect diaphragm paralysis; and to locate lung masses. The specific procedure performed under fluoroscopy will guide those respective nursing interventions (e.g., see nursing interventions described in the Lung Biopsy Procedures section).

Pulmonary Angiography

Pulmonary angiography is used to investigate congenital abnormalities of the pulmonary vascular tree and thromboembolic disease of the lungs, such as pulmonary emboli, when less invasive testing is inconclusive or catheter-based interventions such as angioplasty are anticipated (Agnelli & Becattini, 2010). To visualize the pulmonary vessels, a radiopaque agent is injected through a catheter, which has been initially inserted into a vein (e.g., jugular, subclavian, brachial, or femoral vein) and then threaded into the pulmonary artery. Contraindications include allergy to the radiopaque dye, pregnancy, and bleeding abnormalities, whereas potential complications include acute renal failure, acidosis, cardiac dysrhythmias, and bleeding (Pagana & Pagana, 2011).

Nursing Interventions

Prior to the angiography, the nurse should verify that informed consent has been obtained; assess for known allergies that may suggest allergies to radiopaque dye (e.g., iodine and shellfish); assess anticoagulation status and renal function; ensure that the patient has not eaten or had anything to drink preprocedurally as prescribed (normally for 6 to 8 hours); and administer preprocedure medications that may include antianxiety medications, secretion-reducing agents, and antihistamines. The nurse should instruct patients that they may experience a warm flushing sensation or chest pain during the injection of the dye. If an arterial puncture is necessary, the affected extremity will need to be immobilized for a certain amount of time depending on the size of the sheath that was used and the type of arterial closure device employed. Following the procedure, the nurse should closely monitor vital signs, level of consciousness, oxygen saturation, and the vascular access site for bleeding or hematoma, and perform frequent assessment of neurovascular status (Potter & Perry, 2010).

Radioisotope Diagnostic Procedures (Lung Scans)

Several types of lung scans—$\dot{V}/\dot{Q}$ scan, gallium scan, and positron emission tomography (PET)—are used to assess normal lung functioning, pulmonary vascular supply, and gas exchange. Pregnancy is a contraindication for these scans.

A $\dot{V}/\dot{Q}$ lung scan is performed by injecting a radioactive agent into a peripheral vein and then obtaining a scan of the chest to detect radiation. The isotope particles pass through the right side of the heart and are distributed into the lungs in proportion to the regional blood flow, making it possible to trace and measure blood perfusion through the lung. This procedure is used clinically to measure the integrity of the pulmonary vessels relative to blood flow and to evaluate blood flow abnormalities, as seen in pulmonary emboli. The imaging time is 20 to 40 minutes, during which the patient lies under the camera with a mask fitted over the nose and mouth. This is followed by the ventilation component of the scan. The patient takes a deep breath of a mixture of oxygen and radioactive gas, which diffuses throughout the lungs. A scan is performed to detect ventilation abnormalities in patients who have regional differences in ventilation. It may be helpful in the diagnosis of bronchitis, asthma, inflammatory fibrosis, pneumonia, emphysema, and lung cancer. Ventilation without perfusion is seen with pulmonary emboli.

A gallium scan is a radioisotope lung scan used to detect inflammatory conditions; abscesses; adhesions; and the presence, location, and size of tumors. It is used to stage bronchogenic cancer and to document tumor regression after chemotherapy or radiation. Gallium is injected intravenously (IV), and scans are taken at intervals (e.g., 6, 24, and 48 hours) to evaluate gallium uptake by the pulmonary tissues.

PET is a radioisotope study with advanced diagnostic capabilities that is used to evaluate lung nodules for malignancy. PET can detect and display metabolic changes in tissue, distinguish normal tissue from diseased tissue (such as in cancer), differentiate viable from dead or dying tissue, show regional blood flow, and determine the distribution and fate of medications in the body. PET is more accurate in detecting malignancies than CT and has equivalent accuracy in detecting malignant nodules when compared with invasive procedures such as thoracoscopy. Images from PET scans are now being superimposed on CT and MRI films to enhance the accuracy of diagnosis (Pagana & Pagana, 2011).

Nursing Interventions

For each of these nuclear scans, the nurse should educate the patient on what to expect. IV access is required. Sometimes, an enema is prescribed prior to a gallium scan to decrease its uptake in the gastrointestinal tract. A chest x-ray should be performed prior to a $\dot{V}/\dot{Q}$ scan. Patients should be told that $\dot{V}/\dot{Q}$ and gallium scans require only a small amount of radioisotopes; therefore, radiation safety measures are not indicated. Normally, the patient may eat or drink prior to $\dot{V}/\dot{Q}$ or gallium scans. Multiple factors can hinder the uptake of radioactive agents used for a PET scan. The nurse should instruct the patient to avoid caffeine, alcohol, and tobacco for 24 hours prior to the PET scan and abstain from food and fluids for 4 hours prior to the scan. Accurate results depend on an empty bladder; thus, a Foley catheter may be indicated. The nurse should encourage fluid intake postprocedurally to facilitate the elimination of radioisotopes in the urine (Pagana & Pagana, 2011).

Endoscopic Procedures

Endoscopic procedures include bronchoscopy, thoracoscopy, and thoracentesis.

Bronchoscopy

Bronchoscopy is the direct inspection and examination of the larynx, trachea, and bronchi through either a flexible fiberoptic bronchoscope or a rigid bronchoscope (Fig. 20-13). The fiberoptic scope is used more frequently in current practice.

Procedure

The purposes of diagnostic bronchoscopy are (1) to visualize tissues and determine the nature, location, and extent of the pathologic process; (2) to collect secretions for analysis and to obtain a tissue sample for diagnosis; (3) to determine whether

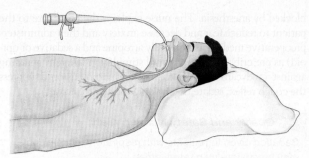

Fiberoptic bronchoscopy

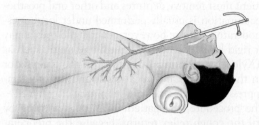

Rigid bronchoscopy

FIGURE 20-13 • Endoscopic bronchoscopy permits visualization of bronchial structures. The bronchoscope is advanced into bronchial structures orally. Bronchoscopy permits the clinician not only to diagnose but also to treat various lung problems.

a tumor can be resected surgically; and (4) to diagnose sources of hemoptysis.

Therapeutic bronchoscopy is used to (1) remove foreign bodies or secretions from the tracheobronchial tree, (2) control bleeding, (3) treat postoperative atelectasis, (4) destroy and excise lesions, and (5) provide brachytherapy (endobronchial radiation therapy). It has also been used to insert stents to relieve airway obstruction that is caused by tumors or miscellaneous benign conditions or that occurs as a complication of lung transplantation.

The fiberoptic bronchoscope is a thin, flexible bronchoscope that can be directed into the segmental bronchi. Because of its small size, its flexibility, and its excellent optical system, it allows increased visualization of the peripheral airways and is ideal for diagnosing pulmonary lesions. Fiberoptic bronchoscopy allows biopsy of previously inaccessible tumors and can be performed at the bedside. It also can be performed through endotracheal or tracheostomy tubes of patients on ventilators. Cytologic examinations can be performed without surgical intervention.

The rigid bronchoscope is a hollow metal tube with a light at its end. It is used mainly for removing foreign substances, investigating the source of massive hemoptysis, or performing endobronchial surgical procedures. Rigid bronchoscopy is performed in the operating room, not at the bedside.

Possible complications of bronchoscopy include a reaction to the local anesthetic, infection, aspiration, bronchospasm, hypoxemia, pneumothorax, bleeding, and perforation (Pagana & Pagana, 2011; Potter & Perry, 2010).

Nursing Interventions

Before the procedure, informed consent is obtained from the patient. Food and fluids are withheld for 4 to 8 hours before the test to reduce the risk of aspiration when the cough reflex is blocked by anesthesia. The nurse explains the procedure to the patient to reduce fear and decrease anxiety and then administers preoperative medications (usually atropine and a sedative or opioid) as prescribed to inhibit vagal stimulation (thereby guarding against bradycardia, dysrhythmias, and hypotension), suppress the cough reflex, sedate the patient, and relieve anxiety.

Quality and Safety Nursing Alert

Sedation given to patients with respiratory insufficiency may precipitate respiratory arrest.

The patient must remove dentures and other oral prostheses. The examination is usually performed under local anesthesia or moderate sedation; however, general anesthesia may be used for rigid bronchoscopy. A topical anesthetic such as lidocaine (Xylocaine) is normally sprayed on the pharynx or dropped on the epiglottis and vocal cords and into the trachea to suppress the cough reflex and minimize discomfort.

After the procedure, the patient must take nothing by mouth until the cough reflex returns, because the preoperative sedation and local anesthesia impair the protective laryngeal reflex and swallowing. Once the patient demonstrates a cough reflex, the nurse may offer ice chips and eventually fluids. In the older adult patient, the nurse assesses for confusion and lethargy, which may be owing to the large doses of lidocaine administered during the procedure. The nurse also monitors the patient's respiratory status and observes for hypoxia, hypotension, tachycardia, dysrhythmias, hemoptysis, and dyspnea. Any abnormality is reported promptly. A small amount of blood-tinged sputum and fever may be expected within the first 24 hours (Pagana & Pagana, 2011). The patient is not discharged from the recovery area until adequate cough reflex and respiratory status are present. The nurse instructs the patient and caregivers to report any shortness of breath or bleeding immediately.

Thoracoscopy

Thoracoscopy is a diagnostic procedure in which the pleural cavity is examined with an endoscope and fluid and tissues can be obtained for analysis (Fig. 20-14).

Procedure

This procedure is performed in the operating room, normally under anesthesia. Small incisions are made into the pleural cavity in an intercostal space, at the location indicated by clinical and diagnostic findings. The fiberoptic mediastinoscope is inserted into the pleural cavity, any fluid present is aspirated, and the pleural cavity is inspected through the instrument. After the procedure, a chest tube may be inserted to facilitate re-expansion of the lung.

Thoracoscopy is primarily indicated in the diagnostic evaluation and treatment of pleural effusions, pleural disease, and tumor staging. Biopsies of the lesions and resection of tissues can be performed under visualization for diagnosis.

Thoracoscopic procedures have expanded with the availability of video monitoring, which permits improved visualization of the lung. Video-assisted thoracoscopy (VATS) may be used in the diagnosis and treatment of empyema, pleural effusion, pulmonary and pleural masses, and pneumothorax. Although VATS does not replace the need for thoracotomy

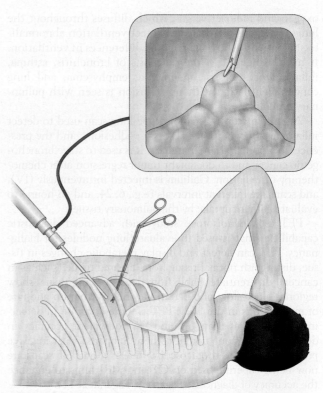

FIGURE 20-14 • Endoscopic thoracoscopy. Like bronchoscopy, thoracoscopy uses fiber-optic instruments and video cameras for visualizing thoracic structures. Unlike bronchoscopy, thoracoscopy usually requires the surgeon to make a small incision before inserting the endoscope. A combined diagnostic–treatment procedure, thoracoscopy includes excising tissue for biopsy.

in the treatment of some lung cancers, its use continues to expand, because it is less invasive than open surgical procedures and hospitalization and recovery are shorter.

Nursing Interventions

The nurse should follow routine preoperative practices, such as ensuring that informed consent is obtained and that the patient remains NPO (has nothing by mouth) prior to the procedure. Postoperatively, the nurse should monitor vital signs, pain level, and respiratory status, and should look for signs of bleeding and infection at the incisional site. Shortness of breath may indicate a pneumothorax and should be reported immediately. If a chest tube was inserted during the procedure, monitoring of the chest drainage system and chest tube insertion site is essential (see Chapter 21).

Thoracentesis

In some respiratory disorders, pleural fluid may accumulate. Thoracentesis (aspiration of fluid and air from the pleural space) is performed for diagnostic or therapeutic reasons. Purposes of the procedure include removal of fluid and, very rarely, air from the pleural cavity; aspiration of pleural fluid for analysis; pleural biopsy; and instillation of medication into the pleural space. Studies of pleural fluid include Gram stain culture and sensitivity, acid-fast staining and culture, differential cell count, cytology, pH, total protein, lactic dehydrogenase, glucose, amylase, triglycerides, and cancer markers such as carcinoembryonic antigen (CEA). Nursing implications for thoracentesis are outlined in Chart 20-11.

GUIDELINES
Assisting the Patient Undergoing Thoracentesis

Chart
20-11

Equipment
- Thoracentesis tray (should include standard supplies needed to perform procedure)
- Sterile gloves
- Antiseptic solution
- Local anesthetic
- Sterile collection bottles, laboratory requisition forms, and labels

Implementation

Action

1. Ascertain in advance that a chest x-ray or ultrasound has been ordered and completed and the consent form has been signed.

2. Verify patient's identity using at least two identifiers, not including the patient's room number. Verify purpose of procedure and procedure site; assess patient for allergies to latex, antiseptic, or local anesthetic; and review coagulation status (prothrombin time/INR [international normalized ratio] and platelet count).

3. Inform the patient about the nature of the procedure as well as:
   a. The importance of remaining immobile
   b. Pressure sensations to be experienced
   c. That minimal discomfort is anticipated after the procedure

4. Obtain baseline vital signs, oxygen saturation, pain level, and respiratory status. Administer sedation if prescribed.

5. Position the patient comfortably with adequate supports. If possible, place the patient upright or in one of the following positions:
   a. Sitting on the edge of the bed with the feet supported and arms on a padded over-the-bed table
   b. Straddling a chair with arms and head resting on the back of the chair
   c. Lying on the unaffected side with the head of the bed elevated 30 to 45 degrees if unable to assume a sitting position

Rationale

1. Chest x-ray films are used to localize fluid and air in the pleural cavity and to aid in determining the puncture site. When fluid is loculated (isolated in a pocket of pleural fluid), ultrasound scans are performed to help select the best site for needle aspiration.

2. Verification maintains patient safety and prevents potential complications such as allergic reactions and bleeding.

3. An explanation helps to orient the patient to the procedure, assists the patient to mobilize resources, and provides an opportunity to ask questions and verbalize anxiety.

5. The upright position facilitates the removal of fluid that usually localizes at the base of the thorax. It expands the ribs and widens the intercostal space to aid needle insertion A position of comfort helps the patient to relax and prevents patient movement that could contribute to potential complications.

4. Provides preprocedure assessment data to guide sedation administration and postprocedure assessment. Sedation enables the patient to cooperate with the procedure and promotes relaxation.

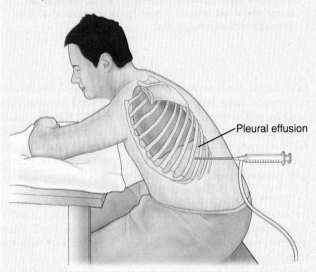

Pleural effusion

(continues on page 490)

Chart 20-11

GUIDELINES

Assisting the Patient Undergoing Thoracentesis (continued)

Action	Rationale
6. Support and reassure the patient during the procedure. a. Prepare the patient for the cold sensation of skin antiseptic solution and for a pressure sensation from infiltration of local anesthetic agent. b. Encourage the patient to refrain from coughing.	6. Sudden and unexpected movement, such as coughing, by the patient can damage the visceral pleura and lung.
7. Expose the entire chest. The site for aspiration is visualized by chest x-ray and percussion. If fluid is in the pleural cavity, the thoracentesis site is determined by the chest x-ray, ultrasound scan, or fluoroscopy and physical findings, with attention to the site of maximal dullness on percussion.	7. If air is in the pleural cavity, the thoracentesis site is usually in the second or third intercostal space in the midclavicular line, because air rises in the thorax.
8. The procedure is performed under aseptic conditions. After the skin is cleansed, the physician uses a small-caliber needle to inject a local anesthetic slowly into the intercostal space.	8. An intradermal wheal is raised slowly; rapid injection causes pain. The parietal pleura is very sensitive and should be well infiltrated with anesthetic before the physician passes the thoracentesis needle through it.
9. The physician advances the thoracentesis needle with the syringe attached. When the pleural space is reached, suction may be applied with the syringe. a. A 20-mL syringe with a three-way stopcock is attached to the needle (one end of the adapter is attached to the needle and the other to the tubing leading to a receptacle that receives the fluid being aspirated). b. If a considerable quantity of fluid is removed, the needle is held in place on the chest wall with a small hemostat.	9. The use of a thoracentesis needle allows proper insertion. a. When a large quantity of fluid is withdrawn, a three-way stopcock serves to keep air from entering the pleural cavity. b. The hemostat steadies the needle on the chest wall. Sudden pleuritic chest pain or shoulder pain may indicate that the needle point is irritating the visceral or the diaphragmatic pleura.
10. After the needle is withdrawn, pressure is applied over the puncture site and a small, airtight, sterile dressing is fixed in place.	10. Pressure helps to stop bleeding, and the airtight dressing protects the site and prevents air from entering the pleural cavity.
11. Advise the patient that a chest x-ray will be obtained after thoracentesis and activity will be limited for the first hour.	11. A chest x-ray verifies that there is no pneumothorax.
12. Record the total amount of fluid withdrawn from the procedure and document the nature of the fluid, its color, and its viscosity. If indicated, prepare samples of fluid for laboratory evaluation. A specimen container with formalin may be needed for a pleural biopsy.	12. The fluid may be clear, serous, bloody, or purulent and provides clues to the pathology. Bloody fluid may indicate malignancy, whereas purulent fluid usually indicates an infection.
13. Monitor the patient at intervals for increasing respiratory rate; asymmetry in respiratory movement; dyspnea; diminished breath sounds; anxiety or restlessness; tightness in chest; uncontrollable cough; blood-tinged, frothy mucus; a rapid pulse; and signs of hypoxemia.	13. Pneumothorax, tension pneumothorax, subcutaneous emphysema, and pyogenic infection are complications of a thoracentesis. Pulmonary edema or cardiac distress can occur after a sudden shift in mediastinal contents when large amounts of fluid are aspirated.

Biopsy

Biopsy—the excision of a small amount of tissue—may be performed to permit examination of cells from the upper and lower respiratory structures and adjacent lymph nodes. Local, topical, or moderate sedation, or general anesthesia, may be administered, depending on the site and the procedure.

Pleural Biopsy

Pleural biopsy is accomplished by needle biopsy of the pleura, thoracoscopy, or pleuroscopy, a visual exploration through a fiberoptic pleuroscope inserted into the pleural space or through a thoracotomy. Pleural biopsy is performed when there is pleural exudate of undetermined origin or when there is a need to culture or stain the tissue to identify tuberculosis or fungi.

Lung Biopsy Procedures

Lung biopsy is performed to obtain tissue for examination when other diagnostic testing indicates potential interstitial

lung disease, such as cancer, infection, or sarcoidosis. Several nonsurgical lung biopsy techniques are used because they yield accurate information with low morbidity: transbronchial brushing or needle aspiration, transbronchial lung biopsy, and percutaneous (through-the-skin) needle biopsy. Possible complications for all methods include pneumothorax, pulmonary hemorrhage, and empyema (Pagana & Pagana, 2011).

Procedure

In transbronchial brushing, a fiberoptic bronchoscope is introduced into the bronchus under fluoroscopy. A small brush attached to the end of a flexible wire is inserted through the bronchoscope. Under direct visualization, the area under suspicion is brushed back and forth, causing cells to slough off and adhere to the brush. The catheter port of the bronchoscope may be used to irrigate the lung tissue with saline solution to secure material for additional studies. The brush is removed from the bronchoscope, and a slide is made for examination under the microscope. The brush may be cut off and sent to the pathology laboratory for analysis. This procedure is especially useful in the immunologically compromised patient.

In transbronchial needle aspiration, a catheter with a needle is inserted into the tissue through the bronchoscope and aspirated, whereas in transbronchial lung biopsy, biting or cutting forceps are introduced by a fiberoptic bronchoscope to excise the tissue.

In percutaneous needle biopsy, a cutting needle or a spinal-type needle is used to obtain a tissue specimen for histologic study under fluoroscopic or CT guidance. Analgesia may be administered before the procedure. The skin over the biopsy site is cleansed and anesthetized, and a small incision is made. The biopsy needle is inserted through the incision into the pleura with the patient holding his or her breath in midexpiration. The surgeon guides the needle into the periphery of the lesion and obtains a tissue sample from the mass.

Nursing Interventions

After the procedure, recovery and home care are similar to those for bronchoscopy and thoracoscopy. Nursing care involves monitoring the patient for complications such as shortness of breath, bleeding, or infection. In preparation for discharge, the patient and family are instructed to report pain, shortness of breath, visible bleeding, redness of the biopsy site, or purulent drainage (pus) to the health care provider immediately. Patients who have undergone biopsy are often anxious because of the need for the biopsy and the potential findings; the nurse must consider this in providing postbiopsy care and patient education.

Lymph Node Biopsy

The scalene lymph nodes, which are enmeshed in the deep cervical pad of fat overlying the scalenus anterior muscle, drain the lungs and mediastinum and may show histologic changes from intrathoracic disease. If these nodes are palpable on physical examination, a scalene node biopsy may be performed. A biopsy of these nodes may be performed to detect spread of pulmonary disease to the lymph nodes and to establish a diagnosis or prognosis in such diseases as Hodgkin lymphoma, sarcoidosis, fungal disease, tuberculosis, and carcinoma.

Procedure

Mediastinoscopy is the endoscopic examination of the mediastinum for exploration and biopsy of mediastinal lymph nodes that drain the lungs; this examination does not require a thoracotomy. Biopsy is usually performed through a suprasternal incision. Mediastinoscopy is carried out to detect mediastinal involvement of pulmonary malignancy and to obtain tissue for diagnostic studies of other conditions (e.g., sarcoidosis).

An anterior mediastinotomy is thought to provide better exposure and diagnostic possibilities than a mediastinoscopy. An incision is made in the area of the second or third costal cartilage. The mediastinum is explored, and biopsies are performed on any lymph nodes found. Chest tube drainage is required after the procedure. Mediastinotomy is particularly valuable to determine whether a pulmonary lesion is resectable.

Nursing Interventions

Postprocedure care focuses on providing adequate oxygenation, monitoring for bleeding, and providing pain relief. The patient may be discharged a few hours after the chest drainage system is removed. The nurse should instruct the patient and family about monitoring for changes in respiratory status, taking into consideration the impact of anxiety about the potential findings of the biopsy on their ability to remember those instructions.

Critical Thinking Exercises

1 **ebp** You are caring for a 78-year-old woman who is 2 days postoperative for a cholecystectomy. She has refused to take pain medication due to fears of developing an addiction and as a result is reluctant to advance her activity. On assessment, you note an increase in respiratory rate, the use of accessory muscles, a decrease in SpO_2, and crackles to bilateral lower lobes. Based on your knowledge of respiratory function, what pulmonary complications could these findings reflect and why? What additional types of assessment will you perform? How will the findings influence your understanding of these changes? Discuss the evidence-based interventions that could have been initiated to prevent this patient's clinical deterioration.

2 A 42-year-old African American man who has recently been diagnosed with lung cancer is anxious about his diagnosis. He tells you that he has never smoked and as a result wants to know how he could have developed lung cancer. What components of his health history are important for you to ascertain to assess factors that may have contributed to his diagnosis of lung cancer? What questions will you ask to explore the psychosocial impact of this diagnosis on his life? As you proceed with the history, your patient becomes short of breath while answering your questions. How will you modify your interaction with this patient and prioritize your assessment based on your observations?

3 **pcc** A 68-year-old woman is admitted to your unit from the emergency department for hemoptysis. During your assessment, the patient asks you to explain why you are asking so many questions about the nature of the bloody sputum. How will you respond? She is reluctant to consent to the bronchoscopy procedure scheduled for the next day. What information will you give her about the purpose of the procedure and what to expect before, during, and after the procedure to decrease her anxiety? What will the priority nursing assessments be after the procedure and why?

4 A 32-year-old woman who was admitted with acute shortness of breath and chest pain from a pulmonary embolism has been stabilized and transferred to your unit. Currently a nursing student, she tells you that she overheard the doctors say that she had a $\dot{V}/\dot{Q}$ imbalance. She asks you to explain what this means. She also wants to better understand the differences between the diagnostic tests that she had during her admission, which included ABGs, chest x-ray, chest CT, and a $\dot{V}/\dot{Q}$ scan, and wonders why she did not have a pulmonary angiogram. Describe the major differences between these tests and related nursing implications.

Brunner Suite Resources

Explore these additional resources to enhance learning for this chapter:
• NCLEX-Style Questions and Other Resources on thePoint, http://thePoint.lww.com/Brunner13e
• Study Guide
• PrepU
• Clinical Handbook
• Handbook of Laboratory and Diagnostic Tests

References

Books

Bickley, L. S. (2009). *Bates' guide to physical examination and history taking* (10th ed.). Philadelphia: Lippincott Williams & Wilkins.

Chulay, M., & Burns, S. (2010). *AACN essentials of critical care nursing* (2nd ed.). New York: McGraw-Hill Medical.

Ferrell, B. R., & Coyle, N. (2010). *Oxford textbook of palliative nursing* (3rd ed.). New York: Oxford University Press.

Pagana, K. S., & Pagana, T. J. (2011). *Mosby's diagnostic and laboratory test reference* (10th ed.). St. Louis: Mosby Elsevier.

Porth, C. M. (2011). *Essentials of pathophysiology* (3rd ed.). Philadelphia: Lippincott Williams & Wilkins.

Potter, P. A., & Perry, A. G. (2010). *Clinical nursing skills and techniques* (7th ed.). St. Louis: Mosby Elsevier.

Wrede-Seaman, L. (2009). *Symptom management algorithms: A handbook for palliative care* (3rd ed.). Yakima, WA: Intellicard.

Journals and Electronic Documents

Agnelli, G., & Becattini, C. (2010). Acute pulmonary embolism. *New England Journal of Medicine, 363*(3), 266–274.

Cox, B. (2010). Developing an assessment tool. *Primary Health Care, 20*(4), 26–28.

Higginson, R., & Jones, B. (2009). Respiratory assessment in critically ill patients: Airway and breathing. *British Journal of Nursing, 18*(8), 456–461.

Massey, D., & Meredith, T. (2010). Respiratory assessment 1: Why do it and how to do it? *British Journal of Cardiac Nursing, 5*(11), 537–541.

Shellock, F. G., & Spinazzi, A. (2008). MRI safety update 2008: Part 2: Screening patients for MRI. *American Journal of Roentgenology, 191*(4), 1140–1149.

Resources

American Association for Respiratory Care (AARC), www.aarc.org

American Lung Association, www.lungusa.org

Cystic Fibrosis Foundation, www.cff.org

GeneTests, National Center for Biotechnology Information, www.geneclinics.org

Genetic Alliance, www.geneticalliance.org

National Heart, Lung, and Blood Institute, National Institutes of Health, www.nhlbi.nih.gov

National Organization for Rare Disorders (NORD), www.rarediseases.org

OMIM: Online Mendelian Inheritance in Man, www.ncbi.nlm.nih.gov/omim

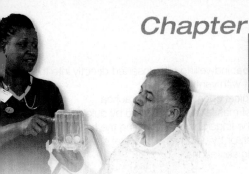
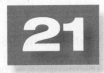

Respiratory Care Modalities

Learning Objectives

On completion of this chapter, the learner will be able to:

1 Describe the nursing management of patients receiving oxygen therapy, incentive spirometry, small-volume nebulizer therapy, chest physiotherapy, and breathing retraining.
2 Describe the patient education and home care considerations for patients receiving oxygen therapy.
3 Describe the nursing care of a patient with an endotracheal tube and a patient with a tracheostomy.
4 Demonstrate the procedure of tracheal suctioning.
5 Use the nursing process as a framework for care of patients who are mechanically ventilated.

6 Describe the process of weaning the patient from mechanical ventilation.
7 Describe the significance of preoperative nursing assessment and patient education for the patient who is going to have thoracic surgery.
8 Explain the principles of chest drainage and the nursing responsibilities related to the care of the patient with a chest drainage system.
9 Use the nursing process as a framework for care of a patient who has had a thoracotomy.

Glossary

airway pressure release ventilation (APRV): mode of mechanical ventilation that allows unrestricted, spontaneous breaths throughout the ventilatory cycle; on inspiration the patient receives a preset level of continuous positive airway pressure, and pressure is periodically released to aid expiration

assist–control (A/C) ventilation: mode of mechanical ventilation in which the patient's breathing pattern may trigger the ventilator to deliver a preset tidal volume; in the absence of spontaneous breathing, the machine delivers a controlled breath at a preset minimum rate and tidal volume

chest drainage system: the use of a chest tube and closed drainage system to re-expand the lung and to remove excess air, fluid, and blood

chest percussion: manually cupping hands over the chest wall and using vibration to mobilize secretions by mechanically dislodging viscous or adherent secretions in the lungs

chest physiotherapy (CPT): therapy used to remove bronchial secretions, improve ventilation, and increase the efficiency of the respiratory muscles; types include postural drainage, chest percussion, and vibration

continuous mandatory ventilation (CMV): mode of mechanical ventilation in which the ventilator completely controls the patient's ventilation according to preset tidal volumes and respiratory rate; because of problems with synchrony, it is rarely used except in paralyzed or anesthetized patients

continuous positive airway pressure (CPAP): positive pressure applied throughout the respiratory cycle to a spontaneously breathing patient to promote alveolar and airway stability; may be administered with endotracheal or tracheostomy tube or by mask

endotracheal intubation: insertion of a breathing tube through the nose or mouth into the trachea

fraction of inspired oxygen (FiO$_2$): concentration of oxygen delivered (1.0 = 100% oxygen)

hypoxemia: decrease in arterial oxygen tension in the blood

hypoxia: decrease in oxygen supply to the tissues and cells

incentive spirometry: method of deep breathing that provides visual feedback to help the patient inhale deeply and slowly and achieve maximum lung inflation

intermittent mandatory ventilation (IMV): mode of mechanical ventilation that provides a combination of mechanically assisted breaths and spontaneous breaths

mechanical ventilator: a positive- or negative-pressure breathing device that supports ventilation and oxygenation

pneumothorax: partial or complete collapse of the lung due to positive pressure in the pleural space

positive end-expiratory pressure (PEEP): positive pressure maintained by the ventilator at the end of exhalation (instead of a normal zero pressure) to increase functional residual capacity and open collapsed alveoli; improves oxygenation with lower fraction of inspired oxygen

postural drainage: positioning the patient to allow drainage from all lobes of the lungs and airways

pressure support ventilation (PSV): mode of mechanical ventilation in which preset positive pressure is delivered with spontaneous breaths to decrease work of breathing

proportional assist ventilation (PAV): mode of mechanical ventilation that provides partial ventilatory support in proportion to the patient's inspiratory efforts; decreases the work of breathing

respiratory weaning: process of gradual, systematic withdrawal or removal of ventilator, breathing tube, and oxygen

(continues on page 494)

synchronized intermittent mandatory ventilation (SIMV): mode of mechanical ventilation in which the ventilator allows the patient to breathe spontaneously while providing a preset number of breaths to ensure adequate ventilation; ventilated breaths are synchronized with spontaneous breathing

thoracotomy: surgical opening into the chest cavity

tracheostomy tube: indwelling tube inserted directly into the trachea to assist with ventilation

tracheotomy: surgical opening into the trachea

vibration: a type of massage administered by quickly tapping the chest with the fingertips or alternating the fingers in a rhythmic manner, or by using a mechanical device to assist in mobilizing lung secretions

---

Numerous treatment modalities are used when caring for patients with respiratory conditions. The choice of modality is based on the oxygenation disorder and whether there is a problem with gas ventilation, diffusion, or both. Therapies range from simple and noninvasive (oxygen and nebulizer therapy, chest physiotherapy [CPT], breathing retraining) to complex and highly invasive treatments (intubation, mechanical ventilation, surgery). Assessment and management of the patient with respiratory disorders are best accomplished when the approach is multidisciplinary and collaborative.

NONINVASIVE RESPIRATORY THERAPIES

Oxygen Therapy

Oxygen therapy is the administration of oxygen at a concentration greater than that found in the environmental atmosphere. At sea level, the concentration of oxygen in room air is 21%. The goal of oxygen therapy is to provide adequate transport of oxygen in the blood while decreasing the work of breathing and reducing stress on the myocardium.

Oxygen transport to tissues depends on factors such as cardiac output, arterial oxygen content, concentration of hemoglobin, and metabolic requirements. These factors must be kept in mind when oxygen therapy is considered. (Respiratory physiology and oxygen transport are discussed in Chapter 20.)

Indications

A change in the patient's respiratory rate or pattern may be one of the earliest indicators of the need for oxygen therapy. These changes may result from hypoxemia or hypoxia. **Hypoxemia**, a decrease in the arterial oxygen tension in the blood, is manifested by changes in mental status (progressing through impaired judgment, agitation, disorientation, confusion, lethargy, and coma), dyspnea, increase in blood pressure, changes in heart rate, dysrhythmias, central cyanosis (late sign), diaphoresis, and cool extremities. Hypoxemia usually leads to **hypoxia**, a decrease in oxygen supply to the tissues and cells which can also be caused by problems outside the respiratory system. Severe hypoxia can be life threatening.

The signs and symptoms signaling the need for oxygen may depend on how suddenly this need develops. With rapidly developing hypoxia, changes occur in the central nervous system because the neurologic centers are very sensitive to oxygen deprivation. The clinical picture may resemble that of alcohol intoxication, with the patient exhibiting lack of coordination and impaired judgment. With long-standing hypoxia (as seen in chronic obstructive pulmonary disease [COPD] and chronic heart failure), fatigue, drowsiness, apathy, inattentiveness, and delayed reaction time may occur. The need for oxygen is assessed by arterial blood gas analysis, pulse oximetry, and clinical evaluation. More information about hypoxia is presented in Chart 21-1.

Chart 21-1 **Types of Hypoxia**

Hypoxia can occur from either severe pulmonary disease (inadequate oxygen supply) or from extrapulmonary disease (inadequate oxygen delivery) affecting gas exchange at the cellular level. The four general types of hypoxia are hypoxemic hypoxia, circulatory hypoxia, anemic hypoxia, and histotoxic hypoxia.

Hypoxemic Hypoxia

Hypoxemic hypoxia is a decreased oxygen level in the blood resulting in decreased oxygen diffusion into the tissues. It may be caused by hypoventilation, high altitudes, ventilation–perfusion mismatch that may include disorders of dead space (e.g., pulmonary embolism) and shunts in which the alveoli are collapsed and cannot provide oxygen to the blood (e.g., atelectasis), and pulmonary diffusion defects. It is corrected by increasing alveolar ventilation or providing supplemental oxygen.

Circulatory Hypoxia

Circulatory hypoxia is hypoxia resulting from inadequate capillary circulation. It may be caused by decreased cardiac output, local vascular obstruction, low-flow states such as shock, or cardiac arrest. Although tissue partial pressure of oxygen (PO_2) is reduced, arterial oxygen (PaO_2) remains normal. Circulatory hypoxia is corrected by identifying and treating the underlying cause.

Anemic Hypoxia

Anemic hypoxia is a result of decreased effective hemoglobin concentration, which causes a decrease in the oxygen-carrying capacity of the blood. It is rarely accompanied by hypoxemia. Carbon monoxide poisoning, because it reduces the oxygen-carrying capacity of hemoglobin, produces similar effects but is not strictly anemic hypoxia, because hemoglobin levels may be normal.

Histotoxic Hypoxia

Histotoxic hypoxia occurs when a toxic substance, such as cyanide, interferes with the ability of tissues to use available oxygen.

Complications

Oxygen is a medication, and except in emergency situations it is administered only when prescribed by a provider with prescriptive authority. As with other medications, the nurse administers oxygen with caution and carefully assesses its effects on each patient.

In general, patients with respiratory disorders are given oxygen therapy only to increase the arterial oxygen pressure (PaO_2) back to the patient's normal baseline, which may vary from 60 to 95 mm Hg. In terms of the oxyhemoglobin dissociation curve (see Chapter 20), arterial hemoglobin at these levels is 80% to 98% saturated with oxygen; higher **fraction of inspired oxygen (FiO_2)** flow values add no further significant amounts of oxygen to the red blood cells or plasma. Instead of helping, increased amounts of oxygen may produce toxic effects on the lungs and central nervous system or may depress ventilation (see later discussion).

It is important to observe for subtle indicators of inadequate oxygenation when oxygen is administered by any method. Therefore, the nurse assesses the patient frequently for confusion, restlessness progressing to lethargy, diaphoresis, pallor, tachycardia, tachypnea, and hypertension. Intermittent or continuous pulse oximetry is used to monitor oxygen levels.

Oxygen Toxicity

Oxygen toxicity may occur when too high a concentration of oxygen (greater than 50%) is administered for an extended period (longer than 48 hours) (Urden, Stacy, & Lough, 2010). It is caused by overproduction of oxygen free radicals, which are by-products of cell metabolism.

If oxygen toxicity is untreated, these radicals can severely damage or kill cells. Antioxidants such as vitamin E, vitamin C, and beta-carotene may help defend against oxygen free radicals. The dietitian can adjust the patient's diet so that it is rich in antioxidants; supplements are also available for patients who have a decreased appetite or who are unable to eat.

Signs and symptoms of oxygen toxicity include substernal discomfort, paresthesias, dyspnea, restlessness, fatigue, malaise, progressive respiratory difficulty, refractory hypoxemia, alveolar atelectasis, and alveolar infiltrates evident on chest x-rays.

Prevention of oxygen toxicity is achieved by using oxygen only as prescribed. If high concentrations of oxygen are necessary, it is important to minimize the duration of administration and reduce its concentration as soon as possible. Often, **positive end-expiratory pressure (PEEP)** or continuous positive airway pressure (CPAP) is used with oxygen therapy to reverse or prevent microatelectasis, thus allowing a lower percentage of oxygen to be used. The level of PEEP that allows the best oxygenation without hemodynamic compromise is known as "best PEEP."

Suppression of Ventilation

In many patients with COPD, the stimulus for respiration is a decrease in blood oxygen rather than an elevation in carbon dioxide levels. The administration of a high concentration of oxygen removes the respiratory drive that has been created largely by the patient's chronic low oxygen tension. The resulting decrease in alveolar ventilation can cause a progressive increase in arterial carbon dioxide pressure ($PaCO_2$). This hypoventilation can, in rare cases, lead to acute respiratory failure secondary to carbon dioxide narcosis, acidosis, and death. Oxygen-induced hypoventilation is prevented by administering oxygen at low flow rates (1 to 2 L/min) and by closely monitoring the respiratory rate and the oxygen saturation as measured by pulse oximetry (SpO_2) (Urden et al., 2010).

Other Complications

Because oxygen supports combustion, there is always a danger of fire when it is used. It is important to post "No Smoking" signs when oxygen is in use, particularly in facilities that are not smoke free. Oxygen therapy equipment is also a potential source of bacterial cross-infection; therefore, the nurse (or respiratory therapist) changes the tubing according to infection control policy and the type of oxygen delivery equipment.

Methods of Oxygen Administration

Oxygen is dispensed from a cylinder or a piped-in system. A reduction gauge is necessary to reduce the pressure to a working level, and a flow meter regulates the flow of oxygen in liters per minute (L/min). When oxygen is used at high flow rates, it should be moistened by passing it through a humidification system to prevent it from drying the mucous membranes of the respiratory tract.

The use of oxygen concentrators is another means of providing varying amounts of oxygen, especially in the home setting. These devices are relatively portable, easy to operate, and cost-effective but require more maintenance than tank or liquid systems. Newer models can deliver oxygen flows from 1 to 10 L/min and provide an FiO_2 of about 40% (Cairo & Pilbeam, 2010).

Many different oxygen devices are used (Table 21-1). The amount of oxygen delivered is expressed as a percentage concentration (e.g., 70%). The appropriate form of oxygen therapy is best determined by arterial blood gas levels (see Chapter 13), which indicate the patient's oxygenation status.

Oxygen delivery systems are classified as low-flow or high-flow delivery systems. Low-flow systems contribute partially to the inspired gas the patient breathes, which means that the patient breathes some room air along with the oxygen. These systems do not provide a constant or precise concentration of inspired oxygen. The amount of inspired oxygen changes as the patient's breathing changes. Examples of low-flow systems are included in Table 21-1. In contrast, high-flow systems provide the total inspired air. A specific percentage of oxygen is delivered independent of the patient's breathing. High-flow systems are indicated for patients who require a constant and precise amount of oxygen. Examples of these systems can also be found in Table 21-1.

A nasal cannula is used when the patient requires a low to medium concentration of oxygen for which precise accuracy is not essential. This method allows the patient to move about in bed, talk, cough, and eat without interrupting oxygen flow. Flow rates in excess of 4 to 6 L/min may lead to swallowing of air or may cause irritation and drying of the nasal and pharyngeal mucosa.

The oropharyngeal catheter is rarely used but may be prescribed for short-term therapy to administer low to moderate

TABLE 21-1	**Oxygen Administration Devices**			
Device	**Suggested Flow Rate (L/min)**	**O₂ Percentage Setting**	**Advantages**	**Disadvantages**
Low-Flow Systems				
Cannula	1–2	23–30	Lightweight, comfortable, inexpensive, continuous use with meals and activity	Nasal mucosal drying, variable FiO₂
	3–5	30–40		
	6	42		
Oropharyngeal catheter	1–6	23–42	Inexpensive, does not require a tracheostomy	Nasal mucosa irritation; catheter should be changed frequently to alternate nostril
Mask, simple	6–8	40–60	Simple to use, inexpensive	Poor fitting, variable FiO₂, must remove to eat
Mask, partial rebreathing	8–11	50–75	Moderate O₂ concentration	Warm, poorly fitting, must remove to eat
Mask, nonrebreathing	12	80–100	High O₂ concentration	Poorly fitting, must remove to eat
High-Flow Systems				
Transtracheal catheter	¼–4	60–100	More comfortable, concealed by clothing, less oxygen liters per minute needed than nasal cannula	Requires frequent and regular cleaning, requires surgical intervention
Mask, Venturi	4–6	24, 26, 28	Provides low levels of supplemental O₂	Must remove to eat
	6–8	30, 35, 40	Precise FiO₂, additional humidity available	
Mask, aerosol	8–10	30–100	Good humidity, accurate FiO₂	Uncomfortable for some
Tracheostomy collar	8–10	30–100	Good humidity, comfortable, fairly accurate FiO₂	
T-piece	8–10	30–100	Same as tracheostomy collar	Heavy with tubing
Face tent	8–10	30–100	Good humidity, fairly accurate FiO₂	Bulky and cumbersome
Oxygen-Conserving Devices				
Pulse dose (or demand)	10–40 mL/breath		Deliver O₂ only on inspiration, conserve 50%–75% of O₂ used	Must carefully evaluate function individually

concentrations of oxygen. The catheter should be changed every 8 hours, alternating nostrils to prevent nasal irritation and infection.

When oxygen is administered via cannula or catheter, the percentage of oxygen reaching the lungs varies with the depth and rate of respirations, particularly if the nasal mucosa is swollen or if the patient is a mouth breather.

Oxygen masks come in several forms. Each is used for different purposes (Fig. 21-1). *Simple masks* are used to administer low to moderate concentrations of oxygen. The body of the mask itself gathers and stores oxygen between breaths. The patient exhales directly through openings or ports in the body of the mask. If oxygen flow ceases, the patient can draw air in through these openings around the mask edges. Although widely used, these masks cannot be used for controlled oxygen concentrations and must be adjusted for proper fit. They should not press too tightly against the skin, because this can cause a sense of claustrophobia as well as skin breakdown; adjustable elastic bands are provided to ensure comfort and security.

Partial rebreathing masks have a reservoir bag that must remain inflated during both inspiration and expiration. The nurse adjusts the oxygen flow to ensure that the bag does not collapse during inhalation. A high concentration of oxygen can be delivered because both the mask and the bag serve as reservoirs for oxygen. Oxygen enters the mask through small-bore tubing that connects at the junction of the mask and bag. As the patient inhales, gas is drawn from the mask, from the bag, and potentially from room air through the exhalation

ports. As the patient exhales, the first third of the exhalation fills the reservoir bag. This is mainly dead space and does not participate in gas exchange in the lungs. Therefore, it has a high oxygen concentration. The remainder of the exhaled gas is vented through the exhalation ports. The actual percentage of oxygen delivered is influenced by the patient's ventilatory pattern (Cairo & Pilbeam, 2010).

Nonrebreathing masks are similar in design to partial rebreathing masks except that they have additional valves. A one-way valve located between the reservoir bag and the base of the mask allows gas from the reservoir bag to enter the mask on inhalation but prevents gas in the mask from flowing back into the reservoir bag during exhalation. One-way valves located at the exhalation ports prevent room air from entering the mask during inhalation. They also allow the patient's exhaled gases to exit the mask on exhalation. As with the partial rebreathing mask, it is important to adjust the oxygen flow so that the reservoir bag does not completely collapse on inspiration. In theory, if the nonrebreathing mask fits the patient snugly and both side exhalation ports have one-way valves, it is possible for the patient to receive 100% oxygen, making the nonrebreathing mask a high-flow oxygen system. However, because it is difficult to get an exact fit from the mask on every patient, and some nonrebreathing masks have only one one-way exhalation valves, it is almost impossible to ensure 100% oxygen delivery, making it a low-flow oxygen system.

The *Venturi mask* is the most reliable and accurate method for delivering precise concentrations of oxygen

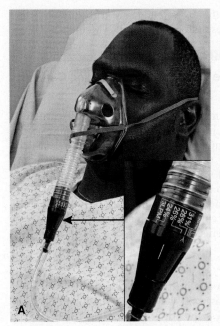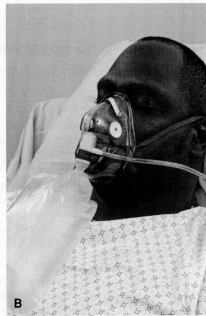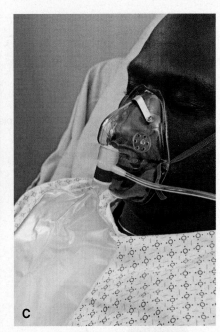

FIGURE 21-1 • Types of oxygen masks used to deliver varying concentrations of oxygen. **A.** Venturi mask. **B.** Nonrebreathing mask. **C.** Partial rebreathing mask.

through noninvasive means. The mask is constructed in a way that allows a constant flow of room air blended with a fixed flow of oxygen. It is used primarily for patients with COPD because it can accurately provide appropriate levels of supplemental oxygen, thus avoiding the risk of suppressing the hypoxic drive.

The Venturi mask uses the Bernoulli principle of air entrainment (trapping the air like a vacuum), which provides a high airflow with controlled oxygen enrichment. For each liter of oxygen that passes through a jet orifice, a fixed proportion of room air is entrained. A precise volume of oxygen can be delivered by varying the size of the jet orifice and adjusting the flow of oxygen. Excess gas leaves the mask through the two exhalation ports, carrying with it the exhaled carbon dioxide. This method allows a constant oxygen concentration to be inhaled regardless of the depth or rate of respiration.

The mask should fit snugly enough to prevent oxygen from flowing into the patient's eyes. The nurse checks the patient's skin for irritation. It is necessary to remove the mask so that the patient can eat, drink, and take medications, at which time supplemental oxygen is provided through a nasal cannula.

 Concept Mastery Alert

Oxygen delivery systems are classified as either low-flow or high-low systems. Whereas a low-flow oxygen delivery system may imprecisely deliver high concentrations of oxygen (e.g., up to 100% via a nonrebreathing mask), the Venturi mask, which is a high-flow system, is specifically designed to deliver precise but lower concentrations of oxygen (e.g., between 24% and 40% oxygen).

The *transtracheal oxygen catheter* is inserted directly into the trachea and is indicated for patients with chronic oxygen

therapy needs. These catheters are more comfortable, less dependent on breathing patterns, and less obvious than other oxygen delivery methods. Because no oxygen is lost into the surrounding environment, the patient achieves adequate oxygenation at lower rates, making this method less expensive and more efficient.

The *T-piece* connects to the endotracheal tube and is useful in weaning patients from mechanical ventilation (Fig. 21-2).

Other oxygen devices include *aerosol masks, tracheostomy collars* (see Fig. 21-2), and *face tents*, all of which are used with aerosol devices (nebulizers) that can be adjusted for oxygen concentrations from 27% to 100% (0.27 to 1.00). If the gas mixture flow falls below patient demand, room air is pulled in, diluting the concentration. The aerosol mist must be available for the patient during the entire inspiratory phase.

Although most oxygen therapy is administered as continuous flow oxygen, new methods of oxygen conservation are coming into use. The *demand oxygen delivery system* (DODS) interrupts the flow of oxygen during exhalation, when it is otherwise mostly wasted. Several versions of the DODS are being evaluated for their effectiveness. Studies show that DODS models conserve oxygen and maintain oxygen saturation better than continuous flow oxygen systems when the respiratory rate increases (Langenhof & Fichter, 2005).

Hyperbaric oxygen therapy is the administration of oxygen at pressures greater than 1 atm. As a result, the amount of oxygen dissolved in plasma is increased, which increases oxygen levels in the tissues. During therapy, the patient is placed in a small (single patient use) or large (multiple patient use) cylinder chamber. Hyperbaric oxygen therapy is used to treat conditions such as air embolism, carbon monoxide poisoning, gangrene, tissue necrosis, and hemorrhage. Although controversial, hyperbaric oxygen has also been used to treat multiple sclerosis (Bennett & Heard, 2010),

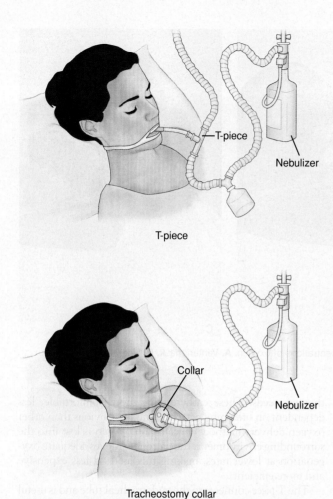

T-piece

Tracheostomy collar

FIGURE 21-2 • T-pieces and tracheostomy collars are devices used when weaning patients from mechanical ventilation.

diabetic foot ulcers (Feldman-Idov, Melamed, & Ore, 2011), closed head trauma, acute myocardial infarction, and unstable angina (Bennett, Lehm, & Jepson, 2011), as well as slow-to-heal bone fractures (Bennett, Stanford, & Turner, 2012). Potential side effects include ear trauma, central nervous system disorders, oxygen toxicity, and anxiety in patients with claustrophobia.

Gerontologic Considerations

The respiratory system changes throughout the aging process, and it is important for nurses to be aware of these changes when assessing patients who are receiving oxygen therapy. As the respiratory muscles weaken and the large bronchi and alveoli become enlarged, the available surface area of the lungs decreases, resulting in reduced ventilation and respiratory gas exchange. The number of functional cilia is also reduced, decreasing ciliary action and the cough reflex. As a result of osteoporosis and calcification of the costal cartilages, chest wall compliance is decreased. Patients may display increased chest rigidity and respiratory rate and decreased PaO_2 and lung expansion. Nurses should be aware that the older adult is at risk for aspiration and infection related to these changes. In addition, patient education regarding adequate nutrition is essential because appropriate dietary intake

can help diminish the excess buildup of carbon dioxide and maintain optimal respiratory functioning (Meiner, 2010).

Nursing Management

Promoting Home and Community-Based Care

Educating Patients About Self-Care

At times, oxygen must be administered to the patient at home. The nurse instructs the patient or family in the methods for administering oxygen safely and informs the patient and family that oxygen is available in gas, liquid, and concentrated forms. The gas and liquid forms come in portable devices so that the patient can leave home while receiving oxygen therapy. Humidity must be provided while oxygen is used (except with portable devices) to counteract the dry, irritating effects of compressed oxygen on the airway (Chart 21-2).

Continuing Care

Home visits by a home health nurse or respiratory therapist may be arranged based on the patient's status and needs. It is important to assess the patient's home environment, the patient's physical and psychological status, and the need for further education. The nurse reinforces educational points on how to use oxygen safely and effectively, including fire safety tips. To maintain a consistent quality of care and to maximize the patient's financial reimbursement for home oxygen therapy, the nurse ensures that the prescription given by the primary care provider (PCP) includes the diagnosis, the prescribed oxygen flow, and conditions for use (e.g., continuous use, nighttime use only). Because oxygen is a medication, the nurse reminds the patient receiving long-term oxygen therapy and the family about the importance of keeping follow-up appointments with the patient's PCP. The patient is instructed to see his or her PCP every 6 months or more often, if indicated. Arterial blood gas measurements and laboratory tests are repeated annually or more often if the patient's condition changes.

Incentive Spirometry (Sustained Maximal Inspiration)

Incentive spirometry is a method of deep breathing that provides visual feedback to encourage the patient to inhale slowly and deeply to maximize lung inflation and prevent or reduce atelectasis. The purpose of an incentive spirometer is to ensure that the volume of air inhaled is increased gradually as the patient takes deeper and deeper breaths.

Incentive spirometers are available in two types: volume or flow. In the volume type, the tidal volume is set using the manufacturer's instructions. The patient takes a deep breath through the mouthpiece, pauses at peak lung inflation, and then relaxes and exhales. Taking several normal breaths before attempting another with the incentive spirometer helps avoid fatigue. The volume is periodically increased as tolerated.

In the flow type, the volume is not preset. The spirometer contains a number of movable balls that are pushed up by the force of the breath and held suspended in the air while the patient inhales. The amount of air inhaled and the flow

Chart 21-2	HOME CARE CHECKLIST Oxygen Therapy		
At the completion of home care education, the patient or caregiver will be able to:		**PATIENT**	**CAREGIVER**
• State proper care of and administration of oxygen to patient:			
• State primary care provider's prescription for oxygen and the manner in which it is to be used.		✔	✔
• Indicate when a humidifier should be used.		✔	✔
• Identify signs and symptoms indicating the need for change in oxygen therapy.		✔	✔
• Describe precautions and safety measures to be used when oxygen is in use.		✔	✔
• Know *NOT* to smoke while using oxygen.		✔	✔
• Post "No smoking—oxygen in use" signs on doors.		✔	✔
• Notify local fire department and electric company of oxygen use in home.		✔	✔
• Keep oxygen tank at least 15 feet away from matches, candles, gas stove, or other source of flame.		✔	✔
• Keep oxygen tank 5 feet away from television, radio, and other appliances.		✔	✔
• Keep oxygen tank out of direct sunlight.		✔	✔
• When traveling in automobile, place oxygen tank on floor behind front seat.		✔	✔
• If traveling by airplane, notify air carrier of need for oxygen at least 2 weeks in advance.		✔	✔
• State how and when to place an order for more oxygen.		✔	✔
• Describe a diet that meets energy demands.		✔	✔
• Maintain equipment properly:			
• Demonstrate correct adjustment of prescribed flow rate.		✔	✔
• Describe how to clean and when to replace oxygen tubing.		✔	✔
• Identify when a portable oxygen delivery device should be used.		✔	✔
• Demonstrate safe and appropriate use of portable oxygen delivery device.		✔	✔
• Identify causes of malfunction of equipment and when to call for replacement of equipment.		✔	✔
• Describe the importance of determining that all electrical outlets are working properly.		✔	✔

of the air are estimated by how long and how high the balls are suspended.

Indications

Incentive spirometry is used after surgery, especially thoracic and abdominal surgery, to promote the expansion of the alveoli and to prevent or treat atelectasis.

Nursing Management

Nursing management of the patient using incentive spirometry includes placing the patient in the proper position, educating the patient on the technique for using the incentive spirometer, setting realistic goals for the patient, and recording the results of the therapy (Chart 21-3). Ideally, the patient assumes a sitting or semi-Fowler's position to enhance diaphragmatic excursion; however, this procedure may be performed with the patient in any position.

Small-Volume Nebulizer (Mini-Nebulizer) Therapy

The small-volume nebulizer is a handheld apparatus that disperses a moisturizing agent or medication, such as a bron-

chodilator or mucolytic agent, into microscopic particles and delivers it to the lungs as the patient inhales. The small-volume nebulizer is usually air driven by means of a compressor through connecting tubing. In some instances, the nebulizer is oxygen driven rather than air driven. To be effective, a visible mist must be available for the patient to inhale.

Chart 21-3	PATIENT EDUCATION Performing Incentive Spirometry

- The inspired air helps inflate the lungs. The ball or weight in the spirometer rises in response to the intensity of the intake of air. The higher the ball rises, the deeper the breath.
- Assume a semi-Fowler's position or an upright position before initiating therapy.
- Use diaphragmatic breathing.
- Place the mouthpiece of the spirometer firmly in the mouth, breathe air in (inspire) through the mouth, and hold the breath at the end of inspiration for about 3 seconds. Exhale slowly through the mouthpiece.
- Coughing during and after each session is encouraged. Splint the incision when coughing postoperatively.
- Perform the procedure approximately 10 times in succession, repeating the 10 breaths with the spirometer each hour during waking hours.

Indications

Indications for the use of a small-volume nebulizer include difficulty in clearing respiratory secretions, reduced vital capacity with ineffective deep breathing and coughing, and unsuccessful trials of simpler and less costly methods for clearing secretions, delivering aerosol, or expanding the lungs (Cairo & Pilbeam, 2010). The patient must be able to generate a deep breath. Diaphragmatic breathing (Chart 21-4) is a helpful technique to prepare for proper use of the small-volume nebulizer. Small-volume nebulizers are frequently used for patients with COPD to dispense inhaled medications, and they are commonly used at home on a long-term basis.

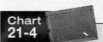

Chart 21-4

PATIENT EDUCATION
Breathing Exercises

General Instructions

- Breathe slowly and rhythmically to exhale completely and empty the lungs completely.
- Inhale through the nose to filter, humidify, and warm the air before it enters the lungs.
- If you feel out of breath, breathe more slowly by prolonging the exhalation time.
- Keep the air moist with a humidifier.

Diaphragmatic Breathing

Goal: To use and strengthen the diaphragm during breathing

- Place one hand on the abdomen (just below the ribs) and the other hand on the middle of the chest to increase the awareness of the position of the diaphragm and its function in breathing.
- Breathe in slowly and deeply through the nose, letting the abdomen protrude as far as possible.
- Breathe out through pursed lips while tightening (contracting) the abdominal muscles.
- Press firmly inward and upward on the abdomen while breathing out.
- Repeat for 1 minute; follow with a rest period of 2 minutes.
- Gradually increase duration up to 5 minutes, several times a day (before meals and at bedtime).

Pursed-Lip Breathing

Goal: To prolong exhalation and increase airway pressure during expiration, thus reducing the amount of trapped air and the amount of airway resistance

- Inhale through the nose while slowly counting to 3—the amount of time needed to say "Smell a rose."
- Exhale slowly and evenly against pursed lips while tightening the abdominal muscles. (Pursing the lips increases intra-tracheal pressure; exhaling through the mouth offers less resistance to expired air.)
- Count to 7 slowly while prolonging expiration through pursed lips—the length of time to say "Blow out the candle."
- While sitting in a chair:
  Fold arms over the abdomen.
  Inhale through the nose while counting to 3 slowly.
  Bend forward and exhale slowly through pursed lips while counting to 7 slowly.
- While walking:
  Inhale while walking two steps.
  Exhale through pursed lips while walking four or five steps.

Nursing Management

The nurse instructs the patient to breathe through the mouth, taking slow, deep breaths, and then to hold the breath for a few seconds at the end of inspiration to increase intrapleural pressure and reopen collapsed alveoli, thereby increasing functional residual capacity. The nurse encourages the patient to cough and to monitor the effectiveness of the therapy. The nurse instructs the patient and family about the purpose of the treatment, equipment setup, medication additive, and proper cleaning and storage of the equipment.

Chest Physiotherapy

Chest physiotherapy (CPT) includes postural drainage, chest percussion and vibration, and breathing retraining. In addition, educating the patient about effective coughing technique is an important part of CPT. The goals of CPT are to remove bronchial secretions, improve ventilation, and increase the efficiency of the respiratory muscles.

■ Postural Drainage (Segmented Bronchial Drainage)

Postural drainage allows the force of gravity to assist in the removal of bronchial secretions. The secretions drain from the affected bronchioles into the bronchi and trachea and are removed by coughing or suctioning. Postural drainage is used to prevent or relieve bronchial obstruction caused by accumulation of secretions.

Because the patient usually sits in an upright position, secretions are likely to accumulate in the lower parts of the lungs. Several other positions (Fig. 21-3) are used so that the force of gravity helps move secretions from the smaller bronchial airways to the main bronchi and trachea. Each position contributes to effective drainage of a different lobe of the lungs; lower and middle lobe bronchi drain more effectively when the head is down, whereas the upper lobe bronchi drain more effectively when the head is up. The secretions then are removed by coughing. The nurse instructs the patient to inhale bronchodilators and mucolytic agents, if prescribed, before postural drainage, because these medications improve drainage of the bronchial tree.

Nursing Management

The nurse should keep in mind the medical diagnosis, the lung lobes or segments involved, the cardiac status, and any structural deformities of the chest wall and spine. Auscultation of the chest before and after the procedure is used to identify the areas that need drainage and assess the effectiveness of treatment. The nurse educates family members who will assist the patient at home to evaluate breath sounds before and after treatment. The nurse explores strategies that will enable the patient to assume the indicated positions at home. This may require the creative use of objects readily available at home, such as pillows, cushions, or cardboard boxes.

Postural drainage is usually performed two to four times daily, before meals (to prevent nausea, vomiting, and aspiration) and

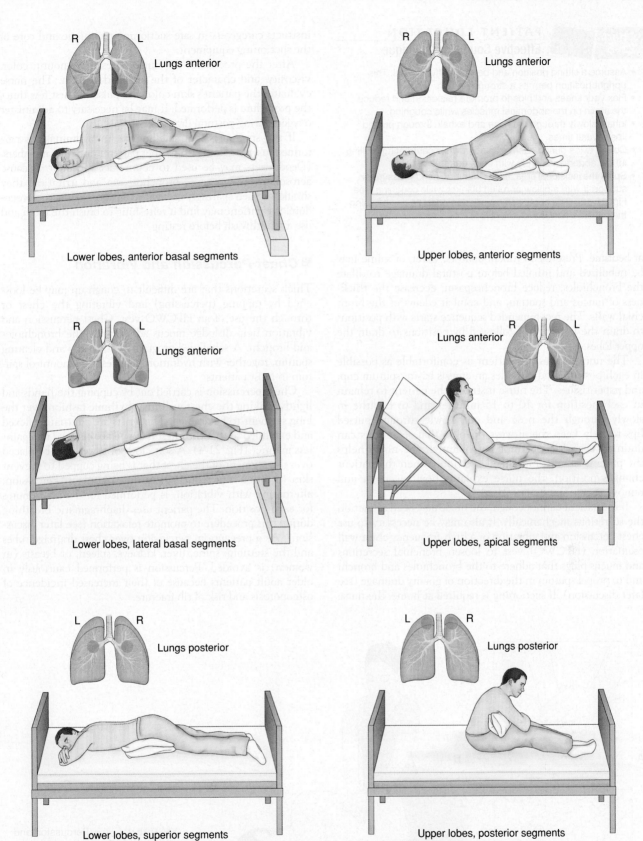

FIGURE 21-3 • Postural drainage positions and the areas of lung drained by each position.

Chart
21-5

PATIENT EDUCATION
Effective Coughing Technique

- Assume a sitting position and bend slightly forward. This upright position permits a stronger cough.
- Flex your knees and hips to promote relaxation and reduce the strain on the abdominal muscles while coughing.
- Inhale slowly through the nose and exhale through pursed lips several times.
- Cough twice during each exhalation while contracting (pulling in) the abdomen sharply with each cough.
- Splint the incisional area, if any, with firm hand pressure or support it with a pillow or rolled blanket while coughing (see Fig. 21-12). (The nurse can initially demonstrate this by using the patient's hands.)

at bedtime. Prescribed bronchodilators, water, or saline may be nebulized and inhaled before postural drainage to dilate the bronchioles, reduce bronchospasm, decrease the thickness of mucus and sputum, and combat edema of the bronchial walls. The recommended sequence starts with positions to drain the lower lobes, followed by positions to drain the upper lobes.

The nurse makes the patient as comfortable as possible in each position and provides an emesis basin, sputum cup, and paper tissues. The nurse instructs the patient to remain in each position for 10 to 15 minutes and to breathe in slowly through the nose and out slowly through pursed lips to help keep the airways open so that secretions can drain. If a position cannot be tolerated, the nurse helps the patient assume a modified position. When the patient changes position, the nurse explains how to cough and remove secretions (Chart 21-5).

If the patient cannot cough, the nurse may need to suction the secretions mechanically. It also may be necessary to use chest percussion and vibration or a high-frequency chest wall oscillation (HFCWO) vest to loosen bronchial secretions and mucus plugs that adhere to the bronchioles and bronchi and to propel sputum in the direction of gravity drainage (see later discussion). If suctioning is required at home, the nurse

instructs caregivers in safe suctioning technique and care of the suctioning equipment.

After the procedure, the nurse notes the amount, color, viscosity, and character of the expelled sputum. The nurse evaluates the patient's skin color and pulse the first few times the procedure is performed. It may be necessary to administer oxygen during postural drainage.

If the sputum is foul smelling, postural drainage is performed in a room away from other patients or family members. (Deodorizers may be used to counteract the odor. Because aerosol sprays can cause bronchospasm and irritation, they should be used sparingly and with caution.) After the procedure, the patient may find it refreshing to brush the teeth and use a mouthwash before resting.

■ Chest Percussion and Vibration

Thick secretions that are difficult to cough up may be loosened by tapping (percussing) and vibrating the chest or through the use of an HFCWO vest. Chest percussion and vibration help dislodge mucus adhering to the bronchioles and bronchi. A scheduled program of coughing and clearing sputum, together with hydration, reduces the amount of sputum in most patients.

Chest percussion is carried out by cupping the hands and lightly striking the chest wall in a rhythmic fashion over the lung segment to be drained. The wrists are alternately flexed and extended so that the chest is cupped or clapped in a painless manner (Fig. 21-4). A soft cloth or towel may be placed over the segment of the chest that is being cupped to prevent skin irritation and redness from direct contact. Percussion, alternating with vibration, is performed for 3 to 5 minutes for each position. The patient uses diaphragmatic breathing during this procedure to promote relaxation (see later discussion). As a precaution, percussion over chest drainage tubes and the sternum, spine, liver, kidneys, spleen, or breasts (in women) is avoided. Percussion is performed cautiously in older adult patients because of their increased incidence of osteoporosis and risk of rib fracture.

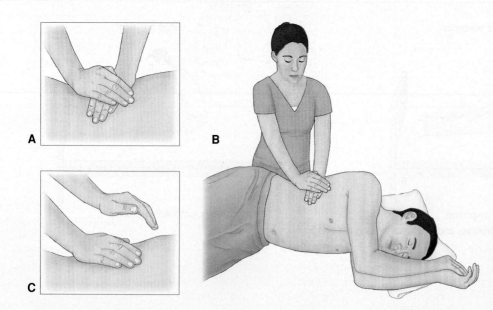

A

B

C

FIGURE 21-4 • Percussion and vibration. **A.** Proper hand position for vibration. **B.** Proper technique for vibration. The wrists and elbows remain stiff; the vibrating motion is produced by the shoulder muscles. **C.** Proper hand position for percussion.

Vibration is the technique of applying manual compression and tremor to the chest wall during the exhalation phase of respiration (see Fig. 21-4). This helps increase the velocity of the air expired from the small airways, thus freeing mucus. After three or four vibrations, the patient is encouraged to cough, contracting the abdominal muscles to increase the effectiveness of the cough.

The number of times the percussion and coughing cycle is repeated depends on the patient's tolerance and clinical response. The nurse evaluates breath sounds before and after the procedures.

An inflatable HFCWO vest (Fig. 21-5) may be used to provide chest therapy. The vest uses air pulses to compress the chest wall 8 to 18 times/sec, causing secretions to detach from the airway wall and enabling the patient to expel them by coughing. Patients prescribed vest therapy are generally more satisfied with this mode of treatment delivery than patients who receive manual CPT. Furthermore, research suggests that the vest is equally effective to manual CPT; however, the mode of therapy selected should consider the patient's specific needs and preferences (Mahajan, Diette, Hatipoglu, et al., 2011; Morrison & Agnew, 2011). Chest therapy may also be delivered using specialized beds. These beds feature programmable mattresses that deliver vibropercussion and may rotate the upper torso up to 45 degrees to help mobilize pulmonary secretions (Marini & Wheeler, 2010).

To increase the effectiveness of coughing, a flutter valve may be used, especially by patients who have cystic fibrosis. The flutter valve looks like a pipe but has a cap covering the bowl, which contains a steel ball. When the patient exhales actively into the valve, movement of the ball causes pressure oscillations, thereby decreasing viscosity of the mucus, allowing it to move within the airways and be coughed out.

Nursing Management

When performing CPT, the nurse ensures that the patient is comfortable, is not wearing restrictive clothing, and has not just eaten. The nurse gives medication for pain, as prescribed, before percussion and vibration and splints any incision and provides pillows for support as needed. The positions are varied, but focus is placed on the affected areas. On completion

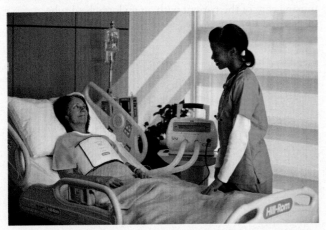

FIGURE 21-5 • High-frequency chest wall oscillation (HFCWO) vest. © 2013 Hill-Rom Services, Inc. Reprinted with permission— all rights reserved.

of the treatment, the nurse assists the patient to assume a comfortable position.

If an HFCWO vest is being used, the patient may assume whatever position is most comfortable and may even continue to perform light activity during therapy within the length of the compressed air hose. The patient does not need to assume specific positions for the vest to be effective.

The nurse must stop treatment if any of the following occur: increased pain, increased shortness of breath, weakness, lightheadedness, or hemoptysis. Therapy is indicated until the patient has normal respirations, can mobilize secretions, and has normal breath sounds, and until the chest x-ray findings are normal.

Promoting Home and Community-Based Care

Educating Patients About Self-Care

CPT is frequently indicated at home for patients with COPD, bronchiectasis, or cystic fibrosis. The techniques are the same as described previously; however, gravity drainage is achieved by placing the hips over a box, a stack of magazines, or pillows (unless a hospital bed is available). The nurse instructs the patient and family in the positions and techniques of percussion and vibration so that therapy can be continued in the home. In addition, the nurse instructs the patient to maintain an adequate fluid intake and air humidity to prevent secretions from becoming thick and tenacious. It also is important to educate the patient to recognize early signs of infection, such as fever and a change in the color or character of sputum.

Continuing Care

CPT may be carried out during visits by a home care nurse. The nurse also assesses the patient's physical status, understanding of the treatment plan, adherence with recommended therapy, and the effectiveness of therapy. Patient and family education is reinforced during these visits. The nurse reports to the patient's primary provider any deterioration in the patient's physical status or inability to clear secretions.

■ *Breathing Retraining*

Breathing retraining consists of exercises and breathing practices that are designed to achieve more efficient and controlled ventilation and to decrease the work of breathing. Breathing retraining is especially indicated in patients with COPD and dyspnea. These exercises promote maximal alveolar inflation and muscle relaxation; relieve anxiety; eliminate ineffective, uncoordinated patterns of respiratory muscle activity; slow the respiratory rate; and decrease the work of breathing (Facchiano, Hoffman, & Núñez, 2011). Slow, relaxed, rhythmic breathing also helps to control the anxiety that occurs with dyspnea. Specific breathing exercises include diaphragmatic and pursed-lip breathing (see Chart 21-4).

Diaphragmatic breathing can become automatic with sufficient practice and concentration. Pursed-lip breathing, which improves oxygen transport, helps induce a slow, deep breathing pattern and assists the patient to control breathing, even during periods of stress. This type of breathing helps prevent airway collapse secondary to loss of lung elasticity in emphysema. The nurse instructs the patient in diaphragmatic breathing and pursed-lip breathing, as described in Chart 21-4. Breathing exercises should be practiced in several positions because air distribution and pulmonary circulation vary with the position of the chest.

Many patients require additional oxygen, using a low-flow method, while performing breathing exercises. Emphysema-like changes in the lung occur as part of the natural aging process of the lung; therefore, breathing exercises are appropriate for all older adult patients, whether hospitalized or not, who are sedentary, even without primary lung disease.

Nursing Management

The nurse instructs the patient to breathe slowly and rhythmically in a relaxed manner and to exhale completely to empty the lungs. The patient is instructed to always inhale through the nose because this filters, humidifies, and warms the air. If short of breath, the patient should be instructed to concentrate on prolonging the length of exhalation; this helps avoid initiating a cycle of increasing shortness of breath and panic.

The nurse instructs the patient that an adequate dietary intake promotes gas exchange and increases energy levels. It is important to obtain adequate nutrition without overeating by consuming small, frequent meals and snacks. Having ready-prepared meals and favorite foods available helps encourage nutrient consumption. Gas-producing foods such as beans, legumes, broccoli, cabbage, and brussels sprouts should be avoided to prevent gastric distress. Because many patients lack the energy to eat, they should be instructed to rest before and after meals to conserve energy.

AIRWAY MANAGEMENT

Adequate ventilation depends on free movement of air through the upper and lower airways. In many disorders, the airway becomes narrowed or blocked as a result of disease, bronchoconstriction (narrowing of the airway by contraction of muscle fibers), a foreign body, or secretions. Maintaining a patent (open) airway is achieved through meticulous airway management, whether in an emergency situation, such as airway obstruction, or in long-term management, as in caring for a patient with an endotracheal or a tracheostomy tube.

Emergency Management of Upper Airway Obstruction

Upper airway obstruction has a variety of causes. Acute upper airway obstruction may be caused by food particles, vomitus, blood clots, or anything that obstructs the larynx or trachea. It also may occur from enlargement of tissue in the wall of the airway, as in epiglottitis, obstructive sleep apnea, laryngeal edema, laryngeal carcinoma, or peritonsillar abscess, or from thick secretions. Pressure on the walls of the airway, as occurs in retrosternal goiter, enlarged mediastinal lymph nodes, hematoma around the upper airway, and thoracic aneurysm, also may result in upper airway obstruction.

The patient with an altered level of consciousness from any cause is at risk for upper airway obstruction because of loss of the protective reflexes (cough and swallowing) and loss of the tone of the pharyngeal muscles, which causes the tongue to fall back and block the airway.

The nurse makes the following rapid observations to assess for signs and symptoms of upper airway obstruction:

- *Inspection:* Is the patient conscious? Is there any inspiratory effort? Does the chest rise symmetrically? Is there use or retraction of accessory muscles? What is the skin color? Are there any obvious signs of deformity or obstruction (trauma, food, teeth, vomitus)? Is the trachea midline?
- *Palpation:* Do both sides of the chest rise equally with inspiration? Are there any specific areas of tenderness, fracture, or subcutaneous emphysema (crepitus)?
- *Auscultation:* Is there any audible air movement, stridor (inspiratory sound), or wheezing (expiratory sound)? Are breath sounds present over the lower trachea and all lobes?

As soon as an upper airway obstruction is identified, the nurse takes emergency measures (Chart 21-6). (See Chapter 22 or Chapter 72 for more details on managing a foreign body airway obstruction.)

Endotracheal Intubation

Endotracheal intubation involves passing an endotracheal tube through the mouth or nose into the trachea (Fig. 21-6). Intubation provides a patent airway when the patient is having respiratory distress that cannot be treated with simpler methods and is the method of choice in emergency care. Endotracheal intubation is a means of providing an airway for patients who cannot maintain an adequate airway on their own (e.g., patients who are comatose, patients with upper airway obstruction), for patients needing mechanical ventilation, and for suctioning secretions from the pulmonary tree.

An endotracheal tube usually is passed with the aid of a laryngoscope by specifically trained medical, nursing, or respiratory therapy personnel (see Chapter 72). Once the tube is inserted, a cuff is inflated to prevent air from leaking around the outer part of the tube in order to minimize the possibility of aspiration and secure the tube. Chart 21-7 discusses the nursing care of the patient with an endotracheal tube.

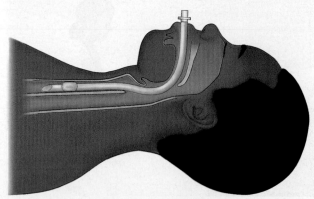

FIGURE 21-6 • Endotracheal tube in place. The tube has been inserted using the oral route. The cuff has been inflated to maintain the tube's position and to minimize the risk of aspiration.

Chart 21-6 | Clearing an Upper Airway Obstruction

Attempt to Open the Airway

Perform the head-tilt/chin-lift maneuver by placing one hand on the forehead and placing the fingers of the other hand underneath the jaw and lifting upward and forward. This action pulls the tongue away from the back of the pharynx.

Attempt to Clear the Airway

- Assess the patient by observing the chest and listening and feeling for the movement of air.
- Use a cross-finger technique to open the mouth and observe for obvious obstructions such as secretions, blood clots, or food particles.
- If no passage of air is detected, begin cardiopulmonary resuscitation (CPR).

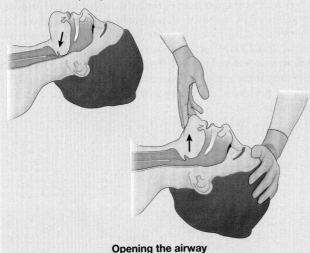

Opening the airway

Bag and Mask Resuscitation

- Apply the mask to the patient's face and create a seal by pressing the thumb of the nondominant hand on the bridge of the nose and the index finger on the chin.
- Using the rest of the fingers on that hand, pull on the chin and the angle of the mandible to maintain the head in extension.
- Use the dominant hand to inflate the lungs by squeezing the bag to its full volume.

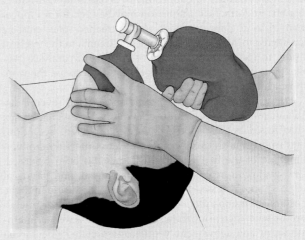

Resuscitation via bag and mask apparatus

Adapted from American Heart Association. (2010). *Basic life support for healthcare providers: Student manual*. Dallas, TX: Author.

Chart 21-7 | Care of the Patient With an Endotracheal Tube

Immediately After Intubation

1. Check symmetry of chest expansion.
2. Auscultate breath sounds of anterior and lateral chest bilaterally.
3. Obtain order for chest x-ray to verify proper tube placement.
4. Check cuff pressure every 6–8 hours.
5. Monitor for signs and symptoms of aspiration.
6. Ensure high humidity; a visible mist should appear in the T-piece or ventilator tubing.
7. Administer oxygen concentration as prescribed by the primary care provider.
8. Secure the tube to the patient's face with tape, and mark the proximal end for position maintenance.
   a. Cut proximal end of tube if it is longer than 7.5 cm (3 inches) to prevent kinking.
   b. Insert an oral airway or mouth device to prevent the patient from biting and obstructing the tube.
9. Use sterile suction technique and airway care to prevent iatrogenic contamination and infection.
10. Continue to reposition patient every 2 hours and as needed to prevent atelectasis and to optimize lung expansion.
11. Provide oral hygiene and suction the oropharynx whenever necessary.

Extubation (Removal of Endotracheal Tube)

1. Explain procedure.
2. Have self-inflating bag and mask ready in case ventilatory assistance is required immediately after extubation.
3. Suction the tracheobronchial tree and oropharynx, remove tape, and then deflate the cuff.
4. Give 100% oxygen for a few breaths, then insert a new, sterile suction catheter inside tube.
5. Have the patient inhale. At peak inspiration, remove the tube, suctioning the airway through the tube as it is pulled out.

Note: In some hospitals, this procedure can be performed by respiratory therapists; in others, by nurses. Check hospital policy.

Care of Patient Following Extubation

1. Give heated humidity and oxygen by facemask and maintain the patient in a sitting or high Fowler's position.
2. Monitor respiratory rate and quality of chest excursions. Note stridor, color change, and change in mental alertness or behavior.
3. Monitor the patient's oxygen level using a pulse oximeter.
4. Keep patient NPO (nothing by mouth), or give only ice chips for next few hours.
5. Provide mouth care.
6. Educate the patient about how to perform coughing and deep-breathing exercises.

Complications can occur from pressure exerted by the cuff on the tracheal wall. Cuff pressures should be maintained between 15 and 20 mm Hg (Morton, Fontaine, Hudak, et al., 2009). High cuff pressure can cause tracheal bleeding, ischemia, and pressure necrosis, whereas low cuff pressure can increase the risk of aspiration pneumonia. Routine deflation of the cuff is not recommended because of the increased risk of aspiration and hypoxia. Tracheobronchial secretions are suctioned through the tube. Warmed, humidified oxygen should always be introduced through the tube, whether the patient is breathing spontaneously or is receiving ventilatory support. Endotracheal intubation may be used for no longer than 14 to 21 days, by which time a tracheostomy must be considered to decrease irritation of and trauma to the tracheal lining, to reduce the incidence of vocal cord paralysis (secondary to laryngeal nerve damage), and to decrease the work of breathing (Wiegand, 2011).

Endotracheal and tracheostomy tubes have several disadvantages. The tubes cause discomfort. The cough reflex is depressed because glottis closure is hindered. Secretions tend to become thicker because the warming and humidifying effect of the upper respiratory tract has been bypassed. The swallowing reflexes (glottic, pharyngeal, and laryngeal reflexes) are depressed because of prolonged disuse and the mechanical trauma produced by the endotracheal or tracheostomy tube, increasing the risk of aspiration as well as microaspiration and subsequent ventilator-associated pneumonia (VAP) (Hamilton & Grap, 2012). In addition, ulceration and stricture of the larynx or trachea may develop. Of great concern to the patient is the inability to talk and to communicate needs.

Unintentional or premature removal of the tube is a potentially life-threatening complication of endotracheal intubation. Removal of the tube is a frequent problem in intensive care units (ICUs) and occurs mainly during nursing care or by the patient. Nurses must instruct and remind patients and family members about the purpose of the tube and the dangers of removing it. Baseline and ongoing assessment of the patient and of the equipment ensures effective care. Providing comfort measures, including opioid analgesia and sedation, can improve the patient's tolerance of the endotracheal tube.

> ▶ **Quality and Safety Nursing Alert**
>
> Inadvertent removal of an endotracheal tube can cause laryngeal swelling, hypoxemia, bradycardia, hypotension, and even death. Measures must be taken to prevent premature or inadvertent removal.

To prevent tube removal by the patient, the nurse should explain to the patient and family the purpose of the tube, distract the patient through one-to-one interaction or with television, and maintain comfort measures. If the patient cannot move the arms and hands to the endotracheal tube, restraints are not needed. If the patient is alert, oriented, able to follow directions, and cooperative to the point that it is highly unlikely that he or she will remove the endotracheal tube, restraints are not needed. However, if the nurse determines there is a risk that the patient may try to remove the tube, the least invasive method of restraints (e.g., soft wrist restraints)

may be appropriate with a primary provider's order (check agency policy). The rationale for use of restraints should be documented, and the patient's significant others should receive explanations why restraints are necessary. Close monitoring of the patient is essential to ensure safety and prevent harm. The use of restraints is generally limited to no more than 24 hours (Sole, Klein, & Moseley, 2013).

Tracheostomy

A **tracheotomy** is a surgical procedure in which an opening is made into the trachea. The indwelling tube inserted into the trachea is called a **tracheostomy tube** (Fig. 21-7). A tracheostomy (the stoma that is the product of the tracheotomy) may be either temporary or permanent.

A tracheotomy is used to bypass an upper airway obstruction, to allow removal of tracheobronchial secretions, to permit the long-term use of mechanical ventilation, to prevent aspiration of oral or gastric secretions in the unconscious or paralyzed patient (by closing off the trachea from the esophagus), and to replace an endotracheal tube. Many disease processes and emergency conditions make a tracheotomy necessary.

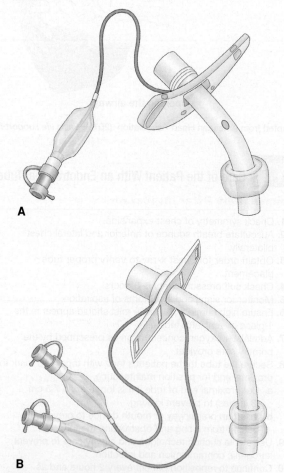

FIGURE 21-7 • Tracheostomy tubes. **A.** Fenestrated tube, which allows patient to talk. **B.** Double-cuffed tube. Inflating the two cuffs alternately can help prevent tracheal damage.

Procedure

The surgical procedure is usually performed in the operating room or in an ICU, where the patient's ventilation can be well controlled and optimal aseptic technique can be maintained. A surgical opening is made between the second and third tracheal rings. After the trachea is exposed, a cuffed tracheostomy tube of an appropriate size is inserted. The cuff is an inflatable attachment to the tracheostomy tube that is designed to occlude the space between the tracheal walls and the tube, to permit effective mechanical ventilation, and to minimize the risk of aspiration. See Figure 21-7 for the different types of tracheostomy tubes.

The tracheostomy tube is held in place by tapes fastened around the patient's neck. Usually, a square of sterile gauze is placed between the tube and the skin to absorb drainage and reduce the risk of infection.

Complications

Complications may occur early or late in the course of tracheostomy tube management. They may even occur years after the tube has been removed. Early complications include bleeding, pneumothorax, air embolism, aspiration, subcutaneous or mediastinal emphysema, recurrent laryngeal nerve damage, and posterior tracheal wall penetration. Long-term complications include airway obstruction from accumulation of secretions or protrusion of the cuff over the opening of the tube, infection, rupture of the innominate artery, dysphagia, tracheoesophageal fistula, tracheal dilation, tracheal ischemia, and necrosis. Tracheal stenosis may develop after the tube is removed. Chart 21-8 outlines measures nurses can take to prevent complications.

Nursing Management

The patient requires continuous monitoring and assessment. The newly made opening must be kept patent by proper suctioning of secretions. After the vital signs are stable, the patient is placed in a semi-Fowler's position to facilitate ventilation, promote drainage, minimize edema, and prevent strain on the suture lines. Analgesia and sedative agents must be administered with caution because of the risk of suppressing the cough reflex.

Major objectives of nursing care are to alleviate the patient's apprehension and to provide an effective means of communication. The nurse keeps paper and pencil or a Magic Slate® and the call light within the patient's reach at all times to ensure a means of communication. Chart 21-9 summarizes the care of the patient with a tracheostomy tube.

Suctioning the Tracheal Tube (Tracheostomy or Endotracheal Tube)

When a tracheostomy or endotracheal tube is in place, it is usually necessary to suction the patient's secretions because of the decreased effectiveness of the cough mechanism. Tracheal suctioning is performed when adventitious breath sounds are detected or whenever secretions are obviously present. Unnecessary suctioning can initiate bronchospasm and cause mechanical trauma to the tracheal mucosa.

All equipment that comes into direct contact with the patient's lower airway must be sterile to prevent sepsis. Chart 21-10 presents the procedure for suctioning a patient with a tracheostomy tube. In patients who are mechanically ventilated, an in-line suction catheter may be used to allow rapid suction when needed and to minimize cross-contamination by airborne pathogens. An in-line suction device allows the patient to be suctioned without being disconnected from the ventilator circuit. In-line suctioning (also called *closed suctioning*) decreases hypoxemia, sustains PEEP, and can decrease patient anxiety associated with suctioning (Sole et al., 2013). Because in-line suctioning protects staff from patient secretions, it can be performed without using personal protective gear.

Managing the Cuff

The cuff on an endotracheal or tracheostomy tube should be inflated if the patient requires mechanical ventilation or is at high risk for aspiration. The pressure within the cuff should be the lowest possible pressure that allows delivery of adequate tidal volumes and prevents pulmonary aspiration. Usually, the pressure is maintained at less than 25 mm Hg to prevent injury and at more than 15 mm Hg to prevent aspiration (Wiegand, 2011). Cuff pressure must be monitored by the respiratory therapist or nurse at least every 8 hours by attaching a handheld pressure gauge to the pilot balloon of the tube or by using the minimal leak volume or minimal occlusion volume technique. With long-term intubation, higher pressures may be needed to maintain an adequate seal.

Promoting Home and Community-Based Care

Educating Patients About Self-Care

If the patient is pending discharge to the home setting with a tracheostomy tube, the nurse should ensure that suction and other appropriate equipment is at place in the home prior to discharge. The nurse also instructs the patient and family about daily care, including techniques to prevent infection, as well as measures to take in an emergency. The nurse provides the patient and family with a list of community contacts for education and support needs.

Continuing Care

A referral for home care is indicated for ongoing assessment of the patient and of the ability of the patient and family

---

Chart 21-8

Preventing Complications Associated With Endotracheal and Tracheostomy Tubes

- Administer adequate warmed humidity.
- Maintain cuff pressure at appropriate level.
- Suction as needed per assessment findings.
- Maintain skin integrity. Change tape and dressing as needed or per protocol.
- Auscultate lung sounds.
- Monitor for signs and symptoms of infection, including temperature and white blood cell count.
- Administer prescribed oxygen and monitor oxygen saturation.
- Monitor for cyanosis.
- Maintain adequate hydration of the patient.
- Use sterile technique when suctioning and performing tracheostomy care.

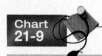

GUIDELINES

Chart 21-9   Care of the Patient With a Tracheostomy Tube

Equipment
- Sterile and clean gloves
- Hydrogen peroxide
- Normal saline solution or sterile water
- Basin

- Cotton-tipped applicators
- Split gauze dressing
- Tracheostomy ties (e.g., twill tape, Velcro)
- Type of tube prescribed, if the tube is to be changed

Implementation

Actions	Rationale
1. Provide patient and family instruction on the key points for tracheostomy care, beginning with how to inspect the tracheostomy dressing for moisture or drainage. A cuffed tube (air injected into cuff) is required during mechanical ventilation. A low-pressure cuff is most commonly used. Patients requiring long-term use of a tracheostomy tube and who can breathe spontaneously commonly use an uncuffed, metal tube.	The tracheostomy dressing is changed as needed to keep the skin clean and dry. To prevent potential breakdown, moist or soiled dressings should not remain on the skin. A cuffed tube prevents air from leaking during positive-pressure ventilation and also prevents tracheal aspiration of gastric contents. An adequate seal is indicated by the disappearance of any air leakage from the mouth or tracheostomy or by the disappearance of the harsh, gurgling sound of air coming from the throat. Low-pressure cuffs exert minimal pressure on the tracheal mucosa and thus reduce the danger of tracheal ulceration and stricture.
2. Perform hand hygiene.	Hand hygiene reduces bacteria on hands.
3. Explain procedure to patient and family as appropriate.	A patient with a tracheostomy is apprehensive and requires ongoing assurance and support.
4. Put on clean gloves; remove and discard the soiled dressing in a biohazard container.	Observing body substance isolation reduces cross-contamination from soiled dressings.
5. Prepare sterile supplies, including hydrogen peroxide, normal saline solution or sterile water, cotton-tipped applicators, dressing, and ties.	Having necessary supplies and equipment readily available allows the procedure to be completed efficiently.
6. Put on sterile gloves. (Some primary care providers approve clean technique for long-term tracheostomy patients in the home.)	Sterile equipment minimizes transmission of surface flora to the sterile respiratory tract. Clean technique may be used in the home because of decreased exposure to potential pathogens.
7. Cleanse the wound and the plate of the tracheostomy tube with sterile cotton-tipped applicators moistened with hydrogen peroxide. Rinse with sterile saline solution.	Hydrogen peroxide is effective in loosening crusted secretions. Rinsing prevents skin residue.
8. Soak inner cannula in peroxide or sterile saline, per manufacturer's instructions; rinse with saline solution; and inspect to be sure all dried secretions have been removed. Dry and reinsert inner cannula or replace with a new disposable inner cannula.	Soaking loosens and removes secretions from the inner lumen of the tracheostomy tube. Retained secretions could harbor bacteria, leading to infection. Some plastic tracheostomy tubes may be damaged by using peroxide.
9. Place clean tracheostomy ties in position to secure the tracheostomy tube by inserting one end of the tie through the side opening of the outer cannula. Take the ties around the back of the patient's neck and thread them through the opposite opening of the outer cannula. Bring both ends around so that they meet on one side of the neck. Tighten the ties until only two fingers can be comfortably inserted under them. Secure with a knot. For a new tracheostomy, two people should assist with tie changes. Remove soiled ties after the new ties are in place.	This anchoring technique is needed because the tracheostomy tube can be dislodged by movement or by a forceful cough if left unsecured. A dislodged tracheostomy tube is difficult to reinsert, and respiratory distress may occur. Dislodgement of the tube with a new tracheostomy is a medical emergency.
10. Remove old tracheostomy ties and discard them in a biohazard container after the new ties are in place.	Tracheostomy ties with old secretions may harbor bacteria.
11. Although some long-term tracheostomies with healed stomas may not require a dressing, other tracheostomies do. In such cases, use a sterile tracheostomy dressing, fitting it securely under the tracheostomy ties and flange of tracheostomy tube so that the incision is covered, as shown below.	Healed tracheostomies with minimal secretions do not need a dressing. Dressings that will shred are not used around a tracheostomy because of the risk that pieces of material, lint, or thread may get into the tube, and eventually into the trachea, causing obstruction or abscess formation. Special dressings that do not have a tendency to shred are used.

Chart 21-9 Care of the Patient With a Tracheostomy Tube (continued)

A. The cuff of the tracheostomy tube fits smoothly and snugly in the trachea in a way that promotes circulation but seals off the escape of secretions and air surrounding the tube. **B.** For a dressing change, a 4- × 4-inch gauze pad may be folded (cutting would promote shredding, placing the patient at risk for aspiration) around the tracheostomy tube. **C.** The tracheostomy tube may then be stabilized by slipping the tracheostomy ties through the neck plate slots of the tracheostomy tube. The ties may be fastened to the side of the neck to eliminate the discomfort of lying on the knot.

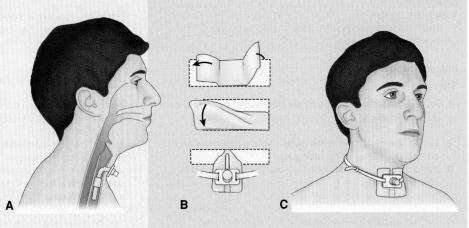

to provide appropriate and safe care. The home care nurse assesses the patient's and family's ability to cope with the physical changes and psychological issues associated with having a tracheostomy. Minimizing the amount of dust or particles in the air and providing adequate humidification may make it easier for the patient to breathe. Dust and particles in the air can be decreased by removing drapes and upholstered furniture; using air filters; and washing floors, dusting, and vacuuming frequently. The nurse identifies resources and makes referrals for appropriate services to assist the patient and family to manage the tracheostomy tube at home.

Mechanical Ventilation

Mechanical ventilation may be required for a variety of reasons: to control the patient's respirations during surgery or treatment, to oxygenate the blood when the patient's ventilatory efforts are inadequate, and to rest the respiratory muscles, among others. Many patients placed on a ventilator can breathe spontaneously, although the effort needed to do so may be exhausting.

A **mechanical ventilator** is a positive- or negative-pressure breathing device that can maintain ventilation and oxygen delivery for a prolonged period. Caring for a patient on mechanical ventilation has become an integral part of nursing care in critical care or general medical-surgical units, extended care facilities, and the home. Nurses, physicians, and respiratory therapists must understand each patient's specific pulmonary needs and work together to set realistic goals. Positive patient outcomes depend on an understanding of the principles of mechanical ventilation and the patient's care needs as well as open communication among members of the health care team about the goals of therapy, weaning plans, and the patient's tolerance of changes in ventilator settings.

Indications

If a patient has evidence of respiratory failure or a compromised airway, endotracheal intubation and mechanical ventilation are indicated. This clinical evidence may be corroborated by a continuous decrease in oxygenation (PaO_2), an increase in arterial carbon dioxide levels ($PaCO_2$), and a persistent acidosis (decreased pH); however, if the patient's status appears emergent, then waiting for these laboratory results prior to ensuring these ventilator support measures is imprudent (Amitai & Sinert, 2011). Conditions such as thoracic or abdominal surgery, drug overdose, neuromuscular disorders, inhalation injury, COPD, multiple trauma, shock, multisystem failure, and coma may lead to respiratory failure and the need for mechanical ventilation. General indications for mechanical ventilation are displayed in Chart 21-11. A patient with apnea that is not readily reversible also is a candidate for mechanical ventilation.

Classification of Ventilators

Mechanical ventilators were traditionally classified according to the method by which they supported ventilation. The two general categories are negative-pressure and positive-pressure ventilators (Fig. 21-8 displays commonly used positive-pressure ventilators). Negative-pressure ventilators (e.g., "iron lungs," chest cuirass) are older modes of ventilatory support that are rarely utilized today.

Positive-Pressure Ventilators

Positive-pressure ventilators inflate the lungs by exerting positive pressure on the airway, pushing air in, similar to a bellows mechanism, and forcing the alveoli to expand during inspiration. Expiration occurs passively. Endotracheal intubation or tracheostomy is usually necessary. These ventilators are widely used in the hospital setting and are increasingly used in the home for patients with primary lung disease. Three types of positive-pressure ventilators are classified by the method of ending the inspiratory phase of respiration: volume cycled, pressure cycled, and high-frequency oscillatory support (Amitai & Sinert, 2011). The fourth type, noninvasive positive-pressure ventilation (NIPPV), does not require intubation.

Chart 21-10

Performing Tracheal Suction

Equipment
- Suction catheters
- Gloves (sterile and nonsterile), gown, mask, and goggles for eye protection

- Basin for sterile normal saline solution for irrigation
- Manual resuscitation bag with supplemental oxygen
- Suction source

Implementation

Step	Rationale
1. Assess the patient's lung sounds and oxygen saturation via pulse oximeter.	Assessment data indicate the need for suctioning and allow the nurse to monitor the effect of suction on the patient's level of oxygenation.
2. Explain the procedure to the patient before beginning and offer reassurance during suctioning.	The patient may be apprehensive about choking and about an inability to communicate.
3. Perform hand hygiene. Put on nonsterile gloves, goggles, gown, and mask.	Hand hygiene reduces bacteria on hands. Nonsterile gloves, goggles, gown, and mask serve as personal protective equipment (PPE) because they protect the clinician from becoming infected with pathogens.
4. Turn on suction source (pressure should not exceed 120 mm Hg for an open system and 160 mm Hg for a closed system).	Suction pressure should be set high enough to be effective without causing trauma to the tissues.
5. Open suction catheter kit.	Having equipment ready prevents interruption of the procedure.
6. Fill basin with sterile water.	This provides sterile solution for clearing suction catheter of secretions.
7. Put sterile glove on dominant hand.	Equipment that will contact the patient's lower airway must remain sterile to prevent infection.
8. Ventilate the patient with manual resuscitation bag and high-flow oxygen for about 30 seconds or turn on suction mode of ventilator (if available) to hyperoxygenate the patient.	This prevents hypoxia during suctioning.
9. Pick up suction catheter in sterile gloved hand and connect to suction.	This prevents contamination of sterile catheter.
10. Insert suction catheter at least as far as the end of the tube without applying suction, just far enough to stimulate the cough reflex.	Inserting the catheter without applying suction permits insertion without causing trauma to the tissues.
11. Apply suction while withdrawing and gently rotating the catheter 360 degrees (no longer than 10–15 seconds).	Prolonged suctioning may result in hypoxia and dysrhythmias, leading to cardiac arrest.
12. Reoxygenate and inflate the patient's lungs for several breaths with manual resuscitation bag, or allow ventilator to reoxygenate patient for several breaths using suction mode.	This prevents hypoxia during procedure and restores oxygen supply.
13. Rinse catheter by suctioning a few milliliters of sterile water solution from the basin between suction attempts.	This keeps suction catheter patent.
14. Repeat steps 8–13 until the airway is clear.	This ensures removal of all tracheal secretions.
15. Suction oropharyngeal cavity after completing tracheal suctioning.	This avoids contamination of trachea with oropharyngeal secretions and organisms.
16. Rinse suction tubing and discard catheter, gloves, and basin appropriately. Dispose of PPE as directed by facility's policies.	Safe disposal of equipment avoids cross-contamination.
17. Assess the patient's lung sounds and oxygen saturation via pulse oximeter after procedure.	Assessment provides information about effectiveness of procedure.
18. Document the amount, color, and consistency of secretions.	Documentation allows monitoring of patient's status over time.

Adapted from Nance-Floyd, B. (2011). Tracheostomy care: An evidence-based guide to suctioning and dressing changes. *American Nurse Today*, *6*(7), 14–16; and Oversend, T. J., Anderson, C. M., Brooks, D., et al. (2009). Updating the evidence base for suctioning adult patients: A systematic review. *Canadian Respiratory Journal*, *16*(3), e6–e17.

Volume-Cycled Ventilators

Volume-cycled ventilators deliver a preset volume of air with each inspiration. Once this preset volume is delivered to the patient, the ventilator cycles off and exhalation occurs passively. From breath to breath, the volume of air delivered by the ventilator is relatively constant, ensuring consistent, adequate breaths despite varying airway pressures. A major disadvantage to using volume-cycled ventilators is that patients may experience barotrauma because the pressures required to deliver the breaths may be excessive (Amitai & Sinert, 2011)

Pressure-Cycled Ventilators

When the pressure-cycled ventilator cycles on, it delivers a flow of air (inspiration) until it reaches a preset pressure, and then cycles off, and expiration occurs. The major limitation is the volume of air or oxygen can vary as the patient's airway

Chart 21-11   Indications for Mechanical Ventilation

Laboratory Values

PaO_2 <55 mm Hg
$PaCO_2$ >50 mm Hg and pH <7.32
Vital capacity <10 mL/kg
Negative inspiratory force <25 cm H_2O
FEV_1 <10 mL/kg

Clinical Manifestations

Apnea or bradypnea
Respiratory distressed with confusion
Increased work of breathing not relieved by other interventions
Confusion with need for airway protection
Circulatory shock

Adapted from Amitai, A., & Sinert, R. H. (2011). *Ventilator manage-ment.* Available at: emedicine.medscape.com/article/810126-overview#aw2qqb6b6

resistance or compliance changes. As a result, the tidal volume delivered may be inconsistent, possibly compromising ventilation.

High-Frequency Oscillatory Support Ventilators

These types of ventilators deliver very high respiratory rates (i.e., 180 to 900 breaths/minute) that are accompanied by very low tidal volumes and high airway pressures (hence the name *high-frequency oscillatory support*). These small pulses of oxygen-enriched air move down the center of the airways, allowing alveolar air to exit the lungs along the margins of the airways. This ventilatory mode is used to open the alveoli in situations characterized by closed small airways, such as atelectasis and acute respiratory distress syndrome (ARDS) (see Chapter 23), and it is also thought to protect the lung from pressure injury (Stewart, Jagelman, & Webster, 2011).

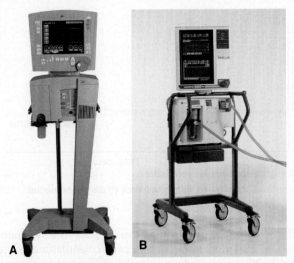

FIGURE 21-8 • Positive-pressure ventilators. **A.** The AVEA can be used to both ventilate and monitor neonatal, pediatric, and adult patients. It can also deliver noninvasive ventilation with Heliox to adult and pediatric patients. Courtesy of VIASYS Healthcare, Inc., Yorba Linda, CA. **B.** The Puritan-Bennett 840 Ventilator System has volume, pressure, and mixed modes designed for adult, pediatric, and infant ventilation. Courtesy of Tyco Healthcare/Nellcor Puritan Bennett, Pleasanton, CA.

Noninvasive Positive-Pressure Ventilation

NIPPV is a method of positive-pressure ventilation that can be given via facemasks that cover the nose and mouth, nasal masks, or other oral or nasal devices such as the nasal pillow (a small nasal cannula that seals around the nares to maintain the prescribed pressure). NIPPV eliminates the need for endotracheal intubation or tracheostomy and decreases the risk of nosocomial infections such as pneumonia. The most comfortable mode for the patient is pressure-controlled ventilation with pressure support. This eases the work of breathing and enhances gas exchange. The ventilator can be set with a minimum backup rate for patients with periods of apnea.

Patients are candidates for NIPPV if they have acute or chronic respiratory failure, acute pulmonary edema, COPD, chronic heart failure, or a sleep-related breathing disorder. The technique also may be used at home to improve tissue oxygenation and to rest the respiratory muscles while patients sleep at night. NIPPV is contraindicated for those who have experienced respiratory arrest, serious dysrhythmias, cognitive impairment, or head or facial trauma. NIPPV may also be used for obstructive sleep apnea, for patients at the end of life, and for those who do not want endotracheal intubation but may need short- or long-term ventilatory support (Bauman, 2009; Jallu & Salzman, 2011).

Continuous positive airway pressure (CPAP) provides positive pressure to the airways throughout the respiratory cycle. Although it can be used as an adjunct to mechanical ventilation with a cuffed endotracheal tube or tracheostomy tube to open the alveoli, it is also used with a leak-proof mask to keep alveoli open, thereby preventing respiratory failure. CPAP is the most effective treatment for obstructive sleep apnea because the positive pressure acts as a splint, keeping the upper airway and trachea open during sleep. To use CPAP, the patient must be breathing independently.

Bilevel positive airway pressure (BiPAP) ventilation offers independent control of inspiratory and expiratory pressures while providing pressure support ventilation (PSV). It delivers two levels of positive airway pressure provided via a nasal or oral mask, nasal pillow, or mouthpiece with a tight seal and a portable ventilator. Each inspiration can be initiated either by the patient or by the machine if it is programmed with a backup rate. The backup rate ensures that the patient receives a set number of breaths per minute. BiPAP is most often used for patients who require ventilatory assistance at night, such as those with severe COPD or sleep apnea. Tolerance is variable; BiPAP usually is most successful with highly motivated patients.

Ventilator Modes

Ventilator mode refers to how breaths are delivered to the patient. The most commonly used modes are continuous mandatory, assist–control (A/C), intermittent mandatory ventilation (IMV), synchronized intermittent mandatory ventilation (SIMV), PSV, and airway pressure release ventilation (APRV) (Fig. 21-9).

Continuous mandatory ventilation (CMV) provides full ventilatory support by delivering a preset tidal volume and respiratory rate. This mode of ventilation is indicated for patients who are apneic. **Assist–control (A/C) ventilation**

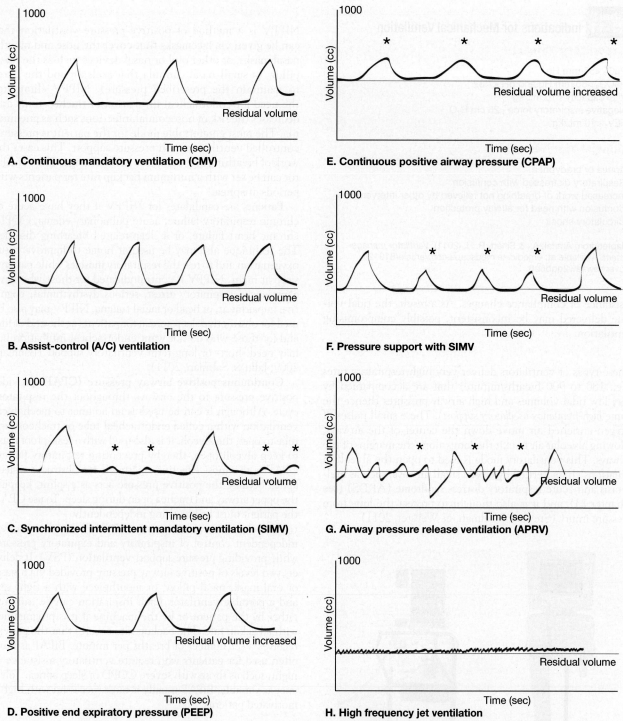

FIGURE 21-9 • Modes of mechanical ventilation with airflow waveforms. Inhalations marked with an asterisk (*) are spontaneous.

is similar to CMV in that the ventilator will deliver preset tidal volumes at a preset rate of respirations. However, if the patient initiates a breath between the machine's breaths, the ventilator delivers at the preset volume (assisted breath). Therefore, every breath is the preset volume.

Intermittent mandatory ventilation (IMV) provides a combination of mechanically assisted breaths and spontaneous breaths. Mechanical breaths are delivered at preset intervals and a preselected tidal volume, regardless of the patient's

efforts. Although the patient can increase the respiratory rate by initiating inspiration between ventilator-delivered breaths, these spontaneous breaths are limited to the tidal volume generated by the patient. IMV allows patients to use their own muscles for ventilation to help prevent muscle atrophy. It lowers mean airway pressure, which can assist in preventing barotrauma. However, "fighting the ventilator" or "bucking the ventilator" (i.e., trying to exhale when the ventilator is delivering a breath) may be increased.

Synchronized intermittent mandatory ventilation (SIMV) also delivers a preset tidal volume and number of breaths per minute. Between ventilator-delivered breaths, the patient can breathe spontaneously with no assistance from the ventilator on those extra breaths. Because the ventilator senses patient breathing efforts and does not initiate a breath in opposition to the patient's efforts, fighting the ventilator is reduced. As the patient's ability to breathe spontaneously increases, the preset number of ventilator breaths is decreased and the patient does more of the work of breathing. Like IMV, SIMV can be used to provide full or partial ventilatory support. Nursing interventions for patients receiving IMV or SIMV include monitoring progress by recording respiratory rate, minute volume, spontaneous and machine-generated tidal volume, FiO$_2$, and arterial blood gas levels.

Pressure support ventilation (PSV) applies a pressure plateau to the airway throughout the patient-triggered inspiration to decrease resistance within the tracheal tube and ventilator tubing. Pressure support is reduced gradually as the patient's strength increases. An SIMV backup rate may be added for extra support. The nurse must closely observe the patient's respiratory rate and tidal volumes on initiation of PSV. It may be necessary to adjust the pressure support to avoid tachypnea or large tidal volumes.

Airway pressure release ventilation (APRV) is a time-triggered, pressure-limited, time-cycled mode of mechanical ventilation that allows unrestricted, spontaneous breathing throughout the ventilatory cycle. The inflation period is long, and breaths may be initiated spontaneously as well as by the ventilator. APRV allows alveolar gas to be expelled through the lungs' natural recoil. APRV has the important advantages of causing less ventilator-induced lung injury and fewer adverse effects on cardiocirculatory function and being associated with lower need for sedation and neuromuscular blockade (Maung & Kaplan, 2011).

Proportional assist ventilation (PAV) provides partial ventilatory support in which the ventilator generates pressure in proportion to the patient's inspiratory efforts. With every breath, the ventilator synchronizes with the patient's ventilatory efforts. The more inspiratory pressure the patient generates, the more pressure the ventilator generates, amplifying the patient's inspiratory effort without any specific preselected target pressure or volume. It generally adds "additional muscle" to the patient's effort; the depth and frequency of breaths are controlled by the patient (Stewart et al., 2011).

Other modes of mechanical ventilation that incorporate computerized control of ventilation are being developed. In some of these modes, the ventilator constantly monitors many variables and adjusts gas delivery during individual breaths; these within-breath adjustment systems include automatic tube compensation, volume-ensured pressure support, and proportional support ventilation. In other modes, the ventilator evaluates gas delivery during one breath and uses that information to adjust the next breath; these between-breath adjustment systems can be made to ensure a preset tidal volume by adjusting pressure, up to a preset maximum, and include pressure volume support, pressure-regulated volume control, and adaptive support ventilation.

Chart 21-12 Initial Ventilator Settings

The following guide is an example of the steps involved in operating a mechanical ventilator. The nurse, in collaboration with the respiratory therapist, always reviews the manufacturer's instructions, which vary according to the equipment, before beginning mechanical ventilation.

1. Set the machine to deliver the tidal volume required (10–15 mL/kg).
2. Adjust the machine to deliver the lowest concentration of oxygen to maintain normal PaO$_2$ (80–100 mm Hg). This setting may be high initially but will gradually be reduced based on arterial blood gas results.
3. Record peak inspiratory pressure.
4. Set mode (assist–control or synchronized intermittent mandatory ventilation) and rate according to the order given by the primary provider. (See the glossary for definitions of modes of mechanical ventilation.) Set positive end-expiratory pressure (PEEP) and pressure support if ordered.
5. Adjust sensitivity so that the patient can trigger the ventilator with a minimal effort (usually 2 mm Hg negative inspiratory force).
6. Record minute volume and obtain arterial blood gases (ABGs) to measure carbon dioxide partial pressure (PaCO$_2$), pH, and PaO$_2$ after 20 minutes of continuous mechanical ventilation.
7. Adjust setting (FiO$_2$ and rate) according to results of ABG analysis to provide normal values or those set by the primary provider.
8. If there is poor coordination between the breathing rhythms of the patient and the ventilator (i.e., if the patient is "fighting" or "bucking the ventilator"), assess for hypoxia and manually ventilate on 100% oxygen with a resuscitation bag.

Adapted from Marini, J. J., & Wheeler, A. P. (2010). *Critical care medicine* (4th ed.). Philadelphia: Lippincott Williams & Wilkins.

Adjusting the Ventilator

The ventilator is adjusted so that the patient is comfortable and breathes synchronously (i.e., "in sync") with the machine. Minimal alteration of the normal cardiovascular and pulmonary dynamics is desired. If the volume ventilator is adjusted appropriately, the patient's arterial blood gas values will be satisfactory and there will be little or no cardiovascular compromise. Chart 21-12 describes initial ventilator settings.

Monitoring the Equipment

The ventilator needs to be monitored to make sure that it is functioning properly and that the settings are appropriate. Although the nurse may not be primarily responsible for adjusting the settings on the ventilator or measuring ventilator parameters (these are usually responsibilities of the respiratory therapist), the nurse is responsible for the patient and therefore needs to evaluate how the ventilator affects the patient's overall status.

When monitoring the ventilator, the nurse notes the following:

- Controlling mode (e.g., A/C ventilation, SIMV)
- Tidal volume and rate settings (tidal volume is usually set at 6 to 12 mL/kg [ideal body weight]; rate is usually set at 12 to 16 breaths/min)
- FiO$_2$ setting

- Inspiratory pressure reached and pressure limit (Normal is 15 to 20 cm H_2O; this increases if there is increased airway resistance or decreased compliance.)
- Sensitivity (A 2-cm H_2O inspiratory force should trigger the ventilator.)
- Inspiratory-to-expiratory ratio (usually 1:3 [1 second of inspiration to 3 seconds of expiration] or 1:2)
- Minute volume (tidal volume × respiratory rate, usually 6 to 8 L/min)
- Sigh settings (usually set at 1.5 times the tidal volume and ranging from 1 to 3 per hour), if applicable
- Water in the tubing, disconnection or kinking of the tubing
- Humidification (humidifier filled with water) and temperature
- Alarms (turned on and functioning properly)
- PEEP and pressure support level, if applicable (with PEEP usually set at 5 to 15 cm H_2O) (Carlson, 2009; Urden et al., 2010)

NURSING PROCESS

The Patient Receiving Mechanical Ventilation

Assessment

The nurse plays a vital role in assessing the patient's status and the functioning of the ventilator. In assessing the patient, the nurse evaluates the patient's physiologic status and how he or she is coping with mechanical ventilation. Physical assessment includes systematic assessment of all body systems, with an in-depth focus on the respiratory system. Respiratory assessment includes vital signs, respiratory rate and pattern, breath sounds, evaluation of spontaneous ventilatory effort, and potential evidence of hypoxia (e.g., skin color). Increased adventitious breath sounds may indicate a need for suctioning. The nurse also evaluates the settings and functioning of the mechanical ventilator, as described previously.

Assessment also addresses the patient's neurologic status and effectiveness of coping with the need for assisted ventilation and the changes that accompany it. The nurse assesses the patient's comfort level and ability to communicate as well. Because weaning from mechanical ventilation requires adequate nutrition, it is important to assess the patient's gastrointestinal system and nutritional status.

Diagnosis

Nursing Diagnoses

Based on the assessment data, major nursing diagnoses may include:

- Impaired gas exchange related to underlying illness, ventilator setting adjustments, or weaning
- Ineffective airway clearance related to increased mucus production associated with presence of the tube in trachea or continuous positive-pressure mechanical ventilation
- Risk for trauma and infection related to endotracheal intubation or tracheostomy
- Impaired physical mobility related to ventilator dependency

- Impaired verbal communication related to endotracheal tube or tracheostomy tube
- Defensive coping and powerlessness related to ventilator dependency

Collaborative Problems/Potential Complications

Based on the assessment data, potential complications may include the following (Table 21-2):

- Ventilator problems (increase in peak airway pressure or decrease in pressure or loss of volume)
- Alterations in cardiac function
- Barotrauma (trauma to the trachea or alveoli secondary to positive pressure) and pneumothorax
- Pulmonary infection (e.g., VAP; see Chart 21-13)
- Sepsis

Planning and Goals

The major goals for the patient may include achievement of optimal gas exchange, maintenance of a patent airway, absence of trauma or infection, attainment of optimal mobility, adjustment to nonverbal methods of communication, acquisition of successful coping measures, and absence of complications.

Nursing Interventions

Nursing care of the patient who is mechanically ventilated requires expert technical and interpersonal skills. Nursing interventions are similar regardless of the setting; however, the frequency of interventions and the stability of the patient vary from setting to setting. Nursing interventions for the patient who is mechanically ventilated are not uniquely different from those for patients with other pulmonary disorders, but astute nursing assessment and a therapeutic nurse–patient relationship are critical. The specific interventions used by the nurse are determined by the underlying disease process and the patient's response.

Two general nursing interventions that are important in the care of the patient who is mechanically ventilated are pulmonary auscultation and interpretation of arterial blood gas measurements. The nurse is often the first to note changes in physical assessment findings or significant trends in blood gases that signal the development of a serious problem (e.g., pneumothorax, tube displacement, pulmonary embolus).

Enhancing Gas Exchange

The purpose of mechanical ventilation is to optimize gas exchange by maintaining alveolar ventilation and oxygen delivery. The alteration in gas exchange may be caused by the underlying illness or by mechanical factors related to adjustment of the machine to the patient. The health care team, including the nurse, physician, and respiratory therapist, continually assesses the patient for adequate gas exchange, signs and symptoms of hypoxia, and response to treatment. Therefore, the nursing diagnosis of impaired gas exchange is, by its complex nature, multidisciplinary and collaborative. The team members must share goals and information freely. All other goals directly or indirectly relate to this primary goal.

Nursing interventions to promote optimal gas exchange include judicious administration of analgesic agents to relieve pain without suppressing the respiratory drive and

TABLE 21-2 Troubleshooting Problems With Mechanical Ventilation

Problem	Cause	Solution
Ventilator Problems		
Increase in peak airway pressure	Coughing or plugged airway tube	Suction airway for secretions; empty condensation fluid from circuit.
	Patient "fighting" ventilator Decreasing lung compliance	Adjust sensitivity. Manually ventilate patient. Assess for hypoxia or bronchospasm. Check arterial blood gas values. Sedate only if necessary.
	Tubing kinked Pneumothorax Atelectasis or bronchospasm	Check tubing; reposition patient; insert oral airway if necessary. Manually ventilate patient; notify primary provider. Clear secretions.
Decrease in pressure or loss of volume	Increase in compliance	None
	Leak in ventilator or tubing; cuff on tube/humidifier not tight	Check entire ventilator circuit for patency. Correct leak.
Patient Problems		
Cardiovascular compromise	Decrease in venous return due to application of positive pressure to lungs	Assess for adequate volume status by measuring heart rate, blood pressure, central venous pressure, pulmonary capillary wedge pressure, and urine output; notify primary care provider if values are abnormal.
Barotrauma/pneumothorax	Application of positive pressure to lungs; high mean airway pressures lead to alveolar rupture	Notify primary provider. Prepare patient for chest tube insertion. Avoid high pressure settings for patients with COPD, ARDS, or history of pneumothorax.
Pulmonary infection	Bypass of normal defense mechanisms; frequent breaks in ventilator circuit; decreased mobility; impaired cough reflex	Use meticulous aseptic technique. Provide frequent mouth care. Optimize nutritional status.

COPD, chronic obstructive pulmonary disease; ARDS, acute respiratory distress syndrome.

frequent repositioning to diminish the pulmonary effects of immobility. The nurse also monitors for adequate fluid balance by assessing for the presence of peripheral edema, calculating daily intake and output, and monitoring daily weights. The nurse administers medications prescribed to control the primary disease and monitors for their side effects.

Promoting Effective Airway Clearance
Continuous positive-pressure ventilation increases the production of secretions regardless of the patient's underlying condition. The nurse assesses for the presence of secretions by lung auscultation at least every 2 to 4 hours. Measures to clear the airway of secretions include suctioning, CPT, frequent position changes, and increased mobility as soon as possible. Frequency of suctioning should be determined by patient assessment. If excessive secretions are identified by inspection or auscultation techniques, suctioning should be performed. Sputum is not produced continuously or every 1 to 2 hours but as a response to a pathologic condition. Therefore, there is no rationale for routine suctioning of all patients every 1 to 2 hours. Although suctioning is used to aid in the clearance of secretions, it can damage the airway mucosa and impair cilia action.

The sigh mechanism on the ventilator may be adjusted to deliver at least 1 to 3 sighs per hour at 1.5 times the tidal volume if the patient is receiving A/C ventilation. Periodic sighs prevent atelectasis and the further retention of secretions. Because of the risk for hyperventilation and trauma to pulmonary tissue from excess ventilator pressure (barotrauma, pneumothorax), the sigh feature is not used frequently. If the SIMV mode is being used, the mandatory ventilations act as sighs because they are of greater volume than the patient's spontaneous breaths.

Humidification of the airway via the ventilator is maintained to help liquefy secretions so that they are more easily removed. Bronchodilators may be indicated to dilate the bronchioles in patients with acute lung injury or COPD and are classified as adrenergic or anticholinergic. Adrenergic bronchodilators (see Chapter 24) are mostly inhaled and work by stimulating the beta-receptor sites, mimicking the effects of epinephrine in the body. The desired effect is smooth muscle relaxation, which dilates the constricted bronchial tubes. Anticholinergic bronchodilators produce airway relaxation by blocking cholinergic-induced bronchoconstriction. Patients receiving bronchodilator therapy of either type should be monitored for adverse effects, including dizziness, nausea, decreased oxygen saturation, hypokalemia, increased heart rate, and urine retention. Mucolytic agents may also be indicated in these patients to liquefy secretions so that they are more easily mobilized. Nursing management of patients receiving mucolytic therapy includes assessment for an adequate cough reflex, sputum characteristics, and (in patients not receiving mechanical ventilation) improvement in incentive spirometry. Side effects include nausea, vomiting, bronchospasm, stomatitis (oral ulcers), urticaria, and rhinorrhea (runny nose) (Marini & Wheeler, 2010).

Preventing Trauma and Infection
Maintaining the endotracheal or tracheostomy tube is an essential part of airway management. The nurse positions the ventilator tubing so that there is minimal pulling or distortion of the tube in the trachea, reducing the risk of trauma to the trachea. Cuff pressure is monitored every 6 to 8 hours to maintain the pressure at less than 25 mm Hg (optimal cuff pressure is 15 to 20 mm Hg) (Weigand, 2011). The nurse assesses for the presence of a cuff leak at the same time.

Patients with an endotracheal or tracheostomy tube do not have the normal defenses of the upper airway. In addition, these patients frequently have multiple additional body system disturbances that lead to immunocompromise. Tracheostomy care is performed at least every 8 hours, and more frequently if needed, because of the increased risk of infection. The ventilator circuit tubing and in-line suction tubing are replaced periodically, according to infection control guidelines, to decrease the risk of infection.

The nurse administers oral hygiene frequently because the oral cavity is a primary source of contamination of the lungs in the patient who is intubated and compromised (American Thoracic Society, 2005). The presence of a nasogastric tube in the patient who is intubated can increase the risk of aspiration, leading to nosocomial pneumonia. The nurse positions the patient with the head elevated above the stomach as much as possible. (Chart 21-13 provides an overview of strategies to prevent VAP.)

Promoting Optimal Level of Mobility

Being connected to a ventilator limits the patient's mobility. Immobility in patients who are mechanically ventilated is associated with decreases in muscle strength and increases in length of hospital stay, as well as increased mortality rates (Perme & Chandrashekar, 2009). The nurse helps the patient whose condition has become stable to get out of bed and move to a chair as soon as possible. If the patient is unable to get out of bed, the nurse encourages performance of active range-of-motion exercises at least every 6 to 8 hours. If the patient cannot perform these exercises, the nurse performs passive range-of-motion exercises at least every 8 hours to prevent contractures and venous stasis.

Promoting Optimal Communication

It is important to develop alternative methods of communication for the patient who is receiving mechanical ventilation. The nurse assesses the patient's communication abilities to evaluate for limitations. Questions to consider when assessing the ability of the patient who is ventilator dependent to communicate include the following:

- Is the patient conscious and able to communicate? Can the patient nod or shake his or her head?
- Is the patient's mouth unobstructed by the tube so that words can be mouthed?
- Is the patient's dominant hand strong and available for writing? For example, if the patient is right-handed, the intravenous (IV) line should be placed in the left arm if possible so that the right hand is free.
- Is the patient a candidate for a fenestrated tracheostomy tube or a one-way speaking valve (such as Passy-Muir valve® or Olympic Trach-Talk®) that permits talking?

Once the patient's limitations are known, the nurse offers several appropriate communication approaches: lip or speech reading (use single key words), pad and pencil or Magic Slate®, communication board, gesturing, sign language, or electric larynx. The use of a "talking" or fenestrated tracheostomy tube or one-way valve may be suggested to the primary provider, which would allow the patient to talk while on the ventilator. The nurse makes sure that the patient's eyeglasses, hearing aid, sign interpreter, and language translator are available if needed to enhance the patient's ability to communicate.

Some communication methods may be frustrating to the patient, family, and nurse; these need to be identified and minimized. A speech therapist can assist in determining the most appropriate method.

Promoting Coping Ability

Dependence on a ventilator is frightening to both the patient and the family and disrupts even the most stable families. Encouraging the family to verbalize their feelings about the ventilator, the patient's condition, and the environment in general is beneficial. Explaining procedures every time they are performed helps reduce anxiety and familiarizes the patient with ventilator procedures. To restore a sense of control, the nurse encourages the patient to participate in decisions about care, schedules, and treatment when possible. The patient may become withdrawn or depressed while receiving mechanical ventilation, especially if its use is prolonged (Chart 21-14). To promote effective coping, the nurse informs the patient about progress when appropriate. It is important to provide diversions such as watching television, playing music, or taking a walk (if appropriate and possible). Stress reduction techniques (e.g., a back rub, relaxation measures) relieve tension and help the patient deal with anxieties and fears about both the condition and the dependence on the ventilator.

Monitoring and Managing Potential Complications

Alterations in Cardiac Function. Alterations in cardiac output may occur as a result of positive-pressure ventilation. The positive intrathoracic pressure during inspiration compresses

---

Chart 21-13 **Collaborative Practice Interventions to Prevent Ventilator-Associated Pneumonia**

Current best practices can include the implementation of specific evidence-based bundle interventions that, when used together (i.e., as a "bundle"), improve patient outcomes. This chart outlines specific parameters for the ventilator-bundled collaborative interventions that have been found to reduce ventilator-associated pneumonia (VAP).

What are the five key elements of the central venous line bundle?

- Elevation of the head of the bed (30–45 degrees)
- Daily "sedation vacations" and assessment of readiness to extubate (see below)
- Peptic ulcer disease prophylaxis (with histamine-2 receptor antagonists, such as ranitidine [Zantac])
- Deep venous thrombosis (DVT) prophylaxis (see below)
- Daily oral care with chlorhexidine (0.12% oral rinses)

What is meant by daily "sedation vacations," and how does this tie into assessing readiness to extubate?

- Protocols should be developed so that sedative doses are purposely decreased at a time of the day when it is possible to assess the patient's neurologic readiness for extubation.
- Vigilance must be employed during the time that sedative doses are lower to ensure that the patient does not self-extubate.

What effect does DVT prophylaxis have on preventing VAP?

- The exact relationship is unclear. However, when appropriate, evidence-based methods to ensure DVT prophylaxis are applied (see Chapter 30), then the rates of VAP also drops.

Adapted from Institute for Healthcare Improvement. (2011). *Implement the IHI ventilator bundle.* Available at: http://www.ihi.org/knowledge/Pages/Changes/ImplementtheVentilatorBundle.aspx

NURSING RESEARCH PROFILE

| Chart 21-14 | What It Is Like to Live on a Ventilator |

Briscoe, W., & Woodgate, R. (2010). Sustaining self: The lived experience of transition to long-term ventilation. *Qualitative Health Research, 20*(1), 57–67.

Purpose

Advances in medical treatments and technologies have contributed to improved survival and decreased mortality rates for individuals suffering from chronic neurologic and respiratory diseases. Some patients progress to chronic respiratory failure (CRF) and eventually require long-term mechanical ventilation (LTMV), which is defined as the use of a ventilator by a patient for greater than 6 hours a day for more than 3 weeks post acute illness—despite attempts to be weaned off ventilator support. This study examined the emotional challenges and lived experience of CRF participants' transition from spontaneous breathing to LTMV.

Design

This qualitative study was conducted in a Canadian western province and utilized interpretive phenomenology, a research method that explores the lived experiences of individuals and how they interpret those experiences. The sample consisted of 11 participants who were recruited from an outpatient respiratory clinic and a long-term care facility. All participants met the following inclusion criteria: minimum age of 18 years; able to speak, read, and write English; on LTMV; had transitioned to LTMV 6 months prior to the start of the study; and were able to recall and communicate their experience. Participants took part in detailed, semistructured interviews, lasting a total of 60–120 minutes. Data were collected through audio recordings and field notes. Words and phrases were analyzed, giving rise to shared themes.

Findings

The researchers uncovered six major themes that depicted the participants' lived experience of transitioning to LTMV: (1) sustaining self, (2) tyranny of symptoms, (3) self in peril, (4) awakening to a paradox, (5) struggling for autonomy, and (6) life goes on with a reclaimed self. The participants lived with CRF, suffering from symptoms associated with poor ventilation and oxygenation. At the end point of CRF and admission to the intensive care unit, they had to choose between life or death, and the choice of life meant going on LTMV. Initially, participants struggled with basic communication with others, issues of autonomy, and the right for self-determination. They also had to adjust their lifestyles to accommodate the restrictions inherent with mechanical ventilation. Nonetheless, LTMV provided them with a new lease on life. With newfound energy from improved ventilation and oxygenation, participants began to redefine themselves and learned to live with the limitations imposed by mechanical ventilation. At the end of their transitional journey, participants reclaimed themselves as autonomous beings, acknowledging that life must go on.

Nursing Implications

The transition of patients with CRF to LTMV occurs in an acute care setting. Nurses can help facilitate this transition by utilizing therapeutic communication and shaping nursing interventions to encourage patient autonomy. On a multidisciplinary level, nurses can serve as patient advocates, collaborating with physicians, respiratory therapists, physical therapists, social workers, and other health care professionals to create care plans to optimize wellness and promote patients' right for self-determination.

---

the heart and great vessels, thereby reducing venous return and cardiac output. This is usually corrected during exhalation when the positive pressure is off. The patient may have decreased cardiac output and resultant decreased tissue perfusion and oxygenation.

To evaluate cardiac function, the nurse first observes for signs and symptoms of hypoxia (restlessness, apprehension, confusion, tachycardia, tachypnea, pallor progressing to cyanosis, diaphoresis, transient hypertension, and decreased urine output). If a pulmonary artery catheter is in place, cardiac output, cardiac index, and other hemodynamic values can be used to assess the patient's status.

Barotrauma and Pneumothorax. Excessive positive pressure can cause lung damage, or barotrauma, which may result in a spontaneous **pneumothorax**, which may quickly develop into a tension pneumothorax, further compromising venous return, cardiac output, and blood pressure (see Chapter 23 for discussion of pneumothorax). The nurse considers any sudden changes in oxygen saturation or the onset of respiratory distress to be a life-threatening emergency requiring immediate action.

Pulmonary Infection. The patient is at high risk for infection, as described earlier. The nurse reports fever or a change in the color or odor of sputum to the primary provider for follow-up. (See Chapter 23 for discussion of pneumonia.)

Promoting Home and Community-Based Care

Increasingly, patients are being cared for in extended care facilities or at home while receiving mechanical ventila-

tion, with a tracheostomy tube, or receiving oxygen therapy. Patients receiving home ventilator care usually have a chronic neuromuscular condition or COPD. Providing the opportunity for ventilator-dependent patients to return home to live with their families in familiar surroundings can be a positive experience. The ultimate goal of home ventilator therapy is to enhance the patient's quality of life, not simply to support or prolong life.

Educating Patients About Self-Care. Caring for the patient with mechanical ventilator support at home can be accomplished successfully. A home care team consisting of the nurse, physician, respiratory therapist, social service or home care agency, and equipment supplier is needed. The home is evaluated to determine whether the electrical equipment needed can be operated safely. Chart 21-15 summarizes the basic assessment criteria needed for successful home care.

Once the decision to initiate mechanical ventilation at home is made, the nurse prepares the patient and family for home care. The nurse educates the patient and family about the ventilator, suctioning, tracheostomy care, signs of pulmonary infection, cuff inflation and deflation, and assessment of vital signs. Education begins in the hospital and continues at home. Nursing responsibilities include evaluating the patient's and family's understanding of the information presented.

The nurse educates the family about cardiopulmonary resuscitation, including mouth-to-tracheostomy tube (instead

Chart 21-15 Criteria for Successful Home Ventilator Care

The decision to proceed with home ventilation therapy is usually based on the following parameters.

Patient Criteria

• The patient has a chronic underlying pulmonary or neuromuscular disorder.
• The patient's clinical pulmonary status is stable.
• The patient is willing to go home on mechanical ventilation.

Home Criteria

• The home environment is conducive to care of the patient.
• The electrical facilities are adequate to operate all equipment safely.
• The home environment is controlled, without drafts in cold weather and with proper ventilation in warm weather.
• Space is available for cleaning and storing ventilator equipment.

Family Criteria

• Family members are competent, dependable, and willing to spend the time required for proper training as primary caregivers.
• Family members understand the diagnosis and prognosis.
• Family has sufficient financial and supportive resources and can obtain professional support if necessary.

of mouth-to-mouth) breathing. The nurse also explains how to handle a power failure, which usually involves converting the ventilator from an electrical power source to a battery power source. Conversion is automatic in most types of home ventilators and lasts approximately 1 hour. The nurse instructs the family on the use of a manual self-inflation bag should it be necessary. Chart 21-16 lists some of the patient's and family's responsibilities.

Continuing Care. A home care nurse monitors and evaluates how well the patient and family are adapting to providing care in the home. The nurse assesses the adequacy of the patient's ventilation and oxygenation as well as airway patency. The nurse addresses any unique adaptation problems that the patient may have and listens to the patient's and family's anxieties and frustrations, offering support and encouragement where possible. The home care nurse helps identify and contact community resources that may assist in home management of the patient with mechanical ventilation.

The technical aspects of the ventilator are managed by vendor follow-up. A respiratory therapist usually is assigned to the patient and makes frequent home visits to evaluate the patient and perform a maintenance check of the ventilator.

Transportation services are identified in case the patient requires transportation in an emergency. These arrangements must be made before an emergency arises.

Chart 21-16 HOME CARE CHECKLIST — Ventilator Care

At the completion of home care education, the patient or caregiver will be able to:	PATIENT	CAREGIVER
• State proper care of patient on ventilator:		
• Observe physical signs such as color, secretions, breathing pattern, and state of consciousness.		✔
• Perform physical care such as suctioning, postural drainage, and ambulation.		✔
• Observe the tidal volume and pressure manometer regularly. Intervene when they are abnormal (i.e., suction if airway pressure increases).		✔
• Provide a communication method for the patient (e.g., pad and pencil, electric larynx, talking tracheostomy tube, sign language).		✔
• Monitor vital signs as directed.		✔
• Use a predetermined signal to indicate when feeling short of breath or in distress.	✔	
• Care for and maintain equipment properly:		
• Check the ventilator settings twice each day and whenever the patient is removed from the ventilator.		✔
• Adjust the volume and pressure alarms if needed.		✔
• Fill humidifier as needed and check its level three times a day.		✔
• Empty water in tubing as needed.	✔	✔
• Use a clean humidifier when circuitry is changed.		✔
• Keep exterior of ventilator clean and free of any objects.		✔
• Change external circuitry once a week or more often as indicated.		✔
• Report malfunction or strange noises immediately.	✔	✔

Evaluation

Expected patient outcomes may include the following:

1. Exhibits adequate gas exchange, as evidenced by normal breath sounds, acceptable arterial blood gas levels, and vital signs
2. Demonstrates adequate ventilation with minimal mucus accumulation
3. Is free of injury or infection, as evidenced by normal temperature, white blood cell count, and clear sputum
4. Is mobile within limits of ability
   a. Gets out of bed to chair, bears weight, or ambulates as soon as possible
   b. Performs range-of-motion exercises every 6 to 8 hours
5. Communicates effectively through written messages, gestures, or other communication strategies
6. Copes effectively
   a. Verbalizes fears and concerns about condition and equipment
   b. Participates in decision making when possible
   c. Uses stress reduction techniques when necessary
7. Absence of complications
   a. Absence of cardiac compromise, as evidenced by stable vital signs and adequate urine output
   b. Absence of pneumothorax, as evidenced by bilateral chest excursion, normal chest x-ray, and adequate oxygenation
   c. Absence of pulmonary infection, as evidenced by normal temperature, clear pulmonary secretions, and negative sputum cultures

Weaning the Patient From the Ventilator

Respiratory weaning, the process of withdrawing the patient from dependence on the ventilator, takes place in three stages: the patient is gradually removed from the ventilator, then from either the endotracheal or tracheostomy tube, and finally from oxygen. Weaning from mechanical ventilation is performed at the earliest possible time consistent with patient safety. The decision must be made from a physiologic rather than a mechanical viewpoint. A thorough understanding of the patient's clinical status is required in making this decision. Weaning is started when the patient is hemodynamically stable and recovering from the acute stage of medical and surgical problems and when the cause of respiratory failure is sufficiently reversed (Girard, Kress, Fuchs, et al., 2008). Chart 21-17 presents information about patient care during weaning from mechanical ventilation.

Successful weaning involves collaboration among the primary provider, respiratory therapist, and nurse. Each health care provider must understand the scope and function of other team members in relation to patient weaning to conserve the patient's strength, use resources efficiently, and maximize successful outcomes.

Criteria for Weaning

Careful assessment is required to determine whether the patient is ready to be removed from mechanical ventilation. If the patient is stable and showing signs of improvement or reversal of the disease or condition that caused the need for

---

Chart 21-17 — **Care of the Patient Being Weaned From Mechanical Ventilation**

- Assess patient for weaning criteria:
  a. Vital capacity: 10–15 mL/kg
  b. Maximum inspiratory pressure (MIP) at least –20 cm H_2O
  c. Tidal volume: 7–9 mL/kg
  d. Minute ventilation: 6 L/min
  e. Rapid/shallow breathing index: Below 100 breaths/minute/L; PaO_2 >60 mm Hg with FiO_2 <40%
- Monitor activity level, assess dietary intake, and monitor results of laboratory tests of nutritional status. Reestablishing independent spontaneous ventilation can be physically exhausting. It is crucial that the patient have enough energy reserves to succeed.
- Assess the patient's and family's understanding of the weaning process, and address any concerns about the process. Explain that the patient may feel short of breath initially and provide encouragement as needed. Reassure the patient that he or she will be attended closely and that if the weaning attempt is not successful, it can be tried again later.
- Implement the weaning method as prescribed (e.g., continuous positive airway pressure [CPAP], T-piece).
- Monitor vital signs, pulse oximetry, electrocardiogram, and respiratory pattern constantly for the first 20–30 minutes and every 5 minutes after that until weaning is complete. Monitoring the patient closely provides ongoing indications of success or failure.
- Maintain a patent airway; monitor arterial blood gas levels and pulmonary function tests. Suction the airway as needed.
- In collaboration with the primary provider, terminate the weaning process if adverse reactions occur. These include a heart rate increase of 20 bpm, systolic blood pressure increase of 20 mm Hg, a decrease in oxygen saturation to <90%, respiratory rate <8 or >20 breaths/min, ventricular dysrhythmias, fatigue, panic, cyanosis, erratic or labored breathing, paradoxical chest movement.
- If the weaning process continues, measure tidal volume and minute ventilation every 20–30 minutes; compare with the patient's desired values, which have been determined in collaboration with the primary provider.
- Assess for psychological dependence if the physiologic parameters indicate that weaning is feasible and the patient still resists. Possible causes of psychological dependence include fear of dying and depression from chronic illness. It is important to address this issue before the next weaning attempt.

---

mechanical ventilation, weaning indices should be assessed (see Chart 21-17).

Stable vital signs and arterial blood gases are also important predictors of successful weaning. Once readiness has been determined, the nurse records baseline measurements of weaning indices to monitor progress.

Patient Preparation

To maximize the chances of success of weaning, the nurse must consider the patient as a whole, taking into account factors that impair the delivery of oxygen and elimination of carbon dioxide as well as those that increase oxygen demand (e.g., sepsis, seizures, thyroid imbalances) or decrease the patient's overall strength (e.g., inadequate nutrition, neuromuscular disease). Adequate psychological preparation is necessary before and during the weaning process.

Methods of Weaning

Successful weaning depends on the combination of adequate patient preparation, available equipment, and an interdisciplinary approach to solve patient problems (see Chart 21-17). All usual modes of ventilation can be used for weaning.

CPAP (also known as spontaneous mode ventilation in this context) allows the patient to breathe spontaneously while applying positive pressure throughout the respiratory cycle to keep the alveoli open and promote oxygenation. Providing CPAP during spontaneous breathing also offers the advantage of an alarm system and may reduce patient anxiety if the patient has been taught that the machine is keeping track of breathing. It also maintains lung volumes and improves the patient's oxygenation status. CPAP is often used in conjunction with PSV. Nurses should carefully assess for tachypnea, tachycardia, reduced tidal volumes, decreasing oxygen saturations, and increasing carbon dioxide levels.

When the patient can breathe spontaneously, weaning trials using a T-piece for the patient with an endotracheal tube or tracheostomy mask for the patient with a tracheostomy tube (see Fig. 21-2) are normally conducted with the patient disconnected from the ventilator, receiving humidified oxygen only and performing all work of breathing. Because patients do not have to overcome the resistance of the ventilator, they may find this mode more comfortable, or they may become anxious as they breathe with no support from the ventilator. During these trial periods, the nurse monitors the patient closely and provides encouragement. This method of weaning is usually used when the patient is awake and alert, is breathing without difficulty, has good gag and cough reflexes, and is hemodynamically stable. During the weaning process, the patient is maintained on the same or a higher oxygen concentration than when receiving mechanical ventilation. While the patient is using the T-piece or tracheostomy mask, he or she is observed for signs and symptoms of hypoxia, increasing respiratory muscle fatigue, or systemic fatigue. These include restlessness, increased respiratory rate (greater than 35 breaths/min), the use of accessory muscles, tachycardia with premature ventricular contractions, and paradoxical chest movement (asynchronous breathing, chest contraction during inspiration and expansion during expiration). Fatigue or exhaustion is initially manifested by an increased respiratory rate associated with a gradual reduction in tidal volume; later there is a slowing of the respiratory rate.

If the patient appears to be tolerating the T-piece/tracheostomy mask trial, a second set of arterial blood gas measurements is drawn 20 minutes after the patient has been on spontaneous ventilation at a constant FiO_2 PSV. (Alveolar–arterial equilibration takes 15 to 20 minutes to occur.)

Signs of exhaustion and hypoxia correlated with deterioration in the blood gas measurements indicate the need for ventilatory support. The patient is placed back on the ventilator each time signs of fatigue or deterioration develop.

If clinically stable, the patient usually can be extubated within 2 or 3 hours after weaning and allowed spontaneous ventilation by means of a mask with humidified oxygen. Patients who have had prolonged ventilatory assistance usually require more gradual weaning; it may take days or even weeks. They are weaned primarily during the day and placed back on the ventilator at night to rest.

Because patients respond in different manners to weaning methods, there is no definitive way to assess which method is best. Regardless of the weaning method being used, ongoing assessment of respiratory status is essential to monitor patient progress.

Successful weaning from the ventilator is supplemented by intensive pulmonary care. The following methods are used: oxygen therapy; arterial blood gas evaluation; pulse oximetry; bronchodilator therapy; CPT; adequate nutrition, hydration, and humidification; blood pressure measurement; and incentive spirometry. Daily spontaneous breathing trials may be used to evaluate the patient's ability to breathe without ventilatory support. If the patient is receiving IV sedatives (e.g., propofol, midazolam), current guidelines recommend that the patient's sedative dose be decreased by 25% to 50% prior to weaning, called a *sedation vacation* (Girard et al., 2008). In order to decrease agitation in patients who do not tolerate withdrawal of sedation, dexmedetomidine (Precedex) may be initiated for spontaneous breathing trials without causing significant respiratory depression (Arpino, Kalafatas, & Thompson, 2008). A patient may still have borderline pulmonary function and need vigorous supportive therapy before his or her respiratory status returns to a level that supports activities of daily living.

Removal of the Tracheostomy Tube

Removal of the tracheostomy tube is considered when the patient can breathe spontaneously; maintain an adequate airway by effectively coughing up secretions, swallow, and move the jaw. Secretion clearance and aspiration risks are assessed to determine whether active pharyngeal and laryngeal reflexes are intact.

Once the patient can clear secretions adequately, a trial period of mouth breathing or nose breathing is conducted. This can be accomplished by several methods. The first method requires changing to a smaller size tube to increase the resistance to airflow or plugging the tracheostomy tube (deflating the cuff first). The smaller tube is sometimes replaced by a cuffless tracheostomy tube, which allows the tube to be plugged at lengthening intervals to monitor patient progress. A second method involves changing to a fenestrated tube (a tube with an opening or window in its bend). This permits air to flow around and through the tube to the upper airway and enables talking. A third method involves switching to a smaller tracheostomy button (stoma button). A tracheostomy button is a plastic tube approximately 1 inch long that helps keep the windpipe open after the larger tracheostomy tube has been removed. Finally, when the patient demonstrates the ability to maintain a patent airway, the tube can be removed. An occlusive dressing is placed over the stoma, which heals in several days to weeks.

Weaning From Oxygen

The patient who has been successfully weaned from the ventilator, cuff, and tube and has adequate respiratory function is then weaned from oxygen. The FiO_2 is gradually reduced until the PaO_2 is in the range of 70 to 100 mm Hg while the patient is breathing room air. If the PaO_2 is less than 70 mm Hg on room air, supplemental oxygen is recommended. To be eligible for financial reimbursement from the Centers for Medicare and Medicaid Services (CMS) for in-home oxygen, the patient must have a PaO_2 of less than 55 mm Hg while awake and at rest (CMS, 1993).

Nutrition

Success in weaning the patient who is long-term ventilator dependent requires early and aggressive but judicious nutritional support. The respiratory muscles (diaphragm and especially intercostals) become weak or atrophied after just a few days of mechanical ventilation and may be catabolized for energy, especially if nutrition is inadequate. Compensation for inadequate nutrition must be undertaken with care; excessive intake can increase production of carbon dioxide and the demand for oxygen and lead to prolonged ventilator dependence and difficulty in weaning (Casaer, Mesotten, Hermans, et al., 2011). Because the metabolism of fat produces less carbon dioxide than the metabolism of carbohydrates, it was long presumed that a high-fat and limited carbohydrate diet would be most therapeutic; however, evidence-based findings do not support its efficacy (Casaer et al., 2011; Weijs, Stapel, de Groot, et al., 2012). Adequate protein intake is important in increasing respiratory muscle strength. Protein intake should be approximately 25% of total daily kilocalories, or 1.2 to 1.5 g/kg/day. Daily nutrition should be closely monitored.

Soon after the patient is admitted, a consultation with a dietitian or nutrition support team should be arranged to plan the best form of nutritional replacement. Adequate nutrition may decrease the duration of mechanical ventilation and prevent other complications, especially sepsis. Sepsis can occur if bacteria enter the bloodstream and release toxins that, in turn, cause vasodilation and hypotension, fever, tachycardia, increased respiratory rate, and coma. Aggressive treatment of sepsis is essential to reverse this threat to survival and to promote weaning from the ventilator when the patient's condition improves.

THE PATIENT UNDERGOING THORACIC SURGERY

Respiratory care modalities are particularly important for the patient undergoing thoracic surgery. Frequently, patients undergoing such surgery have obstructive pulmonary disease or other chronic disease. Careful preoperative preparation, assessment, and postoperative management are crucial for successful patient outcomes because these patients may have a narrow range between their physical tolerance for certain activities and their limitations, which, if exceeded, can lead to distress. Various types of thoracic surgical procedures are performed to relieve disease conditions such as lung abscesses, lung cancer, cysts, benign tumors, and emphysema (Chart 21-18). An exploratory **thoracotomy** (creation of a surgical opening into the thoracic cavity) may be performed to diagnose lung or chest disease. A biopsy may be performed in this procedure with a small amount of lung tissue removed for analysis; the chest incision is then closed.

The objectives of preoperative assessment and care for the patient undergoing thoracic surgery are to ascertain the patient's functional reserve, to determine whether the patient is likely to survive and recover from the surgery, and to ensure that the patient is in optimal condition for surgery.

Preoperative Management

Assessment and Diagnostic Findings

The nurse performs chest auscultation to assess breath sounds in all regions of the lungs (see Chapter 20). It is important to note whether breath sounds are normal, indicating a free flow of air in and out of the lungs. (In the patient with emphysema, the breath sounds may be markedly decreased or even absent on auscultation.) The nurse notes crackles and wheezes and assesses for hyperresonance and decreased diaphragmatic motion. Unilateral diminished breath sounds and rhonchi can be the result of occlusion of the bronchi by mucus plugs. The nurse assesses for retained secretions during auscultation by asking the patient to cough. It is important to note any signs of rhonchi or wheezing. The patient history and assessment should include the following questions:

- What signs and symptoms (cough, sputum expectorated [amount and color], hemoptysis, chest pain, dyspnea) are present?
- If there is a smoking history, how long has the patient smoked? Does the patient smoke currently? How many packs a day?
- What is the patient's cardiopulmonary tolerance while resting, eating, bathing, and walking?
- What is the patient's breathing pattern? How much exertion is required to produce dyspnea?
- Does the patient need to sleep in an upright position or with more than two pillows?
- What is the patient's general physiologic status (e.g., general appearance, mental alertness, behavior, nutritional status)?
- What other medical conditions exist (e.g., allergies, cardiac disorders, diabetes)?

Numerous tests are performed to determine the patient's preoperative status and to assess the patient's physical assets and limitations. Many patients are seen by their surgeons in the office, and many diagnostic tests and examinations are performed on an outpatient basis. The decision to perform any pulmonary resection is based on the patient's cardiovascular status and pulmonary reserve. Pulmonary function studies (especially lung volume and vital capacity) are performed to determine whether the planned resection will leave sufficient functioning lung tissue. Arterial blood gas values are assessed to provide a more complete picture of the functional capacity of the lung. Exercise tolerance tests are useful to determine whether the patient who is a candidate for pneumonectomy can tolerate removal of one of the lungs.

Preoperative studies provide a baseline for comparison during the postoperative period and detect additional abnormalities. Studies may include a bronchoscopic examination (a lighted scope is inserted into the airways to examine the bronchi), chest x-ray, magnetic resonance imaging, electrocardiogram (ECG) (for arteriosclerotic heart disease, conduction defects), nutritional assessment, determination of blood urea nitrogen and serum creatinine levels (to assess renal function), determination of glucose tolerance or blood glucose level (to check for diabetes), serum electrolytes and protein levels, blood volume determinations, and complete blood cell count.

Chart 21-18 **Thoracic Surgeries and Procedures**

Pneumonectomy

The removal of an entire lung (pneumonectomy) is performed chiefly for cancer when the lesion cannot be removed by a less extensive procedure. It also may be performed for lung abscesses, bronchiectasis, or extensive unilateral tuberculosis. The removal of the right lung is more dangerous than the removal of the left, because the right lung has a larger vascular bed and its removal imposes a greater physiologic burden.

A posterolateral or anterolateral thoracotomy incision is made, sometimes with resection of a rib. The pulmonary artery and the pulmonary veins are ligated and severed. The main bronchus is divided and the lung removed. The bronchial stump is stapled, and usually no drains are used because the accumulation of fluid in the empty hemithorax prevents mediastinal shift.

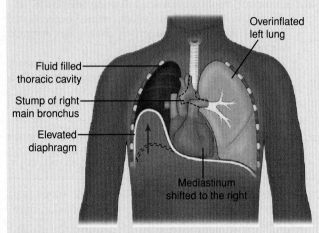

Fluid filled thoracic cavity
Stump of right main bronchus
Elevated diaphragm
Overinflated left lung
Mediastinum shifted to the right

Pneumonectomy

Lobectomy

When the pathology is limited to one area of a lung, a lobectomy (removal of a lobe of a lung) is performed. Lobectomy, which is more common than pneumonectomy, may be carried out for bronchogenic carcinoma, giant emphysematous blebs or bullae, benign tumors, metastatic malignant tumors, bronchiectasis, and fungal infections.

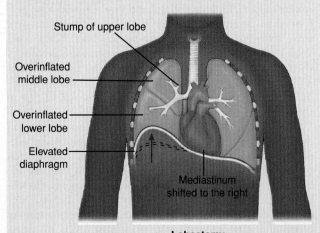

Stump of upper lobe
Overinflated middle lobe
Overinflated lower lobe
Elevated diaphragm
Mediastinum shifted to the right

Lobectomy

The surgeon makes a thoracotomy incision. Its exact location depends on the lobe to be resected. When the pleural space is entered, the involved lung collapses and the lobar vessels and the bronchus are ligated and divided. After the lobe is removed, the remaining lobes of the lung are re-expanded. Usually, two chest catheters are inserted for drainage. The upper tube is for air removal; the lower one is for fluid drainage. Sometimes, only one catheter is needed. The chest tube is connected to a chest drainage apparatus for several days.

Segmentectomy (Segmental Resection)

Some lesions are located in only one segment of the lung. Bronchopulmonary segments are subdivisions of the lung that function as individual units. They are held together by delicate connective tissue. Disease processes may be limited to a single segment. Care is used to preserve as much healthy and functional lung tissue as possible, especially in patients who already have limited cardiopulmonary reserve. Single segments can be removed from any lobe; the right middle lobe, which has only two small segments, invariably is removed entirely. On the left side, corresponding to a middle lobe, is a "lingular" segment of the upper lobe. This can be removed as a single segment or by lingulectomy. This segment frequently is involved in bronchiectasis.

Wedge Resection

A wedge resection of a small, well-circumscribed lesion may be performed without regard to the location of the intersegmental planes. The pleural cavity usually is drained because of the possibility of an air or blood leak. This procedure is performed for diagnostic lung biopsy and for the excision of small peripheral nodules.

Bronchoplastic or Sleeve Resection

Bronchoplastic resection is a procedure in which only one lobar bronchus, together with a part of the right or left bronchus, is excised. The distal bronchus is reanastomosed to the proximal bronchus or trachea.

Lung Volume Reduction

Lung volume reduction is a surgical procedure involving the removal of 20%–30% of a patient's lung through a midsternal incision or video thoracoscopy. The diseased lung tissue is identified on a lung perfusion scan. This surgery leads to significant improvements in dyspnea, exercise capacity, quality of life, and survival of a subgroup of people with end-stage emphysema (Oey, Morgan, Spyt, et al., 2010).

Video Thoracoscopy

A video thoracoscopy is an endoscopic procedure that allows the surgeon to look into the thorax without making a large incision. The procedure is performed to obtain specimens of tissue for biopsy, to treat recurrent spontaneous pneumothorax, and to diagnose either pleural effusions or pleural masses. Thoracoscopy has also been found to be an effective diagnostic and therapeutic alternative for the treatment of mediastinal disorders (Solaini, Prusciano, Bagioni, et al., 2008). Some advantages of video thoracoscopy are rapid diagnosis and treatment of some conditions, a decrease in postoperative complications, and a shortened hospital stay.

Preoperative Nursing Management

Improving Airway Clearance

The underlying lung condition often is associated with increased respiratory secretions. Before surgery, the airway is cleared of secretions to reduce the possibility of postoperative atelectasis or infection. Chart 21-19 lists the risk factors for postoperative atelectasis and pneumonia. Strategies to reduce the risk of atelectasis and infection include humidification, postural drainage, and chest percussion after bronchodilators are administered, if prescribed. The nurse estimates the volume of sputum if the patient expectorates large amounts of secretions. Such measurements are carried out to determine whether and when the amount decreases. Antibiotics are administered as prescribed for infection, which can cause excessive secretions.

Educating the Patient

Increasingly, patients are admitted on the day of surgery, which does not provide much time for preoperative assessment or education. Nurses in all settings must take an active role in educating the patient and relieving anxiety. The nurse informs the patient about what to expect, from administration of anesthesia to thoracotomy and the likely use of chest tubes and a drainage system in the postoperative period. The patient is also informed about the usual postoperative administration of oxygen to facilitate breathing and the possible use of a ventilator. It is essential to explain the importance of frequent turning to promote drainage of lung secretions. Instruction in the use of incentive spirometry begins before surgery to familiarize the patient with its correct use. The nurse educates the patient on the use of diaphragmatic and pursed-lip breathing, and the patient should begin practicing these techniques (see Charts 21-3 and 21-4).

| Chart 21-19 | **RISK FACTORS**
 Surgery-Related Atelectasis and Pneumonia |

Preoperative Risk Factors

- Increased age
- Obesity
- Poor nutritional status
- Smoking history
- Abnormal pulmonary function tests
- Preexisting lung disease
- Emergency surgery
- History of aspiration
- Comorbid states
- Preexisting disability

Intraoperative Risk Factors

- Thoracic incision
- Prolonged anesthesia

Postoperative Risk Factors

- Immobilization
- Supine position
- Decreased level of consciousness
- Inadequate pain management
- Prolonged intubation/mechanical ventilation
- Presence of nasogastric tube
- Inadequate preoperative education

Because a coughing schedule is necessary in the postoperative period to promote the clearance or removal of secretions, the nurse instructs the patient in the technique of coughing and warns the patient that the coughing routine may be uncomfortable. The nurse educates the patient about how to splint the incision with the hands, a pillow, or a folded towel (see Chart 21-5).

Encouraging the use of forced expiratory technique (FET) may be helpful for the patient with diminished expiratory flow rates or for the patient who refuses to cough because of severe pain. FET is the expulsion of air through an open glottis. This technique stimulates pulmonary expansion and assists in alveolar inflation (Fink, 2007). The nurse instructs the patient as follows:

- Take a deep diaphragmatic breath and exhale forcefully against your hand in a quick, distinct pant, or huff.
- Practice doing small huffs and progress to one strong huff during exhalation.

Patients should be informed preoperatively that blood and other fluids may be administered, oxygen will be administered, and vital signs will be checked often for several hours after surgery. If a chest tube is needed, the patient should be informed that it will drain the fluid and air that normally accumulate after chest surgery. The patient and family are informed that the patient may be admitted to the ICU for 1 to 2 days after surgery, that the patient may experience pain at the incision site, and that medication is available to relieve pain and discomfort.

Relieving Anxiety

The nurse listens to the patient to evaluate his or her feelings about the illness and proposed treatment. The nurse also determines the patient's motivation to return to normal or baseline function. The patient may reveal significant concerns: fear of hemorrhage because of bloody sputum, fear of discomfort from a chronic cough and chest pain, fear of ventilator dependence, or fear of death because of dyspnea and the underlying disease (e.g., tumor).

The nurse helps the patient to address fears and to cope with the stress of surgery by correcting any misconceptions, supporting the patient's decision to undergo surgery, reassuring the patient that the incision will "hold," and dealing honestly with questions about pain and discomfort and the patient's treatment. The management and control of pain begin before surgery, when the nurse informs the patient that many postoperative problems can be overcome by following certain routines related to deep breathing, coughing, turning, and moving. Non-opioid preemptive analgesic agents (e.g., acetaminophen and nonsteroidal anti-inflammatory drugs [NSAIDs]) may also be prescribed to help decrease the dose of postoperative opioid agents. This also helps to facilitate deep-breathing techniques and return to normal respiratory function. If patient-controlled analgesia (PCA) or patient-controlled epidural analgesia (PCEA) is to be used after surgery, the nurse instructs the patient in its use.

Postoperative Management

After surgery, the vital signs are checked frequently. Oxygen is administered by a mechanical ventilator, nasal cannula, or mask for as long as necessary. A reduction in lung capacity requires a period of physiologic adjustment, and fluids may be given at a low hourly rate to prevent fluid overload and pulmonary edema. After the patient is conscious and the vital signs have stabilized, the head of the bed may be elevated 30 to 45 degrees. Careful positioning of the patient is important. After pneumonectomy, a patient is usually turned every hour from the back to the operative side and should not be completely turned to the unoperated side. This allows the fluid left in the space to consolidate and prevents the remaining lung and the heart from shifting (mediastinal shift) toward the operative side. The patient with a lobectomy may be turned to either side, and a patient with a segmental resection usually is not turned onto the operative side unless the surgeon prescribes this position.

Medication for pain is needed for several days after surgery; it is usually a combination of epidural analgesia, PCA, and scheduled or as-needed oral analgesics. Because coughing can be painful, the patient should be encouraged to splint the chest as taught in the preoperative period. Exercises are resumed early in the postoperative period to facilitate lung ventilation. The nurse assesses for signs of complications, including cyanosis, dyspnea, and acute chest pain. These may indicate atelectasis and should be reported immediately. Increased temperature or white blood cell count may indicate an infection, and pallor and increased pulse may indicate internal hemorrhage. Dressings are assessed for fresh bleeding.

Mechanical Ventilation

Depending on the nature of the surgery, the patient's underlying condition, the intraoperative course, and the depth of anesthesia, the patient may require mechanical ventilation after surgery. The primary provider is responsible for determining and ordering the ventilator settings and modes, as well as determining the overall method and pace of weaning. It is important to assess the patient's tolerance and weaning progress. Early extubation from mechanical ventilation can lead to earlier removal of arterial lines.

Chest Drainage

A crucial intervention for improving gas exchange and breathing in the postoperative period is the proper management of chest drainage and the **chest drainage system**. After thoracic surgery, chest tubes and a closed drainage system are used to re-expand the involved lung and to remove excess air, fluid, and blood. Chest drainage systems also are used in treatment of spontaneous pneumothorax and trauma resulting in pneumothorax. Table 21-3 describes and compares the main features of these systems, and Chart 21-20 explains the setup and management of chest drainage systems. Chart 21-21 discusses actions that may prevent cardiopulmonary complications after thoracic surgery.

The normal breathing mechanism operates on the principle of negative pressure. The pressure in the chest cavity normally is lower than the pressure of the atmosphere, causing air to move into the lungs during inspiration. Whenever the chest is opened, there is a loss of negative pressure, which results in collapse of the lung. The collection of air, fluid, or other substances in the chest can compromise cardiopulmonary function and can also cause the lung to collapse. Pathologic substances that collect in the pleural space include fibrin or clotted blood, liquids (serous fluids, blood, pus, chyle), and gases (air from the lung, tracheobronchial tree, or esophagus).

Chest tubes may be inserted to drain fluid or air from any of the three compartments of the thorax (the right and left pleural spaces and the mediastinum). The pleural space, located between the visceral and parietal pleura, normally contains 20 mL or less of fluid, which helps lubricate the visceral and parietal pleura (Porth & Matfin, 2009). Surgical incision of the chest wall almost always causes some degree of pneumothorax (air accumulating in the pleural space) or hemothorax (buildup of serous fluid or blood in the pleural space). Air and fluid collect in the pleural space, restricting lung expansion and reducing gas exchange. Placement of a chest tube in the pleural space restores the negative

TABLE 21-3 Comparison of Chest Drainage Systems*		
Types of Chest Drainage Systems	**Description**	**Comments**
Traditional Water Seal Also referred to as wet suction	Has three chambers: a collection chamber, water seal chamber (middle chamber), and wet suction control chamber	Requires that sterile fluid be instilled into water seal and suction chambers Has positive- and negative-pressure release valves Intermittent bubbling indicates that the system is functioning properly. Additional suction can be added by connecting system to a suction source.
Dry Suction Water Seal Also referred to as dry suction	Has three chambers: a collection chamber, water seal chamber (middle chamber), and wet suction control chamber	Requires that sterile fluid be instilled in water seal chamber at 2-cm level No need to fill suction chamber with fluid Suction pressure is set with a regulator. Has positive- and negative-pressure release valves Has an indicator to signify that the suction pressure is adequate Quieter than traditional water seal systems
Dry Suction Also referred to as one-way valve system	Has a one-way mechanical valve that allows air to leave the chest and prevents air from moving back into the chest	No need to fill suction chamber with fluid; thus, can be set up quickly in an emergency Works even if knocked over, making it ideal for patients who are ambulatory

*If no fluid drainage is expected, a drainage collection device may not be needed.

GUIDELINES

Chart 21-20

Setup and Management of Chest Drainage Systems

Equipment
- Chest tube insertion tray (contains chest tube, scalpel, gloves)
- Antiseptic solution
- Local anesthetic agent
- Chest drainage system
- Adhesive tape

Implementation

Actions	Rationale
1. If using a chest drainage system with a water seal, fill the water seal chamber with sterile water to the level specified by the manufacturer.	Water seal drainage allows air and fluid to escape into a drainage chamber. The water acts as a seal and keeps the air from being drawn back into the pleural space.
2. When using suction in chest drainage systems with a water seal, fill the suction control chamber with sterile water to the 20-cm level or as prescribed. In systems without a water seal, set the regulator dial to the appropriate suction level.	The water level regulator dial setting determines the degree of suction applied.
3. Attach the drainage catheter exiting the thoracic cavity to the tubing coming from the collection chamber. Tape securely with adhesive tape.	In chest drainage units, the system is closed. The only connection is the one to the patient's catheter.
4. If suction is used, connect the suction control chamber tubing to the suction unit. If using a wet suction system, turn on the suction unit and increase pressure until slow but steady bubbling appears in the suction control chamber. If using a chest drainage system with a dry suction control chamber, turn the regulator dial to 20 cm H_2O.	With a wet suction system, the degree of suction is determined by the amount of water in the suction control chamber and is not dependent on the rate of bubbling or the pressure gauge setting on the suction unit. With a dry suction control chamber, the regulator dial replaces the water.

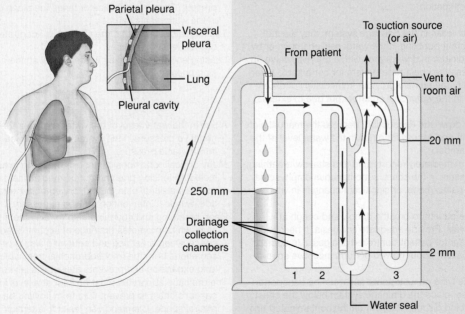

Example of a disposable chest drainage system.

5. Mark the drainage from the collection chamber with tape on the outside of the drainage unit. Mark hourly/daily increments (date and time) at the drainage level.	This marking shows the amount of fluid loss and how fast fluid is collecting in the drainage chamber. It serves as a basis for determining the need for blood replacement, if the fluid is blood. Visibly bloody drainage will appear in the chamber in the immediate postoperative period but should gradually becomes serous. If the patient is bleeding as heavily as 100 mL every 15 minutes, check the drainage every few minutes. A reoperation or autotransfusion may be needed. The transfusion of blood collected in the drainage chamber must be reinfused within 4–6 hours. Usually, however, drainage decreases progressively in the first 24 hours.
6. Ensure that the drainage tubing does not kink, loop, or interfere with the patient's movements.	Kinking, looping, or pressure on the drainage tubing can produce back pressure, which may force fluid back into the pleural space or impede its drainage.

(continues on page 526)

**Chart
21-20**

Setup and Management of Chest Drainage Systems (continued)

Actions	Rationale
7. Encourage the patient to assume a comfortable position with good body alignment. With the lateral position, make sure that the patient's body does not compress the tubing. The patient should be turned and repositioned every 1.5–2 hours. Provide adequate analgesia.	Frequent position changes promote drainage, and good body alignment helps prevent postural deformities and contractures. Proper positioning also helps breathing and promotes better air exchange. Analgesics may be needed to promote comfort.
8. Assist the patient with range-of-motion exercises for the affected arm and shoulder several times daily. Provide adequate analgesia.	Exercise helps to prevent ankylosis of the shoulder and to reduce postoperative pain and discomfort. Analgesics may be needed to relieve pain.
9. Gently "milk" the tubing in the direction of the drainage chamber as needed.	"Milking" prevents the tubing from becoming obstructed by clots and fibrin. Constant attention to maintaining the patency of the tube facilitates prompt expansion of the lung and minimizes complications.
10. Make sure there is fluctuation ("tidaling") of the fluid level in the water seal chamber (in wet systems), or check the air leak indicator for leaks (in dry systems with a one-way valve). *Note:* Fluid fluctuations in the water seal chamber or air leak indicator area will stop when: **a.** The lung has re-expanded **b.** The tubing is obstructed by blood clots, fibrin, or kinks **c.** A loop of tubing hangs below the rest of the tubing **d.** Suction motor or wall suction is not working properly	Fluctuation of the water level in the water seal shows effective connection between the pleural cavity and the drainage chamber and indicates that the drainage system remains patent. Fluctuation is also a gauge of intrapleural pressure in systems with a water seal (wet and dry, but not with the one-way valve).
11. With a dry system, assess for the presence of the indicator (bellows or float device) when setting the regulator dial to the desired level of suction.	An air leak indicator shows changes in intrathoracic pressure in dry systems with a one-way valve. Bubbles will appear if a leak is present. The air leak indicator takes the place of fluid fluctuations in the water seal chamber.
12. Observe for air leaks in the drainage system; they are indicated by constant bubbling in the water seal chamber, or by the air leak indicator in dry systems with a one-way valve. In addition, assess the chest tube system for correctable external leaks. Notify the primary provider immediately of excessive bubbling in the water seal chamber not due to external leaks.	The indicator shows that the vacuum is adequate to maintain the desired level of suction. Leaking and trapping of air in the pleural space can result in tension pneumothorax.
13. When turning down the dry suction, depress the manual high-negativity vent, and assess for a rise in the water level of the water seal chamber.	A rise in the water level of the water seal chamber indicates high negative pressure in the system that could lead to increased intrathoracic pressure.
14. Observe and immediately report rapid and shallow breathing, cyanosis, pressure in the chest, subcutaneous emphysema, symptoms of hemorrhage, or significant changes in vital signs.	Many clinical conditions can cause these signs and symptoms, including tension pneumothorax, mediastinal shift, hemorrhage, severe incisional pain, pulmonary embolus, and cardiac tamponade. Surgical intervention may be necessary.
15. Encourage the patient to breathe deeply and cough at frequent intervals. Provide adequate analgesia. If needed, request an order for patient-controlled analgesia. In addition, educate the patient about how to perform incentive spirometry.	Deep breathing and coughing help to raise the intrapleural pressure, which promotes drainage of accumulated fluid in the pleural space. Deep breathing and coughing also promote removal of secretions from the tracheobronchial tree, which in turn promotes lung expansion and prevents atelectasis (alveolar collapse).
16. If the patient is lying on a stretcher and must be transported to another area, place the drainage system below the chest level. If the tubing disconnects, cut off the contaminated tips of the chest tube and tubing, insert a sterile connector in the cut ends, and reattach to the drainage system. Do *not* clamp the chest tube during transport.	The drainage apparatus must be kept at a level lower than the patient's chest to prevent fluid from flowing backward into the pleural space. Clamping can result in a tension pneumothorax.
17. When assisting in the chest tube's removal, instruct the patient to perform a gentle Valsalva maneuver or to breathe quietly. The chest tube is then clamped and quickly removed. Simultaneously, a small bandage is applied and made airtight with petrolatum gauze covered by a 4- × 4-inch gauze pad and thoroughly covered and sealed with nonporous tape.	The chest tube is removed as directed when the lung is re-expanded (usually 24 hours to several days), depending on the cause of the pneumothorax. During tube removal, the chief priorities are preventing air from entering the pleural cavity as the tube is withdrawn and preventing infection.

Preventing Postoperative Cardiopulmonary
Complications After Thoracic Surgery

Patient Management

- Auscultate lung sounds and assess for rate, rhythm, and depth.
- Monitor oxygenation with pulse oximetry.
- Monitor electrocardiogram for rate and rhythm changes.
- Assess capillary refill, skin color, and status of the surgical dressing.
- Encourage and assist the patient to turn, cough, and take deep breaths.

Chest Drainage Management

- Verify that all connection tubes are patent and connected securely.
- Assess that the water seal is intact when using a wet suction system, and assess the regulator dial in dry suction systems.
- Monitor characteristics of drainage, including color, amount, and consistency. Assess for significant increases or decreases in drainage output.
- Note fluctuations in the water seal chamber for wet suction systems and the air leak indicator in dry suction systems.
- Keep system below the patient's chest level.
- Assess suction control chamber for bubbling in wet suction systems.
- Keep suction at prescribed level.
- Maintain appropriate fluid in water seal in wet suction systems.
- Keep air vent open when suction is off.

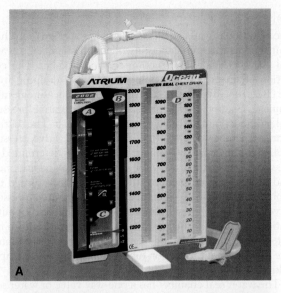

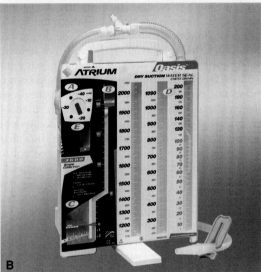

FIGURE 21-10 • Chest drainage systems. **A.** The Atrium Ocean is an example of a water seal chest drain system composed of a drainage chamber and water seal chamber. The suction control is determined by the height of the water column in that chamber (usually 20 cm). *A,* suction control chamber; *B,* water seal chamber; *C,* air leak zone; *D,* collection chamber. **B.** The Atrium Oasis is an example of a dry suction water seal system that uses a mechanical regulator for vacuum control, a water seal chamber, and a drainage chamber. *A,* dry suction regulator; *B,* water seal chamber; *C,* air leak monitor; *D,* collection chamber; *E,* suction monitor bellows. Photos used with permission from Atrium Medical Corporation, Hudson, NH.

intrathoracic pressure needed for lung re-expansion after surgery or trauma.

The mediastinal space is an extrapleural space that lies between the right and left thoracic cavities and contains the large blood vessels, heart, mainstem bronchus, and thymus gland. If fluid accumulates here, the heart can become compressed and stop beating, causing death. Mediastinal chest tubes can be inserted either anteriorly or posteriorly to the heart to drain blood after surgery.

There are two types of chest tubes: small-bore and large-bore catheters. Small-bore catheters (7 Fr to 12 Fr) have a one-way valve apparatus to prevent air from moving back into the chest. They can be inserted through a small skin incision. Large-bore catheters, which range in size up to 40 Fr, are usually connected to a chest drainage system to collect any pleural fluid and monitor for air leaks. After the chest tube is positioned, it is sutured to the skin and connected to a drainage apparatus to remove the residual air and fluid from the pleural or mediastinal space. This results in the re-expansion of remaining lung tissue.

Chest Drainage Systems

Chest drainage systems have a suction source, a collection chamber for pleural drainage, and a mechanism to prevent air from reentering the chest with inhalation (Fig. 21-10). Various types of chest drainage systems are available for use in removal of air and fluid from the pleural space and re-expansion of the lungs. Chest drainage systems come with either wet (water seal) or dry suction control. In wet suction systems, the amount of suction is determined by the amount of water instilled in the suction chamber. The amount of bubbling in the suction chamber indicates the strength of the suction. Wet systems use a water seal to prevent air from moving back into the chest on inspiration. Dry systems use a one-way valve and may have a suction control dial in place of the water. Both systems can operate by gravity drainage, without a suction source.

 Quality and Safety Nursing Alert

When the wall vacuum is turned off, the drainage system must be open to the atmosphere so that intrapleural air can escape from the system. This can be done by detaching the tubing from the suction port to provide a vent.

Water Seal Systems

The traditional water seal system (or wet suction) for chest drainage has three chambers: a collection chamber, a water seal chamber, and a wet suction control chamber. The collection chamber acts as a reservoir for fluid draining from the chest tube. It is graduated to permit easy measurement of drainage. Suction may be added to create negative pressure and promote drainage of fluid and removal of air. The suction control chamber regulates the amount of negative pressure applied to the chest. The amount of suction is determined by the water level. It is usually set at 20 cm H_2O; adding more fluid results in more suction. After the suction is turned on, bubbling appears in the suction chamber. A positive-pressure valve is located at the top of the suction chamber that automatically opens with increases in positive pressure within the system. Air is automatically released through a positive-pressure relief valve if the suction tubing is inadvertently clamped or kinked.

The water seal chamber has a one-way valve or water seal that prevents air from moving back into the chest when the patient inhales. There is an increase in the water level with inspiration and a return to the baseline level during exhalation; this is referred to as tidaling. Intermittent bubbling in the water seal chamber is normal, but continuous bubbling can indicate an air leak. Bubbling and tidaling do not occur when the tube is placed in the mediastinal space; however, fluid may pulsate with the patient's heartbeat. If the chest tube is connected to gravity drainage only, suction is not used. The pressure is equal to the water seal only. Two-chamber chest drainage systems (water seal chamber and collection chamber) are available for use with patients who need only gravity drainage.

The water level in the water seal chamber reflects the negative pressure present in the intrathoracic cavity. A rise in the water level indicates negative pressure in the pleural or mediastinal space. Excessive negative pressure can cause trauma to tissue. Most chest drainage systems have an automatic means to prevent excessive negative pressure. By pressing and holding a manual high-negativity vent (usually located on the top of the chest drainage system) until the water level in the water seal chamber returns to the 2-cm mark, excessive negative pressure is avoided, preventing damage to tissue.

▶ *Quality and Safety Nursing Alert*

If the chest tube and drainage system become disconnected, air can enter the pleural space, producing a pneumothorax. To prevent pneumothorax if the chest tube is inadvertently disconnected from the drainage system, a temporary water seal can be established by immersing the chest tube's open end in a bottle of sterile water.

Dry Suction Water Seal Systems

Dry suction water seal systems, also referred to as dry suction, have a collection chamber for drainage, a water seal chamber, and a dry suction control chamber. The water seal chamber is filled with water to the 2-cm level. Bubbling in this area can indicate an air leak. The dry suction control chamber contains a regulator dial that conveniently regulates vacuum to the chest drain. Water is not needed for suction in these

systems. Without the bubbling in the suction chamber, the machine is quieter. However, if the container is knocked over, the water seal may be lost.

Once the tube is connected to the suction source, the regulator dial allows the desired level of suction to be set; the suction is increased until an indicator appears. The indicator has the same function as the bubbling in the traditional water seal system—that is, it indicates that the vacuum is adequate to maintain the desired level of suction. Some drainage systems use a bellows (a chamber that can be expanded or contracted) or an orange-colored float device as an indicator of when the suction control regulator is set.

When the water in the water seal rises above the 2-cm level, intrathoracic pressure increases. Dry suction water seal systems have a manual high-negativity vent located on top of the drain. The manual high-negativity vent is pressed until the indicator appears (either a float device or bellows) and the water level in the water seal returns to the desired level, indicating that the intrathoracic pressure is decreased.

▶ *Quality and Safety Nursing Alert*

The manual vent should not be used to lower the water level in the water seal when the patient is on gravity drainage (no suction) because intrathoracic pressure is equal to the pressure in the water seal.

Dry Suction Systems With a One-Way Valve

A third type of chest drainage system is dry suction with a one-way mechanical valve. This system has a collection chamber, a one-way mechanical valve, and a dry suction control chamber. The valve permits air and fluid to leave the chest but prevents their movement back into the pleural space. This model lacks a water seal chamber and therefore can be set up quickly in emergency situations, and the dry control drain still works even if it is knocked over. This makes the dry suction systems useful for the patient who is ambulating or being transported. However, without the water seal chamber, there is no way to tell by inspection whether the pressure in the chest has changed, even though an air leak indicator is present so that the system can be checked. If an air leak is suspected, 30 mL of water is injected into the air leak indicator or the container is tipped so that fluid enters the air leak detection chamber. Bubbles will appear if a leak is present.

If the chest tube has been inserted to re-expand a lung after pneumothorax, or if very little fluid drainage is expected, a one-way valve (Heimlich valve) may be connected to the chest tube. This valve may be attached to a collection bag (Fig. 21-11) or covered with a sterile dressing if no drainage is expected.

Postoperative Nursing Management

Postoperative nursing care of the patient who has undergone thoracic surgery involves close monitoring of the patient's respiratory and cardiovascular status, as well as interventions to prevent complications. The psychological reactions that occur in response to this major surgical procedure and the fears that it often engenders in patients and their families are also addressed. For a detailed plan of nursing care for the patient who has had a thoracotomy, see Chart 21-22.

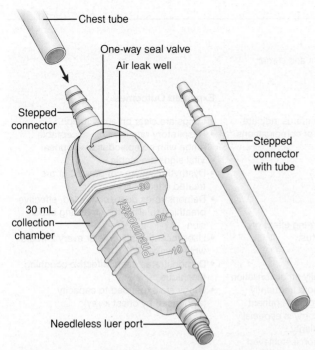

FIGURE 21-11 • One-way (Heimlich) valve, a disposable, single-use chest drainage system with 30 mL collection volume. Used when minimal volume of chest drainage is expected.

Labels: Chest tube, One-way seal valve, Air leak well, Stepped connector, Stepped connector with tube, 30 mL collection chamber, Needleless luer port

Monitoring Respiratory and Cardiovascular Status

The nurse monitors the heart rate and rhythm by auscultation and ECG because episodes of major dysrhythmias are common after thoracic and cardiac surgery. In the immediate postoperative period, an arterial line may be maintained to allow frequent monitoring of arterial blood gases, serum electrolytes, hemoglobin and hematocrit values, and arterial pressure. Central venous pressure may be monitored to detect early signs of fluid volume disturbances; however, central venous pressure monitoring devices are being used less than in the past. Early extubation from mechanical ventilation can also lead to earlier removal of arterial lines. Another important component of postoperative assessment is to note the results of the preoperative evaluation of the patient's lung reserve by pulmonary function testing. A preoperative FEV_1 (the volume of air that the patient can forcibly exhale in 1 second) of more than 2 L or more than 70% of predicted value indicates a good lung reserve. Patients who have a postoperative FEV_1 of less than 40% of predicted value have decreased tidal volume, which places them at risk for respiratory failure, other morbidity, and death.

Improving Gas Exchange and Breathing

Gas exchange is determined by evaluating oxygenation and ventilation. In the immediate postoperative period, this is achieved by measuring vital signs (blood pressure, pulse, and respirations) at least every 15 minutes for the first 1 to 2 hours and then less frequently as the patient's condition stabilizes. Pulse oximetry is used for continuous monitoring of the adequacy of oxygenation. Arterial blood gas measurements are obtained early in the postoperative period to establish a baseline to assess the adequacy of oxygenation and ventilation and the possible retention of carbon dioxide. The frequency

with which postoperative arterial blood gases are measured depends on whether the patient is mechanically ventilated and whether he or she exhibits signs of respiratory distress; these measurements can help determine appropriate therapy. It also is common practice for patients to have an arterial line in place to obtain blood for blood gas measurements and to monitor blood pressure closely. Hemodynamic monitoring may be used to assess hemodynamic stability.

Breathing techniques, such as diaphragmatic and pursed-lip breathing, taught prior to surgery should be performed by the patient every 2 hours to expand the alveoli and prevent atelectasis. Sustained maximal inspiration therapy or incentive spirometry promotes lung inflation, improves the cough mechanism, and allows early assessment of acute pulmonary changes. (See Charts 21-3 and 21-4 for more information.)

If the patient is oriented and blood pressure is stabilized, the head of the bed is elevated 30 to 40 degrees during the immediate postoperative period. This position facilitates ventilation, promotes chest drainage from the lower chest tube, and helps residual air to rise in the upper portion of the pleural space, where it can be removed through the upper chest tube.

The nurse consults with the surgeon about patient positioning to determine the best side-lying position. In general, the patient should be repositioned from back to side frequently and moved from a flat to a semiupright position as soon as tolerated. Most commonly, the patient is instructed to lie on the operative side. However, the patient with unilateral lung pathology may not be able to turn well onto that side because of pain. In addition, positioning the patient with the "good lung" (the nonoperated lung) down allows a better match of ventilation and perfusion and therefore may actually improve oxygenation. The patient's position is changed from flat to semiupright as soon as possible because remaining in one position tends to promote the retention of secretions in the dependent portion of the lungs, and the upright position increases diaphragmatic excursion, enhancing lung expansion. After a pneumonectomy, the operated side should be dependent so that fluid in the pleural space remains below the level of the bronchial stump and the other lung can fully expand.

Improving Airway Clearance

Retained secretions are a threat to the patient after thoracotomy surgery. Trauma to the tracheobronchial tree during surgery, diminished lung ventilation, and diminished cough reflex all result in the accumulation of excessive secretions. If the secretions are retained, airway obstruction occurs. This, in turn, causes the air in the alveoli distal to the obstruction to become absorbed and the affected portion of the lung to collapse. Atelectasis, pneumonia, and respiratory failure may result.

To maintain a patent airway, secretions are suctioned from the tracheobronchial tree before the endotracheal tube is discontinued. Secretions continue to be removed by suctioning until the patient can cough up secretions effectively. Nasotracheal suctioning may be needed to stimulate a deep cough and aspirate secretions that the patient cannot clear by coughing. However, it should be used only after other methods to raise secretions have been unsuccessful (Chart 21-23).

(text continues on page 532)

Chart 21-22

PLAN OF NURSING CARE

Care of the Patient After Thoracotomy

NURSING DIAGNOSIS: Impaired gas exchange related to lung impairment and surgery
GOAL: Improvement of gas exchange and breathing

Nursing Interventions	Rationale	Expected Outcomes

1. Monitor pulmonary status as directed and as needed.
  a. Auscultate breath sounds.
  b. Check rate, depth, and pattern of respirations.
  c. Assess blood gases for signs of hypoxemia or CO_2 retention.
  d. Evaluate patient's color for cyanosis.
	1. Changes in pulmonary status indicate improvement or onset of complications.	• Lungs are clear on auscultation.
		• Respiratory rate is within acceptable range with no episodes of dyspnea.
		• Vital signs are stable.
		• Dysrhythmias are not present or are treated effectively.
		• Demonstrates deep, controlled, effective breathing to allow maximal lung expansion
		• Uses incentive spirometer every 2 hours while awake
		• Demonstrates deep, effective coughing technique
		• Lungs are expanded to capacity (evidenced by chest x-ray).

2. Monitor and record blood pressure, apical pulse, and temperature every 2–4 hours, and central venous pressure (if indicated) every 2 hours.	2. Vital signs aid in evaluating effect of surgery on cardiac status.	
3. Monitor continuous electrocardiogram for pattern and dysrhythmias.	3. Dysrhythmias (especially atrial fibrillation and atrial flutter) are more frequently seen after thoracic surgery. A patient with total pneumonectomy is especially prone to cardiac irregularity.	
4. Elevate head of bed 30–40 degrees when patient is oriented and hemodynamic status is stable.	4. Maximum lung excursion is achieved when patient is as close to upright as possible.	
5. Encourage deep-breathing exercises (see Breathing Retraining section) and effective use of incentive spirometer (sustained maximal inspiration).	5. Helps to achieve maximal lung inflation and to open closed airways	
6. Encourage and promote an effective cough routine to be performed every 1–2 hours during first 24 hours.	6. Coughing is necessary to remove retained secretions.	

7. Assess and monitor the chest drainage system.*
  a. Assess for leaks and patency as needed (see Chart 21–20).
  b. Monitor amount and character of drainage and document every 2 hours. Notify primary provider if drainage is ≥150 mL per hour.
	7. System is used to eliminate any residual air or fluid after thoracotomy.	

NURSING DIAGNOSIS: Ineffective airway clearance related to lung impairment, anesthesia, and pain
GOAL: Improvement of airway clearance and achievement of a patent airway

Nursing Interventions	Rationale	Expected Outcomes
1. Maintain an open airway.	1. Provides for adequate ventilation and gas exchange	• Airway is patent. • Coughs effectively • Splints incision while coughing • Sputum is clear or colorless. • Lungs are clear on auscultation.
2. Perform endotracheal suctioning until patient can cough effectively.	2. Endotracheal secretions are present in excessive amounts in postthoracotomy patients due to trauma to the tracheobronchial tree during surgery, diminished lung ventilation, and cough reflex.	
3. Assess and medicate for pain. Encourage deep-breathing and coughing exercises. Help splint incision during coughing.	3. Helps to achieve maximal lung inflation and to open closed airways. Coughing is painful; incision needs to be supported.	
4. Monitor amount, viscosity, color, and odor of sputum. Notify primary provider if sputum is excessive or contains bright-red blood.	4. Changes in sputum suggest presence of infection or change in pulmonary status. Colorless sputum is not unusual; opacification or coloring of sputum may indicate dehydration or infection.	
5. Administer humidification and small-volume nebulizer therapy as prescribed.	5. Secretions must be moistened and thinned if they are to be raised from the chest with the least amount of effort.	

Chart 21-22

PLAN OF NURSING CARE

Care of the Patient After Thoracotomy (continued)

Nursing Interventions	Rationale	Expected Outcomes
6. Perform postural drainage, percussion, and vibration as prescribed. Do not percuss or vibrate directly over operative site. 7. Auscultate both sides of chest to determine changes in breath sounds.	6. Chest physiotherapy uses gravity to help remove secretions from the lung. 7. Indications for tracheal suctioning are determined by chest auscultation.	

NURSING DIAGNOSIS: Acute pain related to incision, drainage tubes, and the surgical procedure
GOAL: Relief of pain and discomfort

Nursing Interventions	Rationale	Expected Outcomes

1. Evaluate location, character, quality, and severity of pain. Administer analgesic medication as prescribed and as needed. Observe for respiratory effect of opioid. Is patient too somnolent to cough? Are respirations depressed?
2. Maintain care postoperatively in positioning the patient.
  a. Place patient in semi-Fowler's position.
  b. Patients with limited respiratory reserve may not be able to turn on unoperated side.
  c. Assist or turn patient every 2 hours.
3. Assess incision area every 8 hours for redness, heat, induration, swelling, separation, and drainage.
4. Request order for patient-controlled analgesia pump if appropriate for patient.
	1. Pain limits chest excursions and thereby decreases ventilation.
	
	2. The patient who is comfortable and free of pain will be less likely to splint the chest while breathing. A semi-Fowler's position permits residual air in the pleural space to rise to upper portion of pleural space and be removed via the upper chest catheter.
	
	3. These signs indicate possible infection.
	
	4. Allowing patient control over frequency and dose improves comfort and adherence with treatment regimen.
		• Asks for pain medication but verbalizes that he or she expects some discomfort while deep breathing and coughing
		• Verbalizes that he or she is comfortable and not in acute distress
		• No signs of incisional infection evident

NURSING DIAGNOSIS: Anxiety related to outcomes of surgery, pain, technology
GOAL: Reduction of anxiety to a manageable level

Nursing Interventions	Rationale	Expected Outcomes
1. Explain all procedures in understandable language. 2. Assess for pain and medicate, especially before potentially painful procedures. 3. Silence all *unnecessary* alarms on technology (monitors, ventilators). 4. Encourage and support patient while increasing activity level. 5. Mobilize resources (family, clergy, social worker) to help patient cope with outcomes of surgery (diagnosis, change in functional abilities).	1. Explaining what can be expected in understandable terms decreases anxiety and increases cooperation. 2. Premedication before painful procedures or activities improves comfort and minimizes undue anxiety. 3. *Unnecessary* alarms increase the risk of sensory overload and may increase anxiety. *Essential* alarms must be turned on at all times. 4. Positive reinforcement improves patient motivation and independence. 5. A multidisciplinary approach promotes the patient's strengths and coping mechanisms.	• States that anxiety is at a manageable level • Participates with health care team in treatment regimen • Uses appropriate coping skills (verbalization; pain relief strategies; the use of support systems such as family, clergy) • Demonstrates basic understanding of technology used in care

(continues on page 532)

**Chart
21-22**

PLAN OF NURSING CARE

Care of the Patient After Thoracotomy (continued)

NURSING DIAGNOSIS: Impaired physical mobility of the upper extremities related to thoracic surgery
GOAL: Increased mobility of the affected shoulder and arm

Nursing Interventions	Rationale	Expected Outcomes
1. Assist patient with normal range of motion and function of shoulder and trunk. a. Educate about use of breathing exercises to mobilize thorax. b. Encourage skeletal exercises to promote abduction and mobilization of shoulder (see Chart 21-24). c. Assist out of bed to chair as soon as pulmonary and circulatory systems are stable (usually by evening of surgery). 2. Encourage progressive activities according to level of fatigue.	1. Necessary to regain normal mobility of arm and shoulder and to speed recovery and minimize discomfort 2. Increases patient's use of affected shoulder and arm	• Demonstrates arm and shoulder exercises and verbalizes intent to perform them on discharge • Regains previous range of motion in shoulder and arm

NURSING DIAGNOSIS: Risk for imbalanced fluid volume related to the surgical procedure
GOAL: Maintenance of adequate fluid volume

Nursing Interventions	Rationale	Expected Outcomes
1. Monitor and record hourly intake and output. Urine output should be at least 30 mL per hour after surgery. 2. Administer blood component therapy and parenteral fluids and/or diuretics as prescribed to restore and maintain fluid volume.	1. Fluid management may be altered before, during, and after surgery, and patient's response to and need for fluid management must be assessed. 2. Pulmonary edema due to transfusion or fluid overload is an ever-present threat; after pneumonectomy, the pulmonary vascular system has been greatly reduced.	• Patient is adequately hydrated, as evidenced by: • Urine output >30 mL per hour • Vital signs stable, heart rate, and central venous pressure approaching normal • No excessive peripheral edema

NURSING DIAGNOSIS: Deficient knowledge of home care procedures
GOAL: Increased ability to carry out care procedures at home

Nursing Interventions	Rationale	Expected Outcomes
1. Encourage patient to practice arm and shoulder exercises five times daily at home. 2. Instruct patient to practice assuming a functionally erect position in front of a full-length mirror. 3. Instruct patient about home care (see Chart 21-25).	1. Exercise accelerates recovery of muscle function and reduces long-term pain and discomfort. 2. Practice will help restore normal posture. 3. Knowing what to expect facilitates recovery.	• Demonstrates arm and shoulder exercises • Verbalizes need to try to assume an erect posture • Verbalizes the importance of relieving discomfort, alternating walking and rest, performing breathing exercises, avoiding heavy lifting, avoiding undue fatigue, avoiding bronchial irritants, preventing colds or lung infections, getting influenza vaccine, keeping follow-up visits, and stopping smoking

*A patient with a pneumonectomy usually does not have water seal chest drainage because it is desirable that the pleural space fill with an effusion, which eventually obliterates this space. Some surgeons do use a modified water seal system.

The patient is encouraged to cough effectively to maintain a patent airway; ineffective coughing results in exhaustion and retention of secretions (see Chart 21-5). To be effective, the cough must be low-pitched, deep, and controlled. Because it is difficult to cough in a supine position, the patient is helped to a sitting position on the edge of the bed, with the feet resting on a chair. The patient should cough at least every hour during the first 24 hours and when necessary thereafter. If audible crackles are present, it may be necessary to use chest percussion with the cough routine until the lungs are clear. Aerosol therapy is helpful in humidifying and mobilizing secretions so that they can easily be cleared with coughing. To minimize incisional pain during coughing, the nurse supports the incision or encourages the patient to do so (Fig. 21-12). If a patient is identified as being at high risk for postoperative pulmonary complications, then CPT is started

Chart 21-23 Performing Nasotracheal Suction

- Explain procedure to the patient.
- Medicate patient for pain if necessary.
- Place the patient in a sitting or semi-Fowler's position. Make sure the patient's head is not flexed forward. Remove excess pillows if necessary.
- Oxygenate the patient several minutes before initiating the suctioning procedure. Have oxygen source ready nearby during procedure.
- Put on sterile gloves.
- Lubricate catheter with water-soluble gel.
- Gently pass catheter through the patient's nose to the pharynx. If it is difficult to pass the catheter, and repeated suctioning is expected, a soft rubber nasal trumpet may be placed nasopharyngeally to provide easier catheter passage. Check the position of the tip of the catheter by asking the patient to open the mouth to inspect it; the tip of the catheter should be in the lower pharynx.
- Instruct the patient to take a deep breath or stick out the tongue. This action opens the epiglottis and promotes downward movement of the catheter.
- Advance the catheter into the trachea only during inspiration. Listen for cough or for passage of air through the catheter.
- Attach the catheter to suction apparatus. Apply intermittent suction while slowly withdrawing the catheter. Do not let suction exceed 120 mm Hg.
- Do not suction for longer than 10–15 seconds, as dysrhythmias, bradycardia, or cardiac arrest may occur in patients with borderline oxygenation.
- If additional suctioning is needed, withdraw the catheter to the back of the pharynx. Reassure patient and oxygenate for several minutes before resuming suctioning.

immediately (perhaps even before surgery). The techniques of postural drainage, vibration, and percussion help loosen and mobilize the secretions so that they can be coughed up or suctioned.

Following the use of these measures, the nurse listens to both lungs, anteriorly and posteriorly, to determine whether there are any changes in breath sounds. Diminished breath sounds may indicate collapsed or hypoventilated alveoli.

Relieving Pain and Discomfort

Pain after a thoracotomy may be severe, depending on the type of incision and the patient's reaction and ability to cope with pain. Pain can impair the patient's ability to breathe deeply and cough. Preoperatively or postoperatively, an anesthesiologist or anesthetist can perform paravertebral blocks with a long-acting local anesthetic such as bupivacaine (Marcaine) or ropivacaine (Naropin) (Wenk & Schug, 2011). A thoracic epidural catheter may be placed for continuous analgesia or PCEA using a combination of a long-acting local anesthetic and an opioid. As an alternative, a continuous epidural infusion may be combined with IV PCA using an opioid. Bupivacaine or ropivacaine is titrated in the epidural catheter to relieve postoperative pain, improving the patient's mobility and ability to deep breathe and cough. Opioid analgesic agents such as morphine are commonly used in PCA, which allows the patient to control the frequency and total dosage. Preset limits on the pump avoid overdosage. With proper instruction, PCA and PCEA are well tolerated and allow earlier mobilization and cooperation with the treatment regimen. (See Chapter 12 for a more extensive discussion of PCA and pain management.)

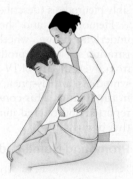

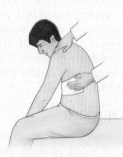

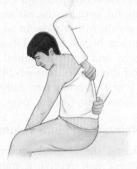

A. Nurse's hands should support the chest incision anteriorly and posteriorly. The patient is instructed to take several deep breaths, inhale, and then cough forcibly.

B. With one hand, the nurse exerts downward pressure on the soulder of the affected side while firmly supporting the area beneath the wound. The patient is instructed to take several deep breaths, inhale, and then cough forcibly.

C. The nurse can wrap a towel or sheet around the patient's chest and hold the ends together, pulling slightly as the patient coughs, and releasing during deep breaths.

D. The patient can be taught to hold a pillow firmly against the incision while coughing. This can be done while lying down or sitting in an upright position.

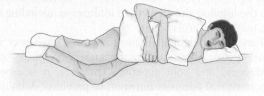

FIGURE 21-12 • Techniques for supporting incision while a patient recovering from thoracic surgery coughs.

It is important to avoid depressing the respiratory system with excessive opioid analgesia. The patient should not be so sedated as to be unable to cough. Incorporating a multimodal approach to pain management with PCEAs and NSAIDs can help to alleviate this problem. Inadequate treatment of pain, however, may also lead to hypoventilation and decreased coughing.

 Concept Mastery Alert

> It is important not to confuse the restlessness of hypoxia with the restlessness caused by pain. Dyspnea, restlessness, increasing respiratory rate, increasing blood pressure, and tachycardia are warning signs of impending respiratory insufficiency. Pulse oximetry is used to monitor oxygenation and to differentiate causes of restlessness.

Lidocaine (Xylocaine) and prilocaine (Citanest) are local anesthetic agents that may be used to treat pain at the site of the chest tube insertion. These medications are administered as topical transdermal analgesics that penetrate the skin; they have also been found to be effective when used together. EMLA cream, which is a mixture of the two medications, may be effective in treating pain from chest tube removal. However, analgesia is not typically indicated when removing chest tubes, because the pain, although severe, is of short duration (usually less than a few minutes) and the analgesia might interfere with respiratory effort.

Promoting Mobility and Shoulder Exercises

Because large shoulder girdle muscles are transected during a thoracotomy, the arm and shoulder must be mobilized by full range of motion of the shoulder. As soon as physiologically possible, usually within 8 to 12 hours, the patient is helped to get out of bed. Although this may be painful initially, the earlier the patient moves, the sooner the pain will subside. In addition to getting out of bed, the patient begins arm and shoulder exercises to restore movement and prevent painful stiffening of the affected arm and shoulder (Chart 21-24). A scheduled regimen of 3 to 4 g of acetaminophen daily can help relieve shoulder pain (Gottschalk, Cohen, Yang, et al., 2006).

Maintaining Fluid Volume and Nutrition

During the surgical procedure or immediately after, the patient may receive a transfusion of blood products (see Chapter 32), followed by a continuous IV infusion. Because a reduction in lung capacity often occurs after thoracic surgery, a period of physiologic adjustment is needed. Fluids should be administered at a low hourly rate and titrated (as prescribed) to prevent overloading the vascular system and precipitating pulmonary edema. The nurse performs careful respiratory and cardiovascular assessments and monitors intake and output, vital signs, and jugular vein distention. The nurse also monitors the infusion site for signs of infiltration, including swelling, tenderness, and redness.

Patients undergoing thoracotomy may have poor nutritional status before surgery because of dyspnea, sputum production, and poor appetite. Therefore, it is especially important that adequate nutrition be provided. A liquid diet is provided as soon as bowel sounds return, and the patient is progressed to a full diet as soon as possible. Small, frequent meals are better tolerated and are crucial to the recovery and maintenance of lung function.

Monitoring and Managing Potential Complications

Complications after thoracic surgery are always a possibility and must be identified and managed early. The nurse monitors the patient at regular intervals for signs of respiratory distress or developing respiratory failure, dysrhythmias, bronchopleural fistula, hemorrhage and shock, atelectasis, and incisional or pulmonary infection.

Respiratory distress is treated by identifying and eliminating its cause while providing supplemental oxygen. If the patient progresses to respiratory failure, intubation and mechanical ventilation are necessary.

Dysrhythmias are often related to the effects of hypoxia or the surgical procedure. They are treated with antiarrhythmic medication and supportive therapy (see Chapter 26). Pulmonary infections or effusion, often preceded by atelectasis, may occur a few days into the postoperative course.

Pneumothorax may occur after thoracic surgery if there is an air leak from the surgical site to the pleural cavity or from the pleural cavity to the environment. Failure of the chest drainage system prevents return of negative pressure in the pleural cavity and results in pneumothorax. In the postoperative patient, pneumothorax is often accompanied by hemothorax. The nurse maintains the chest drainage system and monitors the patient for signs and symptoms of pneumothorax: increasing shortness of breath, tachycardia, increased respiratory rate, and increasing respiratory distress.

Bronchopleural fistula is a serious but rare complication that prevents the return of negative intrathoracic pressure and lung re-expansion. Depending on its severity, it is treated with closed chest drainage, mechanical ventilation, and possibly pleurodesis (described in Chapter 23).

Hemorrhage and shock are managed by treating the underlying cause, whether by reoperation or by administration of blood products or fluids. Pulmonary edema from overinfusion of IV fluids is a significant danger. Early symptoms are dyspnea; crackles; tachycardia; and pink, frothy sputum. This constitutes an emergency and must be reported and treated immediately (see Chapter 29 for further discussion).

Promoting Home and Community-Based Care

Educating Patients About Self-Care

The nurse instructs the patient and family about postoperative care that will be continued at home. The nurse explains signs and symptoms that should be reported to the primary provider. These include the following:

- Change in respiratory status, such as increasing shortness of breath, fever, increased restlessness or other changes in mental or cognitive status, increased respiratory rate, change in respiratory pattern, change in amount or color of sputum
- Bleeding or other drainage from the surgical incision or chest tube exit sites
- Increased chest pain

In addition, respiratory care and other treatment modalities (oxygen; incentive spirometry; CPT; and oral, inhaled, or

Chart
21-24

PATIENT EDUCATION

Performing Arm and Shoulder Exercises

Arm and shoulder exercises are performed after thoracic surgery to restore movement, prevent painful stiffening of the shoulder, and improve muscle power.

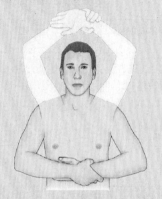

Hold hand of the affected side with the other hand, palms facing in. Raise the arms forward, upward, and then overhead, while taking a deep breath. Exhale while lowering the arms. Repeat five times.

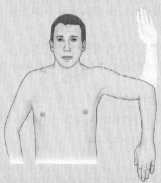

Raise arm sideward, upward, and downward in a waving motion

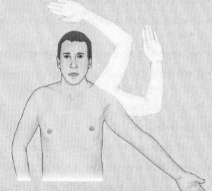

Place arm at side. Raise arm sideward, upward, and then overhead. Repeat five times. These exercises can also be performed while lying in bed.

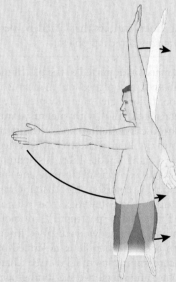

Extend the arm up and back, out to the side and back, down at the side, and back.

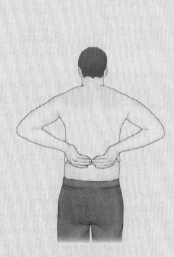

Place hands in small of back. Push elbows as far back as possible.

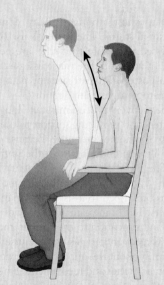

Sit erect in an armchair; place the hands on arms of the chair. Press down on hands, consciously pulling the abdomen in and stretching up from the waist. Inhale while raising the body until elbows are extended completely. Hold this position a moment, and begin exhaling while lowering the body slowly to the original position.

IV medications) may be continued at home. Therefore, the nurse needs to instruct the patient and family in their correct and safe use.

The nurse emphasizes the importance of progressively increased activity. The nurse instructs the patient to ambulate within limits and explains that return of strength is likely to be very gradual. Another important aspect of patient education addresses shoulder exercises. The patient is instructed

to do these exercises five times daily. Additional patient education is described in Chart 21-25.

Continuing Care

Depending on the patient's physical status and the availability of family assistance, a home care referral may be indicated. The home care nurse assesses the patient's recovery from surgery, with special attention to respiratory status, the surgical

HOME CARE CHECKLIST

Chart 21-25

The Patient With a Thoracotomy

At the completion of home care education, the patient or caregiver will be able to:	PATIENT	CAREGIVER
• Use local heat and oral analgesia to relieve intercostal pain.	✔	✔
• Alternate walking and other activities with frequent rest periods, expecting weakness and fatigue for the first 3 weeks.	✔	✔
• Perform breathing exercises several times daily for the first few weeks at home.	✔	
• Avoid lifting >20 pounds until complete healing has taken place; the chest muscles and incision may be weaker than normal for 3–6 months after surgery.	✔	
• Walk at a moderate pace, gradually and persistently extending walking time and distance.	✔	
• Immediately stop any activity that causes undue fatigue, increased shortness of breath, or chest pain.	✔	
• Avoid bronchial irritants (smoke, fumes, air pollution, aerosol sprays).	✔	✔
• Avoid others with known colds or lung infections.	✔	✔
• Obtain an annual influenza vaccine, and discuss vaccination against pneumonia with the primary provider.	✔	
• Report for follow-up care by the surgeon or clinic as necessary.	✔	✔
• Stop smoking, if applicable, and avoid exposure to secondhand smoke.	✔	✔

incision, chest drainage, pain control, ambulation, and nutritional status. The patient's use of respiratory modalities is assessed to ensure that they are being used correctly and safely. In addition, the nurse assesses the patient's adherence to the postoperative treatment plan and identifies acute or late postoperative complications.

The recovery process may take longer than the patient had expected, and providing support to the patient is an important task for the home care nurse. Because of shorter hospital stays, follow-up appointments with the primary provider are essential. The nurse educates the patient about the importance of keeping follow-up appointments and completing laboratory tests as prescribed to assist the primary provider in evaluating recovery. The home care nurse provides continuous encouragement and education to the patient and family during the process. As recovery progresses, the nurse also reminds the patient and family about the importance of participating in health promotion activities and recommended health screening.

Critical Thinking Exercises

1 A 48-year-old woman is 2 days postoperative on your unit for gastric bypass surgery. She is currently receiving 2 L/min of oxygen by nasal cannula. Her most recent vital signs include the following: oral temperature, 38.2°C (100.8°F); heart rate, 87 bpm; respiratory rate, 26 breaths/min; blood pressure, 144/85; and SpO$_2$, 94%. Pain control has been an issue since surgery despite being on a morphine PCA, with her reporting surgical site pain between a "7" and "10" on a 0 to 10 rating scale over the last 24 hours. Upon auscultation, her breath sounds are clear with decreased breath sounds bilaterally at the bases. Her postoperative incentive spirometry volumes have been between 250 and 500 mL. What is the likely cause of her fever? What diagnostic tests and labs would you anticipate that the PCP might order? How does pain control affect this patient's respiratory

status? Describe nursing interventions that could be performed to prevent or treat this clinical problem.

2 **ebp** A 60-year-old man was admitted to the ICU after being emergently intubated and placed on mechanical ventilation for respiratory failure. He originally presented to the emergency department (ED) with mental status changes secondary to chronic liver failure and a history of alcohol abuse. On day 3 in the ICU, a chest x-ray revealed infiltrates in the patient's right middle lobe, his sputum culture revealed gram-positive cocci in clusters, and his white blood cell count on his complete blood count was 17,500/cu mm. Based upon these findings, the patient was diagnosed with VAP and broad-spectrum IV antibiotics were started. List and discuss the evidence-based interventions associated with the VAP bundle as described by the Institute for Healthcare Improvement (IHI) (see Chart 21-13). How does oral care and subglottic suctioning help prevent VAP?

3 **pq** A 19-year-old man was admitted to a medical-surgical unit after being treated in the ED with an emergently placed chest tube for a large right-sided spontaneous pneumothorax. The chest drainage system is set at 20 cm H$_2$O of suction. Four hours after arriving to the unit, the patient complains of mild respiratory distress. Auscultation of his chest reveals slightly diminished breath sounds on the right, clear sounds on the left, and a "popping noise." There is a "crackling" noise elicited upon palpation of the patient's right lateral chest, and continuous bubbling is noted in the chest drainage system's water seal chamber. Describe the potential causes for bubbling in the water seal chamber of a chest tube drainage system. Based on these findings, what chest tube complication seems most likely? Describe your priority interventions.

Brunner Suite Resources

Explore these additional resources to enhance
learning for this chapter:
  • NCLEX-Style Questions and Other Resources
on thePoint, http://thePoint.lww.com/Brunner13e
• Study Guide
• PrepU
• Clinical Handbook
• Handbook of Laboratory and Diagnostic Tests

References

*Asterisk indicates nursing research.

Books

Cairo, J. M., & Pilbeam, S. P. (2010). *Mosby's respiratory care equipment* (8th ed.). St. Louis: Elsevier Mosby.

Carlson, K. K. (2009). *AACN advanced critical care nursing*. St. Louis: Elsevier Saunders.

Marini, J. J., & Wheeler, A. P. (2010). *Critical care medicine* (4th ed.). Philadelphia: Lippincott Williams & Wilkins.

Meiner, S. E. (2010). *Gerontologic nursing* (4th ed.). St. Louis: Elsevier Mosby.

Morton, P. G., Fontaine, D. K., Hudak, C. M., et al. (2009). *Critical care nursing: A holistic approach* (9th ed.). Philadelphia: Lippincott Williams & Wilkins.

Porth, C. M., & Matfin, G. (2009). *Pathophysiology: Concepts of altered health states* (8th ed.). Philadelphia: Lippincott Williams & Williams.

Sole, M. L., Klein, D. G., & Moseley, M. J. (2013). *Introduction to critical care nursing* (6th ed.). St. Louis: Elsevier Saunders.

Urden, L. D., Stacy, K. M., & Lough, M. E. (2010). *Critical care nursing: Diagnosis and management* (6th ed.). St. Louis: Elsevier Mosby.

Wiegand, D. J. L. (2011). *AACN Procedure Manual for Critical Care* (6th ed.). St. Louis: Elsevier Saunders.

Journals and Electronic Documents

American Thoracic Society. (2005). Guidelines for the management of adults with hospital-acquired, ventilator-associated and health-care associated pneumonia. *American Journal of Respiratory and Critical Care Medicine, 171*(4), 388–416.

Amitai, A., & Sinert, R. H. (2011). *Ventilator management*. Available at: emedicine.medscape.com/article/810126-overview#aw2qqb6b6

Arpino, P. A., Kalafatas, K., & Thompson, B. T. (2008). Feasibility of dexmedetomidine in facilitating extubation in the intensive care unit. *Journal of Clinical Pharmacy and Therapeutics, 33*(1), 25–30.

Bauman, M. (2009). Noninvasive ventilation makes a comeback. *American Nurse Today, 4*(4), 20–24.

Bennett, M., & Heard, R. (2010). Hyperbaric oxygen therapy for multiple sclerosis. *CNS Neuroscience Therapies, 16*(2), 115–124.

Bennett, M., Lehm, J., & Jepson, N. (2011). Hyperbaric oxygen therapy for acute coronary syndrome. *Cochrane Database of Systematic Reviews*, (3), CD004818.

Bennett, M. H., Stanford, R., & Turner, R. (2012). Hyperbaric oxygen therapy for promoting fracture healing and treating fracture non-union. *Cochrane Database of Systematic Reviews*, (1), CD004712.

*Briscoe, W., & Woodgate, R. (2010). Sustaining self: The lived experience of transition to long-term ventilation. *Qualitative Health Research, 20*(1), 57–67.

Casaer, M. P., Mesotten, D., Hermans, G., et al. (2011). Early versus late parenteral nutrition in critically ill adults. *New England Journal of Medicine, 365*(6), 506–517.

Centers for Medicare and Medicaid Services. (1993). *National coverage determination (NCD) for home use of oxygen (240.2)*. Available at: www.cms.gov/medicare-coverage-database/details/ncd-details.aspx?NCDId=169&ncdver=1&DocID=240.2&SearchType=Advanced&bc=IAAAABAAAAAA&

Facchiano, L., Hoffman, S. C., & Núñez, D. E. (2011) A literature review on breathing retraining as a self-management strategy operationalized through Rosswurm and Larrabee's evidence-based practice model. *Journal of the American Academy of Nurse Practitioners, 23*(8), 421–426.

Feldman-Idov, Y., Melamed, Y, Ore, L., et al. (2011). Improvement of ischemic non-healing wounds following hyperoxygenation: The experience at Rambam-Elisha Hyperbaric Center in Israel, 1998-2007. *Israel Association Medical Journal, 13*(9), 524–529.

Fink, J. B. (2007). Forced expiratory technique, directed cough, and autogenic drainage. *Respiratory Care, 52*(9), 1210–1221.

Girard, T. D., Kress, J. P., Fuchs, B. D., et al. (2008). Efficacy and safety of a paired sedation and ventilator weaning protocol for mechanically ventilated patients in intensive care (Awakening and Breathing Controlled trial): A randomized controlled trial. *Lancet, 371*, 126–134.

Gottschalk, A., Cohen, S. P., Yang, S., et al. (2006). Preventing and treating pain after thoracic surgery. *Anesthesiology, 104*(3), 594–600.

Hamilton, V. A., & Grap, M. J. (2012). The role of the endotracheal tube cuff in microaspiration. *Heart & Lung: The Journal of Acute and Critical Care, 41*(2), 167–72.

Jallu, S. S., & Salzman, G. A. (2011). A case-based approach to noninvasive positive pressure ventilation. *Hospital Practice, 39*(3), 168–175.

Langenhof, S., & Fichter, J. (2005). Comparison of two demand oxygen delivery devices for administration of oxygen in COPD. *Chest, 128*(4), 2082–2087.

Mahajan, A. K., Diette, G. B., Hatipoglu, U., et al. (2011). High frequency chest wall oscillation for asthma and chronic obstructive pulmonary disease exacerbations: A randomized sham-controlled clinical trial. *Respiratory Research, 12*, 120. Available at: respiratory-research.com/content/12/1/120.

Maung, A. A., & Kaplan, L. J. (2011). Airway pressure release ventilation in acute respiratory distress syndrome. *Critical Care Clinics, 27*(3), 501–509.

Morrison, L., & Agnew, J. (2011). Oscillating devices for airway clearance in people with cystic fibrosis. *Cochrane Database of Systematic Reviews*, (2), CD006842.

Oey, I. F., Morgan, M. D, Spyt, D. A., et al. (2010). Staged bilateral lung volume reduction surgery: The benefits of a patient-led strategy. *European Journal of Cardio-thoracic Surgery, 37*(4), 846–852.

Perme, C., & Chandrashekar, R. (2009). Early mobility and walking program for patients in intensive care units: Creating a standard of care. *American Journal of Critical Care, 18*(3), 212–221.

Solaini, L., Prusciano, F., Bagioni, P., et al. (2008). Video-assisted thoracic surgery (VATS) of the lung: Analysis of interoperative and postoperative complications over 15 years and review of literature. *Surgical Endoscopy, 22*(2), 298–310.

Stewart, N. I., Jagelman, A. J., & Webster, N. R. (2011). Emerging modes of ventilation in the intensive care unit. *British Journal of Anaesthesia, 107*(1), 74–82.

Weijs, P. J., Stapel, S. N., de Groot, S. D., et al. (2012). Optimal protein and energy nutrition decreases mortality in mechanically ventilated, critically ill patients: A prospective observational cohort study. *Journal of Parenteral and Enteral Nutrition, 36*(1), 60–68.

Wenk, M., & Schug, S. (2011). Perioperative pain management after thoracotomy. *Current Opinion in Anesthesiology, 24*(1), 8–12.

Resources

American Association for Respiratory Care (AARC), www.aarc.org
American Lung Association, www.lungusa.org
American Thoracic Society (ATS), www.thoracic.org
Institute for Healthcare Improvement (IHI), www.ihi.org
National Institutes of Health, National Heart, Lung, and Blood Institute, www.nhlbi.nih.gov/index.htm
National Lung Health Education Program (NLHEP), www.nlhep.org (Has easy-to-read educational resources for patients.)

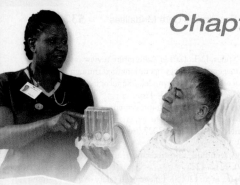

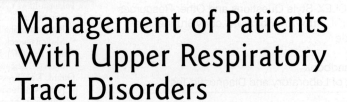

Management of Patients With Upper Respiratory Tract Disorders

Learning Objectives

On completion of this chapter, the learner will be able to:

1 Describe nursing management of patients with upper airway disorders.
2 Compare and contrast the upper respiratory tract infections according to cause, incidence, clinical manifestations, management, and the significance of preventive health care.
3 Use the nursing process as a framework for care of patients with upper airway infection.
4 Describe nursing management of the patient with epistaxis.
5 Use the nursing process as a framework for care of patients undergoing laryngectomy.

Glossary

alaryngeal communication: alternative modes of speaking that do not involve the normal larynx; used by patients whose larynx has been surgically removed

aphonia: impaired ability to use one's voice due to disease or injury to the larynx

apnea: cessation of breathing

dysphagia: difficulties in swallowing

epistaxis: hemorrhage from the nose due to rupture of tiny, distended vessels in the mucous membrane of any area of the nose

herpes simplex: "cold sore"; a cutaneous viral infection with painful vesicles and erosions on the tongue, palate, gingiva, buccal membranes, or lips

laryngectomy: surgical removal of all or part of the larynx and surrounding structures

laryngitis: inflammation of the larynx; may be caused by voice abuse, exposure to irritants, or infectious organisms

nuchal rigidity: stiffness of the neck or inability to bend the neck

pharyngitis: inflammation of the throat; usually viral or bacterial in origin

rhinitis: inflammation of the mucous membranes of the nose; may be infectious, allergic, or inflammatory in origin

rhinitis medicamentosa: rebound nasal congestion commonly associated with overuse of over-the-counter nasal decongestants

rhinorrhea: drainage of a large amount of fluid from the nose

rhinosinusitis: inflammation of the nares and paranasal sinuses, including frontal, ethmoid, maxillary, and sphenoid sinuses; replaces the term *sinusitis*

tonsillitis: inflammation of the tonsils, usually due to an acute infection

xerostomia: dryness of the mouth from a variety of causes

Upper respiratory tract disorders are those that involve the nose, paranasal sinuses, pharynx, larynx, trachea, or bronchi. Many of these conditions are relatively minor, and their effects are limited to mild and temporary discomfort and inconvenience for the patient. However, others are acute, severe, and life threatening and may require permanent alterations in breathing and speaking. Therefore, the nurse must have expert assessment skills, an understanding of the wide variety of disorders that may affect the upper airway, and an awareness of the impact of these alterations on patients. Patient education is an important aspect of nursing care because many of these disorders are treated outside the hospital or at home by patients themselves. When caring for patients with acute, life-threatening disorders, the nurse needs highly developed assessment and clinical management skills, along with a focus on rehabilitation needs.

UPPER AIRWAY INFECTIONS

Upper airway infections (otherwise known as upper respiratory infections or URIs) are the most common cause of illness and affect most people on occasion. Some infections are acute, with symptoms that last several days; others are chronic, with symptoms that may last for weeks or months or recur.

The common cold is the most frequently occurring example of a URI. URIs occur when microorganisms such as viruses and bacteria are inhaled. There are many causative organisms, and people are susceptible throughout life. Viruses, the most common cause of URIs, affect the upper respiratory passages and lead to subsequent mucous membrane inflammation (Williams, 2011). URIs are the most common reason for seeking health care and for absences from school and work.

URIs affect the nasal cavity; ethmoidal air cells; and frontal, maxillary, and sphenoid sinuses; as well as the pharynx, larynx, and trachea. On average, adults typically develop two to four URIs per year because of the wide variety of respiratory viruses that circulate in the community. Although patients are rarely hospitalized for treatment of URIs, nurses working in community settings or long-term care facilities may encounter patients who have these infections. It is important for nurses to recognize the signs and symptoms of URIs and provide appropriate care. Nurses in these settings also can influence patient outcomes through patient education. Special considerations with regard to URIs in older adults are summarized in Chart 22-1.

Chart 22-1

Upper Respiratory Tract Disorders in Older Adults

- Upper respiratory infections in older adults may have more serious consequences if patients have concurrent medical problems that compromise their respiratory or immune status.
- Influenza causes exacerbations of chronic obstructive pulmonary disease and reduced pulmonary function.
- Antihistamines and decongestants used to treat upper respiratory disorders must be used cautiously in older adults because of their side effects and potential interactions with other medications.
- Of Americans 65 years and older, approximately 14.1% have chronic rhinosinusitis (CRS). With anticipated future growth in the older adult population, the need for endoscopic sinus surgery will increase. Older patients with CRS present with symptoms similar to those of younger adults and experience a similar degree of improvement and quality of life after endoscopic sinus surgery.
- The structure of the nose changes with aging; it lengthens and the tip droops from loss of cartilage. This can cause restriction in airflow and predispose older adult patients to geriatric rhinitis, characterized by increased thin, watery sinus drainage. These structural changes may also adversely affect the sense of smell.
- Laryngitis in the older adults is common and may be secondary to gastroesophageal reflux disease. Older adults are more likely to have impaired esophageal peristalsis and a weaker esophageal sphincter. Treatment measures include sleeping with the head of the bed elevated and the use of medications such as histamine-2 receptor blockers (e.g., famotidine [Pepcid], ranitidine [Zantac]) or proton pump inhibitors (omeprazole [Prilosec]).
- Age-related loss of muscle mass and thinning of the mucous membranes can cause structural changes in the larynx that may change characteristics of the voice. In general, the pitch of voice becomes higher in older adult men and lower in older adult women. The voice also "thins" (decreased projection) and may sound tremulous. These changes should be discriminated from signs that could indicate pathological conditions.

Adapted from American College of Otolaryngology. (2012). *Fact sheet: Sinusitis: Special considerations for aging patients.* Available at: www.entnet.org/HealthInformation/agingSinusitisPatients.cfm; and American College of Otolaryngology. (2012). *Fact sheet: The voice and aging.* Available at: www.entnet.org/HealthInformation/Voice-and-Aging.cfm

---

Rhinitis

Rhinitis is a group of disorders characterized by inflammation and irritation of the mucous membranes of the nose. These conditions can have a significant impact on quality of life and contribute to sinus, ear, and sleep problems and learning disorders. Rhinitis often coexists with other respiratory disorders, such as asthma (Wood, 2011). It affects between 10% and 30% of the population worldwide annually (Pawankar, Canonica, Holgate, et al., 2011). Viral rhinitis, especially the common cold, affects approximately one billion individuals yearly (Regan, 2008).

Rhinitis may be acute or chronic, nonallergic or allergic. Allergic rhinitis is further classified as seasonal or perennial rhinitis and is commonly associated with exposure to airborne particles such as dust, dander, or plant pollens in people who are allergic to these substances. Seasonal rhinitis occurs during pollen seasons, and perennial rhinitis occurs throughout the year. (See Chapter 38 for detailed descriptions of allergic disorders, including allergic rhinitis.)

Pathophysiology

Rhinitis may be caused by a variety of factors, including changes in temperature or humidity; odors; infection; age; systemic disease; use of over-the-counter (OTC) and prescribed nasal decongestants; and the presence of a foreign body. Allergic rhinitis may occur with exposure to allergens such as foods (e.g., peanuts, walnuts, brazil nuts, wheat, shellfish, soy, cow's milk, and eggs), medications (e.g., penicillin, sulfa medications, aspirin, and others with the potential to produce an allergic reaction), and particles in the indoor and outdoor environment (Chart 22-2). The most common cause of nonallergic rhinitis is the common cold (Regan, 2008). Drug-induced rhinitis may occur with antihypertensive agents, such as angiotensin-converting enzyme (ACE) inhibitors and beta-blockers; "statins," such as atorvastatin (Lipitor) and simvastatin (Zocor); antidepressants and antipsychotics such as risperidone (Risperdal); aspirin; and some antianxiety medications. Figure 22-1 shows the pathologic processes involved in rhinitis and rhinosinusitis. Other causes of rhinovirus are identified in Table 22-1.

Chart 22-2

Examples of Common Indoor and Outdoor Allergens

Common Indoor Allergens

- Dust mite feces
- Dog dander
- Cat dander
- Cockroach droppings
- Molds

Common Outdoor Allergens

- Trees (e.g., oak, elm, western red cedar, ash, birch, sycamore, maple, walnut, cypress)
- Weeds (e.g., ragweed, tumbleweed, sagebrush, pigweed, cockle weed, Russian thistle)
- Grasses (e.g., timothy, orchard, sweet vernal, bermuda, sour dock, redtop, bluegrass)
- Molds (*Alternaria, Cladosporium, Aspergillus*)

TABLE 22-1	Causes of Rhinosinusitis
Category	**Causes**
Vasomotor	Idiopathic
	Abuse of nasal decongestants (rhinitis medicamentosa)
	Psychological stimulation (anger, sexual arousal)
	Irritants (smoke, air pollution, exhaust fumes, cocaine)
Mechanical	Tumor
	Deviated septum
	Crusting
	Hypertrophied turbinates
	Foreign body
	Cerebrospinal fluid leak
Chronic inflammatory	Polyps (in cystic fibrosis)
	Sarcoidosis
	Wegener's granulomatosis
	Midline granuloma
Infectious	Acute viral infection
	Acute or chronic rhinosinusitis
	Rare nasal infections (syphilis, tuberculosis)
Hormonal	Pregnancy
	Use of oral contraceptives
	Hypothyroidism

Adapted from Settipane, R. A. (2011). Other causes of rhinitis: Mixed rhinitis, rhinitis medicamentosa, hormonal rhinitis, rhinitis of the elderly, and gustatory rhinitis. *Immunology Clinics of North America, 31*(3), 457–467.

Clinical Manifestations

The signs and symptoms of rhinitis include **rhinorrhea** (excessive nasal drainage, runny nose); nasal congestion; nasal discharge (purulent with bacterial rhinitis); sneezing; and pruritus of the nose, roof of the mouth, throat, eyes, and ears. Headache may occur, particularly if rhinosinusitis is also present. Nonallergic rhinitis can occur throughout the year.

Medical Management

The management of rhinitis depends on the cause, which may be identified through the history and physical examination. The nurse asks the patient about recent symptoms as well as possible exposure to allergens in the home, environment, or workplace. If viral rhinitis is the cause, medications may be prescribed to relieve the symptoms. In allergic rhinitis, allergy tests may be performed to identify possible allergens. Depending on the severity of the allergy, desensitizing immunizations and corticosteroids may be required (see Chapter 38 for more details). If symptoms suggest a bacterial infection, an antimicrobial agent is used (see later discussion of rhinosinusitis). Patients with nasal septal deformities or nasal polyps may be referred to an ear, nose, and throat specialist.

Pharmacologic Therapy

Medication therapy for allergic and nonallergic rhinitis focuses on symptom relief. Antihistamines and corticosteroid nasal sprays may be useful. Antihistamines remain the most common treatment and are administered for sneezing, pruritus, and rhinorrhea. (Examples of commonly prescribed antihistamines are discussed in more detail in Chapter 38.) Brompheniramine/pseudoephedrine (Dimetapp) is an example of combination antihistamine/decongestant medications. Cromolyn (NasalCrom), a mast cell stabilizer

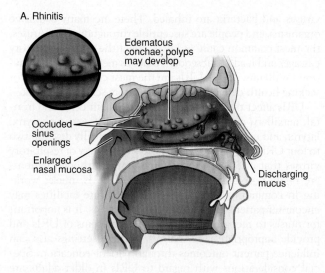

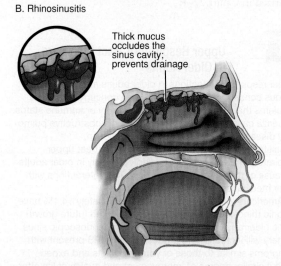

FIGURE 22-1 • Pathophysiologic processes in rhinitis and rhinosinusitis. Although pathophysiologic processes are similar in rhinitis and rhinosinusitis, they affect different structures. **A.** In rhinitis, the mucous membranes lining the nasal passages become inflamed, congested, and edematous. The swollen nasal conchae block the sinus openings, and mucus is discharged from the nostrils. **B.** Rhinosinusitis is also marked by inflammation and congestion, with thickened mucous secretions filling the sinus cavities and occluding the openings.

that inhibits the release of histamine and other chemicals, is also used in the treatment of rhinitis. Oral decongestant agents may be used for nasal obstruction. The use of saline nasal spray can act as a mild decongestant and can liquefy mucus to prevent crusting. Two inhalations of intranasal ipratropium (Atrovent) can be administered in each nostril two to three times per day for symptomatic relief of rhinorrhea. In addition, intranasal corticosteroids may be used for severe congestion, and ophthalmic agents (cromolyn ophthalmic solution 4%) may be used to relieve irritation, itching, and redness of the eyes. Newer allergy treatments include leukotriene modifiers (e.g., montelukast [Singulair], zafirlukast [Accolate], zileuton [Zyflo]), immunoglobulin E modifiers (omalizumab [Xolair]), and immunomodulatory medications, which are also components of asthma treatment guidelines (discussed further in Chapter 24). The choice of medications depends on the symptoms, adverse reactions, adherence factors, risk of drug interactions, and cost to the patient.

Nursing Management

Educating Patients About Self-Care

The nurse instructs the patient with allergic rhinitis to avoid or reduce exposure to allergens and irritants, such as dusts, molds, animals, fumes, odors, powders, sprays, and tobacco smoke. Patient education is essential when assisting the patient in the use of all medications. To prevent possible drug interactions, the patient is cautioned to read drug labels before taking any OTC medication.

The nurse instructs the patient about the importance of controlling the environment at home and at work. Saline nasal sprays or aerosols may be helpful in soothing mucous membranes, softening crusted secretions, and removing irritants. The nurse instructs the patient in correct administration of nasal medications. To achieve maximal relief, the patient is instructed to blow the nose before applying any medication into the nasal cavity. In addition, the patient is taught to keep the head upright; spray quickly and firmly into each nostril away from the nasal septum; and wait at least 1 minute before administering the second spray. The container should be cleaned after each use and should never be shared with other people to avoid cross-contamination.

In the case of infectious rhinitis, the nurse reviews hand hygiene technique with the patient as a measure to prevent transmission of organisms. This is especially important for those in contact with vulnerable populations such as the very young, older adults, or people who are immunosuppressed (e.g., patients with human immunodeficiency virus [HIV] infection, those taking immunosuppressive medications). In older adults and other high-risk populations, the nurse reviews the importance of receiving an influenza vaccination each year to achieve immunity before the beginning of the flu season.

Viral Rhinitis (Common Cold)

Viral rhinitis is the most frequent viral infection in the general population (Regan, 2008). The term *common cold* often is used when referring to a URI that is self-limited and caused by a virus. The term *cold* refers to an infectious, acute inflammation of the mucous membranes of the nasal cavity characterized by nasal congestion, rhinorrhea, sneezing, sore throat, and general malaise. More broadly, the term refers to an acute URI, whereas terms such as *rhinitis*, *pharyngitis*, and *laryngitis* distinguish the sites of the symptoms. The term is also used when the causative virus is influenza (the flu). Colds are highly contagious because virus is shed for about 2 days before the symptoms appear and during the first part of the symptomatic phase.

Colds caused by rhinoviruses tend to occur in the early fall and spring. Other viruses tend to cause winter colds (Centers for Disease Control and Prevention [CDC], 2011). Seasonal changes in relative humidity may affect the prevalence of colds. The most common cold-causing viruses survive better when humidity is low, in the colder months of the year.

Colds are believed to be caused by as many as 200 different viruses (National Institute of Allergy and Infectious Diseases, 2011). Rhinoviruses are the most likely causative organisms. Other viruses implicated in the common cold include coronavirus, adenovirus, respiratory syncytial virus, influenza virus, and parainfluenza virus. Each virus may have multiple strains; as a result, people are susceptible to colds throughout life (Tierney, McPhee, & Papadakis, 2012). Development of a vaccine against the multiple strains of virus is almost impossible. Immunity after recovery is variable and depends on many factors, including a person's natural host resistance and the specific virus that caused the cold. Despite popular belief, cold temperatures and exposure to cold rainy weather do not increase the incidence or severity of the common cold.

Clinical Manifestations

Signs and symptoms of viral rhinitis are low-grade fever, nasal congestion, rhinorrhea and nasal discharge, halitosis, sneezing, tearing watery eyes, "scratchy" or sore throat, general malaise, chills, and often headache and muscle aches. As the illness progresses, cough usually appears. In some people, the virus exacerbates **herpes simplex**, commonly called a *cold sore* (Chart 22-3).

The symptoms of viral rhinitis may last from 1 to 2 weeks. If severe systemic respiratory symptoms occur, it is no longer considered viral rhinitis but one of the other acute URIs. Allergic conditions can affect the nose, mimicking the symptoms of a cold.

Medical Management

Management consists of symptomatic therapy that includes adequate fluid intake, rest, prevention of chilling, and the use of expectorants as needed. Warm salt-water gargles soothe the sore throat, and nonsteroidal anti-inflammatory drugs (NSAIDs), such as aspirin or ibuprofen, relieve aches and pains. Antihistamines are used to relieve sneezing, rhinorrhea, and nasal congestion. Petroleum jelly can soothe irritated, chapped, and raw skin around the nares (National Institute of Allergy and Infectious Diseases, 2011).

Guaifenesin (Mucinex), an expectorant, is available without a prescription and is used to promote removal of secretions. Several antiviral medications are available by prescription, including amantadine (Symmetrel) and rimantadine (Flumadine). These medications can reduce the severity of symptoms and may reduce the duration of the common cold. Antimicrobial agents (antibiotics) should not be used, because they do not affect the virus or reduce the incidence of bacterial complications. In addition, their inappropriate use has been implicated in the development of organisms resistant to therapy.

Topical nasal decongestants (e.g., phenylephrine nasal [Neo-Synephrine], oxymetazoline nasal [Afrin]) should be used with caution. Topical therapy delivers medication directly to the nasal mucosa, and its overuse can produce **rhinitis medicamentosa**, or rebound rhinitis. Most patients treat the common cold with OTC medications that produce moderate clinical benefits, such as relief of symptoms.

In addition, alternative medicines (e.g., echinacea, zinc lozenges, zinc nasal spray) are frequently used to treat the common cold; however, evidence regarding their effectiveness in

Chart 22-3 Colds and Cold Sores (Herpes Simplex Virus)

Herpes labialis is an infection that is caused by herpes simplex virus type 1 (HSV-1). It is characterized by an eruption of small, painful blisters on the skin of the lips, mouth, gums, tongue, or the skin around the mouth. The blisters are commonly referred to as cold sores or fever blisters. Once the person is infected with this virus, it can lie latent in the cells for a period of time. The incubation period is about 2–12 days. Between 50% and 80% of Americans are infected by age 30 years, because HSV-1 is typically transmitted during childhood through non-sexual contact. Herpes labialis is extremely contagious and can be spread through contaminated razors, towels, and dishes. It is activated by overexposure to sunlight or wind, colds, influenza and similar infections, heavy alcohol use, and physical or emotional stress.

Although herpes simplex virus type 2 (HSV-2) typically causes painful vesicular and ulcerative lesions in the genital and anal areas, HSV-1 may also cause genital herpes. Oral–genital contact can spread oral herpes to the genitals (and vice versa). People with active herpetic lesions should avoid oral sex. It is extremely important for patients to understand that the virus can be transmitted by asymptomatic people. Estimates suggest that 80% of people infected are asymptomatic.

Early symptoms of herpes labialis include burning, itching, and increased sensitivity or tingling sensation. These symptoms may occur several days before the appearance of lesions. The lesions appear as macules or papules, progressing to small blisters (vesicles) filled with clear, yellowish fluid. They are raised, red, and painful and can break and ooze. The lesions typically extend through the epidermis and penetrate into the underlying dermis, consistent with a partial-thickness wound. Eventually, yellow crusts slough to reveal pink, healing skin. Typically, the virus is no longer detectable in the lesion or wound 5 days after the vesicle has developed.

Medications used in the management of herpes labialis include acyclovir (Zovirax) and valacyclovir (Valtrex), which help to minimize the symptoms and the duration or length of flare-up. Acetaminophen may be given for analgesia. Topical anesthetics such as lidocaine (Xylocaine) can help in the control of discomfort. Occlusive dressings have been shown to speed the healing process. Not only do such dressings prevent desiccation and scab formation, but they also maintain an aqueous wound environment rich in growth factors and matrix materials. However, occlusive dressings are not practical for lip and mucosal lesions. In this case, alternatives include occlusive ointments such as Herpecin-L or docosanol (Abreva).

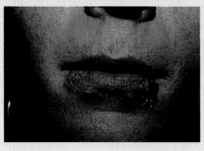

Adapted from Salvaggio, M. R. (2012). *Herpes simplex.* Available at: emedicine.medscape.com/article/218580-overview

shortening the symptomatic phase is limited (Barrett, Brown, Rakel, et al., 2011). The inhalation of steam or heated, humidified air has been a mainstay of home remedies for common cold sufferers; however, the value of this therapy has not been demonstrated.

Nursing Management

Educating Patients About Self-Care

Most viruses can be transmitted in several ways: direct contact with infected secretions, inhalation of large particles from others' coughing or sneezing, or inhalation of small particles (aerosol) that may be suspended in the air for up to an hour. Implementation of appropriate hand hygiene measures (e.g., handwashing or use of alcohol-based antibacterial cleaning agents) remains the most effective measure to prevent transmission of organisms. The nurse educates the patient about how to break the chain of infection with appropriate hand hygiene and the use of tissues to avoid the spread of the virus with coughing and sneezing, and to cough or sneeze into the upper arm if tissues are not readily available. The nurse instructs the patient about methods to treat symptoms of the common cold and provides both verbal and written information to assist in the prevention and management of URIs.

Rhinosinusitis

Rhinosinusitis, formerly called *sinusitis*, is an inflammation of the paranasal sinuses and nasal cavity. The clinical practice guideline for adult sinusitis released by the American Academy of Otolaryngology–Head and Neck Surgery Foundation (Rosenfeld, Andes, Bhattacharyya, et al., 2007) recommends the use of the term *rhinosinusitis* because sinusitis is almost always accompanied by inflammation of the nasal mucosa. Rhinosinusitis affects 1 in 7 Americans. About 31 million people in the United States are diagnosed with this condition each year, resulting in direct annual health care costs of $5.8 billion in ambulatory and emergency services alone (Rosenfeld et al., 2007).

Uncomplicated rhinosinusitis occurs without extension of inflammation outside of the paranasal sinuses and nasal cavity. Rhinosinusitis is classified by duration of symptoms as acute (less than 4 weeks), subacute (4 to 12 weeks), and chronic (more than 12 weeks). Rhinosinusitis can be caused by a bacterial or viral infection.

■ *Acute Rhinosinusitis*

Acute rhinosinusitis is classified as acute bacterial rhinosinusitis (ABRS) or acute viral rhinosinusitis (AVRS). Recurrent acute rhinosinusitis is characterized by four or more acute episodes of ABRS per year (Rosenfeld et al., 2007) and is discussed with chronic rhinosinusitis (CRS).

Pathophysiology

Acute rhinosinusitis usually follows a viral URI or cold, such as an unresolved viral or bacterial infection, or an exacerbation of allergic rhinitis. Normally, the sinus openings into the nasal passages are clear and infections resolve promptly. However, if their drainage is obstructed by a deviated septum or by hypertrophied turbinates, spurs, or nasal polyps or tumors, sinus infection may persist as a smoldering (persistent) secondary infection or progress to an acute suppurative process (causing purulent discharge).

Nasal congestion, caused by inflammation, edema, and transudation of fluid secondary to URI, leads to obstruction of the sinus cavities (see Fig. 22-1). This provides an excellent medium for bacterial growth. Other conditions that can block the normal flow of sinus secretions include abnormal structures of the nose, enlarged adenoids, diving and swimming, tooth infection, trauma to the nose, tumors, and the pressure of foreign objects. Some people are more prone to rhinosinusitis because exposure to environmental hazards such as paint, sawdust, and chemicals may result in chronic inflammation of the nasal passages.

Bacterial organisms account for more than 60% of the cases of acute rhinosinusitis. Typical pathogens include *Streptococcus pneumoniae*, *Haemophilus influenzae*, and less commonly *Staphylococcus aureus*, and *Moraxella catarrhalis* (Brook & Hausfield, 2011; Chow, Benninger, Brook, et al., 2012; Tierney et al., 2012). Biofilms, which consist of organized, heterogenous communities of bacteria, have been found to be 10 to 1,000 times more resistant to antibiotic treatment and more likely to contribute to host resistance when compared with other bacteria. They serve as bacterial reservoirs that can cause systemic illness when released into the circulation. Although antibiotics kill bacteria in the biofilm margin, cells deep in the biofilm are not affected, allowing for regrowth once antibiotic therapy has been discontinued. Pathogens in the upper respiratory tract that form biofilms include those species listed earlier as well as *Pseudomonas aeruginosa*.

Other organisms that are occasionally isolated include *Chlamydia pneumoniae*, *Streptococcus pyogenes*, viruses, and fungi (*Aspergillus fumigatus*). Fungal infections occur most often in immunosuppressed patients.

Clinical Manifestations

Symptoms of ABRS include purulent nasal drainage (anterior, posterior, or both) accompanied by nasal obstruction or a combination of facial pain, pressure, or a sense of fullness (referred to collectively as facial pain–pressure–fullness), or both (Rosenfeld et al., 2007). The facial pain–pressure–fullness may involve the anterior face or the periorbital region. The patient may also report cloudy or colored nasal discharge congestion, blockage, or stuffiness as well as a localized or diffuse headache. Patients with ABRS may present with a high fever (i.e., 39°C [102°F] or higher). In addition, the occurrence of symptoms for 10 days or more after the initial onset of upper respiratory symptoms indicates ABRS (Chow et al., 2012).

The symptoms of AVRS are similar to those of ABRS, except the patient does not present with a high fever, nor with the same intensity of symptoms (e.g., there tends to be an absence of facial pain–pressure–fullness), nor with symptoms that persist for as long a period of time. Symptoms of AVRS occur for fewer than 10 days after the onset of upper respiratory symptoms and do not worsen (Chow et al., 2012).

Assessment and Diagnostic Findings

A careful history and physical examination are performed. The head and neck, particularly the nose, ears, teeth, sinuses, pharynx, and chest, are examined. There may be tenderness to palpation over the infected sinus area. The sinuses are percussed using the index finger, tapping lightly to determine whether the patient experiences pain. Although less frequently performed, transillumination of the affected area may

reveal a decrease in the transmission of light with rhinosinusitis (see Chapter 20). Diagnostic imaging (x-ray, computed tomography [CT], magnetic resonance imaging [MRI]) is not recommended and generally not needed for the diagnosis of acute rhinosinusitis if the patient meets clinical diagnostic criteria (Rosenfeld et al., 2007). When a complication or alternative diagnosis is suspected, CT scans may be indicated because these scans are sensitive to inflammatory changes and bone destruction and identify anatomic variations that can guide sinus surgery if indicated.

To confirm the diagnosis of maxillary and frontal rhinosinusitis and identify the pathogen, sinus aspirates may be obtained. Flexible endoscopic culture techniques and swabbing of the sinuses have been used for this purpose (Chow et al., 2012).

Complications

If untreated, acute rhinosinusitis may lead to severe complications. Local complications include osteomyelitis and mucocele (cyst of the paranasal sinuses). Osteomyelitis requires prolonged antibiotic therapy and at times removal of necrotic bone. Intracranial complications, although rare, include cavernous sinus thrombosis, meningitis, brain abscess, ischemic brain infarction, and severe orbital cellulitis (Tierney et al., 2012). Mucoceles may require surgical treatment to establish intranasal drainage or complete excision with ablation of the sinus cavity. Brain abscesses occur by direct spread and can be life threatening. Frontal epidural abscesses are usually quiescent but can be detected by CT scan.

Medical Management

Treatment of acute rhinosinusitis depends on the cause; a 5- to 7-day course of antibiotics is prescribed for bacterial cases (Chow et al., 2012). The goals of treatment for acute rhinosinusitis are to shrink the nasal mucosa, relieve pain, and treat infection. Because of inappropriate use of antibiotics for nonbacterial illness, including AVRS, and the resulting resistance that has occurred, oral antibiotics are only prescribed when there is sufficient empiric evidence that the patient has ABRS (e.g., high fever or symptoms that persist for at least 10 days or worsening symptoms following a viral respiratory illness).

Antibiotics should be administered as soon as the diagnosis of ABRS is established. Amoxicillin–clavulanic acid (Augmentin) is the antibiotic of choice. For patients who are allergic to penicillin, doxycycline (Vibramycin) or respiratory quinolones such as levofloxacin (Levaquin) or moxifloxacin (Avelox) can be used. Other antibiotics prescribed previously to treat ABRS, including cephalosporins such as cephalexin (Keflex), cefuroxime (Ceftin), cefaclor (Ceclor), and cefixime (Suprax), trimethoprim–sulfamethoxazole (Bactrim, Septra), and macrolides such as clarithromycin (Biaxin) and azithromycin (Zithromax), are no longer recommended because they are not effective in treating antibiotic-resistant organisms that are now more commonly implicated in ABRS (Chow et al., 2012). Intranasal saline lavage is an effective adjunct therapy to antibiotics in that it may relieve symptoms, reduce inflammation, and help clear the passages of stagnant mucus. Neither decongestants nor antihistamines are recommended adjunctive medications for treating ABRS (Chow et al., 2012).

TABLE 22-2 Nasal Corticosteroids and Common Side Effects

Nasal Corticosteroids	Side Effects	Contraindications (for all nasal corticosteroids)
Beclomethasone (Beconase)	Nasal irritation, headache, nausea, lightheadedness, epistaxis, rhinorrhea, watering eyes, sneezing, dry nose and throat	Avoid in patients with recurrent epistaxis, glaucoma, and cataracts. Patients who have been exposed to measles/varicella or who have adrenal insufficiency should avoid these medications.
Budesonide (Rhinocort)	Epistaxis, pharyngitis, cough, nasal irritation, bronchospasm	
Mometasone (Nasonex)	Headache, viral infection, pharyngitis, epistaxis, cough, dysmenorrhea, musculoskeletal pain, arthralgia	
Triamcinolone (Nasacort AQ)	Pharyngitis, epistaxis, cough, headache	

Treatment of AVRS typically involves nasal saline lavage and decongestants (guaifenesin/pseudoephedrine [Entex PSE]). Decongestants or nasal saline sprays can increase patency of the ostiomeatal unit and improve drainage of the sinuses. Topical decongestants should not be used for longer than 3 or 4 days. Oral decongestants must be used cautiously in patients with hypertension. OTC antihistamines, such as diphenhydramine (Benadryl) and cetirizine (Zyrtec), and prescription antihistamines, such as fexofenadine (Allegra), are used if an allergic component is suspected.

Intranasal corticosteroids have been shown to produce complete or marked improvement in acute symptoms of either bacterial or viral rhinosinusitis; however, they are only recommended for use in patients with a previous history of allergic rhinitis (Chow et al., 2012; Rosenfeld et al., 2007). Examples of intranasal corticosteroids, side effects, and contraindications are presented in Table 22-2.

Nursing Management

Educating Patients About Self-Care

Patient education is an important aspect of nursing care for the patient with acute rhinosinusitis. The nurse instructs the patient about symptoms of complications that require immediate follow-up. Referral to the primary provider is indicated if periorbital edema and severe pain on palpation occur. The nurse instructs the patient about methods to promote drainage of the sinuses, including humidification of the air in the home and the use of warm compresses to relieve pressure. The patient is advised to avoid swimming, diving, and air travel during the acute infection. Patients using tobacco are instructed to immediately stop smoking or using any form of tobacco. Most patients use nasal sprays incorrectly, which can lead to several side effects that include nasal irritation, nasal burning, bad taste, and drainage in the throat or even epistaxis. Therefore, if an intranasal corticosteroid is prescribed, it is important to instruct the patient about the correct use of prescribed nasal sprays through demonstration, explanation, and return demonstration to evaluate the patient's understanding of the correct method of administration. The nurse also educates the patient about the side effects of prescribed and OTC nasal sprays and about rebound congestion (rhinitis medicamentosa). Once the decongestant is discontinued, the nasal passages close and congestion results. Appropriate medications to use for pain relief include acetaminophen (Tylenol) and NSAIDs such as ibuprofen (Advil), naproxen sodium (Aleve), and aspirin for adults older than 20 years.

The nurse tells patients with recurrent rhinosinusitis to begin decongestants, such as pseudoephedrine (Sudafed), at the first sign of rhinosinusitis. This promotes drainage and decreases the risk of bacterial infection. Patients should also check with their primary provider or pharmacist before using OTC medications because many cold medications can worsen symptoms or other health problems, specifically hypertension.

The nurse stresses the importance of following the recommended antibiotic regimen because a consistent blood level of the medication is critical to treat the infection. The nurse educates the patient about the early signs of a sinus infection and recommends preventive measures such as following healthy practices and avoiding contact with people with URIs.

The nurse explains to the patient that fever, severe headache, and **nuchal rigidity** (stiffness of the neck or inability to bend the neck) are signs of potential complications. Patients with chronic symptoms of rhinosinusitis who do not have marked improvement in 4 weeks with continuous medical treatment may be candidates for functional endoscopic sinus surgery (FESS, see later discussion) (Regan, 2008).

> **⚑ Quality and Safety Nursing Alert**
>
> Patients with nasotracheal and nasogastric tubes in place are at risk for development of sinus infections. Thus, accurate assessment of patients with these tubes is critical. Removal of the nasotracheal or nasogastric tube as soon as the patient's condition permits allows the sinuses to drain, possibly avoiding septic complications.

▪ Chronic Rhinosinusitis and Recurrent Acute Rhinosinusitis

CRS affects 14% to 16% of the U.S. population and occurs most commonly in young and middle-aged adults (Upton, Welham, Kuo, et al., 2011). It is diagnosed when the patient has experienced 12 weeks or longer of two or more of the following symptoms: mucopurulent drainage, nasal obstruction, facial pain–pressure–fullness, or hyposmia (decreased sense of smell). In about 29% to 36% of patients, CRS is accompanied by nasal polyps (Rosenfeld et al., 2007). Recurrent acute rhinosinusitis is diagnosed when four or more episodes of ABRS occur per year with no signs or symptoms of rhinosinusitis between the episodes. The use of antibiotics in people with recurrent acute rhinosinusitis is even higher than in CRS. Both CRS and recurrent acute rhinosinusitis affect quality of life as well as physical and social function (Rosenfeld et al., 2007).

Pathophysiology

Mechanical obstruction in the ostia of the frontal, maxillary, and anterior ethmoid sinuses (known collectively as the ostiomeatal complex) is the usual cause of CRS and recurrent acute rhinosinusitis. Obstruction prevents adequate drainage of the nasal passages, resulting in accumulation of secretions and an ideal medium for bacterial growth. Persistent blockage in an adult may occur because of infection, allergy, or structural abnormalities. Other associated conditions and factors may include cystic fibrosis, ciliary dyskinesia, neoplastic disorders, gastroesophageal reflux disease, tobacco use, and environmental pollution (Rosenfeld et al., 2007).

Both aerobic and anaerobic bacteria have been implicated in CRS and recurrent rhinosinusitis. Common aerobic bacteria include alpha-hemolytic streptococci, microaerophilic streptococci, and *S. aureus*. Common anaerobic bacteria include gram-negative bacilli, *Peptostreptococcus*, and *Fusobacterium*.

In addition, immunodeficiency should be considered in patients with CRS or acute recurrent rhinosinusitis. Acute fulminant/invasive rhinosinusitis is a life-threatening illness and is commonly attributed to *Aspergillus* in immunocompromised patients. Chronic fungal sinusitis also poses a risk. Chronic invasive fungal sinusitis occurs in immunocompromised patients along with fungus ball/mycetoma and allergic fungal sinusitis—the more common forms of chronic fungal sinusitis—which are considered noninvasive conditions in immunocompromised patients. The fungus ball is characterized by the presence of a noninvasive accumulation of a dense conglomeration of fungal hyphae in one sinus cavity, usually the maxillary sinus. The fungus generally remains contained in the fungus ball, which consists of mucopurulent cheesy or claylike materials within the sinus, but can become invasive when immunosuppression occurs, leading to encephalopathy (Chadrabarti, Denning, Ferguson, et al., 2009). Symptoms include nasal stuffiness, nasal discharge, and facial pain. Vision loss, headache, and cranial nerve palsies have been identified in patients with a sphenoid sinus fungal ball (Hu, Wang, & Yu, 2009).

Clinical Manifestations

Clinical manifestations of CRS include impaired mucociliary clearance and ventilation, cough (because the thick discharge constantly drips backward into the nasopharynx), chronic hoarseness, chronic headaches in the periorbital area, periorbital edema, and facial pain. As a result of chronic nasal congestion, the patient is usually required to breathe through the mouth. Snoring, sore throat, and, in some situations, adenoidal hypertrophy may also occur. Symptoms are generally most pronounced on awakening in the morning. Fatigue and nasal congestion are also common. Many patients experience a decrease in smell and taste and a sense of fullness in the ears.

Assessment and Diagnostic Findings

The health assessment focuses on onset and duration of symptoms. It addresses the quantity and quality of nasal discharge and cough, the presence of pain, factors that relieve or aggravate the pain, and allergies. It is essential to obtain any history of comorbid conditions, including asthma, and history of tobacco use. A history of fever, fatigue, previous episodes and treatments, and previous response to therapies is also obtained.

In the physical assessment, the external nose is evaluated for any evidence of anatomic abnormality. A crooked-appearing external nose may imply septal deviation internally. The nasal mucous membranes are assessed for erythema, pallor, atrophy, edema, crusting, discharge, polyps, erosions, and septal perforations or deviations. Appropriate lighting improves visualization of the nasal cavity and should be used in every examination. Pain on examination of the teeth, with tapping with a tongue blade, suggests tooth infection (Bickley & Szilagyi, 2009).

Assessment of the posterior oropharynx may reveal purulent or mucoid discharge, which is indicative of an infection caused by CRS. The patient's eyes are examined for conjunctival erythema, tearing, photophobia, and edema of the lids. Additional assessment techniques include transillumination of the sinuses and palpation of the sinuses. The frontal and maxillary sinuses are palpated, and the patient is asked whether this produces tenderness. The pharynx is inspected for erythema and discharge and palpated for cervical node adenopathy (Rosenfeld et al., 2007).

Imaging studies such as x-ray, sinoscopy, ultrasound, CT scanning, and MRI may be used in the diagnosis of CRS. X-ray is an inexpensive and readily available tool to assess disorders of the paranasal sinuses. A CT scan of the paranasal sinuses can identify mucosal abnormalities, sinus ostial obstruction, anatomic variants, sinonasal polyposis, and neoplastic disease. In addition, nasal endoscopy allows for visualization of the posterior nasal cavity, nasopharynx, and sinus drainage pathways and can identify posterior septal deviation and polyps. Osseous destruction, extrasinus extension of the disease process, and local invasion suggest malignancy (Rosenfeld et al., 2007). (See Chapter 21 for further discussion of CT, MRI, and x-ray.)

Complications

Complications of CRS, although uncommon, include severe orbital cellulitis, subperiosteal abscess, cavernous sinus thrombosis, meningitis, encephalitis, and ischemic infarction. CRS can lead to intracranial infection either by direct spread through bone or via venous channels, resulting in epidural abscess, subdural empyema, meningitis, and brain abscess. Clinical sequelae can include personality changes with frontal lobe abscesses, headache, symptoms of elevated intracranial pressure to include alterations of consciousness, visual changes, focal neurologic deficits, seizures, and, ultimately, coma and death.

Frontal rhinosinusitis can lead to osteomyelitis of the frontal bones. Patients typically present with headache, fever, and a characteristic doughy edema over the involved bone. Ethmoid rhinosinusitis may result in orbital cellulitis, which usually begins with edema of the eyelids and rapidly progresses to ptosis (droopy eyelid), proptosis (bulging eye), chemosis (edema of the bulbar conjunctiva), and diminished extraocular movements. Patients are usually febrile and acutely ill and require immediate attention, because pressure on the optic nerve can lead to loss of vision and spread of infection can lead to intracranial infection. Cavernous sinus thrombophlebitis can result from extension of infection along venous channels from the orbit, ethmoid or frontal sinuses, or nose. Symptoms may include altered consciousness, lid edema, and proptosis, as well as third, fourth, and sixth cranial nerve palsies.

Medical Management

Medical management of CRS and recurrent acute rhinosinusitis is similar to that of acute rhinosinusitis. Early identification of risk factors guides the selection of treatment and leads to early intervention and ultimately better patient outcomes. General measures include encouraging adequate hydration and recommending the use of OTC nasal saline sprays, analgesics such as acetaminophen or NSAIDs, and decongestants such as oxymetazoline and pseudoephedrine (Aring & Chan, 2011; Brook, 2012). Patients are instructed to sleep with the head of the bed elevated and to avoid exposure to cigarette smoke and fumes. Patients are cautioned to avoid caffeine and alcohol, which can cause dehydration.

Prescribed medications may be necessary. First-line antibiotics include amoxicillin-clavulanic acid, erythromycin–sulfisoxazole (Eryzole), and second-generation antibiotics such as cefuroxime or cefixime (Brook, 2012). The course of antibiotic treatment for CRS and recurrent ABRS is typically as long as 2 to 4 weeks to effectively eradicate the offending organism, and may be indicated for up to 12 months in some cases (Brook, 2012). Corticosteroid nasal sprays such as fluticasone (Flonase) or beclomethasone (Beconase AQ) may be indicated in patients with concomitant allergic rhinitis or nasal polyps. Patients with allergic rhinitis may also benefit from the addition of a mast cell stabilizer such as cromolyn. For patients with concomitant asthma, leukotriene inhibitors such as montelukast and zafirlukast may be used (Brook, 2012).

Surgical Management

If standard medical therapy fails and symptoms persist, FESS may be indicated to correct structural deformities that obstruct the ostia (openings) of the sinuses. FESS is a minimally invasive surgical procedure that is associated with reduced postoperative discomfort and improvement in the patient's quality of life. In particular, FESS is associated with either complete or moderate relief of symptoms in more than 80% of patients (Brook, 2012). Some of the specific procedures performed include excising and cauterizing nasal polyps, correcting a deviated septum, incising and draining the sinuses, aerating the sinuses, and removing tumors. Antimicrobial agents may be administered before and after surgery. Computer-assisted or computer-guided surgery is used to increase the precision of the surgical procedure and to minimize complications (Patel, 2012).

Surgical intervention may be required in acute invasive fungal rhinosinusitis to excise the fungus ball and necrotic tissue and drain the sinuses. Patients require aggressive surgical débridement and drainage as well as systemic antifungal medications.

Nursing Management

Patients usually perform care measures for rhinosinusitis at home; therefore, nursing management consists mainly of patient education.

Educating Patients About Self-Care

Many people with sinus infections tend to blow their nose frequently and with force to clear their nasal passages. Doing so often increases the symptoms; therefore, the patient is instructed to blow the nose gently and to use tissue to remove the nasal drainage. Increasing fluid intake, applying local heat (hot wet packs), and elevating the head of the bed promote drainage of the sinuses. The nurse also instructs the patient about the importance of following the prescribed medication regimen. Instructions on the early signs of a sinus infection are provided, and preventive measures are reviewed. The nurse instructs the patient about signs and symptoms that require follow-up and provides these instructions verbally and in writing. Instructions in alternate formats (e.g., large font, patient's language) may be needed to increase the patient's understanding and adherence to the treatment plan. The nurse encourages the patient to follow up with his or her primary provider if symptoms persist.

> **▶ Quality and Safety Nursing Alert**
>
> URIs, specifically CRS and recurrent acute rhinosinusitis, may be linked to primary or secondary immune deficiency or treatment with immunosuppressive therapy (i.e., for cancer or organ transplantation). Typical symptoms may be blunted or absent due to immunosuppression. Immunocompromised patients are at increased risk for acute or chronic fungal infections; these infections can progress rapidly and become life threatening. Thus, assessment, early reporting of symptoms to the patient's primary provider, and immediate initiation of treatment are essential.

Pharyngitis

■ Acute Pharyngitis

Acute **pharyngitis** is a sudden painful inflammation of the pharynx, the back portion of the throat that includes the posterior third of the tongue, soft palate, and tonsils. It is commonly referred to as a sore throat. In the United States, it is estimated that approximately 11 million people experience pharyngitis each year (Choby, 2009). Because of environmental exposure to viral agents and poorly ventilated rooms, the incidence of viral pharyngitis peaks during winter and early spring in regions that have warm summers and cold winters. Viral pharyngitis spreads easily in the droplets of coughs and sneezes, as well as from unclean hands that have been exposed to the contaminated fluids.

Pathophysiology

Viral infection causes most cases of acute pharyngitis. Responsible viruses include the adenovirus, influenza virus, Epstein-Barr virus, and herpes simplex virus. Bacterial infection accounts for the remainder of cases. Ten percent of adults with pharyngitis have group A beta-hemolytic streptococcus (GABHS), which is commonly referred to as group A streptococcus (GAS) or streptococcal pharyngitis. Streptococcal

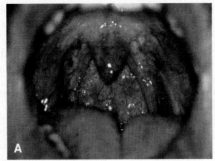 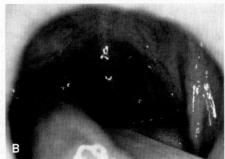

FIGURE 22-2 • Pharyngitis—inflammation without exudate. **A.** Redness and vascularity of the pillars and uvula are mild to moderate. **B.** Redness is diffuse and intense. Each patient would probably complain of a sore throat. From the Wellcome Trust, National Medical Slide Bank, London, UK.

pharyngitis warrants the use of antibiotic treatment. When GAS causes acute pharyngitis, the condition is known as strep throat. The body responds by triggering an inflammatory response in the pharynx. This results in pain, fever, vasodilation, edema, and tissue damage, manifested by redness and swelling in the tonsillar pillars, uvula, and soft palate. A creamy exudate may be present in the tonsillar pillars (Fig. 22-2). Other bacterial organisms implicated in acute pharyngitis include groups B and G streptococci, *Neisseria gonorrhoeae, Mycoplasma pneumoniae, C. pneumoniae, Arcanobacterium haemolyticum,* and HIV (Gerber, Baltimore, Eaton, et al., 2009).

Uncomplicated viral infections usually subside promptly, within 3 to 10 days after onset. However, pharyngitis caused by more virulent bacteria, such as GAS, is a more severe illness. If left untreated, the complications can be severe and life threatening. Complications include rhinosinusitis, otitis media, peritonsillar abscess, mastoiditis, and cervical adenitis. In rare cases, the infection may lead to bacteremia, pneumonia, meningitis, rheumatic fever, and nephritis.

Clinical Manifestations

The signs and symptoms of acute pharyngitis include a fiery-red pharyngeal membrane and tonsils, lymphoid follicles that are swollen and flecked with white-purple exudate, enlarged and tender cervical lymph nodes, and no cough. Fever (higher than 38.3°C [101°F]), malaise, and sore throat also may be present. Occasionally, patients with GAS pharyngitis exhibit vomiting, anorexia, and a scarlatina-form rash with urticaria known as scarlet fever.

People who have streptococcal pharyngitis suddenly develop a painful sore throat 1 to 5 days after being exposed to the streptococcus bacteria. They usually report malaise, fever (with or without chills), headache, myalgia, painful cervical adenopathy, and nausea. The tonsils appear swollen and erythematous, and they may or may not have an exudate. The roof of the mouth is often erythematous and may demonstrate petechiae. Bad breath is common.

Assessment and Diagnostic Findings

Accurate diagnosis of pharyngitis is essential to determine the cause (viral or bacterial) and to initiate treatment early. Rapid antigen detection testing (RADT) uses swabs that collect specimens from the posterior pharynx and tonsil. RADT is reported to be 90% to 95% sensitive, thus facilitating earlier treatment and earlier symptom improvement and reductions in pathogen transmission. Negative results

should be confirmed by a throat culture (Choby, 2009). In most communities, preliminary culture reports are available in 24 hours. Once a definitive diagnosis of GAS is made, administration of appropriate antibiotics hastens symptom resolution and reduces the transmission of the illness.

Medical Management

Viral pharyngitis is treated with supportive measures because antibiotics have no effect on the causal organism. Bacterial pharyngitis is treated with a variety of antimicrobial agents.

Pharmacologic Therapy

If the cause of pharyngitis is bacterial, penicillin is usually the treatment of choice. Penicillin V potassium given for 5 days is the regimen of choice. Traditionally, penicillin was administered as a single injection; however, oral forms are used more often and are as effective and less painful than injections. Penicillin injections are recommended only if there is a concern that the patient will not comply with therapy (Tierney et al., 2012).

For patients who are allergic to penicillin or have organisms that are resistant to erythromycin (one fifth of GAS and most *S. aureus* organisms are resistant to penicillin and erythromycin), cephalosporins and macrolides (clarithromycin and azithromycin) may be used. Once-daily azithromycin may be given for only 3 days due to its long half-life (Tierney et al., 2012). A 5- or 10-day course of cephalosporin may be prescribed. Five-day administration of cefpodoxime and cefuroxime has also been successful in producing bacteriologic cures.

Severe sore throats can also be relieved by analgesic medications, as prescribed. For example, aspirin or acetaminophen can be taken at 4- to 6-hour intervals; if required, acetaminophen with codeine can be taken three or four times daily. In severe cases, gargles with benzocaine may relieve symptoms.

Nutritional Therapy

A liquid or soft diet is provided during the acute stage of the disease, depending on the patient's appetite and the degree of discomfort that occurs with swallowing. Cool beverages, warm liquids, and flavored frozen desserts such as ice pops are often soothing. Occasionally, the throat is so sore that liquids cannot be taken in adequate amounts by mouth. In severe situations, intravenous (IV) fluids may be needed. Otherwise, the patient is encouraged to drink as much fluid as possible (at least 2 to 3 L/day).

Nursing Management

Nursing care for patients with viral pharyngitis focuses on symptomatic management. For patients who demonstrate signs of strep throat and have a history of rheumatic fever, who have scarlet fever, or who have symptoms suggesting peritonsillar abscess, nursing care focuses on prompt initiation and correct administration of prescribed antibiotic therapy. The nurse instructs the patient about signs and symptoms that warrant prompt contact with the primary provider. These include dyspnea, drooling, inability to swallow, and inability to fully open the mouth.

The nurse instructs the patient to stay in bed during the febrile stage of illness and to rest frequently once up and about. Used tissues should be disposed of properly to prevent the spread of infection. The nurse (or the patient or family member, if the patient is not hospitalized) should examine the skin once or twice daily for possible rash, because acute pharyngitis may precede some other communicable diseases (e.g., rubella).

Depending on the severity of the pharyngitis and the degree of pain, warm saline gargles or throat irrigations are used. The benefits of this treatment depend on the degree of heat that is applied. The nurse educates the patient about these procedures and about the recommended temperature of the solution, which should be high enough to be effective and as warm as the patient can tolerate, usually 40.6°C to 43.3°C (105°F to 110°F). Irrigating the throat may reduce spasm in the pharyngeal muscles and relieve soreness of the throat.

An ice collar also can relieve severe sore throats. Mouth care may promote the patient's comfort and prevent the development of fissures (cracking) of the lips and oral inflammation when bacterial infection is present. The nurse instructs the patient to resume activity gradually and to delay returning to work or school until after 24 hours of antibiotic therapy. A full course of antibiotic therapy is indicated in patients with strep infection because of the potential complications such as nephritis and rheumatic fever, which may have their onset 2 or 3 weeks after the pharyngitis has subsided. The nurse instructs the patient and family about the importance of taking the full course of therapy and informs them about the symptoms to watch for that may indicate complications.

In addition, the nurse instructs the patient about preventive measures that include not sharing eating utensils, glasses, napkins, food, or towels; cleaning telephones after use; using a tissue to cough or sneeze; disposing of used tissues appropriately; and avoiding exposure to tobacco and secondhand smoke. The nurse also instructs the patient with pharyngitis, especially streptococcal pharyngitis, to replace his or her toothbrush with a new one.

▌ *Chronic Pharyngitis*

Chronic pharyngitis is a persistent inflammation of the pharynx. It is common in adults who work in dusty surroundings, use their voice to excess, suffer from chronic cough, or habitually use alcohol and tobacco.

There are three types of chronic pharyngitis:
- Hypertrophic—characterized by general thickening and congestion of the pharyngeal mucous membrane

- Atrophic—probably a late stage of the first type (the membrane is thin, whitish, glistening, and at times wrinkled)
- Chronic granular—characterized by numerous swollen lymph follicles on the pharyngeal wall

Clinical Manifestations

Patients with chronic pharyngitis complain of a constant sense of irritation or fullness in the throat, mucus that collects in the throat and can be expelled by coughing, and difficulty swallowing. This is often associated with intermittent postnasal drip that causes minor irritation and inflammation of the pharynx. A sore throat that is worse with swallowing in the absence of pharyngitis suggests the possibility of thyroiditis, and patients with this symptom are referred for evaluation for possible thyroiditis.

Medical Management

Treatment of chronic pharyngitis is based on relieving symptoms; avoiding exposure to irritants; and correcting any upper respiratory, pulmonary, gastrointestinal, or cardiac condition that might be responsible for a chronic cough.

Nasal congestion may be relieved by short-term use of nasal sprays or medications containing ephedrine sulfate (Kondon's Nasal) or phenylephrine. For a patient with a history of allergy, one of the antihistamine decongestant medications, such as pseudoephedrine or brompheniramine/pseudoephedrine, is prescribed orally every 4 to 6 hours. Aspirin (for patients older than 20 years) or acetaminophen is recommended for its analgesic properties.

For adults with chronic pharyngitis, tonsillectomy may be an effective option. For further information, see the Tonsillitis and Adenoiditis section.

Nursing Management

Educating Patients About Self-Care

The nurse recommends avoidance of alcohol, tobacco, secondhand smoke, and exposure to cold or to environmental or occupational pollutants. The patient may minimize exposure to pollutants by wearing a disposable facemask. The nurse encourages the patient to drink plenty of fluids. Gargling with warm saline solution may relieve throat discomfort. Lozenges keep the throat moistened.

Tonsillitis and Adenoiditis

The tonsils are composed of lymphatic tissue and are situated on each side of the oropharynx. The faucial or palatine tonsils and lingual tonsils are located behind the pillars of fauces and tongue, respectively. They frequently serve as the site of acute infection (**tonsillitis**). Acute tonsillitis can be confused with pharyngitis. Chronic tonsillitis is less common and may be mistaken for other disorders such as allergy, asthma, and rhinosinusitis.

The adenoids or pharyngeal tonsils consist of lymphatic tissue near the center of the posterior wall of the nasopharynx. Infection of the adenoids frequently accompanies acute tonsillitis. Frequently occurring bacterial pathogens include GABHS, the most common organism. The most common viral pathogen is Epstein-Barr virus, although cytomegalovirus may also cause tonsillitis and adenoiditis. Often thought of as a childhood disorder, tonsillitis can occur in adults.

Clinical Manifestations

The symptoms of tonsillitis include sore throat, fever, snoring, and difficulty swallowing. Enlarged adenoids may cause mouth breathing, earache, draining ears, frequent head colds, bronchitis, foul-smelling breath, voice impairment, and noisy respiration. Unusually enlarged adenoids fill the space behind the posterior nares, making it difficult for the air to travel from the nose to the throat and resulting in nasal obstruction. Infection can extend to the middle ears by way of the auditory (eustachian) tubes and may result in acute otitis media, which can lead to spontaneous rupture of the tympanic membranes (eardrums) and further extension of the infection into the mastoid cells, causing acute mastoiditis. The infection also may reside in the middle ear as a chronic, low-grade, smoldering process that eventually may cause permanent deafness.

Assessment and Diagnostic Findings

The diagnosis of acute tonsillitis is primarily clinical, with attention given to whether the illness is viral or bacterial in nature. As in acute pharyngitis, RADT is quick and convenient; however, it is less sensitive than the throat swab culture.

A thorough physical examination is performed and a careful history is obtained to rule out related or systemic conditions. The tonsillar site is cultured to determine the presence of bacterial infection. When cytomegalovirus infection is present, the differential diagnosis should include HIV, hepatitis A, and rubella. In adenoiditis, if recurrent episodes of suppurative otitis media result in hearing loss, comprehensive audiometric assessment is warranted (see Chapter 64).

Medical Management

Tonsillitis is treated with supportive measures that include increased fluid intake, analgesics, salt-water gargles, and rest. Bacterial infections are treated with penicillin (first-line therapy) or cephalosporins. Viral tonsillitis is not effectively treated with antibiotic therapy.

Tonsillectomy and adenoidectomy continue to be commonly performed surgical procedures, with evolving surgical techniques aimed at reducing complications and improving postoperative recovery. Patients who experience no adverse events for 6 hours have a low overall risk of later bleeding and other complications (Tierney et al., 2012). Adults who have undergone a tonsillectomy to treat recurrent streptococcal infections experience a decrease in the number of episodes of streptococcal or other throat infections or days with throat pain.

Tonsillectomy or adenoidectomy is indicated if the patient has had repeated episodes of tonsillitis despite antibiotic therapy; hypertrophy of the tonsils and adenoids that could cause obstruction and obstructive sleep apnea (OSA); repeated attacks of purulent otitis media; and suspected hearing loss due to serous otitis media that has occurred in association with enlarged tonsils and adenoids. Indications for adenoidectomy include chronic nasal airway obstruction, chronic rhinorrhea, obstruction of the eustachian tube with related ear infections, and abnormal speech. Surgery is also indicated if the patient has developed a peritonsillar abscess that occludes

the pharynx, making swallowing difficult and endangering the patency of the airway (particularly during sleep). The presence of persistent tonsillar asymmetry should prompt an excisional biopsy to rule out lymphoma (Tierney et al., 2012). Antibiotic therapy may be initiated for patients undergoing tonsillectomy or adenoidectomy. Therapy may include oral penicillin or a cephalosporin (e.g., cefdinir [Omnicef] or moxifloxacin [Avelox]).

Nursing Management

Providing Postoperative Care

Continuous nursing observation is required in the immediate postoperative and recovery periods because of the risk of hemorrhage, which may also compromise the patient's airway (Regan & Nevius, 2012). In the immediate postoperative period, the most comfortable position is prone, with the patient's head turned to the side to allow drainage from the mouth and pharynx. The nurse must not remove the oral airway until the patient's gag and swallowing reflexes have returned. The nurse applies an ice collar to the neck, and a basin and tissues are provided for the expectoration of blood and mucus.

Symptoms of postoperative complications include fever, throat pain, ear pain, and bleeding. Pain can be effectively controlled with analgesic medications. Postoperative bleeding may be seen as bright red blood if the patient expectorates it before swallowing it. If the patient swallows the blood, it becomes brown because of the action of the acidic gastric juice. If the patient vomits large amounts of dark blood or bright-red blood at frequent intervals, or if the pulse rate and temperature rise and the patient is restless, the nurse notifies the surgeon immediately. The nurse should have the following items ready for examination of the surgical site for bleeding: a light, a mirror, gauze, curved hemostats, and a waste basin.

Occasionally, suture or ligation of a bleeding vessel is required. In such cases, the patient is taken to the operating room and given general anesthesia. After ligation, continuous nursing observation and postoperative care are required, as in the initial postoperative period. If there is no bleeding, water and ice chips may be given to the patient as soon as desired. The patient is instructed to refrain from too much talking and coughing, because these activities can produce throat pain. (See Chapter 19 for further discussion of postoperative nursing care.)

Educating Patients About Self-Care

Tonsillectomy and adenoidectomy are usually performed as outpatient surgery, and the patient is sent home from the recovery room once awake, oriented, and able to drink liquids and void. The patient and family must understand the signs and symptoms of hemorrhage. Bleeding may occur up to 8 days after surgery. The nurse instructs the patient about use of liquid acetaminophen with or without codeine for pain control and explains that the pain will subside during the first 3 to 5 days. The nurse informs the patient about the need to take the full course of any prescribed antibiotic.

Alkaline mouthwashes and warm saline solutions are useful in coping with the thick mucus and halitosis that may be present after surgery. The nurse should explain to the patient that a sore throat, stiff neck, minor ear pain, and vomiting may occur in the first 24 hours. The patient should eat an adequate diet with soft foods, which are more easily swallowed than hard foods. The patient should avoid spicy, hot, acidic, or rough foods. Milk and milk products (ice cream and yogurt) may be restricted because they make removal of mucus more difficult for some patients. The nurse instructs the patient about the need to maintain good hydration. The patient is advised to avoid vigorous tooth brushing or gargling because these activities can cause bleeding. The nurse encourages the use of a cool-mist vaporizer or humidifier in the home postoperatively. The patient should avoid smoking and heavy lifting or exertion for 10 days.

Peritonsillar Abscess

Peritonsillar abscess (also called *quinsy*) is the most common major suppurative complication of sore throat. It most commonly afflicts adults between the ages of 20 to 40 years, with the incidence roughly the same between men and women (Tan, 2012). This collection of purulent exudate between the tonsillar capsule and the surrounding tissues, including the soft palate, may develop after an acute tonsillar infection that progresses to a local cellulitis and abscess. Several bacteria are typically implicated in the pathogenesis of these abscesses, including *S. pyogenes, S. aureus, Neisseria* species, and *Corynebacterium* species (Tan, 2012). In more severe cases, the infection can spread over the palate and to the neck and chest. Edema can cause airway obstruction, which can be life threatening and is a medical emergency. Peritonsillar abscess can be life threatening with mediastinitis, intracranial abscess, and empyemas resulting from spread of infection. Early detection and aggressive management are essential (Tan, 2012).

Clinical Manifestations

The patient with a peritonsillar abscess is acutely ill with a severe sore throat, fever, trismus (inability to open the mouth), and drooling. Inflammation of the medial pterygoid muscle that lies lateral to the tonsil results in spasm, severe pain, and difficulty in opening the mouth fully. The pain may be so intense that the patient has difficulty swallowing saliva. The patient's breath often smells rancid. Other symptoms include a raspy voice, odynophagia (a severe sensation of burning, squeezing pain while swallowing), **dysphagia** (difficulty swallowing), and otalgia (pain in the ear). Odynophagia is caused by the inflammation of the superior constrictor muscle of the pharynx that forms the lateral wall of the tonsil. This causes pain on lateral movement of the head. The patient may also have tender and enlarged cervical lymph nodes. Examination of the oropharynx reveals erythema of the anterior pillar and soft palate as well as a purulent tonsil on the side of the peritonsillar abscess. The tonsil is pushed inferomedially, and the uvula is shifted contralaterally (Tan, 2012).

Assessment and Diagnostic Findings

Emergency department (ED) physicians frequently are the providers who diagnose patients with peritonsillar abscesses. When this occurs in the ED setting, the ED physician decides whether aspiration—an invasive procedure—should be carried out based on the patient's clinical picture. Intraoral ultrasound and transcutaneous cervical ultrasound are used in the diagnosis of peritonsillar cellulitis and abscesses.

Medical Management

Antimicrobial agents and corticosteroid therapy are used for treatment of peritonsillar abscess. Antibiotics (usually penicillin) are extremely effective in controlling the infection, and if they are prescribed early in the course of the disease, the abscess may resolve without needing to be incised. However, if the abscess does not resolve, treatment choices include needle aspiration, incision and drainage under local or general anesthesia, and drainage of the abscess with simultaneous tonsillectomy. Following needle aspiration (discussed later) intramuscular administration of clindamycin (Cleocin) can be used in the outpatient setting, thus reducing both antibiotic and hospital costs. The use of topical anesthetic agents and throat irrigations may be prescribed to promote comfort along with administration of prescribed analgesic agents.

Patients with complications require hospitalization for IV antibiotics, imaging studies, observation, and proper airway management. Rarely, the patient with a peritonsillar abscess presents with acute airway obstruction and requires immediate airway management. Procedures may include intubation, cricothyroidotomy, or tracheotomy (Tan, 2012).

Surgical Management

Needle aspiration may be preferred over a more extensive procedure due to its high efficacy, low cost, and patient tolerance. The mucous membrane over the swelling is first sprayed with a topical anesthetic and then injected with a local anesthetic. Single or repeated needle aspirations are performed to decompress the abscess. Alternatively, the abscess may be incised and drained. These procedures are performed best with the patient in the sitting position to make it easier to expectorate the pus and blood that accumulate in the pharynx. The patient experiences almost immediate relief. Incision and drainage is also an effective option but is more painful than needle aspiration.

Tonsillectomy is considered for patients who are poor candidates for needle aspiration or incision and drainage. The risk of hemorrhage following tonsillectomy to treat peritonsillar abscess is higher than that of elective tonsillectomy and may be due to the patient's previous use of aspirin for pain relief.

Nursing Management

If the patient requires intubation, cricothyroidotomy, or tracheotomy to treat airway obstruction, the nurse assists with the procedure and provides support to the patient before, during, and after the procedure. The nurse also assists with the needle aspiration when indicated.

The nurse encourages the patient to use prescribed topical anesthetic agents and assists with throat irrigations or the frequent use of mouthwashes or gargles, using saline or alkaline solutions at a temperature of 40.6°C to 43.3°C (105°F to 110°F). Gentle gargling after the procedure with a cool normal saline gargle may relieve discomfort. The patient must be upright and clearly expectorate forward. The nurse instructs the patient to gargle *gently* at intervals of 1 or 2 hours for 24 to 36 hours. Liquids that are cool or at room temperature are usually well tolerated. Adequate fluids must be provided to treat dehydration and prevent its recurrence.

The nurse also observes the patient for complications and instructs the patient about signs and symptoms of complications that require prompt attention by the patient's primary provider. At discharge, the nurse provides verbal and written instructions regarding foods to avoid, when to return to work, and the need to refrain from or cease smoking. The need for continuation of good oral hygiene is also reinforced.

Laryngitis

Laryngitis, an inflammation of the larynx, often occurs as a result of voice abuse or exposure to dust, chemicals, smoke, and other pollutants or as part of a URI. It also may be caused by isolated infection involving only the vocal cords. Laryngitis is also associated with gastroesophageal reflux (referred to as reflux laryngitis).

Laryngitis is very often caused by the pathogens that cause the common cold and pharyngitis; the most common cause is a virus, and laryngitis is often associated with allergic rhinitis or pharyngitis. Bacterial invasion may be secondary. The onset of infection may be associated with exposure to sudden temperature changes, dietary deficiencies, malnutrition, or an immunosuppressed state. Viral laryngitis is common in the winter and is easily transmitted to others.

Clinical Manifestations

Signs of acute laryngitis include hoarseness or **aphonia** (complete loss of voice) and severe cough. Chronic laryngitis is marked by persistent hoarseness. Other signs of acute laryngitis include sudden onset made worse by cold dry wind. The throat feels worse in the morning and improves when the patient is indoors in a warmer climate. At times, the patient presents with a dry cough and a dry, sore throat that worsens in the evening hours. If allergies are present, the uvula will be visibly edematous. Many patients also complain of a "tickle" in the throat that is made worse by cold air or cold liquids.

Medical Management

Management of acute laryngitis includes resting the voice, avoiding irritants (including smoking), resting, and inhaling cool steam or an aerosol. If the laryngitis is part of a more extensive respiratory infection caused by a bacterial organism or if it is severe, appropriate antibacterial therapy is instituted. The majority of patients recover with conservative treatment; however, laryngitis tends to be more severe in older adult patients and may be complicated by pneumonia.

For chronic laryngitis, the treatment includes resting the voice, eliminating any primary respiratory tract infection, eliminating smoking, and avoiding secondhand smoke. Corticosteroids, such as beclomethasone, may be given. These preparations have few systemic or long-lasting effects and may reduce local inflammatory reactions. Treatment for reflux laryngitis typically involves use of proton pump inhibitors such as omeprazole (Prilosec) given once daily.

Nursing Management

The nurse instructs the patient to rest the voice and to maintain a well-humidified environment. If laryngeal secretions are present during acute episodes, expectorant agents are suggested, along with a daily fluid intake of 2 to 3 L to thin secretions. The nurse instructs the patient about the importance of taking prescribed medications, including proton pump inhibitors, and using continuous positive airway therapy at bedtime, if prescribed for OSA. In cases involving infection, the nurse informs the patient that the symptoms of laryngitis often extend a week to 10 days after completion of antibiotic therapy. The nurse instructs the patient about signs and symptoms that require contacting the patient's primary provider. These signs and symptoms include loss of voice with sore throat that makes swallowing saliva difficult, hemoptysis, and noisy respirations. Continued hoarseness after voice rest or laryngitis that persists for longer than 5 days must be reported because of the possibility of malignancy.

NURSING PROCESS

The Patient With Upper Airway Infection

Assessment

A health history may reveal signs and symptoms of headache, sore throat, pain around the eyes and on either side of the nose, difficulty in swallowing, cough, hoarseness, fever, stuffiness, and generalized discomfort and fatigue. Determining when the symptoms began, what precipitated them, what if anything relieves them, and what aggravates them is part of the assessment. The nurse should also determine any history of allergy or the existence of a concomitant illness. Inspection may reveal swelling, lesions, or asymmetry of the nose as well as bleeding or discharge. The nurse inspects the nasal mucosa for abnormal findings such as increased redness, swelling, exudate, and nasal polyps, which may develop in chronic rhinitis. The mucosa of the nasal turbinates may also be swollen (boggy) and pale bluish-gray. The nurse palpates the frontal and maxillary sinuses for tenderness, which suggests inflammation, and then inspects the throat by having the patient open the mouth wide and take a deep breath. Redness, asymmetry, or evidence of drainage, ulceration, or enlargement of the tonsils and pharynx are abnormal. Palpation of the neck lymph nodes for enlargement and tenderness is necessary.

Diagnosis

Nursing Diagnoses

Based on the assessment data, major nursing diagnoses may include the following:

- Ineffective airway clearance related to excessive mucus production secondary to retained secretions and inflammation
- Acute pain related to upper airway irritation secondary to an infection
- Impaired verbal communication related to physiologic changes and upper airway irritation secondary to infection or swelling
- Deficient fluid volume related to decreased fluid intake and increased fluid loss secondary to diaphoresis associated with a fever
- Deficient knowledge regarding prevention of URIs, treatment regimen, surgical procedure, or postoperative care

Collaborative Problems/Potential Complications

Based on the assessment data, potential complications include:

- Sepsis
- Meningitis or brain abscess
- Peritonsillar abscess, otitis media, or rhinosinusitis

Planning and Goals

The major goals for the patient may include maintenance of a patent airway, relief of pain, maintenance of effective means of communication, normal hydration, knowledge of how to prevent upper airway infections, and absence of complications.

Nursing Interventions

Maintaining a Patent Airway

An accumulation of secretions can block the airway in patients with an upper airway infection. As a result, changes in the respiratory pattern occur, and the work of breathing increases to compensate for the blockage. The nurse can implement several measures to loosen thick secretions or to keep the secretions moist so that they can be easily expectorated. Increasing fluid intake helps thin the mucus. The use of room vaporizers or steam inhalation also loosens secretions and reduces inflammation of the mucous membranes. To enhance drainage from the sinuses, the nurse instructs the patient about positioning; this depends on the location of the infection or inflammation. For example, drainage for rhinosinusitis or rhinitis is achieved in the upright position. In some conditions, topical or systemic medications, when prescribed, help relieve nasal or throat congestion.

Promoting Comfort

URIs usually produce localized discomfort. In rhinosinusitis, pain may occur in the area of the sinuses, or a general headache may be produced. In pharyngitis, laryngitis, or tonsillitis, a sore throat occurs. The nurse encourages the patient to take analgesics, such as acetaminophen with codeine, as prescribed, to relieve this discomfort. A pain intensity rating scale (see Chapter 12) may be used to assess effectiveness of pain relief measures. Other helpful measures include topical anesthetic agents for symptomatic relief of herpes simplex blisters (see Chart 22-3) and sore throats, hot packs to relieve the congestion of rhinosinusitis and promote drainage, and warm water gargles or irrigations to relieve the pain of a sore throat. The nurse encourages rest to relieve the generalized discomfort and fever that accompany many upper airway conditions (especially rhinitis, pharyngitis, and laryngitis). For postoperative care after tonsillectomy and adenoidectomy, an ice collar may reduce swelling and decrease bleeding.

Promoting Communication

Upper airway infections may result in hoarseness or loss of speech. The nurse instructs the patient to refrain from speaking as much as possible and, if possible, to communicate in writing instead. Additional strain on the vocal cords may delay full return of the voice. The nurse encourages the patient and family to use alternative forms of communication, such as a memo pad or a bell to signal for assistance.

Encouraging Fluid Intake

Upper airway infections lead to fluid loss. Sore throat, malaise, and fever may interfere with a patient's willingness to eat and drink. The nurse provides a list of easily ingested foods to increase caloric intake during the acute phase of illness. These include soups, gelatin, pudding, yogurt, cottage cheese, high-protein drinks, water, ice, and ice pops. The nurse encourages the patient to drink 2 to 3 L of fluid per day during the acute stage of airway infection, unless contraindicated, to thin the secretions and promote drainage. Liquids (hot or cold) may be soothing, depending on the disorder.

Promoting Home and Community-Based Care

Educating Patients About Self-Care. Prevention of most upper airway infections is challenging because of the many potential causes. But because most URIs are transmitted by hand-to-hand contact, the nurse educates the patient and family about techniques to minimize the spread of infection to others, including implementing hand hygiene measures. The nurse advises the patient to avoid exposure to people who are at risk for serious illness if respiratory infection is transmitted (older adults, immunosuppressed people, and those with chronic health problems).

The nurse instructs patients and their families about strategies to relieve symptoms of URIs and reinforces the need to complete the treatment regimen, particularly when antibiotics are prescribed.

Continuing Care. Referral for home care is rare. However, it may be indicated for people whose health status was compromised before the onset of the respiratory infection and for those who cannot manage self-care without assistance. In such circumstances, the home care nurse assesses the patient's respiratory status and progress in recovery. The nurse may advise older adult patients and those at increased risk from a respiratory infection to consider annual influenza and pneumococcal vaccination. A follow-up appointment with the primary provider may be indicated for patients with compromised health status to ensure that the respiratory infection has resolved.

Monitoring and Managing Potential Complications

Although major complications of URIs are rare, the nurse must be aware of them and assess the patient for them. Because most patients with URIs are managed at home, patients and their families must be instructed to monitor for signs and symptoms and to seek immediate medical care if the patient's condition does not improve or if the patient's physical status appears to be worsening.

Sepsis or meningitis may occur in patients with compromised immune status or in those with an overwhelming bacterial infection. The patient with a URI and family members are instructed to seek medical care if the patient's condition fails to improve within several days after the onset of symptoms, if unusual symptoms develop, or if the patient's condition deteriorates. They are instructed about signs and symptoms that require further attention: persistent or high fever, increasing shortness of breath, confusion, and increasing weakness and malaise. The patient with sepsis requires expert care to treat the infection, stabilize vital signs, and prevent or treat septicemia and shock. Deterioration of the patient's condition necessitates intensive care measures (e.g., hemodynamic monitoring and administration of vasoactive medications, IV fluids, nutritional support, corticosteroids) to monitor the patient's status and to support the patient's vital signs. High doses of antibiotics may be administered to treat the causative organism. The nurse's role is to monitor the patient's vital signs, hemodynamic status, and laboratory values; administer needed treatment; alleviate the patient's physical discomfort; and provide explanations, education, and emotional support to the patient and family.

Peritonsillar abscess may develop after an acute infection of the tonsils. The patient requires treatment to drain the abscess and receives antibiotics for infection and topical anesthetic agents and throat irrigations to relieve pain and sore throat. Follow-up is necessary to ensure that the abscess resolves; tonsillectomy may be required. The nurse assists the patient in administering throat irrigations and instructs the patient and family about the importance of adhering to the prescribed treatment regimen and recommended follow-up appointments.

In some severe situations, peritonsillar abscess may progress to meningitis or brain abscess. The nurse assesses for changes in mental status ranging from subtle personality changes through drowsiness to coma, nuchal rigidity, and focal neurologic signs that signal increasing cerebral edema around the abscess (see Chapter 69). Seizures, typically tonic–clonic, occur in this setting. Intensive care measures are necessary. High doses of antibiotics may be used to treat the causative organism. The nurse's role is similar to caring for the patient with sepsis in an intensive care setting. The nurse monitors the patient's neurologic status and reports changes immediately.

Otitis media and rhinosinusitis may develop with URI. The patient and family are instructed about the signs and symptoms of otitis media and rhinosinusitis and about the importance of follow-up with the primary practitioner to ensure adequate evaluation and treatment of these conditions.

Evaluation

Expected patient outcomes may include the following:

1. Maintains a patent airway by managing secretions
   a. Reports decreased congestion
   b. Assumes best position to facilitate drainage of secretions
   c. Uses self-care measures appropriately and consistently to manage secretions during the acute phase of illness
2. Reports relief of pain and discomfort using pain intensity scale
   a. Uses comfort measures: analgesics, hot packs, gargles, rest
   b. Demonstrates adequate oral hygiene
3. Demonstrates ability to communicate needs, wants, level of comfort
4. Maintains adequate fluid and nutrition intake
5. Utilizes strategies to prevent upper airway infections and allergic reactions
   a. Demonstrates hand hygiene technique
   b. Identifies the value of the influenza vaccine
6. Demonstrates an adequate level of knowledge and performs self-care adequately
7. Becomes free of signs and symptoms of infection
   a. Exhibits normal vital signs (temperature, pulse, respiratory rate)
   b. Absence of purulent drainage
   c. Free of pain in ears, sinuses, and throat
   d. Absence of signs of inflammation
8. Absence of complications
   a. No signs of sepsis: fever, hypotension, deterioration of cognitive status
   b. Vital signs and hemodynamic status normal
   c. No evidence of neurologic involvement
   d. No signs of development of peritonsillar abscess
   e. Resolution of URI without development of otitis media or rhinosinusitis
   f. No signs and symptoms of brain abscess

OBSTRUCTION AND TRAUMA OF THE UPPER RESPIRATORY AIRWAY

Obstruction During Sleep

Obstructive sleep apnea (OSA) is a disorder characterized by recurrent episodes of upper airway obstruction and a reduction in ventilation. It is defined as cessation of breathing (**apnea**) during sleep usually caused by repetitive upper airway obstruction. It is believed that between 2% and 4% of women and 4% and 9% of men in the United States have OSA, and that up to 80% are not diagnosed (Downey, 2012). OSA interferes with people's ability to obtain adequate rest, thus affecting memory, learning, and decision making.

Risk factors for OSA include obesity, male gender, postmenopausal status, and advanced age. The major risk factor is obesity; a larger neck circumference and increased amounts of peripharyngeal fat narrow and compress the upper airway. Other associated factors include alterations in the upper airway, such as structural changes (e.g., tonsillar hypertrophy, abnormal posterior positioning of one or both jaws, and variations in craniofacial structures) that contribute to the collapsibility of the upper airway (Downey, 2012).

Pathophysiology

The pharynx is a collapsible tube that can be compressed by the soft tissues and structures surrounding it. The tone of the muscles of the upper airway is reduced during sleep. Mechanical factors such as reduced diameter of the upper airway or dynamic changes in the upper airway during sleep may result in obstruction. These sleep-related changes may predispose to upper airway collapse when small amounts of negative pressure are generated during inspiration.

Repetitive apneic events result in hypoxia (decreased oxygen saturation) and hypercapnia (increased concentration of carbon dioxide), which triggers a sympathetic response. As a consequence, patients with OSA have a high prevalence of hypertension. In addition, OSA is associated with an increased risk of myocardial infarction and stroke (cerebrovascular accident), which may be mitigated with appropriate treatment (Downey, 2012).

Clinical Manifestations

OSA is characterized by frequent and loud snoring with breathing cessation for 10 seconds or longer, for at least five episodes per hour, followed by awakening abruptly with a loud snort as the blood oxygen level drops. Patients with sleep apnea may have anywhere from five apneic episodes per hour to several hundred per night.

Chart
22-4

ASSESSMENT

Assessing for Obstructive Sleep Apnea

Be alert for the following signs and symptoms of obstructive sleep apnea:

• Excessive daytime sleepiness
• Frequent nocturnal awakening
• Insomnia
• Loud snoring
• Morning headaches
• Intellectual deterioration
• Personality changes, irritability
• Impotence
• Systemic hypertension
• Dysrhythmias
• Pulmonary hypertension, cor pulmonale
• Polycythemia
• Enuresis

Classic signs and symptoms of OSA include the "3 S's"—namely, snoring, sleepiness, and significant-other report of sleep apnea episodes. Common signs and symptoms of OSA are presented in Chart 22-4. Symptoms typically progress with increases in weight and aging (Downey, 2012). Patients are typically unaware of nocturnal upper airway obstruction during sleep. They frequently complain of insomnia, including difficulty in going to sleep, nighttime awakenings, and early morning awakenings with an inability to go back to sleep, as well as chronic fatigue and hypersomnolence (daytime sleepiness). When obtaining the health history, the nurse asks the patient about sleeping during normal activities such as eating or talking. Patients with this symptom are considered to have pathologic hypersomnolence (Downey, 2012).

Assessment and Diagnostic Findings

The diagnosis of sleep apnea is based on clinical features plus a polysomnographic finding (sleep study), which is the definitive test for OSA. The test is an overnight study that measures multiple physiologic signals to include those related to sleep (electroencephalogram, electro-oculogram, segmental electrocardiogram), respiration (airflow, thoracoabdominal effort, and oximetry), and cardiac dysrhythmia (electrocardiogram).

Medical Management

Patients usually seek medical treatment because their sleeping partners express concern or because they experience excessive sleepiness at inappropriate times or settings (e.g., while driving a car). A variety of treatments are used. Weight loss, avoidance of alcohol, positional therapy (using devices that prevent patients from sleeping on their backs), and oral appliances are the first steps (American Sleep Apnea Association, 2011; Park, Ramar, & Olson, 2011). In more severe cases involving hypoxemia and severe hypercapnia, the treatment includes continuous positive airway pressure (CPAP) or bilevel positive airway pressure (BiPAP) therapy with supplemental oxygen via nasal cannula. CPAP is used to prevent airway collapse, whereas BiPAP makes breathing easier and results in a lower average airway pressure. (The use of CPAP is discussed in more detail in Chapter 21.)

Surgical Management

Surgical procedures also may be performed to correct OSA. Simple tonsillectomy may be effective for patients with larger tonsils when deemed clinically necessary, or when other options have failed or are refused by patients (Aurora, Casey, Kristo, et al., 2010). Uvulopalatopharyngoplasty is the resection of pharyngeal soft tissue and removal of approximately 15 mm of the free edge of the soft palate and uvula. Effective in about 50% of patients, it is more effective in eliminating snoring than apnea. Nasal septoplasty may be performed for gross anatomic nasal septal deformities. Maxillomandibular surgery may be performed to advance the maxilla and mandible forward in order to enlarge the posterior pharyngeal region (Park et al., 2011). Tracheostomy relieves upper airway obstruction but has numerous adverse effects, including speech difficulties and increased risk of infections. These procedures, as well as other maxillofacial surgeries, are reserved for patients with life-threatening dysrhythmias or severe disability who have not responded to conventional therapy (Tierney et al., 2012).

Pharmacologic Therapy

Some medications are useful in managing symptoms associated with OSA. Modafinil (Provigil) has been used to reduce daytime sleepiness (Park et al., 2011). Protriptyline (Triptil) given at bedtime may increase the respiratory drive and improve upper airway muscle tone. Medroxyprogesterone acetate (Provera) and acetazolamide (Diamox) have been used for sleep apnea associated with chronic alveolar hypoventilation; however, their benefits have not been well established. The patient must understand that these medications are not a substitute for CPAP or BiPAP. Administration of low-flow nasal oxygen at night can help relieve hypoxemia in some patients but has little effect on the frequency or severity of apnea.

Nursing Management

The patient with OSA may not recognize the potential consequences of the disorder. Therefore, the nurse explains the disorder in terms that are understandable to the patient and relates symptoms (daytime sleepiness) to the underlying disorder. The nurse also instructs the patient and family about treatments, including the correct and safe use of CPAP, BiPAP, and oxygen therapy, if prescribed. The nurse educates the patient about the risk of untreated OSA and the benefits of treatment approaches.

Epistaxis (Nosebleed)

Epistaxis, a hemorrhage from the nose, is caused by the rupture of tiny, distended vessels in the mucous membrane of any area of the nose. Rarely does epistaxis originate in the densely vascular tissue over the turbinates. Most commonly, the site is the anterior septum, where three major blood vessels enter the nasal cavity: (1) the anterior ethmoidal artery on the forward part of the roof (Kiesselbach's plexus), (2) the sphenopalatine artery in the posterosuperior region, and (3) the internal maxillary branches (the plexus of veins located at the back of the lateral wall under the inferior turbinate).

Several risk factors are associated with epistaxis (Chart 22-5).

RISK FACTORS

Epistaxis

- Local infections (vestibulitis, rhinitis, rhinosinusitis)
- Systemic infections (scarlet fever, malaria)
- Drying of nasal mucous membranes
- Nasal inhalation of corticosteroids (e.g., beclomethasone) or illicit drugs (e.g., cocaine)
- Trauma (digital trauma, blunt trauma, fracture, forceful nose blowing)
- Arteriosclerosis
- Hypertension
- Tumor (sinus or nasopharynx)
- Thrombocytopenia
- Use of aspirin
- Liver disease
- Redu-Osler-Weber syndrome (hereditary hemorrhagic telangiectasia)

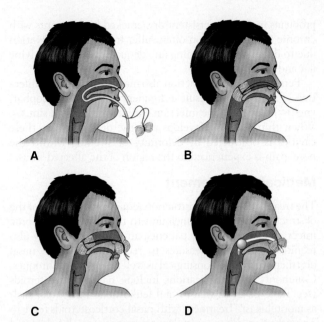

FIGURE 22-3 • Packing to control bleeding from the posterior nose. **A.** Catheter is inserted and packing is attached. **B.** Packing is drawn into position as the catheter is removed. **C.** Strip is tied over a bolster to hold the packing in place with an anterior pack installed "accordion pleat" style. **D.** Alternative method, using a balloon catheter instead of gauze packing.

Medical Management

Management of epistaxis depends on its cause and the location of the bleeding site. A nasal speculum, penlight, or headlight may be used to identify the site of bleeding in the nasal cavity. Most nosebleeds originate from the anterior portion of the nose. Initial treatment may include applying direct pressure. The patient sits upright with the head tilted forward to prevent swallowing and aspiration of blood and is directed to pinch the soft outer portion of the nose against the midline septum for 5 or 10 minutes continuously. Application of nasal decongestants (phenylephrine, one or two sprays) to act as vasoconstrictors may be necessary. If these measures are unsuccessful in stopping the bleeding, the nose must be examined using good illumination and suction to determine the site of bleeding. Visible bleeding sites may be cauterized with silver nitrate or electrocautery (high-frequency electrical current). A supplemental patch of Surgicel or Gelfoam may be used (Tierney et al., 2012).

Alternatively, a cotton tampon may be used to try to stop the bleeding. Suction may be used to remove excess blood and clots from the field of inspection. The search for the bleeding site should shift from the anteroinferior quadrant to the anterosuperior, then to the posterosuperior, and finally to the posteroinferior area. The field is kept clear by using suction and by shifting the cotton tampon.

If the origin of the bleeding cannot be identified, the nose may be packed with gauze impregnated with petrolatum jelly or antibiotic ointment; a topical anesthetic spray and decongestant agent may be used before the gauze packing is inserted, or a balloon-inflated catheter may be used (Fig. 22-3). Alternatively, a compressed nasal sponge may be used. Once the sponge becomes saturated with blood or is moistened with a small amount of saline, it will expand and produce tamponade to halt the bleeding. The packing may remain in place for 3 to 4 days if necessary to control bleeding (Nguyen, 2011). Antibiotics may be prescribed because of the risk of iatrogenic rhinosinusitis and toxic shock syndrome.

Nursing Management

The nurse monitors the patient's vital signs, assists in the control of bleeding, and provides tissues and an emesis basin to allow the patient to expectorate any excess blood. It is common for patients to be anxious in response to a nosebleed. Blood loss on clothing and handkerchiefs can be frightening, and the nasal examination and treatment are uncomfortable. Assuring the patient in a calm, efficient manner that bleeding can be controlled can help reduce anxiety. The nurse continuously assesses the patient's airway and breathing as well as vital signs. On rare occasions, a patient with significant hemorrhage requires IV infusions of crystalloid solutions (normal saline) as well as cardiac and pulse oximetry monitoring.

Educating Patients About Self-Care

Once the bleeding is controlled, the nurse instructs the patient to avoid vigorous exercise for several days and to avoid hot or spicy foods and tobacco, because this may cause vasodilation and increase the risk of rebleeding. Discharge education includes reviewing ways to prevent epistaxis: avoiding forceful nose blowing, straining, high altitudes, and nasal trauma (including nose picking). Adequate humidification may prevent drying of the nasal passages. The nurse explains how to apply direct pressure to the nose with the thumb and the index finger for 15 minutes in the case of a recurrent nosebleed. If recurrent bleeding cannot be stopped, the patient is instructed to seek additional medical attention.

Nasal Obstruction

The passage of air through the nostrils is frequently obstructed by a deviation of the nasal septum, hypertrophy of the turbinate bones, or the pressure of nasal polyps. Chronic nasal congestion forces the patient to breathe through the mouth, thus producing dryness of the oral mucosa and associated problems including persistent dry, cracked lips. Patients with chronic nasal congestion often suffer from sleep deprivation due to difficulty maintaining an adequate airway while lying flat and during sleep.

Persistent nasal obstruction also may lead to chronic infection of the nose and result in frequent episodes of nasopharyngitis. Frequently, the infection extends to the nasal sinuses. When rhinosinusitis develops and the drainage from these cavities is obstructed by deformity or swelling within the nose, pain is experienced in the region of the affected sinus.

Medical Management

The treatment of nasal obstruction requires the removal of the obstruction, followed by measures to treat whatever chronic infection exists. In many patients, an underlying allergy also requires treatment. Measures to reduce or alleviate nasal obstruction include nonsurgical as well as surgical techniques. Commonly used medications include nasal corticosteroids (see Table 22-2) as well as oral leukotriene inhibitors, such as montelukast. Treatment with nasal corticosteroids for 1 to 3 months is usually successful for treatment of small polyps and may even reduce the need for surgical intervention. A short course of oral corticosteroids (6-day course of prednisone) may be beneficial in the treatment of nasal obstruction due to polyps (Tierney et al., 2012). Additional medications may include antibiotics for the treatment of underlying infection or antihistamines for management of allergies. Hypertrophied turbinates may be treated by applying an astringent agent to shrink them.

A more aggressive approach in treating nasal obstruction caused by turbinate hypertrophy involves surgical reduction of the hypertrophy. Surgical procedures used to treat obstructive nasal conditions are collectively known as functional rhinoplasty. Technical advances with newer techniques provide a number of options for reconstruction and reshaping of the nose.

Nursing Management

When a surgical procedure is indicated, most often it is performed on an outpatient basis. The nurse explains the procedure to the patient. Postoperatively, the nurse elevates the head of the bed to promote drainage and to alleviate discomfort from edema. Frequent oral hygiene is encouraged to overcome dryness caused by breathing through the mouth. Before discharge from the outpatient or same-day surgical unit, the patient is instructed to avoid blowing the nose with force during the postoperative recovery period. The patient is also instructed about the signs and symptoms of bleeding and infection and when to contact the primary provider. The patient is provided with written postoperative instructions, including emergency phone numbers.

Fractures of the Nose

The location of the nose makes it susceptible to injury. Nasal fracture is the most common facial fracture and the most common fracture in the body (Becker, 2012). Fractures of the nose usually result from a direct assault. Nasal fractures may affect the ascending process of the maxilla and the septum. The torn mucous membrane results in a nosebleed. Compli-

cations include hematoma, infection, abscess, and avascular or septic necrosis. However, as a rule, serious consequences usually do not occur.

Clinical Manifestations

The signs and symptoms of a nasal fracture are pain, bleeding from the nose externally and internally into the pharynx, swelling of the soft tissues adjacent to the nose, periorbital ecchymosis, nasal obstruction, and deformity. The patient's nose may have an asymmetric appearance that may not be obvious until the edema subsides.

Assessment and Diagnostic Findings

The nose is examined internally to rule out the possibility that the injury may be complicated by a fracture of the nasal septum and a submucosal septal hematoma. Intranasal examination is performed in all cases to rule out septal hematoma (Tierney et al., 2012). Because of the swelling and bleeding that occur with a nasal fracture, an accurate diagnosis can be made only after the swelling subsides.

Clear fluid draining from either nostril suggests a fracture of the cribriform plate with leakage of cerebrospinal fluid. Usually, careful inspection or palpation discloses any deviations of the bone or disruptions of the nasal cartilages. An x-ray may reveal displacement of the fractured bones and may help rule out extension of the fracture into the skull.

Medical Management

A nasal fracture very often produces bleeding from the nasal passage. As a rule, bleeding is controlled with the use of packing. Cold compresses are used to prevent or reduce edema. For the patient who has sustained enough trauma to break the nose or any facial bone, the emergency medical team must consider the possibility of a cervical spine fracture. Therefore, it is essential to ensure a patent airway and to rule out a cervical spine fracture (see Chapter 68). Uncomplicated nasal fractures may be treated initially with antibiotics, analgesic agents, and a decongestant nasal spray.

Treatment of nasal fractures is aimed at restoring nasal function and returning the appearance of the nose to baseline. The patient is referred to a specialist to evaluate the need to realign the bones. Although improved outcomes are obtained when reduction of the fracture is performed during the first 3 hours after the injury, this is often not possible because of the edema. If immediate reduction of the fracture is not possible, it is performed within 3 to 7 days. Timing is important when treating nasal fractures because further delay in treatment may result in significant bone healing, which ultimately may require surgical intervention that includes rhinoplasty to reshape the external appearance of the nose. A septorhinoplasty is performed when the nasal septum needs to be repaired. In patients who develop a septal hematoma, the physician drains the hematoma through a small incision. A septal hematoma that is not drained can lead to permanent deformity of the nose.

Nursing Management

Immediately after the fracture, the nurse applies ice and encourages the patient to keep the head elevated. The nurse instructs the patient to apply ice packs to the nose to decrease swelling. The patient who experiences bleeding from the nose (epistaxis) is usually frightened and anxious and needs reassurance. The packing inserted to stop the bleeding may be uncomfortable and unpleasant, and obstruction of the nasal passages by the packing forces the patient to breathe through the mouth. This in turn causes the oral mucous membranes to become dry. Mouth rinses help to moisten the mucous membranes and to reduce the odor and taste of dried blood in the oropharynx and nasopharynx. The use of analgesic agents such as acetaminophen or NSAIDs (i.e., ibuprofen or naproxen) is encouraged. When removing the cotton pledgets, the nurse carefully inspects the mucosa for lacerations or a septal hematoma. The nurse instructs the patient to avoid sports activities for 6 weeks.

Laryngeal Obstruction

Obstruction of the larynx because of edema is a serious, often fatal, condition. The larynx is a stiff box that will not stretch. It contains a narrow space between the vocal cords (glottis), through which air must pass. Swelling of the laryngeal mucous membranes may close off the opening tightly, leading to life-threatening hypoxia or suffocation. Edema of the glottis occurs rarely in patients with acute laryngitis, occasionally in patients with urticaria, and more frequently in patients with severe inflammation of the throat, as in scarlet fever. It is an occasional cause of death in severe anaphylaxis (angioedema).

Hereditary angioedema is also characterized by episodes of life-threatening laryngeal edema. Laryngeal edema in people with hereditary angioedema can occur at any age, although young adults are at greatest risk. Some causes of laryngeal obstruction are given in Table 22-3.

Foreign bodies frequently are aspirated into the pharynx, the larynx, or the trachea and cause a twofold problem. First, they obstruct the air passages and cause difficulty in breathing, which may lead to asphyxia; later, they may be drawn

farther down, entering the bronchi or a bronchial branch and causing symptoms of irritation, such as a croupy cough, expectoration of blood or mucus, or labored breathing. The physical signs and x-ray findings may confirm the diagnosis.

Clinical Manifestations

The patient's clinical presentation and x-ray findings confirm the diagnosis of laryngeal obstruction. The patient may demonstrate lowered oxygen saturation; however, normal oxygen saturation should not be interpreted as a sign that the obstruction is not significant. The use of accessory muscles to maximize airflow may occur and is often manifested by retractions in the neck or abdomen during inspirations. Patients who demonstrate these symptoms are at an immediate risk of collapse, and respiratory support (i.e., mechanical ventilation or positive-pressure ventilation) is considered.

Assessment and Diagnostic Findings

A thorough history can be very useful in diagnosing and treating the patient with a laryngeal obstruction. However, emergency measures to secure the patient's airway should not be delayed to obtain a history or perform tests. If possible, the nurse obtains a history from the patient or family about heavy alcohol or tobacco consumption, current medications, history of airway problems, recent infections, pain or fever, dental pain or poor dentition, and any previous surgeries, radiation therapy, or trauma.

Rarely, patients with nasogastric tubes in place develop a postcricoid ulceration (referred to as nasogastric tube syndrome). This ulceration affects the posterior cricoarytenoid muscles, causing vocal cord abduction paralysis and ultimately upper airway obstruction (Marcus, Caine, Hamdan, et al., 2006).

Medical Management

Medical management is based on the initial evaluation of the patient and the need to ensure a patent airway. If the airway is obstructed by a foreign body and signs of asphyxia are apparent, immediate treatment is necessary. Emergent maneuvers to clear an airway obstruction were presented in Chart 21-6 in Chapter 21. If all efforts are unsuccessful, an immediate tracheotomy is necessary (see Chapter 21 for further discussion). If the obstruction is caused by edema resulting from an allergic reaction, treatment may include immediate administration of subcutaneous epinephrine and a corticosteroid (see Chapter 38). Ice may be applied to the neck in an effort to reduce edema. Continuous pulse oximetry is essential in the patient who has experienced acute upper airway obstruction.

Cancer of the Larynx

Cancer of the larynx accounts for approximately half of all head and neck cancers. The American Cancer Society (ACS, 2012) estimates that about 12,360 new cases and 3,650 deaths occur annually, with a 5-year relative survival rate that ranges from 32% to 90%, depending upon the location of the tumor and its stage at the time of diagnosis (ACS, 2011). Cancer of the larynx is most common in people older than 65 years and is four times more common in men (ACS, 2011) (Chart 22-6).

TABLE 22-3   Causes of Laryngeal Obstruction

Precipitating Event	Mechanism of Obstruction
History of allergies; exposure to medications, latex, foods (peanuts, tree nuts [e.g., walnuts, pecans]), bee stings	Anaphylaxis
Foreign body	Inhalation/ingestion of meat or other food items, coin, chewing gum, balloon fragments, drug packets (ingested to avoid criminal arrest)
Heavy alcohol consumption; heavy tobacco use	Obstruction from tumor
Family history of airway problems	Suggests angioedema (type I hypersensitivity reaction)
Use of angiotensin-converting enzyme inhibitor	Increased risk of angioedema of the mucous membranes
Recent throat pain or recent fever	Infectious process
History of surgery or previous tracheostomy	Possible subglottic stenosis
History of nasogastric tube placement	Nasogastric tube syndrome

Almost all malignant tumors of the larynx arise from the surface epithelium and are classified as squamous cell carcinoma. Approximately 55% of patients with laryngeal cancer present with involved lymph nodes at the time of diagnosis, with bilateral lesions present in 16% of patients (De Vita, Hellman, & Rosenberg, 2011). Recurrence occurs usually within the first 2 to 3 years after diagnosis. The presence of disease after 5 years is often secondary to a new primary malignancy. The incidence of distant metastasis with squamous cell carcinoma of the head and neck (including larynx cancer) is relatively low.

Clinical Manifestations

Hoarseness of more than 2 weeks' duration occurs in the patient with cancer in the glottic area because the tumor impedes the action of the vocal cords during speech. The voice may sound harsh, raspy, and lower in pitch. Affected voice sounds are not always early signs of subglottic or supraglottic cancer, however. The patient may complain of a persistent cough or sore throat and pain and burning in the throat, especially when consuming hot liquids or citrus juices. A lump may be felt in the neck. Later symptoms include dysphagia, dyspnea (difficulty breathing), unilateral nasal obstruction or discharge, persistent hoarseness, persistent ulceration, and foul breath. Cervical lymph adenopathy, unintentional weight loss, a general debilitated state, and pain radiating to the ear may occur with metastasis.

Assessment and Diagnostic Findings

An initial assessment includes a complete history and physical examination of the head and neck. This includes identification of risk factors, family history, and any underlying medical conditions. An indirect laryngoscopy, using a flexible endoscope, is initially performed in the otolaryngologist's office to visually evaluate the pharynx, larynx, and possible tumor. Mobility of the vocal cords is assessed; if normal movement is limited, the growth may affect muscle, other tissue, and even the airway. The lymph nodes of the neck and the thyroid gland are palpated for enlargement.

Diagnostic procedures that may be used include fine-needle aspiration (FNA) biopsy, a barium swallow, endoscopy, CT or MRI scan, and a positron emission tomography (PET) scan (ACS, 2011). FNA biopsy may be done as an initial screening procedure to obtain samples of any enlarged lymph nodes in the neck. A barium swallow may be done if the patient initially presents with a chief complaint of difficulty in swallowing, to outline any structural anomalies of the neck that could pinpoint a tumor. However, if a tumor of the larynx is suspected on an initial examination, a direct laryngoscopic examination is indicated. Laryngoscopy is performed under local or general anesthesia to evaluate all areas of the larynx. In some cases, intraoperative examination obtained by direct microscopic visualization and palpation of the vocal folds may yield a more accurate diagnosis. Samples of the suspicious tissue are obtained for analysis (ACS, 2011).

The classification, including stage of the tumor (i.e., size and histology of the tumor, presence and extent of cervical lymph node involvement) and location of the tumor serve as a basis for treatment. CT scanning and MRI are used to assess regional adenopathy and soft tissues and to stage and determine the extent of a tumor. MRI is also helpful in post-treatment follow-up to detect a recurrence. PET scanning may also be used to detect recurrence of the laryngeal tumor after treatment.

Medical Management

The goals of treatment of laryngeal cancer include cure; preservation of safe, effective swallowing; preservation of useful voice; and avoidance of permanent tracheostoma (Tierney et al., 2012). Treatment options include surgery, radiation therapy, and adjuvant chemoradiation therapy. The prognosis depends on the tumor location (i.e., supraglottic, glottis, subglottic), as well as the tumor grade and stage (i.e., using the TNM system; see Chapter 15). The treatment plan also depends on whether the cancer is an initial diagnosis or a recurrence. In addition, before treatment begins, a complete dental examination is performed to rule out any oral disease. A consultation with a dental oncologist may be warranted. Any dental problems are resolved, if possible, before surgery and radiotherapy (Gilbert, Devries-Aboud, Winquist, et al., 2009).

For patients with early-stage tumors (i.e., stages I and II) and lesions without lymph node involvement, external-beam radiation therapy or conservation surgery (i.e., less invasive surgery, such as vocal cord stripping or cordectomy) may be effective. Other indicated surgical procedures may include transoral endoscopic laser excision or partial laryngectomy (Gilbert et al., 2009). Patients with stage III and IV tumors that are resectable may be advised to have either total laryngectomies with or without postoperative radiation therapy or radiation therapy with concurrent adjuvant chemotherapy (with single-agent cisplatin) and surgical resection aimed at preserving some of the larynx (i.e., organ preservation surgery). Patients with late-stage tumors that extend through cartilage and into soft tissues are generally advised to have total laryngectomies with postoperative radiation therapy (Gilbert et al., 2009).

Patients and their physicians must carefully consider the various side effects and complications associated with the different treatment modalities. The presence of lymph node involvement in the neck can affect the outcome. Supraglottic tumors metastasize early and bilaterally even when there appears to be no lymph node involvement at the time of diagnosis. When the neck lymph nodes are involved, the treatment includes surgery, chemoradiation, or both (Tierney et al., 2012).

Surgical Management

The overall goals for the patient undergoing surgical treatment include minimizing the effects of surgery on speech, swallowing, and breathing while maximizing the cure of the cancer. Several different curative procedures are available that can offer voice-sparing results while achieving a positive cure rate for the patient who has an early laryngeal carcinoma. Surgical options include vocal cord stripping, cordectomy, laser surgery, partial laryngectomy, or total laryngectomy (De Vita et al., 2011).

Vocal Cord Stripping

Stripping of the vocal cord is used to treat dysplasia, hyperkeratosis, and leukoplakia and is often curative for these lesions. The procedure involves removal of the mucosa of the edge of the vocal cord, using an operating microscope. Early vocal cord lesions are initially treated with radiation therapy.

Cordectomy

Cordectomy, which is an excision of the vocal cord, is usually performed via transoral laser. This procedure is used for lesions limited to the middle third of the vocal cord. The resulting voice quality is related to the extent of tissue removed.

Laser Surgery

Laser microsurgery is well known to have several advantages for treatment of early glottic cancers. Treatment and recovery are shorter, with fewer side effects, and treatment may be less costly than for other forms of therapy (De Vita et al., 2011). Microelectrodes are useful for surgical resection of smaller laryngeal carcinomas. The carbon dioxide (CO_2) laser can be used for the treatment of many laryngeal tumors, with the exception of large vascular tumors. When compared with the results of other treatments for early laryngeal cancer, laser microsurgery is considered to be the method of choice based on patient outcomes (De Vita et al., 2011).

Partial Laryngectomy

A partial laryngectomy (laryngofissure–thyrotomy) is often used for patients in the early stages of cancer in the glottic area when only one vocal cord is involved. The surgery is associated with a very high cure rate. It may also be performed for recurrence when high-dose radiation has failed. A portion of the larynx is removed, along with one vocal cord and the tumor; all other structures remain. The airway remains intact, and the patient is expected to have no difficulty swallowing. The voice quality may change, or the patient may sound hoarse.

Total Laryngectomy

Complete removal of the larynx (total **laryngectomy**) can provide a cure in most advanced laryngeal cancers, when the tumor extends beyond the vocal cords, or for cancer that recurs or persists after radiation therapy. In a total laryngectomy, the laryngeal structures are removed, including the hyoid bone, epiglottis, cricoid cartilage, and two or three rings of the trachea. The tongue, pharyngeal walls, and most of the trachea are preserved. A total laryngectomy results in permanent loss of the voice and a change in the airway, requiring a permanent tracheostomy (Fig. 22-4). Occasionally, patients continue to have a laryngectomy tube in the stoma. Laryngectomy tubes are similar in appearance to tracheostomy tubes; however, a laryngectomy tube can be distinguished from a tracheostomy tube because the patient is unable to speak or breathe when the laryngectomy tube

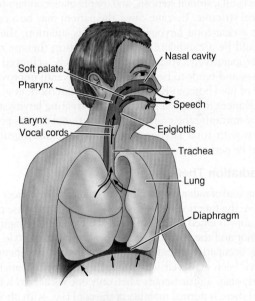

A

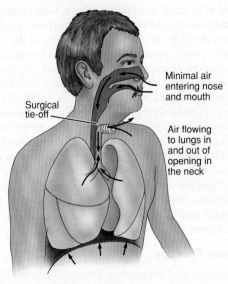

B

FIGURE 22-4 • Total laryngectomy produces a change in airflow for breathing and speaking. **A.** Normal airflow. **B.** Airflow after total laryngectomy.

is occluded. Patients who have a total laryngectomy require alternatives to normal speech; these may include a prosthetic device, such as a Blom-Singer valve, to speak without aspirating.

Surgery is more difficult when the lesion involves the midline structures or both vocal cords. With or without neck dissection, a total laryngectomy requires a permanent tracheal stoma because the larynx that provides the protective sphincter is no longer present. The tracheal stoma prevents the aspiration of food and fluid into the lower respiratory tract. The patient has no voice but has normal swallowing. A total laryngectomy changes the manner in which airflow is used for breathing and speaking, as depicted in Figure 22-4. The patient has significant loss of the natural voice and the need to breathe through an opening (stoma) created in the lower neck. Complications that may occur include a salivary leak, wound infection from the development of a pharyngocutaneous fistula, stomal stenosis, and dysphagia secondary to esophageal stricture. In some cases, the patient may be a candidate for a near-total laryngectomy. In this situation, the patient would be a candidate for chemoradiation therapy regimens postoperatively. Voice preservation can be achieved in most cases and tends to be associated with overall improved quality of life (Boscolo-Rizzo, Maronato, Marchiori, et al., 2008). Advances in surgical techniques for treating laryngeal cancer may minimize the cosmetic and functional deficits previously seen with total laryngectomy. Some microlaryngeal surgery can be performed endoscopically.

Radiation Therapy

The goal of radiation therapy is to eradicate the cancer and preserve the function of the larynx. The decision to use radiation therapy is based on several factors, including the staging of the tumor and the patient's overall health status, lifestyle (including occupation), and personal preference. Excellent results have been achieved with radiation therapy in patients with early-stage glottic tumors when only one vocal cord is involved and there is normal mobility of the cord (i.e., with phonation), as well as in small supraglottic lesions. One of the benefits of radiation therapy is that patients retain a near-normal voice. A few may develop chondritis (inflammation of the cartilage) or stenosis; a small number may later require laryngectomy.

Radiation therapy may also be used preoperatively to reduce the tumor size. Radiation therapy is combined with surgery in advanced laryngeal cancer as adjunctive therapy to surgery or chemotherapy and as a palliative measure.

Complications from radiation therapy are a result of external radiation to the head and neck area, which may also include the parotid gland, which is responsible for mucus production. Symptoms may include acute mucositis, ulceration of the mucous membranes, pain, **xerostomia** (dry mouth), loss of taste, dysphasia, fatigue, and skin reactions. Later complications may include laryngeal necrosis, edema, and fibrosis (see Chapter 15).

Speech Therapy

The patient who undergoes a laryngectomy and the patient's family face potentially complex challenges, including significant changes in the ability to communicate. To minimize anxiety and frustration on the part of the patient and family, the loss or alteration of speech is discussed with them. To plan

postoperative communication strategies and speech therapy, the speech therapist or pathologist conducts a preoperative evaluation (Gilbert et al., 2009). During this time, the nurse discusses with the patient and family the methods of communication that will be available in the immediate postoperative period. These include writing, lip speaking and reading, and communication or word boards. A system of communication is established with the patient, family, nurse, and physician and is implemented consistently after surgery.

In addition, a long-term postoperative communication plan for **alaryngeal communication** is developed. The three most common techniques of alaryngeal communication are esophageal speech, artificial larynx (electric larynx), and tracheoesophageal puncture. Training in these techniques begins once medical clearance is obtained from the physician.

Esophageal Speech

Esophageal speech was the primary method of alaryngeal speech taught to patients until the 1980s. The patient needs the ability to compress air into the esophagus and expel it, setting off a vibration of the pharyngeal esophageal segment. The technique can be taught once the patient begins oral feedings, approximately 1 week after surgery. First, the patient learns to belch and is reminded to do so an hour after eating. Then, the technique is practiced repeatedly. Later, this conscious belching action is transformed into simple explosions of air from the esophagus for speech purposes. The speech therapist continues to work with the patient to make speech intelligible and as close to normal as possible. Because it takes a long time to become proficient, the success rate is low (Kazi, Pawar, Sayed, et al., 2010).

Artificial Larynx

If esophageal speech is not successful, or until the patient masters the technique, an electric larynx may be used for communication. This battery-powered apparatus projects sound into the oral cavity. When the mouth forms words (articulation), the sounds from the electric larynx become audible words. The voice that is produced sounds mechanical, and some words may be difficult to understand. The advantage is that the patient is able to communicate with relative ease while working to become proficient at either esophageal or tracheoesophageal puncture speech.

Tracheoesophageal Puncture

The third technique of alaryngeal speech is tracheoesophageal puncture (Fig. 22-5). This technique for voice restoration is simple and has few complications. It is associated with high phonation success, good phonation quality, and steady long-term results. This technique is the most widely used because the speech associated with it most resembles normal speech (the sound produced is a combination of esophageal speech and voice), and it is easily achieved either during the initial surgery to treat the tumor or at a later date (ACS, 2011). A valve is placed in the tracheal stoma to divert air into the esophagus and out the mouth. Once the puncture is surgically created and has healed, a voice prosthesis (Blom-Singer) is fitted over the puncture site. A speech therapist teaches the patient how to produce sounds. Moving the tongue and lips to form the sound into words produces speech as before. To prevent airway obstruction, the prosthesis is removed and cleaned when mucus builds up.

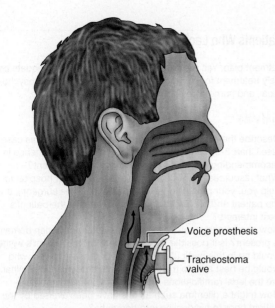

Voice prosthesis

Tracheostoma
valve

FIGURE 22-5 • Schematic representation of tracheoesophageal puncture speech. Air travels from the lung through a puncture in the posterior wall of the trachea into the esophagus and out the mouth. A voice prosthesis is fitted over the puncture site.

NURSING PROCESS

The Patient Undergoing Laryngectomy

Assessment

The nurse obtains a health history and assesses the patient's physical, psychosocial, and spiritual domains. The health history focuses on the following symptoms: hoarseness, sore throat, dyspnea, dysphagia, and pain or burning in the throat. The physical assessment includes a thorough head and neck examination with an emphasis on the patient's airway. In addition, the neck and thyroid are palpated for swelling, nodularity, or adenopathy.

The nurse also assesses the patient's general state of nutrition, including height and weight and body mass index and reviews laboratory values that assist in determining the patient's nutritional status (albumin, protein, glucose, and electrolyte levels). If treatment includes surgery, the nurse must know the nature of the surgery to plan appropriate care. If the patient is expected to have no voice as a result of the surgical procedure, a preoperative evaluation by the speech therapist is essential. The patient's ability to hear, see, read, and write is assessed. Visual impairment and functional illiteracy may create additional problems with communication and may require creative approaches to ensure that the patient is able to communicate any needs. Because alcohol abuse is a risk factor for cancer of the larynx, the patient's pattern of alcohol intake must be assessed. Patients who are accustomed to daily consumption of alcohol are at risk for alcohol withdrawal syndrome (delirium tremens) when alcohol intake is stopped suddenly.

In addition, the nurse assesses the psychological readiness of the patient and family (Chart 22-7). The fear of a diagnosis of cancer is compounded by the possibility of permanent voice loss and, in some cases, some degree of disfigurement. The nurse evaluates the patient's and family's knowledge of the planned surgical procedure and expected postoperative course and assesses their coping methods and support systems. The nurse assesses the patient's spirituality needs based on the patient's individual preferences, beliefs, and culture.

Diagnosis

Nursing Diagnoses

Based on the assessment data, major nursing diagnoses may include the following:

- Deficient knowledge about the surgical procedure and postoperative course
- Anxiety related to the diagnosis of cancer and impending surgery
- Ineffective airway clearance related to excess mucus production secondary to surgical alterations in the airway
- Impaired verbal communication related to anatomic deficit secondary to removal of the larynx and to edema
- Imbalanced nutrition: less than body requirements, related to inability to ingest food secondary to swallowing difficulties
- Disturbed body image and low self-esteem secondary to major neck surgery, change in appearance, and altered structure and function
- Self-care deficit related to pain, weakness, fatigue, musculoskeletal impairment related to surgical procedure and postoperative course

Collaborative Problems/Potential Complications

Based on the assessment data, potential complications may include the following:

- Respiratory distress (hypoxia, airway obstruction, tracheal edema)
- Hemorrhage, infection, and wound breakdown
- Aspiration
- Tracheostomal stenosis

Planning and Goals

The major goals for the patient may include attainment of an adequate level of knowledge, reduction in anxiety, maintenance of a patent airway (patient is able to handle own secretions), effective use of alternative means of communication, attainment of optimal levels of nutrition and hydration, improvement in body image and self-esteem, improved self-care management, and absence of complications.

Nursing Interventions

Providing Preoperative Patient Education

The diagnosis of laryngeal cancer often produces misconceptions and fears. Many people assume that loss of speech and disfigurement are inevitable with this condition. Once the physician explains the diagnosis and discusses treatment options with the patient and family, the nurse clarifies any misconceptions by identifying the location of the larynx, its function, the nature of the planned surgical procedure, and its effect on speech. Further, the patient's ability to sing, laugh, and whistle will be lost. Informational materials (written and audiovisual) about the surgery are given to the patient and family for review and reinforcement. If a complete

ETHICAL DILEMMA
Chart 22-7
Who Makes Difficult Health Care Decisions for Patients Who Lack Capacity?

Case Scenario

As a nurse working on a medical-surgical unit, you are caring for an 82-year-old man with a new diagnosis of advanced stage IV cancer of the larynx. The surgeon recommends a total laryngectomy for this patient to better control the disease. Although the patient lives at home, he has mild to moderate Alzheimer's disease and has recently experienced significant weight loss; he is debilitated and frail. He has a history of tobacco abuse and continues to smoke one pack of cigarettes per day. He is a widower with two living adult children: one daughter and one son. Because of his dementia, the patient is not considered competent to sign consent for his total laryngectomy. The patient's daughter has informed the surgeon that she will not agree to sign surgical consent for a total laryngectomy. The daughter has asked to speak with you regarding her concerns. She tells you that she knows for certain that her father would not want this surgery and would want to live at home and not in a skilled nursing facility. She is very concerned about the possible outcome of the surgery and states, "Who will take care of Dad after this? I work full-time, have three children to care for, and no husband. There is no one to help him recover from this." The patient's son agrees with the recommendation for a total laryngectomy and would be willing to sign surgical consent, but he lives out of state and cannot travel at this time. He is estranged from his sister. The patient does not have a designated health care surrogate or power of attorney.

Discussion

This patient has been diagnosed with a life-threatening illness and needs surgical intervention for control of the disease. He is unable to make medical decisions due to his dementia; in the absence of a spouse, his children are now responsible to function as his health care surrogates. He is unable to care for himself at home postoperatively. His children disagree regarding the recommended

treatment plan. Yet, the patient is entitled to receive adequate and timely treatment for his illness and appropriate physical, psychological, and home care should he undergo this procedure.

Analysis

- Describe the ethical principles that are in conflict in this case (see Chart 3-3). Which principle should have preeminence in recommending the best treatment plan for the patient?
- What resources might be available to you in your hospital to help you, your professional colleagues (e.g., the surgeon), and the patient and his family determine what is in the patient's best interests?
- How can you advocate for a patient's autonomy when dementia is present? Is it possible to determine what the patient's wishes would be in this particular situation? Of those involved, who would be best able to make this type of determination? What are the legal ramifications of this type of family dispute?
- How might a dilemma such as this have been averted by the patient prior to his decline into dementia?
- For whom do you feel an obligation to advocate for in this situation—the patient, the daughter, the son, or perhaps the surgeon? Does any one of these people merit your primary focus of concern, according to the American Nurses Association (2001) Code of Ethics?

Reference

American Nurses Association. (2001). *Code of ethics for nurses with interpretive statements*. Washington, DC: American Nurses Publishing, American Nurses Foundation/American Nurses Association.

Resources

See Chapter 3, Chart 3-6 for ethics resources.

---

laryngectomy is planned, the patient must understand that the natural voice will be lost, but that special training can provide a means for communicating. The patient needs to know that until training is started, communication will be possible by using the call light, by writing, or by using a special communication board. The interdisciplinary team conducts an initial assessment of the patient and family. In addition to the nurse in charge of the patient's care and the physician, the team might include an advanced practice nurse or nurse practitioner, speech therapist, respiratory therapist, social worker, dietitian, and home care nurse. The services of a spiritual advisor are made available to the patient and family, as appropriate.

The nurse also reviews equipment and treatments for postoperative care with the patient and family, teaches important coughing and deep-breathing exercises, and helps the patient perform return demonstrations. The nurse clarifies the patient's role in the postoperative and rehabilitation periods. The family's needs must also be addressed because family members are often responsible for complex care of the patient in the home.

Reducing Anxiety

Because surgery of the larynx is performed most often for a malignant tumor, the patient may have many questions: Will

the surgeon be able to remove all of the tumor? Is it cancer? Will I die? Will I choke? Will I suffocate? Will I ever speak again? What will I look like? Because of these and other questions, the psychological preparation of the patient is as important as the physical preparation.

Any patient undergoing surgery may have many fears. In laryngeal surgery, these fears may relate to the diagnosis of cancer and the possibility of permanent loss of the voice and disfigurement. The nurse provides the patient and family with opportunities to ask questions, verbalize feelings, and discuss perceptions. The nurse should address any questions and misconceptions the patient and family have. During the preoperative or postoperative period, a visit from someone who has had a laryngectomy may reassure the patient that people are available to assist and that rehabilitation is possible.

In the immediate postoperative period, the nurse attempts to spend uninterrupted time with the patient that is focused on building trust and reducing the patient's anxiety. Active listening provides an environment that promotes open communication and allows the patient to verbalize feelings. Clear instructions and explanations are given to the patient and family in a calm, reassuring manner. The nurse listens attentively, encourages the patient, and identifies and reduces environmental stressors. The nurse seeks to learn from the patient what activities promote feelings of comfort and assists the patient in such activities (e.g., listening to music, reading). Relaxation techniques such as guided imagery and meditation are often helpful. The nurse remains with the patient during episodes of severe anxiety and includes the patient in decision making.

Maintaining a Patent Airway

The nurse helps maintain a patent airway by positioning the patient in the semi-Fowler's or Fowler's position after recovery from anesthesia. This position decreases surgical edema and promotes lung expansion. Observing the patient for restlessness, labored breathing, apprehension, and increased pulse rate helps identify possible respiratory or circulatory problems. The nurse assesses the patient's lung sounds and reports changes that may indicate impending complications. Medications that depress respiration, particularly opioids, should be used cautiously. However, adequate use of analgesic medications is essential for pain relief because postoperative pain can result in shallow breathing and an ineffective cough (see Chapter 12 for discussion of pain management). The nurse encourages the patient to turn, cough, and take deep breaths. If necessary, suctioning may be performed to remove secretions, but disruption of suture lines must be avoided. The nurse also encourages and assists the patient with early ambulation to prevent atelectasis, pneumonia, and deep vein thrombosis. Pulse oximetry is used to monitor the patient's oxygen saturation level.

If a total laryngectomy was performed, a laryngectomy tube will most likely be in place. In some instances a laryngectomy tube is not used; in others it is used temporarily; and in many it is used permanently. The laryngectomy tube, which is shorter than a tracheostomy tube but has a larger diameter, is the patient's only airway. The care of this tube is similar to that for a tracheostomy tube (see Chapter 21). The nurse changes the inner cannula (if present) every 8 hours if it is disposable. Although nondisposable tubes are used infrequently, if one is used, the nurse cleans the inner cannula every 8 hours or more often as needed. If a tracheostomy tube without an inner cannula is used, humidification and suctioning of this tube are essential to prevent formation of mucus plugs. If a T-shaped laryngectomy tube is used, both sides of the T-tube should be suctioned to prevent obstruction due to copious secretions. The nurse should also use secure tracheostomy ties to prevent tube dislodgement. The nurse cleans the stoma daily with soap and water or another prescribed solution and a soft cloth or gauze, taking care to prevent water and soap or solution from entering the stoma. If a non–oil-based antibiotic ointment is prescribed, it is applied around the stoma and suture line. If crusting appears around the stoma, the crusts are removed with sterile tweezers and additional ointment is applied.

Wound drains, inserted during surgery, may be in place to assist in removal of fluid and air from the surgical site. Suction also may be used, but cautiously, to avoid trauma to the surgical site and incision. The nurse observes, measures, and records drainage. When drainage is less than 30 mL/day for 2 consecutive days, the physician usually removes the drains.

Frequently, the patient coughs up large amounts of mucus through this opening. Because air passes directly into the trachea without being warmed and moistened by the upper respiratory mucosa, the tracheobronchial tree compensates by secreting excessive amounts of mucus. Therefore, the patient has frequent coughing episodes and may develop a brassy-sounding, mucus-producing cough. The nurse reassures the patient that these problems will diminish in time as the tracheobronchial mucosa adapts to the altered physiology.

After the patient coughs, the tracheostomy opening must be wiped clean and clear of mucus. A simple gauze dressing, washcloth, or even paper towel (because of its size and absorbency) worn below the tracheostomy may serve as a barrier to protect the clothing from the copious mucus that the patient may initially expel.

One of the most important factors in decreasing cough, mucus production, and crusting around the stoma is adequate humidification of the environment. Mechanical humidifiers and aerosol generators (nebulizers) increase the humidity and are important for the patient's comfort. The laryngectomy tube may be removed when the stoma is well healed, within 3 to 6 weeks after surgery. The nurse teaches the patient how to clean and change the tube (see Chapter 21) and remove secretions.

Promoting Alternative Communication Methods

Establishing an effective means of communication is usually the ultimate goal in the rehabilitation of the laryngectomy patient. To understand and anticipate the patient's postoperative needs, the nurse works with the patient, speech therapist, and family to encourage the use of alternative communication methods. These means of communication are established preoperatively and must be used consistently by all personnel who come in contact with the patient postoperatively. The patient is now unable to use an intercom system. A call bell or hand bell must be placed within easy reach of the patient. A Magic Slate is often used for communication, and the nurse documents which hand the patient uses for writing so that the opposite arm can be used for IV infusions. (To ensure the patient's privacy, the nurse discards notes used for communication.) If the patient cannot write, a picture-word-phrase board, handheld electronic devices, or hand signals can be used.

Writing everything or communicating through gestures can be very time consuming and frustrating. The patient must be given adequate time to communicate his or her needs. The patient may become impatient and angry when not understood.

Promoting Adequate Nutrition and Hydration

Postoperatively, the patient may not be permitted to eat or drink for at least 7 days (Ackerberg, 2011). Alternative sources of nutrition and hydration include IV fluids, enteral feedings through a nasogastric or gastrostomy tube, and parenteral nutrition.

When the patient is ready to start oral feedings, a speech therapist or radiologist may conduct a swallow study (a video fluoroscopy radiology procedure) to evaluate the patient's risk of aspiration. Once the patient is cleared for oral feedings, the nurse explains that thick liquids will be used first because they are easy to swallow. Different swallowing maneuvers are attempted with various food consistencies. Once the patient is cleared for food intake, the nurse stays with the patient during initial oral feedings and keeps a suction setup at the bedside for needed suctioning. The nurse instructs the patient to avoid sweet foods, which increase salivation and suppress the appetite. Solid foods are introduced as tolerated. The patient is instructed to rinse the mouth with warm water or mouthwash after oral feedings and to brush the teeth frequently.

Because taste and smell are so closely related, taste sensations are altered for a while after surgery because inhaled air passes directly into the trachea, bypassing the nose and the olfactory end organs. In time, however, the patient usually accommodates to this change and olfactory sensation adapts, often with return of interest in eating. The nurse observes the patient for any difficulty in swallowing, particularly when eating resumes, and reports its occurrence to the physician.

The patient's weight and laboratory data are monitored to ensure that nutritional and fluid intake are adequate. In addition, skin turgor and vital signs are assessed for signs of decreased fluid volume.

Promoting Positive Body Image and Self-Esteem

Disfiguring surgery and an altered communication pattern are threats to a patient's body image and self-esteem. The reaction of family members and friends is a major concern for the patient. The nurse encourages the patient to express feelings about the changes brought about by surgery, particularly feelings related to fear, anger, depression, and isolation. Encouraging the use of previous effective coping strategies may be helpful. Referral to a support group, such as the International Association of Laryngectomees (IAL), WebWhispers, and I Can Cope (through the ACS) may help the patient and family deal with the changes in their lives. Information about these support groups can be found in the Resource section at the end of the chapter.

Promoting Self-Care Management

A positive approach along with promotion of self-care activities is important when caring for the patient. The patient should begin participating in self-care activities as soon as possible. The nurse assesses the patient's readiness for decision making and encourages the patient to participate actively in performing care. The nurse provides positive reinforcement when the patient makes an effort in self-care. The nurse needs to be a good listener and a support to the family, especially when explaining the tubes, dressings, and drains that are in place postoperatively.

Monitoring and Managing Potential Complications

The potential complications after laryngectomy include respiratory distress and hypoxia, hemorrhage, infection, wound breakdown, aspiration, and tracheostomal stenosis.

Respiratory Distress and Hypoxia. The nurse monitors the patient for signs and symptoms of respiratory distress and hypoxia, particularly restlessness, irritation, agitation, confusion, tachypnea, the use of accessory muscles, and decreased oxygen saturation on pulse oximetry (SpO_2). Any change in respiratory status requires immediate intervention. Hypoxia may cause restlessness and an initial rise in blood pressure; this is followed by hypotension and somnolence. Cyanosis is a late sign of hypoxia. Obstruction needs to be ruled out immediately by suctioning and by having the patient cough and breathe deeply. Hypoxia and airway obstruction, if not treated immediately, are life threatening.

Other nursing measures include repositioning of the patient to ensure an open airway and administering oxygen as prescribed and used with caution in patients with chronic obstructive pulmonary disease. The nurse should always be prepared for possible intubation and mechanical ventilation. The nurse must be knowledgeable about the hospital's emergency code protocols and skilled in the use of emergency equipment. The nurse must remain with the patient at all times during respiratory distress and initiate a call to the rapid response team as necessary.

Hemorrhage. Bleeding from the drains at the surgical site or with tracheal suctioning may signal the occurrence of hemorrhage. The nurse promptly notifies the surgeon of any active bleeding, which can occur at a variety of sites, including the surgical site, drains, and trachea. Rupture of the carotid artery is especially dangerous. Should this occur, the nurse must apply direct pressure over the artery, summon assistance, and provide emotional support to the patient until the vessel is ligated. The nurse monitors vital signs for changes, particularly increased pulse rate, decreased blood pressure, and rapid deep respirations. Cold, clammy, pale skin may indicate active bleeding. IV fluids and blood components may be administered and other measures implemented to prevent or treat hemorrhagic shock. (Management of the patient with shock is discussed in detail in Chapter 14.)

Infection. The nurse monitors the patient for signs of postoperative infection. These include an increase in temperature and pulse, a change in the type of wound drainage, and increased areas of redness or tenderness at the surgical site. Other signs include purulent drainage, odor, and increased wound drainage. The nurse monitors the patient's white blood cell (WBC) count; a rise in WBCs may indicate the body's effort to combat infection. In older adult patients, infection can be present without an increase in the patient's WBC count; therefore, the nurse must monitor the patient for more subtle signs, such as lethargy, weakness, and decreased appetite (Tingström, Milberg, Sund-Levander, et al., 2010). WBCs are suppressed in the patient with decreased immune function (e.g., patients with HIV infection, or those receiving chemotherapy or radiation therapy); this predisposes the patient to a severe infection and sepsis. Antimicrobial (antibiotic) medications must be administered as scheduled. All suspicious drainage is cultured, and the patient may be placed in isolation as indicated. Strategies are implemented to minimize the exposure of the patient to microorganisms and their spread to others. The nurse reports any significant change in the patient's status to the surgeon.

Wound Breakdown. Wound breakdown caused by infection, poor wound healing, development of a fistula, radiation therapy, or tumor growth can create a life-threatening emergency. The carotid artery, which is close to the stoma, may rupture from erosion if the wound does not heal properly. The nurse observes the stoma area for wound breakdown, hematoma, and bleeding and reports their occurrence to the surgeon. If wound breakdown occurs, the patient must be monitored carefully and identified as at high risk for carotid hemorrhage.

Aspiration. The patient who has undergone a laryngectomy is at risk for aspiration and aspiration pneumonia due to depressed cough, the sedating effects of anesthetic and analgesic medications, alteration in the airway, impaired swallowing, and the administration of tube feedings. The nurse assesses for the presence of nausea and administers antiemetic medications, as prescribed. The nurse keeps a suction setup available in the hospital and instructs the family to do so at home for use if needed. Patients receiving tube feedings are positioned with the head of the bed at 30 degrees or higher during feedings and for 30 to 45 minutes after tube feedings. Patients receiving oral feedings are positioned with the head of the bed in an upright position for 30 to 45 minutes after feedings. For patients with a nasogastric or gastrostomy tube, the placement of the tube and residual gastric volume must be checked before each feeding. High amounts of residual volume (greater than 50% of previous intake) indicate delayed gastric emptying; this can lead to reflux and aspiration (Metheny, Mills, & Stewart, 2012). Signs or symptoms of aspiration are reported to the physician immediately.

Tracheostomal Stenosis. Tracheostomal stenosis is an abnormal narrowing of the trachea or the tracheostomy stoma. Infection at the stoma site, excessive traction on the tracheostomy tube by the connecting tubing, and persistent high tracheostomy cuff pressure are risk factors for tracheostomal stenosis. The incidence of this condition varies widely, and it is often preventable. The nurse assesses the patient's stoma for signs and symptoms of infection and reports any evidence of this to the physician immediately. Tracheostomy care is performed routinely. The nurse assesses the connecting tubing (e.g., ventilation tubing) and secures the tubing to avoid excessive traction on the patient's tracheostomy. The nurse ensures that the tracheostomy cuff is deflated (for a patient with a cuffed tube) except for short periods, such as when the patient is eating or taking medications.

Promoting Home and Community-Based Care

Educating Patients About Self-Care. The nurse has an important role in the recovery and rehabilitation of the patient who has had a laryngectomy. To facilitate the patient's ability to manage self-care, discharge instruction begins as soon as the patient is able to participate. Nursing care and patient education in the hospital, outpatient setting, and rehabilitation or

long-term care facility must take into consideration the many emotions, physical changes, and lifestyle changes experienced by the patient. In preparing the patient to go home, the nurse assesses the patient's readiness to learn and the level of knowledge about self-care management. The nurse also reassures the patient and family that most self-care management strategies can be mastered. The patient needs to learn a variety of self-care behaviors, including tracheostomy and stoma care, wound care, and oral hygiene. The nurse also instructs the patient about the need for adequate dietary intake, safe hygiene, and recreational activities.

Tracheostomy and Stoma Care. The nurse provides specific instructions to the patient and family about what to expect with a tracheostomy and its management. The nurse instructs the patient and caregiver how to perform suctioning and emergency measures and tracheostomy and stoma care. The nurse stresses the importance of humidification at home and instructs the family to obtain and set up a humidification system before the patient returns home. (See Chapter 21 for details about tracheostomy care.)

Hygiene and Safety Measures. The nurse instructs the patient and family about safety precautions that are needed because of the changes in structure and function resulting from the surgery. Special precautions are needed in the shower to prevent water from entering the stoma. Wearing a loose-fitting plastic bib over the tracheostomy or simply holding a hand over the opening is effective. Swimming is not recommended because a person with a laryngectomy can drown without submerging his or her face. Barbers and beauticians need to be alerted so that hair sprays, loose hair, and powder do not get near the stoma, because they can block or irritate the trachea and possibly cause infection. These self-care points are summarized in Chart 22-8.

Chart 22-8

HOME CARE CHECKLIST

The Patient With a Laryngectomy

At the completion of home care education, the patient or caregiver will be able to:	PATIENT	CAREGIVER
• Demonstrate methods to clear the airway and handle secretions.	✔	✔
• Explain the rationale for maintaining adequate humidification with a humidifier or nebulizer.	✔	✔
• Demonstrate how to clean the skin around the stoma and how to use ointments and tweezers to remove encrustations.	✔	✔
• State the rationale for wearing a loose-fitting protective cloth at the stoma.	✔	✔
• Discuss the need to avoid cold air from air-conditioning and the environment to prevent irritation of the airway.	✔	✔
• Demonstrate safe technique in changing the laryngectomy/tracheostomy tube.	✔	✔
• Identify the signs and symptoms of wound infection and state what to do about them.	✔	✔
• Describe safety or emergency measures to implement in case of breathing difficulty or bleeding.	✔	✔
• State the rationale for wearing or carrying special medical identification and ways to obtain help in an emergency.	✔	✔
• Explain the importance of covering the stoma when showering or bathing.	✔	✔
• Identify fluid and caloric needs.	✔	✔
• Describe mouth care and discuss its importance.	✔	✔
• Demonstrate alternative communication methods.	✔	✔
• Identify support groups and agency resources.	✔	✔
• State the need for regular checkups and reporting of any problems immediately.	✔	✔

The nurse educates the patient and caregiver about the signs and symptoms of infection and identifies indications that require contacting the physician after discharge. A discussion regarding cleanliness and infection control behaviors is essential. The nurse educates the patient and family to use hand hygiene before and after caring for the tracheostomy, to use tissue to remove mucus, and to dispose of soiled dressings and equipment properly. If the patient's surgery included cervical lymph node dissection, the nurse instructs the patient about how to perform exercises to strengthen the shoulder and neck muscles.

Recreation and exercise are important for the patient's well-being and quality of life, and all but very strenuous exercise can be enjoyed safely. Avoidance of strenuous exercise and fatigue is important because the patient will have more difficulty speaking when tired, which can be discouraging. Additional safety points to address include the need for the patient to wear or carry medical identification, such as a bracelet or card, to alert medical personnel to the special requirements for resuscitation should this need arise. If resuscitation is needed, direct mouth-to-stoma ventilation should be performed. For home emergency situations, prerecorded emergency messages for police, the fire department, or other rescue services can be kept near the phone to be used quickly.

The nurse instructs and encourages the patient to perform oral care frequently to prevent halitosis and infection.

If the patient is receiving radiation therapy, synthetic saliva may be required because of decreased saliva production. The nurse instructs the patient to drink water or sugar-free liquids throughout the day and to use a humidifier at home. Brushing the teeth or dentures and rinsing the mouth several times a day will assist in maintaining proper oral hygiene.

Continuing Care. Referral for home care is an important aspect of postoperative care for the patient who has had a laryngectomy and will assist the patient and family in the transition to the home. The home care nurse assesses the patient's general health status and the ability of the patient and family to care for the stoma and tracheostomy. The nurse assesses the surgical incisions, nutritional and respiratory status, and adequacy of pain management. The nurse assesses for signs and symptoms of complications and the patient's and family's knowledge of signs and symptoms to be reported to the physician. During the home visit, the nurse identifies and addresses other learning needs and concerns of the patient and family, such as adaptation to physical, lifestyle, and functional changes, as well as the patient's progress with learning and using new communication strategies (Chart 22-9). The nurse assesses the patient's psychological status as well. The home care nurse reinforces previous instructions and provides reassurance and support to the patient and family caregivers as needed.

Chart 22-9

NURSING RESEARCH PROFILE

The Impact of Total Laryngectomy: The Patient's Perspective

Noonan, B., & Haggerty, J. (2010). The impact of total laryngectomy: The patient's perspective. *Oncology Nursing Forum, 37*(3), 293–301.

Purpose

Patients who undergo total laryngectomy for treatment of laryngeal cancer experience significant psychological, physical, social, and emotional challenges. The purpose of this study was to describe the experience of a total laryngectomy from the patient's perspective.

Design

This descriptive qualitative study investigated the impact a total laryngectomy had on patients' lives, moods, and self-reported physical health. Ten participants (eight male, two female) who had a total laryngectomy between 6 months and 7 years before data collection commenced, spoke English, and communicated using tracheoesophageal speech were purposively recruited for this study from one hospital in the Republic of Ireland. Data were collected by semistructured, open-ended 40–60 minute interviews in the participants' homes or the investigator's hospital office, based upon participants' preferences. Data were analyzed with descriptive content analysis.

Findings

Participants identified difficulties and concerns postlaryngectomy that were categorized as functional difficulties and psychological concerns. Functional difficulties included physical symptoms and speech difficulties. Physical symptoms that

participants identified as difficult to contend with included sputum or phlegm production, difficulty swallowing, limitations eating in public, a need for careful eating, recurrent candidal infections, and low energy levels. Some speech difficulties identified included difficulties with speech, clumsy communication, very awkward speech, speech "not the same," "can't chat," and speech that was "slow in coming." Psychological concerns included symptoms of depression as well as feelings of regret tempered by expressions of personal resolve.

Nursing Implications

The findings of this study provide nurses with insights into problems and concerns faced by patients who have undergone total laryngectomy. Difficulty with sputum production and a need for frequent suctioning was a concern expressed by the participants in this study. In addition, difficulty with speech and the quality of speech was a major concern expressed by these participants, even though all of them had voice restored with transesophageal speech. Presumably, the loss of one's natural voice affects one's quality of life. Although all participants reported depression, depression lessened with increased time. Interestingly, however, psychological distress was not limited to the immediate postoperative period. Despite these symptoms of psychological distress, most participants reported a strong resolve for life and a positive outlook on the future.

These findings indicate that patients who have undergone total laryngectomy need support during the preoperative period, the postoperative period, the rehabilitation period, and beyond. Strategies for support and management of patients' concerns, including collaborative care and referral as needed following a total laryngectomy, should be a priority for nurses and the health care team.

The person who has had a laryngectomy should have regular physical examinations and seek advice concerning any problems related to recovery and rehabilitation. The nurse also reminds the patient to participate in health promotion activities and health screening and about the importance of keeping scheduled appointments with the physician, speech therapist, and other health care providers.

Evaluation

Expected patient outcomes may include the following:

1. Demonstrates an adequate level of knowledge, verbalizing an understanding of the surgical procedure and performing self-care adequately
2. Demonstrates less anxiety
   a. Expresses a sense of hope
   b. Is aware of available community organizations and agencies that provide patient education and support groups
   c. Participates in support group for people with a laryngectomy
3. Maintains a clear airway and handles own secretions; also demonstrates practical, safe, and correct technique for cleaning and changing the tracheostomy or laryngectomy tube
4. Acquires effective communication techniques
   a. Uses assistive devices and strategies for communication (Magic Slate, call bell, picture board, sign language, speech reading, handheld electronic devices)
   b. Follows the recommendations of the speech therapist
   c. Demonstrates ability to communicate with new communication strategy
   d. Reports availability of prerecorded messages to summon emergency assistance by telephone
5. Maintains adequate nutrition and adequate fluid intake
6. Exhibits improved body image, self-esteem, and self-concept
   a. Expresses feelings and concerns
   b. Participates in self-care and decision making
   c. Accepts information about support group
7. Adheres to rehabilitation and home care program
   a. Practices recommended speech therapy
   b. Demonstrates proper methods for caring for stoma and laryngectomy or tracheostomy tube (if present)
   c. Verbalizes understanding of symptoms that require medical attention
   d. States safety measures to take in emergencies
   e. Performs oral hygiene as prescribed
8. Absence of complications
   a. Demonstrates a patent airway
   b. No bleeding from surgical site and minimal bleeding from drains; vital signs (blood pressure, temperature, pulse, respiratory rate) are normal
   c. No redness, tenderness, or purulent drainage at surgical site
   d. No wound breakdown
   e. Clear breath sounds; oxygen saturation level within acceptable range; chest x-ray clear
   f. No indications of infection, stenosis, or obstruction of tracheal stoma

Critical Thinking Exercises

1 **pq** A 21-year-old female nursing student comes to the student health clinic with complaints of a sore throat. She states that she had a fever last night but does not have an elevated temperature at present. She states she has not been feeling well and is tired "all the time" but attributes these symptoms to studying late into the night for midterm examinations this week. She states she has difficulty swallowing and has not had anything to eat or drink for 2 days. She says she does not want to miss her clinical because she does not want to have to make it up. What further questions do you have regarding her symptoms? What is your priority focus for your physical examination? What diagnostic tests and treatments may you anticipate?

2 **ebp** A 59-year-old man presents to the family health clinic because of increased fatigue and difficulty staying awake during the day. His wife, who accompanies him, tells you that he "stops breathing and then makes unusual loud noises" at night and has generally become more irritable. The patient is obese, with a body mass index of 38. You suspect that this patient may have OSA. What risk factors for OSA will your health history focus on? What are the common signs and symptoms of OSA? Describe how a patient with OSA is diagnosed and the treatment(s) that might be prescribed. What is the strength of the evidence that commonly prescribed therapies (such as CPAP) may be effective in alleviating symptoms and improving quality of life for patients with OSA?

3 **pq** You are a spectator at a baseball game. A pitched baseball forcefully hits the batter in the face, striking him in the nose. You rush to aid the batter and suspect that there is a fractured nose. Briefly describe what you would do in this situation. What are your priority assessments? What are the signs and symptoms of a fractured nose? What are your priority interventions?

4 As a home health nurse, you are caring for a 75-year-old male patient who has undergone a total laryngectomy for the treatment of cancer of the larynx. You are responsible to provide patient education regarding tracheostomy care and gastric tube feedings. The overall plan is for the patient to begin to assume responsibility for his own care and to consider speech therapy. The patient lives alone in a rural area and has no next of kin nearby. What are your priorities in terms of assessment of this patient? What is your plan to address the patient's fear, anxiety, communication, and nutrition needs?

Brunner Suite Resources

Explore these additional resources to enhance learning for this chapter:
- NCLEX-Style Questions and Other Resources on thePoint, http://thePoint.lww.com/Brunner13e
- Study Guide
- PrepU
- Clinical Handbook
- Handbook of Laboratory and Diagnostic Tests

References

*Asterisk indicates nursing research.

Books

Bickley, L. S., & Szilagyi, P. G. (2009). *Bates' guide to physical examination and history taking* (10th ed.). Philadelphia: Lippincott Williams & Wilkins.

De Vita, V., Hellman, S., & Rosenberg, S. (Eds.). (2011). *Cancer: Principles and practice of oncology* (9th ed.). Philadelphia: Lippincott Williams & Wilkins.

Gilbert, R., Devries-Aboud, M., Winquist, E., et al. (2009). *The management of head and neck cancer in Ontario: Organizational and clinical practice guideline recommendations.* Toronto, Ontario: Cancer Care Ontario.

Tierney, L., McPhee, S. J., & Papadakis, M. (Eds.). (2012). *Current medical diagnosis and treatment* (51st ed.). New York: McGraw-Hill.

Journals and Electronic Documents

Ackerberg, T. (2011). Nutritional management after total laryngectomy. *South African Journal of Clinical Nutrition, 24*(2), 107–108.

American Cancer Society. (2011). *What are the risk factors for laryngeal and hypopharyngeal cancers?* Available at: www.cancer.org/Cancer/Laryngealand-HypopharyngealCancer/DetailedGuide/laryngeal-and-hypopharyngeal-cancer-risk-factors

American Cancer Society. (2012). *Cancer facts and figures.* Available at: www.cancer.org/Research/CancerFactsFigures/index

American Sleep Apnea Association. (2011). *Obstructive sleep apnea.* Available at: www.sleepapnea.org/learn/sleep-apnea/obstructive-sleep-apnea.html

Aring, A., & Chan, M. (2011). Acute rhinosinusitis in adults. *American Family Physician, 83*(9), 1057–1063.

Aurora, R., Casey, K., Kristo, D., et al. (2010). Practice parameters for the surgical modifications of the upper airway for obstructive sleep apnea in adults. *Sleep, 33*(10), 1408–1413.

Barrett, B., Brown, R., Rakel, D., et al. (2011). Placebo effects and the common cold: A randomized controlled trial. *Annals of Family Medicine, 9*(4), 312–322.

Becker, D. (2012). *Nasal and septal fractures.* Available at: emedicine.medscape.com/article/878595-overview

Boscolo-Rizzo, P., Maronato, F., Marchiori, C., et al. (2008). Long-term quality of life after total laryngectomy and postoperative radiotherapy versus concurrent chemoradiotherapy for laryngeal preservation. *Laryngoscope, 118*(2), 300–306.

Brook, I. (2012). *Chronic sinusitis.* Available at: emedicine.medscape.com/article/232791-overview

Brook, I., & Hausfield, J. (2011). Microbiology of acute and chronic maxillary sinusitis in smokers and nonsmokers. *Annals of Otology, Rhinology, Laryngology, 120*(11), 707–717.

Centers for Disease Control and Prevention. (2011). *Common cold (viral rhinitis).* Available at: www.intelihealth.com/IH/ihtIH/WSIHW000/9339/10974.htm

Chadrabarti, A., Denning, D., Ferguson, B., et al. (2009). Fungal rhinosinusitis: A categorization and definitional schema addressing current controversies. *Laryngoscope, 119*(9), 1809–1818.

Choby, B. (2009). Diagnosis and treatment of streptococcal pharyngitis. *American Family Physician, 79*(5), 383–390.

Chow, A. W., Benninger, M. S., Brook, I., et al. (2012). IDSA clinical practice guideline for acute bacterial rhinosinusitis in children and adults. *Clinical Infectious Diseases, 58*(4), e72–e112.

Downey, R. (2012). *Obstructive sleep apnea.* Available at: emedicine.medscape.com/article/295807-overview

Gerber, M., Baltimore, R., Eaton, C., et al. (2009). Preventing rheumatic fever and diagnosis in the treatment of acute streptococcal pharyngitis. *Circulation, 119*(11), 1541–1551.

Hu, L., Wang, D., & Yu, H. (2009). Isolated sphenoid fungal sinusitis and vision loss: The case for early intervention. *Journal of Laryngology and Otology, 123*(2), 1–4.

Kazi, R., Pawar, P., Sayed, S. I., et al. (2010). Perspectives on voice rehabilitation following total laryngectomy. *European Journal of Cancer Care, 19*(6), 703–705.

Marcus, E., Caine, Y., Hamdan, K., et al. (2006). Nasogastric tube syndrome: A life-threatening laryngeal obstruction in a 72-year-old patient. *Age & Ageing, 35*(5), 538–539.

*Metheny, N., Mills, A., & Stewart, B. (2012). Monitoring for intolerance to gastric tube feedings: A national survey. *American Journal of Critical Care, 21*(2), 33–40.

National Institute of Allergy and Infectious Diseases. (2011). *Common cold.* Available at: www3.niaid.nih.gov/healthscience/healthtopics/colds/

Nguyen, Q. A. (2011). *Epistaxis.* Available at: emedicine.medscape.com/article/863220-overview

*Noonan, B., & Haggerty, J. (2010). The impact of total laryngectomy: The patient's perspective. *Oncology Nursing Forum, 37*(3), 293–301.

Park, J., Ramar, L., & Olson, E. (2011). Update on definition, consequences and management of obstructive sleep apnea. *Mayo Clinic Proceedings, 86*(6), 549–555.

Patel, A. (2012). *Functional endoscopic sinus surgery.* Available at: emedicine.medscape.com/article/863420-oveview

Pawankar, R., Canonica, G., Holgate, S., et al. (2011). *World Allergy Organization: WAO white book on allergy 2011-2012: Executive summary.* Available at: www.worldallergy.org/publications/wao_white_book.pdf

Regan, E., & Nevius, K. (2012). Getting back in touch with tonsillectomy. *OR Nurse, 6*(2), 16–24.

Regan, N. (2008). Diagnosing rhinitis: Viral and allergic characteristics. *Nurse Practitioner, 33*(9), 20–27.

Rosenfeld, R. M., Andes, D., Bhattacharyya, M., et al. (2007). Clinical practice guideline: Adult sinusitis. *Otolaryngology Head & Neck Surgery, 137*(3 Suppl.), S1–S31.

Tan, A. J. (2012). *Peritonsillar abscess in emergency medicine.* Available at: emedicine.medscape.com/article/764188-overview

*Tingström, P., Milberg, A., Sund-Levander, M., et al. (2010). Early and nonspecific signs and symptoms of infection in institutionalized elderly: Perceptions of nursing assistants. *Journal of Caring Sciences, 24*(1), 24–31.

Upton, D., Welham, N., Kuo, J., et al. (2011) Chronic rhinosinusitis with nasal polyps: A proteomic analysis. *Annals of Otology, Rhinology & Laryngology, 120*(12), 780–786.

Williams, R. (2011). *Upper respiratory infection.* Available at: www.localhealth.com/article/upper-respiratory-infection

Wood, S. (2011). Nasal congestion & rhinitis. *Practice Nurse, 41*(7), 11–15.

Resources

American Academy of Allergy, Asthma & Immunology (AAAAI), www.aaaai.org

American Academy of Otolaryngology–Head and Neck Surgery, www.entnet.org

American Cancer Society, www.cancer.org

American Lung Association, www.lungusa.org

American Sleep Apnea Association (ASAA), www.sleepapnea.org/info/index.html

International Association of Laryngectomees (IAL), www.theial.com/ial/

National Cancer Institute (NCI), www.cancernet.nci.nih.gov

National Comprehensive Cancer Network (NCCN), www.nccn.org/about/contact.asp

National Heart, Lung, and Blood Institute (NHBLI), www.nhlbi.nih.gov

National Institute of Allergy and Infectious Diseases (NIAID), www.niaid.nih.gov

National Sleep Foundation, www.sleepfoundation.org

WebWhispers, www.webwhispers.org

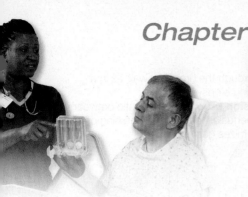

23

Management of Patients With Chest and Lower Respiratory Tract Disorders

Glossary

acute lung injury: an umbrella term for hypoxemic respiratory failure; acute respiratory distress syndrome is a severe form of acute lung injury

acute respiratory distress syndrome (ARDS): nonspecific pulmonary response to a variety of pulmonary and nonpulmonary insults to the lung; characterized by interstitial infiltrates, alveolar hemorrhage, atelectasis, decreased compliance, and refractory hypoxemia

asbestosis: diffuse lung fibrosis resulting from exposure to asbestos fibers

aspiration: inhalation of either oropharyngeal or gastric contents into the lower airways

atelectasis: collapse or airless condition of the alveoli caused by hypoventilation, obstruction to the airways, or compression

central cyanosis: bluish discoloration of the skin or mucous membranes due to hemoglobin carrying reduced amounts of oxygen

consolidation: lung tissue that has become more solid in nature due to collapse of alveoli or infectious process (pneumonia)

cor pulmonale: "heart of the lungs"; enlargement of the right ventricle from hypertrophy or dilation or as a secondary response to disorders that affect the lungs

empyema: accumulation of purulent material in the pleural space

fine-needle aspiration: insertion of a needle through the chest wall to obtain cells of a mass or tumor; usually performed under fluoroscopy or chest computed tomography guidance

hemoptysis: the coughing up of blood from the lower respiratory tract

hemothorax: partial or complete collapse of the lung due to blood accumulating in the pleural space; may occur after surgery or trauma

induration: an abnormally hard lesion or reaction, as in a positive tuberculin skin test

open lung biopsy: biopsy of lung tissue performed through a limited thoracotomy incision

orthopnea: shortness of breath when reclining or in the supine position

pleural effusion: abnormal accumulation of fluid in the pleural space

pleural friction rub: localized grating or creaking sound caused by the rubbing together of inflamed parietal and visceral pleurae

pleural space: the area between the parietal and visceral pleurae; a potential space

pneumothorax: partial or complete collapse of the lung due to positive pressure in the pleural space

pulmonary edema: increase in the amount of extravascular fluid in the lung

pulmonary embolism: obstruction of the pulmonary vasculature with an embolus; embolus may be due to blood clot, air bubbles, or fat droplets

purulent: consisting of, containing, or discharging pus

restrictive lung disease: disease of the lung that causes a decrease in lung volumes

tension pneumothorax: pneumothorax characterized by increasing positive pressure in the pleural space with each breath; this is an emergency situation, and the positive pressure needs to be decompressed or released immediately

(continues on page 570)

thoracentesis: insertion of a needle into the pleural space to remove fluid that has accumulated and decrease pressure on the lung tissue; may also be used diagnostically to identify potential causes of a pleural effusion

transbronchial: through the bronchial wall, as in a transbronchial lung biopsy
ventilation–perfusion ratio ($\dot{V}/\dot{Q}$): the ratio between ventilation and perfusion in the lung; matching of ventilation to perfusion optimizes gas exchange

Conditions affecting the chest and lower respiratory tract range from acute problems to chronic disorders. Many of these disorders are serious and often life threatening. Patients with lower respiratory tract disorders require care from nurses with astute assessment and clinical management skills as well as knowledge of evidence-based practice. Nurses must also understand the impact of the particular disorder on the patient's quality of life and ability to carry out usual activities of daily living. Patient and family education is an important nursing intervention in the management of all lower respiratory tract disorders.

ATELECTASIS

Atelectasis refers to closure or collapse of alveoli and often is described in relation to x-ray findings and/or clinical signs and symptoms. It is one of the most commonly encountered abnormalities seen on a chest x-ray (Stark, 2012). Atelectasis may be acute or chronic and may cover a broad range of pathophysiologic changes, from microatelectasis (which is not detectable on chest x-ray) to macroatelectasis with loss of segmental, lobar, or overall lung volume. The most commonly described atelectasis is acute atelectasis, which occurs most often in the postoperative setting or in people who are immobilized and have a shallow, monotonous breathing pattern (Lamar, 2012). Excess secretions or mucus plugs may also cause obstruction of airflow and result in atelectasis in an area of the lung. Atelectasis also is observed in patients with a chronic airway obstruction that impedes or blocks the flow of air to an area of the lung (e.g., obstructive atelectasis in the patient with lung cancer that is invading or compressing the airways). This type of atelectasis is more insidious and slower in onset (Johnson & Conde, 2012; Stark, 2012).

Pathophysiology

Atelectasis may occur in adults as a result of reduced ventilation (nonobstructive atelectasis) or any blockage that obstructs passage of air to and from the alveoli (obstructive atelectasis), thus reducing alveolar ventilation (Stark, 2012). Obstructive atelectasis is the most common type and results from reabsorption of gas (trapped alveolar air is absorbed into the bloodstream); no additional air can enter into the alveoli because of the blockage. As a result, the affected portion of the lung becomes airless and the alveoli collapse. Causes of atelectasis include foreign body, tumor or growth in an airway, altered breathing patterns, retained secretions, pain, alterations in small airway function, prolonged supine positioning, increased abdominal pressure, reduced lung volumes due to musculoskeletal or neurologic disorders, restrictive defects, and specific surgical procedures (e.g., upper abdominal, thoracic, or open heart surgery) (Johnson & Conde, 2012).

Patients are at high risk for atelectasis postoperatively because of several factors. A monotonous, low tidal breathing pattern may cause small airway closure and alveolar collapse. This can result from the effects of anesthesia or analgesic agents, supine positioning, splinting of the chest wall because of pain, or abdominal distention. Secretion retention, airway obstruction, and an impaired cough reflex may also occur, or patients may be reluctant to cough because of pain (Johnson & Conde, 2012). Figure 23-1 shows the mechanisms and consequences of acute atelectasis in postoperative patients.

Atelectasis resulting from bronchial obstruction by secretions may also occur in patients with impaired cough mechanisms (e.g., musculoskeletal or neurologic disorders) as well as in those who are debilitated and bedridden. In addition, atelectasis may develop because of excessive pressure on the lung tissue (i.e., compressive atelectasis), which restricts normal lung expansion on inspiration (Stark, 2012). Such pressure can be produced by fluid accumulating within the pleural space (**pleural effusion**), air in the pleural space (**pneumothorax**), or blood in the pleural space (**hemothorax**). The **pleural space** is the area between the parietal and the visceral pleurae. Pressure may also be produced by a pericardium distended with fluid (pericardial effusion), tumor growth within the thorax, or an elevated diaphragm.

Clinical Manifestations

The development of atelectasis usually is insidious. Signs and symptoms include increasing dyspnea, cough, and sputum production.

In acute atelectasis involving a large amount of lung tissue (lobar atelectasis), marked respiratory distress may be observed. In addition to the previously mentioned signs and symptoms, tachycardia, tachypnea, pleural pain, and **central cyanosis** (a bluish skin hue that is a late sign of hypoxemia) may be anticipated. Patients characteristically have difficulty breathing in the supine position and are anxious.

In chronic atelectasis, signs and symptoms are similar to those of acute atelectasis. The chronic nature of the alveolar collapse predisposes patients to infection distal to the obstruction. Therefore, the signs and symptoms of a pulmonary infection also may be present.

Assessment and Diagnostic Findings

When clinically significant atelectasis develops, it is generally characterized by increased work of breathing and hypoxemia. Decreased breath sounds and crackles are heard over the affected area. A chest x-ray may suggest a diagnosis of atelectasis before clinical symptoms appear; the x-ray may reveal patchy infiltrates or consolidated areas. Depending on the degree of hypoxemia, pulse oximetry (SpO_2) may demonstrate a low saturation of hemoglobin with oxygen (less than 90%) or a lower-than-normal partial pressure of arterial oxygen (PaO_2).

Physiology ···:·· Pathophysiology

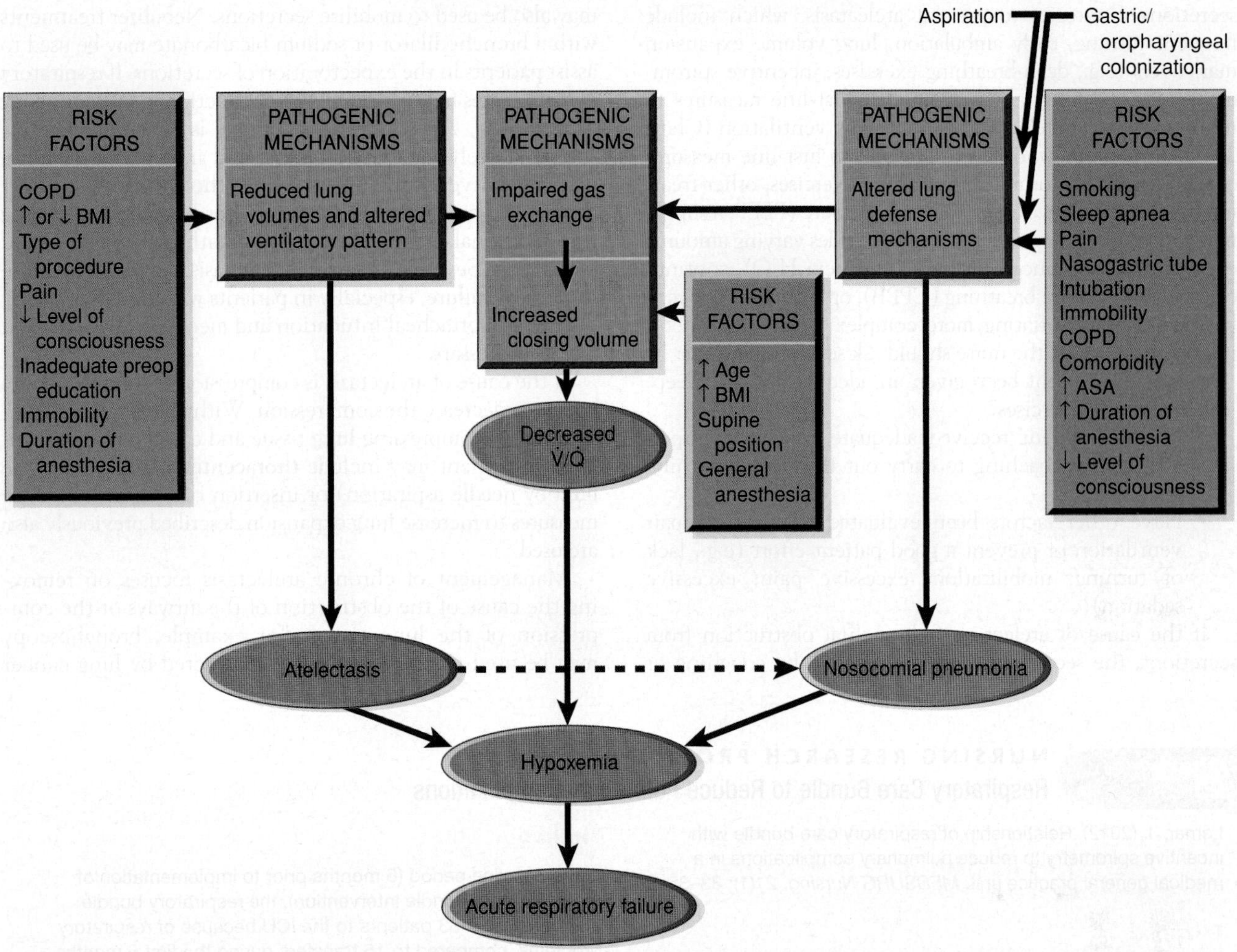

FIGURE 23-1 • Relationship of risk factors, pathogenic mechanisms, and consequences of acute atelectasis in the postoperative patient. ASA, acetylsalicylic acid; COPD, chronic obstructive pulmonary disease; BMI, body mass index; (V̇/Q̇), ventilation–perfusion ratio. From the work of Jo Ann Brooks-Brunn, DNS, RN, FAAN, FCCP, Indiana University Medical Center, Indianapolis.

▶ Quality and Safety Nursing Alert

Tachypnea, dyspnea, and mild to moderate hypoxemia are hallmarks of the severity of atelectasis.

Prevention

Nursing measures to prevent atelectasis include frequent turning, early mobilization, and strategies to expand the lungs and to manage secretions. Voluntary deep-breathing maneuvers (at least every 2 hours) assist in preventing and treating atelectasis. The performance of these maneuvers requires the patient to be alert and cooperative. Patient education and reinforcement are key elements to the success of these interventions. The use of incentive spirometry or voluntary deep breathing enhances lung expansion, decreases the potential for airway closure, and may generate a cough. Secretion management techniques include directed cough, suctioning, aerosol nebulizer treatments followed by chest physiotherapy (postural drainage and chest percussion), and bronchoscopy.

In some settings, a metered-dose inhaler is used to dispense a bronchodilator rather than an aerosol nebulizer. Chart 23-1 summarizes measures used to prevent atelectasis.

Chart 23-1   Preventing Atelectasis

- Change patient's position frequently, especially from supine to upright position, to promote ventilation and prevent secretions from accumulating.
- Encourage early mobilization from bed to chair followed by early ambulation.
- Encourage appropriate deep breathing and coughing to mobilize secretions and prevent them from accumulating.
- Educate/reinforce appropriate technique for incentive spirometry.
- Administer prescribed opioids and sedatives judiciously to prevent respiratory depression.
- Perform postural drainage and chest percussion, if indicated.
- Institute suctioning to remove tracheobronchial secretions, if indicated.

Management

The goal of treatment is to improve ventilation and remove secretions. Strategies to prevent atelectasis, which include frequent turning, early ambulation, lung volume expansion maneuvers (e.g., deep-breathing exercises, incentive spirometry), and coughing, also serve as the first-line measures to minimize or treat atelectasis by improving ventilation (Chart 23-2). In patients who do not respond to first-line measures or who cannot perform deep-breathing exercises, other treatments such as positive end-expiratory pressure (PEEP; a simple mask and one-way valve system that provides varying amounts of expiratory resistance, usually 10 to 15 cm H_2O), continuous positive pressure breathing (CPPB), or bronchoscopy may be used. Before initiating more complex, costly, and labor-intensive therapies, the nurse should ask several questions:

- Has the patient been given an adequate trial of deep-breathing exercises?
- Has the patient received adequate education, supervision, and coaching to carry out the deep-breathing exercises?
- Have other factors been evaluated that may impair ventilation or prevent a good patient effort (e.g., lack of turning, mobilization; excessive pain; excessive sedation)?

If the cause of atelectasis is bronchial obstruction from secretions, the secretions must be removed by coughing or suctioning to allow air to reenter that portion of the lung. Chest physiotherapy (chest percussion and postural drainage) may also be used to mobilize secretions. Nebulizer treatments with a bronchodilator or sodium bicarbonate may be used to assist patients in the expectoration of secretions. If respiratory care measures fail to remove the obstruction, a bronchoscopy is performed. Although bronchoscopy is an excellent measure to acutely remove secretions and increase ventilation, it is imperative for the nurse to assist the patient with maintaining the patency of the airways after bronchoscopy, using the traditional techniques of deep breathing, coughing, and suctioning. Severe or massive atelectasis may lead to acute respiratory failure, especially in patients with underlying lung disease. Endotracheal intubation and mechanical ventilation may be necessary.

If the cause of atelectasis is compression of lung tissue, the goal is to decrease the compression. With a large pleural effusion that is compressing lung tissue and causing alveolar collapse, treatment may include **thoracentesis** (removal of the fluid by needle aspiration) or insertion of a chest tube. The measures to increase lung expansion described previously also are used.

Management of chronic atelectasis focuses on removing the cause of the obstruction of the airways or the compression of the lung tissue. For example, bronchoscopy may be used to open an airway obstructed by lung cancer

---

Chart 23-2

NURSING RESEARCH PROFILE
Respiratory Care Bundle to Reduce Pulmonary Complications

Lamar, J. (2012). Relationship of respiratory care bundle with incentive spirometry to reduce pulmonary complications in a medical general practice unit. *MEDSURG Nursing, 21*(1), 33–36.

Purpose

The purpose of this study was to evaluate the effectiveness of a respiratory care bundle that included the use of incentive spirometry at reducing respiratory complications in medical patients.

Design

A quasi-experimental design was used to compare a respiratory bundle intervention to standard care on reducing respiratory complications. The intervention was initiated on a 31-bed medical general care unit while standard care that continued on a 30-bed medical unit designated the control. The respiratory care bundle intervention included two regimens to distinguish between cognitively and physically independent patients versus dependent patients. Independent patients received an incentive spirometer and an oral care packet of toothbrush and toothpaste. Patients were taught how to use the incentive spirometer and were instructed to use the spirometer 10 times every 2 hours and to brush their teeth twice daily. The dependent patient intervention required nurses to elevate the head of the patient's bed to 30–45 degrees, reposition the patient every 2 hours, and provide oral care once per shift. The standard care (control group) patients followed the institution's daily oral care policy. Three time points were used for data collection: 6-month period before initiation of the intervention and 6 and 12 months after implementation. Outcome data collected included the number of patient transfers to the ICU due to respiratory reasons and rapid response team calls for respiratory problems.

Findings

In the baseline period (6 months prior to implementation of the respiratory bundle intervention), the respiratory bundle unit transferred 33 patients to the ICU because of respiratory problems, compared to 15 transfers during the first 6 months of intervention and 5 transfers during the second 6 months of intervention. Rapid response calls for respiratory reasons decreased by 13% during the 12-month intervention period. Rapid response calls in the control unit increased 10% over the same time period. Using chi-square analysis, there was a statistically significant reduction in respiratory response calls on the intervention unit as compared to the control unit ($p < .001$). Incidental benefits of this study included a marked reduction in ICU transfers, which had a positive impact on patient care as well as the cost of care. A serendipitous finding was a significant reduction in the incidence of pressure ulcers on the intervention unit as compared to other units in the hospital. This also resulted in a cost savings.

Nursing Implications

This study demonstrates the importance of basic nursing care to ensure good patient outcomes. Patients admitted to the intervention unit benefited from a systematic application of basic nursing care (e.g., deep breathing, turning, good oral hygiene). Patient outcomes from the use of incentive spirometry has not been studied in the general medical patient population, and study results in surgical patients have been mixed. The application of basic nursing care had a positive impact on the intervention group (e.g., decrease in ICU transfers) and demonstrates the importance of basic nursing care in our "high-tech" health care environment.

or a nonmalignant lesion, and the procedure may involve cryotherapy or laser therapy. If the atelectasis is a result of obstruction caused by lung cancer, an airway stent or radiation therapy to shrink a tumor may be used to open the airways and provide ventilation to the collapsed area. However, reopening the airways and reaerating the area of the lung may not be possible in patients who have experienced chronic, long-term collapse. In some cases, surgical management may be indicated.

RESPIRATORY INFECTIONS

Acute Tracheobronchitis

Acute tracheobronchitis, an acute inflammation of the mucous membranes of the trachea and the bronchial tree, often follows infection of the upper respiratory tract (see Chapter 22). Patients with viral infections have decreased resistance and can readily develop a secondary bacterial infection. Adequate treatment of upper respiratory tract infection is one of the major factors in the prevention of acute bronchitis.

Pathophysiology

In acute tracheobronchitis, the inflamed mucosa of the bronchi produces mucopurulent sputum, often in response to infection by *Streptococcus pneumoniae*, *Haemophilus influenzae*, or *Mycoplasma pneumoniae*. In addition, a fungal infection (e.g., *Aspergillus*) may also cause tracheobronchitis. A sputum culture is essential to identify the specific causative organism. In addition to infection, inhalation of physical and chemical irritants, gases, or other air contaminants can also cause acute bronchial irritation. A subcategory of tracheobronchitis is ventilator-associated tracheobronchitis, which is a common illness in chronically ventilated patients. If managed appropriately, ventilator-associated pneumonia (VAP) may be prevented (Niederman, 2011).

Clinical Manifestations

Initially, the patient has a dry, irritating cough and expectorates a scanty amount of mucoid sputum. The patient may report sternal soreness from coughing and have fever or chills, night sweats, headache, and general malaise. As the infection progresses, the patient may be short of breath, have noisy inspiration and expiration (inspiratory stridor and expiratory wheeze), and produce **purulent** (pus-filled) sputum. In severe tracheobronchitis, blood-streaked secretions may be expectorated as a result of the irritation of the mucosa of the airways.

Medical Management

Antibiotic treatment may be indicated depending on the symptoms, sputum purulence, and results of the sputum culture and sensitivity. Antihistamines usually are not prescribed, because they can cause excessive drying and make secretions more difficult to expectorate. Fluid intake is increased to thin the viscous and tenacious secretions. Copious, purulent secretions that cannot be cleared by coughing

place patients at risk for increasing airway obstruction and the development of more severe lower respiratory tract infections, such as pneumonia. Suctioning and bronchoscopy may be needed to remove secretions. Rarely, endotracheal intubation may be necessary in cases of acute tracheobronchitis leading to acute respiratory failure, such as in patients who are severely debilitated or who have coexisting diseases that also impair the respiratory system.

In most cases, treatment of tracheobronchitis is largely symptomatic. Increasing the vapor pressure (moisture content) in the air reduces airway irritation. Cool vapor therapy or steam inhalations may help relieve laryngeal and tracheal irritation. Moist heat to the chest may relieve the soreness and pain, and mild analgesics may be prescribed.

Nursing Management

Acute tracheobronchitis is usually treated in the home setting. A primary nursing function is to encourage bronchial hygiene, such as increased fluid intake and directed coughing to remove secretions. The nurse encourages and assists the patient to sit up frequently to cough effectively and to prevent retention of mucopurulent sputum. If the patient is taking antibiotics for an underlying infection, the need to complete the full course of antibiotics prescribed is emphasized. Fatigue is a consequence of tracheobronchitis; therefore, the nurse cautions the patient against overexertion, which can induce a relapse or exacerbation of the infection. The patient is advised to rest.

Pneumonia

Pneumonia is an inflammation of the lung parenchyma caused by various microorganisms, including bacteria, mycobacteria, fungi, and viruses. *Pneumonitis* is a more general term that describes an inflammatory process in the lung tissue that may predispose or place the patient at risk for microbial invasion. Pneumonia and influenza are the most common causes of death from infectious diseases in the United States. Pneumonia accounted for close to 51,000 deaths in the United States in 2009 and 1.1 million discharges from hospitals (Centers for Disease Control and Prevention [CDC], 2012b). Combined, influenza and pneumonia were the eighth leading cause of death in the United States in 2010, accounting for 53,692 deaths (CDC, 2012b; Murphy, Jiaquan, & Kochanek, 2012).

Classification

Pneumonia can be classified into four types: community-acquired pneumonia (CAP), health care–associated pneumonia (HCAP), hospital-acquired pneumonia (HAP), and VAP (American Thoracic Society & Infectious Diseases Society of America, 2005; File, 2012). HCAP was added as a category in 2005 to identify patients at increased risk for multidrug-resistant (MDR) pathogens versus community-acquired pathogens (File, 2012). In the past, hospital-acquired, ventilator-associated, and health care–associated pneumonias were all called *nosocomial pneumonias*. Chart 23-3 describes the different classifications and definitions of pneumonias. Other subcategories of HCAPs are those in the

<table>
<tr><td colspan="2">

Chart 23-3 **Classifications and Definitions of Pneumonias**

</td></tr>
</table>

- *Community-acquired pneumonia (CAP):* Pneumonia occurring in the community or ≤48 hours of hospital admission in patients who do not meet the criteria for health care–associated pneumonia (HCAP)
- *Health care–associated pneumonia (HCAP):* Pneumonia occurring in a nonhospitalized patient with extensive health care contact with one or more of the following:
  - Hospitalization for ≥2 days in an acute care facility within 90 days of infection
  - Residence in a nursing home or long-term care facility
  - Antibiotic therapy, chemotherapy, or wound care within 30 days of current infection
  - Hemodialysis treatment at a hospital or clinic
  - Home infusion therapy or home wound care
  - Family member with infection due to multidrug-resistant bacteria
- *Hospital-acquired pneumonia (HAP):* Pneumonia occurring ≥48 hours after hospital admission that did not appear to be incubating at the time of admission
- *Ventilator-associated pneumonia (VAP):* A type of HAP that develops ≥48 hours after endotracheal tube intubation

Adapted from American Thoracic Society & Infectious Diseases Society of America. (2005). Guidelines for the management of adults with hospital-acquired, ventilator-associated, and healthcare-associated pneumonia. *American Journal of Respiratory and Critical Care Medicine, 171*(4), 388–416; and File, T. (2012). Risk factors and prevention of hospital-acquired, ventilator-associated and healthcare-associated pneumonia in adults. *UpToDate.* Last updated June 26, 2012. Available at: www.uptodate.com

<table>
<tr><td colspan="2">

Chart 23-4 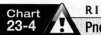 **RISK FACTORS** **Pneumonia Based Upon Pathogen Type**

</td></tr>
</table>

Risk Factors for Infection With Penicillin-Resistant and Drug-Resistant Pneumococci

- Age >65 years
- Alcoholism
- Beta-lactam therapy (e.g., cephalosporins) in past 3 months
- Immunosuppressive disorders
- Multiple medical comorbidities
- Exposure to a child in a day care facility

Risk Factors for Infection With Enteric Gram-Negative Bacteria

- Residency in a long-term care facility
- Underlying cardiopulmonary disease
- Multiple medical comorbidities
- Recent antibiotic therapy

Risk Factors for Infection With *Pseudomonas aeruginosa*

- Structural lung disease (e.g., bronchiectasis)
- Corticosteroid therapy
- Broad-spectrum antibiotic therapy (>7 days in the past month)
- Malnutrition

immunocompromised host and aspiration pneumonia. There is overlap in how specific pneumonias are classified, because they may occur in differing settings. Risk factors associated for specific pathogens are shown in Chart 23-4.

Community-Acquired Pneumonia

CAP occurs either in the community setting or within the first 48 hours after hospitalization or institutionalization. The need for hospitalization for CAP depends on the severity of the pneumonia. The causative pathogens for CAP by site of care are shown in Table 23-1. The specific etiologic pathogen is identified in about 50% of cases. More than five million cases of CAP are reported each year, with more than 915,000 episodes in adults 65 years and older (Al-Qadi, Al-Alwan, Opal, et al., 2010).

S. pneumoniae (pneumococcus) is the most common cause of CAP in people younger than 60 years without comorbidity and in those 60 years and older with comorbidity (Wunderink & Niederman, 2012). *S. pneumoniae,* a gram-positive organism that resides naturally in the upper respiratory tract, colonizes the upper respiratory tract and can cause disseminated invasive infections, pneumonia and other lower respiratory tract infections, and upper respiratory tract infections such as otitis media and rhinosinusitis. It may occur as a lobar or bronchopneumonic form in patients of any age and may follow a recent respiratory illness.

H. influenzae causes a type of CAP that frequently affects older adults and those with comorbid illnesses (e.g., chronic obstructive pulmonary disease [COPD], alcoholism, and diabetes). The presentation is indistinguishable from that

TABLE 23-1 **Community-Acquired Pneumonia Microbial Causes by Site of Care***

	Hospitalized Patients	
Outpatients	**Non-ICU**	**ICU**
Streptococcus pneumoniae	*S. pneumoniae*	*S. pneumoniae*
Mycoplasma pneumoniae	*M. pneumoniae*	*Staphylococcus aureus*
Haemophilus influenzae	*Chlamydophila pneumoniae*	*Legionella*
C. pneumoniae	*H. influenzae*	Gram-negative bacilli
Respiratory viruses	*Legionella*	*H. influenzae*
	Respiratory viruses	

ICU, intensive care unit.
*Listed in descending order of frequency at each site.
Adapted from Loscalzo, J. (2010). *Harrison's pulmonary and critical care medicine.* New York: McGraw-Hill.

of other forms of bacterial CAP and may be subacute, with cough or low-grade fever for weeks before diagnosis.

Mycoplasma pneumonia is caused by M. *pneumoniae*. Mycoplasma pneumonia is spread by infected respiratory droplets through person-to-person contact. Patients can be tested for mycoplasma antibodies. The inflammatory infiltrate is primarily interstitial rather than alveolar. It spreads throughout the entire respiratory tract, including the bronchioles, and has the characteristics of a bronchopneumonia. Earache and bullous myringitis are common. Impaired ventilation and diffusion may occur.

Viruses are the most common cause of pneumonia in infants and children but are relatively uncommon causes of CAP in adults. In immunocompromised adults, cytomegalovirus is the most common viral pathogen, followed by herpes simplex virus, adenovirus, and respiratory syncytial virus. The acute stage of a viral respiratory infection occurs within the ciliated cells of the airways, followed by infiltration of the tracheobronchial tree. With pneumonia, the inflammatory process extends into the alveolar area, resulting in edema and exudation. The clinical signs and symptoms of a viral pneumonia are often difficult to distinguish from those of a bacterial pneumonia.

Health Care–Associated Pneumonia

An important distinction of HCAP is that the causative pathogens are often MDR. Consequently, identifying this type of pneumonia in areas such as the emergency department is crucial. Because HCAP is often difficult to treat, initial antibiotic treatment must not be delayed. Initial antibiotic treatment for HCAP is often different from that for CAP due to the possibility of MDR bacteria (Loscalzo, 2010; Wunderink & Niederman, 2012).

Hospital-Acquired Pneumonia

HAP develops 48 hours or more after admission and does not appear to be incubating at the time of admission. VAP can be considered a subtype of HAP, as the only differentiating factor is the presence of an endotracheal tube (see later discussion of VAP). Certain factors may predispose patients to HAP because of impaired host defenses (e.g., severe acute or chronic illness), a variety of comorbid conditions, supine positioning and aspiration, coma, malnutrition, prolonged hospitalization, hypotension, and metabolic disorders. Hospitalized patients are also exposed to potential bacteria from other sources (e.g., respiratory therapy devices and equipment, transmission of pathogens by the hands of health care personnel). Numerous intervention-related factors also may play a role in the development of HAP (e.g., therapeutic agents leading to central nervous system depression with decreased ventilation, impaired removal of secretions, or potential aspiration; prolonged or complicated thoracoabdominal procedures, which may impair mucociliary function and cellular host defenses; endotracheal intubation (VAP); prolonged or inappropriate use of antibiotics; the use of nasogastric tubes). In addition, immunocompromised patients are at particular risk. HAP is associated with a high mortality rate, in part because of the virulence of the organisms, the resistance to antibiotics, and the patient's underlying disorder.

The common organisms responsible for HAP include the *Enterobacter* species, *Escherichia coli*, *H. influenzae*, *Klebsiella* species, *Proteus*, *Serratia marcescens*, *Pseudomonas aeruginosa*, methicillin-sensitive or methicillin-resistant *Staphylococcus aureus* (MRSA), and *S. pneumoniae*. Most patients with HAP are colonized by multiple organisms. Pseudomonal pneumonia occurs in patients who are debilitated, those with altered mental status, and those with prolonged intubation or with tracheostomy. Staphylococcal pneumonia can occur through inhalation of the organism or spread through the hematogenous route. It is often accompanied by bacteremia and positive blood cultures. Its mortality rate is high. Specific strains of staphylococci are resistant to all available antimicrobial agents except vancomycin (Bartlett, Auwaerter, & Pham, 2012; Liu, Bayer, Cosgrove, et al., 2011). Overuse and misuse of antimicrobial agents are major risk factors for the emergence of these resistant pathogens. Because MRSA is highly virulent, steps must be taken to prevent its spread. Patients with MRSA are isolated in a private room, and contact precautions (gown, mask, gloves, and antibacterial soap) are used. The number of people in contact with affected patients is minimized, and appropriate precautions must be taken when transporting these patients within or between facilities.

The usual presentation of HAP is a new pulmonary infiltrate on chest x-ray combined with evidence of infection such as fever, respiratory symptoms, purulent sputum, or leukocytosis. Pneumonias from *Klebsiella* or other gram-negative organisms (*E. coli*, *Proteus*, *Serratia*) are characterized by destruction of lung structure and alveolar walls, **consolidation** (tissue that solidifies as a result of collapsed alveoli or infectious process such as pneumonia), and bacteremia. Older adult patients and those with alcoholism, chronic lung disease, or diabetes are at particular risk (File, 2012). Development of a cough or increased cough and sputum production are common presentations, along with low-grade fever and general malaise. In debilitated or dehydrated patients, sputum production may be minimal or absent. Pleural effusion, high fever, and tachycardia are common.

Ventilator-Associated Pneumonia

As noted earlier, VAP can be thought of as a subtype of HAP; however, in such cases, the patient has been endotracheally intubated and has received mechanical ventilatory support for at least 48 hours. VAP is the most common infection seen in intensive care units (ICUs); it accounts for 25% of the infections occurring in critically ill patients (Ashraf & Ostrosky-Zeichner, 2012). It contributes significantly to the morbidity and mortality of ICU patients, with an estimated attributable mortality rate of 8% to 15% (Ashraf & Ostrosky-Zeichner, 2012). VAP is the most costly infectious complication in ICU patients and has been estimated to cost at least $40,000 per patient and increases length of stay (Blot, Lisboa, Angles, et al., 2011). The etiologic bacteriologic agents associated with VAP typically differ based on the timing of the occurrence of the infection relative to the start of mechanical ventilation. VAP occurring within 96 hours of the onset of mechanical ventilation is usually due to antibiotic-sensitive bacteria that colonize the patient prior to hospital admission, whereas VAP developing after 96 hours of ventilatory support is more often associated with MDR bacteria. Prevention remains the key to reducing the burden of VAP (Kollef, 2012). (See Chart 21-13 in Chapter 21 for overview of bundled interventions aimed at preventing VAP.)

Pneumonia in the Immunocompromised Host

Pneumonia in immunocompromised hosts includes *Pneumocystis* pneumonia (PCP), fungal pneumonias, and *Mycobacterium tuberculosis*. The organism that causes PCP is now known as *Pneumocystis jiroveci* instead of *Pneumocystis carinii*. The acronym PCP still applies because it can be read "**P**neumo**c**ystis **p**neumonia."

Pneumonia in the immunocompromised host occurs with the use of corticosteroids or other immunosuppressive agents, chemotherapy, nutritional depletion, the use of broad-spectrum antimicrobial agents, acquired immunodeficiency syndrome (AIDS), genetic immune disorders, and long-term advanced life support technology (mechanical ventilation). It is seen with increasing frequency because affected patients constitute a growing portion of the population; however, pneumonias that typically occur in immunocompromised people may also occur in immunocompetent people. Patients with compromised immune systems commonly develop pneumonia from organisms of low virulence. In addition, increasing numbers of patients with impaired defenses develop HAP from gram-negative bacilli (*Klebsiella, Pseudomonas, E. coli,* Enterobacteriaceae, *Proteus, Serratia*) (Wunderink & Niederman, 2012).

Pneumonia in immunocompromised hosts may be caused by the organisms also observed in CAP or HAP (*S. pneumoniae, S. aureus, H. influenzae, P. aeruginosa, M. tuberculosis*). PCP is rarely observed in immunocompetent hosts and is often an initial AIDS-defining complication, although it is no longer the most common pulmonary diagnosis in these patients (Wunderink & Niederman, 2012). Whether patients are immunocompromised or immunocompetent, the clinical presentation of pneumonia is similar. PCP has a subtle onset, with progressive dyspnea, fever, and a nonproductive cough.

Aspiration Pneumonia

Aspiration pneumonia refers to the pulmonary consequences resulting from entry of endogenous or exogenous substances into the lower airway. The most common form of aspiration pneumonia is bacterial infection from aspiration of bacteria that normally reside in the upper airways. Aspiration pneumonia may occur in the community or hospital setting. Common pathogens are anaerobes, *S. aureus, Streptococcus* species, and gram-negative bacilli (Loscalzo, 2010). Substances other than bacteria may be aspirated into the lung, such as gastric contents, exogenous chemical contents, or irritating gases. This type of aspiration or ingestion may impair the lung defenses, cause inflammatory changes, and lead to bacterial growth and a resulting pneumonia. (See later discussion of aspiration.)

Pathophysiology

Normally, the upper airway prevents potentially infectious particles from reaching the sterile lower respiratory tract. Pneumonia arises from normal flora present in patients whose resistance has been altered or from aspiration of flora present in the oropharynx; patients often have an acute or chronic underlying disease that impairs host defenses. Pneumonia may also result from bloodborne organisms that enter the pulmonary circulation and are trapped in the pulmonary capillary bed.

Pneumonia affects both ventilation and diffusion. An inflammatory reaction can occur in the alveoli, producing an exudate that interferes with the diffusion of oxygen and carbon dioxide. White blood cells, mostly neutrophils, also migrate into the alveoli and fill the normally air-filled spaces. Areas of the lung are not adequately ventilated because of secretions and mucosal edema that cause partial occlusion of the bronchi or alveoli, with a resultant decrease in alveolar oxygen tension. Bronchospasm may also occur in patients with reactive airway disease. Because of hypoventilation, a ventilation-perfusion ($\dot{V}/\dot{Q}$) mismatch occurs in the affected area of the lung. Venous blood entering the pulmonary circulation passes through the underventilated area and travels to the left side of the heart poorly oxygenated. The mixing of oxygenated and unoxygenated or poorly oxygenated blood eventually results in arterial hypoxemia.

If a substantial portion of one or more lobes is involved, the disease is referred to as lobar pneumonia. The term *bronchopneumonia* is used to describe pneumonia that is distributed in a patchy fashion, having originated in one or more localized areas within the bronchi and extending to the adjacent surrounding lung parenchyma. Bronchopneumonia is more common than lobar pneumonia (Fig. 23-2).

Risk Factors

Being knowledgeable about the factors and circumstances that commonly predispose people to pneumonia helps identify patients at high risk for the disease (File, 2012). Table 23-2 describes risk factors for pneumonia; additional risk factors are travel or exposure to certain environments and residence in a long-term care facility. Increasing numbers of patients who have compromised defenses against infections are susceptible to pneumonia. Some types of pneumonia,

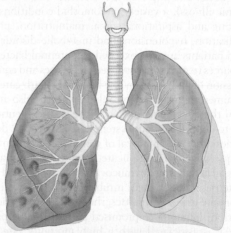

Bronchopneumonia   Lobar pneumonia

FIGURE 23-2 • Distribution of lung involvement in bronchial and lobar pneumonia. In bronchopneumonia (*left*), patchy areas of consolidation occur. In lobar pneumonia (*right*), an entire lobe is consolidated.

TABLE 23-2 Risk Factors and Preventive Measures for Pneumonia	
Risk Factor	**Preventive Measure**
Conditions that produce mucus or bronchial obstruction and interfere with normal lung drainage (e.g., cancer, cigarette smoking, chronic obstructive pulmonary disease)	Promote coughing and expectoration of secretions. Encourage smoking cessation.
Immunosuppressed patients and those with a low neutrophil count (neutropenic)	Initiate special precautions against infection.
Smoking (cigarette smoke disrupts both mucociliary and macrophage activity)	Encourage smoking cessation.
Prolonged immobility and shallow breathing pattern	Reposition frequently and promote lung expansion exercises and coughing. Initiate suctioning and chest physical therapy if indicated.
Depressed cough reflex (due to medications, a debilitated state, or weak respiratory muscles); aspiration of foreign material into the lungs during a period of unconsciousness (head injury, anesthesia, depressed level of consciousness), or abnormal swallowing mechanism	Reposition frequently to prevent aspiration and administer medications judiciously, particularly those that increase risk for aspiration. Perform suctioning and chest physical therapy if indicated.
Nothing-by-mouth (NPO) status; placement of nasogastric, orogastric, or endotracheal tube	Promote frequent oral hygiene. Minimize risk for aspiration by checking placement of tube and proper positioning of patient.
Supine positioning in patients unable to protect their airway	Elevate head of bed at least 30 degrees.
Antibiotic therapy (in very ill people, the oropharynx is likely to be colonized by gram-negative bacteria)	Monitor patients receiving antibiotic therapy for signs and symptoms of pneumonia.
Alcohol intoxication (because alcohol suppresses the body's reflexes, may be associated with aspiration, and decreases white cell mobilization and tracheobronchial ciliary motion)	Encourage reduced or moderate alcohol intake (in case of alcohol stupor, position patient to prevent aspiration).
General anesthetic, sedative, or opioid preparations that promote respiratory depression, which causes a shallow breathing pattern and predisposes to the pooling of bronchial secretions and potential development of pneumonia	Observe the respiratory rate and depth during recovery from general anesthesia and before giving medications. If respiratory depression is apparent, withhold the medication and contact the primary provider.
Advanced age, because of possible depressed cough and glottic reflexes and nutritional depletion	Promote frequent turning, early ambulation and mobilization, effective coughing, breathing exercises, and nutritious diet.
Respiratory therapy with improperly cleaned equipment	Make sure that respiratory equipment is cleaned properly; participate in continuous quality improvement monitoring with the respiratory care department.
Transmission of organisms from health care providers	Use strict hand hygiene and gloves. Implement health care provider education.

such as those caused by viral infections, occur in previously healthy people, often after a viral illness.

Pneumonia occurs in patients with certain underlying disorders such as heart failure, diabetes, alcoholism, COPD, and AIDS (File, 2012; Wunderink & Niederman, 2012). Certain diseases also have been associated with specific pathogens. For example, staphylococcal pneumonia has been noted after epidemics of influenza, and patients with COPD are at increased risk for development of pneumonia caused by pneumococci or *H. influenzae*. In addition, cystic fibrosis is associated with respiratory infection caused by pseudomonal and staphylococcal organisms, and PCP has been associated with AIDS. Pneumonias occurring in hospitalized patients often involve organisms not usually found in CAP, including enteric gram-negative bacilli and *S. aureus*.

Clinical Manifestations

Pneumonia varies in its signs and symptoms depending on the type, causal organism, and presence of underlying disease. However, it is not possible to diagnose a specific form or classification of pneumonia by clinical manifestations alone. The patient with streptococcal (pneumococcal) pneumonia usually has a sudden onset of chills, rapidly rising fever (38.5° to 40.5°C [101° to 105°F]), and pleuritic chest pain that is aggravated by deep breathing and coughing. The patient is

severely ill, with marked tachypnea (25 to 45 breaths/min), accompanied by other signs of respiratory distress (e.g., shortness of breath, the use of accessory muscles in respiration). A relative bradycardia (a pulse–temperature deficit in which the pulse is slower than that expected for a given temperature) may suggest viral infection, mycoplasma infection, or infection with a *Legionella* organism.

Some patients exhibit an upper respiratory tract infection (nasal congestion, sore throat), and the onset of symptoms of pneumonia is gradual and nonspecific. The predominant symptoms may be headache, low-grade fever, pleuritic pain, myalgia, rash, and pharyngitis. After a few days, mucoid or mucopurulent sputum is expectorated. In severe pneumonia, the cheeks are flushed and the lips and nail beds demonstrate central cyanosis (a late sign of poor oxygenation [hypoxemia]).

The patient may exhibit **orthopnea** (shortness of breath when reclining or in the supine position), preferring to be propped up or sitting in bed leaning forward (orthopneic position) in an effort to achieve adequate gas exchange without coughing or breathing deeply. Appetite is poor, and the patient is diaphoretic and tires easily. Sputum is often purulent; however, this is not a reliable indicator of the etiologic agent. Rusty, blood-tinged sputum may be expectorated with streptococcal (pneumococcal), staphylococcal, and *Klebsiella* pneumonia.

Signs and symptoms of pneumonia may also depend on a patient's underlying condition. Different signs occur in patients with conditions such as cancer, and in those who are undergoing treatment with immunosuppressant medications, which decrease the resistance to infection. Such patients have fever, crackles, and physical findings that indicate consolidation of lung tissue, including increased tactile fremitus (vocal vibration detected on palpation), percussion dullness, bronchial breath sounds, egophony (when auscultated, the spoken "E" becomes a loud, nasal-sounding "A"), and whispered pectoriloquy (whispered sounds are easily auscultated through the chest wall). These changes occur because sound is transmitted better through solid or dense tissue (consolidation) than through normal air-filled tissue; these sounds are described in Chapter 20.

Purulent sputum or slight changes in respiratory symptoms may be the only sign of pneumonia in patients with COPD. Determining whether an increase in symptoms is an exacerbation of the underlying disease process or an additional infectious process may be difficult.

Assessment and Diagnostic Findings

The diagnosis of pneumonia is made by history (particularly of a recent respiratory tract infection), physical examination, chest x-ray, blood culture (bloodstream invasion [bacteremia] occurs frequently), and sputum examination. The sputum sample is obtained by having patients do the following: (1) rinse the mouth with water to minimize contamination by normal oral flora, (2) breathe deeply several times, (3) cough deeply, and (4) expectorate the raised sputum into a sterile container.

More invasive procedures may be used to collect specimens. Sputum may be obtained by nasotracheal or orotracheal suctioning with a sputum trap or by fiberoptic bronchoscopy (see Chapter 20). Bronchoscopy is often used in patients with acute severe infection, in patients with chronic or refractory infection, in immunocompromised patients when a diagnosis cannot be made from an expectorated or induced specimen, and in mechanically ventilated patients.

Prevention

Pneumococcal vaccination reduces the incidence of pneumonia, hospitalizations for cardiac conditions, and deaths in the general older adult population. A one-time vaccination of pneumococcal polysaccharide vaccine (PPSV) is recommended for all patients 65 years and older and those with chronic diseases. A second PPSV revaccination dose is recommended for all adults 65 years and older who were previously vaccinated with one dose if 5 years or more have elapsed since the previous dose. For those who were first vaccinated at 65 years or older, only one dose is required regardless of medical condition (CDC, 2011). Other preventive measures are summarized in Table 23-2.

Medical Management

Pharmacologic Therapy

The treatment of pneumonia includes administration of the appropriate antibiotic as determined by the results of a culture and sensitivity. However, the causative organ-

ism is not identified in half of CAP cases when therapy is initiated (Loscalzo, 2010). Guidelines are used to guide antibiotic choice; however, the resistance patterns, prevalence of causative organisms, patient risk factors, treatment setting (inpatient vs. outpatient), and costs and availability of newer antibiotic agents must all be considered. See Table 23-3 for treatment of patients with pneumonia due to specific pathogens.

Inpatients should be switched from intravenous (IV) to oral therapy when they are hemodynamically stable, are improving clinically, are able to take medications/fluids by mouth, and have a normally functioning gastrointestinal tract. As soon as patients are clinically stable, have no medical problems, and have a safe environment for continued care, they should be discharged from the hospital. Clinical stability is defined as temperature less than or equal to 37.8°C (100°F), heart rate less than or equal to 100 bpm, respiratory rate less than or equal to 24 breaths/min, systolic blood pressure greater than or equal to 90 mm Hg, and oxygen saturation greater than or equal to 90%, with ability to maintain oral intake and normal (baseline) mental status.

In suspected HAP, treatment is usually initiated with a broad-spectrum IV antibiotic and may be monotherapy or combination therapy. For patients with no known multidrug resistance, monotherapy with ceftriaxone (Rocephin), ampicillin/sulbactam (Unasyn), levofloxacin (Levaquin), or ertapenem (Invanz) is used. With known multidrug resistance, a three-drug combination therapy may be used; this drug regimen may include an antipseudomonal cephalosporin or ceftazidime (Fortaz) or antipseudomonal carbapenem or piperacillin/tazobactam (Zosyn) plus antipseudomonal fluoroquinolone or aminoglycoside plus linezolid (Zyvox) or vancomycin (Vancocin). The patient's status must be assessed 72 hours after the initiation of therapy, and antibiotics should be discontinued or modified based on the culture results. Of concern is the rampant rise in respiratory pathogens that are resistant to available antibiotics. Examples include vancomycin-resistant enterococcus (VRE), MRSA, and drug-resistant *S. pneumoniae*. Clinicians tend to use antibiotics aggressively; broad-spectrum agents may be used when narrow-spectrum agents are more appropriate. Mechanisms to monitor and minimize the inappropriate use of antibiotics are in place. Education of clinicians about the use of evidence-based guidelines in the treatment of respiratory infection is important, and some institutions have implemented algorithms to assist clinicians in choosing the appropriate antibiotics. Monitoring and surveillance of susceptibility patterns for pathogens are also important.

Other Therapeutic Regimens

Antibiotics are ineffective in viral upper respiratory tract infections and pneumonia, and their use may be associated with adverse effects. Treatment of viral infections with antibiotics is a major reason for the overuse of these medications in the United States. Antibiotics are indicated with a viral respiratory infection *only* if a secondary bacterial pneumonia, bronchitis, or rhinosinusitis is present. With the exception of the use of antimicrobial therapy, treatment of viral pneumonia is the same as that for bacterial pneumonia.

TABLE 23-3   Commonly Encountered Pneumonias

Type (Causal Organism)	Epidemiology	Clinical Features	Treatment	Complications/Comments
Community-Acquired Pneumonia				
Streptococcal pneumonia (*Streptococcus pneumoniae*)	Most prevalent in winter months More frequent occurrence in African Americans	Abrupt onset, toxic appearance, pleuritic chest pain; usually involves ≥1 lobes	*PCN sensitive:* PCN, amoxicillin (Amoxil), ceftriaxone (Rocephin), cefotaxime (Claforan), cefpodoxime (Vantin), cefprozil (Cefzil) or a macrolide *PCN resistant:* levofloxacin (Levaquin), moxifloxacin (Avelox), vancomycin (Vancocin) or linezolid (Zyvox)	Shock, pleural effusion, superinfections, pericarditis, and otitis media
	Incidence greatest in older adults and in patients with COPD, heart failure, alcoholism, asplenia, diabetes, and after influenza Leading infectious cause of illness worldwide among young children, people with underlying chronic health conditions, and older adults *Mortality rate (in hospitalized adults with invasive disease): 14%*	Lobar infiltrate common on chest x-ray or bronchopneumonia pattern		
Haemophilus influenzae (*Haemophilus influenzae*)	Incidence greatest in alcoholics, older adults, patients in long-term care facilities and nursing homes, patients with diabetes or COPD, and children <5 y of age Accounts for 5%–20% of community-acquired pneumonias *Mortality rate: 30%*	Frequently insidious onset associated with upper respiratory tract infection 2–6 wk before onset of illness; fever, chills, productive cough; usually involves ≥1 lobes Bacteremia is common. Infiltrate, occasional bronchopneumonia pattern on chest x-ray.	Doxycycline (Vibramycin), 2nd- or 3rd-generation cephalosporin or a fluoroquinolone	Lung abscess, pleural effusion, meningitis, arthritis, pericarditis, epiglottitis
Legionnaires' disease (*Legionella pneumophila*)	Highest occurrence in summer and fall May cause disease sporadically or as part of an epidemic Incidence greatest in middle-aged and older men, smokers, patients with chronic diseases, those receiving immunosuppressive therapy, and those in close proximity to excavation sites Accounts for 15% of community-acquired pneumonias *Mortality rate: 15–50%*	Flulike symptoms; high fevers, mental confusion, headache, pleuritic pain, myalgias, dyspnea, productive cough, hemoptysis, leukocytosis Bronchopneumonia, unilateral or bilateral disease, lobar consolidation	Azithromycin (Zithromax) or a fluoroquinolone	Hypotension, shock, and acute renal failure
Mycoplasma pneumoniae (*Mycoplasma pneumoniae*)	Increase in fall and winter Responsible for epidemics of respiratory illness	Onset is usually insidious. Patients not usually as ill as in other pneumonias. Sore throat, nasal congestion, ear pain, headache, low-grade fever, pleuritic pain, myalgias, diarrhea, erythematous rash, pharyngitis. Interstitial infiltrates on chest x-ray.	Macrolide or doxycycline	Aseptic meningitis, meningoencephalitis, transverse myelitis, cranial nerve palsies, pericarditis, myocarditis
	Most common type of atypical pneumonia Accounts for 20% of community-acquired pneumonias; more common in children and young adults *Mortality rate: <0.1%*			

(continues on page 580)

TABLE 23-3 **Commonly Encountered Pneumonias** (continued)

Type (Causal Organism)	Epidemiology	Clinical Features	Treatment	Complications/ Comments
Viral pneumonia (influenza viruses types A, B adenovirus, parainfluenza, cytomegalovirus, coronavirus, varicella-zoster)	Incidence greatest in winter months Epidemics occur every 2–3 y. Most common causative organisms in adults; other organisms in children (e.g., cytomegalovirus, respiratory syncytial virus) Accounts for 20% of community-acquired pneumonias	Patchy infiltrate, small pleural effusion on chest x-ray In most patients, influenza begins as an acute upper respiratory infection; others have bronchitis, pleurisy, and so on, and still others develop gastrointestinal symptoms.	Treated symptomatically; treat in high-risk patients; oseltamivir (Tamiflu) or zanamivir (Relenza) (+ other agents depending upon dominant strain [type of virus]) Does not respond to treatment with currently available antimicrobials	Superimposed bacterial infection, bronchopneumonia
Chlamydial pneumonia (*Chlamydophila pneumoniae*)	Reported mainly in college students, military recruits, and older adults May be a common cause of community-acquired pneumonia or observed in combination with other pathogens Mortality rate is low because the majority of cases are relatively mild. Older adults with coexistent infections, comorbidities, and reinfections may require hospitalization.	Hoarseness, fever, chills, pharyngitis, rhinitis, nonproductive cough, myalgias, arthralgias Single infiltrate on chest x-ray; pleural effusion possible	Macrolide or doxycycline	Reinfection and acute respiratory failure

Hospital-Acquired and Health Care–Associated Pneumonias

Type (Causal Organism)	Epidemiology	Clinical Features	Treatment	Complications/ Comments
Pseudomonas pneumonia (*Pseudomonas aeruginosa*)	Incidence greatest in those with preexisting lung disease, cancer (particularly leukemia); those with homograft transplants, burns; debilitated people; and patients receiving antimicrobial therapy and treatments such as tracheostomy, suctioning, and in postoperative settings. Almost always of nosocomial origin. Accounts for 15% of hospital-acquired pneumonias *Mortality rate: 40%–60%*	Diffuse consolidation on chest x-ray; toxic appearance: fever, chills, productive cough, relative bradycardia, leukocytosis	*Sensitivity tests guide choice:* ceftazidime (Fortaz), ciprofloxacin (Cipro), cefepime (Maxipime), aztreonam (Azactam), imipenem/cilastatin (Primaxin), meropenem (Merrem), piperacillin (Pipracil), +/− an aminoglycoside	Lung cavitation; has capacity to invade blood vessels, causing hemorrhage and lung infarction; usually requires hospitalization
Staphylococcal pneumonia (*Staphylococcus aureus*)	Incidence greatest in immunocompromised patients, IV drug users, and as a complication of epidemic influenza Commonly nosocomial in origin Accounts for 10%–30% of hospital-acquired pneumonias *Mortality rate: 25%–60%* MRSA may also cause community-based infection.	Severe hypoxemia, cyanosis, necrotizing infection. Bacteremia is common.	MSSA: oxacillin or nafcillin MRSA or PCN allergy: vancomycin or linezolid	Pleural effusion/ pneumothorax, lung abscess, empyema, meningitis, endocarditis Frequently requires hospitalization. Treatment must be vigorous and prolonged because disease tends to destroy lung tissue.

Type (Causal Organism)	Epidemiology	Clinical Features	Treatment	Complications/ Comments
Klebsiella pneumonia (*Klebsiella pneumoniae* [Friedländer's bacillus-encapsulated gram-negative aerobic bacillus])	Incidence greatest in older adults; alcoholics; patients with chronic disease, such as diabetes, heart failure, COPD; patients in chronic care facilities and nursing homes Accounts for 2%–5% of community-acquired and 10%–30% of hospital-acquired pneumonias *Mortality rate:* 40%–50%	Tissue necrosis occurs rapidly. Toxic appearance: fever, cough, sputum production, bronchopneumonia, lung abscess. Lobar consolidation, bronchopneumonia pattern on chest x-ray.	*Hospital acquired:* cefepime, ceftazidime, imipenem, meropenem, or piperacillin/ tazobactam plus an aminoglycoside or a fluoroquinolone; *Community acquired:* a levofloxacin plus ciprofloxacin or nitrofurantoin (Macrodantin) or nitrofurantoin macrocrystals	Multiple lung abscesses with cyst formation, empyema, pericarditis, pleural effusion; may be fulminating, progressing to fatal outcome
Pneumonia in the Immunocompromised Host				
Pneumocystis pneumonia (*Pneumocystis jiroveci*)	Incidence greatest in patients with AIDS and patients receiving immunosuppressive therapy for cancer, organ transplantation, and other disorders Frequently seen with cytomegalovirus infection Mortality rate 15%–20% in hospitalized patients and fatal if not treated	Pulmonary infiltrates on chest x-ray; nonproductive cough, fever, dyspnea	Trimethoprim/sulfamethoxazole (TMP-SMZ)	Respiratory failure
Fungal pneumonia (*Aspergillus fumigatus*)	Incidence greatest in immunocompromised and neutropenic patients *Mortality rate:* 15%–20%	Cough, hemoptysis, infiltrates, fungus ball on chest x-ray	Voriconazole (Vfend); for invasive disease: amphotericin B or liposomal amphotericin B (L-AMB) or caspofungin (Cancidas) Lobectomy for fungus ball	Dissemination to brain, myocardium, and thyroid gland
Tuberculosis (*Mycobacterium tuberculosis*)	Incidence increased in indigent, immigrant, and prison populations; people with AIDS; and the homeless *Mortality rate:* <1% (depending on comorbidity)	Weight loss, fever, night sweats, cough, sputum production, hemoptysis, nonspecific infiltrate (lower lobe), hilar node enlargement, pleural effusion on chest x-ray	Isoniazid (INH) + rifampin (Rifadin) + ethambutol (Myambutol) + pyrazinamide (PZA) (see section on TB and Table 23-4)	Reinfection and acute respiratory infection
Pneumonia From Aspiration				
Anaerobic bacteria (*S. pneumoniae*, *H. influenzae*, *S. aureus*)	*Risk:* reduced consciousness, dysphagia, disorders of upper GI tract; mechanical disruption of glottic closure (endotracheal tube, tracheostomy, nasogastric feeding)	Abrupt onset of dyspnea, low-grade fever, cough, predisposing condition for aspiration	Clindamycin (Cleocin) +/– a fluoroquinolone	Identification of potential aspirate is important for treatment.

PCN, penicillin; COPD, chronic obstructive pulmonary disease; IV, intravenous; MSSA, methicillin-sensitive *Staphylococcus aureus*; MRSA, methicillin resistant *Staphylococcus aureus*; AIDS, acquired immunodeficiency syndrome; TB, tuberculosis; GI, gastrointestinal.
Adapted from American Thoracic Society & Infectious Diseases Society of America. (2005). Guidelines for the management of adults with hospital-acquired, ventilator-associated, and healthcare-associated pneumonia. *American Journal of Respiratory and Critical Care Medicine, 171*(4), 388–416; and Bartlett, R., Auwaerter, P., & Pham, P. (2012). *John Hopkins ABX guide* (3rd ed.). Burlington, MA: Jones & Bartlett Learning.

Treatment of viral pneumonia is primarily supportive. Hydration is a necessary part of therapy, because fever and tachypnea may result in insensible fluid losses. Antipyretics may be used to treat headache and fever; antitussive medications may be used for the associated cough. Warm, moist inhalations are helpful in relieving bronchial irritation. Antihistamines may provide benefit with reduced sneezing and rhinorrhea. Nasal decongestants may also be used to treat symptoms and improve sleep; however, excessive use can cause rebound nasal congestion. Bed rest is prescribed until the infection shows signs of clearing. If hospitalized, the patient is observed carefully until the clinical condition improves.

If hypoxemia develops, oxygen is administered. Pulse oximetry or arterial blood gas analysis is used to determine the need for oxygen and to evaluate the effectiveness of the therapy. Arterial blood gases may be used to obtain a baseline measure of the patient's oxygenation and acid–base status; however, pulse oximetry is used to continuously monitor the patient's oxygen saturation and response to therapy. More aggressive respiratory support measures include administration of high concentrations of oxygen (fraction of inspired oxygen [FiO_2]), endotracheal intubation, and mechanical ventilation. Different modes of mechanical ventilation may be required (see Chapter 21).

Gerontologic Considerations

Pneumonia in older adult patients may occur as a primary diagnosis or as a complication of a chronic disease. Pulmonary infections in older people frequently are difficult to treat and result in a higher mortality rate than in younger people. In a study of CAP in patients 65 years and older, increasing age impacted mortality. The 30-day mortality rate was 5%, 11%, and 24% in patients 65 to 74 years of age, 75 to 84 years of age, and 85 years of age or greater, respectively (Kothe, Bauer, Marre, et al., 2008). General deterioration, weakness, abdominal symptoms, anorexia, confusion, tachycardia, and tachypnea may signal the onset of pneumonia. The diagnosis of pneumonia may be missed because the classic symptoms of cough, chest pain, sputum production, and fever may be absent or masked in older adult patients. In addition, the presence of some signs may be misleading. Abnormal breath sounds, for example, may be caused by microatelectasis that occurs as a result of decreased mobility, decreased lung volumes, or other respiratory function changes. Chest x-rays may be needed to differentiate chronic heart failure, which is often seen in older adults, from pneumonia as the cause of clinical signs and symptoms.

Supportive treatment includes hydration (with caution and with frequent assessment because of the risk of fluid overload in older adults); supplemental oxygen therapy; and assistance with deep breathing, coughing, frequent position changes, and early ambulation. All of these are particularly important in the care of older adult patients with pneumonia. To reduce or prevent serious complications of pneumonia in older adults, vaccination against pneumococcal and influenza infections is recommended.

Complications

Shock and Respiratory Failure

Severe complications of pneumonia include hypotension and septic shock and respiratory failure (especially with gram-negative bacterial disease in older adult patients). These complications are encountered chiefly in patients who have received no specific treatment or inadequate or delayed treatment. These complications are also encountered when the infecting organism is resistant to therapy, when a comorbid disease complicates the pneumonia, or when the patient is immunocompromised. (See Chapter 14 for further discussion of management of the patient with septic shock.)

Pleural Effusion

Parapneumonic pleural effusions occur in at least 30% of bacterial pneumonias (Bartlett et al., 2012). A parapneumonic effusion is any pleural effusion associated with bacterial pneumonia, lung abscess, or bronchiectasis. After the pleural effusion is detected on a chest x-ray, a thoracentesis may be performed to remove the fluid, which is sent to the laboratory for analysis. There are three stages of parapneumonic pleural effusions based on pathogenesis: uncomplicated, complicated, and thoracic empyema. An **empyema** occurs when thick, purulent fluid accumulates within the pleural space, often with fibrin development and a loculated (walled-off) area where the infection is located (see later discussion). A chest tube may be inserted to treat pleural infection by establishing proper drainage of the empyema. Sterilization of the empyema cavity requires 4 to 6 weeks of antibiotics, and sometimes surgical management is required.

NURSING PROCESS

The Patient With Pneumonia

Assessment

Nursing assessment is critical in detecting pneumonia. Fever, chills, or night sweats in a patient who also has respiratory symptoms should alert the nurse to the possibility of bacterial pneumonia. Respiratory assessment further identifies the clinical manifestations of pneumonia: pleuritic-type pain, fatigue, tachypnea, the use of accessory muscles for breathing, bradycardia or relative bradycardia, coughing, and purulent sputum. The nurse monitors the patient for the following: changes in temperature and pulse; amount, odor, and color of secretions; frequency and severity of cough; degree of tachypnea or shortness of breath; changes in physical assessment findings (primarily assessed by inspecting and auscultating the chest); and changes in the chest x-ray findings.

In addition, it is important to assess older adult patients for unusual behavior, altered mental status, dehydration, excessive fatigue, and concomitant heart failure.

Diagnosis

Nursing Diagnoses

Based on the assessment data, major nursing diagnoses may include the following:

- Ineffective airway clearance related to copious tracheobronchial secretions
- Fatigue and activity intolerance related to impaired respiratory function
- Risk for deficient fluid volume related to fever and a rapid respiratory rate
- Imbalanced nutrition: less than body requirements
- Deficient knowledge about the treatment regimen and preventive measures

Collaborative Problems/Potential Complications

Based on the assessment data, collaborative problems or potential complications that may occur include the following:

- Continuing symptoms after initiation of therapy
- Sepsis and septic shock
- Respiratory failure
- Atelectasis
- Pleural effusion
- Confusion

Planning and Goals

The major goals may include improved airway patency, increased activity, maintenance of proper fluid volume, maintenance of adequate nutrition, an understanding of the treatment protocol and preventive measures, and absence of complications.

Nursing Interventions

Improving Airway Patency

Removing secretions is important because retained secretions interfere with gas exchange and may slow recovery. The nurse encourages hydration (2 to 3 L/day), because adequate hydration thins and loosens pulmonary secretions. Humidification may be used to loosen secretions and improve ventilation. A high-humidity facemask (using either compressed air or oxygen) delivers warm, humidified air to the tracheobronchial tree, helps liquefy secretions, and relieves tracheobronchial irritation. Coughing can be initiated either voluntarily or by reflex. Lung expansion maneuvers, such as deep breathing with an incentive spirometer, may induce a cough. To improve airway patency, the nurse encourages the patient to perform an effective, directed cough, which includes correct positioning, a deep inspiratory maneuver, glottic closure, contraction of the expiratory muscles against the closed glottis, sudden glottic opening, and an explosive expiration. In some cases, the nurse may assist the patient by placing both hands on the lower rib cage (either anterior or posterior) to focus the patient on a slow deep breath, and then manually assisting the patient by applying constant, external pressure during the expiratory phase.

Chest physiotherapy (percussion and postural drainage) is important in loosening and mobilizing secretions (see Chapter 21). Indications for chest physiotherapy include sputum retention not responsive to spontaneous or directed cough, a history of pulmonary problems previously treated with chest physiotherapy, continued evidence of retained secretions (decreased or abnormal breath sounds, change in vital signs), abnormal chest x-ray findings consistent with atelectasis or infiltrates, and deterioration in oxygenation. The patient is placed in the proper position to drain the involved lung segments, then the chest is percussed and vibrated either manually or with a mechanical percussor. Other devices, such as the Flutter device (Axcan Pharma), assist in secretion removal. The nurse may consult the respiratory therapist for volume expansion protocols and secretion management protocols that help direct the respiratory care of the patient and match the patient's needs with appropriate treatment schedules.

After each position change, the nurse encourages the patient to breathe deeply and cough. If the patient is too weak to cough effectively, the nurse may need to remove the mucus by nasotracheal suctioning (see Chapter 21). It may take time for secretions to mobilize and move into the central airways for expectoration. Therefore, it is important for the nurse to monitor the patient for cough and sputum production after the completion of chest physiotherapy.

The nurse also administers and titrates oxygen therapy as prescribed or via protocols. The effectiveness of oxygen therapy is monitored by improvement in clinical signs and symptoms, patient comfort, and adequate oxygenation values as measured by pulse oximetry or arterial blood gas analysis.

Promoting Rest and Conserving Energy

The nurse encourages the debilitated patient to rest and avoid overexertion and possible exacerbation of symptoms. The patient should assume a comfortable position to promote rest and breathing (e.g., semi-Fowler's position) and should change positions frequently to enhance secretion clearance and pulmonary ventilation and perfusion. Outpatients must be instructed to avoid overexertion and to engage in only moderate activity during the initial phases of treatment.

Promoting Fluid Intake

The respiratory rate of patients with pneumonia increases because of the increased workload imposed by labored breathing and fever. An increased respiratory rate leads to an increase in insensible fluid loss during exhalation and can lead to dehydration. Therefore, unless contraindicated, increased fluid intake (at least 2 L/day) is encouraged. Hydration must be achieved more slowly and with careful moni-

toring in patients with preexisting conditions such as heart failure (see Chapter 29).

Maintaining Nutrition

Many patients with shortness of breath and fatigue have a decreased appetite and consume only fluids. Fluids with electrolytes (commercially available drinks, such as Gatorade) may help provide fluid, calories, and electrolytes. Small, frequent meals may be advisable. Other nutritionally enriched drinks or shakes may be helpful. In addition, IV fluids and nutrients may be administered if necessary.

Promoting Patients' Knowledge

The patient and family are instructed about the cause of pneumonia, management of symptoms, signs and symptoms that should be reported to the primary provider or nurse, and the need for follow-up. The patient also needs information about factors (both patient risk factors and external factors) that may have contributed to development of pneumonia and strategies to promote recovery and prevent recurrence. If the patient is hospitalized, he or she is instructed about the purpose and importance of management strategies that have been implemented and about the importance of adhering to them during and after the hospital stay. Explanations should be given simply and in language that the patient can understand. If possible, written instructions and information should be provided, and alternative formats should be provided for patients with hearing or vision loss, if necessary. Because of the severity of symptoms, the patient may require that instructions and explanations be repeated several times.

Monitoring and Managing Potential Complications

Continuing Symptoms After Initiation of Therapy. The patient is observed for response to antibiotic therapy; patients usually begin to respond to treatment within 24 to 48 hours after antibiotic therapy is initiated. If the patient started taking antibiotics before evaluation by culture and sensitivity of the causative organisms, antibiotics may need to be changed once the results are available. The patient is monitored for changes in physical status (deterioration of condition or resolution of symptoms) and for persistent recurrent fever, which may be a result of medication allergy (signaled possibly by a rash); medication resistance or slow response (greater than 48 hours) of the susceptible organism to therapy; pleural effusion; or pneumonia caused by an unusual organism, such as *P. jiroveci* or *Aspergillus fumigatus*. Failure of the pneumonia to resolve or persistence of symptoms despite changes on the chest x-ray raises the suspicion of other underlying disorders, such as lung cancer. As described previously, lung cancers may invade or compress airways, causing an obstructive atelectasis that may lead to pneumonia.

In addition to monitoring for continuing symptoms of pneumonia, the nurse also monitors for other complications, such as septic shock and multiple organ dysfunction syndrome (MODS) and atelectasis, which may develop during the first few days of antibiotic treatment.

Shock and Respiratory Failure. The nurse assesses for signs and symptoms of septic shock and respiratory failure by evaluating the patient's vital signs, pulse oximetry values, and hemodynamic monitoring parameters. The nurse reports signs of deteriorating patient status and assists in administering IV fluids and medications prescribed to combat shock. Intubation and mechanical ventilation may be required if respiratory failure occurs. (Sepsis and septic shock are described in detail in Chapter 14, and care of the patient receiving mechanical ventilation is described in Chapter 21.)

Pleural Effusion. If pleural effusion develops and thoracentesis is performed to remove fluid, the nurse assists in the procedure and explains it to the patient. After thoracentesis, the nurse monitors the patient for pneumothorax or recurrence of pleural effusion. If a chest tube needs to be inserted, the nurse monitors the patient's respiratory status. (See Chapter 21 for more information on care of patients with chest tubes.)

Confusion. A patient with pneumonia is assessed for confusion and other more subtle changes in cognitive status. Confusion and changes in cognitive status resulting from pneumonia are poor prognostic signs (File, 2012). Confusion may be related to hypoxemia, fever, dehydration, sleep deprivation, or developing sepsis. The patient's underlying comorbid conditions may also play a part in the development of confusion. Addressing and correcting underlying factors as well as ensuring patient safety are important nursing interventions.

Promoting Home and Community-Based Care
Educating Patients About Self-Care. Depending on the severity of the pneumonia, treatment may occur in the hospital or in the outpatient setting. Patient education is crucial regardless of the setting, and the proper administration of antibiotics is important. In some instances, the patient may be treated initially with IV antibiotics as an inpatient and then discharged to continue the IV antibiotics at home. A seamless system of care must be maintained for the patient from hospital to home; this includes communication between the nurses caring for the patient in both settings.

If oral antibiotics are prescribed, the nurse educates the patient about their proper administration and potential side effects. The patient should be instructed about symptoms that require contacting the primary provider: difficulty breathing, worsening cough, recurrent/increasing fever, and medication intolerance.

After the fever subsides, the patient may gradually increase activities. Fatigue and weakness may be prolonged after pneumonia, especially in older adults. The nurse encourages breathing exercises to promote secretion clearance and volume expansion. A patient who is being treated as an outpatient should be contacted by the health care team or instructed to contact the primary provider 24 to 48 hours after starting therapy. The patient is also instructed to return to the clinic or primary provider's office for a follow-up chest x-ray and physical examination. Often, improvement in chest x-ray findings lags behind improvement in clinical signs and symptoms.

The nurse encourages the patient to stop smoking. Smoking inhibits tracheobronchial ciliary action, which is the first line of defense of the lower respiratory tract. Smoking also irritates the mucous cells of the bronchi and inhibits the function of alveolar macrophage (scavenger) cells. The patient is instructed to avoid stress, fatigue, sudden changes in temperature, and excessive alcohol intake, all of which lower resistance to pneumonia. The nurse reviews with the patient the principles of adequate nutrition and rest, because one episode of pneumonia may make a patient susceptible to recurring respiratory tract infections.

Continuing Care. A patient who is severely debilitated or who cannot care for him- or herself may require referral for

home care. During home visits, the nurse assesses the patient's physical status, monitors for complications, assesses the home environment, and reinforces previous education. The nurse evaluates the patient's adherence to the therapeutic regimen (i.e., taking medications as prescribed; performing breathing exercises; consuming adequate fluid and dietary intake; and avoiding smoking, alcohol, and excessive activity). The nurse stresses to the patient and family the importance of monitoring for complications or exacerbation of the pneumonia. The nurse encourages the patient to obtain an influenza vaccination at the prescribed times, because influenza increases susceptibility to secondary bacterial pneumonia, especially that caused by staphylococci, *H. influenzae,* and *S. pneumoniae.* The nurse also urges the patient to receive the PPSV against *S. pneumoniae* according to CDC recommendations (see previous discussion on PPSV).

Evaluation
Expected patient outcomes may include the following:
1. Demonstrates improved airway patency, as evidenced by adequate oxygenation by pulse oximetry or arterial blood gas analysis, normal temperature, normal breath sounds, and effective coughing
2. Rests and conserves energy by limiting activities and remaining in bed while symptomatic and then slowly increasing activities
3. Maintains adequate hydration, as evidenced by an adequate fluid intake and urine output and normal skin turgor
4. Consumes adequate dietary intake, as evidenced by maintenance or increase in body weight without excess fluid gain
5. Verbalizes increased knowledge about management strategies
6. Complies with management strategies
7. Exhibits no complications
   a. Exhibits acceptable vital signs, pulse oximetry, and arterial blood gas measurements
   b. Reports productive cough that diminishes over time
   c. Has absence of signs or symptoms of sepsis, septic shock, respiratory failure, or pleural effusion
   d. Remains oriented and aware of surroundings
   e. Maintains or increases weight
8. Complies with treatment protocol and prevention strategies

Aspiration

Aspiration is inhalation of foreign material (e.g., oropharyngeal or stomach contents) into the lungs. It is a serious complication that can cause pneumonia and result in the following clinical picture: tachycardia, dyspnea, central cyanosis, hypertension, hypotension, and potentially death. It can occur when the protective airway reflexes are decreased or absent due to a variety of factors (Chart 23-5).

Pathophysiology

The primary factors responsible for death and complications after aspiration are the volume and character of the aspirated

Chart 23-5	⚠	**RISK FACTORS** **Aspiration**

- Seizure activity
- Brain injury
- Decreased level of consciousness from trauma, drug or alcohol intoxication, excessive sedation, or general anesthesia
- Flat body positioning
- Stroke
- Swallowing disorders
- Cardiac arrest

Adapted from American Association of Critical-Care Nurses. (2012). AACN practice alert: Prevention of aspiration. *AACN Bold Voices, 4*(4), 11–14; and Bartlett, J. (2012). Aspiration pneumonia in adults. *UpTo-Date*. Last updated June 21, 2012. Available at: www.uptodate.com

contents. Aspiration pneumonia develops after inhalation of colonized oral or pharyngeal material. The pathologic process involves an acute inflammatory response to bacteria and bacterial products. Most commonly, the bacteriologic findings include gram-positive cocci, gram-negative rods, and occasionally anaerobic bacteria (Bartlett, 2012).

A full stomach contains solid particles of food. If these are aspirated, the problem then becomes one of mechanical blockage of the airways and secondary infection. During periods of fasting, the stomach contains acidic gastric juice, which, if aspirated, can be very destructive to the alveoli and capillaries. Fecal contamination (more likely seen in intestinal obstruction) increases the likelihood of death, because the endotoxins produced by intestinal organisms may be absorbed systemically, or the thick proteinaceous material found in the intestinal contents may obstruct the airway, leading to atelectasis and secondary bacterial invasion.

Esophageal conditions may also be associated with aspiration pneumonia. These include dysphagia, esophageal strictures, neoplasm or diverticula, tracheoesophageal fistula, and gastroesophageal reflux disease.

Prevention

The risk of aspiration is indirectly related to the level of consciousness of the patient. Aspiration of small amounts of material from the buccal (oral) cavity is not uncommon, particularly during sleep; however, disease as a result of aspiration does not occur in healthy persons because the material is cleared by the mucociliary tree and the macrophages. Witnessed aspiration of large volumes occurs occasionally; however, small-volume clinically silent aspiration is more common (American Association of Critical Care Nurses [AACN], 2012). Prevention is the primary goal when caring for patients at risk for aspiration.

▶ *Quality and Safety Nursing Alert*

When a nonfunctioning nasogastric tube allows the gastric contents to accumulate in the stomach, a condition known as silent aspiration may result. Silent aspiration often occurs unobserved and may be more common than suspected. If untreated, massive inhalation of gastric contents develops in a period of several hours.

Compensating for Absent Reflexes

Aspiration may occur if the patient cannot adequately coordinate protective glottic, laryngeal, and cough reflexes. This hazard is increased if the patient has a distended abdomen, is supine, has the upper extremities immobilized in any manner, receives local anesthetic agents to the oropharyngeal or laryngeal area for diagnostic procedures, has been sedated, or has had long-term intubation.

Patients with altered consciousness or those receiving mechanical ventilation or tube feedings should be placed in a semirecumbent position with the head of the bed at a 30- to 45-degree angle, unless contraindicated (AACN, 2012). Sedation should be used as sparingly as possible.

For patients with known swallowing dysfunction or those recently extubated following prolonged endotracheal intubation, a swallowing assessment is necessary. This assessment is often done by a speech therapist. Besides positioning the patient semirecumbent or upright prior to eating, other helpful techniques may include suggesting a soft diet and encouraging the patient to take small bites. The patient should be instructed to keep the chin tucked and the head turned with repeated swallowing. Although body positioning and changing the consistency of food are reasonable prophylactic measures, efficacy has not been demonstrated in controlled clinical trials (AACN, 2012).

When vomiting, people can normally protect their airway by sitting up or turning on the side and coordinating breathing, coughing, gag, and glottic reflexes. If these reflexes are active, an oral airway should not be inserted. If an airway is in place, it should be pulled out the moment the patient gags so as not to stimulate the pharyngeal gag reflex and promote vomiting and aspiration. Suctioning of oral secretions with a catheter should be performed with minimal pharyngeal stimulation.

For patients with an endotracheal tube and feeding tube, the endotracheal cuff pressure should be maintained at greater than 20 cm H_2O (but less than 30 cm H_2O to minimize injury) to prevent leakage of secretions from around the cuff into the lower respiratory tract. In addition, hypopharyngeal suctioning is recommended before the cuff is deflated (AACN, 2012).

Assessing Feeding Tube Placement

Tube feedings must be given only when it is certain that the feeding tube is positioned correctly in the stomach. Many patients receive enteral feeding directly into the duodenum through a small-bore flexible feeding tube or surgically implanted tube. (See Chapter 45 for discussion of confirming placement of enteral tubes and administration of tube feedings.)

Identifying Delayed Stomach Emptying

A full stomach can cause aspiration because of increased intragastric or extragastric pressure. The following may delay emptying of the stomach: intestinal obstruction; increased gastric secretions in gastroesophageal reflex disease; increased gastric secretions during anxiety, stress, or pain; and abdominal distention due to paralytic ileus, ascites, peritonitis, the use of opioids or sedatives, severe illness, or vaginal delivery. (See Chapter 45 for discussion of management of patients receiving gastric tube feedings.)

Managing Effects of Prolonged Intubation

Prolonged endotracheal intubation or tracheostomy can depress the laryngeal and glottic reflexes because of disuse. Patients with prolonged tracheostomies are encouraged to phonate and exercise their laryngeal muscles. For patients who have had long-term intubation or tracheostomies, it may be helpful to have a speech therapist experienced in swallowing disorders work with the patient to address swallowing problems, as noted previously.

Severe Acute Respiratory Syndrome

Severe acute respiratory syndrome (SARS) is a viral respiratory illness caused by a coronavirus, called *SARS-associated coronavirus*. It was first reported in Asia in 2003 and quickly spread to countries in North America, South America, Europe, and Asia. The World Health Organization (WHO) reported that 8,098 people worldwide became sick with SARS during the 2003 outbreak, and 774 died (CDC, 2013). Since 2004, there have been no reported cases of SARS transmission anywhere in the world (CDC, 2013).

SARS develops in people who either have close contact with a person who has been diagnosed with the disease or a history of travel or residence in an area with known cases. The SARS-associated coronavirus is transmitted via respiratory droplets when an infected person coughs or sneezes; the droplets may be deposited on the mucous membranes (mouth, nose, eyes) of a nearby person. The virus may also be spread when a person touches a surface or object contaminated by the droplets and then touches his or her mucous membranes. The virus may be transmitted in other ways, including sewage and water; however, these methods of transmission are unclear at this time (CDC, 2013).

Characteristic symptoms of SARS are a fever (greater than 38°C [100.4°F]), coughing, and difficulty breathing. Additional symptoms include headache, overall feeling of discomfort, body aches, and diarrhea. Most patients develop pneumonia. The incubation period is usually 2 to 7 days, although longer periods have been reported. Risk factors associated with poor outcomes include older age, comorbid conditions (e.g., diabetes, chronic hepatitis B, COPD), atypical symptoms, elevated serum lactate dehydrogenase on admission, and acute renal failure. Currently, no treatment except supportive care is recommended (CDC, 2013).

Infection control measures designed to limit transmission of SARS are a priority. In health care settings, the general CDC guidelines for infection control in health care facilities should be followed; in addition, specific strategies for SARS should be in place, including the use of negative pressure isolation rooms, personal protective equipment, hand hygiene, environmental cleaning and disinfection techniques, and source control measures to contain patients' secretions. (See the CDC entry in the Resource section at end of this chapter for link to additional information on SARS.)

Pulmonary Tuberculosis

Tuberculosis (TB) is an infectious disease that primarily affects the lung parenchyma. It also may be transmitted to other parts of the body, including the meninges, kidneys, bones, and lymph nodes. The primary infectious agent, *M. tuberculosis,* is an acid-fast aerobic rod that grows slowly and is sensitive to heat and ultraviolet light. *Mycobacterium bovis* and *Mycobacterium avium* have rarely been associated with the development of a TB infection.

TB is a worldwide public health problem that is closely associated with poverty, malnutrition, overcrowding, substandard housing, and inadequate health care. Mortality and morbidity rates continue to rise; *M. tuberculosis* infects an estimated one third of the world's population and remains the leading cause of death from infectious disease in the world. According to the WHO, there were an estimated 8.8 million cases and an estimated 1.1 million deaths from TB in 2010 (WHO, 2011).

In the United States, 11,182 cases of TB were reported in 2010 (CDC, 2012d). Factors that prevent elimination of TB in the United States include the prevalence of TB among foreign-born residents, delays in detecting and reporting cases of TB, the lack of protection of contacts of people with infectious cases of TB, the presence of a substantial number of people with latent TB, and maintaining clinical and public health expertise in this disease (CDC, 2012d).

Transmission and Risk Factors

TB spreads from person to person by airborne transmission. An infected person releases droplet nuclei (usually particles 1 to 5 mcm in diameter) through talking, coughing, sneezing, laughing, or singing. Larger droplets settle; smaller droplets remain suspended in the air and are inhaled by a susceptible person. Chart 23-6 lists risk factors for TB. Chart 23-7 summarizes the CDC's recommendations for prevention of TB transmission in health care settings.

Pathophysiology

TB begins when a susceptible person inhales mycobacteria and becomes infected. The bacteria are transmitted through the airways to the alveoli, where they are deposited and begin to multiply. The bacilli also are transported via the lymph system and bloodstream to other parts of the body (kidneys, bones, cerebral cortex) and other areas of the lungs (upper lobes). The body's immune system responds by initiating an inflammatory reaction. Phagocytes (neutrophils and macrophages) engulf many of the bacteria, and TB-specific lymphocytes lyse (destroy) the bacilli and normal tissue. This tissue reaction results in the accumulation of exudate in the alveoli, causing bronchopneumonia. The initial infection usually occurs 2 to 10 weeks after exposure.

Granulomas, new tissue masses of live and dead bacilli, are surrounded by macrophages, which form a protective wall. They are then transformed to a fibrous tissue mass, the central portion of which is called a *Ghon tubercle*. The material (bacteria and macrophages) becomes necrotic, forming a cheesy mass. This mass may become calcified and form a collagenous scar. At this point, the bacteria become dormant, and there is no further progression of active disease.

After initial exposure and infection, active disease may develop because of a compromised or inadequate immune system response. Active disease also may occur with reinfection and activation of dormant bacteria. In this case, the

Chart 23-6 ⚠ RISK FACTORS
Tuberculosis

- Close contact with someone who has active TB. Inhalation of airborne nuclei from an infected person is proportional to the amount of time spent in the same air space, the proximity of the person, and the degree of ventilation.
- Immunocompromised status (e.g., those with HIV infection, cancer, transplanted organs, and prolonged high-dose corticosteroid therapy)
- Substance abuse (IV/injection drug users and alcoholics)
- Any person without adequate health care (the homeless; impoverished; minorities, particularly children <15 years and young adults between ages 15 and 44 years)
- Preexisting medical conditions or special treatment (e.g., diabetes, chronic renal failure, malnourishment, selected malignancies, hemodialysis, transplanted organ, gastrectomy, jejunoileal bypass)
- Immigration from countries with a high prevalence of TB (southeastern Asia, Africa, Latin America, Caribbean)
- Institutionalization (e.g., long-term care facilities, psychiatric institutions, prisons)
- Living in overcrowded, substandard housing
- Being a health care worker performing high-risk activities: administration of aerosolized pentamidine and other medications, sputum induction procedures, bronchoscopy, suctioning, coughing procedures, caring for the immunosuppressed patient, home care with the high-risk population, and administering anesthesia and related procedures (e.g., intubation, suctioning)

Adapted from Centers for Disease Control and Prevention. (2012c). *TB fact sheets-infection control and prevention; TB in specific populations.* Available at www.cdc.gov/tb/publications/factsheets/default.htm; and World Health Organization. (2011). *Global tuberculosis control 2011.* Geneva: WHO Press.

Ghon tubercle ulcerates, releasing the cheesy material into the bronchi. The bacteria then become airborne, resulting in further spread of the disease. Then, the ulcerated tubercle heals and forms scar tissue. This causes the infected lung to become more inflamed, resulting in further development of bronchopneumonia and tubercle formation.

Unless this process is arrested, it spreads slowly downward to the hilum of the lungs and later extends to adjacent lobes. The process may be prolonged and is characterized by long remissions when the disease is arrested, followed by periods of renewed activity. Approximately 10% of people who are initially infected develop active disease. Some people develop reactivation TB (also called *adult-type progressive TB*). Reactivation TB represents 90% of adult cases in the non–human immunodeficiency virus (HIV)-infected population. The reactivation of a dormant focus occurring during the primary infection is the cause. It most commonly occurs in the lungs, usually in the apical or posterior segments of the upper lobes or the superior segments of the lower lobes (Basgov, Fordham von Reyn, & Baron, 2012).

Clinical Manifestations

The signs and symptoms of pulmonary TB are insidious. Most patients have a low-grade fever, cough, night sweats, fatigue, and weight loss. The cough may be nonproductive, or mucopurulent sputum may be expectorated. Hemoptysis also may occur. Both the systemic and the pulmonary symptoms are chronic and may have been present for weeks to

Chart 23-7 Centers for Disease Control and Prevention Recommendations for Preventing Transmission of Tuberculosis in Health Care Settings

1. Early identification and treatment of persons with active TB
   a. Maintain a high index of suspicion for TB to identify cases rapidly.
   b. Promptly initiate effective multidrug anti-TB therapy based on clinical and drug-resistance surveillance data.
2. Prevention of spread of infectious droplet nuclei by source control methods and by reduction of microbial contamination of indoor air
   a. Initiate AFB isolation precautions immediately for all patients who are suspected or confirmed to have active TB and who may be infectious. AFB isolation precautions include the use of a private room with negative pressure in relation to surrounding areas and a minimum of six air exchanges per hour. Air from the room should be exhausted directly to the outside. The use of ultraviolet lamps and/or high-efficiency particulate air filters to supplement ventilation may be considered.
   b. Persons entering the AFB isolation room should use disposable particulate respirators that fit snugly around the face.
   c. Continue AFB isolation precautions until there is clinical evidence of reduced infectiousness (i.e., cough has substantially decreased, and the number of organisms on sequential sputum smears is decreasing). If drug resistance is suspected or confirmed, continue AFB precautions until the sputum smear is negative for AFB.
   d. Use special precautions during cough-inducing procedures.
3. Surveillance for TB transmission
   a. Maintain surveillance for TB infection among health care workers (HCWs) by routine, periodic tuberculin skin testing. Recommend appropriate preventive therapy for HCWs when indicated.
   b. Maintain surveillance for TB cases among patients and HCWs.
   c. Promptly initiate contact investigation procedures among HCWs, patients, and visitors exposed to an untreated, or ineffectively treated, patient with infectious TB for whom appropriate AFB procedures are not in place. Recommend appropriate therapy or preventive therapy for contacts with disease or TB infection without current disease. Therapeutic regimens should be chosen based on the clinical history and local drug-resistance surveillance data.

Adapted from Centers for Disease Control and Prevention. (2012c). *TB fact sheet-infection control and prevention.* Available at www.cdc.gov/tb/publications/factsheets/default.htm.

months. Older adult patients usually present with less pronounced symptoms than younger patients. Extrapulmonary disease occurs in up to 16% of cases in the United States. In patients infected with HIV, extrapulmonary disease is more prevalent.

Assessment and Diagnostic Findings

Once a patient presents with a positive skin test, blood test, or sputum culture for acid-fast bacilli (AFB; see later discussion on these), additional assessments must be done. These tests include a complete history, physical examination, tuberculin skin test, chest x-ray, and drug susceptibility testing.

Clinical manifestations of fever, anorexia, weight loss, night sweats, fatigue, cough, and sputum production prompt a more thorough assessment of respiratory function—for example, assessing the lungs for consolidation by evaluating breath sounds (diminished, bronchial sounds; crackles), fremitus, and egophony. If the patient is infected with TB, the chest x-ray usually reveals lesions in the upper lobes. For all patients, the initial M. *tuberculosis* isolate should be tested for drug resistance. Drug susceptibility patterns should be repeated at 3 months for patients who do not respond to therapy (CDC, 2012c).

Tuberculin Skin Test

The Mantoux method is used to determine whether a person has been infected with the TB bacillus and is used widely in screening for latent M. *tuberculosis* infection. The Mantoux method is a standardized, intracutaneous injection procedure and should be performed only by those trained in its administration and reading. Tubercle bacillus extract (tuberculin), purified protein derivative (PPD), is injected into the intradermal layer of the inner aspect of the forearm, approximately 4 inches below the elbow (Fig. 23-3). Intermediate-strength PPD, in a tuberculin syringe with a half-inch 26- or 27-gauge needle, is used. The needle, with the bevel facing up, is inserted beneath the skin. Then, 0.1 mL of PPD is injected, creating an elevation in the skin, a well-demarcated wheal 6 to 10 mm in diameter. The site, antigen name, strength, lot number, date, and time of the test are recorded. The test result is read 48 to 72 hours after injection. Tests read after 72 hours tend to underestimate the true size of **induration** (hardening). A delayed localized reaction indicates that the person is sensitive to tuberculin.

A reaction occurs when both induration and erythema (redness) are present. After the area is inspected for induration, it is lightly palpated across the injection site, from the area of normal skin to the margins of the induration. The diameter of the induration (not erythema) is measured in millimeters at its widest part (see Fig. 23-3), and the size of the induration is documented. Erythema without induration is not considered significant.

The size of the induration determines the significance of the reaction. A reaction of 0 to 4 mm is considered not significant. A reaction of 5 mm or greater may be significant in people who are considered to be at risk. It is defined as positive in patients who are HIV positive or have HIV risk factors and are of unknown HIV status, in those who are close contacts of someone with active TB, and in those who have chest x-ray results consistent with TB. An induration of 10 mm or greater is usually considered significant in people who have normal or mildly impaired immunity. A significant reaction indicates past exposure to M. *tuberculosis* or vaccination with bacille Calmette-Guérin (BCG) vaccine. The BCG vaccine is given to produce a greater resistance to development of TB. It is effective in up to 76% of people who receive it. The BCG vaccine is used in Europe and Latin America but not routinely in the United States.

A significant (positive) reaction does not necessarily mean that active disease is present in the body. More than 90% of people who are tuberculin-significant reactors do not develop clinical TB. However, all significant reactors are candidates for active TB. In general, the more intense the reaction, the greater the likelihood of an active infection.

A nonsignificant (negative) skin test does not exclude TB infection or disease, because patients who are immunosuppressed cannot develop an immune response that is adequate to produce a positive skin test. This is referred to as anergy.

QuantiFERON-TB Gold Test

The QuantiFERON-TB Gold (QFT-G) test is an enzyme-linked immunosorbent assay (ELISA) that detects the release of interferon-gamma by white blood cells when the blood of a patient with TB is incubated with peptides similar to those in M. *tuberculosis*. The results of the QFT-G test are available in less than 24 hours and are not affected by prior vaccination with BCG (Loscalzo, 2010). Additional rapid tests for TB include the QuantiFERON-TB Gold in-tube test (QFT-GIT), the T-SPOT TB test (T-Spot), and the Xpert MTB/RIF, which was endorsed by the WHO in 2011 (CDC, 2010; WHO, 2011).

Sputum Culture

The presence of AFB on a sputum smear may indicate disease but does not confirm the diagnosis of TB because some AFB are not M. *tuberculosis*. A culture is done to confirm the diagnosis. For all patients, the initial M. *tuberculosis* isolate should be tested for drug resistance.

Gerontologic Considerations

TB may have atypical manifestations in older adult patients, whose symptoms may include unusual behavior and altered mental status, fever, anorexia, and weight loss. In many older adult patients, the tuberculin skin test produces no reaction (loss of immunologic memory) or delayed reactivity for up to

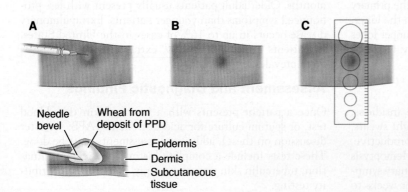

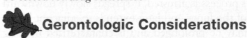

Needle bevel — Wheal from deposit of PPD

— Epidermis
— Dermis
— Subcutaneous tissue

FIGURE 23-3 • The Mantoux test for tuberculosis. **A.** Correct technique for inserting the needle involves depositing the purified protein derivative (PPD) subcutaneously with the needle bevel facing upward. **B.** The reaction to the Mantoux test usually consists of a wheal, a hivelike, firm welt. **C.** To determine the extent of the reaction, the wheal is measured using a commercially prepared gauge. Interpretation of the Mantoux test is discussed in the text.

1 week (recall phenomenon). A second skin test is performed in 1 to 2 weeks.

Medical Management

Pulmonary TB is treated primarily with anti-TB agents for 6 to 12 months. A prolonged treatment duration is necessary to ensure eradication of the organisms and to prevent relapse. The continuing and increasing resistance of M. *tuberculosis* to TB medications is a worldwide concern and challenge in TB therapy. Several types of drug resistance must be considered when planning effective therapy:

- *Primary drug resistance:* Resistance to one of the first-line anti-TB agents in people who have not had previous treatment
- *Secondary or acquired drug resistance:* Resistance to one or more anti-TB agents in patients undergoing therapy
- *Multidrug resistance:* Resistance to two agents, isoniazid (INH) and rifampin. The populations at greatest risk for multidrug resistance are those who are HIV positive, institutionalized, or homeless.

The increasing prevalence of drug resistance points out the need to begin TB treatment with four or more medications, to ensure completion of therapy, and to develop and evaluate new anti-TB medications.

In current TB therapy, four first-line medications are used (Table 23-4): INH, rifampin (Rifadin), pyrazinamide (PZA), and ethambutol (Myambutol). Combination medications, such as INH and rifampin (Rifamate) or INH, pyrazinamide, and rifampin (Rifater) and medications administered twice a week (e.g., rifapentine [Priftin]) are available to help improve patient adherence. However, these medications are more costly. Capreomycin (Capastat), ethionamide (Trecator), para-aminosalicylate sodium, and cycloserine (Seromycin) are second-line medications. Additional potentially effective medications include other aminoglycosides, quinolones, rifabutin, and clofazimine (Lamprene).

Recommended treatment guidelines for newly diagnosed cases of pulmonary TB have remained consistent since 2003 and have two phases: an initial treatment phase and a continuation phase (Bartlett et al., 2012; CDC, 2003). The initial phase consists of a multiple-medication regimen

TABLE 23-4 First-Line Antituberculosis Medications for Active Disease

Commonly Used Agents	Adult Daily Dosage*	Most Common Side Effects	Drug Interactions[†]	Remarks*
Isoniazid (INH)	5 mg/kg (300 mg maximum daily)	Peripheral neuritis, hepatic enzyme elevation, hepatitis, hypersensitivity	Phenytoin—synergistic Antabuse Alcohol	Bactericidal Pyridoxine is used as prophylaxis for neuritis. Monitor AST and ALT.
Rifampin (Rifadin)	10 mg/kg (600 mg maximum daily)	Hepatitis, febrile reaction, purpura (rare), nausea, vomiting	Rifampin increases metabolism of oral contraceptives, quinidine, corticosteroids, coumarin derivatives and methadone, digoxin, oral hypoglycemics. PAS may interfere with absorption of rifampin.	Bactericidal Orange urine and other body secretions Discoloring of contact lenses Monitor AST and ALT.
Rifabutin (Mycobutin)	5 mg/kg (300 mg maximum daily)		Avoid protease inhibitors.	
Rifapentine (Priftin)	10 mg/kg (600 mg twice weekly)	Hepatotoxicity, thrombocytopenia		Orange-red coloration of body secretions, contact lenses, dentures Use with caution in older adults or in those with renal disease.
Pyrazinamide	15–30 mg/kg (2 g maximum daily)*	Hyperuricemia, hepatotoxicity, skin rash, arthralgias, GI distress		Bactericidal Monitor uric acid, AST, and ALT.
Ethambutol (Myambutol)	15–25 mg/kg (1.6 g maximum daily dose)*	Optic neuritis (may lead to blindness; very rare at 15 mg/kg), skin rash		Bacteriostatic Use with caution with renal disease or when eye testing is not feasible. Monitor visual acuity, color, and discrimination.[‡]
Combinations: INH + rifampin (e.g., Rifamate)	150-mg and 300-mg caps (2 caps daily)			

AST, aspartate transaminase; ALT, alanine transaminase; PAS, para-aminosalicylic acid; GI, gastrointestinal.
*Check product labeling for detailed information on dose, contraindications, drug interactions, adverse reactions, and monitoring.
[†]Refer to current literature, particularly on rifampin, because it increases hepatic microenzymes and therefore interacts with many drugs.
[‡]Initial examination should be performed at start of treatment.
Adapted from Bartlett, R., Auwaerter, P., & Pham, P. (2012). *John Hopkins ABX guide* (3rd ed.). Burlington, MA: Jones & Bartlett Learning; and Centers for Disease Control and Prevention. (2003). Treatment of tuberculosis. *MMWR Morbidity and Mortality Weekly Report, 52*(RR-11), 1–77.

of INH, rifampin, pyrazinamide, and ethambutol plus vitamin B_6 50 mg. All are taken once a day and are oral medications (Bartlett et al., 2012). This initial intensive-treatment regimen is administered daily for 8 weeks, after which options for the continuation phase of treatment include INH and rifampin or INH and rifapentine. The continuation regimen lasts for an additional 4 or 7 months. The 4-month period is used for the large majority of patients (CDC, 2003). The 7-month period is recommended for patients with cavitary pulmonary TB whose sputum culture after the initial 2 months of treatment is positive, for those whose initial phase of treatment did not include PZA, and for those being treated once weekly with INH and rifapentine whose sputum culture is positive at the end of the initial phase of treatment. People are considered noninfectious after 2 to 3 weeks of continuous medication therapy. The total number of doses taken, not simply the duration of treatment, more accurately determines whether a course of therapy has been completed.

INH also may be used as a prophylactic (preventive) measure for people who are at risk for significant disease, including:

- Household family members of patients with active disease
- Patients with HIV infection who have a PPD test reaction with 5 mm of induration or more
- Patients with fibrotic lesions suggestive of old TB detected on a chest x-ray and a PPD reaction with 5 mm of induration or more
- Patients whose current PPD test results show a change from former test results, suggesting recent exposure to TB and possible infection (skin test converters)
- Users of IV/injection drugs who have PPD test results with 10 mm of induration or more
- Patients with high-risk comorbid conditions and a PPD result with 10 mm of induration or more

Other candidates for preventive INH therapy are those 35 years or younger who have PPD test results with 10 mm of induration or more and one of the following criteria:

- Foreign-born individuals from countries with a high prevalence of TB
- High-risk, medically underserved populations
- Institutionalized patients

Prophylactic INH treatment involves taking daily doses for 6 to 12 months. Liver enzymes, blood urea nitrogen (BUN), and creatinine levels are monitored monthly. Sputum culture results are monitored for AFB to evaluate the effectiveness of treatment and the patient's adherence to the treatment regimen.

Nursing Management

Nursing management includes promoting airway clearance, advocating adherence to the treatment regimen, promoting activity and nutrition, and preventing transmission.

Promoting Airway Clearance

Copious secretions obstruct the airways in many patients with TB and interfere with adequate gas exchange. Increasing the fluid intake promotes systemic hydration and serves as an effective expectorant. The nurse instructs the patient about correct positioning to facilitate airway drainage (postural drainage; described in Chapter 21).

Promoting Adherence to Treatment Regimen

The multiple-medication regimen that the patient must follow can be quite complex. Understanding of the medications, schedule, and side effects is important. The nurse educates the patient that TB is a communicable disease and that taking medications is the most effective means of preventing transmission. The major reason treatment fails is that patients do not take their medications regularly and for the prescribed duration. This may be due to side effects or the complexity of the treatment regimen.

The nurse educates the patient to take the medication either on an empty stomach or at least 1 hour before meals, because food interferes with medication absorption (although taking medications on an empty stomach frequently results in gastrointestinal upset). Patients taking INH should avoid foods that contain tyramine and histamine (tuna, aged cheese, red wine, soy sauce, yeast extracts), because eating them while taking INH may result in headache, flushing, hypotension, lightheadedness, palpitations, and diaphoresis. Patients should also avoid alcohol because of the high potential for hepatoxic effects.

In addition, rifampin can alter the metabolism of certain other medications, making them less effective. These medications include beta-blockers, oral anticoagulants such as warfarin (Coumadin), digoxin, quinidine, corticosteroids, oral hypoglycemic agents, oral contraceptives, theophylline, and verapamil (Calan, Isoptin). This issue should be discussed with the primary provider and pharmacist so that medication dosages can be adjusted accordingly. The nurse informs the patient that rifampin may discolor contact lenses and that the patient may want to wear eyeglasses during treatment. The nurse monitors for other side effects of anti-TB medications, including hepatitis, neurologic changes (hearing loss, neuritis), and rash. Liver enzymes, BUN, and serum creatinine levels are monitored to detect changes in liver and kidney function. Sputum culture results are monitored for AFB to evaluate the effectiveness of the treatment regimen and adherence to therapy.

The nurse instructs the patient about the risk of drug resistance if the medication regimen is not strictly and continuously followed. The nurse carefully monitors vital signs and observes for spikes in temperature or changes in the patient's clinical status. Caregivers of patients who are not hospitalized are taught to monitor the patient's temperature and respiratory status. Changes in the patient's respiratory status are reported to the primary provider.

Promoting Activity and Adequate Nutrition

Patients with TB are often debilitated from prolonged chronic illness and impaired nutritional status. The nurse plans a progressive activity schedule that focuses on increasing activity tolerance and muscle strength. Anorexia, weight loss, and malnutrition are common in patients with TB. The patient's willingness to eat may be altered by fatigue from excessive coughing; sputum production; chest pain; generalized debilitated state; or cost, if the patient has few resources. Identifying facilities (e.g., shelters, soup kitchens, Meals on Wheels) that provide meals in the patient's neighborhood may increase the likelihood that the patient with limited resources and energy will have access to a more nutritious intake. A nutritional plan that allows for small, frequent meals may be required. Liquid nutritional supplements may assist in meeting basic caloric requirements.

Preventing Transmission of Tuberculosis Infection

To prevent transmission of TB to others, the nurse carefully instructs the patient about important hygiene measures, including mouth care, covering the mouth and nose when coughing and sneezing, proper disposal of tissues, and hand hygiene. TB is a disease that must be reported to the health department so that people who have been in contact with the affected patient during the infectious stage can undergo screening and possible treatment, if indicated.

In addition to the risk of transmission of TB infection to other people, it can also be spread to other parts of the body of affected patients. Spread or dissemination of TB infection to nonpulmonary sites of the body is known as miliary TB. It is the result of invasion of the bloodstream by the tubercle bacillus. Usually, it results from late reactivation of a dormant infection in the lung or elsewhere. The origin of the bacilli that enter the bloodstream is either a chronic focus that has ulcerated into a blood vessel or multitudes of miliary tubercles lining the inner surface of the thoracic duct. The organisms migrate from these foci into the bloodstream, are carried throughout the body, and disseminate throughout all tissues, with tiny miliary tubercles developing in the lungs, spleen, liver, kidneys, meninges, and other organs.

The clinical course of miliary TB may vary from an acute, rapidly progressive infection with high fever to a slowly developing process with low-grade fever, anemia, and debilitation. At first, there may be no localizing signs except an enlarged spleen and a reduced number of leukocytes. However, within a few weeks, the chest x-ray reveals small densities scattered diffusely throughout both lung fields; these are the miliary tubercles, which gradually grow.

The possibility of spread to nonpulmonary sites in the body requires careful monitoring for this very serious form of TB. The nurse monitors vital signs and observes for spikes in temperature as well as changes in renal and cognitive function. Few physical signs may be elicited on physical examination of the chest, but at this stage, the patient has a severe cough and dyspnea. Treatment of miliary TB is the same as for pulmonary TB.

Lung Abscess

A lung abscess is necrosis of the pulmonary parenchyma caused by microbial infection (Bartlett et al., 2012). It is generally caused by aspiration of anaerobic bacteria. By definition, in a lung abscess, the chest x-ray demonstrates a cavity of at least 2 cm. Patients who are at risk for aspiration of foreign material and development of a lung abscess include those with impaired cough reflexes who cannot close the glottis and those with swallowing difficulties. Other at-risk patients include those with central nervous system disorders (e.g., seizure, stroke), drug addiction, alcoholism, esophageal disease, or compromised immune function; patients without teeth and those receiving nasogastric tube feedings; and patients with an altered state of consciousness due to anesthesia.

Pathophysiology

Most lung abscesses are a complication of bacterial pneumonia or are caused by aspiration of oral anaerobes into the lung. Abscesses also may occur secondary to mechanical or functional obstruction of the bronchi by a tumor, foreign body, or bronchial stenosis, or from necrotizing pneumonias, TB, pulmonary embolism (PE), or chest trauma.

Most lung abscesses are found in areas of the lung that may be affected by aspiration. The site of the lung abscess is related to gravity and is determined by position. For patients who are confined to bed, the posterior segment of an upper lobe and the superior segment of the lower lobe are the most common areas. However, atypical presentations may occur, depending on the position of the patient when the aspiration occurred.

Initially, the cavity in the lung may or may not extend directly into a bronchus. Eventually, the abscess becomes surrounded, or encapsulated, by a wall of fibrous tissue. The necrotic process may extend until it reaches the lumen of a bronchus or the pleural space and establishes communication with the respiratory tract, the pleural cavity, or both. If the bronchus is involved, the purulent contents are expectorated continuously in the form of sputum. If the pleura is involved, an empyema results. A communication or connection between the bronchus and pleura is known as a bronchopleural fistula.

The organisms frequently associated with lung abscesses are *S. aureus*, *Klebsiella*, and other gram-negative species (Bartlett et al., 2012). However, anaerobic organisms may also be present. The organisms vary depending on the underlying predisposing factors.

Clinical Manifestations

The clinical manifestations of a lung abscess may vary from a mild productive cough to acute illness. Most patients have a fever and a productive cough with moderate to copious amounts of foul-smelling, sometimes bloody, sputum. The fever and cough may develop insidiously and may have been present for several weeks before diagnosis. Leukocytosis may be present. Pleurisy or dull chest pain, dyspnea, weakness, anorexia, and weight loss are common.

Assessment and Diagnostic Findings

Physical examination of the chest may reveal dullness on percussion and decreased or absent breath sounds with an intermittent **pleural friction rub** (grating or creaking sound) on auscultation. Crackles may be present. Confirmation of the diagnosis is made by chest x-ray, sputum culture, and, in some cases, fiberoptic bronchoscopy. The chest x-ray reveals an infiltrate with an air–fluid level. A computed tomography (CT) scan of the chest may be required to provide more detailed images of different cross-sectional areas of the lung.

Prevention

The following measures reduce the risk of lung abscess:
- Appropriate antibiotic therapy before any dental procedures in patients who must have teeth extracted while their gums and teeth are infected

- Adequate dental and oral hygiene, because anaerobic bacteria play a role in the pathogenesis of lung abscess
- Appropriate antimicrobial therapy for patients with pneumonia

Medical Management

The findings of the history, physical examination, chest x-ray, and sputum culture indicate the type of organism and the treatment required. Adequate drainage of the lung abscess may be achieved through postural drainage and chest physiotherapy. Patients should be assessed for an adequate cough. Some patients require insertion of a percutaneous chest catheter for long-term drainage of the abscess. Therapeutic use of bronchoscopy to drain an abscess is uncommon. A diet high in protein and calories is necessary, because chronic infection is associated with a catabolic state, necessitating increased intake of calories and protein to facilitate healing. Surgical intervention is rare, but pulmonary resection (lobectomy) is performed if massive **hemoptysis** (coughing up of blood) occurs or if there is little or no response to medical management.

IV antimicrobial therapy depends on the results of the sputum culture and sensitivity and is administered for an extended period. Standard treatment for an anaerobic lung infection is clindamycin (Cleocin). Large IV doses are usually required, because the antibiotic must penetrate the necrotic tissue and the fluid in the abscess. The IV dose is continued until symptoms improve.

Long-term therapy with oral antibiotics replaces IV therapy after the patient shows signs of improvement (usually 3 to 5 days). Improvement is demonstrated by normal temperature, decreased white blood cell count, and improvement on chest x-ray (resolution of surrounding infiltrate, reduction in cavity size, and absence of fluid). Oral administration of antibiotic therapy is continued for an additional 4 to 12 weeks and sometimes longer. If treatment is stopped too soon, a relapse may occur (Bartlett et al., 2012).

Nursing Management

The nurse administers antibiotics and IV treatments as prescribed and monitors for adverse effects. Chest physiotherapy is initiated as prescribed to facilitate drainage of the abscess. The nurse educates the patient to perform deep-breathing and coughing exercises to help expand the lungs. To ensure proper nutritional intake, the nurse encourages a diet that is high in protein and calories. The nurse also offers emotional support, because the abscess may take a long time to resolve.

Promoting Home and Community-Based Care

Educating Patients About Self-Care

A patient who has had surgery may return home before the wound closes entirely or with a drain or tube in place. In these cases, the nurse educates the patient or caregivers about how to change the dressings to prevent skin excoriation and odor, how to monitor for signs and symptoms of infection, and how to care for and maintain the drain or tube. The nurse also reminds the patient to perform deep-breathing and coughing exercises every 2 hours during the day and shows caregivers how to perform chest percussion and postural drainage to facilitate expectoration of lung secretions.

Continuing Care

A patient whose condition requires therapy at home may need referral for home care. During home visits, the nurse assesses the patient's physical condition, nutritional status, and home environment, as well as the ability of the patient and family to carry out the therapeutic regimen. Patient education is reinforced, and nutritional counseling is provided with the goal of attaining and maintaining an optimal state of nutrition. To prevent relapses, the nurse emphasizes the importance of completing the antibiotic regimen and of following suggestions for rest and appropriate activity. If IV antibiotic therapy is to continue at home, the services of home care nurses may be arranged to initiate IV therapy and to evaluate its administration by the patient or family.

Although most outpatient IV therapy is administered in the home setting, the patient may visit a nearby clinic or provider's office for this treatment. In some cases, patients with lung abscess may have ignored their health. Therefore, the nurse should use this opportunity to address health promotion strategies and health screening with the patient.

PLEURAL CONDITIONS

Pleural conditions are disorders that involve the membranes covering the lungs (visceral pleura) and the surface of the chest wall (parietal pleura) or disorders affecting the pleural space.

Pleurisy

Pathophysiology

Pleurisy (pleuritis) refers to inflammation of both layers of the pleurae (parietal and visceral). Pleurisy may develop in conjunction with pneumonia or an upper respiratory tract infection, TB, or collagen disease; after trauma to the chest, pulmonary infarction, or PE; in patients with primary or metastatic cancer; and after thoracotomy. The parietal pleura has nerve endings, and the visceral pleura does not. When the inflamed pleural membranes rub together during respiration (intensified on inspiration), the result is severe, sharp, knife-like pain.

Clinical Manifestations

The key characteristic of pleuritic pain is its relationship to respiratory movement. Taking a deep breath, coughing, or sneezing worsens the pain. Pleuritic pain is limited in distribution rather than diffuse; it usually occurs only on one side. The pain may become minimal or absent when the breath is held. It may be localized or radiate to the shoulder or abdomen. Later, as pleural fluid develops, the pain decreases.

Assessment and Diagnostic Findings

In the early period, when little fluid has accumulated, a pleural friction rub can be heard with the stethoscope, only to disappear later as more fluid accumulates and separates the inflamed pleural surfaces. Diagnostic tests may include chest x-rays, sputum analysis, thoracentesis to obtain a specimen of pleural fluid for examination, and, less commonly, a pleural biopsy.

Medical Management

The objectives of treatment are to discover the underlying condition causing the pleurisy and to relieve the pain. As the underlying disease (pneumonia, infection) is treated, the pleuritic inflammation usually resolves. At the same time, the patient must be monitored for signs and symptoms of pleural effusion, such as shortness of breath, pain, assumption of a position that decreases pain, and decreased chest wall excursion.

Prescribed analgesic agents and topical applications of heat or cold provide symptomatic relief. A nonsteroidal anti-inflammatory drug may provide pain relief while allowing the patient to take deep breaths and cough more effectively. If the pain is severe, an intercostal nerve block may be required.

Nursing Management

Because the patient has pain on inspiration, the nurse offers suggestions to enhance comfort, such as turning frequently onto the affected side to splint the chest wall and reduce the stretching of the pleurae. The nurse also educates the patient to use the hands or a pillow to splint the rib cage while coughing.

Pleural Effusion

Pleural effusion, a collection of fluid in the pleural space, is rarely a primary disease process; it is usually secondary to other diseases (Loscalzo, 2010). Normally, the pleural space contains a small amount of fluid (5 to 15 mL), which acts as a lubricant that allows the pleural surfaces to move without friction (Fig. 23-4). Pleural effusion may be a complication of heart failure, TB, pneumonia, pulmonary infections (particularly viral infections), nephrotic syndrome, connective tissue disease, PE and neoplastic tumors. The most common malignancy associated with a pleural effusion is bronchogenic carcinoma.

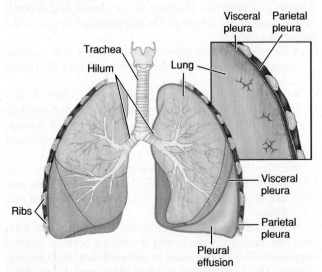

FIGURE 23-4 • In pleural effusion, an abnormal volume of fluid collects in the pleural space, causing pain and shortness of breath. Pleural effusion is usually secondary to other disease processes.

Pathophysiology

In certain disorders, fluid may accumulate in the pleural space to a point at which it becomes clinically evident. This almost always has pathologic significance. The effusion can be a relatively clear fluid, or it can be bloody or purulent. An effusion of clear fluid may be a transudate or an exudate. A transudate (filtrate of plasma that moves across intact capillary walls) occurs when factors influencing the formation and reabsorption of pleural fluid are altered, usually by imbalances in hydrostatic or oncotic pressures. The finding of a transudative effusion generally implies that the pleural membranes are not diseased. A transudative effusion most commonly results from heart failure. An exudate (extravasation of fluid into tissues or a cavity) usually results from inflammation by bacterial products or tumors involving the pleural surfaces.

Clinical Manifestations

Usually, the clinical manifestations are caused by the underlying disease. Pneumonia causes fever, chills, and pleuritic chest pain, whereas a malignant effusion may result in dyspnea, difficulty lying flat, and coughing. The severity of symptoms is determined by the size of the effusion, the speed of its formation, and the underlying lung disease. A large pleural effusion causes dyspnea (shortness of breath). A small to moderate pleural effusion causes minimal or no dyspnea.

Assessment and Diagnostic Findings

Assessment of the area of the pleural effusion reveals decreased or absent breath sounds; decreased fremitus; and a dull, flat sound on percussion. In the case of an extremely large pleural effusion, the assessment reveals a patient in acute respiratory distress. Tracheal deviation away from the affected side may also be apparent.

Physical examination, chest x-ray, chest CT, and thoracentesis confirm the presence of fluid. In some instances, a lateral decubitus x-ray is obtained. For this x-ray, the patient lies on the affected side in a side-lying position. A pleural effusion can be diagnosed because this position allows for the "layering out" of the fluid, and an air–fluid line is visible.

Pleural fluid is analyzed by bacterial culture, Gram stain, AFB stain (for TB), red and white blood cell counts, chemistry studies (glucose, amylase, lactate dehydrogenase, protein), cytologic analysis for malignant cells, and pH. A pleural biopsy also may be performed as a diagnostic tool.

Medical Management

The objectives of treatment are to discover the underlying cause of the pleural effusion; to prevent reaccumulation of fluid; and to relieve discomfort, dyspnea, and respiratory compromise. Specific treatment is directed at the underlying cause (e.g., heart failure, pneumonia, cirrhosis). If the pleural fluid is an exudate, more extensive diagnostic procedures are performed to determine the cause. Treatment for the primary cause is then instituted.

Thoracentesis is performed to remove fluid, to obtain a specimen for analysis, and to relieve dyspnea and respiratory compromise (see Chapter 20). Thoracentesis may be performed under ultrasound guidance. Depending on the size of the pleural effusion, the patient may be treated by removing the fluid during the thoracentesis procedure or by inserting a chest tube connected to a water-seal drainage system or suction to evacuate the pleural space and re-expand the lung.

However, if the underlying cause is a malignancy, the effusion tends to recur within a few days or weeks. Repeated thoracenteses result in pain, depletion of protein and electrolytes, and sometimes pneumothorax. Once the pleural space is adequately drained, a chemical pleurodesis may be performed to obliterate the pleural space and prevent reaccumulation of fluid. Pleurodesis may be performed using either a thoracoscopic approach or a chest tube. A chemically irritating agent (e.g., talc or another chemical irritant) is instilled or aerosolized into the pleural space. With the chest tube approach, after the agent is instilled, the chest tube is clamped for 60 to 90 minutes and the patient is assisted to assume various positions to promote uniform distribution of the agent and to maximize its contact with the pleural surfaces. The tube is unclamped as prescribed, and chest drainage may be continued several days longer to prevent reaccumulation of fluid and to promote the formation of adhesions between the visceral and parietal pleurae.

Other treatments for pleural effusions caused by malignancy include surgical pleurectomy, insertion of a small catheter attached to a drainage bottle for outpatient management (PleurX catheter [CareFusion]), or implantation of a pleuroperitoneal shunt. A pleuroperitoneal shunt consists of two catheters connected by a pump chamber containing two one-way valves. Fluid moves from the pleural space to the pump chamber and then to the peritoneal cavity. The patient manually pumps on the reservoir daily to move fluid from the pleural space to the peritoneal space.

Nursing Management

The nurse's role in the care of patients with a pleural effusion includes supporting the medical regimen. The nurse prepares and positions the patient for thoracentesis and offers support throughout the procedure. The nurse is responsible for making sure the thoracentesis fluid amount is recorded and sent for appropriate laboratory testing. If a chest tube drainage and water-seal system is used, the nurse is responsible for monitoring the system's function and recording the amount of drainage at prescribed intervals. Nursing care related to the underlying cause of the pleural effusion is specific to the underlying condition. (See Chapter 21 for a discussion of care of the patient with a chest tube.)

If a chest tube is inserted for talc instillation, pain management is a priority and the nurse helps the patient assume positions that are the least painful. However, frequent turning and movement are important to facilitate adequate spreading of the talc over the pleural surface. The nurse evaluates the patient's pain level and administers analgesic agents as prescribed and as needed.

If the patient is to be managed as an outpatient with a pleural catheter for drainage, the nurse educates the patient and family about management and care of the catheter and drainage system.

Empyema

An empyema is an accumulation of thick, purulent fluid within the pleural space, often with fibrin development and a loculated (walled-off) area where infection is located.

Pathophysiology

Most empyemas occur as complications of bacterial pneumonia or lung abscess. They also result from penetrating chest trauma, hematogenous infection of the pleural space, nonbacterial infections, and iatrogenic causes (after thoracic surgery or thoracentesis). At first the pleural fluid is thin, with a low leukocyte count, but it frequently progresses to a fibropurulent stage and, finally, to a stage where it encloses the lung within a thick exudative membrane (loculated empyema).

Clinical Manifestations

The patient is acutely ill and has signs and symptoms similar to those of an acute respiratory infection or pneumonia (fever, night sweats, pleural pain, cough, dyspnea, anorexia, weight loss). If the patient is immunocompromised, the symptoms may be vague. If the patient has received antimicrobial therapy, the clinical manifestations may be less obvious.

Assessment and Diagnostic Findings

Chest auscultation demonstrates decreased or absent breath sounds over the affected area, and there is dullness on chest percussion as well as decreased fremitus. The diagnosis is established by chest CT. Usually, a diagnostic thoracentesis is performed, often under ultrasound guidance.

Medical Management

The objectives of treatment are to drain the pleural cavity and to achieve complete expansion of the lung. The fluid is drained, and appropriate antibiotics (usually begun by the IV route) in large doses are prescribed based on the causative organism. Sterilization of the empyema cavity requires 4 to 6 weeks of antibiotics. Drainage of the pleural fluid depends on the stage of the disease and is accomplished by one of the following methods:

- Needle aspiration (thoracentesis) with a thin percutaneous catheter, if the volume is small and the fluid is not too purulent or too thick
- Tube thoracostomy (chest drainage using a large-diameter intercostal tube attached to water-seal drainage [see Chapter 21]) with fibrinolytic agents instilled through the chest tube in patients with loculated or complicated pleural effusions
- Open chest drainage via thoracotomy, including potential rib resection, to remove the thickened pleura, pus, and debris and to remove the underlying diseased pulmonary tissue

With long-standing inflammation, an exudate can form over the lung, trapping it and interfering with its normal expansion. This exudate must be removed surgically (decortication). The drainage tube is left in place until the pus-filled space is obliterated completely. The complete obliteration of the pleural space is monitored by serial chest x-rays, and the patient should be informed that treatment may be long term (weeks to months). Patients are frequently discharged from the hospital with a chest tube in place, with instructions to monitor fluid drainage at home.

Nursing Management

Resolution of empyema is a prolonged process. The nurse helps the patient cope with the condition and instructs the patient in lung-expanding breathing exercises to restore normal respiratory function. The nurse also provides care specific to the method of drainage of the pleural fluid (e.g., needle aspiration, closed chest drainage, rib resection and drainage). When the patient is discharged home with a drainage tube or system in place, the nurse instructs the patient and family on care of the drainage system and drain site, measurement and observation of drainage, signs and symptoms of infection, and how and when to contact the primary provider. (See The Patient Undergoing Thoracic Surgery section in Chapter 21.)

Pulmonary Edema (Noncardiogenic)

Pulmonary edema is defined as abnormal accumulation of fluid in the lung tissue, the alveolar space, or both. It is a severe, life-threatening condition. Pulmonary edema can be classified as cardiogenic or noncardiogenic. (See Chapter 29 for further discussion of cardiogenic pulmonary edema.) Noncardiogenic pulmonary edema occurs due to damage of the pulmonary capillary lining. It may be due to direct injury to the lung (e.g., chest trauma, aspiration, smoke inhalation), hematogenous injury to the lung (e.g., sepsis, pancreatitis, multiple transfusions, cardiopulmonary bypass), or injury plus elevated hydrostatic pressures. Management of noncardiogenic pulmonary edema mirrors that of cardiogenic pulmonary edema (see Chapter 29); however, hypoxemia may persist despite high concentrations of supplemental oxygen, due to the intrapulmonary shunting of blood.

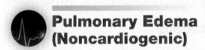

Acute Respiratory Failure

Respiratory failure is a sudden and life-threatening deterioration of the gas exchange function of the lung and indicates failure of the lungs to provide adequate oxygenation or ventilation for the blood. Acute respiratory failure is defined as a decrease in arterial oxygen tension (PaO_2) to less than 50 mm Hg (hypoxemia) and an increase in arterial carbon dioxide tension ($PaCO_2$) to greater than 50 mm Hg (hypercapnia), with an arterial pH of less than 7.35 (Loscalzo, 2010).

It is important to distinguish between acute and chronic respiratory failure. Chronic respiratory failure is defined as deterioration in the gas exchange function of the lung that has developed insidiously or has persisted for a long period after an episode of acute respiratory failure. The absence of acute symptoms and the presence of a chronic respiratory acidosis suggest the chronicity of the respiratory failure. Two causes of chronic respiratory failure are COPD (discussed

in Chapter 24) and neuromuscular diseases (discussed in Chapter 70). Patients with these disorders develop a tolerance to the gradually worsening hypoxemia and hypercapnia. However, patients with chronic respiratory failure can develop acute failure. For example, a patient with COPD may develop an exacerbation or infection that causes additional deterioration of gas exchange. The principles of management of acute versus chronic respiratory failure are different; the following discussion is limited to acute respiratory failure.

Pathophysiology

In acute respiratory failure, the ventilation or perfusion mechanisms in the lung are impaired. Ventilatory failure mechanisms leading to acute respiratory failure include impaired function of the central nervous system (i.e., drug overdose, head trauma, infection, hemorrhage, sleep apnea), neuromuscular dysfunction (i.e., myasthenia gravis, Guillain-Barré syndrome, amyotrophic lateral sclerosis, spinal cord trauma), musculoskeletal dysfunction (i.e., chest trauma, kyphoscoliosis, malnutrition), and pulmonary dysfunction (i.e., COPD, asthma, cystic fibrosis).

Oxygenation failure mechanisms leading to acute respiratory failure include pneumonia, acute respiratory distress syndrome, heart failure, COPD, PE, and **restrictive lung diseases** (diseases that cause decrease in lung volumes).

In the postoperative period, especially after major thoracic or abdominal surgery, inadequate ventilation and respiratory failure may occur because of several factors. During this period, for example, acute respiratory failure may be caused by the effects of anesthetic, analgesic, and sedative agents, which may depress respiration (as described earlier) or enhance the effects of opioids and lead to hypoventilation. Pain may interfere with deep breathing and coughing. A ventilation–perfusion mismatch is the usual cause of respiratory failure after major abdominal, cardiac, or thoracic surgery.

Clinical Manifestations

Early signs are those associated with impaired oxygenation and may include restlessness, fatigue, headache, dyspnea, air hunger, tachycardia, and increased blood pressure. As the hypoxemia progresses, more obvious signs may be present, including confusion, lethargy, tachycardia, tachypnea, central cyanosis, diaphoresis, and finally respiratory arrest. Physical findings are those of acute respiratory distress, including the use of accessory muscles, decreased breath sounds if the patient cannot adequately ventilate, and other findings related specifically to the underlying disease process and cause of acute respiratory failure.

  Concept Mastery Alert

In the early phase of acute respiratory failure, vague signs and symptoms such as restlessness, fatigue, and headache make it difficult to determine what the patient is experiencing. However, as oxygenation becomes more impaired, hypoxemia increases and leads to more obvious signs. Pain usually is not present. Some patients may progress through these phases over several hours, whereas others may progress within seconds.

Medical Management

The objectives of treatment are to correct the underlying cause and to restore adequate gas exchange in the lung. Endotracheal intubation and mechanical ventilation may be required to maintain adequate ventilation and oxygenation while the underlying cause is corrected.

Nursing Management

Nursing management of patients with acute respiratory failure includes assisting with intubation and maintaining mechanical ventilation (described in Chapter 21). Patients are usually managed in the ICU. The nurse assesses the patient's respiratory status by monitoring the level of responsiveness, arterial blood gases, pulse oximetry, and vital signs. In addition, the nurse assesses the entire respiratory system and implements strategies (e.g., turning schedule, mouth care, skin care, range of motion of extremities) to prevent complications. The nurse also assesses the patient's understanding of the management strategies that are used and initiates some form of communication to enable the patient to express concerns and needs to the health care team.

Finally, the nurse addresses the problems that led to the acute respiratory failure. As the patient's status improves, the nurse assesses the patient's knowledge of the underlying disorder and provides education as appropriate to address the disorder.

Acute Respiratory Distress Syndrome

Acute respiratory distress syndrome (ARDS) can be thought of as a spectrum of disease, from its milder form (**acute lung injury**) to its most severe form of fulminate, life-threatening ARDS. This clinical syndrome is characterized by a severe inflammatory process causing diffuse alveolar damage that results in sudden and progressive pulmonary edema, increasing bilateral infiltrates on chest x-ray, hypoxemia unresponsive to oxygen supplementation regardless of the amount of PEEP, and the absence of an elevated left atrial pressure (Dushianthan, Grott, Postle, et al., 2011). Patients often demonstrate reduced lung compliance. A wide range of factors are associated with the development of ARDS (Chart 23-8), including direct injury to the lungs (e.g., smoke inhalation) or indirect insult

---

Chart 23-8 Etiologic Factors Related to Acute Respiratory Distress Syndrome

- Aspiration (gastric secretions, drowning, hydrocarbons)
- Drug ingestion and overdose
- Hematologic disorders (disseminated intravascular coagulopathy, massive transfusions, cardiopulmonary bypass)
- Prolonged inhalation of high concentrations of oxygen, smoke, or corrosive substances
- Localized infection (bacterial, fungal, viral pneumonia)
- Metabolic disorders (pancreatitis, uremia)
- Shock (any cause)
- Trauma (pulmonary contusion, multiple fractures, head injury)
- Major surgery
- Fat or air embolism
- Sepsis

---

to the lungs (e.g., shock). ARDS has been associated with a mortality rate ranging from 36% to 44% (Dushianthan et al., 2011). The major cause of death in ARDS is nonpulmonary MODS, often with sepsis.

Pathophysiology

Inflammatory triggers initiate the release of cellular and chemical mediators, causing injury to the alveolar capillary membrane in addition to other structural damage to the lungs. Severe ventilation–perfusion mismatching occurs. Alveoli collapse because of the inflammatory infiltrate, blood, fluid, and surfactant dysfunction. Small airways are narrowed because of interstitial fluid and bronchial obstruction. Lung compliance may markedly decrease, resulting in decreased functional residual capacity and severe hypoxemia. The blood returning to the lung for gas exchange is pumped through the nonventilated, nonfunctioning areas of the lung, causing shunting. This means that blood is interfacing with nonfunctioning alveoli and gas exchange is markedly impaired, resulting in severe, refractory hypoxemia. Figure 23-5 shows the sequence of pathophysiologic events leading to ARDS.

Clinical Manifestations

Initially, ARDS closely resembles severe pulmonary edema. The acute phase of ARDS is marked by a rapid onset of severe dyspnea that usually occurs less than 72 hours after the precipitating event (Dushianthan et al., 2011). Arterial hypoxemia that does not respond to supplemental oxygen is characteristic. Findings on chest x-ray are similar to those seen with cardiogenic pulmonary edema and are visible as bilateral infiltrates that quickly worsen. The acute lung

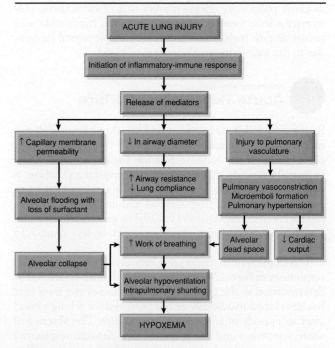

FIGURE 23-5 • Pathogenesis and pathophysiology of acute respiratory distress syndrome.

injury then progresses to fibrosing alveolitis with persistent, severe hypoxemia. The patient also has increased alveolar dead space (ventilation to alveoli but poor perfusion) and decreased pulmonary compliance ("stiff lungs," which are difficult to ventilate). Clinically, the patient is thought to be in the recovery phase if the hypoxemia gradually resolves, the chest x-ray improves, and the lungs become more compliant.

Assessment and Diagnostic Findings

On physical examination, intercostal retractions and crackles may be present as the fluid begins to leak into the alveolar interstitial space. Common diagnostic tests performed in patients with potential ARDS include plasma brain natriuretic peptide (BNP) levels, echocardiography, and pulmonary artery catheterization. The BNP level is helpful in distinguishing ARDS from cardiogenic pulmonary edema. Transthoracic echocardiography may be used if the BNP is not conclusive.

Medical Management

The primary focus in the management of ARDS includes identification and treatment of the underlying condition. Aggressive, supportive care must be provided to compensate for the severe respiratory dysfunction. This supportive therapy almost always includes endotracheal intubation and mechanical ventilation. In addition, circulatory support, adequate fluid volume, and nutritional support are important. Supplemental oxygen is used as the patient begins the initial spiral of hypoxemia. As the hypoxemia progresses, intubation and mechanical ventilation are instituted. The concentration of oxygen and ventilator settings and modes are determined by the patient's status. This is monitored by arterial blood gas analysis, pulse oximetry, and bedside pulmonary function testing.

Providing ventilatory PEEP support is a critical part of the treatment of ARDS. PEEP usually improves oxygenation, but it does not influence the natural history of the syndrome. The use of PEEP helps increase functional residual capacity and reverse alveolar collapse by keeping the alveoli open, resulting in improved arterial oxygenation and a reduction in the severity of the ventilation–perfusion imbalance. By using PEEP, a lower FiO_2 may be required. The goal is a PaO_2 greater than 60 mm Hg or an oxygen saturation level of greater than 90% at the lowest possible FiO_2. (See Chapter 21 for a discussion of PEEP and modes of mechanical ventilation.)

Systemic hypotension may occur in ARDS as a result of hypovolemia secondary to leakage of fluid into the interstitial spaces and depressed cardiac output from high levels of PEEP therapy. Hypovolemia must be carefully treated without causing further overload. Inotropic or vasopressor agents may be required. Additional treatments may include prone positioning, high-frequency oscillatory ventilation, and low-dose corticosteroids that are administered within the first 14 days of the onset of manifestations (Dushianthan et al., 2011).

Pharmacologic Therapy

There is no specific pharmacologic treatment for ARDS except supportive care. Neuromuscular blocking agents, sedatives,

and analgesics may be used to improve patient–ventilator synchronization and help to decrease severe hypoxemia (see later discussion in Ventilator Considerations section). Inhaled nitric oxide (an endogenous vasodilator) may help to reduce ventilation–perfusion mismatch and improve oxygenation. Multiple therapies are undergoing clinical evaluation but are not yet approved or supported for widespread clinical use (Dushianthan et al., 2011).

Nutritional Therapy

Adequate nutritional support is vital in the treatment of ARDS. Patients with ARDS require 35 to 45 kcal/kg/day to meet caloric requirements. Enteral feeding is the first consideration; however, parenteral nutrition also may be required.

Nursing Management

General Measures

A patient with ARDS is critically ill and requires close monitoring in an ICU. Most of the respiratory modalities discussed in Chapter 21 are used in this situation (oxygen administration, nebulizer therapy, chest physiotherapy, endotracheal intubation or tracheostomy, mechanical ventilation, suctioning, bronchoscopy). Frequent assessment of the patient's status is necessary to evaluate the effectiveness of treatment.

In addition to supporting the medical plan of care, the nurse considers other needs of the patient. Positioning is important. The nurse turns the patient frequently to improve ventilation and perfusion in the lungs and enhance secretion drainage. However, the nurse must closely monitor the patient for deterioration in oxygenation with changes in position. Oxygenation in patients with ARDS is sometimes improved in the prone position. This position may be evaluated for improvement in oxygenation and used in special circumstances. Devices and specialty beds are available to assist the nurse in placing the patient in a prone position.

The patient is extremely anxious and agitated because of the increasing hypoxemia and dyspnea. It is important to reduce the patient's anxiety because anxiety increases oxygen expenditure by preventing rest. Rest is essential to limit oxygen consumption and reduce oxygen needs.

Ventilator Considerations

If the patient is intubated and receiving mechanical ventilation with PEEP, several considerations must be addressed. PEEP, which causes increased end-expiratory pressure, is an unnatural pattern of breathing and feels strange to the patient. The patients may be anxious and "fight" the ventilator. Nursing assessment is important to identify problems with ventilation that may be causing the anxiety reaction: tube blockage by kinking or retained secretions, other acute respiratory problems (e.g., pneumothorax, pain), a sudden decrease in the oxygen level, the level of dyspnea, or ventilator malfunction. In some cases, sedation may be required to decrease the patient's oxygen consumption, allow the ventilator to provide full support of ventilation, and decrease the patient's anxiety. Sedatives that may be used are lorazepam (Ativan), midazolam (Versed), dexmedetomidine (Precedex), propofol (Diprivan), and short-acting barbiturates.

If the PEEP level cannot be maintained despite the use of sedatives, neuromuscular blocking agents (paralytic agents) may be administered to paralyze the patient. Examples of these agents include pancuronium (Pavulon), vecuronium (Norcuron), atracurium (Tracrium), and rocuronium (Zemuron). The resulting paralysis allows the patient to be ventilated more easily. With paralysis, the patient appears to be unconscious; loses motor function; and cannot breathe, talk, or blink independently. However, the patient retains sensation and is awake and able to hear. The nurse must reassure the patient that the paralysis is a result of the medication and is temporary. Paralysis should be used for the shortest possible time and never without adequate sedation and pain management.

Peripheral nerve stimulators are used to assess nerve impulse transmissions at the neuromuscular junction of select skeletal muscles when neuromuscular blocking agents are used. A "train-of-four" test may be used to measure the level of neuromuscular blockade. With this test, four consecutive stimuli are delivered along the path of a nerve, and the response of the muscle is measured in order to evaluate whether or not stimuli are effectively blocked. Four equal muscle contractions, seen as "twitches," will result if there is no neuromuscular blockade. However, if neuromuscular blockade is present, there will be a loss of twitch height and number, which will indicate the degree of blockade. If all four stimulations result in an absence of twitches, it is estimated that 100% of the receptors are blocked (Mosby's Nursing Consult, 2012).

The use of neuromuscular blocking agents has many dangers and side effects. The nurse must be sure the patient does not become disconnected from the ventilator, because respiratory muscles are paralyzed and the patient will be apneic. Consequently, the nurse ensures that the patient is closely monitored; all ventilator and patient alarms must be on at all times. Eye care is important as well, because the patient cannot blink, increasing the risk of corneal abrasions. Neuromuscular blockers predispose the patient to venous thromboembolism (VTE), muscle atrophy, and skin breakdown.

> ◤ **Quality and Safety Nursing Alert**
>
> Nursing assessment is essential to minimize the complications related to neuromuscular blockade. The patient may have discomfort or pain but cannot communicate these sensations.

Analgesia must be administered concurrently with neuromuscular blocking agents (Siegel, 2010). The nurse must anticipate the patient's needs regarding pain and comfort. The nurse checks the patient's position to ensure it is comfortable and in normal alignment and talks to, and not about, the patient while in the patient's presence.

In addition, the nurse must describe the purpose and effects of the neuromuscular blocking agents to the patient's family. If family members are unaware that these agents have been administered, they may become distressed by the change in the patient's status.

Pulmonary Hypertension

Pulmonary hypertension (PH) is characterized by elevated pulmonary arterial pressure and secondary right heart ventricular failure (Rubin & Hopkins, 2012). It may be suspected in a patient with dyspnea with exertion without other clinical manifestations. Unlike systemic blood pressure, the pulmonary pressures cannot be measured indirectly. In the absence of these measurements, clinical recognition becomes the only indicator of PH. However, PH is a condition that is often not clinically evident until late in its progression.

The classification of this disease has been updated recently. Previously, patients were classified as having primary or secondary PH (Rubin & Hopkins, 2012). Currently, patients are classified by the WHO into five groups based upon the mechanism of PH (Rubin & Hopkins, 2012; Simonneau, Robbins, Beghetti, et al., 2009) (Chart 23-9).

Pathophysiology

Conditions such as collagen vascular disease, congenital heart disease, anorexigens (specific appetite depressants), chronic use of stimulants, portal hypertension, and HIV infection increase the risk of PH in susceptible patients. Vascular injury occurs with endothelial dysfunction and vascular smooth muscle dysfunction, which leads to disease progression (vascular smooth muscle hypertrophy, adventitial and intimal proliferation [thickening of the wall], and advanced vascular lesion formation). Normally, the pulmonary vascular bed can

Chart 23-9	**Clinical Classification of Pulmonary Hypertension**

Group 1: Pulmonary Arterial Hypertension (PAH)

- Sporadic idiopathic PAH
- Heritable idiopathic PAH
- Drug and toxin-induced PAH
- PAH due to diseases such as connective tissues disorders, HIV infection, portal hypertension, congenital heart disease

Group 2: Pulmonary Hypertension (PH) due to left heart disease

- Systolic dysfunction
- Diastolic dysfunction
- Valvular heart disease

Group 3: Pulmonary Hypertension (PH) due to lung diseases or hypoxemia

- Chronic obstructive pulmonary disease
- Interstitial lung disease
- Mixed restrictive and obstructive lung disease
- Sleep disordered breathing

Group 4: Chronic thromboembolic pulmonary hypertension (CTEPH)

- Due to thromboembolic occlusion of the proximal or distal pulmonary vasculature

Group 5: Pulmonary Hypertension (PH) with unclear multifactorial mechanisms

- Hematologic disorders
- Systemic disorders (e.g., sarcoidosis)
- Metabolic disorders

Adapted from Simonneau, G, Robbins, I., Beghetti, M., et al. (2009). Updated clinical classification of pulmonary hypertension. *Journal of the American College of Cardiology, 54*(1 Suppl. 1), S43–S54.

handle the blood volume delivered by the right ventricle. It has a low resistance to blood flow and compensates for increased blood volume by dilation of the vessels in the pulmonary circulation. However, if the pulmonary vascular bed is destroyed or obstructed, as in PH, the ability to handle whatever flow or volume of blood it receives is impaired, and the increased blood flow then increases the pulmonary artery pressure. As the pulmonary arterial pressure increases, the pulmonary vascular resistance also increases. Both pulmonary artery constriction (as in hypoxemia or hypercapnia) and a reduction of the pulmonary vascular bed (which occurs with PE) result in increased pulmonary vascular resistance and pressure. This increased workload affects right ventricular function. The myocardium ultimately cannot meet the increasing demands imposed on it, leading to right ventricular hypertrophy (enlargement and dilation) and failure. Passive hepatic congestion may also develop.

Clinical Manifestations

Dyspnea, the main symptom of PH, occurs at first with exertion and eventually at rest. Substernal chest pain also is common. Other signs and symptoms include weakness, fatigue, syncope, occasional hemoptysis, and signs of right-sided heart failure (peripheral edema, ascites, distended neck veins, liver engorgement, crackles, heart murmur). Anorexia and abdominal pain in the right upper quadrant may also occur.

Assessment and Diagnostic Findings

Diagnostic testing is used to confirm that PH exists, determine its severity, and identify its causes. Initial diagnostic evaluation includes a history, physical examination, chest x-ray, pulmonary function studies, electrocardiogram (ECG), and echocardiogram. Echocardiography can be used to estimate the pulmonary artery systolic pressure and to assess right ventricular size, thickness, and function. It can also evaluate the right atrial size, left ventricular system, and diastolic function as well as valve function. Right heart catheterization is necessary to confirm the diagnosis of PH and to accurately assess the hemodynamic abnormalities. PH is confirmed with a mean pulmonary artery pressure greater than 25 mm Hg. If left heart disease is identified via echocardiography and correlates with the degree of estimated PH, then exercise testing and both a right and left heart catheterization may be done to determine the functional severity of the disease and the abnormalities in pressures (left heart filling, pulmonary vascular resistance, transpulmonary gradient) (Rubin & Hopkins, 2012).

Pulmonary function studies may be normal or show a slight decrease in vital capacity and lung compliance, with a mild decrease in the diffusing capacity. The PaO_2 also is decreased (hypoxemia). The ECG reveals right ventricular hypertrophy, right axis deviation, and tall peaked P waves in inferior leads; tall anterior R waves; and ST-segment depression, T-wave inversion, or both anteriorly. An echocardiogram can assess the progression of the disease and rule out other conditions with similar signs and symptoms. A ventilation–perfusion scan or pulmonary angiography detects defects in pulmonary vasculature, such as PE.

Medical Management

The primary goal of treatment is to manage the underlying condition related to PH if the cause is known. Recommendations regarding therapy are tailored to the patient's individual situation, functional New York Heart Association class, and specific needs (Hopkins & Rubin, 2012). All patients with PH should be considered for the following therapies: diuretics, oxygen, anticoagulation, digoxin, and exercise training. Diuretics and oxygen should be added as needed. Appropriate oxygen therapy (see Chapter 21) reverses the vasoconstriction and reduces the PH in a relatively short time. Most patients with PH do not have hypoxemia at rest but require supplemental oxygen with exercise. Anticoagulation should be considered for patients at risk for intrapulmonary thrombosis. Digoxin may improve right ventricular ejection fraction in some patients and may help to control heart rate; however, patients must be monitored closely for potential complications (Hopkins & Rubin, 2012).

Pharmacologic Therapy

Different classes of medications are used to treat PH; these include calcium channel blockers, prostanoids, endothelin antagonists, and phosphodiesterase-5 inhibitors. The choice of therapeutic agents is based on many facets, including the classification group status of the patient with PH (see Chart 23-9), as well as the cost and the patient's tolerance of the agents (Hopkins & Rubin, 2012). In addition, a vasoreactivity test may be done to identify which medication is best suited for the patient with PH; this is done during cardiac catheterization using vasodilating medications such as nitric oxide. A positive vasoreactivity test occurs when there is a decrease of at least 10 mm Hg in the pulmonary artery pressure with an overall pressure that is less than 40 mm Hg in the presence of both an increased or unchanged cardiac output and a minimally decreased or unchanged systemic blood pressure (Hopkins & Rubin, 2012).

Patients with a positive vasoreactivity test may be prescribed calcium channel blockers. Calcium channel blockers have a significant advantage over other medications taken to treat PH in that they may be taken orally and are generally less costly; however, because calcium channel blockers are indicated in only a small percentage of patients, other treatment options, including prostanoids, are often necessary (Rubin & Hopkins, 2012).

Prostanoids mimic the effect of the prostaglandin prostacyclin. Prostacyclin relaxes vascular smooth muscle by stimulating the production of cyclic 3′,5′-adenosine monophosphate (AMP) and inhibits the growth of smooth muscle cells. Prostanoids used to treat PH include epoprostenol (Flolan), treprostinil (Remodulin), and iloprost (Ventavis). Limitations of the prostanoids include their short half-life (epoprostenol's half-life is less than 3 minutes) and variable patient responses to therapy (Hopkins & Rubin, 2012). IV epoprostenol (Flolan) is the most widely studied advanced therapy for PH. It is continuously delivered through a permanently implanted central venous catheter using a portable infusion pump. Although a useful therapy, it requires extensive patient education and caregiver support. Treprostinil can be delivered IV or subcutaneously, although the subcutaneous method causes severe pain at the injection site. A benefit of iloprost (Ventavis) is that it is an inhaled preparation; however, it needs to be administered six to nine times daily. Clinical trials comparing epoprostenol and treprostinil have not been performed (Hopkins & Rubin, 2012).

Endothelin receptor antagonists are vasodilators. Bosentan (Tracleer), an endothelin receptor antagonist, causes vasodilation and is prescribed for its antihypertensive effects in patients with PH. It is administered orally twice a day. Liver function must be monitored in patients using bosentan. Other selective endothelin receptor antagonists include sitaxentan (Thelin) and ambrisentan (Letairis).

The oral medications sildenafil (Revatio, Viagra), tadalafil (Cialis, Adcirca), and vardenafil (Levitra) are potent, specific phosphodiesterase-5 inhibitors that degrade cyclic 3′,5′-guanosine monophosphate (cGMP) and promotes pulmonary vasodilation. These drugs are also prescribed to treat erectile dysfunction (Hopkins & Rubin, 2012).

Surgical Management

Lung transplantation remains an option for a select group of patients with PH who are refractory to medical therapy. Bilateral lung or heart–lung transplantation is the procedure of choice. Atrial septostomy may be considered for selected patients with severe disease (Hopkins & Rubin, 2012); this procedure results in shunting of blood from the right side of the heart to the left, decreasing the strain on the right side of the heart and maintaining left ventricular output.

Nursing Management

The major nursing goal is to identify patients at high risk for PH, such as those with COPD, PE, congenital heart disease, and mitral valve disease so that early treatment can commence. The nurse must be alert for signs and symptoms, administer oxygen therapy appropriately, and instruct the patient and family about the use of home oxygen therapy. In patients treated with prostanoids (e.g., epoprostenol or treprostinil), education about the need for central venous access (epoprostenol), subcutaneous infusion (treprostinil), proper administration and dosing of the medication, pain at the injection site, and potential severe side effects is extremely important. Emotional and psychosocial aspects of this disease must be addressed. Formal and informal support groups for patients and families are extremely valuable.

Pulmonary Heart Disease (Cor Pulmonale)

Cor pulmonale is a condition that results from PH, which causes the right side of the heart to enlarge because of the increased work required to pump blood against high resistance through the pulmonary vascular system. This causes right-sided heart failure (Porth & Matfin, 2009). (See Chapter 29 for further discussion of management of right-sided heart failure.)

Pulmonary Embolism

Pulmonary embolism (PE) refers to the obstruction of the pulmonary artery or one of its branches by a thrombus (or thrombi) that originates somewhere in the venous system or in the right side of the heart. Deep vein thrombosis (DVT), a related condition, refers to thrombus formation in the deep veins, usually in the calf or thigh, but sometimes in the arm, especially in patients with peripherally inserted central catheters. *Venous thromboembolism* is a term that includes both DVT and PE. (DVT is discussed in detail in Chapter 30.)

PE is a common disorder and often is associated with trauma, surgery (orthopedic, major abdominal, pelvic, gynecologic), pregnancy, heart failure, age older than 50 years, hypercoagulable states, and prolonged immobility. It also may occur in apparently healthy people. In the United States, VTE-related deaths are estimated at 300,000 annually; of these, approximately 7% are diagnosed with VTE and treated, 34% are sudden and fatal PE, and 59% have PE undetected until autopsy (Loscalzo, 2010). The outcome in acute PE depends on the presence of preexisting comorbidities and the extent of hemodynamic compromise (Stamm, 2012). Many people who have a first episode of DVT or PE will have a recurrent event (Goldhaber & Bounameaux, 2012). (Risk factors for PE are identified in Chart 30-7 in Chapter 30.)

Pathophysiology

Most commonly, PE is due to a blood clot or thrombus. However, there are other types of emboli: air, fat, amniotic fluid, and septic (from bacterial invasion of the thrombus).

When a thrombus completely or partially obstructs a pulmonary artery or its branches, the alveolar dead space is increased. The area, although continuing to be ventilated, receives little or no blood flow. Therefore, gas exchange is impaired or absent in this area. In addition, various substances are released from the clot and surrounding area that cause regional blood vessels and bronchioles to constrict. This results in an increase in pulmonary vascular resistance—a reaction that compounds the ventilation–perfusion imbalance.

The hemodynamic consequences are increased pulmonary vascular resistance due to the regional vasoconstriction and reduced size of the pulmonary vascular bed. This results in an increase in pulmonary arterial pressure and, in turn, an increase in right ventricular work to maintain pulmonary blood flow. When the work requirements of the right ventricle exceed its capacity, right ventricular failure occurs, leading to a decrease in cardiac output followed by a decrease in systemic blood pressure and the development of shock. Atrial fibrillation also causes PE. An enlarged right atrium in fibrillation causes blood to stagnate and form clots in this area. These clots are prone to travel into the pulmonary circulation.

A massive PE is best defined by the degree of hemodynamic instability rather than the percentage of pulmonary vasculature occlusion. It is described as an occlusion of the outflow tract of the main pulmonary artery or of the bifurcation of the pulmonary arteries. Multiple small emboli can lodge in the terminal pulmonary arterioles, producing multiple small infarctions of the lungs. A pulmonary infarction causes ischemic necrosis of part of the lung.

Clinical Manifestations

Symptoms of PE depend on the size of the thrombus and the area of the pulmonary artery occluded by the thrombus; they may be nonspecific. Dyspnea is the most frequent symptom;

the duration and intensity of the dyspnea depend on the extent of embolization. Chest pain is common and is usually sudden and pleuritic in origin. It may be substernal and may mimic angina pectoris or a myocardial infarction. Other symptoms include anxiety, fever, tachycardia, apprehension, cough, diaphoresis, hemoptysis, and syncope. The most frequent sign is tachypnea (very rapid respiratory rate).

The clinical picture may mimic that of bronchopneumonia or heart failure. In atypical instances, PE causes few signs and symptoms, whereas in other instances, it mimics various other cardiopulmonary disorders. Obstruction of the pulmonary artery results in pronounced dyspnea, sudden substernal pain, rapid and weak pulse, shock, syncope, and sudden death.

Assessment and Diagnostic Findings

Death from acute PE commonly occurs within 1 hour after the onset of symptoms; therefore, early recognition and diagnosis are priorities. Initially, a clinical assessment will focus on the clinical probability of risk, clinical history, symptoms, signs, and testing. Because the symptoms of PE can vary from few to severe, a diagnostic workup is performed to rule out other diseases. The initial diagnostic workup may include chest x-ray, ECG, pulse oximetry, arterial blood gas analysis, and ventilation–perfusion ($\dot{V}/\dot{Q}$) scan. The chest x-ray is usually normal but may show infiltrates, atelectasis, elevation of the diaphragm on the affected side, or a pleural effusion. The chest x-ray is most helpful in excluding other possible causes. In addition to sinus tachycardia, the most frequent ECG abnormality is T-wave inversion in leads V_1 to V_4 (Loscalzo, 2010). If an arterial blood gas analysis is performed, it may show hypoxemia and hypocapnia (from tachypnea); however, arterial blood gas measurements may be normal even in the presence of PE.

Pulmonary angiography is considered the best method to diagnose PE; however, it may not be feasible, cost-effective, or easily performed, especially with critically ill patients. The pulmonary angiogram allows for direct visualization under fluoroscopy of the arterial obstruction and accurate assessment of the perfusion deficit. A specially trained team must be available to perform the procedure, in which a catheter is threaded through the vena cava to the right side of the heart to inject dye, similar to a cardiac catheterization.

The $\dot{V}/\dot{Q}$ scan continues to be used to diagnose PE, especially in facilities that do not use pulmonary angiography or do not have access to a spiral CT scanner. The $\dot{V}/\dot{Q}$ scan is minimally invasive, involving the IV administration of a contrast agent. This scan evaluates different regions of the lung (upper, middle, lower) and allows comparisons of the percentage of ventilation and perfusion in each area. This test has a high sensitivity but can be more cumbersome than a CT scan and is not as accurate as a pulmonary angiogram.

A high suspicion of PE may warrant a spiral CT scan of the lung, D-dimer assay (blood test for evidence of blood clots), and pulmonary arteriogram. Spiral CT of the chest may also assist in the diagnosis. In spiral CT, the examination table advances at a constant rate through the scanner while the x-ray tube rotates continuously around the patient, following a spiral path, thus allowing the gathering of continuous data with no gaps between images. Unlike the traditional CT

scan, the spiral CT scan evaluates slices as narrow as 1 mm, as compared with 5-mm slices obtained by traditional CT scan. This allows for a more accurate visualization of a PE. However, spiral CT has limitations. It cannot be performed at the bedside, so unstable patients must be transported to a CT scanner. In addition, IV infusion of contrast agent is necessary for visualization.

Prevention

For patients at risk for PE, the most effective approach is to prevent DVT. Active leg exercises to avoid venous stasis, early ambulation, and the use of anti-embolism stockings are general preventive measures. Guidelines for prevention and treatment of VTE and PE are available (American College of Chest Physicians [ACCP], 2012). (See Chapter 30 for discussion of VTE prevention.)

Medical Management

Because PE is often a medical emergency, emergency management is of primary concern. After emergency measures have been initiated and the patient is stabilized, the treatment goal is to dissolve (lyse) the existing emboli and prevent new ones from forming. Treatment may include a variety of modalities: general measures to improve respiratory and vascular status, anticoagulation therapy, thrombolytic therapy, and surgical intervention.

Emergency Management

Massive PE is a life-threatening emergency. The immediate objective is to stabilize the cardiopulmonary system. A sudden increase in pulmonary resistance increases the work of the right ventricle, which can cause acute right-sided heart failure with cardiogenic shock. Emergency management consists of the following actions:

- Nasal oxygen is administered immediately to relieve hypoxemia, respiratory distress, and central cyanosis; severe hypoxemia may necessitate emergent endotracheal intubation and mechanical ventilatory support.
- IV infusion lines are inserted to establish routes for medications or fluids that will be needed.
- For hypotension that does not resolve with IV fluids, prompt initiation of vasopressor therapy is recommended, with agents that may include dobutamine, dopamine, or norepinephrine. Norepinephrine is the agent least likely to cause tachycardia (Tapson, 2012).
- A perfusion scan, hemodynamic measurements, and evaluation for hypoxemia (pulse oximetry or arterial blood gas) are performed. Spiral (helical) CT or pulmonary angiography may be performed.
- The ECG is monitored continuously for dysrhythmias and right ventricular failure, which may occur suddenly.
- Blood is drawn for serum electrolytes, complete blood count, and coagulation studies.
- If the patient has suffered massive embolism and is hypotensive, an indwelling urinary catheter is inserted to monitor urinary output.
- Small doses of IV morphine or sedatives are administered to relieve patient anxiety, to alleviate chest discomfort, to improve tolerance of the endotracheal tube, and to ease adaptation to the mechanical ventilator, if necessary.

General Management

Measures are initiated to improve respiratory and vascular status. Oxygen therapy is administered to correct the hypoxemia, relieve the pulmonary vascular vasoconstriction, and reduce the PH. The use of anti-embolism stockings or intermittent pneumatic leg compression devices reduces venous stasis. These measures compress the superficial veins and increase the velocity of blood in the deep veins by redirecting the blood through the deep veins. Elevating the leg (above the level of the heart) also increases venous flow. However, increasing flow may cause a volume challenge to a hemodynamically unstable patient.

Pharmacologic Therapy

Anticoagulation Therapy

Treatment of a nonmassive PE has three phases: initial phase, early maintenance phase, and long-term secondary prevention phase (Goldhaber & Bounameaux, 2012). Low-molecular-weight heparin and fondaparinux (Arixtra) are the cornerstones of therapy, but IV unfractionated heparin may be used during the initial phase (ACCP, 2012).

The early maintenance phase of anticoagulation typically consists of overlapping regimens of heparins or fondaparinux for at least 5 days with an oral vitamin K antagonist (e.g., warfarin [Coumadin]). A 3- to 6-month regimen of long-term maintenance with warfarin is typical but depends on the risks of recurrence and bleeding (ACCP, 2012).

Other heparinoids may also be used for PE. These include dalteparin (Fragmin), tinzaparin (Innohep), lepirudin (Refludan), and argatroban (Novastan). All patients must continue to take some form of anticoagulation for at least 3 to 6 months after the embolic event. (See Chapter 30 for further discussion of anticoagulants.)

Thrombolytic (Fibrinolytic) Therapy

Thrombolytic (fibrinolytic) therapy with recombinant tissue plasminogen activator (tPA) is used in treating massive PE, particularly in patients who are severely compromised (e.g., those who are hypotensive and have significant hypoxemia despite oxygen supplementation) (Loscalzo, 2010). Thrombolytic therapy resolves the thrombi or emboli quickly and restores more normal hemodynamic functioning of the pulmonary circulation, thereby reducing PH and improving perfusion, oxygenation, and cardiac output. However, bleeding is a significant side effect. Contraindications to thrombolytic therapy include a cerebrovascular accident (CVA) within the past 2 months, other active intracranial processes, active bleeding, surgery within 10 days of the thrombotic event, recent labor and delivery, trauma, or severe hypertension. Consequently, thrombolytic agents are advocated only for PE affecting a significant area of blood flow to the lung and causing hemodynamic instability.

Before thrombolytic therapy is started, international normalized ratio (INR), partial thromboplastin time (PTT), hematocrit, and platelet counts are obtained. An anticoagulant is stopped prior to administration of a thrombolytic agent. During therapy, all but essential invasive procedures are avoided because of potential bleeding. If necessary, fresh whole blood, packed red cells, cryoprecipitate, or frozen plasma is administered to replace blood loss and reverse the

bleeding tendency. After the thrombolytic infusion is completed (which varies in duration according to the agent used), anticoagulant therapy is initiated.

Surgical Management

A surgical embolectomy is rarely performed but may be indicated if the patient has a massive PE or hemodynamic instability or if there are contraindications to thrombolytic (fibrinolytic) therapy. Embolectomy can be performed using catheters or surgically. Surgical removal must be performed by a cardiovascular surgical team with the patient on cardiopulmonary bypass. Although surgical embolectomy ensures removal of the clot, it is not without risk (Loscalzo, 2010; Tapson, 2012).

Transvenous catheter embolectomy is a variety of techniques. For a suction embolectomy, a large-lumen catheter is inserted and the thrombus is suctioned by manually applying negative pressure with an aspiration syringe. Rheolytic embolectomy is accomplished by injecting pressurized saline through the catheter's distal tip that macerates the emboli. The saline and clots are then sucked back into the exhaust lumen for disposal. A rotational embolectomy involves a rotating device within the catheter to fragment the thrombus. The fragments are continuously aspirated. In addition, catheter-directed ultrasound combined with low-dose thrombolytic therapy has been studied and may offer benefit (Tapson, 2012).

An inferior vena cava (IVC) filter may be inserted at the time of surgery to protect against a recurrence. IVC filters are not recommended for the initial treatment of patients with PE (ACCP, 2012). The IVC filter provides a screen in the IVC, allowing blood to pass through while large emboli from the pelvis or lower extremities are blocked or fragmented before reaching the lung (Tapson, 2012). Numerous catheters have been developed since the introduction of the original Greenfield filter (Fig. 23-6). The choice of filter depends on the diameter of the IVC as well as the planned duration of

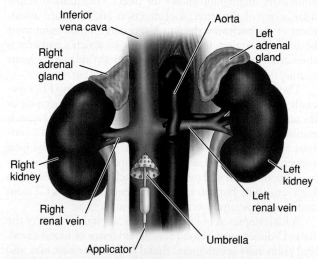

FIGURE 23-6 • An umbrella filter is in place in the inferior vena cava to prevent PE. The filter (compressed within an applicator catheter) is inserted through an incision in the right internal jugular vein. The applicator is withdrawn when the filter fixes itself to the wall of the inferior vena cava after ejection from the applicator.

placement of the filter. Some filters are retrievable and some are nonretrievable (Fedullo, 2012). It is recommended that anticoagulation be continued in patients with an IVC filter if there are no contraindications to its use.

Nursing Management

Minimizing the Risk of Pulmonary Embolism

A key role of the nurse is to identify the patient at high risk for PE and to minimize the risk of PE in all patients. The nurse must have a high degree of suspicion for PE in all patients, but particularly in those with conditions predisposing to a slowing of venous return.

Preventing Thrombus Formation

Preventing thrombus formation is a major nursing responsibility. The nurse encourages ambulation and active and passive leg exercises to prevent venous stasis in patients prescribed bed rest. The nurse instructs the patient to move the legs in a "pumping" exercise so that the leg muscles can help increase venous flow. The nurse also advises the patient not to sit or lie in bed for prolonged periods, not to cross the legs, and not to wear constrictive clothing. Legs should not be dangled or feet placed in a dependent position while the patient sits on the edge of the bed; instead, feet should rest on the floor or on a chair. In addition, IV catheters (for parenteral therapy or measurements of central venous pressure) should not be left in place for prolonged periods.

Assessing Potential for Pulmonary Embolism

All patients are evaluated for risk factors for thrombus formation and PE. The nurse conducts a careful assessment of the patient's health history, family history, and medication record. On a daily basis, the patient is asked about pain or discomfort in the extremities. In addition, the extremities are evaluated for warmth, redness, and inflammation.

Monitoring Thrombolytic (Fibrinolytic) Therapy

The nurse is responsible for monitoring thrombolytic (fibrinolytic) and anticoagulant therapy. Thrombolytic (fibrinolytic) therapy (streptokinase, urokinase, tissue plasminogen activator) causes lysis of deep vein thrombi and PE, which helps dissolve the clots. During thrombolytic infusion, while the patient remains on bed rest, vital signs are assessed every 2 hours and invasive procedures are avoided. Tests to determine INR or PTT are performed 3 to 4 hours after the thrombolytic infusion is started to confirm that the fibrinolytic systems have been activated. (See Chapter 30 for nursing management for the patient receiving anticoagulant or thrombolytic therapy.)

> ⚑ *Quality and Safety Nursing Alert*
>
> Because of the prolonged clotting time, only essential arterial punctures or venipunctures are performed in patients who have received thrombolytics/fibrinolytics, and manual pressure is applied to any puncture site for at least 30 minutes. Pulse oximetry is used to monitor changes in oxygenation. The thrombolytic/fibrinlytic infusion is discontinued immediately if uncontrolled bleeding occurs.

Managing Pain

Chest pain, if present, is usually pleuritic rather than cardiac in origin. A semi-Fowler's position provides a more comfortable position for breathing. However, the nurse must continue to turn patients frequently and reposition them to improve the **ventilation–perfusion ratio ($\dot{V}/\dot{Q}$)** in the lung. The nurse administers opioid analgesic agents as prescribed for severe pain.

Managing Oxygen Therapy

Careful attention is given to the proper use of oxygen. The patient must understand the need for continuous oxygen therapy. The nurse assesses the patient frequently for signs of hypoxemia and monitors the pulse oximetry values to evaluate the effectiveness of the oxygen therapy. Deep breathing and incentive spirometry are indicated for all patients to minimize or prevent atelectasis and improve ventilation. Nebulizer therapy or percussion and postural drainage may be used for management of secretions.

Relieving Anxiety

The nurse encourages the stabilized patient to talk about any fears or concerns related to this frightening episode, answers the patient's and family's questions concisely and accurately, explains the therapy, and describes how to recognize untoward effects early.

Monitoring for Complications

When caring for a patient who has had PE, the nurse must be alert for the potential complication of cardiogenic shock or right ventricular failure subsequent to the effect of PE on the cardiovascular system. (Nursing activities for managing shock are found in Chapter 14; see Chapter 29 for nursing management of right ventricular failure.)

Providing Postoperative Nursing Care

If the patient has undergone surgical embolectomy, the nurse measures the patient's pulmonary arterial pressure and urinary output. The nurse also assesses the insertion site of the arterial catheter for hematoma formation and infection. Maintaining the blood pressure at a level that supports perfusion of vital organs is crucial. To prevent peripheral venous stasis and edema of the lower extremities, the nurse elevates the foot of the bed and encourages isometric exercises, the use of anti-embolism stockings, and walking when the patient is permitted out of bed. Sitting is discouraged, because hip flexion compresses the large veins in the legs.

Promoting Home and Community-Based Care

Educating Patients About Self-Care

Before hospital discharge and at follow-up visits to the clinic, the nurse educates the patient about preventing recurrence and reporting signs and symptoms. Patient education instructions, presented in Chart 23-10, are intended to help prevent recurrences and side effects of treatment.

Continuing Care

During follow-up or home care visits, the nurse monitors the patient's adherence to the prescribed management plan and reinforces previous instructions. The nurse also

Chart 23-10

HOME CARE CHECKLIST
Prevention of Recurrent Pulmonary Embolism

At the completion of home care education, the patient or caregiver will be able to:	PATIENT	CAREGIVER
• Describe the underlying process leading to pulmonary embolism.	✔	✔
• Describe the need for continued anticoagulant therapy after the initial embolism.	✔	✔
• Name the anticoagulant prescribed and identify dosage and schedule of administration.	✔	✔
• Describe potential side effects of coagulation such as bruising and bleeding and identify ways to prevent bleeding: • Avoid the use of sharps (razors, knives, etc.) to prevent cuts; shave with an electric shaver. • Use a toothbrush with soft bristles to prevent gum injury. • Do not take aspirin or antihistamines while taking warfarin sodium (Coumadin). • Always check with the primary provider before taking any medicine, including over-the-counter medications. • Avoid laxatives, because they may affect vitamin K absorption. • Report the occurrence of dark, tarry stools to the primary provider immediately. • Wear an identification bracelet or carry a medicine card stating that you are taking anticoagulants.	✔	✔
• Describe strategies to prevent recurrent deep venous thrombosis and pulmonary emboli: • Continue to wear anti-embolism stockings (compression hose) as long as directed. • Avoid sitting with legs crossed or sitting for prolonged periods of time. • When traveling, change position regularly, walk occasionally, and do active exercises of moving the legs and ankles while sitting. • Drink fluids, especially while traveling and in warm weather, to avoid hemoconcentration due to fluid deficit.	✔	✔
• Describe the signs and symptoms of lower extremity circulatory compromise and potential deep venous thrombosis: calf or leg pain, swelling, pedal edema.	✔	✔
• Describe the signs and symptoms of pulmonary compromise related to recurrent pulmonary embolism.	✔	✔
• Describe how and when to contact the primary provider if symptoms of circulatory compromise or pulmonary compromise are identified.	✔	✔

monitors the patient for residual effects of the PE and recovery. The patient is reminded about the importance of keeping follow-up appointments for coagulation tests and appointments with the primary provider. The nurse also reminds the patient about the importance of participation in health promotion activities (e.g., immunizations) and health screening.

Sarcoidosis

Sarcoidosis is a type of interstitial lung disease (Shigemitsu & Zauma, 2011). It is a multisystem, granulomatous disease of unknown etiology. Although 90% of patients demonstrate thoracic involvement, any organ may be affected (Morgenthau & Iannuzzi, 2011). Sarcoidosis usually presents between 20 and 40 years of age (Loscalzo, 2010). In the United States, the disease is more common in African Americans, and the estimated prevalence is 10 to 20 per 100,000 persons (King, 2011).

Pathophysiology

Sarcoidosis is thought to be a hypersensitivity response to one or more exogenous agents (bacteria, fungi, virus, chemicals) in people with an inherited or acquired predisposition to the disorder. The hypersensitivity response and inflammation results in the formation of a noncaseating granuloma, which is a noninfectious organized collection of macrophages that appear as a nodule. In the lung, granuloma infiltration and fibrosis may occur, resulting in low lung compliance, impaired diffusing capacity, and reduced lung volumes (King, 2011).

Clinical Manifestations

Hallmarks of sarcoidosis are its insidious onset and lack of prominent clinical signs or symptoms. The clinical picture depends on the systems affected. The lung is most commonly involved; signs and symptoms may include dyspnea, cough, hemoptysis, and congestion. Generalized symptoms include anorexia, fatigue, and weight loss. Other signs include uveitis; joint pain; fever; and granulomatous lesions of the skin, liver, spleen, kidney, and central nervous system. The granulomas may disappear or gradually convert to fibrous tissue. With multisystem involvement, patients may also have fatigue, fever, anorexia, and weight loss.

Assessment and Diagnostic Findings

Chest x-rays and CT scans are used to assess pulmonary adenopathy. These may show hilar adenopathy and disseminated miliary and nodular lesions in the lungs. A mediastinoscopy or **transbronchial** biopsy (in which a tissue specimen is obtained through the bronchial wall) may be used to confirm the diagnosis. In rare cases, an **open lung biopsy** is performed. Diagnosis is confirmed by a biopsy that shows noncaseating granulomas. Pulmonary function test results are abnormal if there is restriction of lung function (reduction in total lung capacity). Arterial blood gas measurements may be normal or may show reduced oxygen levels (hypoxemia) and increased carbon dioxide levels (hypercapnia).

Medical Management

Many patients undergo remission without specific treatment. Corticosteroids may be beneficial because of their anti-inflammatory effects. Short-course, moderate-dose therapy with prednisone has been suggested as initial management of symptoms (London, 2011). Corticosteroids have been shown to be useful in patients with ocular and myocardial involvement, skin involvement, extensive pulmonary disease that compromises pulmonary function, hepatic involvement, and hypercalcemia. However, it is not known if steroids alter the long-term course of the disease (London, 2011). When there is inadequate response to prednisone or the dose cannot be decreased, an immune modulator may be added (e.g., methotrexate [Trexall], azathioprine [Imuran], leflunomide [Arava], mycophenolate [CellCept]). No single test monitors the progression or recurrence of sarcoidosis; multiple tests are used to monitor involved systems.

OCCUPATIONAL LUNG DISEASES: PNEUMOCONIOSES

Pneumoconiosis refers to a nonneoplastic alteration of the lung resulting from inhalation of mineral or inorganic dust (e.g., "dusty lung"). Pneumoconioses are caused by inhalation and deposition of mineral dusts in the lungs, resulting in pulmonary fibrosis and parenchymal changes. Usually, extended exposure to irritating or toxic substances accounts for these changes, although severe single exposures may also lead to chronic lung disease. Occupational lung disease is the number one work-related illness in the United States based on its frequency, severity, and preventability (American Lung Association [ALA], 2012). Many people with early pneumoconiosis are asymptomatic, but advanced disease often is accompanied by disability and premature death.

Diseases of the lungs occur in numerous occupations as a result of exposure to several different types of agents, such as mineral dusts, metal dusts, biologic dusts, and toxic fumes. Smoking may compound the problem and may increase the risk of lung cancers in people exposed to the mineral asbestos and other potential carcinogens (ALA, 2012). The effects of inhaling these materials depend on the composition of the substance, its concentration, its ability to initiate an immune response, its irritating properties, the duration of exposure, and the individual's response or susceptibility to the irritant.

These diseases are not treatable once they develop; however, they are preventable. Therefore, a major role for nurses, especially occupational health nurses, is that of advocate for employees. Nurses need to make every effort to promote measures to reduce the exposure of workers to industrial products. Strategies to control exposure should be identified and encouraged; these strategies include the use of protective devices (facemasks, hoods, industrial respirators) to minimize exposure and screening/monitoring of individuals at risk.

Key aspects of any assessment of patients with a potential occupational respiratory history include job and job activities, exposure levels, general hygiene, time frame of exposure, effectiveness of respiratory protection used, and direct versus indirect exposures. Specific information that should be obtained includes the following:

- Exposure to an agent known to cause an occupational disorder
- Length of time from exposure of agent to onset of symptoms
- Congruence of symptoms with those of known exposure-related disorder
- Lack of other more likely explanations of the signs and symptoms

The most common pneumoconioses are silicosis, **asbestosis**, and coal worker's pneumoconiosis (ALA, 2012) (Table 23-5). More than one million workers are exposed to silica each year. Symptoms rarely develop in less than 5 years; however, progression of the disease results in extreme shortness of breath, loss of appetite, chest pains, and potentially respiratory failure (ALA, 2012). Asbestosis is progressive and causes severe scarring of the lung, which leads to fibrosis. The lungs become stiff, making it difficult to breathe or to oxygenate well. The disease may not evidence manifestations until 10 to 40 years after exposure (ALA, 2012). Coal worker's pneumoconiosis is a collection of lung disease caused by exposure to inhaled dusts.

The nurse provides education about preventive measures to patients and their families, assesses patients for a history of exposure to environmental agents, and makes referrals so that pulmonary function can be evaluated and the patient can be treated early in the course of the disease. These diseases have no effective treatment because damage is irreversible. Supportive therapy is aimed at preventing infections and managing complications.

CHEST TUMORS

Tumors of the lung may be benign or malignant. A malignant chest tumor can be primary, arising within the lung, chest wall, or mediastinum or it can be a metastasis from a primary tumor site elsewhere in the body.

Lung Cancer (Bronchogenic Carcinoma)

Lung cancer is the leading cancer killer among men and women in the United States, with almost 161,000 deaths estimated in 2012. Approximately 226,000 new cases of lung cancer are diagnosed annually; 14% of new cancers for men and women involve the lung or bronchus. In approximately 70% of patients with lung cancer, the disease has spread to regional lymphatics and other sites by the time of diagnosis. As a result, the long-term survival rate is low. Overall, the 5-year survival rate is 13% (ACS, 2012a).

Pathophysiology

The most common cause of lung cancer is inhaled carcinogens, most often cigarette smoke (90%); other carcinogens

TABLE 23-5 Occupational Lung Diseases: Pneumoconioses

Disease (Source)	Pathophysiology	Clinical Manifestations
Silicosis (glass manufacturing, foundry work, stone cutting)	Inhaled silica dust produces nodular lesions in the lungs. Nodules enlarge and coalesce. Dense masses form on upper portion of lungs, resulting in loss of pulmonary volume. Fibrotic destruction of pulmonary tissue can lead to restrictive lung disease, emphysema, pulmonary hypertension, and cor pulmonale.	*Acute silicosis:* dyspnea, fever, cough, weight loss *Chronic silicosis:* progressive symptoms indicative of hypoxemia, severe airflow obstruction, and right-sided heart failure
Asbestosis (shipbuilding, building demolition)	Inhaled asbestos fibers enter alveoli and are surrounded by fibrous tissue. Fibrous changes can also affect the pleura, which thicken and develop plaque. These changes lead to restrictive lung disease, with a decrease in lung volume, diminished exchange of oxygen and carbon dioxide, hypoxemia, cor pulmonale, and respiratory failure. It also increases risk of lung cancer, mesothelioma, and pleural effusion.	Progressive dyspnea; persistent, dry cough; mild to moderate chest pain; anorexia; weight loss; malaise; clubbing of the fingers
Coal worker's pneumoconiosis	Encompasses a variety of lung diseases; is also known as black lung disease. Inhaled dusts that are mixtures of coal, kaolin, mica, and silica are deposited in the alveoli and respiratory bronchioles. When macrophages that engulf the dust can no longer be cleared, they aggregate and fibroblasts appear. The bronchioles and alveoli become clogged with dust, dying macrophages, and fibroblasts, leading to formation of coal macules. Fibrotic lesions develop and subsequently localized emphysema develops, with cor pulmonale and respiratory failure.	Chronic cough, dyspnea, and expectoration of black or gray sputum, especially in miners who are smokers with cavitation in the lungs

Adapted from American Lung Association. (2012). *Occupational lung disease fast fact sheet.* Available at www.lungusa.org; and Loscalzo, J. (2010). *Harrison's pulmonary and critical care medicine.* New York: McGraw-Hill.

include radon gas and occupational and environmental agents (Loscalzo, 2010). Lung cancers arise from a single transformed epithelial cell in the tracheobronchial airways, in which the carcinogen binds to and damages the cell's DNA. This damage results in cellular changes, abnormal cell growth, and eventually a malignant cell. As the damaged DNA is passed on to daughter cells, the DNA undergoes further changes and becomes unstable. With the accumulation of genetic changes, the pulmonary epithelium undergoes malignant transformation from normal epithelium eventually to invasive carcinoma. Carcinoma tends to arise at sites of previous scarring (TB, fibrosis) in the lung.

Classification and Staging

For purposes of staging and treatment, most lung cancers are classified into one of two major categories: small cell lung cancer (SCLC) and non–small cell lung cancer (NSCLC). SCLC represents 10% to 15% of tumors; NSCLC represents approximately 85% to 90% of tumors (ACS, 2012b). In NSCLC, the cell types include squamous cell carcinoma (25% to 30%), large cell carcinoma (10% to 15%), and adenocarcinoma (40%), including bronchoalveolar carcinoma. In SCLC, the two general cell types include small cell and combined small cell.

NSCLC is further classified by cell type. Squamous cell cancer is usually more centrally located and arises more commonly in the segmental and subsegmental bronchi. Adenocarcinoma is the most prevalent carcinoma of the lung in both men and women; it occurs peripherally as peripheral masses or nodules and often metastasizes. Large cell carcinoma (also called *undifferentiated carcinoma*) is a fast-growing tumor that tends to arise peripherally. Bronchoalveolar cell cancer is found in the terminal bronchi and alveoli and is usually slower growing compared with other bronchogenic carcinomas.

In addition to classification according to cell type, lung cancers are staged. The stage of the tumor refers to the size of the tumor, its location, whether lymph nodes are involved, and whether the cancer has spread (Lababede, Meziane, & Rice, 2011). NSCLC is staged as I to IV. Stage I is the earliest stage and has the highest cure rate, whereas stage IV designates metastatic spread. Survival rates for NSCLC are shown in Table 23-6. (Diagnostic tools and further information on staging are described in Chapter 15.)

Risk Factors

Environmental factors (i.e., tobacco smoke, secondhand (passive) smoke, environmental and occupational exposures) account for an estimated 75% to 80% of cancer cases and deaths in the United States (ACS, 2012a). Other factors that have been associated with lung cancer include male gender, genetic predisposition, dietary deficits, and underlying respiratory diseases, such as COPD and TB. Some familial predisposition to lung cancer exists, as the incidence of lung cancer in

TABLE 23-6 Five-Year Survival Rates for Lung Cancer

Stage	5-Year Survival Rate (%)
NSCLC	
IA	49
IB	45
IIA	30
IIB	31
IIIA	14
IIIB	5
IV	1
SCLC	
I	31
II	19
III	8
IV	2

NSCLC, non–small cell lung cancer; SCLC, small cell lung cancer.
Adapted from Howlader, N., Noone, A. M., Krapcho, M., et al. (Eds.). (2009). *SEER cancer statistics review, 1975–2009 (vintage 2009 populations).* Bethesda, MD: National Cancer Institute. Available at: seer.cancer.gov/csr/1975_2009_pops09

close relatives of patients with lung cancer is two to three times that in the general population regardless of smoking status.

Tobacco Smoke

The ACS reports that smoking is responsible for approximately 78% of lung cancer in men and 44% in women (ACS, 2012a). The risk of developing lung cancer is about 23 times higher in male smokers and 13 times higher in female smokers compared to lifelong nonsmokers (ACS, 2012a). Risk is determined by the pack-year history (number of packs of cigarettes used each day, multiplied by the number of years smoked), the age of initiation of smoking, the depth of inhalation, and the tar and nicotine levels in the cigarettes smoked. The younger a person is when he or she starts smoking, the greater the risk of developing lung cancer. Smokers who use smokeless products as a supplemental source of nicotine will increase their risk of lung cancer (ACS, 2012a).

Almost all cases of SCLC are due to cigarette smoking. SCLC is rare in people who have never smoked. It is the most aggressive form of lung cancer, grows quickly, and usually starts in the airways in the center of the chest (National Cancer Institute [NCI], 2012).

Secondhand Smoke

Passive smoking has been identified as a cause of lung cancer in nonsmokers. Each year, about 3,400 nonsmoking adults die of lung cancer as a result of secondhand smoke (ACS, 2012a). People who are involuntarily exposed to tobacco smoke in a closed environment (house, automobile, building) have an increased risk of lung cancer when compared with unexposed nonsmokers.

Environmental and Occupational Exposure

Various carcinogens have been identified in the atmosphere, including motor vehicle emissions and pollutants from refineries and manufacturing plants. Evidence suggests that the incidence of lung cancer is greater in urban areas as a result of the buildup of pollutants and motor vehicle emissions.

Radon is a colorless, odorless gas found in soil and rocks. For many years, it has been associated with uranium mines, but it is now known to seep into homes through ground rock. High levels of radon have been associated with the development of lung cancer, especially when combined with cigarette smoking. Homeowners are advised to have radon levels checked in their houses and to arrange for special venting if the levels are high.

Chronic exposure to industrial carcinogens, such as arsenic, asbestos, mustard gas, chromates, coke oven fumes, nickel, oil, and radiation, has been associated with the development of lung cancer. Laws have been passed to control exposure to these carcinogens in the workplace.

Clinical Manifestations

Often, lung cancer develops insidiously and is asymptomatic until late in its course. The signs and symptoms depend on the location and size of the tumor, the degree of obstruction, and the existence of metastases to regional or distant sites.

The most frequent symptom of lung cancer is cough or change in a chronic cough. People frequently ignore this symptom and attribute it to smoking or a respiratory infec-

tion. The cough may start as a dry, persistent cough, without sputum production. When obstruction of airways occurs, the cough may become productive due to infection.

> ### ► Quality and Safety Nursing Alert
>
> A cough that changes in character should arouse suspicion of lung cancer.

Dyspnea is prominent in patients early in their disease. Causes of dyspnea may include tumor occlusion of the airway or lung parenchyma, pleural effusion, pneumonia, or complications of treatment. Hemoptysis or blood-tinged sputum may be expectorated. Chest or shoulder pain may indicate chest wall or pleural involvement by a tumor. Pain also is a late manifestation and may be related to metastasis to the bone.

In some patients, a recurring fever is an early symptom in response to a persistent infection in an area of pneumonitis distal to the tumor. In fact, cancer of the lung should be suspected in people with repeated unresolved upper respiratory tract infections. If the tumor spreads to adjacent structures and regional lymph nodes, the patient may present with chest pain and tightness, hoarseness (involving the recurrent laryngeal nerve), dysphagia, head and neck edema, and symptoms of pleural or pericardial effusion. The most common sites of metastases are lymph nodes, bone, brain, contralateral lung, adrenal glands, and liver (Fig. 23-7). Nonspecific symptoms of weakness, anorexia, and weight loss also may be present.

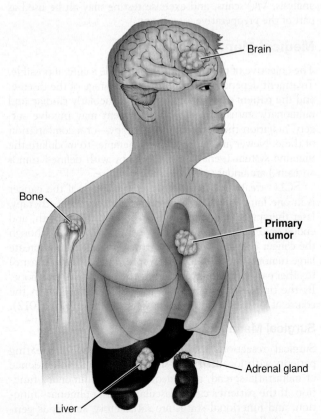

FIGURE 23-7 • Frequent sites of lung cancer metastasis.

Assessment and Diagnostic Findings

If pulmonary symptoms occur in heavy smokers, cancer of the lung should always be considered. A chest x-ray is performed to search for pulmonary density, a solitary pulmonary nodule (coin lesion), atelectasis, and infection. CT scans of the chest are used to identify small nodules not easily visualized on the chest x-ray and also to serially examine areas for lymphadenopathy.

Sputum cytology is rarely used to make a diagnosis of lung cancer. Fiberoptic bronchoscopy is commonly used; it provides a detailed study of the tracheobronchial tree and allows for brushings, washings, and biopsies of suspicious areas. For peripheral lesions not amenable to bronchoscopic biopsy, a transthoracic **fine-needle aspiration** may be performed under CT guidance to aspirate cells from a suspicious area.

A variety of scans may be used to assess for metastasis of the cancer. These may include bone scans, abdominal scans, positron emission tomography (PET) scans, and liver ultrasound. CT scan of the brain, magnetic resonance imaging (MRI), and other neurologic diagnostic procedures are used to detect central nervous system metastases. Mediastinoscopy or mediastinotomy may be used to obtain biopsy samples from lymph nodes in the mediastinum. Endobronchial ultrasound biopsy of mediastinal nodes is also used. In some circumstances, an endoscopy with esophageal ultrasound may be used to obtain a transesophageal biopsy of enlarged subcarinal lymph nodes.

If surgery is a potential treatment, the patient is evaluated to determine whether the tumor is resectable and whether the patient can tolerate the physiologic impairment resulting from such surgery. Pulmonary function tests, arterial blood gas analysis, V̇/Q̇ scans, and exercise testing may all be used as part of the preoperative assessment.

Medical Management

The objective of management is to provide a cure, if possible. Treatment depends on the cell type, the stage of the disease, and the patient's physiologic status (particularly cardiac and pulmonary status). In general, treatment may involve surgery, radiation therapy, or chemotherapy—or a combination of these. Newer and more specific therapies to modulate the immune system (gene therapy, therapy with defined tumor antigens) are under study and show promise.

SCLC treatment includes surgery (but only if the cancer is in one lung and there is no metastasis), radiation therapy, laser therapy to open airways blocked by tumor growth, and endoscopic stent placement (to open an airway). Although the cancer cells are small, they grow very quickly and create large tumors. These tumors often spread rapidly (metastasize) to other parts of the body, including the brain, liver, and bone. By the time a patient presents with SCLC, it is late in the course of the disease and metastasis has occurred (NCI, 2012).

Surgical Management

Surgical resection is the preferred method of treating patients with localized non–small cell tumors, no evidence of metastatic spread, and adequate cardiopulmonary function. If the patient's cardiovascular status, pulmonary function, and functional status are satisfactory, surgery is generally well tolerated. However, coronary artery disease,

---

Chart 23-11 Types of Lung Resection

- Lobectomy: a single lobe of the lung is removed
- Bilobectomy: two lobes of the lung are removed
- Sleeve resection: cancerous lobe(s) is removed and a segment of the main bronchus is resected
- Pneumonectomy: removal of entire lung
- Segmentectomy: a segment of the lung is removed*
- Wedge resection: removal of a small, pie-shaped area of the segment*
- Chest wall resection with removal of cancerous lung tissue: for cancers that have invaded the chest wall

*Not recommended as curative resection for lung cancer.

---

pulmonary insufficiency, and other comorbidities may contraindicate surgical intervention. The cure rate of surgical resection depends on the type and stage of the cancer. Surgery is primarily used for NSCLCs, because small cell cancer of the lung grows rapidly and metastasizes early and extensively. Lesions of many patients with bronchogenic cancer are inoperable at the time of diagnosis. Several different types of lung resection may be performed (Chart 23-11). The most common surgical procedure for a small, apparently curable tumor of the lung is lobectomy (removal of a lobe of the lung). In some cases, an entire lung may be removed (pneumonectomy) (see Chapter 21 for further details).

Radiation Therapy

Radiation therapy may offer cure in a small percentage of patients. It is useful in controlling neoplasms that cannot be surgically resected but are responsive to radiation. Irradiation also may be used to reduce the size of a tumor, to make an inoperable tumor operable, or to relieve the pressure of the tumor on vital structures. It can reduce symptoms of spinal cord metastasis and superior vena caval compression. In addition, prophylactic brain irradiation is used in certain patients to treat microscopic metastases to the brain. Radiation therapy may help relieve cough, chest pain, dyspnea, hemoptysis, and bone and liver pain. Relief of symptoms may last from a few weeks to many months and is important in improving the quality of the remaining period of life.

Radiation therapy usually is toxic to normal tissue within the radiation field, and this may lead to complications such as esophagitis, pneumonitis, and radiation lung fibrosis, although the incidence of these complications have decreased over time with improvements in delivery of radiation therapy (Merrill, 2012). These complications may impair ventilatory and diffusion capacity and significantly reduce pulmonary reserve. The patient's nutritional status, psychological outlook, fatigue level, and signs of anemia and infection are monitored throughout the treatment. (See Chapter 15 for management of the patient receiving radiation therapy.)

Chemotherapy

Chemotherapy is used to alter tumor growth patterns, to treat distant metastases or small cell cancer of the lung, and as an adjunct to surgery or radiation therapy. Chemotherapy may provide relief, especially of pain, but it does not usually cure the disease or prolong life to any great degree. Chemotherapy is also accompanied by side effects. It is valuable in reducing pressure symptoms of lung cancer and in treating brain, spinal cord, and pericardial metastasis. (See Chapter 15 for a discussion of chemotherapy for the patient with cancer.)

The choice of agent depends on the growth of the tumor cell and the specific phase of the cell cycle that the medication affects. In combination with surgery, chemotherapy may be administered before surgery (neoadjuvant therapy) or after surgery (adjuvant therapy). Combinations of two or more medications may be more beneficial than single-dose regimens. A variety of agents are used in NSCLC, including platinum analogues (cisplatin [Platinol] and carboplatin [Paraplatin]) and non–platinum-containing agents—taxanes (paclitaxel [Taxol, Onxol], docetaxel [Taxotere]), vinca alkaloids (vinblastine [Velban] and vindesine [Eldisine]), doxorubicin (Adriamycin, Doxil), gemcitabine (Gemzar), vinorelbine (Navelbine), irinotecan (Camptosar), etoposide (Toposar), and pemetrexed (Alimta). Other approved chemotherapeutic agents in oral form are gefitinib (Iressa) and erlotinib (Tarceva), which are epidermal growth factor tyrosine kinase inhibitors. Bevacizumab (Avastin) and cetuximab (Erbitux) are epidermal growth factor receptor inhibitors. Specific guidelines are available for the treatment of differing states of NSCLC through the National Comprehensive Cancer Network (NCCN, 2012). Numerous new agents are being investigated for various types of lung cancer.

Palliative Therapy

Palliative care, concurrent with standard oncologic care for lung cancer, should be considered early in the course of illness for any patient with metastatic cancer or high symptom burden (Smith, Temin, Alesi, et al., 2012). In lung cancer, palliative therapy may include radiation therapy to shrink the tumor to provide pain relief, a variety of bronchoscopic interventions to open a narrowed bronchus or airway, and pain management and other comfort measures. Evaluation and referral for hospice care are important in planning for comfortable and dignified end-of-life care for the patient and family (see Chapter 16 for further discussion).

Treatment-Related Complications

A variety of complications may occur as a result of treatment for lung cancer. Surgical resection may result in respiratory failure, particularly if the cardiopulmonary system is compromised before surgery. Surgical complications and prolonged mechanical ventilation are potential outcomes. Radiation therapy may result in diminished cardiopulmonary function and other complications, such as pulmonary fibrosis, pericarditis, myelitis, and cor pulmonale. Chemotherapy, particularly in combination with radiation therapy, can cause pneumonitis. Pulmonary toxicity is a potential side effect of chemotherapy.

Nursing Management

Nursing care of patients with lung cancer is similar to that for other patients with cancer (see Chapter 15) and addresses the physiologic and psychological needs of the patient. The physiologic problems are primarily due to the respiratory manifestations of the disease. Nursing care includes strategies to ensure relief of pain and discomfort and to prevent complications.

Managing Symptoms

The nurse educates the patient and family about the potential side effects of the specific treatment and strategies to manage them. Strategies for managing such symptoms as dyspnea, fatigue, nausea and vomiting, and anorexia help the patient and family cope with therapeutic measures.

Relieving Breathing Problems

Airway clearance techniques are key to maintaining airway patency through the removal of excess secretions. This may be accomplished through deep-breathing exercises, chest physiotherapy, directed cough, suctioning, and in some instances bronchoscopy. Bronchodilator medications may be prescribed to promote bronchial dilation. As the tumor enlarges or spreads, it may compress a bronchus or involve a large area of lung tissue, resulting in an impaired breathing pattern and poor gas exchange. At some stage of the disease, supplemental oxygen will probably be necessary.

Nursing measures focus on decreasing dyspnea by encouraging the patient to assume positions that promote lung expansion and to perform breathing exercises for lung expansion and relaxation. Patient education about energy conservation and airway clearance techniques is also necessary. Many of the techniques used in pulmonary rehabilitation can be applied to patients with lung cancer. Depending on the severity of disease and the patient's wishes, a referral to a pulmonary rehabilitation program may be helpful in managing respiratory symptoms.

Reducing Fatigue

Fatigue is a devastating symptom that affects quality of life in patients with cancer. It is commonly experienced by patients with lung cancer and may be related to the disease itself, the cancer treatment and complications (e.g., anemia), sleep disturbances, pain and discomfort, hypoxemia, poor nutrition, or the psychological ramifications of the disease (e.g., anxiety, depression). (See Chapter 15 for nursing strategies to promote energy conservation and reduce fatigue.)

Providing Psychological Support

Another important part of the nursing care of patients with lung cancer is provision of psychological support and identification of potential resources for the patient and family. Often, the nurse must help the patient and family deal with the following:

- The poor prognosis and relatively rapid progression of this disease
- Informed decision making regarding the possible treatment options
- Methods to maintain the patient's quality of life during the course of this disease
- End-of-life treatment options

Gerontologic Considerations

At the time of diagnosis of lung cancer, most patients are older than 65 years and have stage III or IV disease (Gore, Movsas, Santana-Davila, et al., 2012). Although age is not a significant prognostic factor for overall survival and response to treatment for either NSCLC or SCLC, older patients have specific needs. The presence of comorbidities and the patient's cognitive, functional, nutritional, and social status are important issues to consider with the patient of advanced age (Gore et al., 2012). Depending on the comorbidities and functional status of older adult patients, chemotherapy agents, doses, and cycles may need to be adjusted to maintain quality of life.

Tumors of the Mediastinum

Tumors of the mediastinum include neurogenic tumors, tumors of the thymus, lymphomas, germ cell tumors, cysts, and mesenchymal tumors. These tumors may be malignant or benign. They are usually described in relation to location: anterior, middle, or posterior masses or tumors.

Clinical Manifestations

Nearly all symptoms of mediastinal tumors result from the pressure of the mass against important intrathoracic organs. Symptoms may include cough, wheezing, dyspnea, anterior chest or neck pain, bulging of the chest wall, heart palpitations, angina, other circulatory disturbances, central cyanosis, superior vena cava syndrome (i.e., swelling of the face, neck, and upper extremities), marked distention of the veins of the neck and the chest wall (evidence of the obstruction of large veins of the mediastinum by extravascular compression or intravascular invasion), and dysphagia and weight loss from pressure or invasion into the esophagus (Muller, 2012).

Assessment and Diagnostic Findings

Chest x-rays are the major method used initially to diagnose mediastinal tumors and cysts. A CT scan is the standard diagnostic test for assessment of the mediastinum and surrounding structures. MRI, as well as PET, may be used in some circumstances (Muller, 2012).

Medical Management

If the tumor is malignant and has infiltrated the surrounding tissue and complete surgical removal is not feasible, radiation therapy, chemotherapy, or both are used.

Many mediastinal tumors are benign and operable. The location of the tumor (anterior, middle, or posterior compartment) in the mediastinum dictates the type of incision. The common incision used is a median sternotomy; however, a thoracotomy may be used, depending on the location of the tumor. Additional approaches include a bilateral anterior thoracotomy (clamshell incision) and video-assisted thoracoscopic surgery (see Chapter 21). The care is the same as for any patient undergoing thoracic surgery. Major complications include hemorrhage, injury to the phrenic or recurrent laryngeal nerve, and infection.

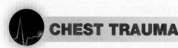 **CHEST TRAUMA**

Thoracic injuries account for 20% to 25% of deaths due to trauma and contribute to 25% to 50% of the remaining deaths. Approximately 16,000 deaths per year in the United States alone are attributable to chest trauma. Thoracic injuries are a contributing factor in up to 75% of all trauma-related deaths (CDC, 2012a). The increased incidence of

penetrating chest injury and improved prehospital and perioperative care have resulted in an increasing number of critically injured but potentially salvageable patients presenting to trauma centers.

Major chest trauma may occur alone or in combination with multiple other injuries. Chest trauma is classified as either blunt or penetrating. Blunt chest trauma results from sudden compression or positive pressure inflicted to the chest wall. Penetrating trauma occurs when a foreign object penetrates the chest wall.

Blunt Trauma

Overall, blunt thoracic injuries are directly responsible for 20% to 25% of all trauma deaths (Mancini, 2012). Although blunt chest trauma is more common than penetrating trauma, it is often difficult to identify the extent of the damage because the symptoms may be generalized and vague. In addition, patients may not seek immediate medical attention, which may complicate the problem.

Pathophysiology

The most common causes of blunt chest trauma are motor vehicle crashes (trauma from steering wheel, seat belt), falls, and bicycle crashes (trauma from handlebars). Types of blunt chest trauma include chest wall fractures, dislocations, and barotraumas (including diaphragmatic injuries); injuries of the pleura, lungs, and aerodigestive tracts; and blunt injuries of the heart, great arteries, veins, and lymphatics (Mancini, 2012). Injuries to the chest are often life threatening and result in one or more of the following pathologic states:

- Hypoxemia from disruption of the airway; injury to the lung parenchyma, rib cage, and respiratory musculature; massive hemorrhage; collapsed lung; and pneumothorax
- Hypovolemia from massive fluid loss from the great vessels, cardiac rupture, or hemothorax
- Cardiac failure from cardiac tamponade, cardiac contusion, or increased intrathoracic pressure

These pathologic states frequently result in impaired ventilation and perfusion leading to acute renal failure, hypovolemic shock, and death.

Assessment and Diagnostic Findings

Because time is critical in treating chest trauma, the patient must be assessed immediately to determine the following: time elapsed since injury occurred, mechanism of injury, level of responsiveness, specific injuries, estimated blood loss, recent drug or alcohol use, and prehospital treatment. Initial assessment of thoracic injuries includes assessment for airway obstruction, tension pneumothorax, open pneumothorax, massive hemothorax, flail chest, and cardiac tamponade. These injuries are life threatening and require immediate treatment. Secondary assessment includes assessment for simple pneumothorax, hemothorax, pulmonary contusion, traumatic aortic rupture, tracheobronchial disruption, esophageal perforation, traumatic diaphragmatic injury, and penetrating wounds to the mediastinum. Although listed as secondary, these injuries may be life threatening as well.

The physical examination includes inspection of the airway, thorax, neck veins, and breathing difficulty. Specifics include assessing the rate and depth of breathing for abnormalities such as stridor, cyanosis, nasal flaring, the use of accessory muscles, drooling, and overt trauma to the face, mouth, or neck. The chest is assessed for symmetric movement, symmetry of breath sounds, open chest wounds, entrance or exit wounds, impaled objects, tracheal shift, distended neck veins, subcutaneous emphysema, and paradoxical chest wall motion. In addition, the chest wall is assessed for bruising, petechiae, lacerations, and burns. The vital signs and skin color are assessed for signs of shock. The thorax is palpated for tenderness and crepitus, and the position of the trachea is also assessed.

The initial diagnostic workup includes a chest x-ray, CT scan, complete blood count, clotting studies, type and cross-match, electrolytes, oxygen saturation, arterial blood gas analysis, and ECG. The patient is completely undressed to avoid missing additional injuries that may complicate care. Many patients with injuries involving the chest have associated head and abdominal injuries that require attention. Ongoing assessment is essential to monitor the patient's response to treatment and to detect early signs of clinical deterioration.

Medical Management

The goals of treatment are to evaluate the patient's condition and to initiate aggressive resuscitation. An airway is immediately established with oxygen support and, in some cases, endotracheal intubation and ventilatory support. Reestablishing fluid volume and negative intrapleural pressure and draining intrapleural fluid and blood are essential.

The potential for massive blood loss and exsanguination with blunt or penetrating chest injuries is high because of injury to the great blood vessels. Many patients die at the scene of the injury or are in shock by the time help arrives. Agitation and irrational and combative behavior are signs of decreased oxygen delivery to the cerebral cortex. Strategies to restore and maintain cardiopulmonary function include ensuring an adequate airway and ventilation; stabilizing and reestablishing chest wall integrity; occluding any opening into the chest (open pneumothorax); and draining or removing any air or fluid from the thorax to relieve pneumothorax, hemothorax, or cardiac tamponade. Hypovolemia and low cardiac output must be corrected. Many of these treatment efforts, along with the control of hemorrhage, are carried out simultaneously at the scene of the injury or in the emergency department. Depending on the success of efforts to control the hemorrhage in the emergency department, the patient may be taken immediately to the operating room. Principles of management are essentially those pertaining to care of the postoperative thoracic patient (see Chapter 21).

■ *Sternal and Rib Fractures*

Sternal fractures are most common in motor vehicle crashes with a direct blow to the sternum via the steering wheel. Rib fractures are the most common type of chest trauma, occurring in more than 50% of patients admitted with blunt chest injury (Mancini, 2012). Most rib fractures are benign and are treated conservatively; ribs 4 through 10 are most fre-

quently involved. Fractures of the first three ribs are rare but can result in a high mortality rate because they are associated with laceration of the subclavian artery or vein. Fractures of the lower ribs are associated with injury to the spleen and liver, which may be lacerated by fragmented sections of the rib. Older adult patients with three or more rib fractures have been shown to have a fivefold increased mortality rate and a fourfold increased incidence of pneumonia (Mancini, 2012).

Clinical Manifestations

Patients with sternal fractures have anterior chest pain, overlying tenderness, ecchymosis, crepitus, swelling, and possible chest wall deformity. For patients with rib fractures, clinical manifestations are similar: severe pain, point tenderness, and muscle spasm over the area of the fracture that are aggravated by coughing, deep breathing, and movement. The area around the fracture may be bruised. To reduce the pain, the patient splints the chest by breathing in a shallow manner and avoids sighs, deep breaths, coughing, and movement. This reluctance to move or breathe deeply results in diminished ventilation, atelectasis (collapse of unaerated alveoli), pneumonitis, and hypoxemia. Respiratory insufficiency and failure can be the outcomes of such a cycle.

Assessment and Diagnostic Findings

The patient must be closely evaluated for underlying cardiac injuries. A crackling, grating sound in the thorax (subcutaneous crepitus) may be detected with auscultation. The diagnostic workup may include a chest x-ray, rib films of a specific area, ECG, continuous pulse oximetry, and arterial blood gas analysis.

Medical Management

Medical management is directed toward relieving pain, avoiding excessive activity, and treating any associated injuries. Surgical fixation is rarely necessary unless fragments are grossly displaced and pose a potential for further injury.

The goals of treatment for rib fractures are to control pain and to detect and treat the injury. Sedation is used to relieve pain and to allow deep breathing and coughing. Care must be taken to avoid oversedation and suppression of respiratory drive. Alternative strategies to relieve pain include an intercostal nerve block and ice over the fracture site. A chest binder may be used as supportive treatment to provide stability to the chest wall and may decrease pain. The patient is instructed to apply the binder snugly enough to provide support, but not to impair respiratory excursion. Usually, the pain abates in 5 to 7 days, and discomfort can be relieved with epidural analgesia, patient-controlled analgesia, or nonopioid analgesia. Most rib fractures heal in 3 to 6 weeks. The patient is monitored closely for signs and symptoms of associated injuries.

■ *Flail Chest*

Flail chest is frequently a complication of blunt chest trauma from a steering wheel injury. It occurs when three or more adjacent ribs (multiple contiguous ribs) are fractured at two or more sites, resulting in free-floating rib segments. It may also result as a combination fracture of ribs and costal cartilages or sternum. As a result, the chest wall loses stability,

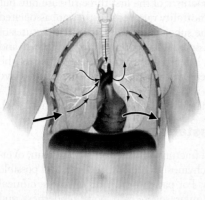
A. Inspiration

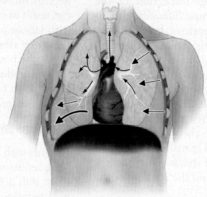
B. Expiration

FIGURE 23-8 • Flail chest is caused by a free-floating segment of rib cage resulting from multiple rib fractures. **A.** Paradoxical movement on inspiration occurs when the flail rib segment is sucked inward and the mediastinal structures shift to the unaffected side. The amount of air drawn into the affected lung is reduced. **B.** On expiration, the flail segment bulges outward and the mediastinal structures shift back to the affected side.

causing respiratory impairment and usually severe respiratory distress.

Pathophysiology

During inspiration, as the chest expands, the detached part of the rib segment (flail segment) moves in a paradoxical manner (pendelluft movement) in that it is pulled inward during inspiration, reducing the amount of air that can be drawn into the lungs. On expiration, because the intrathoracic pressure exceeds atmospheric pressure, the flail segment bulges outward, impairing the patient's ability to exhale. The mediastinum then shifts back to the affected side (Fig. 23-8). This paradoxical action results in increased dead space, a reduction in alveolar ventilation, and decreased compliance. Retained airway secretions and atelectasis frequently accompany flail chest. The patient has hypoxemia, and if gas exchange is greatly compromised, respiratory acidosis develops as a result of carbon dioxide retention. Hypotension, inadequate tissue perfusion, and metabolic acidosis often follow as the paradoxical motion of the mediastinum decreases cardiac output.

Medical Management

As with rib fracture, treatment of flail chest is usually supportive. Management includes providing ventilatory support, clearing secretions from the lungs, and controlling pain. Specific management depends on the degree of respiratory dysfunction. If only a small segment of the chest is involved, the objectives are to clear the airway through positioning, coughing, deep breathing, and suctioning to aid in the expansion of the lung, and to relieve pain by intercostal nerve blocks, high thoracic epidural blocks, or cautious use of IV opioids.

For mild to moderate flail chest injuries, the underlying pulmonary contusion is treated by monitoring fluid intake and appropriate fluid replacement while relieving chest pain. Pulmonary physiotherapy focusing on lung volume expansion and secretion management techniques are performed. The patient is closely monitored for further respiratory compromise.

For severe flail chest injuries, endotracheal intubation and mechanical ventilation are required to provide internal pneumatic stabilization of the flail chest and to correct abnormalities in gas exchange. This helps to treat the underlying pulmonary contusion, serves to stabilize the thoracic cage to allow the fractures to heal, and improves alveolar ventilation

and intrathoracic volume by decreasing the work of breathing. This treatment modality requires endotracheal intubation and ventilator support. Differing modes of ventilation are used depending on the patient's underlying disease and specific needs (see Chapter 21).

In rare circumstances, surgery may be required to more quickly stabilize the flail segment. This may be used for patients who are difficult to ventilate or for high-risk patients with underlying lung disease who may be difficult to wean from mechanical ventilation. Recent evidence finds that internal rib fixation—a surgical procedure that places clips, bars, or plates on the broken ribs to stabilize the flail segments—may shorten the time required for mechanical ventilation (Wendling, 2011).

Regardless of the type of treatment, the patient is carefully monitored by serial chest x-rays, arterial blood gas analysis, pulse oximetry, and bedside pulmonary function monitoring. Pain management is key to successful treatment. Patient-controlled analgesia, intercostal nerve blocks, epidural analgesia, and intrapleural administration of opioids may be used to relieve or manage thoracic pain.

■ *Pulmonary Contusion*

Pulmonary contusion is a common thoracic injury and is frequently associated with flail chest. It is defined as damage to the lung tissues resulting in hemorrhage and localized edema. It is associated with chest trauma when there is rapid compression and decompression to the chest wall (i.e., blunt trauma). Pulmonary contusion represents a spectrum of lung injury characterized by the development of infiltrates and various degrees of respiratory dysfunction and sometimes respiratory failure. It is often cited as the most common potentially life-threatening chest injury; however, mortality is often attributed to other associated injuries. Pulmonary contusion may not be evident initially on examination but develops in the posttraumatic period; it may involve a small portion of one lung, a massive section of a lung, one entire lung, or both lungs. Depending on the extent of injury, this type of trauma may be associated with a mortality rate greater than 50% (Mancini, 2012).

Pathophysiology

The primary pathologic defect is an abnormal accumulation of fluid in the interstitial and intra-alveolar spaces. It is thought that injury to the lung parenchyma and its capillary network results in a leakage of serum protein and plasma. The leaking serum protein exerts an osmotic pressure that enhances loss of fluid from the capillaries. Blood, edema, and cellular debris (from cellular response to injury) enter the lung and accumulate in the bronchioles and alveoli, where they interfere with gas exchange. An increase in pulmonary vascular resistance and pulmonary artery pressure occurs. The patient has hypoxemia and carbon dioxide retention. Occasionally, a contused lung occurs on the other side of the point of body impact; this is called a *contrecoup contusion* (Kaewlai, Avery, Asrani, et al., 2008).

Clinical Manifestations

Pulmonary contusion may be mild, moderate, or severe. The clinical manifestations vary from decreased breath sounds, tachypnea, tachycardia, chest pain, hypoxemia, and blood-tinged secretions to more severe tachypnea, tachycardia, crackles, frank bleeding, severe hypoxemia (cyanosis), and respiratory acidosis. Changes in sensorium, including increased agitation or combative irrational behavior, may be signs of hypoxemia.

In addition, patients with moderate pulmonary contusion have a large amount of mucus, serum, and frank blood in the tracheobronchial tree; patients often have a constant cough but cannot clear the secretions. Patients with severe pulmonary contusion have signs and symptoms that mirror ARDS, which may include central cyanosis; agitation; combativeness; and productive cough with frothy, bloody secretions.

Assessment and Diagnostic Findings

The efficiency of gas exchange is determined by pulse oximetry and arterial blood gas measurements. Pulse oximetry is also used to measure oxygen saturation continuously. The initial chest x-ray may show no changes; changes may not appear for 1 or 2 days after the injury and appear as pulmonary infiltrates on chest x-ray.

Medical Management

Treatment priorities include maintaining the airway, providing adequate oxygenation, and controlling pain. In mild pulmonary contusion, adequate hydration via IV fluids and oral intake is important to mobilize secretions. However, fluid intake must be closely monitored to avoid hypervolemia. Volume expansion techniques, postural drainage, physiotherapy including coughing, and endotracheal suctioning are used to remove the secretions. Pain is managed by intercostal nerve blocks or by opioids via patient-controlled analgesia or other methods. Usually, antimicrobial therapy is administered because the damaged lung is susceptible to infection. Supplemental oxygen is usually given by mask or cannula for 24 to 36 hours.

In patients with moderate pulmonary contusion, bronchoscopy may be required to remove secretions. Intubation and mechanical ventilation with PEEP (see Chapter 21) may also be necessary to maintain the pressure and keep the lungs inflated. A nasogastric tube is inserted to relieve gastrointestinal distention.

In patients with severe contusion, who may develop respiratory failure, aggressive treatment with endotracheal intuba-

tion and ventilatory support, diuretics, and fluid restriction may be necessary. Antimicrobial medications may be prescribed for the treatment of pulmonary infection. This is a common complication of pulmonary contusion (especially pneumonia in the contused segment) because the fluid and blood that extravasates into the alveolar and interstitial spaces serve as an excellent culture medium.

Penetrating Trauma

Any organ or structure within the chest is potentially susceptible to traumatic penetration. These organs include the chest wall, lung and pleura, tracheobronchial system, esophagus, diaphragm, and major thoracic blood vessels, as well as heart and other mediastinal structures. Common injuries include pneumothorax and cardiac tamponade.

Medical Management

The objective of immediate management is to restore and maintain cardiopulmonary function. After an adequate airway is ensured and ventilation is established, examination for shock and intrathoracic and intra-abdominal injuries is necessary. The patient is undressed completely so that additional injuries are not missed. (See Chapter 72 for discussion of primary and secondary survey.) There is a high risk of associated intra-abdominal injuries with stab wounds below the level of the fifth anterior intercostal space. Death can result from exsanguinating hemorrhage or intra-abdominal sepsis.

The diagnostic workup includes a chest x-ray, chemistry profile, arterial blood gas analysis, pulse oximetry, and ECG. The patient's blood is typed and cross-matched in case blood transfusion is required. After the status of the peripheral pulses is assessed, a large-bore IV line is inserted. An indwelling catheter is inserted to monitor urinary output. A nasogastric tube is inserted and connected to low suction to prevent aspiration, minimize leakage of abdominal contents, and decompress the gastrointestinal tract.

Hemorrhagic shock is treated simultaneously with colloid solutions, crystalloids, or blood, as indicated by the patient's condition. Diagnostic procedures are carried out as dictated by the needs of the patient (e.g., CT scans of chest or abdomen, flat plate x-ray of the abdomen, abdominal tap to check for bleeding) (see Chapter 14).

A chest tube is inserted into the pleural space in most patients with penetrating wounds of the chest to achieve rapid and continuing re-expansion of the lungs. The insertion of the chest tube frequently results in a complete evacuation of the blood and air. The chest tube also allows early recognition of continuing intrathoracic bleeding, which would make surgical exploration necessary. If the patient has a penetrating wound of the heart or great vessels, the esophagus, or the tracheobronchial tree, surgical intervention is required.

Pneumothorax

Pneumothorax occurs when the parietal or visceral pleura is breached and the pleural space is exposed to positive atmospheric pressure. Normally, the pressure in the pleural space is negative or subatmospheric; this negative pressure is required to maintain lung inflation. When either pleura is breached, air enters the pleural space, and the lung or a portion of it collapses.

Types of Pneumothorax

Types of pneumothorax include simple, traumatic, and tension pneumothorax.

Simple Pneumothorax

A simple, or spontaneous, pneumothorax occurs when air enters the pleural space through a breach of either the parietal or visceral pleura. Most commonly, this occurs as air enters the pleural space through the rupture of a bleb or a bronchopleural fistula. A spontaneous pneumothorax may occur in an apparently healthy person in the absence of trauma due to rupture of an air-filled bleb, or blister, on the surface of the lung, allowing air from the airways to enter the pleural cavity. It may be associated with diffuse interstitial lung disease and severe emphysema.

Traumatic Pneumothorax

A traumatic pneumothorax occurs when air escapes from a laceration in the lung itself and enters the pleural space or from a wound in the chest wall. It may result from blunt trauma (e.g., rib fractures), penetrating chest or abdominal trauma (e.g., stab wounds or gunshot wounds), or diaphragmatic tears. Traumatic pneumothorax may occur during invasive thoracic procedures (i.e., thoracentesis, transbronchial lung biopsy, insertion of a subclavian line) in which the pleura is inadvertently punctured, or with barotrauma from mechanical ventilation.

A traumatic pneumothorax resulting from major injury to the chest is often accompanied by hemothorax (collection of blood in the pleural space resulting from torn intercostal vessels, lacerations of the great vessels, or lacerations of the lungs). Often both blood and air are found in the chest cavity (hemopneumothorax) after major trauma. Chest surgery can be classified as a traumatic pneumothorax as a result of the entry into the pleural space and the accumulation of air and fluid in the pleural space.

Open pneumothorax is one form of traumatic pneumothorax. It occurs when a wound in the chest wall is large enough to allow air to pass freely in and out of the thoracic cavity with each attempted respiration. Because the rush of air through the wound in the chest wall produces a sucking sound, such injuries are termed *sucking chest wounds*. In such patients, not only does the lung collapse, but the structures of the mediastinum (heart and great vessels) also shift toward the uninjured side with each inspiration and in the opposite direction with expiration. This is termed *mediastinal flutter* or *swing*, and it produces serious circulatory problems.

▶ **Quality and Safety Nursing Alert**

Traumatic open pneumothorax calls for emergency interventions. Stopping the flow of air through the opening in the chest wall is a lifesaving measure.

Tension Pneumothorax

A **tension pneumothorax** occurs when air is drawn into the pleural space from a lacerated lung or through a small opening or wound in the chest wall. It may be a complication of other types of pneumothorax. In contrast to open pneumothorax, the air that enters the chest cavity with each inspiration is trapped; it cannot be expelled during expiration through the air passages or the opening in the chest wall. In effect, a one-way valve or ball valve mechanism occurs where air enters the pleural space but cannot escape. With each breath, tension (positive pressure) is increased within the affected pleural space. This causes the lung to collapse and the heart, the great vessels, and the trachea to shift toward the unaffected side of the chest (mediastinal shift). Both respiration and circulatory function are compromised because of the increased intrathoracic pressure, which decreases venous return to the heart, causing decreased cardiac output and impairment of peripheral circulation. In extreme cases, the pulse may be undetectable—this is known as pulseless electrical activity.

Clinical Manifestations

The signs and symptoms associated with pneumothorax depend on its size and cause. Pain is usually sudden and may be pleuritic. The patient may have only minimal respiratory distress with slight chest discomfort and tachypnea with a small simple or uncomplicated pneumothorax. If the pneumothorax is large and the lung collapses totally, acute respiratory distress occurs. The patient is anxious, has dyspnea and air hunger, has increased use of the accessory muscles, and may develop central cyanosis from severe hypoxemia.

In assessing the chest for any type of pneumothorax, the nurse assesses tracheal alignment, expansion of the chest, breath sounds, and percussion of the chest. In a simple pneumothorax, the trachea is midline, expansion of the chest is decreased, breath sounds may be diminished or absent, and percussion of the chest may reveal normal sounds or hyperresonance depending on the size of the pneumothorax. In a tension pneumothorax, the trachea is shifted away from the affected side, chest expansion may be decreased or fixed in a hyperexpansion state, breath sounds are diminished or absent, and percussion to the affected side is hyperresonant. The clinical picture is one of air hunger, agitation, increasing hypoxemia, central cyanosis, hypotension, tachycardia, and profuse diaphoresis. Figure 23-9 compares open and tension pneumothorax.

Medical Management

Medical management of pneumothorax depends on its cause and severity. The goal of treatment is to evacuate the air or blood from the pleural space. A small chest tube (28 Fr) is inserted near the second intercostal space; this space is used because it is the thinnest part of the chest wall, minimizes the danger of contacting the thoracic nerve, and leaves a less visible scar. If a patient also has a hemothorax, a large-diameter chest tube (32 Fr or greater) is inserted, usually in the fourth or fifth intercostal space at the midaxillary line. The tube is directed posteriorly to drain the fluid and air. Once the chest tube or tubes are inserted and suction is applied (usually to 20 mm Hg suction), effective decompression of the pleural cavity (drainage of blood or air) occurs.

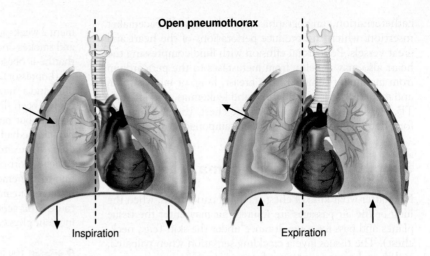

Open pneumothorax

Inspiration   Expiration

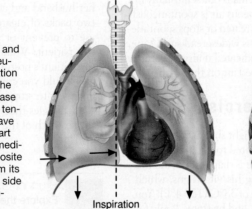

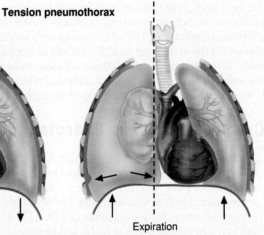

Tension pneumothorax

Inspiration   Expiration

FIGURE 23-9 • Open pneumothorax (*top*) and tension pneumothorax (*bottom*). In open pneumothorax, air enters the chest during inspiration and exits during expiration. A slight shift of the affected lung may occur because of a decrease in pressure as air moves out of the chest. In tension pneumothorax, air enters but cannot leave the chest. As the pressure increases, the heart and great vessels are compressed and the mediastinal structures are shifted toward the opposite side of the chest. The trachea is pushed from its normal midline position toward the opposite side of the chest, and the unaffected lung is compressed.

If an excessive amount of blood enters the chest tube in a relatively short period, an autotransfusion may be needed. This technique involves taking the patient's own blood that has been drained from the chest, filtering it, and then transfusing it back into the vascular system.

In such an emergency, anything may be used that is large enough to fill the chest wound—a towel, a handkerchief, or the heel of the hand. If conscious, the patient is instructed to inhale and strain against a closed glottis. This action assists in re-expanding the lung and ejecting the air from the thorax. In the hospital, the opening is plugged by sealing it with gauze impregnated with petrolatum. A pressure dressing is applied. Usually, a chest tube connected to water-seal drainage is inserted to remove air and fluid. Antibiotics usually are prescribed to combat infection from contamination.

The severity of open pneumothorax depends on the amount and rate of thoracic bleeding and the amount of air in the pleural space. The pleural cavity can be decompressed by needle aspiration (thoracentesis) or by chest tube drainage of the blood or air. The lung is then able to re-expand and resume the function of gas exchange. As a rule of thumb, the chest wall is opened surgically (thoracotomy) if more than 1,500 mL of blood is aspirated initially by thoracentesis (or is the initial chest tube output) or if chest tube output continues at greater than 200 mL per hour (Shahani, 2011). The urgency with which the blood must be removed is determined by the degree of respiratory compromise. An emer-

gency thoracotomy may also be performed in the emergency department if a cardiovascular injury secondary to chest or penetrating trauma is suspected. The patient with a possible tension pneumothorax should immediately be given a high concentration of supplemental oxygen to treat the hypoxemia, and pulse oximetry should be used to monitor oxygen saturation. In an emergency situation, a tension pneumothorax can be decompressed or quickly converted to a simple pneumothorax by inserting a large-bore needle (14-gauge) at the second intercostal space, midclavicular line on the affected side. This relieves the pressure and vents the positive pressure to the external environment. A chest tube is then inserted and connected to suction to remove the remaining air and fluid, reestablish the negative pressure, and re-expand the lung. If the lung re-expands and air leakage from the lung parenchyma stops, further drainage may be unnecessary. If a prolonged air leak continues despite chest tube drainage to underwater seal, surgery may be necessary to close the leak.

Cardiac Tamponade

Cardiac tamponade is compression of the heart resulting from fluid or blood within the pericardial sac. It usually is caused by blunt or penetrating trauma to the chest. A penetrating wound of the heart is associated with a high mortality rate. Cardiac tamponade also may follow diagnostic cardiac catheterization, angiographic procedures, and pacemaker insertion, which can produce perforations of the heart and great vessels. Pericardial effusion with fluid compressing the heart also may develop from metastases to the pericardium from malignant tumors of the breast, lung, or mediastinum and may occur with lymphomas and leukemias, renal failure, TB, and high-dose radiation to the chest. (See Chapter 29 for a detailed discussion of cardiac tamponade.)

Subcutaneous Emphysema

No matter what kind of chest trauma a patient has, when the lung or the air passages are injured, air may enter the tissue planes and pass for some distance under the skin (e.g., neck, chest). The tissues give a crackling sensation when palpated, and the subcutaneous air produces an alarming appearance as the face, neck, body, and scrotum become misshapen by subcutaneous air. Subcutaneous emphysema is of itself usually not a serious complication. The subcutaneous air is spontaneously absorbed if the underlying air leak is treated or stops spontaneously. In severe cases in which there is widespread subcutaneous emphysema, a tracheostomy is indicated if airway patency is threatened by pressure of the trapped air on the trachea.

Critical Thinking Exercises

1 **pq** While you are working the night shift, a 56-year-old homeless man with diabetes is admitted to your unit for an infected foot ulcer. You note that he is diaphoretic and has a persistent cough as you are taking his vital signs, which are normal except for a temperature of 38°C (100.4°F). You ask him if he usually sweats at night, and he states, "only for the past couple of months." He says his cough began around the same time as his night sweats and that he occasionally produces sputum that is tannish-green with streaks of red. What other priority assessments might you consider for this patient? What respiratory diseases may he be at risk for, and which are most consistent with his clinical manifestations? Are these communicable diseases? If so, what type of precautions should you take, both for him and for you? What kind of follow-up would be necessary those he has come in contact with inside and outside of the hospital?

2 **pq** An 85-year-old woman is being admitted to your unit from a long-term care facility. She had a CVA 5 years ago with subsequent persistent right-sided flaccid paralysis. She has a gastrostomy tube that is clamped. From the brief report you received, you know she was receiving enteral tube feedings at 60 mL per hour. She is supine in bed, is awake, and her face is flushed. She has the following vital signs: BP, 104/60; pulse, 110 bpm; respiratory rate, 30 breaths/min; temperature, 38.8°C (101.8°F). What risk factors does she have for developing pneumonia? What type of breath sounds might you expect to hear when auscultating her lungs? Identify five priority nursing interventions to treat her nursing diagnosis of Ineffective airway clearance.

3 A 62-year-old man presents to the emergency department with a history of sudden onset of shortness of breath, anxiety, and difficulty ambulating. He had a knee replacement 2 weeks ago. He reports a history of high blood pressure and smokes one pack of cigarettes per day, and you observe that he is obese. His medications include aspirin, metoprolol (Lopressor), another "blood pressure pill," a "cholesterol pill," and a "new pill" he got to "thin his blood" after surgery. He has been slow to ambulate following discharge from the hospital but has been doing some rehabilitation exercises. He said he had felt pain in his leg for the past 3 days while doing his exercises. He reports that he woke up suddenly tonight short of breath, was scared, and had his wife bring him to the emergency department. What risk factors does he have for cardiopulmonary disease? What is the potential cause of his acute problem? What signs will you look for during your physical examination of this patient?

4 **ebp** You are on a surgical unit caring for a 58-year-old woman who has undergone a right middle lobectomy for lung cancer. The patient has no history of smoking, but her husband and adult son who live with her both smoke two packs of cigarettes daily. What strategies would you use to prevent or minimize pulmonary complications in this patient? What parameters would you use to monitor the patient's postoperative respiratory status? What strategies would you consider to encourage the patient's family members to stop smoking? What is the evidence base for the strategies that you consider? How would you evaluate the strength of the evidence?

Brunner Suite Resources
Explore these additional resources to enhance learning for this chapter:
• NCLEX-Style Questions and Other Resources on thePoint, http://thePoint.lww.com/Brunner13e
• Study Guide
• PrepU
• Clinical Handbook
• Handbook of Laboratory and Diagnostic Tests

References

*Asterisk indicates nursing research.

Books

American Cancer Society. (2012a). *Cancer facts & figures 2012*. Atlanta, GA: Author.
Bartlett, R., Auwaerter, P., & Pham, P. (2012). *Johns Hopkins ABX guide* (3rd ed.). Burlington, MA: Jones & Bartlett Learning.
Loscalzo, J. (2010). *Harrison's pulmonary and critical care medicine*. New York: McGraw-Hill.
National Comprehensive Cancer Network. (2012). *NCCN guidelines version 3.2012: Non-small cell lung cancer*. National Comprehensive Cancer Network, Inc.
Porth, C. M., & Matfin, G. (2009). *Pathophysiology: Concepts of altered health states* (8th ed.). Philadelphia: Lippincott Williams & Wilkins.
World Health Organization. (2011). *Global tuberculosis control 2011*. Geneva: WHO Press.

Journals and Electronic Documents

Al-Qadi, M. O., Al-Alwan, A., Opal, S. M., et al. (2010). Community acquired pneumonia. *Medicine & Health/Rhode Island*, 93(7), 196–200.

American Association of Critical-Care Nurses. (2012). AACN practice alert: Prevention of aspiration. *AACN Bold Voices, 4*(4), 11–14.

American Cancer Society. (2012b). *Lung cancer overview.* Available at: www.cancer.org/cancer/lungcancer

American College of Chest Physicians. (2012). Antithrombotic therapy and prevention of thrombosis, 9th ed.: American College of Chest Physicians evidence-based clinical practice guidelines. *Chest, 141*(2), 1S–70S.

American Lung Association. (2012). *Occupational lung disease fast fact sheet.* Available at: www.lungusa.org

American Thoracic Society & Infectious Diseases Society of America. (2005). Guidelines for the management of adults with hospital-acquired, ventilator-associated, and healthcare-associated pneumonia. *American Journal of Respiratory and Critical Care Medicine, 171*(4), 388–416.

Ashraf, M., & Ostrosky-Zeichner, L. (2012). Ventilatory-associated pneumonia: A review. *Hospital Practice, 40*(1), 93–105.

Bartlett, J. (2012). Aspiration pneumonia in adults. *UpToDate.* Available at: www.uptodate.com

Basgov, N., Forham von Reyn, C., & Baron, E. (2012). Clinical manifestations of pulmonary tuberculosis. *UpToDate.* Available at: www.uptodate.com

Blot, S., Lisboa, T., Angles, R., et al. (2011). Prevention of VAP: Is zero rate possible? *Clinics in Chest Medicine, 32*(3), 591–599.

Centers for Disease Control and Prevention. (2003). Treatment of tuberculosis. *MMWR Morbidity and Mortality Weekly Report, 52*(RR-11), 1–77.

Centers for Disease Control and Prevention. (2010). Updated guidelines for using interferon gamma release assays to detect Mycobacterium tuberculosis infection—United States, 2010. *MMWR Morbidity and Mortality Weekly Report, 59*(RR-5), 1–13.

Centers for Disease Control and Prevention. (2011). *Pneumococcal polysaccharide vaccine (PPSV): CDC answers your questions.* Available at: www.cdc.gov/vaccines

Centers for Disease Control and Prevention. (2012a). *Accidents or unintentional injuries.* Available at: www.cdc.gov/nchs/FASTATS/acc-inj.htm

Centers for Disease Control and Prevention. (2012b). *Pneumonia.* Available at www.cdc.gov/features/pneumonia

Centers for Disease Control and Prevention. (2012c). *TB fact sheet-infection control and prevention.* Available at www.cdc.gov/tb/publications/factsheets/default.htm.

Centers for Disease Control and Prevention. (2012d). *Tuberculosis (TB): Data and statistics.* Available at: www.cdc.gov/tb/statistics/default.htm

Centers for Disease and Prevention. (2013). *Severe acute respiratory syndrome (SARS).* Last updated April 15, 2013. Available at www.cdc.gov/sars/index/html

Dushianthan, A., Grott, M., Postle A., et al. (2011). Acute respiratory distress syndrome and acute lung injury. *Postgraduate Medicine Journal, 87*(1031), 612–622.

Fedullo, P. (2012). Placement of inferior vena cava filters and their complications. *UpToDate.* Last updated June 21, 2012. Available at: www.uptodate.com

File, T. (2012). Risk factors and prevention of hospital-acquired, ventilator-associated and healthcare-associated pneumonia in adults. *UpToDate.* Last updated June 26, 2012. Available at: www.uptodate.com

Goldhaber, S., & Bounameaux, H. (2012). Pulmonary embolism and deep vein thrombosis. *Lancet, 379*(9828), 1835–1846.

Gore, E., Movsas. B., Santana-Davila, R., et al. (2012). Evaluation and management of elderly patients with lung cancer. *Seminars in Radiation Oncology, 22*(4), 304–310.

Hopkins, W., & Rubin, L. (2012). Treatment of pulmonary hypertension in adults. *UpToDate.* Last updated August 16, 2012. Available at: www.uptodate.com

Johnson, M., & Conde, M. (2012). Overview of the management of postoperative pulmonary complications. *UpToDate.* Last updated September 14, 2012. Available at: www.uptodate.com

Kaewlai, R., Avery, L., Asrani, A., et al. (2008). Multidetector CT of blunt thoracic trauma. *RadioGraphics: The Journal of CME in Radiology, 28*(6), 1555–1570.

King, T. (2011). Clinical manifestations and diagnosis of sarcoidosis. *UpToDate.* Last updated April 18, 2011. Available at: www.uptodate.com

Kollef, M. (2012). Prevention of ventilator-associated pneumonia or ventilator-associated complications: A worthy, yet challenging goal. *Critical Care Medicine, 40*(1), 271–277.

Kothe, H., Bauer, T., Marre, R., et al. (2008). Competence Network for Community-Acquired Pneumonia Study Group: Outcome of community acquired pneumonia: Influence of age, residence status and antimicrobial. *European Respiratory Journal, 32*(1), 139–146.

Lababede, O., Meziane, M., & Rice, T. (2011). Seventh edition of the cancer staging manual and stage grouping of lung cancer. *Chest, 139*(1), 183–189.

*Lamar, J. (2012). Relationship of respiratory care bundle with incentive spirometry to reduced pulmonary complications in a medical general practice unit. *MEDSURG Nursing, 21*(1), 33–36.

Liu, C., Bayer, A., Cosgrove, S., et al. (2011). Clinical practice guidelines by the Infectious Diseases Society of America for the treatment of methicillin-resistant Staphylococcus aureus infections in adults and children. *Clinical Infectious Diseases, 52*(1), 1–38.

London, S. (2011). Less therapy may be better in pulmonary sarcoidosis. *Chest Physician, 6*(2), 13.

Mancini, M. (2012). Blunt chest trauma. *Medscape.* Updated January 10, 2012. Available at: www.medscape.com/article/428723-overview

Merrill, W. (2012). Radiation-induced lung injury. *UpToDate.* Last updated August 3, 2012. Available at: www.uptodate.com

Morgenthau, A., & Iannuzzi, M. (2011). Recent advances in sarcoidosis. *Chest, 139*(1), 174–182.

Mosby's Nursing Consult. (2012). *Mosby's skills: Peripheral nerve stimulator.* Available password-protected at: mns.elsevierperformancemanager.com/NursingSkills

Muller, N. (2012). Evaluation of mediastinal mass. *UpToDate.* Last updated January 6, 2012. Available at: www.uptodate.com

Murphy, S., Jiaquan, X., & Kochanek, K. D. (2012). Deaths: Preliminary data for 2010. *National Vital Statistics Reports, 60*(4).

National Cancer Institute. (2012). *Small cell lung cancer treatment (PDQ®).* Available at: www.cancer.gov/cancertopics/pdq/treatment/small-cell-lung

Niederman, M. (2011). Preface: Respiratory tract infections: Advances in diagnosis, management and prevention. *Clinics in Chest Medicine, 32*(3), xiii–xiv.

Rubin, L., & Hopkins, W. (2012). Clinical features and diagnosis of pulmonary hypertension in adults. *UpToDate.* Last updated September 11, 2012. Available at: www.uptodate.com

Shahani, R. (2011). Penetrating chest trauma treatment and management. *Medscape.* Updated May 12, 2011. Available at: www.medscape.com/article/425698-treatment

Shigemitsu, H., & Zauma, A. (2011). Sarcoidosis and interstitial pulmonary fibrosis: Two distinct disorders or two ends of the same spectrum. *Current Opinion in Pulmonary Medicine, 17*(5), 303–307.

Siegel, H. (2010). Analytic reviews: Managing the agitated patient in the ICU: Sedation, analgesia, and neuromuscular blockade. *Journal of Intensive Care Medicine, 25*(4), 187–204.

Simonneau, G., Robbins, I., Beghetti, M., et al. (2009). Updated clinical classification of pulmonary hypertension. *Journal of the American College of Cardiology, 54*(1 Suppl.), S43–S54.

Smith, T. J., Temin, S., Alesi, E. R., et al. (2012). American Society of Clinical Oncology provisional clinical opinion: The integration of palliative care into standard oncology care. *Journal of Clinical Oncology, 30*(8), 880–887.

Stamm, J. (2012). Risk stratification for acute pulmonary embolism. *Critical Care Clinics, 28*(2), 305–321.

Stark, P. (2012). Atelectasis: Types and pathogenesis in adults. *UpToDate.* Last updated March 27, 2012. Available at: www.uptodate.com

Tapson, V. (2012). Treatment of acute pulmonary embolism. *UpToDate.* Last updated April 3, 2012. Available at: www.uptodate.com

Wendling, P. (2011). Rib fixation in flail chest may shorten ventilation. *Chest Physician, 6*(3), 10.

Wunderink, R., & Niederman, M. (2012). Update in respiratory infections 2011. *American Journal of Respiratory and Critical Care Medicine, 185*(12), 1261–1265.

Resources

Agency for Healthcare Quality and Research (AHRQ), www.ahrq.gov
American Association for Respiratory Care (AARC), www.aarc.org
American Cancer Society, www.cancer.org
American College of Chest Physicians, www.chestnet.org
American Lung Association, www.lungusa.org
American Thoracic Society (ATS), www.thoracic.org
Centers for Disease Control and Prevention (CDC), www.cdc.gov; www.cdc.gov/ncidod/sars
National Cancer Institute (NCI), www.cancer.gov
National Heart, Lung, and Blood Institute (NHLBI), www.nhlbi.nih.gov
Occupational Safety and Health Administration (OSHA), www.osha.gov
Pulmonary Hypertension Association (PHA), www.phassociation.org
Respiratory Nursing Society (RNS), www.respiratorynursingsociety.org

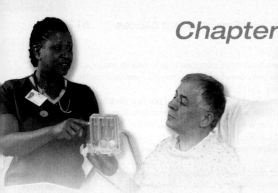

Chapter

24

Management of Patients With Chronic Pulmonary Disease

Learning Objectives

On completion of this chapter, the learner will be able to:

1 Describe the pathophysiology of chronic obstructive pulmonary disease (COPD).
2 Discuss the major risk factors for developing COPD and nursing interventions to minimize or prevent these risk factors.
3 Use the nursing process as a framework for care of patients with COPD.

4 Develop an education plan for patients with COPD.
5 Describe the pathophysiology of bronchiectasis and relate it to signs and symptoms of bronchiectasis.
6 Identify medical and nursing management of bronchiectasis.
7 Describe the pathophysiology of asthma.
8 Discuss the medications used in asthma management.
9 Describe asthma self-management strategies.
10 Describe the pathophysiology of cystic fibrosis.

Glossary

air trapping: incomplete emptying of alveoli during expiration due to loss of lung tissue elasticity (emphysema), bronchospasm (asthma), or airway obstruction

alpha$_1$-antitrypsin deficiency: genetic disorder resulting from deficiency of alpha$_1$-antitrypsin, a protective agent for the lung; increases patient's risk for developing panacinar emphysema even in the absence of smoking

asthma: a disease with multiple precipitating mechanisms resulting in a common clinical outcome of reversible airflow obstruction

bronchiectasis: chronic, irreversible dilation of the bronchi and bronchioles that results from destruction of muscles and elastic connective tissue; dilated airways become saccular and are a medium for chronic infection

chronic bronchitis: a disease of the airways defined as the presence of cough and sputum production for at least a combined total of 3 months in each of 2 consecutive years

chronic obstructive pulmonary disease: disease state characterized by airflow limitation that is not fully reversible;

sometimes referred to as chronic airway obstruction or chronic obstructive lung disease

desaturate: a precipitous drop in the saturation of hemoglobin with oxygen

emphysema: a disease of the airways characterized by destruction of the walls of overdistended alveoli

metered-dose inhaler: patient-activated medication canister that provides aerosolized medication that the patient inhales into the lungs

polycythemia: increase in the red blood cell concentration in the blood; in COPD, the body attempts to improve oxygen carrying capacity by producing increasing amounts of red blood cells

spirometry: pulmonary function tests that measure specific lung volumes (e.g., FEV$_1$, FVC) and rates (FEF$_{25-75\%}$); may be measured before and after bronchodilator administration

---

Chronic pulmonary disorders are a leading cause of morbidity and mortality in the United States. Nurses care for patients with chronic pulmonary disease across the spectrum of care, from outpatient and home care to emergency department (ED), critical care, and hospice settings. To care for these patients, nurses not only need to have astute assessment and clinical management skills, but they also need knowledge of how these disorders can affect quality of life. In addition, the nurse's knowledge of palliative and end-of-life care is important for applicable patients. Patient and family education is an important nursing intervention to enhance self-management in patients with any chronic pulmonary disorder.

Chronic Obstructive Pulmonary Disease

Chronic obstructive pulmonary disease (COPD) is a preventable and treatable slowly progressive respiratory disease of airflow obstruction involving the airways, pulmonary parenchyma, or both (Global Initiative for Chronic Obstructive Lung Disease [GOLD], 2010; Qaseem, Wilt, Weinberger, et al., 2011). The parenchyma includes any form of lung tissue, including bronchioles, bronchi, blood vessels, interstitium, and alveoli. The airflow limitation or obstruction in COPD is not fully reversible. Most patients with COPD present with

618

overlapping signs and symptoms of emphysema and chronic bronchitis, which are two distinct disease processes.

COPD may include diseases that cause airflow obstruction (e.g., emphysema, chronic bronchitis) or any combination of these disorders. Other diseases such as cystic fibrosis (CF), bronchiectasis, and asthma are classified as chronic pulmonary disorders. Asthma is considered a distinct, separate disorder and is classified as an abnormal airway condition characterized primarily by reversible inflammation. COPD can coexist with asthma. Both of these diseases have the same major symptoms; however, symptoms are generally more variable in asthma than in COPD. This chapter discusses COPD as a disease and describes chronic bronchitis and emphysema as distinct disease states, providing a foundation for understanding the pathophysiology of COPD. Bronchiectasis, asthma, and CF are discussed separately.

In 2011, COPD and associated respiratory diseases were estimated to affect 24 million adults and was the third leading cause of death in the United States (National Heart, Lung, and Blood Institute [NHLBI], 2011). Whereas mortality from other major causes of death has been decreasing, deaths from COPD have continued to rise. COPD affects more than 5% of the adult population in the United States. An estimated 27 million adults have COPD, including 14 million diagnosed and more than 12 million undiagnosed adults (NHLBI, 2010). Mortality from COPD among women has dramatically increased since World War II; since 2005, more women than men died of COPD. From 1999 through 2007, COPD hospitalization rates declined for both men and women, but COPD death rates declined only for men (Akinbami & Liu, 2011). The annual direct cost of COPD, asthma, and pneumonia was $66 billion in 2010, with indirect costs of $19 billion (NHLBI, 2010).

Pathophysiology

People with COPD commonly become symptomatic during the middle adult years, and the incidence of the disease increases with age. Although certain aspects of lung function normally decrease with age—for example, vital capacity and forced expiratory volume in 1 second (FEV_1)—COPD accentuates and accelerates these physiologic changes as described later. In COPD, the airflow limitation is both progressive and associated with the lungs' abnormal inflammatory response to noxious particles or gases. The inflammatory response occurs throughout the proximal and peripheral airways, lung parenchyma, and pulmonary vasculature (GOLD, 2010). Because of the chronic inflammation and the body's attempts to repair it, changes and narrowing occur in the airways. In the proximal airways (trachea and bronchi greater than 2 mm in diameter), changes include increased numbers of goblet cells and enlarged submucosal glands, both of which lead to hypersecretion of mucus. In the peripheral airways (bronchioles less than 2 mm diameter), inflammation causes thickening of the airway wall, peribronchial fibrosis, exudate in the airway, and overall airway narrowing (obstructive bronchiolitis). Over time, this ongoing injury-and-repair process causes scar tissue formation and narrowing of the airway lumen (GOLD, 2010). Inflammatory and structural changes also occur in the lung parenchyma (respiratory bronchioles and alveoli). Alveolar wall destruction leads to loss of alveolar attachments and a decrease in elastic recoil. Finally, the chronic inflammatory process affects the pulmonary vasculature and causes thickening of the lining of the vessel and hypertrophy of smooth muscle, which may lead to pulmonary hypertension (GOLD, 2010).

Processes related to imbalances of substances (proteinases and antiproteinases) in the lung may also contribute to airflow limitation. When activated by chronic inflammation, proteinases and other substances may be released, damaging the parenchyma of the lung. These parenchymal changes may also occur as a consequence of inflammation or environmental or genetic factors (e.g., alpha$_1$-antitrypsin deficiency).

Chronic Bronchitis

Chronic bronchitis, a disease of the airways, is defined as the presence of cough and sputum production for at least 3 months in each of 2 consecutive years. Although *chronic bronchitis* is a clinically and epidemiologically useful term, it does not reflect the major impact of airflow limitation on morbidity and mortality in COPD (GOLD, 2010). In many cases, smoke or other environmental pollutants irritate the airways, resulting in inflammation and hypersecretion of mucus. Constant irritation causes the mucus-secreting glands and goblet cells to increase in number, leading to increased mucus production. Mucus plugging of the airway reduces ciliary function. Bronchial walls also become thickened, further narrowing the bronchial lumen (Fig. 24-1). Alveoli adjacent to the bronchioles may become damaged and fibrosed, resulting in altered function of the alveolar macrophages. This is significant because the macrophages play an important role in destroying foreign particles, including bacteria. As a result, the patient becomes more susceptible to respiratory infection. A wide range of viral, bacterial, and mycoplasmal infections can produce acute episodes of bronchitis. Exacerbations of chronic bronchitis are most likely to occur during the winter when viral and bacterial infections are more prevalent.

Emphysema

In **emphysema**, impaired oxygen and carbon dioxide exchange results from destruction of the walls of overdistended alveoli. *Emphysema* is a pathologic term that describes an abnormal distention of the airspaces beyond the terminal bronchioles and destruction of the walls of the alveoli (GOLD, 2010). In addition, a chronic inflammatory response may induce disruption of the parenchymal tissues. This end-stage process progresses slowly for many years. As the walls of the alveoli are destroyed (a process accelerated by recurrent infections), the alveolar surface area in direct contact with the pulmonary capillaries continually decreases. This causes an increase in dead space (lung area where no gas exchange can occur) and impaired oxygen diffusion, which leads to hypoxemia. In the later stages of disease, carbon dioxide elimination is impaired, resulting in increased carbon dioxide tension in arterial blood (hypercapnia) leading to respiratory acidosis. As the alveolar walls continue to break down, the pulmonary capillary bed is reduced in size. Consequently, resistance to pulmonary blood flow is increased, forcing the right ventricle to maintain a higher blood pressure in the pulmonary artery. Hypoxemia may further increase pulmonary artery pressures (pulmonary hypertension). Cor pulmonale, one of the complications of emphysema, is right-sided heart failure brought on by long-term high blood pressure in the pulmonary arteries. This high pressure in the pulmonary arteries and right ventricle lead to

NORMAL BRONCHUS   CHRONIC BRONCHITIS

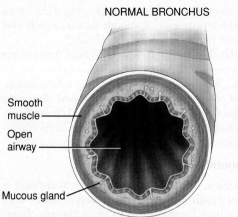

Smooth muscle

Open airway

Mucous gland

Inflammation

Increased number of mucous glands

Excess mucus causing chronic cough

FIGURE 24-1 • Pathophysiology of chronic bronchitis as compared to a normal bronchus. The bronchus in chronic bronchitis is narrowed and has impaired airflow due to multiple mechanisms: inflammation, excess mucus production, and potential smooth muscle constriction (bronchospasm).

back up of blood in the venous system, resulting in dependent edema, distended neck veins, or pain in the region of the liver (see Chapter 29 for further discussion).

There are two main types of emphysema, based on the changes taking place in the lung (Fig. 24-2). Both types may occur in the same patient. In the panlobular (panacinar) type of emphysema, there is destruction of the respiratory bronchiole, alveolar duct, and alveolus. All airspaces within the lobule are essentially enlarged, but there is little inflammatory disease. A hyperinflated (hyperexpanded) chest, marked dyspnea on exertion, and weight loss typically occur. To move air into and out of the lungs, negative pressure is required during inspiration, and an adequate level of positive pressure must be attained and maintained during expiration. Instead of being an involuntary passive act, expiration becomes active and requires muscular effort.

In the centrilobular (centroacinar) form, pathologic changes take place mainly in the center of the secondary lobule, preserving the peripheral portions of the acinus (i.e., the terminal airway unit where gas exchange occurs). Frequently,

there is a derangement of ventilation–perfusion ratios, producing chronic hypoxemia, hypercapnia, **polycythemia** (i.e., an increase in red blood cells), and episodes of right-sided heart failure. This leads to central cyanosis and respiratory failure. The patient also develops peripheral edema.

Risk Factors

Risk factors for COPD include environmental exposures and host factors (Chart 24-1). The most important environmental risk factor for COPD worldwide is cigarette smoking. A dose–response relationship exists between the intensity of smoking (pack-year history) and the decline in pulmonary function. Other environmental risk factors include smoking pipes, cigars, and other types of tobacco. Passive smoking (i.e., secondhand smoke) also contributes to respiratory symptoms and COPD (GOLD, 2010). Smoking depresses the activity of scavenger cells and affects the respiratory tract's ciliary cleansing mechanism, which keeps breathing passages free of inhaled irritants, bacteria, and other foreign matter. When smoking damages this cleansing mechanism, airflow is obstructed and air becomes trapped behind the obstruction. The alveoli greatly distend, which diminishes lung capacity. Smoking also irritates the goblet cells and mucous glands, causing an increased accumulation of mucus, which in turn produces more irritation, infection, and damage to the lung (U.S. Department of Health and Human Services [HHS], 2010a). In addition, carbon monoxide (a by-product of smoking) combines with hemoglobin to form carboxyhemoglobin. Hemoglobin that is bound by carboxyhemoglobin

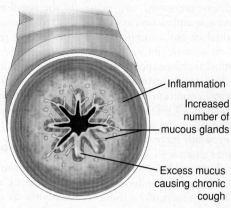

Panlobular emphysema (PLE)

Normal

Centrilobular emphysema (CLE)

FIGURE 24-2 • Changes in alveolar structure in centrilobular and panlobular emphysema. In panlobular emphysema, the bronchioles, alveolar ducts, and alveoli are destroyed, and the airspaces within the lobule are enlarged. In centrilobular emphysema, the pathologic changes occur in the lobule, whereas the peripheral portions of the acinus are preserved.

Chart 24-1 ⚠	**RISK FACTORS**
	Chronic Obstructive Pulmonary Disease

- Exposure to tobacco smoke accounts for an estimated 80%–90% of cases of chronic obstructive pulmonary disease
- Passive smoking (i.e., secondhand smoke)
- Increased age
- Occupational exposure—dust, chemicals
- Indoor and outdoor air pollution
- Genetic abnormalities, including a deficiency of alpha$_1$-antitrypsin, an enzyme inhibitor that normally counteracts the destruction of lung tissue by certain other enzymes

Adapted from Global Initiative for Chronic Obstructive Pulmonary Disease. (2011). *Global strategy for the diagnosis, management and prevention of COPD.* Available at: www.goldcopd.org

cannot carry oxygen efficiently. Other environmental risk factors for COPD include prolonged and intense exposure to occupational dusts and chemicals, indoor air pollution (e.g., using biomass stoves for cooking, heating in poorly ventilated dwellings), and outdoor air pollution (GOLD, 2010).

Host risk factors include a person's genetic makeup. One well-documented genetic risk factor is a deficiency of alpha$_1$-antitrypsin, an enzyme inhibitor that protects the lung parenchyma from injury. Of patients with COPD, 1% to 2% are found to have severe alpha$_1$-antitrypsin deficiency (Loscalzo, 2010). This deficiency predisposes young people to rapid development of lobular emphysema, even in the absence of smoking. Among Caucasians, **alpha$_1$-antitrypsin deficiency** is one of the most common genetically linked lethal diseases. COPD may also result from gene–environment interactions (GOLD, 2010). Genetically susceptible people are sensitive to environmental factors (e.g., smoking, air pollution, infectious agents, and allergens) and eventually develop chronic obstructive symptoms. Carriers must be identified so that they can modify environmental risk factors to delay or prevent overt symptoms of disease. Genetic counseling should be offered. Alpha-protease inhibitor replacement therapy, which slows the progression of the disease, is available for patients with this genetic defect and for those with severe disease. However, this infusion therapy is costly and is required on an ongoing basis.

Other genetic risk factors may predispose a patient to COPD. Work is ongoing to identify specific variants of genes hypothesized to be involved in the development of COPD. These may include specific phenotypes to several chromosomal regions in families with multiple members developing early-onset COPD.

Clinical Manifestations

Although the natural history of COPD is variable, it is generally a progressive disease characterized by three primary symptoms: chronic cough, sputum production, and dyspnea (GOLD, 2010). These symptoms often worsen over time. Chronic cough and sputum production often precede the development of airflow limitation by many years. However, not all people with cough and sputum production develop COPD. The cough may be intermittent and may be unproductive in some patients (GOLD, 2010). Dyspnea may be severe and interfere with the patient's activities. It is usually progressive, is worse with exercise, and is persistent. As COPD progresses, dyspnea may occur at rest. Weight loss is common, because dyspnea interferes with eating and the work of breathing is energy depleting. As the work of breathing increases over time, the accessory muscles are recruited in an effort to breathe. Patients with COPD are at risk for respiratory insufficiency and respiratory infections, which in turn increase the risk of acute and chronic respiratory failure.

In patients with COPD who have a primary emphysematous component, chronic hyperinflation leads to the "barrel chest" thorax configuration. This configuration results from a more fixed position of the ribs in the inspiratory position (due to hyperinflation) and from loss of lung elasticity (Fig. 24-3). Retraction of the supraclavicular fossae occurs on inspiration, causing the shoulders to heave upward (Fig. 24-4). In advanced emphysema, the abdominal muscles may also contract on inspiration.

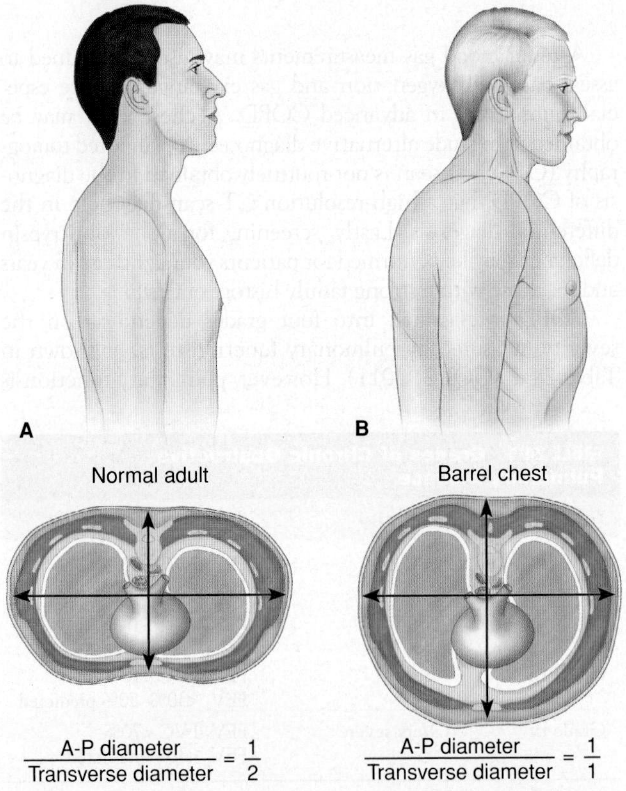

A

B

Normal adult

Barrel chest

$$\frac{\text{A-P diameter}}{\text{Transverse diameter}} = \frac{1}{2}$$

$$\frac{\text{A-P diameter}}{\text{Transverse diameter}} = \frac{1}{1}$$

FIGURE 24-3 • Characteristics of normal chest wall and chest wall in emphysema. **A.** The normal chest wall and its cross-section. **B.** The barrel-shaped chest of emphysema and its cross-section.

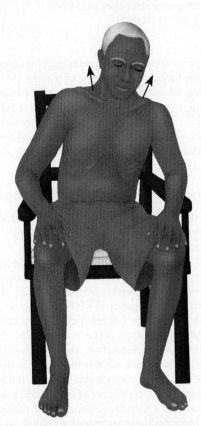

FIGURE 24-4 • Typical posture of a person with chronic obstructive pulmonary disease—primarily emphysema. The person tends to lean forward and uses the accessory muscles of respiration to breathe, forcing the shoulder girdle upward and causing the supraclavicular fossae to retract on inspiration.

ASSESSMENT

Chart 24-2

Assessing Patients With Chronic Obstructive Pulmonary Disease

Health History

- Has the patient been exposed to risk factors (types, intensity, duration)?
- Does the patient have a past medical history of respiratory diseases/problems, including asthma, allergy, sinusitis, nasal polyps, or respiratory infections?
- Does the patient have a family history of chronic obstructive pulmonary disease or other chronic respiratory diseases?
- How long has the patient had respiratory difficulty?
- What is the pattern of symptom development?
- Does exertion increase the dyspnea? What type of exertion?
- What are the limits of the patient's tolerance for exercise?
- At what times during the day does the patient complain most of fatigue and shortness of breath?
- Does the patient describe any discomfort or pain in any part of the body? If so, where does it occur, how intense is this pain, when does it occur, and does it interfere with activities of daily living? Is there any intervention that helps to alleviate the pain or discomfort?
- Which eating and sleeping habits have been affected?
- What is the impact of respiratory disease on quality of life?
- What does the patient know about the disease and his or her condition?
- What is the patient's smoking history (primary and secondary)?
- Is there occupational exposure to smoke or other pollutants?
- What are the triggering events (e.g., exertion, strong odors, dust, exposure to animals)?
- Does the patient have a history of exacerbations or previous hospitalizations for respiratory problems?
- Are comorbidities present?

- How appropriate are current medical treatments?
- Does the patient have available social and family support?
- What is the potential for reducing risk factors (e.g., smoking cessation)?

Physical Assessment

- What position does the patient assume during the interview?
- What are the pulse and the respiratory rates?
- What is the character of respirations? Even and without effort? Other?
- Can the patient complete a sentence without having to take a breath?
- Does the patient contract the abdominal muscles during inspiration?
- Does the patient use accessory muscles of the shoulders and neck when breathing?
- Does the patient take a long time to exhale (prolonged expiration)?
- Is central cyanosis evident?
- Are the patient's neck veins engorged?
- Does the patient have peripheral edema?
- Is the patient coughing?
- What are the color, amount, and consistency of the sputum?
- Is clubbing of the fingers present?
- What types of breath sounds (i.e., clear, diminished or distant, crackles, wheezes) are heard? Describe and document findings and locations.
- Are there any sensory deficits?
- Is there short- or long-term memory impairment?
- Is there increasing stupor?
- Is the patient apprehensive?

There are systemic or extrapulmonary manifestations of COPD. These include musculoskeletal wasting (see Chapter 5 for discussion of nutrition assessment and Chapter 45 for discussion of nutrition therapy), metabolic syndrome (see Chapter 27), and depression (a frequent comorbidity that accompanies chronic debilitating illnesses). These clinical manifestations beyond the lungs must also be assessed and treated (Nussbaumer-Ochsner & Rabe, 2011).

Assessment and Diagnostic Findings

The nurse obtains a thorough health history from patients with known or potential COPD. Chart 24-2 lists the key factors to assess. Pulmonary function studies are used to help confirm the diagnosis of COPD, determine disease severity, and monitor disease progression. **Spirometry** is used to evaluate airflow obstruction, which is determined by the ratio of FEV_1 to forced vital capacity (FVC). Spirometric results are expressed as an absolute volume and as a percentage of the predicted value using appropriate normal values for gender, age, and height. With obstruction, the patient either has difficulty exhaling or cannot forcibly exhale air from the lungs, reducing the FEV_1. Spirometry is also used to determine reversibility of obstruction after the use of bronchodilators (GOLD, 2010). Spirometry is initially performed, the patient is given an inhaled bronchodilator treatment according to a standard protocol, and then spirometry is repeated. The patient demonstrates a degree of reversibility if the pulmonary function values improve after administration of the bronchodilator.

Arterial blood gas measurements may also be obtained to assess baseline oxygenation and gas exchange and are especially important in advanced COPD. A chest x-ray may be obtained to exclude alternative diagnoses. A computed tomography (CT) chest scan is not routinely obtained in the diagnosis of COPD, but a high-resolution CT scan may help in the differential diagnosis. Lastly, screening for alpha$_1$-antitrypsin deficiency may be performed for patients younger than 45 years and for those with a strong family history of COPD.

COPD is classified into four grades depending on the severity measured by pulmonary function tests, as shown in Table 24-1 (GOLD, 2011). However, pulmonary function is

TABLE 24-1 Grades of Chronic Obstructive Pulmonary Disease

Grade	Severity	Pulmonary Function
Grade I	Mild	FEV_1/FVC <70% FEV_1 ≥80% predicted
Grade II	Moderate	FEV_1/FVC <70% FEV_1 50%–80% predicted
Grade III	Severe	FEV_1/FVC <70% FEV_1 <30%–50% predicted
Grade IV	Very severe	FEV_1/FVC <70% FEV_1 <30% predicted

FEV_1, forced expiratory volume in 1 second; FVC, forced vital capacity.
Adapted from Global Initiative for Chronic Obstructive Pulmonary Disease. (2011). *Global strategy for the diagnosis, management and prevention of COPD*. Available at: www.goldcopd.org

NURSING RESEARCH PROFILE

Chart 24-3 Pain and Quality of Life With Chronic Obstructive Pulmonary Disease

Borge, C. R., Wahl, A. K., & Moum, T. (2011). Pain and quality of life with chronic obstructive pulmonary disease. *Heart and Lung, 40*(3), e90–e101.

Purpose

The purpose of this study was to explore the prevalence and intensity of pain, its location, and how demographic and clinical variables may be related to pain in patients with COPD. In addition, the association of pain and quality of life (QOL) was explored.

Design

This descriptive study was based on data from a cross-sectional study investigating symptoms of depression, anxiety, fatigue, sleep quality, pain, QOL, and self-efficacy in patients with COPD. The investigators identified a potential 502 patients with COPD at a clinic. Of these, 387 patients with all stages of COPD were recruited via mail for the study, and 168 accepted the invitation. Fourteen participants were eventually dropped from the study because they did not return questionnaires, missed appointments, or withdrew from the study. The final sample of 154 participants was equally distributed by gender, and the mean age was 64.6 years. The subjects were asked to perform spirometry and complete three questionnaires (Brief Pain Inventory, Respiratory Quality of Life Questionnaire [disease specific], and Quality of Life Scale [global]).

Findings

A total of 111, or 72%, of participants shaded the location of pain on an outline body diagram. Pain was most frequently reported in the shoulder, followed by lumbar region, legs, back, chest, neck, thighs, and head. Based on pain intensity and interference scores (anchors of "0" and "10," with "10" representing highest pain score), the mean pain intensity score was 3.7 (standard deviation [SD] = 1.9) with a range of 0.25 to 8.8, whereas the mean pain interference score was 3.9 (SD = 2.3) with a range of 0 to 9.1. The top five pain interference items included interference with the following during the past 24 hours: normal work, walking ability, general activity, relationships to other people, and sleep. Comorbidities, pain intensity, and pain interference were positively and significantly related to disease-specific QOL. Using hierarchic multiple regression analysis with 12 variables (age, gender, smoking, living alone, education, duration of COPD, comorbidity, body mass index, lung function, pain intensity, pain interference, disease-specific QOL), there was a strong direct effect ($P < .001$) of disease-specific QOL on global QOL. This model explained 24% of the variance in global QOL.

Nursing Implications

Pain as a symptom in the patient with COPD has received little attention. The nurse should assess pain in the inpatient and outpatient setting by identifying its location and intensity, and ascertaining how it interferes with the patient's activities of daily living. A focus on relieving pain (both nonpharmacologic and pharmacologic mechanisms) may help to reduce breathlessness and anxiety, improve mobility, and impact the patient's disease-specific QOL. Further research is needed to improve our knowledge and treatment of pain in patients with COPD.

---

not the only way to assess or classify COPD; pulmonary function is evaluated in conjunction with symptoms, health status impairment with COPD, and the potential for exacerbations. Factors that determine the clinical course and survival of patients with COPD include history of cigarette smoking, passive smoking exposure, age, rate of decline of FEV_1, hypoxemia, pulmonary artery pressure, resting heart rate, weight loss, reversibility of airflow obstruction, and comorbidities. See Chart 24-3 regarding pain and quality of life with COPD.

In diagnosing COPD, several differential diagnoses must be ruled out. The primary differential diagnosis is asthma. It may be difficult to differentiate between a patient with COPD and one with chronic asthma. Other diseases that must be considered in the differential diagnosis include heart failure, bronchiectasis, tuberculosis, obliterative bronchiolitis, and diffuse panbronchiolitis (GOLD, 2010). Key factors in determining the diagnosis are the patient's history and responsiveness to bronchodilators.

Complications

Respiratory insufficiency and failure are major life-threatening complications of COPD. The acuity of the onset and the severity of respiratory failure depend on baseline pulmonary function, pulse oximetry or arterial blood gas values, comorbid conditions, and the severity of other complications of COPD. Respiratory insufficiency and failure may be chronic (with severe COPD) or acute (with severe bronchospasm or pneumonia in a patient with severe COPD). Acute respiratory insufficiency and failure may necessitate ventilatory support until other acute complications, such as infection, can be treated. (See Chapter 21 for management of the patient requiring ventilatory support.) Other complications of COPD include pneumonia, chronic atelectasis, pneumothorax, and pulmonary arterial hypertension (cor pulmonale).

Medical Management

Risk Reduction

For patients with stable disease, treatment aims to reduce risk and symptoms. Approximately 8 million people in the United States have chronic illnesses related to smoking; this costs the nation $193 billion in health care expenses and lost productivity each year (HHS, 2010a). Smoking cessation is the single most cost-effective intervention to reduce the risk of developing COPD and to stop its progression (GOLD, 2010; HHS, 2010b). However, smoking cessation is difficult to achieve and even more difficult to sustain in the long term. Nurses are key in promoting smoking cessation and educating patients about its importance. Patients diagnosed with COPD who continue to smoke must be encouraged and assisted to quit. Factors associated with continued smoking vary among patients and may include the strength of the nicotine addiction, continued exposure to smoking-associated stimuli (at work or in social settings), stress, depression, and habit.

Because multiple factors are associated with continued smoking, successful cessation often requires multiple strategies.

Health care providers should promote cessation by explaining the risks of smoking and personalizing the "at-risk" message to the patient. After giving a strong warning about smoking, health care providers should work with the patient to set a definite "quit date." Referral to a smoking cessation program may be helpful. Follow-up within 3 to 5 days after the quit date to review progress and to address any problems is associated with an increased rate of success; this should be repeated as needed. Continued reinforcement with a modality that is individualized to the patient and his or her lifestyle (e.g., telephone calls, texting, e-mail or clinic visits) is beneficial. Relapses should be analyzed, and the patient and health care provider should jointly identify possible solutions to prevent future backsliding. It is important to emphasize successes rather than failures. Nicotine replacement—a first-line pharmacotherapy that reliably increases long-term smoking abstinence rates—comes in a variety of forms (gum, inhaler, nasal spray, transdermal patch, sublingual tablet, or lozenge). Bupropion SR (Wellbutrin, Zyban) and nortriptyline (Aventyl), both antidepressants, may also increase long-term quit rates. Other pharmacologic agents include the antihypertensive agent clonidine (Catapres); however, its side effects limit its use. Varenicline (Chantix), a nicotinic acetylcholine receptor partial agonist, may assist in smoking cessation (GOLD, 2010). Patients who are not appropriate candidates for such pharmacotherapy include those with medical contraindications, light smokers (fewer than 10 cigarettes per day), pregnant women, and adolescent smokers.

Smoking cessation can begin in a variety of health care settings—outpatient clinic, nursing center, pulmonary rehabilitation center, community, hospital, and in the home. Regardless of the setting, nurses have the opportunity to educate patients about the risks of smoking and the benefits of smoking cessation. Various materials, resources, and programs developed by several organizations (e.g., Agency for Healthcare Research and Quality, Centers for Disease Control and Prevention [CDC], National Cancer Institute, American Lung Association, American Cancer Society) are available to assist with this effort.

Pharmacologic Therapy

Bronchodilators

Bronchodilators relieve bronchospasm by altering smooth muscle tone and reduce airway obstruction by allowing increased oxygen distribution throughout the lungs and improving alveolar ventilation. Although regular use of bronchodilators that act primarily on the airway smooth muscle does not modify the decline of function or the prognosis of COPD, their use is central in the management of COPD (GOLD, 2010). These agents can be delivered through a metered-dose inhaler (MDI) or other type of inhaler, by nebulization, or via the oral route in pill or liquid form. Bronchodilators are often administered regularly throughout the day as well as on an as-needed basis. They may also be used prophylactically to prevent breathlessness by having the patient

TABLE 24-2	Aerosol Delivery Devices	
Devices/Drugs	**Optimal Technique**	**Therapeutic Issues**
Metered-dose inhaler (MDI) Beta$_2$-agonists Corticosteroids Cromolyn sodium Anticholinergics	Actuation* during a slow (30 L/min or 3–5 s) deep inhalation, followed by 10-s breathhold	Slow inhalation and coordination of actuation may be difficult for some patients. Patients may incorrectly stop inhalation at actuation. Deposition of 50%–80% of actuated dose in the oropharynx. Mouth washing and spitting is effective in reducing the amount of drug swallowed and absorbed systemically.
Breath-actuated MDI Beta$_2$-agonists	Tight seal around mouthpiece and slightly more rapid inhalation than standard MDI (see above) followed by 10-s breathhold	May be particularly useful for patients unable to coordinate inhalation and actuation. May also be useful for older patients. Patients may incorrectly stop inhalation at actuation. Cannot be used with currently available spacer/valved-holding chamber (VHC) devices.
Dry powder inhaler Beta$_2$-agonists Corticosteroids Anticholinergics	Rapid (1–2 s) deep inhalation. Minimally effective inspiratory flow is device dependent.	Dose is lost if patient exhales through device after actuating. Delivery may be greater or lesser than MDIs, depending on device and technique. Delivery is more flow dependent in devices with highest internal resistance. Rapid inhalation promotes greater deposition in larger central airways. Mouth washing and spitting are effective in reducing amount of drug swallowed and absorbed systemically.
Spacer or VHC	Slow (30 L/min or 3–5 s) deep inhalation, followed by 10-s breathhold immediately following actuation. Actuate only once into spacer/VHC per inhalation. Rinse plastic VHCs once a month with low concentration of liquid household dishwashing detergent (1:5,000 or 1–2 drops per cup of water) and let drip dry.	Indicated for patients who have difficulty performing adequate MDI technique. May be bulky. Simple tubes do not obviate coordinating actuation and inhalation. VHCs are preferred. Spacers or VHCs may increase delivery of inhalational corticosteroids to the lungs.
Nebulizer Beta$_2$-agonists Corticosteroids Cromolyn sodium Anticholinergics	Slow tidal breathing with occasional deep breaths. Tightly fitting facemask for those unable to use mouthpiece.	Less dependent on patient's coordination and cooperation. May be expensive, time consuming, and bulky; output depends on device and operating parameters (fill volume, driving gas flow); internebulizer and intranebulizer output variances are significant. The use of a facemask reduces delivery to lungs by 50%. Choice of delivery system depends on resources, availability, and clinical judgment of clinician caring for patient. There is potential for infections if device is not cleaned properly.

*Actuation refers to release of dose of medication with inhalation.
Adapted from Expert Panel Report 3. (2007). *Guidelines for the diagnosis and management of asthma* (pp. 31–32). NIH Publication No. 08-5846. National Asthma Education and Prevention Program. Summary Report. Bethesda, MD: U.S. Department of Health and Human Services, National Heart, Lung, and Blood Institute.

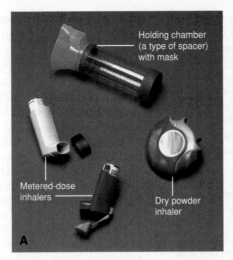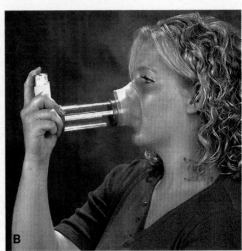

Holding chamber
(a type of spacer)
with mask

Metered-dose
inhalers

Dry powder
inhaler

FIGURE 24-5 • **A.** Examples of metered-dose inhalers and spacers. **B.** A metered-dose inhaler and spacer in use.

use them before participating in or completing an activity, such as eating or walking.

Several devices are available to deliver medication via an aerosolized method. These include MDIs, breath-actuated MDIs, dry powder inhalers, spacer or valved-holding chambers, and nebulizers. Key aspects of each are described in Table 24-2. A **metered-dose inhaler** is a pressurized device that contains an aerosolized powder of medication. A precise amount of medication is released with each activation of the canister. Patients must be instructed in the correct use of the device. A spacer or valved-holding chamber may also be used to enhance deposition of the medication in the lung and help the patient coordinate activation of the MDI with inspiration. Spacers come in several designs, but all are attached to the MDI and have a mouthpiece on the opposite end (Fig. 24-5). Specific package insert information is available for different types of aerosol delivery devices.

Several classes of bronchodilators are used, including beta-adrenergic agonists (short- and long acting), anticholinergic agents (short- and long acting), methylxanthines, and combination agents (GOLD, 2011; Niewoehner, 2010). These medications may be used in combination to optimize bronchodilation. Long-acting B_2-agonist bronchodilators are more convenient for patient use as compared to short-acting B_2-agonist bronchodilators. Examples of these medications are described in Table 24-3. Nebulized medications also known as wet nebulizers (nebulization of medication via an air compressor) may also be effective in patients who cannot use an MDI properly or who prefer this method of administration. However, wet nebulizers are more expensive than other devices and require appropriate cleaning and maintenance (GOLD, 2010).

Bronchodilators are key for symptom management in stable COPD (Qaseem et al., 2011). Before these agents are used, the following information should be considered. Inhaled

TABLE 24-3	**Common Types of Bronchodilator Medications for Chronic Obstructive Pulmonary Disease**			
	Method of Administration			
Class/Drug (Trade Name)	**Inhaler***	**Nebulizer**	**Oral**	**Duration of Action†**
Beta₂-Adrenergic Agonist Agents				
salbutamol, albuterol (Proventil, Ventolin)	X	X	X	Short
metoproterenol sulfate (Alupent)	X	X	X	Short
terbutaline (Brethine)	X			Short
formoterol (Foradil)	X			Long
salmeterol (Serevent Diskus)	X			Long
indacaterol (Arcapta Neohaler)	X			Long
Anticholinergic Agents				
ipratropium bromide (Atrovent)	X	X		Short
tiotropium bromide (Spiriva HandiHaler)	X			Long
Combination Short-Acting Beta-2 Adrenergic Agonist and Anticholinergic Agents				
fenoterol/ipratropium (Duovent)	X	X		
salbutamol/ipratropium (Combivent)	X	X		
Methylxanthines				
aminophylline (Phyllocontin, Truphylline)			X	Variable
theophylline (Theo-Dur, Slo-Bid)			X	Variable

*Inhaler may include metered-dose inhaler, powdered inhalation with inhaler, or discus.
†Short acting, 4–6 h; long acting, 12+ h.

therapy is preferred, and the choice of bronchodilator depends on availability and individual response in terms of symptom relief and side effects. Inhaled therapy may be prescribed on an as-needed or regular basis to reduce symptoms. Long-acting bronchodilators are more convenient for patients to use, and combining bronchodilators with different durations of action and different mechanisms may optimize symptom management (GOLD, 2010). Even patients who do not show a significant response to a short-acting bronchodilator test may benefit symptomatically from long-term bronchodilator treatment.

Corticosteroids

Although inhaled and systemic corticosteroids may improve the symptoms of COPD, they do not slow the decline in lung function. Their effects are less dramatic than in asthma. A short trial course of oral corticosteroids may be prescribed for patients to determine whether pulmonary function improves and symptoms decrease. Long-term treatment with oral corticosteroids is not recommended in COPD and can cause steroid myopathy, leading to muscle weakness, decreased ability to function, and, in advanced disease, respiratory failure (GOLD, 2010). Inhaled corticosteroids are frequently prescribed in COPD. Used in combination with a long-acting beta-agonist, inhaled corticosteroids may reduce exacerbations by an additional 10% as compared to either therapy used alone (Niewoehner, 2010).

Medication regimens used to manage COPD are based on disease severity. For grade I (mild) COPD, a short-acting bronchodilator may be prescribed. For grade II or III COPD, a short-acting bronchodilator and regular treatment with one or more long-acting bronchodilators may be used. For grade III or IV (severe or very severe) COPD, medication therapy includes regular treatment with one or more bronchodilators and/or inhaled corticosteroids for repeated exacerbations. Combination long-term beta$_2$-agonists plus corticosteroids in one inhaler may be appropriate; examples include formoterol/budesonide (Symbicort) and salmeterol/fluticasone (Advair Diskus) (GOLD, 2010; Qaseem et al., 2011).

Other Medications

Other pharmacologic treatments that may be used in COPD include alpha$_1$-antitrypsin augmentation therapy, antibiotic agents, mucolytic agents, antitussive agents, vasodilators, and narcotics. Vaccines are also effective in that they prevent exacerbations by preventing respiratory infections. For instance, influenza vaccines can reduce serious morbidity and death in patients with COPD by approximately 50% (GOLD, 2010; Qaseem et al., 2011). It is recommended that people limit their risk through influenza vaccination and smoking cessation. Pneumococcal vaccination also reduces the incidence of pneumonia, hospitalizations for cardiac conditions, and deaths in the general older adult population. Pneumococcal pneumonia is responsible for approximately 175,000 hospitalizations per year (National Foundation for Infectious Disease, 2010). A one-time dose of pneumococcal polysaccharide vaccine (PPSV) is recommended for all patients 65 years or older and those with chronic diseases (CDC, 2011b; GOLD, 2010). A second PPSV revaccination dose is recommended for all adults 65 years and older who were previously vaccinated with one dose if 5 years or more have elapsed since the previous dose. For those who were first vaccinated at 65 years or older, only one dose is required regardless of medical condition (CDC, 2011b).

Management of Exacerbations

An exacerbation of COPD is defined as an event in the natural course of the disease characterized by acute changes (worsening) in the patient's respiratory symptoms beyond the normal day-to-day variations. An exacerbation also leads to change in medication (GOLD, 2011). Primary causes of an acute exacerbation include tracheobronchial infection and air pollution. However, the cause of approximately one third of severe exacerbations cannot be identified (GOLD, 2010). In 2011, roflumilast (Daliresp) was approved by the U.S. Food and Drug Administration (FDA) as a treatment to reduce the risk of exacerbations in patients with severe COPD associated with chronic bronchitis and a history of exacerbations. Roflumilast—the first and only selective phosphodiesterase-4 (PDE4) inhibitor that is FDA approved—is an oral tablet taken once daily. Although the specific mechanism by which roflumilast exerts its therapeutic action in patients with COPD is not well defined, it is thought to be related to the effects of increased intracellular cyclic 3',5'-adenosine monophosphate (cAMP) in lung cells (FDA, 2011).

Treatment of an exacerbation requires identifying the primary cause (if possible) and administering the specific treatment. Optimization of bronchodilator medications is first-line therapy and involves identifying the best medication or combinations of medications taken on a regular schedule for a specific patient. Depending on the signs and symptoms, corticosteroids, antibiotic agents, oxygen therapy, and intensive respiratory interventions may also be used. Indications for hospitalization for acute exacerbation of COPD include severe dyspnea that does not respond adequately to initial therapy, confusion or lethargy, respiratory muscle fatigue, paradoxical chest wall movement, peripheral edema, worsening or new onset of central cyanosis, persistent or worsening hypoxemia, and the need for noninvasive or invasive assisted mechanical ventilation (GOLD, 2010). The outcome from an exacerbation of COPD is closely related to the development of respiratory acidosis, the presence of significant comorbidities, and the need for noninvasive or invasive positive pressure ventilatory support.

The GOLD guidelines (2010) provide indications for assessment, hospital admission, and possible critical care admission for patients with exacerbations of COPD. Indications for hospitalization include marked increase in intensity of symptoms, severe underlying COPD, onset of new physical signs (i.e., the use of accessory muscles, paradoxical chest wall movement, worsening or new onset of central cyanosis, peripheral edema, signs of right heart failure, reduced alertness), failure to respond to initial medical management, older age, and insufficient home support.

On the patient's arrival at the ED, the first line of treatment is supplemental oxygen therapy and rapid assessment to determine if the exacerbation is life threatening (GOLD, 2010). A short-acting inhaled bronchodilator may be used to assess response to treatment. Oral or intravenous (IV) corticosteroids, in addition to bronchodilators, are recommended in the hospital management of a COPD exacerbation. Antibiotics also benefit patients because bacterial infections often follow viral infections.

General Principles of Oxygen Therapy

Oxygen therapy can be administered as long-term continuous therapy, during exercise, or to prevent acute dyspnea during an exacerbation. The goal of supplemental oxygen therapy is to increase the baseline resting partial pressure of arterial oxygen (PaO_2) to at least 60 mm Hg at sea level and an arterial oxygen saturation (SaO_2) to at least 90% (GOLD, 2010). Long-term oxygen therapy (more than 15 hours per day) has also been shown to improve quality of life, reduce pulmonary arterial pressure and dyspnea, and improve survival (GOLD, 2010). Long-term oxygen therapy is usually introduced in very severe COPD, and indications generally include a PaO_2 of 55 mm Hg or less or evidence of tissue hypoxia and organ damage such as cor pulmonale, secondary polycythemia, edema from right-sided heart failure, or impaired mental status (GOLD, 2010; Qaseem et al., 2011). For patients with exercise-induced hypoxemia, oxygen supplementation during exercise may improve performance. No evidence supports the idea that short bursts of oxygen before or after exercise provide any symptomatic relief (GOLD, 2010). Patients who are hypoxemic while awake are likely to be so during sleep. Therefore, nighttime oxygen therapy is recommended as well, and the prescription for oxygen therapy is for continuous, 24-hour use. Intermittent oxygen therapy is indicated for patients who **desaturate** (i.e., experience a precipitous drop in hemoglobin molecule saturation with oxygen) only during activities of daily living, exercise, or sleep.

The main objective in treating patients with hypoxemia and hypercapnia is to give sufficient oxygen to improve oxygenation. Patients with COPD who require oxygen may have respiratory failure that is caused primarily by a ventilation–perfusion mismatch. These patients respond to oxygen therapy and should be treated to keep the resting oxygen saturation above 90%. However, a small subset of patients with COPD and chronic hypercapnia (elevated partial pressure of arterial carbon dioxide [$PaCO_2$] levels) may be more oxygen sensitive; their respiratory failure is caused more by alveolar hypoventilation. Administering too much oxygen can result in the retention of carbon dioxide. Patients with alveolar hypoventilation cannot increase ventilation to adjust for this increased load, and increasing hypercapnia occurs. Monitoring and assessment are essential in the care of patients with COPD on supplemental oxygen. Pulse oximetry is helpful in assessing response to therapy but does not assess $PaCO_2$ levels. Optimal oxygenation of patients is important while monitoring for any possible complications of oxygen supplementation.

> ◤ *Quality and Safety Nursing Alert*
>
> Oxygen therapy is variable in patients with COPD; its aim in COPD is to achieve an acceptable oxygen level without a fall in the pH (increasing hypercapnia).

Surgical Management

Bullectomy

A bullectomy is a surgical option for select patients with bullous emphysema. Bullae are enlarged airspaces that do not contribute to ventilation but occupy space in the thorax; these areas may be surgically excised. These bullae compress areas of the lung and may impair gas exchange. Bullectomy may help reduce dyspnea and improve lung function. It can be performed via a video-assisted thoracoscope or a limited thoracotomy incision (see Chapter 21).

Lung Volume Reduction Surgery

Treatment options for patients with advanced or end-stage COPD (grade IV) with a primary emphysematous component are limited, although lung volume reduction surgery is a palliative surgical option that is approved by Medicare in selected patients. This includes patients with homogenous disease or disease that is focused in one area and not widespread throughout the lungs. Lung volume reduction surgery involves the removal of a portion of the diseased lung parenchyma. This reduces hyperinflation and allows the functional tissue to expand, resulting in improved elastic recoil of the lung and improved chest wall and diaphragmatic mechanics. This type of surgery does not cure the disease nor improve life expectancy; however, it may decrease dyspnea, improve lung function and exercise tolerance, and improve the patient's overall quality of life (GOLD, 2010).

Bronchoscopic lung volume reduction therapies that are performed in parts of Europe are under investigation in clinical research protocols in the United States. These bronchoscopic procedures were developed to collapse areas of emphysematous lung and thus improve aeration of the functional lung tissue. Techniques include endobronchial placement of a one-way valve that allows air and mucus to exit the treated area but does not allow air to reenter. Another technique achieves biologic lung volume reduction through bronchoscopic instillation of a sealant or gel into the airway of the hyperinflated lung tissue. Because air can no longer enter the airway, the lung tissue beyond the sealed airway collapses over time. Lastly, thermal ablation involves administering steam vapor directly to the segmental airway via a bronchoscope. The resultant inflammatory response in the airway leads to occlusion and atelectasis of the targeted lung tissue segment. Also under study is the endobronchial placement of a drug-eluting stent through the bronchial wall to decompress hyperinflated areas of the lung. In studies, most of these bronchoscopic techniques improve quality-of-life measures but do not demonstrate improved physiologic or exercise tolerance benefits (Berger, DeCamp, Criner, et al., 2010).

Lung Transplantation

Lung transplantation is a viable option for definitive surgical treatment of end-stage emphysema. It has been shown to improve quality of life and functional capacity in a select group of patients with COPD. Limited not only by the shortage of donor organs, it is also a costly procedure with financial implications for months to years because of complications and the need for costly immunosuppressive medication regimens (GOLD, 2010).

Pulmonary Rehabilitation

Pulmonary rehabilitation for patients with COPD is well established and widely accepted as a means to alleviate symptoms and optimize functional status (American Association of Cardiovascular and Pulmonary Rehabilitation, 2011; Birnbaum, 2011).

The primary goals of rehabilitation are to reduce symptoms, improve quality of life, and increase physical and emotional participation in everyday activities (GOLD, 2010). The benefits of this therapy include improvement of exercise capacity, reduction of the perceived intensity of breathlessness, improvement in health-related quality of life, reduction in the number of hospitalizations and days in the hospital, and reduction of the anxiety and depression associated with COPD (GOLD, 2010). Pulmonary rehabilitation services are multidisciplinary and include assessment, education, smoking cessation, physical reconditioning, nutritional counseling, skills training, and psychological support. Patients are taught methods to alleviate symptoms. Breathing exercises, as well as retraining and exercise programs, are used to improve functional status.

Pulmonary rehabilitation is appropriate for patients with grades II through IV COPD (GOLD, 2010). The minimum length of an effective program is 6 weeks; the longer the program, the more effective the results (GOLD, 2010; Qaseem et al., 2011). Programs vary in duration and may be conducted in inpatient, outpatient, or home settings. Program selection depends on the patient's physical, functional, and psychosocial status; insurance coverage; availability of programs; and preference. Pulmonary rehabilitation may also be used therapeutically in other disorders besides COPD, including asthma, CF, lung cancer, interstitial lung disease, thoracic surgery, and lung transplantation. Despite their proven efficacy, it was only in the past decade that these services were approved for coverage by Medicare and other payers. Medicare covers a comprehensive program, but specific criteria must be met. These criteria can be barriers for patient referral as well as initiation of programs in the inpatient or outpatient setting (Birnbaum, 2011).

Patient Education

Nurses play a key role in identifying potential candidates for pulmonary rehabilitation and in facilitating and reinforcing the material learned in the rehabilitation program. Not all patients have access to a formal rehabilitation program. However, nurses can be instrumental in educating patients and families as well as facilitating specific services, such as respiratory therapy education, physical therapy for exercise and breathing retraining, occupational therapy for conserving energy during activities of daily living, and nutritional counseling. Patient education is a major component of pulmonary rehabilitation and includes a broad variety of topics.

Depending on the length and setting of the educational program, topics may include normal anatomy and physiology of the lung, pathophysiology and changes with COPD, medications and home oxygen therapy, nutrition, respiratory therapy treatments, symptom alleviation, smoking cessation, sexuality and COPD, coping with chronic disease, communicating with the health care team, and planning for the future (advance directives, living wills, informed decision making about health care alternatives). Education, including that relating to smoking cessation, should be incorporated into all aspects of care for COPD and in many settings (physicians' offices, clinics, hospitals, home and community health care settings, and comprehensive rehabilitation programs).

Breathing Exercises

The breathing pattern of most people with COPD is shallow, rapid, and inefficient; the more severe the disease, the more inefficient the breathing pattern. With practice, this type of upper chest breathing can be changed to diaphragmatic breathing, which reduces the respiratory rate, increases alveolar ventilation, and sometimes helps expel as much air

as possible during expiration (see Chapter 21 for technique). Pursed-lip breathing helps slow expiration, prevents collapse of small airways, and helps the patient control the rate and depth of respiration. It also promotes relaxation, enabling the patient to gain control of dyspnea and reduce feelings of panic.

Activity Pacing

People with COPD have decreased exercise tolerance during specific periods of the day, especially in the morning on arising, because bronchial secretions have collected in the lungs during the night while the patient was lying down. The patient may have difficulty bathing or dressing and may become fatigued. Activities that require the arms to be supported above the level of the thorax may produce fatigue or respiratory distress but may be tolerated better after the patient has been up and moving around for an hour or more. The nurse can help the patient reduce these limitations by planning self-care activities and determining the best times for bathing, dressing, and other daily activities.

Self-Care Activities

As gas exchange, airway clearance, and the breathing pattern improve, the patient is encouraged to assume increasing participation in self-care activities. The patient is taught to coordinate diaphragmatic breathing with activities such as walking, bathing, bending, or climbing stairs. The patient should bathe, dress, and take short walks, resting as needed to avoid fatigue and excessive dyspnea. Fluids should always be readily available, and the patient should begin to drink fluids without having to be reminded. If management of secretions is a problem and some type of postural drainage or airway clearance maneuver is to be performed at home, the nurse or respiratory therapist instructs and supervises the patient before discharge or in an outpatient setting.

Physical Conditioning

People with COPD of all grades may benefit from exercise training programs. These benefits may include increased exercise tolerance and decreased dyspnea and fatigue (GOLD, 2010). Physical conditioning techniques include breathing exercises and general exercises intended to conserve energy and increase pulmonary ventilation. Graded exercises and physical conditioning programs using treadmills, stationary bicycles, and measured level walks can improve symptoms and increase work capacity and exercise tolerance. Any physical activity that can be performed regularly is helpful. Walking aids may be beneficial (GOLD, 2010). Lightweight portable oxygen systems are available for ambulatory patients who require oxygen therapy during physical activity.

Oxygen Therapy

Oxygen supplied to the home comes in compressed gas, liquid, or concentrator systems. Portable oxygen systems allow the patient to exercise, work, and travel. To help the patient adhere to the oxygen prescription, the nurse explains the proper flow rate and required number of hours for oxygen use as well as the dangers of arbitrary changes in flow rate or duration of therapy. The nurse also reassures the patient that oxygen is not "addictive" and explains the need for regular evaluations of blood oxygenation by pulse oximetry or arterial blood gas analysis.

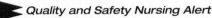

Nutritional Therapy

Nutritional assessment and counseling are important for patients with COPD. Nutritional status is reflected in severity of symptoms, degree of disability, and prognosis. Significant weight loss is often a major problem; however, excessive weight can also be problematic, although it occurs less often. Most people have difficulty gaining and maintaining weight. A thorough assessment of caloric needs and counseling about meal planning and supplementation is part of the rehabilitation process. Continual monitoring of weight and interventions as necessary are important parts of the care of patients with COPD.

Coping Measures

Any factor that interferes with normal breathing quite naturally induces anxiety, depression, and changes in behavior. Constant shortness of breath and fatigue may make the patient irritable and apprehensive to the point of panic. Restricted activity (and reversal of family roles due to loss of employment), the frustration of having to work to breathe, and the realization that the disease is prolonged and unrelenting may cause the patient to become angry, depressed, and demanding. Sexual function may be compromised, which also diminishes self-esteem. The nurse should provide education and support to spouses or significant others and families, because the caregiver role in end-stage COPD can be challenging.

Nursing Management

Assessing the Patient

Assessment involves obtaining information about current symptoms as well as previous disease manifestations. See Chart 24-2 for sample questions that may be used to obtain a clear history of the disease process. In addition to the history, the nurse reviews the results of available diagnostic tests. (Visit thePoint to view a Clinical Simulation Case Study of Nursing Management of a Patient With COPD.)

Achieving Airway Clearance

Bronchospasm, which occurs in many pulmonary diseases, reduces the caliber of the small bronchi and may cause dyspnea, static secretions, and infection. Bronchospasm can sometimes be detected on auscultation with a stethoscope when wheezing or diminished breath sounds are heard. Increased mucus production, along with decreased mucociliary action, contributes to further reduction in the caliber of the bronchi and results in decreased airflow and decreased gas exchange. This is further aggravated by the loss of lung elasticity that occurs with COPD (GOLD, 2010). These changes in the airway require that the nurse monitor the patient for dyspnea and hypoxemia. If bronchodilators or corticosteroids are prescribed, the nurse must administer the medications properly and be alert for potential side effects. The relief of bronchospasm is confirmed by measuring improvement in expiratory flow rates and volumes (the force of expiration, how long it takes to exhale, and the amount of air exhaled) as well as by assessing the dyspnea and making sure that it has lessened.

Diminishing the quantity and viscosity of sputum can clear the airway and improve pulmonary ventilation and gas exchange. All pulmonary irritants should be eliminated or reduced, particularly cigarette smoke, which is the most persistent source of pulmonary irritation. The nurse instructs the patient in directed or controlled coughing, which is more effective and reduces the fatigue associated with undirected forceful coughing. Directed coughing consists of a slow, maximal inspiration followed by breath-holding for several seconds and then two or three coughs. "Huff" coughing may also be effective. The technique consists of one or two forced exhalations (huffs) from low to medium lung volumes with the glottis open.

Chest physiotherapy with postural drainage, intermittent positive pressure breathing, increased fluid intake, and bland aerosol mists (with normal saline solution or water) may be useful for some patients with COPD. The use of these measures must be based on the response and tolerance of each patient.

Improving Breathing Patterns

Ineffective breathing patterns and shortness of breath are due to the modified respiratory mechanics of the chest wall and lung resulting from **air trapping** (i.e., incomplete emptying of alveoli during expiration), ineffective diaphragmatic movement, airway obstruction, the metabolic cost of breathing, and stress. Inspiratory muscle training and breathing retraining may help improve breathing patterns. Training in diaphragmatic breathing reduces the respiratory rate, increases alveolar ventilation, and sometimes helps expel as much air as possible during expiration. Pursed-lip breathing helps slow expiration, prevent collapse of small airways, and control the rate and depth of respiration. It also promotes relaxation, which allows patients to gain control of dyspnea and reduce feelings of panic.

Improving Activity Tolerance

Patients with COPD experience progressive activity and exercise intolerance that may lead to disability. Education is focused on rehabilitative therapies to promote independence in executing activities of daily living. These may include pacing activities throughout the day or using supportive devices to decrease energy expenditure. The nurse evaluates the patient's activity tolerance and limitations and uses education strategies to promote independent activities of daily living. The patient may be a candidate for exercise training to strengthen the muscles of the upper and lower extremities and to improve exercise tolerance and endurance. The use of walking aids may be recommended to improve activity levels and ambulation (GOLD, 2010). Other health care professionals (rehabilitation therapist, occupational therapist, physical therapist) may be consulted as additional resources.

Monitoring and Managing Potential Complications

The nurse must assess for various complications of COPD, such as life-threatening respiratory insufficiency and failure, as well as respiratory infection and chronic atelectasis, which may increase the risk of respiratory failure. The nurse monitors for cognitive changes (personality and behavioral changes, memory impairment), increasing dyspnea, tachypnea, and tachycardia, which may indicate increasing hypoxemia and impending respiratory failure.

The nurse monitors pulse oximetry values to assess the patient's need for oxygen and administers supplemental oxygen as prescribed. The nurse also instructs the patient about signs and symptoms of respiratory infection that may worsen hypoxemia and reports changes in the patient's physical and cognitive status to the primary provider.

Bronchopulmonary infections must be controlled to diminish inflammatory edema and to permit recovery of normal ciliary action. Minor respiratory infections that are of no consequence to people with normal lungs can be life threatening to people with COPD. Infection compromises lung function and is a common cause of respiratory failure in people with COPD. In COPD, infection may be accompanied by subtle changes. The nurse instructs the patient to report any signs of infection, such as a fever or change in sputum color, character, consistency, or amount. Any worsening of symptoms (increased tightness of the chest, increased dyspnea, fatigue) also suggests infection and must be reported. Viral infections are hazardous to the patient because they are often followed by infections caused by bacterial organisms, such as *Streptococcus pneumoniae* and *Haemophilus influenzae*.

To prevent infection, the nurse encourages the patient with COPD to be immunized against influenza and pneumococcal pneumonia, because the patient is prone to respiratory infection. In addition, because each patient reacts differently to external exposures (significant air pollution, high or low temperatures, high humidity, strong smells), the nurse must assess the patient's actual and potential triggers that cause bronchospasm so that avoidance or a treatment plan can be established.

Pneumothorax is a potential complication of COPD and can be life threatening in patients with COPD who have minimal pulmonary reserve. Patients with severe emphysematous changes can develop large bullae, which may rupture and cause a pneumothorax. Development of a pneumothorax may be spontaneous or related to an activity such as severe coughing or large intrathoracic pressure changes. If a rapid onset of shortness of breath occurs, the nurse should quickly evaluate the patient for potential pneumothorax by assessing the symmetry of chest movement, differences in breath sounds, and pulse oximetry.

Over time, pulmonary hypertension may occur as a result of chronic hypoxemia, which causes the pulmonary arteries to constrict and thus leads to this complication. Pulmonary hypertension may be prevented by maintaining adequate oxygenation through an adequate hemoglobin level, improved ventilation–perfusion of the lungs, or continuous administration of supplemental oxygen (if needed).

Promoting Home and Community-Based Care

Educating Patients About Self-Care

When providing education about self-management, the nurse must assess the knowledge of patients and family members about self-care and the therapeutic regimen. The nurse should also consider whether they are comfortable with this knowledge. Familiarity with prescribed medications' potential side effects is essential. In addition, patients and family members need to learn the early signs and symptoms of infection and other complications so that they seek appropriate health care promptly.

> ### Quality and Safety Nursing Alert
>
> Education is essential and should be tailored to the stage of COPD.

A major area of patient education involves setting and accepting realistic short-term and long-range goals. If the COPD is mild (i.e., grade I), the objectives of treatment are to increase exercise tolerance and prevent further loss of pulmonary function. If the COPD is severe (i.e., grade III), the objectives are to preserve current pulmonary function and relieve symptoms as much as possible. It is important to plan and share the goals and expectations of treatment with the patient. Both the patient and the care provider need patience to achieve these goals.

The nurse instructs the patient to avoid extremes of heat and cold. Heat increases the body temperature, thereby raising oxygen requirements, and cold tends to promote bronchospasm. Air pollutants such as fumes, smoke, dust, and even talcum, lint, and aerosol sprays may initiate bronchospasm. High altitudes aggravate hypoxemia.

A patient with COPD should adopt a lifestyle of moderate activity, ideally in a climate with minimal shifts in temperature and humidity. As much as possible, the patient should avoid emotional disturbances and stressful situations that might trigger a coughing episode. The medication regimen can be quite complex; patients receiving aerosol medications by an MDI or other type of inhaler may be particularly challenged. The nurse must review educational information and have the patient demonstrate correct MDI use before discharge, during follow-up visits to a caregiver's office or clinic, and during home visits (Chart 24-4).

Smoking cessation goes hand in hand with lifestyle changes, and reinforcing the patient's efforts is a key nursing activity. Smoking cessation is the single most important

	PATIENT EDUCATION
Chart 24-4	**Use of Metered-Dose Inhaler**

To administer medication:

- Remove the cap and hold the inhaler upright.
- Shake the inhaler.
- Tilt your head back slightly and breathe out slowly and all the way.
- Position the inhaler approximately 1–2 inches away from the open mouth, or use a spacer/holding chamber. When using a medicine chamber, place the lips around the mouthpiece.
- Start breathing in slowly through your mouth, and press down on the inhaler one time. If using a chamber, first press down on the inhaler and within 5 seconds begin to breathe in slowly.
- Breathe in slowly and deeply for as long as possible.
- Hold your breath as you count to 10 slowly (10 seconds) to allow the medication to reach down into your airways.
- Repeat puffs as directed, allowing 15–30 seconds between puffs for quick-acting medications. There is no need to wait for other medications.
- Apply the cap to the metered-dose inhaler (MDI) for storage.
- After inhalation, rinse mouth with water when using a corticosteroid-containing MDI.

Adapted from Expert Panel Report 3. (2007). *Guidelines for the diagnosis and management of asthma*. Bethesda, MD: National Asthma Education and Prevention Program, National Institutes of Health.

therapeutic intervention for patients with COPD. There are many strategies, including prevention, cessation with or without oral or topical patch medications, and behavior modification techniques (HHS, 2010b).

Numerous educational materials are available to assist nurses in educating patients with COPD. Potential resources include those of organizations such as the American Lung Association, the American Association of Cardiovascular and Pulmonary Rehabilitation, the American Thoracic Society, the American College of Chest Physicians, and the American Association for Respiratory Care.

Continuing Care

Referral for home care is important to enable assessment of the patient's home environment and physical and psychological status, to evaluate the patient's adherence to a prescribed regimen, and to assess the patient's ability to cope with changes in lifestyle and physical status. Home care visits provide an opportunity to reinforce the information and activities learned in the inpatient or outpatient pulmonary rehabilitation program and to have the patient and family demonstrate correct administration of medications and oxygen, if indicated, and performance of exercises. If the patient does not have access to a formal pulmonary rehabilitation program, the nurse provides the education and breathing retraining necessary to optimize the patient's functional status.

The nurse directs patients to community resources, such as pulmonary rehabilitation programs and smoking cessation programs, to help improve patients' ability to cope with their chronic condition and the therapeutic regimen and to provide a sense of worth, hope, and well-being. In addition, the nurse reminds the patient and family about the importance of participating in general health promotion activities and health screening.

Patients with COPD have indicated that information about their end-of-life needs is limited. Consequently, the nurse must address quality of life and issues surrounding the end of life in patients with end-stage COPD. Areas to discuss regarding end of life care may include symptom management, quality of life, satisfaction with care, information/communication, the use of care professionals, the use of care facilities, hospital admission, and place of death (Heffner, 2011). It is crucial that patients know what to expect as the disease progresses. In addition, they should have information about their role in decisions regarding aggressiveness of care near the end of life and access to specialists who may help them and their families. As the disease course progresses, a holistic assessment of physical and psychological needs should be undertaken at each hospitalization, clinic visit, or home visit. This helps gauge the patient's assessment of the progression of the disease and its impact on quality of life and guides planning for future interventions and management.

Chart 24-5 provides further information on providing nursing care for the patient with COPD.

Bronchiectasis

Bronchiectasis is a chronic, irreversible dilation of the bronchi and bronchioles that results from destruction of muscles and elastic connective tissue. Under the new definition of

COPD, it is considered a disease process separate from COPD (GOLD, 2010). Bronchiectasis may be caused by a variety of conditions, including:

- Airway obstruction
- Diffuse airway injury
- Complications of long-term pulmonary infections
- Congenital disorders
- Genetic disorders such as CF
- Abnormal host defense (e.g., ciliary dyskinesia or humoral immunodeficiency)
- Idiopathic causes

People may be predisposed to bronchiectasis as a result of recurrent respiratory infections in early childhood, measles, influenza, tuberculosis, or immunodeficiency disorders.

Pathophysiology

The inflammatory process associated with pulmonary infections damages the bronchial wall, causing a loss of its supporting structure and resulting in thick sputum that ultimately obstructs the bronchi. The walls become permanently distended and distorted, impairing mucociliary clearance. In saccular bronchiectasis, each dilated peribronchial tube amounts to a lung abscess, the exudate of which drains freely through the bronchus. Bronchiectasis is usually localized, affecting a segment or lobe of a lung, most frequently the lower lobes.

The retention of secretions and subsequent obstruction ultimately cause the alveoli distal to the obstruction to collapse (atelectasis). Inflammatory scarring or fibrosis replaces functioning lung tissue. In time, the patient develops respiratory insufficiency with reduced vital capacity, decreased ventilation, and an increased ratio of residual volume to total lung capacity. There is impairment in the match of ventilation to perfusion (ventilation–perfusion imbalance) and hypoxemia.

Clinical Manifestations

Characteristic symptoms of bronchiectasis include chronic cough and the production of purulent sputum in copious amounts. Many patients with this disease have hemoptysis. Clubbing of the fingers also is common because of respiratory insufficiency. Patients usually have repeated episodes of pulmonary infection.

Assessment and Diagnostic Findings

Bronchiectasis is not readily diagnosed because the symptoms can be mistaken for those of simple chronic bronchitis. A definite sign is a prolonged history of productive cough, with sputum consistently negative for tubercle bacilli. The diagnosis is established by a CT scan, which reveals bronchial dilation. The advent of high-resolution CT scanning makes it possible to diagnose this disease during its earlier stages.

Medical Management

Treatment objectives are to promote bronchial drainage, to clear excessive secretions from the affected portion of the lungs, and to prevent or control infection. Postural drainage is part of all treatment plans, because draining of the bronchiectatic areas by gravity reduces the amount of secretions and the degree of infection. Sometimes, mucopurulent sputum must

(text continues on page 636)

PLAN OF NURSING CARE

Care of the Patient With Chronic Obstructive Pulmonary Disease

Chart
24-5

NURSING DIAGNOSIS: Impaired gas exchange and Ineffective airway clearance due to chronic inhalation of toxins
GOAL: Improvement in gas exchange

Nursing Interventions	Rationale	Expected Outcomes

1. Evaluate current smoking status, educate regarding smoking cessation, and facilitate efforts to quit.
  a. Evaluate current smoking habits of patient and family.
  b. Educate regarding hazards of smoking and relationship to COPD.
  c. Evaluate previous smoking cessation attempts.
  d. Provide educational materials.
  e. Refer to a smoking cessation program or resource.
2. Evaluate current exposure to occupational toxins or pollutants and indoor/outdoor pollution.
  a. Evaluate current exposures to occupational toxins, indoor and outdoor air pollution (e.g., smog, toxic fumes, chemicals).
  b. Emphasize primary prevention to occupational exposures. This is best achieved by elimination or reduction of exposures in the workplace.
  c. Educate regarding types of indoor and outdoor air pollution (e.g., biomass fuel burned for cooking and heating in poorly ventilated buildings, outdoor air pollution).
  d. Advise patient to monitor public announcements regarding air quality.
	1. Smoking causes permanent damage to the lungs and diminishes the lungs' protective mechanisms. Airflow is obstructed, secretions are increased, and lung capacity is reduced. Continued smoking increases morbidity and mortality in COPD and is also a risk factor for lung cancer.
	
	2. Chronic inhalation of both indoor and outdoor toxins causes damage to the airways and impairs gas exchange.
		• Identifies the hazards of cigarette smoking
		• Identifies resources for smoking cessation
		• Enrolls in smoking cessation program
		• Reports success in stopping smoking
		• Verbalizes types of inhaled toxins
		• Minimizes or eliminates exposures
		• Monitors public announcements regarding air quality and minimizes or eliminates exposures during episodes of severe pollution

---

NURSING DIAGNOSIS: Impaired gas exchange related to ventilation–perfusion inequality
GOAL: Improvement in gas exchange

Nursing Interventions	Rationale	Expected Outcomes

1. Administer bronchodilators as prescribed.
  a. Inhalation is the preferred route.
  b. Observe for side effects: tachycardia, dysrhythmias, central nervous system excitation, nausea, and vomiting.
  c. Assess for correct technique of metered-dose inhaler (MDI) or other type of administration.
2. Evaluate effectiveness of nebulizer or MDI treatments.
  a. Assess for decreased shortness of breath, decreased wheezing or crackles, loosened secretions, and decreased anxiety.
  b. Ensure that treatment is given before meals to avoid nausea and to reduce fatigue that accompanies eating.
3. Instruct and encourage patient in diaphragmatic breathing and effective coughing.
	1. Bronchodilators dilate the airways. The medication dosage is carefully adjusted for each patient, in accordance with clinical response.
	
	2. Combining medication with aerosolized bronchodilators is typically used to control bronchoconstriction in an acute exacerbation. Generally, however, the MDI with spacer is the preferred route (less cost and time to treatment).
	
	3. These techniques improve ventilation by opening airways to facilitate clearing the airways of sputum. Gas exchange is improved, and fatigue is minimized.
		• Verbalizes need for bronchodilators and for taking them as prescribed
		• Evidences minimal side effects; heart rate near normal, absence of dysrhythmias, normal mentation
		• Reports a decrease in dyspnea
		• Shows an improved expiratory flow rate
		• Uses and cleans respiratory therapy equipment as applicable
		• Demonstrates diaphragmatic breathing and coughing
		• Uses oxygen equipment appropriately when indicated
		• Evidences improved arterial blood gases or pulse oximetry
		• Demonstrates correct technique for use of MDI

Care of the Patient With Chronic Obstructive Pulmonary Disease (continued)

Nursing Interventions	Rationale	Expected Outcomes
4. Administer oxygen by the method prescribed. 　a. Explain rationale and importance to patient. 　b. Evaluate effectiveness; observe for signs of hypoxemia. Notify physician if restlessness, anxiety, somnolence, cyanosis, or tachycardia is present. 　c. Analyze arterial blood gases and compare with baseline values. When arterial puncture is performed and a blood sample is obtained, hold puncture site for 5 minutes to prevent arterial bleeding and development of ecchymoses. 　d. Initiate pulse oximetry to monitor oxygen saturation. 　e. Explain that no smoking is permitted by patient or visitors while oxygen is in use.	4. Oxygen will correct the hypoxemia. Careful observation of the liter flow or the percentage administered and its effect on the patient is important. These patients generally require low-flow oxygen rates of 1–2 L/min. Monitor and titrate to achieve desired PaO_2. Periodic arterial blood gases and pulse oximetry help evaluate adequacy of oxygenation. Smoking may render pulse oximetry inaccurate because the carbon monoxide from cigarette smoke also saturates hemoglobin.	

NURSING DIAGNOSIS: Ineffective airway clearance related to bronchoconstriction, increased mucus production, ineffective cough, bronchopulmonary infection, and other complications

GOAL: Achievement of airway clearance

Nursing Interventions	Rationale	Expected Outcomes
1. Adequately hydrate the patient. 2. Instruct in and encourage the use of diaphragmatic breathing and coughing techniques. 3. Assist in administering nebulizer or MDI. 4. If indicated, perform postural drainage with percussion and vibration in the morning and at night as prescribed. 5. Instruct patient to avoid bronchial irritants such as cigarette smoke, aerosols, extremes of temperature, and fumes. 6. Educate about early signs of infection that are to be reported to the clinician immediately: 　a. Increased sputum production 　b. Change in color of sputum 　c. Increased thickness of sputum 　d. Increased shortness of breath, tightness in chest, or fatigue 　e. Increased coughing 　f. Fever or chills 7. Administer antibiotics as prescribed. 8. Encourage patient to be immunized against influenza and *Streptococcus pneumoniae*.	1. Systemic hydration keeps secretions moist and easier to expectorate. Fluids must be given with caution if right- or left-sided heart failure is present. 2. These techniques help to improve ventilation and mobilize secretions without causing breathlessness and fatigue. 3. This ensures adequate delivery of medication to the airways. 4. This uses gravity to help raise secretions so they can be more easily expectorated or suctioned. 5. Bronchial irritants cause bronchoconstriction and increased mucus production, which then interfere with airway clearance. 6. Minor respiratory infections that are of no consequence to the person with normal lungs can produce fatal disturbances in the lungs of the person with emphysema. Early recognition is crucial. 7. Antibiotics may be prescribed to prevent or treat infection. 8. People with respiratory conditions are prone to respiratory infections and are encouraged to be immunized.	• Verbalizes need to drink fluids • Demonstrates diaphragmatic breathing and coughing • Performs postural drainage correctly • Coughing is minimized. • Does not smoke • Verbalizes that pollens, fumes, gases, dusts, and extremes of temperature and humidity are irritants to be avoided • Identifies signs of early infection • Is free of infection (no fever, no change in sputum, lessening of dyspnea) • Verbalizes need to notify primary provider at the earliest sign of infection • Verbalizes need to stay away from crowds or people with colds in flu season • Discusses flu and pneumonia vaccines with clinician to help prevent infection

(continues on page 634)

**Chart
24-5**

PLAN OF NURSING CARE

Care of the Patient With Chronic Obstructive Pulmonary Disease (continued)

NURSING DIAGNOSIS: Ineffective breathing pattern related to shortness of breath, mucus, bronchoconstriction, and airway irritants
GOAL: Improvement in breathing pattern

Nursing Interventions	Rationale	Expected Outcomes
1. Instruct patient in diaphragmatic and pursed-lip breathing.	1. This helps patient prolong expiration time and decreases air trapping. With these techniques, patient will breathe more efficiently and effectively.	• Practices pursed-lip and diaphragmatic breathing and uses them when short of breath and with activity
2. Encourage alternating activity with rest periods. Allow patient to make some decisions (bath, shaving) about care based on tolerance level.	2. Pacing activities permits patient to perform activities without excessive distress.	• Shows signs of decreased respiratory effort and paces activities • Uses inspiratory muscle trainer as prescribed
3. Encourage the use of an inspiratory muscle trainer if prescribed.	3. This strengthens and conditions the respiratory muscles.	

NURSING DIAGNOSIS: Self-care deficits related to fatigue secondary to increased work of breathing and insufficient ventilation and oxygenation
GOAL: Independence in self-care activities

Nursing Interventions	Rationale	Expected Outcomes
1. Educate patient to coordinate diaphragmatic breathing with activity (e.g., walking, bending).	1. This will allow the patient to be more active and to avoid excessive fatigue or dyspnea during activity.	• Uses controlled breathing while bathing, bending, and walking
2. Encourage patient to begin to bathe self, dress self, walk, and drink fluids. Discuss energy conservation measures.	2. As condition resolves, patient will be able to do more but needs to be encouraged to avoid increasing dependence.	• Paces activities of daily living to alternate with rest periods to reduce fatigue and dyspnea • Describes energy conservation strategies • Performs same self-care activities as before
3. Educate patient about postural drainage if appropriate.	3. This encourages patient to become involved in own care and prepares patient to manage at home.	• Performs postural drainage correctly

NURSING DIAGNOSIS: Activity intolerance due to fatigue, hypoxemia, and ineffective breathing patterns
GOAL: Improvement in activity tolerance

Nursing Interventions	Rationale	Expected Outcomes

1. Support patient in establishing a regular regimen of exercise using treadmill and exercise bicycle, walking, or other appropriate exercises, such as mall walking.
  a. Assess the patient's current level of functioning, and develop exercise plan based on baseline functional status.
  b. Suggest consultation with a physical therapist or pulmonary rehabilitation program to determine an exercise program specific to the patient's capability. Have portable oxygen unit available if oxygen is prescribed for exercise.
	1. Muscles that are deconditioned consume more oxygen and place an additional burden on the lungs. Through regular, graded exercise, these muscle groups become more conditioned, and the patient can do more without getting as short of breath. Graded exercise breaks the cycle of debilitation.	• Performs activities with less shortness of breath
		• Verbalizes need to exercise daily and demonstrates an exercise plan to be carried out at home
		• Walks and gradually increases walking time and distance to improve physical condition
		• Exercises both upper and lower body muscle groups

NURSING DIAGNOSIS: Ineffective coping related to reduced socialization, anxiety, depression, lower activity level, and the inability to work
GOAL: Attainment of an optimal level of coping

Nursing Interventions	Rationale	Expected Outcomes
1. Help the patient develop realistic goals.	1. Developing realistic goals will promote a sense of hope and accomplishment rather than defeat and hopelessness.	• Expresses interest in the future • Participates in the discharge plan • Discusses activities or methods that can be performed to ease shortness of breath
2. Encourage activity to level of symptom tolerance.	2. Activity reduces tension and decreases degree of dyspnea as patient becomes conditioned.	

Chart 24-5

PLAN OF NURSING CARE

Care of the Patient With Chronic Obstructive Pulmonary Disease (continued)

Nursing Interventions	Rationale	Expected Outcomes
3. Educate the patient about relaxation techniques or provide a relaxation tape for the patient. 4. Enroll patient in pulmonary rehabilitation program where available.	3. Relaxation reduces stress, anxiety, and dyspnea and helps patient to cope with disability. 4. Pulmonary rehabilitation programs have been shown to promote a subjective improvement in a patient's status and self-esteem as well as increased exercise tolerance and decreased hospitalizations.	• Uses relaxation techniques appropriately • Expresses interest in a pulmonary rehabilitation program

NURSING DIAGNOSIS: Deficient knowledge about self-management to be performed at home
GOAL: Adherence to therapeutic program and home care

Nursing Interventions	Rationale	Expected Outcomes
1. Help patient identify/develop short- and long-term goals. a. Educate the patient about disease, medications, procedures, and how and when to seek help. b. Refer patient to pulmonary rehabilitation. 2. Give strong message to stop smoking. Discuss smoking cessation strategies. Provide information about resource groups (e.g., SmokEnders, American Cancer Society, American Lung Association).	1. Patient needs to be a partner in developing the plan of care and needs to know what to expect. Education about the condition is one of the most important aspects of care; it will prepare the patient to live and cope with the condition and improve quality of life. 2. Smoking causes permanent damage to the lung and diminishes the lungs' protective mechanisms. Airflow is obstructed, and lung capacity is reduced. Smoking increases morbidity and mortality and is also a risk factor for lung cancer.	• Understands disease and what affects it • Verbalizes the need to preserve existing lung function by adhering to the prescribed program • Understands purposes and proper administration of medications • Stops smoking or enrolls in a smoking cessation program • Identifies when and whom to call for assistance

COLLABORATIVE PROBLEM: Atelectasis
GOAL: Absence of atelectasis on x-ray and physical examination

Nursing Interventions	Rationale	Expected Outcomes
1. Monitor respiratory status, including rate and pattern of respirations, breath sounds, signs and symptoms of respiratory distress, and pulse oximetry. 2. Instruct in and encourage diaphragmatic breathing and effective coughing techniques. 3. Promote the use of lung expansion techniques (e.g., deep-breathing exercises, incentive spirometry) as prescribed.	1. A change in respiratory status, including tachypnea, dyspnea, and diminished or absent breath sounds, may indicate atelectasis. 2. These techniques improve ventilation and lung expansion and ideally improve gas exchange. 3. Deep-breathing exercises and incentive spirometry promote maximal lung expansion.	• Normal (baseline for patient) respiratory rate and pattern • Normal breath sounds for patient • Demonstrates diaphragmatic breathing and effective coughing • Performs deep-breathing exercises, incentive spirometry as prescribed • Pulse oximetry ≥90%

COLLABORATIVE PROBLEM: Pneumothorax
GOAL: Absence of signs and symptoms of pneumothorax

Nursing Interventions	Rationale	Expected Outcomes
1. Monitor respiratory status, including rate and pattern of respirations, symmetry of chest wall movement, breath sounds, signs and symptoms of respiratory distress, and pulse oximetry. 2. Assess pulse. 3. Assess for chest pain and precipitating factors.	1. Dyspnea, tachypnea, tachycardia, acute pleuritic chest pain, tracheal deviation away from the affected side, absence of breath sounds on the affected side, and decreased tactile fremitus may indicate pneumothorax. 2. Tachycardia is associated with pneumothorax and anxiety. 3. Pain may accompany pneumothorax.	• Normal respiratory rate and pattern for patient • Normal breath sounds bilaterally • Normal pulse for patient • Normal tactile fremitus • Absence of pain • Tracheal position is midline • Pulse oximetry ≥90% • Maintains normal oxygen saturation and arterial blood gas measurements

(continues on page 634)

PLAN OF NURSING CARE

Care of the Patient With Chronic Obstructive Pulmonary Disease (continued)

Nursing Interventions	Rationale	Expected Outcomes
4. Palpate for tracheal deviation/shift away from the affected side.	4. Early detection of pneumothorax and prompt intervention will prevent other serious complications.	• Exhibits no hypoxemia and hypercapnia (or returns to baseline values)
5. Monitor pulse oximetry and, if indicated, arterial blood gases.	5. Recognition of deterioration in respiratory function will prevent serious complications.	• Absence of pain • Symmetric chest wall movement • Lungs fully expanded bilaterally on chest x-ray
6. Administer supplemental oxygen therapy, as indicated.	6. Oxygen will correct hypoxemia; administer it with caution.	
7. Administer analgesic agents, as indicated, for chest pain.	7. Pain interferes with deep breathing, resulting in decreased lung expansion.	
8. Assist with chest tube insertion and use pleural drainage system, as prescribed.	8. Removal of air from the pleural space will re-expand the lung.	

COLLABORATIVE PROBLEM: Respiratory failure
GOAL: Absence of signs and symptoms of respiratory failure; no evidence of respiratory failure on laboratory tests

Nursing Interventions	Rationale	Expected Outcomes
1. Monitor respiratory status, including rate and pattern of respirations, breath sounds, and signs and symptoms of acute respiratory distress.	1. Early recognition of deterioration in respiratory function will avert further complications, such as respiratory failure, severe hypoxemia, and hypercapnia.	• Normal respiratory rate and pattern for patient with no acute distress • Recognizes symptoms of hypoxemia and hypercapnia
2. Monitor pulse oximetry and arterial blood gases.	2. Recognition of changes in oxygenation and acid–base balance will guide in correcting and preventing complications.	• Maintains normal arterial blood gases/ pulse oximetry or returns to baseline values
3. Administer supplemental oxygen and initiate mechanisms for mechanical ventilation, as prescribed.	3. Acute respiratory failure is a medical emergency. Hypoxemia is a hallmark sign. Administration of oxygen therapy and mechanical ventilation (if indicated) are critical to survival.	

COLLABORATIVE PROBLEM: Pulmonary arterial hypertension
GOAL: Absence of evidence of pulmonary arterial hypertension on physical examination or laboratory tests

Nursing Interventions	Rationale	Expected Outcomes
1. Monitor respiratory status, including rate and pattern of respirations, breath sounds, pulse oximetry, and signs and symptoms of acute respiratory distress.	1. Dyspnea is the primary symptom of pulmonary arterial hypertension. Other symptoms include fatigue, angina, near-syncope, edema, and palpitations.	• Normal respiratory rate and pattern for patient • Exhibits no signs and symptoms of right-sided failure
2. Assess for signs and symptoms of right-sided heart failure, including peripheral edema, ascites, distended neck veins, crackles, and heart murmur.	2. Right-sided heart failure is a common clinical manifestation of pulmonary arterial hypertension due to increased right ventricular workload.	• Maintains baseline pulse oximetry values and arterial blood gases
3. Administer oxygen therapy, as prescribed.	3. Continuous oxygen therapy is a major component of management of pulmonary arterial hypertension; it prevents hypoxemia, thereby reducing pulmonary vascular constriction (resistance) secondary to hypoxemia.	

be removed by bronchoscopy. Chest physiotherapy, including percussion and postural drainage, is important in the management of secretions. Smoking cessation is important, because smoking impairs bronchial drainage by paralyzing ciliary action, increasing bronchial secretions, and causing inflammation of the mucous membranes, resulting in hyperplasia of the mucous glands.

Antibiotics are the cornerstone therapy for bronchiectasis management. Antimicrobial therapy choice is based on the results of sensitivity studies on organisms cultured from spu-

tum; however, empiric coverage (i.e., broad-spectrum antibiotics that are effective in treating commonly implicated pathogens) is often prescribed initially, pending results of sputum cultures. For patients with infrequent exacerbations, antibiotics are used only during acute episodes. Because infection with *Pseudomonas aeruginosa* is associated with a greater rate of lung function deterioration, more aggressive oral or IV antibiotic therapy may be used for a longer duration (Loscalzo, 2010). Patients should be vaccinated against influenza and pneumococcal pneumonia. Bronchodilators, which may be prescribed for patients who also have reactive airway disease, may also assist with secretion management.

Surgical intervention, although used infrequently, may be indicated for patients who continue to expectorate large amounts of sputum and have repeated bouts of pneumonia and hemoptysis despite adherence to treatment regimens. The disease must involve only one or two areas of the lung that can be removed without producing respiratory insufficiency. The goals of surgical treatment are to conserve normal pulmonary tissue and to avoid infectious complications. Diseased tissue is removed, provided that postoperative lung function will be adequate. It may be necessary to remove a segment of a lobe (segmental resection), a lobe (lobectomy), or, rarely, an entire lung (pneumonectomy). (See Chapter 21 for further information.) Segmental resection is the removal of an anatomic subdivision of a pulmonary lobe. The chief advantage is that only diseased tissue is removed, and healthy lung tissue is conserved.

The surgery is preceded by a period of careful preparation. The objective is to obtain a dry (free of infection) tracheobronchial tree to prevent complications (atelectasis, pneumonia, bronchopleural fistula, and empyema). This is accomplished by postural drainage or, depending on the location, by direct suction through a bronchoscope. A course of antibacterial therapy may be prescribed. After surgery, care is the same as for any patient who has undergone chest surgery (see Chapter 21).

Nursing Management

Nursing management focuses on alleviating symptoms and helping patients clear pulmonary secretions. Patient education targets eliminating smoking and other factors that increase the production of mucus and hamper its removal. Patients and families are taught to perform postural drainage and to avoid exposure to people with upper respiratory or other infections. If the patient experiences fatigue and dyspnea, he or she is informed about strategies to conserve energy while maintaining as active a lifestyle as possible. The patient is educated about the early signs of respiratory infection and the progression of the disorder so that appropriate treatment can be implemented promptly. The presence of a large amount of mucus may decrease the patient's appetite and result in an inadequate dietary intake; therefore, the patient's nutritional status is assessed and strategies are implemented to ensure an adequate diet.

Asthma

Asthma is a chronic inflammatory disease of the airways that causes airway hyperresponsiveness, mucosal edema, and mucus production. This inflammation ultimately leads to recurrent episodes of asthma symptoms: cough, chest tightness, wheezing, and dyspnea (Fig. 24-6). In the United States, asthma affects more than 25 million people and accounts for approximately 3,500 deaths per year. Medical expenses associated with asthma exceeded $50 billion in 2007 (CDC, 2011a). The most common chronic disease of childhood, asthma can occur at any age. For most patients, asthma is a disruptive disease, affecting school and work attendance, occupational choices, physical activity, and general quality of life.

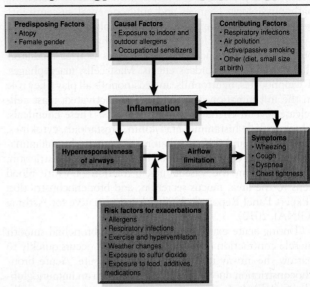

FIGURE 24-6 • Pathophysiology of asthma. Adapted from materials developed for the Global Initiative for Asthma. (2008). *Global strategy for asthma management and prevention.* Available at: www.ginasthma.org.

Despite increased knowledge regarding the pathology of asthma and the development of improved medications and management plans, the death rate from the disease continues to rise. Ethnic and racial disparities affect morbidity and mortality in asthma, which are higher in inner-city African Americans and Latinos (CDC, 2011c). Contributing to these disparities are epidemiology and risk factors; genetics and molecular aspects; inner-city environments; limited community assets; health care access, delivery, and quality; and lack of insurance coverage.

Unlike other obstructive lung diseases, asthma is largely reversible, either spontaneously or with treatment. Patients with asthma may experience symptom-free periods alternating with acute exacerbations that last from minutes to hours or days.

Allergy is the strongest predisposing factor for asthma. Chronic exposure to airway irritants or allergens also increases the risk of asthma. Common allergens can be seasonal (grass, tree, and weed pollens) or perennial (e.g., mold, dust, roaches, animal dander). Common triggers for asthma symptoms and exacerbations include airway irritants (e.g., air pollutants, cold, heat, weather changes, strong odors or perfumes, smoke, occupational exposure), foods (e.g., shellfish, nuts), exercise, stress, hormonal factors, medications, viral respiratory tract infections, and gastroesophageal reflux. Most people who have asthma are sensitive to a variety of triggers.

Pathophysiology

The underlying pathology in asthma is reversible diffuse airway inflammation that leads to long-term airway narrowing. This narrowing, which is exacerbated by various changes in the airway, includes bronchoconstriction, airway edema, airway hyperresponsiveness, and airway remodeling. The interaction of these factors determines the clinical manifestations and severity of asthma (Expert Panel Report 3, 2007; Holgate, 2011). Over the course of a lifetime, the impact of increasing pathophysiologic changes and environmental susceptibility lead to an irreversible disease process (Holgate, 2011).

Asthma is a complex disease process that involves numerous inflammatory and structural cells as well as mediators that lead to the disorder's effects. Mast cells, macrophages, T lymphocytes, neutrophils, and eosinophils all play a key role in the inflammation of asthma. When activated, mast cells release several chemicals called *mediators*. These chemicals, which include histamine, bradykinin, prostanoids, cytokines, leukotrienes, and other mediators, perpetuate the inflammatory response, causing increased blood flow, vasoconstriction, fluid leak from the vasculature, attraction of white blood cells to the area, mucus secretion, and bronchoconstriction (Expert Panel Report 3, 2007; Global Initiative for Asthma [GINA], 2010).

During acute exacerbations of asthma, bronchial smooth muscle contraction or bronchoconstriction occurs quickly to narrow the airway in response to an exposure. Acute bronchoconstriction due to allergens results from an immunoglobulin E (IgE)-dependent release of mediators from mast cells; these mediators include histamine, tryptase, leukotrienes, and prostaglandins that directly contract the airway. There are also non–IgE-mediated responses and proinflammatory cytokines (Expert Panel Report 3, 2007). In addition, alpha- and beta$_2$-adrenergic receptors of the sympathetic nervous system located in the bronchi play a role. When the alpha-adrenergic receptors are stimulated, bronchoconstriction occurs. The balance between alpha- and beta$_2$-adrenergic receptors is controlled primarily by cAMP. Beta$_2$-adrenergic stimulation results in increased levels of cAMP, which inhibits the release of chemical mediators and causes bronchodilation.

As asthma becomes more persistent, the inflammation progresses and other factors may be involved in airflow limitation. These include airway edema, mucus hypersecretion, and the formation of mucus plugs. In addition, airway "remodeling" (i.e., structural changes) may occur in response to chronic inflammation, causing further airway narrowing.

Clinical Manifestations

The three most common symptoms of asthma are cough, dyspnea, and wheezing. In some instances, cough may be the only symptom. An asthma attack often occurs at night or early in the morning, possibly because of circadian variations that influence airway receptor thresholds.

An asthma exacerbation may begin abruptly but most frequently is preceded by increasing symptoms over the previous few days. There is cough, with or without mucus production. At times, the mucus is so tightly wedged in the narrowed airway that the patient cannot cough it up. There may be generalized wheezing (the sound of airflow through narrowed airways), first on expiration and then possibly during inspiration as well. Generalized chest tightness and dyspnea occur. Expiration requires effort and becomes prolonged. As the exacerbation progresses, diaphoresis, tachycardia, and a widened pulse pressure may occur along with hypoxemia and central cyanosis (a late sign of poor oxygenation). Although severe, life-threatening hypoxemia can occur in asthma, it is relatively uncommon. The hypoxemia is secondary to a

ventilation–perfusion mismatch and readily responds to supplemental oxygenation.

Symptoms of exercise-induced asthma include maximal symptoms during exercise, absence of nocturnal symptoms, and sometimes only a description of a "choking" sensation during exercise.

Assessment and Diagnostic Findings

To establish the diagnosis, the clinician must determine that episodic symptoms of airflow obstruction are present, airflow is at least partially reversible, and other causes have been excluded. A positive family history and environmental factors, including seasonal changes, high pollen counts, mold, pet dander, climate changes (particularly cold air), and air pollution, are primarily associated with asthma. In addition, asthma is associated with a variety of occupation-related chemicals, foods, and compounds. Comorbid conditions that may accompany asthma include gastroesophageal reflux disease, drug-induced asthma, and allergic bronchopulmonary aspergillosis. Other possible allergic reactions that may accompany asthma include eczema, rashes, and temporary edema. Specific questions in the assessment that may help to evaluate the individual's asthma control include:

- Has your asthma awakened you at night or in the early morning?
- Have you needed your quick-acting relief medication more than usual?
- Have you needed unscheduled care for your asthma—a call to the physician's office, office visit, emergency department?
- Has your asthma impacted your normal activities at school/work/sports?

During acute episodes, sputum and blood tests may disclose eosinophilia (elevated levels of eosinophils). Serum levels of IgE may be elevated if allergy is present. Arterial blood gas analysis and pulse oximetry reveal hypoxemia during acute attacks. Initially, hypocapnia and respiratory alkalosis are present. As the patient's condition worsens and he or she becomes more fatigued, the PaCO$_2$ may increase. Because carbon dioxide is 20 times more diffusible than oxygen, it is rare for PaCO$_2$ to be normal or elevated in a person who is breathing very rapidly.

Quality and Safety Nursing Alert

Normal PaCO$_2$ during an asthma attack may be a signal of impending respiratory failure.

During an exacerbation, the FEV$_1$ and FVC are markedly decreased but improve with bronchodilator administration (demonstrating reversibility). Pulmonary function is usually normal between exacerbations. The occurrence of a severe, continuous reaction is referred to as status asthmaticus and is considered life threatening (see later discussion).

Asthma severity is considered in the selection of the initial type, amount, and schedule of treatment (Expert Panel Report 3, 2007; GINA, 2010). Disease severity is classified by current impairment and future risk of adverse events. Impairment is defined by the following factors: nighttime awakenings, the need for short-acting bronchodilators for symptom relief, work/school days missed, ability to engage in normal activities, and quality of life. Lung function is evaluated by spirometry. Assessment of risk of future adverse events is evaluated by numbers of exacerbations, the need for ED care or hospitalizations in the past year, demographic data (gender, ethnicity, nonuse of prescribed inhaled corticosteroid therapy, existing smoking), psychosocial factors and attitudes, and beliefs about taking medication (Expert Panel Report 3, 2007).

Prevention

Patients with recurrent asthma should undergo tests to identify the substances that precipitate the symptoms. Possible causes are dust, dust mites, roaches, certain types of cloth, pets, horses, detergents, soaps, certain foods, molds, and pollens. If the attacks are seasonal, pollens can be strongly suspected. Patients are instructed to avoid the causative agents whenever possible. Knowledge is the key to quality asthma care. Evaluation of impairment and risk are primary methods that help ensure control.

Occupational asthma refers to asthma induced by exposure in the work environment to dusts, vapors, or fumes, with or without a preexisting diagnosis of asthma. An estimated 15% of new asthma cases in the United States are related to workplace exposures (Cowl, 2011). Work-related asthma should be part of the differential diagnosis of every case of adult-onset asthma. A detailed work history evaluation is key to identifying occupational asthma. Immediate treatment is aimed at removing or decreasing the exposure in the patient's environment and following the patient on an ongoing basis. Standard asthma medications may be prescribed to minimize bronchoconstriction and airway inflammation. In certain cases, patients may be impaired or disabled from the disease. Compensation systems are in place to protect a worker; however, these systems are often slow and complex to navigate (Cowl, 2011).

Complications

Complications of asthma may include status asthmaticus, respiratory failure, pneumonia, and atelectasis. Airway obstruction, particularly during acute asthmatic episodes, often results in hypoxemia, requiring the administration of oxygen and the monitoring of pulse oximetry and arterial blood gases. Fluids are administered because people with asthma are frequently dehydrated from diaphoresis and insensible fluid loss with hyperventilation.

Medical Management

Immediate intervention may be necessary because continuing and progressive dyspnea leads to increased anxiety, aggravating the situation. The Expert Panel 3 *Guidelines for the Diagnosis and Management of Asthma* (2007) and GINA (2010) recommendations are based on the concept of severity and control of asthma along with the domains of impairment and risk as keys to improving care. Primary treatment concerns are impairment of lung function and normal life and risk of exacerbations, decline in lung function, and adverse effects from medications (Expert Panel Report 3, 2007).

Pharmacologic Therapy

Figure 24-7 shows the pharmacologic treatment of asthma using a stepwise approach. There are two general classes of asthma medications: quick-relief medications for immediate treatment of asthma symptoms and exacerbations and long-acting medications to achieve and maintain control of persistent asthma (Tables 24-4 and 24-5). Because the underlying pathology of asthma is inflammation, control of persistent asthma is accomplished primarily with regular use of anti-inflammatory medications. These medications have systemic side effects when used over the long term. The route of choice for administration of these medications is an MDI or other type of inhaler, because it allows for topical administration (see Chart 24-4 and Table 24-2).

Quick-Relief Medications

Short-acting beta₂-adrenergic agonists (albuterol [AccuNeb, Proventil, Ventolin], levalbuterol [Xopenex HFA], and pirbuterol [Maxair]) are the medications of choice for relief of acute symptoms and prevention of exercise-induced asthma. They are used to relax smooth muscle.

Anticholinergics (e.g., ipratropium [Atrovent]) inhibit muscarinic cholinergic receptors and reduce intrinsic vagal tone of the airway. These may be used in patients who do not tolerate short-acting beta₂-adrenergic agonists.

Long-Acting Control Medications

Corticosteroids are the most potent and effective anti-inflammatory medications currently available. They are broadly effective in alleviating symptoms, improving airway function, and decreasing peak flow variability. Initially, an inhaled form is used. A spacer should be used with inhaled corticosteroids, and patients should rinse their mouth after administration to prevent thrush, a common complication associated with use of inhaled corticosteroids. A systemic preparation may be used to gain rapid control of the disease; to manage severe, persistent asthma; to treat moderate to severe exacerbations; to accelerate recovery; and to prevent recurrence.

Cromolyn sodium (Crolom, NasalCrom) and *nedocromil* (Alocril, Tilade) are mild to moderate anti-inflammatory agents and are considered alternative medications for treatment. These medications stabilize mast cells. They also are effective on a prophylactic basis to prevent exercise-induced asthma or in unavoidable exposure to known triggers. These medications are contraindicated in acute asthma exacerbations.

Long-acting beta₂-adrenergic agonists are used with anti-inflammatory medications to control asthma symptoms, particularly those that occur during the night. These agents are also effective in the prevention of exercise-induced asthma. Long-acting beta₂-adrenergic agonists are not indicated for immediate relief of symptoms. Theophylline (Slo-Bid, Theo-Dur) is a mild to moderate bronchodilator that is usually used in addition to inhaled corticosteroids, mainly for relief of nighttime asthma symptoms. Salmeterol (Serevent Diskus) and formoterol (Foradil Aerolizer) have duration of bronchodilation of at least 12 hours. They are used with other medications in long-term control of asthma.

Leukotriene modifiers (inhibitors), or *antileukotrienes*, are a class of medications that include montelukast (Singulair), zafirlukast (Accolate), and zileuton (Zyflo). Leukotrienes, which are synthesized from membrane phospholipids through a cascade of enzymes, are potent bronchoconstrictors that also dilate blood vessels and alter permeability. Leukotriene inhibitors act either by interfering with leukotriene synthesis

(text continues on page 643)

Intermittent Asthma	**Persistent Asthma: Daily Medication** Consult with asthma specialist if step 4 care or higher is required. Consider consultation at step 3.

Step 1

Preferred:

SABA PRN

Step 2

Preferred:
Low-dose ICS

Alternative:

Cromolyn, LTRA, nedocromil, or theophylline

Step 3

Preferred:
Low-dose ICS + LABA
OR
Medium-dose ICS

Alternative:
Low-dose ICS + either LTRA, theophylline, or zileuton

Step 4

Preferred:
Medium-dose ICS + LABA

Alternative:
Medium-dose ICS + either LTRA, theophylline, or zileuton

Step 5

Preferred:
High-dose ICS + LABA

AND

Consider omalizumab for patients who have allergies

Step 6

Preferred:
High-dose ICS + LABA + oral corticosteroid

AND

Consider omalizumab for patients who have allergies

Step up if needed

(first, check adherence, environmental control, and comorbid conditions)

Assess control

Step down if possible

(and asthma is well controlled at least 3 months)

Each step: Patient education, environmental control, and management of comorbidities.
Steps 2-4: Consider subcutaneous allergen immunotherapy for patients who have allergic asthma (see notes).

Quick-Relief Medication for All Patients

- SABA as needed for symptoms. Intensity of treatment depends on severity of symptoms: up to 3 treatments at 20-minute intervals as needed. Short course of oral systemic corticosteroids may be needed.
- Use of SABA >2 days a week for symptom relief (not prevention of EIB) generally indicates inadequate control and the need to step up treatment.

Key: **Alphabetical order is used when more than one treatment option is listed within either preferred or alternative therapy.** EIB, exercise-induced bronchospasm; ICS, inhaled corticosteroid; LABA, inhaled long-acting beta$_2$-agonist; LTRA, leukotriene receptor antagonist; SABA, inhaled short-acting beta$_2$-agonist

Notes:

- The stepwise approach is meant to assist, not replace, the clinical decision making required to meet individual patient needs.

- If alternative treatment is used and response is inadequate, discontinue it and use the preferred treatment before stepping up.

- Zileuton is a less desirable alternative due to limited studies as adjunctive therapy and the need to monitor liver function. Theophylline requires monitoring of serum concentration levels.

- In step 6, before oral systemic corticosteroids are introduced, a trial of high-dose ICS + LABA + either LTRA, theophylline, or zileuton may be considered, although this approach has not been studied in clinical trials.

- Steps 1, 2, and 3 preferred therapies are based on evidence A; step 3 alternative therapy is based on evidence A for LTRA, evidence B for theophylline, and evidence D for zileuton. Step 4 preferred therapy is based on evidence B, and alternative therapy is based on evidence B for LTRA and theophylline and evidence D for zileuton. Step 5 preferred therapy is based on evidence B. Step 6 preferred therapy is based on (EPR—2 1997) and evidence B for omalizumab.

- Immunotherapy for steps 2-4 is based on evidence B for house-dust mites, animal danders, and pollens; evidence is weak or lacking for molds and cockroaches. Evidence is strongest for immunotherapy with single allergens. The role of allergy in asthma is greater in children than in adults.

- Clinicians who administer immunotherapy or omalizumab should be prepared and equipped to identify and treat anaphylaxis that may occur.

FIGURE 24-7 • Stepwise approach for managing asthma in youths 12 years and older and adults. Redrawn from Expert Panel Report 3. (2007). *Guidelines for the diagnosis and management of asthma* (p. 343). NIH Publication No. 08-5846. National Asthma Education and Prevention Program. Summary Report. Bethesda, MD: U.S. Department of Health and Human Services, National Heart, Lung, and Blood Institute.

TABLE 24-4   Long-Term Medications for Treatment of Asthma (Controller Medications)

Medication	Indications/Mechanisms	Potential Adverse Effects	Nursing Considerations
Inhaled Corticosteroids beclomethasone dipropionate (QVAR) beclomethasone (Beconase-AQ) budesonide (Pulmicort) ciclesonide (Alvesco) flunisolide (AeroBid) fluticasone (Flovent) mometasone furoate (Asmanex) triamcinolone acetonide (Azmacort)	*Indications* Long-term prevention of symptoms; suppression, control, and reversal of inflammation Reduce need for oral corticosteroid *Mechanisms* Anti-inflammatory; block late reaction to allergen and reduce airway hyperresponsiveness Inhibit cytokine production, adhesion protein activation, and inflammatory cell migration and activation; reverse beta-2 receptor down-regulation; inhibit microvascular leakage	Cough, dysphonia, oral thrush (candidiasis), headache In high doses, systemic effects may occur (e.g., adrenal suppression, osteoporosis, skin thinning, and easy bruising).	Instruct patient in correct use of MDI and use of spacer/holding chamber devices. Instruct patient to rinse mouth after inhalation to reduce local side effects.
Systemic Corticosteroids methylprednisolone (Medrol) prednisolone (Prelone) prednisone (Deltasone, Orasone)	*Indications* For short-term (3–10 d) "burst": to gain prompt control of inadequately controlled persistent asthma For long-term prevention of symptoms in severe persistent asthma: suppression, control, and reversal of inflammation *Mechanisms* Same as inhaled corticosteroids.	*Short-term use:* reversible abnormalities in glucose metabolism, increased appetite, fluid retention, weight gain, mood alteration, hypertension, peptic ulcer, and rarely aseptic necrosis *Long-term use:* adrenal axis suppression, growth suppression, dermal thinning, hypertension, diabetes, Cushing syndrome, cataracts, muscle weakness, and, in rare instances, impaired immune function Consideration should be given to comorbidities that could be worsened by systemic corticosteroids.	Instruct patient about possible side effects and the importance of taking the medication as prescribed (usually a single dose in the morning daily or on an alternate-day schedule, which may produce less adrenal suppression).
Long-Acting Beta₂-Agonists *Inhaled* salmeterol (Serevent Diskus) formoterol (Foradil Aerolizer)	*Indications* Long-term prevention of symptoms, added to ICS Prevention of exercise-induced bronchospasm *Mechanisms* Bronchodilation; smooth muscle relaxation following adenylate cyclase activation and increase in cAMP, producing functional antagonism of bronchoconstriction Compared to SABA, salmeterol (but not formoterol) has slower onset of action (15–30 min). Both salmeterol and formoterol have longer duration (>12 h) compared to SABA.	Should *not* be used to treat acute symptoms or exacerbations Decreased protection against exercise-induced bronchospasm may occur with regular use. Tachycardia, muscle tremor, hypokalemia, ECG changes with overdose. A diminished bronchoprotective effect may occur within 1 week of chronic therapy. Potential risk of uncommon, severe, life-threatening, or fatal exacerbation	Reinforce to patient that these medications should *not* be used to treat acute asthma symptoms or exacerbations. Instruct patient about correct use of MDI or aerolizer inhaler.
Oral albuterol (Proventil) sustained release		Inhaled route is preferred to oral route because LABAs are longer acting and have fewer side effects than oral sustained-release agents.	
Methylxanthines theophylline (Slo-Bid, Theo-Dur) sustained-release tablets and capsules	*Indications* Long-term control and prevention of symptoms in mild persistent asthma or as adjunctive with ICS, in moderate or persistent asthma	Dose-related acute toxicities include tachycardia, nausea and vomiting, tachyarrhythmias (SVT), central nervous system stimulation, headache, seizures, hematemesis, hyperglycemia, and hypokalemia.	Maintain steady-state serum concentrations between 5 and 15 mcg/mL.

(continues on page 642)

TABLE 24-4 Long-Term Medications for Treatment of Asthma (Controller Medications) (continued)

Medication	Indications/Mechanisms	Potential Adverse Effects	Nursing Considerations
	Mechanisms Bronchodilation; smooth muscle relaxation from phosphodiesterase inhibition and possibly adenosine antagonism May affect eosinophilic infiltration into bronchial mucosa as well as decreased T-lymphocyte numbers in epithelium Increases diaphragm contractility and mucociliary clearance	Adverse effects at usual therapeutic doses include insomnia, gastric upset, aggravation of ulcer or reflux, and difficulty in urination in older males who have prostatism. Not generally recommended for exacerbations. There is minimal evidence for added benefit to optimal doses of SABA. Serum concentration monitoring is mandatory. Available as sustained-release tablets and capsules	Be aware that absorption and metabolism may be affected by numerous factors that can produce significant changes in steady-state serum theophylline concentrations. Instruct patients to discontinue if they experience toxicity. Inform patients about the importance of blood tests to monitor serum concentration. Instruct patient to check with primary provider before taking any new medication.
Combined Medication			
fluticasone/salmeterol (Advair)	*DPI* 100 mcg/50 mcg 250 mcg/50 mcg 500 mcg/50 mcg *HFA* 45 mcg/21 mcg 115 mcg/21 mcg 230 mcg/21 mcg	Lowest dose of DPI or HFA used for patients whose asthma is not controlled on low- to medium-dose ICS Higher doses of DPI or HFA used for patients whose asthma is not controlled on medium- to high-dose ICS	
budesonide/formoterol (Symbicort)	*HFA MDI* 80 mcg/4.5 mcg 160 mcg/4.5 mcg	Lower dose used for patients who have asthma not controlled on low- to medium-dose ICS Higher dose used for patients who have asthma not controlled on medium- to high-dose ICS	
Cromolyn and Nedocromil			
Cromolyn sodium (Crolom, NasalCrom, Intal) nedocromil (Alocril, Tilade)	*Indications* Long-term prevention of symptoms in mild persistent asthma; may modify inflammation Preventive treatment prior to exposure to exercise or known allergen *Mechanisms* Anti-inflammatory; blocks *early* and late reaction to allergen Stabilizes mast cell membranes and inhibits activation and release of mediators from eosinophils and epithelial cells Inhibits acute response to exercise, cold dry air, and SO$_2$	Cough and irritation 15%–20% of patients complain of an unpleasant taste from nedocromil. Dose of cromolyn by MDI may be inadequate to affect airway hyperresponsiveness. Nebulizer delivery may be preferred for some patients. Safety is the primary advantage of these agents. One dose before exercise or exposure to allergen provides effective prophylaxis for 1–2 h. Not as effective for exercise-induced bronchospasm as short-acting beta$_2$-agonist.	Inform patient that 4–6-wk trial may be needed to determine maximum benefit. Instruct patient about correct use of inhaler.
Leukotriene Modifiers			
Leukotriene Receptor Antagonists montelukast (Singulair)	*Mechanism* Selective competitive inhibitor of CysLT1 receptor *Indications* Long-term control and prevention of symptoms in mild persistent asthma for patients ≥1 y of age May also be used with ICS as combination therapy in moderate persistent asthma	May attenuate EIB in some patients, but less effective than ICS therapy LTRA + LABA should not be used as a substitute for ICS + LABA. No specific adverse effects have been identified. Available in tablets and granules.	Instruct patient to take at least 1 h before meals or 2 h after meals. Inform patient that zafirlukast can inhibit the metabolism of warfarin. INRs should be monitored if patient is taking both medications.
zafirlukast (Accolate)	Long-term control and prevention of symptoms in mild persistent asthma; may also be used with ICS as combination therapy in moderate persistent asthma	Cases of reversible hepatitis have been reported along with rare cases of irreversible hepatic failure resulting in death and liver transplantation. Available in tablets	Instruct patients to discontinue use if they experience signs and symptoms of liver dysfunction (right upper quadrant pain, pruritus, lethargy, jaundice, nausea), and to notify their primary provider.

Medication	Indications/Mechanisms	Potential Adverse Effects	Nursing Considerations
5-Lipoxygenase Inhibitor			
zileuton (Zyflo)	*Mechanism* Inhibits the production of leukotrienes from arachidonic acid, both LTB and the cysteinyl leukotrienes *Indications* Long-term control and prevention of symptoms in mild persistent asthma for patients May be used with ICS as combination therapy in moderate persistent asthma in patients	Elevation of liver enzymes has been reported. Limited case reports of reversible hepatitis and hyperbilirubinemia.	Inform patient that zileuton can inhibit the metabolism of warfarin and theophylline. Therefore, the doses of these medications should be monitored accordingly. Educate patient about the importance of monitoring medication levels and tests of liver function.
Immunomodulators			
omalizumab (Xolair)	*Indications* Long-term control and prevention of symptoms in adults with moderate or severe persistent allergic asthma inadequately controlled with ICS *Mechanisms* Monoclonal antibody (anti-IgE) that binds to circulating IgE, preventing it from binding to the high-affinity receptors on basophils and mast cells Decreases mast cell mediator release from allergen exposure	Administered by subcutaneous injection Anaphylaxis has been reported in 0.2% of treated patients. Pain, bruising, and skin reactions (itching, redness, stinging) at injection sites Dose is administered either every 2 or 4 wk and depends on the patient's body weight and IgE level before therapy. A maximum of 150 mg can be administered in 1 injection. Medication needs to be stored under refrigeration at 2–8°C (35.6–46.4°F). It is unknown if patients will develop significant antibody titers to the drug with long-term administration.	Monitor patients for allergic reactions or anaphylaxis following administration. Be prepared to initiate emergency treatment if anaphylaxis occurs. Instruct patient about signs and symptoms that indicate allergic reaction and immediate action to take. Remind patient to continue to take other medications prescribed for treatment of asthma.

MDI, metered-dose inhaler; ICS, inhaled corticosteroid; cAMP, cyclic 3′,5′-adenosine monophosphate; ECG, electrocardiogram; SABA, inhaled short-acting $beta_2$-agonist; LABA, long-acting $beta_2$-agonist; SVT, supraventricular tachycardia; DPI, dry powder inhaler; HFA, hydrofluoroalkane; SO_2, sulfur dioxide; CysLT1, cysteinyl leukotriene receptor 1; EIB, exercise-induced bronchospasm; LTRA, leukotriene receptor antagonist; INR, international normalized ratio; LTB, leukotriene B; IgE, immunoglobulin E.

or by blocking the receptors where leukotrienes exert their action. They may provide an alternative to inhaled corticosteroids for mild persistent asthma, or they may be added to a regimen of inhaled corticosteroids in more severe asthma to attain further control.

Immunomodulators prevent binding of IgE to the high-affinity receptors of basophils and mast cells. Omalizumab (Xolair) is a monoclonal antibody and may be used for patients with allergies and severe persistent asthma.

Numerous asthma biologic agents are in development. Most of these target a specific cell or mediator and may only be appropriate for a small subset of patients. The future of asthma may be stratification of specific pathway-selective phenotypes in patients; thus, treatment in the future may include individually tailored medications (Holgate, 2011; Szefler, 2011).

Management of Exacerbations

Asthma exacerbations are best managed by early treatment and education, including the use of written action plans as part of any overall effort to educate patients about self-management techniques, especially those with moderate or severe persistent asthma or with a history of severe exacerbations (Expert Panel Report 3, 2007). Quick-acting $beta_2$-adrenergic agonist medications are first used for prompt relief of airflow obstruction. Systemic corticosteroids may be necessary to decrease airway inflammation in patients who fail to respond to inhaled beta-adrenergic medications. In some patients, oxygen supplementation may be required to relieve hypoxemia associated with moderate to severe exacerbations. In addition, response to treatment may be monitored by serial measurements of lung function.

Evidence from clinical trials suggests that antibiotic therapy, whether administered routinely or when suspicion of bacterial infection is low, is not beneficial for asthma exacerbations (Expert Panel Report 3, 2007; GINA, 2010). Antibiotics may be appropriate in the treatment of acute asthma exacerbations in patients with comorbid conditions (e.g., fever and purulent sputum, evidence of pneumonia, suspected bacterial sinusitis).

Despite insufficient data supporting or refuting the benefits of using a written asthma action plan as compared to medical management alone, the 2007 Expert Panel Report 3 recommends the use of a written asthma action plan to educate patients about self-management (Fig. 24-8). Plans can be based on either symptoms or peak flow measurements. They should focus on daily management as well as the recognition and handling of worsening symptoms. Patient self-management and early recognition of problems lead to more efficient communication with health care providers about asthma exacerbations (Expert Panel Report 3, 2007).

TABLE 24-5 Quick-Relief Medications for Treatment of Asthma

Medication	Indications/Mechanisms	Potential Adverse Effects	Nursing Considerations
Inhaled Short-Acting Beta₂-Agonists			
albuterol (AccuNeb, Proventil HFA, Ventolin HFA) levalbuterol HFA (Xopenex HFA) metaproterenol sulfate (Alupent)	*Indications* Relief of acute symptoms; quick-relief medication Preventive treatment for exercise-induced bronchospasm *Mechanisms* Bronchodilation; binds to the beta-2 adrenergic receptor, producing smooth muscle relaxation and decreased bronchoconstriction	Tachycardia, muscle tremor, hypokalemia, increased lactic acid, headache, and hyperglycemia. Inhaled route causes few systematic adverse effects. Patients with preexisting cardiovascular disease, especially older adults, may have adverse cardiovascular reactions with inhaled therapy. Lack of effect or need for regular use indicates inadequate asthma control.	Instruct patient in correct use of inhaled agents and how to evaluate amount of remaining medication in metered-dose inhaler. Recommend periodic cleaning of device. Inform patient about possible adverse effects and need to inform primary provider about increased use of medication to control symptoms.
Anticholinergics			
ipratropium (Atrovent)	*Indications* Relief of acute bronchospasm *Mechanisms* Bronchodilation; inhibition of muscarinic cholinergic receptors Reduction of vagal tone of airways May decrease mucous gland secretion	Dryness of mouth and respiratory secretions; may cause increased wheezing in some patients Does not block exercise-induced bronchospasm Is not effective in long-term control of asthma	Instruct patient in correct use of inhaled agents. Ensure adequate fluid intake. Assess patient for hypersensitivity to atropine, soybeans, peanuts; glaucoma; prostatic hypertrophy.
Corticosteroids			
Systemic methylprednisolone (Medrol) prednisolone (Prelone) prednisone (Deltasone, Orasone)	*Indications* For moderate or severe exacerbations to prevent progression of exacerbation, reverse inflammation, speed recovery, and reduce rate of relapse *Mechanisms* Anti-inflammatory; block reaction to allergen and reduce hyperresponsiveness; inhibit cytokine production, adhesion protein activation, and inflammatory cell migration and activation; reverses beta-2 receptor down-regulation	Blood glucose abnormalities, increased appetite, fluid retention, weight gain, mood alteration, hypertension, peptic ulcer Consideration must be given to comorbidities that may be worsened by systemic corticosteroids.	Explain to patient that action is often rapid in onset, although resolution of symptoms may take 3–10 d. Instruct patient about possible side effects and the importance of taking the medication as prescribed.

HFA, hydrofluoroalkane; CFC, chlorofluorocarbon.

Peak Flow Monitoring

Peak flow meters measure the highest airflow during a forced expiration (Fig. 24-9). Daily peak flow monitoring is recommended for patients who meet one or more of the following criteria: have moderate or severe persistent asthma, have poor perception of changes in airflow or worsening symptoms, have unexplained response to environmental or occupational exposures, or at the discretion of the clinician and patient (Expert Panel Report 3, 2007). Peak flow monitoring helps measure asthma severity and, when added to symptom monitoring, indicates the current degree of asthma control.

The patient is instructed in the proper technique (Chart 24-6), particularly about using maximal effort; peak flows are monitored for 2 or 3 weeks after receipt of optimal asthma therapy. Then, the patient's "personal best" value is measured. The green (80% to 100% of personal best), yellow (60% to 80%), and red (less than 60%) zones are determined, and specific actions are delineated for each zone, enabling the patient to monitor and manipulate his or her own therapy after careful instruction (Expert Panel Report 3, 2007).

The Expert Panel Report 3 (2007) recommends that peak flow monitoring be considered an adjunct to asthma management for patients with moderate to severe persistent asthma. Peak flow monitoring plans may enhance communication between the patient and health care providers and may increase the patient's awareness of disease status and control.

Nursing Management

The immediate nursing care of patients with asthma depends on the severity of symptoms. The patient may be treated successfully as an outpatient if asthma symptoms are relatively mild or may require hospitalization and intensive care if symptoms are acute and severe. The patient and family are often frightened and anxious because of the patient's dyspnea. Therefore, a calm approach is an important aspect of care. The nurse assesses the patient's respiratory status by monitoring the severity of symptoms, breath sounds, peak flow, pulse oximetry, and vital signs.

The nurse generally performs the following interventions:
- Obtains a history of allergic reactions to medications before administering medications
- Identifies medications the patient is taking
- Administers medications as prescribed and monitors the patient's responses to those medications. These medications may include an antibiotic if the patient has an underlying respiratory infection.
- Administers fluids if the patient is dehydrated

Asthma Action Plan

For: _____   Doctor: _____   Date: _____
Doctor's Phone Number _____   Hospital/Emergency Department Phone Number _____

GREEN ZONE

Doing Well
- No cough, wheeze, chest tightness, or shortness of breath during the day or night
- Can do usual activites

And, if a peak flow meter is used,
Peak flow: more than _____
(80% or more of my best peak flow)
My best peak flow is: _____

Take these long-term-control medicines each day (include an anti-inflammatory).

Medicine	How much to take	When to take it

Identify and avoid and control the things that make your asthma worse, like (list here):

_____

Before exercise, if prescribed, take: ☐ 2 or ☐ 4 puffs _____   5 to 60 minutes before exercise

YELLOW ZONE

Asthma Is Getting Worse
- Cough, wheeze, chest tightness, or shortness of breath, or
- Waking at night due to asthma, or
- Can do some, but not all, usual activites

-Or-
Peak flow: _____ to _____
(50% to 79% of my best peak flow)

First ▷ Add: quick-relief medicine—and keep taking your GREEN ZONE medicine.

_____ ☐ 2 or ☐ 4 puffs, every 20 minutes for up to 1 hour
(short-acting beta₂-agonist) ☐ Nebulizer, once

If applicable, remove yourself from the thing that made your asthma worse.

Second ▷ If your symptoms (and peak flow, if used) return to GREEN ZONE after 1 hour of above treatment:
Continue monitoring to be sure you stay in the green zone.
-Or-
If your symptoms (and peak flow, if used) do not return to GREEN ZONE after 1 hour of above treatment:
☐ Take: _____ ☐ 2 or ☐ 4 puffs or ☐ Nebulizer
(short-acting beta₂-agonist)
☐ Add: _____ mg per day For _____ (3-10) days
(oral corticosteroid)
☐ Call the doctor: _____, ☐before/☐ within _____ hours after taking the oral corticosteroid.
(phone)

RED ZONE

Medical Alert!
- Very short of breath, or
- Quick-relief medicines have not helped, or
- Cannot do usual activites, or
- Symptoms are same or get worse after 24 hours in Yellow Zone

-Or-
Peak flow: less than _____
(50% of my best peak flow)

Take this medicine:

☐ _____ ☐ 4 or ☐6 puffs or ☐ Nebulizer
(short-acting beta₂-agonist)

☐ _____ mg
(oral corticosteroid)

Then call your doctor NOW. Go to the hospital or call an ambulance if:
- You are still in the red zone after 15 minutes AND
- You have not reached your doctor.

DANGER SIGNS
- Trouble walking and talking due to shortness of breath
- Lips or fingernails are blue

▷ ■ Take ☐4 or ☐6 puffs of your quick-relief medicine AND
■ Go to the hospital or call for an ambulance _____ NOW!
(phone)

FIGURE 24-8 • Asthma action plan. Redrawn from Expert Panel Report 3. (2007). *Guidelines for the diagnosis and management of asthma* (p. 119). NIH Publication No. 08-5846. National Asthma Education and Prevention Program. Bethesda, MD: U.S. Department of Health and Human Services, National Heart, Lung, and Blood Institute.

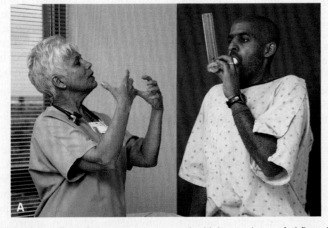
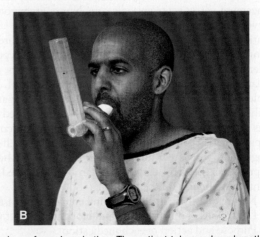

FIGURE 24-9 • Peak flow meters measure the highest volume of airflow during a forced expiration. The patient takes a deep breath and places lips around the mouthpiece (**A**), and then exhales hard and fast (**B**). Volume may be measured in color-coded zones: the green zone signifies 80% to 100% of personal best; yellow, 60% to 80%; and red, less than 60%. If peak flow falls below the red zone, the patient should take the appropriate actions prescribed by his or her primary provider.

Chart 24-6	HOME CARE CHECKLIST
	Use of Peak Flow Meter

At the completion of home care instruction, the patient or caregiver will be able to:	PATIENT	CAREGIVER
• Describe the rationale for using a peak flow meter in asthma management.	✔	✔
• Explain how peak flow monitoring is used along with symptoms to determine severity of asthma.	✔	✔
• Demonstrate steps for using the peak flow meter correctly.	✔	
• Move the indicator to the bottom of the numbered scale.	✔	
• Stand up.	✔	
• Take a deep breath, and fill the lungs completely.	✔	
• Place mouthpiece in mouth, and close lips around mouthpiece. (Do not put tongue inside opening.)	✔	
• Blow out hard and fast with a single blow.	✔	
• Record the number achieved on the indicator. If patient coughs or a mistake is made in the process, do it again.	✔	
• Repeat steps 1–5 two more times, and write the highest number in the asthma diary.	✔	
• Explain how to determine the "personal best" peak flow reading.	✔	✔
• Describe the significance of the color zones for peak flow monitoring.	✔	✔
• Demonstrate how to clean the peak flow meter.	✔	✔
• Discuss how and when to contact the primary provider about changes or decreases in peak flow values.	✔	✔

If the patient requires intubation because of acute respiratory failure, the nurse assists with the intubation procedure, continues close monitoring of the patient, and keeps the patient and family informed about procedures. (See Chapter 21 for discussion of intubation and mechanical ventilation.) (Visit thePoint to view a Clinical Simulation Case Study of Nursing Management of the Adult with Asthma.)

Promoting Home and Community-Based Care

Educating Patients About Self-Care

Implementation of basic asthma management principles at the community level is a major challenge. Strategies include education of health care providers, establishment of programs for asthma education (for patients and providers), the use of outpatient follow-up care for patients, and a focus on chronic management versus acute episodic care. Nurses are pivotal to achievement of these objectives.

Patient education is a critical component of care for patients with asthma. Multiple inhalers, different types of inhalers, antiallergy therapy, antireflux medications, and avoidance measures are essential for long-term control. This complex therapy requires a partnership between the patient and the health care providers to determine the desired outcomes and to formulate a plan to achieve those outcomes. The patient then carries out daily therapy as part of self-care management, with input and guidance by his or her health care providers. Before a partnership can be established, the patient must understand the following:

- Nature of asthma as a chronic inflammatory disease
- Definitions of inflammation and bronchoconstriction
- Purpose and action of each medication
- Triggers to avoid and how to avoid them
- Proper inhalation technique
- How to perform peak flow monitoring (see Chart 24-6)

- How to implement an asthma action plan (see Fig. 24-8)
- When to seek assistance, and how to do so

An assortment of excellent educational materials is available from the NHLBI and other sources (GINA, 2010). The nurse should obtain current educational materials for the patient based on the patient's diagnosis, causative factors, educational level, and cultural background. If a patient has a coexisting sensory impairment (i.e., vision loss or hearing impairment), materials should be provided in an alternative format.

Continuing Care

Nurses who have contact with patients in the hospital, clinic, school, or office use the opportunity to assess the patient's respiratory status and ability to manage self-care to prevent serious exacerbations. Nurses emphasize adherence to the prescribed therapy, preventive measures, and the need to keep follow-up appointments with health care providers. Home visits to assess the home environment for allergens may be indicated for patients with recurrent exacerbations. Nurses refer patients to community support groups. In addition, nurses remind patients and families about the importance of health promotion strategies and recommended health screening.

Status Asthmaticus

An asthma exacerbation can range from mild to severe with potential respiratory arrest (GINA, 2010). The term *status asthmaticus* is sometimes used to describe rapid onset, severe, and persistent asthma that does not respond to conventional therapy. The attacks can occur with little or no warning and can progress rapidly to asphyxiation. Infection, anxiety, nebulizer abuse, dehydration, increased adrenergic blockage, and nonspecific irritants may contribute to these episodes. An acute episode may be precipitated by hypersensitivity to aspirin.

Pathophysiology

The basic characteristics of asthma (inflammation of bronchial mucosa, constriction of the bronchiolar smooth muscle, and thickened secretions) decrease the diameter of the bronchi and occur in status asthmaticus. The most common scenario is severe bronchospasm, with mucus plugging leading to asphyxia. A ventilation–perfusion abnormality results in hypoxemia. There is a reduced PaO_2 and initial respiratory alkalosis, with a decreased $PaCO_2$ and an increased pH. As status asthmaticus worsens, the $PaCO_2$ increases and the pH decreases, reflecting respiratory acidosis.

Concept Mastery Alert

Understanding the sequence of the pathophysiologic processes in status asthmaticus is important for understanding assessment findings. Respiratory *alkalosis* occurs initially because the patient hyperventilates and $PaCO_2$ decreases. As the condition continues, air becomes trapped in the narrowed airways and carbon dioxide is retained, leading to respiratory *acidosis*.

Clinical Manifestations

The clinical manifestations are the same as those seen in severe asthma; signs and symptoms include labored breathing, prolonged exhalation, engorged neck veins, and wheezing. However, the extent of wheezing does not indicate the severity of the attack. As the obstruction worsens, the wheezing may disappear; this is frequently a sign of impending respiratory failure.

Assessment and Diagnostic Findings

The severity of an exacerbation may be evaluated by a general assessment of the patient (degree of breathlessness, ability to talk, positioning of patient, level of alertness or cognitive function), physical assessment (respiratory rate, the use of accessory muscles, presence of central cyanosis, auscultatory findings, pulse, and pulsus paradoxus), and laboratory evaluation (peak expiratory flow after a bronchodilator, PaO_2 and $PaCO_2$, and pulse oximetry). Pulmonary function studies are the most accurate means of assessing an acute, severe airway obstruction. Arterial blood gas measurement and/or pulse oximetry are obtained if the patient cannot perform pulmonary function maneuvers because of severe obstruction or fatigue, or if the patient does not respond to treatment. Respiratory alkalosis (low $PaCO_2$) is the most common finding in patients with an ongoing asthma exacerbation and is due to hyperventilation.

Quality and Safety Nursing Alert

In status asthmaticus, increasing $PaCO_2$ (to normal levels or levels indicating respiratory acidosis) is a danger sign signifying impending respiratory failure.

Medical Management

Close monitoring of the patient and objective reevaluation for response to therapy are key in status asthmaticus. In the emergency setting, the patient is treated initially with a short-acting beta₂-adrenergic agonist and subsequently a short course of systemic corticosteroids, especially if the patient does not respond to the short-acting beta₂-adrenergic agonist. Corticosteroids are critical in the therapy of status asthmaticus and are used to decrease the intense airway inflammation and swelling. Short-acting inhaled beta₂-adrenergic agonists provide the most rapid relief from bronchospasm. An MDI with or without a spacer may be used for nebulization of the medications. The patient usually requires supplemental oxygen and IV fluids for hydration. Oxygen therapy is initiated to treat dyspnea, central cyanosis, and hypoxemia. High-flow supplemental oxygen is best delivered using a partial or complete nonrebreathing mask. Sedatives are contraindicated. Magnesium sulfate, a calcium antagonist, may be administered to induce smooth muscle relaxation; the magnesium can relax smooth muscle and hence cause bronchodilation by competing with calcium at calcium-mediated smooth muscle binding sites. Adverse effects of magnesium sulfate may include facial warmth, flushing, tingling, nausea, central nervous system depression, respiratory depression, and hypotension.

If there is no response to repeated treatments, hospitalization is required. Other criteria for hospitalization include poor pulmonary function test results and deteriorating blood gas levels (respiratory acidosis), which may indicate that the patient is tiring and will require mechanical ventilation. Most patients do not need mechanical ventilation, but it is used for patients in respiratory failure, for those who tire and are too fatigued by the attempt to breathe, and for those whose condition does not respond to initial treatment.

For a very select group of patients with uncontrolled severe asthma, bronchial thermoplasty may be considered. Bronchial thermoplasty is the first nondrug therapy for the treatment of severe, uncontrolled asthma. It consists of controlled radiofrequency heating of the central airways through a bronchoscope. The thermal energy reduces the amount of smooth muscle involved in bronchospasm and potentially decreases the severity and frequency of symptoms. This therapy is invasive and relatively new; therefore, only select centers have the ability to perform this procedure, and it should only be considered in a select group of patients (Thomson, Rubin, Niven, et al., 2011).

Death from asthma is associated with several risk factors, including the following (Expert Panel Report 3, 2007):

- Past history of severe exacerbation (e.g., intubation or intensive care unit admission)
- Two or more hospitalizations for asthma within the past year
- Three or more emergency care visits for asthma in the past year
- Hospitalization or emergency care visit for asthma in the past month
- Use of more than two canisters of short-acting beta-agonist inhalers per month
- Difficulty in perceiving asthma symptoms or severity of exacerbations
- Lack of written asthma action plan
- Concurrent cardiovascular disease, COPD, or chronic psychiatric disease
- Low socioeconomic status or inner-city residence
- Illicit drug use

Nursing Management

The main focus of nursing management is to actively assess the airway and the patient's response to treatment. The nurse should be prepared for the next intervention if the patient does not respond to treatment.

The nurse constantly monitors the patient for the first 12 to 24 hours, or until the severe exacerbation resolves. The nurse also assesses the patient's skin turgor for signs of dehydration. Fluid intake is essential to combat dehydration, to loosen secretions, and to facilitate expectoration. Nurses administer IV fluids as prescribed, up to 3 to 4 L/day, unless contraindicated. Blood pressure and cardiac rhythm should be monitored continuously during the acute phase and until the patient stabilizes and responds to therapy. The patient's energy needs to be conserved, and his or her room should be quiet and free of respiratory irritants, including flowers, tobacco smoke, perfumes, or odors of cleaning agents. Nonallergenic pillows should be used. Once the exacerbation is resolved, the factors that precipitated the exacerbation should be identified and strategies for their future avoidance implemented. In addition, the patient's medication plan should be reviewed.

Cystic Fibrosis

CF is the most common fatal autosomal recessive disease among the Caucasian population. A person must inherit a defective copy of the CF gene (one from each parent) to have CF. Each year, 1,000 new cases of CF are diagnosed, and more than 70% of patients are diagnosed by 2 years of age. Approximately 30,000 children and adults in the United States have CF, and there are 70,000 cases worldwide (Cystic Fibrosis Foundation [CFF], 2011). CF is found less frequently among Hispanic, Asian, and African Americans. CF was once considered a fatal childhood disease; however, the median expected survival age is now in the late 30s (CFF, 2011).

Although most patients are diagnosed by age 2 years, this disease may not be diagnosed until later in life (CFF, 2011). Respiratory symptoms are frequently the major manifestation of CF when it is diagnosed later in life. However, many patients will not demonstrate the classic symptoms of CF, which may potentially cause a diagnostic dilemma.

Pathophysiology

CF is caused by mutations or dysfunction in the protein cystic fibrosis transmembrane conductance regulator (CFTR), which normally transports chloride ions across epithelial cell membranes. Gene mutations affect transport of these ions, leading to CF, which is characterized by thick, viscous secretions in the lungs, pancreas, liver, intestine, and reproductive tract as well as increased salt content in sweat gland secretions. The most common mutation is deltaF508; however, more than 1,500 mutations have been identified (Warwick & Elston, 2011). The numerous mutations of the *CFTR* gene create multiple variations in the presentation and progression of the disease.

The ability to detect the common mutations of this gene allows for routine screening for CF and the detection of carriers of the disease. Genetic counseling is an important part of health care for couples at risk (see Chapter 8). People who are heterozygous for CF (i.e., have one defective gene and one normal gene) do not have the disease but can be carriers and pass the defective gene on to their children. If both parents are carriers, their risk of having a child with CF is one in four (25%) with each pregnancy. Genetic testing should be offered to adults with a positive family history of CF and to partners of people with CF who are planning a pregnancy or seeking prenatal counseling. Currently, genetic testing for CF is not recommended for the general population. The hallmark pathology of CF is bronchial mucus plugging, inflammation, and eventual bronchiectasis. Commonly, the bronchiectasis begins in the upper lobes and progresses to involve all lobes.

Clinical Manifestations

The pulmonary manifestations of CF include a productive cough, wheezing, hyperinflation of the lung fields on chest x-ray, and pulmonary function test results consistent with obstructive disease of the airways. Chronic respiratory inflammation and infection are caused by impaired mucus clearance. Colonization of the airways with pathogenic bacteria usually occurs early in life. *Staphylococcus aureus* and *H. influenzae* are common organisms during early childhood. As the disease progresses, *P. aeruginosa* is ultimately isolated from the sputum of most patients. Upper respiratory manifestations of the disease include sinusitis and nasal polyps.

Nonpulmonary manifestations include gastrointestinal problems (e.g., pancreatic insufficiency, recurrent abdominal pain, biliary cirrhosis, vitamin deficiencies, recurrent pancreatitis, and weight loss), CF-related diabetes, and genitourinary problems (male and female infertility). (See Chapter 50 for a discussion of pancreatitis.)

Assessment and Diagnostic Findings

The diagnosis of CF requires a clinical picture consistent with the CF phenotype and laboratory evidence of CFTR dysfunction. Key assessment findings include:

- Chronic sinopulmonary disease as manifested by chronic cough and sputum production, persistent infection consistent with typical CF pathogens, and x-ray evidence of bronchiectasis and chronic sinusitis, often with nasal polyps
- Gastrointestinal tract and nutritional abnormalities (pancreatic insufficiency, meconium ileus or distal intestinal obstruction syndrome, failure to thrive or chronic malnutrition)
- Male urogenital problems as manifested by congenital bilateral absence of the vas deferens and obstructive azoospermia

Medical Management

CF requires both acute and chronic therapy. Because chronic bacterial infection of the airways occurs in CF, control of infections is essential to treatment. For acute airway exacerbations, aggressive therapy involves airway clearance and antibiotics based on results of sputum cultures. The majority of patients are colonized with *P. aeruginosa*, and the duration of antibiotic treatment varies. The CFF states that there is insufficient evidence to recommend an optimal duration of treatment for an acute exacerbation of pulmonary disease (Flume, Mogayzel, Robinson, et al., 2010). In an acute exacerbation, airway clearance treatments may be used three to four times per day.

The therapeutic options for chronic disease management of CF have undergone tremendous changes. Cornerstones of treatment include airway clearance measures, the mucolytic dornase alfa, nebulized antibiotics, oral antibiotics, inhaled hypertonic saline, nutritional support, and exercise (Warwick & Elston, 2011).

Airway clearance is a key intervention, and various pulmonary techniques are used to enhance secretion clearance. Examples include manual postural drainage and chest physical therapy; high-frequency chest wall oscillation; autogenic drainage (a combination of breathing techniques at different lung volume levels to move the secretions to where they can be huff-coughed out); and other devices that assist in airway clearance, such as masks that generate positive expiratory pressure (PEP masks) and "flutter devices" (devices that provide an oscillatory expiratory pressure pattern with positive expiratory pressure and assist with expectoration of secretions).

Dornase alfa (Pulmozyme) is a nebulized medication administered to degrade the large amount of deoxyribonucleic acid (DNA) that accumulates within CF mucus. This agent helps decrease the viscosity of the sputum and promotes expectoration of secretions. It is recommended for patients with moderate to severe disease (severity of lung disease classification is based on predicted FEV_1 percentage) (Mogayzel & Flume, 2011).

Nebulized antibiotics are used for chronic colonization of the lung. Nebulization provides high intrapulmonary drug concentrations and minimal systemic absorption. Acute infections are treated with a variety of antibiotics. Such infections remain a major cause of mortality related to pulmonary exacerbations in adults with CF. Antibiotics such as the macrolide azithromycin (Zithromax) may be used (Warwick & Elston, 2011). Inhaled hypertonic saline may be used in the chronic treatment of CF. Inhalations increase hydration of the airway surface liquid in patients with CF and improve airway clearance. Regular inhalations have been shown to improve FEV_1, decrease frequency of pulmonary exacerbations, and improve quality of life (Warwick & Elston, 2011).

Nearly 90% of patients with CF have pancreatic exocrine insufficiency and require oral pancreatic enzyme supplementation with meals (Warwick & Elston, 2011). Given the fat malabsorption in CF and increased caloric needs due to the work of breathing, nutritional counseling and weight monitoring are extremely important. Supplements of fat-soluble vitamins A, D, E, and K are also used.

Other therapeutic measures may be necessary as well. Anti-inflammatory agents may be used to treat inflammatory response in the airways. The CFF states that there is insufficient evidence for the use of routine inhaled or oral corticosteroids. However, long-term use of nonsteroidal anti-inflammatory agents is recommended to slow the loss of lung function (Flume et al., 2010). Inhaled bronchodilators may be used in patients who have a significant bronchoconstrictive component as indicated by spirometry before and after bronchodilator therapy.

In clinical trials, several interventions are being studied for the treatment of CF. These include gene therapy, CFTR modulation, restoration of airway surface liquid, anti-inflammatories, and new antibiotics (CFF, 2011).

As the pulmonary deterioration advances, supplemental oxygen is used to treat the progressive hypoxemia that occurs with CF. It helps correct the hypoxemia and may minimize the complications seen with chronic hypoxemia (pulmonary hypertension). Lung transplantation is an option for a small, selected population of patients with CF. A double-lung transplantation technique is used because of chronic infection of both lungs in end-stage CF. Because there is a long waiting list for lung transplants, many patients die while waiting for suitable lungs for transplantation.

Nursing Management

Nursing management is crucial to the interdisciplinary approach required for care of adults with CF. Nursing care includes helping patients manage pulmonary symptoms and prevent complications. Specific measures include strategies that promote removal of pulmonary secretions, chest physiotherapy (including postural drainage, chest percussion, and vibration), and breathing exercises (which are implemented and taught to the patient and family when the patient is very young). The patient is reminded of the need to reduce risk factors associated with respiratory infections (e.g., exposure to crowds or to people with known infections). In addition, the patient is taught the early signs and symptoms of respiratory infection and disease progression that indicate the need to notify a primary provider.

The nurse emphasizes the importance of an adequate fluid and dietary intake to promote removal of secretions and to ensure an adequate nutritional status. Because CF is a lifelong disorder, patients often have learned to modify their daily activities to accommodate their symptoms and treatment modalities. As the disease progresses, periodic reassessment of the home environment may be warranted to identify modifications required to address changes in the patient's needs, increasing dyspnea and fatigue, and nonpulmonary symptoms.

As with any chronic disease, palliative care and end-of-life issues and concerns need to be addressed with the patient when warranted. For the patient whose disease is progressing and who is developing increasing hypoxemia, preferences for end-of-life care should be discussed, documented, and honored (see Chapter 16). Patients and family members require support as they face a shortened lifespan and an uncertain future.

Critical Thinking Exercises

1 **PG** In the ED, a 63-year-old man tells the triage nurse that he has no insurance or doctor because he lost his job 3 years ago as a warehouse worker. He presents with a chief complaint of increased shortness of breath and a change in the quantity and color of his sputum. He says that he usually has little sputum in the morning and that it is clear, but in the last week it has become yellow in color, continues all day, and is difficult to cough out. He has become progressively short of breath over the past 5 years to the point where he could no longer work. He is dyspneic at rest while sitting on the examination table. He denies asthma, respiratory problems, allergies, and any occupational exposures. What are your focused priorities with this patient? For instance, what additional questions would you ask him? What are some of the physical examination findings you might observe or assess? What other tests might be ordered to continue to evaluate this patient and why? What resources might be appropriate for this patient before he leaves the hospital?

2 Allan, a 40-year-old man, presents to your clinic because of episodic shortness of breath. He has a full-time job in a body shop, which he started 16 months ago. He says that he can hear himself wheeze and has a dry cough at times. He says that he seems to get better over the weekend but gets progressively worse during the week. He recently had a 2-week vacation and felt great the whole time. His wife thinks that he just doesn't like his job. He has smoked two packs of cigarettes per day for more than 20 years but has tried to quit several times. His wife smokes as well. He thinks that his respiratory problems are due to smoking. Provide examples of open-ended questions that you might ask Allan to gain more information about his breathing problems. What potential nursing diagnoses come to mind, given his presentation? What educational interventions might be appropriate for Allan and why?

3 A 37-year-old black woman with a history of asthma presents to the ED with tachypnea and acute shortness of breath with audible wheezing. She says that she had taken her prescribed inhaler two times at home with no relief in symptoms. She called her doctor but could not get an appointment. She says she is scared and that she is going to die. Physical examination reveals tachycardia at 110 bpm and tachypnea at 40 breaths/min with signs of accessory muscle use. Auscultation reveals decreased breath sounds with inspiratory and expiratory wheezes. Her SaO_2 is 92% on room air. When you ask her what type of inhaler she uses, she cannot remember. She is given a nebulizer treatment with albuterol and normal saline × 2. Two hours later, her heart rate is 108 bpm, her respiratory rate is 24 breaths/min, and she is breathing more easily. The ED physician is ready to release her from the ED for follow-up by her primary provider. What type of education and resources would benefit this patient?

4 A 21-year-old male college student with CF is admitted to your unit from the ED. He obtains his routine CF care closer to his home, which is 200 miles away; he is a new patient to your hospital. He has become progressively short of breath over the past week, and his roommate brought him to the hospital because he "looked sick." In short and choppy phrases, the young man tells you that he is extremely short of breath and that it has been getting worse; he is having paroxysms of coughing. You note that the cough is productive, with thick, yellow sputum, and that he is febrile. His roommate says that he has not been following his usual routine of CF care (airway clearance and nebulized medications) for the past 2 weeks or so and that he thinks he has lost weight. What pathophysiology is associated with these signs and symptoms? What medical and nursing interventions might be used to decrease or alleviate these signs and symptoms? What is the strength of the evidence that supports these interventions? What members of the health care team would you consult and why?

Brunner Suite Resources

Explore these additional resources to enhance learning for this chapter:
- NCLEX-Style Questions and Other Resources on **thePoint**, http://thePoint.lww.com/Brunner13e
- Study Guide
- PrepU
- Clinical Handbook
- Handbook of Laboratory and Diagnostic Tests

References

*Asterisk indicates nursing research.

Books

American Association of Cardiovascular and Pulmonary Rehabilitation. (2011). *Guidelines for pulmonary rehabilitation programs* (4th ed.). Champaign, IL: Human Kinetics.

Expert Panel Report 3. (2007). *Guidelines for the diagnosis and management of asthma*. National Asthma Education and Prevention Program. NIH Publication No. 08-5846. Bethesda, MD: U.S. Department of Health and Human Services, National Heart, Lung, and Blood Institute.

Loscalzo, J. (2010). *Harrison's pulmonary and critical care medicine*. New York: McGraw-Hill.

National Heart, Lung, and Blood Institute. (2010). *Fact book fiscal year 2010*. Bethesda, MD: National Institutes of Health.

U.S. Department of Health and Human Services (HHS). (2010a). *How tobacco smoke causes disease: The biology and behavioral basis for smoking-attributable disease*. Rockville, MD: Author.

Journals and Electronic Documents

Asthma

Centers for Disease Control and Prevention. (2011a). *Fast stats sheet: Asthma*. Atlanta, GA: National Center for Health Statistics. Available at: www.cdc.gov/nchs/fastats/asthma.htm.

Centers for Disease Control and Prevention. (2011c). *Vital signs: Asthma in the US: Growing every year*. Atlanta, GA: National Center for Health Statistics. Available at: www.cdc.gov/VitalSigns/Asthma

Cowl, C. T. (2011). Occupational asthma: Review of assessment, treatment, and compensation. *Chest, 139*(3), 674–681.

Global Initiative for Asthma. (2010). *Global strategy for asthma management and prevention*. Available at: www.ginasthma.org

Holgate, S. T. (2011). Pathophysiology of asthma: What has our current understanding taught us about new therapeutic approaches? *Journal of Allergy and Clinical Immunology, 128*(3), 495–505.

Szefler, S. J. (2011). Advancing asthma care: The glass is only half full! *Journal of Allergy and Clinical Immunology, 128*(3), 485–494.

Thomson, N. C., Rubin, A. S., Niven, R. M., et al. (2011). Long-term (5 year) safety of bronchial thermoplasty: Asthma Intervention Research (AIR) trial. *BioMed Central. BMC Pulmonary Medicine, 11*(8), Available at: www.biomedcentral.com/1471-2466/11/8

Chronic Obstructive Pulmonary Disease

Akinbami, L. J., & Liu, X. (2011). *Chronic obstructive pulmonary disease among adults aged 18 and over in the United States, 1998-2009*. NCHS Data Brief No. 63. Hyattsville, MD: National Center for Health Statistics.

Berger, R. L., DeCamp, M. M., Criner, G. J., et al. (2010). Lung volume reduction therapies for advanced emphysema: An update. *Chest, 138*(2), 407–417.

Birnbaum, S. (2011). Pulmonary rehabilitation: A classic tune with a new beat, but is anyone listening? *Chest 139*(6), 1498–1502.

*Borge, C. R., Wahl, A. K., & Moum, T. (2011). Pain and quality of life with chronic obstructive pulmonary disease. *Heart and Lung, 40*(3), e90–e101.

Centers for Disease Control and Prevention. (2011b). *Pneumococcal polysaccharide vaccine (PPSV): CDC answers your questions*. Available at: www.cdc.gov/vaccines

Global Initiative for Chronic Obstructive Lung Disease. (2010). *Global strategy for the diagnosis, management and prevention of COPD*. Available at: www.goldcopd.org

Global Initiative for Chronic Obstructive Pulmonary Disease. (2011). *Global strategy for the diagnosis, management and prevention of COPD*. Available at: www.goldcopd.org

Heffner, J. E. (2011). Advance care planning in chronic obstructive pulmonary disease: Barriers and opportunities. *Current Opinion in Pulmonary Medicine, 17*(2), 103–109.

National Foundation for Infectious Diseases. (2010). *Pneumococcal disease: Hard to say it: Easy to get vaccinated.* Available at: www.nfid.org/

National Heart, Lung, and Blood Institute. (2011). *COPD awareness continues to rise, new NIH survey finds.* Available at: www.nhlbi.nih.gov/news/press-releases/2011/copd-awareness-continues-to-rise-new-nih-survey-finds.html

Niewoehner, D. E. (2010). Outpatient management of severe COPD. *New England Journal of Medicine, 362*(15), 1407–1416.

Nussbaumer-Ochsner, Y., & Rabe, K. (2011). Systemic manifestations of COPD. *Chest, 139*(1), 165–173.

Qaseem, A., Wilt, T. J., Weinberger, S. E., et al. (2011). Diagnosis and management of stable chronic obstructive pulmonary disease: A clinical practice guideline update from the American College of Physicians, American College of Chest Physicians, American Thoracic Society, and European Respiratory Society. *Annals of Internal Medicine, 155*(3), 179–191.

U.S. Department of Health and Human Services. (2010b). *Ending the tobacco epidemic: A tobacco control strategic action plan for the U.S. Department of Health and Human Services.* Washington, DC: Office of the Assistant Secretary for Health.

U.S. Food and Drug Administration. (2011). *FDA approves new drug to treat chronic obstructive pulmonary disease.* Available at: www.fda.gov/NewsEvents/Newsroom/PressAnnouncements/ucm244989.htm

Cystic Fibrosis
Cystic Fibrosis Foundation. (2011). About cystic fibrosis. Available at: www.cff.org/AboutCF/

Flume, P. A., Mogayzel, P. J., Robinson, K. A., et al. (2010). Cystic fibrosis pulmonary guidelines: Treatment of pulmonary exacerbations. *American Journal of Respiratory and Critical Care Medicine, 180*(3), 802–809.

Mogayzel, P. J., & Flume, P. A. (2011). Update in cystic fibrosis 2010. *American Journal of Respiratory and Critical Care Medicine, 183*(12), 1620–1624.

Warwick, G., & Elston C. (2011). Improving outcomes in patients with cystic fibrosis. *Practitioner, 255*(174), 29–32.

Resources

Agency for Healthcare Research and Quality (AHRQ), www.ahrq.gov

Alpha-1 Association, www.alpha1.org

American Academy of Allergy, Asthma, and Immunology (AAAAI), www.aaaai.org

American Association for Respiratory Care (AARC), www.aarc.org

American Association of Cardiovascular and Pulmonary Rehabilitation (AACVPR), www.aacvpr.org

American Cancer Society, www.cancer.org

American College of Chest Physicians (ACCP), www.chestnet.org

American Lung Association, www.lungusa.org

American Thoracic Society (ATS), www.thoracic.org

Centers for Disease Control and Prevention (CDC), www.cdc.gov

Cystic Fibrosis Foundation, www.cff.org

National Cancer Institute (NCI), cancer.gov

National Heart, Lung, and Blood Institute (NHLBI), www.nhlbi.nih.gov

U.S. Department of Health and Human Services (HHS), www.hhs.gov or www.healthfinder.gov

Cardiovascular and Circulatory Function

A PATIENT WHO HAS INTERMITTENT CLAUDICATION AND ULCERATION

Mr. Black, age 63 years, has a history of peripheral arterial occlusive disease (2 years), hypertension, hypercholesterolemia, type 2 diabetes, and smoking. He eats low-fat foods and has cut back on smoking to half a pack of cigarettes a day. His home-monitored blood glucose levels range from 180 to 215 mg/dL. Because he has severe calf pain after walking, he now walks only two blocks a day—one block from home and one block back. He now receives medical treatment for a nonhealing ulcer on the plantar aspect of his left foot. He questions why he is told that he should walk when it causes pain and wonders how it may affect the healing of his ulcer.

QSEN Competency Focus: *Evidence-Based Practice*

The complexities inherent in today's health care system challenge nurses to demonstrate integration of specific interdisciplinary core competencies. These competencies are aimed at ensuring the delivery of safe, quality patient care (Institute of Medicine, 2003). The concepts from the Quality and Safety Education for Nurses (QSEN) Institute (2012) provide a framework for the knowledge, skills, and attitudes (KSAs) required for nurses to demonstrate competency in these key areas, which include *patient-centered care, interdisciplinary teamwork and collaboration, evidence-based practice, quality improvement, safety,* and *informatics*.

Evidence-Based Practice Definition: Integrate best current evidence with clinical expertise and patient/family preferences and values for delivery of optimal health care.

RELEVANT PRE-LICENSURE KSAs	APPLICATION AND REFLECTION
Knowledge	
Discriminate between valid and invalid reasons for modifying evidence-based clinical practice based on clinical expertise or patient/family preferences.	What is the strength of the evidence that suggests that walking is therapeutic for patients with peripheral arterial occlusive disease? Is the pain that Mr. Black is experiencing a reason for him to stop walking? Identify the pathophysiologic relationships between his multiple comorbidities, the pain he experiences, and the presence of his nonhealing ulcer. How might his continued smoking, albeit less than it had been, also affect his disease processes?
Skills	
Consult with clinical experts before deciding to deviate from evidence-based protocols.	Identify members of the health care team you would consult with to help you craft the most appropriate, individualized plan of care for Mr. Black.
Attitudes	
Acknowledge own limitations in knowledge and clinical expertise before determining when to deviate from evidence-based best practices.	Reflect on the complexity of the interrelationships between Mr. Black's many comorbid conditions. Think about your own desire to relieve a patient's pain. How might your desire to make Mr. Black comfortable potentially hamper his odds of achieving his best outcomes?

Cronenwett, L., Sherwood, G., Barnsteiner, J., et al. (2007). Quality and safety education for nurses. *Nursing Outlook, 55*(3), 122–131.
Institute of Medicine. (2003). *Health professions education: A bridge to quality.* Washington, DC: National Academies Press.
QSEN Institute. (2012). *Competencies: Prelicensure KSAs.* Available at: qsen.org/competencies/pre-licensure-ksas

Read More About This Case

More information about this case study and the relationships between nursing diagnoses, interventions, and expected outcomes is available online. Visit thePoint for Applying Concepts From NANDA-I, NIC, and NOC.

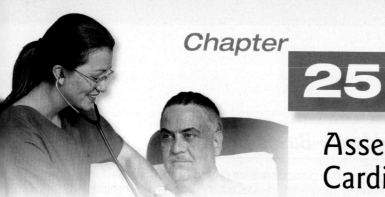

Chapter

25

Assessment of Cardiovascular Function

Glossary

acute coronary syndrome: refers to rupture of an atheromatous plaque in a diseased coronary artery, which rapidly form an obstructive thrombus

afterload: the amount of resistance to ejection of blood from the ventricle

apical impulse: impulse normally palpated at the fifth intercostal space, left midclavicular line; caused by contraction of the left ventricle; also called the *point of maximal impulse*

atrioventricular (AV) node: secondary pacemaker of the heart, located in the right atrial wall near the tricuspid valve

baroreceptors: nerve fibers located in the aortic arch and carotid arteries that are responsible for control of the blood pressure

cardiac catheterization: an invasive procedure used to measure cardiac chamber pressures and assess patency of the coronary arteries

cardiac conduction system: specialized heart cells strategically located throughout the heart that are responsible for methodically generating and coordinating the transmission of electrical impulses to the myocardial cells

cardiac output: amount of blood pumped by each ventricle in liters per minute

cardiac stress test: a test used to evaluate the functioning of the heart during a period of increased oxygen demand; test may be initiated by exercise or medications

contractility: ability of the cardiac muscle to shorten in response to an electrical impulse

depolarization: electrical activation of a cell caused by the influx of sodium into the cell while potassium exits the cell

diastole: period of ventricular relaxation resulting in ventricular filling

ejection fraction: percentage of the end-diastolic blood volume ejected from the ventricle with each heartbeat

hemodynamic monitoring: the use of pressure monitoring devices to directly measure cardiovascular function

hypertension: blood pressure that is persistently greater than 140/90 mm Hg

hypotension: a decrease in blood pressure to less than 100/60 mm Hg that compromises systemic perfusion

murmurs: sounds created by abnormal, turbulent flow of blood in the heart

myocardial ischemia: condition in which heart muscle cells receive less oxygen than needed

myocardium: muscle layer of the heart responsible for the pumping action of the heart

normal heart sounds: sounds produced when the valves close; normal heart sounds are S_1 (atrioventricular valves) and S_2 (semilunar valves)

opening snaps: abnormal diastolic sound generated during opening of a rigid atrioventricular valve leaflet

postural (orthostatic) hypotension: a significant drop in blood pressure (20 mm Hg systolic or more) after an upright posture is assumed

preload: degree of stretch of the cardiac muscle fibers at the end of diastole

pulmonary vascular resistance: resistance to blood flow out of the right ventricle created by the pulmonary circulatory system

pulse deficit: the difference between the apical and radial pulse rates

radioisotopes: unstable atoms that give off small amounts of energy in the form of gamma rays as they decay; used in cardiac nuclear medicine studies

repolarization: return of the cell to resting state, caused by reentry of potassium into the cell while sodium exits the cell

S_1: the first heart sound produced by closure of the atrioventricular (mitral and tricuspid) valves

S₂: the second heart sound produced by closure of the semilunar (aortic and pulmonic) valves

S₃: an abnormal heart sound detected early in diastole as resistance is met to blood entering either ventricle; most often due to volume overload associated with heart failure

S₄: an abnormal heart sound detected late in diastole as resistance is met to blood entering either ventricle during atrial contraction; most often caused by hypertrophy of the ventricle

sinoatrial (SA) node: primary pacemaker of the heart, located in the right atrium

stroke volume: amount of blood ejected from one of the ventricles per heartbeat

summation gallop: abnormal sounds created by the presence of an S₃ and S₄ during periods of tachycardia

systemic vascular resistance: resistance to blood flow out of the left ventricle created by the systemic circulatory system

systole: period of ventricular contraction resulting in ejection of blood from the ventricles into the pulmonary artery and aorta

systolic click: abnormal systolic sound created by the opening of a calcified aortic or pulmonic valve during ventricular contraction

telemetry: the process of continuous electrocardiographic monitoring by the transmission of radio waves from a battery-operated transmitter worn by the patient

---

More than 82 million Americans have one or more types of cardiovascular disease (CVD), including hypertension, coronary artery disease (CAD), heart failure (HF), stroke, and congenital cardiovascular defects (American Heart Association [AHA], 2012). Because of the prevalence of CVD, nurses practicing in any setting across the continuum of care, whether in the home, office, hospital, long-term care facility, or rehabilitation facility, must be able to assess the cardiovascular system. Key components of assessment include a health history, physical assessment, and monitoring of a variety of laboratory and diagnostic test results. This assessment provides the data necessary to identify nursing diagnoses, formulate an individualized plan of care, evaluate the response of the patient to the care provided, and revise the plan as needed.

Anatomic and Physiologic Overview

An understanding of the structure and function of the heart in health and in disease is essential to develop cardiovascular assessment skills.

Anatomy of the Heart

The heart is a hollow, muscular organ located in the center of the thorax, where it occupies the space between the lungs (mediastinum) and rests on the diaphragm. It weighs approximately 300 g (10.6 oz); the weight and size of the heart are influenced by age, gender, body weight, extent of physical exercise and conditioning, and heart disease. The heart pumps blood to the tissues, supplying them with oxygen and other nutrients.

The heart is composed of three layers (Fig. 25-1). The inner layer, or endocardium, consists of endothelial tissue and lines the inside of the heart and valves. The middle layer, or **myocardium**, is made up of muscle fibers and is responsible for the pumping action. The exterior layer of the heart is called the *epicardium*.

The heart is encased in a thin, fibrous sac called the *pericardium*, which is composed of two layers. Adhering to the epicardium is the visceral pericardium. Enveloping the visceral pericardium is the parietal pericardium, a tough fibrous tissue that attaches to the great vessels, diaphragm, sternum, and vertebral column and supports the heart in the mediastinum. The space between these two layers (pericardial space) is normally filled with about 20 mL of fluid, which lubricates the surface of the heart and reduces friction during systole.

Heart Chambers

The pumping action of the heart is accomplished by the rhythmic relaxation and contraction of the muscular walls of its two top chambers (atria) and two bottom chambers (ventricles). During the relaxation phase, called **diastole**, all four chambers relax simultaneously, which allows the ventricles to fill in preparation for contraction. Diastole is commonly referred to as the period of ventricular filling. **Systole** refers to the events in the heart during contraction of the atria and the ventricles. Unlike diastole, atrial and ventricular systole are not simultaneous events. Atrial systole occurs first, just at the end of diastole, followed by ventricular systole. This synchronization allows the ventricles to completely fill prior to ejection of blood from their chambers.

The right side of the heart, made up of the right atrium and right ventricle, distributes venous blood (deoxygenated blood) to the lungs via the pulmonary artery (pulmonary circulation) for oxygenation. The pulmonary artery is the only artery in the body that carries deoxygenated blood. The right atrium receives venous blood returning to the heart from the superior vena cava (head, neck, and upper extremities), inferior vena cava (trunk and lower extremities), and coronary sinus (coronary circulation). The left side of the heart, composed of the left atrium and left ventricle, distributes oxygenated blood to the remainder of the body via the aorta (systemic circulation). The left atrium receives oxygenated blood from the pulmonary circulation via four pulmonary veins. The flow of blood through the four heart chambers is shown in Figure 25-1.

The varying thicknesses of the atrial and ventricular walls relate to the workload required by each chamber. The myocardial layer of both atria is much thinner than that of the ventricles because there is little resistance as blood flows out of the atria and into the ventricles during diastole. In contrast, the ventricular walls are much thicker than the atrial walls. During ventricular systole, the right and left ventricles must overcome resistance to blood flow from the pulmonary and

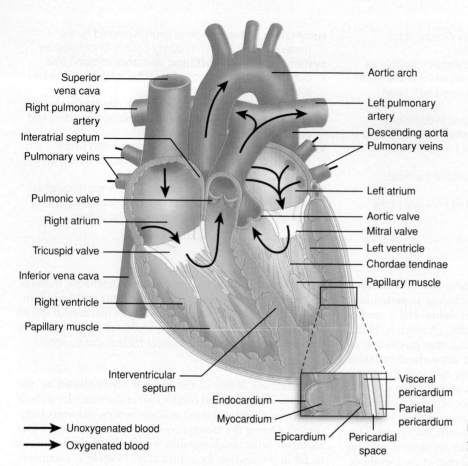

Superior
vena cava

Right pulmonary
artery

Interatrial septum

Pulmonary veins

Pulmonic valve

Right atrium

Tricuspid valve

Inferior vena cava

Right ventricle

Papillary muscle

Aortic arch

Left pulmonary
artery

Descending aorta
Pulmonary veins

Left atrium

Aortic valve
Mitral valve
Left ventricle
Chordae tendinae
Papillary muscle

Interventricular
septum

Endocardium
Myocardium

Epicardium   Pericardial
space

Visceral
pericardium

Parietal
pericardium

➡ Unoxygenated blood
➡ Oxygenated blood

FIGURE 25-1 • Structure of the heart. *Arrows* show course of blood flow through the heart chambers.

systemic circulatory systems, respectively. The left ventricle is two to three times more muscular than the right ventricle. It must overcome high aortic and arterial pressures, whereas the right ventricle contracts against a low-pressure system within the pulmonary arteries and capillaries (Woods, Froelicher, Motzer, et al., 2009). Figure 25-2 identifies the pressures in each of these areas.

The heart lies in a rotated position within the chest cavity. The right ventricle lies anteriorly (just beneath the sternum), and the left ventricle is situated posteriorly. As a result of this close proximity to the chest wall, the pulsation created during normal ventricular contraction, called the **apical impulse** (also called the *point of maximal impulse* [PMI]), is easily detected. In the normal heart, the PMI is

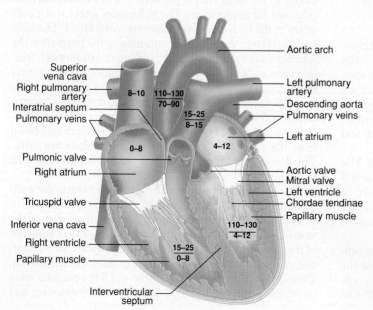

Superior
vena cava
Right pulmonary
artery
Interatrial septum
Pulmonary veins

Pulmonic valve
Right atrium

Tricuspid valve

Inferior vena cava
Right ventricle
Papillary muscle

Interventricular
septum

Aortic arch

Left pulmonary
artery
Descending aorta
Pulmonary veins

Left atrium

Aortic valve
Mitral valve
Left ventricle
Chordae tendinae
Papillary muscle

8–10   110–130
        70–90

15–25
8–15

0–8   4–12

110–130
4–12

15–25
0–8

FIGURE 25-2 • Great vessel and chamber pressures. Pressures are identified in millimeters of mercury (mm Hg) as mean pressure or systolic over diastolic pressure.

located at the intersection of the midclavicular line of the left chest wall and the fifth intercostal space (Bickley, 2009; Woods et al., 2009).

Heart Valves

The four valves in the heart permit blood to flow in only one direction. The valves, which are composed of thin leaflets of fibrous tissue, open and close in response to the movement of blood and pressure changes within the chambers. There are two types of valves: AV and semilunar.

Atrioventricular Valves

The AV valves separate the atria from the ventricles. The tricuspid valve, so named because it is composed of three cusps or leaflets, separates the right atrium from the right ventricle. The mitral or bicuspid (two cusps) valve lies between the left atrium and the left ventricle (see Fig. 25-1).

During diastole, the tricuspid and mitral valves are open, allowing the blood in the atria to flow freely into the relaxed ventricles. As ventricular systole begins, the ventricles contract and blood flows upward into the cusps of the tricuspid and mitral valves, causing them to close. As the pressure against these valves increases, two additional structures, the papillary muscles and the chordae tendineae, maintain valve closure. The papillary muscles, located on the sides of the ventricular walls, are connected to the valve leaflets by the chordae tendineae, which are thin fibrous bands. During ventricular systole, contraction of the papillary muscles causes the chordae tendineae to become taut, keeping the valve leaflets approximated and closed. This action prevents backflow of blood into the atria (regurgitation) as blood is ejected out into the pulmonary artery and aorta.

Semilunar Valves

The two semilunar valves are composed of three leaflets, which are shaped like half-moons. The valve between the right ventricle and the pulmonary artery is called the *pulmonic valve*. The valve between the left ventricle and the aorta is called the *aortic valve*. The semilunar valves are closed during diastole. At this point, the pressure in the pulmonary artery and aorta decreases, causing blood to flow back toward the semilunar valves. This action fills the cusps with blood and closes the valves. The semilunar valves are forced open during ventricular systole as blood is ejected from the right and left ventricles into the pulmonary artery and aorta.

Coronary Arteries

The left and right coronary arteries and their branches supply arterial blood to the heart. These arteries originate from the aorta just above the aortic valve leaflets. The heart has high metabolic requirements, extracting approximately 70% to 80% of the oxygen delivered (other organs extract, on average, 25%) (Woods et al., 2009). Unlike other arteries, the coronary arteries are perfused during diastole. With a normal heart rate of 60 to 80 bpm, there is ample time during diastole for myocardial perfusion. However, as heart rate increases, diastolic time is shortened, which may not allow adequate time for myocardial perfusion. As a result, patients are at risk for **myocardial ischemia** (inadequate oxygen supply) during tachycardias (heart rate greater than 100 bpm), especially patients with CAD.

The left coronary artery has three branches. The artery from the point of origin to the first major branch is called the *left main coronary artery*. Two branches arise from the left main coronary artery: the left anterior descending artery, which courses down the anterior wall of the heart, and the circumflex artery, which circles around to the lateral left wall of the heart.

The right side of the heart is supplied by the *right coronary artery*, which travels to the inferior wall of the heart. The posterior wall of the heart receives its blood supply by an additional branch from the right coronary artery called the *posterior descending artery* (see Fig. 27-2 in Chapter 27).

Superficial to the coronary arteries are the coronary veins. Venous blood from these veins returns to the heart primarily through the coronary sinus, which is located posteriorly in the right atrium.

Myocardium

The myocardium is the middle, muscular layer of the atrial and ventricular walls. It is composed of specialized cells called *myocytes*, which form an interconnected network of muscle fibers. These fibers encircle the heart in a figure-of-eight pattern, forming a spiral from the base (top) of the heart to the apex (bottom). During contraction, this muscular configuration facilitates a twisting and compressive movement of the heart that begins in the atria and moves to the ventricles. The sequential and rhythmic pattern of contraction, followed by relaxation of the muscle fibers, maximizes the volume of blood ejected with each contraction. This cyclical pattern of myocardial contraction is controlled by the conduction system.

Function of the Heart

Cardiac Electrophysiology

The **cardiac conduction system** generates and transmits electrical impulses that stimulate contraction of the myocardium. Under normal circumstances, the conduction system first stimulates contraction of the atria and then the ventricles. The synchronization of the atrial and ventricular events allows the ventricles to fill completely before ventricular ejection, thereby maximizing cardiac output. Three physiologic characteristics of two types of specialized electrical cells, the nodal cells and the Purkinje cells, provide this synchronization:

- *Automaticity*: ability to initiate an electrical impulse
- *Excitability*: ability to respond to an electrical impulse
- *Conductivity*: ability to transmit an electrical impulse from one cell to another

Both the **sinoatrial (SA) node** (the primary pacemaker of the heart) and the **atrioventricular (AV) node** (the secondary pacemaker of the heart) are composed of nodal cells. The SA node is located at the junction of the superior vena cava and the right atrium (Fig. 25-3). The SA node in a normal resting adult heart has an inherent firing rate of 60 to 100 impulses per minute; however, the rate changes in response to the metabolic demands of the body (Weber & Kelley, 2010).

The electrical impulses initiated by the SA node are conducted along the myocardial cells of the atria via specialized tracts called *internodal pathways*. The impulses cause

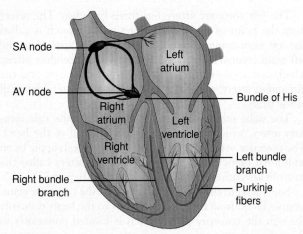

FIGURE 25-3 • Cardiac conduction system. AV, atrioventricular; SA, sinoatrial.

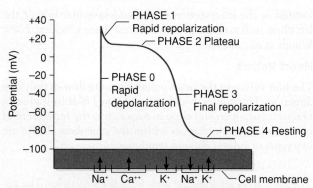

FIGURE 25-4 • Cardiac action potential of a fast-response Purkinje fiber. The *arrows* indicate the approximate time and direction of movement of each ion influencing membrane potential. Ca++ movement out of the cell is not well defined but is thought to occur during phase 4.

electrical stimulation and subsequent contraction of the atria. The impulses are then conducted to the AV node, which is located in the right atrial wall near the tricuspid valve (see Fig. 25-3). The AV node coordinates the incoming electrical impulses from the atria and after a slight delay (allowing the atria time to contract and complete ventricular filling) relays the impulse to the ventricles.

Initially, the impulse is conducted through a bundle of specialized conducting tissue, referred to as the bundle of His, which then divides into the right bundle branch (conducting impulses to the right ventricle) and the left bundle branch (conducting impulses to the left ventricle). To transmit impulses to the left ventricle—the largest chamber of the heart—the left bundle branch divides into the left anterior and left posterior bundle branches. Impulses travel through the bundle branches to reach the terminal point in the conduction system, called the *Purkinje fibers*. These fibers are composed of Purkinje cells, specialized to rapidly conduct the impulses through the thick walls of the ventricles. This is the point at which the myocardial cells are stimulated, causing ventricular contraction.

The heart rate is determined by the myocardial cells with the fastest inherent firing rate. Under normal circumstances, the SA node has the highest inherent rate (60 to 100 impulses per minute), the AV node has the second-highest inherent rate (40 to 60 impulses per minute), and the ventricular pacemaker sites have the lowest inherent rate (30 to 40 impulses per minute) (Woods et al., 2009). If the SA node malfunctions, the AV node generally takes over the pacemaker function of the heart at its inherently lower rate. Should both the SA and the AV nodes fail in their pacemaker function, a pacemaker site in the ventricle will fire at its inherent bradycardic rate of 30 to 40 impulses per minute.

Cardiac Action Potential

The nodal and Purkinje cells (electrical cells) generate and transmit impulses across the heart, stimulating the cardiac myocytes (working cells) to contract. Stimulation of the myocytes occurs due to the exchange of electrically charged particles, called *ions*, across channels located in the cell membrane. The channels regulate the movement and speed of specific ions—namely, sodium, potassium, and calcium—as they

enter and exit the cell. Sodium rapidly enters into the cell through sodium fast channels, in contrast to calcium, which enters the cell through calcium slow channels. In the resting or polarized state, sodium is the primary extracellular ion, whereas potassium is the primary intracellular ion. This difference in ion concentration means that the inside of the cell has a negative charge compared to the positive charge on the outside. This relationship changes during cellular stimulation, when sodium or calcium crosses the cell membrane into the cell and potassium ions exit into the extracellular space. This exchange of ions creates a positively charged intracellular space and a negatively charged extracellular space that characterizes the period known as **depolarization**. Once depolarization is complete, the exchange of ions reverts to its resting state; this period is known as **repolarization**. The repeated cycle of depolarization and repolarization is called the *cardiac action potential*.

As shown in Figure 25-4, the cardiac action potential has five phases:

- *Phase 0:* Cellular depolarization is initiated as positive ions influx into the cell. During this phase, the atrial and ventricular myocytes rapidly depolarize as sodium moves into the cells through sodium fast channels. The myocytes have a fast response action potential. In contrast, the cells of the SA and AV node depolarize when calcium enters these cells through calcium slow channels. These cells have a slow response action potential.
- *Phase 1:* Early cellular repolarization begins during this phase as potassium exits the intracellular space.
- *Phase 2:* This phase is called the *plateau phase* because the rate of repolarization slows. Calcium ions enter the intracellular space.
- *Phase 3:* This phase marks the completion of repolarization and return of the cell to its resting state.
- *Phase 4:* This phase is considered the resting phase before the next depolarization.

Refractory Periods

Myocardial cells must completely repolarize before they can depolarize again. During this time, the cells are in a refractory period. There are two phases of the refractory period: the effective (or absolute) refractory period and the relative refractory period. During the effective refractory period, the cell is completely unresponsive to any electrical stimulus; it is incapable of initiating an early depolarization. The effective refractory period corresponds with the time in phase 0 to the middle of phase 3 of the action potential. The relative refractory period corresponds with the short time at the end of phase 3. During the relative refractory period, if an electrical stimulus is stronger than normal, the cell may depolarize prematurely. Early depolarizations of the atrium or ventricle cause premature contractions, placing the patient at risk for dysrhythmias. Premature ventricular contractions in certain situations, such as the presence of myocardial ischemia, are of concern because these early ventricular depolarizations can trigger life-threatening dysrhythmias, including ventricular tachycardia or ventricular fibrillation. Several circumstances make the heart more susceptible to early depolarization during the relative refractory period, thus increasing the risk for serious dysrhythmias. (These dysrhythmias and others are discussed in detail in Chapter 26.)

Cardiac Hemodynamics

An important determinant of blood flow in the cardiovascular system is the principle that fluid flows from a region of higher pressure to one of lower pressure (see Fig. 25-2). The pressures responsible for blood flow in the normal circulation are generated during systole and diastole.

Cardiac Cycle

The cardiac cycle refers to the events that occur in the heart from the beginning of one heartbeat to the next. The number of cardiac cycles completed in a minute depends on the heart rate. Each cardiac cycle has three major sequential events: diastole, atrial systole, and ventricular systole. These events cause blood to flow through the heart due to changes in chamber pressures and valvular function during diastole and systole. During diastole, all four heart chambers are relaxed. As a result, the AV valves are open and the semilunar valves are closed. Pressures in all of the chambers are the lowest during diastole, which facilitates ventricular filling. Venous blood returns to the right atrium from the superior and inferior vena cava, then into the right ventricle. On the left side, oxygenated blood returns from the lungs via the four pulmonary veins into the left atrium and ventricle.

Toward the end of this diastolic period, atrial systole occurs as the atrial muscles contract in response to an electrical impulse initiated by the SA node. Atrial systole increases the pressure inside the atria, ejecting the remaining blood into the ventricles. Atrial systole augments ventricular blood volume by 15% to 25% and is sometimes referred to as the atrial kick (Woods et al., 2009). At this point, ventricular systole begins in response to propagation of the electrical impulse that began in the SA node some milliseconds earlier.

Beginning with ventricular systole, the pressure inside the ventricles rapidly increases, forcing the AV valves to close. As a result, blood ceases to flow from the atria into the ventricles, and regurgitation (backflow) of blood into the atria is prevented. The rapid increase of pressure inside the right and left ventricles forces the pulmonic and aortic valves to open, and blood is ejected into the pulmonary artery and aorta, respectively. The exit of blood is at first rapid; then, as the pressure in each ventricle and its corresponding artery equalizes, the flow of blood gradually decreases. At the end of systole, pressure within the right and left ventricles rapidly decreases. As a result, pulmonary arterial and aortic pressures decrease, causing closure of the semilunar valves. These events mark the onset of diastole, and the cardiac cycle is repeated.

Chamber pressures can be measured with the use of special monitoring catheters and equipment. This technique is called *hemodynamic monitoring*. Methods of hemodynamic monitoring are covered in more detail at the end of this chapter.

Cardiac Output

Cardiac output refers to the total amount of blood ejected by one of the ventricles in liters per minute. The cardiac output in a resting adult is 4 to 6 L/min but varies greatly depending on the metabolic needs of the body. Cardiac output is computed by multiplying the stroke volume by the heart rate. **Stroke volume** is the amount of blood ejected from one of the ventricles per heartbeat. The average resting stroke volume is about 60 to 130 mL (Woods et al., 2009).

Effect of Heart Rate on Cardiac Output. The cardiac output responds to changes in the metabolic demands of the tissues associated with stress, physical exercise, and illness. To compensate for these added demands, the cardiac output is enhanced by increases in both stroke volume and heart rate. Changes in heart rate are due to inhibition or stimulation of the SA node mediated by the parasympathetic and sympathetic divisions of the autonomic nervous system. The balance between these two reflex control systems normally determines the heart rate. Branches of the parasympathetic nervous system travel to the SA node by the vagus nerve. Stimulation of the vagus nerve slows the heart rate. The sympathetic nervous system increases heart rate by innervation of the beta-1 receptor sites located within the SA node. The heart rate is increased by the sympathetic nervous system through an increased level of circulating catecholamines (secreted by the adrenal gland) and by excess thyroid hormone, which produces a catecholaminelike effect.

In addition, the heart rate is affected by central nervous system and baroreceptor activity. **Baroreceptors** are specialized nerve cells located in the aortic arch and in both right and left internal carotid arteries (at the point of bifurcation from the common carotid arteries). The baroreceptors are sensitive to changes in blood pressure (BP). During significant elevations in BP (**hypertension**), these cells increase their rate of discharge, transmitting impulses to the cerebral medulla. This action initiates parasympathetic activity and inhibits sympathetic response, lowering the heart rate and the BP. The opposite is true during **hypotension** (low BP). Less baroreceptor stimulation during periods of hypotension prompts a decrease in parasympathetic activity and enhances sympathetic responses. These compensatory mechanisms attempt to elevate the BP through vasoconstriction and increased heart rate.

Effect of Stroke Volume on Cardiac Output. Stroke volume is primarily determined by three factors: preload, afterload, and contractility.

Preload refers to the degree of stretch of the ventricular cardiac muscle fibers at the end of diastole. The end of diastole is the period when filling volume in the ventricles is the highest and the degree of stretch on the muscle fibers is the greatest. The volume of blood within the ventricle at the end of diastole determines preload, which directly affects stroke volume. Therefore, preload is commonly referred to as left ventricular end-diastolic pressure. As the volume of blood returning to the heart increases, muscle fiber stretch also increases (increased preload), resulting in stronger contraction and a greater stroke volume. This relationship, referred to as the Frank-Starling (or Starling) law of the heart, is maintained until the physiologic limit of the muscle is reached.

The Frank-Starling law is based on the fact that, within limits, the greater the length or stretch of the cardiac muscle cells (sarcomeres), the greater the degree of shortening that occurs. This result is caused by increased interaction between the thick and thin filaments within the cardiac muscle cells. Preload is decreased by a reduction in the volume of blood returning to the ventricles. Diuresis, venodilating agents (e.g., nitrates), excessive loss of blood, or dehydration (excessive loss of body fluids from vomiting, diarrhea, or diaphoresis) reduce preload. Preload is increased by increasing the return of circulating blood volume to the ventricles. Controlling the loss of blood or body fluids and replacing fluids (i.e., blood transfusions and intravenous [IV] fluid administration) are examples of ways to increase preload.

Afterload, or resistance to ejection of blood from the ventricle, is the second determinant of stroke volume. The resistance of the systemic BP to left ventricular ejection is called **systemic vascular resistance**. The resistance of the pulmonary BP to right ventricular ejection is called **pulmonary vascular resistance**. There is an inverse relationship between afterload and stroke volume. For example, afterload is increased by arterial vasoconstriction, which leads to decreased stroke volume. The opposite is true with arterial vasodilation, in which case afterload is reduced because there is less resistance to ejection, and stroke volume increases.

Contractility refers to the force generated by the contracting myocardium. Contractility is enhanced by circulating catecholamines, sympathetic neuronal activity, and certain medications (e.g., digoxin [Lanoxin], dopamine [Intropin], or dobutamine [Dobutrex]). Increased contractility results in increased stroke volume. Contractility is depressed by hypoxemia, acidosis, and certain medications (e.g., beta-adrenergic blocking agents such as atenolol [Tenormin]).

The heart can achieve an increase in stroke volume (e.g., during exercise) if preload is increased (through increased venous return), if contractility is increased (through sympathetic nervous system discharge), and if afterload is decreased (through peripheral vasodilation with decreased aortic pressure).

The percentage of the end-diastolic blood volume that is ejected with each heartbeat is called the **ejection fraction**. The ejection fraction of the normal left ventricle is 55% to 65% (Woods et al., 2009). The right ventricular ejection fraction is rarely measured. The ejection fraction is used as a measure of myocardial contractility. An ejection fraction of less than 40% indicates that the patient has decreased left ventricular function and likely requires treatment for HF (refer to Chapter 29 for further discussion).

 Gerontologic Considerations

Changes in cardiac structure and function occur with age. A loss of function of the cells throughout the conduction system leads to a slower heart rate. The size of the heart increases due to hypertrophy (thickening of the heart walls), which reduces the volume of blood that the chambers can hold. Hypertrophy also changes the structure of the myocardium, reducing the strength of contraction. Both of these changes negatively affect cardiac output. The valves, due to stiffening, no longer close properly. The resulting backflow of blood creates heart murmurs, a common finding in older adults (Bickley, 2009; Boltz, Capezuti, Fulmer, et al., 2012; Woods et al., 2009).

The heart of an older person cannot compensate quickly to increases in metabolic demands due to stress, exercise, or illness. In these situations, older adults may become symptomatic with fatigue, shortness of breath, or palpitations and present with new physical examination findings (Boltz et al., 2012). The structural and functional changes with aging and associated history and physical examination findings are summarized in Table 25-1.

Gender Considerations

Structural differences between the hearts of men and women have significant implications. The heart of a woman tends to be smaller than that of a man. The coronary arteries of a woman are also narrower in diameter than a man's arteries. When atherosclerosis occurs, these differences make procedures such as cardiac catheterization and angioplasty technically more difficult.

Women typically develop CAD 10 years later than men, as women have the benefit of the female hormone estrogen and its cardioprotective effects. The three major effects of estrogen are (1) an increase in high-density lipoprotein (HDL) that transports cholesterol out of arteries; (2) a reduction in low-density lipoprotein (LDL) that deposits cholesterol in the artery; and (3) dilatation of the blood vessels, which enhance blood flow to the heart. As women reach menopause, around 50 years of age, estrogen levels slowly disappear and place women at higher risk for CAD. By age 65, women's CAD risk is equivalent to that of men.

In the past hormone therapy was routinely prescribed for postmenopausal women with the belief that it would deter the onset and progression of CAD. However, based on results from the multisite, prospective, longitudinal Women's Health Initiative study, the AHA no longer recommends the use of hormone therapy as a prevention strategy for women. In the most recently published AHA guidelines for primary prevention of CAD in women, the use of hormone therapy (estrogen) is noted to be ineffective and potentially harmful (Mosca, Benjamin, Berra, et al., 2011).

TABLE 25-1	Age-Related Changes of the Cardiac System		
Cardiovascular Structure	**Structural Changes**	**Functional Changes**	**History and Physical Findings**
Atria	↑ Size of left atrium Thickening of the endocardium	↑ Atrial irritability	Irregular heart rhythm from atrial dysrhythmias
Left ventricle	Endocardial fibrosis Myocardial thickening (hypertrophy) Infiltration of fat into myocardium	Left ventricle stiff and less compliant Progressive decline in cardiac output ↑ Risk for ventricular dysrhythmias Prolonged systole	Fatigue ↓ Exercise tolerance Signs and symptoms of heart failure or ventricular dysrhythmias Point of maximal impulse palpated lateral to the midclavicular line ↓ Intensity S_1, S_2; split S_2 S_4 may be present.
Valves	Thickening and rigidity of AV valves Calcification of aortic valve	Abnormal blood flow across valves during cardiac cycle	Murmurs may be present. Thrill may be palpated if significant murmur is present.
Conduction system	Connective tissue collects in SA node, AV node, and bundle branches ↓ Number of SA node cells ↓ Number of AV, bundle of His, and right and left bundle branch cells	Slower SA node rate of impulse discharge Slowed conduction across AV node and ventricular conduction system	Bradycardia Heart block ECG changes consistent with slowed conduction (↑ PR interval, widened QRS complex)
Sympathetic nervous system	↓ Response to beta-adrenergic stimulation	↓ Adaptive response to exercise: contractility and heart rate slower to respond to exercise demands Heart rate takes more time to return to baseline	Fatigue Diminished exercise tolerance ↓ Ability to respond to stress
Aorta and arteries	Stiffening of vasculature ↓ Elasticity and widening of aorta Elongation of aorta, displacing the brachiocephalic artery upward	Left ventricular hypertrophy	Progressive increase in systolic BP; slight ↑ in diastolic BP Widening pulse pressure Pulsation visible above right clavicle
Baroreceptor response	↓ Sensitivity of baroreceptors in the carotid artery and aorta to transient episodes of hypertension and hypotension	Baroreceptors unable to regulate heart rate and vascular tone, causing slow response to postural changes in body position	Postural BP changes and reports of feeling dizzy, fainting when moving from lying to sitting or standing position

AV, atrioventricular; SA, sinoatrial; ECG, electrocardiographic; BP, blood pressure.
Adapted from Aronow, W. S., Fleg, J. L., Pepine, C. J., et al. (2011). ACCF/AHA 2011 expert consensus document on hypertension in the elderly: A report of the American College of Cardiology Foundation Task Force on Clinical Expert Consensus Documents. *Journal of the American College of Cardiology, 57*(20), 2434–2506; Bickley, L. S. (2009). *Bates' guide to physical examination and history taking* (9th ed.). Philadelphia: Lippincott Williams & Wilkins; and Boltz, M., Capezuti, E., Fulmer, T., et al. (2012). *Evidence-based geriatric nursing: Protocols for best practice* (4th ed.). New York: Springhouse.

Assessment of the Cardiovascular System

The frequency and extent of the nursing assessment of cardiovascular function are based on several factors, including the severity of the patient's symptoms, the presence of risk factors, the practice setting, and the purpose of the assessment. An acutely ill patient with CVD who is admitted to the emergency department (ED) or coronary intensive care unit (ICU) requires a very different assessment than a person who is being examined for a chronic stable condition. Although the key components of the cardiovascular assessment remain the same, the assessment priorities vary according to the needs of the patient. For example, an ED nurse performs a rapid and focused assessment of a patient in which **acute coronary syndrome** (ACS), rupture of an atheromatous plaque in a diseased coronary artery, is suspected. Diagnosis and treatment must be started within minutes of arrival to the ED. The physical assessment is ongoing and concentrates on evaluating the patient for ACS complications, such as dysrhythmias and HF, and determining the effectiveness of medical treatment.

Health History

The patient's ability to recognize cardiac symptoms and to know what to do when they occur is essential for effective self-care management. All too often, a patient's new symptoms or those of progressing cardiac dysfunction go unrecognized. This results in prolonged delays in seeking lifesaving treatment. Major barriers to seeking prompt medical care include lack of knowledge about the symptoms of heart disease, attributing symptoms to a benign source, denying symptom significance, and feeling embarrassed about having symptoms (Moser, Kimble, Alberts, et al., 2007). Therefore, during the health history, the nurse needs to determine if the patient and involved family members are able to recognize symptoms of an acute cardiac problem, such as ACS or HF, and seek timely treatment for these symptoms. Responses to this level of inquiry will help the nurse individualize the plan for patient and family education.

Common Symptoms

The signs and symptoms experienced by people with CVD are related to dysrhythmias and conduction problems (see Chapter 26); CAD (see Chapter 27); structural, infectious, and inflammatory disorders of the heart (see Chapter 28); and complications of CVD such as HF and cardiogenic shock (see Chapters 29 and 14, respectively). These disorders have many signs and symptoms in common; therefore, the nurse must be skillful at recognizing these signs and symptoms so that patients are given timely and often lifesaving care.

The following are the most common signs and symptoms of CVD, with related medical diagnoses in parentheses:

- Chest pain or discomfort (angina pectoris, ACS, dysrhythmias, valvular heart disease)
- Shortness of breath or dyspnea (ACS, cardiogenic shock, HF, valvular heart disease)
- Peripheral edema, weight gain, abdominal distention due to enlarged spleen and liver or ascites (HF)
- Palpitations (tachycardia from a variety of causes, including ACS, caffeine or other stimulants, electrolyte imbalances, stress, valvular heart disease, ventricular aneurysms)
- Unusual fatigue, sometimes referred to as vital exhaustion (an early warning symptom of ACS, HF, or valvular heart disease, characterized by feeling unusually tired or fatigued, irritable, and dejected)
- Dizziness, syncope, or changes in level of consciousness (cardiogenic shock, cerebrovascular disorders, dysrhythmias, hypotension, postural hypotension, vasovagal episode)

Chest Pain

Chest pain and chest discomfort are common symptoms that may be caused by a number of cardiac and noncardiac problems. Table 25-2 summarizes the characteristics and patterns of common causes of chest pain or discomfort. To differentiate among these causes of pain, the nurse asks the patient to identify the quantity (0 = no pain to 10 = worst pain), location, and quality of pain. The nurse assesses for radiation of the pain to other areas of the body and determines if associated signs and symptoms are present, such as diaphoresis or nausea. It is important to identify the events that precipitate the onset of symptoms, the duration of the symptoms, and measures that aggravate or relieve the symptoms.

The nurse should keep the following important points in mind when assessing patients reporting chest pain or discomfort:

- The location of chest symptoms is not well correlated with the cause of the pain. For example, substernal chest pain can result from a number of causes as outlined in Table 25-2.
- The severity or duration of chest pain or discomfort does not predict the seriousness of its cause. For example, when asked to rate pain using a 0 to 10 scale, patients experiencing esophageal spasm may rate their chest pain as a 10. In contrast, patients having an acute myocardial infarction (MI), which is a potentially life-threatening event, may report having moderate pain rated as a 4 to 6 on the pain scale.
- More than one clinical cardiac condition may occur simultaneously. During an MI, patients may report chest

pain from myocardial ischemia, shortness of breath from HF, and palpitations from dysrhythmias. Both HF and dysrhythmias can be complications of an acute MI. (See Chapter 27 for discussion of clinical manifestations of ACS, including MI.)

Past Health, Family, and Social History

The health history provides an opportunity for the nurse to assess patients' understanding of their personal risk factors for coronary artery, peripheral vascular, and cerebrovascular diseases (see Chart 27-1 in Chapter 27) and any measures that they are taking to modify these risks. Risk factors are classified by the extent to which they can be modified by changing one's lifestyle or modifying personal behaviors.

In an effort to determine how the patient perceives his or her current health status, the nurse must ask some of the following questions:

- How is your health? Have you noticed any changes from last year? From 5 years ago?
- Do you have a cardiologist or primary provider? How often do you go for checkups?
- What health concerns do you have?
- Do you have a family history of genetic disorders that place you at risk for CVD (Chart 25-1)? What are your risk factors for heart disease (see Chart 27-1 in Chapter 27)?
- What do you do to stay healthy and take care of your heart?

Patients who do not understand that their behaviors or diagnoses pose a threat to their health may be less motivated to make lifestyle changes or to manage their illness effectively. However, patients who perceive that their modifiable risk factors for heart disease affect their health and believe that they have the power to modify or change them may be more likely to change these behaviors. The AHA has published guidelines that identify interventions and treatment goals for each of the cardiac risk factors (Smith, Benjamin, Bonow, et al., 2011). (Chapter 27 provides an overview of this information.)

Medications

Nurses collaborate with primary providers and pharmacists to obtain a complete list of the patient's medications, including dose and frequency. Vitamins, herbals, and other over-the-counter medications are included on this list. During this aspect of the health assessment, the nurse asks the following questions to ensure that the patient is safely and effectively taking the prescribed medications.

- What are the names and doses of your medications?
- What is the purpose of each of these medications?
- How and when are these medications taken? Do you ever skip a dose or forget to take them?
- Are their any special precautions associated with any of these medications?
- What symptoms or problems do you need to report to your doctor?

Aspirin is a common nonprescription medication that improves outcomes in patients with CAD when taken daily (Levine, Bates, Blankenship, et al., 2011). However, if patients are not aware of this benefit, they may be inclined to stop taking aspirin if they think it is a trivial medication.

TABLE 25-2   Assessing Chest Pain

Location	Character	Duration	Precipitating Events and Aggravating Factors	Alleviating Factors
Angina Pectoris **ACS (unstable angina, MI)** Usual distribution of pain with myocardial ischemia Jaw Epigastrium Right side Back Less common sites of pain with myocardial ischemia	*Angina:* Uncomfortable pressure, squeezing, or fullness in substernal chest area Can radiate across chest to the medial aspect of one or both arms and hands, jaw, shoulders, upper back, or epigastrium Radiation to arms and hands, described as numbness, tingling, or aching *ACS:* Same as angina pectoris Pain or discomfort ranges from mild to severe Associated with shortness of breath, diaphoresis, palpitations, unusual fatigue, and nausea or vomiting	*Angina:* 5–15 min *ACS:* >15 min	*Angina:* Physical exertion, emotional upset, eating large meal, or exposure to extremes in temperature *ACS:* Emotional upset or unusual physical exertion occurring within 24 h of symptom onset Can occur at rest or while asleep	*Angina:* Rest, nitroglycerin, oxygen *ACS:* Morphine, reperfusion of coronary artery with thrombolytic (fibrinolytic) agent or percutaneous coronary intervention
Pericarditis	Sharp, severe substernal or epigastric pain Can radiate to neck, arms, and back Associated symptoms include fever, malaise, dyspnea, cough, nausea, dizziness, and palpitations	Intermittent	Sudden onset Pain increases with inspiration, swallowing, coughing, and rotation of trunk	Sitting upright, analgesia, anti-inflammatory medications
Pulmonary Disorders (pneumonia, pulmonary embolism)	Sharp, severe substernal or epigastric pain arising from inferior portion of pleura (referred to as pleuritic pain) Patient may be able to localize the pain	≥30 min	Follows an infectious or noninfectious process (MI, cardiac surgery, cancer, immune disorders, uremia) Pleuritic pain increases with inspiration, coughing, movement, and supine positioning Occurs in conjunction with community- or hospital-acquired lung infections (pneumonia) or venous thromboembolism (pulmonary embolism)	Treatment of underlying cause
Esophageal Disorders (hiatal hernia, reflux esophagitis or spasm)	Substernal pain described as sharp, burning, or heavy Often mimics angina Can radiate to neck, arm, or shoulders	5–60 min	Recumbency, cold liquids, exercise	Food or antacid Nitroglycerin

(continues on page 664)

TABLE 25-2 **Assessing Chest Pain** (continued)

Location	Character	Duration	Precipitating Events and Aggravating Factors	Alleviating Factors
Anxiety and Panic Disorders	Pain described as stabbing to dull ache Associated with diaphoresis, palpitations, shortness of breath, tingling of hands or mouth, feeling of unreality, or fear of losing control	Peaks in 10 min	Can occur at any time including during sleep Can be associated with a specific trigger	Removal of stimulus, relaxation, medications to treat anxiety or underlying disorder
Musculoskeletal Disorders (costochondritis)	Sharp or stabbing pain localized in anterior chest Most often unilateral Can radiate across chest to epigastrium or back	Hours to days	Most often follows respiratory tract infection with significant coughing, vigorous exercise, or posttrauma Some cases are idiopathic. Exacerbated by deep inspiration, coughing, sneezing, and movement of upper torso or arms	Rest, ice, or heat Analgesic or anti-inflammatory medications

ACS, acute coronary syndrome; MI, myocardial infarction.

Adapted from Bickley, L. S. (2009). *Bates' guide to physical examination and history taking* (9th ed.). Philadelphia: Lippincott Williams & Wilkins; DeVon, H. A., Ryan, C. J., Rankin, S. H., et al. (2010). Classifying subgroups of patients with symptoms of acute coronary syndrome: A cluster analysis. *Research in Nursing and Health, 33,* 386–397; and Woods, S. L., Froelicher, E. S., Motzer, S. A., et al. (2009). *Cardiac nursing* (6th ed.). Philadelphia: Lippincott Williams & Wilkins.

Chart 25-1

GENETICS IN NURSING PRACTICE
Cardiovascular Disorders

Several cardiovascular disorders are associated with genetic abnormalities. Some examples are:

- Familial hypercholesterolemia
- Hypertrophic cardiomyopathy
- Long QT syndrome
- Hereditary hemochromatosis
- Elevated homocysteine levels

Nursing Assessments

Family History Assessment

- Assess all patients with cardiovascular symptoms for coronary artery disease (CAD), regardless of age (early-onset CAD occurs).
- Assess family history of sudden death in people who may or may not have been diagnosed with CAD (especially of early onset).
- Ask about sudden death in a previously asymptomatic child, adolescent, or adult.
- Ask about other family members with biochemical or neuromuscular conditions (e.g., hemochromatosis or muscular dystrophy).

- Assess whether DNA mutation or other genetic testing has been performed on an affected family member.

Patient Assessment

- Assess for signs and symptoms of hyperlipidemias (xanthomas, corneal arcus, abdominal pain of unexplained origin).
- Assess for muscular weakness.

Management Issues Specific to Genetics

- If indicated, refer for further genetic counseling and evaluation so that the family can discuss inheritance, risk to other family members, and availability of genetic testing, as well as gene-based interventions.
- Offer appropriate genetic information and resources (e.g., Genetic Alliance Web site, American Heart Association).
- Provide support to families newly diagnosed with genetics-related cardiovascular disease.

Genetics Resources

See Chapter 8, Chart 8-6 for genetics resources.

A careful medication history often uncovers common medication errors and causes for nonadherence to the medication regimen.

Nutrition

Dietary modifications, exercise, weight loss, and careful monitoring are important strategies for managing three major cardiovascular risk factors: hyperlipidemia, hypertension, and diabetes. Diets that are restricted in sodium, fat, cholesterol, or calories are commonly prescribed. The nurse obtains the following information:

- The patient's current height and weight (to determine body mass index [BMI]); waist measurement (assessment for obesity); BP; and any laboratory test results such as blood glucose, glycosylated hemoglobin (diabetes), total blood cholesterol, HDL and LDL levels, and triglyceride levels (hyperlipidemia)
- How often the patient self-monitors BP, blood glucose, and weight as appropriate to the medical diagnoses
- The patient's level of awareness regarding his or her target goals for each of the risk factors and any problems achieving or maintaining these goals
- What the patient normally eats and drinks in a typical day and any food preferences (including cultural or ethnic preferences)
- Eating habits (canned or commercially prepared foods vs. fresh foods, restaurant cooking vs. home cooking, assessing for high-sodium foods, dietary intake of fats)
- Who shops for groceries and prepares meals

Elimination

Typical bowel and bladder habits need to be identified. Nocturia (awakening at night to urinate) is common in patients with HF. Fluid collected in gravity-dependent tissues (extremities) during the day (i.e., edema) redistributes into the circulatory system once the patient is recumbent at night. The increased circulatory volume is excreted by the kidneys (increased urine production).

When straining during defecation, the patient bears down (the Valsalva maneuver), which momentarily increases pressure on the baroreceptors. This triggers a vagal response, causing the heart rate to slow and resulting in syncope in some patients. Straining during urination can produce the same response.

Because many cardiac medications can cause gastrointestinal side effects or bleeding, the nurse asks about bloating, diarrhea, constipation, stomach upset, heartburn, loss of appetite, nausea, and vomiting. Screening for bloody urine or stools should be done for patients taking platelet-inhibiting medications such as aspirin and clopidogrel (Plavix); platelet aggregation inhibitors such as abciximab (ReoPro), eptifibatide (Integrilin), and tirofiban (Aggrastat); and anticoagulants such as low-molecular-weight heparin (e.g., dalteparin [Fragmin], enoxaparin [Lovenox]), heparin, or warfarin (Coumadin).

Activity and Exercise

Changes in the patient's activity tolerance are often gradual and may go unnoticed. The nurse determines if there are recent changes by comparing the patient's current activity level with that performed in the past 6 to 12 months. New symptoms or a change in the usual symptoms during activity is a significant finding. Activity-induced angina or shortness of breath may indicate CAD. These CAD-related symptoms occur when myocardial ischemia is present, due to an inadequate arterial blood supply to the myocardium, in the setting of increased demand (e.g., exercise, stress, or anemia). Patients experiencing these kinds of symptoms need to seek medical attention. Fatigue, associated with a low left ventricular ejection fraction (less than 40%) and certain medications (e.g., beta-adrenergic blocking agents), can result in activity intolerance. Patients with fatigue may benefit from having their medications adjusted and learning energy conservation techniques.

Additional areas to explore include the presence of architectural barriers in the home (stairs, multilevel home); the patient's participation in cardiac rehabilitation; and his or her current exercise pattern including intensity, duration, and frequency.

Sleep and Rest

Clues to worsening cardiac disease, especially HF, can be revealed by sleep-related events. Patients with worsening HF often experience *orthopnea*, a term used to indicate the need to sit upright or stand to avoid feeling short of breath. Patients experiencing orthopnea will report that they need to sleep upright in a chair or add extra pillows to their bed. Sudden awakening with shortness of breath, called *paroxysmal nocturnal dyspnea*, is an additional symptom of worsening HF. This nighttime symptom is caused by the reabsorption of fluid from dependent areas of the body (arms and legs) back into the circulatory system within hours of lying in bed. This sudden fluid shift increases preload and places increased demand on the heart of patients with HF, causing sudden pulmonary congestion.

Self-Perception and Self-Concept

Self-perception and self-concept are both related to the cognitive and emotional processes that people use to formulate their beliefs and feelings about themselves. Having a chronic cardiac illness, such as HF, or experiencing an acute cardiac event, such as an MI, can alter an individual's self-perception and self-concept. The nurse must understand that patients' beliefs and feelings about their health are key determinants in adherence to health regimen recommendations and recovery after an acute cardiac event (Heydari, Ahrari, & Vaghee, 2011). To reduce the risk of future cardiovascular-related health problems, patients are asked to make difficult lifestyle changes, such as quitting smoking. Patients who have misperceptions about the health consequences of their illness are at risk for nonadherence to these recommended lifestyle changes. The health history is used to discover how patients perceive their health by asking questions that may include the following:

- What is your cardiac condition?
- How has this illness changed your feelings about your health?
- What do you think caused this illness?
- What consequences do you think this illness will have on your physical activity, work, social relationships, and role in your family?
- How much of an influence do you think you have on controlling this illness?

The patient's responses to these questions can guide the nurse in planning interventions to ensure that the patient is prepared to manage the illness and that adequate services are in place to support the patient's recovery and self-management needs.

Roles and Relationships

Hospital stays for cardiac disorders have shortened, with many invasive diagnostic cardiac procedures, such as cardiac catheterization and percutaneous coronary intervention (PCI), being performed as outpatient procedures. Therefore, the nurse in the hospital setting needs to assess the support systems that the patient may tap into post discharge.

To assess support systems, the nurse needs to ask: Who is the primary caregiver? With whom does the patient live? Are there adequate services in place to provide a safe home environment? The nurse also assesses for any significant effects the cardiac illness has had on the patient's role in the family. Are there adequate finances and health insurance? The answers to these questions help the nurse develop a plan to meet the patient's home care needs.

Sexuality and Reproduction

Although people recovering from cardiac illnesses or procedures are often concerned about sexual activity, they are unlikely to ask their nurse or other health care provider for information to help them resume their normal sex life. Therefore, the nurse needs to initiate a discussion about sexuality with the patient.

The most commonly cited reasons for changes in sexual activity are fear of another heart attack or sudden death; untoward symptoms such as angina, dyspnea, or palpitations; and problems with impotence or depression. In men, impotence may develop as a side effect of cardiac medications (e.g., beta-blockers); some men will stop taking their medication as a result. Other medications may be substituted, so patients should be encouraged to discuss this problem with their health care providers. Often, patients and their partners do not have adequate information about the physical demands related to sexual activity and ways in which these demands can be modified. The physiologic demands associated with sexual activity range between 3 and 5 metabolic equivalents (METs), which is similar to the METs expended during mild to moderate activity. The variation in METs expended reflects the individual patient's age, level of physical fitness, and presence of CVD (Levine, Steinke, Bakaeen, et al., 2012). Sharing this information may make the patient and his or her partner more comfortable about resuming sexual activity.

A reproductive history is necessary for women of childbearing age, particularly those with seriously compromised cardiac function. The reproductive history includes information about previous pregnancies, plans for future pregnancies, oral contraceptive use (especially in women older than 35 years who smoke), menopausal status, and the use of hormone therapy.

Coping and Stress Tolerance

Anxiety, depression, and stress are known to influence both the development of and recovery from CAD and HF. High levels of anxiety are associated with an increased incidence of CAD and in-hospital complication rates after MI.

Patients with a diagnosis of an acute MI and depression have an increased risk of rehospitalization, death, more frequent angina, more physical limitations, and poorer quality of life compared with patients without depression (Brown, Stewart, Stump, et al., 2011). Although the association between depression and CAD is not completely understood, both biologic factors (e.g., platelet abnormalities, inflammatory responses) and lifestyle factors may contribute to the development of CAD. Patients who are depressed are less motivated to adhere to recommended lifestyle changes and medical regimens necessary to prevent future cardiac events, such as an MI (Bigger & Glassman, 2010).

Patients with CAD or HF should be assessed for depression. Patients who have depression exhibit common signs and symptoms, such as feelings of worthlessness or guilt, problems falling asleep or staying asleep, having little interest or pleasure in doing things that they usually enjoy, having difficulty concentrating, restlessness, and recent changes in appetite or weight. A quick and simple screening tool recommended by the AHA is the two-question Patient Health Questionnaire (PHQ-2) (Bigger & Glassman, 2010). The nurse asks the patient the following:

Over the past 2 weeks, how often have you been bothered by either of the following problems?
- Little interest or pleasure in doing things
- Feeling down, depressed, or hopeless

The nurse scores the patient's responses to each question by assigning 0 for "not at all," 1 for "several days," 2 for "more than half the days," or 3 for "nearly every day." The PHQ-2 score ranges from 0 to 6. Patients with a score of 3 or higher may be experiencing major depression and should be referred for further evaluation and treatment.

Stress initiates a variety of responses, including increased levels of catecholamines and cortisol, and has been strongly linked to cardiovascular events, such as an MI. Therefore, patients need to be assessed for sources of stress; the nurse should ask about recent or ongoing stressors, previous coping styles and effectiveness, and the patient's perception of his or her current mood and coping ability. A widely used tool used to measure life stress is the Social Readjustment Rating Scale (Homes & Rahe, 1967). Examples of items on this scale include death of a spouse, divorce, and change in responsibilities at work. Each item is assigned a score of 11 to 100. Patients identify the items that happened to them in the previous year. Patients with a score less than 150 have a slight risk for future illness, whereas a score of 150 to 299 indicates a moderate risk. A score of 300 or higher indicates a high risk for future illness. Consultation with a psychiatric advanced practice nurse, psychologist, psychiatrist, or social worker is indicated for anxious or depressed patients or those patients having difficulty coping with their cardiac illness.

Physical Assessment

Physical assessment is conducted to confirm information obtained from the health history, to establish the patient's current or baseline condition, and, in subsequent assessments, to evaluate the patient's response to treatment. Once the initial physical assessment is completed, the frequency of future assessments is determined by the purpose of the encounter and the patient's condition. For example, a focused cardiac assessment may be performed each time the patient is seen in the outpatient setting, whereas patients in the acute care setting may require a more extensive assessment at least every 8 hours. During the physical assessment, the nurse evaluates the cardiovascular system for any deviations from normal with regard to the following (examples of abnormalities are in parentheses):

- The heart as a pump (reduced pulse pressure, displaced PMI from fifth intercostal space midclavicular line, gallop sounds, murmurs)
- Atrial and ventricular filling volumes and pressures (elevated jugular venous distension, peripheral edema, ascites, crackles, postural changes in BP)
- Cardiac output (reduced pulse pressure, hypotension, tachycardia, reduced urine output, lethargy, or disorientation)
- Compensatory mechanisms (peripheral vasoconstriction, tachycardia).

General Appearance

This part of the assessment evaluates the patient's level of consciousness (alert, lethargic, stuporous, comatose) and mental status (oriented to person, place, time; coherence). Changes in level of consciousness and mental status may be attributed to inadequate perfusion of the brain from a compromised cardiac output or thromboembolic event (stroke). Patients are observed for signs of distress, which include pain or discomfort, shortness of breath, or anxiety.

The nurse notes the size of the patient (normal, overweight, underweight, or cachectic). The patient's height and weight are measured to calculate BMI (weight in kilograms/square of the height in meters), as well as the waist circumference (see Chapter 5). These measures are used to determine if obesity (BMI greater than 30 kg/m^2) and abdominal fat (males: waist greater than 40 inches; females: waist greater than 35 inches) are placing the patient at risk for CAD.

Assessment of the Skin and Extremities

Examination of the skin includes all body surfaces, starting with the head and finishing with the lower extremities. Skin color, temperature, and texture are assessed for acute and chronic problems with arterial or venous circulation. Table 25-3 summarizes common skin findings in patients with CVD. The most noteworthy changes include the following:

- Signs and symptoms of acute obstruction of arterial blood flow in the extremities, referred to as the six P's, are *pain*, *pallor*, *pulselessness*, *paresthesia*, *poikilothermia* (coldness), and *paralysis*. During the first few hours after invasive cardiac procedures (e.g., cardiac catheterization, PCI, or cardiac electrophysiology testing), affected extremities should be assessed frequently for these acute vascular changes.
- Hematoma, or a localized collection of clotted blood in the tissue, may be observed in patients who have undergone invasive cardiac procedures. Major blood vessels of the arms and legs may be used for catheter insertion. During these procedures, systemic anticoagulation with heparin is necessary, and bruising or small hematomas may occur at the catheter access site. However, large hematomas are a serious complication that

can compromise circulating blood volume and cardiac output. Patients who have undergone these procedures must have catheter access sites frequently observed until hemostasis is adequately achieved.
- Edema is an abnormal accumulation of fluid in dependent areas of the body. Edema of the feet, ankles, or legs is called *peripheral edema*. Sacral edema can be observed in the sacral area of patients on bed rest. The nurse assesses the patient for edema by using the thumb to place firm pressure over the dorsum of each foot, behind each medial malleolus, over the shins or sacral area for 5 seconds. *Pitting edema* is the term used to describe an indentation in the skin created by this pressure (see Fig. 29-2 in Chapter 29). The degree of pitting edema relies on the clinician's judgment of depth of edema and time the indentation remains after release of pressure. Pitting edema is graded as absent (0) or as present on a scale from slight (1+ = up to 2 mm) to very marked (4+ = more than 8 mm) (Weber & Kelley, 2010). It is important that clinicians use a consistent scale in order to ensure reliable clinical measurements and management. Peripheral edema is a common finding in patients with HF and peripheral vascular diseases, such as deep vein thrombosis or chronic venous insufficiency.
- Prolonged capillary refill time indicates inadequate arterial perfusion to the extremities. To test capillary refill time, the nurse compresses the nail bed briefly to occlude perfusion and the nail bed blanches. Then, the nurse releases pressure and determines the time it takes to restore perfusion. Normally, reperfusion occurs within 2 seconds, as evidenced by the return of color to the nail bed. Prolonged capillary refill time indicates compromised arterial perfusion, a problem associated with cardiogenic shock and HF.
- Clubbing of the fingers and toes indicates chronic hemoglobin desaturation and is associated with congenital heart disease.
- Hair loss, brittle nails, dry or scaling skin, atrophy of the skin, skin color changes, and ulcerations are indicative of chronically reduced oxygen and nutrient supply to the skin observed in patients with arterial or venous insufficiency (see Chapter 30 for a complete description of these conditions) (Weber & Kelley, 2010).

Blood Pressure

Systemic arterial BP is the pressure exerted on the walls of the arteries during ventricular systole and diastole. It is affected by factors such as cardiac output; distention of the arteries; and the volume, velocity, and viscosity of the blood. A normal BP in adults is considered a systolic BP less than 120 mm Hg over a diastolic BP less than 80 mm Hg. High BP, or hypertension, is defined by having a systolic BP that is consistently greater than 140 mm Hg or a diastolic BP greater than 90 mm Hg. Hypotension refers to an abnormally low systolic and diastolic BP that can result in lightheadedness or fainting. (See Chapter 31 for additional definitions, measurement, and management.)

Pulse Pressure

The difference between the systolic and the diastolic pressures is called the *pulse pressure*. It is a reflection of stroke

TABLE 25-3	Common Skin Findings Associated With Cardiovascular Disease
Findings	**Associated Causes and Conditions**
Clubbing of the fingers or toes (thickening of the skin under the fingers or toes)	Chronic hemoglobin desaturation most often due to congenital heart disease, advanced pulmonary diseases
Cool/cold skin and diaphoresis	Low cardiac output (e.g., cardiogenic shock, acute myocardial infarction) causing sympathetic nervous system stimulation with resultant vasoconstriction
Cold, pain, pallor of the fingertips or toes	Intermittent arteriolar vasoconstriction (Raynaud's disease). Skin may change in color from white, blue, and red accompanied by numbness, tingling, and burning pain.
Cyanosis, central (a bluish tinge observed in the tongue and buccal mucosa)	Serious cardiac disorders (pulmonary edema, cardiogenic shock, congenital heart disease) result in venous blood passing through the pulmonary circulation without being oxygenated.
Cyanosis, peripheral (a bluish tinge, most often of the nails and skin of the nose, lips, earlobes, and extremities)	Peripheral vasoconstriction, allowing more time for the hemoglobin molecules to become desaturated. It can be caused by exposure to cold environment, anxiety, or ↓ cardiac output.
Ecchymosis or bruising (a purplish-blue color fading to green, yellow, or brown)	Blood leaking outside of the blood vessels Excessive bruising is a risk for patients on anticoagulants or platelet-inhibiting medications.
Edema, lower extremities (collection of fluid in the interstitial spaces of the tissues)	Heart failure and vascular problems (PAD, chronic venous insufficiency, deep vein thrombosis, thrombophlebitis)
Hematoma (localized collection of clotted blood in the tissue)	Bleeding after catheter removal/tissue injury in patients on anticoagulant/ antithrombotic agents
Pallor (↓ skin color in fingernails, lips, oral mucosa, and lower extremities)	Anemia or ↓ arterial perfusion. Suspect PAD if feet develop pallor after elevating legs 60 degrees from a supine position.
Rubor (a reddish-blue discoloration of the legs, seen within 20 sec to 2 min after placing in a dependent position)	Filling of dilated capillaries with deoxygenated blood, indicative of PAD
Ulcers, feet and ankles: Superficial, irregular ulcers at medial malleolus. Red to yellow granulation tissue.	Rupture of small skin capillaries from chronic venous insufficiency
Ulcers, feet and ankles: Painful, deep, round ulcers on feet or from exposure to pressure. Pale to black wound base.	Prolonged ischemia to tissues due to PAD. Can lead to gangrene.
Thinning of skin around a pacemaker or an implantable cardioverter defibrillator	Erosion of the device through the skin
Xanthelasma (yellowish, raised plaques observed along nasal portion of eyelids)	Elevated cholesterol levels (hypercholesterolemia)

PAD, peripheral arterial disease.
Adapted from Bickley, L. S. (2009). *Bates' guide to physical examination and history taking* (9th ed.). Philadelphia: Lippincott Williams & Wilkins; and Woods, S. L., Froelicher, E. S., Motzer, S. A., et al. (2009). *Cardiac nursing* (6th ed.). Philadelphia: Lippincott Williams & Wilkins.

volume, ejection velocity, and systemic vascular resistance. Pulse pressure, which normally is 30 to 40 mm Hg, indicates how well the patient maintains cardiac output. The pulse pressure increases in conditions that elevate the stroke volume (anxiety, exercise, bradycardia), reduce systemic vascular resistance (fever), or reduce distensibility of the arteries (atherosclerosis, aging, hypertension). Decreased pulse pressure reflects reduced stroke volume and ejection velocity (shock, HF, hypovolemia, mitral regurgitation) or obstruction to blood flow during systole (mitral or aortic stenosis). A pulse pressure of less than 30 mm Hg signifies a serious reduction in cardiac output and requires further cardiovascular assessment (Woods et al., 2009).

Postural Blood Pressure Changes

There is a gravitational redistribution of approximately 300 to 800 mL of blood into the lower extremities and the gastrointestinal system immediately upon standing. These changes reduce venous return to the heart, compromising preload that ultimately reduces stroke volume and cardiac output. As a consequence, the autonomic nervous system is activated. The sympathetic nervous system increases heart rate and enhances peripheral vasoconstriction, whereas parasympathetic activity of the heart via the vagus nerve is decreased.

These compensatory mechanisms stabilize arterial BP (Freeman, Wieling, Axelrod, et al., 2011).

Normal postural responses that occur when a person moves from a lying to a standing position include (1) a heart rate increase of 5 to 20 bpm above the resting rate; (2) an unchanged systolic pressure, or a slight decrease of up to 10 mm Hg; and (3) a slight increase of 5 mm Hg in diastolic pressure.

Postural (orthostatic) hypotension is a sustained decrease of at least 20 mm Hg in systolic BP or 10 mm Hg in diastolic BP within 3 minutes of moving from a lying or sitting to a standing position (Freeman et al., 2011). It is usually accompanied by dizziness, lightheadedness, or syncope.

Postural hypotension in patients with CVD is most often due to a significant reduction in preload, which compromises cardiac output. Reduced preload, which is reflective of intravascular volume depletion, is caused by dehydration from overdiuresis, bleeding (due to antiplatelet or anticoagulant medications or post intravascular procedures), or medications that dilate the blood vessels (e.g., nitrates and antihypertensive agents). In these situations, the usual mechanisms needed to maintain cardiac output (increased heart rate and peripheral vasoconstriction) cannot compensate for the significant loss in intravascular volume. As a result, the BP drops

Adapted from Woods, S. L., Froelicher, E. S., Motzer, S. A., et al. (2009). *Cardiac nursing* (6th ed.). Philadelphia: Lippincott Williams & Wilkins.

ASSESSMENT
Assessing Patients for Postural Hypotension

The following steps are recommended when assessing patients for postural hypotension:

- Position the patient supine for 10 minutes before taking the initial blood pressure (BP) and heart rate measurements.
- Reposition the patient to a sitting position with legs in the dependent position, wait 2 minutes, then reassess both BP and heart rate measurements.
- If the patient is symptom free or has no significant decreases in systolic or diastolic BP, assist the patient into a standing position, obtain measurements immediately, and recheck in 2 minutes; continue measurements every 2 minutes for a total of 10 minutes to rule out postural hypotension.
- Return the patient to a supine position if postural hypotension is detected or if the patient becomes symptomatic.
- Document heart rate and BP measured in each position (e.g., supine, sitting, and standing) and any signs or symptoms that accompany the postural changes.

and heart rate increases with changes from lying or sitting to upright positions (see Chart 25-2).

The following is an example of BP and heart rate measurements in a patient with postural hypotension:

Supine: BP 120/70 mm Hg, heart rate 70 bpm
Sitting: BP 100/55 mm Hg, heart rate 90 bpm
Standing: BP 98/52 mm Hg, heart rate 94 bpm

Arterial Pulses

The arteries are palpated to evaluate the pulse rate, rhythm, amplitude, contour, and obstruction to blood flow.

Pulse Rate

The normal pulse rate varies from a low of 50 bpm in healthy, athletic young adults to rates well in excess of 100 bpm after exercise or during times of excitement. Anxiety frequently raises the pulse rate during the physical examination. If the rate is higher than expected, the nurse should reassess the pulse near the end of the physical examination, when the patient may be more relaxed.

Pulse Rhythm

The rhythm of the pulse is normally regular. Minor variations in regularity of the pulse may occur with respirations. The pulse rate may increase during inhalation and slow during exhalation due to changes in blood flow to the heart during the respiratory cycle This phenomenon, called *sinus arrhythmia,* occurs most commonly in children and young adults.

For the initial cardiac examination, or if the pulse rhythm is irregular, the heart rate should be counted by auscultating the apical pulse, located at the PMI, for a full minute while simultaneously palpating the radial pulse. Any discrepancy between contractions heard and pulses felt is noted. Disturbances of rhythm (dysrhythmias) often result in a **pulse deficit**, which is a difference between the apical and radial pulse rates. Pulse deficits commonly occur with atrial fibrillation, atrial flutter, and premature ventricular contractions. These dysrhythmias stimulate the ventricles to contact prematurely, before diastole is finished. As a result, these early

ventricular contractions produce a smaller stroke volume, which can be heard during auscultation but do not produce a palpable pulse (see Chapter 26 for a detailed discussion of these dysrhythmias).

Pulse Amplitude

The pulse amplitude, indicative of the BP in the artery, is used to assess peripheral arterial circulation. The nurse assesses pulse amplitude bilaterally and describes and records the amplitude of each artery. The simplest method characterizes the pulse as absent, diminished, normal, or bounding. Scales are also used to rate the strength of the pulse. The following is an example of a 0-to-4 scale:

0: Not palpable or absent
+1: Diminished—weak, thready pulse; difficult to palpate; obliterated with pressure
+2: Normal—cannot be obliterated
+3: Moderately increased—easy to palpate, full pulse; cannot be obliterated
+4: Markedly increased—strong, bounding pulse; may be abnormal

The numerical classification is subjective; therefore, when documenting the pulse amplitude, specify location of the artery and scale range (e.g., "left radial +3/+4") (Weber & Kelley, 2010).

If the pulse is absent or difficult to palpate, the nurse can use a continuous wave Doppler. This portable ultrasound device has a transducer that is placed over the artery. The transducer emits and receives ultrasound beams. Rhythmic changes are heard as blood cells flow through patent arteries, whereas obstruction to blood flow is evidenced by no changes in sound. (Ultrasound techniques are discussed in more detail in Chapter 30.)

Pulse Contour

The contour of the pulse conveys important information. In patients with stenosis of the aortic valve, the valve opening is narrowed, reducing the amount of blood ejected into the aorta. The pulse pressure is narrow, and the pulse feels feeble. In aortic insufficiency, the aortic valve does not close completely, allowing blood to flow back from the aorta into the left ventricle. The rise of the pulse wave is abrupt and strong, and its fall is precipitous—a "collapsing" or "water hammer" pulse. The true contour of the pulse is best appreciated by palpating over the carotid artery rather than the distal radial artery, because the dramatic characteristics of the pulse wave may be distorted when the pulse is transmitted to smaller vessels.

Palpation of Arterial Pulses

To assess peripheral circulation, the nurse locates and evaluates all arterial pulses. Arterial pulses are palpated at points where the arteries are near the skin surface and are easily compressed against bones or firm musculature. Pulses are detected over the right and left temporal, common carotid, brachial, radial, femoral, popliteal, dorsalis pedis, and posterior tibial arteries (see Fig. 30-2 in Chapter 30). A reliable assessment of the pulses depends on accurate identification of the location of the artery and careful palpation of the area. Light palpation is essential; firm finger pressure can obliterate the temporal, dorsalis pedis, and posterior tibial pulses and confuse the examiner. In approximately 10% of patients, the dorsalis pedis pulses are not palpable (Woods et al., 2009). In such circumstances, both are usually absent and the posterior tibial arteries alone provide adequate blood supply to the feet. Arteries in the extremities are often palpated simultaneously to facilitate comparison of quality.

> ▶ *Quality and Safety Nursing Alert*
>
> **Do not simultaneously palpate both the temporal and carotid arteries, because it is possible to decrease the blood flow to the brain.**

Jugular Venous Pulsations

Right-sided heart function can be estimated by observing the pulsations of the jugular veins of the neck, which reflects central venous pressure (CVP). CVP is the pressure in the right atria or the right ventricle at the end of diastole. If the internal jugular pulsations are difficult to see, pulsations of the external jugular veins may be noted. These veins are more superficial and are visible just above the clavicles, adjacent to the sternocleidomastoid muscles.

In patients who have normal blood volume (euvolemia), the jugular veins are normally visible in the supine position with the head of the bed elevated to 30 degrees (Bickley, 2009). Obvious distention of the veins with the patient's head elevated 45 to 90 degrees indicates an abnormal increase in CVP. This abnormality is observed in patients with right-sided HF, due to hypervolemia, pulmonary hypertension, and pulmonary stenosis; less commonly with obstruction of blood flow in the superior vena cava; and rarely with acute massive pulmonary embolism.

Heart Inspection and Palpation

The heart is examined by inspection, palpation, and auscultation of the precordium or anterior chest wall that covers the heart and lower thorax. A systematic approach is used to examine the precordium in the following six areas. Figure 25-5 identifies these important landmarks:

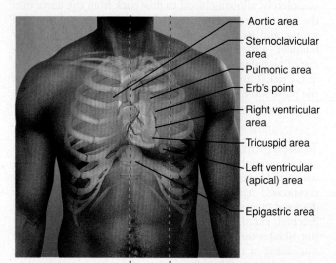

Midsternum Midclavicular line

FIGURE 25-5 • Areas of the precordium to be assessed when evaluating heart function. Numerals identify ribs of adjacent intercostal spaces.

1. *Aortic area*—second intercostal space to the right of the sternum. To determine the correct intercostal space, the nurse first finds the angle of Louis by locating the bony ridge near the top of the sternum, at the junction of the sternum and the manubrium. From this angle, the second intercostal space is located by sliding one finger to the left or right of the sternum. Subsequent intercostal spaces are located from this reference point by palpating down the rib cage.
2. *Pulmonic area*—second intercostal space to the left of the sternum
3. *Erb's point*—third intercostal space to the left of the sternum
4. *Tricuspid area*—fourth and fifth intercostal spaces to the left of the sternum
5. *Mitral (apical) area*—left fifth intercostal space at the midclavicular line
6. *Epigastric area*—below the xiphoid process

For most of the examination, the patient lies supine, with the head of the bed slightly elevated. A right-handed examiner stands at the right side of the patient, a left-handed examiner at the left side.

Each area of the precordium is inspected for pulsations and is then palpated. An apical impulse is a normal finding observed in young patients and adults who have thin chest walls.

The apical impulse may be felt as a light pulsation, 1 to 2 cm in diameter. It is felt at the onset of the first heart sound and lasts for only half of ventricular systole (see the next section for a discussion of heart sounds). The nurse uses the palm of the hand to locate the apical impulse initially and the fingerpads to assess its size and quality. Palpation of the apical pulse may be facilitated by repositioning the patient to the left lateral position, which puts the heart in closer contact with the chest wall (Fig. 25-6).

There are several abnormalities that the nurse may find during palpation of the precordium. Normally, the apical impulse is palpable in only one intercostal space; palpability in two or more adjacent intercostal spaces indicates left ventricular enlargement. An apical impulse below the fifth intercostal space or lateral to the midclavicular line usually denotes left ventricular enlargement from left ventricular failure. If the apical impulse can be palpated in two distinctly separate areas and the pulsation movements are paradoxical (not simultaneous), a ventricular aneurysm may be suspected. A broad and forceful apical impulse is known as a left ventricular heave or lift because it appears to lift the hand from the chest wall during palpation.

A vibration or purring sensation may be felt over areas where abnormal, turbulent blood flow is present. It is best detected by using the palm of the hand. This vibration is called a *thrill* and is associated with a loud murmur. Depending on the location of the thrill, it may be indicative of serious valvular heart disease; an atrial or ventricular septal defect (abnormal opening); or stenosis of a large artery, such as the carotid artery.

Heart Auscultation

A stethoscope is used to auscultate each of the locations identified in Figure 25-5, with the exception of the epigastric area. The purpose of cardiac auscultation is to determine

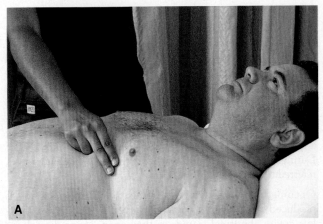
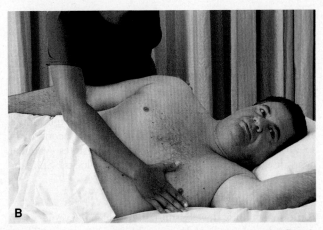

FIGURE 25-6 • Palpating the apical impulse. **A.** Remain on the patient's right side, and ask the patient to remain supine. Use the finger pads to palpate the apical impulse in the mitral area (fourth or fifth intercostal space at the midclavicular line). **B.** You may ask the patient to roll to the left side to better feel the impulse using the palmar surfaces of your hand. Photos from Weber, J. W., & Kelley, J. (2014). *Health assessment in nursing* (5th ed.). Philadelphia: Lippincott Williams & Wilkins.

heart rate and rhythm and evaluate heart sounds. The apical area is auscultated for 1 minute to determine the apical pulse rate and the regularity of the heartbeat. Normal and abnormal heart sounds detected during auscultation are described next.

Normal Heart Sounds

Normal heart sounds, referred to as S_1 and S_2, are produced by closure of the AV valves and the semilunar valves, respectively. The period between S_1 and S_2 corresponds with ventricular systole (Fig. 25-7). When the heart rate is within the normal range, systole is much shorter than the period between S_2 and S_1 (diastole). However, as the heart rate increases, diastole shortens.

Normally, S_1 and S_2 are the only sounds heard during the cardiac cycle (Bickley, 2009).

S_1—First Heart Sound. Tricuspid and mitral valve closure creates the first heart sound (S_1). The word "lub" is used to replicate its sound. S_1 is usually heard the loudest at the apical area. S_1 is easily identifiable and serves as the point of reference for the remainder of the cardiac cycle.

The intensity of S_1 increases during tachycardias or with mitral stenosis. In these circumstances, the AV valves are wide open during ventricular contraction. The accentuated S_1 occurs as the AV valves close with greater force than normal. Similarly, dysrhythmias can vary the intensity of S_1 from beat to beat due to lack of synchronized atrial and ventricular contraction.

S2—Second Heart Sound. Closure of the pulmonic and aortic valves produces the second heart sound (S_2), commonly referred to as the "dub" sound. The aortic component of S_2 is heard the loudest over the aortic and pulmonic areas. However, the pulmonic component of S_2 is a softer sound and is heard best over the pulmonic area.

Although these valves close almost simultaneously, the pulmonic valve lags slightly behind the aortic valve. In some individuals, it is possible to distinguish between the closure of the aortic and pulmonic valves. When this situation occurs,

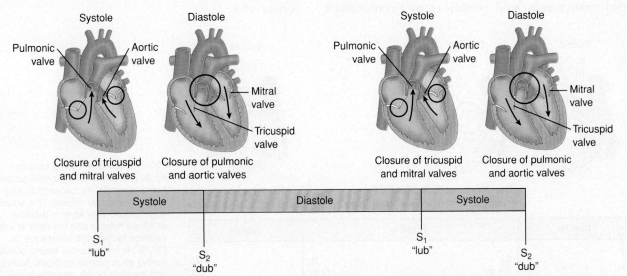

FIGURE 25-7 • Normal heart sounds. The first heart sound (S_1) is produced by closure of the mitral and tricuspid valves ("lub"). The second heart sound (S_2) is produced by closure of the aortic and pulmonic valves ("dub"). *Arrows represent the direction of blood flow.*

the patient is said to have a split S_2. Normal physiologic splitting of S_2 is accentuated on inspiration and disappears on expiration. During inspiration, there is a decrease in intrathoracic pressure and subsequent increase in venous return to the right atrium and ventricle. The right ventricle takes a little longer to eject this extra volume, which causes the pulmonic valve to close a little later than normal. Splitting of S_2 that remains constant during inspiration and expiration is an abnormal finding. Abnormal splitting of the second heart sound can be caused by a variety of disease states (valvular heart disease, septal defects, bundle branch blocks). Splitting of S_2 is best heard over the pulmonic area.

Abnormal Heart Sounds

Abnormal sounds develop during systole or diastole when structural or functional heart problems are present. These sounds are called S_3 or S_4 gallops, opening snaps, systolic clicks, and murmurs. S_3 and S_4 gallop sounds are heard during diastole. These sounds are created by the vibration of the ventricle and surrounding structures as blood meets resistance during ventricular filling. The term *gallop* evolved from the cadence that is produced by the addition of a third or fourth heart sound, similar to the sound of a galloping horse. Gallop sounds are very low-frequency sounds and are heard with the bell of the stethoscope placed very lightly against the chest.

S_3—**Third Heart Sound.** An S_3 ("DUB") is heard early in diastole during the period of rapid ventricular filling as blood flows from the atrium into a noncompliant ventricle. It is heard immediately after S_2. "Lub-dub-DUB" is used to imitate the abnormal sound of a beating heart when an S_3 is present. It represents a normal finding in children and adults up to 35 or 40 years of age. In these cases, it is referred to as a physiologic S_3 (Fig. 25-8). In older adults, an S_3 is a significant finding, suggesting HF. It is best heard with the bell of the stethoscope. If the right ventricle is involved, a right-sided S_3 is heard over the tricuspid area with the patient in a supine position. A left-sided S_3 is best heard over the apical area with the patient in the left lateral position.

S_4—**Fourth Heart Sound.** S_4 ("LUB") occurs late in diastole (see Fig. 25-8). S_4 heard just before S_1 is generated during atrial contraction as blood forcefully enters a noncompliant

ventricle. This resistance to blood flow is due to ventricular hypertrophy caused by hypertension, CAD, cardiomyopathies, aortic stenosis, and numerous other conditions. "LUB lub-dub" is the mnemonic used to imitate this gallop sound. S_4, produced in the left ventricle, is auscultated using the bell of the stethoscope over the apical area with the patient in the left lateral position. A right-sided S_4, although less common, is heard best over the tricuspid area with the patient in supine position. There are times when both S_3 and S_4 are present, creating a quadruple rhythm, which sounds like "LUB lub-dub DUB." During tachycardia, all four sounds combine into a loud sound, referred to as a **summation gallop**.

Opening Snaps and Systolic Clicks. Normally, no sound is produced when valves open. However, diseased valve leaflets create abnormal sounds as they open during diastole or systole. **Opening snaps** are abnormal diastolic sounds heard during opening of an AV valve. For example, mitral stenosis can cause an opening snap, which is an unusually high-pitched sound very early in diastole. This sound is caused by high pressure in the left atrium that abruptly displaces or "snaps" open a rigid valve leaflet. Timing helps to distinguish an opening snap from the other gallop sounds. It occurs too long after S_2 to be mistaken for a split S_2 and too early in diastole to be mistaken for an S_3. The high-pitched, snapping quality of the sound is another way to differentiate an opening snap from an S_3. Hearing a murmur or the sound of turbulent blood flow is expected following the opening snap. An opening snap is heard best using the diaphragm of the stethoscope placed medial to the apical area and along the lower left sternal border.

In a similar manner, stenosis of one of the semilunar valves creates a short, high-pitched sound in early systole, immediately after S_1. This sound, called a **systolic click**, is the result of the opening of a rigid and calcified aortic or pulmonic valve during ventricular contraction. Mid- to late systolic clicks may be heard in patients with mitral or tricuspid valve prolapse as the malfunctioning valve leaflet is displaced into the atrium during ventricular systole. Murmurs are expected to be heard following these abnormal systolic sounds. These sounds are the loudest in the areas directly over the malfunctioning valve.

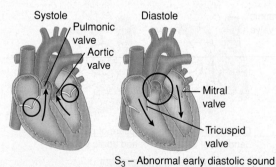

S_3 – Abnormal early diastolic sound during period of rapid ventricular filling

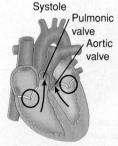

S_4 – Abnormal late diastolic sound during atrial systole

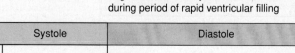

FIGURE 25-8 • Gallop sounds. An S_3 ("DUB") is an abnormal sound heard immediately following S_2 (closure of semilunar valves). This sound is generated very early in diastole as blood flowing into the right or left ventricle is met with resistance. S_4 ("LUB") is an abnormal sound created during atrial systole as blood flowing into the right or left ventricle is met with resistance. *Arrows* represent the direction of blood flow.

Chart 25-3   Characteristics of Heart Murmurs

Heart murmurs are described in terms of location, timing, intensity, pitch, quality, and radiation. These characteristics provide information needed to determine the cause of the murmur and its clinical significance.

Location

Pinpointing the location of the murmur helps to determine the underlying structures that are involved in generating the abnormal sounds. The locations described in Figure 25-5 are used to identify where the loudest sounds are detected. The description should include the exact location from which the sound emanates, such as the location of the intercostal space and other important landmarks (right or left sternal border; midsternal, midclavicular, anterior axillary, or midaxillary lines). For example, a ventricular septal defect can be located at the left sternal border in the third and fourth intercostal spaces.

Timing

A murmur is described in terms of when it occurs during the cardiac cycle (systole or diastole). Murmurs are further differentiated by identifying exactly when during systole or diastole they are heard. A skilled clinician can detect that the murmur is occurring during early, mid-, or late systole or diastole. Some murmurs have sounds that occur in both systole and diastole.

Intensity

A grading system is used to describe the intensity or loudness of a murmur.

Grade 1: Very faint and difficult for the inexperienced clinician to hear

Grade 2: Quiet but readily perceived by the experienced clinician
Grade 3: Moderately loud
Grade 4: Loud and may be associated with a thrill
Grade 5: Very loud; heard when stethoscope is partially off the chest; associated with a thrill
Grade 6: Extremely loud; detected with the stethoscope off the chest; associated with a thrill

Pitch

Pitch describes the sound frequency, identified as high, medium, or low pitched. High-pitched murmurs are heard best with the stethoscope's diaphragm, whereas low-pitched sounds are detected using the bell of the stethoscope placed lightly on the chest wall.

Quality

Quality describes the sound that the murmur resembles. Murmurs can produce a rumbling, blowing, whistling, harsh, or musical sound. For example, murmurs caused by mitral or tricuspid regurgitation have a blowing quality, whereas mitral stenosis generates a rumbling sound.

Radiation

Radiation refers to the transmission of the murmur from the point of maximal intensity to other areas in the upper chest. The examiner determines if radiation is present by listening carefully to areas of the heart adjacent to the point where the murmur is the loudest. If radiation is present, the exact location is described. A murmur associated with aortic stenosis, for example, can radiate into the neck, down the left sternal border, and into the apical area.

Murmurs. Murmurs are created by turbulent flow of blood in the heart. The causes of the turbulence may be a critically narrowed valve, a malfunctioning valve that allows regurgitant blood flow, a congenital defect of the ventricular wall, a defect between the aorta and the pulmonary artery, or an increased flow of blood through a normal structure (e.g., with fever, pregnancy, hyperthyroidism). Murmurs are characterized and consequently described by several characteristics, including their timing in the cardiac cycle, location on the chest wall, intensity, pitch, quality, and pattern of radiation (Chart 25-3).

Friction Rub. A harsh, grating sound that can be heard in both systole and diastole is called a *friction rub*. It is caused by abrasion of the inflamed pericardial surfaces from pericarditis. Because a friction rub may be confused with a murmur, care should be taken to identify the sound and to distinguish it from murmurs that may be heard in both systole and diastole. A pericardial friction rub can be heard best using the diaphragm of the stethoscope, with the patient sitting up and leaning forward.

Auscultation Procedure

During auscultation, the patient remains supine and the examining room is as quiet as possible. A stethoscope with both diaphragm and bell functions is necessary for accurate auscultation of the heart.

Using the diaphragm of the stethoscope, the examiner starts at the apical area and progresses upward along the left sternal border to the pulmonic and aortic areas. Alternatively, the examiner may begin the examination at the aortic and pulmonic areas and progress downward to the apex of the heart. Initially, S_1 is identified and evaluated with respect to its intensity and splitting. Next, S_2 is identified, and its intensity and any splitting are noted. After concentrating on S_1 and S_2, the examiner listens for extra sounds in systole and then in diastole.

Sometimes it helps to ask the following questions: Do I hear snapping or clicking sounds? Do I hear any high-pitched blowing sounds? Is this sound in systole, or diastole, or both? The examiner again proceeds to move the stethoscope to all of the designated areas of the precordium, listening carefully for these sounds. Finally, the patient is turned on the left side and the stethoscope is placed on the apical area, where an S_3, an S_4, and a mitral murmur are more readily detected.

Once an abnormality is heard, the entire chest surface is reexamined to determine the exact location of the sound and its radiation. The patient may be concerned about the prolonged examination and must be supported and reassured. The auscultatory findings, particularly murmurs, are documented by identifying the following characteristics (see Chart 25-3): location on chest wall, timing, intensity, pitch, quality, and radiation.

Interpretation of Heart Sounds

Interpreting heart sounds requires detailed knowledge of cardiac physiology and pathophysiology. However, all nurses should have adequate knowledge and skill to recognize normal heart sounds (S_1, S_2) and the presence of abnormal sounds. When assessment is at this very basic level of practice, abnormal findings are reported for further evaluation and treatment. More advanced skills are required of nurses caring for critically ill patients with CVD or those nurses functioning in advanced practice roles. Nurses in these roles readily identify abnormal heart sounds, recognize the diagnostic significance of their findings, and use their assessment skills to evaluate patients' responses to medical interventions. For example, these highly skilled nurses monitor heart sounds in patients with HF to detect the resolution of an S_3 after treatment with a diuretic.

Assessment of Other Systems

Lungs

The details of respiratory assessment are described in Chapter 20. Findings frequently exhibited by patients with cardiac disorders include the following:

Hemoptysis: Pink, frothy sputum is indicative of acute pulmonary edema.

Cough: A dry, hacking cough from irritation of small airways is common in patients with pulmonary congestion from HF.

Crackles: HF or atelectasis associated with bed rest, splinting from ischemic pain, or the effects of analgesic, sedative, or anesthetic agents often results in the development of crackles. Typically, crackles are first noted at the bases (because of gravity's effect on fluid accumulation and decreased ventilation of basilar tissue), but they may progress to all portions of the lung fields.

Wheezes: Compression of the small airways by interstitial pulmonary edema may cause wheezing. Beta-adrenergic blocking agents (beta-blockers), such as propranolol (Inderal), may cause airway narrowing, especially in patients with underlying pulmonary disease.

Abdomen

For the patient with a cardiovascular disorder, several components of the abdominal examination are relevant:

Abdominal distension: A protuberant abdomen with bulging flanks indicates ascites. Ascites develops in patients with right ventricular or biventricular HF (both right- and left-sided HF). In the failing right heart, abnormally high chamber pressures impede the return of venous blood. As a result, the liver and spleen become engorged with excessive venous blood (hepatosplenomegaly). As pressure in the portal system rises, fluid shifts from the vascular bed into the abdominal cavity. Ascitic fluid, found in the dependent or lowest points in the abdomen, will shift with position changes.

Hepatojugular reflux: This test is performed when right ventricular or biventricular HF is suspected. The patient is positioned so that the jugular venous pulse is visible in the lower part of the neck. While observing the jugular venous pulse, firm pressure is applied over the right upper quadrant of the abdomen for 30 to 60 seconds. An increase of 1 cm or more in jugular venous pressure is indicative of a positive hepatojugular reflux. This positive test aids in confirming the diagnosis of HF.

Bladder distention: Urine output is an important indicator of cardiac function. Reduced urine output may indicate inadequate renal perfusion or a less serious problem such as one caused by urinary retention. When urine output is decreased, the patient must be assessed for a distended bladder or difficulty voiding. The bladder may be assessed with an ultrasound scanner (see Figure 53-8 in Chapter 53) or the suprapubic area palpated for an oval mass and percussed for dullness, indicative of a full bladder.

 Gerontologic Considerations

When performing a cardiovascular examination on an older patient, the nurse may note such differences as more readily palpable peripheral pulses because of decreased elasticity of the arteries and a loss of adjacent connective tissue. Palpation of the precordium in older adults is affected by the changes in the shape of the chest. For example, a cardiac impulse may not be palpable in patients with chronic obstructive pulmonary disease, because these patients usually have an increased anterior–posterior chest diameter. Kyphoscoliosis, a spinal deformity that occurs in many older adult patients, may move the cardiac apex downward so that palpation of the apical impulse is obscured.

Hypertension is a common problem in older adults that results from age-related stiffening of the aorta and other large arteries. As people age, their systolic BP gradually increases, whereas when they reach late middle age, the diastolic BP plateaus (Aronow, Fleg, Pepine, et al., 2011). Isolated systolic hypertension occurs most commonly among older adults and is associated with significant cardiovascular morbidity and mortality. Orthostatic hypotension, a result of impaired baroreceptor function that normally regulates BP, places older adults at risk for falls. Prolonged bed rest, dehydration, and many cardiovascular medications (e.g., beta-blockers, angiotensin-converting enzyme inhibitors, angiotensin receptor blockers, diuretics, nitrates) are additional risk factors that heighten the risk for orthostatic hypotension.

An S_4 that is associated with hypertension is common in older adults. It is thought to be due to a decrease in compliance of the left ventricle. The S_2 is usually split. At least 60% of older patients have murmurs, the most common being a soft systolic ejection murmur resulting from sclerotic changes of the aortic leaflets (Bickley, 2009) (see Table 25-1).

Diagnostic Evaluation

A wide range of diagnostic studies may be performed in patients with cardiovascular conditions. The nurse should educate the patient on the purpose, what to expect, and any possible side effects related to these examinations prior to testing. The nurse should note trends in results because they provide information about disease progression as well as the patient's response to therapy.

Laboratory Tests

Samples of the patient's blood are sent to the laboratory for the following reasons:
- To assist in making a diagnosis
- To screen for risk factors associated with CAD

- To establish baseline values before initiating other diagnostic tests, procedures, or therapeutic interventions
- To monitor response to therapeutic interventions
- To assess for abnormalities in the blood that affect prognosis

Normal values for laboratory tests may vary depending on the laboratory and the health care institution. This variation is due to the differences in equipment and methods of measurement across organizations.

Cardiac Biomarker Analysis

The diagnosis of MI is made by evaluating the history and physical examination, the 12-lead electrocardiogram (ECG), and the results of laboratory tests that measure serum cardiac biomarkers. Myocardial cells that become necrotic from prolonged ischemia or trauma release specific enzymes (creatine kinase [CK]), CK isoenzymes (CK-MB), and proteins (myoglobin, troponin T, and troponin I). These substances leak into the interstitial spaces of the myocardium and are carried by the lymphatic system into general circulation. As a result, abnormally high levels of these substances can be detected in serum blood samples. (See Chapter 27 for further discussion of cardiac biomarker analysis.)

Blood Chemistry, Hematology, and Coagulation Studies

Table 25-4 provides information about some common serum laboratory tests and the implications for patients with CVD. Discussion of lipid, brain (B-type) natriuretic peptide (BNP), C-reactive protein (CRP), and homocysteine measurements follows.

Lipid Profile

Cholesterol, triglycerides, and lipoproteins are measured to evaluate a person's risk of developing CAD, especially if there is a family history of premature heart disease, or to diagnose a specific lipoprotein abnormality. Cholesterol and triglycerides are transported in the blood by combining with plasma proteins to form lipoproteins (LDLs and HDLs). The risk of CAD increases as the ratio of LDL to HDL or the ratio of total cholesterol to HDL increases. Although cholesterol levels remain relatively constant over 24 hours, the blood specimen for the lipid profile should be obtained after a 12-hour fast.

Cholesterol Levels. Cholesterol (normal level is less than 200 mg/dL) is a lipid required for hormone synthesis and cell membrane formation. It is found in large quantities in brain and nerve tissue. Two major sources of cholesterol are diet (animal products) and the liver, where cholesterol is synthesized. Elevated cholesterol levels are known to increase the risk of CAD. Factors that contribute to variations in cholesterol levels include age, gender, diet, exercise patterns, genetics, menopause, tobacco use, and stress levels.

LDLs (normal level is less than 160 mg/dL) are the primary transporters of cholesterol and triglycerides into the cell. One harmful effect of LDL is the deposition of these substances in the walls of arterial vessels. Elevated LDL levels are associated with a greater incidence of CAD. In people with known CAD or diabetes, the primary goal for lipid management is reduction of LDL levels to less than 70 mg/dL (Smith et al., 2011).

HDLs (normal range in men is 35 to 70 mg/dL; in women, 35 to 85 mg/dL) have a protective action. They transport cholesterol away from the tissue and cells of the arterial wall to the liver for excretion. Therefore, there is an inverse relationship between HDL levels and risk of CAD. Factors that lower HDL levels include smoking, diabetes, obesity, and physical inactivity. In patients with CAD, a secondary goal of lipid management is the increase of HDL levels to more than 40 mg/dL (Smith et al., 2011).

Triglycerides. Triglycerides (normal range is 100 to 200 mg/dL), composed of free fatty acids and glycerol, are stored in the adipose tissue and are a source of energy. Triglyceride levels increase after meals and are affected by stress. Diabetes, alcohol use, and obesity can elevate triglyceride levels. These levels have a direct correlation with LDL and an inverse one with HDL.

Brain (B-Type) Natriuretic Peptide

BNP is a neurohormone that helps regulate BP and fluid volume. It is primarily secreted from the ventricles in response to increased preload with resulting elevated ventricular pressure. The level of BNP in the blood increases as the ventricular walls expand from increased pressure, making it a helpful diagnostic, monitoring, and prognostic tool in the setting of HF. Because this serum laboratory test can be quickly obtained, BNP levels are useful for prompt diagnosis of HF in settings such as the ED. Elevations in BNP can occur from a number of other conditions such as pulmonary embolus, MI, and ventricular hypertrophy. Therefore, the clinician correlates BNP levels with abnormal physical assessment findings and other diagnostic tests before making a definitive diagnosis of HF. A BNP level greater than 100 pg/mL is suggestive of HF.

C-Reactive Protein

CRP is a protein produced by the liver in response to systemic inflammation. Inflammation is thought to play a role in the development and progression of atherosclerosis. The high-sensitivity CRP (hs-CRP) test is used as an adjunct to other tests to predict CVD risk. People with high hs-CRP levels (3 mg/L or greater) may be at greatest risk for CVD compared to people with moderate (1 to 3 mg/L) or low (less than 1 mg/L) hs-CRP levels (Woods et al., 2009).

Homocysteine

Homocysteine, an amino acid, is linked to the development of atherosclerosis because it can damage the endothelial lining of arteries and promote thrombus formation. Therefore, an elevated blood level of homocysteine is thought to indicate a high risk for CAD, stroke, and peripheral vascular disease, although it is not an independent predictor of CAD. Genetic factors and a diet low in folate, vitamin B_6, and vitamin B_{12} are associated with elevated homocysteine levels. A 12-hour fast is necessary before drawing a blood sample for an accurate serum measurement. Test results are interpreted as optimal (less than 12 mcmol/L), borderline (12 to 15 mcmol/L), and high risk (greater than 15 mcmol/L) (Woods et al., 2009).

Chest X-Ray and Fluoroscopy

A chest x-ray is obtained to determine the size, contour, and position of the heart. It reveals cardiac and pericardial

TABLE 25-4   Common Serum Laboratory Tests and Implications for Patients With Cardiovascular Disease

Laboratory Test Reference Range	Implications
Blood Chemistries	
Blood urea nitrogen (BUN): 10–20 mg/dL	BUN and creatinine are end products of protein metabolism excreted by the kidneys. Elevated BUN reflects reduced renal perfusion from decreased cardiac output or intravascular fluid volume deficit as a result of diuretic therapy or dehydration.
Calcium (Ca^{++}): 8.6–10.2 mg/dL	Calcium is necessary for blood coagulability, neuromuscular activity, and automaticity of the nodal cells (sinus and atrioventricular nodes). *Hypocalcemia:* Decreased calcium levels slow nodal function and impair myocardial contractility. The latter effect increases the risk for heart failure. *Hypercalcemia:* Increased calcium levels can occur with the administration of thiazide diuretics because these medications reduce renal excretion of calcium. Hypercalcemia potentiates digitalis toxicity, causes increased myocardial contractility, and increases the risk for varying degrees of heart block and sudden death from ventricular fibrillation.
Creatinine: 0.7–1.4 mg/dL	Both BUN and creatinine are used to assess renal function, although creatinine is a more sensitive measure. Renal impairment is detected by an increase in both BUN and creatinine. A normal creatinine level and an elevated BUN suggest an intravascular fluid volume deficit.
Magnesium (Mg^{++}): 1.3–2.3 mEq/L	Magnesium is necessary for the absorption of calcium, maintenance of potassium stores, and metabolism of adenosine triphosphate. It plays a major role in protein and carbohydrate synthesis and muscular contraction. *Hypomagnesemia:* Decreased magnesium levels are due to enhanced renal excretion of magnesium from the use of diuretic or digitalis therapy. Low magnesium levels predispose patients to atrial or ventricular tachycardias. *Hypermagnesemia:* Increased magnesium levels are commonly caused by the use of cathartics or antacids containing magnesium. Increased magnesium levels depress contractility and excitability of the myocardium, causing heart block and, if severe, asystole.
Potassium (K^{+}): 3.5–5 mEq/L	Potassium has a major role in cardiac electrophysiologic function. *Hypokalemia:* Decreased potassium levels due to administration of potassium-excreting diuretics can cause many forms of dysrhythmias, including life-threatening ventricular tachycardia or ventricular fibrillation, and predispose patients taking digitalis preparations to digitalis toxicity. *Hyperkalemia:* Increased potassium levels can result from an increased intake of potassium (e.g., foods high in potassium or potassium supplements), decreased renal excretion of potassium, the use of potassium-sparing diuretics (e.g., spironolactone), or the use of angiotensin-converting enzyme inhibitors that inhibit aldosterone function. Serious consequences of hyperkalemia include heart block, asystole, and life-threatening ventricular dysrhythmias.
Sodium (Na^{+}): 135–145 mEq/L	Low or high serum sodium levels do not directly affect cardiac function. *Hyponatremia:* Decreased sodium levels indicate fluid excess and can be caused by heart failure or administration of thiazide diuretics. *Hypernatremia:* Increased sodium levels indicate fluid deficits and can result from decreased water intake or loss of water through excessive sweating or diarrhea.
Coagulation Studies	Injury to a vessel wall or tissue initiates the formation of a thrombus. This injury activates the coagulation cascade, the complex interactions among phospholipids, calcium, and clotting factors that convert prothrombin to thrombin. The coagulation cascade has two pathways: the intrinsic and extrinsic pathways. Coagulation studies are routinely performed before invasive procedures, such as cardiac catheterization, electrophysiology testing, and cardiac surgery.
Partial thromboplastin time (PTT): 60–70 s Activated partial thromboplastin time (aPTT): 20–39 s	PTT or aPTT measures the activity of the intrinsic pathway and is used to assess the effects of unfractionated heparin. A therapeutic range is 1.5–2.5 times baseline values. Adjustment of heparin dose is required for aPTT <50 s (↑ dose) or >100 s (↓ dose).
Prothrombin time (PT): 9.5–12 s	PT measures the extrinsic pathway activity and is used to monitor the level of anticoagulation with warfarin (Coumadin).
International normalized ratio (INR): 1	The INR, reported with the PT, provides a standard method for reporting PT levels and eliminates the variation of PT results from different laboratories. The INR, rather than the PT alone, is used to monitor the effectiveness of warfarin. The therapeutic range for INR is 2–3.5, although specific ranges vary based on diagnosis.
Hematologic Studies	
Complete blood count (CBC)	The CBC identifies the total number of white and red blood cells and platelets, and measures hemoglobin and hematocrit. The CBC is carefully monitored in patients with cardiovascular disease.
Hematocrit Male: 42%–52% Female: 35%–47% Hemoglobin Male: 13–18 g/dL Female: 12–16 g/dL	The hematocrit represents the percentage of red blood cells found in 100 mL of whole blood. The red blood cells contain hemoglobin, which transports oxygen to the cells. Low hemoglobin and hematocrit levels have serious consequences for patients with cardiovascular disease, such as more frequent angina episodes or acute myocardial infarction.
Platelets: 150,000–450,000/mm^3	Platelets are the first line of protection against bleeding. Once activated by blood vessel wall injury or rupture of atherosclerotic plaque, platelets undergo chemical changes that form a thrombus. Several medications inhibit platelet function, including aspirin, clopidogrel (Plavix), and intravenous glycoprotein IIb/IIIa inhibitors (abciximab [ReoPro], eptifibatide [Integrilin], and tirofiban [Aggrastat]). When these medications are administered, it is essential to monitor for thrombocytopenia (low platelet counts).
White blood cell (WBC) count: 4,500–11,000/mm^3	WBC counts are monitored in immunocompromised patients, including patients with heart transplants or in situations where there is concern for infection (e.g., after invasive procedures or surgery).

Adapted from Woods, S. L., Froelicher, E. S., Motzer, S. A., et al. (2009). *Cardiac nursing* (6th ed.). Philadelphia: Lippincott Williams & Wilkins.

calcifications and demonstrates physiologic alterations in the pulmonary circulation. Although it does not help diagnose acute MI, it can help diagnose some complications (e.g., HF). Correct placement of pacemakers and pulmonary artery catheters is also confirmed by chest x-ray.

Fluoroscopy is an x-ray imaging technique that allows visualization of the heart on a screen. It shows cardiac and vascular pulsations and unusual cardiac contours. This technique uses a movable x-ray source, which makes it a useful aid for positioning transvenous pacing electrodes and for guiding the insertion of arterial and venous catheters during cardiac catheterization and other cardiac procedures.

Electrocardiography

The ECG is a graphic representation of the electrical currents of the heart. The ECG is obtained by placing disposable electrodes in standard positions on the skin of the chest wall and extremities (see Chapter 26 for electrode placement). Recordings of the electrical current flowing between two electrodes is made on graph paper or displayed on a monitor. Several different recordings can be obtained by using a variety of electrode combinations, called *leads*. Simply stated, a lead is a specific view of the electrical activity of heart. The standard ECG is composed of 12 leads or 12 different views, although it is possible to record 15 or 18 leads.

The 12-lead ECG is used to diagnose dysrhythmias, conduction abnormalities, and chamber enlargement, as well as myocardial ischemia, injury, or infarction. It can also suggest cardiac effects of electrolyte disturbances (high or low calcium and potassium levels) and the effects of antiarrhythmic medications. A 15-lead ECG adds three additional chest leads across the right precordium and is used for early diagnosis of right ventricular and left posterior (ventricular) infarction. The 18-lead ECG adds three posterior leads to the 15-lead ECG and is useful for early detection of myocardial ischemia and injury. To enhance interpretation of the ECG, the patient's age, gender, BP, height, weight, symptoms, and medications (especially digitalis and antiarrhythmic agents) are noted on the ECG requisition. (See Chapter 26 for a more detailed discussion of ECG.)

Continuous Electrocardiographic Monitoring

Continuous ECG monitoring is the standard of care for patients who are at high risk for dysrhythmias. This form of cardiac monitoring detects abnormalities in heart rate and rhythm. Many systems have the capacity to monitor for changes in ST segments, which are used to identify the presence of myocardial ischemia or injury (see Chapter 27). Two types of continuous ECG monitoring techniques are used in health care settings: hardwire cardiac monitoring, found in EDs, critical care units, and progressive care units; and telemetry, found in general nursing care units or outpatient cardiac rehabilitation programs. Hardwire cardiac monitoring and telemetry systems vary in sophistication; however, most systems have the following features in common:

- Monitor more than one ECG lead simultaneously
- Monitor ST segments (ST-segment depression is a marker of myocardial ischemia; ST-segment elevation provides evidence of an evolving MI)
- Provide graded visual and audible alarms (based on priority, asystole merits the highest grade of alarm)

- Interpret and store alarms
- Trend data over time
- Print a copy of rhythms from one or more specific ECG leads over a set time (called a *rhythm strip*)

⚑ Quality and Safety Nursing Alert

Patients placed on continuous ECG monitoring must be informed of its purpose and cautioned that it does not detect shortness of breath, chest pain, or other ACS symptoms. Thus, patients are instructed to report new or worsening symptoms immediately.

Hardwire Cardiac Monitoring

Hardwire cardiac monitoring is used to continuously observe the heart for dysrhythmias and conduction disorders using one or two ECG leads. A real-time ECG is displayed on a bedside monitor and at a central monitoring station. In critical care units, additional components can be added to the bedside monitor to continuously monitor hemodynamic parameters (noninvasive BP, arterial pressures, pulmonary artery pressures), respiratory parameters (respiratory rate, oxygen saturation), and ST segments for myocardial ischemia.

Telemetry

In addition to hardwire cardiac monitoring, the ECG can be continuously observed by **telemetry**—the transmission of radio waves from a battery-operated transmitter to a central bank of monitors. The primary benefit of using telemetry is that the system is wireless, which allows patients to ambulate while one or two ECG leads are monitored. The patient has electrodes placed on the chest with a lead cable that connects to the transmitter. The transmitter can be placed in a disposable pouch and worn around the neck, or simply secured to the patient's clothing. Most transmitter batteries are changed every 24 to 48 hours.

Lead Systems

The number of electrodes needed for hardwire cardiac monitoring and telemetry is dictated by the lead system used in the clinical setting. Electrodes need to be securely and accurately placed on the chest wall. Chart 25-4 provides helpful hints on how to apply these electrodes. There are three-, four-, or five-lead systems available for ECG monitoring. The type of lead system used determines the number of lead options for monitoring. For example, the five-lead system provides up to seven different lead selections. Unlike the other two systems, the five-lead system can monitor the activity of the anterior wall of the left ventricle. Figure 25-9 presents diagrams of electrode placement.

The two ECG leads most often selected for continuous ECG monitoring are leads II and V_1. Lead II provides the best visualization of atrial depolarization (represented by the P wave). Lead V_1 best records ventricular depolarization and is most helpful when monitoring for certain dysrhythmias (e.g., premature ventricular contractions, tachycardias, bundle branch blocks) (see Chapter 26).

Ambulatory Electrocardiography

Ambulatory electrocardiography is a form of continuous ECG monitoring used for diagnostic purposes in the outpatient

Chart 25-4 Applying Electrodes

The monitoring system requires an adequate electrical signal to analyze the patient's cardiac rhythm. When applying electrodes, the following recommendations should be followed to optimize skin adherence and conduction of the heart's electrical current:

- Débride the skin surface of dead cells with soap and water and dry well (or as recommended by the manufacturer).
- Clip (do not shave) hair from around the electrode site, if needed.
- If the patient is diaphoretic (sweaty), apply a small amount of benzoin to the skin, avoiding the area under the center of the electrode.
- Connect the electrodes to the lead wires prior to placing them on the chest (connecting lead wires when electrodes are in place may be uncomfortable for some patients).
- Peel the backing off the electrode, and check to make sure the center is moist with electrode gel.
- Locate the appropriate lead placement, and apply the electrode to the skin, securing it in place with light pressure.
- Change the electrodes every 24–48 hours (or as recommended by the manufacturer), examine the skin for irritation, and apply the electrodes to different locations.
- If the patient is sensitive to the electrodes, use hypoallergenic electrodes.

Adapted from Drew, B. J., Califf, R. M., Funk, M., et al. (2005). AHA scientific statement: Practice standards for electrocardiographic monitoring in hospital settings: An American Heart Association scientific statement from the Councils on Cardiovascular Nursing, Clinical Cardiology, and Cardiovascular Disease in the Young: Endorsed by the International Society of Computerized Electrocardiology and the American Association of Critical Care Nurses. *Journal of Cardiovascular Nursing, 20*(2), 76–106.

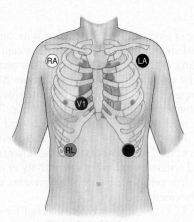

RA – Right arm (white)
LA – Left arm (black)
RL – Right leg (green)
LL – Left leg (red)
V1 – Chest or precordium (brown)

FIGURE 25-9 • Electrode placement used in continuous electrocardiographic monitoring for three-lead system, placement on RA, LA, and LL; four-lead system, placement on RA, LA, RL, and LL; five-lead system, placement on RA, LA, RL, LL, and V1.

setting. Electrodes (number varies based on model used) are connected with lead wires to a cable that is inserted into a portable recorder (i.e., Holter monitor) that records the ECG onto a digital memory device. The patient wears the recorder for 24 hours to detect dysrhythmias or myocardial ischemia that may occur during waking hours or sleep. The patient keeps a diary, noting the time of any symptoms or performance of unusual activities. Data from the digital memory device are uploaded into a computer for analysis, and rhythms that need further evaluation by a clinician are identified. Ambulatory electrocardiography is used to identify the etiology of symptoms (e.g., syncope, palpitations) that may be caused by dysrhythmias, to detect episodes of myocardial ischemia, and to evaluate effectiveness of cardiac medications (e.g., antiarrhythmic medications, nitrates) or pacemaker function.

Transtelephonic Monitoring

Another method of evaluating the ECG of a patient at home is by transtelephonic monitoring. The patient attaches a specific lead system for transmitting the signals and places a landline telephone mouthpiece over the transmitter box. The ECG is recorded and evaluated at a remote location, such as a physician's office or community agency. This method is often used for diagnosing dysrhythmias and to evaluate pacemaker and implantable cardioverter defibrillator function.

Wireless Mobile Cardiac Monitoring Systems

This technology allows health care professionals to monitor and transmit the ECG of patients outside of the hospital or office setting continuously. The wireless method has several advantages when compared with Holter and transtelephonic monitoring. It is lightweight and can monitor the patient 24 hours a day, 7 days a week. Patients wear a small sensing device that transmits each heartbeat to a small monitor. When a dysrhythmia is detected, the system automatically transmits the patient's ECG to a monitoring center either through the patient's telephone line when at home or through wireless communications systems when outside of the home. This system enhances detection and early treatment of dysrhythmias that might otherwise be diagnosed only after the patient develops serious symptoms.

Nursing Interventions for Cardiac Monitoring

Several nursing interventions facilitate acquisition of accurate data and ensure patient safety when using various forms of cardiac monitoring. The nurse should change electrodes according to the manufacturer's recommendations using proper skin preparation. During electrode changes, the skin should be assessed for allergic responses (itchy, reddened skin) to the adhesive or electrode gel. If present, the electrodes should be replaced with hypoallergenic electrodes. In addition, in order to avoid skin breakdown, electrode placement should be rotated (see Fig. 25-9).

The nurse should ensure that electrodes and lead connections are positioned correctly. Improper positioning can result in an inaccurate ECG tracing that mimics ischemia or dysrhythmias. Two leads should be selected that provide the best tracing for dysrhythmia monitoring, which are usually lead II and the chest lead V_1. In addition, the nurse should keep the ECG recordings free of artifact, which is an abnormal ECG pattern caused by muscular activity, patient movement, electrical interference, or lead cable or electrode malfunction. Artifact can mimic dysrhythmias and cause unnecessary alarms. To avoid artifact, the nurse should prepare the patient's skin as recommended by the manufacturer and avoid placing electrodes over bony areas of the chest. Electrical equipment in use around the patient should be inspected to be certain that it is functioning properly and has been recently checked by the medical engineering department per organization policy, because improperly functioning equipment may also cause artifact.

The nurse must respond to and correct all monitors immediately. Inoperative (inop) monitoring alarms—used to communicate that electrodes have fallen off, that leads are loose, or that the system's battery power is low (e.g., telemetry)—are just as significant as the alarms that indicate the patient is tachycardic, bradycardic, and experiencing another potentially life-threatening dysrhythmia. Timely responses to all alarms can prevent serious consequences, including death.

Hospital-acquired infections may be prevented by keeping lead wire cables and transmitter equipment clean, per organizational policy. A patient should never be connected to monitoring equipment that has not been thoroughly cleaned between patients. If a patient is scheduled for a device implant, such as a pacemaker, electrodes should not be placed over the planned incision site. Likewise, electrodes should never be placed over an incision, implanted device, open wounds, or inflamed skin.

Electrodes should be removed once monitoring is discontinued and skin cleansed to remove excess electrode gel and adhesive. Metal-containing electrodes must be removed before sending a patient for magnetic resonance angiography (MRA).

Telemetry transmitters and other monitoring equipment should be maintained according to the manufacturer's recommendations. Monitoring devices of any type should not be submerged in water. A monitoring device may break if dropped; therefore, it should be secured to the patient's gown or clothing (Baranchuk, Shaw, Alanazi, et al., 2009; Evenson & Farnsworth, 2010; Graham & Cvach, 2010; Hannibal, 2011).

Cardiac Stress Testing

Normally, the coronary arteries dilate to four times their usual diameter in response to increased metabolic demands for oxygen and nutrients. However, coronary arteries affected by atherosclerosis dilate less, compromising blood flow to the myocardium and causing ischemia. Therefore, abnormalities in cardiovascular function are more likely to be detected during times of increased demand, or "stress." The **cardiac stress test** procedures—the exercise stress test and the pharmacologic stress test—are noninvasive ways to evaluate the response of the cardiovascular system to stress. The stress test helps determine the following: (1) presence of CAD, (2) cause of chest pain, (3) functional capacity of the heart after an MI or heart surgery, (4) effectiveness of antianginal or antiarrhythmic medications, (5) occurrence of dysrhythmias, and (6) specific goals for a physical fitness program. Contraindications to stress testing include severe aortic stenosis, acute myocarditis or pericarditis, severe hypertension, suspected left main CAD, HF, and unstable angina. Because complications of stress testing can be life threatening (MI, cardiac arrest, HF, and severe dysrhythmias), testing facilities must have staff and equipment ready to provide treatment, including advanced cardiac life support.

Stress testing is often combined with echocardiography or radionuclide imaging, techniques used to capture images of the heart. Cardiac imaging is performed during the resting state and immediately after stress testing.

Exercise Stress Testing

Procedure

During an exercise stress test, the patient walks on a treadmill (most common), pedals a stationary bicycle, or uses an arm crank (Myers, Arena, & Franklin, 2009). Exercise intensity progresses according to established protocols. The protocol selected for the test is based on the purpose of the test and the physical fitness level and health of the patient (Woods et al., 2009). During the test, the following are monitored: two or more ECG leads for heart rate, rhythm, and ischemic changes; BP; skin temperature; physical appearance; perceived exertion; and symptoms, including chest pain, dyspnea, dizziness, leg cramping, and fatigue. The test is terminated when the target heart rate is achieved or if the patient experiences signs of myocardial ischemia. Further diagnostic testing, such as a cardiac catheterization, may be warranted if the patient develops chest pain, extreme fatigue, a decrease in BP or pulse rate, serious dysrhythmias, or ST-segment changes on the ECG during the stress test.

Nursing Interventions

In preparation for the exercise stress test, the patient is instructed to fast for 4 hours before the test and to avoid stimulants such as tobacco and caffeine. Medications may be taken with sips of water. The primary provider may instruct the patient not to take certain cardiac medications, such as beta-adrenergic blocking agents, before the test. Clothes and sneakers or rubber-soled shoes suitable for exercising are to be worn. The nurse prepares the patient for the stress test by describing how the stress test is performed, the type of monitoring equipment used, the rationale for insertion of an IV catheter, and what symptoms to report. The exercise method is reviewed, and patients are asked to put forth their best exercise effort. If the test is to be performed with echocardiography or radionuclide imaging (described in the next section), this information is reviewed as well. After the test, the patient is monitored for 10 to 15 minutes. Once stable, patients may resume their usual activities.

Pharmacologic Stress Testing

Procedure

Patients who are physically disabled or deconditioned will not be able to achieve their target heart rate by exercising on a treadmill or bicycle. Two vasodilating agents, dipyridamole (Persantine) and adenosine (Adenocard), administered IV, are used to mimic the effects of exercise by maximally dilating the coronary arteries. The effects of dipyridamole last about 15 to 30 minutes. The side effects are related to its vasodilating action and include chest discomfort, dizziness, headache, flushing, and nausea. Adenosine has similar side effects, although patients report these symptoms as more severe. Adenosine has an extremely short half-life (less than 10 seconds), so any severe effects subside rapidly. Dipyridamole and adenosine are the agents of choice used in conjunction with radionuclide imaging techniques. Theophylline and other xanthines, such as caffeine, block the effects of dipyridamole and adenosine and must be avoided before these pharmacologic stress tests.

Dobutamine may also be used if the patient cannot exercise. Dobutamine, a synthetic sympathomimetic agent, increases heart rate, myocardial contractility, and BP, thereby increasing the metabolic demands of the heart. It is the agent of choice when echocardiography is used because of its effects on altering myocardial wall motion (due to enhanced contractility). Dobutamine is also used for patients who have bronchospasm or pulmonary disease and cannot tolerate having doses of theophylline withheld.

Nursing Interventions

In preparation for the pharmacologic stress test, the patient is instructed not to eat or drink anything for at least 4 hours before the test. This includes chocolate, caffeine, caffeine-free coffee, tea, carbonated beverages, or medications that contain caffeine (e.g., Anacin). If caffeine is ingested before a dipyridamole or adenosine stress test, the test will have to be rescheduled. Patients taking aminophylline, theophylline, or dipyridamole are instructed to stop taking these medications for 24 to 48 hours before the test (if tolerated). The patient is informed about the transient sensations that may occur during infusion of the vasodilating agent, such as flushing or nausea, which will disappear quickly. The patient is instructed to report the occurrence of any other symptoms during the test to the cardiologist or nurse. The stress test may take about 1 hour, or up to 3 hours if imaging is performed.

Echocardiography

Transthoracic Echocardiography

Echocardiography is a noninvasive ultrasound test that is used to measure the ejection fraction and examine the size, shape, and motion of cardiac structures. It is particularly useful for diagnosing pericardial effusions; determining chamber size and the etiology of heart murmurs; evaluating the function of heart valves, including prosthetic heart valves; and evaluating ventricular wall motion.

Procedure

Echocardiography involves transmission of high-frequency sound waves into the heart through the chest wall and the recording of the return signals. With the traditional transthoracic approach, the ultrasound is generated by a handheld transducer applied to the front of the chest. The transducer picks up the echoes and converts them to electrical impulses that are recorded and displayed on a monitor. It creates sophisticated, spatially correct images of the heart. An ECG is recorded simultaneously to assist in interpretation of the echocardiogram.

With the use of Doppler techniques, an echocardiogram can also show the direction and velocity of the blood flow through the heart. These techniques are used to assess for "leaking valves," conditions referred to as valvular regurgitation, and will also detect abnormal blood flow between the septum of the left and right heart.

Echocardiography may be performed with an exercise or pharmacologic stress test. Images are obtained at rest and then immediately after the target heart rate is reached. Myocardial ischemia from decreased perfusion during stress causes abnormalities in ventricular wall motion and is easily detected by echocardiography. A stress test using echocardiography is considered positive if abnormalities in ventricular wall motion are detected during stress but not during rest. These findings are highly suggestive of CAD and require further evaluation, such as a cardiac catheterization.

Nursing Interventions

Before transthoracic echocardiography, the nurse informs the patient about the test, explaining that it is painless. Echocardiographic monitoring is performed while a transducer that emits sound waves is moved over the surface of the chest wall. Gel applied to the skin helps transmit the sound waves. Periodically, the patient is asked to turn onto the left side or hold a breath. The test takes about 30 to 45 minutes. If the patient is to undergo an exercise or pharmacologic stress test with echocardiography, information on stress testing is also reviewed with the patient.

Transesophageal Echocardiography

Procedure

A significant limitation of transthoracic echocardiography is the poor quality of the images produced. Ultrasound loses its clarity as it passes through tissue, lung, and bone. An alternate technique involves threading a small transducer through the mouth and into the esophagus. This technique, called *transesophageal echocardiography* (TEE), provides clearer images because ultrasound waves pass through less tissue. A topical anesthetic agent and moderate sedation are used during TEE because of the discomfort associated with the positioning of the transducer in the esophagus (refer to Chapter 18 for further discussion of moderate sedation). Once the patient is comfortable, the transducer is inserted into the mouth and the patient is asked to swallow several times until it is positioned in the esophagus.

The high-quality imaging obtained during TEE makes this technique an important first-line diagnostic tool for evaluating patients with many types of CVD, including HF, valvular heart disease, dysrhythmias, and many other conditions that place the patient at risk for atrial or ventricular thrombi. Pharmacologic stress testing using dobutamine and TEE can also be performed. It is frequently used during cardiac surgery to continuously monitor the response of the heart to the surgical procedure (e.g., valve replacement or coronary artery bypass). Complications are uncommon during TEE; however, if they do occur, they are serious. These complications are caused by sedation and impaired swallowing resulting from the topical anesthesia (respiratory depression and aspiration) and by insertion and manipulation of the transducer into the esophagus and stomach (vasovagal response or esophageal perforation). The patient must be assessed before TEE for a history of dysphagia or radiation therapy to the chest, which increases the likelihood of complications.

Nursing Interventions

Prior to the test, the nurse provides preprocedure education and ensures that the patient has a clear understanding of what the test entails and why it is being performed, instructs the patient not to eat or drink anything for 6 hours prior to the study, and checks to make sure that informed consent has been obtained. The nurse also inserts an IV line or assesses an existing IV for patency and asks the patient to remove full or partial dentures. During the test, the nurse provides emotional support and monitors level of consciousness, BP, ECG, respiration, and oxygen saturation (SpO₂). During the recovery period, the patient must maintain bed rest with the head of the bed elevated to 45 degrees. Following the moderate sedation policy of the agency, the nurse monitors the patient for dyspnea and assesses vital signs, SpO₂, level of consciousness, and gag reflex as recommended. Food and oral fluids are withheld until the patient is fully alert and the effects of the topical anesthetic agent are reversed, usually 2 hours after the procedure; if the gag reflex is intact, the nurse begins feeding with sips of water, then advances to the preprocedure diet. The patient is informed that a sore throat may be present for the next 24 hours; he or she is instructed to report the presence of a persistent sore throat, shortness of breath, or difficulty swallowing. If the procedure is performed in an outpatient setting, a family member or friend must be available to transport the patient home from the test site.

Radionuclide Imaging

Radionuclide imaging studies involve the use of radioisotopes to noninvasively evaluate coronary artery perfusion, to detect myocardial ischemia and infarction, and to assess left ventricular function. **Radioisotopes** are unstable atoms that give off small amounts of energy in the form of gamma rays as they decay. When radioisotopes are injected into the bloodstream, the energy emitted can be detected by a gamma scintillation camera positioned over the body.

Myocardial Perfusion Imaging

Procedure

Myocardial perfusion imaging is used in combination with stress testing to compare images obtained when the heart is resting to images of the heart in a stressed state resulting from exercise or medications. Results of this test aid in determining if CAD is the cause of chest pain or other CAD-related symptoms. It is commonly performed after an acute MI to determine if arterial perfusion to the heart is compromised during activity and to evaluate the extent of myocardial damage.

The imaging is performed in two stages. Usually, the resting images are taken first. An IV is inserted to administer the radioisotope, and electrodes are placed on the chest to monitor the heart rate and rhythm. Patients are positioned on their backs with their arms over their heads under the imaging camera. The procedure takes approximately 30 minutes. The second scan is repeated following the exercise or pharmacologic stress test.

An area of the myocardium that shows no perfusion or reduced perfusion is said to have a "defect" present. Comparing resting images with images taken after the stress test help differentiate ischemic myocardium from infarct-related myocardium. After an MI, there will be a defect present in the infarcted area of the heart that remains the same size during exercise and rest. This is called a *fixed defect*, indicating that there is no perfusion in that area of the myocardium. Defects that appear or that get larger after the stress test images are taken indicate reduced perfusion to that area of the heart. Because the defect disappears with rest, it is called a *reversible defect*. Reversible defects constitute positive stress test findings. Typically, cardiac catheterization is recommended after a positive test result to determine the severity of obstructions to blood flow caused by CAD.

Nursing Interventions

The patient undergoing nuclear imaging techniques with stress testing should be prepared for the type of stressor to be used (exercise or medication) and provided with details of what to expect during imaging. Prior to the study, the nurse inserts an IV line or assesses an existing IV for patency. The patient may be concerned about receiving a radioactive substance and needs to be reassured that these tracers are safe—the radiation exposure is similar to that of other diagnostic x-ray studies. No postprocedure radiation precautions are necessary.

Test of Ventricular Function and Wall Motion

Equilibrium radionuclide angiocardiography (ERNA), also known as multiple-gated acquisition (MUGA) scanning, is a common noninvasive technique that uses a conventional scintillation camera interfaced with a computer to record images of the heart during several hundred heartbeats. The computer processes the data and allows for sequential viewing of the functioning heart. The sequential images are analyzed to evaluate left ventricular function, wall motion, and ejection fraction.

The patient is reassured that there is no known radiation danger and is instructed to remain motionless during the scan.

Computed Tomography

Procedure

Cardiovascular computed tomography (CT) scanning is a form of cardiac imaging that uses x-rays to provide accurate anatomic images of the four chambers of the heart, valves, arteries, veins, and pericardium. It is not commonly used to evaluate myocardial perfusion or valvular function.

CT scanning is performed by placing the patient on a table that moves into a structure that holds the x-ray and scanning equipment. Images are created through analysis of data obtained during the scan by using complex mathematical and computer algorithms (Woods et al., 2009). These images are used to evaluate bypass graft patency, congenital heart lesions, and left and right ventricular wall thickness, as well as to localize cardiac tumors and masses. The CT scan is contraindicated in pregnancy and in patients with renal insufficiency. The contrast agent used during the CT scan is excreted through the kidneys; therefore, renal function should be assessed prior to the scan. IV hydration before and after the scan may be indicated to minimize the effect of the contrast on renal function. If the patient has a history of hypersensitivity to contrast agents, premedication with steroids and antihistamines is indicated (Woods et al., 2009).

CT angiography is performed using IV contrast agents to enhance the x-rays and improve visualization of the lumen of the arteries for stenosis. One of the limiting factors in the use of CT angiography is the fact that the motion created by respirations and cardiac rate and rhythm affects the quality of the imaging. Patients may receive beta-blockers prior to the scan to control heart rate and rhythm. The patient is instructed to hold his or her breath periodically throughout the scan.

CT scans, using electron beam computed tomography (EBCT), are used to determine the amount of calcium deposits in the coronary arteries that may be indicative of atherosclerosis. From this scan, a calcium score is derived that predicts the likelihood of cardiac events, such as MI, or the need for a revascularization procedure in the future. Currently, coronary calcium measurement is thought to be a reasonable test to consider in patients with low to intermediate risk for future CAD-related events. Results of the test may help to reclassify them to higher risk and thus intensify primary prevention measures (Greenland, Alpert, Beller, et al., 2010).

Nursing Interventions

The nurse provides details of the procedure to help prepare the patient for the test. The patient is positioned on a table, and the scanner rotates around the table during the test. The procedure is noninvasive and painless. However, to obtain adequate images, the patient must lie completely still during the scanning process. An IV is necessary if contrast is to be used to enhance the images. The patient should be told to expect transient flushing, metallic taste, nausea, or bradycardia during the contrast infusion.

Positron Emission Tomography

Positron emission tomography (PET) is a commonly used noninvasive nuclear cardiovascular imaging technique. It is used to evaluate the severity of CAD by evaluating myocardial perfusion. In addition, it evaluates left ventricular function and the extent of damage caused by MI. The results of this test help clinicians establish a treatment plan for CAD (e.g., coronary artery bypass surgery, PCI) (Woods et al., 2009).

The nurse should assess patients for fear of closed spaces or claustrophobia. Patients should be reassured that medications are given to help them relax. Patients should also be reassured that radiation exposure is at safe and acceptable levels, similar to those of other diagnostic x-ray studies.

Procedure

During a PET scan, radioisotopes are administered by injection; one compound is used to determine blood flow in the myocardium, and another determines the metabolic function. The PET camera provides detailed three-dimensional images of the distributed compounds. The viability of the myocardium is determined by comparing the extent of glucose metabolism in the myocardium to the degree of blood flow. For example, ischemic but viable tissue will show decreased blood flow and elevated metabolism. For a patient with this finding, revascularization through surgery or angioplasty will probably be indicated to improve heart function. Restrictions of food intake before the test vary among institutions, but because PET evaluates glucose metabolism, the patient's blood glucose level should be within the normal range before testing.

Nursing Interventions

The nurse should instruct the patient to refrain from using tobacco and ingesting caffeine for 4 hours before the PET procedure. To prepare the patient for the test, the nurse inserts an IV or assesses the existing IV catheter for patency, and then describes the procedure to the patient. A radioisotope is injected into the IV. It takes about an hour for the tracer to absorb into the body. Electrodes are placed on the chest to monitor the heart rate and rhythm. The patient lies on a narrow table that is positioned inside a large tubelike scanner. The test takes 90 minutes to complete. During this time, the patient must lie still so that clear images of the heart can be obtained.

Magnetic Resonance Angiography

Procedure

MRA is a noninvasive, painless technique that is used to examine both the physiologic and anatomic properties of the heart. MRA uses a powerful magnetic field and computer-generated pictures to image the heart and great vessels. It is valuable in diagnosing diseases of the aorta, heart muscle, and pericardium, as well as congenital heart lesions. The application of this technique to the evaluation of coronary artery anatomy is limited because the quality of the images are distorted by respirations, the beating heart, and certain implanted devices (stents and surgical clips). In addition, this technique cannot adequately visualize the small distal coronary arteries as accurately as conventional angiography performed during a cardiac catheterization. Therefore, the latter technique remains the gold standard for the diagnosis of CAD (Bluemke, Achenbach, Budoff, et al., 2008).

Nursing Interventions

Because of the magnetic field used during MRA, patients must be screened for contraindications for its use. MRA cannot be performed on patients who have a pacemaker, metal plates, prosthetic joints, or other metallic implants that can become dislodged if exposed to MRA. Patients are instructed to remove any jewelry, watches, or other metal items (e.g., ECG leads). Transdermal patches that contain a heat-conducting aluminized layer (e.g., NicoDerm, Androderm, Transderm Nitro, Transderm Scop, Catapres-TTS) must be removed before MRA to prevent burning of the skin. During MRA, the patient is positioned supine on a table that is placed into an enclosed imager or tube containing the magnetic field. A patient who is claustrophobic may need to receive a mild sedative before undergoing an MRA. An intermittent clanking or thumping that can be annoying is generated by the magnetic coils, so the patient may be offered a headset to listen to music. The scanner is equipped with a microphone so that the patient can communicate with the staff. The patient is instructed to remain motionless during the scan.

Cardiac Catheterization

Cardiac catheterization is an invasive diagnostic procedure in which radiopaque arterial and venous catheters are advanced into the right and left heart. As noted previously, it is the gold standard diagnostic test for CAD (Bluemke et al., 2008). Catheter advancement is guided by fluoroscopy. Catheters are inserted through the blood vessels percutaneously, or via a cutdown procedure if the patient has poor vascular access. Pressures and oxygen saturation levels in the four heart chambers are measured.

Cardiac catheterization is performed to diagnose CAD; assess coronary artery patency; determine the extent of atherosclerosis; and determine whether revascularization procedures, including PCI or coronary artery bypass surgery, may be of benefit to the patient (see Chapter 27). Cardiac catheterization is also performed to diagnose pulmonary artery hypertension and valvular heart disease. During cardiac catheterization, the patient has one or more IV lines in place for the administration of sedative agents, fluids, heparin, and other medications. BP and ECG monitoring is necessary to observe for hemodynamic instability or dysrhythmias. The myocardium can become ischemic and trigger dysrhythmias as catheters are positioned in the coronary arteries or during injection of radiopaque contrast agents. Resuscitation equipment must be readily available, and staff must be prepared to provide advanced cardiac life support measures as necessary.

Radiopaque contrast agents are used to visualize the coronary arteries. Some contrast agents contain iodine, and the patient is assessed before the procedure for previous reactions to contrast agents or allergies to iodine-containing substances (e.g., seafood). If the patient has a suspected or known allergy to the substance, antihistamines or methylprednisolone (Solu-Medrol) may be administered before the procedure. In addition, the following blood tests are performed to identify abnormalities that may complicate recovery: blood urea nitrogen (BUN) and creatinine levels, international normalized ratio and prothrombin time, activated thromboplastin time, hematocrit and hemoglobin values, platelet count, and electrolyte levels.

Patients undergoing cardiac catheterization who have comorbid conditions—including diabetes, HF, preexisting renal disease, hypotension, dehydration, or advanced age—are at risk for contrast agent–induced nephropathy (defined as an increase in the baseline serum creatinine by 25% or more within 2 days of the procedure) (Raingruber, Kirkland-Walsh, Chahon, et al., 2011). Although this form of acute renal failure is usually reversible, temporary dialysis may be necessary. Preventive strategies for high-risk patients include preprocedure and postprocedure hydration with IV infusions of saline or sodium bicarbonate and the antioxidant acetylcysteine (Mucomyst) (Levine et al., 2011).

Cardiac catheterization is commonly performed on an outpatient basis and requires 2 to 6 hours of bed rest after the procedure before the patient is allowed to ambulate. Variations in time to ambulation are related to the size of the catheter used during the procedure, the site of catheter insertion (femoral or radial artery), the patient's anticoagulation status, and other variables (e.g., advanced age, obesity, bleeding disorder). The use of smaller (4 or 6 Fr) catheters is associated with shorter recovery times.

Several options are used to achieve arterial hemostasis after catheter removal. Compression devices specifically designed for use with the transradial artery approach are available. For example, the Termuo TR Band™, positioned over the artery, has a device that puts pressure against the artery after it is inflated with air. It remains in place for about 2 hours.

For the femoral approach, manual pressure may be used alone or in combination with mechanical compression devices such as the FemoStop™ (placed over the puncture site for 30 minutes). Percutaneously deployed devices are also available. These devices are positioned at the femoral arterial puncture site after completion of the procedure. They deploy a saline-soaked gelatin sponge (QuickSeal), collagen (VasoSeal), sutures (Perclose, Techstar), or a combination of both collagen and sutures (Angio-Seal). Other products that expedite arterial hemostasis include external patches (Syvek Patch, Clo-Sur P.A.D.). These products are placed over the puncture site as the catheter is removed and manual pressure is applied for 4 to 10 minutes. Once hemostasis is achieved, the patch is covered with a dressing that remains in place for 24 hours. A number of factors, such as the patient's condition, cost, institutional availability of these devices, and the physician's preference, determine which closure devices are used.

Major benefits of the percutaneously deployed vascular closure devices include reliable, immediate hemostasis and a shorter time on bed rest without a significant increase in bleeding or other complications. Rare complications associated with these devices include bleeding around the closure device, infection, and arterial obstruction.

Patients hospitalized for angina or acute MI who require cardiac catheterization usually return to their hospital rooms for recovery. In some cardiac catheterization laboratories, a PCI (discussed in Chapter 27) may be performed immediately during the catheterization if indicated.

Right Heart Catheterization

Right heart catheterization usually precedes left heart catheterization. It involves the passage of a catheter from an antecubital or femoral vein into the right atrium, right ventricle, pulmonary artery, and pulmonary arterioles. Pressures and oxygen saturation levels from each of these areas are obtained and recorded. Although right heart catheterization is considered relatively safe, potential complications include dysrhythmias, venous spasm, infection of the insertion site, cardiac perforation, and, rarely, cardiac arrest.

Left Heart Catheterization

Left heart catheterization is performed to evaluate the aortic arch and its major branches, patency of the coronary arteries, and the function of the left ventricle and mitral and aortic valves. Left heart catheterization is performed by retrograde catheterization of the left ventricle. In this approach, the physician usually inserts the catheter into the right brachial artery or a femoral artery and advances it into the aorta and left ventricle. Potential complications include dysrhythmias, MI, perforation of the heart or great vessels, and systemic embolization.

During a left heart catheterization, angiography is also performed. Angiography is an imaging technique that involves the injection of a radiopaque contrast agent into the arterial catheter. The contrast agent is filmed as it passes through the chambers of the heart, aortic arch, and its major arteries. These films allow for comparison of the structure and function of the heart over time.

Coronary angiography is performed to observe the coronary artery anatomy and evaluate the degree of atherosclerosis. A catheter is positioned into the right and left coronary arteries so that the radiopaque contrast agent can be injected directly into each artery. Ventriculography, another angiographic technique, is also performed to evaluate the size and function of the left ventricle. After the catheter is in position, a large amount of radiopaque contrast agent (30 mL) is rapidly injected into the ventricle.

After the procedure, the catheter is carefully withdrawn and arterial hemostasis is achieved using manual pressure or other techniques described previously.

Nursing Interventions

Nursing responsibilities before cardiac catheterization include:
- Instructing the patient to fast, usually for 8 to 12 hours, before the procedure
- Informing patient that if catheterization is to be performed as an outpatient procedure, a friend, family member, or other responsible person must transport the patient home
- Informing the patient about the expected duration of the procedure and advising that it will involve lying on a hard table for less than 2 hours
- Reassuring the patient that IV medications are given to maintain comfort
- Informing the patient about sensations that will be experienced during the catheterization. Knowing what to expect can help the patient cope with the experience. The nurse explains that an occasional pounding sensation (palpitation) may be felt in the chest because of extra heartbeats that almost always occur, particularly when the catheter tip touches the endocardium. The patient may be asked to cough and to breathe deeply, especially after the injection of contrast agent. Coughing may help disrupt a dysrhythmia and clear the contrast agent from the arteries. Breathing deeply and holding the breath help lower the diaphragm for better visualization of heart structures. The injection of a contrast agent into either side of the heart may produce a flushed feeling throughout the body and a sensation similar to the need to void, which subsides in 1 minute or less.
- Encouraging the patient to express fears and anxieties. The nurse provides education and reassurance to reduce apprehension.

Nursing responsibilities after cardiac catheterization are dictated by hospital policy and primary provider preferences and may include:
- Observing the catheter access site for bleeding or hematoma formation and assessing peripheral pulses in the affected extremity (dorsalis pedis and posterior tibial pulses in the lower extremity, radial pulse in the upper extremity) every 15 minutes for 1 hour, every 30 minutes for 1 hour, and hourly for 4 hours or until discharge. BP and heart rate are also assessed during these same time intervals. However, a recent study did not find an association between changes in these vital signs and bleeding complications (Mert, Intepeler, Bengu, et al., 2012). These results suggest that the best method for discovering bleeding is through frequent nursing assessments of the catheter access site (Chart 25-5).
- Evaluating temperature, color, and capillary refill of the affected extremity during these same time intervals. The patient is assessed for affected extremity pain, numbness, or tingling sensations that may indicate arterial insufficiency. The best technique to use is to compare the examination findings between the affected and unaffected extremities. Any changes are reported promptly.
- Screening carefully for dysrhythmias by observing the cardiac monitor or by assessing the apical and peripheral pulses for changes in rate and rhythm. A vasovagal reaction, consisting of bradycardia, hypotension, and nausea, can be precipitated by a distended bladder or by discomfort from manual pressure that is applied during removal of an arterial or venous catheter. The vasovagal response is reversed by promptly elevating the lower extremities above the level of the heart, infusing a bolus of IV fluid, and administering IV atropine to treat the bradycardia.
- Maintaining bed rest for 2 to 6 hours after the procedure. If manual pressure or a mechanical device was used during a femoral artery approach, the patient remains on bed rest for up to 6 hours with the affected leg straight and the head of the bed elevated no greater than 30 degrees (Weigand, 2011). For comfort, the patient may be turned from side to side with the affected extremity straight. If a percutaneous vascular closure device or patch was deployed, the nurse checks local nursing care standards and anticipates that the patient will have fewer activity restrictions. The patient may be permitted to ambulate within 2 hours (Hammel, 2009). If the radial artery was accessed, the patient remains on bed rest for 2 to 3 hours or until the effects of sedation have dissipated. The patient may sit up in bed. A hemostasis band or pressure dressing may be applied over the catheter access site. Analgesic medication is administered as prescribed for discomfort. Patients are instructed to avoid repetitive movement of the affected extremity for 24 to 48 hours (Durham, 2012). Patients are instructed to avoid sleeping on the affected arm for 24 hours.
- Instructing the patient to report chest pain and bleeding or sudden discomfort from the catheter insertion sites promptly
- Monitoring the patient for contrast agent–induced nephropathy by observing for elevations in serum creatinine levels. Oral and IV hydration is used to increase urinary output and flush the contrast agent from the urinary tract; accurate oral and IV intake and urinary output are recorded.
- Ensuring patient safety by instructing the patient to ask for help when getting out of bed the first time after the procedure. The patient is monitored for bleeding from

NURSING RESEARCH PROFILE

Chart 25-5
Monitoring and Identifying Bleeding Following Percutaneous Coronary Intervention

Mert, H., Intepeler, S. S., Bengu, N., et al. (2012). Efficacy of frequent blood pressure and heart rate monitoring for early identification of bleeding following percutaneous coronary intervention. *International Journal of Nursing Practice, 18,* 52–59.

Purpose

An important nursing intervention following percutaneous coronary intervention (PCI) is to assess for procedure-related complications. For example, undetected bleeding from an arterial catheter insertion site can have devastating consequences. To minimize this risk, traditional nursing practice involves obtaining frequent vital signs, which is a time-intensive task for a busy nurse. Typically, blood pressure (BP) and heart rate (HR) are taken on arrival to the patient care unit, then every 15 minutes for 1 hour, every 30 minutes for 1 hour, then hourly for 4 hours. However, there is little evidence in the literature that can be used to define best practice for nursing assessment of this population. The purpose of this study was to determine the efficacy of routine intervals for BP and HR measurement for identification of bleeding complications in patients post PCI.

Design

This descriptive study was conducted in a university hospital. It was comprised of 1,292 participants who were predominately men (71.9%) and had a mean age of 61.4 years. Almost two thirds of the sample (62.8%) underwent a cardiac catheterization, and the remaining (37.2%) had a percutaneous transluminal coronary angioplasty. The femoral artery was cannulated in the majority of these patients (92.8%). Vital signs and assessment for bleeding were initiated upon arrival to the postprocedure recovery unit and continued for the first hour after ambulation.

Findings

There was evidence of bleeding in 118 (9.1%) of the participants. Only 17 (1.3%) participants experienced a small hematoma, all measuring <2 inches, whereas 96 (7.4%) had oozing from the catheter insertion site. In 1,214 cases (94%), the nurses detected the presence of bleeding. There were no significant differences found between the mean systolic and diastolic BP and HR before and during bleeding episodes in these participants. Participants with and without bleeding complications were similar in age, gender, and history of hypertension. A small percentage of participants with or without a bleeding complication had abnormal BPs (hypertension or hypotension) and abnormal HRs (tachycardia or bradycardia). In this cohort, there were no significant differences between the abnormal HR and BP of participants with or without bleeding at time of arrival to the patient care unit and 15, 45, and 60 minutes post PCI. At 30 minutes post PCI, abnormal BP (elevated systolic BP) was significantly higher in participants with bleeding versus no bleeding (152 [11.8%] vs. 43 [3.3%]). After adjusting for age, gender, and history of hypertension, the differences between BP and HR values taken at various time points were not predictive of bleeding complications.

Nursing Implications

Nursing practice needs to be evidence based. Results of this study found that frequent monitoring of BP and HR every 15 minutes for the first hour after PCI may not be an effective method for detecting bleeding complications in this population. Nurses' time may be better served by individualizing the frequency of vital signs based on each patient's condition, which will give nurses more opportunities to assess the catheter insertion site and affected extremity for bleeding.

the catheter access site and for orthostatic hypotension, indicated by complaints of dizziness or lightheadedness (Wiegand, 2011; Woods et al., 2009).

For patients being discharged from the hospital on the same day as the procedure, additional instructions are provided (Chart 25-6).

Chart 25-6
PATIENT EDUCATION
Self-Management After Cardiac Catheterization

After discharge from the hospital for cardiac catheterization, patients should follow these guidelines for self-care:

- *If the artery in your arm or wrist artery was used:* For the next 48 hours, avoid lifting anything heavier than 5 pounds and avoid repetitive movement of your affected hand and wrist.
- *If the artery in your groin was used:* For the next 24 hours, do not bend at the waist, strain, or lift heavy objects.
- Do not submerge the puncture site in water. Avoid tub baths, but shower as desired.
- Talk with your primary provider about when you may return to work, drive, or resume strenuous activities.
- If bleeding occurs, sit (arm or wrist approach) or lie down (groin approach) and apply firm pressure to the puncture site for 10 minutes. Notify your primary provider as soon as possible and follow instructions. If there is a large amount of bleeding, call 911. Do not drive to the hospital.

- Call your primary provider if any of the following occur: swelling, new bruising or pain from your procedure puncture site, temperature of 101°F or more.
- If test results show that you have coronary artery disease, talk with your primary provider about options for treatment, including cardiac rehabilitation programs in your community.
- Talk with your primary provider about lifestyle changes to reduce your risk for further or future heart problems, such as quitting smoking, lowering your cholesterol level, initiating dietary changes, beginning an exercise program, or losing weight.
- Your primary provider may prescribe one or more new medications depending on your risk factors (medications to lower your blood pressure or cholesterol; aspirin or clopidogrel to prevent blood clots). Take all of your medications as instructed. If you feel that any of them are causing side effects, call your primary provider immediately. Do not stop taking any medications before talking to your primary provider.

Adapted from Durham, K. A. (2012). Cardiac catheterization through the radial artery. *American Journal of Nursing, 112*(1), 49–56; and Woods, S. L., Froelicher, E. S., Motzer, S. A., et al. (2009). *Cardiac nursing* (6th ed.). Philadelphia: Lippincott Williams & Wilkins.

Electrophysiologic Testing

The electrophysiology study (EPS) is an invasive procedure that plays a major role in the diagnosis and management of serious dysrhythmias. EPS may be indicated for patients with syncope, palpitations, or both, and for survivors of cardiac arrest from ventricular fibrillation (sudden cardiac death) (Woods et al., 2009). EPS is used to distinguish atrial from ventricular tachycardias when the determination cannot be made from the 12-lead ECG; to evaluate how readily a life-threatening dysrhythmia (e.g., ventricular tachycardia, ventricular fibrillation) can be induced; to evaluate AV node function; to evaluate the effectiveness of antiarrhythmic medications in suppressing the dysrhythmia; or to determine the need for other therapeutic interventions, such as a pacemaker, implantable cardioverter defibrillator, or radiofrequency ablation. (See Chapter 26 for a detailed discussion of EPS.)

 Hemodynamic Monitoring

Critically ill patients require continuous assessment of their cardiovascular system to diagnose and manage their complex medical conditions. This type of assessment is achieved by the use of direct pressure monitoring systems, referred to as **hemodynamic monitoring**. Common forms include CVP, pulmonary artery pressure, and intra-arterial BP monitoring. Patients requiring hemodynamic monitoring are cared for in critical care units. Some progressive care units also admit stable patients with CVP or intra-arterial BP monitoring. To perform hemodynamic monitoring, a CVP, pulmonary artery, or arterial catheter is introduced into the appropriate blood vessel or heart chamber. It is connected to a pressure monitoring system that has several components, including:

- A disposable flush system, composed of IV normal saline solution (which may include heparin), tubing, stopcocks, and a flush device, which provides continuous and manual flushing of the system. Dextrose-containing solutions are no longer indicated because of the risk of infection (O'Grady, Alexander, Burns, et al., 2011).
- A pressure bag placed around the flush solution that is maintained at 300 mm Hg of pressure. The pressurized flush system delivers 3 to 5 mL of solution per hour through the catheter to prevent clotting and backflow of blood into the pressure monitoring system.

- A transducer to convert the pressure coming from the artery or heart chamber into an electrical signal
- An amplifier or monitor, which increases the size of the electrical signal for display on an oscilloscope

Nurses caring for patients who require hemodynamic monitoring receive training prior to using this sophisticated technology. The nurse helps ensure safe and effective care by adhering to the following guidelines:

- Ensuring that the system is set up and maintained properly. For example, the pressure monitoring system must be kept patent and free of air bubbles.
- Checking that the stopcock of the transducer is positioned at the level of the atrium before the system is used to obtain pressure measurements. This landmark is referred to as the phlebostatic axis (Fig. 25-10). The nurse uses a marker to identify this level on the chest wall, which provides a stable reference point for subsequent pressure readings.
- Establishing the zero reference point in order to ensure that the system is properly functioning at atmospheric pressure. This process is accomplished by placing the stopcock of the transducer at the phlebostatic axis, opening the transducer to air, and activating the zero function key on the bedside monitor. Measurements of CVP, BP, and pulmonary artery pressures can be made with the head of the bed elevated up to 60 degrees; however, the system must be repositioned to the phlebostatic axis to ensure an accurate reading (Woods et al., 2009).

Complications from the use of hemodynamic monitoring systems are uncommon and can include pneumothorax, infection, and air embolism. The nurse observes for signs of pneumothorax during the insertion of catheters using a central venous approach (CVP and pulmonary artery catheters). The longer any of these catheters are left in place (after 72 to 96 hours), the greater the risk of infection. Air emboli can be introduced into the vascular system if the stopcocks attached to the pressure transducers are mishandled during blood drawing, administration of medications, or other procedures that require opening the system to air. Therefore, nurses handling this equipment must demonstrate competence prior to independently caring for a patient requiring hemodynamic monitoring.

Catheter-related bloodstream infections are the most common preventable complication associated with hemody-

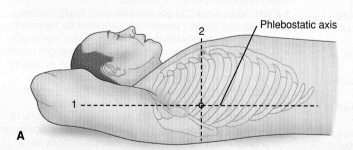
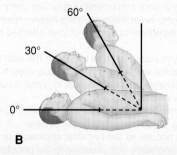

FIGURE 25-10 • A. The phlebostatic axis is the reference point for the atrium when the patient is positioned supine. It is the intersection of two lines on the chest wall: (*1*) the midaxillary line drawn between the anterior and posterior surfaces of the chest and (*2*) the line drawn through the fourth intercostal space. Its location is identified with a skin marker. The stopcock of the transducer used in hemodynamic monitoring is "leveled" at this mark prior to taking pressure measurements. **B.** Measurements can be taken with the head of the bed (HOB) elevated up to 60 degrees. Note the phlebostatic axis changes as the HOB is elevated; thus, the stopcock and transducer must be repositioned after each position change.

namic monitoring systems. Comprehensive guidelines for the prevention of these infections have been published by Centers for Disease Control and Prevention (CDC) (O'Grady et al., 2011). To minimize the risk of infection, a group of evidence-based interventions, called a *care bundle,* should be implemented (see Chart 14-2).

The CDC has additional infection control guidelines that pertain to the ongoing care of these patients, including skin care, dressing changes, and pressure monitoring systems that are outlined in Table 25-5.

Central Venous Pressure Monitoring

CVP is a measurement of the pressure in the vena cava or right atrium. The pressure in the vena cava, right atrium, and right ventricle are equal at the end of diastole; thus, the CVP also reflects the filling pressure of the right ventricle

(preload). The normal CVP is 2 to 6 mm Hg. It is measured by positioning a catheter in the vena cava or right atrium and connecting it to a pressure monitoring system. The CVP is most valuable when it is monitored over time and correlated with the patient's clinical status. A CVP greater than 6 mm Hg indicates an elevated right ventricular preload. There are many problems that can cause an elevated CVP, but the most common problem is hypervolemia (excessive fluid circulating in the body) or right-sided HF. In contrast, a low CVP (less than 2 mm Hg) indicates reduced right ventricular preload, which is most often from hypovolemia. Dehydration, excessive blood loss, vomiting or diarrhea, and overdiuresis can result in hypovolemia and a low CVP. This diagnosis can be substantiated when a rapid IV infusion of fluid causes the CVP to increase.

Before insertion of a CVP catheter, the site is prepared as recommended by the CDC (see Chart 14-2). The preferred site is the subclavian vein; the femoral vein is generally avoided (O'Grady et al., 2011). A local anesthetic agent is used. During this sterile procedure, the physician threads a single-lumen or multilumen catheter through the vein into the vena cava just above or within the right atrium. Once the CVP catheter is inserted, it is secured and a dry sterile dressing is applied. Position of the catheter is confirmed by a chest x-ray.

Nursing Interventions

The frequency of CVP measurements is dictated by the patient's condition and the treatment plan. In addition to obtaining pressure readings, the CVP catheter is used for infusing IV fluids, administering IV medications, and drawing blood specimens. Nursing care of the patient with a CVP catheter is outlined in Table 25-5.

Pulmonary Artery Pressure Monitoring

Pulmonary artery pressure monitoring is used in critical care for assessing left ventricular function, diagnosing the etiology of shock, and evaluating the patient's response to medical interventions (e.g., fluid administration, vasoactive medications). A pulmonary artery catheter and a pressure monitoring system are used. A variety of catheters are available for cardiac pacing, oximetry, cardiac output measurement, or a combination of functions. Pulmonary artery catheters are balloon-tipped, flow-directed catheters that have distal and proximal lumens (Fig. 25-11). The distal lumen has a port that opens into the pulmonary artery. Once connected by its hub to the pressure monitoring system, it is used to measure continuous pulmonary artery pressures. The proximal lumen has a port that opens into the right atrium. It is used to administer IV medications and fluids or to monitor right atrial pressures (i.e., CVP). Each catheter has a balloon inflation hub and valve. A syringe is connected to the hub, which is used to inflate or deflate the balloon with air (1.5-mL capacity). The valve opens and closes the balloon inflation lumen.

A pulmonary artery catheter with specialized capabilities has additional components. For example, the thermodilution catheter has three additional features that enable it to measure cardiac output: a thermistor connector attached to the cardiac output computer of the bedside monitor, a proximal injectate port used for injecting fluids when obtaining the

TABLE 25-5 **Nursing Interventions to Prevent Catheter-Related Bloodstream Infections**

Topic	Intervention
Hand hygiene	• Wash hands with soap and water or use alcohol-based hand rubs before and after contact with the catheter for any reason.
Dressing	• Wear clean or sterile gloves when changing the dressing. • Cleanse the skin during dressing changes with a >0.5% chlorhexidine preparation with alcohol. • Dress the site with sterile gauze or sterile, transparent, semipermeable dressing to cover the catheter site. If the patient is diaphoretic or if the site is bleeding or oozing, use a gauze dressing until it is resolved. • Change gauze dressings every 2 days or transparent dressings at least every 7 days and whenever dressings become damp, loosened, or visibly soiled. • Do not use topical antibiotic ointment or creams on insertion sites.
Catheter site	• Assess the site regularly—visually when changing the dressing or by palpation through an intact dressing. Remove the dressing for a thorough assessment if the patient has tenderness at the insertion site, fever without obvious source, or other signs of local or bloodstream infection.
Pressure monitoring system	• Keep all components of the pressure monitoring system sterile. • Replace transducers, tubing, continuous-flush device, and flush solution every at 96-hour intervals. • Do not infuse dextrose containing solutions through the monitoring system.
Bathing	• Do not submerge the catheter or catheter site in water. • Showering is permitted if the catheter and related tubing are placed in an impermeable cover.
Patient education	• Ask patients to report any new discomforts from the catheter site.

Adapted from O'Grady, N. P., Alexander, A., Burns, L., et al. (2011). *2011 guidelines for the prevention of intravascular catheter-related infections.* Available at: www.cdc.gov/hicpac/bsi/bsi-guidelines-2011.html

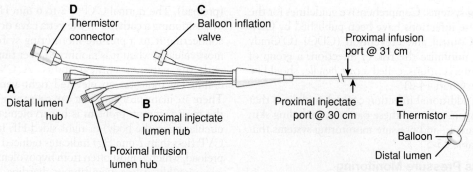

FIGURE 25-11 • The pulmonary artery catheter used for obtaining pressure measurements and cardiac output. **A.** The pressure monitoring system is connected to the distal lumen hub. **B.** Intravenous solutions are infused through the proximal infusion and injectate lumen hubs. **C.** An air-filled syringe connected to the balloon inflation valve is used for balloon inflation during catheter insertion and pulmonary artery wedge pressure measurements. **D.** To obtain cardiac output, the thermistor connector is inserted into the cardiac output component of the bedside cardiac monitor, and 5 to 10 mL of normal saline is injected in 4 seconds into the proximal injectate port. **E.** The thermistor located near the balloon is used to calculate the cardiac output. Redrawn courtesy of Baxter Healthcare Corporation, Edwards Critical Care Division, Santa Ana, California.

cardiac output, and a thermistor (positioned near the distal port) (see Fig. 25-11).

The pulmonary artery catheter, covered with a sterile sleeve, is inserted into a large vein, preferably the subclavian, through a sheath. As noted previously, the femoral vein is avoided; insertion techniques and protocols mirror those used for inserting a CVP catheter (see previous discussion) (O'Grady et al., 2011). The sheath is equipped with a side port for infusing IV fluids and medications. The catheter is then passed into the vena cava and right atrium. In the right atrium, the balloon tip is inflated, and the catheter is carried rapidly by the flow of blood through the tricuspid valve into the right ventricle, through the pulmonic valve, and into a branch of the pulmonary artery. When the catheter reaches the pulmonary artery, the balloon is deflated and the catheter is secured with sutures (Fig. 25-12). Fluoroscopy may be used during insertion to visualize the progression of the catheter through the right heart chambers to the pulmonary artery. This procedure can be performed in the operating room, in the cardiac catheterization laboratory, or at the bedside in the critical care unit. During insertion of the pulmonary artery catheter, the bedside monitor is observed for pressure and waveform changes, as well as dysrhythmias, as the catheter progresses through the right heart to the pulmonary artery.

Once the catheter is in position, the following are measured: right atrial, pulmonary artery systolic, pulmonary artery diastolic, mean pulmonary artery, and pulmonary artery wedge pressures (see Fig. 25-2 for normal chamber pressures). Monitoring of the pulmonary artery diastolic and pulmonary artery wedge pressures is particularly important in critically ill patients because they are used to evaluate left ventricular filling pressures (i.e., left ventricular preload).

It is important to note that the pulmonary artery wedge pressure is achieved by inflating the balloon tip, which causes it to float more distally into a smaller portion of the pulmonary artery until it is wedged into position. This is an occlusive maneuver that impedes blood flow through that segment of the pulmonary artery. Therefore, the wedge pressure is measured immediately and the balloon deflated promptly to restore blood flow.

> ◣ *Quality and Safety Nursing Alert*
>
> After measuring the pulmonary artery wedge pressure, the nurse ensures that the balloon is deflated and that the catheter has returned to its normal position. This important intervention is verified by evaluating the pulmonary artery pressure waveform displayed on the bedside monitor.

Nursing Interventions

Catheter site care is essentially the same as for a CVP catheter. Similar to CVP measurement, the transducer must be positioned at the phlebostatic axis to ensure accurate readings (see Fig. 25-10). Serious complications include pulmonary artery rupture, pulmonary thromboembolism, pulmonary infarction, catheter kinking, dysrhythmias, and air embolism.

Intra-Arterial Blood Pressure Monitoring

Intra-arterial BP monitoring is used to obtain direct and continuous BP measurements in critically ill patients who have severe hypertension or hypotension. Arterial catheters are also useful when arterial blood gas measurements and blood samples need to be obtained frequently.

The radial artery is the usual site selected. However, placement of a catheter into the radial artery can further impede perfusion to an area that has poor circulation. As a result, the tissue distal to the cannulated artery can become ischemic or necrotic. Patients with diabetes, peripheral vascular disease, hypotension, IV vasopressors, or previous surgery are at highest risk for this complication. Traditionally, collateral circulation to the involved extremity was assessed by using the Allen test. To perform the Allen test, the hand is elevated and the patient is asked to make a fist for 30 seconds. The nurse compresses the radial and ulnar arteries simultaneously, causing the hand to blanch. After the patient opens the fist, the nurse releases the pressure on the ulnar artery. If blood flow is restored (hand turns pink) within 6 seconds, the circulation to the hand may be adequate enough to tolerate placement of a radial artery catheter. Current evidence now suggests that Doppler

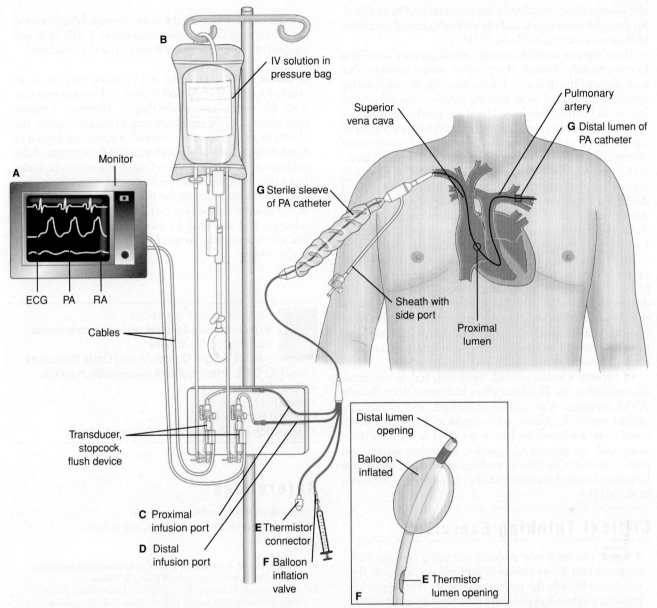

FIGURE 25-12 • Pulmonary artery (PA) catheter and pressure monitoring systems. Bedside monitor that connects with cables (**A**) to the pressure monitoring systems (includes intravenous [IV] solution in a pressure bag, IV tubing, and two transducers with stopcocks and flush devices) (**B**). This system connects to the proximal infusion port that opens in the right atria (**C**) and is used to infuse fluids or medications and monitor central venous pressures and the distal infusion port (**D**). This port opens in the PA and is used to monitor PA pressures. **E.** The thermistor connector is attached to the bedside cardiac monitor to obtain cardiac output. **F.** An air-filled syringe is attached to the balloon inflation valve during catheter insertion and measurement of PA wedge pressure. **G.** PA catheter positioned in the pulmonary artery. Note the sterile sleeve over the PA catheter. The PA catheter is threaded through the sheath until it reaches the desired position in the PA. The side port on the sheath is used to infuse medications or fluids. ECG, electrocardiogram; RA, right atrium.

ultrasonography, digit pressure measurement, and plethysmography are more reliable methods for assessing circulation to the hand (Woods et al., 2009).

Nursing Interventions

Site preparation and care are the same as for CVP catheters. The catheter flush solution is the same as for pulmonary artery catheters. A transducer is attached, and pressures are measured in millimeters of mercury (mm Hg). The nurse monitors the patient for complications, which include local obstruction with distal ischemia, external

hemorrhage, massive ecchymosis, dissection, air embolism, blood loss, pain, arteriospasm, and infection.

Minimally Invasive Cardiac Output Monitoring Devices

Monitoring cardiac output using the pulmonary artery catheter has been the standard of practice in critical care since its inception almost 50 years ago. Its use has diminished recently with the availability of new, less invasive devices. Three different types of devices are commercially available. Selection of a specific device for clinical use is determined by availability, provider preferences, and the patient's clinical condition (Alhasemi, Cecconi, & Hofer, 2011).

Pulse pressure analysis uses an arterial pressure waveform to continuously estimate the patient's stroke volume. One such device, the Edwards Lifesciences Vigileo monitoring system, is connected to an existing radial or femoral arterial line via its FloTrac transducer. Using age, gender, body surface area, and BP of the patient, this device calculates continuous cardiac output and other parameters used in the management of critically ill patients. The major drawback to this device is that in order for it to capture accurate data, it must first capture optimal arterial waveforms. Therefore, this type of device has limited usefulness in patients with poor waveform signals, various dysrhythmias, hemodynamic instability, and those who may be concomitantly using an intra-aortic balloon pump (Alhasemi et al., 2011) (see Chapter 29).

Esophageal Doppler probes are used to noninvasively estimate cardiac output. The esophageal probe measures blood flow velocity within a cross-sectional area of the descending aorta to calculate cardiac output. The use of this device in the perioperative setting has been shown to improve patient outcomes, including decreased lengths of hospital stay and an overall decrease in rates of complications (Alhasemi et al., 2011).

In patients who are sedated, intubated, and on mechanical ventilation, the Fick principle, which uses carbon dioxide (CO_2) measures, is an additional method used to estimate cardiac output. To obtain cardiac output in this select patient population, a rebreathing loop is attached to the ventilator along with an infrared CO_2 sensor, an airflow sensor, and pulse oximeter. Continuous readings of cardiac output may be updated every 3 minutes with use of this device (Alhasemi et al., 2011).

Critical Thinking Exercises

1 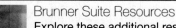 You are a new graduate practicing on a medical inpatient unit where change of shift report is given at the bedside to include the patient and family. This approach provides a valuable opportunity for you to observe patients and include them in the plan of care. Many patients on this unit are admitted with HF. What key physical assessment findings and laboratory data that indicate improvement in the patient's condition need to be discussed during report? What findings might suggest that the patient's condition is worsening? What questions would you ask the patient and family members to help you assess their understanding of HF self-management? Because you have limited time to conduct beside report, how will you prioritize the information that you need to hand off to the oncoming nurse?

2 Many of the patients in your practice as a nurse for a home care agency are older adults and have CVD. A new patient of yours, a 68-year-old woman recovering from a left hip replacement, complains of feeling more tired than usual and has intermittent episodes of right arm numbness and neck pain. You immediately report these symptoms to the patient's primary provider, who orders a cardiac workup consisting of a number of laboratory and diagnostic tests to

rule out CAD. What are the most common laboratory and diagnostic tests that are used to diagnose CAD? How will you prepare your patient for these tests and procedures?

3 **ebp** ECG monitoring is a common practice in all types of inpatient units and is used to keep patients safe from life-threatening dysrhythmias. However, frequent false alarms can be overwhelming to nurses, causing the alarms to go unnoticed or ignored, a condition known as alarm fatigue. Discuss the evidence and the strength of the evidence that identifies alarm fatigue as a serious problem. From this evidence, describe ECG monitoring best practices aimed at minimizing the risk of alarm fatigue. Include in this description the skin care, electrode placement, lead selection and rationale for monitoring, and alarms that you will individualize to meet the ECG monitoring needs of the patient.

Brunner Suite Resources
Explore these additional resources to enhance learning for this chapter:
• NCLEX-Style Questions and Other Resources on **thePoint**, http://thePoint.lww.com/Brunner13e
• Study Guide
• PrepU
• Clinical Handbook
• Handbook of Laboratory and Diagnostic Tests

References

*Asterisk indicates nursing research.
**Double asterisk indicates classic reference.

Books

Bickley, L. S. (2009). *Bates' guide to physical examination and history taking* (9th ed.). Philadelphia: Lippincott Williams & Wilkins.

Boltz, M., Capezuti, E., Fulmer, T., et al. (2012). *Evidence-based geriatric nursing: Protocols for best practice* (4th ed.). New York: Springhouse.

Weber, J., & Kelley, J. (2010). *Health assessment in nursing* (4th ed.). Philadelphia: Lippincott Williams & Wilkins.

Wiegand, D. L. (2011). *AACN procedure manual for critical care* (6th ed). St. Louis: Saunders.

Woods, S. L., Froelicher, E. S., Motzer, S. A., et al. (2009). *Cardiac nursing* (6th ed.). Philadelphia: Lippincott Williams & Wilkins.

Journals and Electronic Documents

Alhasemi, J. A., Cecconi, M., & Hofer, C. K. (2011). Cardiac output monitoring: An integrative perspective. *Annual Update in Intensive Care and Emergency Medicine, 978*(3), 443–457.

American Heart Association. (2012). *Heart disease and stroke statistics—2012 update.* Available at: www.americanheart.org

Aronow, W. S., Fleg, J. L., Pepine, C. J., et al. (2011). ACCF/AHA 2011 expert consensus document on hypertension in the elderly: A report of the American College of Cardiology Foundation Task Force on Clinical Expert Consensus Documents. *Journal of the American College of Cardiology, 57*(20), 2434–2506.

Baranchuk, A., Shaw, C., Alanazi, H., et al. (2009). Electrocardiography pitfalls and artifacts: The 10 commandments. *Critical Care Nurse, 29*(1), 67–73.

Bigger, J. T., & Glassman, A. H. (2010). The American Heart Association science advisory on depression and coronary heart disease: An exploration of the issues raised. *Cleveland Clinic Journal of Medicine, 77*(Suppl. 3), S12–S19.

Bluemke, D. A., Achenbach, S., Budoff, M., et al. (2008). Noninvasive coronary artery imaging: Magnetic resonance angiography and multidetector computed tomography angiography: A scientific statement from the American Heart Association Committee on Cardiovascular Imaging and Intervention of the Council on Cardiovascular Radiology and Intervention, and the Council on Clinical Cardiology and Cardiovascular Disease in the Young. *Circulation, 118*(5), 586–606.

Brown, J. M., Stewart, J. C., Stump, T. E., & Callahan, C. M. (2011). Risk of coronary heart disease events over 15 years among older adults with depressive symptoms. *American Journal of Geriatric Psychiatry, 19*(8), 721–729.

*DeVon, H. A., Ryan, C. J., Rankin, S. H., et al. (2010). Classifying subgroups of patients with symptoms of acute coronary syndrome: A cluster analysis. *Research in Nursing and Health, 33*(5), 386–397.

**Drew, B. J., Califf, R. M., Funk, M., et al. (2005). AHA scientific statement: Practice standards for electrocardiographic monitoring in hospital settings: An American Heart Association scientific statement from the Councils on Cardiovascular Nursing, Clinical Cardiology, and Cardiovascular Disease in the Young: Endorsed by the International Society of Computerized Electrocardiology and the American Association of Critical Care Nurses. *Journal of Cardiovascular Nursing, 20*(2), 76–106.

Durham, K. A. (2012). Cardiac catheterization through the radial artery. *American Journal of Nursing, 112*(1), 49–56.

Evenson, L., & Farnsworth, M. (2010). Skilled cardiac monitoring at the bedside: An algorithm for success. *Critical Care Nurse, 30*(5), 14–22.

Freeman, R., Wieling, W., Axelrod, F. B., et al. (2011). Consensus statement on the definition of orthostatic hypotension, neurally mediated syncope and the postural tachycardia syndrome. *Clinical Autonomic Research, 21*(2), 69–72.

Graham, C. K., & Cvach, M. (2010). Monitor alarm fatigue: Standardizing use of physiological monitors and decreasing nuisance alarms. *American Journal of Critical Care, 19*(1), 28–34.

Greenland, P., Alpert, J. S., Beller, G. A., et al. (2010). 2010 ACCF/AHA guideline for assessment of cardiovascular risk in asymptomatic adults: A report of the American College of Cardiology Foundation/American Heart Association Task Force on Practice Guidelines. *Journal of the American College of Cardiology, 56*(25), 50–103.

Hammel, W. (2009). Femoral artery closure after cardiac catheterization. *Critical Care Nurse, 29*(1), 39–46.

Hannibal, G. B. (2011). Monitor alarms and alarm fatigue. *AACN Advanced Critical Care, 22*(4), 418–420.

*Heydari, A., Ahrari, S., & Vaghee, S. (2011). The relationship between self-concept and adherence to therapeutic regimens in patients with heart failure. *Journal of Cardiovascular Nursing, 26*(6), 475–480.

**Homes, T. H., & Rahe, R. H. (1967). The Social Readjustment Rating Scale. *Journal of Psychosomatic Research, 11*(2), 213–218.

Levine, G. N., Bates, E. R., Blankenship, J. C., et al. (2011). 2011 ACCF/AHA/SCAI guideline for percutaneous coronary intervention: A report of the American College of Cardiology Foundation/American Heart Association Task Force on Practice Guidelines and the Society for Cardiovascular Angiography and Interventions. *Circulation, 124*(23), 574–651.

Levine, G. N., Steinke, E. E., Bakaeen, F. G., et al. (2012). Sexual activity and cardiovascular disease: A scientific statement from the American Heart Association. *Circulation, 125*(8), 1058–1072.

Mert, H., Intepeler, S. S., Bengu, N., et al. (2012). Efficacy of frequent blood pressure and heart rate monitoring for early identification of bleeding following percutaneous coronary intervention. *International Journal of Nursing Practice, 18*, 52–59.

Mosca, L., Benjamin, E. J., Berra, K., et al. (2011). Effectiveness-based guidelines for the prevention of cardiovascular disease in women—2011: A guideline from the American Heart Association. *Circulation, 123*(11), 1243–1262.

Moser, D. K., Kimble, L. P., Alberts, M. J., et al. (2007). Reducing delay in seeking treatment by patients with acute coronary syndrome and stroke: A scientific statement from the American Heart Association Council on Cardiovascular Nursing and Stroke Council. *Circulation, 114*(2), 168–182.

Myers, J., Arena, R., & Franklin, B. (2009). Recommendations for clinical exercise laboratories: A scientific statement from the American Heart Association. *Circulation, 119*(24), 3144–3161.

O'Grady, N. P., Alexander, A., Burns, L., et al. (2011) *2011 guidelines for the prevention of intravascular catheter-related infections.* Available at: www.cdc.gov/hicpac/bsi/bsi-guidelines-2011.html

Raingruber, B., Kirkland-Walsh, H., Chahon, N., et al. (2011). Using the Mehran Risk Scoring Tool to predict risk for contrast medium–induced nephropathy in patients undergoing percutaneous angiography. *Critical Care Nurse, 31*(1), 17–22.

Smith, S. C., Benjamin, E. J., Bonow, R. O., et al. (2011). AHA/ACCF secondary prevention and risk reduction therapy for patients with coronary and other atherosclerotic vascular disease: 2011 update: A guideline from the American Heart Association and American College of Cardiology Foundation. *Circulation, 124*, 2458–2473.

Resources

American Heart Association, www.americanheart.org

Medi-Smart Cardiovascular Nursing Resources, www.medi-smart.com/cardiac.htm

New York Cardiac Center, nycardiaccenter.org

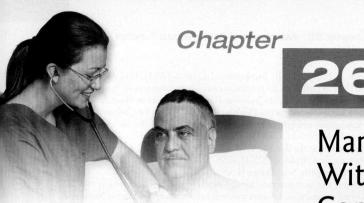

Chapter

26

Management of Patients With Dysrhythmias and Conduction Problems

Learning Objectives

On completion of this chapter, the learner will be able to:

1 Correlate the components of the normal electrocardiogram (ECG) with physiologic events of the heart.
2 Define the ECG as a waveform that represents the cardiac electrical event in relation to the lead (placement of electrodes).
3 Analyze elements of an ECG rhythm strip: ventricular and atrial rate, ventricular and atrial rhythm, QRS complex and shape, QRS duration, P wave and shape, PR interval, and P:QRS ratio.
4 Identify the ECG criteria, causes, and management of several dysrhythmias, including conduction disturbances.

5 Use the nursing process as a framework for care of patients with dysrhythmias.
6 Compare the different types of pacemakers, their uses, possible complications, and nursing implications.
7 Describe the nursing management of patients with implantable cardiac devices.
8 Describe the key points of using a defibrillator.
9 Describe the purpose of an implantable cardioverter defibrillator, the types available, and the nursing implications.
10 Describe invasive methods to diagnose and treat recurrent dysrhythmias and discuss the nursing implications.

Glossary

ablation: removal of material from the surface of an object; in the context of cardiology, it is the purposeful destruction of heart muscle cells, usually in an attempt to control a dysrhythmia

antiarrhythmic medication: a medication that suppresses or prevents a dysrhythmia

artifact: distorted, irrelevant, and extraneous electrocardiographic (ECG) waveforms

automaticity: ability of the cardiac cells to initiate an electrical impulse

cardioversion: electrical current administered in synchrony with the patient's own QRS complex to stop a dysrhythmia

chronotropy: rate of impulse formation

conduction: transmission of electrical impulses from one cell to another

defibrillation: electrical current administered to stop a dysrhythmia, not synchronized with the patient's QRS complex

depolarization: process by which cardiac muscle cells change from a more negatively charged to a more positively charged intracellular state

dromotropy: conduction velocity

dysrhythmia: disorder of the formation or conduction (or both) of the electrical impulse within the heart, altering the heart rate, heart rhythm, or both and potentially causing altered blood flow (also referred to as arrhythmia)

elective replacement indicator (ERI): a signal produced by a pacemaker when it is interrogated to indicate a near-depleted battery

implantable cardioverter defibrillator (ICD): a device implanted into the chest to treat dysrhythmias

inotropy: force of myocardial contraction

P wave: the part of an ECG that reflects conduction of an electrical impulse through the atrium; atrial depolarization

paroxysmal: a dysrhythmia that has a sudden onset and/or termination and is usually of short duration

PP interval: the duration between the beginning of one P wave and the beginning of the next P wave; used to calculate atrial rate and rhythm

PR interval: the part of an ECG that reflects conduction of an electrical impulse from the sinoatrial node through the atrioventricular node

proarrhythmic: an agent (e.g., a medication) that causes or exacerbates a dysrhythmia

QRS complex: the part of an ECG that reflects conduction of an electrical impulse through the ventricles; ventricular depolarization

QT interval: the part of an ECG that reflects the time from ventricular depolarization through repolarization

repolarization: process by which cardiac muscle cells return to a more negatively charged intracellular condition, their resting state

RR interval: the duration between the beginning of one QRS complex and the beginning of the next QRS complex; used to calculate ventricular rate and rhythm

sinus rhythm: electrical activity of the heart initiated by the sinoatrial node

ST segment: the part of an ECG that reflects the end of the QRS complex to the beginning of the T wave

supraventricular tachycardia (SVT): a rhythm that originates in the conduction system above the ventricles

T wave: the part of an ECG that reflects repolarization of the ventricles

TP interval: the part of an ECG that reflects the time between the end of the T wave and the beginning of the next P wave; used to identify the isoelectric line

U wave: the part of an ECG that may reflect Purkinje fiber repolarization; usually, it is not seen unless a patient's serum potassium level is low

ventricular tachycardia (VT): a rhythm that originates in the ventricles

---

Without a regular rate and rhythm, the heart may not perform efficiently as a pump to circulate oxygenated blood and other life-sustaining nutrients to all of the body's tissues and organs (including the heart itself). With an irregular or erratic rhythm, the heart is considered to be dysrhythmic (sometimes called *arrhythmic*). This is a potentially dangerous condition.

Nurses may encounter patients with many different types of dysrhythmias in all health care settings, including primary care settings, skilled nursing facilities, rehabilitation settings, and hospitals. Some dysrhythmias are acute and others chronic; some require emergent interventions while others may not. Because patients with dysrhythmias are so frequently encountered in so many settings, nurses must be able to identify and provide appropriate first-line treatment of dysrhythmias.

DYSRHYTHMIAS

Dysrhythmias are disorders of the formation or conduction (or both) of the electrical impulse within the heart. These disorders can cause disturbances of the heart rate, the heart rhythm, or both. Dysrhythmias may initially be evidenced by the hemodynamic effect they cause (e.g., a change in conduction may change the pumping action of the heart and cause decreased blood pressure). Dysrhythmias are diagnosed by analyzing the electrocardiographic (ECG) waveform. Their treatment is based on the frequency and severity of symptoms produced. Dysrhythmias are named according to the site of origin of the impulse and the mechanism of formation or conduction involved (Chart 26-1). For example, an

impulse that originates in the sinoatrial (SA) node and at a slow rate is called *sinus bradycardia*.

Normal Electrical Conduction

The electrical impulse that stimulates and paces the cardiac muscle normally originates in the SA node, also called the *sinus node*, an area located near the superior vena cava in the right atrium. Usually, the electrical impulse occurs at a rate of 60 to 100 times a minute in the adult. The electrical impulse quickly travels from the SA node through the atria to the atrioventricular (AV) node (Fig. 26-1); this process is known as **conduction**. The electrical stimulation of the muscle cells of the atria causes them to contract. The structure of the AV node slows the electrical impulse, giving the atria time to contract and fill the ventricles with blood. This part of atrial contraction is frequently referred to as the atrial kick and accounts for nearly one third of the volume ejected during ventricular contraction (Fuster, Walsh, & Harrington, 2011). The electrical impulse then travels very quickly through the bundle of His to the right and left bundle branches and the Purkinje fibers, located in the ventricular muscle. The electrical stimulation of the muscle cells of the ventricles in turn causes the mechanical contraction of the ventricles (systole). The cells repolarize and the ventricles then relax (diastole). The electrical impulse causes the mechanical contraction of the heart muscle that follows.

The electrical stimulation is called **depolarization**, and the mechanical contraction is called *systole*. Electrical relaxation is called **repolarization**, and mechanical relaxation is called *diastole*. The process from sinus node electrical impulse generation through ventricular repolarization completes the electromechanical circuit, and the cycle begins again. (See Chapter 25 for a more complete explanation of cardiac function.)

Influences on Heart Rate and Contractility

The heart rate is influenced by the autonomic nervous system, which consists of sympathetic and parasympathetic fibers. Sympathetic nerve fibers (also referred to as adrenergic fibers) are attached to the heart and arteries as well as several other areas in the body. Stimulation of the sympathetic system increases heart rate (positive **chronotropy**), conduction through the AV node (positive **dromotropy**), and the force of myocardial contraction (positive **inotropy**). Sympathetic stimulation also constricts peripheral blood vessels, therefore increasing blood pressure. Parasympathetic nerve fibers

---

Chart 26-1   **Identifying Cardiac Rhythms**

Sites of Origin

Sinus node
Atria
Atrioventricular node or junction
Ventricles

Mechanisms of Formation or Conduction

Normal (idio) rhythm
Bradycardia
Tachycardia
Dysrhythmia
Flutter
Fibrillation
Premature complexes
Conduction blocks

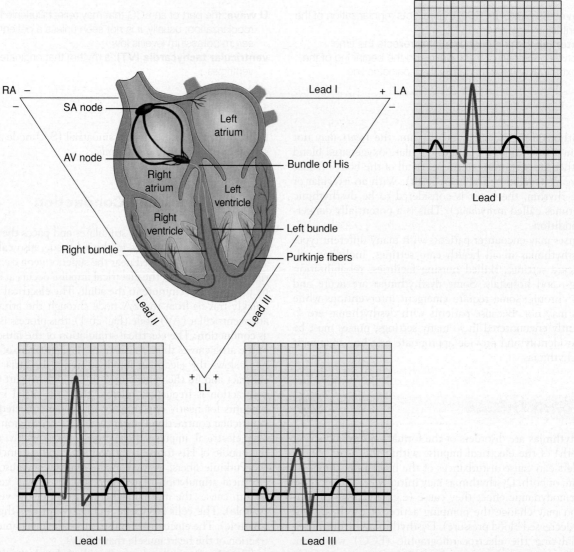

FIGURE 26-1 • Relationship of electrocardiographic (ECG) complex, lead system, and electrical impulse. The heart conducts electrical activity, which the ECG measures and shows. The configurations of electrical activity displayed on the ECG vary depending on the lead (or view) of the ECG and on the rhythm of the heart. Therefore, the configuration of a normal rhythm tracing from lead I will differ from the configuration of a normal rhythm tracing from lead II, lead II will differ from lead III, and so on. The same is true for abnormal rhythms and cardiac disorders. To make an accurate assessment of the heart's electrical activity or to identify where, when, and what abnormalities occur, the ECG needs to be evaluated from every lead, not just from lead II. Here the different areas of electrical activity are identified by color. RA, right arm; LA, left arm; SA, sinoatrial; AV, atrioventricular; LL, left leg.

are also attached to the heart and arteries. Parasympathetic stimulation reduces the heart rate (negative chronotropy), AV conduction (negative dromotropy), and the force of atrial myocardial contraction. The decreased sympathetic stimulation results in dilation of arteries, thereby lowering blood pressure.

Manipulation of the autonomic nervous system may increase or decrease the incidence of dysrhythmias. Increased sympathetic stimulation (e.g., caused by exercise, anxiety, fever, or administration of catecholamines, such as dopamine [Intropin], aminophylline, or dobutamine [Dobutrex]) may increase the incidence of dysrhythmias. Decreased sympathetic stimulation (e.g., with rest, anxiety reduction methods such as therapeutic communication or meditation, or administration of beta-adrenergic blocking agents) may decrease the incidence of dysrhythmias.

The Electrocardiogram

The electrical impulse that travels through the heart can be viewed by means of electrocardiography, the end product of which is an electrocardiogram, or ECG. Each phase of the cardiac cycle is reflected by specific waveforms on the screen of a cardiac monitor or on a strip of ECG graph paper.

Obtaining an Electrocardiogram

An ECG is obtained by placing electrodes on the body at specific areas. Electrodes come in various shapes and sizes, but they all have two components: (1) an adhesive substance that attaches to the skin to secure the electrode in place and (2) a substance that reduces the skin's electrical impedance, the resistance to electrical signal conduction and detection of the electrical current. Gently abrading the skin with a clean dry gauze pad helps to expose the inner conductive layer of epidermis, which will reduce skin impedance. Although cleansing the skin with alcohol removes any oily residue from the skin, it also increases the skin's electrical impedance and hinders detection of the cardiac electrical signal. If the amount of chest hair prevents the electrode from having good contact with the skin and there is no other place to position the electrode, the hair may need to be clipped. Poor electrode adhesion will cause significant **artifact** (distorted, irrelevant, and extraneous ECG waveforms), which may distort capturing an accurate ECG waveform.

The number and placement of the electrodes depend on the type of ECG being obtained. Most continuous monitors use two to five electrodes, usually placed on the limbs and the chest. These electrodes create an imaginary line, called a *lead*, which serves as a reference point from which the electrical activity is viewed. A lead is like an eye of a camera—it has a narrow peripheral field of vision, looking only at the electrical activity directly in front of it. Therefore, the ECG waveforms that appear on the paper and cardiac monitor represent the electrical current in relation to the lead (see Fig. 26-1). A change in the waveform can be caused by a change in the electrical current (where it originates or how it is conducted) or by a change in the lead.

Electrodes are attached to cable wires, which are connected to one of the following:

- An ECG machine placed at the patient's side for an immediate recording (standard 12-lead ECG)
- A cardiac monitor at the patient's bedside for continuous reading; this kind of monitoring, usually called *hardwire monitoring*, is used in intensive care units
- A small box that the patient carries and that continuously transmits the ECG information by radiowaves to a central monitor located elsewhere (called *telemetry*)
- A small, lightweight tape recorder–like machine (called *ambulatory ECG monitoring* or a *Holter monitor*) that the patient wears and that continuously records the ECG, which is later viewed and analyzed with a scanner.

A patient may undergo an electrophysiology (EP) study in which electrodes are placed inside the heart in order to obtain an intracardiac ECG. This is used not only to diagnose the dysrhythmia but also to determine the most effective treatment plan. However, because an EP study is invasive, it is performed in the hospital and may require that the patient be admitted. (A more in-depth discussion is found later in this chapter.)

During open heart surgery, temporary pacemaker wires may be lightly sutured to the epicardium and brought through the chest wall. These wires may be used not only for temporary pacing but also, when connected to the V lead cable, to obtain an atrial ECG, which can be helpful in the differential diagnosis of tachydysrhythmias (McRae, Chan, & Imperial-Perez, 2010).

The placement of electrodes for continuous monitoring, telemetry, or Holter monitoring varies with the type of technology, the purpose of monitoring, and the standards of the health care facility. For a standard 12-lead ECG, 10 electrodes (6 on the chest and 4 on the limbs) are placed on the body (Fig. 26-2). To prevent interference from the electrical activity of skeletal muscle, the limb electrodes are usually placed on

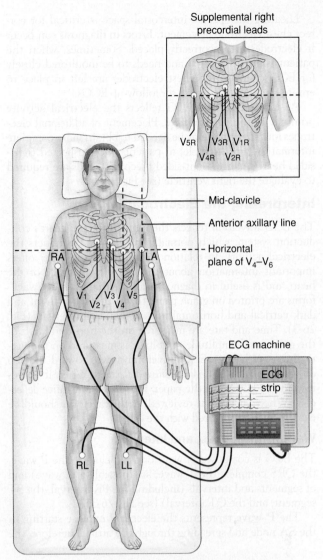

FIGURE 26-2 • ECG electrode placement. The standard left precordial leads are V_1—fourth intercostal space, right sternal border; V_2—fourth intercostal space, left sternal border; V_3—diagonally between V_2 and V_4; V_4—fifth intercostal space, left midclavicular line; V_5—same level as V_4, anterior axillary line; V_6 (not illustrated)—same level as V_4 and V_5, midaxillary line. The right precordial leads, placed across the right side of the chest, are the mirror opposite of the left leads. RA, right arm; LA, left arm; RL, right leg; LL, left leg. Adapted from Molle, E. A., Kronenberger, J., West-Stack, C., et al. (2005). *Lippincott Williams & Wilkins' pocket guide to medical assisting* (2nd ed.). Philadelphia: Lippincott Williams & Wilkins.

areas that are not bony and that do not have significant movement. These limb electrodes provide the first six leads: leads I, II, III, aVR (augmented voltage right arm), aVL (augmented voltage left arm), and aVF (augmented voltage left leg/foot). The six chest electrodes are applied to the chest at very specific areas. The chest electrodes provide the V or precordial leads, V_1 through V_6. To locate the fourth intercostal space and the placement of V_1, the sternal angle and then the sternal notch, which is about 1 or 2 inches below the sternal angle, are located. When the fingers are moved to the patient's immediate right, the second rib can be palpated. The second intercostal space is the indentation felt just below the second rib.

Locating the specific intercostal space is critical for correct chest electrode placement. Errors in diagnosis can occur if electrodes are incorrectly placed. Sometimes, when the patient is in the hospital and needs to be monitored closely for ECG changes, the chest electrodes are left in place to ensure the same placement for follow-up ECGs.

A standard 12-lead ECG reflects the electrical activity primarily in the left ventricle. Placement of additional electrodes for other leads may be needed to obtain more complete information. For example, in patients with suspected right-sided heart damage, right-sided precordial leads are required to evaluate the right ventricle (see Fig. 26-2).

Interpreting the Electrocardiogram

The ECG waveform reflects the function of the heart's conduction system, which normally initiates and conducts the electrical activity, in relation to the lead. The ECG offers important information about the electrical activity of the heart and is useful in diagnosing dysrhythmias. ECG waveforms are printed on graph paper that is divided by light and dark vertical and horizontal lines at standard intervals (Fig. 26-3). Time and rate are measured on the horizontal axis of the graph, and amplitude or voltage is measured on the vertical axis. When an ECG waveform moves toward the top of the paper, it is called a *positive deflection*. When it moves toward the bottom of the paper, it is called a *negative deflection*. When an ECG is reviewed, each waveform should be examined and compared with the others.

Waves, Complexes, and Intervals

The ECG is composed of waveforms (including the P wave, the QRS complex, the T wave, and possibly a U wave) and of segments and intervals (including the PR interval, the ST segment, and the QT interval) (see Fig. 26-3).

The **P wave** represents the electrical impulse starting in the SA node and spreading through the atria. Therefore, the P wave represents atrial depolarization. It is normally 2.5 mm or less in height and 0.11 seconds or less in duration.

The **QRS complex** represents ventricular depolarization. Not all QRS complexes have all three waveforms. The Q wave is the first negative deflection after the P wave. The Q wave is normally less than 0.04 seconds in duration and less than 25% of the R-wave amplitude. The R wave is the first positive deflection after the P wave, and the S wave is the first negative deflection after the R wave. When a wave is less than 5 mm in height, small letters (q, r, s) are used; when a wave is taller than 5 mm, capital letters (Q, R, S) are used to label the waves. The QRS complex is normally less than 0.12 seconds in duration.

The **T wave** represents ventricular repolarization (when the cells regain a negative charge; also called the *resting state*). It follows the QRS complex and is usually the same direction as the QRS complex. Atrial repolarization also occurs but is not visible on the ECG because it occurs at the same time as ventricular depolarization (i.e., the QRS).

The **U wave** is thought to represent repolarization of the Purkinje fibers; although this wave is rare, it sometimes appears in patients with hypokalemia (low potassium levels), hypertension, or heart disease. If present, the U wave follows the T wave and is usually smaller than the P wave. If tall, it may be mistaken for an extra P wave.

The **PR interval** is measured from the beginning of the P wave to the beginning of the QRS complex and represents the time needed for sinus node stimulation, atrial depolarization, and conduction through the AV node before ventricular depolarization. In adults, the PR interval normally ranges from 0.12 to 0.20 seconds in duration.

The **ST segment**, which represents early ventricular repolarization, lasts from the end of the QRS complex to the beginning of the T wave. The beginning of the ST segment is usually identified by a change in the thickness or angle of the terminal portion of the QRS complex. The end of the ST

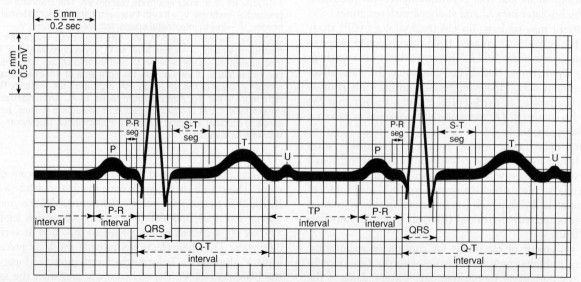

FIGURE 26-3 • ECG graph and commonly measured components. Each small box represents 0.04 seconds on the horizontal axis and 1 mm or 0.1 millivolt on the vertical axis. The PR interval is measured from the beginning of the P wave to the beginning of the QRS complex; the QRS complex is measured from the beginning of the Q wave to the end of the S wave; the QT interval is measured from the beginning of the Q wave to the end of the T wave; and the TP interval is measured from the end of the T wave to the beginning of the next P wave.

segment may be more difficult to identify because it merges into the T wave. The ST segment is normally isoelectric (see later discussion of TP interval). It is analyzed to identify whether it is above or below the isoelectric line, which may be, among other signs and symptoms, a sign of cardiac ischemia (see Chapter 27).

The **QT interval**, which represents the total time for ventricular depolarization and repolarization, is measured from the beginning of the QRS complex to the end of the T wave. The QT interval varies with heart rate, gender, and age; therefore, the measured interval needs to be corrected (QT$_c$) for these variables through specific calculations. The QT$_c$ may be automatically calculated by the ECG technology, or a nurse may use an ECG interpretation book or other resource that contains a chart of these calculations. The QT interval is usually 0.32 to 0.40 seconds in duration if the heart rate is 65 to 95 bpm. If the QT interval becomes prolonged, the patient may be at risk for a lethal ventricular dysrhythmia called *torsades de pointes*. Although many hospitalized patients would benefit from QT monitoring, one study indicated that nurses frequently do not have the skill to perform this assessment properly (Pickham, Shinn, Chan, et al., 2012).

The **TP interval** is measured from the end of the T wave to the beginning of the next P wave—an isoelectric period (see Fig. 26-3). When no electrical activity is detected, the line on the graph remains flat; this is called the *isoelectric line*. The ST segment is compared with the TP interval to detect ST segment changes.

The **PP interval** is measured from the beginning of one P wave to the beginning of the next P wave. The PP interval is used to determine atrial rate and rhythm. The **RR interval** is measured from one QRS complex to the next QRS complex. The RR interval is used to determine ventricular rate and rhythm (Fig. 26-4).

Determining Heart Rate from the Electrocardiogram

Heart rate can be obtained from the ECG strip by several methods. A 1-minute strip contains 300 large boxes and 1,500 small boxes. Therefore, an easy and accurate method of determining heart rate with a regular rhythm is to count the number of small boxes within an RR interval and divide 1,500 by that number. If, for example, there are 10 small boxes between two R waves, the heart rate is 1,500/10, or 150 bpm; if there are 25 small boxes, the heart rate is 1,500/25, or 60 bpm (see Fig. 26-4A).

An alternative but less accurate method for estimating heart rate, which is usually used when the rhythm is irregular, is to count the number of RR intervals in 6 seconds and multiply that number by 10. The top of the ECG paper is usually marked at 3-second intervals, which is 15 large boxes horizontally (see Fig. 26-4B). The RR intervals are counted, rather than QRS complexes, because a computed heart rate based on the latter might be inaccurately high.

The same methods may be used for determining atrial rate, using the PP interval instead of the RR interval.

Determining Heart Rhythm from the Electrocardiogram

The rhythm is often identified at the same time the rate is determined. The RR interval is used to determine ventricular rhythm and the PP interval to determine atrial rhythm. If the intervals are the same or if the difference between the intervals is less than 0.8 seconds throughout the strip, the rhythm is called *regular*. If the intervals are different, the rhythm is called *irregular*.

Analyzing the Electrocardiogram Rhythm Strip

The ECG must be analyzed in a systematic manner to determine the patient's cardiac rhythm and to detect dysrhythmias and conduction disorders, as well as evidence of myocardial ischemia, injury, and infarction. Chart 26-2 is an example of a method that can be used to analyze the patient's rhythm.

Once the rhythm has been analyzed, the findings are compared with and matched to the ECG criteria for dysrhythmias

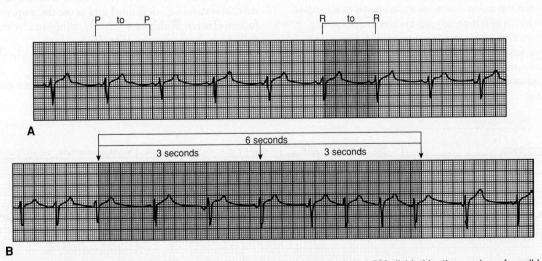

FIGURE 26-4 • A. Ventricular and atrial heart rate determination with a regular rhythm: 1,500 divided by the number of small boxes between two P waves (atrial rate) or between two R waves (ventricular rate). In this example, there are 25 small boxes between both the R waves and the P waves, so the heart rate is 60 bpm. **B.** Heart rate determination if the rhythm is irregular. There are approximately seven RR intervals in 6 seconds, so there are about 70 RR intervals in 60 seconds (7 × 10 = 70). The ventricular heart rate is 70 bpm.

Chart 26-2 Interpreting Dysrhythmias: Systematic Analysis of the Electrocardiogram

When examining an electrocardiogram (ECG) rhythm strip to learn more about a patient's dysrhythmia:

1. Determine the ventricular rate.
2. Determine the ventricular rhythm.
3. Determine QRS duration.
4. Determine whether the QRS duration is consistent throughout the strip. If not, identify other duration.
5. Identify QRS shape; if not consistent, then identify other shapes.
6. Identify P waves; is there a P in front of every QRS?
7. Identify P-wave shape; identify whether it is consistent or not.
8. Determine the atrial rate.
9. Determine the atrial rhythm.
10. Determine each PR interval.
11. Determine if the PR intervals are consistent, irregular but with a pattern to the irregularity, or just irregular.
12. Determine how many P waves for each QRS (P:QRS ratio).

In many cases, the nurse may use a checklist and document the findings next to the appropriate ECG criterion.

to determine a diagnosis. It is important for the nurse not only to identify the dysrhythmia but also to assess the patient to determine the physiologic effect of the dysrhythmia and identify possible causes. Treatment of a dysrhythmia is based on clinical evaluation of the patient with identification of the dysrhythmia's etiology and effect, not on its presence alone.

Most cardiac monitoring has functionality that includes that ability to continuously monitor the rhythm and alert health care personnel with an auditory and visual alarm when a significant change in the rhythm occurs. However, a high rate of triggered alarms, especially if they are caused by artifact, may lead to "monitor alarm fatigue," which has been linked to nurses ignoring, disabling, or silencing alarms (Graham & Cvach, 2010)—this puts patients at risk of having dysrhythmias ignored.

Quality and Safety Nursing Alert

It is vital that the nurse assesses the cause(s) of a cardiac monitor's alarm and then adjusts the alarm default settings and individualizes the alarm parameter limits and levels. The assessment should also include an evaluation and discussion with the primary provider to validate that the patient needs to remain on continuous cardiac monitoring.

Normal Sinus Rhythm

Normal **sinus rhythm** occurs when the electrical impulse starts at a regular rate and rhythm in the SA node and travels through the normal conduction pathway. Normal sinus rhythm has the following characteristics (Fig. 26-5):

Ventricular and atrial rate: 60 to 100 bpm in the adult

Ventricular and atrial rhythm: Regular

QRS shape and duration: Usually normal, but may be regularly abnormal

P wave: Normal and consistent shape; always in front of the QRS

PR interval: Consistent interval between 0.12 and 0.20 seconds

P:QRS ratio: 1:1

Although normal sinus rhythm is generally indicative of good cardiovascular health, a resting heart rate that exceeds 90 bpm is associated with a higher risk of all-cause mortality and cardiovascular events (Perret-Guillaume, Joly, & Benetos, 2009). Patients with this increased baseline heart rate should receive a full medical workup and be counseled about lifestyle modification, especially maintaining a regular physical activity program.

 Types of Dysrhythmias

Dysrhythmias include sinus, atrial, junctional, and ventricular dysrhythmias and their various subcategories.

Sinus Node Dysrhythmias

Sinus Bradycardia

Sinus bradycardia occurs when the SA node creates an impulse at a slower-than-normal rate. Causes include lower metabolic needs (e.g., sleep, athletic training, hypothyroidism), vagal stimulation (e.g., from vomiting, suctioning, severe pain), medications (e.g., calcium channel blockers, amiodarone, beta-blockers), idiopathic sinus node dysfunction, increased intracranial pressure, and coronary artery disease, especially myocardial infarction (MI) of the inferior wall. Unstable and symptomatic bradycardia is frequently due to hypoxemia. Other possible causes include acute altered mental status (e.g., delirium) and acute decompensated heart failure (Fuster, Walsh et al., 2011). Sinus bradycardia has the following characteristics (Fig. 26-6):

Ventricular and atrial rate: Less than 60 bpm in the adult

Ventricular and atrial rhythm: Regular

QRS shape and duration: Usually normal, but may be regularly abnormal

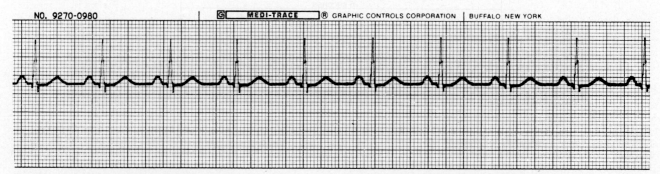

FIGURE 26-5 • Normal sinus rhythm in lead II.

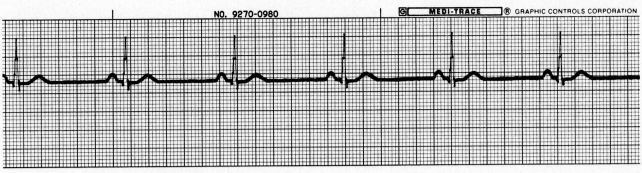

FIGURE 26-6 • Sinus bradycardia in lead II.

P wave: Normal and consistent shape; always in front of the QRS

PR interval: Consistent interval between 0.12 and 0.20 seconds

P:QRS ratio: 1:1

All characteristics of sinus bradycardia are the same as those of normal sinus rhythm, except for the rate. The patient is assessed to determine the hemodynamic effect and the possible cause of the dysrhythmia. If the decrease in heart rate results from stimulation of the vagus nerve, such as with bearing down during defecation or vomiting, attempts are made to prevent further vagal stimulation. If the bradycardia is caused by a medication such as a beta-blocker, the medication may be withheld. If the slow heart rate causes significant hemodynamic changes resulting in shortness of breath, acute alteration of mental status, angina, hypotension, ST-segment changes, or premature ventricular complexes (PVCs), treatment is directed toward increasing the heart rate. If the slow heart rate is due to sinus node dysfunction (previously known as sick sinus syndrome), which most often occurs in people older than 50 years, decreased exercise capacity, fatigue, unexplained confusion, or memory loss may result (Fuster, Walsh et al., 2011). *Tachy-brady syndrome* is the term used when bradycardia alternates with tachycardia.

Medical Management. Management depends on the cause and symptoms. Resolving the causative factors may be the only treatment needed. If the bradycardia is symptomatic (e.g., shakiness, hypotension, syncope), 0.5 mg of atropine given rapidly as an intravenous (IV) bolus every 3 to 5 minutes to a maximum total dose of 3 mg is the medication of choice. Rarely, catecholamines and emergency transcutaneous pacing are implemented when the rhythm is unresponsive to atropine.

Atropine blocks vagal stimulation, thus allowing a normal rate to occur. However, it should be avoided in cardiac transplant patients because it may cause a paradoxical AV block (see later discussion on AV block) (Morrison, Deakin, Morley, et al., 2010). Rather, theophylline 100 to 200 mg may be administered slowly IV to patients with bradycardia who have had a cardiac transplantation, as well as those who have had an acute inferior MI or spinal cord injury (Morrison et al., 2010).

Sinus Tachycardia

Sinus tachycardia occurs when the sinus node creates an impulse at a faster-than-normal rate. Causes may include the following:

- Physiologic or psychological stress (e.g., acute blood loss, anemia, shock, hypervolemia, hypovolemia, heart failure, pain, hypermetabolic states, fever, exercise, anxiety)
- Medications that stimulate the sympathetic response (e.g., catecholamines, aminophylline, atropine), stimulants (e.g., caffeine, nicotine), and illicit drugs (e.g., amphetamines, cocaine, Ecstasy)
- Enhanced automaticity of the SA node and/or excessive sympathetic tone with reduced parasympathetic tone that is out of proportion to physiologic demands, a condition called *inappropriate sinus tachycardia*
- Autonomic dysfunction, which results in a type of sinus tachycardia referred to as postural orthostatic tachycardia syndrome (POTS). Patients with POTS have tachycardia without hypotension within 5 to 10 minutes of standing or with head-upright tilt testing.

Sinus tachycardia has the following characteristics (Fig. 26-7):

Ventricular and atrial rate: Greater than 100 bpm in the adult, but usually less than 120 bpm

Ventricular and atrial rhythm: Regular

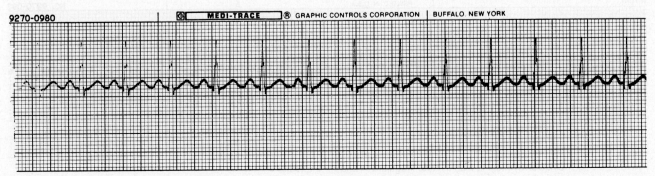

FIGURE 26-7 • Sinus tachycardia in lead II.

QRS shape and duration: Usually normal, but may be regularly abnormal

P wave: Normal and consistent shape; always in front of the QRS, but may be buried in the preceding T wave

PR interval: Consistent interval between 0.12 and 0.20 seconds

P:QRS ratio: 1:1

All aspects of sinus tachycardia are the same as those of normal sinus rhythm, except for the rate. Sinus tachycardia does not start or end suddenly (i.e., it is nonparoxysmal). As the heart rate increases, the diastolic filling time decreases, possibly resulting in reduced cardiac output and subsequent symptoms of syncope and low blood pressure. If the rapid rate persists and the heart cannot compensate for the decreased ventricular filling, the patient may develop acute pulmonary edema.

Medical Management. Medical management of sinus tachycardia is determined by the severity of symptoms and directed at identifying and abolishing its cause. If the tachycardia is persistent and causing hemodynamic instability, synchronized cardioversion is the treatment of choice (see later discussion). Otherwise, vagal maneuvers or administration of adenosine may be considered. Beta-blockers and calcium channel blockers (Table 26-1), although rarely used, may also be considered in a narrow-QRS tachycardia. If the tachycardia has a wide QRS, then adenosine is considered only if the QRS is monomorphic (uniform shape) and the ventricular rhythm is regular. Otherwise, procainamide, amiodarone, and sotalol are the options in wide QRS tachycardia (see later discussion of all of these medications). Catheter ablation (discussed later in this chapter) of the SA node may be used in cases of persistent inappropriate sinus tachycardia unresponsive to other treatments. Treatment for POTS may include increased fluid and sodium intake and the use of graduated compression stockings to prevent pooling of blood in the lower extremities (Fuster, Walsh et al., 2011).

Sinus Arrhythmia

Sinus arrhythmia occurs when the sinus node creates an impulse at an irregular rhythm; the rate usually increases with inspiration and decreases with expiration. Nonrespiratory causes include heart disease and valvular disease, but these are rare. Sinus arrhythmia has the following characteristics (Fig. 26-8):

Ventricular and atrial rate: 60 to 100 bpm in the adult

Ventricular and atrial rhythm: Irregular

QRS shape and duration: Usually normal, but may be regularly abnormal

P wave: Normal and consistent shape; always in front of the QRS

PR interval: Consistent interval between 0.12 and 0.20 seconds

P:QRS ratio: 1:1

Medical Management. Sinus arrhythmia does not cause any significant hemodynamic effect and therefore is not typically treated.

Atrial Dysrhythmias

Premature Atrial Complex

A premature atrial complex (PAC) is a single ECG complex that occurs when an electrical impulse starts in the atrium before the next normal impulse of the sinus node. The PAC may be caused by caffeine, alcohol, nicotine, stretched atrial myocardium (e.g., as in hypervolemia), anxiety, hypokalemia (low potassium level), hypermetabolic states (e.g., with pregnancy), or atrial ischemia, injury, or infarction. PACs are often seen with sinus tachycardia. PACs have the following characteristics (Fig. 26-9):

Ventricular and atrial rate: Depends on the underlying rhythm (e.g., sinus tachycardia)

Ventricular and atrial rhythm: Irregular due to early P waves, creating a PP interval that is shorter than the others. This is sometimes followed by a longer-than-normal PP interval, but one that is less than twice the normal PP interval. This type of interval is called a *noncompensatory pause*.

QRS shape and duration: The QRS that follows the early P wave is usually normal, but it may be abnormal (aberrantly conducted PAC). It may even be absent (blocked PAC).

P wave: An early and different P wave may be seen or may be hidden in the T wave; other P waves in the strip are consistent.

PR interval: The early P wave has a shorter-than-normal PR interval, but still between 0.12 and 0.20 seconds.

P:QRS ratio: Usually 1:1

PACs are common in normal hearts. The patient may say, "My heart skipped a beat." A pulse deficit (a difference between the apical and radial pulse rate) may exist.

Medical Management. If PACs are infrequent, no treatment is necessary. If they are frequent (more than six per minute), this may herald a worsening disease state or the onset of more serious dysrhythmias, such as atrial fibrillation. Medical management is directed toward treating the underlying cause (e.g., reduction of caffeine intake, correction of hypokalemia).

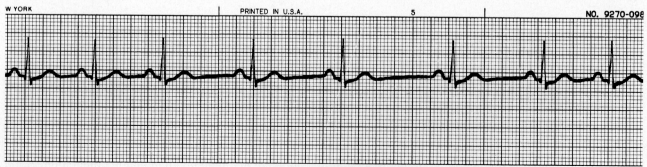

FIGURE 26-8 • Sinus arrhythmia in lead II. Note irregular RR and PP intervals.

TABLE 26-1 Summary of Antiarrhythmic Medications*

Class*	Action	Drug Names	Side Effects	Nursing Interventions
IA	Moderate depression of depolarization; prolongs repolarization Treats and prevents atrial and ventricular dysrhythmias	quinidine (Quinaglute, Quinidex, Cardioquin) procainamide (Pronestyl, Procan SR) disopyramide (Norpace)	Decreased cardiac contractility Prolonged QRS, QT Proarrhythmic Hypotension with IV administration Diarrhea with quinidine, constipation with disopyramide Cinchonism with quinidine Lupuslike syndrome with procainamide Anticholinergic effects: dry mouth, urinary hesitancy with disopyramide	Observe for HF. Monitor BP with IV administration. Monitor QRS duration for increase >50% from baseline. Monitor for prolonged QT. Monitor N-acetyl procainamide (NAPA) laboratory values during procainamide therapy. If administered for atrial fibrillation, ensure patient has been pretreated with a medication to control AV conduction.
IB	Minimal depression of depolarization; shortened repolarization Treats ventricular dysrhythmias	lidocaine (Xylocaine) mexiletine (Mexitil) tocainide (Tonocard)	CNS changes (e.g., confusion, lethargy) Bradycardia GI distress Tremors	Monitor for CNS changes and tremors. Discuss with primary provider decreasing lidocaine dose in older adult patients and patients with cardiac/liver dysfunction.
IC	Marked depression of depolarization; little effect on repolarization Treats atrial and ventricular dysrhythmias	flecainide (Tambocor) propafenone (Rythmol)	Proarrhythmic HF Dizziness, visual disturbances, dyspnea	Decrease dose with renal dysfunction and strict vegetarian diets. Avoid use in patients with structural heart disease (e.g., coronary artery disease and heart failure).
II	Decreases automaticity and conduction Treats atrial and ventricular dysrhythmias	acebutolol (Sectral)§ atenolol (Tenormin) bisoprolol/HCTZ (Ziac, Zebeta) esmolol (Brevibloc)§ labetalol (Trandate) metoprolol (Lopressor, Toprol-XL) nadolol (Corgard) nebivolol (Bystolic) propranolol (Inderal)§ sotalol (Betapace; Sorine; also has class III actions)§	Bradycardia, AV block Decreased contractility Bronchospasm Nausea Asymptomatic and symptomatic hypotension Masks hypoglycemia and thyrotoxicosis CNS disturbances (e.g., confusion, dizziness, fatigue, depression)	Monitor heart rate, PR interval, signs and symptoms of HF, especially in those also taking calcium channel blockers. Monitor blood glucose level in patients with type 2 diabetes. Caution the patient about abrupt withdrawal to avoid tachycardia, hypertension, and myocardial ischemia.
III	Prolongs repolarization Amiodarone treats and prevents ventricular and atrial dysrhythmias, especially in patients with ventricular dysfunction. Dofetilide and ibutilide treat and prevent atrial dysrhythmias.	amiodarone (Cordarone) dofetilide (Tikosyn) ibutilide (Corvert)	Pulmonary toxicity (amiodarone) Corneal microdeposits (amiodarone) Photosensitivity (amiodarone) Bradycardia Hypotension, especially with IV administration Polymorphic ventricular dysrhythmias (rare with amiodarone) Nausea and vomiting Potentiates digoxin (amiodarone) See beta-blockers above (sotalol).	Make sure patient is sent for baseline pulmonary function tests (amiodarone). Closely monitor patient. Assess for contraindications prior to administration. Monitor QT duration. Continuous ECG monitoring with initiation of dofetilide and ibutilide. Monitor renal function.
IV	Blocks calcium channel Treats and prevents paroxysmal atrial dysrhythmias†	verapamil (Calan, Isoptin) diltiazem (Cardizem, Dilacor, Tiazac, Diltia, Cartia)	Bradycardia, AV blocks Hypotension with IV administration HF, peripheral edema Constipation, dizziness, headache, nausea	Monitor heart rate, PR interval. Monitor blood pressure closely with IV administration. Monitor for signs and symptoms of HF. Do not crush sustained-release medications.

IV, intravenous; HF, heart failure; BP, blood pressure; AV, atrioventricular; CNS, central nervous system; GI, gastrointestinal; HCTZ, hydrochlorothiazide; ECG, electrocardiogram.

*Based on Vaughn-Williams classification.

†There are other calcium channel blockers, but they are not approved or used for dysrhythmias.

§Beta-blocker with labeled use for dysrhythmias.

Adapted from American Heart Association. (2010). *Advanced cardiac life support provider manual*. Dallas: American Heart Association; American Society of Health System Pharmacists. (2012). *AHFS drug information*. Bethesda, MD: Author; and Fuster, V., Walsh, R. A., & Harrington, R. A. (Eds.). (2011). *Hurst's the heart* (13th ed.). New York: McGraw-Hill.

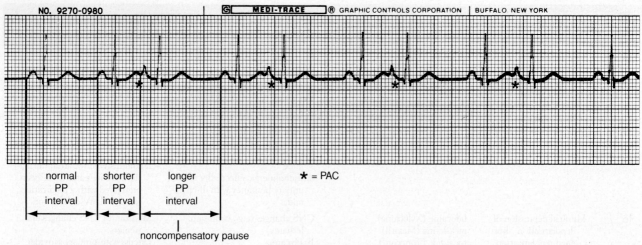

normal
PP
interval

shorter
PP
interval

longer
PP
interval

noncompensatory pause

★ = PAC

FIGURE 26-9 • Premature atrial complexes (PACs) in lead II. Note that the pause following the PAC is longer than the normal PP interval but shorter than twice the normal PP interval.

Atrial Flutter

Atrial flutter occurs because of a conduction defect in the atrium and causes a rapid, regular atrial rate, usually between 250 and 400 bpm. Because the atrial rate is faster than the AV node can conduct, not all atrial impulses are conducted into the ventricle, causing a therapeutic block at the AV node. This is an important feature of this dysrhythmia. If all atrial impulses were conducted to the ventricle, the ventricular rate would also be 250 to 400 bpm, which would result in ventricular fibrillation, a life-threatening dysrhythmia. Atrial flutter often occurs in patients with chronic obstructive pulmonary disease, pulmonary hypertension, valvular disease, and thyrotoxicosis, as well as following open heart surgery and repair of congenital cardiac defects (Fuster, Walsh et al., 2011).

Atrial flutter has the following characteristics (Fig. 26-10):

Ventricular and atrial rate: Atrial rate ranges between 250 and 400 bpm; ventricular rate usually ranges between 75 and 150 bpm.

Ventricular and atrial rhythm: The atrial rhythm is regular; the ventricular rhythm is usually regular but may be irregular because of a change in the AV conduction.

QRS shape and duration: Usually normal, but may be abnormal or may be absent

P wave: Saw-toothed shape; these waves are referred to as F waves

PR interval: Multiple F waves may make it difficult to determine the PR interval.

P:QRS ratio: 2:1, 3:1, or 4:1

Medical Management. Medical management involves the use of vagal maneuvers or administration of adenosine (Adenocard, Adenoscan), which cause sympathetic block and slowing of conduction in the AV node, and may terminate the tachycardia or at least allow better visualization of flutter waves. Adenosine should be rapidly administered IV, followed by a 20-mL saline flush and elevation of the arm with the IV line to promote rapid circulation of the medication. If the tachycardia does not terminate within 2 minutes, then a larger dose of adenosine may be given (Morrison et al., 2010).

Atrial flutter can cause serious signs and symptoms, such as chest pain, shortness of breath, and low blood pressure. Electrical cardioversion (discussed later) is often successful in converting the rhythm to sinus rhythm. If the dysrhythmia has lasted longer than 48 hours and a transesophageal echocardiogram has not confirmed the absence of atrial clots, then adequate anticoagulation, using the same criteria as for atrial fibrillation, may be indicated before cardioversion or ablation. Medications used to slow the ventricular response rate include beta-blockers, nondihydropyridine calcium channel blockers, and digitalis, alone or in combination (see Table 26-1). Catheter ablation rather than antiarrhythmic medications is now the long-term treatment of choice. Atrial flutter should be treated with antithrombotic therapy in the same manner as with atrial fibrillation (Crandall, Bradley, Packer, et al., 2009) (see later discussion).

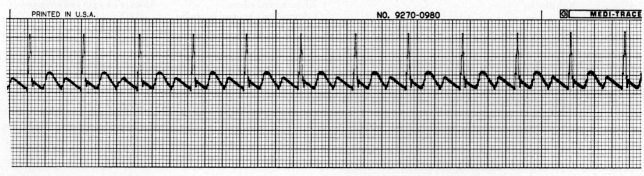

FIGURE 26-10 • Atrial flutter in lead II.

**Chart
26-3**   **Atrial Fibrillation Classification System**

Type	Description
Paroxysmal	Recurrent, with sudden onset and termination; lasts ≤7 days
Persistent	Continuous, lasting >7 days
Long-standing persistent	Continuous, lasting >1 year
Permanent	Persistent, but decision has been made not to restore or maintain sinus rhythm

Adapted from Calkins, H., Kuck, K. H., Cappato, R., et al. (2012). 2012 HRS/EHRA/ECAS expert consensus statement on catheter and surgical ablation of atrial fibrillation: Recommendations for patient selection, procedural techniques, patient management and follow-up, definitions, endpoints, and research trial design. *Heart Rhythm, 9*(4), 632–696.

Atrial Fibrillation

Atrial fibrillation is an uncoordinated atrial electrical activation that causes a rapid, disorganized, and uncoordinated twitching of atrial musculature. The ventricular rate response depends on the ability of the AV node to conduct the atrial impulses, the level of sympathetic and parasympathetic tone, presence of accessory pathways, and effects of any medications (Fuster, Rydén, Cannom, et al., 2011). For example, regular RR intervals in atrial fibrillation may indicate the presence of complete AV block. The lack of consistency in describing the pattern of atrial fibrillation has led to the use of numerous labels (e.g., acute, chronic, **paroxysmal** [i.e., if it occurs suddenly], persistent, and permanent). The recommended classification system is noted in Chart 26-3. Note that the use of "chronic atrial fibrillation" is not included; because it lacks a standard definition, using this label should be avoided (Calkins, Kuck, Cappoto, et al., 2012).

Atrial fibrillation is the most common sustained dysrhythmia, occurring in more than 2 million people in the United States (Schnabel, Sullivan, Levy, et al., 2009). The exact cause of atrial fibrillation is unknown; however, autonomic foci and multiple reentry phenomena are involved, most often originating not in the atrium but in nearby tissue (e.g., the pulmonary vein) (Crandall et al., 2009). Risk factors for atrial fibrillation are noted in Chart 26-4.

Atrial fibrillation may occur in the postoperative period of any major surgery, but especially open heart surgery (Cramm, Kirchof, Lip, et al., 2010). It may also occur in structural heart

**Chart
26-4**   ⚠   **RISK FACTORS
Atrial Fibrillation**

- Increasing age
- Male gender
- Higher body mass index
- Systolic blood pressure ≥160 mm Hg
- Hypertension
- PR interval ≥160 milliseconds
- Clinically significant heart murmur (i.e., grade 3 or higher)
- Heart failure

Adapted from Schnabel, R. B., Sullivan, L. M., Levy, D., et al. (2009). Development of a risk score for atrial fibrillation (Framingham Heart Study): A community-based cohort study. *Lancet, 373*(9665), 739–745.

disease, such as valvular heart disease (most often mitral or tricuspid); inflammatory or infiltrative disease (pericarditis, myocarditis, amyloidosis); dilated, hypertrophic, and restrictive cardiomyopathy; coronary artery disease; hypertension; congenital disorder (especially atrial septal defect); and heart failure (diastolic or systolic) (Fuster, Rydén et al., 2011). The dysrhythmia also may be found in people with hyperthyroidism, pheochromocytoma, pulmonary hypertension and embolism, obstructive sleep apnea, and acute moderate to heavy ingestion of alcohol ("holiday heart" syndrome), as well as following pulmonary or open heart surgery (Fuster, Rydén et al., 2011). Neurogenic atrial fibrillation that occurs with subarachnoid hemorrhage and nonhemorrhagic stroke is caused by increased vagal or sympathetic stimulation. Sometimes atrial fibrillation occurs in people younger than 60 years with no underlying pathophysiology and is called *lone atrial fibrillation* (Fuster, Rydén et al., 2011). Many studies have indicated that atrial fibrosis is involved in persistent atrial fibrillation, which has led to the investigation of substances such as endothelin 1, C-reactive protein, and interleukin 6 as biomarkers for atrial fibrillation (Estes, Sacco, Al-Khatib, et al., 2011).

Atrial fibrillation is growing in prevalence and is linked to increased risk of stroke, dementia, and premature death (Estes et al., 2011). Hospital admissions for atrial fibrillation increased by 66% over the past 20 years, and occurrence of the dysrhythmia increases the length and cost of the hospital stay (Fuster, Rydén et al., 2011).

Atrial fibrillation has the following characteristics (Fig. 26-11):

Ventricular and atrial rate: Atrial rate is 300 to 600 bpm; ventricular rate is usually 120 to 200 bpm in untreated atrial fibrillation.

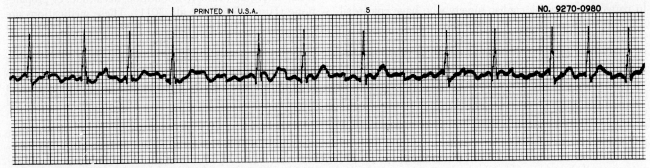

PRINTED IN U.S.A.   5   NO. 9270-0980

FIGURE 26-11 • Atrial fibrillation in lead II.

Ventricular and atrial rhythm: Highly irregular

QRS shape and duration: Usually normal, but may be abnormal

P wave: No discernible P waves; irregular undulating waves that vary in amplitude and shape are seen and referred to as fibrillatory or f waves

PR interval: Cannot be measured

P:QRS ratio: Many:1

A rapid and irregular ventricular response reduces the time for ventricular filling, resulting in a smaller stroke volume. Because atrial fibrillation causes a loss in AV synchrony (the atria and ventricles contract at different times), the atrial kick (the last part of diastole and ventricular filling, which accounts for 25% to 30% of the cardiac output) is also lost. This may lead to irregular palpitations and symptoms of heart failure such as shortness of breath, fatigue, exercise intolerance, and malaise. Patients may be asymptomatic or experience significant hemodynamic collapse (hypotension, chest pain, pulmonary edema, and altered level of consciousness), especially if they also have hypertension, mitral stenosis, hypertrophic cardiomyopathy, or some form of restrictive heart failure (Fuster, Rydén et al., 2011). There is usually a pulse deficit—a numeric difference between apical and radial pulse rates. The shorter time in diastole reduces the time available for coronary artery perfusion, thereby increasing the risk of myocardial ischemia with the onset of chest discomfort. The erratic atrial contraction, altered blood flow, and the atrial myocardial dysfunction promote the formation of thrombi, especially within the left atrium, increasing the risk of an embolic event.

In addition, a high ventricular rate response during atrial fibrillation can lead to dilated ventricular cardiomyopathy. The rapid ventricular rate can also lead to mitral valve dysfunction, mitral regurgitation, and intraventricular conduction delay. Controlling the ventricular rate may avoid and correct these effects.

Medical Management. The clinical evaluation of atrial fibrillation should include a history and physical examination (to identify pattern of atrial fibrillation, associated symptoms, and any underlying conditions); 12-lead ECG (to identify the presence of ventricular hypertrophy, pre-excitation from accessory pathways, intraventricular conduction defects, and history of MI); echocardiogram (to assess cardiac chamber size, thickness, and function; to identify potential causes, such as cardiomyopathy or valvular dysfunction; and to identify the presence of a thrombus); and blood tests to assess thyroid, renal, and hepatic function when the ventricular rate is difficult to control (Fuster, Rydén et al., 2011). In patients undergoing cardiac surgery who have epicardial wires attached, obtaining an atrial ECG assists in diagnosing atrial fibrillation and differentiating it from other common dysrhythmias, such as an accelerated junctional rhythm (McRae et al., 2010). Additional tests may include a chest x-ray (to evaluate pulmonary vasculature), exercise test (to assess rate control as well as myocardial ischemia), Holter or event monitoring, and an EP study. The physical examination may reveal an irregular pulse, irregular jugular venous pulsations, and irregular S₁ heart sounds.

Treatment of atrial fibrillation depends on the cause, pattern, and duration of the dysrhythmia, the ventricular

response rate, and the patient's type and severity of symptoms, as well as the patient's age and comorbidities. Rhythm control (conversion to sinus rhythm) versus rate control is a clinical decision in the initial and ongoing treatment for atrial fibrillation. Prospective studies have found that controlling the heart rate (resting heart rate less than 80 bpm) is equivalent to controlling the rhythm in terms of quality of life, frequency of hospitalization for heart failure, and incidence of stroke (Fuster, Rydén et al., 2011; Wyse, Waldo, DiMarco, et al., 2002). However, if atrial fibrillation persists in some patients, such as those who are younger or have heart failure, electrical and structural remodeling may then prevent sinus rhythm restoration from ever occurring. Therefore, management of atrial fibrillation may not only be different in different patients, but it also may change over time for any one patient.

In some patients, atrial fibrillation converts to sinus rhythm within 24 hours and without treatment. Hospitalization may not be necessary. Electrical cardioversion is indicated for patients with atrial fibrillation that is hemodynamically unstable and does not quickly respond to medications, unless they have concomitant digitalis toxicity or hypokalemia. Because of the high risk of embolization of atrial thrombi, cardioversion of atrial fibrillation that has lasted longer than 48 hours should be avoided unless the patient has received warfarin for at least 3 to 4 weeks prior to cardioversion. Alternatively, the absence of a mural thrombus can be confirmed by transesophageal echocardiogram, and heparin can be administered immediately prior to cardioversion.

 Concept Mastery Alert

The patient with atrial fibrillation is at high risk for thrombus formation. When electrical cardioversion is indicated, the nurse may anticipate that a transesophageal echocardiogram may be performed to evaluate for possible atrial thrombi.

Because atrial function may be impaired for several weeks after cardioversion, warfarin is indicated for at least 4 weeks after the procedure. Patients may be given amiodarone (Cordarone), flecainide (Tambocor), ibutilide (Corvert), propafenone (Rythmol), or sotalol (Betapace) prior to cardioversion to enhance the success of cardioversion and prevent relapse of the atrial fibrillation (Fuster, Rydén et al., 2011).

Medications that may be administered to achieve pharmacologic cardioversion to sinus rhythm include amiodarone, dofetilide (Tikosyn), ibutilide, flecainide, or propafenone (Fuster, Rydén et al., 2011). These medications are most effective if given within 7 days of the onset of atrial fibrillation. Because of the incidence of torsade de pointes, which is a type of ventricular tachycardia (VT), the use of ibutilide warrants ECG monitoring for at least 4 hours after its administration. The use of dofetilide also requires patient hospitalization for monitoring of the QT interval and renal function.

If the QRS is wide and the ventricular rhythm is very fast and irregular, atrial fibrillation with an accessory pathway should be suspected. An accessory pathway is congenital tissue between the atria, His bundle, AV node, Purkinje fibers, or ventricular myocardium. This anomaly is known as Wolff-Parkinson-White (WPW) syndrome. Electrical cardioversion is the treatment of choice for atrial fibrillation in the presence of WPW syndrome that causes hemodynamic instability. Medications that block AV conduction (e.g., digoxin, diltiazem [Cardizem], and verapamil) [Calan]) should be avoided in WPW because they can increase the ventricular rate. If the patient is hemodynamically stable, procainamide (Pronestyl), propafenone, flecainide, and amiodarone are recommended to restore sinus rhythm (Fuster, Rydén et al., 2011). Catheter ablation is performed for long-term management.

To control the heart rate in persistent atrial fibrillation, a beta-blocker (propranolol [Inderal], atenolol [Tenormin], metoprolol [Lopressor], or esmolol [Brevibloc]) or a nondihydropyridine calcium channel blocker (diltiazem or verapamil) is recommended (Fuster, Rydén et al., 2011). However, people with impaired ventricular function should not receive verapamil, those with bronchospasm should not receive a beta-blocker, and those with AV block should not receive any of these medications. IV digoxin or amiodarone may be used for rate control in patients with heart failure or left ventricular dysfunction but without an accessory pathway. IV procainamide or ibutilide is an alternative for rate control in patients with an accessory pathway. In pregnant women, digoxin, a beta-blocker, or a nondihydropyridine calcium channel blocker may be used for rate control. If medications fail to control the heart rate or cause significant side effects, catheter ablation may be indicated (Fuster, Rydén et al., 2011).

Persistent atrial fibrillation can cause sinus node dysfunction and alteration in the atrial musculature and contractile function (atrial stunning), which may persist for days or weeks following conversion to sinus rhythm (Crandall et al., 2009). This has implications for the length of recovery time and the duration of anticoagulation therapy needed after conversion.

Maintenance of sinus rhythm may be obtained with amiodarone, dofetilide, disopyramide (Norpace), flecainide, propafenone, or sotalol (Fuster, Rydén et al., 2011). Patients with specific characteristics who have been observed in the hospital may be given a medication to self-administer outside of the hospital if they have a recurrence, an approach referred to as "pill in the pocket" (Fuster, Rydén et al., 2011; Saborido, Hockenhull, Bagust, et al., 2010). Several approaches are used to prevent the occurrence of postoperative atrial fibrillation; preoperative administration of a beta-blocker or amiodarone is the most successful (Fuster, Rydén et al., 2011). Pacemaker implantation, catheter ablation, or surgical ablation, also called the *maze procedure* (see later discussion), which requires the patient to be placed on cardiopulmonary bypass, may be indicated for patients who do not respond to medications. Although implantable atrial defibrillators have been studied, the average energy needed to cardiovert is 3 joules, causing significant and unacceptable discomfort to the patient (Fuster, Rydén et al., 2011).

Antithrombotic therapy is indicated for all patients with atrial fibrillation, especially those who are at risk for an embolic event, such as stroke, and is the only therapy that decreases cardiovascular mortality (Cramm et al., 2010). This type of therapy should be primarily based on the risks

of stroke (Lip, Nieuwlaat, Pisters, et al., 2010) rather than the risk of bleeding (Lip, Frison, Halperin, et al., 2011) in a particular patient (Fuster, Rydén et al., 2011). Patients with significant risk factors for a stroke (history of a previous stroke, transient ischemic attack or embolic event, mitral stenosis, or prosthetic heart valve) may be started on warfarin (Coumadin) therapy (Fuster, Rydén et al., 2011). If the patient has no risk factors, then the patient may be placed on 81 to 325 mg daily aspirin therapy (Fuster, Rydén et al., 2011). If the patient has one moderate risk factor (hypertension, diabetes, 75 years or older, or an ejection fraction of 35% or less [see Chapter 25]), aspirin or warfarin therapy may be initiated (Fuster, Rydén et al., 2011). If the patient has more than one moderate risk factor, warfarin therapy may be initiated (Fuster, Rydén et al., 2011). Another study indicated that antithrombotic therapy should be initiated if the patient has one, if female, or two, if male, of the following risk factors: 64 to 74 years of age, or a history of hypertension, heart failure, diabetes, or vascular disease (e.g., peripheral arterial disease), a previous MI, or an aortic plaque (Lip et al., 2010).

If immediate anticoagulation is necessary, the patient may be placed on heparin until the warfarin level is therapeutic, usually defined as an international normalized ratio (INR) between 2 and 3. If a patient sustains an ischemic stroke or is at high risk, the antithrombotic therapy may be increased with an INR goal between 3 and 3.5 (Fuster, Rydén et al., 2011). If a patient will be undergoing a procedure that carries a risk of bleeding, anticoagulation therapy may be withheld for up to a week. If more than a week is needed, heparin may be given, although its efficiency is unknown. There are several newer anticoagulants available, such as apixaban (Eliquis), rivaroxaban (Xarelto), and dabigatran (Pradaxa). However, it is believed that there are no profound differences between these drugs in terms of efficacy (Lip, Larsen, Skjøth, et al., 2012).

Recent studies have demonstrated that angiotensin-converting enzyme (ACE) inhibitors and angiotensin receptor blockers (ARBs) decrease the incidence of atrial fibrillation, the number of defibrillation attempts required to restore sinus rhythm, and the number of hospital readmissions (Fuster, Rydén et al., 2011). More studies are needed to clarify the role of ACE inhibitors and ARBs in long-term maintenance of sinus rhythm. In addition, 3-hydroxy-3-methylglutaryl coenzyme A (HMG-CoA) reductase inhibitors (i.e., statins) assist in maintaining sinus rhythm in patients with persistent lone atrial fibrillation (Fuster, Rydén et al., 2011) (see Chapter 27 for discussion of these drugs).

Junctional Dysrhythmias

Premature Junctional Complex

A premature junctional complex is an impulse that starts in the AV nodal area before the next normal sinus impulse reaches the AV node. Premature junctional complexes are less common than PACs. Causes include digitalis toxicity, heart failure, and coronary artery disease. The ECG criteria for premature junctional complex are the same as for PACs, except for the P wave and the PR interval. The P wave may be absent, may follow the QRS, or may occur before the QRS but with a PR interval of less than 0.12 seconds. This

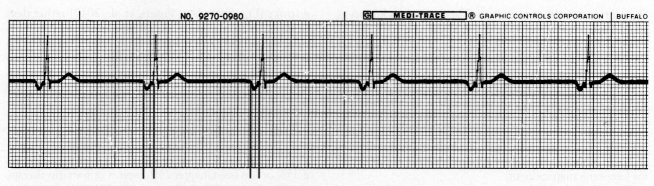

FIGURE 26-12 • Junctional rhythm in lead II; note short PR intervals.

dysrhythmia rarely produces significant symptoms. Treatment for frequent premature junctional complexes is the same as for frequent PACs.

Junctional Rhythm

Junctional or idionodal rhythm occurs when the AV node, instead of the sinus node, becomes the pacemaker of the heart. When the sinus node slows (e.g., from increased vagal tone) or when the impulse cannot be conducted through the AV node (e.g., because of complete heart block), the AV node automatically discharges an impulse. Junctional rhythm not caused by complete heart block has the following characteristics (Fig. 26-12):

Ventricular and atrial rate: Ventricular rate 40 to 60 bpm; atrial rate also 40 to 60 bpm if P waves are discernible
Ventricular and atrial rhythm: Regular
QRS shape and duration: Usually normal, but may be abnormal
P wave: May be absent, after the QRS complex, or before the QRS; may be inverted, especially in lead II
PR interval: If the P wave is in front of the QRS, the PR interval is less than 0.12 seconds.
P:QRS ratio: 1:1 or 0:1

Medical Management

Junctional rhythm may produce signs and symptoms of reduced cardiac output. If this occurs, the treatment is the same as for sinus bradycardia. Emergency pacing may be needed.

Nonparoxysmal Junctional Tachycardia

Junctional tachycardia is caused by enhanced automaticity in the junctional area, resulting in a rhythm similar to junctional rhythm, except at a rate of 70 to 120 bpm. Although this rhythm generally does not have any detrimental hemodynamic effect, it may indicate a serious underlying condition,

such as digitalis toxicity, myocardial ischemia, hypokalemia, or chronic obstructive pulmonary disease. Because junctional tachycardia is caused by increased automaticity, cardioversion is not an effective treatment (Fuster, Walsh et al., 2011).

Atrioventricular Nodal Reentry Tachycardia

Atrioventricular nodal reentry tachycardia (AVNRT) is a common dysrhythmia that occurs when an impulse is conducted to an area in the AV node that causes the impulse to be rerouted back into the same area over and over again at a very fast rate. Each time the impulse is conducted through this area, it is also conducted down into the ventricles, causing a fast ventricular rate. AVNRT that has an abrupt onset and an abrupt cessation with a QRS of normal duration has been termed *paroxysmal atrial tachycardia*. AVNRT also occurs when the duration of the QRS complex is 0.12 seconds or greater and a block in the bundle branch is known to be present. This dysrhythmia may last for seconds or several hours. Factors associated with the development of AVNRT include caffeine, nicotine, hypoxemia, and stress. Underlying pathologies include coronary artery disease and cardiomyopathy; however, it occurs more often in females and not in association with underlying structural heart disease. AVNRT has the following characteristics (Fig. 26-13):

Ventricular and atrial rate: Atrial rate usually 150 to 250 bpm; ventricular rate usually 120 to 200 bpm
Ventricular and atrial rhythm: Regular; sudden onset and termination of the tachycardia
QRS shape and duration: Usually normal, but may be abnormal
P wave: Usually very difficult to discern
PR interval: If the P wave is in front of the QRS, the PR interval is less than 0.12 seconds.
P:QRS ratio: 1:1, 2:1

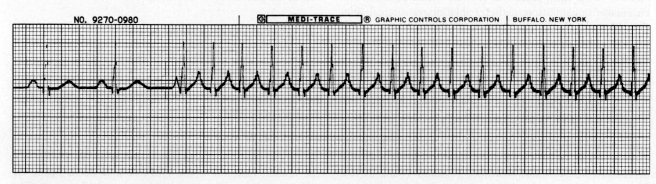

FIGURE 26-13 • AV nodal reentry tachycardia in lead II.

The clinical symptoms vary with the rate and duration of the tachycardia and the patient's underlying condition. The tachycardia usually is of short duration, resulting only in palpitations. A fast rate may also reduce cardiac output, resulting in significant signs and symptoms such as restlessness, chest pain, shortness of breath, pallor, hypotension, and loss of consciousness.

Medical Management. Because AVNRT is generally a benign dysrhythmia, the goal of medical management is to alleviate symptoms and improve quality of life. Patients who become significantly symptomatic and require emergency department visits to terminate the rhythm may want to initiate therapy immediately. However, those with minimum symptoms with an AVRNT that terminates spontaneously or with minimal treatment may choose just to be monitored.

The aim of therapy is to break the reentry of the impulse. Catheter ablation is the initial treatment of choice and is used to eliminate the area that permits the rerouting of the impulse that causes the tachycardia (Calkins et al., 2012). Vagal maneuvers, such as carotid sinus massage (Fig. 26-14), gagging, breath-holding, and immersing the face in ice water, may be used to interrupt AVNRT. These techniques increase parasympathetic stimulation, causing slower conduction through the AV node and blocking the reentry of the rerouted impulse. Some patients use some of these methods to terminate the episode on their own. Because of the risk of a cerebral embolic event, carotid sinus massage is contraindicated in patients with carotid bruits. If the vagal maneuvers are ineffective, the patient may then receive a bolus of adenosine to correct the rhythm; this is nearly 100% effective in terminating AVNRT (Rothman, 2010). Because the effect of adenosine is so short, AVNRT may recur; the first dose may be followed with a larger dose or with a calcium channel blocker, such as verapamil (Calan), followed by one or two additional boluses. Digoxin is not indicated because of it slow onset. If the patient is unstable or does not respond to the medications, cardioversion is the treatment of choice. The patient who is unstable may be given adenosine while preparations for cardioversion are being made. For recurrent sustained AVNRT, treatment with calcium channel blockers such as verapamil and diltia-

zem, class 1a antiarrhythmic agents such as procainamide and disopyramide, class 1c antiarrhythmic agents such as flecainide and propafenone, and class III agents such as sotalol and amiodarone may prevent a recurrence. If the rhythm is infrequent and there is no underlying cardiac structural disorder, a single oral dose of flecainide or a combination of diltiazem and propranolol during an episode of tachycardia may be effective.

If P waves cannot be identified, the rhythm may be called **supraventricular tachycardia (SVT)**, or paroxysmal supraventricular tachycardia (PSVT) if it has an abrupt onset, until the underlying rhythm and resulting diagnosis is determined. SVT and PSVT indicate only that the rhythm is not **ventricular tachycardia (VT)**. SVT could be atrial fibrillation, atrial flutter, or AVNRT, among others. Vagal maneuvers and adenosine may be used to convert the rhythm or at least slow conduction in the AV node to allow visualization of the P waves. If the ECG does not assist in the differentiation of the dysrhythmia, invasive EP testing may be necessary to make the diagnosis.

Ventricular Dysrhythmias

Premature Ventricular Complex

A PVC is an impulse that starts in a ventricle and is conducted through the ventricles before the next normal sinus impulse. PVCs can occur in healthy people, especially with intake of caffeine, nicotine, or alcohol. PVCs may be caused by cardiac ischemia or infarction, increased workload on the heart (e.g., heart failure and tachycardia), digitalis toxicity, hypoxia, acidosis, or electrolyte imbalances, especially hypokalemia.

In a rhythm referred to as bigeminy, every other complex is a PVC. In trigeminy, every third complex is a PVC, and in quadrigeminy, every fourth complex is a PVC. PVCs have the following characteristics (Fig. 26-15):

Ventricular and atrial rate: Depends on the underlying rhythm (e.g., sinus rhythm)

Ventricular and atrial rhythm: Irregular due to early QRS, creating one RR interval that is shorter than the others. The PP interval may be regular, indicating that the PVC did not depolarize the sinus node.

QRS shape and duration: Duration is 0.12 seconds or longer; shape is bizarre and abnormal.

P wave: Visibility of the P wave depends on the timing of the PVC; may be absent (hidden in the QRS or T wave) or in front of the QRS. If the P wave follows the QRS, the shape of the P wave may be different.

PR interval: If the P wave is in front of the QRS, the PR interval is less than 0.12 seconds.

P:QRS ratio: 0:1; 1:1

The patient may feel nothing or may say that the heart "skipped a beat." The effect of a PVC depends on its timing in the cardiac cycle and how much blood was in the ventricles when they contracted. Initial treatment is aimed at correcting the cause.

Medical Management. PVCs usually are not serious. PVCs that are frequent and persistent may be treated with amiodarone or sotalol, but long-term pharmacotherapy for only PVCs is not usually indicated. In patients with an acute MI, recent studies have found that PVCs are not associated with

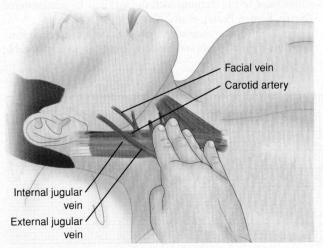

Facial vein
Carotid artery
Internal jugular vein
External jugular vein

FIGURE 26-14 • Carotid sinus massage.

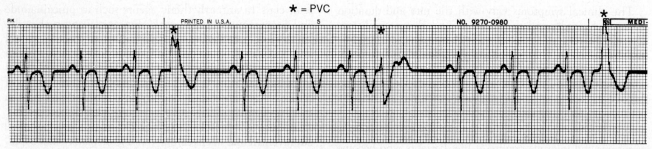

FIGURE 26-15 • Multifocal premature ventricular complexes (PVCs) in quadrigeminy in lead V₁. Note regular PP interval (P wave within PVC).

sudden cardiac death and do not warrant more aggressive therapy (Patton, 2010). In the past, PVCs were considered to be indicative of an increased risk for ensuing VT. However, PVCs that (1) are more frequent than six per minute, (2) are multifocal or polymorphic (having different shapes and rhythms), (3) occur two in a row (pair), and (4) occur on the T wave (the vulnerable period of ventricular depolarization) have not been found to be precursors of VT in patients without structural heart disease (Cardiac Arrhythmia Suppression Trial Investigators, 1989; Patton, 2010). PVCs are not considered a warning for ensuing VT.

Ventricular Tachycardia

VT is defined as three or more PVCs in a row, occurring at a rate exceeding 100 bpm. The causes are similar to those of PVC. Patients with larger MIs and lower ejection fractions are at higher risk of lethal VT (see Chapter 29). VT is an emergency because the patient is usually (although not always) unresponsive and pulseless. VT has the following characteristics (Fig. 26-16):

Ventricular and atrial rate: Ventricular rate is 100 to 200 bpm; atrial rate depends on the underlying rhythm (e.g., sinus rhythm).

Ventricular and atrial rhythm: Usually regular; atrial rhythm may also be regular

QRS shape and duration: Duration is 0.12 seconds or more; bizarre, abnormal shape.

P wave: Very difficult to detect, so the atrial rate and rhythm may be indeterminable.

PR interval: Very irregular, if P waves are seen

P:QRS ratio: Difficult to determine, but if P waves are apparent, there are usually more QRS complexes than P waves.

The patient's tolerance or lack of tolerance for this rapid rhythm depends on the ventricular rate and severity of ventricular dysfunction. However, hemodynamic stability does not predict mortality risk (Pelligrini & Schneiman, 2010).

Medical Management. Several factors determine the initial treatment, including the following: identifying the rhythm as monomorphic (having a consistent QRS shape and rate) or polymorphic (having varying QRS shapes and rhythms), determining the existence of a prolonged QT interval before the initiation of VT, any comorbities, and ascertaining the patient's heart function (normal or decreased). If the patient is stable, continuing the assessment, especially obtaining a 12-lead ECG, may be the only action necessary.

However, the patient may need antiarrhythmic medications, antitachycardia pacing, or direct cardioversion or defibrillation. Procainamide (Pronestyl) may be used for monomorphic stable VT in patients who do not have acute MI or severe HF (Morrison et al., 2010). IV amiodarone is the medication of choice for a patient with impaired cardiac function or acute MI. Sotalol may also be considered for stable monomorphic VT. Although lidocaine had been the medication most commonly used for immediate, short-term therapy, especially for patients with impaired cardiac function, it has no proven short- or long-term efficacy in cardiac arrest (Morrison et al., 2010).

Cardioversion is the treatment of choice for monophasic VT in a symptomatic patient. Defibrillation is the treatment of choice for pulseless VT. Any type of VT in a patient who is unconscious and without a pulse is treated in the same manner as ventricular fibrillation: immediate **defibrillation** is the action of choice. In monitored, witnessed VT when a defibrillator is not immediately available, a precordial thump (a single blow to the sternum with the fist) may be administered (Sayre, Koster, Botha, et al., 2010).

For long-term management, patients with an ejection fraction less than 35% should be considered for an implantable

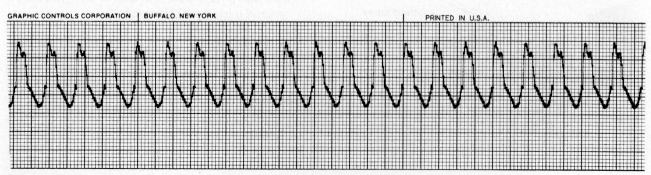

FIGURE 26-16 • Ventricular tachycardia in lead V₁.

cardioverter defibrillator (ICD) (see later discussion). Those with an ejection fraction greater than 35% may be managed with amiodarone. A small percentage of patients with VT have structurally normal hearts and respond well to medications and ablation, and they have an excellent prognosis (Fuster, Walsh et al., 2011). If the ventricular rate is above 200 bpm, then the presence of an accessory pathway should be suspected. If the ventricular rhythm is irregular, atrial fibrillation should be suspected and treated appropriately (Morrison et al., 2010).

Torsades de pointes is a polymorphic VT preceded by a prolonged QT interval, which could be congenital or acquired. Common causes include central nervous system disease; certain medications; or low levels of potassium, calcium, or magnesium. Congenital QT prolongation is another cause. Because this rhythm is likely to cause the patient to deteriorate and become pulseless, immediate treatment is required and includes correction of any electrolyte imbalance, such as administration of IV magnesium. IV isoproterenol (Isuprel) may be used but is contraindicated in the presence of ischemia or hypertension (Morrison et al., 2010). IV beta-blockers or the initiation of overdrive atrial or ventricular pacing (see later discussion) may also be used to treat this dysrhythmia (Morrison et al., 2010).

Ventricular Fibrillation

The most common dysrhythmia in patients with cardiac arrest is ventricular fibrillation, which is a rapid, disorganized ventricular rhythm that causes ineffective quivering of the ventricles. No atrial activity is seen on the ECG. The most common cause of ventricular fibrillation is coronary artery disease and resulting acute MI. Other causes include untreated or unsuccessfully treated VT, cardiomyopathy, valvular heart disease, several **proarrhythmic** medications, acid–base and electrolyte abnormalities, and electrical shock. Another cause is Brugada syndrome, in which the patient (frequently of Asian descent) has a structurally normal heart, few or no risk factors for coronary artery disease, and a family history of sudden cardiac death. Ventricular fibrillation has the following characteristics (Fig. 26-17):

Ventricular rate: Greater than 300 bpm
Ventricular rhythm: Extremely irregular, without a specific pattern
QRS shape and duration: Irregular, undulating waves without recognizable QRS complexes

Medical Management. Ventricular fibrillation is always characterized by the absence of an audible heartbeat, a palpable pulse, and respirations. Because there is no coordinated cardiac activity, cardiac arrest and death are imminent if the dysrhythmia is not corrected. Early defibrillation is critical to survival, with administration of immediate bystander cardiopulmonary resuscitation (CPR) until defibrillation is available. The chance of survival decreases every minute in delay of defibrillation (Jacobs, Sunde, Deakin, et al., 2010). If there is a delay in an emergency services response, CPR may be given while preparing to defibrillate (Jacobs et al., 2010). After the initial defibrillation, five additional cycles of CPR (about 2 minutes of continuous chest compressions in the intubated patient), beginning with chest compression and alternating with a rhythm check and defibrillation, are used to convert ventricular fibrillation to an electrical rhythm that produces a pulse. Cardiocerebral resuscitation for cardiac arrest with continuous chest compressions, interrupted only with defibrillation, and its de-emphasis on the use of positive-pressure ventilation continues to be explored as a better method for improving survival. Epinephrine should be administered as soon as possible after the first unsuccessful defibrillation and then every 3 to 5 minutes. One dose of vasopressin may be administered instead of epinephrine if the cardiac arrest persists. Other antiarrhythmic medications (amiodarone, lidocaine, or possibly magnesium) should be administered as soon as possible after the third defibrillation.

For refractory ventricular fibrillation, amiodarone may be the medication of choice. However, once the patient is intubated, CPR should be given continuously, not in cycles. In addition, underlying and contributing factors are identified and eliminated throughout the event (Morrison et al., 2010).

Current resuscitation guidelines recommend inducing mild hypothermia in comatose adults who experience cardiac arrest. Hypothermia is defined as a core body temperature of 32°C to 34°C (89.6°F to 93.2°F) (Morrison et al., 2010). Induction should be started as soon as possible after circulation is restored, preferably within 60 minutes, and maintained for 12 to 24 hours (Morrison et al., 2010). It is usually initiated by applying ice packs to the axilla and groin, as well as administering iced normal saline or lactated Ringer's IV fluids 30 mL/kg until a cooling machine is obtained.

The nurse caring for a patient with hypothermia (passive or induced) needs to monitor for appropriate level of cooling, sedation, and neuromuscular paralysis to prevent seizures, myoclonus, and shivering. Development of seizures following

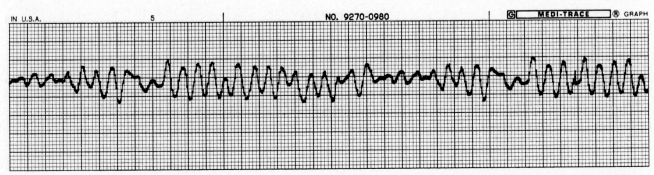

FIGURE 26-17 • Ventricular fibrillation in lead II.

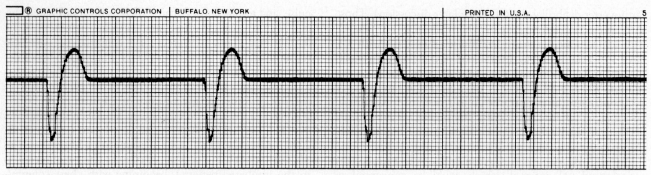

FIGURE 26-18 • Idioventricular rhythm in lead V₁.

resuscitation may indicate severe anoxic brain damage. The nurse also needs to monitor for complications of hypothermia, which include electrolyte imbalance (especially due to the diuresis caused by hypothermia), hypotension, pneumonia, sepsis, hyperglycemia, dysrhythmias, and coagulopathy, especially if the temperature drops below the intended goal. Because of these numerous nursing interventions, patients receive care in intensive care units.

Idioventricular Rhythm

Idioventricular rhythm, also called *ventricular escape rhythm*, occurs when the impulse starts in the conduction system below the AV node. When the sinus node fails to create an impulse (e.g., from increased vagal tone) or when the impulse is created but cannot be conducted through the AV node (e.g., due to complete AV block), the Purkinje fibers automatically discharge an impulse. When idioventricular rhythm is not caused by AV block, it has the following characteristics (Fig. 26-18):

> *Ventricular rate:* Between 20 and 40 bpm; if the rate exceeds 40 bpm, the rhythm is known as accelerated idioventricular rhythm.
> *Ventricular rhythm:* Regular
> *QRS shape and duration:* Bizarre, abnormal shape; duration is 0.12 seconds or more.

Medical Management. Idioventricular rhythm commonly causes the patient to lose consciousness and experience other signs and symptoms of reduced cardiac output. In such cases, the treatment is the same as for asystole and pulseless electrical activity (PEA) if the patient is in cardiac arrest or for bradycardia if the patient is not in cardiac arrest. Interventions include identifying the underlying cause; administering IV epinephrine, atropine, and vasopressor medications; and

initiating emergency transcutaneous pacing. In some cases, idioventricular rhythm may cause no symptoms of reduced cardiac output. However, bed rest is prescribed so as not to increase the cardiac workload.

Ventricular Asystole

Commonly called *flatline*, ventricular asystole (Fig. 26-19) is characterized by absent QRS complexes confirmed in two different leads, although P waves may be apparent for a short duration. There is no heartbeat, no palpable pulse, and no respiration. Without immediate treatment, ventricular asystole is fatal.

Medical Management. Ventricular asystole is treated the same as PEA, focusing on high-quality CPR with minimal interruptions and identifying underlying and contributing factors. The key to successful treatment is a rapid assessment to identify a possible cause, which is known as the Hs and Ts: hypoxia, hypovolemia, hydrogen ion (acid–base imbalance), hypo- or hyperglycemia, hypo- or hyperkalemia, hyperthermia, trauma, toxins, tamponade (cardiac), tension pneumothorax, or thrombus (coronary or pulmonary) (Morrison et al., 2010). After the initiation of CPR, intubation and establishment of IV access are the next recommended actions, with no or minimal interruptions in chest compressions. Once the IV is established, a bolus of IV epinephrine is administered and repeated at 3- to 5-minute intervals. One dose of vasopressin may be administered for the first or second dose of epinephrine. Because of the poor prognosis associated with asystole, if the patient does not respond to these actions and others aimed at correcting underlying causes, resuscitation efforts are usually ended ("the code is called") unless special circumstances (e.g., hypothermia, transportation to a hospital is required) exist.

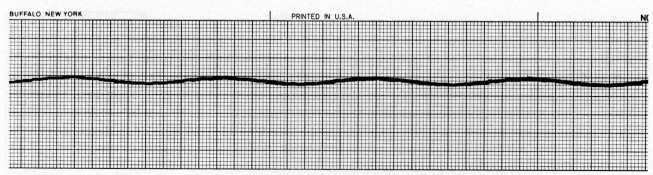

FIGURE 26-19 • Asystole. Always check two different leads to confirm rhythm.

Conduction Abnormalities

When assessing the rhythm strip, the underlying rhythm is first identified (e.g., sinus rhythm, sinus arrhythmia). Then, the PR interval is assessed for the possibility of an AV block. AV blocks occur when the conduction of the impulse through the AV nodal or His bundle area is decreased or stopped. These blocks can be caused by medications (e.g., digitalis, calcium channel blockers, beta-blockers), Lyme disease, myocardial ischemia and infarction, valvular disorders, cardiomyopathy, endocarditis, or myocarditis. If the AV block is caused by increased vagal tone (e.g., long-term athletic training, sleep, coughing, suctioning, pressure above the eyes or on large vessels, anal stimulation), it is commonly accompanied by sinus bradycardia. AV block may be temporary and resolve on its own, or it may be permanent and require permanent pacing.

The clinical signs and symptoms of a heart block vary with the resulting ventricular rate and the severity of any underlying disease processes. Whereas first-degree AV block rarely causes any hemodynamic effect, the other blocks may result in decreased heart rate, causing a decrease in perfusion to vital organs, such as the brain, heart, kidneys, lungs, and skin. A patient with third-degree AV block caused by digitalis toxicity may be stable; another patient with the same rhythm caused by acute MI may be unstable. Health care providers must always keep in mind the need to treat the patient, not the rhythm. The treatment is based on the hemodynamic effect of the rhythm.

First-Degree Atrioventricular Block

First-degree AV block occurs when all the atrial impulses are conducted through the AV node into the ventricles at a rate slower than normal. This conduction disorder has the following characteristics (Fig. 26-20):

Ventricular and atrial rate: Depends on the underlying rhythm

Ventricular and atrial rhythm: Depends on the underlying rhythm

QRS shape and duration: Usually normal, but may be abnormal

P wave: In front of the QRS complex; shows sinus rhythm, regular shape

PR interval: Greater than 0.20 seconds; PR interval measurement is constant.

P:QRS ratio: 1:1

Second-Degree Atrioventricular Block, Type I (Wenckebach)

Second-degree AV block, type I, occurs when there is a repeating pattern in which all but one of a series of atrial impulses are conducted through the AV node into the ventricles (e.g., every four of five atrial impulses are conducted). Each atrial impulse takes a longer time for conduction than the one before, until one impulse is fully blocked. Because the AV node is not depolarized by the blocked atrial impulse, the AV node has time to fully repolarize so that the next atrial impulse can be conducted within the shortest amount of time. Second-degree AV block, type I, has the following characteristics (Fig. 26-21):

Ventricular and atrial rate: Depends on the underlying rhythm, but the ventricular rate is lower than the atrial rate.

Ventricular and atrial rhythm: The PP interval is regular if the patient has an underlying normal sinus rhythm; the RR interval characteristically reflects a pattern of change. Starting from the RR that is the longest, the RR interval gradually shortens until there is another long RR interval.

QRS shape and duration: Usually normal, but may be abnormal

P wave: In front of the QRS complex; shape depends on underlying rhythm

PR interval: The PR interval becomes longer with each succeeding ECG complex until there is a P wave not followed by a QRS. The changes in the PR interval are repeated between each "dropped" QRS, creating a pattern in the irregular PR interval measurements.

P:QRS ratio: 3:2, 4:3, 5:4, and so forth

Second-Degree Atrioventricular Block, Type II

Second-degree AV block, type II, occurs when only some of the atrial impulses are conducted through the AV node into the ventricles. Second-degree AV block, type II, has the following characteristics (Fig. 26-22):

Ventricular and atrial rate: Depends on the underlying rhythm, but the ventricular rate is lower than the atrial rate.

Ventricular and atrial rhythm: The PP interval is regular if the patient has an underlying normal sinus rhythm. The RR interval is usually regular but may be irregular, depending on the P:QRS ratio.

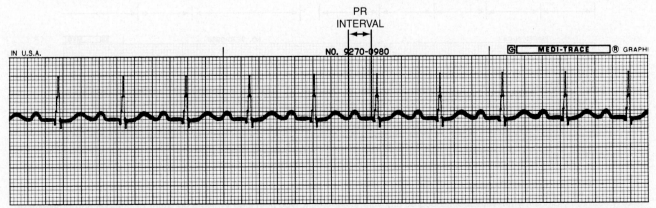

FIGURE 26-20 • Sinus rhythm with first-degree atrioventricular block in lead II. Note that PR is constant but greater than 0.20 seconds.

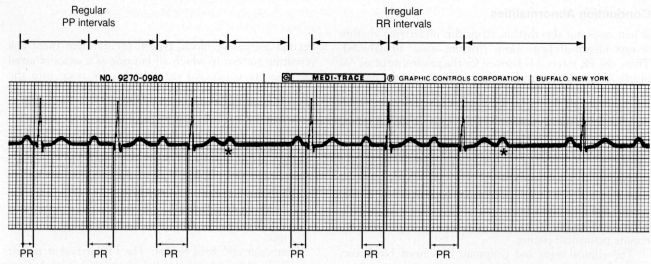

FIGURE 26-21 • Sinus rhythm with second-degree atrioventricular block, type I, in lead II. Note progressively longer PR durations until there is a nonconducted P wave, indicated by the *asterisk* (*).

QRS shape and duration: Usually abnormal, but may be normal

P wave: In front of the QRS complex; shape depends on underlying rhythm

PR interval: The PR interval is constant for those P waves just before QRS complexes.

P:QRS ratio: 2:1, 3:1, 4:1, 5:1, and so forth

Third-Degree Atrioventricular Block

Third-degree AV block occurs when no atrial impulse is conducted through the AV node into the ventricles. In third-degree AV block, two impulses stimulate the heart: one stimulates the ventricles, represented by the QRS complex, and one stimulates the atria, represented by the P wave. P waves may be seen, but the atrial electrical activity is not conducted down into the ventricles to cause the QRS complex, the ventricular electrical activity. Having two impulses stimulate the heart results in a condition referred to as AV dissociation, which may also occur during VT. Complete block (third-degree AV block) has the following characteristics (Fig. 26-23):

Ventricular and atrial rate: Depends on the escape rhythm (idionodal or idioventricular) and underlying atrial rhythm, but the ventricular rate is lower than the atrial rate.

Ventricular and atrial rhythm: The PP interval is regular and the RR interval is regular, but the PP interval is not equal to the RR interval.

QRS shape and duration: Depends on the escape rhythm; with junctional rhythm, QRS shape and duration are usually normal; with idioventricular rhythm, QRS shape and duration are usually abnormal.

P wave: Depends on underlying rhythm

PR interval: Very irregular

P:QRS ratio: More P waves than QRS complexes

Medical Management of Conduction Abnormalities

Based on the cause of the AV block and the stability of the patient, treatment is directed toward increasing the heart rate to maintain a normal cardiac output. If the patient is stable and has no symptoms, no treatment may be indicated or it may simply consist of decreasing or eliminating the cause (e.g., withholding the medication or treatment).

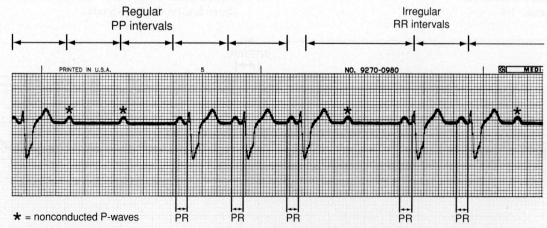

★ = nonconducted P-waves

FIGURE 26-22 • Sinus rhythm with second-degree atrioventricular block, type II, in lead V₁. Note constant PR interval and presence of more P waves than QRS complexes.

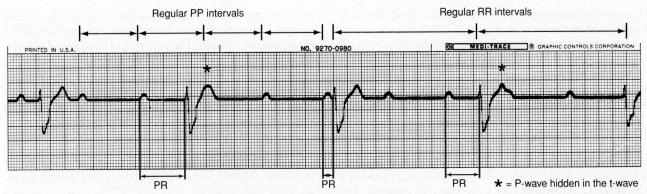

FIGURE 26-23 • Sinus rhythm with third-degree atrioventricular block and idioventricular rhythm in lead V₁. Note irregular PR intervals.

If the causal medication is necessary for treating other conditions and no effective alternative is available, pacemaker implantation may be indicated. The initial treatment of choice is an IV bolus of atropine, although it is not effective in second-degree AV block, type II, or third-degree AV block. If the patient does not respond to atropine, has advanced AV block, or has had an acute MI, temporary transcutaneous pacing may be started. If the patient has no pulse, treatment is the same as for ventricular asystole. A permanent pacemaker may be necessary if the block persists.

NURSING PROCESS

The Patient With a Dysrhythmia

Assessment

Major areas of assessment include possible causes of the dysrhythmia, contributing factors, and the dysrhythmia's effect on the heart's ability to pump an adequate blood volume. When cardiac output is reduced, the amount of oxygen reaching the tissues and vital organs is diminished. This diminished oxygenation produces the signs and symptoms associated with dysrhythmias. If these signs and symptoms are severe or if they occur frequently, the patient may experience significant distress and disruption of daily life.

A health history is obtained to identify any previous occurrences of decreased cardiac output, such as syncope (fainting), lightheadedness, dizziness, fatigue, chest discomfort, and palpitations. Possible causes of the dysrhythmia (e.g., heart disease, chronic obstructive pulmonary disease) need to be identified. All medications, prescribed and over-the-counter (including herbs and nutritional supplements), as well as the route of administration, are reviewed. If a patient is taking an antiarrhythmic medication, assessment for treatment adherence, side effects, adverse reactions, and potential contraindications is necessary. For example, some medications (e.g., digoxin) can cause dysrhythmias. Laboratory results are reviewed to assess levels of medications as well as factors that could contribute to the dysrhythmia (e.g., anemia). A thorough psychosocial assessment is performed to identify the possible effects of the dysrhythmia, the patient's perception and understanding of the dysrhythmia and its treatment, and whether anxiety is a significant contributing factor.

The nurse conducts a physical assessment to confirm the data obtained from the history and to observe for signs of diminished cardiac output during the dysrhythmic event, especially changes in level of consciousness. The nurse assesses the patient's skin, which may be pale and cool. Signs of fluid retention, such as neck vein distention and crackles and wheezes auscultated in the lungs, may be detected. The rate and rhythm of apical and peripheral pulses are also assessed, and any pulse deficit is noted. The nurse auscultates for extra heart sounds (especially S₃ and S₄) and for heart murmurs, measures blood pressure, and determines pulse pressures. A declining pulse pressure indicates reduced cardiac output. One assessment may not disclose significant changes in cardiac output; therefore, the nurse compares multiple assessment findings over time, especially those that occur with and without the dysrhythmia.

Diagnosis

Nursing Diagnoses

Based on the assessment data, major nursing diagnoses may include:

- Decreased cardiac output
- Anxiety related to fear of the unknown
- Deficient knowledge about the dysrhythmia and its treatment

Collaborative Problems/Potential Complications

Potential complications may include the following:

- Cardiac arrest (see Chapter 29)
- Heart failure (see Chapter 29)
- Thromboembolic event, especially with atrial fibrillation (see Chapter 29)

Planning and Goals

The major goals for the patient may include eliminating or decreasing the occurrence of the dysrhythmia (by decreasing contributory factors) to maintain cardiac output; minimizing anxiety; acquiring knowledge about the dysrhythmia, tests used to diagnose the problem, and its treatment; and developing or maintaining self-management skills.

Nursing Interventions

Monitoring and Managing the Dysrhythmia

The nurse evaluates the patient's blood pressure, pulse rate and rhythm, rate and depth of respirations, and breath sounds on an ongoing basis to determine the dysrhythmia's hemodynamic effect. The nurse also asks the patient about episodes of lightheadedness, dizziness, or fainting as part of the ongoing assessment. If a patient with a dysrhythmia is hospitalized, the nurse may obtain a 12-lead ECG, continuously monitor the patient, and analyze rhythm strips to track the dysrhythmia.

Control of the occurrence or the effect of the dysrhythmia, or both, is often achieved with **antiarrhythmic medications**. The nurse assesses and observes for the benefits and adverse effects of each medication. The nurse, in collaboration with the primary provider, also manages medication administration carefully so that a constant serum level of the medication is maintained. The nurse may also conduct a 6-minute walk test as prescribed, which is used to identify the patient's ventricular rate in response to exercise. The patient is asked to walk for 6 minutes, covering as much distance as possible. The nurse monitors the patient for symptoms. At the end, the nurse records the distance covered and the pre- and postexercise heart rate as well as the patient's response.

The nurse assesses for factors that contribute to the dysrhythmia (e.g., oxygen deficits, acid–base and electrolyte imbalances, caffeine, or nonadherence to the medication regimen). The nurse also monitors for ECG changes (e.g., widening of the QRS, prolongation of the QT interval, increased heart rate) that increase the risk of a dysrhythmic event.

Minimizing Anxiety

When the patient experiences episodes of dysrhythmia, the nurse stays with the patient and provides assurance of safety and security while maintaining a calm and reassuring attitude. This assists in reducing anxiety (reducing the sympathetic response) and fosters a trusting relationship with the patient. The nurse seeks the patient's view of the events and discusses the emotional response to the dysrhythmia, encouraging verbalization of feelings and fears, providing supportive or empathetic statements, and assisting the patient to recognize feelings of anxiety, anger, or sadness. The nurse emphasizes successes with the patient to promote a sense of self-management of the dysrhythmia. For example, if a patient is experiencing episodes of dysrhythmia and a medication is administered that begins to reduce the incidence of the dysrhythmia, the nurse communicates that information to the patient and explores the patient's response to this information. In addition, the nurse can help the patient develop a system to identify possible causative, influencing, and alleviating factors (e.g., keeping a diary). The nursing goal is to maximize the patient's control and to make the episode less threatening.

Promoting Home and Community-Based Care

Educating Patients About Self-Care. When educating patients about dysrhythmias, the nurse first assesses the patient's understanding, clarifies misinformation, and then shares needed information in terms that are understandable and in a manner that is not frightening or threatening. The nurse clearly explains treatment options to the patient and family. If necessary, the nurse explains the importance of maintaining therapeutic serum levels of antiarrhythmic medications so that the patient understands why medications should be taken regularly each day and the importance of regular blood testing. If the medication has the potential to alter the heart rate, the patient should be taught how to take his or her pulse before each dose and to notify the primary provider if the pulse is abnormal. In addition, the relationship between a dys-

rhythmia and cardiac output is explained so that the patient recognizes symptoms of the dysrhythmia and the rationale for the treatment regimen. The patient and family need to know what measures to take to decrease the risk of recurrence of the dysrhythmia. If the patient has a potentially lethal dysrhythmia, the nurse establishes with the patient and family a plan of action to take in case of an emergency and, if appropriate, encourages a family member to obtain CPR training.

The patient and family should also be educated about potential risks of the dysrhythmia and their signs and symptoms. For example, the patient with chronic atrial fibrillation should be educated about the possibility of an embolic event.

Continuing Care. A referral for home care usually is not necessary for the patient with a dysrhythmia unless the patient is hemodynamically unstable and has significant symptoms of decreased cardiac output. Home care may be warranted if the patient has significant comorbidities, socioeconomic issues, or limited self-management skills that could increase the risk of nonadherence to the therapeutic regimen. Home care referral may also be indicated if the patient has had an electronic device implanted recently.

Evaluation

Expected patient outcomes may include:

1. Maintains cardiac output
   a. Demonstrates heart rate, blood pressure, respiratory rate, and level of consciousness within normal ranges
   b. Demonstrates no or decreased episodes of dysrhythmia
2. Experiences reduced anxiety
   a. Expresses a positive attitude about living with the dysrhythmia
   b. Expresses confidence in ability to take appropriate actions in an emergency
3. Expresses understanding of the dysrhythmia and its treatment
   a. Explains the dysrhythmia and its effects
   b. Describes the medication regimen and its rationale
   c. Explains the need to maintain a therapeutic serum level of the medication
   d. Describes a plan to eliminate or limit factors that contribute to the dysrhythmia
   e. States actions to take in the event of an emergency

ADJUNCTIVE MODALITIES AND MANAGEMENT

Dysrhythmia treatments depend on whether the disorder is acute or chronic, as well as on the cause of the dysrhythmia and its actual or potential hemodynamic effects.

Acute dysrhythmias may be treated with medications or with external electrical therapy (emergency defibrillation, cardioversion, or pacing). Many antiarrhythmic medications are used to treat atrial and ventricular tachydysrhythmias (see Table 26-1). The choice of medication depends on the specific dysrhythmia and its duration, the presence of structural heart disease (e.g., heart failure), and the patient's response to previous treatment. The nurse is responsible for monitoring and documenting the patient's responses to the medication and for ensuring that the patient has the knowledge and ability to manage the medication regimen.

If medications alone are ineffective in eliminating or decreasing the dysrhythmia, certain adjunctive mechanical therapies are available. The most common therapies are elective cardioversion and defibrillation for acute tachydysrhythmia, and implantable devices (pacemakers for bradycardias and ICDs for chronic tachydysrhythmias). Surgical treatments, although less common, are also available. The nurse is responsible for assessing the patient's understanding of and response to mechanical therapy, as well as the patient's self-management abilities. The nurse explains that the purpose of the device is to help the patient lead a life that is as active and productive as possible.

Cardioversion and Defibrillation

Cardioversion and defibrillation are used to treat tachydysrhythmias by delivering an electrical current that depolarizes a critical mass of myocardial cells. When the cells repolarize, the SA node is usually able to recapture its role as the heart's pacemaker.

 Concept Mastery Alert

One major difference between cardioversion and defibrillation is the timing of the delivery of electrical current. In cardioversion, the delivery of the electrical current is synchronized with the patient's electrical events; in defibrillation, the delivery of the current is immediate and unsynchronized.

The same type of device, called a *defibrillator*, is used for both cardioversion and defibrillation. The electrical voltage required to defibrillate the heart is usually greater than that required for cardioversion and may cause more myocardial damage. Defibrillators are classified as monophasic or biphasic. Monophasic defibrillators deliver current in only one direction and require increased energy loads. Newer biphasic defibrillators deliver the electrical charge from one paddle that then automatically redirects its charge back to the originating paddle. This type of defibrillator uses lower voltage and thus there is less associated myocardial damage.

The electrical current may be delivered externally through the skin with the use of paddles or with conductor pads. The paddles or pads may be placed on the front of the chest (Fig. 26-24) (standard placement), or one may

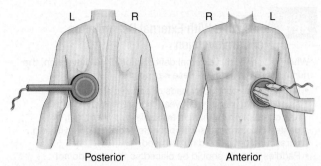

FIGURE 26-25 • Anteroposterior paddle placement for defibrillation.

be placed on the front of the chest and the other, using an adapter with a long handle if using paddles, placed under the patient's back just left of the spine (anteroposterior placement) (Fig. 26-25). If a monophasic defibrillator is used for cardioverting atrial fibrillation, handheld paddles are preferred (Jacobs et al., 2010).

Defibrillator multifunction conductor pads (Fig. 26-26) contain a conductive medium and are connected to the defibrillator to allow for hands-off defibrillation. This method reduces the risk of touching the patient during the procedure and increases electrical safety. Automated external defibrillators (AEDs), which are now found in many public areas, use this type of delivery for the electrical current.

▶ *Quality and Safety Nursing Alert*

When using paddles, the appropriate conductant is applied between the paddles and the patient's skin. Any other type of conductant, such as ultrasound gel, should not be substituted.

Whether using pads or paddles, the nurse must observe two safety measures. First, good contact must be maintained between the pads or paddles and the patient's skin (with a conductive medium between them) to prevent electrical current from leaking through the air (arcing) when the defibrillator is discharged. Second, no one is to be in contact with the patient or with anything that is touching the patient when the defibrillator is discharged, to minimize the chance that electrical current is conducted to anyone other than the patient (Chart 26-5 provides a review of nursing responsibility when a patient is cardioverted or defibrillated).

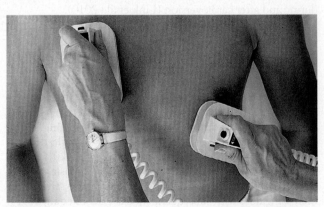

FIGURE 26-24 • Standard paddle placement for defibrillation.

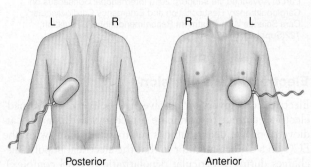

FIGURE 26-26 • Multifunction pads for defibrillation.

Chart 26-5   Assisting With External Defibrillation or Cardioversion

When assisting with external defibrillation or cardioversion, the nurse should remember these key points:

- Multifunction conductor pads or paddles are used, with a conducting medium between the paddles and the skin (the conducting medium is available as a sheet, gel, or paste). Gels or pastes with poor electrical conductivity (e.g., ultrasound gel) should not be used.
- Paddles or pads should be placed so that they do not touch the patient's clothing or bed linen and are not near medication patches or in the direct flow of oxygen.
- Women with large breasts should have the left pad or paddle placed underneath or lateral to the left breast.
- During cardioversion, the monitor leads must be attached to the patient and the defibrillator is set to the synchronized mode ("in sync"). If defibrillating, the defibrillator must *not* be in the synchronized mode (most machines default to the "not-sync" mode).
- When using paddles, 20 to 25 lb of pressure must be used in order to ensure good skin contact.
- When using a manual discharge device, it must not be charged until it is ready to shock; then thumbs and fingers must be kept off the discharge buttons until paddles or pads are on the chest and ready to deliver the electrical charge.
- "Clear!" must be called three times before discharging: As "Clear" is called the first time, the discharger must visually check that he or she is not touching the patient, bed, or equipment; as "Clear" is called the second time, the discharger must visually check that no one else is touching the bed, the patient, or equipment, including the endotracheal tube or adjuncts; and as "Clear" is called the third time, the discharger must perform a final visual check to ensure that everyone is clear of the patient and anything touching the patient.
- The delivered energy and resulting rhythm are recorded.
- Cardiopulmonary resuscitation (CPR) is immediately resumed after the defibrillation charge is delivered, if appropriate, starting with chest compressions.
- If CPR is warranted, after five cycles (about 2 minutes) of CPR, the cardiac rhythm is checked again and another shock is delivered, if indicated. A vasoactive or antiarrhythmic medication is administered as soon as possible after the rhythm check.
- After the event is complete, the skin under the pads or paddles is inspected for burns; if any are detected, the primary provider or a wound care nurse is consulted about appropriate treatment.

Adapted from Jacobs, I., Sunde, K., Deakin, C. D., et al. (2010). Part 6: Defibrillation: 2010 International Consensus on Cardiopulmonary Resuscitation and Emergency Cardiovascular Care Science With Treatment Recommendations. *Circulation, 122*(Suppl. 2), S325–S337; and Morrison, L. J., Deakin, C. D., Morley, P. T., et al. (2010). Part 8: Advanced life support: 2010 International Consensus on Cardiopulmonary Resuscitation and Emergency Cardiovascular Care Science With Treatment Recommendations. *Circulation, 122*(Suppl. 2), S345–S421.

Electrical Cardioversion

Electrical **cardioversion** involves the delivery of a "timed" electrical current to terminate a tachydysrhythmia. In cardioversion, the defibrillator is set to synchronize with the ECG on a cardiac monitor so that the electrical impulse discharges during ventricular depolarization (QRS complex).

The synchronization prevents the discharge from occurring during the vulnerable period of repolarization (T wave), which could result in VT or ventricular fibrillation. The ECG monitor connected to the external defibrillator usually displays a mark or line that indicates sensing of a QRS complex. Sometimes the lead and the electrodes must be changed for the monitor to recognize the patient's QRS complex. When the synchronizer is on, no electrical current is delivered if the defibrillator does not discern a QRS complex. Therefore, it is important to ensure that the patient is connected to the monitor and to select a lead (not "paddles") that has the most appropriate sensing of the QRS. Because there may be a short delay until recognition of the QRS, the discharge buttons of an external manual defibrillator must be held down until the shock has been delivered. In most monitors, the synchronization mode must be reactivated if the initial cardioversion was ineffective and another cardioversion is needed (i.e., the device defaults to unsynchronized defibrillation mode).

If the cardioversion is elective and the dysrhythmia has lasted longer than 48 hours, anticoagulation for a few weeks before cardioversion may be indicated. Digoxin is usually withheld for 48 hours before cardioversion to ensure the resumption of sinus rhythm with normal conduction. The patient is instructed not to eat or drink for at least 4 hours before the procedure. Gel-covered paddles or conductor pads are positioned front and back (anteroposteriorly) for cardioversion. Before cardioversion, the patient receives moderate sedation IV as well as an analgesic medication or anesthesia. Respiration is then supported with supplemental oxygen delivered by a bag-valve mask device with suction equipment readily available. Although patients rarely require intubation, equipment is nearby in case it is needed. The amount of voltage used varies from 50 to 360 joules, depending on the defibrillator's technology, the type and duration of the dysrhythmia, and the size and hemodynamic status of the patient. If ventricular fibrillation occurs after cardioversion, the defibrillator is used to defibrillate the patient (synchronization mode is *not* used) (Link, Atkins, Passman, et al., 2010).

Indications of a successful response are conversion to sinus rhythm, adequate peripheral pulses, and adequate blood pressure. Because of the sedation, airway patency must be maintained and the patient's state of consciousness assessed. Vital signs and oxygen saturation are monitored and recorded until the patient is stable and recovered from sedation and analgesic medications or anesthesia. ECG monitoring is required during and after cardioversion (Link et al., 2010).

Defibrillation

Defibrillation is used in emergency situations as the treatment of choice for ventricular fibrillation and pulseless VT, the most common cause of abrupt loss of cardiac function and sudden cardiac death. Defibrillation is not used for patients who are conscious or have a pulse. The energy setting for the initial and subsequent shocks using a monophasic defibrillator should be set at 360 joules (Jacobs et al., 2010). The energy setting for the initial shock using a biphasic defibrillator may be set at 150 to 200 joules, with the same or an increasing dose with subsequent shocks (Jacobs et al., 2010).

The sooner defibrillation is used, the better the survival rate; if it is used within 1 minute of the onset of VT or ventricular fibrillation, the survival rate is 90%; if it is delayed for 12 minutes, the survival rate is only 2% to 5%. Several studies have demonstrated that early defibrillation performed by lay people in a community setting can increase the survival rate. If immediate CPR is provided and defibrillation is performed within 5 minutes, more adults in ventricular fibrillation may survive with intact neurologic function (Jacobs et al., 2010). The availability and the use of AEDs in public places shorten the interval from collapse to rhythm recognition and defibrillation, which can significantly increase survival (Jacobs et al., 2010).

Epinephrine or vasopressin is administered after defibrillation to make it easier to convert the dysrhythmia to a normal rhythm with the next defibrillation. These medications may also increase cerebral and coronary artery blood flow. Antiarrhythmic medications such as amiodarone (Cordarone, Pacerone), lidocaine (Xylocaine), or magnesium may be administered if ventricular dysrhythmia persists (see Table 26-1). This treatment with continuous CPR, medication administration, and defibrillation continues until a stable rhythm resumes or until it is determined that the patient cannot be revived.

Pacemaker Therapy

A pacemaker is an electronic device that provides electrical stimuli to the heart muscle. Pacemakers are usually used when a patient has a permanent or temporary slower-than-normal impulse formation, or a symptomatic AV or ventricular conduction disturbance. They may also be used to control some tachydysrhythmias that do not respond to medication. Biventricular (both ventricles) pacing, also called *resynchronization therapy,* may be used to treat advanced heart failure that does not respond to medication. Pacemaker technology also may be used in an ICD (e.g., in patients with coronary artery disease and a reduced ejection fraction). (See Chapter 29 for further discussion of heart failure.)

Pacemakers can be permanent or temporary. Temporary pacemakers are used to support patients until they improve or receive a permanent pacemaker (e.g., after acute MI or during open heart surgery). Temporary pacemakers are used only in hospital settings.

Pacemaker Design and Types

Pacemakers consist of two components: an electronic pulse generator and pacemaker electrodes, which are located on leads or wires. The generator contains the circuitry and batteries that determine the rate (measured in beats per minute) and the strength or output (measured in milliamperes [mA]) of the electrical stimulus delivered to the heart. The generator also has circuitry that can detect the intracardiac electrical activity to cause an appropriate response; this component of pacing is called *sensitivity* and is measured in millivolts (mV). Sensitivity is set at the level that the intracardiac electrical activity must exceed to be sensed by the device. Leads, which carry the impulse created by the generator to the heart, can be threaded by fluoroscopy through a major vein into the heart, usually the right

atrium and ventricle (endocardial leads), or they can be lightly sutured onto the outside of the heart and brought through the chest wall during open heart surgery (epicardial wires). The epicardial wires are always temporary and are removed by a gentle tug a few days after surgery. The endocardial leads may be temporarily placed with catheters through a vein (usually the femoral, subclavian, or internal jugular vein [transvenous wires]), usually guided by fluoroscopy. The leads may also be part of a specialized pulmonary artery catheter (see Chapter 29). However, obtaining a pulmonary artery wedge pressure may cause the leads to move out of pacing position. The endocardial and epicardial wires are connected to a temporary generator, which is about the size of a small paperback book. The energy source for a temporary generator is a common household battery. Monitoring for pacemaker malfunctioning and battery failure is a nursing responsibility.

The endocardial leads also may be placed permanently, passed into the heart through the subclavian, axillary, or cephalic vein, and connected to a permanent generator. Most current leads have a fixation mechanism (e.g., a screw) at the end of the lead that allows precise positioning and avoidance of dislodgement. The permanent generator, which often weighs less than 1 oz and is the size of a large book of matches, is usually implanted in a subcutaneous pocket created in the pectoral region, below the clavicle, or behind the breast, especially in young women (Fig. 26-27). This procedure usually takes about 1 hour, and it is performed in a cardiac catheterization laboratory using a local anesthetic and moderate sedation. Close monitoring of the respiratory status is needed until the patient is fully awake.

Permanent pacemaker generators are insulated to protect against body moisture and warmth and have filters that protect them from electrical interference from most household devices, motors, and appliances. Several different energy sources for permanent generators have been used and others

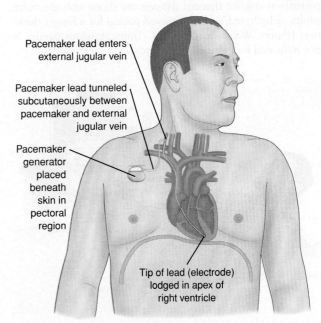

Pacemaker lead enters external jugular vein

Pacemaker lead tunneled subcutaneously between pacemaker and external jugular vein

Pacemaker generator placed beneath skin in pectoral region

Tip of lead (electrode) lodged in apex of right ventricle

FIGURE 26-27 • Implanted transvenous pacing lead (with electrode) and pacemaker generator.

have been investigated, but lithium cell units are most often used today. They last approximately 6 to 12 years, depending on the type of pacemaker, how it is programmed, and how often it is used. Most pacemakers have an **elective replacement indicator (ERI)**, which is a signal that indicates when the battery is approaching depletion. The pacemaker continues to function for several months after the appearance of ERI to ensure that there is adequate time for a battery replacement. Although some batteries are rechargeable, most are not. Because the battery is permanently sealed in the pacemaker, the entire generator must be replaced. To replace a failing generator, the leads are disconnected, the old generator is removed, and a new generator is reconnected to the existing leads and reimplanted in the already existing subcutaneous pocket. Sometimes the leads are also replaced. Battery replacement is usually performed using a local anesthetic. Hospitalization is necessary for implantation or battery replacement; the patient usually can be discharged the next day.

If a patient suddenly develops a bradycardia, is symptomatic but has a pulse, and is unresponsive to atropine, emergency pacing may be started with transcutaneous pacing, which most defibrillators are now equipped to perform. Some AEDs are able to do both defibrillation and transcutaneous pacing. Large pacing ECG electrodes (sometimes the same conductive pads used for cardioversion and defibrillation) are placed on the patient's chest and back. The electrodes are connected to the defibrillator, which is the temporary pacemaker generator (Fig. 26-28). Because the impulse must travel through the patient's skin and tissue before reaching the heart, transcutaneous pacing can cause significant discomfort (burning sensation and involuntary muscle contraction) and is intended to be used only in emergencies for short periods of time. This type of pacing necessitates hospitalization. If the patient is alert, sedation and analgesia may be administered. After transcutaneous pacing, the skin under the electrode should be inspected. Although erythema is to be expected, patients at risk for thermal damage are those who are older adults, dehydrated, or had received pacing for a longer duration (Fuster, Walsh et al., 2011). Transcutaneous pacing is not indicated for pulseless bradycardia.

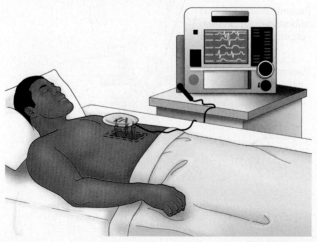

FIGURE 26-28 • Transcutaneous pacemaker with electrode pads connected to the anterior and posterior chest walls.

Pacemaker Generator Functions

Because of the sophistication and wide use of pacemakers, a universal code has been adopted to provide a means of safe communication about their function. The coding is referred to as the NASPE-BPEG code because it is sanctioned by the North American Society of Pacing and Electrophysiology (now known as the Heart Rhythm Society) and the British Pacing and Electrophysiology Group. The complete code consists of five letters and was revised in 2002 (Bernstein, Daubert, Fletcher, et al., 2002). The fourth and fifth letters are used only with permanent pacemakers (Chart 26-6).

The pacemaker paces the atrium and then the ventricle when no ventricular activity is sensed for a period of time (the time is individually programmed into the pacemaker for each patient). A straight vertical line usually can be seen on the ECG when pacing is initiated. The line that represents pacing is called a *pacemaker spike*. The appropriate ECG complex should immediately follow the pacing spike; therefore, a P wave should follow an atrial pacing spike and a QRS complex should follow a ventricular pacing spike. Because the impulse starts in a different place than the patient's normal rhythm, the QRS complex or P wave that responds to pacing looks different from the patient's normal ECG complex. *Capture* is a term used to denote that the appropriate complex followed the pacing spike.

The type of pacemaker generator and the settings selected depend on the patient's dysrhythmia, underlying cardiac function, and age. Pacemakers are generally set to sense and respond to intrinsic activity, which is called *on-demand pacing* (Fig. 26-29). If the pacemaker is set to pace but not to sense, it is called a *fixed* or *asynchronous pacemaker* (Fig. 26-30); this is written in pacing code as AOO or VOO. The pacemaker paces at a constant rate, independent of the patient's intrinsic rhythm. VOO pacing may indicate battery failure.

VVI (V, paces the ventricle; V, senses ventricular activity; I, paces only if the ventricles do not depolarize) pacing causes loss of AV synchrony and atrial kick, which may cause a decrease in cardiac output and an increase in atrial distention and venous congestion. Pacemaker syndrome, causing symptoms such as chest discomfort, shortness of breath, fatigue, activity intolerance, and postural hypotension, is most common with VVI pacing (Gillis, Russo, Ellenbogen, et al., 2012). Atrial pacing and dual-chamber (right atrial and right ventricular) pacing have been found to reduce the incidence of atrial fibrillation, ventricular dysfunction, and heart failure (Gillis et al., 2012).

Single-chamber atrial pacing (AAI) or dual-chamber pacing (DDD) is recommended over VVI in patients with sinus node dysfunction (formerly called *sick sinus syndrome*), the most common cause of bradycardias requiring a pacemaker, and a functioning AV node (Gillis et al., 2012). AAI pacing ensures synchrony between atrial and ventricular stimulation (and therefore contraction), as long as the patient has no conduction disturbances in the AV node. Dual-chamber pacemakers are recommended as the treatment for patients with AV conduction disturbances (Gillis et al., 2012).

Synchronized biventricular pacing, also called *cardiac resynchronized therapy*, has been found to modify the intraventricular, interventricular, and atrioventricular

Chart 26-6 North American Society of Pacing and Electrophysiology and the British Pacing and Electrophysiology Group Code (NASPE-BPEG Code) for Pacemaker Generator Function

- The first letter of the code identifies the chamber or chambers being paced (i.e., the chamber containing a pacing electrode). The letter characters for this code are A (atrium), V (ventricle), or D (dual, meaning both A and V).
- The second letter identifies the chamber or chambers being sensed by the pacemaker generator. Information from the electrode within the chamber is sent to the generator for interpretation and action by the generator. The letter characters are A (atrium), V (ventricle), D (dual), and O (indicating that the sensing function is turned off).
- The third letter of the code describes the type of response that will be made by the pacemaker to what is sensed. The letter characters used to describe this response are I (inhibited), T (triggered), D (dual—inhibited and triggered), and O (none). Inhibited response means that the response of the pacemaker is controlled by the activity of the patient's heart—that is, when the patient's heart beats, the pacemaker does not function, but when the heart does not beat, the pacemaker does function. In contrast, a triggered response means that the pacemaker responds (paces the heart) when it senses intrinsic heart activity.
- The fourth letter of the code is related to a permanent generator's ability to vary the heart rate. This ability is available in most current pacemakers. The possible letters are O,

indicating no rate responsiveness, or R, indicating that the generator has rate modulation (i.e., the pacemaker has the ability to automatically adjust the pacing rate from moment to moment based on parameters such as QT interval, physical activity, acid–base changes, body temperature, rate and depth of respirations, or oxygen saturation). A pacemaker with rate-responsive ability is capable of improving cardiac output during times of increased cardiac demand, such as exercise and decreasing the incidence of atrial fibrillation. All contemporary pacemakers have some type of sensor system that enables them to provide rate-adaptive pacing (Gillis, Russo, Ellenbogen, et al., 2012).

- The fifth letter of the code has two different indications: (1) that the permanent generator has multisite pacing capability with the letters A (atrium), V (ventricle), D (dual), and O (none); or (2) that the pacemaker has an antitachycardia function.
- Commonly, only the first three letters are used for a pacing code. An example of an NASPE-BPEG code is DVI:

  D: Both the atrium and the ventricle have a pacing electrode in place.
  V: The pacemaker is sensing the activity of the ventricle only.
  I: The pacemaker's stimulating effect is inhibited by ventricular activity—in other words, it does not create an impulse when the pacemaker senses that the patient's ventricle is active.

Adapted from Bernstein, A. D., Daubert, J-C., Fletcher, R. D., et al. (2002). The revised NASPE/BPEG generic code for antibradycardia, adaptive-rate, and multisite pacing. *Journal of Pacing and Clinical Electrophysiology, 25*(2), 260–264.

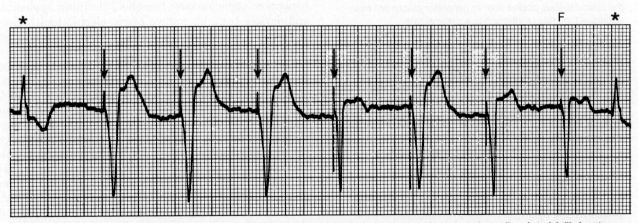

FIGURE 26-29 • Pacing with appropriate sensing (on-demand pacing) in lead V_1. *Arrows* denote pacing spike. *Asterisk* (*) denotes intrinsic (patient's own) beats; therefore, no pacing. F denotes a fusion beat, which is a combination of an intrinsic beat and a paced beat occurring at the same time.

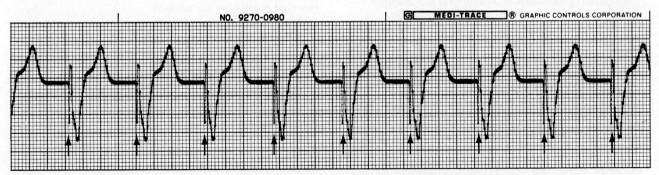

FIGURE 26-30 • Fixed pacing or total loss of sensing pacing in lead V_1. *Arrows* denote pacing spikes.

conduction defects identified with symptomatic moderate to severe left ventricular dysfunction and heart failure (New York Heart Association [NYHA] functional classes III and IV) (Brenyo, Link, Barsheshet, et al., 2011). The generator for biventricular pacing has three leads: one for the right atrium; one for the right ventricle, as with most standard pacemaker generators; and one for the left ventricle, usually placed in the left lateral wall. This therapy improves cardiac function, resulting in decreased heart failure symptoms and an improved quality of life. Biventricular pacing may be used with an ICD.

Complications of Pacemaker Use

Complications associated with pacemakers relate to their presence within the body and improper functioning (Chart 26-7). In the initial hours after a temporary or permanent pacemaker is inserted, the most common complication is dislodgment of the pacing electrode. Minimizing patient activity can help prevent this complication. If a temporary electrode is in place, the extremity through which the catheter has been advanced is immobilized. With a permanent pacemaker,

---

Chart 26-7 Complications from Insertion of a Pacemaker

- Local infection at the entry site of the leads for temporary pacing, or at the subcutaneous site for permanent generator placement. Prophylactic antibiotics and antibiotic irrigation of the subcutaneous pocket prior to generator placement has decreased the rate of infection to a minimal rate.
- Pneumothorax; the use of sheaths marketed as "safe" reduces this risk.
- Bleeding and hematoma at the lead entry sites for temporary pacing, or at the subcutaneous site for permanent generator placement. This usually can be managed with cold compresses and discontinuation of antiplatelet and antithrombotic medications.
- Hemothorax from puncture of the subclavian vein or internal mammary artery
- Ventricular ectopy and tachycardia from irritation of the ventricular wall by the endocardial electrode
- Movement or dislocation of the lead placed transvenously (perforation of the myocardium)
- Phrenic nerve, diaphragmatic (hiccuping may be a sign), or skeletal muscle stimulation if the lead is dislocated or if the delivered energy (mA) is set high. The occurrence of this complication is avoided by testing during device implantation.
- Cardiac perforation resulting in pericardial effusion and, rarely, cardiac tamponade, which may occur at the time of implantation or months later. This condition can be recognized by the change in QRS complex morphology, diaphragmatic stimulation, or hemodynamic instability.
- Twiddler syndrome may occur when the patient manipulates the generator, causing lead dislodgement or fracture of the lead.
- Pacemaker syndrome (hemodynamic instability caused by ventricular pacing and the loss of AV synchrony)

Adapted from Fuster, V., Walsh, R. A., & Harrington, R. A. (Eds.). (2011). *Hurst's the heart* (13th ed.). New York: McGraw-Hill; and Tracy, C. M., Epstein, A. E., Darbar, D., et al. (2012). ACCF/AHA/HRS focused update of the 2008 guidelines for device-based therapy of cardiac rhythm abnormalities: A report of the American College of Cardiology Foundation/American Heart Association Task Force on Practice Guidelines. *Journal of the American College of Cardiology, 60*(14), 1297–1313.

---

the patient is instructed initially to restrict activity on the side of the implantation.

The ECG is monitored very carefully to detect pacemaker malfunction. Improper pacemaker function, which can arise from failure in one or more components of the pacing system, is outlined in Table 26-2. The following data should be noted on the patient's record: model of pacemaker, type of generator, date and time of insertion, location of pulse generator, stimulation threshold, and pacer settings (e.g., rate, energy output [mA], sensitivity [mV], and duration of interval between atrial and ventricular impulses [AV delay]). This information is important for identifying normal pacemaker function and diagnosing pacemaker malfunction.

A patient experiencing pacemaker malfunction may develop bradycardia as well as signs and symptoms of decreased cardiac output. The degree to which these symptoms become apparent depends on the severity of the malfunction, the patient's level of dependency on the pacemaker, and the patient's underlying condition. Pacemaker malfunction is diagnosed by analyzing the ECG. Manipulating the electrodes, changing the generator's settings, or replacing the pacemaker generator or leads (or both) may be necessary.

Inhibition of permanent pacemakers or reversion to asynchronous fixed rate pacing can occur with exposure to strong electromagnetic fields (electromagnetic interference [EMI]). However, recent pacemaker technology allows patients to safely use most household electronic appliances and devices (e.g., microwave ovens, electric tools). Gas-powered engines should be turned off before working on them. Objects that contain magnets (e.g., the earpiece of a phone, large stereo speakers, jewelry) should not be near the generator for longer than a few seconds. Patients are advised to place digital cellular phones at least 6 to 12 inches away from (or on the side opposite of) the pacemaker generator and not to carry them in a shirt pocket. Large electromagnetic fields, such as those produced by magnetic resonance imaging, radio and television transmitter towers and lines, transmission power lines (not the distribution lines that bring electricity into a home), and electrical substations may cause EMI. Patients should be cautioned to avoid such situations or to simply move farther away from the area if they experience dizziness or a feeling of rapid or irregular heartbeats (palpitations). Welding and the use of a chain saw should be avoided. If such tools are used, precautionary steps such as limiting the welding current to a 60- to 130-ampere range or using electric rather than gasoline-powered chain saws are advised.

In addition, the metal of the pacemaker generator may trigger store and library antitheft devices as well as airport and building security alarms; however, these alarm systems generally do not interfere with the pacemaker function. Patients should walk through them quickly and avoid standing in or near these devices. The handheld screening devices used in airports may interfere with the pacemaker. Patients should be advised to ask security personnel to perform a hand search instead of using the handheld screening device. Patients also should be educated to wear or carry medical identification to alert personnel to the presence of the pacemaker.

TABLE 26-2   Assessing Pacemaker Malfunction

Problem	Possible Cause	Nursing Considerations
Loss of capture—complex does *not* follow pacing spike	Inadequate stimulus Lead dislodgement Lead wire fracture Catheter malposition Battery depletion Electronic insulation break Medication change Myocardial ischemia	Check security of all connections; increase milliamperage. Reposition extremity; turn patient to left side. Change battery. Change generator.
Undersensing—pacing spike occurs at preset interval despite patient's intrinsic rhythm	Sensitivity too high Electrical interference (e.g., by a magnet) Faulty generator	Decrease sensitivity. Eliminate interference. Replace generator.
Oversensing—loss of pacing artifact; pacing does not occur at preset interval despite lack of intrinsic rhythm	Sensitivity too low Electrical interference Battery depletion Change in medication	Increase sensitivity. Eliminate interference. Change battery.
Loss of pacing—total absence of pacing spikes	Oversensing Battery depletion Loose or disconnected wires Perforation	Change battery. Check security of all connections. Apply magnet over permanent generator. Obtain 12-lead ECG and portable chest x-ray. Assess for murmur. Contact physician.
Change in pacing QRS shape	Septal perforation	Obtain 12-lead ECG and portable chest x-ray. Assess for murmur. Contact physician.
Rhythmic diaphragmatic or chest wall twitching or hiccuping	Output too high Myocardial wall perforation	Decrease milliamperage. Turn pacer off. Contact physician at once. Monitor closely for decreased cardiac output.

ECG, electrocardiogram.
Adapted from Calkins, H., Kuck, K. H., Cappato, R., et al. (2012). 2012 HRS/EHRA/ECAS expert consensus statement on catheter and surgical ablation of atrial fibrillation: Recommendations for patient selection, procedural techniques, patient management and follow-up, definitions, endpoints, and research trial design. *Heart Rhythm, 9*(4), 632–696.

Pacemaker Surveillance

Pacemaker clinics have been established to monitor patients and to test pulse generators for impending pacemaker battery failure. A computerized device is held over the generator to "interrogate" it with painless radio signals; it detects the generator's settings, battery status and the presence of ERI, pacing threshold, sensing function, lead integrity, pacing data (e.g., number of pacing events), and other stored information. Several factors, such as lead fracture, muscle inhibition, and insulation disruption, also may be assessed depending on the type of pacemaker and the equipment available. If indicated, the pacemaker is turned off for a few seconds, using a magnet or a programmer, while the ECG is recorded to assess the patient's underlying cardiac rhythm. Transtelephonic transmission of the generator's information is another follow-up method. Special equipment is used to transmit information about the patient's pacemaker over the telephone to a receiving system at a pacemaker clinic. The information is converted into tones; equipment at the clinic converts these tones to an electronic signal and records them on an ECG strip. The pacemaker rate and other data concerning pacemaker function are obtained and evaluated by a cardiologist. This simplifies the diagnosis of a failing generator, reassures the patient, and improves management when the patient is physically remote from pacemaker testing facilities. The frequency of the pacemaker checks varies with the patient's age and underlying condition, the degree of pacemaker dependency, the age and type of the device, and the results from previous pacemaker checks (Tracy, Epstein, Darbar, et al., 2012). A typical follow-up schedule is every 2 weeks during the first month, every 4 to 8 weeks for 3 years, and every 4 weeks thereafter.

Implantable Cardioverter Defibrillator

The **implantable cardioverter defibrillator (ICD)** is an electronic device that detects and terminates life-threatening episodes of tachycardia or fibrillation, especially those that are ventricular in origin. Patients at high risk of VT or ventricular fibrillation and who would benefit from an ICD are those who have survived sudden cardiac death syndrome, which usually is caused by ventricular fibrillation, or have experienced spontaneous, symptomatic VT (syncope secondary to VT) not due to a reversible cause (called a *secondary prevention intervention*). The Centers for Medicaid and Medicare Services (CMS, 2005) recommends that people with coronary artery disease who are 40 days post acute MI with moderate to severe left ventricular dysfunction (ejection fraction less than or equal to 35%) are at risk of sudden cardiac death and therefore an ICD is indicated (called a *primary prevention intervention*). The CMS has also approved ICD implantation in patients who have been diagnosed with nonischemic dilated cardiomyopathy for at least 9 months and NYHA functional class II or III heart failure (CMS, 2005). ICDs may also be implanted in patients with symptomatic, recurrent, medication-refractory atrial fibrillation. A recent study indicated that the underutilization of ICDs for primary prevention purposes was most often due to patient preference, indicating a need for patient education

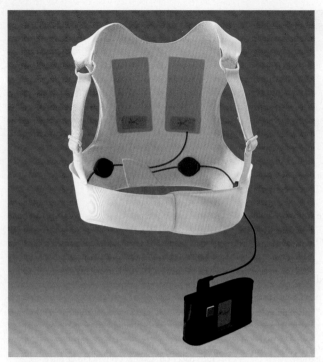

FIGURE 26-31 • The wearable automatic cardioverter defibrillator vest. Courtesy of ZOLL LifeVest.

and exploration of patients' perceived barriers to consenting to this potentially lifesaving intervention (Castellanos, Smith, Varosky, et al., 2012).

Because there may be a waiting period for ICD implantation, patients who are at risk for sudden cardiac death may be prescribed a wearable vestlike automated defibrillator, which works just like an AED in that a shock is delivered less than a minute after a life-threatening rhythm is detected (Zishiri, Cronin, Williams, et al., 2011) (Fig. 26-31). Prior to the delivery of the shock, the vest vibrates and issues an alarm to announce that a shock is imminent. The vest weighs about a pound, is worn under the patient's clothing, and is attached to a monitor with a battery that is worn in a holster or on a shoulder strap. The monitor automatically downloads information once a day, usually in the middle of the night. The vest must be worn at all times, even if the patient is admitted to the hospital and placed on an ECG monitor, and removed only when showering or bathing. The battery needs to be changed every day. Education is provided to the patient by the device manufacturer. However, the nurse should assess the patient's understanding of the education provided and explore any issues that may prevent the patient from wearing it.

An ICD has a generator about the size of a large book of matches and has at least a right ventricular lead that can sense intrinsic electrical activity and deliver an electrical impulse. The implantation procedure, postimplantation care, and length of hospital stay are much like those for insertion of a pacemaker (Fig. 26-32). ICDs are designed to respond to two criteria: a rate that exceeds a predetermined level and a change in the isoelectric line segments. When a dysrhythmia occurs, rate sensors require a set duration of time to sense the dysrhythmia. Then, the device automatically

charges; after a second "look" confirms the dysrhythmia, it delivers the programmed charge through the lead to the heart. The time from dysrhythmia detection to electrical discharge depends on the charging time, which depends on the programmed energy level (Fuster, Walsh et al., 2011). However, in an ICD that has the capability of providing atrial therapies, the device can be programmed to be activated by the patient, giving the patient time to activate the charge at a time and place of his or her choosing. The life of the lithium battery is about 9 years but varies depending on use of the ICD. ICD surveillance is similar to that of the pacemaker; however, it includes stored endocardial ECGs as well as information about the number and frequency of shocks that have been delivered.

Antiarrhythmic medication may be administered with this technology to minimize the occurrence of the tachydysrhythmia and to reduce the frequency of ICD discharge.

Several types of devices are available and may be programmed for multiple treatments (Fuster, Walsh et al., 2011). ICD, the generic name, is used as the abbreviation for these various devices. Each device offers a different delivery sequence, but all are capable of delivering high-energy (high-intensity) defibrillation to treat a tachycardia (atrial or ventricular). The device may deliver up to six shocks if necessary.

Some ICDs can respond with (1) antitachycardia pacing, in which the device delivers electrical impulses at a fast rate in an attempt to disrupt the tachycardia, (2) low-energy (low-intensity) cardioversion, or (3) defibrillation; others may use all three techniques (Fuster, Walsh et al., 2011). Pacing is used to terminate tachycardias caused by a conduction disturbance called *reentry*, which is repetitive restimulation of the heart by the same impulse. An impulse or a series

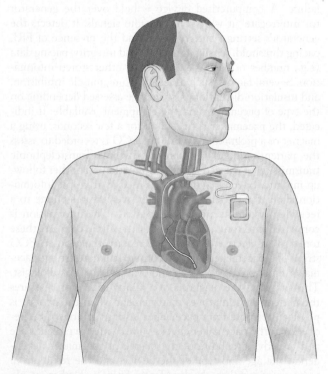

FIGURE 26-32 • The implantable cardioverter defibrillator consists of a generator and a sensing/pacing/defibrillating electrode.

of impulses is delivered to the heart by the device at a fast rate to collide with and stop the heart's reentry conduction impulses, and therefore to stop the tachycardia. Some ICDs also have pacemaker capability if the patient develops bradycardia, which sometimes occurs after treatment of the tachycardia. Usually, the mode is VVI (V, paces the ventricle; V, senses ventricular activity; I, paces only if the ventricles do not depolarize). Some ICDs also treat atrial fibrillation (Fuster, Rydén et al., 2011).

Which device is used and how it is programmed depend on the patient's dysrhythmia(s). The device may be programmed differently for different dysrhythmias (e.g., ventricular fibrillation, VT with a fast ventricular rate, and VT with a slow ventricular rate). As with pacemakers, there is an NASPE-BPEG code for communicating the functions of the ICDs (Bernstein et al., 2002). The first letter represents the chamber or chambers shocked (O, none; A, atrium; V, ventricle; D, both atrium and ventricle). The second letter represents the chamber that can be antitachycardia paced (O, A, V, D, meaning the same as the first letter). The third letter indicates the method used by the generator to detect a tachycardia (E, electrogram; H, hemodynamics). The last letter represents the chambers that have antibradycardia pacing (O, A, V, D, meaning the same as the first and second letters of the ICD code).

Complications of ICD implantation are similar to those associated with pacemaker insertion. The primary complication is surgery-related infection; its risk increases with battery or lead replacement (Fuster, Walsh et al., 2011). A few complications are associated with the technical aspects of the equipment, like those of pacemakers, such as premature battery depletion and dislodged or fractured leads. Inappropriate

delivery of ICD therapy, usually due to oversensing or atrial and sinus tachycardias with a rapid ventricular rate response is the most frequent complication. This requires reprogramming of the device.

Nursing Management

After a permanent electronic device (pacemaker or ICD) is inserted, the patient's heart rate and rhythm are monitored by ECG. The device's settings are noted and compared with the ECG recordings to assess the device's function. For example, pacemaker malfunction is detected by examining the pacemaker spike and its relationship to the surrounding ECG complexes (Fig. 26-33). In addition, cardiac output and hemodynamic stability are assessed to identify the patient's response to pacing and the adequacy of pacing. The appearance or increasing frequency of dysrhythmia is observed and reported to the primary provider. If the patient has an ICD implanted and develops VT or ventricular fibrillation, the ECG should be recorded to note the time between the onset of the dysrhythmia and the onset of the device's shock or antitachycardia pacing.

The incision site where the generator was implanted is observed for bleeding, hematoma formation, or infection, which may be evidenced by swelling, unusual tenderness, drainage, and increased warmth. The patient may complain of continuous throbbing or pain. These symptoms are reported to the primary provider.

A chest x-ray is usually taken after the procedure and prior to discharge to document the position of leads in addition to ensuring that the procedure did not cause a pneumothorax. It is necessary to assess the function of the device throughout

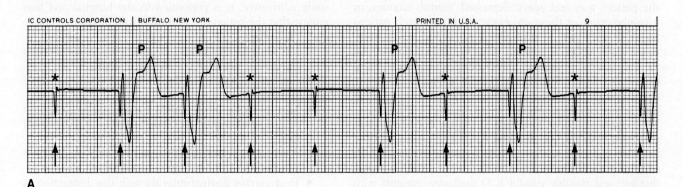

A

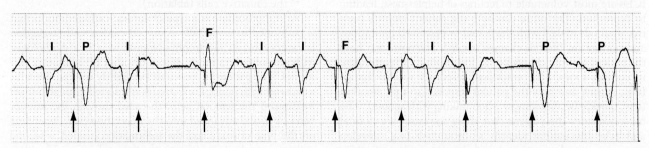

B

FIGURE 26-33 • A. Ventricular pacing in lead V_1 with intermittent loss of capture (a pacing spike not followed by a QRS complex). **B.** Ventricular pacing with loss of sensing (a pacing spike occurring at an inappropriate time). ↑, pacing spike; *, loss of capture; P, pacemaker-induced QRS complex; I, patient's intrinsic QRS complex; F, fusion (a QRS complex formed by a merging of the patient's intrinsic QRS complex and the pacemaker-induced QRS complex).

its lifetime and especially after changes in the patient's medication regimen. For example, antiarrhythmic agents, beta-blockers, and diuretics may increase the pacing threshold, whereas corticosteroids and alpha-adrenergic agents may decrease the pacing threshold; the opposite effect occurs when the patient is taken off these medications.

The patient is also assessed for anxiety, depression, or anger, which may be symptoms of ineffective coping with the implantation. In addition, the level of knowledge and education needs of the patient and family and the history of adherence to the therapeutic regimen should be identified. It is especially important to include the family when providing education and support.

In the peri- and postoperative phases, the nurse carefully observes the patient's responses to the device and provides the patient and family with further education as needed (Chart 26-8). The nurse also assists the patient and family in addressing concerns and in making decisions about self-care and lifestyle changes necessitated by the dysrhythmia and resulting device implantation.

Preventing Infection

The nurse changes the dressing as needed and inspects the insertion site for redness, swelling, soreness, or any unusual drainage. Any change in wound appearance, an increase in the patient's temperature, or an increase in the patient's white blood count should be reported to the primary provider.

Promoting Effective Coping

The patient treated with an electronic device experiences not only lifestyle and physical changes but also emotional changes. At different times during the healing process, the patient may feel angry, depressed, fearful, anxious, or a combination of these emotions. Although each patient uses individual coping strategies (e.g., humor, prayer, communication with a significant other) to manage emotional distress, some strategies may work better than others. Signs that may indicate ineffective coping include social isolation, increased or prolonged irritability or depression, and difficulty in relationships.

To promote effective coping strategies, the nurse must recognize both the patient's and family's perceptions of the situation and their resulting emotional state and assist them to explore their reactions and feelings. Because of the unpredictable and possibly painful ICD discharge, patients with ICDs are most vulnerable to feelings of helplessness, leading to depression. The nurse can help the patient identify positive methods to deal with the actual or perceived limitations and manage any lifestyle changes needed. The nurse may help the patient identify changes (e.g., loss of ability to participate in contact sports), the emotional responses to the change (e.g., anger), and how the patient responds to that emotion (e.g., quickly becomes angry when talking with spouse). The nurse reassures the patient that these responses are normal and helps the patient identify realistic goals (e.g., develop interest in another activity) and develop a plan to attain these goals. The patient and family should be encouraged to talk about their experiences and emotions with each other and the health care team. The nurse may refer the patient and family to a hospital, community, or online support group.

The nurse may also encourage the use of spiritual resources. Based on the patient's interest, the nurse also may educate the patient about easy-to-use stress reduction techniques (e.g., deep-breathing exercises, relaxation) to facilitate coping. Instructing the patient about the ICD may help the patient cope with changes that occur as a result of device implantation (see Chart 26-8).

Promoting Home and Community-Based Care

After device insertion, the patient's hospital stay may be 1 day or less, and follow-up in an outpatient clinic or office is common. The patient's anxiety and feelings of vulnerability may interfere with the ability to learn information provided. The nurse needs to include caregivers in the education and provide printed materials for use by the patient and caregiver. The nurse establishes priorities for learning with the patient and caregiver. Education may include the importance of periodic device monitoring, promoting safety, surgical site care, and avoiding EMI (see Chart 26-8). In addition, the educational plan should include information about activities that are safe and those that may be dangerous. The nurse discusses with the patient and family what they are to do when a shock is delivered. The nurse may facilitate CPR training for the family.

Electrophysiology Studies

An EP study is an invasive procedure used to evaluate and treat various dysrhythmias that have caused cardiac arrest or significant symptoms. It also is indicated for patients with symptoms that suggest a dysrhythmia that has gone undetected and undiagnosed by other methods. Because an EP study is invasive, it is performed in the hospital and may require that the patient be admitted. An EP study is used to do the following:

- Identify the impulse formation and propagation through the cardiac electrical conduction system
- Assess the function or dysfunction of the SA and AV nodal areas
- Identify the location (called *mapping*) and mechanism of dysrhythmogenic (the ability to cause dysrhythmias) foci
- Assess the effectiveness of antiarrhythmic medications and devices for the patient with a dysrhythmia
- Treat certain dysrhythmias through the destruction of the causative cells (**ablation**)

An EP procedure is a type of cardiac catheterization that is performed in a specially equipped cardiac catheterization laboratory by an electrophysiologist, who is a cardiologist with specialized training, assisted by other EP laboratory personnel. The patient is conscious but lightly sedated. Usually, a catheter with multiple electrodes is inserted through a small incision in the femoral vein, threaded through the inferior vena cava, and advanced into the heart; however, depending on the type of study and the information needed, a second catheter may be inserted into the femoral artery. The electrodes are positioned within the heart at specific locations—for instance, in the right atrium near the sinus node, in the coronary sinus, near the tricuspid valve, and at the apex of the right ventricle. The number and placement of electrodes

Chart 26-8

HOME CARE CHECKLIST
Educating the Patient With an Implantable Cardiac Device

At the completion of home care education, the patient and caregiver will be able to:	PATIENT	CAREGIVER
• Avoid infection at the insertion site of the device:		
• Leave the incision uncovered and observe it daily for redness, increased swelling, and heat.	✔	✔
• Take temperature at same time each day; report any increase.	✔	✔
• Avoid wearing tight, restrictive clothing that may cause friction over the insertion site.	✔	
• Initially avoid soaking in the tub and lotion, creams, or powders in the area of the device.	✔	
• Adhere to activity restrictions:		
• Restrict movement of arm until incision heals; do not raise arm above head for 2 weeks.	✔	✔
• Avoid heavy lifting for a few weeks.	✔	✔
• Discuss safety of activities (e.g., driving) with primary provider.	✔	✔
• Recognize that although it may take up to 2–3 weeks to resume normal activities, physical activity does not usually have to be curtailed, with the exception of contact sports.	✔	✔
• Electromagnetic interference: Understand the importance of the following:		
• Avoid large magnetic fields such as those created by magnetic resonance imaging, large motors, arc welding, electrical substations, and so forth. Magnetic fields may deactivate the device, negating its effect on a dysrhythmia.	✔	
• At security gates at airports, government buildings, or other secured areas, show identification card and request a hand (not handheld device) search. Obtain and carry a physician's letter about this requirement.	✔	
• Some electrical and small motor devices, as well as products that contain magnets (e.g., cellular phones), may interfere with the functioning of the cardiac device if the electrical device is placed very close to it. Avoid leaning directly over large electrical devices or motors, or ensure that contact is of brief duration; place cellular phone on opposite side of cardiac device.	✔	
• Household appliances (e.g., microwave ovens) should not cause any concern.	✔	✔
• Promote safety:		
• Describe what to do if symptoms occur, and notify physician if any discharges seem unusual.	✔	✔
• Maintain a log that records discharges of an implantable cardioverter defibrillator (ICD). Record events that precipitate the sensation of shock. This provides important data for the physician to use in readjusting the medical regimen.	✔	✔
• Encourage family members to attend a cardiopulmonary resuscitation class.	✔	✔
• Call 911 for emergency assistance if feeling of dizziness occurs.	✔	✔
• Wear medical identification (e.g., Medic-Alert) that includes physician information.	✔	
• Avoid frightening family or friends with unexpected shocks from an ICD, which will not harm them. Inform family and friends that in the event they are in contact with the patient when a shock is delivered, they may also feel the shock. It is especially important to warn sexual partners that this may occur.	✔	✔
• Carry medical identification with physician's name, type and model number of the device, manufacturer's name, and hospital where device was inserted.	✔	✔
• Follow-up care:		
• Discuss psychological responses to the device implantation, such as changes in self-image, depression due to loss of mobility secondary to driving restrictions, fear of shocks, increased anxiety, concerns that sexual activity may trigger the device, and changes in partner relationship.	✔	✔
• Adhere to appointments that are scheduled to monitor the electronic performance of the cardiac device. This is especially important during the first month after implantation and near the end of the battery life. Remember to take log of ICD discharges to review with physician.	✔	✔
• For patients with pacemakers, check pulse daily. Report *immediately* any sudden slowing or increasing of the pulse rate. This may indicate pacemaker malfunction.	✔	✔

depend on the type of study being conducted. These electrodes allow the electrical signal to be recorded from within the heart (intracardiogram).

The electrodes also allow the clinician to introduce a pacing stimulus to the intracardiac area at a precisely timed interval and rate, thereby stimulating the area (programmed stimulation). An area of the heart may be paced at a rate much faster than the normal rate of **automaticity**, the rate at which impulses are spontaneously formed (e.g., in the sinus node). This allows the pacemaker to become an artificial focus of automaticity and to assume control (overdrive suppression). Then, the pacemaker is stopped suddenly, and the time it takes for the sinus node to resume control is assessed. A prolonged time indicates dysfunction of the sinus node.

One of the main purposes of programmed stimulation is to assess the ability of the area surrounding the electrode to cause a reentry dysrhythmia. One or a series of premature impulses is delivered to an area in an attempt to cause the tachydysrhythmia. Because the precise location of the suspected area and the specific timing of the pacing needed are unknown, the electrophysiologist uses several different techniques to cause the dysrhythmia during the study. If the dysrhythmia can be reproduced by programmed stimulation, it is called *inducible*. Once a dysrhythmia is induced, a treatment plan is determined and implemented. If, on the follow-up EP study, the tachydysrhythmia cannot be induced, then the treatment is determined to be effective. Different medications may be administered and combined with electrical devices (pacemaker, ICD) to determine the most effective treatment to suppress the dysrhythmia.

Patient care, patient education, and associated complications of an EP study are similar to those associated with cardiac catheterization (see Chapter 25). The study is usually about 2 hours in length; however, if the electrophysiologist conducts not only a diagnostic procedure but also treatment, the study can take up to 6 hours. During the procedure, patients benefit from a calm, reassuring approach.

Patients who are to undergo an EP study may be anxious about the procedure and its outcome. A detailed discussion involving the patient, the family, and the electrophysiologist usually occurs to ensure that the patient can give informed consent and to reduce the patient's anxiety about the procedure. Before the procedure, the patient should receive instructions about the procedure and its usual duration, the environment where the procedure is performed, and what to expect. Although an EP study is not painful, it does cause discomfort and can be tiring. It may also cause feelings that were experienced when the dysrhythmia occurred in the past. In addition, patients are educated about what will be expected of them (e.g., lying very still during the procedure, reporting symptoms or concerns).

The patient should also know that the dysrhythmia may occur during the procedure. It often stops on its own; if it does not, treatment is given to restore the patient's normal rhythm. The dysrhythmia may have to be terminated using cardioversion or defibrillation, but this is performed under more controlled circumstances than if performed in an emergency.

Postprocedural care is similar to that for cardiac catheterization, including restriction of activity to promote hemostasis at the insertion site. To identify any complications and to ensure healing, the patient's vital signs and the appearance of the insertion site are assessed frequently. Because an artery is not always used, there is a lower incidence of vascular complications than with other catheterization procedures. Cardiac arrest may occur, but the incidence is low (less than 1%) (Fuster, Walsh et al., 2011).

Cardiac Conduction Surgery

Atrial and ventricular tachycardias that do not respond to medications and are not suitable for antitachycardia pacing may be treated by methods that include a maze procedure and ablation. Hospitalization is required for both procedures.

Maze Procedure

The maze procedure is an open heart surgical procedure for refractory atrial fibrillation. Small transmural incisions are made throughout the atria. The resulting formation of scar tissue prevents reentry conduction of the electrical impulse. Because the procedure requires significant time and cardiopulmonary bypass, its use is reserved only for those patients undergoing cardiac surgery for other reason (e.g., coronary artery bypass) (Fuster, Walsh et al., 2011). In addition, some patients need a permanent pacemaker after the surgery.

Catheter Ablation Therapy

Catheter ablation destroys specific cells that are the cause or central conduction route of a tachydysrhythmia. It is performed with or after an EP study. Usual indications for ablation are AVNRT, a recurrent atrial dysrhythmia (especially atrial fibrillation), or VT unresponsive to previous therapy (or for which the therapy produced significant side effects).

Ablation is also indicated to eliminate accessory AV pathways or bypass tracts that exist in the hearts of patients with preexcitation syndromes such as WPW. During normal embryonic development, all connections between the atria and ventricles disappear, except for that between the AV node and the bundle of His. In some people, embryonic connections of normal heart muscle between the atria and ventricles remain, providing an accessory pathway or a tract through which the electrical impulse can bypass the AV node. These pathways can be located in several different areas. If the patient develops atrial fibrillation, the impulse may bypass the slow conduction in the AV node and be directly conducted into the ventricle at a rate of 300 times per minute or more, which can lead to ventricular fibrillation and sudden cardiac death. Preexcitation syndromes are identified by specific ECG findings (Thanavaro & Thanavaro, 2010). For example, in WPW syndrome, there is a shortened PR interval, slurring (called a *delta wave*) of the initial QRS deflection, and prolonged QRS duration (Fig. 26-34).

Ablation is most often accomplished by using radiofrequency (RF), which involves placing a special catheter at or near the origin of the dysrhythmia. High-frequency, low-energy sound waves are passed through the catheter, causing

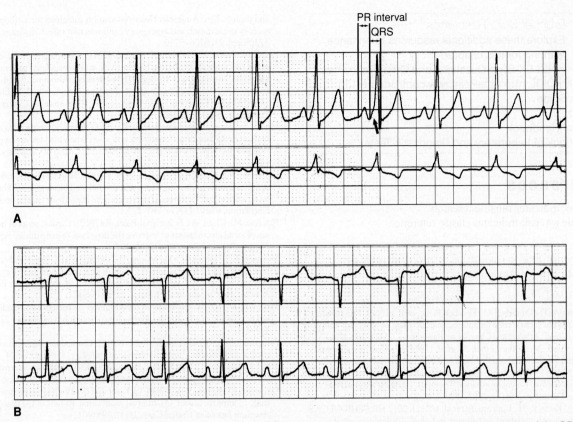

FIGURE 26-34 • Wolff-Parkinson-White syndrome. **A.** Sinus rhythm. Note the short PR interval, slurred initial upstroke of the QRS complex (delta wave, at the *arrow*), and prolonged QRS duration, upper lead II, lower lead V₁. **B.** Rhythm strip of same patient following ablation, upper lead V₁, lower lead II. ECG strips courtesy of Linda Ardini and Catherine Berkmeyer, Inova Fairfax Hospital, Falls Church, VA.

thermal injury and cellular changes that result in localized destruction and scarring. The tissue damage is more specific to the dysrhythmic tissue, with less trauma to the surrounding cardiac tissue than occurs with electrical ablation. Although RF ablation has less risk of causing AV block, it has been associated with myocardial perforation and cardiac tamponade. Ablation may also be accomplished using a different special catheter to apply extremely cold temperature to destroy selected cardiac cells, called *cryoablation*. Cryoablation causes less endocardial irritation and thrombosis but also takes longer (Calkins et al., 2012). During the ablation procedure, defibrillation pads, an automatic blood pressure cuff, and a pulse oximeter are used, and an indwelling urinary catheter is inserted. The patient is usually given moderate sedation (see Chapter 18). An EP study is performed to induce the dysrhythmia. The ablation catheter is placed at the origin of the dysrhythmia, and the ablation procedure is performed. Multiple ablations may be necessary. Successful ablation is achieved when the dysrhythmia can no longer be induced. The patient is monitored for another 30 to 60 minutes and then retested to ensure that the dysrhythmia does not recur.

Postprocedural care on a step-down unit is similar to that for an EP study, except that the patient is monitored more closely, depending on the time needed for recovery from sedation. Major risks of catheter ablation include pericardial tamponade, phrenic nerve injury, stroke, pulmonary vein stenosis, and atrioesophageal fistulas (Fuster, Rydén et al., 2011).

Critical Thinking Exercises

1 **ebp** You are working as an occupational health nurse in a paper mill. One of the mill workers comes into your office to have a wood sliver removed from her hand. Your standard protocol is to take vital signs on all health office visits. The worker's vital signs include the following: blood pressure, 110/72 mm Hg; heart rate, 30 bpm; respiratory rate, 16 breaths/min. What are some possible causes of this heart rate? Identify other key factors that would need to be included in your assessment to help identify the cause of the dysrhythmia. What nursing interventions are needed? What is the evidence base that supports these nursing interventions? Discuss the strength of the evidence and the criteria used to evaluate the strength of the evidence.

2 **pq** You are conducting a home care visit on a 70-year-old man who recently had an ICD inserted. Identify the priority assessments that you need to complete during this visit related to the ICD. What other factors need to be assessed?

3 **ebp** You are employed as a nurse in a college health office. The Dean of Students comes to your office and asks you about the need to purchase an AED. What information would you require prior to answering that question? Discuss the evidence that supports your answer. Discuss processes that would need to be developed and any educational factors that would need to be considered in implementing an AED program.

Brunner Suite Resources

Explore these additional resources to enhance learning for this chapter:
- NCLEX-Style Questions and Other Resources on thePoint, http://thePoint.lww.com/Brunner13e
- Study Guide
- PrepU
- Clinical Handbook
- Handbook of Laboratory and Diagnostic Tests

References

*Asterisk indicates nursing research.
**Double asterisk indicates classic reference.

Book

Fuster, V., Walsh, R. A., & Harrington, R. A. (Eds.). (2011). *Hurst's the heart* (13th ed.). New York: McGraw-Hill.

Journals and Electronic Documents

**Bernstein, A. D., Daubert, J-C., Fletcher, R. D., et al. (2002). The revised NASPE/BPEG generic code for antibradycardia, adaptive-rate, and multisite pacing. *Journal of Pacing and Clinical Electrophysiology, 25*(2), 260–264.

Brenyo, A., Link, M. S., Barsheshet, A., et al. (2011). Cardiac resynchronization therapy reduces left atrial volume and the risk of atrial tachyarrhythmias in MADIT-CRT (Multicenter Automatic Defibrillator Implantation Trial with Cardiac Resynchronization Therapy). *Journal of the American College of Cardiology, 58*(16), 1682–1689.

Calkins, H., Kuck, K. H., Cappato, R., et al. (2012). 2012 HRS/EHRA/ECAS expert consensus statement on catheter and surgical ablation of atrial fibrillation: Recommendations for patient selection, procedural techniques, patient management and follow-up, definitions, endpoints, and research trial design. *Heart Rhythm, 9*(4), 632–696.

**Cardiac Arrhythmia Suppression Trial Investigators. (1989). The Cardiac Arrhythmia Suppression Trial. *New England Journal of Medicine, 321*(25), 1754–1756.

Castellanos, J. M., Smith, L. M., Varosky, P. D., et al. (2012). Referring physicians' discordance with the primary prevention implantable cardioverter-defibrillator guidelines: A national survey. *Heart Rhythm, 9*(6), 874–881.

Centers for Medicare and Medicaid Services. (January 27, 2005). *Administrative file CAG: Decision memorandum: Implantable cardioverter defibrillators (# 00157R3)*. Available at: www.cms.gov

Cramm, A. J., Kirchhof, P., Lip, G. U., et al. (2010). Guidelines for the management of atrial fibrillation. *European Heart Journal, 31*(19), 2369–2429.

Crandall, M. A., Bradley, D. J., Packer D. L., et al. (2009). Contemporary management of atrial fibrillation: Update on anticoagulation and invasive management strategies. *Mayo Clinic Proceedings, 84*(7), 643–662.

Estes, N. A., Sacco, R. L., Al-Khatib, S. M., et al. (2011). American Heart Association Atrial Fibrillation Research Summit: A conference report from the American Heart Association. *Circulation, 124*(3), 363–372.

Fuster, V., Rydén L. E., Cannom D. S., et al. (2011). ACCF/AHA/HRS focused updates incorporated into the ACC/AHA/ESC 2006 guidelines for the management of patients with atrial fibrillation: A report of the American College of Cardiology Foundation/American Heart Association Task Force on Practice Guidelines developed in partnership with the European Society of Cardiology and in collaboration with the European Heart Rhythm Association and the Heart Rhythm Society. *Journal of the American College of Cardiology, 57*(11), 223–242.

Gillis, A. M., Russo, A. M., Ellenbogen, K.A., et al. (2012). HRS/ACCF expert consensus statement on pacemaker device and mode selection. *Journal of American College of Cardiology, 60*(7), 682–703.

Graham, K. C., & Cvach, M. (2010). Monitor alarm fatigue: Standardizing use of physiological monitors and decreasing nuisance alarms. *American Journal of Critical Care, 19*(1), 28–34.

Jacobs, I., Sunde, K., Deakin, C. D., et al. (2010). Part 6: Defibrillation: 2010 International Consensus on Cardiopulmonary Resuscitation and Emergency Cardiovascular Care Science With Treatment Recommendations. *Circulation, 122*(Suppl. 2), S325–S337.

Link, M. S., Atkins, D. L., Passman, H. R., et al. (2010). Part 6: Electrical therapies: Automated external defibrillators, defibrillation, cardioversion,

and pacing: 2010 American Heart Association guidelines for cardiopulmonary resuscitation and emergency cardiovascular care. *Circulation, 122*(Suppl. 2), S706–S719.

Lip, G. Y., Frison, L., Halperin, J. L., et al. (2011). Comparative validation of a novel risk score for predicting bleeding risk in anticoagulated patients with atrial fibrillation: The HAS-BLED (Hypertension, Abnormal Renal/Liver Function, Stroke, Bleeding History or Predisposition, Labile INR, Elderly, Drugs/Alcohol Concomitantly) score. *Journal of the American College of Cardiology, 57*(2), 173–180.

Lip, G. Y., Larsen, T. B., Skjøth, F., et al. (2012). Indirect comparisons of new oral anticoagulant drugs for efficacy and safety when used for stroke prevention in atrial fibrillation. *Journal of the American College of Cardiology, 60*(2), 738–746.

Lip, G. Y., Nieuwlaat, R., Pisters, R., et al. (2010). Refining clinical risk stratification for predicting stroke and thromboembolism in atrial fibrillation using a novel risk factor-based approach. The Euro Heart Survey on Atrial Fibrillation. *Chest, 137*(2), 263–272.

*McRae, M., Chan, A., & Imperial-Perez, F. (2010). Cardiac surgical nurses' use of atrial electrograms to improve the diagnoses of arrhythmia. *American Journal of Critical Care, 19*(2), 124–133.

Morrison, L. J., Deakin, C. D., Morley, P. T., et al. (2010). Part 8: Advanced life support: 2010 International Consensus on Cardiopulmonary Resuscitation and Emergency Cardiovascular Care Science With Treatment Recommendations. *Circulation, 122*(Suppl. 2), S345–S421.

Patton, K. K. (2010). The riddle of nonsustained ventricular tachycardia and sudden cardiac death. Are we approaching a solution? *Circulation, 22*(5), 449–451.

Pelligrini, C. A., & Schneiman, M. M. (2010). Clinical management of ventricular tachycardia. *Current Problems in Cardiology, 35*(9), 453–504.

Perret-Guillaume, C., Joly, L., & Benetos, A. (2009). Heart rate as a risk factor for cardiovascular disease. *Progress in Cardiovascular Disease, 52*(1), 6–10.

*Pickham, D., Shinn, J. A., Chan, G. K., et al. (2012). Quasi-experimental study to improve nurses' QT-interval monitoring: Results of QTIP study. *American Journal of Critical Care, 21*(3), 195–201.

Rothman, S. A. (2010). Antiarrhythmic drug therapy in supraventricular tachycardia. *Cardiac Electrophysiology Clinics, 2*(3), 379–391.

Saborido, C. M., Hockenhull, J., Bagust, A., et al. (2010). Systematic review and cost effectiveness evaluation of 'pill-in-the-pocket' strategy for paroxysmal atrial fibrillation compared to episodic in-hospital treatment or continuous antiarrhythmic drug therapy. *Health Technology Assessment, 14*(31), 1–75.

Sayre, M. R., Koster, R.W., Botha, M., et al. (2010). Part 5: Adult basic life support: 2010 International Consensus on Cardiopulmonary Resuscitation and Emergency Cardiovascular Care Science With Treatment Recommendations. *Circulation, 122*(Suppl. 2), S298–S324.

Schnabel, R. B., Sullivan, L. M., Levy, D., et al. (2009). Development of a risk score for atrial fibrillation (Framingham Heart Study): A community-based cohort study. *Lancet, 373*(9665), 739–745.

Thanavaro, J. I., & Thanavaro, S. (2010). Clinical presentation and treatment of atrial fibrillation in Wolff-Parkinson-White syndrome. *Heart & Lung, 39*(2), 131–136.

Tracy, C. M., Epstein, A. E., Darbar, D., et al. (2012). ACCF/AHA/HRS focused update of the 2008 guidelines for device-based therapy of cardiac rhythm abnormalities: A report of the American College of Cardiology Foundation/American Heart Association Task Force on Practice Guidelines. *Journal of the American College of Cardiology, 60*(14), 1297–1313.

**Wyse, D. G., Waldo, A. L., DiMarco, J. P., et al. (2002). A comparison of rate control and rhythm control in patients with atrial fibrillation. *New England Journal of Medicine, 347*(23), 1825–1833.

Zishiri, E., Cronin, E., & Williams, S., et al. (2011). Use of the wearable cardioverter defibrillator and survival after coronary artery revascularization in patients with left ventricular dysfunction. *Circulation, 124*(21), A9816.

Resources

American Association of Critical-Care Nurses, www.aacn.org
American Association of Heart Failure Nurses (AAHFN), aahfn.org
American College of Cardiology (ACC), www.acc.org
American Heart Association, National Center, www.americanheart.org
Heart Rhythm Society, www.hrsonline.org
National Institute on Aging (NIA), www.nia.nih.gov
National Institutes of Health, National Heart, Lung, Blood Institute, Health Information Center, www.nhlbi.nih.gov

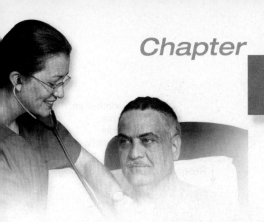

Chapter 27

Management of Patients With Coronary Vascular Disorders

Learning Objectives

On completion of this chapter, the learner will be able to:

1 Describe the pathophysiology, clinical manifestations, and treatment of coronary atherosclerosis.
2 Describe the pathophysiology, clinical manifestations, and treatment of angina pectoris.
3 Use the nursing process as a framework for care of patients with angina pectoris.
4 Describe the pathophysiology, clinical manifestations, and treatment of myocardial infarction.
5 Use the nursing process as a framework for care of a patient with acute coronary syndrome.
6 Describe percutaneous coronary interventional and coronary artery revascularization procedures.
7 Describe the nursing care of a patient who has had a percutaneous coronary interventional procedure for treatment of coronary artery disease.
8 Use the nursing process as a framework for care of a patient who has undergone cardiac surgery.

Glossary

acute coronary syndrome (ACS): signs and symptoms that indicate unstable angina or acute myocardial infarction
angina pectoris: chest pain brought about by myocardial ischemia
atheroma: fibrous cap composed of smooth muscle cells that forms over lipid deposits within arterial vessels and protrudes into the lumen of the vessel, narrowing the lumen and obstructing blood flow; also called *plaque*
atherosclerosis: abnormal accumulation of lipid deposits and fibrous tissue within arterial walls and the lumen
contractility: ability of the cardiac muscle to shorten in response to an electrical impulse
coronary artery bypass graft (CABG): a surgical procedure in which a blood vessel from another part of the body is grafted onto the occluded coronary artery below the occlusion in such a way that blood flow bypasses the blockage
high-density lipoprotein (HDL): a protein-bound lipid that transports cholesterol to the liver for excretion in the bile; composed of a higher proportion of protein to lipid than low-density lipoprotein; exerts a beneficial effect on the arterial wall
ischemia: insufficient tissue oxygenation
low-density lipoprotein (LDL): a protein-bound lipid that transports cholesterol to tissues in the body; composed

of a lower proportion of protein to lipid than high-density lipoprotein; exerts a harmful effect on the arterial wall
metabolic syndrome: a cluster of metabolic abnormalities including insulin resistance, obesity, dyslipidemia, and hypertension that increase the risk of cardiovascular disease
myocardial infarction (MI): death of heart tissue caused by lack of oxygenated blood flow
percutaneous coronary intervention (PCI): a procedure in which a catheter is placed in a coronary artery, and one of several methods is employed to reduce blockage within the artery
percutaneous transluminal coronary angioplasty (PTCA): a type of percutaneous coronary intervention in which a balloon is inflated within a coronary artery to break an atheroma and open the vessel lumen, improving coronary artery blood flow
stent: a metal mesh that provides structural support to a coronary vessel, preventing its closure
sudden cardiac death: abrupt cessation of effective heart activity
thrombolytic: a pharmacologic agent that breaks down blood clots; alternatively referred to as a fibrinolytic
troponin: a cardiac muscle biomarker; measurement is used as an indicator of heart muscle injury

---

Cardiovascular disease is the leading cause of death in the United States for men and women of all racial and ethnic groups (Roger, Go, Lloyd-Jones, et al., 2011). Research related to the identification of and treatment for cardiovascular disease includes all segments of the population affected by cardiac conditions, including women, children, and people of diverse racial and ethnic backgrounds. The results of ongoing research are used by nurses to identify specific prevention and treatment strategies in these populations.

CORONARY ARTERY DISEASE

Coronary artery disease (CAD) is the most prevalent type of cardiovascular disease in adults. For this reason, nurses must recognize various manifestations of coronary artery conditions and evidence-based methods for assessing, preventing, and treating these disorders.

Coronary Atherosclerosis

The most common cause of cardiovascular disease in the United States is **atherosclerosis**, an abnormal accumulation of lipid, or fatty substances, and fibrous tissue in the lining of arterial blood vessel walls. These substances block and narrow the coronary vessels in a way that reduces blood flow to the myocardium. Atherosclerosis involves a repetitious inflammatory response to injury of the artery wall and subsequent alteration in the structural and biochemical properties of the arterial walls. New information that relates to the development of atherosclerosis has increased the understanding of treatment and prevention of this progressive and potentially life-threatening process.

Pathophysiology

The inflammatory response involved with the development of atherosclerosis begins with injury to the vascular endothelium and progresses over many years (McCance, Huether, Brashers, et al., 2010). The injury may be initiated by smoking, hypertension, hyperlipidemia, and other factors. The endothelium undergoes changes and stops producing the normal antithrombotic and vasodilating agents. The presence of inflammation attracts inflammatory cells, such as monocytes (macrophages). The macrophages ingest lipids, becoming "foam cells" that transport the lipids into the arterial wall. Some of the lipid is deposited on the arterial wall, forming fatty streaks. Activated macrophages also release biochemical substances that can further damage the endothelium by contributing to the oxidation of low-density lipoprotein (LDL). The oxidized LDL is toxic to the endothelial cells and fuels progression of the atherosclerotic process (Porth, 2011).

Following the transport of lipid into the arterial wall, smooth muscle cells proliferate and form a fibrous cap over a core filled with lipid and inflammatory infiltrate. These deposits, called **atheromas**, or plaques, protrude into the lumen of the vessel, narrowing it and obstructing blood flow (Fig. 27-1). Plaque may be stable or unstable, depending on the degree of inflammation and thickness of the fibrous cap. If the fibrous cap over the plaque is thick and the lipid pool remains relatively stable, it can resist the stress of blood flow and vessel movement. If the cap is thin and inflammation is ongoing, the lesion becomes what is called *vulnerable plaque*. At this point, the lipid core may grow, causing the fibrous plaque to rupture. A ruptured plaque attracts platelets and causes thrombus formation. A thrombus may then obstruct blood flow, leading to acute coronary syndrome (ACS), which may result in an acute **myocardial infarction (MI)**. When an MI occurs, a portion of the heart muscle no longer receives blood flow and becomes necrotic.

The anatomic structure of the coronary arteries makes them particularly susceptible to the mechanisms of atherosclerosis. As Figure 27-2 shows, the three major coronary arteries have multiple branches. Atherosclerotic lesions most often form where the vessels branch, suggesting a hemodynamic component that favors their formation (Porth, 2011). Although heart disease is most often caused by atherosclerosis of the coronary arteries, other phenomena may also decrease blood flow to the heart. Examples include vasospasm (sudden constriction or narrowing) of a coronary artery and profound hypotension.

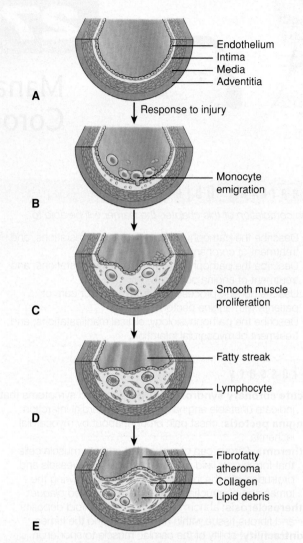

FIGURE 27-1 • A, B: Atherosclerosis begins as monocytes and lipids enter the intima of an injured vessel. Smooth muscle cells proliferate within the vessel wall (**C**), contributing to the development of fatty accumulations and atheroma (**D**). As the plaque enlarges, the vessel narrows and blood flow decreases (**E**). The plaque may rupture and a thrombus might form, obstructing blood flow.

Clinical Manifestations

CAD produces symptoms and complications according to the location and degree of narrowing of the arterial lumen, thrombus formation, and obstruction of blood flow to the myocardium. This impediment to blood flow is usually progressive, causing an inadequate blood supply that deprives the cardiac muscle cells of oxygen needed for their survival. The condition is known as **ischemia**. **Angina pectoris** refers to chest pain that is brought about by myocardial ischemia. Angina pectoris usually is caused by significant coronary atherosclerosis. If the decrease in blood supply is great enough, of long enough duration, or both, irreversible damage and death of myocardial cells may result. Over time, irreversibly damaged myocardium undergoes degeneration and is replaced by scar tissue, causing various degrees of myocardial dysfunction. Significant myocardial damage may result in persistently low cardiac output and heart failure where the heart cannot

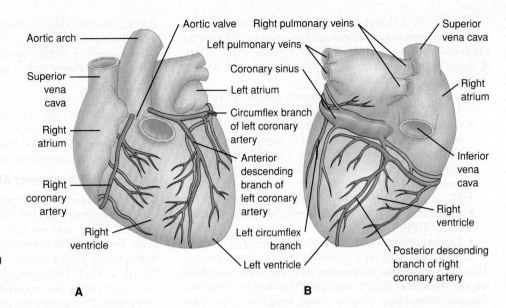

FIGURE 27-2 • The coronary arteries supply the heart muscle with oxygenated blood, adjusting the flow according to metabolic needs. **A.** Anterior view of the heart. **B.** Posterior view of heart.

support the body's needs for blood. A decrease in blood supply from CAD may even cause the heart to abruptly stop beating (**sudden cardiac death**).

The most common manifestation of myocardial ischemia is the onset of chest pain. However, the classic epidemiologic study of the people in Framingham, Massachusetts, showed that nearly 15% of men and women who had coronary events, which included unstable angina, MIs, or sudden cardiac death events, were totally asymptomatic prior to the coronary event (Kannel, 1986). Patients with myocardial ischemia may present to an emergency department (ED) or clinic with a variety of symptoms other than chest pain. Some complain of epigastric distress and pain that radiates to the jaw or left arm. Patients who are older or have a history of diabetes or heart failure may report shortness of breath. Many women have been found to have atypical symptoms, including indigestion, nausea, palpitations, and numbness (Overbaugh, 2009). Prodromal symptoms may occur (i.e., angina a few hours to days before the acute episode), or a major cardiac event may be the first indication of coronary atherosclerosis.

Risk Factors

Epidemiologic studies point to several factors that increase the probability that a person will develop heart disease. Major risk factors are listed in Chart 27-1. Although many people with CAD have one or more risk factors, some do not have classic risk factors. Elevated **low-density lipoprotein (LDL)** cholesterol, also known as bad cholesterol, is a well-known risk factor and the primary target of cholesterol-lowering therapy. People at highest risk for having a cardiac event are those with known CAD or those with diabetes, peripheral arterial disease, abdominal aortic aneurysm, or carotid artery disease. The latter diseases are referred to as CAD risk equivalents, because patients with these diseases have the same risk for a cardiac event as patients with CAD. The likelihood of having a cardiac event is also affected by factors such as age, gender, systolic blood pressure, smoking history, level of total cholesterol, and level of **high-density lipoprotein (HDL)**, also known as good cholesterol. The Framingham Risk Calculator

is a tool commonly used to estimate the risk for having a cardiac event within the next 10 years (Arsenault, Pibarot, & Despres, 2009). This tool is designed for adults 20 years and older. The calculation is performed using the individual's risk factor data, including age, gender, total cholesterol, HDL cholesterol, smoking status, systolic blood pressure, and need for antihypertensive medication.

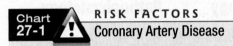

Chart 27-1   **RISK FACTORS**
Coronary Artery Disease

A nonmodifiable risk factor is a circumstance over which a person has no control. A modifiable risk factor is one over which a person may exercise control, such as by changing a lifestyle or personal habit or by using medication. A risk factor may operate independently or in tandem with other risk factors. The more risk factors a person has, the greater the likelihood of coronary artery disease (CAD). Those at risk are advised to seek regular medical examinations and to engage in heart-healthy behavior (a deliberate effort to reduce the number and extent of risks).

Nonmodifiable Risk Factors

Family history of CAD (first-degree relative with cardiovascular disease at 55 years of age or younger for men and at 65 years of age or younger for women)
Increasing age (more than 45 years for men; more than 55 years for women)
Gender (men develop CAD at an earlier age than women)
Race (higher incidence of heart disease in African Americans than in Caucasians)

Modifiable Risk Factors

Hyperlipidemia
Cigarette smoking, tobacco use
Hypertension
Diabetes
Metabolic syndrome
Obesity
Physical inactivity

In addition, a cluster of metabolic abnormalities known as **metabolic syndrome** has emerged as a major risk factor for cardiovascular disease (Alberti, Eckel, Grundy, et al., 2009). A diagnosis of this syndrome includes three of the following conditions:

- Insulin resistance (fasting plasma glucose more than 100 mg/dL or abnormal glucose tolerance test)
- Central obesity (waist circumference more than 35 inches in females, more than 40 inches in males)
- Dyslipidemia (triglycerides more than 150 mg/dL, HDL less than 50 mg/dL in females, less than 40 mg/dL in males)
- Blood pressure persistently greater than 130/85 mm Hg
- Proinflammatory state (high levels of C-reactive protein [CRP])
- Prothrombotic state (high fibrinogen level)

Many people with type 2 diabetes fit this clinical picture. Theories suggest that in patients who are obese, excessive adipose tissue may secrete mediators that lead to metabolic changes. Adipokines (adipose tissue cytokines), free fatty acids, and other substances are known to modify insulin action and contribute to atherogenic changes in the cardiovascular system (Fig. 27-3).

CRP is known to be an inflammatory marker for cardiovascular risk, including acute coronary events and stroke. The liver produces CRP in response to a stimulus such as tissue injury, and high levels of this protein may occur in people with diabetes and those who are likely to have an acute coronary

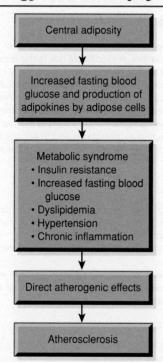

Physiology ··· Pathophysiology

Central adiposity

↓

Increased fasting blood glucose and production of adipokines by adipose cells

↓

Metabolic syndrome
- Insulin resistance
- Increased fasting blood glucose
- Dyslipidemia
- Hypertension
- Chronic inflammation

↓

Direct atherogenic effects

↓

Atherosclerosis

FIGURE 27-3 • Pathophysiology of cardiovascular disease in metabolic syndrome. Central adiposity plays a major role in the development of metabolic syndrome. Adipokines (such as leptin) and other hormones and metabolites are thought to contribute to the development of metabolic abnormalities. The eventual effect of these processes is the promotion of atherosclerosis.

event (Devaraj, Valleggi, Siegel, et al., 2010). To determine overall cardiovascular risk, clinicians may view high sensitivity C-reactive protein (hs-CRP) test results together with other screening tools such as measurements of lipid levels.

Prevention

Four modifiable risk factors—cholesterol abnormalities, tobacco use, hypertension, and diabetes—have been cited as major risk factors for CAD and its complications. As a result, they receive much attention in health promotion programs.

Controlling Cholesterol Abnormalities

The *Third Report of the Expert Panel on Detection, Evaluation, and Treatment of High Blood Cholesterol in Adults* (ATP III), published first in 2001 and updated in subsequent years, lists the clinical guidelines for cholesterol testing and management (Institute for Clinical Systems Improvement [ICSI], 2011a). These guidelines address primary prevention (preventing the occurrence of CAD) and secondary prevention (preventing the progression of CAD). The association of a high blood cholesterol level with heart disease is well established, and the metabolism of fats is known to be an important contributor to the development of heart disease. Fats, which are insoluble in water, are encased in water-soluble lipoproteins that allow them to be transported within the circulatory system. The various lipoproteins are categorized by their protein content, which is measured in density. The density increases when more protein is present. Four elements of fat metabolism—total cholesterol, LDL, HDL, and triglycerides—are known to affect the development of heart disease. Cholesterol is processed by the gastrointestinal (GI) tract into lipoprotein globules called *chylomicrons*. These are reprocessed by the liver as lipoproteins (Fig. 27-4). This is a physiologic process necessary for the formation of lipoprotein-based cell membranes and other important metabolic processes. When an excess of LDL is produced, LDL particles adhere to receptors in the arterial endothelium. Here, macrophages ingest them, contributing to plaque formation.

All adults 20 years and older should have a fasting lipid profile (total cholesterol, LDL, HDL, and triglycerides) performed at least once every 5 years, and more often if the profile is abnormal. Patients who have had an acute event (e.g., MI), a percutaneous coronary intervention (PCI), or a coronary artery bypass graft (CABG) require assessment of their LDL cholesterol level within a few months of the event or procedure, because LDL levels may be low immediately after the acute event or procedure. Subsequently, lipids should be monitored every 6 weeks until the desired level is achieved and then every 4 to 6 months. A fasting lipid profile should demonstrate the following values (Alberti et al., 2009):

- LDL cholesterol less than 100 mg/dL (less than 70 mg/dL for very high-risk patients)
- Total cholesterol less than 200 mg/dL
- HDL cholesterol greater than 40 mg/dL for males and greater than 50 mg/dL for females
- Triglyceride less than 150 mg/dL

LDL is the target of current therapy because of its strong association with advancing CAD. The total cholesterol level is also a clear predictor of coronary events. HDL is known as good cholesterol because it transports other lipoproteins such

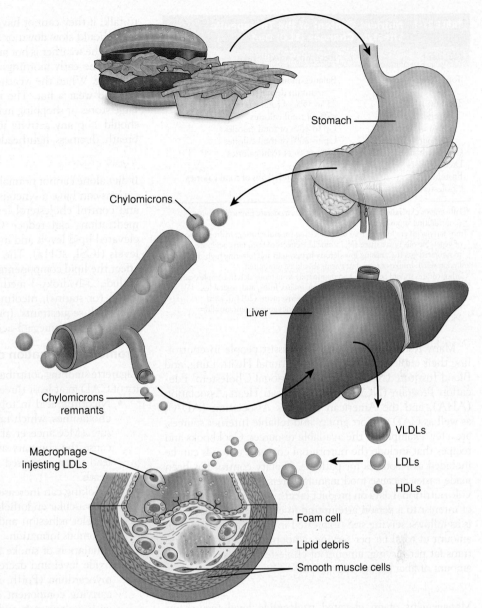

FIGURE 27-4 • Lipoproteins and the development of atherosclerosis. As dietary cholesterol and saturated fat are processed by the gastrointestinal tract, chylomicrons enter the blood. They are broken down into chylomicron remnants in the capillaries. The liver processes them into lipoproteins. When these are released into the circulation, excess low-density lipoproteins (LDLs) adhere to receptors on the intimal wall. Macrophages also ingest LDLs and transport them into the vessel wall, beginning the process of plaque formation. HDLs, high-density lipoproteins; VLDLs, very-low-density lipoproteins.

Labels in figure: Stomach; Chylomicrons; Liver; Chylomicrons remnants; Macrophage injesting LDLs; VLDLs; LDLs; HDLs; Foam cell; Lipid debris; Smooth muscle cells

as LDL to the liver, where they can be degraded and excreted. Because of this, a high HDL level is a strong negative risk factor for heart disease (i.e., it protects against heart disease).

Triglyceride is made up of fatty acids and is transported through the blood by a lipoprotein. Although an elevated triglyceride level (more than 200 mg/dL) may be genetic in origin, it also can be caused by obesity, physical inactivity, excessive alcohol intake, high-carbohydrate diets, diabetes, kidney disease, and certain medications, such as oral contraceptives and corticosteroids.

 Concept Mastery Alert

It is important to remember the different types of cholesterol and the role of each as a risk factor for heart disease. HDL is the "good cholesterol," and higher levels are better; LDL is the "bad cholesterol," and lower levels are better.

Dietary Measures

Table 27-1 provides recommendations of the Therapeutic Lifestyle Changes (TLC) diet, a diet low in saturated fat and high in soluble fiber (ICSI, 2011a). These general recommendations may need to be adjusted for the individual patient who has other nutritional needs, such as the patient who has diabetes. In addition, referral to a dietitian can help the patient in following the appropriate TLC diet. Other TLC recommendations include weight loss, cessation of tobacco use, and increased physical activity.

The Mediterranean diet, another diet that promotes vegetables and fish and restricts red meat, is also reported to reduce mortality from cardiovascular disease (Miller, Stone, Ballantyne, et al., 2011). People who adopt strict vegetarian diets can significantly reduce blood lipids, blood glucose, body mass index, and blood pressure. However, very intensive dietary programs such as these may not be acceptable to all patients who need to modify risk factors.

TABLE 27-1   Nutrient Content of the Therapeutic Lifestyle Changes (TLC) Diet

Nutrient	Recommended Intake
Total calories*	Balance intake and expenditure to maintain desirable weight.
Total fat	25%–35% of total calories
Saturated fat†	<7% of total calories
Polyunsaturated fat	Up to 10% of total calories
Monounsaturated fat	Up to 20% of total calories
Carbohydrate‡	50%–60% of total calories
Dietary fiber	20–30 g/d
Protein	Approximately 15% of total calories
Cholesterol	<200 mg/d

*Daily energy expenditure should include at least moderate physical activity (contributing approximately 200 kcal/d).

†Trans fatty acids are formed from the processing (manufacturing, hydrogenation) of vegetable oils into a more solid form. The effects of trans fatty acids are similar to saturated fats (i.e., raising low-density lipoprotein and lowering high-density lipoprotein). Intake of trans-fatty acids should be minimized.

‡Carbohydrates should be derived predominantly from foods rich in complex carbohydrates, including grains, especially whole grains, fruits, and vegetables.

Adapted from Institute for Clinical Systems Improvement. (2011a). *Lipid management in adults*. Available at: www.guidelines.gov/content.aspx?id=36062&search=lipid+management

Many resources are available to assist people in controlling their cholesterol levels. The National Heart, Lung, and Blood Institute (NHLBI) and its National Cholesterol Education Program (NCEP), the American Heart Association (AHA), and the American Diabetes Association (ADA), as well as CAD support groups and reliable Internet sources, are a few examples of the available resources. Cookbooks and recipes that include the nutritional contents of foods can be included as resources for patients. Dietary control has been made easier because food manufacturers are required to provide nutritional data on product labels. The label information of interest to a person attempting to eat a heart-healthy diet is as follows: serving size (expressed in household measures), amount of total fat per serving, amount of saturated fat and trans fat per serving, amount of cholesterol per serving, and amount of fiber per serving.

Physical Activity

Management of an elevated triglyceride level focuses on weight reduction and increased physical activity. Regular, moderate physical activity increases HDL levels and reduces triglyceride levels, decreasing the incidence of coronary events and reducing overall mortality risk. The goal for most adults is to engage in moderate-intensity aerobic activity of at least 150 minutes per week or vigorous-intensity aerobic activity of at least 75 minutes per week, or an equivalent combination (Schoenborn & Stommel, 2011). The nurse helps the patient to set realistic goals for physical activity. For example, inactive patients can start with activity that lasts 3 minutes, such as parking farther from a building to increase daily walking time. For sustained activity, patients should begin with a 5-minute warm-up period before stretching to prepare the body for exercise. They should end the exercise with a 5-minute cool-down period in which they gradually reduce the intensity of the activity to prevent a sudden decrease in cardiac output. Patients should be instructed to engage in an activity or variety of activities that interest them to maintain motivation. They should also be taught to exercise to an intensity that does not preclude their ability to talk; if they cannot have a conversation while exercising, they should slow down or switch to a less intensive activity. When the weather is hot and humid, patients should exercise during the early morning, or indoors, and wear loose-fitting clothing. When the weather is cold, they should layer clothing and wear a hat. The nurse can also suggest walking in large stores or shopping malls in inclement weather. Patients should stop any activity if chest pain, unusual shortness of breath, dizziness, lightheadedness, or nausea occurs.

Medications

If diet alone cannot normalize serum cholesterol levels, medications can have a synergistic effect with the prescribed diet and control cholesterol levels (Table 27-2). Lipid-lowering medications can reduce CAD mortality in patients with elevated lipid levels and in at-risk patients with normal lipid levels (ICSI, 2011a). The six types of lipid-lowering agents affect the lipid components somewhat differently; these types include 3-hydroxy-3-methylglutaryl coenzyme A (HMG-CoA) (or statins), nicotinic acids, fibric acids (or fibrates), bile acid sequestrants (or resins), cholesterol absorption inhibitors, and omega-3-acid ethyl esters.

Promoting Cessation of Tobacco Use

Cigarette smoking contributes to the development and severity of CAD in at least three ways:

- Nicotinic acid in tobacco triggers the release of catecholamines, which raise the heart rate and blood pressure (McCance et al., 2010). Nicotinic acid can also cause the coronary arteries to constrict. These effects lead to an increased risk of CAD and sudden cardiac death.
- Smoking can increase the oxidation of LDL, damaging the vascular endothelium (Porth, 2011). This increases platelet adhesion and leads to a higher probability of thrombus formation.
- Inhalation of smoke increases the blood carbon monoxide level and decreases the supply of oxygen to the myocardium (Porth, 2011). Hemoglobin, the oxygen-carrying component of blood, combines more readily with carbon monoxide than with oxygen. Myocardial ischemia and reduced contractility can result.

A person at increased risk for heart disease is encouraged to stop tobacco use through any means possible: educational programs, counseling, consistent motivation and reinforcement messages, support groups, and medications. Some people have found complementary therapies (e.g., acupuncture, guided imagery, hypnosis) to be helpful. People who stop smoking reduce their risk of heart disease within the first year, and the risk continues to decline as long as they refrain from smoking (Office of the U.S. Surgeon General, 2010).

The use of medications such as the nicotine patch (NicoDerm CQ, Habitrol), varenicline (Chantix), or bupropion (Zyban) may assist with stopping the use of tobacco (U.S. Food and Drug Administration, 2010). Products containing nicotine have some of the same effects as smoking: catecholamine release (increasing heart rate and blood pressure) and increased platelet adhesion. These medications should be used for a short time and at the lowest effective doses.

Exposure to other smokers' smoke (passive or secondhand smoke) is believed to cause heart disease in nonsmokers

TABLE 27-2 Medications Affecting Lipoprotein Metabolism

Medications	Therapeutic Effects	Considerations
HMG-CoA Reductase Inhibitors (Statins)		
Atorvastatin (Lipitor) Simvastatin (Zocor)	↓ Total cholesterol ↓ LDL ↑ HDL ↓ TGs Inhibit enzyme involved in lipid synthesis (HMG-CoA) Favorable effects on vascular endothelium, including anti-inflammatory and antithrombotic effects	Frequently given as initial therapy for significantly elevated cholesterol and LDL levels Myalgia and arthralgia are common adverse effects Myopathy and possible rhabdomyolysis are possible serious effects Monitor liver function tests Contraindicated in liver disease Check for drug interactions Indication for use now includes ACS and stroke Administer in evening
Nicotinic Acids		
Niacin extended release (Niaspan) Niacin sustained release (Slo-Niacin)	↓ LDL ↑ HDL ↓ TGs ↓ Lipolysis in adipose tissue and lipoprotein synthesis in the liver	May be used as adjunct to a statin when the lipid goal has not been achieved and TG levels are elevated Adverse effects include flushing, upper GI distress, hepatotoxicity Monitor liver function tests Contraindicated in liver disease and peptic ulcer disease Dose needs to be titrated to achieve therapeutic dosage
Fibric Acids (Fibrates)		
Fenofibrate (TriCor) Gemfibrozil (Lopid)	↑ HDL ↓ TGs ↓ Synthesis of TGs and other lipids	Adverse effects include diarrhea, flatulence, rash, myalgia Serious adverse effects include pancreatitis, hepatotoxicity, and rhabdomyolysis Contraindicated in severe renal and liver disease Use with caution in patients who are also taking statins
Bile Acid Sequestrants		
Cholestyramine (Questran) Colestipol (Colestid)	↓ LDL Slight ↑ HDL Oxidize cholesterol into bile acids, which ↓ fat absorption	Most often used as adjunct therapy when statins alone have not been effective in controlling lipid levels Side effects include constipation, abdominal pain, GI bleeding May decrease absorption of other drugs Taken before meals
Cholesterol Absorption Inhibitor		
Ezetimibe (Zetia)	↓ LDL Inhibits absorption of cholesterol in small intestine	Better tolerated than bile acid sequestrants Used in combination with other agents, such as statins Side effects include abdominal pain, arthralgia, myalgia Contraindicated in liver disease
Omega-3-Acid Ethyl Esters		
Fish oil capsules	↓ TGs Inhibit TG production in liver	May be used alone or in combination with other agents Side effects include GI distress, taste perversion, rash, and back pain

HMG-CoA, 3-hydroxy-3-methylglutaryl coenzyme A; ↓ decrease, ↑ increase; LDL, low-density lipoprotein; HDL, high-density lipoprotein; TGs, triglycerides; ACS, acute coronary syndrome; GI, gastrointestinal.

Adapted from Institute for Clinical Systems Improvement. (2011a). *Lipid management in adults.* Available at: www.guidelines.gov/content.aspx?id=36062&search=lipid+management

(Office of the U.S. Surgeon General, 2010). Oral contraceptive use by women who smoke is inadvisable, because these medications significantly increase the risk of CAD and sudden cardiac death.

Managing Hypertension

Hypertension is defined as blood pressure measurements that repeatedly exceed 140/90 mm Hg. The risk of cardiovascular disease increases as blood pressure increases, and people with a blood pressure greater than 120/80 mm Hg are considered prehypertensive and at risk (ICSI, 2011b). Long-standing elevated blood pressure may result in increased stiffness of the vessel walls, leading to vessel injury and a resulting inflam-

matory response within the intima. Inflammatory mediators then lead to the release of growth-promoting factors that cause vessel hypertrophy and hyperresponsiveness. These changes result in acceleration and aggravation of atherosclerosis. Hypertension also increases the work of the left ventricle, which must pump harder to eject blood into the arteries. Over time, the increased workload causes the heart to enlarge and thicken (i.e., hypertrophy) and may eventually lead to heart failure.

Early detection of high blood pressure and adherence to a therapeutic regimen can prevent the serious consequences associated with untreated elevated blood pressure, including CAD. (See Chapter 31 for a detailed discussion of hypertension.)

Controlling Diabetes

Diabetes is known to accelerate the development of heart disease. For many patients with diabetes, cardiovascular disease is identified as the cause of death (ICSI, 2012a). Hyperglycemia fosters dyslipidemia, increased platelet aggregation, and altered red blood cell function, which can lead to thrombus formation. These metabolic alterations may impair endothelial cell–dependent vasodilation and smooth muscle function, promoting the development of atherosclerosis. Treatment with insulin, metformin (Glucophage), and other therapeutic interventions that lower plasma glucose levels can lead to improved endothelial function and patient outcomes. (See Chapter 51 for a detailed discussion of diabetes.)

Gender

Heart disease has long been recognized as a cause of morbidity and mortality in men, but it has not been as readily recognized and treated in women until recently. Cardiovascular events in women occur an average of 10 years later in life than they do in men; in women older than 75 years, the incidence of CAD is approximately equal to that in men (Roger et al., 2011). Women also tend to have a higher incidence of complications from cardiovascular disease and a higher mortality. In addition, women tend to not recognize the symptoms of CAD as early as men, and they wait longer to report their symptoms and seek medical assistance (Overbaugh, 2009).

The age difference between women and men newly diagnosed with CAD was traditionally thought to be related to estrogen. Menopause is now recognized as a milestone in the aging process, during which risk factors tend to accumulate. Cardiovascular disease may be well developed by the time of menopause despite the supposed protective effects of estrogen (Mosca, Benjamin, Berra, et al., 2011). Although hormone therapy (HT) (formerly referred to as hormone replacement therapy) for menopausal women was once promoted as preventive therapy for CAD, research does not support HT as an effective means of prevention. HT decreases menopausal symptoms and the risk of osteoporosis-related bone fractures; however, it also has been associated with an increased incidence of CAD, breast cancer, deep vein thrombosis, stroke, and pulmonary embolism. Current guidelines do not recommend HT for primary or secondary prevention of CAD. However, women do respond well to other preventive measures, such as management of serum lipids (Mosca et al., 2011).

In the past, women who possibly had coronary vascular events were less likely than men to be referred for coronary artery diagnostic procedures such as heart catheterization or treatment with invasive interventions (e.g., PCI). However, as a result of better education of health care professionals and the general public, gender differences now have less influence on diagnosis and treatment. Despite this, when compared with men, women continue to have poorer outcomes, with increased morbidity and mortality after coronary events and interventions (Parry, Watt-Watson, Hodnett, et al., 2010). Women also have poorer results related to symptom relief. These differences may be due to older age, more comorbid conditions, smaller coronary arteries, and differences in the distribution of plaque in the coronary arteries.

Chart 27-2 Types of Angina

- **Stable angina:** predictable and consistent pain that occurs on exertion and is relieved by rest and/or nitroglycerin
- **Unstable angina** (also called *preinfarction angina* or *crescendo angina*): symptoms increase in frequency and severity; may not be relieved with rest or nitroglycerin
- **Intractable or refractory angina:** severe incapacitating chest pain
- **Variant angina** (also called *Prinzmetal's angina*): pain at rest with reversible ST-segment elevation; thought to be caused by coronary artery vasospasm
- **Silent ischemia:** objective evidence of ischemia (such as electrocardiographic changes with a stress test), but patient reports no pain

---

Angina Pectoris

Angina pectoris is a clinical syndrome usually characterized by episodes or paroxysms of pain or pressure in the anterior chest. The cause is insufficient coronary blood flow, resulting in a decreased oxygen supply when there is increased myocardial demand for oxygen in response to physical exertion or emotional stress. In other words, the need for oxygen exceeds the supply.

Pathophysiology

Angina is usually caused by atherosclerotic disease. Almost invariably, angina is associated with a significant obstruction of at least one major coronary artery. Normally, the myocardium extracts a large amount of oxygen from the coronary circulation to meet its continuous demands. When demand increases, flow through the coronary arteries needs to be increased. When there is blockage in a coronary artery, flow cannot be increased and ischemia results. The types of angina are listed in Chart 27-2. Several factors are associated with typical anginal pain:

- Physical exertion, which precipitates an attack by increasing myocardial oxygen demand
- Exposure to cold, which causes vasoconstriction and elevated blood pressure, with increased oxygen demand
- Eating a heavy meal, which increases the blood flow to the mesenteric area for digestion, thereby reducing the blood supply available to the heart muscle; in a severely compromised heart, shunting of blood for digestion can be sufficient to induce anginal pain
- Stress or any emotion-provoking situation, causing the release of catecholamines, which increases blood pressure, heart rate, and myocardial workload

Unstable angina is not closely associated with these listed factors. It may occur at rest. See the later discussion of unstable angina in Acute Coronary Syndrome and Myocardial Infarction section.

Clinical Manifestations

Ischemia of the heart muscle may produce pain or other symptoms, varying from mild indigestion to a choking or heavy sensation in the upper chest. The severity ranges from discomfort to agonizing pain. The pain may be accompanied by severe apprehension and a feeling of impending death. It is often felt deep in the chest behind the sternum (retrosternal area). Typically, the pain or discomfort is poorly localized and may radiate to the neck, jaw, shoulders, and inner aspects of the upper arms, usually the left arm. The patient often feels tightness or a heavy choking or strangling sensation that has a viselike, insistent quality. The patient with diabetes may not have severe pain with angina because diabetic neuropathy can blunt nociceptor transmission, dulling the perception of pain. Women may have different symptoms than men, possibly because coronary disease in women tends to be more diffuse in its distribution within the coronary arteries (Overbaugh, 2009).

A feeling of weakness or numbness in the arms, wrists, and hands, as well as shortness of breath, pallor, diaphoresis, dizziness or lightheadedness, and nausea and vomiting, may accompany the pain. An important characteristic of angina is that it subsides with rest or administering nitroglycerin. In many patients, anginal symptoms follow a stable, predictable pattern.

Unstable angina is characterized by attacks that increase in frequency and severity and are not relieved by rest and administering nitroglycerin. Patients with unstable angina require medical intervention.

Gerontologic Considerations

The older adult with angina may not exhibit a typical pain profile because of the diminished pain transmission that can occur with aging. Often the presenting symptom in older adults is dyspnea. Sometimes there are no symptoms ("silent" CAD), making recognition and diagnosis a clinical challenge. Older patients should be encouraged to recognize their chest pain–like symptom (e.g., weakness) as an indication that they should rest or take prescribed medications. Pharmacologic stress testing and cardiac catheterization may be used to diagnose CAD in older patients. Medications used to manage angina are administered cautiously in older adults because they are associated with an increase risk of adverse reactions (Aschenbrenner & Venable, 2012). Invasive procedures (e.g., PCI) that were once considered too risky in older adults may

be considered; when these procedures are performed, many older adults benefit from symptom relief and longer survival (Ionescu, Amuchastegui, Ionescu, et al., 2010).

Assessment and Diagnostic Findings

The diagnosis of angina begins with the patient's history related to the clinical manifestations of ischemia. A 12-lead electrocardiogram (ECG) may show changes indicative of ischemia, such as T-wave inversion (Porth, 2011). Laboratory studies are performed; these generally include cardiac biomarker testing to rule out ACS (refer to the Acute Coronary Syndrome and Myocardial Infarction section). The patient may undergo an exercise or pharmacologic stress test in which the heart is monitored continuously by an ECG, echocardiogram, or both. The patient may also be referred for a nuclear scan or invasive procedure (e.g., cardiac catheterization, coronary angiography).

Medical Management

The objectives of the medical management of angina are to decrease the oxygen demand of the myocardium and to increase the oxygen supply. Medically, these objectives are met through pharmacologic therapy and control of risk factors. Alternatively, reperfusion procedures may be used to restore the blood supply to the myocardium. These include PCI procedures (e.g., percutaneous transluminal coronary angioplasty [PTCA] and intracoronary stents) and CABG. (See later discussion.)

Pharmacologic Therapy

Table 27-3 summarizes drug therapy.

Nitroglycerin

Nitrates are a standard treatment for angina pectoris. Nitroglycerin is a potent vasodilator that improves blood flow to the heart muscle and relieves pain. Nitroglycerin dilates

TABLE 27-3 Summary of Medications Used to Treat Angina	
Medications	**Major Indications**
Nitrates	
Nitroglycerin (Nitrostat, Nitro-Bid)	Short- and long-term reduction of myocardial oxygen consumption through selective vasodilation
Beta-Adrenergic Blocking Agents (Beta-Blockers)	
Metoprolol (Lopressor, Toprol) Atenolol (Tenormin)	Reduction of myocardial oxygen consumption by blocking beta-adrenergic stimulation of the heart
Calcium Ion Antagonists (Calcium Channel Blockers)	
Amlodipine (Norvasc) Diltiazem (Cardizem, Tiazac)	Negative inotropic effects; indicated in patients not responsive to beta-blockers; used as primary treatment for vasospasm
Antiplatelet Medications	
Aspirin Clopidogrel (Plavix) Prasugrel (Effient) Glycoprotein IIb/IIIa agents: Abciximab (ReoPro) Eptifibatide (Integrilin)	Prevention of platelet aggregation
Anticoagulants	
Heparin (unfractionated) Low-molecular-weight heparins: Enoxaparin (Lovenox) Dalteparin (Fragmin)	Prevention of thrombus formation

primarily the veins and, to a lesser extent, the arteries. Dilation of the veins causes venous pooling of blood throughout the body. As a result, less blood returns to the heart, and filling pressure (preload) is reduced. If the patient is hypovolemic (does not have adequate circulating blood volume), the decrease in filling pressure can cause a significant decrease in cardiac output and blood pressure.

Nitrates also relax the systemic arteriolar bed, lowering blood pressure and decreasing afterload. These effects decrease myocardial oxygen requirements, bringing about a more favorable balance between supply and demand.

Nitroglycerin may be given by several routes: sublingual tablet or spray, oral capsule, topical agent, and intravenous (IV) administration. Sublingual nitroglycerin is generally placed under the tongue or in the cheek (buccal pouch) and ideally alleviates the pain of ischemia within 3 minutes. With sublingual nitroglycerin, the nurse should check the patient's medication history for drugs that may lead to dry mouth and mucous membranes and thus impair the absorption of the drug. Chart 27-3 provides more information on self-administration of sublingual nitroglycerin. Oral preparations and topical patches are used to provide sustained effects. A regimen in which the patches are applied in the morning and removed at bedtime allows for a nitrate-free period to prevent the development of tolerance.

A continuous or intermittent IV infusion of nitroglycerin may be administered to the hospitalized patient with recurring signs and symptoms of ischemia or after a revascularization procedure. The rate of infusion is titrated to the patient's pain level and blood pressure. It usually is not administered if the systolic blood pressure is less than 90 mm Hg. Generally, after the patient is symptom-free, the nitroglycerin may be switched to an oral or topical preparation within 24 hours. A common adverse effect of nitroglycerin is headache, which may limit the use of this drug in some patients.

Beta-Adrenergic Blocking Agents

Beta-blockers such as metoprolol (Lopressor, Toprol) reduce myocardial oxygen consumption by blocking beta-adrenergic sympathetic stimulation to the heart. The result is a reduction in heart rate, slowed conduction of impulses through the conduction system, decreased blood pressure, and reduced myocardial **contractility** (force of contraction). Because of these effects, beta-blockers balance the myocardial oxygen needs (demands) and the amount of oxygen available (supply). This helps control chest pain and delays the onset of ischemia during work or exercise. Beta-blockers reduce the incidence of recurrent angina, infarction, and cardiac mortality. The dose can be titrated to achieve a resting heart rate of 50 to 60 bpm.

Cardiac side effects and possible contraindications include hypotension, bradycardia, advanced atrioventricular block, and acute heart failure. If a beta-blocker is given IV for an acute cardiac event, the ECG, blood pressure, and heart rate are monitored closely after the medication has been administered. Side effects include depressed mood, fatigue, decreased libido, and dizziness. Patients taking beta-blockers are cautioned not to stop taking them abruptly, because angina may worsen and MI may develop. Beta-blocker therapy should be decreased gradually over several days before being discontinued. Patients with diabetes who take beta-blockers are instructed to monitor their blood glucose levels as prescribed because beta-blockers can mask signs of hypoglycemia. Beta-blockers that are not cardioselective also affect the beta-adrenergic receptors in the bronchioles, causing bronchoconstriction, and therefore are contraindicated in patients with significant chronic pulmonary disorders, such as asthma.

Calcium Channel Blocking Agents

Calcium channel blockers have a variety of effects on the ischemic myocardium. These agents decrease sinoatrial node automaticity and atrioventricular node conduction, resulting in a slower heart rate and a decrease in the strength of myocardial contraction (negative inotropic effect). These effects decrease the workload of the heart. Calcium channel blockers also increase myocardial oxygen supply by dilating the smooth muscle wall of the coronary arterioles; they decrease myocardial oxygen demand by reducing systemic arterial pressure and the workload of the left ventricle.

The calcium channel blockers most commonly used are amlodipine (Norvasc) and diltiazem (Cardizem). In addition to their use to treat angina, they are commonly prescribed for hypertension. Hypotension may occur after the administration of any of the calcium channel blockers, particularly when administered IV. Other side effects may include atrioventricular block, bradycardia, and constipation.

PHARMACOLOGY
Self-Administration of Nitroglycerin

Most patients with angina pectoris must self-administer nitroglycerin on an as-needed basis. A key nursing role in such cases is educating patients about the medication and how to take it. Sublingual nitroglycerin comes in tablet and spray forms.

- Instruct the patient to make sure the mouth is moist, the tongue is still, and saliva is not swallowed until the nitroglycerin tablet dissolves. If the pain is severe, the patient can crush the tablet between the teeth to hasten sublingual absorption.
- Advise the patient to carry the medication at all times as a precaution. However, because nitroglycerin is very unstable, it should be carried securely in its original container (e.g., capped dark glass bottle); tablets should never be removed and stored in metal or plastic pillboxes.
- Explain that nitroglycerin is volatile and is inactivated by heat, moisture, air, light, and time. Instruct the patient to renew the nitroglycerin supply every 6 months.

- Inform the patient that the medication should be taken in anticipation of any activity that may produce pain. Because nitroglycerin increases tolerance for exercise and stress when taken prophylactically (i.e., before angina-producing activity, such as exercise, stair-climbing, or sexual intercourse), it is best taken before pain develops.
- Recommend that the patient note how long it takes for the nitroglycerin to relieve the discomfort. Advise the patient that if pain persists after taking three sublingual tablets at 5-minute intervals, emergency medical services should be called.
- Discuss possible side effects of nitroglycerin, including flushing, throbbing headache, hypotension, and tachycardia.
- Advise the patient to sit down for a few minutes when taking nitroglycerin to avoid hypotension and syncope.

Antiplatelet and Anticoagulant Medications

Antiplatelet medications are administered to prevent platelet aggregation and subsequent thrombosis, which impedes blood flow through the coronary arteries.

Aspirin. Aspirin prevents platelet aggregation and reduces the incidence of MI and death in patients with CAD. A 162- to 325-mg dose of aspirin should be given to the patient with a new diagnosis of angina and then continued with 81 to 325 mg daily. Patients should be advised to continue aspirin even if they concurrently take other analgesics such as acetaminophen (Tylenol). Because aspirin may cause GI upset and bleeding, the use of histamine-2 (H$_2$) blockers (e.g., famotidine [Pepcid]) or proton pump inhibitors (e.g., omeprazole [Prilosec]) should be considered concomitant with continued aspirin therapy (Aschenbrenner & Venable, 2012).

Thienopyridines. These medications act on different pathways than aspirin to block platelet activation (Fletcher & Thalinger, 2010). However, unlike aspirin, these agents may take a few days to achieve antiplatelet effects. Clopidogrel (Plavix) is commonly prescribed in addition to aspirin in patients at high risk for MI. A new thienopyridine, prasugrel (Effient), may be used in place of clopidogrel during coronary events and interventions. Both carry the risk of bleeding from the GI tract or other sites (Martin, Spinler, & Nutescu, 2011).

Heparin. Unfractionated IV heparin prevents the formation of new blood clots (i.e., it is an anticoagulant). Treating patients with unstable angina with heparin reduces the occurrence of MI. If the patient's signs and symptoms indicate a significant risk for a cardiac event, the patient is hospitalized and may be given an IV bolus of heparin and started on a continuous infusion. The amount of heparin administered is based on the results of the activated partial thromboplastin time (aPTT). Heparin therapy is usually considered therapeutic when the aPTT is 2 to 2.5 times the normal aPTT value.

A subcutaneous injection of low-molecular-weight heparin (LMWH; enoxaparin [Lovenox] or dalteparin [Fragmin]) may be used instead of IV unfractionated heparin to treat patients with unstable angina or non–ST-segment elevation myocardial infarction (NSTEMI) (Wright, Anderson, Adams, et al., 2011). LMWH provides effective and stable anticoagulation, potentially reducing the risk of rebound ischemic events, and eliminating the need to monitor aPTT results. LMWHs may be beneficial before and during PCIs as well as for ACS.

Because unfractionated heparin and LMWH increase the risk of bleeding, the patient is monitored for signs and symptoms of external and internal bleeding, such as low blood pressure, increased heart rate, and decreased serum hemoglobin and hematocrit. The patient receiving heparin is placed on bleeding precautions, which include:

- Applying pressure to the site of any needle puncture for a longer time than usual
- Avoiding intramuscular (IM) injections
- Avoiding tissue injury and bruising from trauma or use of constrictive devices (e.g., continuous use of an automatic blood pressure cuff)

A decrease in platelet count or evidence of thrombosis may indicate heparin-induced thrombocytopenia (HIT), an antibody-mediated reaction to heparin that may result in thrombosis (Fennessy-Cooney, 2011). Patients who have received heparin within the past 3 months and those who have been receiving unfractionated heparin for 5 to 15 days are at high risk for HIT. (See Chapter 33 for further discussion of HIT.)

Glycoprotein IIb/IIIa Agents. IV administration of glycoprotein (GP) IIb/IIIa agents, such as abciximab (ReoPro) or eptifibatide (Integrilin), is indicated for hospitalized patients with unstable angina and as adjunct therapy for PCI. These agents prevent platelet aggregation by blocking the GP IIb/IIIa receptors on the platelets, preventing adhesion of fibrinogen and other factors that crosslink platelets to each other and thus form intracoronary clots. As with heparin, bleeding is the major side effect, and bleeding precautions should be initiated.

Oxygen Administration

Oxygen therapy is usually initiated at the onset of chest pain in an attempt to increase the amount of oxygen delivered to the myocardium and to decrease pain. The therapeutic effectiveness of oxygen is determined by observing the rate and rhythm of respirations and the color of skin and mucous membranes. Blood oxygen saturation is monitored by pulse oximetry; the normal oxygen saturation (SpO$_2$) level is greater than 90%.

NURSING PROCESS

The Patient With Angina Pectoris

Assessment

The nurse gathers information about the patient's symptoms and activities, especially those that precede and precipitate attacks of angina pectoris. Appropriate questions are listed in Chart 27-4. The answers to these questions form the basis for designing an effective program of treatment and prevention. In addition to assessing angina pectoris or its equivalent, the nurse also assesses the patient's risk factors for CAD, the patient's response to angina, the patient's and family's understanding of the diagnosis, and adherence to the current treatment plan.

Diagnosis

Nursing Diagnoses

Based on the assessment data, major nursing diagnoses may include:

- Risk for decreased cardiac tissue perfusion
- Anxiety related to cardiac symptoms and possible death
- Deficient knowledge about the underlying disease and methods for avoiding complications
- Noncompliance, ineffective management of therapeutic regimen related to failure to accept necessary lifestyle changes

Collaborative Problems/Potential Complications

Potential complications may include the following:

- ACS and/or MI (described later in this chapter)
- Dysrhythmias and cardiac arrest (see Chapters 26 and 29)
- Heart failure (see Chapter 29)
- Cardiogenic shock (see Chapter 14)

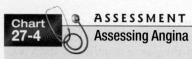

Chart 27-4

ASSESSMENT

Assessing Angina

Ask the following:

- "Where is the pain (or prodromal symptoms)? Can you point to it?"
- "Can you feel the pain anywhere else?"
- "How would you describe the pain?"
- "Is it like the pain you had before?"
- "Can you rate the pain on a 0 to 10 scale, with 10 being the most pain?"
- "When did the pain begin?"
- "How long does it last?"
- "What brings on the pain?"
- "What helps the pain go away?"
- "Do you have any other symptoms with the pain?"

Planning and Goals

Major patient goals include immediate and appropriate treatment when angina occurs, prevention of angina, reduction of anxiety, awareness of the disease process and understanding of the prescribed care, adherence to the self-care program, and absence of complications.

Nursing Interventions

Treating Angina

If the patient reports pain (or cardiac ischemia is suggested by prodromal symptoms, which may include sensations of indigestion or nausea, choking, heaviness, weakness or numbness in the upper extremities, dyspnea, or dizziness), the nurse takes immediate action. The patient experiencing angina is directed to stop all activities and sit or rest in bed in a semi-Fowler's position to reduce the oxygen requirements of the ischemic myocardium. The nurse assesses the patient's angina, asking questions to determine whether the angina is the same as the patient typically experiences. A change may indicate a worsening of the disease or a different cause. The nurse then continues to assess the patient, measuring vital signs and observing for signs of respiratory distress. If the patient is in the hospital, a 12-lead ECG is usually obtained and assessed for ST-segment and T-wave changes. If the patient has been placed on cardiac monitoring with continuous ST-segment monitoring, the ST segment is assessed for changes.

Nitroglycerin is administered sublingually, and the patient's response is assessed (relief of chest pain and effect on blood pressure and heart rate). If the chest pain is unchanged or is lessened but still present, nitroglycerin administration is repeated up to three doses. Each time blood pressure, heart rate, and the ST segment (if the patient is on a monitor with ST-segment monitoring capability) are assessed. The nurse administers oxygen therapy if the patient's respiratory rate is increased or if the oxygen saturation level is decreased. Oxygen is usually administered at 2 L/min by nasal cannula, even without evidence of desaturation, although there is no current evidence of a positive effect on patient outcome. If the pain is significant and continues after these interventions, the patient is further evaluated for acute MI and may be transferred to a higher-acuity nursing unit.

Reducing Anxiety

Patients with angina often fear loss of their roles within society and the family. They may also fear that the pain (or the pro-

dromal symptoms) may lead to an MI or death. Exploring the implications that the diagnosis has for the patient and providing information about the illness, its treatment, and methods of preventing its progression are important nursing interventions. Various stress reduction methods, such as guided imagery or music therapy, should be explored with the patient. Addressing the spiritual needs of the patient and family may also assist in allaying anxieties and fears (Chang, Aggie, Dusek, et al., 2010).

Preventing Pain

The nurse reviews the assessment findings, identifies the level of activity that causes the patient's pain or prodromal symptoms, and plans the patient's activities accordingly. If the patient has pain frequently or with minimal activity, the nurse alternates the patient's activities with rest periods. Balancing activity and rest is an important aspect of the educational plan for the patient and family.

Promoting Home and Community-Based Care

Educating Patients About Self-Care. The program for educating the patient with angina is designed so that the patient and family understand the illness, identify the symptoms of myocardial ischemia, state the actions to take when symptoms develop, and discuss methods to prevent chest pain and the advancement of CAD. The goals of education are to reduce the frequency and severity of anginal attacks, to delay the progress of the underlying disease if possible, and to prevent complications. The factors outlined in Chart 27-5 are important in educating the patient with angina pectoris.

The self-care program is prepared in collaboration with the patient and family or friends. Activities should be planned to minimize the occurrence of anginal episodes. The patient needs to understand that any pain unrelieved within 15 minutes by the usual methods, including nitroglycerin (see Chart 27-3), should be treated at the closest ED; the patient should call 911 for assistance.

Continuing Care. For patients with disabilities or special needs, arrangements are made for a home care nurse when appropriate. The home care nurse assists the patient with scheduling and keeping follow-up appointments. The patient may need reminders about follow-up monitoring, including periodic laboratory testing. In addition, the home care nurse may monitor the patient's adherence to dietary restrictions and to prescribed antianginal medications, including nitroglycerin. If the patient has severe anginal symptoms, the nurse may assess the home environment and recommend modifications that diminish the occurrence of anginal episodes. For instance, if a patient cannot climb stairs without experiencing ischemia, the home care nurse may help the patient plan daily activities that minimize stair-climbing.

Evaluation

Expected patient outcomes may include:

1. Reports that pain is relieved promptly
   a. Recognizes symptoms
   b. Takes immediate action
   c. Seeks medical assistance if pain persists or changes in quality
2. Reports decreased anxiety
   a. Expresses acceptance of diagnosis
   b. Expresses control over choices within medical regimen

HOME CARE CHECKLIST

Chart 27-5 | Managing Angina Pectoris

At the completion of home care education, the patient or caregiver will be able to:	PATIENT	CAREGIVER
• Reduce the probability of an episode of anginal pain by balancing rest with activity.	✔	
• Participate in a regular daily program of activities that do not produce chest discomfort, shortness of breath, or undue fatigue.	✔	
• Follow the prescribed exercise regimen.	✔	
• Recognize that temperature extremes (particularly cold) may induce anginal pain; therefore, avoid exercise in temperature extremes.	✔	
• Alternate activity with periods of rest.	✔	
• Use appropriate resources for support during emotionally stressful times (e.g., counselor, nurse, clergy, physician).	✔	✔
• Avoid using medications or any over-the-counter substances (e.g., diet pills, nasal decongestants) that can increase the heart rate and blood pressure without first discussing with a health care provider.	✔	✔
• Stop smoking and the use of other forms of tobacco, and avoid secondhand smoke (because smoking increases the heart rate, blood pressure, and blood carbon monoxide levels).	✔	✔
• Follow a diet low in saturated fat, high in fiber, and, if indicated, lower in calories.	✔	✔
• Achieve and maintain normal blood pressure.	✔	
• Achieve and maintain normal blood glucose levels.	✔	
• Take medications, especially aspirin and beta-blockers, as prescribed.	✔	
• Carry nitroglycerin at all times; state when and how to use it; identify its side effects.	✔	✔
• Make and keep follow-up appointments.	✔	✔
• Report increase in symptoms to health care provider.	✔	✔

c. Does not exhibit signs and symptoms that indicate a high level of anxiety
3. Understands ways to avoid complications and is free of complications
   a. Describes the process of angina
   b. Explains reasons for measures to prevent complications
   c. Exhibits stable ECG
   d. Experiences no signs and symptoms of acute MI
4. Adheres to self-care program
   a. Takes medications as prescribed
   b. Keeps health care appointments
   c. Implements plan to reduce risk factors

Acute Coronary Syndrome and Myocardial Infarction

Acute coronary syndrome (ACS) is an emergent situation characterized by an acute onset of myocardial ischemia that results in myocardial death (i.e., MI) if definitive interventions do not occur promptly. (Although the terms *coronary occlusion*, *heart attack*, and *myocardial infarction* are used synonymously, the preferred term is *myocardial infarction*.) The spectrum of ACS includes unstable angina, NSTEMI, and ST-segment elevation myocardial infarction (STEMI).

Pathophysiology

In unstable angina, there is reduced blood flow in a coronary artery, often due to rupture of an atherosclerotic plaque. A clot begins to form on top of the coronary lesion, but the artery is not completely occluded. This is an acute situation that can result in chest pain and other symptoms that may be referred to as preinfarction angina because the patient will likely have an MI if prompt interventions do not occur.

In an MI, plaque rupture and subsequent thrombus formation result in complete occlusion of the artery, leading to ischemia and necrosis of the myocardium supplied by that artery. Vasospasm (sudden constriction or narrowing) of a coronary artery, decreased oxygen supply (e.g., from acute blood loss, anemia, or low blood pressure), and increased demand for oxygen (e.g., from a rapid heart rate, thyrotoxicosis, or ingestion of cocaine) are other causes of MI. In each case, a profound imbalance exists between myocardial oxygen supply and demand.

The area of infarction develops over minutes to hours. As the cells are deprived of oxygen, ischemia develops, cellular injury occurs, and the lack of oxygen results in infarction, or the death of cells. The expression "time is muscle" reflects the urgency of appropriate treatment to improve patient outcomes. Each year in the United States, 785,000 people have acute MIs and many of these people die as a result (Roger et al., 2011). Many of those who die never reach a hospital.

Various descriptions are used to further identify an MI: the type (NSTEMI, STEMI), the location of the injury to the ventricular wall (anterior, inferior, posterior, or lateral wall), and the point in time within the process of infarction (acute, evolving, or old). The differentiation between NSTEMI and STEMI are determined by diagnostic tests and are explained later in this chapter.

The 12-lead ECG identifies the type and location of the MI, and other ECG indicators, such as a Q wave and patient history, identify the timing. Regardless of the location, the goals of medical therapy are to relieve symptoms, prevent or minimize myocardial tissue death, and prevent complications. The pathophysiology of CAD and the risk factors involved were discussed earlier in this chapter.

Clinical Manifestations

Chest pain that occurs suddenly and continues despite rest and medication is the presenting symptom in most patients with ACS. Some of these patients have prodromal symptoms or a previous diagnosis of CAD, but about half report no previous symptoms (Overbaugh, 2009). Patients may present with a combination of symptoms, including chest pain, shortness of breath, indigestion, nausea, and anxiety. They may have cool, pale, and moist skin. Their heart rate and respiratory rate may be faster than normal. These signs and symptoms, which are caused by stimulation of the sympathetic nervous system, may be present for only a short time or may persist. In many cases, the signs and symptoms of MI cannot be distinguished from those of unstable angina; hence, the evolution of the term *acute coronary syndrome*.

Assessment and Diagnostic Findings

The diagnosis of ACS is generally based on the presenting symptoms (Chart 27-6); the 12-lead ECG and laboratory tests (e.g., serial cardiac biomarkers) are performed to clarify whether the patient has unstable angina, NSTEMI, or STEMI (ICSI, 2012b). The prognosis depends on the severity of coronary artery obstruction and the presence and extent of myocardial damage. Physical examination is always conducted, but the examination alone does not confirm the diagnosis.

Patient History

The patient history includes the description of the presenting symptom (e.g., pain), the history of previous cardiac and other illnesses, and the family history of heart disease. The history should also include information about the patient's risk factors for heart disease.

Electrocardiogram

The 12-lead ECG provides information that assists in ruling out or diagnosing an acute MI. It should be obtained within 10 minutes from the time a patient reports pain or arrives in the ED. By monitoring serial ECG changes over time, the location, evolution, and resolution of an MI can be identified and monitored.

The ECG changes that occur with an MI are seen in the leads that view the involved surface of the heart. The expected ECG changes are T-wave inversion, ST-segment elevation, and development of an abnormal Q wave (Fig. 27-5). Because infarction evolves over time, the ECG also changes over time. The first ECG signs of an acute MI are usually seen in the T wave and ST segment (Porth, 2011). As the area of injury becomes ischemic, myocardial repolarization is altered and delayed, causing the T wave to invert. Myocardial injury also causes ST-segment changes. The ST segment is normally flat on the ECG tracing. The injured myocardial cells depolarize normally but repolarize more rapidly than normal cells, causing the ST segment to rise at least 1 mm above the isoelectric line (the area between the T wave and the next P wave is used as the reference for the isoelectric line). This change is measured 0.06 to 0.08 seconds after the end of the QRS—a point called the *J point* (Sinz & Navarro, 2011) (Fig. 27-6). An elevation in the ST segment in two contiguous leads is a key diagnostic indicator for MI (i.e., STEMI).

The appearance of abnormal Q waves is another indication of MI. Q waves develop within 1 to 3 days because there is no depolarization current conducted from necrotic tissue

---

Chart 27-6

⚕ ASSESSMENT

Assessing for Acute Coronary Syndrome or Acute Myocardial Infarction

Be alert for the following signs and symptoms:

Cardiovascular

- Chest pain or discomfort not relieved by rest or nitroglycerin; palpitations. Heart sounds may include S_3, S_4, and new onset of a murmur.
- Increased jugular venous distention may be seen if the myocardial infarction (MI) has caused heart failure.
- Blood pressure may be elevated because of sympathetic stimulation or decreased because of decreased contractility, impending cardiogenic shock, or medications.
- Irregular pulse may indicate atrial fibrillation.
- In addition to ST-segment and T-wave changes, the electrocardiogram may show tachycardia, bradycardia, or other dysrhythmias.

Respiratory

Shortness of breath, dyspnea, tachypnea, and crackles if MI has caused pulmonary congestion. Pulmonary edema may be present.

Gastrointestinal

Nausea, indigestion, and vomiting

Genitourinary

Decreased urinary output may indicate cardiogenic shock.

Skin

Cool, clammy, diaphoretic, and pale appearance due to sympathetic stimulation may indicate cardiogenic shock.

Neurologic

Anxiety, restlessness, and lightheadedness may indicate increased sympathetic stimulation or a decrease in contractility and cerebral oxygenation. The same symptoms may also herald cardiogenic shock.

Psychological

Fear with feeling of impending doom, or denial that anything is wrong.

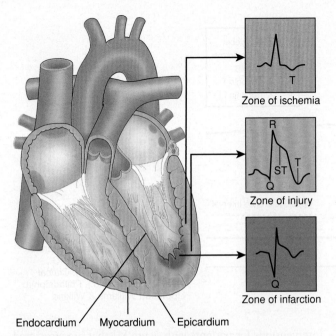

Zone of ischemia

Zone of injury

Zone of infarction

Endocardium Myocardium Epicardium

FIGURE 27-5 • Effects of ischemia, injury, and infarction on an electrocardiogram recording. Ischemia causes inversion of the T wave because of altered repolarization. Cardiac muscle injury causes elevation of the ST segment. Later, Q waves develop because of the absence of depolarization current from the necrotic tissue and opposing currents from other parts of the heart.

(Porth, 2011). The lead system then views the flow of current from other parts of the heart. A new and significant Q wave is 0.04 seconds or longer and 25% of the R wave depth. An acute MI may also cause a significant decrease in the height of the R wave. During an acute MI, injury and ischemic changes are usually present. An abnormal Q wave may be present without ST-segment and T-wave changes, which indicates an old, not acute, MI. For some patients, there are no persistent ST elevation or other ECG changes; therefore, an NSTEMI is diagnosed by blood levels of cardiac biomarkers.

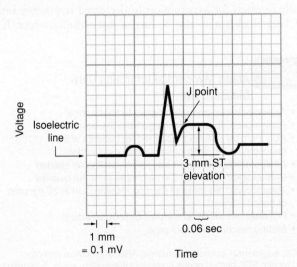

J point

Voltage

Isoelectric line

3 mm ST elevation

1 mm = 0.1 mV

0.06 sec

Time

FIGURE 27-6 • Using the electrocardiogram to diagnose acute myocardial infarction (MI). (ST-segment elevation is measured 0.06 to 0.08 seconds after the J point. An elevation of more than 1 mm in contiguous leads is indicative of acute MI.)

Using the information presented, patients are diagnosed with one of the following forms of ACS:

- *Unstable angina:* The patient has clinical manifestations of coronary ischemia, but ECG and cardiac biomarkers show no evidence of acute MI.
- *STEMI:* The patient has ECG evidence of acute MI with characteristic changes in two contiguous leads on a 12-lead ECG. In this type of MI, there is significant damage to the myocardium.
- *NSTEMI:* The patient has elevated cardiac biomarkers (e.g., troponin) but no definite ECG evidence of acute MI. In this type of MI, there may be less damage to the myocardium.

During recovery from an MI, the ST segment often is the first ECG indicator to return to normal. Q-wave alterations are usually permanent. An old STEMI is usually indicated by an abnormal Q wave or decreased height of the R wave without ST-segment and T-wave changes.

Echocardiogram

The echocardiogram is used to evaluate ventricular function. It may be used to assist in diagnosing an MI, especially when the ECG is nondiagnostic. The echocardiogram can detect hypokinetic and akinetic wall motion and can determine the ejection fraction (see Chapter 25).

Laboratory Tests

Cardiac enzymes and biomarkers, which include troponin, creatine kinase (CK), and myoglobin, are used to diagnose an acute MI. Cardiac biomarkers can be analyzed rapidly, expediting an accurate diagnosis. These tests are based on the release of cellular contents into the circulation when myocardial cells die. Figure 27-7 shows the time courses of cardiac enzymes and biomarkers.

Troponin

Troponin, a protein found in myocardial cells, regulates the myocardial contractile process. There are three isomers of troponin: C, I, and T. Troponins I and T are specific for cardiac muscle, and these biomarkers are currently recognized as reliable and critical markers of myocardial injury (ICSI, 2012b). An increase in the level of troponin in the serum can be detected within a few hours during acute MI. It remains elevated for a long period, often as long as 3 weeks, and it therefore can be used to detect recent myocardial damage.

Creatine Kinase and Its Isoenzymes

There are three CK isoenzymes: CK-MM (skeletal muscle), CK-MB (heart muscle), and CK-BB (brain tissue). CK-MB is the cardiac-specific isoenzyme; it is found mainly in cardiac cells and therefore increases when there has been damage to these cells. Elevated CK-MB is an indicator of acute MI; the level begins to increase within a few hours and peaks within 24 hours of an infarct.

Myoglobin

Myoglobin is a heme protein that helps transport oxygen. Like the CK-MB enzyme, myoglobin is found in cardiac and skeletal muscle. The myoglobin level starts to increase within 1 to 3 hours and peaks within 12 hours after the onset of symptoms. An increase in myoglobin is not very specific in

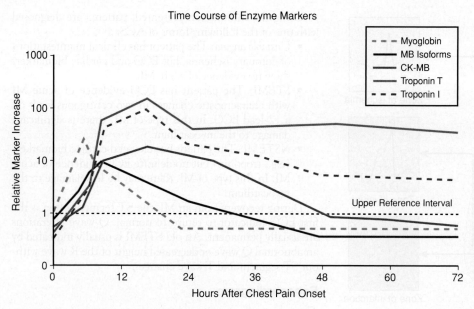

Time Course of Enzyme Markers

FIGURE 27-7 • Peak elevation and duration of serum enzymes and biomarkers after acute myocardial infarction. From Morton, P. G., & Fontaine, D. K. (2009). *Critical care nursing* (9th ed.). Philadelphia: Lippincott Williams & Wilkins.

indicating an acute cardiac event; however, negative results can be used to rule out an acute MI.

Medical Management

The goals of medical management are to minimize myocardial damage, preserve myocardial function, and prevent complications. These goals are facilitated by the use of guidelines developed by the American College of Cardiology (ACC) and the AHA (Chart 27-7). In addition, the Joint Commission (2011) promotes adherence to a set of Core Measures or interventions for patients with acute MI that are associated with improved patient outcomes (Chart 27-8).

The goals for treating patients with acute MI may be achieved by interventions that reestablish coronary flow. Minimizing myocardial damage is also accomplished by reducing myocardial oxygen demand and increasing oxygen supply with medications, oxygen administration, and bed rest. The resolution of pain and ECG changes indicate that demand and supply are in equilibrium; they may also indicate reperfusion. Visualization of blood flow through an open vessel in the catheterization laboratory is evidence of reperfusion.

Initial Management

The patient with suspected MI should immediately receive supplemental oxygen, aspirin, nitroglycerin, and morphine. Morphine is the drug of choice to reduce pain and anxiety. It also reduces preload and afterload, decreasing the work of the heart. The response to morphine is monitored carefully to assess for hypotension or decreased respiratory rate. A beta-blocker may also be used if dysrhythmias occur. If a

---

Chart 27-7 Treatment Guidelines for Acute Myocardial Infarction

- Use rapid transit to the hospital.
- Obtain 12-lead electrocardiogram to be read within 10 minutes.
- Obtain laboratory blood specimens of cardiac biomarkers, including troponin.
- Obtain other diagnostics to clarify the diagnosis.
- Begin routine medical interventions:
  - Supplemental oxygen
  - Nitroglycerin
  - Morphine
  - Aspirin 162–325 mg
  - Beta-blocker
  - Angiotensin-converting enzyme inhibitor within 24 hours
  - Anticoagulation with heparin and platelet inhibitors
- Evaluate for indications for reperfusion therapy:
  - Percutaneous coronary intervention
  - Thrombolytic (fibrinolytic) therapy
- Continue therapy as indicated:
  - IV heparin, low-molecular-weight heparin, bivalirudin, or fondaparinux
  - Clopidogrel (Plavix)
  - Glycoprotein IIb/IIIa inhibitor
  - Bed rest for a minimum of 12–24 hours

Adapted from Institute for Clinical Systems Improvement. (2012b). *Diagnosis and treatment of chest pain and acute coronary syndrome (ACS)*. Available at: www.guideline.gov/content.aspx?id=39320&search=chest+pain+and+acute+coronary+syndrome

---

Chart 27-8 Acute Myocardial Infarction Core Measure Set

- Aspirin administered upon arrival to the hospital
- Aspirin prescribed at discharge from the hospital
- ACE inhibitor or ARB prescribed for patients with concomitant left ventricular systolic dysfunction
- Adult smoking cessation advice/counseling as needed
- Beta-blocker prescribed at discharge from the hospital
- Thrombolytic (fibrinolytic) therapy received within 30 minutes of hospital arrival
- PCI received within 90 minutes of hospital arrival
- Statin prescribed at discharge

ACE, angiotensin-converting enzyme; ARB, angiotensin receptor blocker; PCI, percutaneous coronary intervention; statin, 3-hydroxy-3-methylglutaryl coenzyme A (HMG-CoA).
Adapted from Joint Commission. (2011). *Acute myocardial infarction Core Measure set*. Available at: www.jointcommission.org/assets/1/6/Acute%20Myocardial%20Infarction.pdf

Chart
27-9

ETHICAL DILEMMA

Should Invasive Therapy Be Recommended for Older Adults With Acute Coronary Syndrome?

Case Scenario

An 80-year-old woman is hospitalized with acute coronary syndrome (ACS). When discussing the situation with her two adult sons, the cardiologist recommends emergent cardiac catheterization with a possible percutaneous coronary intervention (PCI). The patient has full capacity to make her own decisions but wishes to defer decision making to her sons regarding treatment decisions. One son worries that she will be subjected to an invasive procedure that is potentially high risk, painful, expensive, and possibly futile. The second son feels that if there is hope of success, then she should have the procedure.

Discussion

Many patients who present with ACS are older adults. They often have chronic conditions such as diabetes or arthritis. Older patients have traditionally been managed conservatively with medications. Currently, however, invasive interventions such as cardiac catheterization and PCI may be recommended. Indeed, studies suggest that older patients may benefit as much, if not more, than younger patients from coronary reperfusion procedures in terms of reduction of death or myocardial infarction (Ionescu, Amuchastegui, Ionescu, et al., 2010).

Analysis

- Describe the ethical principles that are in conflict in this case (see Chart 3-3). Which principle should have preeminence in recommending the best treatment plan for the patient?
- One son apparently wishes that the patient not be subjected to a procedure that may be futile and painful (wishes to ensure nonmaleficence), whereas the other hopes that the patient has the opportunity for a positive outcome (wishes to assure beneficence). Are these two ethical principles necessarily in conflict with each other in this case? How would you approach the patient and her sons to ensure that they receive the information needed to help them reach consensus regarding the decision that is most consistent in preserving the patient's autonomy?
- What resources are available to help you facilitate this discussion with the patient and her sons?

Reference

Ionescu, C. N., Amuchastegui, M., Ionescu, S., et al. (2010) Treatment and outcomes of nonagenarians with ST-elevation. *Journal of Invasive Cardiology, 22*(10), 479–480.

Resources

See Chapter 3, Chart 3-6 for ethics resources.

---

beta-blocker is not needed in the initial management period, it should be introduced within 24 hours of admission, once hemodynamics have stabilized and it is confirmed that the patient has no contraindications (ICSI, 2011c). Unfractionated heparin or LMWH may also be prescribed along with platelet-inhibiting agents to prevent further clot formation.

Emergent Percutaneous Coronary Intervention

The patient with STEMI is taken directly to the cardiac catheterization laboratory for an immediate PCI (if a cardiac catheterization laboratory is on site). The procedure is used to open the occluded coronary artery and promote reperfusion to the area that has been deprived of oxygen. Superior outcomes have been reported with the use of PCI when compared to thrombolytic (also called *fibrinolytic*) agents (ICSI, 2012b; see the Thrombolytics (Fibrinolytics) section). Early PCI has been shown to be effective in patients of all ages, including those older than 75 years (Chart 27-9). The procedure treats the underlying atherosclerotic lesion. Because the duration of oxygen deprivation determines the number of myocardial cells that die, the time from the patient's arrival in the ED to the time PCI is performed should be less than 60 minutes. This is frequently referred to as door-to-balloon time. A cardiac catheterization laboratory and staff must be available if an emergent PCI is to be performed within this short time. The nursing care related to PCI is presented later in this chapter.

Thrombolytics (Fibrinolytics)

Thrombolytic therapy is initiated when primary PCI is not available or the transport time to a PCI-capable hospital is too long. These agents are administered IV according to a specific protocol (Chart 27-10). The thrombolytic agents used most often are alteplase (Activase) and reteplase (r-PA) and tenecteplase (TNKase). The purpose of **thrombolytics** is to dissolve (i.e., lyse)

the thrombus in a coronary artery (thrombolysis), allowing blood to flow through the coronary artery again (reperfusion), minimizing the size of the infarction and preserving ventricular function. However, although thrombolytics may dissolve the thrombus, they do not affect the underlying atherosclerotic lesion. The patient may be referred for a cardiac catheterization and other invasive procedures following the use of thrombolytic therapy. Thrombolytics should not be used if the patient is bleeding or has a bleeding disorder. They should be administered within 30 minutes of presentation to the hospital (ICSI, 2012b). This is frequently referred to as door-to-needle time.

Inpatient Management

Following PCI or thrombolytic therapy, continuous cardiac monitoring is indicated, preferably in a cardiac intensive care unit (ICU). Continuing pharmacologic management includes aspirin, a beta-blocker, and an angiotensin-converting enzyme (ACE) inhibitor. ACE inhibitors prevent the conversion of angiotensin I to angiotensin II. In the absence of angiotensin II, the blood pressure decreases and the kidneys excrete sodium and fluid (diuresis), decreasing the oxygen demand of the heart. The use of ACE inhibitors in patients after MI decreases mortality rates and prevents remodeling of myocardial cells that is associated with the onset of heart failure. Blood pressure, urine output, and serum sodium, potassium, and creatinine levels need to be monitored closely. If an ACE inhibitor is not suitable, an angiotensin receptor blocker (ARB) should be prescribed (ICSI, 2011c). Nicotine replacement therapy and smoking cessation counseling should also be initiated for smokers.

Cardiac Rehabilitation

After the patient with an MI is free of symptoms, an active rehabilitation program is initiated. Cardiac rehabilitation is an important continuing care program for patients with CAD

PHARMACOLOGY
Chart 27-10 Administration of Thrombolytic (Fibrinolytic) Therapy

Indications

- Chest pain >20 minutes, unrelieved by nitroglycerin
- ST-segment elevation in at least two leads that face the same area of the heart
- <6 hours from onset of pain

Absolute Contraindications

- Active bleeding
- Known bleeding disorder
- History of hemorrhagic stroke
- History of intracranial vessel malformation
- Recent major surgery or trauma
- Uncontrolled hypertension
- Pregnancy

Nursing Considerations

- Minimize the number of times the patient's skin is punctured.
- Avoid intramuscular injections.
- Draw blood for laboratory tests when starting the IV line.
- Start IV lines before thrombolytic therapy; designate one line to use for blood draws.
- Avoid continual use of noninvasive blood pressure cuff.
- Monitor for acute dysrhythmias and hypotension.
- Monitor for reperfusion: resolution of angina or acute ST-segment changes.
- Check for signs and symptoms of bleeding: decrease in hematocrit and hemoglobin values, decrease in blood pressure, increase in heart rate, oozing or bulging at invasive procedure sites, back pain, muscle weakness, changes in level of consciousness, complaints of headache.
- Treat major bleeding by discontinuing thrombolytic therapy and any anticoagulants; apply direct pressure and notify the physician immediately.
- Treat minor bleeding by applying direct pressure if accessible and appropriate; continue to monitor.

that targets risk reduction by providing patient and family education, offering individual and group support, and encouraging physical activity and physical conditioning. The goals of rehabilitation for the patient who has had an MI are to extend life and improve the quality of life. The immediate objectives are to limit the effects and progression of atherosclerosis, return the patient to work and a pre-illness lifestyle, enhance the patient's psychosocial and vocational status, and prevent another cardiac event. Research has shown that cardiac rehabilitation programs increase survival, reduce recurrent events and the need for interventional procedures, and improve quality of life (Savage, Sanderson, Brown, et al., 2011).

Physical conditioning is achieved gradually over time. Many times, patients will "overdo it" in an attempt to achieve their goals too rapidly. Patients are observed for chest pain, dyspnea, weakness, fatigue, and palpitations and are instructed to stop exercise if any of these occur. Patients may also be monitored for an increase in heart rate above the target heart rate, an increase in systolic or diastolic blood pressure of more than 20 mm Hg, a decrease in systolic blood pressure, onset or worsening of dysrhythmias, or ST-segment changes on the ECG.

Cardiac rehabilitation programs are categorized into three phases. Phase I begins with the diagnosis of atherosclerosis, which may occur when the patient is admitted to the hospital for ACS. Because of today's brief hospital lengths of stay, mobilization occurs early and patient education focuses on the essentials of self-care rather than instituting behavioral changes for risk reduction. Priorities for in-hospital education include the signs and symptoms that indicate the need to call 911 (seek emergency assistance), the medication regimen, rest–activity balance, and follow-up appointments with the primary provider. The patient is reassured that although CAD is a lifelong disease and must be treated as such, he or she can likely resume a normal life after an MI. The amount and type of activity recommended at discharge depends on the patient's age, his or her condition before the cardiac event, the extent of the disease, the course of the hospital stay, and the development of any complications.

Phase II occurs after the patient has been discharged. The patient attends sessions three times a week for 4 to 6 weeks but may continue for as long as 6 months. The outpatient program consists of supervised, often ECG-monitored, exercise training that is individualized. At each session, the patient is assessed for the effectiveness of and adherence to the treatment. To prevent complications and another hospitalization, the cardiac rehabilitation staff alerts the referring primary provider to any problems. Phase II cardiac rehabilitation also includes educational sessions for patients and families that are given by cardiologists, exercise physiologists, dietitians, nurses, and other health care professionals. These sessions may take place outside a traditional classroom setting. For instance, a dietitian may take a group of patients to a grocery store to examine labels and meat selections or to a restaurant to discuss menu offerings for a heart-healthy diet.

Phase III is a long-term outpatient program that focuses on maintaining cardiovascular stability and long-term conditioning. The patient is usually self-directed during this phase and does not require a supervised program, although it may be offered. The goals of each phase build on the accomplishments of the previous phase.

NURSING PROCESS

The Patient With Acute Coronary Syndrome

Assessment

One of the most important aspects of care of the patient with ACS is the assessment. It establishes the patient's baseline, identifies the patient's needs, and helps determine the priority of those needs. Systematic assessment includes a careful history, particularly as it relates to symptoms: chest pain or discomfort, difficulty breathing (dyspnea), palpitations, unusual fatigue, faintness (syncope), or other possible indicators of myocardial ischemia. Each symptom must be evaluated with regard to time, duration, and the factors that precipitate the symptom and relieve it, and in comparison with previous symptoms. A focused physical assessment is critical to detect complications and any change in patient status. Chart 27-6 identifies important assessments and possible findings.

Two IV lines are typically placed for any patient with ACS to ensure that access is available for administering emergency medications. Medications are administered IV to achieve rapid onset and to allow for timely adjustment. After the patient's condition stabilizes, IV lines may be changed to a saline lock to maintain IV access.

Diagnosis

Nursing Diagnoses

Based on the clinical manifestations, history, and diagnostic assessment data, major nursing diagnoses may include:

- Acute pain related to increased myocardial oxygen demand and decreased myocardial oxygen supply
- Risk for decreased cardiac tissue perfusion related to reduced coronary blood flow
- Risk for imbalanced fluid volume
- Risk for ineffective peripheral tissue perfusion related to decreased cardiac output from left ventricular dysfunction
- Anxiety related to cardiac event and possible death
- Deficient knowledge about post-ACS self-care

Collaborative Problems/Potential Complications

Potential complications may include the following:

- Acute pulmonary edema (see Chapter 29)
- Heart failure (see Chapter 29)
- Cardiogenic shock (see Chapter 14)
- Dysrhythmias and cardiac arrest (see Chapters 26 and 29)
- Pericardial effusion and cardiac tamponade (see Chapter 29)

Planning and Goals

The major goals for the patient include relief of pain or ischemic signs (e.g., ST-segment changes) and symptoms, prevention of myocardial damage, maintenance of effective respiratory function, maintenance or attainment of adequate tissue perfusion, reduced anxiety, adherence to the self-care program, and early recognition of complications. Care of the patient with ACS who has an uncomplicated MI is summarized in the Plan of Nursing Care (Chart 27-11).

Nursing Interventions

Relieving Pain and Other Signs and Symptoms of Ischemia

Balancing myocardial oxygen supply with demand (e.g., as evidenced by the relief of chest pain) is the top priority in the care of the patient with an ACS. Although administering medications as described previously is required to accomplish this goal, nursing interventions are also important. Collaboration among the patient, nurse, and primary provider is critical in evaluating the patient's response to therapy and in altering the interventions accordingly.

Oxygen should be administered along with medication therapy to assist with relief of symptoms. Administration of oxygen raises the circulating level of oxygen to reduce pain associated with low levels of myocardial oxygen. The route of administration (usually by nasal cannula) and the oxygen

flow rate are documented. A flow rate of 2 to 4 L/min is usually adequate to maintain oxygen saturation levels of 96% to 100% unless chronic pulmonary disease is present.

Vital signs are assessed frequently as long as the patient is experiencing pain and other signs or symptoms of acute ischemia. Physical rest in bed with the head of the bed elevated or in a supportive chair helps decrease chest discomfort and dyspnea. Elevation of the head and torso is beneficial for the following reasons:

- Tidal volume improves because of reduced pressure from abdominal contents on the diaphragm and better lung expansion.
- Drainage of the upper lung lobes improves.
- Venous return to the heart (preload) decreases, reducing the work of the heart.

The pain associated with an acute MI reflects an imbalance in myocardial oxygen supply and demand or ineffective myocardial tissue perfusion. The pain also results in increases in heart rate, respiratory rate, and blood pressure. Promptly relieving the pain helps to reestablish this balance, thus decreasing the workload of the heart and minimizing damage to the myocardium. Relief of pain also helps to reduce the patient's anxiety level, which in turn reduces the sympathetic stress response, leading to a decrease in workload of the already stressed heart.

Improving Respiratory Function

Regular and careful assessment of respiratory function detects early signs of pulmonary complications. The nurse monitors fluid volume status to prevent fluid overload and encourages the patient to breathe deeply and change position frequently to maintain effective ventilation throughout the lungs. Pulse oximetry guides the use of oxygen therapy.

Promoting Adequate Tissue Perfusion

Bed or chair rest during the initial phase of treatment helps reduce myocardial oxygen consumption. This limitation on mobility should remain until the patient is pain free and hemodynamically stable. Skin temperature and peripheral pulses must be checked frequently to monitor tissue perfusion.

Reducing Anxiety

Alleviating anxiety and decreasing fear are important nursing functions that reduce the sympathetic stress response. Less sympathetic stimulation decreases the workload of the heart, which may relieve pain and other signs and symptoms of ischemia.

The development of a trusting and caring relationship with the patient is critical in reducing anxiety. Providing information to the patient and family in an honest and supportive manner encourages the patient to be a partner in care and greatly assists in developing a positive relationship. Other interventions that can be used to reduce anxiety include ensuring a quiet environment, preventing interruptions that disturb sleep, and providing spiritual support consistent with the patient's beliefs. The nurse provides frequent opportunities for the patient to privately share concerns and fears. An atmosphere of acceptance helps the patient know that these concerns and fears are both realistic and normal. Alternative therapies such as pet therapy have been shown to relax patients and reduce anxiety (Coakley & Mahoney, 2009). Many hospitals have developed infection control and

PLAN OF NURSING CARE

Chart 27-11

Care of the Patient With an Uncomplicated Myocardial Infarction

NURSING DIAGNOSIS: Ineffective cardiac tissue perfusion related to reduced coronary blood flow
GOAL: Relief of chest pain/discomfort

Nursing Interventions	Rationale	Expected Outcomes
1. Initially assess, document, and report to the physician the following: a. The patient's description of chest discomfort, including location, intensity, radiation, duration, and factors that affect it; other symptoms such as nausea, diaphoresis, or complaints of unusual fatigue b. The effect of coronary ischemia on perfusion to the heart (e.g., change in blood pressure, heart rhythm), to the brain (e.g., changes in level of consciousness), to the kidneys (e.g., decrease in urine output), and to the skin (e.g., color, temperature) 2. Obtain a 12-lead ECG recording during symptomatic events, as prescribed, to assess for ongoing ischemia. 3. Administer oxygen as prescribed. 4. Administer medication therapy as prescribed, and evaluate the patient's response continuously. 5. Ensure physical rest: head of bed elevated to promote comfort; diet as tolerated; the use of bedside commode; the use of stool softener to prevent straining at stool. Provide a restful environment, and allay fears and anxiety by being calm and supportive. Individualize visitation, based on patient response.	1. These data assist in determining the cause and effect of the chest discomfort and provide a baseline with which post-therapy symptoms can be compared. a. There are many conditions associated with chest discomfort. There are characteristic clinical findings of ischemic pain and symptoms. b. Myocardial infarction (MI) decreases myocardial contractility and ventricular compliance and may produce dysrhythmias. Cardiac output is reduced, resulting in reduced blood pressure and decreased organ perfusion. 2. An ECG during symptoms may be useful in the diagnosis of ongoing ischemia. 3. Oxygen therapy increases the oxygen supply to the myocardium. 4. Medication therapy (nitroglycerin, morphine, beta-blocker, aspirin) is the first line of defense in preserving myocardial tissue. 5. Physical rest reduces myocardial oxygen consumption. Fear and anxiety precipitate the stress response; this results in increased levels of endogenous catecholamines, which increase myocardial oxygen consumption.	• Reports beginning relief of chest discomfort and symptoms • Appears comfortable and is free of pain and other signs or symptoms • Respiratory rate, cardiac rate, and blood pressure return to prediscomfort level • Skin warm and dry • Adequate cardiac output as evidenced by: • Stable/improving electrocardiogram (ECG) • Heart rate and rhythm • Blood pressure • Mentation • Urine output • Serum blood urea nitrogen (BUN) and creatinine • Skin color and temperature • No adverse effects from medications

NURSING DIAGNOSIS: Risk for impaired gas exchange related to left ventricular failure
GOAL: Absence of respiratory distress

Nursing Interventions	Rationale	Expected Outcomes
1. Initially, every 4 hours, and with chest discomfort or symptoms, assess, document, and report to the physician abnormal heart sounds (S_3 and S_4 gallop or new murmur), abnormal breath sounds (particularly crackles), decreased oxygenation, and activity intolerance.	1. These data are useful in diagnosing left ventricular failure. Diastolic filling sounds (S_3 and S_4) result from decreased left ventricular compliance associated with MI. Papillary muscle dysfunction (from infarction of the papillary muscle) can result in mitral regurgitation and a reduction in stroke volume. The presence of crackles (usually at the lung bases) may indicate pulmonary congestion from increased left heart pressures. The association of symptoms and activity can be used as a guide for activity prescription and a basis for patient education.	• No shortness of breath, dyspnea on exertion, orthopnea, or paroxysmal nocturnal dyspnea • Respiratory rate <20 breaths/min with physical activity and 16 breaths/min with rest • Skin color and temperature normal • SpO_2, PaO_2, and $PaCO_2$ within normal limits • Heart rate <100 bpm and >60 bpm, with blood pressure within patient's normal limits • Chest x-ray unchanged • Appears comfortable and rested

PLAN OF NURSING CARE

Chart
27-11
Care of the Patient With an Uncomplicated Myocardial Infarction (continued)

NURSING DIAGNOSIS: Risk for ineffective peripheral tissue perfusion related to decreased cardiac output
GOAL: Maintenance/attainment of adequate tissue perfusion

Nursing Interventions	Rationale	Expected Outcomes
1. Initially, every 4 hours, and with chest discomfort, assess, document, and report to the physician the following: a. Hypotension b. Tachycardia and other dysrhythmia c. Activity intolerance d. Mentation changes (use family input) e. Reduced urine output (<0.5 mL/kg/h) f. Cool, moist, cyanotic extremities, decreased peripheral pulses, prolonged capillary refill	1. These data are useful in determining a low cardiac output state.	• Blood pressure within the patient's normal range • Ideally, normal sinus rhythm without dysrhythmia is maintained, or patient's baseline rhythm is maintained between 60 and 100 bpm without further dysrhythmia. • Prescribed activity is well tolerated. • Remains alert and oriented and without cognitive or behavioral change • Appears comfortable • Urine output >0.5 mL/kg/h • Extremities warm and dry with normal color

NURSING DIAGNOSIS: Anxiety related to cardiac event
GOAL: Reduction of anxiety

Nursing Interventions	Rationale	Expected Outcomes
1. Assess, document, and report to the physician the patient's and family's level of anxiety and coping mechanisms.	1. These data provide information about psychological well-being. Causes of anxiety are variable and individual, and may include acute illness, hospitalization, pain, disruption of activities of daily living at home and at work, changes in role and self-image due to illness, and financial concerns. Because anxious family members can transmit anxiety to the patient, the nurse must also identify strategies to reduce the family's fear and anxiety.	• Reports less anxiety • Patient and family discuss their anxieties and fears about illness and death. • Patient and family appear less anxious. • Appears restful, respiratory rate <16 breaths/min, heart rate <100 bpm without ectopic beats, blood pressure within patient's normal limits, skin warm and dry • Participates actively in a progressive rehabilitation program • Practices stress reduction techniques
2. Assess the need for spiritual counseling and refer as appropriate.	2. If a patient finds support in a religion, spiritual counseling may assist in reducing anxiety and fear.	
3. Assess the need for social service referral.	3. Social services can assist with posthospital care and financial concerns.	

NURSING DIAGNOSIS: Deficient knowledge about post-MI self-care
GOAL: Adheres to the home health care program; chooses lifestyle consistent with heart-healthy recommendations
See Chart 27-12.

safety procedures pertaining to the animals, their handlers, and the patients eligible for pet therapy.

Monitoring and Managing Potential Complications

Complications that can occur after acute MI are caused by the damage that occurs to the myocardium and to the conduction system from reduced coronary blood flow. Because these complications can be life threatening, close monitoring for and early identification of their signs and symptoms are critical (see Chart 27-11).

The nurse monitors the patient closely for changes in cardiac rate and rhythm, heart sounds, blood pressure, chest pain, respiratory status, urinary output, skin color and temperature, mental status, ECG changes, and laboratory values. Any changes in the patient's condition must be reported promptly to the physician and emergency measures instituted when necessary.

Promoting Home and Community-Based Care

Educating Patients About Self-Care. The most effective way to increase the probability that the patient will implement a self-care regimen after discharge is to identify the patient's priorities, provide adequate education about heart-healthy living, and facilitate the patient's involvement in a cardiac rehabilitation program (Hall & Lorenc, 2010). Patient participation in the development of an individualized program enhances the potential for an effective treatment plan (Chart 27-12).

Continuing Care. Depending on the patient's condition and the availability of family assistance, a home care referral may be indicated. The home care nurse assists the patient with scheduling and keeping follow-up appointments and with adhering to the prescribed cardiac rehabilitation

HEALTH PROMOTION
Promoting Health After Myocardial Infarction and Other Acute Coronary Syndromes

To extend and improve the quality of life, a patient who has had a myocardial infarction (MI) must make lifestyle adjustments to promote heart-healthy living. With this in mind, the nurse and patient develop a program to help achieve desired outcomes.

Making Lifestyle Modifications During Convalescence and Healing

Adaptation to an MI is an ongoing process and usually requires some modification of lifestyle. Educate patients to make the following specific modifications:

- Avoid any activity that produces chest pain, extreme dyspnea, or undue fatigue.
- Avoid extremes of heat and cold and walking against the wind.
- Lose weight, if indicated.
- Stop smoking and the use of tobacco; avoid secondhand smoke.
- Develop heart-healthy eating patterns, and avoid large meals and hurrying while eating.
- Modify meals to align with the Therapeutic Lifestyle Changes (TLC) or other recommended diets.
- Adhere to medical regimen, especially in taking medications.
- Follow recommendations that ensure blood pressure and blood glucose are in control.
- Pursue activities that relieve and reduce stress.

Adopting an Activity Program

Additionally, the patient needs to undertake a structured program of activity and exercise for long-term rehabilitation. Advise patients to:

- Engage in a regimen of physical conditioning with a gradual increase in activity duration and then a gradual increase in activity intensity.
- Enroll in a cardiac rehabilitation program.
- Walk daily, increasing distance and time as prescribed.
- Monitor pulse rate during physical activity.
- Avoid physical exercise immediately after a meal.
- Alternate activity with rest periods (some fatigue is normal and expected during convalescence).
- Participate in a daily program of exercise that develops into a program of regular exercise for a lifetime.

Managing Symptoms

The patient must learn to recognize and take appropriate action for recurrent symptoms. Make sure that patients know to do the following:

- Call 911 if chest pressure or pain (or prodromal symptoms) is not relieved in 15 minutes by taking 3 nitroglycerin tablets at 5-minute intervals.
- Contact the physician if any of the following occur: shortness of breath, fainting, slow or rapid heartbeat, swelling of feet and ankles.

---

regimen. The patient may need reminders about follow-up monitoring, including periodic laboratory testing, as well as ongoing assessment of cardiac status. In addition, the home care nurse monitors the patient's adherence to dietary restrictions and to prescribed medications. If the patient is receiving home oxygen, the nurse ensures that the patient is using the oxygen as prescribed and that appropriate home safety measures are maintained. If the patient has evidence of heart failure secondary to an MI, appropriate home care guidelines for the patient with heart failure are followed (see Chapter 29).

Evaluation

Expected patient outcomes may include:

1. Experiences relief of angina
2. Has stable cardiac and respiratory status
3. Maintains adequate tissue perfusion
4. Exhibits decreased anxiety
5. Adheres to a self-care program
6. Has no complications

INVASIVE CORONARY ARTERY PROCEDURES

Methods to reperfuse ischemic myocardial tissue when patients are refractory to more conservative management methods include PCIs and CABG surgery, as noted previously. The following sections discuss specific indications for each of these and the nursing management of patients who are having either PCIs or CABGs.

Percutaneous Coronary Interventions

Types of Procedures

Invasive interventional procedures to treat CAD include PTCA and intracoronary stent implantation. These procedures are classified as **percutaneous coronary interventions (PCIs)**, as they are performed through a skin puncture rather than a surgical incision.

Percutaneous Transluminal Coronary Angioplasty

In **percutaneous transluminal coronary angioplasty (PTCA)**, a balloon-tipped catheter is used to open blocked coronary vessels and resolve ischemia. It is used in patients with angina and as an intervention for ACS. Catheter-based interventions can also be used to open blocked CABGs (see later discussion). The purpose of PTCA is to improve blood flow within a coronary artery by compressing the atheroma. The procedure is attempted when the interventional cardiologist believes that PTCA can improve blood flow to the myocardium.

PTCA is carried out in the cardiac catheterization laboratory. Hollow catheters called *sheaths* are inserted, usually in the femoral artery (and sometimes the radial artery), providing a conduit for other catheters. Catheters are then threaded through the femoral artery, up through the aorta, and into the coronary arteries. Angiography is performed using injected radiopaque contrast agents (commonly called *dye*) to identify the location and extent of the blockage. A balloon-tipped dilation catheter is passed through the sheath and positioned over the lesion (Urden, Stacy, & Lough, 2010). The physician determines the catheter position by examining markers on the balloon that can be seen with fluoroscopy. When the

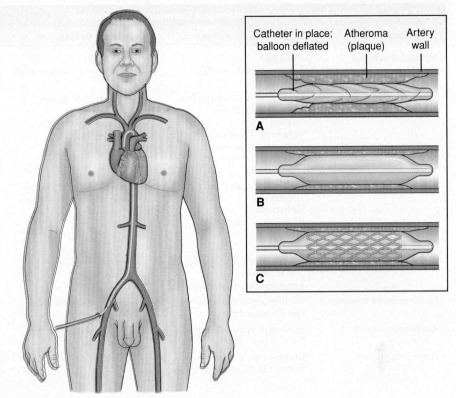

Catheter in place; balloon deflated   Atheroma (plaque)   Artery wall

A

B

C

FIGURE 27-8 • Percutaneous transluminal coronary angioplasty. **A.** A balloon-tipped catheter is passed into the affected coronary artery and placed across the area of the atheroma (plaque). **B.** The balloon is then rapidly inflated and deflated with controlled pressure. **C.** A stent is placed to maintain patency of the artery, and the balloon is removed.

catheter is properly positioned, the balloon is inflated with high pressure for several seconds and then deflated. The pressure compresses and often "cracks" the atheroma (Fig. 27-8). The media and adventitia of the coronary artery are also stretched.

Several inflations and several balloon sizes may be required to achieve the goal, usually defined as an improvement in blood flow and a residual stenosis of less than 20%. Other measures of the success of PTCA are an increase in the artery's lumen and no clinically obvious arterial trauma. Because the blood supply to the coronary artery decreases while the balloon is inflated, the patient may complain of chest pain and the ECG may display ST-segment changes. Intracoronary stents are usually positioned in the intima of the vessel to maintain patency of the artery after the balloon is withdrawn.

Coronary Artery Stent

After PTCA, the area that has been treated may close off partially or completely—a process called *restenosis*. The intima of the coronary artery has been injured and responds by initiating an acute inflammatory process. This process may include release of mediators that leads to vasoconstriction, clotting, and scar tissue formation. A coronary artery stent may be placed to overcome these risks. A **stent** is a metal mesh that provides structural support to a vessel at risk of acute closure. The stent is initially positioned over the angioplasty balloon. When the balloon is inflated, the mesh expands and presses against the vessel wall, holding the artery open. The balloon is withdrawn, but the stent is left permanently in place within the artery (see Fig. 27-8). Eventually, endothelium covers the stent and it is incorporated into the vessel wall. The original stents do not contain medications and are known as bare metal

stents. Some stents are coated with medications, such as sirolimus (Rapamune) or paclitaxel (Taxol), which may minimize the formation of thrombi or scar tissue within the coronary artery lesion. These drug-eluting stents have increased the success of PCI (Greenhalgh, Hockenhull, Rao, et al., 2010). Because of the risk of thrombus formation within the stent, the patient receives antiplatelet medications, usually aspirin and clopidogrel. The clopidogrel is continued for at least a month following placement of a bare metal stent and ideally up to a year following drug-eluting stents (Wright et al., 2011).

Complications

Complications that can occur during a PCI procedure include coronary artery dissection, perforation, abrupt closure, or vasospasm. Additional complications include acute MI, serious dysrhythmias (e.g., ventricular tachycardia), and cardiac arrest. Some of these complications may require emergency surgical treatment. Complications after the procedure may include abrupt closure of the coronary artery and a variety of vascular complications, such as bleeding at the insertion site, retroperitoneal bleeding, hematoma, and arterial occlusion (Bhatty, Cooke, Shettey, et al., 2011). Additionally, there is a risk of acute kidney injury from the contrast agent used during the procedure (Table 27-4).

Postprocedure Care

Patient care is similar to that for a diagnostic cardiac catheterization (see Chapter 25). Patients who are not already hospitalized are admitted the day of the PCI. Those with no complications go home the next day. When the PCI is performed emergently to treat ACS, patients usually go to

TABLE 27-4   Complications After Percutaneous Coronary Interventions

Complication	Clinical Manifestations	Possible Causes	Nursing Actions
Myocardial ischemia	Chest pain Ischemic changes on ECG Dysrhythmias	Thrombosis Restenosis of coronary artery	Administer oxygen and nitroglycerin. Obtain 12-lead ECG. Notify cardiologist.
Bleeding and hematoma formation	Continuation of bleeding from vascular access site Swelling at site Formation of hard lump Pain with leg movement Possible hypotension and tachycardia	Anticoagulant therapy Vascular trauma Inadequate hemostasis Leg movement	Keep patient on bed rest. Apply manual pressure over sheath insertion site. Outline hematoma with marking pen. Notify physician if bleeding continues.
Retroperitoneal hematoma	Back, flank, or abdominal pain Hypotension Tachycardia Restlessness, agitation	Arterial leak of blood into the retroperitoneal space	Notify physician. Stop anticoagulants. Administer IV fluids. Anticipate diagnostic testing (e.g., computed tomography scan). Prepare patient for intervention.
Arterial occlusion	Lost/weakened pulse distal to sheath insertion site Extremity cool, cyanotic, painful	Arterial thrombus or embolus	Notify physician. Anticipate intervention.
Pseudoaneurysm formation	Swelling at vascular access site Pulsatile mass, bruit	Vessel trauma during the procedure	Notify physician. Anticipate intervention.
Arteriovenous fistula formation	Swelling at vascular access site Pulsatile mass, bruit	Vessel trauma during the procedure	Notify physician. Anticipate intervention.
Acute kidney injury	Decreased urine output Elevated BUN, serum creatinine	Nephrotoxic contrast agent	Monitor urine output, BUN, creatinine, electrolytes. Provide adequate hydration. Administer renal protective agents (acetyl-cysteine) before and after procedure as prescribed.

ECG, electrocardiogram; IV, intravenous; BUN, blood urea nitrogen.

a critical care unit and stay in the hospital for a few days. During the PCI, patients receive IV heparin or a thrombin inhibitor (e.g., bivalirudin [Angiomax]) and are monitored closely for signs of bleeding (Vavalle & Rao, 2009). Patients may also receive a GP IIb/IIIa agent (e.g., eptifibatide) for several hours following the PCI to prevent platelet aggregation and thrombus formation in the coronary artery. Hemostasis is achieved, and femoral sheaths may be removed at the end of the procedure by using a vascular closure device (e.g., Angio-Seal, VasoSeal) or a device that sutures the vessels. Hemostasis after sheath removal may also be achieved by direct manual pressure, a mechanical compression device (e.g., C-shaped clamp), or a pneumatic compression device (e.g., FemoStop).

Patients may return to the nursing unit with the large peripheral vascular access sheaths in place. The sheaths are then removed after blood studies (e.g., activated clotting time) indicate that the heparin is no longer active and the clotting time is within an acceptable range. This usually takes a few hours, depending on the amount of heparin given during the procedure. The patient must remain flat in bed and keep the affected leg straight until the sheaths are removed and then for a few hours afterward to maintain hemostasis. Because immobility and bed rest may cause discomfort, treatment may include analgesics and sedation. Sheath removal and the application of pressure on the vessel insertion site may cause the heart rate to slow and the blood pressure to decrease (vasovagal response). A dose of IV atropine is usually given to treat this response.

Some patients with unstable lesions and at high risk for abrupt vessel closure are restarted on heparin after sheath removal, or they receive an IV infusion of a GP IIb/IIIa inhibitor. These patients are monitored closely and may have a delayed recovery period.

After hemostasis is achieved, a pressure dressing is applied to the site. Patients resume self-care and ambulate unassisted within a few hours of the procedure. The duration of immobilization depends on the size of the sheath inserted, the type of anticoagulant administered, the method of hemostasis, the patient's condition, and the physician's preference. On the day after the procedure, the site is inspected and the dressing removed. The patient is instructed to monitor the site for bleeding or development of a hard mass indicative of hematoma.

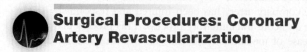

Surgical Procedures: Coronary Artery Revascularization

Advances in diagnostics, medical management, and surgical and anesthesia techniques, as well as the care provided in critical care and surgical units, home care, and rehabilitation programs, have continued to make surgery an effective treatment option for patients with CAD. CAD has been treated by myocardial revascularization since the 1960s, and the most common CABG techniques have been performed for more than 40 years. **Coronary artery bypass graft (CABG)** is a surgical procedure in which a blood vessel is grafted to an occluded coronary artery so that blood can flow beyond the occlusion; it is also called a *bypass graft*.

The major indications for CABG are:
- Alleviation of angina that cannot be controlled with medication or PCI
- Treatment for left main coronary artery stenosis or multivessel CAD
- Prevention of and treatment for MI, dysrhythmias, or heart failure
- Treatment for complications from an unsuccessful PCI

CABG is performed less frequently in women (Parry et al., 2010). Compared with men, women referred for this surgery tend to be older and have more comorbidities such as diabetes. In addition, they have a higher risk of surgical complications and higher operative mortality (Bukkapatnam, Yeo, Li, et al., 2010). Although some women have good outcomes following CABG, men generally have a better rate of graft patency and symptom relief.

The recommendation for CABG for both women and men is determined by a number of factors, including the number of diseased coronary vessels, the degree of left ventricular dysfunction, the presence of other health problems, the patient's symptoms, and any previous treatment. Studies have shown that CABG may be the preferred treatment for patients with triple vessel or left main CAD, because CABG, compared with PCI, results in lower risk of major cardiac or cerebrovascular events (Serruys, Morice, Kappetein, et al., 2009). Studies continue to compare clinical outcomes of CABG and PCI in patients with CAD.

For a patient to be considered for CABG, the coronary arteries to be bypassed must have approximately a 70% occlusion (60% if in the left main coronary artery). If significant blockage is not present, flow through the artery will compete with flow through the bypass, and circulation to the ischemic area of myocardium may not improve. The artery also must be patent beyond the area of blockage or the flow through the bypass will be impeded.

New guidelines recommend that the internal mammary artery should be used for CABG, if possible (Hillis, Smith, Anderson, et al., 2011). Arterial grafts are preferred to venous grafts because they do not develop atherosclerotic changes as quickly and remain patent longer. The surgeon leaves the proximal end of the mammary artery intact and detaches the distal end of the artery from the chest wall. This end of the artery is then grafted to the coronary artery distal to the occlusion. The internal mammary arteries may not be long enough to use for multiple bypasses. Because of this, many CABG procedures are performed with a combination of venous and arterial grafts.

A vein commonly used for CABG is the greater saphenous vein, followed by the lesser saphenous vein (Fig. 27-9). The vein is removed from the leg and grafted to the ascending aorta and to the coronary artery distal to the lesion. Traditionally, a skin incision was made over the length of vein segment, but new techniques allow small leg incisions. Endovascular methods of vein harvesting have reduced complications such as infection and wound dehiscence, which are associated with longer leg incisions (Cadwallader, Walsh, Cooper, et al., 2009). Lower extremity edema continues to be a common adverse effect of vein removal. The degree of edema varies and usually diminishes over time. The patency of vein grafts can be limited. Within 5 to 10 years, atherosclerotic changes often develop in saphenous vein grafts.

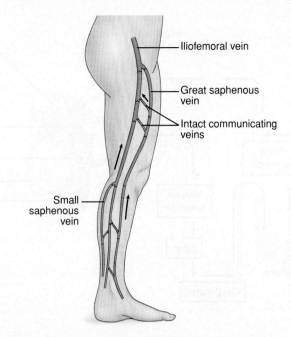

FIGURE 27-9 • The greater and lesser saphenous veins are commonly used in bypass graft procedures.

Traditional Coronary Artery Bypass Graft

CABG procedures are performed with the patient under general anesthesia. In the traditional CABG procedure, the surgeon performs a median sternotomy and connects the patient to the cardiopulmonary bypass (CPB) machine. Next, a blood vessel from another part of the patient's body (e.g., saphenous vein, left internal mammary artery) is grafted distal to the coronary artery lesion, bypassing the obstruction (Fig. 27-10). CPB is then discontinued, chest tubes and epicardial pacing wires are placed, and the incision is closed. The patient is then admitted to a critical care unit.

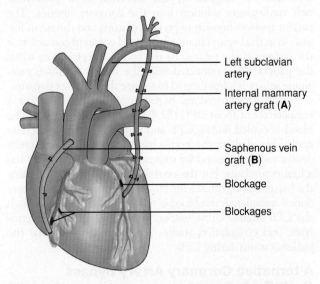

FIGURE 27-10 • Coronary artery bypass grafts. One or more procedures may be performed using various veins and arteries. **A.** Left internal mammary artery, used frequently because of its functional longevity. **B.** Saphenous vein, also used as bypass graft.

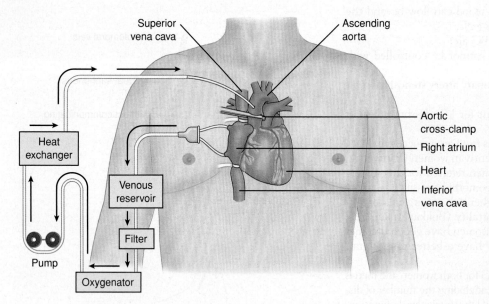

FIGURE 27-11 • The cardiopulmonary bypass system, in which cannulas are placed through the right atrium into the superior and inferior vena cavae to divert blood from the body and into the bypass system. The pump system creates a vacuum, pulling blood into the venous reservoir. The blood is cleared of air bubbles, clots, and particulates by the filter and then is passed through the oxygenator, releasing carbon dioxide and obtaining oxygen. Next, the blood is pulled to the pump and pushed out to the heat exchanger, where its temperature is regulated. The blood is then returned to the body via the ascending aorta.

Cardiopulmonary Bypass

Many cardiac surgical procedures are possible because of CPB (i.e., extracorporeal circulation). The procedure mechanically circulates and oxygenates blood for the body while bypassing the heart and lungs. CPB maintains perfusion to body organs and tissues and allows the surgeon to complete the anastomoses in a motionless, bloodless surgical field.

CPB is accomplished by placing a cannula in the right atrium, vena cava, or femoral vein to withdraw blood from the body. The cannula is connected to tubing filled with an isotonic crystalloid solution. Venous blood removed from the body by the cannula is filtered, oxygenated, cooled or warmed by the machine, and then returned to the body. The cannula used to return the oxygenated blood is usually inserted in the ascending aorta, or it may be inserted in the femoral artery (Fig. 27-11). The heart is stopped by the injection of a potassium-rich cardioplegia solution into the coronary arteries. The patient receives heparin to prevent clotting and thrombus formation in the bypass circuit when blood comes in contact with the surfaces of the tubing. At the end of the procedure when the patient is disconnected from the bypass machine, protamine sulfate is administered to reverse the effects of heparin.

During the procedure, hypothermia is maintained at a temperature of about 28°C (82.4°F) (Urden et al., 2010). The blood is cooled during CPB and returned to the body. The cooled blood slows the body's basal metabolic rate, thereby decreasing the demand for oxygen. Cooled blood usually has a higher viscosity, but the crystalloid solution used to prime the bypass tubing dilutes the blood. When the surgical procedure is completed, the blood is rewarmed as it passes through the CPB circuit. Urine output, arterial blood gases, electrolytes, and coagulation studies are monitored to assess the patient's status during CPB.

Alternative Coronary Artery Bypass Graft Techniques

A number of alternative CABG techniques have been developed that may have fewer complications for some groups of

patients. Off-pump coronary artery bypass (OPCAB) surgery has been used successfully in many patients since the 1990s. OPCAB involves a standard median sternotomy incision, but the surgery is performed without CPB. A beta-adrenergic blocker may be used to slow the heart rate. The surgeon also uses a myocardial stabilization device to hold the site still for the anastomosis of the bypass graft into the coronary artery while the heart continues to beat (Fig. 27-12). Research suggests that OPCAB is associated with reduced short-term postoperative morbidity, including stroke and other complications. However, with on-pump CABG, graft patency rate is higher and long-term mortality may be lower (Shroyer, Grover, Hattler, et al., 2009).

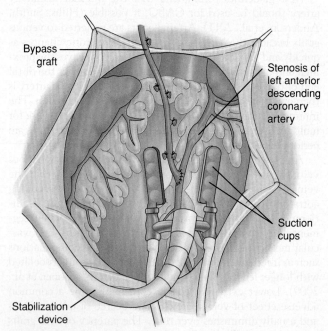

FIGURE 27-12 • Stabilizer device for off-pump coronary artery bypass surgery.

Minimally invasive surgical techniques that eliminate median sternotomy have also been developed. These endoscopic techniques use smaller incisions and a robotic system to place bypass grafts. The patient is placed on CPB via the femoral vessels. Patients who require multiple bypass grafts or grafts to arteries on certain areas of the heart may not be candidates for this technique. Minimally invasive heart surgery has been associated with decreased surgical trauma, shorter length of hospital stay, decreased hospital costs, and overall improvement in patient satisfaction (Iribarne, Karpenko, Russo, et al., 2009).

Complications of Coronary Artery Bypass Graft

CABG may result in complications such as hemorrhage, dysrhythmias, and MI (Table 27-5). The patient may require interventions for more than one complication at a time. Collaboration among nurses, physicians, pharmacists, respiratory therapists, and dietitians is necessary to achieve the desired patient outcomes. Although most patients improve symptomatically following surgery, CABG is not a cure for CAD, and angina, exercise intolerance, or other symptoms experienced before CABG may recur. Medications required before surgery may need to be continued. Lifestyle modifications recommended before surgery remain important to treat the underlying CAD and for the continued viability of the newly implanted grafts.

 Nursing Management

Cardiac surgery patients have many of the same needs and require the same perioperative care as other surgical patients (see Chapters 17 through 19), as well as some special needs.

Preoperative Management

Preoperative education is important; patients and their families may be very anxious as the association of the heart with life and death intensifies their emotions. Before surgery, physical and psychological assessments establish a baseline for future reference. In addition, the patient's understanding of the surgical procedure, informed consent, and adherence to treatment protocols must be evaluated.

Assessing the Patient

Patients are frequently admitted to the hospital the day of the procedure. Therefore, most of the preoperative evaluation is completed in the physician's office and during preadmission testing.

Nursing and medical personnel perform a history and physical examination. Preoperative testing consists of a chest x-ray; ECG; laboratory tests, including coagulation studies; and blood typing and cross-matching. The health assessment focuses on obtaining baseline physiologic, psychological, and social information. Cognitive status is carefully assessed, as patients with impaired cognitive status will need more assistance after surgery and may require subacute care prior to returning home (Harrington, Kraft, Grande, et al., 2011). The patient's and family's learning needs are identified and addressed. Of particular importance are the patient's usual functional level, coping mechanisms, and available support systems. These affect the patient's postoperative course, discharge plans, and rehabilitation.

The preoperative history and health assessment should be thorough and well documented because they provide a basis for postoperative comparison. The nurse assesses the patient for disorders that could complicate or affect the postoperative course, such as diabetes, hypertension, and preexisting disabilities.

The status of the cardiovascular system is determined by reviewing the patient's symptoms, including past and present experiences with chest pain, palpitations, dyspnea, leg pain that occurs with walking (intermittent claudication), and peripheral edema. The patient's history of major illnesses, previous surgeries, medication, and the use of illicit and over-the-counter drugs, herbal supplements, alcohol, and tobacco is also obtained. Particular attention is paid to blood glucose control in patients with diabetes because there is a higher incidence of postoperative complications when glycemic control is poor (Leibowitz, Raizman, Brezis, et al., 2010).

The psychosocial assessment and the assessment of the patient's and family's learning needs are as important as the physical examination. Anticipation of cardiac surgery is a source of great stress to the patient and family, and patients with high anxiety levels have poorer outcomes (Gallagher & McKinley, 2009). However, some anxiety is expected, and the work of worrying can help patients identify priorities and find coping strategies that help them face the threat of surgery. Questions may be asked to obtain the following information:

- Knowledge and understanding of the surgical procedure, postoperative course, and recovery
- Fears and concerns regarding the surgery and future health status
- Coping mechanisms helpful to the patient
- Support systems available during and following hospitalization

Reducing Fear and Anxiety

The nurse gives the patient and family time and opportunity to express their fears. Topics of concern may be pain, changes in body image, fear of the unknown, and fear of disability or death. It may be helpful to describe the sensations that the patient can expect, including the preoperative sedation, surgical anesthesia, and postoperative pain management. The nurse reassures the patient that the fear of pain is normal, that some pain will be experienced, that medication to relieve pain will be provided, and that the patient will be closely monitored. In addition, the nurse instructs the patient to request analgesic medication before the pain becomes severe. If the patient has concerns about scarring from surgery, the nurse encourages him or her to discuss this issue and corrects any misconceptions. The patient and family may want to discuss their fear of the patient dying. After the fear is expressed, the nurse can assure the patient and family that this fear is normal and further explore their feelings.

For patients with extreme anxiety or fear and for whom emotional support and education are not successful, medication may be helpful. The anxiolytic agents most commonly used before cardiac surgery are lorazepam (Ativan) and diazepam (Valium).

Monitoring and Managing Potential Complications

Angina may occur because of increased stress and anxiety related to the forthcoming surgery. The patient who

TABLE 27-5 Potential Complications of Cardiac Surgery

Complication	Cause	Assessment and Management
Cardiac Complications		
Hypovolemia (most common cause of decreased cardiac output after cardiac surgery)	• Net loss of blood and intravascular volume • Vasodilation due to postoperative rewarming • Intravascular fluid loss to the interstitial spaces because surgery and anesthesia increase capillary permeability	• Arterial hypotension, tachycardia, low CVP, and low PAWP are often seen. • Fluid replacement may be prescribed. Replacement fluids include colloid (albumin, hetastarch), packed red blood cells, or crystalloid solution (normal saline, lactated Ringer's solution).
Persistent bleeding	• Cardiopulmonary bypass causes platelet dysfunction, and hypothermia alters clotting mechanisms. • Surgical trauma causes tissues and blood vessels to ooze bloody drainage. • Intraoperative anticoagulant (heparin) therapy • Postoperative coagulopathy may also result from liver dysfunction and depletion of clotting components.	• Accurate measurement of wound bleeding and chest tube blood is essential. Drainage should not exceed 200 mL/h for the first 4–6 hours. Drainage should decrease and stop within a few days, while progressing from serosanguineous to serous. • Serial hemoglobin, hematocrit, and coagulation studies guide therapy. • Administration of blood products: packed red blood cells, fresh frozen plasma, platelet concentrate, recombinant factor VII • Protamine sulfate may be administered to neutralize unfractionated heparin. • Administration of desmopressin acetate (DDAVP) to enhance platelet function • If bleeding persists, the patient may return to the operating room.
Cardiac tamponade	• Fluid and clots accumulate in the pericardial sac, which compress the heart, preventing blood from filling the ventricles.	• Signs and symptoms include arterial hypotension, tachycardia, decreased urine output, and ↑ CVP. Arterial pressure waveform may show pulsus paradoxus (decrease of >10 mm Hg systolic blood pressure during inspiration). • The chest drainage system is checked to eliminate possible kinks or obstructions in the tubing. • Chest x-ray may show a widening mediastinum. • Emergency medical management is required; may include return to surgery.
Fluid overload	• IV fluids and blood products increase circulating volume.	• High CVP and pulmonary artery pressures, as well as crackles, indicate fluid overload. • Diuretics are prescribed, and the rate of IV fluid administration is reduced. • Alternative treatments include continuous renal replacement therapy and dialysis.
Hypothermia	• Low body temperature leads to vasoconstriction, shivering, and arterial hypertension.	• Patient is rewarmed gradually after surgery, decreasing vasoconstriction.
Hypertension	• Results from postoperative vasoconstriction. It may stretch suture lines and cause postoperative bleeding. The condition is usually transient.	• Vasodilators (nitroglycerin [Tridil], nitroprusside [Nipride]) may be used to treat hypertension. Administer cautiously to avoid hypotension.
Tachydysrhythmias	• Increased heart rate is common with perioperative volume changes. Rapid atrial fibrillation commonly occurs during the first few days postoperatively.	• If a tachydysrhythmia is the primary problem, the heart rhythm is assessed and medications (e.g., amiodarone [Cordarone], diltiazem [Cardizem]) may be prescribed. Antidysrhythmic agents (e.g. beta-blockers) are often given before coronary artery bypass graft to minimize the risk. • Carotid massage may be performed by a physician to assist with diagnosing or treating the dysrhythmia. • Cardioversion and defibrillation are alternatives for symptomatic tachydysrhythmias.
Bradycardias	• Decreased heart rate due to surgical trauma and edema affecting the cardiac conduction system	• Many postoperative patients have temporary pacer wires that can be attached to an external pacemaker to stimulate the heart to beat faster. Less commonly, atropine or other medications may be used to increase heart rate.
Cardiac failure	• Myocardial contractility may be decreased perioperatively.	• The nurse observes for and reports signs of heart failure, including hypotension, ↑ CVP, ↑ PAWP, venous distention; labored respirations; and edema. • Medical management includes diuretics and IV inotropic agents.
MI (may occur intraoperatively or postoperatively)	• Portion of the cardiac muscle dies; therefore, contractility decreases. Impaired ventricular wall motion further decreases cardiac output. Symptoms may be masked by the postoperative surgical discomfort or the anesthesia–analgesia regimen.	• Careful assessment to determine the type of pain the patient is experiencing; MI is suspected if the mean blood pressure is low with normal preload. • Serial electrocardiograms and cardiac biomarkers assist in making the diagnosis (alterations may be due to the surgical intervention).

Complication	Cause	Assessment and Management
Pulmonary Complications		
Impaired gas exchange	• During and after anesthesia, patients require mechanical assistance to breathe. • Anesthetic agents stimulate production of mucus, and chest incision pain may decrease the effectiveness of ventilation. • Potential for postoperative atelectasis	• Pulmonary complications are detected during assessment of breath sounds, oxygen saturation levels, arterial blood gases, and ventilator readings. • Extended periods of mechanical ventilation may be required while complications are treated.
Neurologic Complications		
Neurologic changes; stroke	• Thrombi and emboli may cause cerebral infarction, and neurologic signs may be evident when patients recover from anesthesia.	• Inability to follow simple commands within 6 hours of recovery from anesthetic; weakness on one side of body or other neurologic changes may indicate stroke. • Patients who are older or who have renal or hepatic failure may take longer to recover from anesthesia.
Renal Failure and Electrolyte Imbalance		
Acute kidney injury	• May result from hypoperfusion of the kidneys or from injury to the renal tubules by nephrotoxic drugs	• May respond to diuretics or may require continuous renal replacement therapy or dialysis • Fluids, electrolytes, and urine output are monitored frequently. • May result in chronic renal failure and require ongoing dialysis
Electrolyte imbalance	• Postoperative imbalances in potassium, magnesium, sodium, calcium, and blood glucose are related to surgical losses, metabolic changes, and the administration of medications and IV fluids.	• Monitor electrolytes and basic metabolic studies frequently. • Implement treatment to correct electrolyte imbalance promptly (see Chart 27-13).
Other Complications		
Hepatic failure	• Surgery and anesthesia stress the liver. Most common in patients with cirrhosis, hepatitis, or prolonged right-sided heart failure.	• The use of medications metabolized by the liver must be minimized. • Bilirubin and albumin levels are monitored, and nutritional support is provided.
Infection	• Surgery and anesthesia alter the patient's immune system. Multiple invasive devices used to monitor and support the patient's recovery may serve as a source of infection.	• Monitor for signs of possible infection: body temperature, white blood cell and differential counts, incision and puncture sites, urine (clarity, color, and odor), bilateral breath sounds, sputum (color, odor, amount). • Antibiotic therapy may be instituted or modified as necessary. • Invasive devices are discontinued as soon as they are no longer required. Institutional protocols for maintaining and replacing invasive lines and devices are followed to minimize the risk of infection.

CVP, central venous pressure; PAWP, pulmonary artery wedge pressure; ↑, increased; IV, intravenous; MI, myocardial infarction.

develops angina usually responds to typical therapy for angina, most commonly nitroglycerin. Some patients require oxygen and IV nitroglycerin infusions. Physiologically unstable patients may require preoperative management in a critical care unit.

Providing Patient Education

Prior to surgery, patients and their families are given specific instructions. This includes information on how the patient should take or stop specific medications, including anticoagulant agents, antihypertensive medications, and medications that control diabetes. The patient is instructed to shower with an antiseptic solution.

Education also includes information about the hospitalization and surgery. The nurse informs the patient and family about the equipment, tubes, and lines that will be present after surgery and their purposes. They should expect monitors, several IV lines, chest tubes, and a urinary catheter. Explaining the purpose and the approximate time that these devices will be in place helps reassure the patient. Most patients remain intubated and on mechanical ventilation for several hours after surgery. It is important for patients to know that this will prevent them from talking, and the nurse should

reassure them that the staff will be able to assist them with other means of communication.

The nurse takes care to answer the patient's questions about postoperative care and procedures. After the nurse explains deep breathing and coughing, the use of the incentive spirometer, and foot exercises, the nurse practices these procedures with the patient. The benefit of early and frequent ambulation is discussed. The family's questions at this time usually focus on the length of the surgery, who will discuss the results of the procedure with them after surgery, where to wait during the surgery, the visiting procedures for the critical care unit, and how they can support the patient before surgery and in the critical care unit. The nurse should assess the patient's anxiety level before providing education because high levels of anxiety and fear can impact the ability of the patient and family to learn.

Intraoperative Management

The perioperative nurse performs assessments and prepares the patient as described in Chapters 17 and 18. In addition to assisting with the surgical procedure, perioperative nurses are responsible for the comfort and safety of the patient.

Before the chest incision is closed, chest tubes are inserted to evacuate air and drainage from the mediastinum and the thorax. Temporary epicardial pacemaker electrodes may be implanted on the surface of the right atrium and the right ventricle. These epicardial electrodes can be connected to an external pacemaker if the patient has persistent bradycardia perioperatively. Possible intraoperative complications include low cardiac output, dysrhythmias, hemorrhage, MI, stroke, and organ failure from shock, emboli, or adverse drug reactions. Astute intraoperative nursing assessment is critical to prevent, detect, and initiate prompt intervention for these complications.

Postoperative Nursing Management

Initial postoperative care focuses on achieving or maintaining hemodynamic stability and recovery from general anesthesia. Care may be provided in the postanesthesia care unit (PACU) or ICU. The immediate postoperative period for the patient who has undergone cardiac surgery presents many challenges to the health care team. All efforts are made to facilitate the transition from the operating room to the ICU or PACU with minimal risk. Specific information about the surgical procedure and important factors about postoperative management are communicated by the surgical team and anesthesia personnel to the critical care or PACU nurse, who then assumes responsibility for the patient's care. Figure 27-13 presents an overview of the many aspects of postoperative care of the cardiac surgical patient.

After the patient's cardiac status and respiratory status are stable, the patient is transferred to a surgical progressive care unit with telemetry. Care in both the ICU and progressive care unit focuses on monitoring of cardiopulmonary status, pain management, wound care, progressive activity, and nutrition. Education about medications and risk factor modification is emphasized.

A typical plan of postoperative nursing care is presented in Chart 27-13.

Assessing the Patient

When the patient is admitted to the critical care unit or PACU, and hourly for at least every 8 hours thereafter, nursing and medical personnel perform a complete assessment of all systems. It is necessary to assess the following parameters:

Neurologic status: level of responsiveness, pupil size and reaction to light, facial symmetry, movement of the extremities, and hand grip strength

Cardiac status: heart rate and rhythm, heart sounds, pacemaker status, arterial blood pressure, central venous pressure (CVP); in selected patients, hemodynamic parameters: pulmonary artery pressure, pulmonary artery wedge pressure (PAWP), cardiac output and index, systemic and pulmonary vascular resistance, mixed venous oxygen saturation ($S\bar{v}O_2$). A pulmonary artery catheter is often used to monitor these parameters. Alternatively, minimally invasive monitoring of stroke volume, systemic vascular resistance, and cardiac output are calculated through pressures obtained in the arterial line (e.g., Vigileo monitor with FloTrac sensor). (See Chapter 25 for a detailed description of hemodynamic monitoring.)

Respiratory status: chest movement, breath sounds, ventilator settings (e.g., rate, tidal volume, oxygen concentration,

mode such as synchronized intermittent mandatory ventilation, positive end-expiratory pressure, pressure support), respiratory rate, peak inspiratory pressure, arterial oxygen saturation (SaO_2), percutaneous oxygen saturation (SpO_2), end-tidal carbon dioxide (CO_2), pleural chest tube drainage, arterial blood gases. (See Chapters 20 and 21 for detailed descriptions of respiratory assessment and ventilatory management.)

Peripheral vascular status: peripheral pulses; color of skin, nail beds, mucosa, lips, and earlobes; skin temperature; edema; condition of dressings and invasive lines

Renal function: urinary output; serum creatinine and electrolytes

Fluid and electrolyte status: strict intake and output, including all IV fluids and blood products, output from all drainage tubes; clinical and laboratory indicators of imbalance

Pain: nature, type, location, and duration; apprehension; response to analgesics

Assessment also includes checking all equipment and tubes to ensure that they are functioning properly: endotracheal tube, ventilator, end-tidal CO_2 monitor, SpO_2 monitor, pulmonary artery catheter, $S\bar{v}O_2$ monitor, arterial and IV lines, IV infusion devices and tubing, cardiac monitor, pacemaker, chest tubes, and urinary drainage system.

As the patient regains consciousness and progresses through the postoperative period, the nurse also assesses indicators of psychological and emotional status. The patient may exhibit behavior that reflects denial or depression or may experience postoperative delirium. Characteristic signs of delirium include transient perceptual illusions, visual and auditory hallucinations, disorientation, and paranoid delusions (Figueroa-Ramos, Arroyo-Novoa, Lee, et al., 2009).

The family's needs also must be assessed. The nurse ascertains how family members are coping with the situation; determines their psychological, emotional, and spiritual needs; and finds out whether they are receiving adequate information about the patient's condition.

Monitoring for Complications

The patient is continuously assessed for impending complications (see Table 27-5). The nurse and the surgical team function collaboratively to prevent complications, to identify early signs and symptoms of complications, and to institute measures to reverse their progression.

Decreased Cardiac Output. A decrease in cardiac output is always a threat to the patient who has had cardiac surgery, and it can have a variety of causes. Preload alterations occur when too little blood volume returns to the heart as a result of persistent bleeding and hypovolemia. Excessive postoperative bleeding can lead to decreased intravascular volume, hypotension, and low cardiac output. Bleeding problems are common after cardiac surgery because of the effects of CPB, trauma from the surgery, and anticoagulation. Preload can also decrease if there is a collection of fluid and blood in the pericardium (cardiac tamponade), which impedes cardiac filling. Cardiac output is also altered if too much volume returns to the heart, causing fluid overload.

Afterload alterations occur when the arteries are constricted as a result of postoperative hypertension or hypothermia,

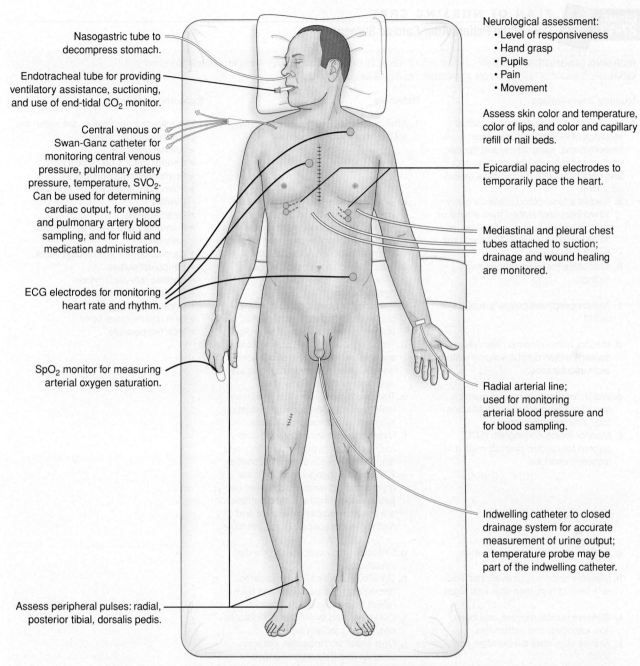

Nasogastric tube to decompress stomach.

Endotracheal tube for providing ventilatory assistance, suctioning, and use of end-tidal CO_2 monitor.

Central venous or Swan-Ganz catheter for monitoring central venous pressure, pulmonary artery pressure, temperature, SVO_2. Can be used for determining cardiac output, for venous and pulmonary artery blood sampling, and for fluid and medication administration.

ECG electrodes for monitoring heart rate and rhythm.

SpO_2 monitor for measuring arterial oxygen saturation.

Assess peripheral pulses: radial, posterior tibial, dorsalis pedis.

Neurological assessment:
• Level of responsiveness
• Hand grasp
• Pupils
• Pain
• Movement

Assess skin color and temperature, color of lips, and color and capillary refill of nail beds.

Epicardial pacing electrodes to temporarily pace the heart.

Mediastinal and pleural chest tubes attached to suction; drainage and wound healing are monitored.

Radial arterial line; used for monitoring arterial blood pressure and for blood sampling.

Indwelling catheter to closed drainage system for accurate measurement of urine output; a temperature probe may be part of the indwelling catheter.

FIGURE 27-13 • Postoperative care of the cardiac surgical patient requires the nurse to be proficient in interpreting hemodynamics, correlating physical assessments with laboratory results, sequencing interventions, and evaluating progress toward desired outcomes.

increasing the workload of the heart. Heart rate alterations from bradycardia, tachycardia, and dysrhythmias can lead to decreased cardiac output, and contractility can be altered in cardiac failure, MI, electrolyte imbalances, and hypoxia.

Fluid Volume and Electrolyte Imbalance. Fluid and electrolyte imbalance may occur after cardiac surgery. Nursing assessment for these complications includes monitoring of intake and output, weight, hemodynamic parameters, hematocrit levels, neck vein distention, edema, breath sounds (e.g., fine crackles, wheezing), and electrolyte levels. The nurse reports changes in serum electrolytes promptly so that treatment

can be instituted. Especially important are dangerously high or dangerously low levels of potassium, magnesium, sodium, and calcium. Elevated blood glucose levels are common in the postoperative period. Administration of IV insulin is recommended in patients both with and without diabetes to achieve the glycemic control necessary to promote wound healing, decrease infection, and improve survival after surgery (Lipshutz & Gropper, 2009).

Impaired Gas Exchange. Impaired gas exchange is another possible complication after cardiac surgery. All body tissues

(text continues on page 764)

PLAN OF NURSING CARE

Chart 27-13

Care of the Patient After Cardiac Surgery

NURSING DIAGNOSIS: Decreased cardiac output related to blood loss and compromised myocardial function
GOAL: Restoration of cardiac output to maintain organ and tissue perfusion

Nursing Interventions	Rationale	Expected Outcomes
1. Monitor cardiovascular status. Serial readings of blood pressure, other hemodynamic parameters, and cardiac rhythm and rate are obtained, recorded, and correlated with the patient's overall condition.	1. Effectiveness of cardiac output is evaluated by continuous monitoring.	• The following parameters are within the patient's normal ranges: • Arterial pressure • Central venous pressure (CVP) • Pulmonary artery pressures • Pulmonary artery wedge pressure (PAWP) • Heart sounds • Pulmonary and systemic vascular resistance • Cardiac output and cardiac index • Peripheral pulses • Cardiac rate and rhythm • Cardiac biomarkers • Urine output • Skin and mucosal color • Skin temperature
a. Assess arterial blood pressure every 15 minutes until stable; then arterial or cuff blood pressure every 1–4 hours × 24 hours; then every 8–12 hours until hospital discharge.	a. Blood pressure is one of the most important physiologic parameters to monitor; vasoconstriction after cardiopulmonary bypass may require treatment with an IV vasodilator.	
b. Auscultate for heart sounds and rhythm.	b. Auscultation provides evidence of pericarditis (precordial rub), dysrhythmias.	
c. Assess peripheral pulses (pedal, tibial, radial).	c. Presence or absence and quality of pulses provide data about cardiac output as well as obstructive lesions.	
d. Monitor hemodynamic parameters to assess cardiac output, volume status, and vascular tone.	d. Rising CVP and PAWP may indicate congestive heart failure or pulmonary edema. Low pressures may indicate need for volume replacement.	
e. Watch for trends in hemodynamics, and note that mechanical ventilation may alter hemodynamics.	e. Trends are more important than isolated readings. Mechanical ventilation increases intrathoracic pressure.	
f. Monitor electrocardiogram (ECG) pattern for cardiac dysrhythmias and ischemic changes.	f. Dysrhythmias may occur with coronary ischemia, hypoxia, bleeding, and acid–base or electrolyte disturbances. ST-segment changes may indicate myocardial ischemia. Pacemaker capture and antiarrhythmic medications are used to maintain heart rate and rhythm and to support blood pressure.	
g. Assess cardiac biomarker results.	g. Elevations may indicate myocardial infarction.	
h. Measure urine output every half hour to 1 hour at first, then with vital signs.	h. Urine output <1 mL/kg/h indicates decreased renal perfusion and may reflect decreased cardiac output.	
i. Observe buccal mucosa, nail beds, lips, earlobes, and extremities.	i. Duskiness and cyanosis may indicate decreased cardiac output.	
j. Assess skin; note temperature and color.	j. Cool moist skin indicates vasoconstriction and decreased cardiac output.	
2. Observe for persistent bleeding: excessive chest tube drainage of blood; hypotension; low CVP; tachycardia. Prepare to administer blood products, IV fluids.	2. Bleeding can result from surgical trauma to tissues, anticoagulant medications, and clotting defects.	• <200 mL/h of drainage through chest tubes during first 4–6 hours • Vital signs stable
3. Observe for cardiac tamponade: hypotension; rising CVP and PAWP, pulsus paradoxus; jugular vein distention; decreasing urinary output. Check for diminished amount of blood in chest drainage collection system. Prepare for reoperation.	3. Cardiac tamponade results from bleeding into the pericardial sac or accumulation of fluid in the sac, which compresses the heart and prevents adequate filling of the ventricles. Decrease in chest drainage may indicate that fluid and clots are accumulating in the pericardial sac.	• CVP and other hemodynamic parameters within normal limits • Urinary output within normal limits • Skin color normal • Respirations unlabored, clear breath sounds • Pain limited to incision
4. Observe for signs of cardiac failure. Prepare to administer diuretics, IV inotropic agents.	4. Cardiac failure results from decreased pumping action of the heart; can cause deficient perfusion to vital organs.	

PLAN OF NURSING CARE

Chart
27-13

Care of the Patient After Cardiac Surgery (continued)

NURSING DIAGNOSIS: Impaired gas exchange related to chest surgery
GOAL: Adequate gas exchange

Nursing Interventions	Rationale	Expected Outcomes
1. Maintain mechanical ventilation until the patient is able to breathe independently. 2. Monitor ABGs, tidal volume, peak inspiratory pressure, and extubation parameters. 3. Auscultate chest for breath sounds. 4. Sedate patient adequately, as prescribed, and monitor respiratory rate and depth. 5. Suction tracheobronchial secretions as needed, using strict aseptic technique. 6. Assist in weaning and endotracheal tube removal. 7. After extubation, promote deep breathing, coughing, and turning. Encourage the use of the incentive spirometer and compliance with breathing treatments. Instruct about incisional splinting with a "cough pillow" to decrease discomfort.	1. Ventilatory support is used to decrease work of the heart, to maintain effective ventilation, and to provide an airway in the event of complications. 2. ABGs and ventilator parameters indicate effectiveness of ventilator and changes that need to be made to improve gas exchange. 3. Crackles indicate pulmonary congestion; decreased or absent breath sounds may indicate pneumothorax, hemothorax, dislodgement of tube. 4. Sedation helps the patient to tolerate the endotracheal tube and to cope with mechanical ventilation. 5. Retention of secretions leads to hypoxia and possible infection. 6. Extubation decreases risk of pulmonary infections and enhances ability of patient to communicate. 7. Aids in keeping airway patent, preventing atelectasis, and facilitating lung expansion	• Airway patent • Arterial blood gases (ABGs) within normal range • Endotracheal tube correctly placed, as evidenced by x-ray • Breath sounds clear bilaterally • Ventilator synchronous with respirations • Breath sounds clear after suctioning/coughing • Nail beds and mucous membranes pink • Mental acuity consistent with amount of sedatives and analgesics received • Oriented to person; able to respond yes and no appropriately • Able to be weaned successfully from ventilator

NURSING DIAGNOSIS: Risk for imbalanced fluid volume and electrolyte imbalance related to alterations in blood volume
GOAL: Fluid and electrolyte balance

Nursing Interventions	Rationale	Expected Outcomes
1. Monitor fluid and electrolyte balance. a. Accurately document intake and output; record urine volume every half hour to 4 hours while in critical care unit; then every 8–12 hours while hospitalized. b. Assess blood pressure, hemodynamic parameters, weight, electrolytes, hematocrit, jugular venous pressure, breath sounds, urinary output, and nasogastric tube drainage. c. Measure postoperative chest drainage; cessation of drainage may indicate kinked or blocked chest tube. Ensure patency and integrity of the drainage system. Maintain autotransfusion system if in use. d. Weigh daily and correlate with intake and output.	1. Adequate circulating blood volume is necessary for optimal cellular activity; fluid and electrolyte imbalance can occur after surgery. a. Provides a method to determine positive or negative fluid balance and fluid requirements b. Provides information about state of hydration c. Excessive blood loss from chest cavity can cause hypovolemia. d. Indicator of fluid balance	• Fluid intake and output balanced • Hemodynamic assessment parameters negative for fluid overload or hypovolemia • Normal blood pressure with position changes • Absence of dysrhythmia • Stable weight • Arterial blood pH 7.35–7.45 • Serum potassium 3.5–5 mEq/L (3.5–5 mmol/L) • Serum magnesium 1.3–2.3 mg/dL (0.62–0.95 mmol/L) • Serum sodium 135–145 mEq/L (135–145 mmol/L) • Serum calcium 8.6–10.2 mg/dL (2.15–2.55 mmol/L) • Serum glucose ≤180 mg/dL

(continues on page 762)

Chart 27-13

PLAN OF NURSING CARE

Care of the Patient After Cardiac Surgery (continued)

Nursing Interventions	Rationale	Expected Outcomes
2. Be alert to changes in serum electrolyte levels.	**2.** A specific concentration of electrolytes is necessary in both extracellular and intracellular body fluids to sustain life.	
a. Hypokalemia (low potassium) *Effects:* Dysrhythmias: premature ventricular contractions, ventricular tachycardia. Observe for specific ECG changes. Administer IV potassium replacement as prescribed.	**a.** *Causes:* Inadequate intake, diuretics, vomiting, excessive nasogastric drainage, perioperative stress response	
b. Hyperkalemia (high potassium) *Effects:* ECG changes, tall peaked T waves, wide QRS, bradycardia. Be prepared to administer diuretic or an ion-exchange resin (sodium polystyrene sulfonate [Kayexalate]); IV sodium bicarbonate, or IV insulin and glucose.	**b.** *Causes:* Increased intake, hemolysis from cardiopulmonary bypass/mechanical assist devices, acidosis, renal insufficiency. The resin binds potassium and promotes intestinal excretion of it. IV sodium bicarbonate drives potassium into the cells from extracellular fluid. Insulin assists the cells with glucose and potassium absorption.	
c. Monitor serum magnesium, sodium, and calcium.	**c.** Low levels of magnesium are associated with dysrhythmias. Low levels of sodium are associated with weakness and neurological symptoms. Low levels of calcium can lead to dysrhythmias and muscle spasm.	
d. Hyperglycemia (high blood glucose) *Effects:* Increased urine output, thirst, impaired healing. Administer insulin as prescribed.	**d.** *Cause:* Stress response to surgery. Affects both patients with diabetes and those without diabetes.	

NURSING DIAGNOSIS: Disturbed sensory perception related to excessive environmental stimulation, sleep deprivation, physiologic imbalance

GOAL: Reduction of symptoms of sensory perceptual imbalance; prevention of postcardiotomy delirium

Nursing Interventions	Rationale	Expected Outcomes

1. Use measures to prevent postcardiotomy delirium:
  a. Explain all procedures and the need for patient cooperation.
  b. Plan nursing care to provide for periods of uninterrupted sleep with patient's normal day–night pattern.
  c. Promote continuity of care.
  d. Orient to time and place frequently. Encourage family to visit.
  e. Assess for medications that may contribute to delirium.
2. Observe for perceptual distortions, hallucinations, disorientation, and paranoid delusions.
	1. Postcardiotomy delirium may result from anxiety, sleep deprivation, increased sensory input, and disorientation to night and day. Normally, sleep cycles are at least 50 minutes long. The first cycle may be as long as 90–120 minutes and then shorten during successive cycles. Sleep deprivation results when the sleep cycles are interrupted or are inadequate in number.
	
	2. Delirium can indicate a serious medical condition such as hypoxia, acid–base imbalance, metabolic abnormalities, and cerebral infarction.
		• Cooperates with procedures
		• Sleeps for long, uninterrupted intervals
		• Oriented to person, place, time
		• Experiences no perceptual distortions, hallucinations, disorientation, delusions

NURSING DIAGNOSIS: Acute pain related to surgical trauma and pleural irritation caused by chest tubes

GOAL: Relief of pain

Nursing Interventions	Rationale	Expected Outcomes
1. Record nature, type, location, intensity, and duration of pain. **2.** Encourage routine pain medication dosing for the first 24–72 hours, and observe for side effects of lethargy, hypotension, tachycardia, respiratory depression.	**1.** Pain and anxiety increase pulse rate, oxygen consumption, and cardiac workload. **2.** Analgesia promotes rest, decreases oxygen consumption caused by pain, and aids patient in performing deep-breathing and coughing exercises; pain medication is more effective when taken before pain is severe.	• States pain is decreasing in severity • Restlessness decreased • Vital signs stable • Participates in deep-breathing and coughing exercises • Verbalizes fewer complaints of pain each day • Positions self; participates in care activities • Gradually increases activity

PLAN OF NURSING CARE

Chart
27-13

Care of the Patient After Cardiac Surgery (continued)

NURSING DIAGNOSIS: Risk for ineffective renal perfusion related to decreased cardiac output, hemolysis, or vasopressor drug therapy
GOAL: Maintenance of adequate renal perfusion

Nursing Interventions	Rationale	Expected Outcomes

1. Assess renal function:
 	
  a. Measure urine output every half hour to 4 hours in critical care, then every 8–12 hours until hospital discharge.
  b. Monitor and report lab results: BUN, serum creatinine, serum electrolytes.
2. Prepare to administer rapid-acting diuretics or inotropic drugs (e.g., dobutamine).
3. Prepare patient for dialysis or continuous renal replacement therapy if indicated.
	1. Renal injury can be caused by deficient perfusion, hemolysis, low cardiac output, and the use of vasopressor agents to increase blood pressure.
	  a. <1 mL/kg/h indicates decreased renal function.
	
	  b. These tests indicate the kidneys' ability to excrete waste products.
	2. These agents promote renal function and increase cardiac output and renal blood flow.
	3. Provides patient with the opportunity to ask questions and prepare for the procedure
		• Urine output consistent with fluid intake; >1 mL/kg/h
		• Urine specific gravity 1.003–1.030
		• Blood urea nitrogen (BUN), creatinine, electrolytes within normal limits

---

NURSING DIAGNOSIS: Ineffective thermoregulation related to infection or postpericardiotomy syndrome
GOAL: Maintenance of normal body temperature

Nursing Interventions	Rationale	Expected Outcomes
1. Assess temperature every hour. 2. Use aseptic technique when changing dressings, suctioning endotracheal tube; maintain closed systems for all IV and arterial lines and for indwelling urinary catheter. 3. Observe for symptoms of postpericardiotomy syndrome. 4. Obtain cultures and other lab work (CBC, ESR); administer antibiotic agents as prescribed. 5. Administer anti-inflammatory agents as directed.	1. Fever can indicate infectious or inflammatory process. 2. Decreases risk of infection 3. Occurs in ~10% of patients after cardiac surgery. 4. Antibiotic agents treat documented infection. 5. Anti-inflammatory agents relieve symptoms of inflammation.	• Normal body temperature • Incisions are free of infection and are healing. • Absence of symptoms of postpericardiotomy syndrome: fever, malaise, pericardial effusion, pericardial friction rub, arthralgia

---

NURSING DIAGNOSIS: Deficient knowledge about self-care activities
GOAL: Ability to perform self-care activities

Nursing Interventions	Rationale	Expected Outcomes

1. Develop education plan for patient and family. Provide specific instructions for the following:
  • Diet and daily weights
  • Activity progression
  • Exercise
  • Deep breathing, coughing, lung expansion exercises
  • Temperature and pulse monitoring
  • Medication regimen
  • Incision care
  • Access to the emergency medical system
2. Provide verbal and written instructions; provide several education sessions for reinforcement and answering questions.
3. Involve family in education sessions.
 	
4. Provide contact information for surgeon and cardiologist and instructions about follow-up visit with surgeon.
5. Make appropriate referrals: home care agency, cardiac rehabilitation program, community support groups.
	1. Each patient has unique learning needs.
	
	2. Repetition promotes learning by allowing for questions and clarification of misinformation.
	3. Family members responsible for home care are usually anxious and require adequate time for learning.
	4. Arrangements for contacts with health care personnel help to allay anxieties.
	
	5. Learning, recovery, and lifestyle changes continue after discharge from the hospital.
		• Patient and family members explain and comply with therapeutic regimen.
		• Patient and family members identify necessary lifestyle changes.
		• Has copy of discharge instructions (in the patient's primary language and at appropriate reading level; has an alternate format if indicated)
		• Keeps follow-up appointments

require an adequate supply of oxygen for survival. To achieve this after surgery, an endotracheal tube with ventilator assistance may be used for hours to days. The assisted ventilation is continued until the patient's blood gas values are acceptable and the patient demonstrates the ability to breathe independently. Patients who are stable after surgery may be extubated as early as 2 to 4 hours after surgery, which reduces their discomfort and anxiety and facilitates patient–nurse communication.

While receiving mechanical ventilation, the patient is continuously assessed for signs of impaired gas exchange: restlessness, anxiety, cyanosis of mucous membranes and peripheral tissues, tachycardia, and fighting the ventilator. Breath sounds are assessed often to detect pulmonary congestion and monitor lung expansion. Arterial blood gases, SpO_2, and end-tidal CO_2 are assessed for decreased oxygen and increased CO_2. Following extubation, aggressive pulmonary interventions, such as turning, coughing, deep breathing, and early ambulation are necessary to prevent atelectasis and pneumonia.

Impaired Cerebral Circulation. Hypoperfusion or microemboli during or following cardiac surgery may produce injury to the brain. Brain function depends on a continuous supply of oxygenated blood. The brain does not have the capacity to store oxygen and must rely on adequate continuous perfusion by the heart. The nurse observes the patient for signs and symptoms of cerebral hypoxia: restlessness, confusion, dyspnea, hypotension, and cyanosis. An assessment of the patient's neurologic status includes level of consciousness, response to verbal commands and painful stimuli, pupil size and reaction to light, facial symmetry, movement of the extremities, and hand grip strength. The nurse documents any indication of a change in status and reports abnormal findings to the surgeon because they may signal the onset of a complication such as a stroke.

Maintaining Cardiac Output

Ongoing evaluation of the patient's cardiac status continues as the nurse monitors the effectiveness of cardiac output through clinical observations and routine measurements: serial readings of blood pressure, heart rate, CVP, arterial pressure, and pulmonary artery pressures.

Renal function is related to cardiac function, as blood pressure and cardiac output drive glomerular filtration; therefore, urinary output is measured and recorded. Urine output of less than 1 mL/kg/h may indicate a decrease in cardiac output or inadequate fluid volume.

Body tissues depend on adequate cardiac output to provide a continuous supply of oxygenated blood to meet the changing demands of the organs and body systems. Because the buccal mucosa, nail beds, lips, and earlobes are sites with rich capillary beds, they are observed for cyanosis or duskiness as possible signs of reduced cardiac output. Distention of the neck veins when the head of the bed is elevated to 30 degrees or more may signal right-sided heart failure. If cardiac output has decreased, the skin becomes cool, moist, and cyanotic or mottled.

Dysrhythmias may develop due to decreased perfusion to or irritation of the myocardium from surgery. The most common dysrhythmias encountered during the postoperative period are atrial fibrillation, bradycardias, tachycardias, and ectopic beats. Continuous observation of the cardiac monitor for dysrhythmias is essential.

The nurse reports any indications of decreased cardiac output promptly. The assessment data is used to determine the cause of the problem. After a diagnosis has been made, the physician and the nurse work collaboratively to restore cardiac output and prevent further complications. When indicated, blood components, fluids, and antidysrhythmics, diuretics, vasodilators, or vasopressors are prescribed. If additional interventions are necessary, such as the placement of an intra-aortic balloon pump, the patient and family are prepared for the procedure.

Promoting Adequate Gas Exchange

To ensure adequate gas exchange, the patency of the endotracheal tube is assessed and maintained. The tube must be secured to prevent it from slipping out or down into the right mainstem bronchus. Suctioning is necessary when crackles or coughing are present. Routinely, 100% oxygen is delivered to the patient from the ventilator before and after suctioning to minimize the risk of hypoxia during the suctioning procedure. Arterial blood gas determinations are compared with baseline data, and changes are reported to the physician promptly.

When the patient's hemodynamic parameters stabilize, body position is changed every 1 to 2 hours. Frequent changes of patient position provide for optimal pulmonary ventilation and perfusion, allowing the lungs to expand more fully.

Physical assessment and arterial blood gas results guide the process of weaning the patient from the ventilator. The nurse assists with the weaning process and eventually with removal of the endotracheal tube. After extubation, the nurse encourages deep breathing and coughing at least every 1 to 2 hours to clear secretions, open the alveolar sacs, and promote effective ventilation. (See Chapter 21 for discussion of weaning the patient from the ventilator.)

Maintaining Fluid and Electrolyte Balance

To promote fluid and electrolyte balance, the nurse carefully assesses intake and output to determine positive or negative fluid balance. It is necessary to record all fluid intake, including IV, nasogastric tube, and oral fluids, as well as all output, including urine, nasogastric drainage, and chest drainage.

Hemodynamic parameters (e.g., blood pressure, CVP, cardiac output) are correlated with intake, output, and weight to determine the adequacy of hydration and cardiac output. Serum electrolytes are monitored, and the patient is observed for signs of potassium, magnesium, sodium, or calcium imbalance.

Indications of dehydration, fluid overload, or electrolyte imbalance are reported promptly, and the physician and nurse work collaboratively to restore fluid and electrolyte balance and monitor the patient's response to therapies.

Minimizing Sensory Perception Imbalance

Some patients exhibit abnormal perceptions and behaviors that occur with varying intensity and duration. The risk of delirium is high in cardiac surgery patients and increases with patients' age (Koster, Hensens, & Schuurmans, 2010). Clinical manifestations of postoperative delirium include restlessness, agitation, visual and auditory hallucinations, and paranoia. The delirium typically appears after a 2- to 5-day stay in an ICU. Patients are assessed for this problem with tools such as the Confusion Assessment Method for the ICU (CAM-ICU) (Nelson, 2009). The CAMU-ICU scale assesses for key indicators of delirium such as disorganized thinking and inattention. When this testing is positive, further assessment of the patient's physiologic and psychological status is required. Presumed causes of postoperative delirium include anxiety, sleep deprivation, increased sensory input, medications, and physiologic problems such as hypoxemia and metabolic imbalance (Urden et al., 2010). Treatment includes correction of identified physiologic problems such as metabolic and electrolyte imbalances. Additionally, behavioral interventions are used (e.g., frequent reorientation). Sedative medications such as haloperidol (Haldol) may help reduce agitation. The delirium often resolves after the patient is transferred from the unit, but nonetheless can be associated with negative outcomes including cognitive and functional decline, longer lengths of hospital stay, and higher mortality (Koster et al., 2010).

For all postoperative patients, basic comfort measures are used in conjunction with prescribed analgesics and sedatives to promote rest. Invasive lines and tubes are discontinued as soon as possible. Patient care is coordinated to provide undisturbed periods of rest. As the patient's condition stabilizes and the patient is disturbed less frequently for monitoring and therapeutic procedures, rest periods can be extended. Uninterrupted sleep is provided as much as possible, especially during the patient's normal hours of sleep.

Careful explanations of all procedures and of the patient's role in facilitating them help keep the patient positively involved throughout the postoperative course. Continuity of care is desirable; a familiar face and a nursing staff with a consistent approach help the patient feel safe. The patient's family should be welcomed at the bedside. A well-designed and individualized plan of nursing care can assist the nursing team in coordinating its efforts for the emotional well-being of the patient.

Relieving Pain

Patients who have had cardiac surgery may have pain in the peri-incisional area or throughout the chest, shoulders, and back. Pain results from trauma to the chest wall and irritation of the pleura by the chest tubes as well as incisional pain from peripheral vein or artery graft harvest sites.

The nurse assesses patients for verbal and nonverbal indicators of pain and records the nature, type, location, and duration of the pain. To reduce the amount of pain, the nurse encourages the patient to accept medication on a regular basis. The addition of adjunctive pain relievers (anti-inflammatory agents, muscle relaxants) to opioids decreases the amount of opioids required for pain relief and increases patient comfort. Patients report the most pain during coughing, turning, and moving. Physical support of the incision with a folded bath blanket or small pillow during deep breathing and coughing helps minimize pain. The patient should then be able to participate in respiratory exercises and to progressively increase self-care. Patient comfort improves after removal of the chest tubes.

Pain produces tension, which may stimulate the central nervous system to release catecholamines, resulting in constriction of the arterioles and increased heart rate. This can cause increased afterload and decreased cardiac output. Opioids alleviate pain and induce sleep and feelings of well-being, which reduces the metabolic rate and oxygen demands. After the administration of opioids, it is necessary to document observations indicating relief of apprehension and pain in the patient's record. The nurse observes the patient for any

adverse effects of opioids, including respiratory depression, hypotension, constipation, ileus, or urinary retention. If serious side effects occur, an opioid antagonist (e.g., naloxone [Narcan]) may be required.

Maintaining Adequate Tissue Perfusion

The nurse routinely palpates peripheral pulses (e.g., pedal, tibial, femoral, radial, brachial) to assess for arterial obstruction. If a pulse is absent in any extremity, the cause may be prior catheterization of that extremity, chronic peripheral vascular disease, or a thromboembolic obstruction. The nurse immediately reports newly identified absence of any pulse.

Thromboembolic events can result from vascular injury, dislodgment of a clot from a damaged valve, loosening of mural thrombi, or coagulation problems. Air embolism can result from CPB or central venous cannulation. Symptoms of embolization vary according to site. The usual embolic sites are the lungs, coronary arteries, mesentery, spleen, extremities, kidneys, and brain. The patient is observed for onset of the following:

- Chest pain and respiratory distress from pulmonary embolus or MI
- Abdominal or back pain from mesenteric emboli
- Pain, cessation of pulses, blanching, numbness, or coldness in an extremity
- One-sided weakness and pupillary changes, as occur in stroke

The nurse promptly reports any of these symptoms.

Venous stasis, which can cause venous thromboembolism (e.g., deep vein thrombosis, pulmonary embolism), may occur after surgery. It can be prevented by using the following measures:

- Apply sequential pneumatic compression devices as prescribed.
- Discourage crossing of legs.
- Avoid elevating the knees on the bed.
- Omit pillows in the popliteal space.
- Begin passive exercises followed by active exercises to promote circulation and prevent venous stasis.

Inadequate renal perfusion can occur as a complication of cardiac surgery. One possible cause is low cardiac output. Trauma to blood cells during CPB can cause hemolysis of red blood cells, which then occlude the renal glomeruli. The use of vasopressor agents to increase blood pressure may constrict the renal arterioles and reduce blood flow to the kidneys.

Nursing management includes accurate measurement of urine output. An output of less than 1 mL/kg/h may indicate hypovolemia or renal insufficiency. The primary provider may prescribe fluids to increase cardiac output and renal blood flow, or IV diuretics may be administered to increase urine output. The nurse should be aware of the patient's blood urea nitrogen, serum creatinine, glomerular filtration rate, and serum electrolyte levels. The nurse should report abnormal levels promptly, because it may be necessary to adjust fluids and the dose or type of medication administered. If efforts to maintain renal perfusion are ineffective, the patient may require continuous renal replacement therapy or dialysis (see Chapter 54).

Maintaining Normal Body Temperature

Patients are usually hypothermic when admitted to the critical care unit following the cardiac surgical procedure. Because induced hypothermia from CPB and anesthesia lower the patient's core temperature, the patient must be gradually warmed to a normal temperature. This is accomplished partially by the patient's own basal metabolic processes and often with the assistance of heated air blanket systems. While the patient is hypothermic, shivering and hypertension are common. Lowering the blood pressure with a vasodilator such as nitroprusside (Nipride) may be necessary. These problems typically resolve as warming occurs.

After cardiac surgery, the patient is at risk for developing elevated body temperature as a result of tissue inflammation or infection. The inflammatory/immune response to surgery includes the release of cytokines that cause fever (Porth, 2011). The resultant increase in metabolic rate increases tissue oxygen demands and increases cardiac workload. Antipyretics and other measures are used to lower body temperature.

Common sites of postoperative infection include the lungs, urinary tract, incisions, and intravascular catheters. Meticulous care is used to prevent contamination at the sites of catheter and tube insertions. Aseptic technique is used when changing dressings and when providing endotracheal tube and catheter care. Clearance of pulmonary secretions is accomplished by frequent repositioning of the patient, suctioning, and chest physical therapy, as well as educating and encouraging the patient to breathe deeply and cough. Prevention of aspiration is another important factor in prevention of postoperative pneumonia (Starks & Harbert, 2011) (see Chart 27-14). Closed systems are used to maintain all IV and arterial lines and the system for endotracheal suction. All invasive lines and tubes are discontinued as soon as possible after surgery.

Postpericardiotomy syndrome may occur in patients who undergo cardiac surgery. The syndrome is characterized by fever, pericardial pain, pleural pain, dyspnea, pericardial effusion, pericardial friction rub, and arthralgia. These signs and symptoms may occur days to weeks after surgery, often after the patient has been discharged from the hospital.

Postpericardiotomy syndrome must be differentiated from other postoperative complications (e.g., infection, incisional pain, MI, pulmonary embolus, bacterial endocarditis, pneumonia, atelectasis). Treatment depends on the severity of the signs and symptoms. Anti-inflammatory agents often produce a dramatic improvement in symptoms.

Promoting Home and Community-Based Care

Educating Patients About Self-Care. Depending on the type of surgery and postoperative progress, the patient may be discharged from the hospital 3 to 5 days after surgery. Following recovery from the surgery, patients can expect fewer symptoms from CAD and an improved quality of life. CABG has been shown to increase the lifespan of high-risk patients, including those with left main artery blockages and left ventricular dysfunction with multivessel blockages (Serruys et al., 2009).

Although the patient may be eager to return home, the patient and family usually are apprehensive about this transition. Family members often express the fear that they are not capable of caring for the patient at home or that they are unprepared to handle complications that may occur.

The nurse helps the patient and family set realistic, achievable goals. An education plan that meets the patient's individual needs is developed with the patient and family. Specific instructions are provided about incision care; signs and symptoms of infection; diet; activity progression and exercise; deep breathing, incentive spirometry, and tobacco use cessation; weight and temperature monitoring; the medication regimen; and follow-up visits with home care nurses, the rehabilitation personnel, the surgeon, and the cardiologist or internist.

Some patients have difficulty learning and retaining information after cardiac surgery. The patient may experience recent memory loss, short attention span, difficulty with simple math, poor handwriting, and visual disturbances. Patients with these difficulties often become frustrated when they try

---

Chart 27-14

NURSING RESEARCH PROFILE

Aspiration Prevention Protocol: Decreasing Postoperative Pneumonia in Heart Surgery Patients

Starks, B., & Harbert, C. (2011). Aspiration prevention protocol: Decreasing postoperative pneumonia in heart surgery patients. *Critical Care Nurse, 31*(5), 38–45.

Purpose

Postoperative pulmonary dysfunction (including atelectasis and pneumonia) is a frequent cause of morbidity and mortality in patients who have open heart surgery. The purpose of this study was to determine if implementation of an aspiration prevention protocol in patients after cardiac surgery would decrease the incidence of postoperative pneumonia.

Design

An aspiration prevention protocol was developed and implemented in a 24-bed intensive care unit using the Plan-Do-Study-Act Model for quality improvement advocated by the Institute for Healthcare Improvement (IHI). The protocol incorporated extending the time that patients received nothing by mouth from 2 hours to at least 6 hours preoperatively and incorporating a postoperative bedside swallowing evaluation by a speech therapist. After the swallow evaluation was completed, nurses implemented a progressive oral intake protocol. A convenience sample of 79

adult patients who had cardiothoracic surgery from April 2008 through October 2008 were enrolled in the study. Historical controls were used to compare rates of pneumonia.

Findings

The interdisciplinary team of nurses, physicians, administrators, and speech therapists who developed and implemented this protocol set a goal that no patients who participated in this protocol would develop postoperative pneumonia. This goal was met; no study participants (*n* = 79) developed pneumonia. However, 11% of historical controls (*n* = 65) developed postoperative pneumonia.

Nursing Implications

The Plan-Do-Study-Act Model encourages team collaboration between nurses and their interdisciplinary colleagues and results in rapid cycle improvement. These rapid cycle improvements enhance quality patient outcomes and ensure patient safety. The development and implementation of this aspiration prevention protocol expeditiously met an ambitious aim to reduce the rate of postoperative pneumonia in patients who had cardiothoracic surgery to nil.

to resume normal activities. The patient and family are reassured that the difficulty is almost always temporary and will subside, usually in 6 to 8 weeks. In the meantime, instructions are given to the patient at a slower pace than normal, and a family member assumes responsibility for making sure that the prescribed regimen is followed.

Continuing Care. Arrangements are made for a home care nurse when appropriate. Because the hospital stay is relatively short, it is particularly important for the nurse to assess the patient's and family's ability to manage care in the home. The home care nurse continues the education process, monitors vital signs and incisions, assesses for signs and symptoms of complications, and provides support for the patient and family. Additional interventions may include dressing changes, diet counseling, and tobacco use cessation strategies. Women may experience a longer recovery and may require additional interventions to manage symptoms (Parry et al., 2010). They also have a higher risk of depression during the postoperative period. Patients and families need to know that cardiac surgery did not cure the patient's underlying heart disease process. Lifestyle changes for risk factor reduction are essential, and medications taken before surgery to control problems such as blood pressure and hyperlipidemia will still be necessary.

The nurse encourages the patient to contact the surgeon, cardiologist, or nurse with problems or questions. This provides the patient and family with reassurance that professional support is available. The patient is expected to have at least one follow-up visit with the surgeon.

Education does not end at the time of discharge from the hospital or home health care. Many patients and families benefit from supportive programs, such as those that focus on cardiac rehabilitation. These programs provide monitored exercise; instructions about diet and stress reduction; information about resuming work, driving, and sexual activity; assistance with tobacco use cessation; and support groups for patients and families. Support groups, such as the AHA-sponsored Mended Hearts, provide information as well as an opportunity for families to share experiences.

Critical Thinking Exercises

1 `pq` A 67-year-old patient has just been diagnosed with metabolic syndrome with hypertension, obesity, dyslipidemia, and insulin resistance. She is asking for more information about this syndrome and what she can do about it. How will you define metabolic syndrome for this patient? What does this diagnosis mean for her future health and health care needs? Knowing that multiple lifestyle changes are recommended, what is your first priority for patient education?

2 `ebp` You are caring for an 88-year-old man who is hospitalized with a diagnosis of syncope. After ambulating in the hall, he tells you that he is having some chest pain and mild shortness of breath. Based on your knowledge of evidence-based guidelines, identify the initial interventions and diagnostic testing that are indicated for patients with these symptoms. Describe how the diagnosis of acute

MI is made. If a diagnosis of STEMI is made, which treatment options may be considered?

3 A 60-year-old woman has just returned to your unit following a heart catheterization and PCI. She appears restless and uncomfortable. What should be included in your initial assessment? What type of monitoring is indicated? Identify serious complications that you should watch for in patients following PCI.

4 You are caring for a 72-year-old man who was recently admitted to the ICU following CABG. His current vital signs are as follows: heart rate, 114 bpm; blood pressure, 88/60 mmHg; CVP, 2 mm Hg. Which other assessment parameters will you evaluate? What type of postoperative interventions do you expect?

 Brunner Suite Resources

Explore these additional resources to enhance learning for this chapter:
- NCLEX-Style Questions and Other Resources on **thePoint**, http://thePoint.lww.com/Brunner13e
- Study Guide
- PrepU
- Clinical Handbook
- Handbook of Laboratory and Diagnostic Tests

References

*Asterisk indicates nursing research.
**Double asterisk indicates classic reference.

Books

Aschenbrenner, D. S., & Venable, S. J. (2012). *Drug therapy in nursing* (4th ed.). Philadelphia: Lippincott Williams & Wilkins.

McCance, K. L., Huether, S. E., Brashers, V. L., et al. (2010). *Pathophysiology. The biologic basis for disease in adults and children* (6th ed.). Maryland Heights, MO: Mosby Elsevier.

Porth, C. M. (2011). *Essentials of pathophysiology* (3rd ed.). Philadelphia: Lippincott Williams & Wilkins.

Sinz, E., & Navarro, K. (2011). *Advanced cardiovascular life support provider manual.* Dallas: American Heart Association.

Urden, L. D., Stacy, K. M., & Lough, M. E. (2010). *Critical care nursing* (6th ed.). St. Louis: Mosby Elsevier.

Journals and Electronic Documents

Alberti, K. G., Eckel, R. H., Grundy, S. M., et al. (2009). Harmonizing the metabolic syndrome. *Circulation, 120*(16), 1640–1645.

Arsenault, B. J., Pibarot, P., & Despres, J. (2009). The quest for the optimal assessment of global cardiovascular risk: Are traditional risk factors and metabolic syndrome partners in crime? *Cardiology, 113*(1), 35–49.

Bhatty, S., Cooke, R., Shettey, R., et al. (2011). Femoral vascular access-site complications in the cardiac catheterization laboratory: Diagnosis and management. *Interventional Cardiology, 3*(4), 503–514.

Bukkapatnam, R. N., Yeo, K. K., Li, Z., et al. (2010). Operative mortality in women and men undergoing coronary artery bypass grafting (from the California Coronary Artery Bypass Grafting Outcomes Reporting Program). *American Journal of Cardiology, 105*(3), 339–342.

Cadwallader, R. A., Walsh, S. R., Cooper, D. G., et al. (2009). Great saphenous vein harvesting: A systematic review and meta-analysis of open versus endoscopic techniques. *Vascular and Endovascular Surgery, 43*(6), 561–566.

Chang, B. H., Aggie, C., Dusek, J. A., et al. (2010). Relaxation response and spirituality: Pathways to improve psychological outcomes in cardiac rehabilitation. *Journal of Psychosomatic Research, 69*(2), 93–100.

Coakley, A. B., & Mahoney, E. K. (2009). Creating a therapeutic and healing environment with a pet therapy program. *Complementary Therapies in Clinical Practice, 15*(3), 141–146.

Devaraj, S., Valleggi, S., Siegel, D., et al. (2010). Role of C-reactive protein in contributing to increased cardiovascular risk in metabolic syndrome. *Current Atherosclerosis Reports, 12*(2), 110–118.

Fennessy-Cooney, M. (2011). HIT heparin-induced thrombocytopenia. *Nurse Practitioner, 36*(6), 31–37.

Figueroa-Ramos, M. I., Arroyo-Novoa, C. M., Lee, K. A., et al. (2009). Sleep and delirium in ICU patients: A review of mechanisms and manifestations. *Intensive Care Medicine, 35*(5), 781–795.

Fletcher, B., & Thalinger, K. K. (2010). Prasugrel as antiplatelet therapy in patients with acute coronary syndromes or undergoing percutaneous coronary intervention. *Critical Care Nurse, 30*(5), 45–54.

*Gallagher, R., & McKinley, S. (2009). Anxiety, depression and perceived control in patients having coronary artery bypass grafts. *Journal of Advanced Nursing, 65*(11), 2386–2396.

Greenhalgh, J., Hockenhull, J., Rao, N., et al. (2010). Drug-eluting stents versus bare metal stents for angina or acute coronary syndromes (review). *Cochrane Database of Systematic Reviews, (5),* CD004587.

Hall, S. L., & Lorenc, T. (2010). Secondary prevention of coronary artery disease. *American Family Physician, 81*(3), 289–296.

*Harrington, M. B., Kraft, M., Grande, L. J., et al. (2011). Independent association between preoperative cognitive status and discharge location after cardiac surgery. *American Journal of Critical Care, 20*(3), 129–137.

Hillis, D. L., Smith, P. K., Anderson, J. L., et al. (2011). 2011 ACCF/AHA guideline for coronary artery bypass graft surgery: Executive summary: A report of the American College of Cardiology Foundation/American Heart Association Task Force on Practice Guidelines. *Circulation, 124*(23), 2610–2642.

Institute for Clinical Systems Improvement. (2011a). *Lipid management in adults.* Available at: www.guideline.gov/content.aspx?id=36062&search=lipid+management

Institute for Clinical Systems Improvement. (2011b). *Medical management of adults with hypertension.* Available at: www.guideline.gov/content.aspx?id=34787&search=hypertension

Institute for Clinical Systems Improvement. (2011c). *Acute coronary syndrome and myocardial infarction.* Available at: www.guideline.gov/content.aspx?id=33192&search=acute+coronary+syndrome+and+myocardial+infarction

Institute for Clinical Systems Improvement. (2012a). *Diagnosis and management of type 2 diabetes mellitus in adults.* Available at: www.guideline.gov/content.aspx?id=36905&search=diabetes+mellitus+adult

Institute for Clinical Systems Improvement. (2012b). *Diagnosis and treatment of chest pain and acute coronary syndrome (ACS).* Available at: www.guideline.gov/content.aspx?id=39320&search=chest+pain+and+acute+coronary+syndrome

Ionescu, C. N., Amuchastegui, M., Ionescu, S., et al. (2010). Treatment and outcomes of nonagenarians with ST-elevation. *Journal of Invasive Cardiology, 22*(10), 479–480.

Iribarne, A., Karpenko, A., Russo, M. J., et al. (2009). Eight-year experience with minimally invasive cardiothoracic surgery. *World Journal of Surgery, 34*(4), 611–615.

Joint Commission. (2011). *Acute myocardial infarction Core Measure set.* Available at: www.jointcommission.org/assets/1/6/Acute%20Myocardial%20Infarction.pdf

**Kannel, W. B. (1986). Silent myocardial ischemia and infarction: Insights from the Framingham Study. *Cardiology Clinics, 4*(4), 583–591.

Koster, S., Hensens, A. G., Schuurmans, M. J., et al. (2010). Consequences of delirium after cardiac operations. *Annals of Thoracic Surgery.* Available at: www.ncbi.nlm.nih.gov/pubmed/21992939

Leibowitz, G., Raizman, E., Brezis, M., et al. (2010). Effects of moderate intensity glycemic control after cardiac surgery. *Annals of Thoracic Surgery, 90*(6), 1825–1832.

Lipshutz, A. K., & Gropper, M. A. (2009). Perioperative glycemic control. *Anesthesiology, 110,* 408–421.

Martin, M. T., Spinler, S. A., & Nutescu, E. A. (2011). Emerging antiplatelet therapies in percutaneous coronary intervention: A focus on prasugrel. *Clinical Therapeutics, 33*(4), 425–442.

Miller, M., Stone, N., Ballantyne, C., et al. (2011). Triglycerides and cardiovascular disease. *Circulation, 123*(20), 2292–2333.

Mosca, L., Benjamin, E. J., Berra, K., et al. (2011). Effectiveness-based guidelines for the prevention of cardiovascular disease in women—2011 update. *Circulation, 123*(11), 1243–1262. Available at: circ.ahajournals.org/content/123/11/1243

**National Cholesterol Education Program (NCEP) Expert Panel on Detection, Evaluation, and Treatment of High Blood Cholesterol in Adults (Adult Treatment Panel III). (2002). Third report on the National Cholesterol Education Program (NCEP) Expert Panel on Detection, Evaluation, and Treatment of High Blood Cholesterol in Adults (Adult Treatment Panel III) final report. *Circulation, 106*(25), 3143–3421.

Nelson, L. (2009). Teaching staff nurses the CAM-ICU for delirium screening. *Critical Care Nursing Quarterly, 32*(2), 137–143.

Office of the U.S. Surgeon General. (2010). *How tobacco smoke causes disease.* Rockville, MD. Available at: www.surgeongeneral.gov/library/tobaccosmoke/report/executivesummary.pdf

Overbaugh, K. J. (2009). Acute coronary syndrome. *American Journal of Nursing, 109*(5), 42–52.

*Parry, M., Watt-Watson, J., Hodnett, E. et al. (2010). Pain experiences of men and women after coronary artery bypass graft surgery. *Journal of Cardiovascular Nursing, 25*(3), E9–E15.

Roger, V. L., Go, A. S., Lloyd-Jones, D. M., et al. (2011). Heart disease and stroke statistics—2011 update. *Circulation, 123*(1), 18–209.

Savage, P. D., Sanderson, B. K., Brown T. M., et al. (2011). Clinical research in cardiac rehabilitation and secondary prevention. *Journal of Cardiopulmonary Rehabilitation and Prevention, 31*(1), 1–6.

Schoenborn, C. A., & Stommel, M. (2011). Adherence to the 2008 adult physical activity guidelines and mortality risk. *American Journal of Preventive Medicine, 40*(5), 514–521.

Serruys, P. W., Morice, M., Kappetein, A. P., et al. (2009). Percutaneous coronary intervention versus coronary-artery bypass grafting for severe coronary artery disease. *New England Journal of Medicine, 360*(10), 961–972.

Shroyer, A. L., Grover, F. L., Hattler, B., et al. (2009). On-pump versus off-pump coronary-artery bypass surgery. *New England Journal of Medicine, 361*(19), 1827–1837.

*Starks, B., & Harbert, C. (2011). Aspiration prevention protocol: Decreasing postoperative pneumonia in heart surgery patients. *Critical Care Nurse, 31*(5), 38–45.

U.S. Food and Drug Administration. (2010). *FDA 101: Smoking cessation products.* Available at: www.fda.gov/forconsumers/consumerupdates/ucm198176.htm

Vavalle, J. P., & Rao, S. V. (2009). Impact of bleeding complications on outcomes after percutaneous coronary interventions. *Interventional Cardiology, 1*(1), 51–62.

Wright, R. S., Anderson, J. L., Adams, C. D., et al. (2011). 2011 ACCF/AHA focused update of the guidelines for the management of patients with unstable angina/non–ST-elevation myocardial infarction (updating the 2007 guideline). *Circulation, 123*(18), 2022–2060. Available at: circ.ahajournals.org/content/123/18/2022

Resources

American Diabetes Association, www.diabetes.org

American Heart Association, www.americanheart.org

Joint Commission, www.jointcommission.org

Mayo Clinic, www.mayoclinic.com/health/DiseasesIndex/DiseasesIndex

Mended Hearts, www.mendedhearts.org

National Cholesterol Education Program, www.nhlbi.nih.gov/about/ncep

National Institutes of Health, National Heart, Lung, and Blood Institute, www.nhlbi.nih.gov

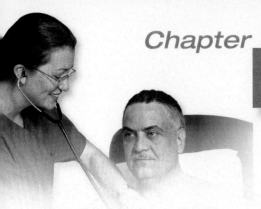

Management of Patients With Structural, Infectious, and Inflammatory Cardiac Disorders

On completion of this chapter, the learner will be able to:

1 Define valvular disorders of the heart and describe the pathophysiology, clinical manifestations, and management of patients with mitral and aortic disorders.
2 Describe types of cardiac valve repair and replacement procedures used to treat valvular problems and care needed by patients who undergo these procedures.
3 Describe the pathophysiology, clinical manifestations, and management of patients with cardiomyopathies.
4 Describe the pathophysiology, clinical manifestations, and management of patients with infections of the heart.
5 Use the nursing process as a framework of care for the patient with a cardiomyopathy and the patient with pericarditis.

allograft: heart valve replacement made from a human heart valve (*synonym:* homograft)

annuloplasty: repair of a cardiac valve's outer ring

aortic valve: semilunar valve located between the left ventricle and aorta

autograft: heart valve replacement made from the patient's own heart valve (e.g., pulmonic valve excised and used as an aortic valve)

bioprosthesis: heart valve replacement made of tissue from an animal heart valve (*synonym:* heterograft)

cardiomyopathy: disease of the heart muscle

chordae tendineae: nondistensible fibrous strands connecting papillary muscles to atrioventricular (mitral, tricuspid) valve leaflets

chordoplasty: repair of chordae tendineae

commissurotomy: splitting or separating fused cardiac valve leaflets

heterograft: heart valve replacement made of tissue from an animal heart valve (*synonym:* bioprosthesis)

homograft: heart valve replacement made from a human heart valve (*synonym:* allograft)

leaflet repair: repair of a cardiac valve's movable "flaps" (leaflets)

mitral valve: atrioventricular valve located between the left atrium and left ventricle

orthotopic transplantation: the recipient's heart is removed and a donor heart is grafted into the same site

prolapse (of a valve): stretching of an atrioventricular heart valve leaflet into the atrium during systole

pulmonic valve: semilunar valve located between the right ventricle and pulmonary artery

regurgitation: backward flow of blood through a heart valve

stenosis: narrowing or obstruction of a cardiac valve's orifice

total artificial heart: mechanical device used to aid a failing heart, assisting the right and left ventricles

tricuspid valve: atrioventricular valve located between the right atrium and right ventricle

valve replacement: insertion of a device at the site of a malfunctioning heart valve to restore blood flow in one direction through the heart

valvuloplasty: repair of a stenosed or regurgitant cardiac valve by commissurotomy, annuloplasty, leaflet repair, or chordoplasty (or a combination of procedures)

ventricular assist device: mechanical device used to aid a failing right or left ventricle

Structural, infectious, and inflammatory disorders of the heart present many challenges for the patient, family, and health care team. Problems with heart valves, cardiomyopathies, and infectious diseases of the heart alter cardiac output. Treatments for these disorders may be noninvasive, such as medication therapy and activity or dietary modification. Invasive treatments also may be used, such as valve repair or replacement, ventricular assist devices (VADs), total artificial hearts, cardiac transplantation, and other procedures. Nurses have an integral role in the care of patients with structural, infectious, and inflammatory cardiac conditions.

VALVULAR DISORDERS

Valves of the heart control the flow of blood through the heart into the pulmonary artery and aorta by opening and

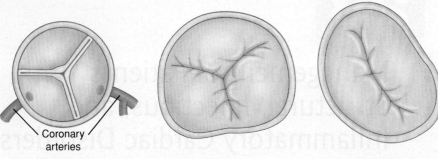

Aortic (semilunar) valve   Tricuspid valve   Mitral valve

FIGURE 28-1 • Valves of the heart (aortic or semilunar, tricuspid, and mitral) in closed positions.

closing in response to blood pressure changes during each cardiac cycle (heart contraction and relaxation).

Atrioventricular valves separate the atria from the ventricles and include the **tricuspid valve**, which separates the right atrium from the right ventricle, and the **mitral valve**, which separates the left atrium from the left ventricle. The tricuspid valve has three leaflets; the mitral valve has two. Both valves have **chordae tendineae** that anchor valve leaflets to papillary muscles of the ventricles.

Semilunar valves are located between the ventricles and their corresponding arteries. The **pulmonic valve** lies between the right ventricle and the pulmonary artery; the **aortic valve** lies between the left ventricle and the aorta. Figure 28-1 shows valves in the closed position. (Also refer to Fig. 25-1 in Chapter 25 to review the structure of a normal heart.)

When any heart valve does not close or open properly, blood flow is affected. When valves do not close completely, blood flows backward through the valve, a condition called **regurgitation**. When valves do not open completely, a condition called **stenosis**, blood flow through the valve is reduced.

Regurgitation and stenosis affect all heart valves. The mitral valve may also **prolapse** (i.e., stretching of the valve leaflet into the atrium during systole). Depending on the severity of symptoms, patients with valve disorders may not require treatment, or they may need to make lifestyle changes, take medications, or require surgical repair or replacement of the valve. Disorders of the mitral and aortic valve cause more symptoms, require treatment, and cause more complications than disorders of the tricuspid and pulmonic valves. Regurgitation and stenosis may occur at the same time in the same or different valves (Fig. 28-2).

Mitral Valve Prolapse

Mitral valve prolapse is a deformity that usually produces no symptoms. Rarely, it progresses and can result in sudden death. This condition occurs in up to 2.5% of the general population and more frequently in women than in men (Bonow, Mann, Zipes, et al., 2012; Nixon, 2011; Otto & Bonow, 2009). The cause may be an inherited connective tissue disorder resulting in enlargement of one or both of the mitral valve leaflets, but in many cases the cause is unknown. The annulus often dilates; chordae tendineae and papillary muscles may elongate or rupture.

Pathophysiology

In mitral valve prolapse, a portion of one or both mitral valve leaflets balloons back into the atrium during systole. Rarely, ballooning stretches the leaflet to the point that the valve does not remain closed during systole. Blood then regurgitates from the left ventricle back into the left atrium. About 15% of patients who develop murmurs eventually experience heart enlargement, atrial fibrillation, pulmonary hypertension, or heart failure (Fuster, Walsh, Harrington, et al., 2011).

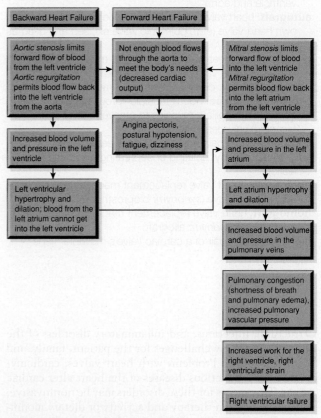

Physiology · ··· · Pathophysiology

Backward Heart Failure	Forward Heart Failure

Aortic stenosis limits forward flow of blood from the left ventricle
Aortic regurgitation permits blood flow back into the left ventricle from the aorta

Not enough blood flows through the aorta to meet the body's needs (decreased cardiac output)

Mitral stenosis limits forward flow of blood into the left ventricle
Mitral regurgitation permits blood flow back into the left atrium from the left ventricle

Increased blood volume and pressure in the left ventricle

Angina pectoris, postural hypotension, fatigue, dizziness

Increased blood volume and pressure in the left atrium

Left ventricular hypertrophy and dilation; blood from the left atrium cannot get into the left ventricle

Left atrium hypertrophy and dilation

Increased blood volume and pressure in the pulmonary veins

Pulmonary congestion (shortness of breath and pulmonary edema), increased pulmonary vascular pressure

Increased work for the right ventricle, right ventricular strain

Right ventricular failure

FIGURE 28-2 • Pathophysiology. Left-sided heart failure as a result of aortic and mitral valvular heart disease and development of right ventricular failure.

Clinical Manifestations

Most people with mitral valve prolapse never have symptoms. A few have fatigue, shortness of breath, lightheadedness, dizziness, syncope, palpitations, chest pain, or anxiety. Fatigue may occur regardless of activity level and amount of rest or sleep. Shortness of breath is not correlated with activity levels or pulmonary function. Atrial or ventricular dysrhythmias may produce the sensation of palpitations, but palpitations have been reported while the heart has been beating normally. Pain, which is often localized to the chest, is not correlated with activity and may last for days. Anxiety may be a response to symptoms; however, some patients report anxiety as the only symptom. Some clinicians speculate that symptoms may be explained by dysautonomia (a dysfunction of the autonomic nervous system that results in increased excretion of catecholamines). No consensus exists about the cause of symptoms (Bonow et al., 2012; Runge, Stouffer, & Patterson, 2011).

Assessment and Diagnostic Findings

Often the first and only sign of mitral valve prolapse is an extra heart sound, referred to as a mitral click. A systolic click is an early sign that a valve leaflet is ballooning into the left atrium. In addition to the mitral click, a murmur of mitral regurgitation may be heard if the valve opens during systole and blood flows back into the left atrium. If mitral regurgitation exists, a patient may experience signs and symptoms of heart failure. Echocardiography is used to diagnose and monitor progression of mitral valve prolapse.

Medical Management

Medical management is directed at controlling symptoms. If dysrhythmias are documented and cause symptoms, the patient is advised to eliminate caffeine and alcohol from the diet and to stop the use of tobacco products. Most patients do not require medication, but some are prescribed antiarrhythmic medications. Prophylactic antibiotics are not recommended prior to dental or invasive procedures (Nishimura, Carabello, Faxon, et al., 2008).

Chest pain that does not respond to nitrates may respond to calcium channel blockers or beta-blockers. Heart failure is treated the same as it would be for any other case of heart failure (see Chapter 29). Patients with severe mitral regurgitation and symptomatic heart failure may require mitral valve repair or replacement (discussed later in this chapter).

Nursing Management

The nurse educates the patient about the diagnosis and the possibility that the condition is hereditary. First-degree relatives (e.g., parents, siblings) may be advised to have echocardiograms. Patients with mitral valve prolapse may be at risk for infective endocarditis from bacteria entering the bloodstream and adhering to abnormal valve structures. The nurse educates the patient how to minimize this risk (see discussion of infective endocarditis later in this chapter).

Because most patients with mitral valve prolapse are asymptomatic, the nurse explains the need to inform the patient's primary provider about any symptoms that may develop. To minimize symptoms, the nurse instructs the patient to avoid caffeine and alcohol. The nurse encourages the patient to read product labels, particularly on over-the-counter products such as cough medicine, because these products may contain alcohol, caffeine, ephedrine, and epinephrine, which may produce dysrhythmias and other symptoms. The nurse also explores possible diet, activity, sleep, and other lifestyle factors that may correlate with symptoms. Treatment of dysrhythmias, chest pain, heart failure, or other complications of mitral valve prolapse is described in Chapters 26 and 29. Women diagnosed with mitral valve prolapse without mitral regurgitation or other complications may complete pregnancies with vaginal deliveries.

Mitral Regurgitation

Mitral regurgitation involves blood flowing back from the left ventricle into the left atrium during systole. Often, edges of mitral valve leaflets do not close completely during systole because leaflets and chordae tendineae have thickened and fibrosed, resulting in their contraction. The most common causes of mitral valve regurgitation in developed countries are degenerative changes of the mitral valve (e.g., mitral valve prolapse) and ischemia of the left ventricle (Bonow et al., 2012; Fuster et al., 2011). The most common cause in developing countries is rheumatic heart disease and its sequelae (Fuster et al., 2011).

Other conditions that lead to mitral regurgitation include myxomatous changes, which enlarge and stretch the left atrium and ventricle, causing leaflets and chordae tendineae to stretch or rupture. Infective endocarditis may cause perforation of a leaflet, or scarring following the infection may cause retraction of leaflets or chordae tendineae. Collagen vascular diseases (e.g., systemic lupus erythematosus), cardiomyopathy, and ischemic heart disease also may result in changes in the left ventricle, causing papillary muscles, chordae tendineae, or leaflets to stretch, shorten, or rupture.

Pathophysiology

Mitral regurgitation may result from problems with one or more leaflets, chordae tendineae, annulus, or papillary muscles. A mitral valve leaflet may shorten or tear, and chordae tendineae may elongate, shorten, or tear. The annulus may be stretched by heart enlargement or deformed by calcification. A papillary muscle may rupture, stretch, or be pulled out of position by changes in the ventricular wall (e.g., scar from a myocardial infarction, ventricular dilation). Papillary muscles may be unable to contract because of ischemia. Regardless of the cause, blood regurgitates into the atrium during systole.

With each beat of the left ventricle, some blood is forced back into the left atrium, adding to blood flowing in from the lungs. This causes the left atrium to stretch and eventually hypertrophy, then dilate. Backward flow of blood from the ventricle decreases blood flow from the lungs into the atrium. As a result, the lungs become congested, eventually adding extra strain to the right ventricle. During diastole, the increased blood volume from the atrium fills the ventricle. The volume overload causes ventricular hypertrophy. Eventually, the ventricle dilates and systolic heart failure develops.

Clinical Manifestations

Chronic mitral regurgitation is often asymptomatic, but acute mitral regurgitation (e.g., resulting from a myocardial infarction) usually manifests as severe congestive heart failure. Dyspnea, fatigue, and weakness are the most common symptoms. Palpitations, shortness of breath on exertion, and cough from pulmonary congestion also occur.

Assessment and Diagnostic Findings

A systolic murmur is a high-pitched, blowing sound at the apex (Hogan-Quigley, Palm, Bickley, 2012). The pulse may be regular and of good volume, or it may be irregular as a result of extrasystolic beats or atrial fibrillation. Echocardiography is used to diagnose and monitor the progression of mitral regurgitation. Transesophageal echocardiography (TEE) provides the best images of the mitral valve.

Medical Management

Management of mitral regurgitation is the same as for heart failure (see Chapter 29). Patients with mitral regurgitation and heart failure benefit from afterload reduction (arterial dilation) by treatment with angiotensin-converting enzyme (ACE) inhibitors such as captopril (Capoten), enalapril (Vasotec), lisinopril (Prinivil, Zestril) or ramipril (Altace), or hydralazine (Apresoline); or angiotensin receptor blockers (ARBs) such as losartan (Cozaar) or valsartan (Diovan); and beta-blockers, such as carvedilol (Coreg). Once symptoms of heart failure develop, the patient needs to restrict his or her activity level to minimize symptoms. Symptoms also are an indicator for surgical intervention by mitral valvuloplasty (i.e., surgical repair of the valve) or valve replacement (discussed later).

Mitral Stenosis

Mitral stenosis is an obstruction to blood flowing from the left atrium into the left ventricle. It most often is caused by rheumatic endocarditis, which progressively thickens mitral valve leaflets and chordae tendineae. Leaflets often fuse together. Eventually, the mitral valve orifice narrows and progressively obstructs blood flow into the ventricle.

Pathophysiology

Normally, the mitral valve orifice is as wide as the diameter of three fingers. In cases of severe stenosis, the orifice narrows to the width of a pencil. The left atrium has difficulty moving blood into the ventricle because of increased resistance by the narrowed orifice. Poor left ventricular filling can cause decreased cardiac output. Increased blood volume in the left atrium causes it to dilate and hypertrophy. Because there is no valve to protect pulmonary veins from backward flow of blood from the atrium, the pulmonary circulation becomes congested. As a result, the right ventricle must contract against abnormally high pulmonary arterial pressure and is subjected to excessive strain. The right ventricle hypertrophies, eventually dilates, and fails. If the heart rate increases, diastole is shortened; thus, the amount of time for forward flow of blood is less, and more blood backs into the pulmonary

veins. Therefore, as the heart rate increases, cardiac output decreases and pulmonary pressures increase.

Clinical Manifestations

The first symptom of mitral stenosis often is dyspnea on exertion (DOE) as a result of pulmonary venous hypertension. Symptoms usually develop after the valve opening is reduced by one third to one half its usual size. Patients may experience progressive fatigue and decreased exercise tolerance as a result of low cardiac output. An enlarged left atrium may create pressure on the left bronchial tree, resulting in a dry cough or wheezing. Patients may expectorate blood (i.e., hemoptysis) or experience palpitations, orthopnea, paroxysmal nocturnal dyspnea (PND), and repeated respiratory infections. As a result of increased blood volume and pressure, the atrium dilates, hypertrophies, and becomes electrically unstable (patients experience atrial dysrhythmias).

Assessment and Diagnostic Findings

The pulse is weak and often irregular because of atrial fibrillation (caused by strain on the atrium). A low-pitched, rumbling diastolic murmur is heard at the apex (Hogan-Quigley et al., 2012). Echocardiography is used to diagnose and quantify the severity of mitral stenosis. Electrocardiography (ECG), exercise testing, and cardiac catheterization with angiography may be used to help determine the severity of mitral stenosis.

Prevention

Prevention of mitral stenosis primarily is minimizing risk of and treatment for bacterial infections (see prevention of endocarditis later in this chapter). Prevention of acute rheumatic fever depends on effective antibiotic treatment of streptococcal pharyngitis (Special Writing Group, 1992). Antibiotic prophylaxis for recurrent rheumatic fever with rheumatic carditis may require 10 or more years of antibiotic coverage (e.g., penicillin G intramuscularly every 4 weeks, penicillin V orally twice daily, sulfadiazine orally daily, or erythromycin orally twice daily) (Bonow, Carabello, Chatterjee, et al., 2008; Bonow et al., 2012; Fuster et al., 2011).

Medical Management

Congestive heart failure is treated as described in Chapter 29. Patients with mitral stenosis may benefit from anticoagulants to decrease the risk of developing atrial thrombus and may require treatment for angina. If atrial fibrillation develops, cardioversion is attempted to restore normal sinus rhythm. If unsuccessful, the ventricular rate is controlled with beta-blockers, digoxin, or calcium channel blockers; furthermore, patients require anticoagulation for thromboembolism prevention. Patients with mitral stenosis are advised to avoid strenuous activities, competitive sports, and pregnancy, all of which increase heart rate. Surgical intervention consists of valvuloplasty, usually a commissurotomy to open or rupture the fused commissures of the valve. Percutaneous transluminal valvuloplasty or valve replacement may be performed.

Aortic Regurgitation

Aortic regurgitation is flow of blood back into the left ventricle from the aorta during diastole. It may be caused by inflammatory lesions that deform aortic valve leaflets or dilation of the aorta, preventing complete closure of the aortic valve. This valvular defect also may result from infective or rheumatic endocarditis, congenital abnormalities, diseases such as syphilis, a dissecting aneurysm that causes dilation or tearing of the ascending aorta, blunt chest trauma, or deterioration of a surgically replaced aortic valve (Bonow et al., 2012; Cohn, 2012; Fuster et al., 2011).

Pathophysiology

Blood from the aorta returns to the left ventricle during diastole, in addition to blood normally delivered by the left atrium. The left ventricle dilates in an attempt to accommodate the increased volume of blood. It also hypertrophies in an attempt to increase muscle strength to expel more blood with above-normal force, thus increasing systolic blood pressure. Arteries attempt to compensate for the higher pressures by reflex vasodilation; peripheral arterioles relax, reducing peripheral resistance and diastolic blood pressure.

Clinical Manifestations

Aortic insufficiency develops without symptoms in most patients. Some patients are aware of a forceful heartbeat, especially in the head or neck. Marked arterial pulsations visible or palpable at carotid or temporal arteries may be present as a result of increased force and volume of blood ejected from a hypertrophied left ventricle. Exertional dyspnea and fatigue follow. Signs and symptoms of progressive left ventricular failure include breathing difficulties (e.g., orthopnea, PND).

Assessment and Diagnostic Findings

A high-pitched, blowing diastolic murmur is heard at the third or fourth intercostal space at the left sternal border (Hogan-Quigley et al., 2012). The pulse pressure (i.e., difference between systolic and diastolic pressures) is considerably widened in patients with aortic regurgitation. One characteristic sign is the water-hammer (Corrigan's) pulse, in which the pulse strikes a palpating finger with a quick, sharp stroke and then suddenly collapses. The diagnosis may be confirmed by echocardiography (preferably transesophageal), cardiac magnetic resonance (CMR) imaging, radionuclide imaging, and cardiac catheterization (Christiansen, Karamitsos, & Myerson, 2011). Patients with symptoms usually have echocardiograms every 6 months, and those without symptoms have echocardiograms every 2 to 3 years (Nixon, 2011; Otto & Bonow, 2009).

Prevention

Prevention of aortic regurgitation is primarily based on prevention of and treatment for bacterial infections (see prevention of endocarditis later in this chapter). The same strategies aimed at preventing acute and recurrent rheumatic fever previously described for the patient with mitral stenosis apply to patients with aortic regurgitation.

Medical Management

The patient is advised to avoid physical exertion, competitive sports, and isometric exercise. Dysrhythmias and heart failure are treated as described in Chapters 26 and 29. The first medications usually prescribed for patients with symptoms of aortic regurgitation are vasodilators such as calcium channel blockers (e.g., felodipine [Plendil], nifedipine [Adalat, Procardia]) and ACE inhibitors (e.g., captopril, enalapril, lisinopril, ramipril) or hydralazine.

> ◣ **Quality and Safety Nursing Alert**
>
> The calcium channel blockers diltiazem (Cardizem) and verapamil (Calan, Isoptin) are contraindicated for patients with aortic regurgitation because they decrease ventricular contractility and may cause bradycardia.

The treatment of choice is aortic valve replacement or valvuloplasty (described later), preferably performed before left ventricular failure occurs. Surgery is recommended for any patient with left ventricular hypertrophy, regardless of the presence or absence of symptoms (Otto & Bonow, 2009).

Aortic Stenosis

Aortic valve stenosis is narrowing of the orifice between the left ventricle and aorta. In adults, stenosis often is a result of degenerative calcifications. Calcifications may be caused by proliferative and inflammatory changes that occur in response to years of normal mechanical stress, similar to changes that occur in atherosclerotic arterial disease. Diabetes, hypercholesterolemia, hypertension, and low levels of high-density lipoprotein cholesterol may be risk factors for degenerative changes of the valve. Congenital leaflet malformations or an abnormal number of leaflets (i.e., one or two rather than three) may be involved. Rheumatic endocarditis may cause adhesions or fusion of the commissures and valve ring, stiffening of the cusps, and calcific nodules on the cusps.

Pathophysiology

Progressive narrowing of the valve orifice occurs, usually over several years to several decades. The left ventricle overcomes obstruction to emptying by contracting more slowly but with more power than normal, forcibly squeezing blood through the smaller orifice. Obstruction to left ventricular outflow increases pressure on the left ventricle, so the ventricular wall thickens (i.e., hypertrophies). When these compensatory mechanisms of the heart begin to fail, clinical signs and symptoms develop (Nixon, 2011; Otto & Bonow, 2009).

Clinical Manifestations

Many patients with aortic stenosis are asymptomatic. When symptoms develop, patients usually first have exertional dyspnea, caused by increased pulmonary venous pressure due to left ventricular failure. Orthopnea, PND, and pulmonary edema also may occur. Reduced blood flow to the brain may cause dizziness and syncope. Angina pectoris is a frequent symptom; it results from increased oxygen demand of the hypertrophied left ventricle with decreased blood supply due to decreased blood flow into the coronary arteries and decreased time in diastole for myocardial perfusion. Blood pressure is usually normal but may be low. Pulse pressure may be low (30 mm Hg or less) because of diminished blood flow.

Assessment and Diagnostic Findings

On physical examination, a loud, rough systolic murmur may be heard over the aortic area and may radiate to the carotid arteries and apex of the left ventricle. The murmur is low-pitched, crescendo–decrescendo, rough, rasping, and vibrating. An S_4 sound may be heard. If the examiner rests a hand over the base of the heart (second intercostal space next to the sternum and above the suprasternal notch) and up along the carotid arteries, a vibration may be felt. The vibration is caused by turbulent blood flow across the narrowed valve orifice. By having the patient lean forward during auscultation and palpation, especially during exhalation, it is possible to accentuate sounds of aortic stenosis (Hogan-Quigley et al., 2012).

Echocardiography, CMR imaging, and computed tomography (CT) scanning are used to diagnose and monitor progression of aortic stenosis. Patients with symptoms usually have echocardiograms every 6 to 12 months, and those without symptoms have echocardiograms every 1 to 5 years (Bonow et al., 2008; Fuster et al., 2011; Nixon, 2011). Evidence of left ventricular hypertrophy may be seen on a 12-lead ECG and an echocardiogram. After stenosis progresses to the point that surgical intervention is considered, left-sided heart catheterization is necessary to measure the severity of the valvular abnormality and to evaluate the coronary arteries. Pressure tracings are taken from the left ventricle and base of the aorta. The systolic pressure in the left ventricle is considerably higher than that in the aorta during systole. Graded exercise studies (stress tests) to assess exercise capacity are performed with caution for patients with aortic stenosis because of the high risk of precipitating ventricular tachycardia or fibrillation (Bonow et al., 2012; Cohn, 2012; Nixon, 2011; Otto & Bonow, 2009).

Prevention

Prevention of aortic stenosis is primarily focused on controlling risk factors for proliferative and inflammatory responses—namely, through treating diabetes, hypertension, cholesterol, and triglycerides and avoiding tobacco products. (See prevention of endocarditis later in this chapter.)

Medical Management

Medications are prescribed to treat dysrhythmia or left ventricular failure (see Chapters 26 and 29). Definitive treatment for aortic stenosis is surgical replacement of the aortic valve. Patients who are symptomatic and are not surgical candidates may benefit from one- or two-balloon percutaneous valvuloplasty procedures with or without transcatheter aortic valve implantation (TAVI) as described later in the chapter.

Nursing Management: Valvular Heart Disorders

The nurse educates the patient with valvular heart disease about the diagnosis, progressive nature of valvular heart disease, and treatment plan. The patient is instructed to report new symptoms or changes in symptoms to the primary provider. The nurse also educates the patient that an infectious agent, usually a bacterium, is able to adhere to a diseased heart valve more readily than to a normal valve. Once attached to the valve, the infectious agent multiplies, resulting in endocarditis and further damage to the valve. In addition, the nurse educates the patient about how to minimize the risk of developing infective endocarditis (discussed later in this chapter).

The nurse measures the patient's heart rate, blood pressure, and respiratory rate, compares these results with previous data, and notes any changes. Heart and lung sounds are auscultated and peripheral pulses palpated. The nurse assesses the patient with valvular heart disease for the following:

- Signs and symptoms of heart failure, such as fatigue, DOE, decreased activity tolerance, an increase in coughing, hemoptysis, multiple respiratory infections, orthopnea, and PND (see Chapter 29)
- Dysrhythmias, by palpating the patient's pulse for strength and rhythm (i.e., regular or irregular) and asking whether the patient has experienced palpitations or felt forceful heartbeats (see Chapter 26)
- Symptoms such as dizziness, syncope, increased weakness, or angina pectoris (see Chapter 27)

The nurse collaborates with the patient to develop a medication schedule and provides education about the name, dosage, actions, adverse effects, and any drug–drug or drug–food interactions of prescribed medications for heart failure, dysrhythmias, angina pectoris, or other symptoms. Specific precautions are emphasized, such as the risk to patients with aortic stenosis who experience angina pectoris and take nitroglycerin. The venous dilation that results from nitroglycerin decreases blood return to the heart, thus decreasing cardiac output and increasing the risk of syncope and decreased coronary artery blood flow. The nurse instructs the patient about the importance of attempting to relieve the symptoms of angina with rest and relaxation before taking nitroglycerin and to anticipate the potential adverse effects.

In addition, the nurse educates the patient to take a daily weight and report gains of 3 pounds in 1 day or 5 pounds in 1 week to the primary provider (American Heart Association, 2011). The nurse may assist the patient with planning activity and rest periods to achieve an acceptable lifestyle. Patients who experience symptoms of pulmonary congestion are advised to rest and sleep sitting in a chair or bed with the head elevated. Care of patients treated with valvuloplasty or surgical valve replacement is described later in this chapter.

SURGICAL MANAGEMENT: VALVE REPAIR AND REPLACEMENT PROCEDURES

Valvuloplasty

Repair, rather than replacement, of a cardiac valve is referred to as **valvuloplasty**. In general, valves that undergo valvuloplasty function longer than prosthetic valve replacements and patients do not require continuous anticoagulation (Bonow et al., 2008; Bonow et al., 2012; Cohn, 2012; Otto & Bonow, 2009). The type of valvuloplasty depends on the cause and type of valve dysfunction. Repair may be made to commissures between the leaflets in a procedure known as **commissurotomy**, to the annulus of the valve by annuloplasty, to leaflets, or to chordae by chordoplasty. TEE usually is performed at the conclusion of a valvuloplasty to evaluate the effectiveness of the procedure.

Most valvuloplasty procedures require general anesthesia and often require cardiopulmonary bypass. However, some procedures do not require general anesthesia or cardiopulmonary bypass and can be performed in a cardiac catheterization laboratory or hybrid room. A hybrid room is an operating room with imaging capability (e.g., fluoroscopy, CT, magnetic resonance imaging) and interventional devices for open, minimally invasive, image-guided and catheter-based procedures (Vallabhajosyula & Bavaria, 2011). Percutaneous partial cardiopulmonary bypass is used in some cardiac catheterization laboratories and hybrid rooms. (Cardiopulmonary bypass is described in Chapter 27.)

Commissurotomy

The most common valvuloplasty procedure is commissurotomy. Each valve has leaflets; the site where the leaflets meet is called the *commissure*. Leaflets may adhere to one another and close the commissure (i.e., stenosis). Less commonly, leaflets fuse in such a way that in addition to stenosis, the leaflets also are prevented from closing completely, resulting in backward flow of blood (i.e., regurgitation). A commissurotomy is the procedure performed to separate the fused leaflets.

Closed Commissurotomy/Balloon Valvuloplasty

Closed commissurotomies do not require cardiopulmonary bypass. The valve is not directly visualized. Closed commissurotomy is more common in developing nations; it is a surgical technique performed in the operating room with the patient under general anesthesia. A midsternal incision is made, a small hole is cut into the heart, and the surgeon's finger or a dilator is used to open the commissure.

Percutaneous balloon valvuloplasty is the technique most commonly performed in the United States for closed commissurotomy. Balloon valvuloplasty is beneficial for mitral valve stenosis in younger patients, for aortic valve stenosis in older patients, and for patients with complex medical conditions that place them at high risk for complications of more extensive surgical procedures. Most often used for mitral and aortic valve stenosis, balloon valvuloplasty also has been used for tricuspid and pulmonic valve stenosis. The procedure is contraindicated for patients with left atrial or ventricular thrombus, severe aortic root dilation, significant mitral valve regurgitation, severe valvular calcification, thoracolumbar scoliosis, rotation of the great vessels, and other cardiac conditions that require open heart surgery (Fuster et al., 2011; Cohn, 2012; Otto & Bonow, 2009).

Balloon valvuloplasty (Fig. 28-3) is performed in the cardiac catheterization laboratory. The patient may receive light or moderate sedation or just a local anesthetic. Mitral balloon valvuloplasty involves advancing one or two catheters into the right atrium, through the atrial septum into the left atrium, across the mitral valve, and into the left ventricle. A

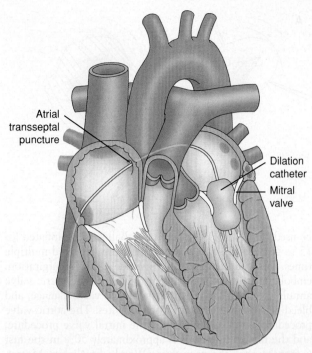

FIGURE 28-3 • Balloon valvuloplasty. Cross-section of heart illustrating the dilation catheter placed through an atrial transseptal puncture and across the mitral valve. The Inoue balloon inflates in three stages: first below the valve, then above, and finally in the valve orifice (this diagram shows the first two sections inflated).

guidewire is placed through each catheter, and the original catheter is removed. In the United States and Europe, most often a specially designed balloon catheter is placed over the guidewire and positioned with the balloon across the mitral valve. The balloon has three sections with progressively greater resistance to inflation. The balloon first expands in the ventricle to help position the catheter at the valve. The second section of the balloon expands above the valve, holding the catheter across the valve. Finally, the middle section of the balloon expands in the valve orifice opening the commissures. Alternately, two balloons are used. Guidewires may be advanced into the aorta to stabilize the balloons' positions. These single-section balloons are inflated simultaneously and expand their entire length. The advantage of two balloons is that each is smaller than the one large balloon often used, making smaller atrial septal defects. As the two balloons are inflated, they usually do not completely occlude the valve, thereby permitting some forward flow of blood during the inflation period. Balloons are inflated with a dilute angiographic solution for 10 to 30 seconds. Multiple inflations usually are required to achieve the desired results.

All patients have some degree of mitral regurgitation after the procedure. Other possible complications include bleeding from the catheter insertion sites, emboli resulting in complications such as strokes, and, rarely, left-to-right atrial shunts through the atrial septal defect created during the procedure.

Aortic balloon valvuloplasty is performed most commonly by introducing a catheter through the aorta, across the aortic valve, and into the left ventricle, although it also may be performed by passing the balloon or balloons through the atrial septum. The one- or two-balloon technique can

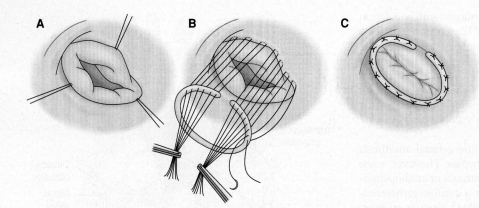

FIGURE 28-4 • Annuloplasty ring insertion. **A.** Mitral valve regurgitation; leaflets do not close. **B.** Insertion of an annuloplasty ring. **C.** Completed valvuloplasty; leaflets close.

be used for treating aortic stenosis. Balloons are inflated for 15 to 60 seconds, and inflation is usually repeated multiple times. Possible complications include aortic regurgitation, emboli, ventricular perforation, rupture of the aortic valve annulus, ventricular dysrhythmia, mitral valve damage, and bleeding from the catheter insertion sites. The aortic valve procedure is not as effective as the mitral valve procedure, and the rate of restenosis is approximately 50% in the first 6 months after the procedure (Woods, Froelicher, Motzer, et al., 2010).

Open Commissurotomy

Open commissurotomies are performed with direct visualization of the valve. The patient is under general anesthesia. A midsternal or left thoracic incision is made. Cardiopulmonary bypass is initiated, and an incision is made into the heart. The valve is exposed, and a scalpel, finger, balloon, or dilator is used to open the commissures.

An added advantage of directly visualizing the valve is that thrombus and calcifications may be identified and removed. If the valve has chordae or papillary muscles, they may be inspected and surgically repaired as necessary.

Annuloplasty

Annuloplasty is repair of the valve annulus (i.e., junction of valve leaflets and muscular heart wall). General anesthesia and cardiopulmonary bypass are required for most annuloplasties. The procedure narrows the diameter of the valve's orifice and is a useful treatment for valvular regurgitation.

There are two annuloplasty techniques. One technique uses an annuloplasty ring (Fig. 28-4), which may be pre-shaped (rigid/semirigid) or flexible. Leaflets of the valve are sutured to a ring, creating an annulus of the desired size. When the ring is in place, tension created by moving blood and the contracting heart is borne by the ring rather than

by the valve or a suture line. The repair prevents progressive regurgitation.

A second technique to tighten the annulus involves taking tucks in leaflets or tacking leaflets to the atrium or each other with sutures. Because the valve's leaflets and suture lines are subjected to direct forces of the blood and heart muscle movement, the repair may degenerate more quickly than one using an annuloplasty ring.

Leaflet Repair

Damage to cardiac valve leaflets may result from stretching, shortening, or tearing. **Leaflet repair** for elongated, ballooning, or other excess tissue leaflets is removal of the extra tissue. Elongated tissue may be folded over onto itself (i.e., tucked) and sutured (i.e., leaflet plication). A wedge of tissue may be cut from the middle of the leaflet and the gap sutured closed (i.e., leaflet resection) (Fig. 28-5). Short leaflets are most often repaired by chordoplasty. After short chordae are released, leaflets often unfurl and resume their normal function (closing the valve during systole). A leaflet may be extended by suturing a piece of pericardium to it. A pericardial or synthetic patch may be used to repair holes in the leaflets.

Chordoplasty

Chordoplasty is repair of chordae tendineae. The mitral valve is involved with chordoplasty (because it has chordae tendineae); the tricuspid valve seldom requires chordoplasty. Stretched, torn, or shortened chordae tendineae may cause regurgitation. Stretched chordae tendineae can be shortened, transposed to the other leaflet, or replaced with synthetic chordae. Torn chordae can be reattached to the leaflet, and shortened chordae can be elongated. Stretched papillary muscles, which may also cause regurgitation, can be shortened or relocated.

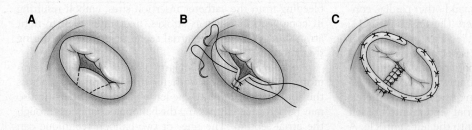

FIGURE 28-5 • Valve leaflet resection and repair with a ring annuloplasty. **A.** Mitral valve regurgitation; the section indicated by *dashed lines* is excised. **B.** Approximation of edges and suturing. **C.** Completed valvuloplasty, leaflet repair, and annuloplasty ring.

Valve Replacement

When valvuloplasty is not a viable alternative (e.g., when the annulus or leaflets of the valve are immobilized by calcifications, severe fibrosis or fusion of leaflets, chordae tendineae, or papillary muscles), **valve replacement** is performed. General anesthesia and cardiopulmonary bypass are used for most valve replacements. Most procedures are performed through a median sternotomy (i.e., incision through the sternum), although the mitral valve may be approached through a right thoracotomy incision.

Mitral, and more rarely aortic, valve replacements may be performed with minimally invasive techniques that do not involve cutting through the length of the sternum. Instead, a 2- to 4-inch incision is made in only the upper or lower half of the sternum or between ribs, or performed percutaneously. Some minimally invasive procedures are robot assisted; surgical instruments are connected to a robot, and the surgeon, watching a video display, uses a joystick to control the robot and surgical instruments. With these procedures, patients have less bleeding, pain, risk of infection, and scarring. Hospital length of stay averages 5 days, and recovery may be as short as 3 to 4 weeks (Bonow et al., 2012; Cohn, 2012; Holmes, Mack, Kaul, et al., 2012).

After the valve is visualized, leaflets of the aortic or pulmonic valve are removed, but some or all of the mitral valve structures (leaflets, chordae, and papillary muscles) are left in place to help maintain the shape and function of the left ventricle after mitral valve replacement. Sutures are placed around the annulus and then through the valve prosthesis. The replacement valve is slid down the suture into position and tied into place (Fig. 28-6). The patient is weaned from cardiopulmonary bypass, the quality of the surgical repair is often assessed with color flow Doppler TEE, and then surgery is completed.

Transcatheter aortic valve implantation (TAVI), a minimally invasive aortic valve replacement procedure, may be performed in a catheterization laboratory or hybrid room. TAVI is indicated for patients with aortic stenosis who are not candidates for surgical valve replacement or have a high surgical risk (Bonow et al., 2012; Fuster et al., 2011; Holmes et al., 2012). With the patient under general anesthesia, a balloon valvuloplasty is performed. Then, a bioprosthetic (tissue) replacement valve (Fig. 28-7) attached to a catheter is inserted percutaneously, positioned at the aortic valve, and implanted (deployed).

Before surgery, the heart gradually adjusted to the pathology; however, surgery abruptly "corrects" the way blood flows through the heart. Complications unique to valve replacement are related to the sudden changes in intracardiac blood pressures. All prosthetic valve replacements create a degree of stenosis when they are implanted in the heart. Usually, the stenosis is mild and does not affect heart function. If valve replacement was for a stenotic valve, blood flow through the heart is often improved. The signs and symptoms of backward heart failure resolve in a few hours or days. If valve replacement was for a regurgitant valve, it may take months for the chamber into which blood had been regurgitating to achieve its optimal postoperative function. Signs and symptoms of heart failure resolve gradually as heart function improves. Patients are at risk for many postoperative complications, such as bleeding, thromboembolism, infection, heart failure, hypertension, dysrhythmias, hemolysis, and mechanical obstruction of the valve.

Two types of valve prostheses may be used: mechanical and tissue valves (see Fig. 28-7).

Mechanical Valves

Mechanical valves are of the bileaflet, tilting-disk, or ball-and-cage design and are thought to be more durable than tissue prosthetic valves; therefore, they often are used for younger patients. These valves also are used for patients with renal failure, hypercalcemia, endocarditis, or sepsis who require valve replacement. For patients with these conditions, mechanical valves do not deteriorate or become infected as easily as tissue valves. Significant complications associated with mechanical valves are thromboemboli and long-term use of required anticoagulants. Some amount of hemolysis also occurs with these valves; usually, it is not clinically significant (Bonow et al., 2012).

Tissue Valves

Tissue valves are of three types: bioprostheses, homografts, and autografts. Tissue valves are less likely than mechanical valves to generate thromboemboli, and long-term anticoagulation is not required. Tissue valves are not as durable as mechanical valves and require replacement more frequently.

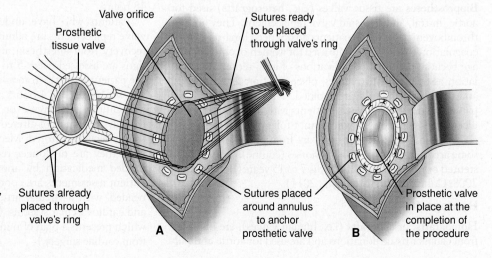

FIGURE 28-6 • Valve replacement. **A.** The native valve is trimmed, and the prosthetic valve is sutured in place. **B.** Once all sutures are placed through the ring, the surgeon slides the prosthetic valve down the sutures and into the natural orifice. Sutures are then tied off and trimmed.

Valve orifice

Prosthetic tissue valve

Sutures ready to be placed through valve's ring

Sutures already placed through valve's ring

Sutures placed around annulus to anchor prosthetic valve

A

Prosthetic valve in place at the completion of the procedure

B

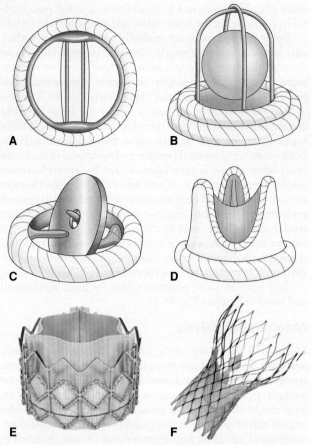

FIGURE 28-7 • Common mechanical and tissue valve replacements. **A.** Bileaflet (St. Jude, mechanical). **B.** Caged ball valve (Starr-Edwards, mechanical). **C.** Tilting-disk valve (Medtronic-Hall, mechanical). **D.** Porcine heterograft valve (Carpenter-Edwards, tissue). **E.** Transcatheter aortic valve (Edwards SAPIEN Transcatheter Heart Valve, tissue). Used with the permission of Edwards Lifesciences LLC, Irvine, CA; Edwards SAPIEN and SAPIEN are trademarks of Edwards Lifesciences Corporation. **F.** Transcatheter aortic valve (Medtronic The CoreValve® System, tissue). Used with the permission of Medtronic. The CoreValve System® is an investigational device and is limited by United States law to investigational use. CoreValve is a registered trademark of Medtronic CV Luxembourg S.a.r.l.).

Bioprostheses

Bioprostheses are tissue valves (e.g., **heterografts**) used for aortic, mitral, and tricuspid valve replacement. They are not thrombogenic; therefore, patients do not need long-term anticoagulation therapy. They are used for women of childbearing age because potential complications of long-term anticoagulation associated with menses, placental transfer to a fetus, and delivery of a child are avoided. They also are used for patients older than 70 years, patients with a history of peptic ulcer disease, and others who cannot tolerate long-term anticoagulation. Most bioprostheses are from pigs (porcine), but some are from cows (bovine) or horses (equine). They may be stented or nonstented. Viability is 7 to 15 years (Bonow et al., 2008; Cohn, 2012; Fuster et al., 2011).

Homografts

Homografts, or **allografts** (i.e., human valves), are obtained from cadaver tissue donations and are used for aortic and pul-

monic valve replacement. The aortic valve and a portion of aorta or the pulmonic valve and a portion of pulmonary artery are harvested and stored cryogenically. Homografts are not always available and are very expensive. They last for about 10 to 15 years (Bonow et al., 2008; Cohn, 2012; Otto & Bonow, 2009).

Autografts

Autografts (i.e., autologous valves) are obtained by excising the patient's own pulmonic valve and a portion of the pulmonary artery for use as the aortic valve. Anticoagulation is unnecessary because the valve is the patient's own tissue and is not thrombogenic. The autograft is an alternative for children (it may grow as the child grows), women of childbearing age, young adults, patients with a history of peptic ulcer disease, and people who cannot tolerate anticoagulation. Aortic valve autografts have remained viable for more than 20 years (Cohn, 2012; Otto & Bonow, 2009).

Most aortic valve autograft procedures are double valve replacement procedures with a homograft pulmonic valve replacement also performed. If pulmonary vascular pressures are normal, some surgeons elect not to replace the pulmonic valve. Patients can recover without a valve between the right ventricle and pulmonary artery.

Nursing Management: Valvuloplasty and Valve Replacement

The nurse assists the patient and family to prepare for the procedure, reinforces and supplements explanations provided by the physician, and provides psychosocial support. (See Chapters 17 through 19 for care of the surgical patient.)

Patients who have undergone percutaneous balloon valvuloplasty with or without percutaneous valve replacement may be admitted to a telemetry unit or intensive care unit (ICU). The nurse assesses for signs and symptoms of heart failure and emboli (see Chapter 29), listens for changes in heart sounds at least every 4 hours, and provides the patient with the same care as for postprocedure cardiac catheterization or percutaneous transluminal coronary angioplasty (see Chapter 27). After undergoing percutaneous balloon valvuloplasty, the patient usually remains in the hospital for 24 to 48 hours.

Patients who have undergone surgical valvuloplasty or valve replacements are admitted to the ICU. Care focuses on recovery from anesthesia and hemodynamic stability. Vital signs are assessed every 5 to 15 minutes and as needed until the patient recovers from anesthesia or sedation and then are assessed every 2 to 4 hours and as needed. Intravenous (IV) medications to increase or decrease blood pressure and to treat dysrhythmias or altered heart rates are administered and their effects monitored. Medications are gradually decreased until they are no longer required or the patient takes the needed medication by another route (e.g., oral, topical). Patient assessments are conducted every 1 to 4 hours and as needed, with particular attention to neurologic, respiratory, and cardiovascular systems. (See Chart 27-13 in Chapter 27, which presents a plan of nursing care for a patient recovering from cardiac surgery.)

After the patient has recovered from anesthesia and sedation, is hemodynamically stable without IV medications, and has stable physical assessment parameters, he or she usually is transferred to a telemetry unit, typically within 24 to 72 hours of surgery. Nursing care continues as for most postoperative patients, including wound care and patient education regarding diet, activity, medications, and self-care. The patient usually is discharged from the hospital in 3 to 7 days.

The nurse educates the patient about anticoagulant therapy, explaining the need for frequent follow-up appointments and blood laboratory studies. Patients who take warfarin (Coumadin) have individualized target international normalized ratios, usually between 2 and 3.5 for mitral valve replacement and 1.8 and 2.2 for aortic valve replacement. Patients who have been treated with an annuloplasty ring or a tissue valve replacement usually require anticoagulation for only 3 months unless there are other risk factors such as atrial fibrillation or a history of thromboembolism. Aspirin is prescribed with warfarin for patients with bioprostheses or at high risk for embolic events (e.g., history of embolic event or having two or more preexisting conditions: diabetes, hypertension, coronary artery disease, congestive heart failure, older than 75 years) (Bonow et al., 2008; Otto & Bonow, 2009). The nurse provides education about all prescribed medications, including the name of medication, dosage, actions, prescribed schedule, potential adverse effects, and any drug–drug or drug–food interactions.

Patients with a mechanical valve prosthesis (including annuloplasty rings and other prosthetic materials used in valvuloplasty) require education to prevent infective endocarditis. Patients may be at risk for infective endocarditis that results from bacteria entering the bloodstream and adhering to abnormal valve structures or prosthetic devices. The nurse educates the patient about how to minimize the risk of developing infective endocarditis (see prevention of endocarditis later in this chapter). Antibiotic prophylaxis is necessary before dental procedures involving manipulation of gingival tissue, the periapical area of the teeth, or perforation of the oral mucosa (not including routine anesthetic injections, placement of orthodontic brackets, or loss of deciduous teeth). Antibiotic therapy should also be used before invasive procedures involving the respiratory tract (e.g., biopsy of respiratory mucosa, tonsillectomy, and adenectomy).

Home care and office or clinic nurses reinforce all new information and self-care instructions with patients and families for 4 to 8 weeks after the procedure. Echocardiograms often are performed 3 to 4 weeks after hospital discharge to further evaluate the effects and results of surgery. The echocardiogram also provides a baseline for future comparison if cardiac symptoms or complications develop. Echocardiograms usually are repeated every 1 to 2 years.

Cardiomyopathy

Cardiomyopathy is disease of the heart muscle that is associated with cardiac dysfunction. It is classified according to the structural and functional abnormalities of the heart muscle: dilated cardiomyopathy (DCM), hypertrophic cardiomyopathy (HCM), restrictive or constrictive cardiomyopathy

(RCM), arrhythmogenic right ventricular cardiomyopathy (ARVC), and unclassified cardiomyopathy (Bonow et al., 2012). A patient may have pathology representing more than one of these classifications, such as a patient with HCM developing dilation and symptoms of DCM. *Ischemic cardiomyopathy* is a term frequently used to describe an enlarged heart caused by coronary artery disease, which is usually accompanied by heart failure (see Chapter 29). In 2006, the American Heart Association proposed a new set of Contemporary Classifications. Under this classification system, cardiomyopathies are divided into two major groups based on predominant organ involvement. These include *primary cardiomyopathies* (genetic, nongenetic, and acquired), which are focused primarily on the heart muscle, and *secondary cardiomyopathies*, which show myocardial involvement secondary to the influence of a vast list of disease processes that include, but are not limited to, amyloidosis, Fabry's disease, sarcoidosis, and scleroderma (Maron, Towbin, Thiene, et al., 2006). This chapter focuses on the primary cardiomyopathies.

Pathophysiology

The pathophysiology of all cardiomyopathies is a series of events that culminate in impaired cardiac output. Decreased stroke volume stimulates the sympathetic nervous system and the renin–angiotensin–aldosterone response, resulting in increased systemic vascular resistance and increased sodium and fluid retention, which place an increased workload on the heart. These alterations can lead to heart failure (see Chapter 29).

Concept Mastery Alert

Sodium is the major electrolyte involved with cardiomyopathy. Cardiomyopathy often leads to heart failure, which develops, in part, from fluid overload. Fluid overload is often associated with elevated sodium levels.

Dilated Cardiomyopathy

DCM is the most common form of cardiomyopathy, with an incidence of five to eight cases per 100,000 people per year (Mann, 2011; Bonow et al., 2012). DCM is distinguished by significant dilation of the ventricles without simultaneous hypertrophy (i.e., increased muscle wall thickness) and systolic dysfunction (Fig. 28-8). The ventricles have elevated systolic and diastolic volumes but a decreased ejection fraction.

More than 75 conditions and diseases may cause DCM, including pregnancy, heavy alcohol intake, viral infection (e.g., influenza), chemotherapeutic medications (e.g., daunorubicin [Cerubidine], doxorubicin [Adriamycin]), and Chagas disease. When the causative factor cannot be identified, the diagnosis is idiopathic DCM, which accounts for the largest subset of patients with DCM (Mann, 2011). Approximately 20% to 30% of all idiopathic DCM can be linked to familial genetics, and as diagnostic testing continues to improve, it is thought that this estimate may increase (Mann, 2011). Because genetic factors may be involved, echocardiography and ECG should be used to screen all first-degree blood relatives (e.g., parents, siblings, and children) for DCM (Bonow et al., 2012).

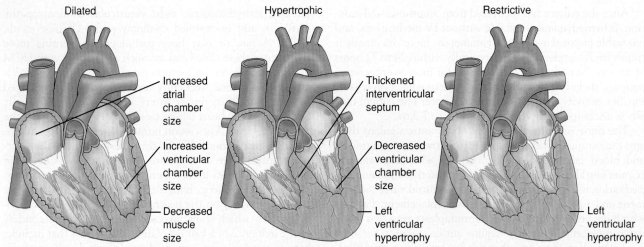

FIGURE 28-8 • Cardiomyopathies that lead to congestive heart failure. Redrawn from Anatomical Chart Company. (2006). *Atlas of pathophysiology* (2nd ed.). Ambler, PA: Lippincott Williams & Wilkins.

Microscopic examination of the muscle tissue shows diminished contractile elements (actin and myosin filaments) of the muscle fibers and diffuse necrosis of myocardial cells. The result is poor systolic function. The structural changes decrease the amount of blood ejected from the ventricle with systole, increasing the amount of blood remaining in the ventricle after contraction. Less blood is then able to enter the ventricle during diastole, increasing end-diastolic pressure and eventually increasing pulmonary and systemic venous pressures. Altered valve function, usually regurgitation, can result from an enlarged stretched ventricle. Poor blood flow through the ventricle may also cause ventricular or atrial thrombi, which may embolize to other locations in the body. Early diagnosis and treatment can prevent or delay significant symptoms and sudden death from DCM.

Restrictive Cardiomyopathy

RCM is characterized by diastolic dysfunction caused by rigid ventricular walls that impair diastolic filling and ventricular stretch (see Fig. 28-8). Systolic function is usually normal. RCM may be associated with amyloidosis (amyloid, a protein substance, is deposited within cells) and other such infiltrative diseases. However, the cause is unknown (i.e., idiopathic) in most cases. Signs and symptoms are similar to constrictive pericarditis and include dyspnea, nonproductive cough, and chest pain. Echocardiography, as well as measurement of pulmonary artery systolic pressure, pulmonary artery wedge pressure, and central venous pressure are used to differentiate the two conditions.

Hypertrophic Cardiomyopathy

HCM is a rare autosomal dominant condition, occurring in men, women, and children (often detected after puberty) with an estimated prevalence rate of 0.05% to 0.2% of the population in the United States (Sander, 2011). Echocardiograms may be performed every year from 12 to 18 years of age and then every 5 years from 18 to 70 years of age in susceptible individuals (i.e., those with a family history of HCM) (Sander, 2011). Doppler echocardiography may also be used to detect HCM and blood flow alterations

(Bonow et al., 2012). HCM also may be idiopathic (i.e., no known cause).

In HCM, the heart muscle asymmetrically increases in size and mass, especially along the septum (see Fig. 28-8). HCM often affects nonadjacent areas of the ventricle. The increased thickness of the heart muscle reduces the size of the ventricular cavities and causes the ventricles to take a longer time to relax after systole. During the first part of diastole, it is more difficult for the ventricles to fill with blood. The atrial contraction at the end of diastole becomes critical for ventricular filling and systolic contraction.

Cardiac muscle cells normally lie parallel to and end to end with each other. The hypertrophied cardiac muscle cells are disorganized, oblique, and perpendicular to each other, decreasing the effectiveness of contractions and possibly increasing the risk of dysrhythmias such as ventricular tachycardia and ventricular fibrillation. In HCM, the coronary arteriole walls are thickened, which decreases the internal diameter of the arterioles. The narrow arterioles restrict the blood supply to the myocardium, causing numerous small areas of ischemia and necrosis. The necrotic areas of the myocardium ultimately fibrose and scar, further impeding ventricular contraction.

Arrhythmogenic Right Ventricular Cardiomyopathy

ARVC occurs when the myocardium of the right ventricle is progressively infiltrated and replaced by fibrous scar and adipose tissue. Initially, only localized areas of the right ventricle are affected, but as the disease progresses, the entire heart is affected. Eventually, the right ventricle dilates and develops poor contractility, right ventricular wall abnormalities, and dysrhythmias. ARVC is an uncommon form of inherited heart muscle disease and often is not recognized. Therefore, the prevalence is largely unknown, although it is estimated to affect about 1 in 5,000 people (Fuster et al., 2011). Palpitations or syncope may develop between 15 and 40 years of age. ARVC should be considered in patients with ventricular tachycardia originating in the right ventricle (i.e., a left bundle branch block configuration on ECG) or sudden death, especially among young athletes (Bonow et al., 2012). ARVC is genetic (i.e., autosomal dominant)

(Basso, Corrado, Marcus, et al., 2009; Fuster et al., 2011). First-degree blood relatives (e.g., parents, siblings, children) should be screened for the disease with a 12-lead ECG, Holter monitor, and echocardiography.

Unclassified Cardiomyopathies

Unclassified cardiomyopathies are different from or have characteristics of more than one of the previously described types and are caused by fibroelastosis, noncompacted myocardium, systolic dysfunction with minimal dilation, and mitochondrial diseases (Bonow et al., 2012). Examples of unclassified cardiomyopathies can include left ventricular noncompaction and stress-induced (Takotsubo) cardiomyopathy.

Clinical Manifestations

Patients with cardiomyopathy may remain stable and without symptoms for many years. As the disease progresses, so do the symptoms. Frequently, dilated or restrictive cardiomyopathy is first diagnosed when the patient presents with signs and symptoms of heart failure (e.g., DOE, fatigue). Patients with cardiomyopathy may also report PND, cough (especially with exertion), and orthopnea, which may lead to a misdiagnosis of bronchitis or pneumonia. Other symptoms include fluid retention, peripheral edema, and nausea, which is caused by poor perfusion of the gastrointestinal system. The patient also may experience chest pain, palpitations, dizziness, nausea, and syncope with exertion. However, with HCM, cardiac arrest (i.e., sudden cardiac death) may be the initial manifestation in young people, including athletes (Bonow et al., 2012; Sander, 2011).

Regardless of type and cause, cardiomyopathy may lead to severe heart failure, lethal dysrhythmias, and death. The mortality rate is highest for African Americans and older adults (Mann, 2011).

Assessment and Diagnostic Findings

Physical examination at early stages may reveal tachycardia and extra heart sounds (e.g., S_3, S_4). Patients with DCM may have diastolic murmurs, and patients with DCM and HCM may have systolic murmurs. With disease progression, examination also reveals signs and symptoms of heart failure (e.g., crackles on pulmonary auscultation, jugular vein distention, pitting edema of dependent body parts, and enlarged liver).

Diagnosis is usually made from findings disclosed by the patient history and by ruling out other causes of heart failure such as myocardial infarction. The echocardiogram is one of the most helpful diagnostic tools because the structure and function of the ventricles can be observed easily. CMR imaging may also be used, particularly to assist with the diagnosis of HCM (Sander, 2011). ECG demonstrates dysrhythmias (atrial fibrillation, ventricular dysrhythmias) and changes consistent with left ventricular hypertrophy (left axis deviation, wide QRS, ST changes, inverted T waves). In ARVC, there often is a small deflection—an epsilon wave—at the end of the QRS. The chest x-ray reveals heart enlargement and possibly pulmonary congestion. Cardiac catheterization is sometimes used to rule out coronary artery disease as a causative factor. Endomyocardial biopsy may be performed to analyze myocardial cells.

Medical Management

Medical management is directed toward identifying and managing possible underlying or precipitating causes; correcting the heart failure with medications, a low-sodium diet, and an exercise/rest regimen (see Chapter 29); and controlling dysrhythmias with antiarrhythmic medications and possibly with an implanted electronic device, such as an implantable cardioverter defibrillator (ICD) (see Chapter 26). Systemic anticoagulation to prevent thromboembolic events is usually recommended. If the patient has signs and symptoms of congestion, fluid intake may be limited to 2 L each day. Patients with HCM should avoid dehydration and may need beta-blockers (atenolol [Tenormin], metoprolol [Lopressor], sotalol [Betapace], propranolol [Inderal]) to maintain cardiac output and minimize the risk of left ventricular outflow tract obstruction during systole. Patients with HCM or RCM may need to limit physical activity and avoid excessive weight gain to avoid a life-threatening dysrhythmia. To date, amiodarone (Cordarone) is the only drug shown to reduce the incidence of arrhythmogenic sudden cardiac death (Sander, 2011).

A pacemaker may be implanted to alter the electrical stimulation of the muscle and prevent the forceful hyperdynamic contractions that occur with HCM. Atrial-ventricular and biventricular pacing have been used to decrease symptoms and obstruction of the left ventricular outflow tract. For some patients with DCM and HCM, biventricular pacing increases the ejection fraction and reverses some of the structural changes in the myocardium.

Nonsurgical septal reduction therapy, also called *alcohol septal ablation*, has been used to treat obstructive HCM. In the cardiac catheterization laboratory, a percutaneous catheter is positioned in one or more of the septal coronary arteries. Once the position is verified, 1 to 5 mL of 96% to 98% ethanol (ethyl alcohol) is injected at a rate of about 1 mL/min to destroy the myocardial cells; it is believed that the ethanol causes dehydration of the cardiac cells (Bonow et al., 2012; Sander, 2011). The slow rate of injection minimizes the risk of heart block and premature ventricular contractions. The procedure produces a septal myocardial infarction. The resulting scar is thinner than the living myocardium had been, so the obstruction is decreased. The patient may develop a left anterior hemibranch block or left bundle branch block. If the patient experiences pain, hydrocodone/acetaminophen (Vicodin) usually is administered. Nitrates and morphine are not used because coronary artery dilation is contraindicated.

Surgical Management

When heart failure progresses and medical treatment is no longer effective, surgical intervention, including heart transplantation, is considered. However, because of the limited number of organ donors, many patients die waiting for transplantation. In some cases, a left ventricular assist device (LVAD) is implanted to support the failing heart until a suitable donor heart becomes available.

Left Ventricular Outflow Tract Surgery

When patients with HCM become symptomatic despite medical therapy and a difference in pressure of 50 mm Hg or more exists between the left ventricle and the aorta, surgery is considered (Gersh, Maron, Bonow, et al., 2011). The most common procedure is a myectomy (sometimes referred to as a myotomy-myectomy), in which some of the heart tissue is excised. Septal tissue approximately 1 cm wide and deep is cut from the enlarged septum below the aortic valve. The length of septum removed depends on the degree of obstruction caused by the hypertrophied muscle.

Instead of a septal myectomy, the surgeon may open the left ventricular outflow tract to the aortic valve by mitral valvuloplasty involving the leaflets, chordae, or papillary muscles, or the patient's mitral valve may be replaced with a low-profile disk valve. The space taken up by the mitral valve is substantially reduced by the valvuloplasty or prosthetic valve, allowing blood to move around the enlarged septum to the aortic valve through the area the mitral valve once occupied. The primary complication of all procedures is dysrhythmia. Additional complications include postoperative surgical complications such as pain, ineffective airway clearance, deep vein thrombosis, risk of infection, and delayed surgical recovery.

Heart Transplantation

Because of advances in surgical techniques and immunosuppressive therapies, heart transplantation is now a therapeutic option for patients with end-stage heart disease. Cyclosporine (Gengraf, Neoral, and Sandimmune) and tacrolimus (Prograf, FK506) are immunosuppressants that decrease the body's rejection of foreign proteins, such as transplanted organs. Unfortunately, these drugs also decrease the body's ability to resist infections, and a satisfactory balance must be achieved between suppressing rejection and avoiding infection. Currently, the number of heart transplantations performed worldwide is estimated to be more than 5,000 procedures annually—a level that is limited by donor availability (Fuster et al., 2011).

Cardiomyopathy, ischemic heart disease, valvular disease, rejection of previously transplanted hearts, and congenital heart disease are the most common indications for transplantation (Fuster et al., 2011). Typical candidates have severe symptoms uncontrolled by medical therapy, no other surgical options, and a prognosis of less than 2 years to live. A multidisciplinary team screens the candidate before recommending the transplantation procedure. The person's age, pulmonary status, other chronic health conditions, psychosocial status, family support, infections, history of other transplantations, adherence to therapeutic regimens, and current health status are considered. When a donor heart becomes available, a computer generates a list of potential recipients on the basis of ABO blood group compatibility, the body sizes of the donor and the potential recipient, age, severity of illness, length of time on the waiting list, and the geographic locations of the donor and potential recipient. Distance is a factor because postoperative function depends on the heart being implanted within 4 hours of harvest from the donor (Costanzo, Dipchand, Starling, et al., 2010). Some patients are candidates for more than one organ transplant (e.g., heart–lung, heart–kidney, heart–liver).

Orthotopic transplantation is the most common surgical procedure for cardiac transplantation. Some surgeons prefer to remove the recipient's heart but leave a portion of the

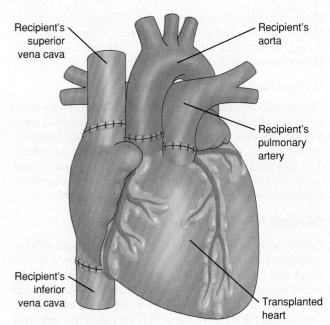

FIGURE 28-9 • Orthotopic method of heart transplantation.

recipient's atria (with the vena cava and pulmonary veins) in place, which is known as the biatrial technique. However, this technique has been modified to a more common approach called the *bicaval technique*. This technique includes removal of the recipient's heart, and the implantation of the donor heart with intact atria at the vena cava and pulmonary veins (Fig. 28-9) (Fuster et al., 2011; Mann, 2011). This newer approach is associated with decreased AV valve regurgitation, dysrhythmias, and conduction abnormalities.

Patients who have had heart transplantations are constantly balancing the risk of rejection with the risk of infection. They must adhere to a complex regimen of diet, medications, activity, follow-up laboratory studies, biopsies of the transplanted heart (to diagnose rejection), and clinic visits. There are three classes of medications that are prescribed for a transplant patient to help minimize rejection: corticosteroids (e.g., prednisone), calcineurin inhibitors (tacrolimus, cyclosporine), and antiproliferative agents (mycophenolate mofetil [CellCept], azathioprine [Imuran], or sirolimus [Rapamune]).

The transplanted heart has no nerve connections (i.e., denervated heart) to the recipient's body, so the sympathetic and vagus nerves do not affect the transplanted heart. The resting rate of the transplanted heart is approximately 70 to 90 bpm, but it increases gradually if catecholamines are in the circulation. Patients must gradually increase and decrease their exercise (i.e., extended warm-up and cool-down periods), because 20 to 30 minutes may be required to achieve the desired heart rate. Atropine does not increase the heart rate of transplanted hearts. Additionally, many heart transplant patients do not experience angina with ischemia and may present with congestive heart failure, silent myocardial infarction, or sudden death without a prior history of coronary artery disease (Fuster et al., 2011).

In addition to rejection and infection, complications may include accelerated atherosclerosis of the coronary arteries (i.e., cardiac allograft vasculopathy, accelerated graft atherosclerosis, transplant coronary artery disease). Both immunologic and nonimmunologic factors cause arterial injury and inflammation of the coronary arteries. The arterial smooth muscle proliferates, and there is hyperplasia of the coronary artery intima, accelerating atherosclerosis along the entire length of the coronary arteries (Bonow et al., 2012; Mann, 2011). Hypertension may occur in patients taking cyclosporine or tacrolimus; the cause has not been identified. Osteoporosis is a frequent side effect of the antirejection medications as well as pretransplantation dietary insufficiency and medications. Patients with a long-term sedentary lifestyle are at greater risk for osteoporosis. Posttransplantation lymphoproliferative disease and cancer of the skin and lips are the most common malignancies after transplantation, possibly caused by immunosuppression. Weight gain, obesity, diabetes, dyslipidemias (e.g., hypercholesterolemia), hypotension, and renal failure, as well as central nervous system, respiratory, and gastrointestinal disturbances, may be adverse effects of corticosteroids or other immunosuppressants. Toxicity from immunosuppressant medications may occur as well. The overall 1-year survival rate for patients with transplanted hearts is approximately 87% (Bonow et al., 2012; Mann, 2011).

In the first year after transplantation, patients respond to the psychosocial stresses imposed by organ transplant in various ways. Most report a better quality of life after transplantation and are able return to activities of daily living with little to no functional limitations (Bonow et al., 2012; Fuster et al., 2011; Mann, 2011). Some experience guilt that someone had to die for them to be able to live, have anxiety about the new heart, experience depression or fear about rejection, or have difficulty with family role changes before and after transplantation (Fuster et al., 2011).

Mechanical Assist Devices and Total Artificial Hearts

The use of cardiopulmonary bypass in cardiovascular surgery and the possibility of performing heart transplantation in patients with end-stage cardiac disease, as well as the desire for a treatment option for patients with such disease who are not transplant candidates, have increased the need for mechanical assist devices. Patients who cannot be weaned from cardiopulmonary bypass and patients in cardiogenic shock may benefit from a period of mechanical heart assistance. The most commonly used device is the intra-aortic balloon pump (see Chapter 29). This pump decreases the work of the heart during contraction but does not perform the actual work of the heart.

Ventricular Assist Devices

More complex devices that actually perform some or all of the pumping function for the heart also are being used. These more sophisticated **ventricular assist devices** (VADs) can circulate as much blood per minute as the heart, if not more (Fig. 28-10). There are short- and long-term devices available, depending on the indication. Each VAD is used to support one ventricle, although in some instances, two VAD pumps may be used for biventricular support. Additionally, some VADs can be combined with an oxygenator; the combination is called *extracorporeal membrane oxygenation*. The oxygenator–VAD combination

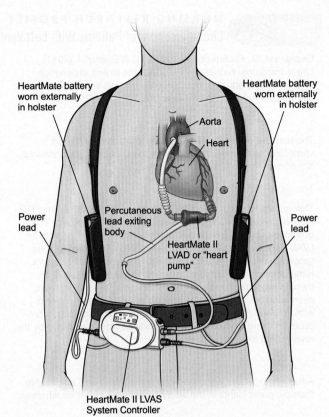

FIGURE 28-10 • Left ventricular assist device. Reprinted with the permission of Thoratec Corporation.

is used for the patient whose heart cannot pump adequate blood through the lungs or the body.

VADs may be used as (1) a "bridge to recovery" for patients who require temporary assistance for reversible ventricular failure, (2) a "bridge to transplant" for patients with end-stage heart failure until a donor organ becomes available for transplant (most common), and (3) "destination therapy" for patients with end-stage heart failure who are not candidates for or decline heart transplantation and have the VAD implanted for permanent use. As patients spend an increased length of time on the transplant list, and as more VADs are becoming approved for destination therapy, VAD patients are being discharged from the hospital with the devices in place. As such, the volume of patients with VADs in the community is rapidly expanding (Fuster et al., 2011; Mann, 2011).

VADs may be external, internal (i.e., implanted) with an external power source, or completely internal, and they may generate a pulsatile or continuous blood flow. There are four types of VADs: pneumatic, electric or electromagnetic, axial flow, and centrifugal. Pneumatic VADs are external or implanted pulsatile devices with a flexible reservoir housed in a rigid exterior. The reservoir usually fills with blood drained from the atrium or ventricle. The device then forces pressurized air into the rigid housing, compressing the reservoir and returning the blood to the circulation, usually into the aorta. Electric or electromagnetic VADs are similar to pneumatic VADs, but instead of using pressurized air to return the blood to the circulation, one or more flat metal plates are pushed against the reservoir. Axial flow VADs use a rotary mechanism (an impeller) to create nonpulsatile blood flow. The impeller

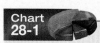

NURSING RESEARCH PROFILE

Chart 28-1

Life Adjustment of Patients With Left Ventricular Assist Device

Overgaard, D., Grufstedt Kjeldgaard, H., & Egerod, I. (2011). Life in transition: A qualitative study of the illness experience and vocational adjustment of patients with left ventricular assist device. *Journal of Cardiovascular Nursing, 27*(5), 394–402.

Purpose

The purpose of this study of patients implanted with a left ventricular assist device (LVAD) was to explore the psychosocial adjustments associated with this therapy.

Design

This qualitative study used the in-depth interview technique. The sample consisted of a convenience sample of 10 patients in the outpatient setting in Denmark who had experienced life with an LVAD between the years of 2008 and 2010. Participants' ages ranged between 18 and 63 years with a mean age of 38 years. Researchers constructed an interview guide that focused on themes related to life stages and their impact on the physical, psychological, social, and vocational adjustments of patients with an LVAD. The data were then managed by qualitative computer software, and concepts and findings were discussed by the researchers to reach consensus.

Findings

Although experiencing a life-altering diagnosis and aggressive therapy, participants in the study coped well with their situation.

Emotions ranged from gratitude and frustration toward the LVAD to hope and fear during preparation for cardiac transplantation. The overall theme showed that these participants with an LVAD succeeded in reestablishing their lives. However, findings from this study suggest that younger patients might need more vocational adjustment than older patients who have a more well-established occupation.

Nursing Implications

Patients who opt for implantation of an LVAD will deal with a plethora of emotions as they work to reestablish their lives. Nurses must be sensitive to the psychological, physical, and social needs of these patients. Patients and families appreciate warm, receptive, friendly nurses. Nurses need to provide patients with as much control over their lives as possible and always treat patients with respect and dignity. Nurses must identify issues important to the patient's quality of life and try to address them whenever possible. Providing patients with control over their routine and tasks are important so that patients can "feel normal." Ventricular assist device programs will often sponsor a support group to encourage and facilitate meetings with other LVAD patients to assist with coping. Additionally, patients appreciate spirituality, humor, peer support, and honesty to help them cope. These patients will rely heavily on support from the health care team, family, and friends.

---

spins rapidly within the VAD, creating a vacuum that pulls blood into the VAD and then pushes the blood out into the systemic circulation—the process is similar to a fan spinning in a tunnel, pulling air in one end of the tunnel and pushing it out the other. Centrifugal VADs are nonpulsatile devices that consist of a single moving impeller that is suspended in the pump housing by a combination of magnetic and hydrodynamic forces. The impeller rotates and pulls blood into the pump housing and ejects the blood out to the systemic circulation (Fuster et al., 2011).

Total Artificial Hearts

Total artificial hearts are designed to replace both ventricles. Some require the removal of the patient's heart to implant the total artificial heart, whereas others do not. Only one total artificial heart has been approved by the U.S. Food and Drug Administration (FDA) as a bridge to transplant, and another is currently FDA approved for destination therapy only. Although there has been some short-term success, the long-term results have been disappointing. Researchers hope to develop a device that can be permanently implanted and will eliminate the need for donated human heart transplantation for end-stage cardiac disease (Mann, 2011).

Complications of VADs and total artificial hearts include bleeding disorders, hemorrhage, thromboemboli, hemolysis, infection, renal failure, right-sided heart failure, multisystem failure, and mechanical failure (Fuster et al., 2011; Mann, 2011; Slaughter, Pagani, Rogers, et al., 2010). Nursing care of patients with these mechanical assist devices focuses on assessment for and minimization of these complications as well as providing emotional support and education about the device and the underlying cardiac disease. As the use of continuous flow devices increases and patients return to

their community and to work, it is imperative that education regarding the potential inability to detect a pulse in these patients is disseminated to families and emergency personnel in the community (Chart 28-1).

NURSING PROCESS

The Patient With Cardiomyopathy

Assessment

Nursing assessment for the patient with cardiomyopathy begins with a detailed history of the presenting signs and symptoms. The nurse identifies possible etiologic factors, such as heavy alcohol intake, recent illness or pregnancy, or history of the disease in immediate family members. If the patient reports chest pain, a thorough review of the pain, including its precipitating factors, is warranted. The review of systems includes the presence of orthopnea, PND, and syncope or dyspnea with exertion. The number of pillows needed to sleep, usual weight, any weight change, and limitations on activities of daily living are assessed. The New York Heart Association Classification for heart failure is determined (see Table 29-1 in Chapter 29). The patient's usual diet is evaluated to determine the need to reduce sodium intake, optimize nutrition, or supplement with vitamins.

Because of the chronicity of cardiomyopathy, the nurse conducts a careful psychosocial history, exploring the impact of the disease on the patient's role within the family and community. Identification of perceived stressors helps the patient and the health care team to implement activities that relieve anxiety related to changes in health status. Very early on, the patient's support systems are identified, and members are encouraged to become involved in the patient's care and therapeutic regimen. The assessment addresses the effect the diagnosis has had on the patient and members of his or her support system and the patient's emotional status. Depression is common in a patient with cardiomyopathy who has developed heart failure.

The physical assessment focuses on signs and symptoms of heart failure. The baseline assessment includes such key components as:

- Vital signs
- Calculation of pulse pressure and identification of pulsus paradoxus
- Current weight and any weight gain or loss
- Detection by palpation of the point of maximal impulse, often shifted to the left
- Cardiac auscultation for a systolic murmur and S_3 and S_4 heart sounds
- Pulmonary auscultation for crackles
- Measurement of jugular vein distention
- Assessment of edema and its severity

Diagnosis

Nursing Diagnoses

Based on the assessment data, major nursing diagnoses may include the following:

- Decreased cardiac output related to structural disorders caused by cardiomyopathy or to dysrhythmia from the disease process and medical treatments
- Risk for ineffective cardiac, cerebral, peripheral, and renal tissue perfusion related to decreased peripheral blood flow (resulting from decreased cardiac output)
- Impaired gas exchange related to pulmonary congestion caused by myocardial failure (resulting from decreased cardiac output)
- Activity intolerance related to decreased cardiac output or excessive fluid volume, or both
- Anxiety related to the change in health status and in role functioning
- Powerlessness related to disease process
- Noncompliance with medication and diet therapies

Collaborative Problems/Potential Complications

Potential complications may include the following:

- Heart failure
- Ventricular dysrhythmias
- Atrial dysrhythmias
- Cardiac conduction defects
- Pulmonary or cerebral embolism
- Valvular dysfunction

These complications are discussed earlier in this chapter and in Chapters 26 and 29.

Planning and Goals

The major goals for patients include improvement or maintenance of cardiac output, increased activity tolerance, reduction of anxiety, adherence to the self-care program, increased sense of power with decision making, and absence of complications.

Nursing Interventions

Improving Cardiac Output and Peripheral Blood Flow

During a symptomatic episode, rest is indicated. Many patients with DCM find that sitting up with their legs down is more comfortable than lying down in a bed. This position is helpful in pooling venous blood in the periphery and reducing preload. Assessing the patient's oxygen saturation at rest and during activity may assist with determining a need for supplemental oxygen. Oxygen usually is administered through a nasal cannula when indicated.

Ensuring that medications are taken as prescribed is important to preserving adequate cardiac output. The nurse may assist the patient with planning a schedule for taking medications and identifying methods to remember to follow it, such as associating the time to take a medication with an activity (e.g., eating a meal, brushing teeth). It is important to ensure that patients with DCM avoid verapamil, that patients with HCM avoid diuretics, and that patients with RCM avoid nifedipine to maintain contractility. In patients with HCM, the inotropic action of digoxin may create or worsen left ventricular outflow track obstruction. Patients with RCM have increased sensitivity to digoxin, and the nurse must anticipate that low doses will be prescribed and assess for digoxin toxicity.

It is also important to ensure that the patient receives or chooses food selections that are appropriate for a low-sodium diet. One way to monitor a patient's response to treatment is to determine the patient's weight every day and identify any significant change. Another indication of the effect of treatment involves assessment of shortness of breath after activity and comparison to before treatment, as well as a change in the number of pillows needed to comfortably sleep. Patients with low cardiac output may need assistance keeping warm and frequently changing position to stimulate circulation and reduce the possibility of skin breakdown. Patients with HCM must be taught to avoid dehydration. One guideline that patients can use for self-assessment is to anticipate the urge to void at least every 4 hours while awake; if the urge to void is not present or the urine is a deep yellow color, more fluid intake is necessary.

Increasing Activity Tolerance and Improving Gas Exchange

The nurse plans the patient's activities so that they occur in cycles, alternating rest with activity periods. This benefits the patient's physiologic status, and it helps educate the patient about the need for planned cycles of rest and activity. For example, after taking a bath or shower, the patient should plan to sit and read a newspaper or engage in other relaxing activities. Suggesting that the patient sit while chopping vegetables, drying his or her hair, or shaving helps the patient learn to balance rest with activity. The nurse also makes sure that the patient recognizes the symptoms indicating the need for rest and actions to take when the symptoms occur. Patients with HCM or RCM must avoid strenuous activity, isometric exercises, and competitive sports.

Reducing Anxiety

Spiritual, psychological, and emotional support may be indicated for patients, families, and significant others. Interventions are directed toward eradicating or alleviating perceived stressors. Patients receive appropriate information about cardiomyopathy and self-management activities. It is important to provide an atmosphere in which patients feel free to verbalize concerns and receive assurance that their concerns are legitimate. If the patient is awaiting transplantation or facing death, it is necessary to allow time to discuss these issues. Providing the patient with realistic hope helps reduce anxiety while he or she awaits a donor heart. The nurse helps the patient, family, and significant others with anticipatory grieving.

Decreasing the Sense of Powerlessness

Patients often go through a grieving process when cardiomyopathy is diagnosed. The patient is assisted in identifying the things in life that he or she has lost (e.g., foods that the patient enjoyed eating but are high in sodium, the ability to engage in an active lifestyle, the ability to play sports, the ability to lift grandchildren) and his or her emotional responses to the loss (e.g., anger, feelings of sadness). The nurse assists the patient in identifying the amount of control that he or she still has over life, such as making food choices, managing medications, and working with the patient's primary provider to achieve the best possible outcomes. A diary in which the patient records food selections and weight may help with understanding the relationship between sodium intake and weight gain and give patients a sense of control over their disease. Some patients can manage a self-titrating diuretic regimen in which they adjust the dose of diuretic to their symptoms.

Promoting Home and Community-Based Care

Educating Patients About Self-Care. A key part of the plan of nursing care involves educating patients about the medication regimen, symptom monitoring, and symptom management. The nurse plays an integral role as the patient learns to balance lifestyle and work while accomplishing therapeutic activities. Helping patients cope with their disease status helps them adjust their lifestyles and implement a self-care program at home. Attainment of a goal, no matter how small, also promotes the patient's sense of well-being.

Continuing Care. The nurse reinforces previous education and performs ongoing assessment of the patient's symptoms and progress. The nurse also assists the patient and family to adjust to lifestyle changes. Patients are taught to read nutrition labels, to maintain a record of daily weights and symptoms, and to organize daily activities to increase activity tolerance. In addition, the nurse assesses the patient's response to recommendations about diet and fluid intake and to the medication regimen and stresses the signs and symptoms that should be reported to the physician. Because of the risk of dysrhythmia, it may be necessary to educate the patient's family about cardiopulmonary resuscitation and the use of an automated external defibrillator (see Chapter 29). Women are often advised to avoid pregnancy, but each case is assessed individually. The nurse assesses the psychosocial needs of the patient and family on an ongoing basis. There may be concerns and fears about the prognosis, changes in lifestyle, effects of medications, and the possibility of others in the family having the same condition; these concerns often increase the patient's anxiety and interfere with effective coping strategies. Establishing trust is vital to the nurse's relationship with these chronically ill patients and their families. This is particularly significant when the nurse is involved with a patient and family in discussions about end-of-life decisions. Patients who have significant symptoms of heart failure or other complications of cardiomyopathy may benefit from a home care referral.

Evaluation

Expected patient outcomes may include:

1. Maintains or improves cardiac function
   a. Exhibits heart and respiratory rates within normal limits
   b. Reports decreased dyspnea and increased comfort; maintains or improves gas exchange
   c. Reports no weight gain; appropriate weight for height
   d. Maintains or improves peripheral blood flow
2. Maintains or increases activity tolerance
   a. Carries out activities of daily living (e.g., brushes teeth, feeds self)
   b. Reports increased tolerance to activity
3. Is less anxious
   a. Discusses prognosis freely
   b. Verbalizes fears and concerns
   c. Participates in support groups if appropriate
   d. Demonstrates appropriate coping mechanisms
4. Decreases sense of powerlessness
   a. Identifies emotional response to diagnosis
   b. Discusses control that he or she has
5. Adheres to self-care program
   a. Takes medications according to prescribed schedule
   b. Modifies diet to accommodate sodium and fluid recommendations
   c. Modifies lifestyle to accommodate activity and rest behavior recommendations
   d. Identifies signs and symptoms to be reported to health care professionals

INFECTIOUS DISEASES OF THE HEART

Any of the heart's three layers may be affected by an infectious process. Infections are named for the layer of the heart most involved in the infectious process: infective endocarditis (endocardium), myocarditis (myocardium), and pericarditis (pericardium). Rheumatic endocarditis is a unique infective endocarditis syndrome. Diagnosis of infection is made primarily on the basis of the patient's symptoms and echocardiography. Ideal management for all infectious diseases is prevention. IV antibiotics usually are necessary once an infection has developed in the heart.

Rheumatic Endocarditis

Acute rheumatic fever, which occurs most often in school-age children, may develop after an episode of group A beta-hemolytic streptococcal pharyngitis (Chart 28-2). Patients with rheumatic fever may develop rheumatic heart disease as evidenced by a new heart murmur, cardiomegaly, pericarditis, and heart failure. Prompt and effective treatment of "strep" throat with antibiotics can prevent development of rheumatic fever. Streptococcus is spread by direct contact with oral or respiratory secretions. Although bacteria are the causative agents, malnutrition, overcrowding, poor

---

**Chart
28-2** **Rheumatic Fever**

Rheumatic fever is a preventable disease. Diagnosing and effectively treating streptococcal pharyngitis can prevent rheumatic fever and, therefore, rheumatic heart disease. Signs and symptoms of streptococcal pharyngitis include:

- Fever (38.9°–40°C [101°–104°F])
- Chills
- Sore throat (sudden in onset)
- Diffuse redness of throat with exudate on oropharynx (may not appear until after the first day)
- Enlarged and tender lymph nodes
- Abdominal pain (more common in children)
- Acute sinusitis and acute otitis media (may cause or result from streptococcal pharyngitis)

If signs and symptoms of streptococcal pharyngitis are present, a throat culture is necessary to make an accurate diagnosis. All patients with throat cultures positive for streptococcal pharyngitis must adhere to the prescribed antibiotic treatment. Penicillin is the most common antibiotic prescribed. Completing the course of prescribed antibiotics minimizes the risk of developing rheumatic fever (and subsequent rheumatic heart disease).

**Chart
28-3** ⚠ **RISK FACTORS
Infective Endocarditis**

- Prosthetic cardiac valves or prosthetic material used for cardiac valve repair
- Implanted cardiac devices (e.g., pacemaker, implanted cardioverter defibrillator)
- History of bacterial endocarditis (even without heart disease)
- Congenital heart disease:
  - Unrepaired cyanotic disease, including patients with palliative shunts and conduits
  - Repaired with prosthetic material or device either by surgery or catheter intervention during the first 6 months after the procedure
  - Repaired with residual defects at the site or adjacent to the site of a prosthetic patch or device
- Cardiac transplant recipients with valvulopathy
- IV drug abuse
- Body piercing (especially oral, nasal, and nipple), branding, and tattooing

Adapted from Wilson, W., Taubert, K. A., Gewitz, M., et al. (2007). The American Heart Association guideline: Prevention of infective endocarditis. *Circulation, 116*(15), 1736–1754.

---

hygiene, and lower socioeconomic status may predispose individuals to rheumatic fever. Incidence of rheumatic fever in the United States and other developed countries generally has decreased (Correa de Sa, Tleyjeh, Anavekar, et al., 2010); however, the exact incidence is difficult to determine because infection may go unrecognized and people may not seek treatment (Fuster et al., 2011). Clinical diagnostic criteria are not standardized, and autopsies are not performed routinely. Further information about rheumatic fever and rheumatic endocarditis can be found in pediatric nursing books.

Infective Endocarditis

Infective endocarditis is a microbial infection of the endothelial surface of the heart. It usually develops in people with prosthetic heart valves, cardiac devices (e.g., pacemaker), or structural cardiac defects (e.g., valve disorders, HCM) (Chart 28-3). It is more common in older people (Correa de Sa et al., 2010), who are more likely to have degenerative or calcific valve lesions, reduced immunologic response to infection, and metabolic alterations associated with aging. Staphylococcal endocarditis infections of valves in the right side of the heart are common among IV drug abusers. Hospital-acquired infective endocarditis occurs most often in patients with debilitating disease or indwelling catheters and in patients who are receiving hemodialysis or prolonged IV fluid or antibiotic therapy. Patients taking immunosuppressive medications or corticosteroids are more susceptible to fungal endocarditis.

Invasive procedures, particularly those involving mucosal surfaces (e.g., those involving manipulation of gingival tissue or periapical regions of teeth), can cause a bacteremia, which rarely lasts more than 15 minutes. However, if a patient has any anatomic cardiac defects or implanted cardiac devices (e.g., prosthetic heart valve, pacemaker, ICD), bacteremia

can cause bacterial endocarditis. Bacteremia also may be caused by IV drug abuse, body piercing (especially oral, nasal, and nipple), branding, and tattooing (Bonow et al., 2008; Bonow et al., 2012; Fuster et al., 2011; Wilson, Taubert, Gewitz, et al., 2007).

Pathophysiology

A deformity or injury of the endocardium leads to accumulation of fibrin and platelets (clot formation) on the endocardium. Infectious organisms, usually staphylococci or streptococci, invade the clot and endocardial lesion. Other causative microorganisms include fungi (e.g., *Candida, Aspergillus*) and Rickettsiae. Infection most frequently results in platelets, fibrin, blood cells, and microorganisms that cluster as vegetations on the endocardium. Vegetations may embolize to other tissues throughout the body. As the clot on the endocardium continues to expand, the infecting organism is covered by new clot and concealed from the body's normal defenses. Infection may erode through the endocardium into underlying structures (e.g., valve leaflets), causing tears or other deformities of valve leaflets, dehiscence of prosthetic valves, deformity of chordae tendineae, or mural abscesses.

Onset of infective endocarditis usually is insidious. Signs and symptoms develop from toxic effects of the infection, destruction of heart valves, and embolization of fragments of vegetative growths on the endocardium. Systemic emboli occur with left-sided heart infective endocarditis; pulmonary emboli occur with right-sided heart infective endocarditis (Bonow et al., 2012; Fuster et al., 2011; Lemmer & Vlahakes, 2010; Wang, 2011).

Clinical Manifestations

Primary presenting symptoms of infective endocarditis are fever and a heart murmur. Fever may be intermittent or absent, especially in patients who are receiving antibiotics or corticosteroids, in those who are older, and in those who have heart failure or renal failure. A heart murmur may be absent initially but develops in almost all patients. Murmurs that worsen over time indicate progressive damage from vegetations or perforation of a valve or rupture of chordae tendineae.

In addition to fever and heart murmur, clusters of petechiae may be found on the body. Small, painful nodules (Osler nodes) may be present in pads of fingers or toes. Irregular, red or purple, painless flat macules (Janeway lesions) may be present on palms, fingers, hands, soles, and toes. Hemorrhages with pale centers (Roth spots) caused by emboli may be observed in fundi of the eyes. Splinter hemorrhages (i.e., reddish-brown lines and streaks) may be seen under the proximal half of fingernails and toenails. Petechiae may appear in conjunctiva and mucous membranes. Cardiomegaly, heart failure, tachycardia, or splenomegaly may occur.

Central nervous system manifestations of infective endocarditis include headache; temporary or transient cerebral ischemia; and strokes, which may be caused by emboli to cerebral arteries. Embolization may be a presenting symptom; it may occur at any time and may involve other organ systems. Embolic phenomena may occur, as discussed in the Rheumatic Endocarditis section.

Heart failure, which may result from perforation of a valve leaflet, rupture of chordae, blood flow obstruction due to vegetations, or intracardiac shunts from dehiscence of prosthetic valves, indicates a poor prognosis with medical therapy alone and a higher surgical risk. Valvular stenosis or regurgitation, myocardial damage, and mycotic (fungal) aneurysms are potential cardiac complications. First-, second-, and third-degree atrioventricular blocks may occur and are often a sign of a valve ring abscess. Emboli, immunologic responses, abscess of the spleen, mycotic aneurysms, cerebritis, and hemodynamic deterioration may cause complications in other organs.

Assessment and Diagnostic Findings

Although characteristics described previously may indicate infective endocarditis, signs and symptoms may indicate other diseases as well. Vague complaints of malaise, anorexia, weight loss, cough, and back and joint pain may be mistaken for influenza. Virulence of the causative organism usually correlates with the speed and degree of symptom development. A definitive diagnosis is made when a microorganism is found in two separate blood cultures, or in a vegetation or abscess. Three sets of blood cultures (with each set including one aerobic and one anaerobic culture) drawn from different venipuncture sites over a 24-hour period (each set at least 12 hours apart), or every 30 minutes if the patient's condition is unstable, should be obtained before administration of any antimicrobial agents (Bonow et al., 2008; Bonow et al., 2012; Fuster et al., 2011). Negative blood cultures do not definitely rule out infective endocarditis. Patients may have elevated white blood cell (WBC) counts. In addition, patients may be anemic, have a positive rheumatoid factor, and an elevated erythrocyte sedimentation rate (ESR) or C-reactive protein. Microscopic hematuria may be present on urinalysis (Bonow et al., 2012).

Echocardiography may assist in diagnosis by demonstrating a mass on a valve, prosthetic valve, or supporting structures and by identifying vegetations, abscesses, new prosthetic valve dehiscence, or new regurgitation. An echocardiogram may reveal development of heart failure. TEE may provide better data than transthoracic imaging (Bonow et al., 2012; Fuster et al., 2011; Lemmer & Vlahakes, 2010; Wiegand, 2011).

Prevention

Although rare, bacterial endocarditis may be life threatening. A key strategy is primary prevention in high-risk patients (e.g., those with previous infective endocarditis, prosthetic heart valves). Antibiotic prophylaxis is recommended for high-risk patients immediately before and sometimes after the following procedures (Nishimura et al., 2008; Wilson et al., 2007):

- Dental procedures that involve manipulation of gingival tissue or periapical area of teeth or perforation of oral mucosa (except routine anesthetic injections through noninfected tissue, placement of orthodontic brackets, loss of deciduous teeth, bleeding from trauma to lips or oral mucosa, dental x-rays, adjustment of orthodontic appliances, and placement of removable prosthodontic or orthodontic appliances)
- Tonsillectomy or adenoidectomy
- Surgical procedures that involve respiratory mucosa
- Bronchoscopy with biopsy or incision of respiratory tract mucosa
- Cystoscopy or urinary tract manipulation for patients with enterococcal urinary tract infections or colonization
- Surgery involving infected skin or musculoskeletal tissue

The type of antibiotic used for prophylaxis varies with the type of procedure and degree of risk. Patients usually are instructed to take 2 g of amoxicillin (Amoxil) orally 1 hour before the procedure. If patients are allergic to penicillin, clindamycin (Cleocin), cephalexin (Keflex), cefazolin (Ancef, Kefzol), ceftriaxone (Rocephin), azithromycin (Zithromax), or clarithromycin (Biaxin) may be used (Bonow et al., 2008; Bonow et al., 2012; Fuster et al., 2011; Otto & Bonow, 2009).

Equally important is ongoing good oral hygiene. Poor dental hygiene can lead to bacteremia, particularly in the setting of a dental procedure. Severity of oral inflammation and infection is a significant factor in the incidence and degree of bacteremia. Regular professional oral care combined with personal oral care may reduce the risk of bacteremia. Personal oral care includes using a soft toothbrush and toothpaste to brush teeth, gums, tongue, and oral mucosa at least twice a day, as well as rinsing the mouth with an antiseptic mouthwash for 30 seconds intermittently between tooth brushing. Patients must be advised to:

- Avoid using toothpicks or other sharp objects in the oral cavity
- Avoid nail biting
- Avoid body piercing, branding, tattooing
- Minimize outbreaks of acne, psoriasis

Female patients are advised not to use intrauterine devices (IUDs). Patients with substance abuse histories are referred to addiction treatment programs. Any fever of more than 7 days' duration is to be reported to a primary provider; patients should not self-medicate with antibiotics or stop taking them before the prescribed dosage has been completed.

Increased vigilance is also required in patients with IV catheters and during invasive procedures. To minimize the risk of infection, nurses must ensure meticulous hand hygiene, site preparation, and aseptic technique during insertion and maintenance procedures. All catheters, tubes, drains, and other devices are removed as soon as they are no longer needed or no longer function.

Medical Management

The objective of treatment is to eradicate invading organisms through adequate doses of an appropriate antimicrobial agent. Antibiotic therapy usually is administered for 2 to 6 weeks every 4 hours or continuously by IV infusion or once daily by intramuscular injection. Parenteral therapy is administered in doses that produce a high serum concentration for a significant period to ensure eradication of the dormant bacteria within dense vegetations. This therapy is often delivered in the patient's home and is monitored by a home care nurse. Serum levels of the antibiotic and blood cultures are monitored to gauge effectiveness of therapy. If there is insufficient bactericidal activity, increased dosages of the antibiotic are prescribed or a different antibiotic is used. Numerous antimicrobial regimens are in use, but penicillin usually is the medication of choice. In fungal endocarditis, an antifungal agent such as amphotericin B (Abelcet, Amphocin) is the usual treatment.

In addition, the patient's temperature is monitored at regular intervals because the course of fever is one indication of treatment effectiveness. However, febrile reactions also may occur as a result of medication. After adequate antimicrobial therapy is initiated, the infective organism is usually eliminated. The patient should begin to feel better, regain an appetite, and have less fatigue. During this time, patients require psychosocial support because although they feel well, they may find themselves confined to the hospital or home with restrictive IV therapy.

Surgical Management

Surgical intervention may be required if the infection does not respond to medications or the patient has prosthetic heart valve endocarditis, has a vegetation larger than 1 cm, or develops complications such as a septal perforation (Bonow et al., 2012; Fuster et al., 2011; Lemmer & Vlahakes, 2010; Otto & Bonow, 2009). Surgical interventions include valve débridement or excision, débridement of vegetations, débridement and closure of an abscess, and closure of a fistula. Aortic or mitral valve débridement, excision, or replacement is required in patients who:

- Develop congestive heart failure despite adequate medical treatment
- Have more than one serious systemic embolic episode
- Develop a valve obstruction
- Develop a periannular (heart valve), myocardial, or aortic abscess
- Have uncontrolled infection, persistent or recurrent infection, or fungal endocarditis

Surgical valve replacement greatly improves the prognosis for patients with severe symptoms from damaged heart valves. The aortic valve may best be treated with an autograft, as described previously. Most patients who have prosthetic valve endocarditis (i.e., infected valve replacements) require valve replacement.

Nursing Management

The nurse monitors the patient's temperature. The patient may have a fever for weeks. The nurse administers antibiotics, antifungals, or antivirals as prescribed or educates the patient to take them as prescribed. Patients need enough fluids to keep their urine light yellow. Fever often causes fatigue; rest periods should be planned and activities spaced to give to rest between activities. Infection control and prevention requires good hand hygiene by both patients and caregivers. Nonsteroidal anti-inflammatory drugs (NSAIDs) may be prescribed as antipyretics or to decrease the discomfort of fever. Patients may be more comfortable with a light layer of linens and exposure of their skin to air. They may be cooled with a fan, tepid water baths, or cloth compresses; if shivering or piloerection occurs, these interventions should be discontinued due to increased oxygen consumption and potential to further increase of body temperature.

Heart sounds are assessed. A new or worsening murmur may indicate dehiscence of a prosthetic valve, rupture of an abscess, or injury to valve leaflets or chordae tendineae. The nurse monitors for signs and symptoms of systemic embolization, or, for patients with right-sided heart endocarditis, for signs and symptoms of pulmonary infarction and infiltrates. In addition, the nurse assesses signs and symptoms of organ damage such as stroke (i.e., cerebrovascular accident or brain attack), meningitis, heart failure, myocardial infarction, glomerulonephritis, and splenomegaly.

Patient care is directed toward management of infection. Long-term IV antimicrobial therapy often is necessary; therefore, many patients have peripherally inserted central catheters or other long-term IV access. All invasive lines and wounds must be assessed daily for redness, tenderness, warmth, swelling, drainage, or other signs of infection. The patient and family are instructed about activity restrictions, medications, and signs and symptoms of infection. Patients with infective endocarditis are at high risk for another episode of infectious endocarditis. The nurse emphasizes the antibiotic prophylaxis described previously. If the patient has undergone surgical treatment, the nurse provides postoperative care and instructions (see Chapters 19 and 27).

As appropriate, the home care nurse supervises and monitors IV antibiotic therapy delivered in the home setting and educates the patient and family about prevention and health promotion. The nurse provides the patient and family with emotional support and facilitates coping strategies during the prolonged course of infection and antibiotic treatment.

Myocarditis

Myocarditis, an inflammatory process involving the myocardium, can cause heart dilation, thrombi on the heart wall (mural thrombi), infiltration of circulating blood cells around the coronary vessels and between the muscle fibers, and degeneration of the muscle fibers themselves. Mortality varies with the severity of symptoms. Most patients with mild symptoms recover completely; however, some patients develop cardiomyopathy and heart failure.

Pathophysiology

Myocarditis usually results from viral (e.g., coxsackievirus A and B, human immunodeficiency virus, influenza A), bacterial, rickettsial, fungal, parasitic, metazoal, protozoal (e.g., Chagas disease), or spirochetal infection. It also may be immune related, occurring after acute systemic infections such as rheumatic fever. It may develop in patients receiving immunosuppressive therapy or in those with infective endocarditis, Crohn's disease, or systemic lupus erythematosus (Mann, 2011; Maron et al., 2006).

Myocarditis may result from an inflammatory reaction to toxins such as pharmacologic agents used in the treatment of other diseases (e.g., anthracyclines for cancer therapy), ethanol, or radiation (especially to the left chest or upper back). It may begin in one small area of the myocardium and then spread throughout the myocardium. The degree of myocardial inflammation and necrosis determines the degree of interstitial collagen and elastin destruction. The greater the destruction, the greater the hemodynamic effect and resulting signs and symptoms. It is thought that DCM and HCM are latent manifestations of myocarditis (Bonow et al., 2012; Fuster et al., 2011).

 Concept Mastery Alert

The most common pathogens involved in myocarditis tend to be viral, whereas in endocarditis they tend to be bacterial.

Clinical Manifestations

The symptoms of acute myocarditis depend on the type of infection, the degree of myocardial damage, and the capacity of the myocardium to recover. Patients may be asymptomatic, with an infection that resolves on its own. However, they may develop mild to moderate symptoms and seek medical attention, often reporting fatigue and dyspnea, syncope, palpitations, and occasional discomfort in the chest and upper abdomen. The most common symptoms are flulike. Patients may also sustain sudden cardiac death or quickly develop severe congestive heart failure.

Assessment and Diagnostic Findings

Assessment of the patient may reveal no detectable abnormalities; as a result, the illness can go undiagnosed. Patients may be tachycardic or may report chest pain. A cardiac catheterization demonstrates normal coronary arteries; however, CMR imaging is being used more often as a diagnostic tool because of its noninvasive approach (Mann, 2011). With contrast, CMR imaging may be diagnostic and can guide clinicians to sites for endocardial biopsies, which may be diagnostic for an organism or its genome, an immune process, or a radiation reaction causing the myocarditis. Patients without any abnormal heart structure (at least initially) may suddenly develop dysrhythmias or ST–T-wave changes. If the patient has structural heart abnormalities (e.g., systolic dysfunction), a clinical assessment may disclose cardiac enlargement, faint heart sounds (especially S_1), a gallop rhythm, or a systolic murmur. The WBC count and ESR may be elevated.

Prevention

Prevention of infectious diseases by means of appropriate immunizations (e.g., influenza, hepatitis) and early treatment appears to be important in decreasing the incidence of myocarditis (Bonow et al., 2012).

Medical Management

Patients are given specific treatment for the underlying cause if it is known (e.g., penicillin for hemolytic streptococci) and are placed on bed rest to decrease cardiac workload. Bed rest also helps decrease myocardial damage and the complications of myocarditis. In young patients with myocarditis, activities, especially athletics, should be limited for a 6-month period or at least until heart size and function have returned to normal. Physical activity is increased slowly, and the patient is instructed to report any symptoms that occur with increasing activity, such as a rapidly beating heart. If heart failure or dysrhythmia develops, management is essentially the same as for all causes of heart failure and dysrhythmias (see Chapters 26 and 29), except that beta-blockers are avoided because they decrease the strength of ventricular contraction (have a negative inotropic effect). Although they are known for their anti-inflammatory effects, NSAIDs should not be used for pain control; they have been shown to be ineffective in relieving the inflammatory process in myocarditis and have been linked to worsening inflammation of the myocardium. This also can contribute to an increased mortality from increased virulence of the pathogen (Mann, 2011).

Nursing Management

The nurse assesses for resolution of tachycardia, fever, and any other clinical manifestations. The cardiovascular assessment focuses on signs and symptoms of heart failure and dysrhythmias. Patients with dysrhythmias should have continuous cardiac monitoring with personnel and equipment readily available to treat life-threatening dysrhythmias.

 Quality and Safety Nursing Alert

Patients with myocarditis are sensitive to digitalis. Nurses must closely monitor these patients for digitalis toxicity, which is evidenced by dysrhythmia, anorexia, nausea, vomiting, headache, and malaise.

Anti-embolism stockings and passive and active exercises should be used because embolization from venous thrombosis and mural thrombi can occur, especially in patients on bed rest.

Pericarditis

Pericarditis refers to an inflammation of the pericardium, which is the membranous sac enveloping the heart. It may be a primary illness, or it may develop during various medical and surgical disorders. For example, pericarditis may occur after pericardectomy (opening of the pericardium) following cardiac surgery. Pericarditis also may occur 10 days to 2 months after acute myocardial infarction (Dressler syndrome) (Bonow et al., 2012; Sparano & Ward, 2011). Pericarditis may be acute, chronic, or recurring. It is classified either as adhesive (constrictive), because the layers of the pericardium become attached to each other and restrict ventricular filling, or by what accumulates in the pericardial sac: serous (serum), purulent (pus), calcific (calcium deposits), fibrinous (clotting proteins), sanguinous (blood), or malignant (cancer). Pericarditis also may be described as exudative or noneffusive.

Pathophysiology

Causes underlying or associated with pericarditis are listed in Chart 28-4. The inflammatory process of pericarditis may lead to an accumulation of fluid in the pericardial sac (pericardial effusion) and increased pressure on the heart, leading to cardiac tamponade (see Chapter 29). Frequent or prolonged episodes of pericarditis also may lead to thickening and decreased elasticity of the pericardium, or scarring may fuse the visceral and parietal pericardium. These conditions restrict the heart's ability to fill with blood (constrictive pericarditis). The pericardium may become calcified, further restricting ventricular expansion during ventricular filling (diastole). With less filling, the ventricles pump less blood, leading to decreased cardiac output and signs and symptoms of heart failure. Restricted diastolic filling may result in increased systemic venous pressure, causing peripheral edema and hepatic failure.

Clinical Manifestations

Pericarditis may be asymptomatic. The most characteristic symptom of pericarditis is chest pain, although pain also may be located beneath the clavicle, in the neck, or in the left trapezius (scapula) region. Pain or discomfort usually remains fairly constant, but it may worsen with deep inspiration and when lying down or turning. The most characteristic clinical manifestation of pericarditis is a creaky or scratchy friction rub heard most clearly at the left lower sternal border.

Chart 28-4 **Causes of Pericarditis**

- Idiopathic or nonspecific causes
- Infection: usually viral (e.g., human immunodeficiency virus, coxsackievirus, influenza); rarely bacterial (e.g., staphylococci, streptococci, meningococci, gonococci, gram-negative rods, *Borrelia* [Lyme disease]; tuberculosis); mycotic (fungal); parasitic
- Disorders of connective tissue: systemic lupus erythematosus, rheumatic fever, rheumatoid arthritis, polyarteritis, scleroderma
- Sarcoidosis
- Hypersensitivity states: immune reactions, medication reactions, serum sickness
- Disorders of adjacent structures: myocardial infarction, dissecting aneurysm, pleural and pulmonary disease (pneumonia)
- Neoplastic disease: caused by metastasis from lung or breast cancer, leukemia and primary (mesothelioma) neoplasms
- Radiation therapy of chest and upper torso (peak occurrence 5–9 months after treatment)
- Trauma: chest injury, cardiac surgery, cardiac catheterization, implantation of pacemaker or implantable cardioverter defibrillator
- Renal failure and uremia

Other signs may include a mild fever, increased WBC count, anemia, and an elevated ESR or C-reactive protein level. Patients may have a nonproductive cough or hiccup. Dyspnea and other signs and symptoms of heart failure may occur as a result of pericardial compression due to constrictive pericarditis or cardiac tamponade. The heart rate may increase to maintain cardiac output.

Assessment and Diagnostic Findings

The diagnosis most often is made on the basis of history, signs, and symptoms. An echocardiogram may detect inflammation, pericardial effusion or tamponade, and heart failure. It may help confirm the diagnosis and may be used to guide pericardiocentesis (needle or catheter drainage of the pericardium). TEE may be useful in diagnosis but may underestimate the extent of pericardial effusions. CT imaging may be the best diagnostic tool for determining size, shape, and location of pericardial effusions and may be used to guide pericardiocentesis. CMR imaging may assist with detection of inflammation and adhesions. Occasionally, a video-assisted pericardioscope-guided biopsy of the pericardium or epicardium is performed to obtain tissue samples for culture and microscopic examination. Because the pericardial sac surrounds the heart, a 12-lead ECG may show concave ST elevations in many, if not all, leads (with no reciprocal changes) and may show depressed PR segments or atrial dysrhythmias.

Medical Management

Objectives of pericarditis management are to determine the cause, administer therapy for treatment and symptom relief, and detect signs and symptoms of cardiac tamponade. When cardiac output is impaired, the patient is placed on bed rest until fever, chest pain, and friction rub have subsided.

Analgesic medications and NSAIDs such as aspirin or ibuprofen (Motrin) may be prescribed for pain relief during the acute phase. These agents also hasten reabsorption of fluid in patients with rheumatic pericarditis. Indomethacin (Indocin) is contraindicated because it may decrease coronary blood flow. Colchicine (Colcrys) or corticosteroids (e.g., prednisone) may be prescribed if the pericarditis is severe or if the patient does not respond to NSAIDs. Colchicine also may be used instead of NSAIDs during the acute phase.

Pericardiocentesis, a procedure in which some pericardial fluid is removed, rarely is necessary. It may be performed to assist in identification of the cause or relieve symptoms, especially if there are signs and symptoms of heart failure or tamponade. Pericardial fluid is cultured if bacterial, tubercular, or fungal disease is suspected; a sample is sent for cytology if neoplastic disease is suspected. A pericardial window, a small opening made in the pericardium, may be performed to allow continuous drainage into the chest cavity. Surgical removal of tough encasing pericardium (pericardiectomy) may be necessary to release both ventricles from constrictive and restrictive inflammation and scarring.

Nursing Management

Patients with acute pericarditis require pain management with analgesics, assistance with positioning, and psychological support. Patients with chest pain often benefit from education and reassurance that the pain is not due to a heart attack. Pain may be relieved with a forward-leaning or sitting position. To minimize complications, the nurse helps the patient with activity restrictions until pain and fever subside. As the patient's condition improves, the nurse encourages gradual increases of activity. However, if pain, fever or friction rub recur, activity restrictions must be resumed. The nurse educates the patient and family about a healthy lifestyle to enhance the patient's immune system.

Nurses caring for patients with pericarditis must be alert to cardiac tamponade (see Chapter 29). The nurse monitors the patient for heart failure. Patients with hemodynamic instability or pulmonary congestion are treated as if they had heart failure (see Chapter 29).

NURSING PROCESS

The Patient With Pericarditis

Assessment

The primary symptom of pericarditis is pain, which is assessed by evaluating the patient in various positions. The nurse tries to identify whether pain is influenced by respiratory movements, while holding an inhaled breath or holding an exhaled breath; by flexion, extension, or rotation of the spine, including the neck; by movements of shoulders and arms; by coughing; or by swallowing. Recognizing events that precipitate or intensify pain may help establish a diagnosis and differentiate pain of pericarditis from pain of myocardial infarction.

When pericardial surfaces lose their lubricating fluid because of inflammation, a pericardial friction rub occurs. The rub is audible on auscultation and is synchronous with the heartbeat. However, it may be elusive and difficult to detect.

◄ Quality and Safety Nursing Alert

A pericardial friction rub is diagnostic of pericarditis. It is a creaky or scratchy sound and is louder at the end of exhalation. Nurses should monitor for pericardial friction rub by placing the diaphragm of the stethoscope tightly against the patient's thorax and auscultating the left sternal edge in the fourth intercostal space, which is the site where the pericardium comes into contact with the left chest wall. The rub may be heard best when a patient is sitting and leaning forward.

If there is difficulty in distinguishing a pericardial friction rub from a pleural friction rub, the patient is asked to hold his or her breath; a pericardial friction rub will continue.

The patient's temperature is monitored frequently. Pericarditis may cause an abrupt onset of fever in a patient who has been afebrile.

Diagnosis

Nursing Diagnosis

Based on the assessment data, the major nursing diagnosis may be:

• Acute pain related to inflammation of the pericardium

Collaborative Problems/Potential Complications

Potential complications may include the following:

• Pericardial effusion
• Cardiac tamponade

Planning and Goals

The patient's major goals may include relief of pain and absence of complications.

Nursing Interventions

Relieving Pain

Relief of pain is achieved by rest. Because sitting upright and leaning forward is the posture that tends to relieve pain, chair rest may be more comfortable. The nurse instructs the patient to restrict activity until pain subsides. As chest pain and friction rub abate, activities of daily living may be resumed gradually. If the patient is taking analgesics, antibiotics, or corticosteroids for pericarditis, his or her responses are monitored and recorded. Patients taking NSAIDs or colchicine are assessed for gastrointestinal adverse effects. If chest pain and friction rub recur, bed rest or chair rest is resumed.

Monitoring and Managing Potential Complications

Pericardial Effusion. Abnormal accumulation of fluid between the pericardial linings (i.e., in the pericardial sac) is called *pericardial effusion* (see Chapter 29). Most patients have no effects or symptoms. However, enough fluid can accumulate to constrict the myocardium, impairing ventricular filling and the myocardium's ability to pump, a condition known as *cardiac tamponade* (discussed below) (Schairer, Biswas, Keteyian, et al., 2011). Failure to identify and treat this problem can lead to death.

Cardiac Tamponade. Signs and symptoms of cardiac tamponade may begin with the patient reporting shortness of breath, chest tightness, or dizziness. The nurse may observe that the patient is becoming progressively more restless. Assessment of blood pressure may reveal a decrease of 10 mm Hg or more in systolic blood pressure during inspiration (pulsus paradoxus). Usually, the systolic pressure decreases and the diastolic pressure remains stable; hence, the pulse pressure narrows. The patient usually has tachycardia, and ECG voltage may be decreased or QRS complexes may alternate in height (electrical alternans). Heart sounds may progress from distant to imperceptible. Blood continues to return to the heart from the periphery but cannot flow into the heart to be pumped back into the circulation. The patient develops jugular vein distention and other signs of rising central venous pressure.

In such situations, the nurse notifies the primary provider immediately and prepares to assist with diagnostic echocardiography and pericardiocentesis (Schairer et al., 2011) (see Chapter 29). The nurse stays with the patient and continues to assess and record signs and symptoms while intervening to decrease patient anxiety.

Promoting Home and Community-Based Care

Because patients, their family members, and health care providers tend to focus on the most obvious needs and issues related to pericarditis, the nurse reminds them about the importance of continuing health promotion and screening practices. The nurse educates patients who have not been involved in these practices in the past about their importance and refers them to appropriate health care providers.

Evaluation

Expected patient outcomes may include:

1. Freedom from pain
   a. Performs activities of daily living without pain, fatigue, or shortness of breath
   b. Temperature returns to normal range
   c. Exhibits no pericardial friction rub
2. Absence of complications
   a. Sustains blood pressure in normal range
   b. Heart sounds strong and can be auscultated
   c. Absence of jugular vein distention

Critical Thinking Exercises

1 **ebp** A 24-year-old female patient tells you that she would like to switch her birth control method from oral contraceptives to an IUD. Knowing that she had a mitral valve replacement the previous year, how would you respond to her request? What complication are you focused on preventing? On what evidence do you base your response? What is the strength of your evidence?

2 **pq** Despite evidence-based medical management, a 49-year-old man with DCM continues to have significant functional limitations. It is recommended that he consult with a cardiologist who specializes in advanced heart failure therapy. The cardiologist recommends that the patient consider heart transplantation and begins the transplant workup; however, the cardiologist feels that the patient should consider an LVAD while he waits on the transplant list. The patient expresses anxiety and fear about the prospect of having a "mechanical" heart and wants to know if he would be able to go home, have a normal life, and go back to work. Based on your knowledge of VADs, how would you respond to these questions? What are the care priorities for this patient?

3 A 35-year-old woman presents to the cardiology clinic with orthopnea, pulmonary edema, dizziness, and syncope. Upon examination, it is noted that she has a loud, rough systolic murmur that radiates into the carotid arteries. She is diagnosed with aortic stenosis and wants to know how to "fix it." What treatment options are available? What education does this patient need to prevent infection?

4 A 55-year-old man presents to the emergency department with chest pain that worsens when lying down and with deep inspirations but is relieved with forward-leaning and sitting positions. A 12-lead ECG is completed and shows ST-segment elevation in all leads. A myocardial infarction is ruled out, and the working diagnosis is pericarditis. When auscultating the patient's heart sounds, what would you expect to hear? For what complications should you be monitoring? When questioned by the patient about what can be done to relieve his pain, how would you respond?

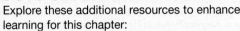

Brunner Suite Resources

Explore these additional resources to enhance learning for this chapter:
- NCLEX-Style Questions and Other Resources on **thePoint**, http://thePoint.lww.com/Brunner13e
- Study Guide
- PrepU
- Clinical Handbook
- Handbook of Laboratory and Diagnostic Tests

References

*Asterisk indicates nursing research.
**Double asterisk indicates classic reference.

Books

Bonow, R. O., Mann, D. L., Zipes, D. P., et al. (Eds.). (2012). *Braunwald's heart disease: A textbook of cardiovascular medicine* (9th ed.). Philadelphia: Saunders Elsevier.

Cohn, L. H. (2012). *Cardiac surgery in the adult* (4th ed.). New York: McGraw-Hill.

Fuster, V., Walsh, R. A., Harrington, R. A., et al. (Eds.). (2011). *Hurst's the heart* (13th ed.). New York: McGraw-Hill.

Hogan-Quigley, B., Palm, M. L., & Bickley, L. S. (2012). *Bates's nursing guide to physical examination and history taking.* Philadelphia: Lippincott Williams & Wilkins.

Lemmer, J. H., & Vlahakes, G. J. (Eds.). (2010). *Handbook of patient care in cardiac surgery* (7th ed.). Philadelphia: Lippincott Williams & Wilkins.

Mann, D. (2011). *Heart failure: A companion to Braunwald's heart disease* (2nd ed.). Philadelphia: Elsevier Saunders.

Nixon, J. V. (Ed.). (2011). *The AHA clinical cardiac consult.* Philadelphia: Lippincott Williams & Wilkins.

Otto, C. M., & Bonow, R. O. (Eds.). (2009). *Valvular heart disease: A companion to Braunwald's heart disease* (3rd ed.). Philadelphia: Saunders Elsevier.

Runge, M. S., Stouffer, G. A., & Patterson, C. (Eds.). (2011). *Netter's cardiology* (2nd ed.). Philadelphia: Saunders Elsevier.

Wiegand, D. L. (Ed.). (2011). *AACN procedure manual for critical care* (6th ed.). Philadelphia: Saunders Elsevier.

Woods, S. L., Froelicher, E. S. S., Motzer, S.U., et al. (2010). *Cardiac nursing* (6th ed.). Philadelphia: Lippincott Williams & Wilkins.

Journals and Electronic Documents

American Heart Association. (2011). *Physical changes to report.* Available at: http://www.heart.org/HEARTORG/Conditions/HeartFailure/Prevention-TreatmentofHeartFailure/Physical-Changes-to-Report_UCM_306356_Article.jsp

Basso, C., Corrado, D., Marcus, F. I., et al. (2009). Arrhythmogenic right ventricular cardiomyopathy. *Lancet, 373,* 1289–1300.

**Bonow, R. O., Carabello, B. A., Chatterjee, K., et al. (2008). 2008 focused update incorporated into the ACC/AHA 2006 guidelines for the management of patients with valvular heart disease: A report of the American College of Cardiology/American Heart Association Task Force on Practice Guidelines (Writing Committee to Revise the 1998 Guidelines for the Management of Patients With Valvular Heart Disease): Developed in collaborations with the Society of Cardiovascular Anesthesiologists: Endorsed by the Society for Cardiovascular Angiography and Interventions and the Society of Thoracic Surgeons. *Circulation, 118*(5), c523–c566.

Christiansen, J. P., Karamitsos, T. D., & Myerson, S. G. (2011). Assessment of valvular heart disease by cardiovascular magnetic resonance imaging: A review. *Heart, Lung and Circulation, 20*(2), 73–82.

Correa de Sa, D. D., Tleyjeh, I. M., Anavekar, N. S., et al. (2010). Epidemiological trends of infective endocarditis: A population-based study in Olmsted County, Minnesota. *Mayo Clinic Proceedings, 85*(5), 422–426.

Costanzo, M. R., Dipchand, A., Starling, R., et al. (2010). The International Society of Heart and Lung Transplantation guidelines for the care of the heart transplant recipients. *Journal of Heart and Lung Transplantation, 29*(8), 914–956.

Gersh, B. J., Maron, B. J., Bonow, R. O., et al. (2011). 2011 ACCF/AHA Guideline for the Diagnosis and Treatment of Hypertrophic Cardiomyopathy:

Executive summary: A report of the American College of Cardiology Foundation/American Heart Association Task Force on Practice Guidelines developed in collaboration with the American Association for Thoracic Surgery, American Society of Echocardiography, American Society of Nuclear Cardiology, Heart Failure Society of America, Heart Rhythm Society, Society for Cardiovascular Angiography and Interventions, and Society of Thoracic Surgeons. *Journal of American College of Cardiology, 58*(25), 2703–2738.

Holmes, D. R., Mack, M. J., Kaul, S., et al. (2012). 2012 ACCF/AATS/SCAI/STS expert consensus document on transcatheter aortic valve replacement. *Annals of Thoracic Surgery, 93*(4), 1340–1395.

**Maron, B. J., Towbin, J. A., Thiene, G., et.al. (2006). Contemporary definitions and classification of the cardiomyopathies: An American Heart Association scientific statement from the Council on Clinical Cardiology, Heart Failure and Transplantation Committee; Quality of Care and Outcomes Research and Functional Genomics and Translational Biology Interdisciplinary Working Groups; and Council on Epidemiology and Prevention. *Circulation, 113*(14), 1807–1816.

**Nishimura, R. A., Carabello, B. A., Faxon, D. P., et al. (2008). ACC/AHA 2008 guideline update on valvular heart disease: Focused update on infective endocarditis. *Journal of the American College of Cardiology, 52*(8), 676–685.

*Overgaard, D., Grufstedt Kjeldgaard, H., & Egerod, I. (2012). Life in transition: A qualitative study of the illness experience and vocational adjustment of patients with left ventricular assist device. *Journal of Cardiovascular Nursing, 27*(5), 394–402.

Sander, G. (2011). Hypertrophic cardiomyopathy. *Medscape.* Available at: emedicine.medscape.com/article/152913-overview

Schairer, J. R., Biswas, S., Keteyian, S., et al. (2011). A systematic approach to evaluation of pericardial effusion and cardiac tamponade. *Cardiology in Review, 19*(5), 233–238.

Slaughter, M. S., Pagani, F. D., Rogers, J. G., et al. (2010). Clinical management of continuous-flow left ventricular assist devices in advanced heart failure. *Journal of Heart and Lung Transplantation, 29*(4), S1–S39.

Sparano, D. M., & Ward, R. P. (2011). Pericarditis and pericardial effusion: Management update. *Current Treatment Options in Cardiovascular Medicine, 13*(6), 543–555.

**Special Writing Group of the Committee on Rheumatic Fever, Endocarditis, and Kawasaki's Disease of the Council on Cardiovascular Disease in the Young of the American Heart Association. (1992). Guidelines for the diagnosis of rheumatic fever. Jones Criteria, 1992 update. *Journal of the American Medical Association, 268*(15), 2069–2973.

Vallabhajosyula, P., & Bavaria, J. E. (2011). Transcatheter aortic valve implantation: Complications and management. *Journal of Heart Valve Disease, 20*(5), 499–509.

Wang, A. (2011). Recent progress in understanding of infective endocarditis. *Current Treatment Options in Cardiovascular Medicine, 13*(6), 586–594.

**Wilson, W., Taubert, K. A., Gewitz, M., et al. (2007). AHA guideline: Prevention of infective endocarditis. *Circulation, 116*(15), 1736–1754.

Resources

American Heart Association, National Center, www.americanheart.org
Cardiomyopathy Association, www.cardiomyopathy.org
Heartmates, www.heartmates.com
National Heart, Lung, and Blood Institute, www.nhlbi.nih.gov

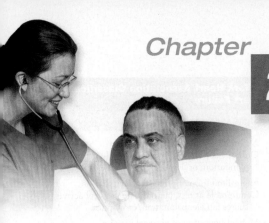

29

Management of Patients With Complications From Heart Disease

Learning Objectives

On completion of this chapter, the learner will be able to:

1 Describe the management of patients with heart failure.
2 Use the nursing process as a framework for care of patients with heart failure.
3 Develop an education plan for patients with heart failure.

4 Describe the medical and nursing management of patients with pulmonary edema.
5 Describe the medical and nursing management of patients with thromboembolism, pericardial effusion, and cardiac arrest.

Glossary

acute decompensated heart failure: acute exacerbation of heart failure, with signs and symptoms of severe respiratory distress and poor systemic perfusion
anuria: urine output of less than 50 mL/24 h
ascites: an accumulation of serous fluid in the peritoneal cavity
cardiac resynchronization therapy (CRT): a treatment for heart failure in which a device paces both ventricles to synchronize contractions
congestive heart failure (CHF): a fluid overload condition (congestion) associated with heart failure
diastolic heart failure: the inability of the heart to pump sufficiently because of an alteration in the ability of the heart to fill; term used to describe a type of heart failure
ejection fraction (EF): percentage of blood volume in the ventricles at the end of diastole that is ejected during systole; a measurement of contractility
heart failure (HF): a clinical syndrome resulting from structural or functional cardiac disorders that impair the ability of a ventricle to fill or eject blood
left-sided heart failure (left ventricular failure): inability of the left ventricle to fill or eject sufficient blood into the systemic circulation

oliguria: diminished urine output; less than 0.5 mL/kg/hr
orthopnea: shortness of breath when laying flat
paroxysmal nocturnal dyspnea (PND): shortness of breath that occurs suddenly during sleep
pericardiocentesis: procedure that involves aspiration of fluid from the pericardial sac
pericardiotomy: surgically created opening of the pericardium
pulmonary edema: abnormal accumulation of fluid in the interstitial spaces and alveoli of the lungs
pulseless electrical activity (PEA): condition in which electrical activity is present on an electrocardiogram, but there is not an adequate pulse or blood pressure
pulsus paradoxus: systolic blood pressure that is more than 10 mm Hg lower during inhalation than during exhalation; difference is normally less than 10 mm Hg
right-sided heart failure (right ventricular failure): inability of the right ventricle to fill or eject sufficient blood into the pulmonary circulation
systolic heart failure: inability of the heart to pump sufficiently because of an alteration in the ability of the heart to contract; term used to describe a type of heart failure

---

Today it is possible to help the patient with heart disease live longer and achieve a high quality of life. Advances in diagnostic procedures, treatments, technologies, and pharmacotherapies allow earlier and more accurate diagnoses and treatment that can begin well before significant debilitation occurs. However, heart disease remains a chronic and often progressive condition that is associated with serious complications. This chapter presents the complications most often associated with heart disorders and the collaborative treatment options for these complications.

HEART FAILURE

Heart failure (HF) is a clinical syndrome resulting from structural or functional cardiac disorders that impair the ability of the ventricles to fill or eject blood. In the past, HF was often referred to as **congestive heart failure (CHF)**, because many patients experience pulmonary or peripheral congestion with edema. Currently, HF is recognized as a clinical syndrome characterized by signs and symptoms of fluid overload or inadequate tissue perfusion. Fluid overload and decreased tissue perfusion result when the heart cannot generate cardiac output (CO) sufficient to meet the body's demands for oxygen and nutrients. The term *heart failure* indicates myocardial disease in which impaired contraction of the heart (systolic dysfunction) or filling of the heart (diastolic dysfunction) may cause pulmonary or systemic congestion. Some cases of HF are reversible, depending on the cause. Most often, HF is a chronic, progressive condition that is managed with lifestyle changes and medications to prevent episodes of **acute decompensated heart failure**. These episodes are characterized by increased symptoms, decreased CO, and low perfusion (Lindenfeld, Albert, Boehmer, et al., 2010). These episodes are also associated with increased hospitalizations, increased health care costs, and decreased quality of life.

Chronic Heart Failure

As with coronary artery disease, the incidence of HF increases with age. Approximately 6 million people in the United States have HF, and 550,000 new cases are diagnosed each year (Roger, Go, Lloyd-Jones, et al., 2012). Although HF can affect people of all ages, it is most common in people older than 75 years. As the U.S. population ages, HF has become an epidemic that challenges the country's health care resources. HF is the most common reason for hospitalization of people older than 65 years and is the second most common reason for visits to a physician's office. The rate of emergency department visits and hospital readmissions for this condition remains very high. Approximately 24% of patients discharged after treatment for HF are readmitted to the hospital within 30 days (Hernandez, Greiner, Fonarow, et al., 2010). The estimated economic burden caused by HF in the United States is more than $39 billion annually in direct and indirect costs and is expected to increase (Norton, Georgiopoulou, Kalogeropoulos, et al., 2011).

The increased incidence of HF reflects not only the aging population but also improvements in treatment and survival rates of people with cardiac diagnoses such as myocardial infarction (MI). Many hospitalizations for HF can be prevented by appropriate outpatient care. Prevention and early intervention to arrest the progression of HF are major U.S. health initiatives (Fonarow, Albert, Curtis, et al., 2010).

Two major types of HF are identified by assessment of left ventricular function, usually by echocardiogram. The most common type is an alteration in ventricular contraction called **systolic heart failure**, which is characterized by a weakened heart muscle. A less common type is **diastolic heart failure**, which is characterized by a stiff and noncompliant heart muscle, making it difficult for the ventricle to fill. An assessment of the **ejection fraction (EF)** is performed by echocardiogram to assist in determining the type of HF. EF is calculated by subtracting the amount of blood present in the left ventricle at the end of systole from the amount present at the end of diastole and calculating the percentage of blood that is ejected. A normal EF is 55% to 65% of the ventricular volume; the ventricle does not completely empty between contractions. The EF is normal in diastolic HF but severely reduced in systolic HF.

TABLE 29-1	New York Heart Association Classification of Heart Failure
Classification	**Signs and Symptoms**
I	No limitation of physical activity Ordinary activity does not cause undue fatigue, palpitation, or dyspnea.
II	Slight limitation of physical activity Comfortable at rest, but ordinary physical activity causes fatigue, palpitation, or dyspnea.
III	Marked limitation of physical activity Comfortable at rest, but less than ordinary activity causes fatigue, palpitation, or dyspnea.
IV	Unable to carry out any physical activity without discomfort Symptoms of cardiac insufficiency at rest If any physical activity is undertaken, discomfort is increased.

Adapted from American Heart Association. (2012). *Classification of functional capacity and objective assessment.* Available at: http://my.americanheart.org/professional/ StatementsGuidelines/ByPublicationDate/PreviousYears/Classification-of-Functional-Capacity-and-Objective-Assessment_UCM_423811_Article.jsp

Although a low EF is a hallmark of systolic HF, the severity of HF is frequently classified according to the patient's symptoms. The New York Heart Association (NYHA) classification of heart failure is described in Table 29-1. The American College of Cardiology and the American Heart Association (ACC/AHA) have developed another HF classification system (Jessup, Abraham, Casey, et al., 2009). This system, described in Table 29-2, takes into consideration the natural history and progressive nature of HF. Treatment guidelines have been developed for each stage, which are discussed later in this chapter.

Etiology

Myocardial dysfunction and HF can be caused by a number of conditions, including coronary artery disease, hypertension, cardiomyopathy, valvular disorders, and renal dysfunction with volume overload (McCance, Huether, Brashers, et al., 2010). Patients with diabetes are also at high risk for HF. Atherosclerosis of the coronary arteries is a primary cause of HF, and coronary artery disease is found in the majority of patients with HF. Ischemia causes myocardial dysfunction because it deprives heart cells of oxygen and causes cellular damage. MI causes focal heart muscle necrosis, the death of myocardial cells, and a loss of contractility; the extent of the infarction correlates with the severity of HF. Revascularization of the coronary artery by a percutaneous coronary intervention (PCI) or by coronary artery bypass surgery (coronary artery bypass graft [CABG]) may improve myocardial oxygenation and ventricular function and prevent more extensive myocardial necrosis that can lead to HF (see Chapter 27).

Systemic or pulmonary hypertension increases afterload (resistance to ejection), which increases cardiac workload and leads to hypertrophy of myocardial muscle fibers. This can be considered a compensatory mechanism because it initially increases contractility. However, sustained hypertension eventually leads to changes that impair the heart's ability to fill properly during diastole, and the hypertrophied ventricles may dilate and fail (Porth, 2011).

TABLE 29-2   American College of Cardiology and American Heart Association Classification of Heart Failure

Classification	Criteria	Patient Characteristics	Treatment Recommendations for Appropriate Patients
Stage A	Patients at high risk for developing left ventricular dysfunction but without structural heart disease or symptoms of HF	Hypertension Atherosclerotic disease Diabetes Obesity	Risk factor control ACE inhibitor or ARB
Stage B	Patients with left ventricular dysfunction or structural heart disease who have not developed symptoms of HF	History of myocardial infarction Left ventricular hypertrophy Low ejection fraction	Implement stage A recommendations, plus: • Beta-blocker
Stage C	Patients with left ventricular dysfunction or structural heart disease with current or prior symptoms of heart disease	Shortness of breath Fatigue Decreased exercise tolerance	Implement stage A and B recommendations, plus: • Diuretics • Sodium restriction • Implantable defibrillator • Cardiac resynchronization therapy
Stage D	Patients with refractory end-stage HF requiring specialized interventions	Symptoms despite maximal medical therapy Recurrent hospitalizations	Implement stage A, B, and C recommendations, plus: • End-of-life care Extraordinary measures: • Cardiac transplantation • Mechanical support

HF, heart failure; ACE, angiotensin-converting enzyme; ARB, angiotensin receptor blocker.
Adapted from Jessup, M., Abraham, W. T., Casey, D. E., et al. (2009). 2009 focused update: ACCF/AHA guidelines for the diagnosis and management of heart failure in adults: A report of the American College of Cardiology Foundation/American Heart Association Task Force on Practice Guidelines. *Circulation, 119*(14), 1977–2016.

Cardiomyopathy is a disease of the myocardium. There are three major types: dilated, hypertrophic, and restrictive or constrictive (see Chapter 28). Dilated cardiomyopathy, the most common type of cardiomyopathy, causes diffuse myocyte necrosis and fibrosis, and commonly leads to HF (Porth, 2011). Dilated cardiomyopathy can be idiopathic (unknown cause), or it can result from an inflammatory process, such as myocarditis, or from a cytotoxic agent, such as alcohol or doxorubicin (Adriamycin). Hypertrophic cardiomyopathy and restrictive cardiomyopathy lead to decreased distensibility and ventricular filling (diastolic failure). Usually, HF due to cardiomyopathy is chronic and progressive. However, cardiomyopathy and HF may resolve following removal of the causative agent (e.g., cessation of alcohol ingestion).

Valvular heart disease is also a cause of HF. The valves ensure that blood flows in one direction. With valvular dysfunction, it becomes increasingly difficult for blood to move forward, increasing pressure within the heart and increasing cardiac workload, leading to HF. (See Chapter 28 for discussion of the effects of valvular heart disease.)

Several systemic conditions, including progressive renal failure, contribute to the development and severity of HF. More than 40% of patients with chronic HF have impaired renal function. The term *cardiorenal syndrome* describes these dual problems that are associated with increased morbidity and mortality (Damman, Voors, Navis, et al., 2011). In addition, cardiac dysrhythmias such as atrial fibrillation may either cause or result from HF; in both instances, the altered electrical stimulation impairs myocardial contraction and decreases the overall efficiency of myocardial function. Other factors, such as hypoxia, acidosis, and electrolyte abnormalities, can worsen myocardial function.

Pathophysiology

Regardless of the etiology, the pathophysiology of HF results in similar pathophysiologic changes and clinical manifes-

tations. Significant myocardial dysfunction usually occurs before the patient experiences signs and symptoms of HF such as shortness of breath, edema, or fatigue.

As HF develops, the body activates neurohormonal compensatory mechanisms. These mechanisms represent the body's attempt to cope with the HF and are responsible for the signs and symptoms that eventually develop (Porth, 2011). Understanding these mechanisms is important because the treatment for HF is aimed at opposing them and relieving symptoms.

Systolic HF results in decreased blood ejected from the ventricle. The decreased blood flow is sensed by baroreceptors in the aortic and carotid bodies. The sympathetic nervous system is then stimulated to release epinephrine and norepinephrine (Fig. 29-1). The purpose of this initial response is to increase heart rate and contractility and support the failing myocardium, but the continued response has multiple negative effects. Sympathetic stimulation causes vasoconstriction in the skin, gastrointestinal tract, and kidneys. A decrease in renal perfusion due to low CO and vasoconstriction then causes the release of renin by the kidneys. Renin converts the plasma protein angiotensinogen to angiotensin I, which then circulates to the lungs. Angiotensin-converting enzyme (ACE) in the lumen of pulmonary blood vessels converts angiotensin I to angiotensin II, a potent vasoconstrictor, which then increases the blood pressure and afterload. Angiotensin II also stimulates the release of aldosterone from the adrenal cortex, resulting in sodium and fluid retention by the renal tubules and an increase in blood volume. These mechanisms lead to the fluid volume overload commonly seen in HF. Angiotensin, aldosterone, and other neurohormones (e.g., endothelin) lead to an increase in preload and afterload, which increases stress on the ventricular wall, causing an increase in cardiac workload. A counter-regulatory mechanism is attempted through the release of natriuretic peptides. Atrial natriuretic peptide (ANP) and B-type natriuretic peptide (BNP; brain type) are released from the overdistended cardiac chambers. These

Physiology ·:·:· Pathophysiology

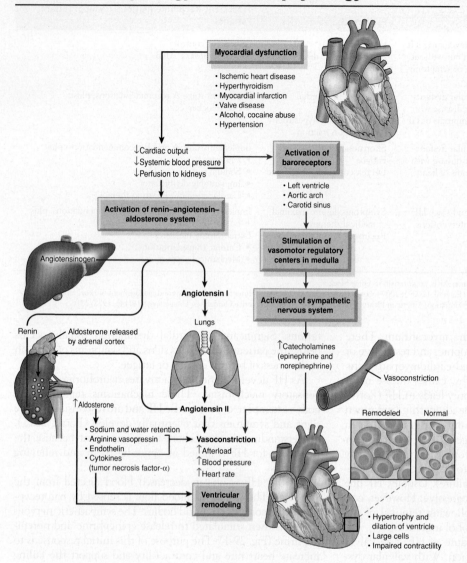

Myocardial dysfunction

- Ischemic heart disease
- Hyperthyroidism
- Myocardial infarction
- Valve disease
- Alcohol, cocaine abuse
- Hypertension

↓Cardiac output
↓Systemic blood pressure
↓Perfusion to kidneys

Activation of baroreceptors

- Left ventricle
- Aortic arch
- Carotid sinus

Activation of renin–angiotensin–aldosterone system

Stimulation of vasomotor regulatory centers in medulla

Angiotensinogen

Angiotensin I

Renin

Aldosterone released by adrenal cortex

Lungs

Activation of sympathetic nervous system

↑Catecholamines (epinephrine and norepinephrine)

Vasoconstriction

↑Aldosterone

Angiotensin II

- Sodium and water retention
- Arginine vasopressin
- Endothelin
- Cytokines (tumor necrosis factor-α)

Vasoconstriction
↑Afterload
↑Blood pressure
↑Heart rate

Remodeled   Normal

Ventricular remodeling

- Hypertrophy and dilation of ventricle
- Large cells
- Impaired contractility

FIGURE 29-1 • The pathophysiology of heart failure. A decrease in cardiac output activates multiple neurohormonal mechanisms that ultimately result in the signs and symptoms of heart failure.

substances promote vasodilation and diuresis. However, their effect is usually not strong enough to overcome the negative effects of the other mechanisms.

As the heart's workload increases, contractility of the myocardial muscle fibers decreases. Decreased contractility results in an increase in end-diastolic blood volume in the ventricle, stretching the myocardial muscle fibers and increasing the size of the ventricle (ventricular dilation). One way the heart compensates for the increased workload is to increase the thickness of the heart muscle (ventricular hypertrophy). However, hypertrophy results in abnormal changes in structure and function of myocardial cells, a process known as ventricular remodeling. Under the influence of neurohormones (e.g., angiotensin II), enlarged myocardial cells become dysfunctional and die early (a process called *apoptosis*), leaving the other normal myocardial cells struggling to maintain CO.

As cardiac cells die and the heart muscle becomes fibrotic, diastolic HF can develop, leading to further dysfunction. A stiff ventricle resists filling, and less blood in the ventricles

causes a further decrease in CO. All of these compensatory mechanisms of HF have been referred to as the "vicious cycle of HF" because low CO leads to multiple mechanisms that make the heart work harder, worsening the HF.

Clinical Manifestations

Many clinical manifestations are associated with HF (Chart 29-1). These signs and symptoms are related to congestion and poor perfusion. The signs and symptoms of HF can also be related to the ventricle that is most affected. **Left-sided heart failure (left ventricular failure)** causes different manifestations than **right-sided heart failure (right ventricular failure)**. In chronic HF, patients may have signs and symptoms of both left and right ventricular failure.

Left-Sided Heart Failure

Pulmonary congestion occurs when the left ventricle cannot effectively pump blood out of the ventricle into the aorta and the systemic circulation. The increased left ventricular

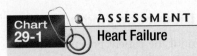

ASSESSMENT
Heart Failure

Be alert for the following signs and symptoms:

Congestion

- Dyspnea
- Orthopnea
- Paroxysmal nocturnal dyspnea
- Cough (recumbent or exertional)
- Pulmonary crackles that do not clear with cough
- Weight gain (rapid)
- Dependent edema
- Abdominal bloating or discomfort
- Ascites
- Jugular venous distention
- Sleep disturbance (anxiety or air hunger)
- Fatigue

Poor Perfusion/Low Cardiac Output

- Decreased exercise tolerance
- Muscle wasting or weakness
- Anorexia or nausea
- Unexplained weight loss
- Lightheadedness or dizziness
- Unexplained confusion or altered mental status
- Resting tachycardia
- Daytime oliguria with recumbent nocturia
- Cool or vasoconstricted extremities
- Pallor or cyanosis

Institute for Clinical Systems Improvement. (2011). *Heart failure in adults.* Available at: www.guidelines.gov/content.aspx?id=34840&search=heart+failure

end-diastolic blood volume increases the left ventricular end-diastolic pressure, which decreases blood flow from the left atrium into the left ventricle during diastole. The blood volume and pressure build up in the left atrium, decreasing flow through the pulmonary veins into the left atrium. Pulmonary venous blood volume and pressure increase in the lungs, forcing fluid from the pulmonary capillaries into the pulmonary tissues and alveoli, causing pulmonary interstitial edema and impaired gas exchange. The clinical manifestations of pulmonary congestion include dyspnea, cough, pulmonary crackles, and low oxygen saturation levels. An extra heart sound, the S₃, or "ventricular gallop," may be detected on auscultation. It is caused by abnormal ventricular filling (Bickley & Szilagyi, 2009).

Dyspnea, or shortness of breath, may be precipitated by minimal to moderate activity (dyspnea on exertion [DOE]); dyspnea also can occur at rest. The patient may report **orthopnea**, difficulty breathing when lying flat. Patients with orthopnea may use pillows to prop themselves up in bed, or they may sit in a chair and even sleep sitting up. Some patients have sudden attacks of dyspnea at night, a condition known as **paroxysmal nocturnal dyspnea (PND)**. Fluid that accumulates in the dependent extremities during the day may be reabsorbed into the circulating blood volume when the patient lies down. Because the impaired left ventricle cannot eject the increased circulating blood volume, the pressure in the pulmonary circulation increases, shifting fluid into the alveoli. The fluid-filled alveoli cannot exchange oxygen and

carbon dioxide. Without sufficient oxygen, the patient experiences dyspnea and has difficulty sleeping.

The cough associated with left ventricular failure is initially dry and nonproductive. Most often, patients complain of a dry hacking cough that may be mislabeled as asthma or chronic obstructive pulmonary disease (COPD). The cough may become moist over time. Large quantities of frothy sputum, which is sometimes pink or tan (blood tinged), may be produced, indicating acute decompensated HF with pulmonary edema.

Adventitious breath sounds may be heard in various areas of the lungs. Usually, bibasilar crackles that do not clear with coughing are detected in the early phase of left ventricular failure. As the failure worsens and pulmonary congestion increases, crackles may be auscultated throughout the lung fields. At this point, oxygen saturation may decrease.

In addition to pulmonary manifestations, the amount of blood ejected from the left ventricle decreases and can lead to inadequate tissue perfusion. The diminished CO has widespread manifestations because not enough blood reaches all of the tissues and organs (low perfusion) to provide the necessary oxygen. The decrease in stroke volume (SV) can also stimulate the sympathetic nervous system to release catecholamines, which further impedes perfusion to many organs, including the kidneys.

As reduced CO and catecholamines decrease blood flow to the kidneys, urine output drops (oliguria). Renal perfusion pressure falls, and the renin–angiotensin–aldosterone system is stimulated to increase blood pressure and intravascular volume. However, when the patient is sleeping, the cardiac workload is decreased, improving renal perfusion, which in some patients leads to frequent urination at night (nocturia).

As HF progresses, decreased output from the left ventricle may cause other symptoms. Decreased gastrointestinal perfusion causes altered digestion. Decreased brain perfusion causes dizziness, lightheadedness, confusion, restlessness, and anxiety due to decreased oxygenation and blood flow. As anxiety increases, so does dyspnea, increasing anxiety and creating a vicious cycle. Stimulation of the sympathetic system also causes the peripheral blood vessels to constrict, so the skin appears pale or ashen and feels cool and clammy.

A decrease in SV causes the sympathetic nervous system to increase the heart rate (tachycardia), often causing the patient to complain of palpitations. The peripheral pulses become weak. Without adequate CO, the body cannot respond to increased energy demands, and the patient becomes easily fatigued and has decreased activity tolerance. Fatigue also results from the increased energy expended in breathing and the insomnia that results from respiratory distress, coughing, and nocturia.

Right-Sided Heart Failure

When the right ventricle fails, congestion in the peripheral tissues and the viscera predominates. This occurs because the right side of the heart cannot eject blood effectively and cannot accommodate all of the blood that normally returns to it from the venous circulation. Increased venous pressure leads to jugular venous distention (JVD) and increased capillary hydrostatic pressure throughout the venous system. Systemic

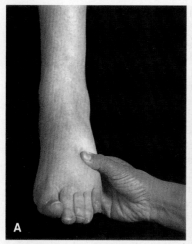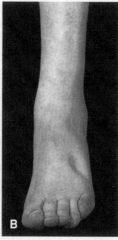

FIGURE 29-2 • Example of pitting edema. **A.** The nurse applies pressure to an area near the ankle. **B.** When the pressure is released, an indentation remains in the edematous tissue. From Bickley, L. S. (2009). *Bates' guide to physical examination and history taking* (10th ed.). Philadelphia: Lippincott Williams & Wilkins.

clinical manifestations include edema of the lower extremities (dependent edema), hepatomegaly (enlargement of the liver), **ascites** (accumulation of fluid in the peritoneal cavity), and weight gain due to retention of fluid.

Edema usually affects the feet and ankles and worsens when the patient stands or sits for a long period. The edema may decrease when the patient elevates the legs. Edema can gradually progress up the legs and thighs and eventually into the external genitalia and lower trunk. Ascites is evidenced by increased abdominal girth and may accompany lower body edema or may be the only edema present. Sacral edema is common in patients who are on bed rest, because the sacral area is dependent. Pitting edema, in which indentations in the skin remain after even slight compression with the fingertips (Fig. 29-2), is generally obvious after retention of at least 4.5 kg (10 lb) of fluid (4.5 L).

Hepatomegaly and tenderness in the right upper quadrant of the abdomen result from venous engorgement of the liver. The increased pressure may interfere with the liver's ability to function (secondary liver dysfunction). As hepatic dysfunction progresses, increased pressure within the portal vessels may force fluid into the abdominal cavity, causing ascites. Ascites may increase pressure on the stomach and intestines and cause gastrointestinal distress. Hepatomegaly may also increase pressure on the diaphragm, causing respiratory distress.

Anorexia (loss of appetite), nausea, or abdominal pain may result from the venous engorgement and venous stasis within the abdominal organs. The generalized weakness that accompanies right-sided HF results from reduced CO and impaired circulation.

 Concept Mastery Alert

Left-sided HF refers to failure of the left ventricle; it results in pulmonary congestion. Right-sided HF, failure of the right ventricle, results in congestion in the peripheral tissues and the viscera.

Assessment and Diagnostic Findings

HF may go undetected until the patient presents with signs and symptoms of pulmonary and peripheral edema. Some of the physical signs that suggest HF may also occur with other diseases, such as renal failure and COPD; therefore, diagnostic testing is essential to confirm a diagnosis of HF.

Assessment of ventricular function is an essential part of the initial diagnostic workup. An echocardiogram is usually performed to determine the EF, identify anatomic features such as structural abnormalities and valve malfunction, and confirm the diagnosis of HF. This information may also be obtained noninvasively by radionuclide ventriculography or invasively by ventriculography as part of a cardiac catheterization procedure. A chest x-ray and a 12-lead electrocardiogram (ECG) are obtained to assist in the diagnosis. Laboratory studies usually performed during the initial workup include serum electrolytes, blood urea nitrogen (BUN), creatinine, liver function tests, thyroid-stimulating hormone, complete blood count (CBC), BNP, and routine urinalysis. The BNP level is a key diagnostic indicator of HF; high levels are a sign of high cardiac filling pressure and can aid in both the diagnosis and management of HF (Institute for Clinical Systems Improvement [ICSI], 2011). The results of these laboratory studies assist in determining the underlying cause and can also be used to establish a baseline to assess effects of treatment. Cardiac stress testing or cardiac catheterization may be performed to determine whether coronary artery disease and cardiac ischemia are causing the HF.

Medical Management

The overall goals of management of HF are to relieve patient symptoms, to improve functional status and quality of life, and to extend survival. The prognosis for HF patients has improved with the use of evidence-based protocols for patient management. Specific interventions are based on the stage of HF. The objectives of medical management include the following (ICSI, 2011):
- Improvement of cardiac function by reducing preload and afterload
- Reduction of symptoms and improvement of functional status
- Stabilization of patient condition and lowering of the risk of hospitalization
- Delay of the progression of HF and extension of life expectancy
- Promotion of a lifestyle conducive to cardiac health

Treatment options vary according to the severity of the patient's condition and may include oral and intravenous (IV) medications, major lifestyle changes, supplemental oxygen, implantation of cardiac devices, and surgical approaches including cardiac transplantation.

Managing the patient with HF begins with providing comprehensive education and counseling to the patient and family. The patient and family must understand the nature of HF and the importance of their participation in the treatment regimen. Lifestyle recommendations include restriction of dietary sodium; avoidance of smoking, including passive smoke; avoidance of excessive fluid and alcohol intake; weight reduction when indicated; and regular exercise. The

TABLE 29-3 Common Medications Used to Treat Heart Failure

Medication	Therapeutic Effects	Key Nursing Considerations
Angiotensin-Converting Enzyme Inhibitors		
Lisinopril (Prinivil) Enalapril (Vasotec)	↓ BP and ↓ afterload Relieves signs and symptoms of HF Prevents progression of HF	Observe for symptomatic hypotension, increased serum K⁺, cough, and worsening renal function.
Angiotensin Receptor Blockers		
Valsartan (Diovan) Losartan (Cozaar)	↓ BP and ↓ afterload Relieves signs and symptoms of HF Prevents progression of HF	Observe for symptomatic hypotension, increased serum K⁺, and worsening renal function.
Hydralazine and Isosorbide Dinitrate (Dilatrate)	Dilates blood vessels ↓ BP and ↓ afterload	Observe for symptomatic hypotension.
Beta-Adrenergic Blocking Agents (Beta-Blockers)		
Metoprolol (Lopressor) Carvedilol (Coreg)	Dilates blood vessels and ↓ afterload ↓ Signs and symptoms of HF Improves exercise capacity	Observe for decreased heart rate, symptomatic hypotension, dizziness, and fatigue.
Diuretics		
Loop diuretic: Furosemide (Lasix)	↓ Fluid volume overload ↓ Signs and symptoms of HF	Observe for electrolyte abnormalities, renal dysfunction, diuretic resistance, and decreased BP. Carefully monitor I&O and daily weight (see Chart 29-2).
Thiazide diuretics: Metolazone (Zaroxolyn) Hydrochlorothiazide (HCTZ)		
Aldosterone antagonist: Spironolactone (Aldactone)	Improves HF symptoms in advanced HF	Observe for hyperkalemia, hyponatremia.
Digitalis		
Digoxin (Lanoxin)	Improves cardiac contractility ↓ Signs and symptoms of HF	Observe for bradycardia and digitalis toxicity.

↓, decreases; BP, blood pressure; HF, heart failure; K⁺, potassium; I&O, input and output.

patient must also know how to recognize signs and symptoms that need to be reported to a health care professional.

Pharmacologic Therapy

Several medications are routinely prescribed for HF, including ACE inhibitors, beta-blockers, and diuretics (Table 29-3). Many of these medications, particularly ACE inhibitors and beta-blockers, improve symptoms and extend survival. Others, such as diuretics, improve symptoms but may not affect survival (Fonarow et al., 2010). Target doses for these medications are identified in the ACC/AHA guidelines, and nurses and physicians work collaboratively toward achieving effective dosing of these medications (Jessup et al., 2009). Calcium channel blockers are no longer recommended for patients with HF because they are associated with worsening failure (ICSI, 2011).

Angiotensin-Converting Enzyme Inhibitors

ACE inhibitors play a pivotal role in the management of systolic HF. They have been found to relieve the signs and symptoms of HF and significantly decrease mortality and morbidity. ACE inhibitors (e.g., lisinopril [Prinivil]) slow the progression of HF, improve exercise tolerance, and decrease the number of hospitalizations for HF (ICSI, 2011). Available as oral and IV medications, ACE inhibitors promote vasodilation and diuresis, ultimately decreasing afterload and preload.

Vasodilation reduces resistance to left ventricular ejection of blood, diminishing the heart's workload and improving ventricular emptying. ACE inhibitors decrease the secretion of aldosterone, which is a hormone that causes the kidneys to retain sodium and water. ACE inhibitors also promote renal excretion of sodium and fluid (while retaining potassium), thereby reducing left ventricular filling pressure and decreasing pulmonary congestion. ACE inhibitors may be the first medication prescribed for patients in mild failure—patients with fatigue or DOE but without signs of fluid overload and pulmonary congestion. These agents are also recommended for prevention of HF in patients at risk due to hypertension and coronary artery disease (Jessup et al., 2009).

ACE inhibitors are started at a low dose that is gradually increased until the optimal dose is achieved and the patient is hemodynamically stable. The final maintenance dose depends on the patient's blood pressure, fluid status, and renal status, as well as the severity of the HF.

Patients receiving ACE inhibitors are monitored for hypotension, hyperkalemia (increased potassium in the blood), and alterations in renal function, especially if they are also receiving diuretics. Because ACE inhibitors cause the kidneys to retain potassium, the patient who is also receiving a diuretic may not need to take oral potassium supplements. However, patients receiving potassium-sparing diuretics (which do not cause potassium loss with diuresis) must be carefully monitored for hyperkalemia. ACE inhibitors may be discontinued if the potassium level remains greater than 5.5 mEq/L or if the serum creatinine rises.

Other adverse effects of ACE inhibitors include a dry, persistent cough that may not respond to cough suppressants. However, cough can also indicate a worsening of ventricular function and failure. Rarely, ACE inhibitors can cause an allergic reaction accompanied by angioedema. If angioedema affects the oropharyngeal area and impairs breathing, the ACE inhibitor must be stopped immediately and emergency care provided.

If the patient cannot continue taking an ACE inhibitor because of development of cough, an elevated creatinine level, or hyperkalemia, an angiotensin receptor blocker (ARB) or a combination of hydralazine and isosorbide dinitrate (Dilatrate) is prescribed (see Table 29-3).

Angiotensin Receptor Blockers

Although the action of ARBs is different from that of ACE inhibitors, ARBs (e.g., valsartan [Diovan]) have similar hemodynamic effects and side effects (ICSI, 2011). Whereas ACE inhibitors block the conversion of angiotensin I to angiotensin II, ARBs block the vasoconstricting effects of angiotensin II at the angiotensin II receptors. ARBs are prescribed for HF patients as an alternative to ACE inhibitors (Jessup et al., 2009).

Hydralazine and Isosorbide Dinitrate

A combination of hydralazine and isosorbide dinitrate may be another alternative for patients who cannot take ACE inhibitors (ICSI, 2011). Nitrates (e.g., isosorbide dinitrate) cause venous dilation, which reduces the amount of blood return to the heart and lowers preload. Hydralazine lowers systemic vascular resistance and left ventricular afterload. This combination of medications is also recommended in HF guidelines and may be more effective for African Americans who do not respond to ACE inhibitors (ICSI, 2011).

Beta-Blockers

Beta-blockers are routinely prescribed in addition to ACE inhibitors. These agents block the adverse effects of the sympathetic nervous system. They relax blood vessels, lower blood pressure, decrease afterload, and decrease cardiac workload. Beta-blockers, such as carvedilol (Coreg) and metoprolol (Lopressor), have been found to improve functional status and reduce mortality and morbidity in patients with HF (ICSI, 2011). In addition, beta-blockers have been recommended for patients with asymptomatic systolic dysfunction, such as those with a decreased EF, to prevent the onset of symptoms of HF. However, the therapeutic effects of these drugs may not be seen for several weeks or even months.

Beta-blockers may produce a number of side effects, including dizziness, hypotension, bradycardia, fatigue, and depression. Side effects are most common in the initial few weeks of treatment. Because of the potential for side effects, beta-blockers are started at a low dose. The dose is titrated up slowly (every few weeks), with close monitoring after each dosage increase. Nurses educate patients about potential symptoms during the early phase of treatment and stress that adjustment to the drug may take several weeks. Nurses must also provide support to patients going through this symptom-provoking phase of treatment. Because beta-blockade can cause bronchiole constriction, these drugs are used with caution in patients with a history of bronchospastic diseases such as asthma. A beta-1–selective beta-blocker (i.e., one that primarily blocks the beta-adrenergic receptor sites in the heart), such as metoprolol, is recommended for these patients (Aschenbrenner & Venable, 2012).

Diuretics

Diuretics are prescribed to remove excess extracellular fluid by increasing the rate of urine produced in patients with signs and symptoms of fluid overload. Loop, thiazide, and aldosterone blocking diuretics may be prescribed for patients with HF. These medications differ in their site of action in the kidney and their effects on renal electrolyte excretion and reabsorption.

Loop diuretics, such as furosemide (Lasix), inhibit sodium and chloride reabsorption mainly in the ascending loop of Henle. HF patients with severe volume overload are generally treated with a loop diuretic first (ICSI, 2011). Thiazide diuretics, such as metolazone (Zaroxolyn), inhibit sodium and chloride reabsorption in the early distal tubules. Both of these classes of diuretics increase potassium excretion; therefore, patients treated with these medications must have their serum potassium levels closely monitored. Both a loop and a thiazide diuretic may be used in patients with severe HF who are unresponsive to a single diuretic. Diuretics may be most effective if the patient assumes a supine position for 1 or 2 hours after taking them. The need for diuretics can be decreased if the patient avoids excessive fluid intake (e.g., more than 2 qt/day) and adheres to a low-sodium diet (e.g., no more than 2 g/day) (Lindenfeld et al., 2010).

Spironolactone (Aldactone) is a potassium-sparing diuretic that blocks the effects of aldosterone in the distal tubule and collecting duct. It effectively reduces mortality and morbidity in patients with moderate to severe HF (ICSI, 2011). Serum creatinine and potassium levels are monitored frequently (e.g., within the first week and then every 4 weeks) when spironolactone is first administered.

The type and dose of diuretic prescribed depend on clinical signs and symptoms and renal function. Careful patient monitoring and dose adjustments are necessary to balance the effectiveness of these medications with the side effects (Chart 29-2). Loop diuretics are administered IV for exacerbations of HF when rapid diuresis is necessary. Diuretics improve the patient's symptoms, provided that renal function is adequate. As HF progresses, cardiorenal syndrome may develop or worsen. Patients with this syndrome are resistant to diuretics and may require other interventions to deal with congestive signs and symptoms (Damman et al., 2011).

Digitalis

For many years, digitalis (digoxin) was considered an essential agent for the treatment of HF, but with the advent of new medications, it is not prescribed as often. Digoxin increases the force of myocardial contraction and slows conduction through the atrioventricular node. It improves contractility, increasing left ventricular output. Although the use of digoxin does not result in decreased mortality rates among patients with HF, it can be effective in decreasing

Chart 29-2

PHARMACOLOGY

Administering and Monitoring Diuretic Therapy

When nursing care involves diuretic therapy for conditions such as heart failure, the nurse needs to administer the medication and monitor the patient's response carefully, as follows:

- Prior to administration of the diuretic, check laboratory results for electrolyte depletion, especially potassium, sodium, and magnesium.
- Prior to administration of the diuretic, check for signs and symptoms of volume depletion, such as postural hypotension, lightheadedness, and dizziness.
- Administer the diuretic at a time conducive to the patient's lifestyle—for example, early in the day to avoid nocturia.
- Monitor urine output during the hours after administration, and analyze intake, output, and daily weights to assess response.
- Continue to monitor serum electrolytes for depletion. Replace potassium with increased oral intake of food rich in potassium or potassium supplements. Replace magnesium as needed.
- Monitor for hyperkalemia in patients receiving potassium-sparing diuretics.
- Continue to assess for signs of volume depletion.
- Monitor creatinine for increased levels indicative of renal dysfunction.
- Monitor for elevated uric acid level and signs and symptoms of gout.
- Assess lungs sounds and edema to evaluate response to therapy.
- Monitor for adverse reactions such as gastrointestinal distress and dysrhythmias.
- Encourage supine position after dose is given to facilitate effects of the diuretic.
- Assist patients to manage urinary frequency and urgency associated with diuretic therapy.

the symptoms of systolic HF and may help prevent hospitalization (ICSI, 2011). Patients with renal dysfunction and older patients should receive smaller doses of digoxin, as it is excreted through the kidneys.

A key concern associated with digoxin therapy is digitalis toxicity. Clinical manifestations of toxicity include anorexia, nausea, visual disturbances, confusion, and bradycardia. The serum potassium level is monitored because the effect of digoxin is enhanced in the presence of hypokalemia and digoxin toxicity may occur. A serum digoxin level is obtained if the patient's renal function changes or there are symptoms of toxicity.

Intravenous Infusions

IV inotropes (milrinone [Primacor], dobutamine [Dobutrex]) increase the force of myocardial contraction; as such, they may be indicated for hospitalized patients with acute decompensated HF. These agents are used for patients who do not respond to routine pharmacologic therapy and are reserved for patients with severe ventricular dysfunction. They are used with caution, as some studies have associated their use with increased mortality (Metra, Bettari, Carubelli, et al., 2011). IV vasodilators such as nitroprusside (Nipride), nitroglycerin, or nesiritide (Natrecor) may also be used in patients with severe decompensated HF (Lindenfeld et al., 2010). Patients

usually require admission to the intensive care unit (ICU) and may also have hemodynamic monitoring with a pulmonary artery catheter or alternative technology (see Chapter 25). Hemodynamic data is used to assess cardiac function and volume status and to guide therapy with inotropes, vasodilators, and diuretics (Urden, Stacy, & Lough, 2010).

Milrinone. Milrinone is a phosphodiesterase inhibitor that delays the release of calcium from intracellular reservoirs and prevents the uptake of extracellular calcium by the cells. This promotes vasodilation, resulting in decreased preload and afterload and reduced cardiac workload. Milrinone is administered IV to patients with severe HF, including patients who are waiting for heart transplantation. Because the drug causes vasodilation, the patient's blood pressure is monitored prior to administration; if the patient is hypovolemic, the blood pressure could drop quickly. The major side effects are hypotension and increased ventricular dysrhythmias. Blood pressure and ECG are monitored closely during and following infusions of milrinone.

Dobutamine. Dobutamine is another IV medication administered to patients with significant left ventricular dysfunction and hypoperfusion. A catecholamine, dobutamine stimulates the beta-1 adrenergic receptors. Its major action is to increase cardiac contractility and renal perfusion to enhance urine output. However, it also increases the heart rate and can precipitate ectopic beats and tachydysrhythmias (Metra et al., 2011).

Medications for Diastolic Dysfunction

Patients with predominant diastolic HF and preserved left ventricular EF are treated differently than patients with systolic HF. Contributing causes such as hypertension and ischemic heart disease are evaluated and treated. These patients do not tolerate tachycardia, because it does not allow time for ventricular filling. Beta-blockers may be used to control tachycardia from atrial fibrillation or other causes (ICSI, 2011).

Other Medications for Heart Failure

Anticoagulants may be prescribed, especially if the patient has a history of atrial fibrillation or a thromboembolic event (Lindenfeld et al., 2010). Antiarrhythmic drugs such as amiodarone (Cordarone) may be prescribed for patients with dysrhythmias, along with evaluation for device therapy with an implantable cardioverter defibrillator (ICD) (see Chapter 26). Medications that manage hyperlipidemia (e.g., statins) are also routinely prescribed. Nonsteroidal anti-inflammatory drugs (NSAIDs) such as ibuprofen (Motrin) should be avoided because they decrease renal perfusion, especially in older adults.

Nutritional Therapy

Following a low-sodium (no more than 2 g/day) diet and avoiding excessive fluid intake are usually recommended. Decreasing dietary sodium reduces fluid retention and the symptoms of peripheral and pulmonary congestion. The purpose of sodium restriction is to decrease the amount of circulating blood volume, which decreases myocardial work. A balance needs to be achieved between the patient's ability to comply with the diet and the recommended dietary restriction. Any change in diet should consider good nutrition as well as the patient's likes, dislikes, and cultural food patterns. Patient adherence is important because dietary indiscretions may result in severe exacerbations of HF requiring hospitalization (ICSI, 2011). However, behavioral changes in this area are difficult for many patients.

Additional Therapy

Supplemental Oxygen

Oxygen therapy may become necessary as HF progresses. The need is based on the degree of pulmonary congestion and resulting hypoxia. Some patients require supplemental oxygen only during periods of activity.

Other Interventions

A number of procedures and surgical approaches may benefit patients with HF. If the patient has underlying coronary artery disease, coronary artery revascularization with PCI or coronary artery bypass surgery (see Chapter 27) may be considered. Ventricular function may improve in some patients when coronary flow is increased.

Patients with HF are at high risk for dysrhythmias, and sudden cardiac death is common among patients with advanced HF. In patients with severe left ventricular dysfunction and the possibility of life-threatening dysrhythmias, placement of an ICD can prevent sudden cardiac death and extend survival (see Chapter 26). Candidates for an ICD include those with an EF less than 35% and with NYHA functional class II or III, including those with and without a history of ventricular dysrhythmias (Jessup et al., 2009).

Patients with HF who do not improve with standard therapy may benefit from **cardiac resynchronization therapy (CRT)**. CRT involves the use of a biventricular pacemaker to treat electrical conduction defects. A prolonged QRS duration on ECG indicates left bundle branch block, which is a type of delayed conduction that is frequently seen in patients with HF. This problem results in dyssynchronous conduction and contraction of the right and left ventricles, which can further decrease EF (Jessup et al., 2009). (See Chapter 26 for discussion of dysrhythmias.) The use of a pacing device with leads placed in the right atrium, right ventricle, and left ventricular cardiac vein can synchronize the contractions of the right and left ventricles (Fig. 29-3). This intervention improves CO, optimizes myocardial energy consumption, reduces mitral regurgitation, and slows the ventricular remodeling process. For selected patients, CRT results in fewer symptoms, increased functional status, and fewer hospitalizations (Goldenberg, Hall, Beck, et al., 2011). Combination devices are available for patients who require CRT and an ICD. (See Chapter 26 for further discussion of care of patients with pacemakers and ICDs.)

Ultrafiltration is an alternative intervention for patients with severe fluid overload. It is reserved for patients with advanced HF who are resistant to diuretic therapy (Fiaccadori, Regolisti, Maggiore, et al., 2011). A dual-lumen central IV catheter is placed, and the patient's blood is circulated through a small bedside filtration machine. Liters of excess fluid and plasma are removed slowly from the patient's intravascular circulating volume over a number of hours. The patient's output of filtration fluid, blood pressure, and hemo-

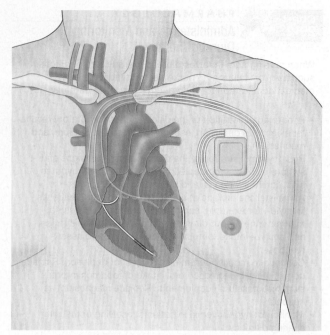

FIGURE 29-3 • Cardiac resynchronization therapy. To pace both ventricles, pacemaker leads are placed in the right atrium and right ventricle; a third lead is threaded through the coronary sinus into a lateral vein on the wall of the left ventricle.

globin (analyzed for hemoconcentration) are monitored as indicators of volume status.

For some patients with end-stage HF, cardiac transplantation is one of the few options for long-term survival. Patients with ACC/AHA stage D HF who may be eligible are referred for consideration of transplantation. Some of these patients require mechanical circulatory assistance with an implanted ventricular assist device as a bridge therapy to cardiac transplantation (see Chapter 28). A left ventricular assist device may also be implanted as permanent therapy for selected patients (Jessup et al., 2009).

Gerontologic Considerations

Several normal age-related changes increase the frequency of HF: increased systolic blood pressure, increased ventricular wall thickness, and increased myocardial fibrosis. Older people may present with atypical signs and symptoms such as fatigue, weakness, and somnolence. Older patients may not always detect or accurately interpret common symptoms of HF such as shortness of breath (Riegel, Dickson, Cameron, et al., 2011). Decreased renal function can make the older patient resistant to diuretics and more sensitive to changes in volume. The administration of diuretics to older men requires nursing surveillance for bladder distention caused by urethral obstruction from an enlarged prostate gland. The bladder may be assessed with an ultrasound scanner or the suprapubic area palpated for an oval mass and percussed for dullness, indicative of bladder fullness. Urinary frequency and urgency may be particularly stressful to older patients, as many have arthritis and limited mobility.

NURSING PROCESS
The Patient With Heart Failure

Despite advances in treatment of HF, morbidity and mortality remain high. Nurses have a major impact on outcomes for patients with HF, especially in the areas of patient education and monitoring.

Assessment

Nursing assessment for the patient with HF focuses on observing for effectiveness of therapy and for the patient's ability to understand and implement self-management strategies. Signs and symptoms of increasing HF are analyzed and reported to the patient's provider so that therapy can be adjusted. The nurse also explores the patient's emotional response to the diagnosis of HF, because it is a chronic and often progressive condition that is commonly associated with depression and other psychosocial issues (Pressler, Subramanian, Perkins, et al., 2011; Sherwood, Blumenthal, Hinderliter, et al., 2011).

Health History

The health history focuses on the signs and symptoms of HF, such as dyspnea, fatigue, and edema. Sleep disturbances, particularly sleep suddenly interrupted by shortness of breath, may be reported. Patients are asked about the number of pillows needed for sleep, edema, abdominal symptoms, altered mental status, activities of daily living, and the activities that cause fatigue. Nurses need to be aware of the variety of clinical manifestations that may indicate worsening HF and assess the patient accordingly (Chart 29-3). While obtaining the patient's history, the nurse assesses the patient's understanding of HF, self-management strategies, and the patient's ability and willingness to adhere to those strategies.

Physical Examination

The patient is observed for restlessness and anxiety that might suggest hypoxia from pulmonary congestion. The patient's level of consciousness is also evaluated for any changes, as low CO can decrease the flow of oxygen to the brain.

The rate and depth of respirations are assessed along with the effort required for breathing. The lungs are auscultated to detect crackles and wheezes. Crackles are produced by the sudden opening of edematous small airways and alveoli. They may be heard at the end of inspiration and are not cleared with coughing (Bickley & Szilagyi, 2009). Wheezing may also be heard in some patients who have bronchospasm along with pulmonary congestion.

The blood pressure is carefully evaluated, because HF patients may present with hypotension or hypertension. Patients may be assessed for orthostatic hypotension, especially if they report lightheadedness, dizziness, or syncope. The heart is auscultated for an S_3 heart sound, which is an early sign that increased blood volume fills the ventricle with each beat. Heart rate and rhythm are also documented, and patients are often placed on continuous ECG monitoring in the hospital setting. When the heart rate is rapid or very slow, the SV decreases and potentially worsens the HF.

JVD is assessed with the patient sitting at a 45-degree angle; distention greater than 3 cm above the sternal angle is considered abnormal and indicative of right ventricular failure. This is an estimate, not a precise measurement, of high central venous pressure (Bickley & Szilagyi, 2009).

The nurse assesses peripheral pulses and rates their volume on a scale from 0 (not palpable) to 3+ (bounding). The skin is also assessed for color and temperature. With significant decreases in SV, there is a decrease in perfusion to the periphery, decreasing the volume of pulses and causing the skin to feel cool and appear pale or cyanotic. The feet and lower legs are examined for edema; if the patient is supine in bed, the sacrum

---

Chart 29-3

NURSING RESEARCH PROFILE
Assessing Signs and Symptoms in Heart Failure Patients

Albert, N., Trochelman, K., Li, J., et al. (2010). Signs and symptoms of heart failure: Are you asking the right questions? *American Journal of Critical Care, 19*(5), 443–453.

Purpose

Clinical manifestations of worsening heart failure (HF) are not always recognized by health care providers or patients, potentially delaying treatment decisions. This study aimed to identify signs and symptoms reported by patients with HF and to determine whether they differed depending on patient demographics, New York Heart Association (NYHA) functional class, or care setting.

Design

A one-page checklist of signs and symptoms of HF was distributed to a convenience sample of 276 adults (112 in hospital and 164 in ambulatory settings) with a diagnosis of systolic HF. Participants were asked to identify all signs and symptoms they were experiencing, not only those commonly associated with HF.

Findings

Shortness of breath, decreased exercise tolerance, orthopnea, profound fatigue, and dizziness were reported most often by

participants with HF in both inpatient and outpatient settings. Dyspnea was reported by participants from all functional classes and in both ambulatory and hospitalized settings. Participants with NYHA functional class IV status reported more atypical manifestations, including nausea, restlessness, and confusion. Profound fatigue was associated with worsening functional class and the need for hospitalization.

Nursing Implications

Dyspnea is commonly believed to be a manifestation of worsening HF; yet, findings from this study suggest that it is commonly experienced by all patients with HF and may not indicate progression of HF. However, profound fatigue may be associated with worsening HF. Furthermore, findings from this study suggest that the sickest HF patients (i.e., those with NYHA functional class IV status) may exhibit atypical manifestations of worsening HF. Nurses need to ask the right questions when assessing patients with HF. It is important to recognize atypical as well as typical signs and symptoms of HF.

and back are also assessed for edema. The upper extremities may also become edematous in some patients. Edema is typically rated on a scale from 0 (no edema) to 4+ (pitting edema).

The abdomen is examined for tenderness and hepatomegaly. The presence of firmness, distention, and possible ascites is noted. The liver may be assessed for hepatojugular reflux. The patient is asked to breathe normally while manual pressure is applied over the right upper quadrant of the abdomen for 30 to 60 seconds. If neck vein distention increases more than 1 cm, the finding is positive for increased venous pressure.

If the patient is hospitalized, the nurse measures urinary output and evaluates it in terms of diuretic use. Intake and output records are rigorously maintained and analyzed. It is important to track whether the patient has excreted excessive volume (i.e., negative fluid balance is generally the goal). The intake and output is then compared with changes in weight. Although diuresis is expected, the HF patient must also be monitored for **oliguria** (diminished urine output, less than 0.5 mL/kg/hr) or **anuria** (urine output less than 50 mL/24 h) because of the risk of renal dysfunction.

The patient is weighed daily in the hospital or at home, at the same time of day, with the same type of clothing, and on the same scale. If there is a significant change in weight (i.e., 2- to 3-lb increase in a day or 5-lb increase in a week), the primary provider is notified and medications are adjusted (e.g., the diuretic dose is increased).

Diagnosis

Nursing Diagnoses

Based on the assessment data, major nursing diagnoses may include the following:

- Activity intolerance related to decreased CO
- Excess fluid volume related to the HF syndrome
- Anxiety-related symptoms related to complexity of the therapeutic regimen
- Powerlessness related to chronic illness and hospitalizations
- Ineffective family therapeutic regimen management

Collaborative Problems/Potential Complications

Potential complications may include the following:

- Hypotension, poor perfusion, and cardiogenic shock (see Chapter 14)
- Dysrhythmias (see Chapter 26)
- Thromboembolism (see Chapter 30)
- Pericardial effusion and cardiac tamponade

Planning and Goals

Major goals for the patient may include promoting activity and reducing fatigue, relieving fluid overload symptoms, decreasing anxiety or increasing the patient's ability to manage anxiety, encouraging the patient to verbalize his or her ability to make decisions and influence outcomes, and educating the patient and family about management of the therapeutic regimen (Doenges, Moorhouse, & Murr, 2010).

Nursing Interventions

Promoting Activity Tolerance

Reduced physical activity caused by HF symptoms leads to physical deconditioning that worsens the patient's symptoms

and exercise tolerance. Prolonged inactivity, which may be self-imposed, should be avoided because of its deconditioning effects and risks, such as pressure ulcers (especially in edematous patients) and venous thromboembolism. An acute illness that exacerbates HF symptoms or requires hospitalization may be an indication for temporary bed rest. Otherwise, some type of physical activity every day should be encouraged. Exercise training has many favorable effects for the HF patient, including increased functional capacity, decreased dyspnea, and improved quality of life (Downing & Balady, 2011). The exercise regimen should include 5 minutes of warm-up activities followed by about 30 minutes of exercise at the prescribed intensity level. A typical program for a patient with HF might include a daily walking regimen, with the duration increased over a 6-week period. The physician, nurse, and patient collaborate to develop a schedule that promotes pacing and prioritization of activities. The schedule should alternate activities with periods of rest and avoid having two significant energy-consuming activities occur on the same day or in immediate succession. Before undertaking physical activity, the patient should be given guidelines similar to those noted in Chart 29-4. Because some patients may be severely debilitated, they may need to limit physical activities to only 3 to 5 minutes at a time, one to four times per day. The patient should increase the duration of the activity, then the frequency, before increasing the intensity of the activity.

Barriers to performing activities are identified, and methods of adjusting an activity are discussed. For example, vegetables can be chopped or peeled while sitting at the kitchen table rather than standing at the kitchen counter. Small, frequent meals decrease the amount of energy needed for digestion while providing adequate nutrition. The nurse helps the patient identify peak and low periods of energy,

Chart 29-4 **HEALTH PROMOTION**

An Exercise Program for Patients With Heart Failure

Before undertaking physical activity, the patient should be given the following guidelines:

- Talk with your primary provider for specific exercise program recommendations.
- Begin with low-impact activities such as walking, cycling, or water exercises.
- Start with warm-up activity followed by sessions that gradually build up to about 30 minutes.
- Follow your exercise period with cool-down activities.
- Avoid performing physical activities outside in extreme hot, cold, or humid weather.
- Wait 2 hours after eating a meal before performing the physical activity.
- Ensure that you are able to talk during the physical activity; if you cannot do so, decrease the intensity of activity.
- Stop the activity if severe shortness of breath, pain, or dizziness develops.

Adapted from Andreuzzi, R. (2010). Does aerobic exercise have a role in the treatment plan of a patient with heart failure. *Internet Journal of American Physician Assistants, 7*(2), 1–29; and Flynn, K. E., Piña, I. L., Whellan, D. J., et al. (2009). Effects of exercise training on health status in patients with chronic heart failure: HF-ACTION randomized controlled trial. *Journal of the American Medical Association, 301*(14), 1451–1459.

planning energy-consuming activities for peak periods. For example, the patient may prepare the meals for the entire day in the morning. Pacing and prioritizing activities help maintain the patient's energy to allow participation in regular physical activity.

The patient's response to activities needs to be monitored. If the patient is hospitalized, vital signs and oxygen saturation level are monitored before, during, and immediately after an activity to identify whether they are within the desired range. Heart rate should return to baseline within 3 minutes following the activity. If the patient is at home, the degree of fatigue felt after the activity can be used to assess the response. If the patient tolerates the activity, short- and long-term goals can be developed to gradually increase the intensity, duration, and frequency of activity.

Adherence to exercise training is essential if the patient is to benefit from it, but it may be difficult for patients with other conditions (e.g., arthritis) and longer duration of HF. Referral to a cardiac rehabilitation program may be indicated, especially for patients newly diagnosed with HF. A supervised program may also benefit those who need a structured environment, significant educational support, regular encouragement, and interpersonal contact.

Managing Fluid Volume

Patients with severe HF may receive IV diuretic therapy; however, patients with less severe symptoms are typically prescribed oral diuretics. Oral diuretics should be administered early in the morning so that diuresis does not interfere with the patient's nighttime rest. Discussing the timing of medication administration is especially important for older patients who may have urinary urgency or incontinence. A single dose of a diuretic may cause the patient to excrete a large volume of fluid shortly after its administration.

The patient's fluid status is monitored closely by auscultating the lungs, monitoring daily body weight, and assisting the patient to adhere to a low-sodium diet by reading food labels and avoiding high-sodium foods such as canned, processed, and convenience foods (Chart 29-5). Weight gain in a patient with HF almost always reflects fluid retention. If the diet includes fluid restriction, the nurse can assist the patient to plan fluid intake throughout the day while respecting the patient's dietary preferences. If the patient is receiving IV fluids and medications, the amount of fluid needs to be monitored closely, and the primary provider or pharmacist can be consulted about the possibility of maximizing the amount of medication in the same volume of IV fluid (e.g., double concentrating to decrease the fluid volume administered).

The patient is positioned or taught how to assume a position that facilitates breathing. The number of pillows may be increased, the head of the bed may be elevated, or the patient may sit in a recliner. In these positions, the venous return to the heart (preload) is reduced, pulmonary congestion is alleviated, and pressure on the diaphragm is minimized. The lower arms are supported with pillows to eliminate the fatigue caused by the pull of the patient's weight on the shoulder muscles.

Because decreased circulation in edematous areas increases the risk of pressure ulcers, the nurse assesses for skin breakdown and institutes preventive measures. Positioning to avoid pressure and frequent changes of position help prevent pressure ulcers.

Controlling Anxiety

Because patients with HF have difficulty maintaining adequate oxygenation, they are likely to develop dyspnea, which may in turn lead to restlessness and anxiety. Complex medical

---

Chart 29-5

HEALTH PROMOTION

Facts About Dietary Sodium

Although the major source of sodium in the average American diet is salt, many types of natural foods contain varying amounts of sodium. Even if no salt is added in cooking and if salty foods are avoided, the daily diet will still contain about 2,000 mg of sodium. Fresh fruits and vegetables are low in sodium and should be encouraged.

Additives in Food

In general, food prepared at home is lower in sodium than restaurant or processed foods. Added food substances (additives), such as sodium alginate, which improves food texture, sodium benzoate, which acts as a preservative, and disodium phosphate, which improves cooking quality in certain foods, increase the sodium intake when included in the daily diet. Therefore, patients on low-sodium diets should be advised to check labels carefully for words such as "salt" or "sodium," especially on canned foods. For example, without looking at the sodium content per serving found on the nutrition labels, when given a choice between a serving of potato chips and a cup of canned cream of mushroom soup, most would think that soup is lower in sodium. However, when the labels are examined, the lower sodium choice is found to be the chips. Although potato chips are *not* recommended in a low-sodium diet, this example illustrates that it is important to read food labels to determine both sodium content and serving size.

Nonfood Sodium Sources

Sodium is contained in municipal water. Water softeners also increase the sodium content of drinking water. Patients on sodium-restricted diets should be cautioned against using nonprescription medications such as antacids, cough syrups, and laxatives. Salt substitutes may be allowed, but it is recognized that they are high in potassium. Over-the-counter medications should not be used without first consulting the patient's primary provider.

Promoting Dietary Adherence

If patients find food unpalatable because of the dietary sodium restrictions and/or the taste disturbances caused by the medications, they may refuse to eat or to adhere with the dietary regimen. For this reason, severe sodium restrictions should be avoided, and diuretic medication should be balanced with the patient's ability to restrict dietary sodium. A variety of flavorings, such as lemon juice, vinegar, and herbs, may be used to improve the taste of the food and facilitate acceptance of the diet. The patient's food preferences should be taken into account—diet counseling and educational handouts can be geared to individual and ethnic preferences—and the family should be involved in the dietary education.

interventions such as implantation of an ICD can also provoke anxiety in patients and families. These sources of anxiety include living with the threat of shocks, role changes, and concerns about the patient's ability to carry out activities of daily living (Van Den Broek, Habibovic, & Pedersen, 2010). The patient's anxiety may intensify at night and interfere with sleep. Emotional stress also stimulates the sympathetic nervous system, causing vasoconstriction, elevated arterial pressure, and increased heart rate. This sympathetic response increases cardiac workload.

When the patient exhibits anxiety, the nurse takes steps to promote physical comfort and provide psychological support. As mentioned previously, the patient may be more comfortable sitting in a recliner. Oxygen may be administered during an acute event to diminish the work of breathing and increase the patient's comfort. In many cases, a family member's presence provides reassurance. Patients with HF rely on their families for many aspects of care; therefore, nurses should assess the needs of family caregivers and provide support to them (Hwang, Fleischmann, Howie-Esquivel, et al., 2011).

Along with reassurance, the nurse can begin educating the patient and family about techniques for controlling anxiety and avoiding anxiety-provoking situations. This includes how to identify factors that contribute to anxiety and how to use relaxation techniques to control anxious feelings. As the patient's anxiety decreases, cardiac function may improve and symptoms of HF may decrease, with overall feelings of relaxation.

> ### ▶ Quality and Safety Nursing Alert
>
> When patients with HF are delirious, confused, or anxious, restraints should be avoided. Restraints are likely to be resisted, and resistance inevitably increases the cardiac workload.

Minimizing Powerlessness

Patients with HF may feel overwhelmed with their diagnosis and treatment regimen, leading to feelings of powerlessness. Contributing factors may include lack of knowledge and lack of opportunity to make decisions, particularly if health care providers or family members do not encourage the patient to participate in the treatment decision-making process.

Nurses should help patients recognize their choices, and that they can positively influence the outcomes of their diagnosis and treatment. Taking time to listen actively to patients encourages them to express their concerns and ask questions. Other strategies include providing the patient with decision-making opportunities, such as when activities are to occur, or encouraging food and fluid choices consistent with the dietary restrictions. Encouragement is provided, progress is identified, and the patient is assisted to differentiate between factors that can and cannot be controlled.

In addition to feelings of powerlessness, patients with HF have a high incidence of depressive symptoms, which are associated with increased morbidity and mortality (Pressler et al., 2011). Because these depressive symptoms are known to increase as the disease worsens, patients with HF need to be screened for depression so that it can be treated, hopefully maintaining the patient's functional status and quality of life.

Assisting Patients and Family to Effectively Manage the Therapeutic Regimen

Therapeutic regimens for HF are complex and require the patient and family to make significant lifestyle changes. Inability to adhere to dietary and pharmacologic recommendations leads to episodes of acute decompensated HF and hospitalization. Nonadherence with prescribed diet and fluid restrictions and medications cause many hospital readmissions.

A number of programs and interventions are available to assist patients and families to effectively manage the HF regimen and to prevent hospitalizations and the associated increased costs and decreased quality of life. These efforts begin with effective patient and family education, which focuses on the importance of medications. Following hospital discharge, patients should see their provider within a week (Hernandez et al., 2010). At the follow-up visit, the patient's response to the HF regimen is assessed and adjusted. Education is also reinforced.

Patients with HF benefit from disease management programs and coordination of care. Nurses are an important part of the various types of outpatient management programs available for HF patients (see later discussion in the Continuing Care section).

Monitoring and Managing Potential Complications

Because HF is a complex and progressive condition, patients are at risk for many complications, including acute decompensated HF, pulmonary edema, renal failure, and life-threatening dysrhythmias. Many potential problems associated with HF therapy relate to the use of diuretics. These problems require ongoing nursing assessment and collaborative intervention:

- Excessive and repeated diuresis can lead to hypokalemia (i.e., potassium depletion). Signs include ventricular dysrhythmias, hypotension, muscle weakness, and generalized weakness. In patients receiving digoxin, hypokalemia can lead to digitalis toxicity, which increases the likelihood of dangerous dysrhythmias. Patients with HF may also develop low levels of magnesium, which can add to the risk of dysrhythmias.
- Hyperkalemia may occur, especially with the use of ACE inhibitors, ARBs, or spironolactone. Hyperkalemia can also lead to profound bradycardia and other dysrhythmias.
- Prolonged diuretic therapy may produce hyponatremia (deficiency of sodium in the blood), which can result in disorientation, weakness, muscle cramps, anorexia, and abdominal discomfort.
- Volume depletion from excessive fluid loss may lead to dehydration and hypotension. ACE inhibitors and beta-blockers may contribute to the hypotension.
- Other problems associated with diuretics include increased serum creatinine (indicative of renal dysfunction) and hyperuricemia (excessive uric acid in the blood), which leads to gout.

Promoting Home and Community-Based Care

Educating Patients About Self-Care. The nurse provides patient education and involves the patient and family in the therapeutic regimen to promote understanding and adherence to the plan. When the patient recognizes that the diagnosis of HF can be successfully managed with lifestyle changes and medications, recurrences of acute HF lessen, unnecessary hospitalizations decrease, and life expectancy increases. The Joint Commission and other agencies have established standards pertaining to the education of patients with HF. Nurses play a key role in instructing patients and their families about medication management, a low-sodium diet, moderate alcohol consumption, activity and exercise recommendations, smoking cessation, how to recognize the signs and symptoms of worsening HF, and when to contact a health care provider (ICSI, 2011). Although nonadherence continues be a challenge in this patient population, interventions that promote adherence include educating the patient and family about effectively managing HF. A basic home education plan for the patient with HF is presented in Chart 29-6. The patient should receive a written copy of the instructions.

The patient's readiness to learn and potential barriers to learning are assessed. Patients with HF may have temporary or ongoing cognitive impairment due to their illness or other factors, increasing the need to rely on family members

(Pressler, Gradus-Pizlo, Chubinski, et al., 2009). An effective treatment plan incorporates both the patient's goals and those of the health care providers. The nurse must consider cultural factors and adapt the education plan accordingly. Patients and families need to be aware of treatment choices and the possible outcomes of specific therapies. They need to understand that effective HF management is influenced by choices made about treatment options and their ability to follow the treatment plan. They also need to be informed that health care providers are available to assist them in reaching their health care goals.

Continuing Care. Successful management of HF requires adherence to a complex medical regimen that includes multiple lifestyle changes for most patients. Assistance may be provided through a number of options that optimize evidence-based recommendations for effective management of HF. These options include home health care services, transitional care programs, HF clinics, and tele-health management programs. Transitional care programs led by advanced practice nurses significantly reduce readmission rates for HF

Chart 29-6 — HOME CARE CHECKLIST
The Patient With Heart Failure

At the completion of home care education, the patient or caregiver will be able to:	PATIENT	CAREGIVER
• Identify heart failure as a chronic disease that can be managed with medications and specific self-management behaviors.	✔	✔
• Take or administer medications daily, exactly as prescribed.	✔	✔
• Monitor effects of medication such as changes in breathing and edema.	✔	✔
• Know signs and symptoms of orthostatic hypotension and how to prevent it.	✔	✔
• Weigh self daily at the same time with same clothes.	✔	
• Restrict sodium intake to no more than 2 g/day: Adapt diet by examining nutrition labels to check sodium content per serving, avoiding canned or processed foods, eating fresh or frozen foods, consulting the written diet plan and the list of permitted and restricted foods, avoiding salt use, and avoiding excesses in eating and drinking.	✔	✔
• Participate in prescribed activity program. • Participate in a daily exercise program. • Increase walking and other activities gradually, provided they do not cause unusual fatigue or dyspnea. • Conserve energy by balancing activity with rest periods. • Avoid activity in extremes of heat and cold, which increase the work of the heart. • Recognize that air-conditioning may be essential in a hot, humid environment.	✔	
• Develop methods to manage and prevent stress. • Avoid tobacco. • Avoid alcohol. • Engage in social and diversional activities.	✔	
• Keep regular appointments with physician or clinic.	✔	✔
• Be alert for symptoms that may indicate recurring heart failure. • Know how to contact primary provider.	✔	✔
• Report immediately to the primary provider or clinic any of the following: • Gain in weight of 2–3 lb (0.9–1.4 kg) in 1 day, or 5 lb (2.3 kg) in 1 week • Unusual shortness of breath with activity or at rest • Increased swelling of ankles, feet, or abdomen • Persistent cough • Loss of appetite • Development of restless sleep; increase in number of pillows needed to sleep • Profound fatigue	✔	✔

patients (Stauffer, Fullerton, Fleming, et al., 2011). Patients meet with an advanced practice nurse before discharge and then receive home visits to assist them with management of their HF.

Depending on the patient's physical status and the availability of family assistance, a home care referral may be indicated for a patient who has been hospitalized. Home visits by trained HF nurses provide assessment and management tailored to specific individualized patient needs. Older patients and those who have long-standing heart disease with compromised physical stamina often require assistance with the transition to home after hospitalization for an acute episode of HF. The home care nurse assesses the physical environment of the home and makes suggestions for adapting the home environment to meet the patient's activity limitations. If stairs are a concern, the patient can plan the day's activities so that stair-climbing is minimized; for some patients, a temporary bedroom may be set up on the main level of the home. The home care nurse works with the patient and family to maximize the benefits of these changes.

The home care nurse also reinforces and clarifies information about dietary changes and fluid restrictions, the need to monitor symptoms and daily body weight, and the importance of obtaining follow-up care with the primary provider's office or clinic. Assistance may be given in scheduling and keeping appointments as well. The patient is encouraged to gradually increase his or her self-care and responsibility for carrying out the therapeutic regimen. Assistance from home health nurses can result in fewer exacerbations of HF, lower costs, and improved quality of life.

Disease management programs are important components in the successful management of HF. ICSI guidelines (2011) recommend patient referral to HF clinics, which provide intensive nursing management along with medical care in a collaborative model. Many of these clinics are managed by advanced practice nurses. Referral to a HF clinic gives the patient ready access to continuing education, professional nursing and medical staff, and timely adjustments to treatment regimens. HF clinics can also provide outpatient treatment (e.g., IV diuretics, laboratory monitoring) as an alternative to hospitalization. Because of the additional support and coordination of care, patients managed through HF clinics have fewer exacerbations of HF, fewer hospitalizations, decreased costs of medical care, and increased quality of life (Jessup et al., 2009).

Other disease management programs are carried out through telemonitoring, using telephones or computers to maintain contact with patients and to obtain patient data. This enables nurses and others to assess and manage patients on a frequent basis, without requiring patients to make frequent visits to health care providers. A variety of techniques ranging from simple telephone monitoring to sophisticated computer and video connections that monitor symptoms, daily weight, vital signs, heart sounds, and breath sounds may be used. Patient data may also include hemodynamics and other parameters transmitted from implantable devices. Studies have shown that tele-health management can decrease costs and hospitalizations for exacerbations of HF (Klersy, De Silvestri, Gabutti, et al., 2011). More research is needed to determine which patients can benefit most

from these interventions (Koehler, Winkler, Schieber, et al., 2011).

End-of-Life Considerations. Because HF is a chronic and often progressive condition, patients and families need to consider issues related to the end of life. Although the prognosis in HF patients may be uncertain, issues often arise sooner or later related to the patient's thoughts and possible concerns about the use of complex treatment options (e.g., ultrafiltration for fluid overload, implantation of a ventricular assist device). Discussions concerning the use of technology, preferences for end-of-life care, and advance directives should take place while the patient is able to participate and express preferences (Jessup et al., 2009). For example, with the expanded use of ICDs in the HF population, patients with ICDs, their families, and their primary providers should receive instructions for ICD inactivation at the end of life to prevent inappropriate discharges (Goldstein, Carlson, Livote, et al., 2010). (See Chapter 16 for further discussion of end-of-life care.)

Evaluation

Expected patient outcomes may include:

1. Demonstrates tolerance for desired activity
   a. Describes adaptive methods for usual activities
   b. Schedules activities to conserve energy and reduce fatigue and dyspnea
   c. Maintains heart rate, blood pressure, respiratory rate, and pulse oximetry within the targeted range
2. Maintains fluid balance
   a. Exhibits decreased peripheral edema
   b. Verbalizes understanding of fluid intake and diuretic use
3. Decreased anxiety
   a. Avoids situations that produce stress
   b. Sleeps comfortably at night
   c. Reports decreased stress and anxiety
   d. Denies symptoms of depression
4. Makes sound decisions regarding care and treatment
   a. Demonstrates ability to influence outcomes
5. Patients and family members adhere to therapeutic regimen
   a. Performs and records daily weights
   b. Limits dietary sodium intake to no more than 2 g/day
   c. Takes medications as prescribed
   d. Reports symptoms of worsening HF
   e. Makes and keeps appointments for follow-up care

  Concept Mastery Alert

For further review, visit thePoint to view an interactive tutorial on HF.

 ## Pulmonary Edema

Pulmonary edema is the abnormal accumulation of fluid in the interstitial spaces and alveoli of the lungs. It is a diagnosis associated with acute decompensated HF that can lead to acute respiratory failure and death.

Pathophysiology

Pulmonary edema is an acute event that results from left ventricular failure. It can occur following acute MI or as an exacerbation of chronic HF. When the left ventricle begins to fail, blood backs up into the pulmonary circulation, causing pulmonary interstitial edema. This may occur quickly in some patients, a condition sometimes called *flash pulmonary edema*. Pulmonary edema can also develop slowly, especially when it is caused by noncardiac disorders such as renal failure and other conditions that cause fluid overload. The pathophysiology is an extreme form of that seen in left-sided HF. The left ventricle cannot handle the volume overload, and blood volume and pressure build up in the left atrium. The rapid increase in atrial pressure results in an acute increase in pulmonary venous pressure, which produces an increase in hydrostatic pressure that forces fluid out of the pulmonary capillaries and into the interstitial spaces and alveoli. Lymphatic drainage of the excess fluid is ineffective.

The fluid within the alveoli mixes with air, producing the classic sign of pulmonary edema—frothy pink (blood-tinged) sputum. The large amounts of alveolar fluid create a diffusion block that severely impairs gas exchange. The result is hypoxemia, which is often severe.

Clinical Manifestations

As a result of decreased cerebral oxygenation, the patient becomes increasingly restless and anxious. Along with a sudden onset of breathlessness and a sense of suffocation, the patient is tachypneic with noisy breathing and low oxygen saturation rates. The skin and mucous membranes may be pale to cyanotic, and the hands may be cool and moist. Tachycardia and JVD are common signs. Incessant coughing may occur, producing increasing quantities of foamy sputum. As pulmonary edema progresses, the patient's anxiety and restlessness increase. The patient may become confused and then stuporous. The patient, nearly suffocated by the blood-tinged, frothy fluid filling the alveoli, is literally drowning in secretions. The situation demands emergent action.

Assessment and Diagnostic Findings

The patient's airway and breathing are assessed to determine the severity of respiratory distress, along with vital signs. The patient is placed on a cardiac monitor, and IV access is confirmed or established for administration of drugs. Laboratory tests are obtained, including electrolytes, BUN and creatinine, and CBC (ICSI, 2011). A chest x-ray is obtained to confirm the extent of pulmonary edema in the lung fields. Abrupt onset of signs of left-sided HF and pulmonary edema may occur without evidence of right-sided HF (e.g., no JVD, no dependent edema).

Prevention

Like many emergent conditions, pulmonary edema is easier to prevent than to treat. To recognize it early, the nurse assesses the degree of dyspnea, auscultates the lung fields and heart sounds, and assesses the degree of peripheral edema. A hacking cough, fatigue, weight gain, development or worsening of edema, and decreased activity tolerance may be early indicators of developing pulmonary edema.

In its early stage, pulmonary edema may be alleviated by increasing dosages of diuretics and by implementing other interventions to decrease preload. For instance, placing the patient in an upright position with the feet and legs dependent reduces left ventricular workload. The treatment regimen and the patient's understanding of and adherence to it are assessed. The long-range approach to preventing pulmonary edema must be directed at identifying and managing its precipitating factors.

Medical Management

Clinical management of a patient with acute pulmonary edema due to left ventricular failure is directed toward reducing volume overload, improving ventricular function, and increasing oxygenation. These goals are accomplished through a combination of oxygen and ventilatory support, IV medication, and nursing assessment and interventions.

Oxygen Therapy

Oxygen is administered in concentrations adequate to relieve hypoxemia and dyspnea. A nonrebreathing mask is used initially. If respiratory failure is severe or persists, noninvasive positive pressure ventilation is the preferred mode of assisted ventilation (Colucci, 2011) (see Chapter 21 for further discussion). For some patients, endotracheal intubation and mechanical ventilation are required. The ventilator can provide positive end-expiratory pressure, which is effective in reducing venous return, decreasing fluid movement from the pulmonary capillaries to the alveoli, and improving oxygenation. Oxygenation is monitored by pulse oximetry and by measurement of arterial blood gases.

Diuretics

Diuretics promote the excretion of sodium and water by the kidneys. Furosemide or another loop diuretic is administered by IV push or as a continuous infusion to produce a rapid diuretic effect. The blood pressure is closely monitored as the urine output increases, because it is possible for the patient to become hypotensive as intravascular volume decreases. The intake and output, daily weights, serum electrolytes, and creatinine are carefully monitored. As the clinical manifestations stabilize, the patient is transitioned to oral diuretics.

Vasodilators

Vasodilators such as IV nitroglycerin or nitroprusside may enhance symptom relief in pulmonary edema (Colucci, 2011). Their use is contraindicated in patients who are hypotensive. Blood pressure is continually assessed in patients receiving IV vasodilator infusions. In the past, morphine was recommended as part of treatment protocols for pulmonary edema because it produced vasodilating effects, reduced patient anxiety, and decreased the work of breathing. However, because its use is associated with increased need for mechanical ventilation, longer hospitalization, and increased mortality, it is no longer recommended (Colucci, 2011).

Nursing Management

Positioning the Patient to Promote Circulation

Proper positioning can help reduce venous return to the heart. The patient is positioned upright, preferably with the legs dangling over the side of the bed. This has the immediate effect of decreasing venous return, decreasing right ventricular SV, and decreasing lung congestion.

Providing Psychological Support

As the ability to breathe decreases, the patient's fear and anxiety rise proportionately, making the condition more severe. Reassuring the patient and providing skillful anticipatory nursing care are integral parts of the therapy. Because the patient is in an unstable condition, the nurse must remain with the patient. The nurse gives the patient simple, concise information in a reassuring voice about what is being done to treat the condition and the expected results.

Monitoring Medications

The patient receiving diuretic therapy may excrete a large volume of urine within minutes after a potent diuretic is administered. A bedside commode may be used to decrease the energy required by the patient and to reduce the resultant increase in cardiac workload induced by getting on and off a bedpan. If necessary, in order to carefully monitor urine output, an indwelling urinary catheter may be inserted.

The patient receiving continuous IV infusions of diuretics and vasoactive medications requires continuous ECG monitoring and frequent measurement of vital signs. Patients who receive continuing therapy require management in an ICU.

OTHER COMPLICATIONS

Cardiogenic Shock

Cardiogenic shock occurs when decreased CO leads to inadequate tissue perfusion and initiation of the shock syndrome. Cardiogenic shock may occur following MI when a large area of myocardium becomes ischemic and hypokinetic. It also can occur as a result of end-stage HF, cardiac tamponade, pulmonary embolism (PE), cardiomyopathy, and dysrhythmias. Cardiogenic shock is a life-threatening condition with a high mortality rate. (See Chapter 14 for detailed information about the pathophysiology and management of cardiogenic shock.)

Medical Management

Goals in the treatment of cardiogenic shock include correcting the underlying problem when possible (e.g., opening the blocked coronary artery), reducing preload and afterload to decrease cardiac workload, improving oxygenation, and restoring tissue perfusion. In addition to standard critical care support with ventilatory and pharmacologic interventions, patients may require mechanical circulatory assistance.

Mechanical Circulatory Assistive Devices

Therapeutic modalities for cardiogenic shock include the use of circulatory assist devices, such as the intra-aortic balloon pump (IABP). The IABP is a catheter with an inflatable balloon at the end. The catheter is usually inserted through the femoral artery and threaded toward the heart, and the balloon is positioned in the descending thoracic aorta (Fig. 29-4). The IABP uses internal counterpulsation through the regular

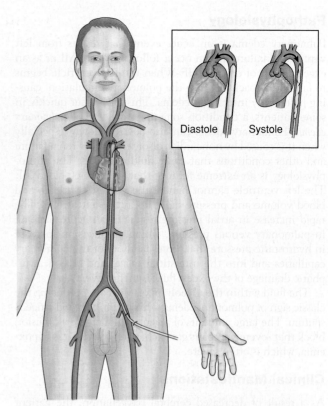

FIGURE 29-4 • The intra-aortic balloon pump inflates at the beginning of diastole, which results in increased perfusion of the coronary and peripheral arteries. It deflates just before systole, which results in a decrease in afterload (resistance to ejection) and in the left ventricular workload.

inflation and deflation of the balloon to augment the pumping action of the heart. It inflates during diastole, increasing the pressure in the aorta during diastole and therefore increasing blood flow through the coronary and peripheral arteries. It deflates just before systole, lessening the pressure within the aorta before left ventricular contraction, decreasing the amount of resistance the heart has to overcome to eject blood and therefore decreasing left ventricular workload. The device is connected to a console that synchronizes the inflation and deflation of the balloon with the ECG or the arterial pressure (as indicators for systole and diastole). Hemodynamic monitoring is often used to determine the patient's response to the IABP.

The IABP provides short-term (days) support for the failing myocardium. Other ventricular assist devices for long-term support of the failing heart are described in Chapter 28.

Nursing Management

The patient in cardiogenic shock requires constant monitoring. Because of the frequency of nursing interventions and the technology required for safe and effective patient management, the patient is treated in an ICU. The critical care nurse must carefully assess the patient, observe the cardiac rhythm, monitor hemodynamic parameters, monitor fluid status, and adjust medications and therapies based on the assessment data. The patient is continuously evaluated for responses to the medical interventions and for the development of complications so that problems can be addressed immediately.

Thromboembolism

Patients with cardiovascular disorders are at risk for the development of arterial and venous thromboemboli. Intracardiac thrombi can form in patients with atrial fibrillation because the atria do not contract forcefully, resulting in slow and turbulent flow, and increasing the likelihood of thrombus formation. Mural thrombi can also form on ventricular walls when contractility is poor. Intracardiac thrombi can break off and travel through the circulation to other structures, including the brain, where they cause a stroke (i.e., cerebrovascular accident). Clots within the cardiac chambers can be detected by an echocardiogram and treated with anticoagulant agents, such as heparin and warfarin (Coumadin).

Decreased mobility and other factors in patients with cardiac disease also can lead to clot formation in the deep veins of the legs. Although signs and symptoms of deep vein thrombosis (DVT) can vary, patients may report leg pain and swelling. These clots can also break off and travel through the inferior vena cava and through the right side of the heart into the pulmonary artery, where they can cause a pulmonary embolus.

Pulmonary Embolism

PE is a potentially life-threatening disorder typically caused by blood clots in the lungs. This disorder poses a particular threat to people with cardiovascular disease (Lindenfeld, et al., 2010). Blood clots that form in the deep veins of the legs and embolize to the lungs can cause a pulmonary infarction where emboli mechanically obstruct the pulmonary vessels, cutting off the blood supply to sections of the lung (Fig. 29-5).

Clinical indicators of PE can vary but typically include dyspnea, pleuritic chest pain, and tachypnea. Other signs include cough, hemoptysis, tachycardia, and hemodynamic instability. Diagnostic tests often include a chest x-ray, ventilation–perfusion lung scan, high-resolution helical computed tomography, or computed tomographic pulmonary angiogram. A blood D-dimer assay is a helpful screening test that identifies whether clotting and fibrinolysis are taking place somewhere in the body.

Patient management begins with cardiopulmonary assessment and intervention. Emboli can cause hypoxic vasoconstriction and the release of inflammatory mediators in the pulmonary vessels, which can ultimately lead to right-sided HF and respiratory failure. Anticoagulant therapy with unfractionated heparin, low-molecular-weight heparin, or fondaparinux (Arixtra) is started when PE is suspected (Qaseem, Chou, Humphrey, et al., 2011). Thrombolytic therapy may be used in patients with massive pulmonary emboli accompanied by hypotension and shock. Following initial therapy, patients are placed on warfarin for at least 6 months. Prevention of DVT and PE is an important aspect of patient management. Pharmacologic interventions are preferred, but mechanical devices (e.g., pneumatic compression devices) are acceptable for patients with contraindications to anticoagulation (e.g., bleeding ulcer) (Qaseem et al., 2011). (Care for patients with PE is further discussed in Chapter 23.)

Pericardial Effusion and Cardiac Tamponade

Pathophysiology

Pericardial effusion (accumulation of fluid in the pericardial sac) may accompany advanced HF, pericarditis, metastatic carcinoma, cardiac surgery, or trauma. Normally, the pericardial sac contains about 20 mL of fluid, which is needed to decrease friction for the beating heart. An increase in pericardial fluid raises the pressure within the pericardial sac and compresses the heart. This has the following effects:

- Elevated pressure in all cardiac chambers
- Decreased venous return due to atrial compression
- Inability of the ventricles to distend and fill adequately

Pericardial fluid may build up slowly without causing noticeable symptoms until a large amount (1 to 2 L) accumulates (Hoit, 2011). However, a rapidly developing effusion (e.g., hemorrhage into the pericardial sac from chest trauma) can quickly stretch the pericardium to its maximum size and cause an acute problem. As pericardial fluid increases, pericardial pressure increases, reducing venous return to the heart and decreasing CO. This can result in cardiac tamponade, which causes low CO and shock.

Clinical Manifestations

The signs and symptoms of pericardial effusion can vary according to whether the problem develops quickly or slowly. In acute cardiac tamponade, the patient suddenly develops chest pain, tachypnea, and dyspnea. JVD results from poor right atrial filling and increased venous pressure. Hypotension occurs from low CO, and heart sounds are often muted. The subacute presentation of a pericardial effusion is less dramatic. The patient may report chest discomfort or a feeling of fullness. The feeling of pressure in the chest may result from stretching of the pericardial sac. These patients have fatigue and edema and also develop dyspnea, JVD, and hypotension over time (Hoit, 2011). Patients with cardiac tamponade typically have tachycardia in response to low CO. In addition to hypotension, patients with cardiac tamponade may develop **pulsus paradoxus**, a systolic blood pressure that is markedly lower during inhalation. Also known as paradoxical pulse, this finding is characterized by an abnormal difference of at least 10 mm Hg in systolic pressure between the point that it is heard during exhalation and the point that it is heard during inhalation. This difference is caused by the variation in cardiac filling that occurs with changes in intrathoracic

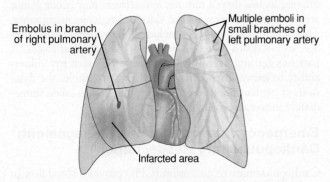

Embolus in branch of right pulmonary artery

Multiple emboli in small branches of left pulmonary artery

Infarcted area

FIGURE 29-5 • Pulmonary emboli may be single or multiple.

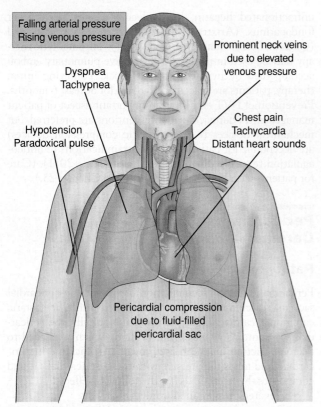

Falling arterial pressure
Rising venous pressure

Dyspnea
Tachypnea

Hypotension
Paradoxical pulse

Prominent neck veins
due to elevated
venous pressure

Chest pain
Tachycardia
Distant heart sounds

Pericardial compression
due to fluid-filled
pericardial sac

FIGURE 29-6 • Assessment findings in cardiac tamponade resulting from pericardial effusion include chest pain or fullness, dyspnea, tachypnea, jugular vein distention, hypotension, paradoxical pulse, tachycardia, and distant heart sounds.

pressure during breathing. The cardinal signs of cardiac tamponade are illustrated in Figure 29-6.

Assessment and Diagnostic Findings

An echocardiogram is performed to confirm the diagnosis and quantify the amount of pericardial fluid. A chest x-ray may show an enlarged cardiac silhouette due to pericardial effusion. The ECG shows tachycardia and may also show low voltage (Hoit, 2011). (See Chapter 27 for discussion of the significance of ECG diagnostics.)

Medical Management

Pericardiocentesis

If cardiac function becomes seriously impaired, **pericardiocentesis** (puncture of the pericardial sac to aspirate pericardial fluid) is performed. During this procedure, the patient is monitored by continuous ECG and frequent vital signs. Emergency resuscitation equipment should be available. The head of the bed is elevated to 45 to 60 degrees, placing the heart in proximity to the chest wall so that the needle can be directly inserted into the pericardial sac. If a peripheral IV line is not already in place, one is inserted, and a slow IV infusion is started in case emergency medications or blood products must be administered. Catheter pericardiocentesis is performed using echocardiography to guide placement of the drainage catheter.

A resulting decrease in central venous pressure and an associated increase in blood pressure after withdrawal of pericardial fluid indicate that the cardiac tamponade has been

relieved. The patient almost always feels immediate relief. If there is a substantial amount of pericardial fluid aspirated, a small catheter may be left in place to drain recurrent accumulation of blood or fluid. Pericardial fluid is sent to the laboratory for examination for tumor cells, bacterial culture, chemical and serologic analysis, and differential blood cell count.

Complications of pericardiocentesis include coronary artery puncture, myocardial trauma, dysrhythmias, pleural laceration, and gastric puncture. After pericardiocentesis, the patient's heart rhythm, blood pressure, venous pressure, and heart sounds are monitored frequently to detect possible recurrence of cardiac tamponade. A follow-up echocardiogram is also performed. If the effusion recurs, repeat aspiration is necessary. Cardiac tamponade may require treatment by open surgical drainage (pericardiotomy).

Pericardiotomy

Recurrent pericardial effusions, usually associated with neoplastic disease, may be treated by a **pericardiotomy** (pericardial window). Under general anesthesia, a portion of the pericardium is excised to permit the exudative pericardial fluid to drain into the lymphatic system. The nursing care following the procedure includes routine postsurgical care (see Chapter 19) in addition to observation for recurrent tamponade.

Cardiac Arrest

In cardiac arrest, the heart is unable to pump and circulate blood to the body's organs and tissues. It is often caused by a dysrhythmia such as ventricular fibrillation, progressive bradycardia, or asystole (i.e., absence of cardiac electrical activity and heart muscle contraction). Cardiac arrest can also occur when electrical activity is present on the ECG but cardiac contractions are ineffective, a condition called **pulseless electrical activity (PEA)**. PEA may be caused by a variety of problems such as profound hypovolemia (e.g., hemorrhage). Diagnoses that are associated with cardiac arrest include MI, massive pulmonary emboli, hyperkalemia, hypothermia, severe hypoxia, and medication overdose. Rapid identification of these problems and prompt intervention can restore circulation in some patients.

Clinical Manifestations

In cardiac arrest, consciousness, pulse, and blood pressure are lost immediately. Breathing usually ceases, but ineffective respiratory gasping may occur. The pupils of the eyes begin dilating in less than a minute, and seizures may occur. Pallor and cyanosis are seen in the skin and mucous membranes. The risk of organ damage, including irreversible brain damage, and of death increases with every minute that passes. A patient's age and overall health determine his or her vulnerability to irreversible damage. As soon as possible, the diagnosis of cardiac arrest must be made and action taken immediately to restore circulation.

Emergency Assessment and Management: Cardiopulmonary Resuscitation

Cardiopulmonary resuscitation (CPR) provides blood flow to vital organs until effective circulation can be reestablished.

Following the recognition of unresponsiveness, a protocol for basic life support is initiated. CPR was first taught in the 1960s; over time, resuscitation protocols have changed with the addition of new knowledge, research, and technology. The 2010 AHA Guidelines for Cardiopulmonary Resuscitation and Emergency Cardiovascular Care direct the current protocols (Field, Hazinski, Sayre, et al., 2010). The process begins with the immediate assessment of the patient and action to call for assistance, as CPR can be performed most effectively with the addition of more health care providers and equipment (e.g., defibrillator). The four basic steps in CPR are as follows:

1. *Recognition of sudden cardiac arrest*. The patient is checked for responsiveness and breathing.
2. *Activation of the Emergency Response System (ERS)*. Within a medical facility, a call is made to alert the emergency response team, often called the "Code 4" or "Code Blue" team. Outside of a medical facility, 911 is called to activate the Emergency Medical Service (EMS).
3. *Performance of high-quality CPR*. If no carotid pulse is detected and no defibrillator is yet available, chest compressions are initiated. Rescue breathing may be added by a health care provider in a ratio of 30 compressions to 2 ventilations.
4. *Rapid cardiac rhythm analysis and defibrillation as soon as it is available*. Patients in ventricular fibrillation must be defibrillated as soon as possible.

Outcomes following CPR are improved by high-quality CPR. Compressions are performed with the patient on a firm surface such as the floor or a cardiac board. The provider, facing the patient's side, places one hand in the center of the chest on the lower half of the sternum and positions the other hand on top of the first hand (Sinz & Navarro, 2011) (Fig. 29-7). The chest is compressed 2 inches at a rate of at least 100 compressions per minute. Complete recoil of the chest is allowed between compressions. Interruptions in CPR to switch providers or check for a pulse are minimized to less than 10 seconds. It is recommended that providers switch every 2 minutes due to the exertion of delivering effective compressions.

Maintaining Airway and Breathing

Rescue breathing is no longer recommended unless health care providers are present; if that is the case, it is then started after chest compressions. The airway is opened using a head-tilt/chin-lift maneuver, and any obvious material in the mouth or throat is removed. An oropharyngeal airway may be inserted if available to help maintain patency of the airway. Rescue ventilations are provided using a bag-valve mask or mouth-mask device. Oxygen is administered at 100% during resuscitation to correct hypoxemia and improve tissue oxygenation. Excessive ventilation is avoided by the 30 to 2 ratio of compressions to ventilations (Sinz & Navarro, 2011).

Defibrillation

As soon as a monitor/defibrillator is available, monitor electrodes are applied to the patient's chest and the heart rhythm is analyzed. When an automated external defibrillator (AED) is used, the device is turned on, the pads are applied to the patient's chest, and the rhythm is analyzed by the defibrillator

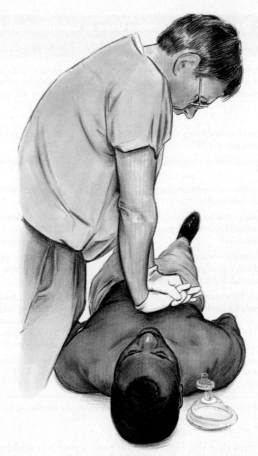

FIGURE 29-7 • Chest compressions in cardiopulmonary resuscitation are performed by placing the heel of one hand in the center of the chest over the sternum and the other hand on top of the first hand. Elbows are kept straight and body weight is used to apply forceful compressions to the lower sternum. The patient should be on a hard surface such as a cardiac board. From Field, Kudenchuk, P. J., O'Connor, R., et al. (2009). *The textbook of emergency cardiovascular care and CPR*. Philadelphia: Lippincott Williams & Wilkins.

to determine whether a shock is indicated. When the ECG shows ventricular fibrillation or pulseless ventricular tachycardia, immediate defibrillation is the treatment of choice. The survival time decreases for every minute that defibrillation is delayed (Field et al., 2010). Following defibrillation, high-quality CPR is resumed immediately. Survival after cardiac arrest has been improved by extensive education of health care providers and by the use of AEDs (Sinz & Navarro, 2011).

Advanced Cardiovascular Life Support

Additional care may be indicated for patients in cardiac arrest. Placement of an advanced airway such as an endotracheal (ET) tube may be performed by a physician, nurse anesthetist, or respiratory therapist during resuscitation to ensure a patent airway and adequate ventilation. Because of the risk of unrecognized esophageal intubation or dislodgement of the ET tube, tracheal intubation must be confirmed by assessment of specific parameters: auscultation of breath sounds, observation of chest expansion, and a carbon dioxide detector. A chest x-ray is always obtained after ET tube placement

TABLE 29-4   Medications Used in Cardiopulmonary Resuscitation

Agent and Action	Indications	Nursing Considerations
Epinephrine—vasopressor used to optimize BP and cardiac output; improves perfusion and myocardial contractility	Given to patients in cardiac arrest caused by asystole, pulseless electrical activity, pulseless VT or VF	• Administer 1 mg every 3–5 minutes by IV push or via IO route. • Follow peripheral IV administration with 20-mL flush and elevate extremity for 10–20 seconds.
Vasopressin—increases systemic vascular resistance and BP	An alternative to epinephrine	• Give 40 U IV one time only.
Norepinephrine—vasopressor given to increase BP	Given for hypotension and shock	• Give 0.1–0.5 mcg/kg/min as IV infusion, preferably through a central line.
Dopamine—vasopressor given to increase BP and contractility	Given for hypotension and shock	• Give 5–10 mcg/kg/min as IV infusion, preferably through a central line.
Atropine—blocks parasympathetic action; increases SA node automaticity and AV conduction	Given to patients with symptomatic bradycardia (i.e., hemodynamically unstable with hypotension)	• Give rapidly as 0.5-mg IV push; may repeat to dose of 3 mg.
Amiodarone—acts on sodium–potassium and calcium channels to prolong action potential and refractory period	Used to treat pulseless VT and VF unresponsive to shock delivery	• Give 300 mg IV; may give second dose of 150 mg in 3–5 minutes.
Sodium bicarbonate ($NaHCO_3$)—corrects metabolic acidosis	Given to correct metabolic acidosis that is refractory to standard advanced cardiac life support interventions (cardiopulmonary resuscitation, intubation, and respiratory management)	• Administer initial dose of 1 mEq/kg IV; then administer dose based on base deficit. • Recognize that to prevent development of rebound metabolic alkalosis, complete correction of acidosis is not indicated.
Magnesium sulfate—promotes adequate functioning of cellular sodium–potassium pump	Given to patients with torsade de pointes, a type of VT	• May give 1–2 g diluted in 10 mL D_5W over 5–20 minutes

BP, blood pressure; VT, ventricular tachycardia; VF, ventricular fibrillation; IV, intravenous; IO, intraosseous; SA, sinoatrial; AV, atrioventricular; D_5W, dextrose 5% in water.

to confirm that the tube is in the proper position within the trachea. Arterial blood gases may also be obtained to assess ventilation and oxygenation.

Specific subsequent advanced support interventions depend on the assessment of the patient's condition and response to therapy. For example, if asystole is detected on the monitor, CPR is continued while IV epinephrine is given and an attempt is made to determine the cause of the arrest, such as severe hypovolemia or hypoxia. Additional medications (Table 29-4) may be indicated for the patient during and after resuscitation.

CPR may be stopped when a pulse and blood pressure are detected, respirations are detected, and the patient responds. CPR efforts may also be stopped when rescuers are exhausted or at risk (e.g., a building is at risk of collapsing), or death is considered to be inevitable. If the patient does not respond to therapies given during the arrest, the resuscitation effort may be stopped by the physician or other provider in charge of the resuscitation. Many factors are considered in the decision, such as the initiating dysrhythmia, potential etiology, length of time for initiation of life support, and the patient's response to treatment.

Follow-Up Monitoring and Care

The care provided to the patient following resuscitation is another determinant of survival. The patient may be transferred to a critical care unit for close monitoring. Continuous ECG monitoring and frequent blood pressure assessments are essential until hemodynamic stability is established. Factors that precipitated the arrest such as dysrhythmias or electrolyte or metabolic imbalances are identified and treated.

Following resuscitation and return of spontaneous circulation, patients who are comatose may benefit from therapeutic hypothermia protocols. These induce a drop in core body temperature to 32°C to 34°C (89.6°F to 93.2°F) for 12 to 24 hours postresuscitation in order to decrease the cerebral metabolic rate and need for oxygen (Sinz & Navarro, 2011). Specific protocols have been developed to guide the use of both external cooling and catheter-based cooling methods and reduce associated complications such as shivering (Logan, Sangkachand, & Funk, 2011).

Advances in cardiac care, such as new techniques for effective resuscitation and postresuscitation hypothermia, have improved outcomes for patients with potentially lethal cardiac disorders, including those with cardiac arrest. Studies have demonstrated better neurologic recovery and overall survival for patients after cardiac arrest, and hope for even better outcomes in the future (Sinz & Navarro, 2011).

Critical Thinking Exercises

1 You are caring for a 78-year-old man who has just been diagnosed with HF. He is asking for more information about his diagnosis and how to manage his condition. How will you define *heart failure*? What does the diagnosis mean for his future health and need for health care? Knowing that changes in medications, diet, and activity will be recommended, what is your plan for educating this patient so that he can optimally managing his disease?

2 **ebp** Your patient is a 55-year-old woman with dilated cardiomyopathy who is hospitalized with acute decompensated HF. Based on your knowledge of evidence-based practice guidelines, list some important pharmacologic and other interventions appropriate for her. Identify the key physical assessment and laboratory parameters that you will need to monitor. Describe evidence-based HF management programs that might improve her functional status and quality of life following discharge.

3 **PQ** Your patient is a 65-year-old man who had a colon resection 3 days ago. At about 2 am, he complains of shortness of breath and pain on inspiration. Describe how you will assess the patient. What are your priority interventions? What diagnostic tests would you expect the medical team to order?

Brunner Suite Resources

Explore these additional resources to enhance learning for this chapter:
• NCLEX-Style Questions and Other Resources on thePoint, http://thePoint.lww.com/Brunner13e
• Study Guide
• PrepU
• Clinical Handbook
• Handbook of Laboratory and Diagnostic Tests

References

*Asterisk indicates nursing research.

Books

Aschenbrenner, D. S., & Venable, S. J. (2012). *Drug therapy in nursing* (4th ed.). Philadelphia: Wolters Kluwer.

Bickley, L. S., & Szilagyi, P. G. (2009). *Bates' guide to physical examination and history taking* (10th ed.). Philadelphia: Lippincott Williams & Wilkins.

Doenges, M. E., Moorhouse, M. F., & Murr, A. C. (2010). *Nursing care plans. Guidelines for individualizing client care across the life span* (8th ed.). Philadelphia: F. A. Davis.

McCance, K. L., Huether, S. E., Brashers, V. L., et al. (2010). *Pathophysiology. The biologic basis for disease in adults and children* (6th ed.). Maryland Heights, MO: Mosby Elsevier.

Porth, C. M. (2011). *Essentials of pathophysiology* (3rd ed.). Philadelphia: Wolters Kluwer.

Sinz, E., & Navarro, K. (2011). *Advanced cardiovascular life support provider manual.* Dallas: American Heart Association.

Urden, L. D., Stacy, K. M., & Lough, M. E. (2010). *Critical care nursing* (6th ed.). St. Louis: Mosby Elsevier.

Journals and Electronic Documents

*Albert, N., Trochelman, K., Li, J., et al. (2010). Signs and symptoms of heart failure: Are you asking the right questions? *American Journal of Critical Care, 19*(5), 443–453.

Colucci, W. S. (2011). *Treatment of acute decompensated heart failure: Components of therapy.* Available at: www.uptodate.com/contents/treatment-of-acute-decompensated-heart-failure-components-of-therapy?source=search_result&search=acute+decompensated+heart+failure&selectedTitle=1%7E150

Damman, K., Voors, A. A., Navis, G., et al. (2011). The cardiorenal syndrome in heart failure. *Progress in Cardiovascular Diseases, 54*(3), 144–153.

Downing, J., & Balady, G. J. (2011). The role of exercise training in heart failure. *Journal of the American College of Cardiology, 58*(6), 561–569.

Fiaccadori, E., Regolisti, G., Maggiore, U., et al. (2011). Ultrafiltration in heart failure. *American Heart Journal, 161*(3), 439–449.

Field, J. M., Hazinski, M. F., Sayre, M. R., et al. (2010). Executive summary: 2010 American Heart Association guidelines for cardiopulmonary

resuscitation and emergency cardiovascular care. *Circulation, 122*(18), S640–S656.

Fonarow, G. C., Albert, N. M., Curtis, A. B., et al. (2010). Improving evidence-based care for heart failure in outpatient cardiology practices: Primary results of the Registry to Improve the Use of Evidence-Based Heart Failure Therapies in the Outpatient Setting (IMPROVE HF). *Circulation, 122*(6), 585–596.

Goldenberg, I., Hall, W. J., Beck, C. A., et al. (2011). Reduction of the risk of recurring heart failure events with cardiac resynchronization therapy. MADIT-CRT (Multicenter Automatic Defibrillator Implantation Trial with Cardiac Resynchronization Therapy). *Journal of the American College of Cardiology, 58*(7), 738–739.

Goldstein, N., Carlson, M., Livote, E., et al. (2010). Management of implantable cardioverter-defibrillators in hospice: A nationwide survey. *Annals of Internal Medicine, 152*(5), 296–299.

Hernandez, A. F., Greiner, M. A., Fonarow, G. C., et al. (2010). Relationship between early physician follow-up and 30-day readmission among Medicare beneficiaries hospitalized for heart failure. *Journal of the American Medical Association, 303*(17), 1716–1722.

Hoit, B. D. (2011). *Cardiac tamponade.* Available at: www.uptodate.com/contents/cardiac-tamponade?source=search_result&search=cardiac+tamponade&selectedTitle=1%7E140

*Hwang, B., Fleischmann, K. E., Howie-Esquivel, J., et al. (2011). Caregiving for patients with heart failure: Impact on patients' families. *American Journal of Critical Care, 20*(6), 431–442.

Institute for Clinical Systems Improvement. (2011). *Heart failure in adults.* Available at: www.guideline.gov/content.aspx?id=34840&search=heart+failure

Jessup, M., Abraham, W. T., Casey, D. E., et al. (2009). 2009 focused update: ACCF/AHA guidelines for the diagnosis and management of heart failure in adults: A report of the American College of Cardiology Foundation/American Heart Association Task Force on Practice Guidelines. *Circulation, 119*(14), 1977–2016.

Klersy, C., De Silvestri, A., Gabutti, G., et al. (2011). Economic impact of remote patient monitoring: An integrated economic model derived from a meta-analysis of randomized controlled trials in heart failure. *European Journal of Heart Failure, 13*(4), 450–459.

Koehler, F., Winkler, S., Schieber, M., et al. (2011). Impact of remote telemedical management on mortality and hospitalizations in ambulatory patients with chronic heart failure. *Circulation, 123*(17), 1873–1880.

Lindenfeld, J., Albert, N. M., Boehmer, J. P., et al. (2010). Evaluation and management of patients with acute decompensated heart failure: HFSA 2010 comprehensive heart failure practice guidelines. *Journal of Cardiac Failure, 16*(6), e134–e156. Available at: www.guidelines.gov/content.aspx?id=23908&search=heart+failure

Logan, A., Sangkachand, P., & Funk, M. (2011). Optimal management of shivering during therapeutic hypothermia after cardiac arrest. *Critical Care Nurse, 31*(6), e18–e30. Available at: http://ccn.aacnjournals.org/content/31/6/e18.full

Metra, M., Bettari, L., Carubelli, V., et al. (2011). Old and new intravenous inotropic agents in the treatment of advanced heart failure. *Progress in Cardiovascular Diseases, 54*(2), 97–106.

Norton, C., Georgiopoulou, V. V., Kalogeropoulos, A. P., et al. (2011). Epidemiology and cost of advanced heart failure. *Progress in Cardiovascular Diseases, 54*(2), 78–85.

*Pressler, S. J., Gradus-Pizlo, I., Chubinski, S. D., et al. (2009). Family caregiver outcomes in heart failure. *American Journal of Critical Care, 18*(2), 149–159.

*Pressler, S. J., Subramanian, U., Perkins, S. M., et al. (2011). Measuring depressive symptoms in heart failure: Validity and reliability of the patient health questionnaire-8. *American Journal of Critical Care, 20*(2), 146–152.

Qaseen, A., Chou, R., Humphrey, L. L., et al. (2011). *Venous thromboembolism prophylaxis in hospitalized patients: A clinical practice guideline from the American College of Physicians.* Available at: guideline.gov/content.aspx?id=34969

Riegel, B., Dickson, V. V., Cameron, J., et al. (2011). Symptom recognition is older adults with heart failure. *Journal of Nursing Scholarship, 42*(1), 92–100.

Roger, V. L., Go, A. S., Lloyd-Jones, D. M., et al. (2012). *Heart disease and stroke statistics—2012 update: A report from the American Heart Association.* Available at: circ.ahajournals.org/content/early/2011/12/15/CIR.0b013e31823ac046.citation/

Sherwood, A., Blumenthal, J. A., Hinderliter, A. L., et al. (2011). Worsening depressive symptoms are associated with adverse clinical outcomes in patients with heart failure. *Journal of the American College of Cardiology, 57*(4), 418–423.

Stauffer, B. D., Fullerton, C., Fleming, N., et al. (2011). Effectiveness and cost of a transitional care program for heart failure: A prospective study with concurrent controls. *Archives of Internal Medicine, 171*(14), 1238–1243.

Van Den Broek, K. C., Habibovic, M., & Pedersen, S. S. (2010). Emotional distress in partners of patients with an implantable cardioverter defibrillator: A systematic review and recommendations for future research. *Pacing and Clinical Electrophysiology, 33*(12), 1442–1450.

Resources

American Heart Association, www.americanheart.org
Heart Failure Society of America (HFSA), www.hfsa.org
National Heart, Lung, and Blood Institute, www.nhlbi.nih.gov

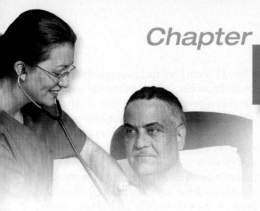

Assessment and Management of Patients With Vascular Disorders and Problems of Peripheral Circulation

Learning Objectives

On completion of this chapter, the learner will be able to:

1 Identify anatomic and physiologic factors that affect peripheral blood flow and tissue oxygenation.
2 Use appropriate parameters for assessment of peripheral circulation.
3 Use the nursing process as a framework of care for patients with vascular insufficiency of the extremities.
4 Compare the various diseases of the arteries and their causes, pathophysiologic changes, clinical manifestations, management, and prevention.

5 Describe the prevention and management of venous thromboembolism.
6 Compare strategies to prevent venous insufficiency, leg ulcers, and varicose veins.
7 Use the nursing process as a framework of care for patients with leg ulcers.
8 Describe the relationship between lymphangitis and lymphedema.

Glossary

anastomosis: junction of two vessels
aneurysm: a localized sac or dilation of an artery formed at a weak point in the vessel wall
angioplasty: an invasive procedure that uses a balloon-tipped catheter to dilate a stenotic area of a blood vessel
ankle-brachial index (ABI): ratio of the ankle systolic pressure to the brachial systolic pressure; an objective measurement of arterial disease that provides quantification of the degree of stenosis
arteriosclerosis: diffuse process whereby the muscle fibers and the endothelial lining of the walls of small arteries and arterioles thicken
atherosclerosis: inflammatory process involving the accumulation of lipids, calcium, blood components, carbohydrates, and fibrous tissue on the intimal layer of a large or medium-sized artery
bruit: sound produced by turbulent blood flow through an irregular, tortuous, stenotic, or dilated vessel

dissection: separation of the weakened elastic and fibromuscular elements in the medial layer of an artery
duplex ultrasonography: combines B-mode grayscale imaging of tissue, organs, and blood vessels with capabilities of estimating velocity changes by the use of a pulsed Doppler
intermittent claudication: a muscular, cramplike pain in the extremities consistently reproduced with the same degree of exercise or activity and relieved by rest
ischemia: deficient blood supply
rest pain: persistent pain in the foot or digits when the patient is resting, indicating a severe degree of arterial insufficiency
rubor: reddish-blue discoloration of the extremities; indicative of severe peripheral arterial damage in vessels that remain dilated and unable to constrict
stenosis: narrowing or constriction of a vessel

Conditions of the vascular system include arterial disorders, venous disorders, lymphatic disorders, and cellulitis. These disorders may be seen in patients in both the inpatient and the outpatient setting. Nursing management depends on an understanding of the vascular system.

Anatomic and Physiologic Overview

Adequate perfusion ensures oxygenation and nourishment of body tissues, and it depends in part on a properly functioning cardiovascular system. Adequate blood flow depends on the efficiency of the heart as a pump, the patency and responsiveness of the blood vessels, and the adequacy of circulating blood volume. Nervous system activity, blood viscosity, and the metabolic needs of tissues influence the rate and adequacy of blood flow.

The vascular system consists of two interdependent systems. The right side of the heart pumps blood through the lungs to the pulmonary circulation, and the left side of the heart pumps blood to all other body tissues through the

819

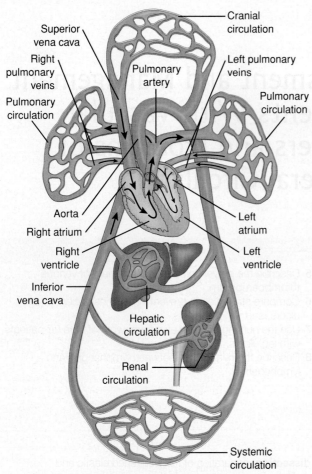

FIGURE 30-1 • Systemic and pulmonary circulation. Oxygen-rich blood from the pulmonary circulation is pumped from the left heart into the aorta and the systemic arteries to the capillaries, where the exchange of nutrients and waste products takes place. The deoxygenated blood returns to the right heart by way of the systemic veins and is pumped into the pulmonary circulation.

systemic circulation. The blood vessels in both systems channel the blood from the heart to the tissues and back to the heart (Fig. 30-1). Contraction of the ventricles is the driving force that moves blood through the vascular system.

Arteries distribute oxygenated blood from the left side of the heart to the tissues, whereas the veins carry deoxygenated blood from the tissues to the right side of the heart. Capillary vessels located within the tissues connect the arterial and venous systems. These vessels permit the exchange of nutrients and metabolic wastes between the circulatory system and the tissues. Arterioles and venules immediately adjacent to the capillaries, together with the capillaries, make up the microcirculation.

The lymphatic system complements the function of the circulatory system. Lymphatic vessels transport lymph (a fluid similar to plasma) and tissue fluids (containing proteins, cells, and cellular debris) from the interstitial space to systemic veins.

Anatomy of the Vascular System

Arteries and Arterioles

Arteries are thick-walled structures that carry blood from the heart to the tissues. The aorta, which has a diameter of

approximately 2.5 cm (1 inch) in the average-sized adult, gives rise to numerous branches, which continue to divide into progressively smaller arteries that are 4 mm (0.16 inch) in diameter. The vessels divide further, diminishing in size to approximately 30 mcm in diameter. These smallest arteries, called *arterioles*, are generally embedded within the tissues (Porth & Matfin, 2009).

The walls of the arteries and arterioles are composed of three layers: the intima, an inner endothelial cell layer; the media, a middle layer of smooth muscle and elastic tissue; and the adventitia, an outer layer of connective tissue. The intima, a very thin layer, provides a smooth surface for contact with the flowing blood. The media makes up most of the vessel wall in the aorta and other large arteries of the body. This layer is composed chiefly of elastic and connective tissue fibers that give the vessels considerable strength and allow them to constrict and dilate to accommodate the blood ejected from the heart during each cardiac cycle (stroke volume) and maintain an even, steady flow of blood. The adventitia is a layer of connective tissue that anchors the vessel to its surroundings. There is much less elastic tissue in the smaller arteries and arterioles, and the media in these vessels is composed primarily of smooth muscle (Porth & Matfin, 2009). Smooth muscle controls the diameter of the vessels by contracting and relaxing. Chemical, hormonal, and neuronal factors influence the activity of smooth muscle. Because arterioles offer resistance to blood flow by altering their diameter, they are often referred to as resistance vessels. Arterioles regulate the volume and pressure in the arterial system and the rate of blood flow to the capillaries. Because of the large amount of smooth muscle in the media, the walls of the arteries are relatively thick, accounting for approximately 25% of the total diameter of the artery.

The intima and the inner third of the smooth muscle layer of the media are in such close contact with the blood that the blood vessels receive their nourishment by direct diffusion. The adventitia and the outer media layers have a limited vascular system for nourishment and require their own blood supply to meet metabolic needs.

Capillaries

The walls of the capillaries, which lack smooth muscle and adventitia, are composed of a single layer of endothelial cells. This thin-walled structure permits rapid and efficient transport of nutrients to the cells and removal of metabolic wastes. The diameter of capillaries ranges from 5 to 10 mcm; this means that red blood cells must alter their shape to pass through these vessels. Changes in a capillary's diameter are passive and are influenced by contractile changes in the blood vessels that carry blood to and from a capillary. The capillary's diameter also changes in response to chemical stimuli. In some tissues, a cuff of smooth muscle, called the *precapillary sphincter*, is located at the arteriolar end of the capillary and is responsible, along with the arteriole, for controlling capillary blood flow (Porth & Matfin, 2009).

Some capillary beds, such as those in the fingertips, contain arteriovenous anastomoses, through which blood passes directly from the arterial to the venous system. These vessels are believed to regulate heat exchange between the body and the external environment.

The distribution of capillaries varies with the type of tissue. For example, skeletal tissue, which has high metabolic requirements, has a denser capillary network than cartilage, which has low metabolic needs.

Veins and Venules

Capillaries join to form larger vessels called *venules,* which join to form veins. The venous system is therefore structurally analogous to the arterial system; venules correspond to arterioles, veins to arteries, and the vena cava to the aorta. Analogous types of vessels in the arterial and venous systems have approximately the same diameters (see Fig. 30-1).

The walls of the veins, in contrast to those of the arteries, are thinner and considerably less muscular. In most veins, the wall makes up only 10% of the diameter, in contrast to 25% in most arteries. In veins, the walls are composed of three layers, like those of arteries; however, in veins, these layers are not as well defined.

The thin, less muscular structure of the vein wall allows these vessels to distend more than arteries. Greater distensibility and compliance permit large volumes of blood to remain in the veins under low pressure. For this reason, veins are referred to as capacitance vessels. Approximately 75% of total blood volume is contained in the veins. The sympathetic nervous system, which innervates the vein musculature, can stimulate the veins to constrict (venoconstriction), thereby reducing venous volume and increasing the volume of blood in the general circulation. Contraction of skeletal muscles in the extremities creates the primary pumping action to facilitate venous blood flow back to the heart (Porth & Matfin, 2009).

Some veins, unlike arteries, are equipped with valves. In general, veins that transport blood against the force of gravity, as in the lower extremities, have one-way bicuspid valves that prevent blood from seeping backward as it is propelled toward the heart. Valves are composed of endothelial leaflets, the competency of which depends on the integrity of the vein wall.

Lymphatic Vessels

The lymphatic vessels are a complex network of thin-walled vessels similar to the blood capillaries. This network collects lymphatic fluid from tissues and organs and transports the fluid to the venous circulation. The lymphatic vessels converge into two main structures: the thoracic duct and the right lymphatic duct. These ducts empty into the junction of the subclavian and the internal jugular veins. The right lymphatic duct conveys lymph primarily from the right side of the head, neck, thorax, and upper arms. The thoracic duct conveys lymph from the remainder of the body. Peripheral lymphatic vessels join larger lymph vessels and pass through regional lymph nodes before entering the venous circulation. The lymph nodes play an important role in filtering foreign particles.

The lymphatic vessels are permeable to large molecules and provide the only means by which interstitial proteins can return to the venous system. With muscular contraction, lymph vessels become distorted to create spaces between the endothelial cells, allowing protein and particles to enter. Muscular contraction of the lymphatic walls and surrounding tissues aids in propelling the lymph toward the venous drainage points (Rockson, 2010).

Function of the Vascular System

Circulatory Needs of Tissues

The amount of blood flow needed by body tissues constantly changes. The percentage of blood flow received by individual organs or tissues is determined by the rate of tissue metabolism, the availability of oxygen, and the function of the tissues. When metabolic requirements increase, blood vessels dilate to increase the flow of oxygen and nutrients to the tissues. When metabolic needs decrease, vessels constrict and blood flow to the tissues decreases. Metabolic demands of tissues increase with physical activity or exercise, local heat application, fever, and infection. Reduced metabolic requirements of tissues accompany rest or decreased physical activity, local cold application, and cooling of the body. If the blood vessels fail to dilate in response to the need for increased blood flow, tissue **ischemia** (deficient blood supply to a body part) results. The mechanism by which blood vessels dilate and constrict to adjust for metabolic changes ensures that normal arterial pressure is maintained (Porth & Matfin, 2009).

As blood passes through tissue capillaries, oxygen is removed and carbon dioxide is added. The amount of oxygen extracted by each tissue differs. For example, the myocardium tends to extract about 50% of the oxygen from arterial blood in one pass through its capillary bed, whereas the kidneys extract only about 7% of the oxygen from the blood that passes through them. The average amount of oxygen removed collectively by all of the body tissues is about 25%. This means that the blood in the vena cava contains about 25% less oxygen than aortic blood. This is known as the systemic arteriovenous oxygen difference (Porth & Matfin, 2009). This difference becomes greater when less oxygen is delivered to the tissues than they need.

Blood Flow

Blood flow through the cardiovascular system always proceeds in the same direction: left side of the heart to the aorta, arteries, arterioles, capillaries, venules, veins, vena cava, and right side of the heart. This unidirectional flow is caused by a pressure difference that exists between the arterial and venous systems. Because arterial pressure (approximately 100 mm Hg) is greater than venous pressure (approximately 40 mm Hg) and fluid always flows from an area of higher pressure to an area of lower pressure, blood flows from the arterial system to the venous system.

The pressure difference (ΔP) between the two ends of the vessel propels the blood. Impediments to blood flow offer the opposing force, which is known as resistance (R). The rate of blood flow is determined by dividing the pressure difference by the resistance:

$$\text{Flow rate} = \Delta P/R$$

This equation clearly shows that when resistance increases, a greater driving pressure is required to maintain the same degree of flow (Porth & Matfin, 2009). In the body, an increase in driving pressure is accomplished by an increase in the force of contraction of the heart. If arterial resistance is chronically elevated, the myocardium hypertrophies (enlarges) to sustain the greater contractile force.

In most long, smooth blood vessels, flow is laminar or streamlined, with blood in the center of the vessel moving slightly faster than the blood near the vessel walls. Laminar flow becomes turbulent when the blood flow rate increases, when blood viscosity increases, when the diameter of the vessel becomes greater than normal, or when segments of the vessel are narrowed or constricted (Porth & Matfin, 2009). Turbulent blood flow creates an abnormal sound, called a **bruit**, which can be heard with a stethoscope.

Blood Pressure

Chapter 31 provides more information on the physiology and measurement of blood pressure.

Capillary Filtration and Reabsorption

Fluid exchange across the capillary wall is continuous. This fluid, which has the same composition as plasma without the proteins, forms the interstitial fluid. The equilibrium between hydrostatic and osmotic forces of the blood and interstitium, as well as capillary permeability, determines the amount and direction of fluid movement across the capillary. Hydrostatic force is a driving pressure that is generated by the blood pressure. Osmotic pressure is the pulling force created by plasma proteins. Normally, the hydrostatic pressure at the arterial end of the capillary is relatively high compared with that at the venous end. This high pressure at the arterial end of the capillaries tends to drive fluid out of the capillary and into the tissue space. Osmotic pressure tends to pull fluid back into the capillary from the tissue space, but this osmotic force cannot overcome the high hydrostatic pressure at the arterial end of the capillary. However, at the venous end of the capillary, the osmotic force predominates over the low hydrostatic pressure, and there is a net reabsorption of fluid from the tissue space back into the capillary (Porth & Matfin, 2009).

Except for a very small amount, fluid that is filtered out at the arterial end of the capillary bed is reabsorbed at the venous end. The excess filtered fluid enters the lymphatic circulation. These processes of filtration, reabsorption, and lymph formation aid in maintaining tissue fluid volume and removing tissue waste and debris. Under normal conditions, capillary permeability remains constant.

Under certain abnormal conditions, the fluid filtered out of the capillaries may greatly exceed the amounts reabsorbed and carried away by the lymphatic vessels. This imbalance can result from damage to capillary walls and subsequent increased permeability, obstruction of lymphatic drainage, elevation of venous pressure, or a decrease in plasma protein osmotic force. Accumulation of excess interstitial fluid that results from these processes is called *edema*.

Hemodynamic Resistance

The most important factor that determines resistance in the vascular system is the vessel radius. Small changes in vessel radius lead to large changes in resistance. The predominant sites of change in the caliber or width of blood vessels, and therefore in resistance, are the arterioles and the precapillary sphincter. Peripheral vascular resistance is the opposition to blood flow provided by the blood vessels. This resistance is proportional to the viscosity or thickness of the blood and the length of the vessel and is influenced by the diameter of the vessels. Under normal conditions, blood viscosity and vessel length do not change significantly, and these factors do not usually play an important role in blood flow. However, a large increase in hematocrit may increase blood viscosity and reduce capillary blood flow.

Peripheral Vascular Regulating Mechanisms

Even at rest, the metabolic needs of body tissues are continuously changing. Therefore, an integrated and coordinated regulatory system is necessary so that blood flow to individual tissues is maintained in proportion to the needs of those tissues. This regulatory mechanism is complex and consists of central nervous system influences, circulating hormones and chemicals, and independent activity of the arterial wall itself.

Sympathetic (adrenergic) nervous system activity, mediated by the hypothalamus, is the most important factor in regulating the caliber and therefore the blood flow of peripheral blood vessels. All vessels are innervated by the sympathetic nervous system except the capillary and precapillary sphincters. Stimulation of the sympathetic nervous system causes vasoconstriction. The neurotransmitter responsible for sympathetic vasoconstriction is norepinephrine (Porth & Matfin, 2009). Sympathetic activation occurs in response to physiologic and psychological stressors. Diminution of sympathetic activity by medications or sympathectomy results in vasodilation.

Other hormones affect peripheral vascular resistance. Epinephrine, released from the adrenal medulla, acts like norepinephrine in constricting peripheral blood vessels in most tissue beds. However, in low concentrations, epinephrine causes vasodilation in skeletal muscles, the heart, and the brain. Angiotensin I, which is formed from the interaction of renin (synthesized by the kidney) and angiotensinogen, a circulating serum protein, is then converted to angiotensin II by an enzyme secreted by the pulmonary vasculature, called *angiotensin-converting enzyme* (ACE). Angiotensin II is a potent vasoconstrictor, particularly of the arterioles. Although the amount of angiotensin II concentrated in the blood is usually small, its profound vasoconstrictive effects are important in certain abnormal states, such as heart failure and hypovolemia (Porth & Matfin, 2009).

Alterations in local blood flow are influenced by various circulating substances that have vasoactive properties. Potent vasodilators include nitric oxide, prostacyclin, histamine, bradykinin, prostaglandin, and certain muscle metabolites. A reduction in available oxygen and nutrients and changes in local pH also affect local blood flow. Proinflammatory cytokines are substances liberated from platelets that aggregate at the site of damaged vessels, causing arteriolar vasoconstriction and continued platelet aggregation at the site of injury (Libby, Ridker, & Hansson, 2009).

Pathophysiology of the Vascular System

Reduced blood flow through peripheral blood vessels characterizes all peripheral vascular diseases. The physiologic effects of altered blood flow depend on the extent to which tissue demands exceed the supply of oxygen and nutrients available. If tissue needs are high, even modestly reduced blood flow may be inadequate to maintain tissue integrity. Tissues then fall prey to ischemia, become malnourished, and ultimately die unless adequate blood flow is restored.

Pump Failure

Inadequate peripheral blood flow occurs when the heart's pumping action becomes inefficient. Left-sided heart failure (left ventricular failure) causes an accumulation of blood in the lungs and a reduction in forward flow or cardiac output, which results in inadequate arterial blood flow to the tissues. Right-sided heart failure (right ventricular failure) causes systemic venous congestion and a reduction in forward flow (see Chapter 29).

Alterations in Blood and Lymphatic Vessels

Intact, patent, and responsive blood vessels are necessary to deliver adequate amounts of oxygen to tissues and to remove metabolic wastes. Arteries can become damaged or obstructed as a result of atherosclerotic plaque, thromboemboli, chemical or mechanical trauma, infections or inflammatory processes, vasospastic disorders, and congenital malformations. A sudden arterial occlusion causes profound and often irreversible tissue ischemia and tissue death. When arterial occlusions develop gradually, there is less risk of sudden tissue death because collateral circulation may develop, giving that tissue the opportunity to adapt to gradually decreased blood flow.

Venous blood flow can be reduced by a thromboembolus obstructing the vein, by incompetent venous valves, or by a reduction in the effectiveness of the pumping action of surrounding muscles. Decreased venous blood flow results in increased venous pressure, a subsequent increase in capillary hydrostatic pressure, net filtration of fluid out of the capillaries into the interstitial space, and subsequent edema. Edematous tissues cannot receive adequate nutrition from the blood and consequently are more susceptible to breakdown, injury, and infection. Obstruction of lymphatic vessels also results in edema. Lymphatic vessels can become obstructed by a tumor or by damage from mechanical trauma or inflammatory processes.

Circulatory Insufficiency of the Extremities

Although many types of peripheral vascular diseases exist, most result in ischemia and produce some of the same symptoms: pain, skin changes, diminished pulse, and possible edema. The type and severity of symptoms depend in part on the type, stage, and extent of the disease process and on the speed with which the disorder develops. Table 30-1 highlights the distinguishing features of arterial and venous insufficiency. In this chapter, peripheral vascular disease is categorized as arterial, venous, or lymphatic.

Gerontologic Considerations

Aging produces changes in the walls of the blood vessels that affect the transport of oxygen and nutrients to the tissues. The intima thickens as a result of cellular proliferation and fibrosis. Elastin fibers of the media become calcified, thin, and fragmented, and collagen accumulates in the intima and the media. These changes cause the vessels to stiffen, which results in increased peripheral resistance, impaired blood flow, and increased left ventricular workload causing hypertrophy, ischemia and failure of the left ventricle, and thrombosis and hemorrhage in microvessels in the brain and kidney (O'Rourke, Safar, & Dzau, 2010).

Assessment of the Vascular System

Health History

The nurse obtains an in-depth description from the patient with peripheral vascular disease of any pain and its precipitating factors. A muscular, cramp-type pain, discomfort, or fatigue in the extremities consistently reproduced with the same degree of exercise or activity and relieved by rest is experienced by patients with peripheral arterial insufficiency. Referred to as **intermittent claudication**, this pain, discomfort, or fatigue is caused by the inability of the arterial system to provide adequate blood flow to the tissues in the

TABLE 30-1	Characteristics of Arterial and Venous Insufficiency and Resulting Ulcers	
Characteristic	**Arterial**	**Venous**
General Characteristics		
Pain	Intermittent claudication to sharp, unrelenting, constant	Aching, cramping
Pulses	Diminished or absent	Present, but may be difficult to palpate through edema
Skin characteristics	Dependent rubor—elevation pallor of foot; dry, shiny skin; cool-to-cold temperature; loss of hair over toes and dorsum of foot; nails thickened and ridged	Pigmentation in gaiter area (area of medial and lateral malleolus), skin thickened and tough, may be reddish blue, frequently with associated dermatitis
Ulcer Characteristics		
Location	Tip of toes, toe webs, heel or other pressure areas if confined to bed	Medial malleolus, lateral malleolus, or anterior tibial area
Pain	Very painful	Minimal pain if superficial or may be very painful
Depth of ulcer	Deep, often involving joint space	Superficial
Shape	Circular	Irregular border
Ulcer base	Pale to black and dry gangrene	Granulation tissue—beefy red to yellow fibrinous in chronic long-term ulcer
Leg edema	Minimal unless extremity kept in dependent position constantly to relieve pain	Moderate to severe

face of increased demands for nutrients and oxygen during exercise. As the tissues are forced to complete the energy cycle without adequate nutrients and oxygen, muscle metabolites and lactic acid are produced. Pain is experienced as the metabolites aggravate the nerve endings of the surrounding tissue. Typically, about 50% of the arterial lumen or 75% of the cross-sectional area must be obstructed before intermittent claudication is experienced. When the patient rests and thereby decreases the metabolic needs of the muscles, the pain subsides. The progression of the arterial disease can be monitored by documenting the amount of exercise or the distance the patient can walk before pain is produced. Persistent pain in the forefoot (i.e., the anterior portion of the foot) when the patient is resting indicates a severe degree of arterial insufficiency and a critical state of ischemia. Known as **rest pain**, this discomfort is often worse at night and may interfere with sleep. This pain frequently requires that the extremity be lowered to a dependent position to improve perfusion to the distal tissues.

The site of arterial disease can be deduced from the location of claudication, because pain occurs in muscle groups distal to the diseased vessel. Calf pain may accompany reduced blood flow through the superficial femoral or popliteal artery, whereas pain in the hip or buttock may result from reduced blood flow in the abdominal aorta or the common iliac or hypogastric arteries.

Physical Assessment

A thorough assessment of the patient's skin color and temperature and the character of the peripheral pulses is important in the diagnosis of arterial disorders.

Inspection of the Skin

Adequate blood flow warms the extremities and gives them a rosy coloring. Inadequate blood flow results in cool and pale extremities. Further reduction of blood flow to these tissues, which occurs when the extremity is elevated, for example, results in an even whiter or more blanched appearance (e.g., pallor). **Rubor**, a reddish-blue discoloration of the extremities, may be observed within 20 seconds to 2 minutes after the extremity is placed in the dependent position. Rubor suggests severe peripheral arterial damage in which vessels that cannot constrict remain dilated. Even with rubor, the extremity begins to turn pale with elevation. Cyanosis, a bluish tint of the skin, is manifested when the amount of oxygenated hemoglobin contained in the blood is reduced.

Additional changes resulting from a chronically reduced nutrient supply include loss of hair, brittle nails, dry or scaling skin, atrophy, and ulcerations. Edema may be apparent bilaterally or unilaterally and is related to the affected extremity's chronically dependent position because of severe rest pain. Gangrenous changes appear after prolonged, severe ischemia and represent tissue necrosis.

Palpation of Pulses

Determining the presence or absence, as well as the quality, of peripheral pulses is important in assessing the status of peripheral arterial circulation (Fig. 30-2). Palpation of pulses is subjective, and the examiner may mistake his or her own pulse for that of the patient. To prevent this, the examiner should use light touch and avoid using only the index finger for palpation, because this finger has the strongest arterial pulsation of all the fingers. The thumb should not be used for the same reason. Absence of a pulse may indicate that the site of **stenosis** (narrowing or constriction) is proximal to that location. Occlusive arterial disease impairs blood flow and can reduce or obliterate palpable pulsations in the extremities. Pulses should be palpated bilaterally and simultaneously, comparing both sides for symmetry in rate, rhythm, and quality.

Diagnostic Evaluation

Various tests may be performed to identify and diagnose abnormalities that can affect the vascular structures (arteries, veins, and lymphatics).

Doppler Ultrasound Flow Studies

When pulses cannot be reliably palpated, a handheld continuous wave (CW) Doppler ultrasound device may be used to hear (insonate) the blood flow in vessels. This handheld device emits a continuous signal through the patient's tissues. The signals are reflected by ("echo off") the moving blood cells and are received by the device. The filtered-output Doppler signal is then transmitted to a loudspeaker or headphones, where it can be heard for interpretation. Because CW Doppler emits a continuous signal, all vascular structures in the path of the sound beam are insonated, and differentiating arterial from venous flow and detecting the site of a stenosis may be difficult. The depth at which blood flow can be detected by Doppler is determined by the frequency (in megahertz [MHz]) it generates. The lower the frequency, the deeper the tissue penetration; a 5- to 10-MHz probe may be used to evaluate the peripheral arteries.

To evaluate the lower extremities, the patient is placed in the supine position with the head of the bed elevated 20 to 30 degrees; the legs are externally rotated, if possible, to permit adequate access to the medial malleolus. Acoustic gel is applied to the patient's skin to permit uniform transmission of the ultrasound wave. The tip of the Doppler transducer is positioned at a 45- to 60-degree angle over the expected location of the artery and angled slowly to identify arterial blood flow. Excessive pressure is avoided because severely diseased arteries can collapse with even minimal pressure.

Because the transducer can detect blood flow in advanced arterial disease states, especially if collateral circulation has developed, identifying a signal documents only the presence of blood flow. The patient's provider must be notified of the absence of a signal if one had been detected previously.

CW Doppler is more useful as a clinical tool when combined with ankle blood pressures, which are used to determine the **ankle-brachial index (ABI)** (Fig. 30-3). The ABI is the ratio of the systolic blood pressure in the ankle to the systolic blood pressure in the arm. It is an objective indicator of arterial disease that allows the examiner to quantify the degree of stenosis. With increasing degrees of arterial narrowing, there is a progressive decrease in systolic pressure distal to the involved sites.

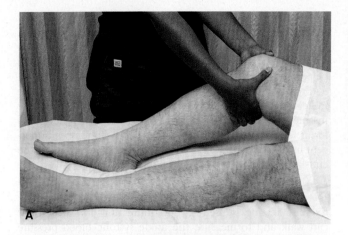

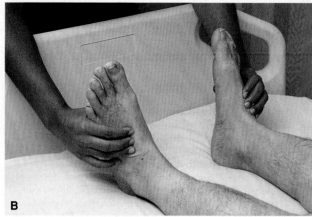

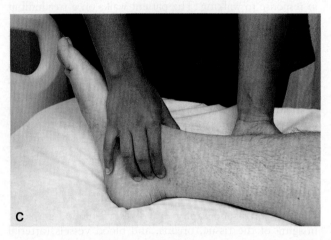

FIGURE 30-2 • Assessing peripheral pulses. **A.** Popliteal pulse. **B.** Dorsalis pedis pulse. **C.** Posterior tibial pulse. From Weber, J., & Kelley, J. (2014). *Health assessment in nursing* (5th ed.). Philadelphia: Lippincott Williams & Wilkins.

The first step in determining the ABI is to have the patient rest in a supine position (not seated) for approximately 5 minutes. An appropriate-sized blood pressure cuff (typically, a 10-cm cuff) is applied to the patient's ankle above the malleolus. After identifying an arterial signal at the posterior tibial

and dorsalis pedis arteries, the systolic pressures are obtained in both ankles. Diastolic pressures in the ankles cannot be measured with Doppler. If pressure in these arteries cannot be measured, pressure can be measured in the peroneal artery, which can also be assessed at the ankle (Fig. 30-4).

Doppler ultrasonography is used to measure brachial pressures in both arms. Both arms are evaluated because the patient may have an asymptomatic stenosis in the subclavian artery, causing brachial pressure on the affected side to be 20 mm Hg or more lower than systemic pressure. The abnormally low pressure should not be used for assessment.

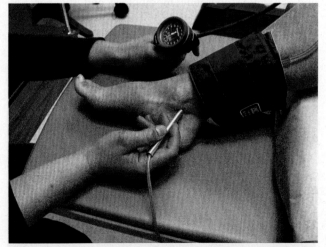

FIGURE 30-3 • Continuous wave Doppler ultrasound detects blood flow in peripheral vessels. Combined with computation of ankle or arm pressures, this diagnostic technique helps health care providers characterize the nature of peripheral vascular disease. Photograph courtesy of Kim Cantwell-Gab.

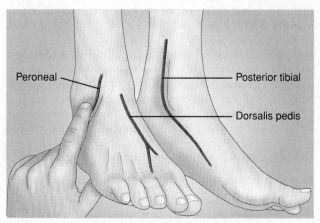

FIGURE 30-4 • Location of peroneal artery; lateral malleolus.

Chart 30-1 Avoiding Common Errors in Calculating Ankle-Brachial Index

Take the following precautions to ensure an accurate ankle-brachial index (ABI) calculation:

- *Use correctly sized blood pressure (BP) cuffs.* To obtain accurate BP measurements, use a cuff with a bladder width at least 40% and length at least 80% of the limb circumference.
- *On the nursing plan of care, document the BP cuff sizes used* (e.g., "12-cm adult BP cuff used for brachial pressures; 10-cm pediatric BP cuff used for ankle pressures"). This minimizes the risk of shift-to-shift discrepancies in ABIs.
- *Use sufficient BP cuff inflation.* To ensure complete closure of the artery and the most accurate measurements, inflate cuffs 20 to 30 mm Hg beyond the point at which the last arterial signal is detected.
- *Do not deflate BP cuffs too rapidly.* Try to maintain a deflation rate of 2 to 4 mm Hg/s for patients without dysrhythmias and 2 mm Hg/s or slower for patients with dysrhythmias. Deflating the cuff more rapidly may miss the patient's highest pressure and result in recording an erroneous (low) BP measurement.
- *Suspect medial calcific sclerosis any time an ABI is 1.20 or greater or ankle pressure is more than 250 mm Hg.* Medial calcific sclerosis is associated with diabetes, chronic renal failure, and hyperparathyroidism. It produces falsely elevated ankle pressures by hardening the media of the arteries, making the vessels noncompressible.
- *Be suspicious of arterial pressures recorded at less than 40 mm Hg.* This may mean the venous signal has been mistaken for the arterial signal. If the arterial pressure, which is normally 120 mm Hg, is measured at less than 40 mm Hg, ask a colleague to double-check the findings before recording this as an arterial pressure.

To calculate ABI, the highest ankle systolic pressure for each foot is divided by the higher of the two brachial systolic pressures (Chart 30-1). The ABI can be computed for a patient with the following systolic pressures:

Right brachial: 160 mm Hg
Left brachial: 120 mm Hg
Right posterior tibial: 80 mm Hg
Right dorsalis pedis: 60 mm Hg
Left posterior tibial: 100 mm Hg
Left dorsalis pedis: 120 mm Hg

The highest systolic pressure for each ankle (80 mm Hg for the right, 120 mm Hg for the left) would be divided by the highest brachial pressure (160 mm Hg):

Right: 80/160 mm Hg = 0.50 ABI
Left: 120/160 mm Hg = 0.75 ABI

In general, systolic pressure in the ankle of a healthy person is the same or slightly higher than the brachial systolic pressure, resulting in an ABI of about 1.0 (no arterial insufficiency). Patients with claudication usually have an ABI of 0.90 to 0.50 (mild to moderate insufficiency); patients with ischemic rest pain have an ABI of less than 0.50; and patients with severe ischemia or tissue loss have an ABI of 0.40 or less (Mohler, Gornik, Gerhard-Herman, et al., 2012).

Nursing Implications

Nurses should perform a baseline ABI on any patient with decreased pulses or any patient 50 years or older with a history of diabetes or smoking (Mohler et al., 2012). Patients who undergo an arterial interventional procedure or surgery should have ABIs performed per their institution's protocols. In addition, if there is a change in the clinical status of a patient, such as a sudden cold or painful limb, an ABI should be performed.

Preprocedurally, nurses should educate patients about the indications for ABI and what to expect. Patients should be instructed to avoid smoking or drinking caffeinated beverages for at least 2 hours prior to testing (if it is done on a nonurgent basis). There may be some discomfort involved when the cuffs are inflated.

Exercise Testing

Exercise testing is used to determine how long a patient can walk and to measure the ankle systolic blood pressure in response to walking. The patient walks on a treadmill at 1.5 mph with a 12% incline for a maximum of 5 minutes. Most patients can complete the test unless they have severe cardiac, pulmonary, or orthopedic problems or a physical disability. A normal response to the test is little or no drop in ankle systolic pressure after exercise. However, in a patient with true vascular claudication, the ankle pressure drops. Combining this hemodynamic information with the walking time helps the primary provider determine whether intervention is necessary. The nurse should reassure the patient that the treadmill test will not require running; rather, the test requires walking on a slight incline.

Duplex Ultrasonography

Duplex ultrasonography involves B-mode grayscale imaging of the tissue, organs, and blood vessels (arterial and venous) and permits estimation of velocity changes by use of a pulsed Doppler (Fig. 30-5). Color flow techniques, which can identify vessels, may be used to shorten the examination time. Duplex ultrasound may be used to determine the level and extent of venous disease as well as chronicity of the disease. Using B mode and Doppler, it is possible to image and assess blood flow, evaluate flow of the distal vessels, locate the disease (stenosis versus occlusion), and determine anatomic morphology and the hemodynamic significance of plaque causing stenosis. Duplex ultrasound findings help in planning therapy and monitoring its

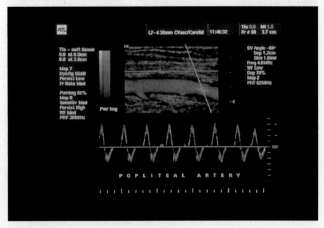

FIGURE 30-5 • Color flow duplex image of popliteal artery with normal triphasic Doppler flow.

outcomes. The test is noninvasive and usually requires no patient preparation. Patients who undergo abdominal vascular duplex ultrasound, however, should be advised to not eat or drink (i.e., NPO status) for at least 6 hours prior to the examination to decrease production of bowel gas that can interfere with the exam. The equipment is portable, making it useful anywhere for initial diagnosis, screening, or follow-up evaluations.

Computed Tomography Scanning

Computed tomography (CT) scanning provides cross-sectional images of soft tissue and visualizes the area of volume changes to an extremity and the compartment where changes take place. CT of a lymphedematous arm or leg, for example, demonstrates a characteristic honeycomb pattern in the subcutaneous tissue. In multidetector computed tomography (MDCT), a spiral CT scanner and rapid intravenous (IV) infusion of contrast agent are used to image very thin sections of the target area, and the results are configured in three dimensions so that the image closely resembles an angiogram. The scan head moves circumferentially around the patient as the patient passes through the scanner, creating a series of overlapping images that are connected to one another in a continuous spiral. Currently, 64-"slice" scanners, which have 64 visual pictures per rotation, are available in most imaging centers; these provide improved volume coverage speed and/or longitudinal spatial resolution, resulting in improved images. Scan times are short. However, the patient is exposed to x-rays, and a contrast agent is injected to visualize the blood vessels. Using computer software, the slicelike images are reconstructed into three-dimensional images that can be rotated and viewed from multiple angles. The high volume of contrast agent injected into a peripheral vein may contraindicate the use of MDCT in children and patients with significantly impaired renal function (Keeling, Farrelly, Carr, et al., 2011).

Nursing Implications

Patients with impaired renal function scheduled for MDCT may require preprocedural treatment to prevent contrast-induced nephropathy. This may include oral or IV hydration 12 hours preprocedure; administration of oral N-acetylcysteine, which acts as an antioxidant; and/or administration of sodium bicarbonate, which alkalinizes urine and protects against free radical damage (Rundback, Nahl, & Yoo, 2011). The nurse should monitor the patient's urinary output postprocedurally, which should be at least 0.5 mL/kg/h. Acute renal failure may occur within 48 to 72 hours postprocedure; therefore, the nurse should follow up with the patient's primary provider should they occur (see Chapter 44 for discussion of acute renal failure). Patients who have known iodine or shellfish allergies may need premedication with steroids and histamine blockers.

Angiography

An arteriogram produced by angiography may be used to confirm the diagnosis of occlusive arterial disease when surgery or other interventions are considered. It involves injecting a radiopaque contrast agent directly into the arterial system to visualize the vessels. The location of a

vascular obstruction or an **aneurysm** (abnormal dilation of a blood vessel) and the collateral circulation can be demonstrated. Typically, the patient experiences a temporary sensation of warmth as the contrast agent is injected, and local irritation may occur at the injection site. Infrequently, a patient may have an immediate or delayed allergic reaction to the iodine contained in the contrast agent. Manifestations include dyspnea, nausea and vomiting, sweating, tachycardia, and numbness of the extremities. Any such reaction must be reported to the interventionalist at once; treatment may include the administration of epinephrine, antihistamines, or corticosteroids. Additional risks include vessel injury, acute arterial occlusion, bleeding, or contrast nephropathy.

Magnetic Resonance Angiography

Magnetic resonance angiography (MRA) is performed with a standard magnetic resonance imaging (MRI) scanner and special software programmed to isolate the blood vessels. The resulting images resemble a standard angiogram, but the images can be rotated and viewed from multiple angles.

Nursing Implications

MRI is contraindicated in patients with any metal implants or devices, including old tattoos, which may contain trace elements (newer materials used in tattoos such as nitinol and titanium are MRI compatible). The nurse should educate the patient regarding what to expect during and after the procedure. The patient should be prepared to lie on a cold, hard table that slides into an enclosed small tube. The nurse should instruct the patient that he or she will hear noises, including banging and popping sounds that will occur periodically. Patients with a history of claustrophobia may be prescribed a sedative prior to the procedure. Patients should be instructed to close their eyes before entering the tube, and to keep them closed, as this may decrease claustrophobic symptoms. Patients should be reassured that they will be provided with a panic button that they may press if they feel a need to stop the procedure. MRA procedures require the use of IV contrast dye; therefore, nursing implications following MRI are the same as those for MDCT (discussed in CT section).

Contrast Phlebography (Venography)

Also known as venography, contrast phlebography involves injecting a radiopaque contrast agent into the venous system. If a thrombus exists, the x-ray image reveals an unfilled segment of vein in an otherwise completely filled vein. Injection of the contrast agent may cause brief but painful inflammation of the vein. The test is generally performed if the patient is to undergo thrombolytic therapy; however, duplex ultrasonography is considered the standard for diagnosing lower extremity venous thrombosis (Zierler, 2009). The nurse should instruct the patient anticipating a contrast phlebogram that he or she will receive contrast dye through a peripheral vein and will be monitored for 2 hours post venogram for access site oozing or hematoma. The guidelines for nursing care following venogram are the same as those for MDCT (see earlier discussion).

Lymphoscintigraphy

Lymphoscintigraphy involves injection of a radioactively labeled colloid subcutaneously in the second interdigital space. The extremity is then exercised to facilitate the uptake of the colloid by the lymphatic system, and serial images are obtained at preset intervals.

Nursing Implications

The nurse should educate the patient regarding what to expect. For instance, the blue dye typically used for this procedure may stain the injection site. If the patient has a lymphatic leak, as can occur with groin incisions, there may be blue drainage from the incision until the dye clears from the system, which may take several days.

ARTERIAL DISORDERS

Arterial disorders cause ischemia and tissue necrosis. These disorders may occur because of chronically progressive pathologic changes to the arterial vasculature (e.g., atherosclerotic changes) or due to an acute loss of blood flow to tissues (e.g., aneurysm rupture).

Arteriosclerosis and Atherosclerosis

Arteriosclerosis (hardening of the arteries) is the most common disease of the arteries. It is a diffuse process whereby the muscle fibers and the endothelial lining of the walls of small arteries and arterioles become thickened. **Atherosclerosis** involves a different process, affecting the intima of large and medium-sized arteries. These changes consist of the accumulation of lipids, calcium, blood components, carbohydrates, and fibrous tissue on the intimal layer of the artery. These accumulations are referred to as atheromas or plaques.

Although the pathologic processes of arteriosclerosis and atherosclerosis differ, rarely does one occur without the other, and the terms are often used interchangeably. Atherosclerosis is a generalized disease of the arteries, and when it is present in the extremities, it is usually present elsewhere in the body (Porth & Matfin, 2009).

Pathophysiology

The most common direct results of atherosclerosis in arteries include narrowing (stenosis) of the lumen, obstruction by thrombosis, aneurysm, ulceration, and rupture. Its indirect results are malnutrition and the subsequent fibrosis of the organs that the sclerotic arteries supply with blood. All actively functioning tissue cells require an abundant supply of nutrients and oxygen and are sensitive to any reduction in the supply of these nutrients. If such reductions are severe and permanent, the cells undergo ischemic necrosis (death of cells due to deficient blood flow) and are replaced by fibrous tissue, which requires much less blood flow.

Atherosclerosis can develop at any point in the body, but certain sites are more vulnerable, such as regions where arteries bifurcate or branch into smaller vessels, with males having more below-the-knee pathology than females (Ortmann, Nuesch, Traupe, et al., 2012). In the proximal

lower extremity, these include the distal abdominal aorta, the common iliac arteries, the orifice of the superficial femoral and profunda femoris arteries, and the superficial femoral artery in the adductor canal, which is particularly narrow. Distal to the knee, atherosclerosis can occur anywhere along the artery.

Although many theories exist about the development of atherosclerosis, no single theory explains the pathogenesis completely; however, tenets of several theories are incorporated into the reaction-to-injury theory. According to this theory, vascular endothelial cell injury results from prolonged hemodynamic forces, such as shearing stresses and turbulent flow, irradiation, chemical exposure, or chronic hyperlipidemia. Injury to the endothelium increases the aggregation of platelets and monocytes at the site of the injury. Smooth muscle cells migrate and proliferate, allowing a matrix of collagen and elastic fibers to form (Cronenwett & Johnston, 2010).

Atherosclerotic lesions are of two types: fatty streaks and fibrous plaque:

- Fatty streaks are yellow and smooth, protrude slightly into the lumen of the artery, and are composed of lipids and elongated smooth muscle cells. These lesions have been found in the arteries of people of all age groups, including infants. It is not clear whether fatty streaks predispose a person to the formation of fibrous plaques or whether they are reversible. They do not usually cause clinical symptoms.
- Fibrous plaques are composed of smooth muscle cells, collagen fibers, plasma components, and lipids. They are white to white-yellow and protrude in various degrees into the arterial lumen, sometimes completely obstructing it. These plaques are found predominantly in the abdominal aorta and the coronary, popliteal, and internal carotid arteries, and they are believed to be progressive lesions (Fig. 30-6).

Gradual narrowing of the arterial lumen stimulates the development of collateral circulation (Fig. 30-7). Collateral circulation arises from preexisting vessels that enlarge to reroute blood flow around a hemodynamically significant stenosis or occlusion. Collateral flow allows continued perfusion to the tissues, but it is often inadequate to meet increased metabolic demand, and ischemia results.

Risk Factors

Many risk factors are associated with atherosclerosis (Chart 30-2). Although it is not entirely clear whether modification of these risk factors prevents the development of cardiovascular disease, evidence indicates that it may slow the process. The National Heart, Lung, and Blood Institute's observational study of genetic determinants of peripheral arterial disease (PAD) found that low lifetime physical activity is positively correlated with PAD. Contrary to previous opinion, this study also found that female gender is an independent risk factor for PAD (Wilson, Sadrzadeh-Rafie, Myers, et al., 2011).

The use of tobacco products may be one of the most important risk factors in the development of atherosclerotic lesions. Nicotine in tobacco decreases blood flow to the extremities and increases heart rate and blood pressure

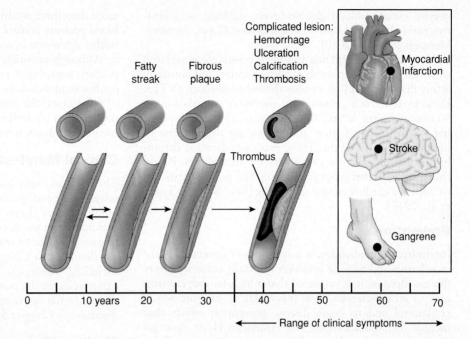

FIGURE 30-6 • Schematic concept of the progression of atherosclerosis. Fatty streaks constitute one of the earliest lesions of atherosclerosis. Many fatty streaks regress, whereas others progress to fibrous plaques and eventually to atheroma, which may be complicated by hemorrhage, ulceration, calcification, or thrombosis and may produce myocardial infarction, stroke, or gangrene.

by stimulating the sympathetic nervous system, causing vasoconstriction. It also increases the risk of clot formation by increasing the aggregation of platelets. Carbon monoxide, a toxin produced by burning tobacco, combines more readily with hemoglobin than oxygen, depriving the tissues of oxygen. There is evidence that smoking decreases high-density lipoprotein (HDL) levels and alters the ratios between HDL and low-density lipoprotein (LDL), HDL and triglycerides, and HDL and total cholesterol levels (see Chapter 27 for discussion of HDL and LDL and their association with atherosclerosis). The amount of tobacco

used—inhaled or chewed—is directly related to the extent of the disease, and cessation of tobacco use reduces the risks. Passive smoking due to secondhand smoke, either mainstream smoke (inhaled by the smoker and exhaled after lung filtration) or sidestream smoke (from the smoldering cigarette), has also been found to have a relationship in the development of atherosclerosis (Vardavas & Panagiotakos, 2009). Many other factors, such as obesity, stress, and lack of exercise, have been identified as contributing to the disease process.

C-reactive protein (CRP) is a sensitive marker of cardiovascular inflammation, both systemically and locally. Slight increases in serum CRP levels are associated with an increased risk of damage in the vasculature, especially if these increases are accompanied by other risk factors, including increasing age, female gender, hypertension, hypercholesterolemia,

FIGURE 30-7 • Development of channels for collateral blood flow in response to occlusion of the right common iliac artery and the terminal aortic bifurcation.

> **Chart 30-2** ⚠
>
> **RISK FACTORS**
> ## Atherosclerosis and Peripheral Arterial Disease
>
> **Modifiable Risk Factors**
>
> - Nicotine use (i.e., tobacco smoking or chewing)
> - Diet (contributing to hyperlipidemia)
> - Hypertension
> - Diabetes (speeds the atherosclerotic process by thickening the basement membranes of both large and small vessels)
> - Hyperlipidemia
> - Stress
> - Sedentary lifestyle
> - Elevated C-reactive protein
> - Hyperhomocysteinemia
>
> **Nonmodifiable Risk Factors**
>
> - Increasing age
> - Female gender
> - Familial predisposition/genetics

obesity, elevated blood glucose levels, smoking, or a positive family history of cardiovascular disease (Lippi, Favaloro, Montagnana, et al., 2010).

Hyperhomocysteinemia has been positively correlated with the risk of peripheral, cerebrovascular, and coronary artery disease as well as venous thromboembolism (VTE). Homocysteine is a protein that promotes coagulation by increasing factor V and factor XI activity while depressing protein C activation and increasing the binding of lipoprotein (a) in fibrin. These processes increase thrombin formation and the propensity for thrombosis. Folate therapy for hyperhomocysteinemia has not been shown to improve cardiovascular outcomes (Sen, Mishra, Tyagi, et al., 2010).

Prevention

Intermittent claudication is a symptom of generalized atherosclerosis and may be a marker of occult coronary artery disease. Because it is suspected that a high-fat diet contributes to atherosclerosis, it is reasonable to measure serum cholesterol and to begin disease prevention efforts that include diet modification. The American Heart Association recommends reducing the amount of fat ingested in a healthy diet, substituting unsaturated fats for saturated fats, and decreasing cholesterol intake to reduce the risk of cardiovascular disease.

Certain medications that supplement dietary modification and exercise are used to reduce blood lipid levels. The Adult Treatment Panel's *Third Report of the National Cholesterol Education Program* (NCEP ATP III) has established guidelines for treating hyperlipidemia, with the primary goal of LDL levels less than 100 mg/dL. LDL levels less than 70 mg/dL are recommended for patients with a history of diabetes, cigarette smoking, atherosclerosis, or hypertension (Paraskevas, Mikhailidis, & Veith, 2011). Secondary goals include achieving total cholesterol levels less than 200 mg/dL and triglyceride levels less than 150 mg/dL. Medications classified as 3-hydroxy-3-methylglutaryl coenzyme A (HMG-CoA) reductase inhibitors (statins), including but not limited to atorvastatin (Lipitor), lovastatin (Mevacor), pravastatin (Pravachol), simvastatin (Zocor), fluvastatin (Lescol), and rosuvastatin (Crestor), are currently first-line treatment because they reduce the incidence of major cardiovascular events (Paraskevas et al., 2011). Several other classes of medications used to reduce lipid levels include bile acid sequestrants (cholestyramine [Questran], colesevelam [WelChol], colestipol [Colestid]), nicotinic acid (niacin [Niacor, Niaspan]), fibric acid inhibitors (gemfibrozil [Lopid], fenofibrate [Tricor]), and cholesterol absorption inhibitors (ezetimibe [Zetia]). Patients receiving long-term therapy with these medications require close monitoring.

Hypertension, which may accelerate the rate at which atherosclerotic lesions form in high-pressure vessels, can lead to a cerebrovascular accident (CVA or stroke), ischemic renal disease, severe PAD, or coronary artery disease. Hypertension is a major risk factor for the development of PAD. The Women's Health Study found a two- to threefold increase in the risk of PAD if the patients had systolic hypertension (Powell, Glynn, Buring, et al., 2011). The majority of patients with hypertension require more than two antihypertensive agents to reach goal blood pressure, and at least one third require more than three antihypertensive agents to achieve effective blood pressure control (Dusing, 2010). (See Chapter 31 for further discussion of antihypertensive agents.)

Although no single risk factor has been identified as the primary contributor to the development of atherosclerotic cardiovascular disease, it is clear that the greater the number of risk factors, the greater the risk of atherosclerosis. Elimination of all controllable risk factors, particularly the use of nicotine products, is strongly recommended.

Clinical Manifestations

The clinical signs and symptoms resulting from atherosclerosis depend on the organ or tissue affected. Coronary atherosclerosis (heart disease), angina, and acute myocardial infarction are discussed in Chapter 27. Cerebrovascular diseases, including transient ischemic attacks and stroke, are discussed in Chapter 67. Atherosclerosis of the aorta, including aneurysm, and atherosclerotic lesions of the extremities are discussed later in this chapter. Renovascular disease (renal artery stenosis and end-stage renal disease) is discussed in Chapter 54.

Medical Management

The management of atherosclerosis involves modification of risk factors, a controlled exercise program to improve circulation and its functioning capacity, medication therapy, and interventional or surgical graft procedures.

Surgical Management

Vascular surgical procedures are divided into two groups: inflow procedures, which improve blood supply from the aorta into the femoral artery, and outflow procedures, which provide blood supply to vessels below the femoral artery. Inflow surgical procedures are described with diseases of the aorta and outflow procedures with peripheral arterial occlusive disease.

Radiologic Interventions

Several interventional radiologic techniques are important adjunctive therapies to surgical procedures. If an isolated lesion or lesions are identified during the arteriogram, **angioplasty**, also called *percutaneous transluminal angioplasty* (PTA), may be performed. After the patient receives a local anesthetic agent, a balloon-tipped catheter is maneuvered across the area of stenosis. Although some clinicians theorize that PTA improves blood flow by overstretching (and thereby dilating) the elastic fibers of the nondiseased arterial segment, most believe that the procedure widens the arterial lumen by "cracking" and flattening the plaque against the vessel wall (see Chapter 27). Complications from PTA include hematoma formation, embolus, **dissection** (separation of the intima) of the vessel, acute arterial occlusion, and bleeding. To decrease the risk of reocclusion, stents (small mesh tubes made of nitinol, titanium, or stainless steel) may be inserted to support the walls of blood vessels and prevent collapse immediately after balloon inflation (Fig. 30-8). A variety of stents and stent grafts may be used for short-segment stenoses. Complications associated with stent or stent graft use include distal embolization, intimal damage (dissection), and dislodgment. The advantage of angioplasty,

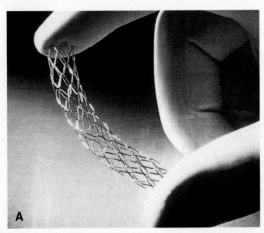
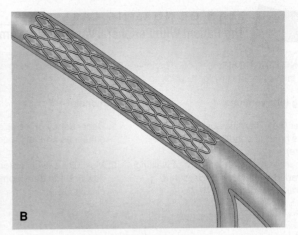

FIGURE 30-8 • **A.** Flexible stent. Courtesy of Medtronics, Peripheral Division, Santa Rosa, California. **B.** Representation of a common iliac artery with a Wallstent.

stents, and stent grafts is the decreased length of hospital stay required for the treatment; many of the procedures are performed on an outpatient basis.

Nursing Management

An overview of the care of a patient with peripheral arterial problems is provided in Chart 30-3.

Improving Peripheral Arterial Circulation

Arterial blood supply to a body part can be enhanced by positioning the part below the level of the heart. For the lower extremities, this is accomplished by elevating the head of the patient's bed or by having the patient use a reclining chair or sit with the feet resting on the floor.

 Concept Mastery Alert

For patients with PAD, blood flow to the lower extremities needs to be enhanced; therefore, the nurse encourages keeping the lower extremities in a neutral or dependent position. In contrast, for patients with venous insufficiency, blood return to the heart needs to be enhanced, so the lower extremities are elevated.

The nurse can assist the patient with walking or other moderate or graded isometric exercises that may be prescribed to promote blood flow and encourage the development of collateral circulation. The nurse instructs the patient to walk to the point of pain, rest until the pain subsides, and then resume walking so that endurance can be increased as collateral circulation develops. Pain can serve as a guide in determining the appropriate amount of exercise. The onset of pain indicates that the tissues are not receiving adequate oxygen, signaling the patient to rest before continuing activity. A regular exercise program can result in increased walking distance before the onset of claudication. The amount of exercise a patient can tolerate before the onset of pain is determined to provide a baseline for evaluation.

Not all patients with peripheral vascular disease should exercise. Before recommending any exercise program, the patient's primary provider should be consulted. Conditions that worsen with exercise include leg ulcers, cellulitis, gangrene, or acute thrombotic occlusions.

Promoting Vasodilation and Preventing Vascular Compression

Arterial dilation promotes increased blood flow to the extremities and is therefore a goal for patients with PAD. However, if the arteries are severely sclerosed, inelastic, or damaged, dilation is not possible. For this reason, measures to promote vasodilation, such as medications or surgery, may be only minimally effective.

Nursing interventions may involve applications of warmth to promote arterial flow and instructions to the patient to avoid exposure to cold temperatures, which causes vasoconstriction. Adequate clothing and warm temperatures protect the patient from chilling. If chilling occurs, a warm bath or drink is helpful. A hot water bottle or heating pad may be applied to the patient's abdomen, causing vasodilation throughout the lower extremities.

 Quality and Safety Nursing Alert

Patients are instructed to test the temperature of bath water and to avoid using hot water bottles and heating pads on the extremities. It is safer to apply a hot water bottle or a heating pad to the abdomen; this can cause reflex vasodilation in the extremities.

In patients with vasospastic disorders (e.g., Raynaud's disease), heat may be applied directly to ischemic extremities using a warmed or electric blanket; however, the temperature of the heat source must not exceed body temperature. Even at low temperatures, trauma to the tissues can occur in ischemic extremities.

Quality and Safety Nursing Alert

Excess heat may increase the metabolic rate of the extremities and increase the need for oxygen beyond that provided by the reduced arterial flow through the diseased artery. Heat must be used with great caution!

Nicotine from tobacco products causes vasospasm and can thereby dramatically reduce circulation to the extremities. Tobacco smoke also impairs transport and cellular use

Chart 30-3

PLAN OF NURSING CARE
The Patient With Peripheral Vascular Problems

NURSING DIAGNOSIS: Ineffective peripheral tissue perfusion related to compromised circulation
GOAL: Increased arterial blood supply to extremities

Nursing Interventions	Rationale	Expected Outcomes
1. Lower the extremities below the level of the heart (if condition is arterial in nature). 2. Encourage moderate amount of walking or graded extremity exercises if no contraindications exist.	1. Dependency of lower extremities enhances arterial blood supply. 2. Muscular exercise promotes blood flow and the development of collateral circulation.	• Has extremities warm to touch • Has extremities with improved color • Experiences decreased muscle pain with exercise

GOAL: Decrease in venous congestion

Nursing Interventions	Rationale	Expected Outcomes
1. Elevate extremities above heart level (if condition is venous in nature). 2. Discourage standing still or sitting for prolonged periods. 3. Encourage walking.	1. Elevation of extremities counteracts gravity, promotes venous return, and prevents venous stasis. 2. Prolonged standing still or sitting promotes venous stasis. 3. Walking promotes venous return by activating the "muscle pump."	• Elevates lower extremities as prescribed • Has decreased edema of extremities • Avoids prolonged standing still or sitting • Gradually increases walking time daily

GOAL: Promotion of vasodilation and prevention of vascular compression

Nursing Interventions	Rationale	Expected Outcomes
1. Maintain warm temperature and avoid chilling. 2. Discourage use of tobacco products. 3. Counsel in ways to avoid emotional upsets; stress management. 4. Encourage avoidance of constrictive clothing and accessories. 5. Encourage avoidance of crossing the legs. 6. Administer vasodilator medications and adrenergic blocking agents as prescribed, with appropriate nursing considerations.	1. Warmth promotes arterial flow by preventing the vasoconstriction effects of chilling. 2. Nicotine in all tobacco products causes vasospasm, which impedes peripheral circulation. 3. Emotional stress causes peripheral vasoconstriction by stimulating the sympathetic nervous system. 4. Constrictive clothing and accessories impede circulation and promote venous stasis. 5. Crossing the legs causes compression of vessels with subsequent impediment of circulation, resulting in venous stasis. 6. Vasodilators relax smooth muscle; adrenergic blocking agents block the response to sympathetic nerve impulses or circulating catecholamines.	• Protects extremities from exposure to cold • Avoids all tobacco products • Uses stress management program to minimize emotional upset • Avoids constricting clothing and accessories • Avoids crossing legs • Takes medication as prescribed

NURSING DIAGNOSIS: Chronic pain related to impaired ability of peripheral vessels to supply tissues with oxygen
GOAL: Relief of pain

Nursing Interventions	Rationale	Expected Outcomes
1. Promote increased circulation through exercise (e.g., walking program, upper extremity exercises, water aerobics, using stationary bicycle). 2. Administer analgesic agents as prescribed, with appropriate nursing considerations.	1. Enhancement of peripheral circulation increases the oxygen supplied to the muscle and decreases the accumulation of metabolites that cause muscle spasms. 2. Analgesic agents help reduce pain and allow the patient to participate in activities and exercises that promote circulation.	• Uses measures to increase arterial blood supply to extremities • Uses analgesic agents as prescribed

PLAN OF NURSING CARE

Chart 30-3

The Patient With Peripheral Vascular Problems (continued)

NURSING DIAGNOSIS: Risk for impaired skin integrity related to compromised circulation
GOAL: Attainment/maintenance of tissue integrity

Nursing Interventions	Rationale	Expected Outcomes
1. Instruct in ways to avoid trauma to extremities.	1. Poorly nourished tissues are susceptible to trauma and bacterial invasion; healing of wounds is delayed or inhibited due to poor tissue perfusion.	• Inspects skin daily for evidence of injury or ulceration • Avoids trauma and irritation to skin • Wears protective shoes • Adheres to meticulous hygiene regimen • Eats a healthy diet that contains adequate protein and vitamins A and C
2. Encourage wearing protective shoes and padding for pressure areas; wear new shoes for short period of time and then inspect feet for signs of injury.	2. Protective shoes and padding prevent foot injuries and blisters.	
3. Encourage meticulous hygiene: bathing with neutral soaps, applying lotions, and carefully trimming nails.	3. Neutral soaps and lotions prevent drying and cracking of skin; avoid lotion between toes because the increased moisture can lead to maceration of tissue.	
4. Caution to avoid scratching or vigorous rubbing.	4. Scratching and rubbing can cause skin abrasions and bacterial invasion.	
5. Promote good nutrition; adequate intake of vitamins A and C, protein, and zinc; and control of obesity.	5. Good nutrition promotes healing and prevents tissue breakdown.	

NURSING DIAGNOSIS: Deficient knowledge regarding self-care activities
GOAL: Adherence to the self-care program

Nursing Interventions	Rationale	Expected Outcomes
1. Include family/significant others in education.	1. Adherence to the self-care program is enhanced when the patient receives support from family and from appropriate self-help groups and agencies.	• Practices frequent position changes as prescribed • Practices postural exercises as prescribed • Takes medications as prescribed • Avoids vasoconstrictors • Uses measures to prevent trauma • Uses stress management program • Accepts condition as chronic but amenable to therapies that will decrease symptoms
2. Provide written instructions about foot care, leg care, and exercise program.	2. Written instructions serve as reminder and reinforcement of information.	
3. Assist to obtain properly fitting clothing, shoes, and stockings.	3. Constrictive clothing and accessories impede circulation and promote venous stasis.	
4. Refer to self-help groups as indicated, such as smoking cessation clinics or stress management, weight management, and exercise program.	4. Reducing risk factors may reduce symptoms or slow disease progression.	

of oxygen and increases blood viscosity. Patients with arterial insufficiency who smoke or chew tobacco must be fully informed of the effects of nicotine on circulation and encouraged to stop. In a meta-analysis of 42 clinical studies with more than 15,000 patients, it was found that advice and support from nurses could increase patients' likelihood of quitting smoking. In one study, a structured smoking cessation intervention that included three visits, an educational video and written materials, and a follow-up telephone call by a nurse increased the quit rate from 2% to 4% when compared to those patients that received only advice from a physician (Rice & Stead, 2009).

Emotional upsets stimulate the sympathetic nervous system, resulting in peripheral vasoconstriction. Emotional stress can be minimized to some degree by avoiding stressful situations when possible or by consistently following a stress management program. Counseling services or relaxation training may be indicated for people who cannot cope effectively with situational stressors.

Constrictive clothing and accessories such as tight socks or shoelaces may impede circulation to the extremities and promote venous stasis and therefore should be avoided. Crossing the legs for more than 15 minutes at a time should be discouraged because it compresses vessels in the legs.

Relieving Pain

Frequently, the pain associated with peripheral arterial insufficiency is chronic, continuous, and disabling. It limits activities, affects work and responsibilities, disturbs sleep, and alters the patient's sense of well-being. Patients may be depressed, irritable, and unable to exert the energy necessary to execute prescribed therapies, making pain relief even more difficult. Analgesic agents such as hydrocodone plus acetaminophen (Vicodin), oxycodone alone (OxyContin), oxycodone plus acetylsalicylic acid (Percodan), or oxycodone plus acetaminophen (Percocet) may be helpful in reducing pain so that the patient can participate in therapies that can increase circulation and ultimately relieve pain more effectively.

Maintaining Tissue Integrity

Poorly perfused tissues are susceptible to damage and infection. When lesions develop, healing may be delayed or inhibited because of the poor blood supply to the area. Infected, nonhealing ulcerations of the extremities can be debilitating and may require prolonged and often expensive treatments. Amputation of an ischemic limb may eventually be necessary. Measures to prevent these complications must be a high priority and vigorously implemented.

Trauma to the extremities must be avoided. Advising the patient to wear sturdy, well-fitting shoes or slippers to prevent foot injury and blisters may be helpful, and recommending neutral soaps and body lotions may prevent drying and cracking of skin. However, the nurse should instruct the patient not to apply lotion between the toes, because the increased moisture can lead to maceration of tissue. Scratching and vigorous rubbing can abrade skin and create sites for bacterial invasion; therefore, feet should be patted dry. Stockings should be clean and dry. Fingernails and toenails should be carefully trimmed straight across and sharp corners filed to follow the contour of the nail. If the nails cannot be trimmed safely, it is necessary to consult a podiatrist, who can also remove corns and calluses. Special shoe inserts may be needed to prevent calluses from recurring. All signs of blisters, ingrown toenails, infection, or other problems should be reported to health care professionals for treatment and follow-up. Patients with diminished vision and those with disabilities that limit mobility of the arms or legs may require assistance in periodically examining the lower extremities for trauma or evidence of inflammation or infection.

Good nutrition promotes healing and prevents tissue breakdown and is therefore included in the overall therapeutic program for patients with peripheral vascular disease. Eating a diet that contains adequate protein and vitamins is necessary for patients with arterial insufficiency. Key nutrients play specific roles in wound healing. Vitamin C is essential for collagen synthesis and capillary development. Vitamin A enhances epithelialization and collagen formation. Zinc is necessary for the synthesis of granulation tissue and re-epithelialization, and it also has anti-inflammatory effects (Collins & Eilinder, 2012). Obesity strains the heart, increases venous congestion, and reduces circulation; therefore, a weight reduction plan may be necessary for some patients. A diet low in lipids may be indicated for patients with atherosclerosis.

Chart 30-4

NURSING RESEARCH PROFILE
Peripheral Arterial Disease: Application of the Chronic Care Model

Lovell, M., Myers, K., Forbes, T. L., et al. (2011). Peripheral arterial disease: Application of the Chronic Care Model. *Journal of Vascular Nursing, 29*(4), 147–152.

Purpose

Peripheral arterial disease (PAD) is a common, chronic atherosclerotic vascular disease that is associated with a high risk of myocardial infarction, stroke, and death. The Chronic Care Model (CCM) is based on the premise that improvement in the care of chronic diseases requires an approach that involves patient, provider, and system-level interventions. The aim of this study was to determine if a multidisciplinary vascular risk management clinic that utilized tenets of the CCM could improve risk factor management and health outcomes for patients with PAD.

Design

This prospective study solicited patients with PAD (*N* = 103) from a large vascular surgery clinic in suburban London, Ontario, if they were not on antiplatelet therapy and if they had suboptimal blood pressure control and elevated lipid profiles. Participants ranged in age from 39 to 79 years; 61% were men. The program was organized by an experienced vascular nurse utilizing the elements of the CCM. Participants were assessed initially and at 3- to 6-month follow-up periods by two vascular internists with a special interest in PAD. Demographic data were collected in addition to cardiovascular risk factors, surgical history, and family history during the initial visit. Key blood laboratory tests were done initially and during follow-up visits to monitor the effectiveness of risk reduction interventions. A dietician and a smoking cessation nurse were available at every visit to counsel patients. The nurse dedicated to supervise the program was available to the participants for questions or concerns. Participants were provided pamphlets and information sheets on PAD, walking, exercise, and the Dietary Approaches to Stopping Hypertension (DASH) heart-healthy diet. Copies of participants' blood work and blood pressure were provided during their follow-up visits.

Findings

Of the 103 participants, 56.3% were smokers, 53.9% had blood pressures >140 mm Hg systolic or 90 mm Hg diastolic, and 80.2% had low-density lipoprotein (LDL) levels >77 mg/dL upon study enrollment. After an average follow-up of 528 days, there was a significant reduction in both systolic and diastolic blood pressures, with 59.8% patients at or below target BP levels (*p* < 0.001). The LDL was significantly reduced from 111.8 to 83.1 mg/dL, with 47.5% of the patients at or below the recommended LDL level (*p* < 0.001). Only 16% of the participants who were smokers at commencement of the study successfully quit, even though they had access to smoking cessation counseling at every clinic visit and via telephone in follow-up care. There were no changes or trends noted with fasting blood glucose or weight over the course of the study.

Nursing Implications

This study confirms previous findings that risk factors for PAD can be improved if there is a dedicated team of interdisciplinary health care professionals working together and consistent with the tenets of the CCM. This study provides a guide in development of a successful PAD CCM that may be replicated by other vascular clinics that have a willing team of health care professionals. Promotion of disease self-management is a key principle to attaining positive outcomes. Nurses are at the forefront of patient care and play an essential role in the coordination of care, providing patient education and helping empower patients to take ownership of their health.

Gerontologic Considerations

In older adults, symptoms of PAD may be more pronounced than in younger people. In older patients who are inactive, gangrene may be the first sign of disease (Olin, Allie, Belkin, et al., 2010). These patients may have adjusted their lifestyle to accommodate the limitations imposed by the disease and may not walk far enough to develop symptoms of claudication. Circulation is decreased, although this is not apparent to the patient until trauma occurs. At this point, gangrene develops when minimal arterial flow is impaired further by edema formation resulting from the traumatic event.

Intermittent claudication may occur after walking only one half to one block or after walking up a slight incline. Any prolonged pressure on the foot can cause pressure areas that become ulcerated, infected, and gangrenous. The outcomes of arterial insufficiency can include reduced mobility and activity as well as a loss of independence. Older people with reduced mobility are less likely to remain in the community setting, have higher rates of hospitalizations, and experience a poorer quality of life (Olin & Sealove, 2010).

Promoting Home and Community-Based Care

The self-care program is planned with the patient so that activities that promote arterial and venous circulation, relieve pain, and promote tissue integrity are acceptable. The patient and family are helped to understand the reasons for each aspect of the program, the possible consequences of nonadherence, and the importance of keeping follow-up appointments (Chart 30-4). Long-term care of the feet and legs is of prime importance in the prevention of trauma, ulceration, and gangrene. Chart 30-5 provides detailed patient instructions for foot and leg care.

Peripheral Arterial Occlusive Disease

Arterial insufficiency of the extremities occurs most often in men and is a common cause of disability. The legs are most frequently affected; however, the upper extremities may be involved. The age of onset and the severity are influenced by the type and number of atherosclerotic risk factors (see

Chart 30-5 HOME CARE CHECKLIST Foot and Leg Care in Peripheral Vascular Disease		
At the completion of home care education, the patient or caregiver will be able to:	**PATIENT**	**CAREGIVER**
• Demonstrate daily foot bathing: Wash between toes with mild soap and lukewarm water, then rinse thoroughly and pat rather than rub dry.	✔	✔

• Recognize the dangers of thermal injury.
  • Wear clean, loose, soft cotton socks (they are comfortable, allow air to circulate, and absorb moisture)
  • In cold weather, wear extra socks in extra-large shoes.
  • Avoid heating pads, whirlpools, and hot tubs.
  • Avoid sunburn.
	✔	

• Identify safety concerns.
  • Inspect feet daily with a mirror for redness, dryness, cuts, blisters, and so forth.
  • Always wear soft shoes or slippers when out of bed.
  • Trim nails straight across after showering.
  • Consult podiatrist to trim nails if vision is decreased and for care of corns, blisters, and ingrown nails.
  • Clear pathways in house to prevent injury.
  • Avoid wearing thong sandals.
  • Use lamb's wool between toes if they overlap or rub each other.
	✔	✔

• Demonstrate the use of comfort measures.
  • Wear leather shoes with an extra-depth toe box. Synthetic shoes do not allow air to circulate.
  • If feet become dry and scaly, use cream with lanolin. Never put cream between toes.
  • If feet perspire, especially between toes, use powder daily and/or lamb's wool between toes to promote drying.
	✔	

• Demonstrate strategies to decrease risk of constricting blood vessels.
  • Avoid circular compression around feet or knees—for example, by applying knee-high stockings or tight socks.
  • Do not cross legs at knees.
  • Stop using all tobacco products (i.e., smoking or chewing) because nicotine causes vasoconstriction and vasospasm.
  • Avoid applying tight, constricting bandages.
  • Participate in a regular walking exercise program to stimulate circulation.
	✔	

• Recognize when to seek medical attention.
  • Contact health care provider at the onset of skin breakdown such as abrasions, blisters, fungus infection (athlete's foot), or pain.
  • Do not use any medication on feet or legs unless prescribed.
  • Avoid using iodine, alcohol, corn-/wart-removing compound, or adhesive products before checking with health care provider.
	✔	✔

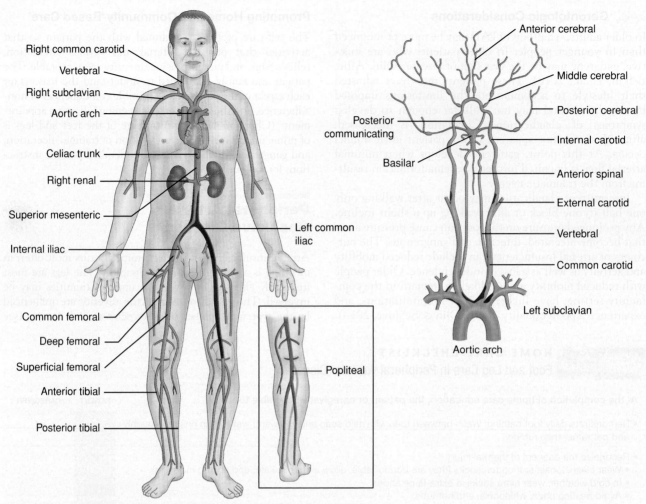

FIGURE 30-9 • Common sites of atherosclerotic obstruction in major arteries.

Chart 30-2). In PAD, obstructive lesions are predominantly confined to segments of the arterial system extending from the aorta below the renal arteries to the popliteal artery (Fig. 30-9). Distal occlusive disease is frequently seen in patients with diabetes and in older patients (Olin et al., 2010).

Clinical Manifestations

The hallmark symptom is intermittent claudication. This pain may be described as aching, cramping, or inducing fatigue or weakness that occurs with the same degree of exercise or activity and is relieved with rest. The pain commonly occurs in muscle groups distal to the area of stenosis or occlusion. As the disease progresses, the patient may have a decreased ability to walk the same distance as before or may notice increased pain with ambulation. When the arterial insufficiency becomes severe, the patient has rest pain. This pain is associated with critical ischemia of the distal extremity and is described as persistent, aching, or boring; it may be so excruciating that it is unrelieved by opioids and can be disabling. Ischemic rest pain is usually worse at night and often wakes the patient. Elevating the extremity or placing it in a horizontal position increases the pain, whereas placing the extremity in a dependent position reduces the pain. Some patients sleep with the affected leg hanging over the

side of the bed. Some patients sleep in a reclining chair in an attempt to prevent or relieve the pain.

Assessment and Diagnostic Findings

A sensation of coldness or numbness in the extremities may accompany intermittent claudication and is a result of reduced arterial flow. The extremity is cool and pale when elevated or ruddy and cyanotic when placed in a dependent position. Skin and nail changes, ulcerations, gangrene, and muscle atrophy may be evident. Bruits may be auscultated with a stethoscope. Peripheral pulses may be diminished or absent.

Examination of the peripheral pulses is an important part of assessing arterial occlusive disease. Unequal pulses between extremities or the absence of a normally palpable pulse is a sign of PAD.

The presence, location, and extent of arterial occlusive disease are determined by a careful history of the symptoms and by physical examination. The color and temperature of the extremity are noted and the pulses palpated. The nails may be thickened and opaque, and the skin may be shiny, atrophic, and dry, with sparse hair growth. The assessment includes comparison of the right and left extremities.

The diagnosis of peripheral arterial occlusive disease may be made using CW Doppler and ABIs, treadmill testing for claudication, duplex ultrasonography, or other imaging studies described previously.

Medical Management

Generally, patients feel better and have fewer symptoms of claudication after they participate in an exercise program. In fact, patients who participated in a home-based walking program where they could freely choose their cadence walked an additional 11 minutes beyond their medically prescribed time per training session (Gardner, Parker, Montgomery, et al., 2011). These findings suggest that home-based programs may be a viable and efficacious option for patients unable to participate in a structured, on-site, supervised exercise program. If a walking program is combined with weight reduction and cessation of tobacco use, patients often can further improve their activity tolerance. Patients should not be promised that their symptoms will be relieved if they stop tobacco use, however, because claudication may persist, and they may lose their motivation to stop using tobacco. In addition to these interventions, arm-ergometer exercise training effectively improves physical fitness, central cardiorespiratory function, and walking capacity in patients with PAD claudication symptoms (Bronas, Treat-Jacobson, & Leon, 2011).

Pharmacologic Therapy

Pentoxifylline (Trental) and cilostazol (Pletal) are approved by the U.S. Food and Drug Administration (FDA) for the treatment of symptomatic claudication. However, the beneficial response to pentoxifylline is small, and the overall data are insufficient to support its widespread use (Olin & Sealove, 2010). Pentoxifylline increases erythrocyte flexibility, lowers blood fibrinogen concentrations, and inhibits neutrophil adhesion and activation. Cilostazol, a phosphodiesterase III inhibitor, is a vasodilator that inhibits platelet aggregation. This agent is contraindicated in patients with a history of congestive heart failure or an ejection fraction less than 40% (Olin & Sealove, 2010).

Antiplatelet agents such as aspirin or clopidogrel (Plavix) prevent the formation of thromboemboli, which can lead to myocardial infarction and stroke. Aspirin has been shown to reduce the risk of cardiovascular events (e.g., myocardial infarction, stroke, and cardiovascular death) in patients with vascular disease; however, adverse events associated with aspirin use include gastrointestinal upset or bleeding.

Statins improve endothelial function in patients with PAD; however, there is conflicting research regarding whether or not statins decrease claudication symptoms in patients or improve pain-free walking time in patients with PAD (Hiatt, Hirsch, Creager, et al., 2010). These medications have beneficial effects on vascular inflammation, plaque stabilization, endothelial dysfunction, and thrombosis but have not improved overall mortality rates in patients without known vascular risk factors (Ray, Seshasai, Erqou, et al., 2010).

Surgical Management

Surgery is reserved for treatment of severe and disabling claudication or when the limb is at risk for amputation because of tissue necrosis. The choice of the surgical procedure depends on the degree and location of the stenosis or occlusion. Other important considerations are the overall health of the patient and the length of the procedure that can be tolerated. For patients whose overall health is so compromised that they cannot tolerate an extensive vascular surgical procedure, it is sometimes necessary to provide the palliative therapy of primary amputation rather than arterial bypass. If endarterectomy is performed, an incision is made into the artery and the atheromatous obstruction is removed (Fig. 30-10).

Bypass grafts are performed to reroute the blood flow around the stenosis or occlusion. Before bypass grafting, the surgeon determines where the distal **anastomosis** (site where the vessels are surgically joined) will be placed. The distal outflow vessel must be at least 50% patent for the graft to remain patent. If the atherosclerotic occlusion is below the inguinal ligament in the superficial femoral artery, the surgical procedure of choice is the femoral-to-popliteal graft. This procedure is further classified as above-knee and below-knee grafts, referring to the location of the distal anastomosis.

Lower leg or ankle vessels with occlusions may also require grafts. Occasionally, the popliteal artery is completely occluded and only collateral vessels maintain perfusion. The distal anastomosis may be made onto any of the tibial arteries (posterior tibial, anterior tibial, or peroneal arteries) or the dorsalis pedis or plantar artery. The distal anastomosis site is determined by the ease of exposure of the vessel in surgery and by which vessel provides the best flow to the distal limb. These grafts require the use of native vein (i.e., autologous—the patient's own vein) to ensure patency. The greater or lesser saphenous vein or a combination of one of the saphenous veins and an upper extremity vein such as the cephalic vein is used to provide the required length.

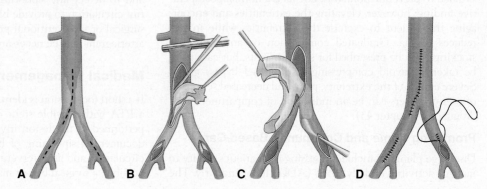

FIGURE 30-10 • In an aortoiliac endarterectomy, the vascular surgeon identifies the diseased area **(A)**, clamps off the blood supply to the vessel **(B)**, removes the plaque **(C)**, and sutures the vessel shut **(D)**, after which blood flow is restored. Adapted with permission from Cronenwett, J. L., & Johnston, K. W. (2010). *Rutherford's vascular surgery* (7th ed., Vols. I and II). Philadelphia: Elsevier.

How long the graft remains patent is determined by several factors, including the size of the graft, graft location, and development of intimal hyperplasia at anastomosis sites (Stillman, Pearce, Talavera, et al., 2012). Bypass grafts may be synthetic or use autologous vein. Several synthetic materials are available for use as a peripheral bypass graft: woven or knitted Dacron or expanded polytetrafluoroethylene (PTFE, such as Gore-Tex or Impra). Cryopreserved saphenous veins and umbilical veins are also available. Infection can be a problem that threatens survival of the graft and almost always requires its removal.

If a vein graft is the surgical choice, care must be taken in the operating room not to damage the vein after harvesting (removing the vein from the patient's body). The vein is occluded at one end and inflated with a heparinized solution to check for leakage and competency. The graft is then placed in a heparinized solution to keep it from becoming dry and brittle.

Nursing Management

Nursing care for patients with peripheral vascular disease is reviewed in Chart 30-3 and in the previous Nursing Management section.

Maintaining Circulation

The primary objective in the postoperative period is to maintain adequate circulation through the arterial repair. Pulses, Doppler assessment, color and temperature, capillary refill, and sensory and motor function of the affected extremity are checked and compared with those of the other extremity; these values are recorded initially every 15 minutes and then at progressively longer intervals if the patient's status remains stable. Doppler evaluation of the vessels distal to the bypass graft should be performed for all postoperative vascular patients, because it is more sensitive than palpation for pulses. The ABI is monitored at least once every 8 hours for the first 24 hours and then once each day until discharge (not usually assessed with pedal artery bypasses). An adequate circulating blood volume should be established and maintained. Disappearance of a pulse that was present may indicate thrombotic occlusion of the graft; the surgeon is immediately notified.

Monitoring and Managing Potential Complications

Continuous monitoring of urine output, central venous pressure, mental status, and pulse rate and volume permits early recognition and treatment of fluid imbalances. Bleeding can result from the heparin administered during surgery or from an anastomotic leak. A hematoma may form as well.

Leg crossing and prolonged extremity dependency are avoided to prevent thrombosis. Edema is a normal postoperative finding; however, elevating the extremities and encouraging the patient to exercise the extremities while in bed reduces edema. Graduated compression or anti-embolism stockings may be prescribed for some patients, but care must be taken to avoid compressing distal vessel bypass grafts. Severe edema of the extremity, pain, and decreased sensation of toes or fingers can be an indication of compartment syndrome (see Chapter 43).

Promoting Home and Community-Based Care

Discharge planning includes assessing the patient's ability to manage activities of daily living (ADLs) independently. The nurse determines whether the patient has a network of family and friends to assist with ADLs. The patient is encouraged to make the lifestyle changes necessitated by the onset of a chronic disease, including pain management and modifications in diet, activity, and hygiene (skin care). The nurse ensures that the patient has the knowledge and ability to assess for any postoperative complications such as infection, occlusion of the artery or graft, and decreased blood flow. The nurse assists the patient in developing and implementing a plan to stop using tobacco.

Upper Extremity Arterial Occlusive Disease

Arterial occlusions occur less frequently in the upper extremities (arms) than in the legs and cause less severe symptoms because the collateral circulation is significantly better in the arms. The arms also have less muscle mass and are not subjected to the workload of the legs.

Clinical Manifestations

Stenosis and occlusions in the upper extremity result from atherosclerosis or trauma. The stenosis usually occurs at the origin of the vessel proximal to the vertebral artery, setting up the vertebral artery as the major contributor of flow. The patient typically complains of arm fatigue and pain with exercise (forearm claudication), inability to hold or grasp objects (e.g., combing hair, placing objects on shelves above the head), and occasionally difficulty driving.

The patient may develop a "subclavian steal" syndrome characterized by reverse flow in the vertebral and basilar artery to provide blood flow to the arm. This syndrome may cause vertebrobasilar (cerebral) symptoms, including vertigo, ataxia, syncope, or bilateral visual changes.

Assessment and Diagnostic Findings

Assessment findings include coolness and pallor of the affected extremity, decreased capillary refill, and a difference in arm blood pressures of more than 20 mm Hg (Zierler, 2009). Noninvasive studies performed to evaluate for upper extremity arterial occlusions include upper and forearm blood pressure determinations and duplex ultrasonography to identify the anatomic location of the lesion and to evaluate the hemodynamics of the blood flow. Transcranial Doppler evaluation is performed to evaluate the intracranial circulation and to detect any siphoning of blood flow from the posterior circulation to provide blood flow to the affected arm. If a surgical or interventional procedure is planned, a diagnostic arteriogram may be necessary.

Medical Management

If a short focal lesion is identified in an upper extremity artery, a PTA with possible stent or stent graft placement may be performed. If the lesion involves the subclavian artery with documented siphoning of blood flow from the intracranial circulation and an interventional radiologic procedure is not possible, a surgical bypass may be performed.

Nursing Management

Nursing assessment involves bilateral comparison of upper arm blood pressures (obtained by stethoscope and Doppler), radial, ulnar, and brachial pulses, motor and sensory function, temperature, color changes, and capillary refill every 2 hours. Disappearance of a pulse or Doppler flow that had been present may indicate an acute occlusion of the vessel, and the primary provider is notified immediately.

After surgery, the arm is kept at heart level or elevated, with the fingers at the highest level. Pulses are monitored with Doppler assessment of the arterial flow every hour for 4 hours and then every shift. Blood pressure (obtained by stethoscope and Doppler) is also assessed every hour for 4 hours and then every shift. Motor and sensory function, warmth, color, and capillary refill are monitored with each arterial flow (pulse) assessment.

> ### ▶ Quality and Safety Nursing Alert
>
> Before surgery and for 24 hours after surgery, the patient's arm is kept at heart level and protected from cold, venipunctures or arterial sticks, tape, and constrictive dressings.

Discharge planning is similar to that for the patient with peripheral arterial occlusive disease. Chart 30-3 describes nursing care for patients with peripheral vascular disease.

Aortoiliac Disease

If collateral circulation has developed, patients with a stenosis or occlusion of the aortoiliac segment may be asymptomatic, or they may complain of buttock or low back discomfort associated with walking. Men may experience impotence. These patients may have decreased or absent femoral pulses.

Medical Management

The treatment of aortoiliac disease is essentially the same as that for atherosclerotic peripheral arterial occlusive disease. A minimally invasive procedure, such as bilateral common iliac stents, may be attempted if the aorta has a less than 50% diameter reduction (Mwipatayi, Thomas, Wong, et al., 2011). If there is significant aortic disease, the surgical procedure of choice is the aortoiliac graft. If possible, the distal graft is anastomosed to the iliac artery, and the entire surgical procedure is performed within the abdomen. If the iliac vessels are diseased, the distal anastomosis is made to the femoral arteries (aortobifemoral graft). Bifurcated woven or knitted Dacron grafts are preferred for this surgical procedure.

Nursing Management

Preoperative assessment, in addition to the standard parameters (see Chapter 17), includes evaluating the brachial, radial, ulnar, femoral, posterior tibial, and dorsalis pedis pulses to establish a baseline for follow-up after arterial lines are placed and postoperatively. Patient education includes an overview of the procedure to be performed, the preparation for surgery, and the anticipated postoperative plan of care. Sights, sounds, and sensations that the patient may experience are discussed.

Postoperative care includes monitoring for signs of thrombosis in arteries distal to the surgical site. The nurse assesses color and temperature of the extremity, capillary refill time, sensory and motor function, and pulses by palpation and Doppler initially every 15 minutes and then at progressively longer intervals if the patient's status remains stable. Any dusky or bluish discoloration, coldness, decrease in sensory or motor function, or decrease in pulse quality is reported immediately to the primary provider.

Postoperative care also includes monitoring urine output and ensuring that output is at least 0.5 mL/kg/h. Renal function may be impaired as a result of hypoperfusion from hypotension, ischemia to the renal arteries during the surgical procedure, hypovolemia, or embolization of the renal artery or renal parenchyma. Vital signs, pain, and intake and output are monitored with the pulse and extremity assessments. Results of laboratory tests are monitored and reported to the primary provider. Abdominal assessment for bowel sounds and paralytic ileus is performed at least every 8 hours. Bowel sounds may not return before the third postoperative day. The absence of bowel sounds, absence of flatus, and abdominal distention are indications of paralytic ileus. Manual manipulation of the bowel during surgery may have caused bruising, resulting in decreased peristalsis. Nasogastric suction may be necessary to decompress the bowel until peristalsis returns. A liquid bowel movement before the third postoperative day may indicate bowel ischemia, which may occur when the mesenteric blood supply (celiac, superior mesenteric, or inferior mesenteric arteries) is occluded. Ischemic bowel usually causes increased pain and a markedly elevated white blood cell count (20,000 to 30,000 cells/mm^3).

Aneurysms

An aneurysm is a localized sac or dilation formed at a weak point in the wall of the artery (Fig. 30-11). It may be classified by its shape or form. The most common forms of aneurysms are saccular and fusiform. A saccular aneurysm projects from only one side of the vessel. If an entire arterial segment becomes dilated, a fusiform aneurysm develops. Very small aneurysms due to localized infection are called *mycotic aneurysms*.

Historically, the cause of abdominal aortic aneurysm, the most common type of degenerative aneurysm, has been attributed to atherosclerotic changes in the aorta. Other causes of aneurysm formation are listed in Chart 30-6. Aneurysms are serious because they can rupture, leading to hemorrhage and death.

■ Thoracic Aortic Aneurysm

Approximately 85% of all cases of thoracic aortic aneurysm are caused by atherosclerosis. They occur most frequently in men between the ages of 50 and 70 years, and are estimated to affect 10 of every 100,000 older adults. The thoracic area is the most common site for a dissecting aneurysm. Previous reports estimated that about one third of patients with thoracic aneurysms die of rupture of the aneurysm. However, recent literature suggests an improvement in the mortality rate; in particular, the mortality rate for patients treated at

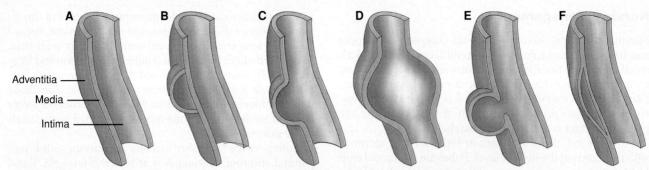

FIGURE 30-11 • Characteristics of arterial aneurysm. **A.** Normal artery. **B.** False aneurysm—actually a pulsating hematoma. The clot and connective tissue are outside the arterial wall. **C.** True aneurysm. One, two, or all three layers of the artery may be involved. **D.** Fusiform aneurysm—symmetric, spindle-shaped expansion of entire circumference of involved vessel. **E.** Saccular aneurysm—a bulbous protrusion of one side of the arterial wall. **F.** Dissecting aneurysm—this usually is a hematoma that splits the layers of the arterial wall.

high-volume aortic centers is estimated at 4% to 9% (Coady, Ikonomidis, Cheung, et al., 2010).

Clinical Manifestations

Symptoms are variable and depend on how rapidly the aneurysm dilates and how the pulsating mass affects surrounding intrathoracic structures. Some patients are asymptomatic. In most cases, pain is the most prominent symptom. The pain is usually constant and boring but may occur only when the person is supine. Other conspicuous symptoms are dyspnea, the result of pressure of the aneurysm sac against the trachea, a main bronchus, or the lung itself; cough, frequently paroxysmal and with a brassy quality; hoarseness, stridor, or weakness or complete loss of the voice (aphonia), resulting from pressure against the laryngeal nerve; and dysphagia (difficulty in swallowing) due to impingement on the esophagus by the aneurysm.

Assessment and Diagnostic Findings

When large veins in the chest are compressed by the aneurysm, the superficial veins of the chest, neck, or arms become dilated, and edematous areas on the chest wall and cyanosis are often evident. Pressure against the cervical sympathetic

---

Chart 30-6 | **Etiologic Classification of Arterial Aneurysms**

Congenital: Primary connective tissue disorders (Marfan syndrome, Ehlers-Danlos syndrome) and other diseases (focal medial agenesis, tuberous sclerosis, Turner syndrome, Menkes syndrome)

Mechanical (hemodynamic): Poststenotic and arteriovenous fistula and amputation related

Traumatic (pseudoaneurysms): Penetrating arterial injuries, blunt arterial injuries, pseudoaneurysms

Inflammatory (noninfectious): Associated with arteritis (Takayasu disease, giant cell arteritis, systemic lupus erythematosus, Behçet syndrome, Kawasaki disease) and periarterial inflammation (i.e., pancreatitis)

Infectious (mycotic): Bacterial, fungal, spirochetal infections

Pregnancy-related degenerative: Nonspecific, inflammatory variant

Anastomotic (postarteriotomy) and graft aneurysms: Infection, arterial wall failure, suture failure, graft failure

Adapted from Rutherford, R. B. (2005). *Vascular surgery* (6th ed., Vols. 1 and 2). Philadelphia: W. B. Saunders.

---

chain can result in unequal pupils. Diagnosis of a thoracic aortic aneurysm is principally made by chest x-ray, computed tomography angiography (CTA), and transesophageal echocardiography (TEE).

Medical Management

Treatment is based on whether the aneurysm is symptomatic, is expanding in size, is caused by an iatrogenic injury, contains a dissection, and involves branch vessels. General measures such as controlling blood pressure and correcting risk factors may be helpful. It is important to control blood pressure in patients with dissecting aneurysms. Preoperatively, the systolic pressure is maintained at approximately 90 to 120 mm Hg in order to maintain a mean arterial pressure at 65 to 75 mm Hg with a beta-blocker such as esmolol (Brevibloc) or metoprolol (Lopressor). Occasionally, antihypertensive agents such as hydralazine (Apresoline) are used for this purpose. Sodium nitroprusside (Nipride) may be used by continuous IV drip to emergently lower the blood pressure, as it has a rapid onset and short action of duration and is easily titrated (Pearce, Annambhotla, Kaufman, et al., 2012). The goal of surgery is to repair the aneurysm and restore vascular continuity with a vascular graft. Intensive monitoring is usually required after this type of surgery, and the patient is cared for in the critical care unit. These patients have a 3% to 4% chance of developing paraplegia (Coady et al., 2010).

Repair of thoracic aneurysms using endovascular grafts placed percutaneously in an interventional suite (e.g., interventional radiology, cardiac catheterization laboratory) or an operating room may decrease postoperative recovery time and decrease complications compared with traditional surgical techniques. Thoracic endografts are made of Gore-Tex or PTFE material reinforced with nitinol or titanium stents. These endovascular grafts are inserted into the thoracic aorta via various vascular access routes, usually the brachial or femoral artery. Because a large surgical incision is not necessary to gain vascular access, the overall patient recovery time tends to be shorter than with open surgical repair. Despite the absence of aortic cross-clamping, there is still a 1.6% chance of paraplegia as a potential complication (Dolinger & Strider, 2010). To decrease the chances of paraplegia, lumbar spinal drains are usually placed in patients undergoing an endovascular repair of thoracic aortic aneurysms. Cerebrospinal fluid drainage is performed to decrease the arterial to cerebral spinal fluid gradient, thereby improving spinal perfusion. What appears to be most important in preventing neurologic deficit is to maintain the cerebrospinal fluid pressure between 10 to 15 mm Hg and to keep the mean arterial pressure greater than 90 mm Hg for the first 48 hours postoperatively (Dolinger & Strider, 2010).

Abdominal Aortic Aneurysm

The most common cause of abdominal aortic aneurysm is atherosclerosis. This condition affects men two to six times more often than women, is two to three times more common in Caucasian versus black men, and is most prevalent in older adult patients (Cronenwett & Johnston, 2010). Most of these aneurysms occur below the renal arteries (infrarenal aneurysms). Untreated, the eventual outcome may be rupture and death.

Pathophysiology

All aneurysms involve a damaged media layer of the vessel. This may be caused by congenital weakness, trauma, or disease. After an aneurysm develops, it tends to enlarge. Risk factors include genetic predisposition, tobacco use, and hypertension; more than half of patients with aneurysms have hypertension.

Clinical Manifestations

Only about 40% of patients with abdominal aortic aneurysms have symptoms. Some patients complain that they can feel their heart beating in their abdomen when lying down, or they may say that they feel an abdominal mass or abdominal throbbing. If the abdominal aortic aneurysm is associated with thrombus, a major vessel may be occluded or smaller distal occlusions may result from emboli. Small cholesterol, platelet, or fibrin emboli may lodge in the interosseous or digital arteries, causing cyanosis and mottling of the toes.

Assessment and Diagnostic Findings

The most important diagnostic indication of an abdominal aortic aneurysm is a pulsatile mass in the middle and upper abdomen. About 80% of these aneurysms can be palpated. A systolic bruit may be heard over the mass. Duplex ultrasonography or CTA is used to determine the size, length, and location of the aneurysm. When the aneurysm is small, ultrasonography is conducted at 6-month intervals until the aneurysm reaches a size so that surgery to prevent rupture is of more benefit than the possible complications of a surgical procedure. Some aneurysms remain stable over many years of monitoring.

 Gerontologic Considerations

Most abdominal aortic aneurysms occur in patients between 60 and 90 years of age. Rupture is likely with coexisting hypertension and with aneurysms more than 6 cm wide. In most cases at this point, the chances of rupture are greater than the chance of death during surgical repair. If the older patient is considered at moderate risk for complications related to surgery or anesthesia, the aneurysm is not repaired until it is at least 5.5 cm (2 inches) wide (Mitchell, 2012).

Medical Management

Pharmacologic Therapy

If the aneurysm is stable in size based on serial duplex ultrasound scans, the blood pressure is closely monitored over time, because there is an association between increased blood pressure and aneurysm rupture (Cronenwett & Johnston, 2010). Antihypertensive agents, including diuretics, beta-blockers, ACE inhibitors, angiotensin II receptor antagonists, and calcium channel blockers, are frequently prescribed to maintain the patient's blood pressure within acceptable limits (see Chapter 31).

Surgical Management

An expanding or enlarging abdominal aortic aneurysm is likely to rupture. Surgery is the treatment of choice for abdominal aortic aneurysms more than 5.5 cm (2 inches) wide or those that are enlarging; the standard treatment has been open surgical repair of the aneurysm by resecting the vessel and sewing a bypass graft in place. The mortality rate associated with elective aneurysm repair—a major surgical procedure—is reported to be 1% to 4% (Cronenwett & Johnston, 2010).

An alternative for treating an infrarenal abdominal aortic aneurysm is endovascular grafting, which involves the transluminal placement and attachment of a sutureless aortic graft prosthesis across an aneurysm (Fig. 30-12). This procedure can be performed under local or regional anesthesia. Endovascular grafting of abdominal aortic aneurysms may be performed if the patient's abdominal aorta and iliac arteries are not extremely tortuous, small, calcified, or filled with thrombi. Results from multiple, prospective studies suggest comparable mortality rates between patients with aneurysms treated by endovascular grafting and those treated with surgical repair,

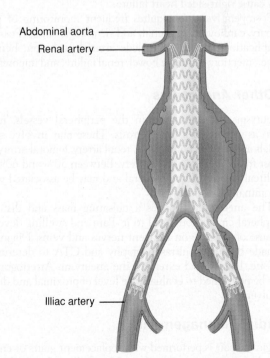

Abdominal aorta

Renal artery

Illiac artery

FIGURE 30-12 • Endograft repair of an abdominal aortic aneurysm.

with similar 2-year survival rates (Cronenwett & Johnston, 2010). Potential complications include bleeding, hematoma, or wound infection at the arterial insertion site; distal ischemia or embolization; dissection or perforation of the aorta; graft thrombosis or infection; break of the attachment system; graft migration; proximal or distal graft leaks; delayed rupture; and bowel ischemia.

Nursing Management

Before surgery, nursing assessment is guided by anticipating a rupture and by recognizing that the patient may have cardiovascular, cerebral, pulmonary, and renal impairment from atherosclerosis. The functional capacity of all organ systems should be assessed. Medical therapies designed to stabilize physiologic function should be promptly implemented.

Signs of impending rupture include severe back or abdominal pain, which may be persistent or intermittent. Abdominal pain is often localized in the middle or lower abdomen to the left of the midline. Low back pain may be present because of pressure of the aneurysm on the lumbar nerves. Indications of a rupturing abdominal aortic aneurysm include constant, intense back pain; falling blood pressure; and decreasing hematocrit. Rupture into the peritoneal cavity is rapidly fatal. A retroperitoneal rupture of an aneurysm may result in hematomas in the scrotum, perineum, flank, or penis. Signs of heart failure or a loud bruit may suggest a rupture into the vena cava. If the aneurysm adheres to the adjacent vena cava, the vena cava may become damaged when rupture or leak of the aneurysm occurs. Rupture into the vena cava results in higher-pressure arterial blood entering the lower-pressure venous system and causing turbulence, which is heard as a bruit. The high blood pressure and increased blood volume returning to the right side of the heart from the vena cava may cause right-sided heart failure.

Postoperative care requires frequent monitoring of pulmonary, cardiovascular, renal, and neurologic status. Possible complications of surgery include arterial occlusion, hemorrhage, infection, ischemic bowel, renal failure, and impotence.

■ Other Aneurysms

Aneurysms may also arise in the peripheral vessels, most often as a result of atherosclerosis. These may involve such vessels as the subclavian artery, renal artery, femoral artery, or (most frequently) popliteal artery. Between 50% and 60% of popliteal aneurysms are bilateral and may be associated with abdominal aortic aneurysms.

The aneurysm produces a pulsating mass and disturbs peripheral circulation distal to it. Pain and swelling develop because of pressure on adjacent nerves and veins. Diagnosis is made by duplex ultrasonography and CTA to determine the size, length, and extent of the aneurysm. Arteriography may be performed to evaluate the level of proximal and distal involvement.

Medical Management

Surgical repair is performed with replacement grafts or endovascular repair using a stent graft or wall graft, which is a Dacron or PTFE graft with external structures made from a variety of materials (e.g., nitinol, titanium, stainless steel) for additional support.

Nursing Management

The patient who has had an endovascular repair must lie supine for 6 hours; the head of the bed may be elevated up to 45 degrees after 2 hours. The patient needs to use a bedpan or urinal while on bed rest. Vital signs and Doppler assessment of peripheral pulses are performed initially every 15 minutes and then at progressively longer intervals if the patient's status remains stable. The access site (usually the femoral or iliac artery) is assessed when vital signs and pulses are monitored. The nurse assesses for bleeding, pulsation, swelling, pain, and hematoma formation. Skin changes of the lower extremity, lumbar area, or buttocks that might indicate signs of embolization, such as extremely tender, irregularly shaped, cyanotic areas, as well as any changes in vital signs, pulse quality, bleeding, swelling, pain, or hematoma, are immediately reported to the primary provider.

The patient's temperature should be monitored every 4 hours, and any signs of postimplantation syndrome should be reported. Postimplantation syndrome typically begins within 24 hours of stent graft placement and consists of a spontaneously occurring fever, leukocytosis, and, occasionally, transient thrombocytopenia. This condition has been attributed to complex immunologic changes, although the exact etiology is unknown. The symptoms are thought to be related to the activation of cytokines (Arnaoutoglou, Kouvelos, Milionis, et al., 2011). They can be managed with a mild analgesic (e.g., acetaminophen [Tylenol]) or an anti-inflammatory agent (e.g., ibuprofen [Motrin]) and usually subside within a week.

Because of the increased risk of hemorrhage, the primary provider is also notified of persistent coughing, sneezing, vomiting, or systolic blood pressure greater than 180 mm Hg. Most patients can resume their preprocedure diet and are encouraged to drink fluids. An IV infusion may be continued until the patient can drink normally. Fluids are important to maintain blood flow through the arterial repair site and to assist the kidneys with excreting IV contrast agents and other medications used during the procedure. Six hours after the procedure, the patient may be able to roll from side to side and may be able to ambulate with assistance to the bathroom. Once the patient can take adequate fluids orally, the IV infusion may be discontinued.

Dissecting Aorta

Occasionally, in an aorta diseased by arteriosclerosis, a tear develops in the intima or the media degenerates, resulting in a dissection (see Fig. 30-11). Arterial dissections are three times more common in men than in women and occur most commonly in the 50- to 70-year age group (Dixon, 2011).

Pathophysiology

Arterial dissections (separations) are commonly associated with poorly controlled hypertension, blunt chest trauma, and cocaine use. The profound increase in sympathetic response caused by cocaine use creates an increase in the force of left ventricular contraction that causes heightened shear forces upon the aortic wall leading to disruption of the intima (Singh, Khaja, & Alpert, 2010). Dissection is caused by rupture in the intimal layer. A rupture may occur through adventitia or into the lumen through the intima, allowing blood to reenter the main channel and resulting in chronic dissection (e.g., pseudoaneurysm) or occlusion of branches of the aorta.

As the separation progresses, the arteries branching from the involved area of the aorta shear and occlude. The tear occurs most commonly in the region of the aortic arch, with the highest mortality rate associated with ascending aortic dissection (Dixon, 2011). The dissection of the aorta may progress backward in the direction of the heart, obstructing the openings to the coronary arteries or producing hemopericardium (effusion of blood into the pericardial sac) or aortic insufficiency, or it may extend in the opposite direction, causing occlusion of the arteries supplying the gastrointestinal tract, kidneys, spinal cord, and legs.

Clinical Manifestations

Onset of symptoms is usually sudden. Severe and persistent pain, described as tearing or ripping, may be reported. The pain is in the anterior chest or back and extends to the shoulders, epigastric area, or abdomen. Aortic dissection may be mistaken for an acute myocardial infarction, which could confuse the clinical picture and initial treatment. Cardiovascular, neurologic, and gastrointestinal symptoms are responsible for other clinical manifestations, depending on the location and extent of the dissection. The patient may appear pale. Sweating and tachycardia may be detected. Blood pressure may be elevated or markedly different from one arm to the other if dissection involves the orifice of the subclavian artery on one side.

Assessment and Diagnostic Findings

Arteriography, multidetector computed tomography angiography (MDCTA), TEE, duplex ultrasonography, and MRA, while limited in terms of expediency during an emergency situation, may aid in the diagnosis.

Medical Management

The medical or surgical treatment of a dissecting aorta depends on the type of dissection present and follows the general principles outlined for the treatment of thoracic aortic aneurysms.

Nursing Management

A patient with a dissecting aorta requires the same nursing care as a patient with an aortic aneurysm requiring surgical intervention, as described earlier in this chapter. Interventions described in Chart 30-3 are also appropriate.

Arterial Embolism and Arterial Thrombosis

Acute vascular occlusion may be caused by an embolus or acute thrombosis. Acute arterial occlusions may result from iatrogenic injury, which can occur during insertion of invasive catheters such as those used for arteriography, PTA or stent placement, or an intra-aortic balloon pump, or it may occur as a result of IV drug abuse. Other causes include trauma from a fracture, crush injury, and penetrating wounds that disrupt the arterial intima. The accurate diagnosis of an arterial occlusion as embolic or thrombotic in origin is necessary to initiate appropriate treatment.

Pathophysiology

Arterial emboli arise most commonly from thrombi that develop in the chambers of the heart as a result of atrial fibrillation, myocardial infarction, infective endocarditis, or chronic heart failure. These thrombi become detached and are carried from the left side of the heart into the arterial system, where they lodge in and obstruct an artery that is smaller than the embolus. Emboli may also develop in advanced aortic atherosclerosis because the atheromatous plaques ulcerate or become rough. Acute thrombosis frequently occurs in patients with preexisting ischemic symptoms.

Clinical Manifestations

Symptoms of arterial emboli depend primarily on the size of the embolus, organ involvement, and the state of collateral vessels. The immediate effect is cessation of distal blood flow. The blockage can progress distal and proximal to the site of the obstruction. Secondary vasospasm can contribute to the ischemia. The embolus can fragment or break apart, resulting in occlusion of distal vessels. Emboli tend to lodge at arterial bifurcations and areas narrowed by atherosclerosis. Cerebral, mesenteric, renal, and coronary arteries are often involved in addition to the large arteries of the extremities.

The symptoms of acute arterial embolism in extremities with poor collateral flow are acute, severe pain and a gradual loss of sensory and motor function. The six Ps associated with acute arterial embolism are *p*ain, *p*allor, *p*ulselessness, *p*aresthesia, *p*oikilothermia (coldness), and *p*aralysis. Eventually, superficial veins may collapse because of decreased blood flow to the extremity. Because of ischemia, the part of the extremity distal to the occlusion is markedly colder and paler than the part proximal to the occlusion.

Arterial thrombosis can also acutely occlude an artery. A thrombosis is a slowly developing clot that usually occurs where the arterial wall has become damaged, generally as a result of atherosclerosis. Thrombi may also develop in an arterial aneurysm. The manifestations of an acute thrombotic arterial occlusion are similar to those described for embolic occlusion. However, treatment is more difficult with a thrombus because the arterial occlusion has occurred in a degenerated vessel and requires more extensive reconstructive surgery to restore flow than is required with an embolic event.

Assessment and Diagnostic Findings

An arterial embolus is usually diagnosed on the basis of the sudden nature of the onset of symptoms and an apparent source for the embolus. Two-dimensional transthoracic echocardiography or TEE, chest x-ray, and electrocardiography (ECG) may reveal underlying cardiac disease. Noninvasive duplex and Doppler ultrasonography can determine the presence and extent of underlying atherosclerosis, and arteriography may be performed.

Medical Management

Management of arterial thrombosis depends on its cause. Management of acute embolic occlusion usually requires surgery because time is of the essence. Because the onset of the event is acute, collateral circulation has not developed, and the patient quickly moves through the list of six Ps to paralysis, the most advanced stage. Heparin therapy is initiated immediately to prevent further development of emboli and to prevent the extension of existing thrombi. Typically, an initial IV bolus of 60 U/kg body weight is administered, followed by a continuous infusion of 12 U/kg/h until the patient undergoes interventional treatment or surgery.

Minimally Invasive Interventional Management

Emergency embolectomy is the procedure of choice if the involved extremity is viable (Fig. 30-13). Arterial emboli are usually treated by insertion of an embolectomy catheter. The catheter is passed through a groin incision into the affected artery and advanced past the occlusion. The catheter balloon is inflated with sterile saline solution, and the thrombus is extracted as the catheter is withdrawn. This procedure involves incising the vessel and removing the clot.

Endovascular Management

Percutaneous mechanical thrombectomy devices may also be used for the treatment of an acute thrombosis. All endovascular devices necessitate obtaining access to the patient's arterial system and inserting a catheter into the patient's artery to obtain access to the thrombus. The approach is similar to that used for angiograms in that it is made through the groin to the femoral artery. Some devices require that a small incision be made into the patient's artery. These devices may use (1) a jet of fluid to disrupt the thrombus and then aspirate the particles; (2) a rotating, sinusoidal-shaped wire that mixes a thrombolytic agent that simultaneously dissolves the clot; or (3) high-frequency, low-energy ultrasound to dissolve an occlusive thrombus. Complications arising from the use of any of the endovascular devices may include arterial dissection or distal artery embolization.

Pharmacologic Therapy

When the patient has adequate collateral circulation, treatment may include IV anticoagulation with heparin, which can prevent the thrombus from spreading and reduce muscle necrosis. Intra-arterial thrombolytic medications are used to dissolve the embolus. Fibrin-specific thrombolytic medications (e.g., tissue plasminogen activator [t-PA, alteplase, Activase] and single-chain urokinase-type plasminogen activator [scu-PA, prourokinase]) do not deplete circulating fibrinogen and plasminogen, which prevents the development of systemic fibrinolysis. Other thrombolytic medications are reteplase (r-PA, Retavase) and tenecteplase (TNKase) (Rivera-Bou, Cabanas, Villanueva, et al., 2012). Although these agents differ in their pharmacokinetics, they are administered in a similar manner: A catheter is advanced under x-ray visualization to the clot, and the thrombolytic agent is infused.

Thrombolytic therapy should not be used when there are known contraindications to therapy or when the extremity cannot tolerate the several additional hours of ischemia that it takes for the agent to lyse (disintegrate) the clot. Contraindications to peripheral thrombolytic therapy include active internal bleeding, cerebrovascular hemorrhage, recent major surgery, uncontrolled hypertension, and pregnancy.

Nursing Management

Before an intervention or surgery, the patient remains on bed rest with the affected extremity level or slightly dependent (15 degrees). The affected part is kept at room temperature and protected from trauma. Heating and cooling pads are contraindicated because ischemic extremities are easily traumatized by alterations in temperature. If possible, tape and ECG electrodes should not be used on the extremity; sheepskin and foot cradles are used to protect an affected leg from mechanical trauma (Gist, Tio-Matos, Falzgraf, et al., 2009).

If the patient is treated with thrombolytic therapy, the dose is based on the patient's weight. The patient is admitted to a critical care unit for continuous monitoring. Vital signs are taken initially every 15 minutes and then at progressively longer intervals if the patient's status remains stable. The patient is closely monitored for bleeding. The nurse minimizes the number of punctures for inserting IV lines and obtaining blood samples, avoids intramuscular injections, prevents any possible tissue trauma, and applies pressure at least twice as long as usual after any puncture is performed. If t-PA is used for the treatment, heparin is usually administered to prevent another thrombus from forming at the site of the lesion. The t-PA activates plasminogen on the thrombus, but it does not decrease the clotting factors as much as other thrombolytic therapies, so patients receiving t-PA can make new thrombi more readily than if they receive other thrombolytics.

During the postoperative period, the nurse collaborates with the surgeon about the patient's appropriate activity level based on the patient's condition. Generally, every effort is made to encourage the patient to move the

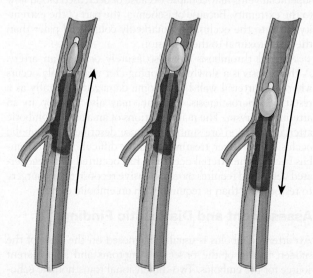

FIGURE 30-13 • Extraction of an embolus by balloon-tipped embolectomy catheter. The deflated balloon-tipped catheter is advanced past the embolus, inflated, and then gently withdrawn, carrying the embolic material with it. Adapted with permission from Rutherford, R. B. (2005). *Vascular surgery* (6th ed., Vols. I and II). Philadelphia: Elsevier.

extremity to stimulate circulation and prevent stasis. Anticoagulant therapy may be continued after surgery to prevent thrombosis of the affected artery and to diminish the development of subsequent thrombi at the initiating site. The nurse assesses for evidence of local and systemic hemorrhage, including mental status changes, which can occur when anticoagulants are administered. Pulses, Doppler signals, ABI, and motor and sensory function are assessed every hour for the first 24 hours, because significant changes may indicate reocclusion. Metabolic abnormalities, renal failure, and compartment syndrome may be complications after an acute arterial occlusion.

Raynaud's Phenomenon and Other Acrosyndromes

Raynaud's phenomenon is a form of intermittent arteriolar vasoconstriction that results in coldness, pain, and pallor of the fingertips or toes. There are two forms of this disorder. Primary or idiopathic Raynaud's (Raynaud's disease) occurs in the absence of an underlying disease. Secondary Raynaud's (Raynaud's syndrome) occurs in association with an underlying disease, usually a connective tissue disorder, such as systemic lupus erythematosus, rheumatoid arthritis, or scleroderma; trauma; or obstructive arterial lesions. Symptoms may result from a defect in basal heat production that eventually decreases the ability of cutaneous vessels to dilate. Episodes may be triggered by emotional factors or by unusual sensitivity to cold. Raynaud's phenomenon is most common in women between 16 and 40 years of age (Bakst, Merola, Franks, et al., 2008). Acrocyanosis was previously thought to be a variant of Raynaud's phenomenon because both are aggravated by cold and emotional stress and both present with blue discoloration of the fingers and hyperhidrosis (excessive sweating).

The prognosis for patients with Raynaud's phenomenon varies; some slowly improve, some become progressively worse, and others show no change. Raynaud's symptoms may be mild so that treatment is not required. However, secondary Raynaud's is characterized by vasospasm and fixed blood vessel obstructions that may lead to ischemia, ulceration, and gangrene. Acrocyanosis is a poorly understood phenomenon that may be benign and require little or no treatment, or the patient may have chronic pain and ulcerations.

Clinical Manifestations

The classic clinical picture of Raynaud's reveals pallor brought on by sudden vasoconstriction. The skin then becomes bluish (cyanotic) because of pooling of deoxygenated blood during vasospasm. As a result of exaggerated reflow (hyperemia) due to vasodilation, a red color (rubor) is produced when oxygenated blood returns to the digits after the vasospasm stops. The characteristic sequence of color change of Raynaud's phenomenon is described as white, blue, and red. Numbness, tingling, and burning pain occur as the color changes. The manifestations tend to be bilateral and symmetric and may involve toes and fingers.

Acrocyanosis is differentiated from Raynaud's by a relative persistence of skin color changes, symmetry, and an absence of the paroxysmal pallor that is found with Raynaud's. Almost all patients with acrocyanosis have marked clamminess and hyperhidrosis of their hands and feet, which tend to worsen in warmer temperatures while the color changes improve. Finger color normalizes when the hands are transferred from the dependent to horizontal position (Kurklinsky, Miller, & Rooke, 2011).

Medical Management

Avoiding the particular stimuli (e.g., cold, tobacco) that provoke vasoconstriction is a primary factor in controlling Raynaud's phenomenon. Calcium channel blockers (nifedipine [Procardia], amlodipine [Norvasc]) may be effective in relieving symptoms. Sympathectomy (interrupting the sympathetic nerves by removing the sympathetic ganglia or dividing their branches) may help some patients.

Avoidance of exposure to cold and trauma and implementing measures to improve local circulation are the primary focus of treatment for acrocyanosis. Calcium channel blockers have not been useful in treating acrocyanosis (Kurlinsky et al., 2011).

Nursing Management

The nurse instructs the patient with Raynaud's or acrocyanosis to avoid situations that may be stressful or unsafe. Stress management classes may be helpful. Exposure to cold must be minimized, and in areas where the fall and winter months are cold, the patient should wear layers of clothing when outdoors. Hats and mittens or gloves should be worn at all times when outside. Fabrics specially designed for cold climates (e.g., Thinsulate) are recommended. Patients should warm up their vehicles before getting in so that they can avoid touching a cold steering wheel or door handle, which could elicit an attack. During summer, a sweater should be available when entering air-conditioned rooms.

Patients are often concerned about serious complications, such as gangrene and amputation; however, these complications are uncommon unless the patient has another underlying disease causing arterial occlusions. Patients should avoid all forms of nicotine; nicotine gum or patches used to help people quit smoking may induce attacks.

Patients should be cautioned to handle sharp objects carefully to avoid injuring their fingers. In addition, patients should be informed about the postural hypotension that may result from medications, such as calcium channel blockers, used to treat Raynaud's phenomenon.

VENOUS DISORDERS

Venous disorders cause reduction in venous blood flow, causing blood stasis. This may then cause a host of pathologic changes, including coagulation defects, edema formation and tissue breakdown, and an increased susceptibility to infections.

Venous Thromboembolism

Deep vein thrombosis (DVT) and pulmonary embolism (PE) collectively make up the condition called *venous thromboembolism.* The incidence of VTE is 10% to 20% in general medical patients and up to 80% in critically ill patients. Studies suggest that 5% to 10% of all in-hospital deaths are a direct result of PE (Qaseem, Chou, Humphrey, et al., 2011). VTE is frequently not diagnosed, however, because DVT and PE are often clinically silent. It is estimated that as many as 30% of patients hospitalized with VTE develop long-term postthrombotic complications. Hospital lengths of stay are shorter, which means that the majority of symptomatic thromboembolic complications in surgical patients occur after hospital discharge.

Pathophysiology

Superficial veins, such as the greater saphenous, lesser saphenous, cephalic, basilic, and external jugular veins, are thick-walled muscular structures that lie just under the skin. Deep veins are thin walled and have less muscle in the media. They run parallel to arteries and bear the same names as the arteries. Deep and superficial veins have valves that permit unidirectional flow back to the heart. The valves lie at the base of a segment of the vein that is expanded into a sinus. This arrangement permits the valves to open without coming into contact with the wall of the vein, permitting rapid closure when the blood starts to flow backward. Other kinds of veins are known as perforating veins. These vessels have valves that allow one-way blood flow from the superficial system to the deep system.

Although the exact cause of VTE remains unclear, three factors, known as Virchow's triad, are believed to play a significant role in its development: endothelial damage, venous stasis, and altered coagulation (Chart 30-7). Damage to the intimal lining of blood vessels creates a site for clot formation. Direct trauma to the veins may occur with fractures or dislocation, diseases of the veins, and chemical irritation of the vein from IV medications or solutions. Venous stasis occurs when blood flow is reduced, as in heart failure or shock; when veins are dilated, as an effect of some medication therapies; and when skeletal muscle contraction is reduced, as in immobility, paralysis of the extremities, or anesthesia. Moreover, bed rest reduces blood flow in the legs by at least 50% (Porth & Matfin, 2009). Altered coagulation occurs most commonly in patients for whom anticoagulant medications have been abruptly withdrawn. Oral contraceptive use, elevated CRP levels (Lippi et al., 2010), and several blood dyscrasias (abnormalities) also can lead to hypercoagulability, with prevalence depending on the ethnicity of the patient. For example, factor V Leiden and prothrombin G20210A mutation is more prevalent in Caucasians, whereas antithrombin III deficiency, protein C deficiency and protein S deficiency are found more commonly in patients of Southeast Asian descent. An increase in factor VIII concentrations is more common among African Americans (Alfirevic & Alfirevic, 2010). Pregnancy is also considered a hypercoagulable state, as it is accompanied by an increase in clotting factors that may not return to baseline until longer than 6 weeks postpartum, increasing the risk of thrombosis. In addition, there is a 50% decrease in venous outflow due to hormonally decreased venous capacitance and reduced venous outflow due to compression from the uterus (Bagaria & Bagaria, 2011).

| **Chart 30-7** | **RISK FACTORS** Deep Vein Thrombosis and Pulmonary Embolism |

Endothelial Damage

- Trauma
- Surgery
- Pacing wires
- Central venous catheters
- Dialysis access catheters
- Local vein damage
- Repetitive motion injury

Venous Stasis

- Bed rest or immobilization
- Obesity
- History of varicosities
- Spinal cord injury
- Age (>65 years)

Altered Coagulation

- Cancer
- Pregnancy
- Oral contraceptive use
- Protein C deficiency
- Protein S deficiency
- Antiphospholipid antibody syndrome
- Factor V Leiden defect
- Prothrombin G20210A defect
- Hyperhomocysteinemia
- Elevated factors II, VIII, IX, XI
- Antithrombin III deficiency
- Polycythemia
- Septicemia

Formation of a thrombus frequently accompanies phlebitis, which is an inflammation of the vein walls. When a thrombus develops initially in the veins as a result of stasis or hypercoagulability but without inflammation, the process is referred to as phlebothrombosis. Venous thrombosis can occur in any vein, but it occurs more often in the veins of the lower extremities. The superficial and deep veins of the extremities may be affected.

Upper extremity venous thrombosis accounts for up to 11% of all cases of DVT. It typically involves more than one venous segment, with the subclavian vein the most frequently affected (Czihal & Hoffmann, 2011). In addition, upper extremity venous thrombosis is more common in patients with IV catheters or in patients with an underlying disease that causes hypercoagulability. Internal trauma to the vessels may result from pacemaker leads, chemotherapy ports, dialysis catheters, or parenteral nutrition lines. The lumen of the vein may be decreased as a result of the catheter or from external compression, such as by neoplasms or an extra cervical rib. Effort thrombosis of the upper extremity is caused by repetitive motion (e.g., in competitive swimmers, tennis players, and construction workers) that irritates the vessel wall, causing inflammation and subsequent thrombosis.

Venous thrombi are aggregates of platelets attached to the vein wall that have a tail-like appendage containing fibrin, white blood cells, and many red blood cells. The "tail"

Chart 30-8 Complications of Venous Thrombosis

Chronic venous occlusion
Pulmonary emboli from dislodged thrombi
Valvular destruction:

- Chronic venous insufficiency
- Increased venous pressure
- Varicosities
- Venous ulcers

Venous obstruction:

- Increased distal pressure
- Fluid stasis
- Edema
- Venous gangrene

---

can grow or can propagate in the direction of blood flow as successive layers of the thrombus form. A propagating venous thrombosis is dangerous because parts of the thrombus can break off and occlude the pulmonary blood vessels. Fragmentation of the thrombus can occur spontaneously as it dissolves naturally, or it can occur with an elevated venous pressure, as may occur after standing suddenly or engaging in muscular activity after prolonged inactivity. After an episode of acute DVT, recanalization (i.e., reestablishment of the lumen of the vessel) typically occurs. Lack of recanalization within the first 6 months after DVT appears to be an important predictor of postthrombotic syndrome, which is one complication of venous thrombosis (Prandoni & Kahn, 2009) (see later discussion). Other complications of venous thrombosis are listed in Chart 30-8.

Clinical Manifestations

A major challenge in recognizing DVT is that the signs and symptoms are nonspecific. The exception is phlegmasia cerulea dolens (massive iliofemoral venous thrombosis), in which the entire extremity becomes massively swollen, tense, painful, and cool to the touch. The large DVT creates severe and sudden venous hypertension that leads to tissue ischemia with resultant translocation of fluid into the interstitial space. Venous gangrene occurs in 40% to 60% of cases and is associated with a poor prognosis for survival (Suwanabol, Tefera, & Schwarze, 2010).

Deep Veins

Clinical manifestations of obstruction of the deep veins include edema and swelling of the extremity because the outflow of venous blood is inhibited. The affected extremity may feel warmer than the unaffected extremity, and the superficial veins may appear more prominent. Tenderness, which usually occurs later, is produced by inflammation of the vein wall and can be detected by gently palpating the affected extremity. In some cases, signs and symptoms of a PE are the first indication of DVT.

Superficial Veins

Thrombosis of superficial veins produces pain or tenderness, redness, and warmth in the involved area. The risk of the superficial venous thrombi becoming dislodged or fragmenting into emboli is very low because most of them dissolve

spontaneously. This condition can be treated at home with bed rest, elevation of the leg, analgesic agents, and, possibly, anti-inflammatory medication.

Assessment and Diagnostic Findings

Careful assessment is invaluable in detecting early signs of venous disorders of the lower extremities. Patients with a history of varicose veins, hypercoagulation, neoplastic disease, cardiovascular disease, or recent major surgery or injury are at high risk. Other patients at high risk include those who are obese or older adults and women taking oral contraceptives (Zhu, Martinez, & Emmerich, 2009).

When performing the nursing assessment, key concerns include limb pain, a feeling of heaviness, functional impairment, ankle engorement, and edema; increase in the surface temperature of the leg, particularly the calf or ankle; and areas of tenderness or superficial thrombosis (i.e., cordlike venous segment). The amount of swelling in the extremity can be determined by measuring the circumference of the affected extremity at various levels (i.e., thigh to ankle) with a tape measure and comparing one extremity with the other at the same level to determine size differences. If both extremities are swollen, a size difference may be difficult to detect. Homan's sign (pain in the calf after the foot is sharply dorsiflexed) is *not* a reliable sign for DVT because it can be elicited in any painful condition of the calf and has no clinical value in assessment for DVT.

Prevention

Patients with a prior history of VTE are at increased risk of a new episode; the rate of recurrence is approximately 25% within 5 years (Zhu et al., 2009). VTE can be prevented, especially if patients who are considered at high risk are identified and preventive measures are instituted without delay. Preventive measures include the application of graduated compression stockings, the use of intermittent pneumatic compression devices, and encouragement of early mobilization and leg exercises. An additional method to prevent venous thrombosis in surgical patients is administration of subcutaneous unfractionated or low-molecular-weight heparin (LMWH). Patients should be advised to make lifestyle changes as appropriate, which may include weight loss, smoking cessation, and regular exercise.

Medical Management

The objectives of treatment for DVT are to prevent the thrombus from growing and fragmenting (thus risking PE), recurrent thromboemboli, and postthrombotic syndrome (discussed later in the chapter) (Key & Kasthuri, 2010). Anticoagulant therapy (administration of a medication to delay the clotting time of blood, prevent the formation of a thrombus in postoperative patients, and forestall the extension of a thrombus after it has formed) can meet these objectives. However, anticoagulants cannot dissolve a thrombus that has already formed. Combining anticoagulation therapy with mechanical and ultrasonic-assisted thrombolytic therapy may eliminate venous obstruction, maintain venous patency, and prevent postthrombotic syndrome by early removal of the thrombus (Polillo, Brower, Benson, et al., 2011).

TABLE 30-2 **Summary of Anticoagulants and Thrombolytics Used to Treat Venous Thromboemboli**

Medication	Major Indications
Unfractionated Heparin	
Heparin	Anticoagulation in patients with current VTE or VTE prophylaxis in patients at risk
Low-Molecular-Weight Heparin	
Dalteparin (Fragmin)	Prophylaxis in patients at risk for VTE or at risk for extension of current VTE
Enoxaparin (Lovenox)	Treatment of current VTE and prophylaxis in patients at risk for VTE or at risk for extension of current VTE
Oral Anticoagulant	
Warfarin (Coumadin)	Anticoagulation in patients with current VTE
Factor Xa Inhibitor	
Fondaparinux (Arixtra)	Prophylaxis in surgical patients at risk for VTE
Oral Factor Xa Inhibitor	
Rivaroxaban (Xarelto)	Fixed-dose regimen for treating acute deep vein thrombosis and for VTE prophylaxis
Dabigatran (Pradaxa)	Fixed-dose regimen for treating acute deep vein thrombosis
Thrombolytic (Fibrinolytic)	
Alteplase (Activase, t-PA)	Fibrinolysis/dissolution of existing VTE
Reteplase (Retavase)	
Tenecteplase (TNKase)	
Urokinase (Abbokinase)	
Direct Thrombin Inhibitor	
Lepirudin (Refludan)	Treatment for heparin-induced thrombocytopenia
Argatroban (Novastan)	

VTE, venous thromboembolism.

Pharmacologic Therapy

Medications for preventing or reducing blood clotting within the vascular system are indicated in patients with thrombophlebitis, recurrent embolus formation, and persistent leg edema from heart failure (Table 30-2). They are also indicated in older patients with a hip fracture that may result in lengthy immobilization. Contraindications for anticoagulant therapy are noted in Chart 30-9.

Unfractionated Heparin

Unfractionated heparin is administered subcutaneously to prevent development of DVT, or by intermittent or continuous IV infusion using weight-adjusted dosing guidelines along with a vitamin K antagonist (e.g., warfarin [Coumadin]) for 5 days to prevent the extension of a thrombus and the development of new thrombi (Holbrook, Schulman, Witt, et al., 2012). Medication dosage is regulated by monitoring the activated partial thromboplastin time (aPTT), the international normalized ratio (INR), and the platelet count.

Low-Molecular-Weight Heparin

Subcutaneous LMWHs that may include medications such as dalteparin and enoxaparin are effective treatments for some cases of DVT. These agents have longer half-lives than unfractionated heparin, so doses can be given in one or two subcutaneous injections each day. Doses are adjusted

Chart 30-9 **PHARMACOLOGY**

Contraindications to Anticoagulant Therapy

- Patient history of nonadherence to medications
- Bleeding from the following systems:
  Gastrointestinal
  Genitourinary
  Respiratory
  Reproductive
- Hemorrhagic blood dyscrasias
- Aneurysms
- Severe trauma
- Alcoholism
- Recent or impending surgery of the eye, spinal cord, or brain
- Severe hepatic or renal disease
- Recent cerebrovascular hemorrhage
- Infections
- Open ulcerative wounds
- Occupations that involve a significant hazard for injury
- Recent childbirth

according to weight. LMWHs prevent the extension of a thrombus and development of new thrombi, and they are associated with fewer bleeding complications and lower risks of heparin-induced thrombocytopenia (HIT) than unfractionated heparin. Because there are several preparations, the dosing schedule must be based on the product used and the protocol at each institution. The cost of LMWH is higher than that of unfractionated heparin; however, LMWH may be used safely in pregnant women, and patients who take it may be more mobile and have an improved quality of life.

Oral Anticoagulants

Warfarin is a vitamin K antagonist that is indicated for extended anticoagulant therapy. Routine coagulation monitoring is essential to ensure that a therapeutic response is obtained and maintained over time. Interactions with a range of other medications can reduce or enhance the anticoagulant effects of warfarin, as can variable intake of foods containing vitamin K (see Chart 33-12 in Chapter 33). Warfarin has a narrow therapeutic window, and there is a slow onset of action. Treatment is initially supported with concomitant parenteral anticoagulation with heparin until the warfarin demonstrates anticoagulant effectiveness.

Factor Xa Inhibitors

Fondaparinux (Arixtra) selectively inhibits factor Xa. This agent is given daily subcutaneously at a fixed dose, has a half-life of 17 hours, and is excreted unchanged via the kidneys (and therefore must be used with caution in patients with renal insufficiency). It has no effect on routine tests of coagulation, such as the aPTT or activated clotting time (ACT), so routine coagulation monitoring is unnecessary. Fondaparinux is approved for prophylaxis during major orthopedic surgery, such as hip or knee arthroplasties, and has been found to be effective for treatment of VTE. A new oral factor Xa inhibitor—dabigatran (Pradaxa), which was FDA approved to reduce the risk of stroke and systemic embolism in patients with nonvalvular atrial fibrillation—was recently licensed for prevention of VTE after planned knee or hip surgery (Van Es, Eerenberg, Kamphuisen, et al., 2011). Dabigatran should be given twice daily with lesser dosages for those patients with renal impairment or disease. There is no need for routine coagulation laboratory monitoring or laboratory test–guided dosage adjustments; however, if measured, aPTT levels may be prolonged approximately 1.5 to 2 times (Gulseth, Wittkowsky, Fanikos, et al., 2011). Rivaroxaban (Xarelto) is another oral factor Xa inhibitor available for DVT prophylaxis that may be taken orally once daily, with reduced dosages administered to patients with renal disorders. Additional oral anticoagulants that directly inhibit factor Xa are undergoing clinical trials and could be imminently available in the United States.

Thrombolytic (Fibrinolytic) Therapy

Catheter-directed thrombolytic (fibrinolytic) therapy lyses and dissolves thrombi in at least 50% of patients. Thrombolytic therapy (e.g., alteplase) is given within the first 3 days after acute thrombosis. Therapy initiated beyond 14 days after the onset of symptoms is significantly less effective. The advantages of thrombolytic therapy include less long-term damage to the venous valves and a reduced incidence of post-thrombotic syndrome and chronic venous insufficiency. Most of the reported complications associated with thrombolytic therapy are related to hemorrhage; the U.S. National Venous Registry reported the incidence of intracranial hemorrhage at less than 1%, retroperitoneal hematoma at approximately 1%, and musculoskeletal, genitourinary, and gastrointestinal bleeds at approximately 3%, although most incidents of bleeding were minor and at the access site (Patterson, Hinchlifee, Loftus, et al., 2010).

Endovascular Management

Endovascular management is necessary for DVT when anticoagulant or thrombolytic therapy is contraindicated (see Chart 30-9), the danger of PE is extreme, or venous drainage is so severely compromised that permanent damage to the extremity is likely. A thrombectomy may be necessary. This mechanical method of clot removal may involve using intraluminal catheters with a balloon or other devices. Some of these spin to break the clot, and others use oscillation to break up the clot to facilitate removal. Ultrasound-assisted thrombolysis may be another option. This intervention uses bursts or continuous high-frequency ultrasound waves emanating from the catheters to cause cavitation of the thrombus, making it more permeable to the thrombolytic agent (Polillo et al., 2011). A vena cava filter may be placed at the time of the thrombectomy or thrombolysis; this filter traps large emboli and prevents PE (see Chapter 23). Some retrievable caval filters can be left in place and then retrieved for up to 6 months. In patients with chronic iliac vein compression (e.g., as is seen in May-Thurner syndrome), balloon angioplasty with stent placement may successfully treat the patient's chronic leg symptoms (Suwanabol et al., 2010).

Nursing Management

If the patient is receiving anticoagulant therapy, the nurse must frequently monitor the aPTT, prothrombin time (PT), INR, ACT, hemoglobin and hematocrit values, platelet count, and fibrinogen level, depending on which medication is being given. Close observation is also required to detect bleeding; if bleeding occurs, it must be reported immediately and anticoagulant therapy discontinued.

Assessing and Monitoring Anticoagulant Therapy

To prevent inadvertent infusion of large volumes of unfractionated heparin, which could cause hemorrhage, unfractionated heparin is always administered by continuous IV infusion using an electronic infusion device. Dosage calculations are based on the patient's weight, and any possible bleeding tendencies are detected by a pretreatment clotting profile. If renal insufficiency exists, lower doses of heparin are required. Periodic coagulation tests and hematocrit levels are obtained. Heparin is in the effective, or therapeutic, range when the aPTT is 1.5 times the control.

Oral anticoagulants, such as warfarin, are monitored by the PT or the INR. Because the full anticoagulant effect of warfarin is delayed for 3 to 5 days, it is usually administered concurrently with heparin until desired anticoagulation has been achieved (i.e., when the PT is 1.5 to 2 times normal or the INR is 2.0 to 3.0) (Holbrook et al., 2012).

Monitoring and Managing Potential Complications

Bleeding

The principal complication of anticoagulant therapy is spontaneous bleeding. Bleeding from the kidneys is detected by microscopic examination of the urine and is often the first sign of excessive dosage. Bruises, nosebleeds, and bleeding gums are also early signs. To promptly reverse the effects of heparin, IV injections of protamine sulfate may be administered. Risks of protamine administration include bradycardia and hypotension, which can be minimized by slow administration. Protamine sulfate can be used to reverse the effects of LMWH, but it is less effective with LMWH than with unfractionated heparin. Reversing the anticoagulation effects of warfarin is more difficult, but effective measures that may be prescribed include administration of vitamin K and/or infusion of fresh-frozen plasma or prothrombin concentrate. Oral and low-dose IV vitamin K significantly reduces the INR within 24 hours (Crowther, Ageno, Garcia, et al., 2009).

Thrombocytopenia

HIT may be a complication of heparin therapy (see Chapter 33 for discussion).

Drug Interactions

Because oral anticoagulants (i.e., warfarin) interact with many other medications and herbal and nutritional supplements, close monitoring of the patient's medication schedule is necessary. Many medications and supplements potentiate or inhibit oral anticoagulants; it is always wise to check to see if any medications or supplements are contraindicated with warfarin (see Chart 33-12 in Chapter 33). Contraindications to anticoagulant therapy are summarized in Chart 30-9.

Providing Comfort

Elevation of the affected extremity, graduated compression stockings, and analgesic agents for pain relief are adjuncts to therapy. They help improve circulation and increase comfort. Warm, moist packs applied to the affected extremity reduce the discomfort associated with DVT. The patient is encouraged to walk once anticoagulation therapy has been initiated. The nurse should instruct the patient that walking is better than standing or sitting for long periods. Bed exercises, such as repetitive dorsiflexion of the foot, are also recommended.

Compression Therapy

Stockings

Graduated compression stockings usually are prescribed for patients with venous insufficiency. The amount of pressure gradient is determined by the amount and severity of venous disease. For example, a pressure gradient of 20 to 30 mm Hg is prescribed for patients with asymptomatic varicose veins, whereas at least a pressure gradient of 30 to 40 mm Hg is prescribed for patients with venous stasis ulceration. These stockings should not be confused with anti-embolism stockings (i.e., TED stockings) that provide less compression (12 to 20 mm Hg). Graduated compression stockings are designed to apply 100% of the prescribed pressure gradient at the ankle and pressure that decreases as the stocking approaches the thigh, reducing the caliber of the superficial veins in the leg and increasing flow in the deep veins. These stockings may be knee high, thigh high, or pantyhose.

> ◣ *Quality and Safety Nursing Alert*
>
> Any type of stocking can inadvertently become a tourniquet if applied incorrectly (i.e., rolled tightly at the top). In such instances, the stockings produce—rather than prevent—stasis. For ambulatory patients, graduated compression stockings are removed at night and reapplied before the legs are lowered from the bed to the floor in the morning.

When the stockings are off, the skin is inspected for signs of irritation, and the calves are examined for tenderness. Any skin changes or signs of tenderness are reported. Stockings are contraindicated in patients with severe pitting edema, because they can produce severe pitting at the knee.

🍂 Gerontologic Considerations. Because of decreased strength and manual dexterity, older patients may be unable to apply graduated compression stockings properly. If this is the case, a family member or friend should be taught to assist the patient to apply the stockings so that they do not cause undue pressure on any part of the feet or legs. Frames have been designed to assist patients with applying stockings, and if there is any concern regarding patients' physical abilities, they should be referred to a stocking vendor who can provide examples of and training in the use of stocking assistance devices.

External Compression Devices and Wraps

Short stretch elastic wraps may be applied from the toes to the knee in a 50% spiral overlap. These wraps are available in a two-layer system, which includes an inner layer of soft padding. These wraps are rectangular and become squares on stretching, indicating the appropriate degree of stretch and reducing the possibility of wrapping a leg too loosely or too tightly. Three- and four-layer systems are also available (e.g., Profore, Dyna-Care), but these may be used only once compared with the two-layer system, which can be used multiple times.

Other types of compression are available. The Unna boot, which consists of a paste bandage impregnated with zinc oxide, glycerin, gelatin, and sometimes calamine, is applied without tension in a circular fashion from the base of the toes to the tibial tuberosity with a 50% spiral overlap. The foot must remain dorsiflexed at a 90-degree angle to the leg, thus avoiding excess pressure or trauma to the anterior ankle area. Once the bandage dries, it provides a constant and consistent compression of the venous system. This type of compression may remain in place for as long as 1 week, although it may be too heavy for debilitated patients to handle.

The CircAid, a nonelastic leg wrap with a series of overlapping, interlocking Velcro straps, augments the effect of muscle while the patient is walking. The CircAid is usually worn during the day. Patients may find the CircAid easier to apply and wear than the Unna boot because it is lighter; they can remove it to shower, and it is adjustable. This readily adjustable feature may also be problematic; patients may be tempted to loosen the straps, and the compression achieved may not be adequate.

Intermittent Pneumatic Compression Devices

These devices can be used with elastic or graduated compression stockings to prevent DVT. They consist of an electric controller that is attached by air hoses to plastic knee-high or thigh-high sleeves. The leg sleeves are divided into compartments, which sequentially fill to apply pressure to the ankle, calf, and thigh at 35 to 55 mm Hg of pressure. These devices can increase blood velocity beyond that produced by the stockings. A randomized controlled trial that compared treatment outcomes of two compression bandaging systems to standard care without compression found that up to 80% of all ulcers healed with the use of compression alone (Wong, Andriessen, Lee, et al., 2012). This study found that bandaging combinations are successful in healing ulcers if they employ a compression level of approximately 40 mm Hg in the ankle region of the leg (Wong et al., 2012). Nursing measures in caring for patients who use these devices include ensuring that prescribed pressures are not exceeded, assessing for patient comfort, and ensuring compliance to therapy.

Positioning the Body and Encouraging Exercise

When the patient is on bed rest, the feet and lower legs should be elevated periodically above the level of the heart. This position allows the superficial and tibial veins to empty rapidly and to remain collapsed. Active and passive leg exercises, particularly those involving calf muscles, should be performed to increase venous flow. Early ambulation is most effective in preventing venous stasis. Deep-breathing exercises are beneficial because they produce increased negative pressure in the thorax, which assists in emptying the large veins. Once ambulatory, the patient is instructed to avoid sitting for more than an hour at a time. The goal is to walk at least 10 minutes every 1 to 2 hours. The patient is also instructed to perform active and passive leg exercises as frequently as necessary when he or she cannot ambulate, such as during long car, bus, train, and plane trips.

Promoting Home and Community-Based Care

In addition to instructing the patient how to apply graduated compression stockings and explaining the importance

PATIENT EDUCATION
Taking Anticoagulant Medications

- Take the anticoagulant medication at the same time each day, usually between 8:00 and 9:00 AM.
- Wear or carry identification indicating the anticoagulant medication being taken.
- Keep all appointments for blood tests.
- Because other medications affect the action of the anticoagulant medication, do not take any of the following medications or supplements without consulting with the primary health care provider: vitamins, cold medicines, antibiotics, aspirin, mineral oil, and anti-inflammatory agents, such as ibuprofen (Motrin) and similar medications or herbal or nutritional supplements. The primary provider should be contacted before taking any over-the-counter drugs.
- Avoid alcohol, because it may change the body's response to an anticoagulant medication.
- Avoid food fads, crash diets, or marked changes in eating habits.
- Do not take warfarin (Coumadin) unless directed.
- Do not stop taking warfarin (when prescribed) unless directed.
- When seeking treatment from any health care provider, be sure to inform the caregiver that you are taking an anticoagulant medication.
- Contact your primary provider before having dental work or elective surgery.
- If any of the following signs appear, report them immediately to the primary provider:
  Faintness, dizziness, or increased weakness
  Severe headaches or abdominal pain
  Reddish or brownish urine
  Any bleeding—for example, cuts that do not stop bleeding
  Bruises that enlarge, nosebleeds, or unusual bleeding from any part of the body
  Red or black bowel movements
  Rash
- Avoid injury that can cause bleeding.
- *For women:* Notify the primary provider if you suspect pregnancy.

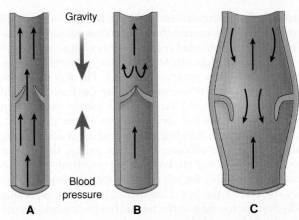

FIGURE 30-14 • Competent valves showing blood flow patterns when the valve is open (**A**) and closed (**B**), allowing blood to flow against gravity. **C.** With faulty or incompetent valves, the blood cannot move toward the heart.

of elevating the legs and exercising adequately, the nurse educates about the prescribed anticoagulant, its purpose, and the need to take the correct amount at the specific times prescribed (Chart 30-10). The patient should also be aware that periodic blood tests are necessary to determine if a change in medication or dosage is required. If the patient fails to adhere to the therapeutic regimen, continuation of the medication therapy should be questioned. A person who refuses to discontinue the use of alcohol should not receive anticoagulants, because chronic alcohol use decreases their effectiveness. In patients with liver disease, the potential for bleeding may be exacerbated by anticoagulant therapy.

Chronic Venous Insufficiency/ Postthrombotic Syndrome

Venous insufficiency results from obstruction of the venous valves in the legs or a reflux of blood through the valves. Superficial and deep leg veins can be involved. Resultant venous hypertension can occur whenever there has been a prolonged increase in venous pressure, such as occurs with

DVT. Because the walls of veins are thinner and more elastic than the walls of arteries, they distend readily when venous pressure is consistently elevated. In this state, leaflets of the venous valves are stretched and prevented from closing completely, causing a backflow or reflux of blood in the veins. Duplex ultrasonography confirms the obstruction and identifies the level of valvular incompetence. Twenty-five to fifty percent of patients who are post DVT that develop deep vein incompetence suffer from postthrombotic syndrome (Henke & Comerota, 2011) (Fig. 30-14).

Clinical Manifestations

Postthrombotic syndrome is characterized by chronic venous stasis, resulting in edema, altered pigmentation, pain, and stasis dermatitis. The patient may notice the symptoms less in the morning and more in the evening. Obstruction or poor calf muscle pumping in addition to valvular reflux must be present for the development of severe postthrombotic syndrome and stasis ulcers. Superficial veins may be dilated. The disorder is long-standing, difficult to treat, and often disabling (Kahn, 2010).

Stasis ulcers develop as a result of the rupture of small skin veins and subsequent ulcerations. When these vessels rupture, red blood cells escape into surrounding tissues and then degenerate, leaving a brownish discoloration of the tissues, called *hemosiderin staining*. The pigmentation and ulcerations usually occur in the lower part of the extremity, in the area of the medial malleolus of the ankle. The skin becomes dry, cracks, and itches; subcutaneous tissues fibrose and atrophy. The risk of injury and infection of the extremities is increased.

Complications

Venous ulceration is the most serious complication of chronic venous insufficiency and can be associated with other conditions affecting the circulation of the lower extremities. Cellulitis or dermatitis may complicate the care of chronic venous insufficiency and venous ulcerations.

Management

Management of the patient with venous insufficiency is directed at reducing venous stasis and preventing ulcerations.

Measures that increase venous blood flow are antigravity activities, such as elevating the leg, and compression of superficial veins with graduated compression stockings.

Elevating the legs decreases edema, promotes venous return, and provides symptomatic relief. The legs should be elevated frequently throughout the day (at least 15 to 20 minutes four times daily). At night, the patient should sleep with the foot of the bed elevated about 15 cm (6 inches). Prolonged sitting or standing in one position is detrimental; walking should be encouraged. When sitting, the patient should avoid placing pressure on the popliteal spaces, as occurs when crossing the legs or sitting with the legs dangling over the side of the bed. Constricting garments, especially socks that are too tight at the top or that leave marks on the skin, should be avoided.

Compression of the legs with graduated compression stockings reduces the pooling of venous blood, enhances venous return to the heart, and is recommended for people with venous insufficiency. It is recommended that stockings with 30 to 40 mm Hg pressure be used during the first year post DVT (Kahn, 2010). Each stocking should fit so that pressure is greater at the foot and ankle and then gradually declines to a lesser pressure at the knee or groin. If the top of the stocking is too tight or becomes twisted, a tourniquet effect is created, which worsens venous pooling. Stockings should be applied after the legs have been elevated for a period, when the amount of blood in the leg veins is at its lowest.

Extremities with venous insufficiency must be carefully protected from trauma; the skin is kept clean, dry, and soft. Signs of ulceration are immediately reported to the health care provider for treatment and follow-up.

Leg Ulcers

A leg ulcer is an excavation of the skin surface that occurs when inflamed necrotic tissue sloughs off. About 70% of all leg ulcers result from chronic venous insufficiency. Lesions due to arterial insufficiency account for approximately 20% of all leg ulcers, with up to 25% lifetime incidence risk among patients with diabetes (Karr, 2011).

Pathophysiology

Inadequate exchange of oxygen and other nutrients in the tissue is the metabolic abnormality that underlies the development of leg ulcers. When cellular metabolism cannot maintain energy balance, cell death (necrosis) results. Alterations in blood vessels at the arterial, capillary, and venous levels may affect cellular processes and lead to the formation of ulcers.

Clinical Manifestations

The characteristics of leg ulcers are determined by the cause of the ulcer. Most ulcers, especially in older patients, have more than one cause. The symptoms depend on whether the problem is arterial or venous in origin (see Table 30-1). The severity of the symptoms depends on the extent and duration of the vascular insufficiency. The ulcer itself appears as an open, inflamed sore. The area may be draining or covered by eschar (dark, hard crust).

Arterial Ulcers

Chronic arterial disease is characterized by intermittent claudication, which is pain caused by activity and relieved after a few minutes of rest. The patient may also complain of digital or forefoot pain at rest. If the onset of arterial occlusion is acute, ischemic pain is unrelenting and rarely relieved even with opioids. Typically, arterial ulcers are small, circular, deep ulcerations on the tips of toes or in the web spaces between the toes. Ulcers often occur on the medial side of the hallux or lateral fifth toe and may be caused by a combination of ischemia and pressure (Fig. 30-15).

Venous Ulcers

Chronic venous insufficiency is characterized by pain described as aching or heavy. The foot and ankle may be edematous. Ulcerations are in the area of the medial or lateral malleolus (gaiter area) and are typically large, superficial, and highly exudative. Venous hypertension causes extravasation of blood, which discolors the area (see Fig. 30-15). Studies report the average venous ulcer requires as long as 6 to 12 months to heal completely and as many as 70% will recur within 5 years of closure (Gillespie, 2010). Patients with neuropathy frequently have ulcerations on the side of the foot over the metatarsal heads. These ulcers are painless and are described in further detail in Chapter 51.

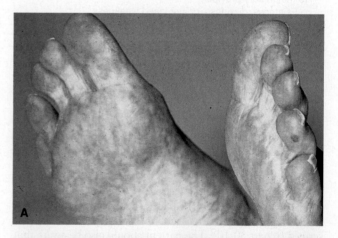

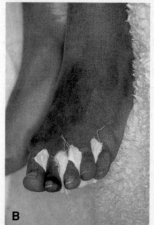
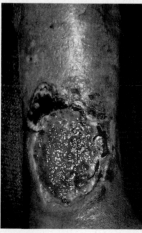

FIGURE 30-15 • A. Ulcers resulting from arterial emboli.
B. Gangrene of the toes resulting from severe arterial ischemia.
C. Ulcer from venous stasis.

Assessment and Diagnostic Findings

Because ulcers have many causes, the cause of each ulcer needs to be identified so that appropriate therapy can be prescribed. The history of the condition is important in determining venous or arterial insufficiency. The pulses of the lower extremities (femoral, popliteal, posterior tibial, and dorsalis pedis) are carefully examined. More conclusive diagnostic aids are Doppler and duplex ultrasound studies, arteriography, and venography. Cultures of the ulcer bed may be necessary to determine whether an infecting agent is the primary cause of the ulcer.

Medical Management

Patients with ulcers can be effectively managed by advanced practice nurses or wound-ostomy-continence nurses in collaboration with physicians. All ulcers have the potential to become infected.

Pharmacologic Therapy

Antiseptic agents, such as povidone-iodine, cadexomer iodine, acetic acid, chlorhexidine, and silver wound products, inhibit growth and development of most skin organisms, are broad spectrum and generate relatively little antimicrobial resistance, and can be used for short periods of time. However, once a wound colonized with pathogens shows signs of infection (e.g., erythema, induration, exudate, edema, wound breakdown, foul odor), a systemic antibiotic is necessary (Lipsky & Hoey, 2009). The specific antibiotic agent selected is based on culture and sensitivity test results. Oral antibiotics usually are prescribed because topical antibiotics have not proven to be effective for leg ulcers.

Compression Therapy

Adequate compression therapy involves the application of external or counter pressure to the lower extremity to facilitate venous return to the heart. The pressure should be applied in a gradient or graduated fashion, with the pressure being somewhat higher at the ankle. Graduated compression stockings are one option; some of these are custom-made to the patient's anatomic specifications. The patient should be instructed to wear the stockings at all times except at night and to reapply the stockings in the morning before getting out of bed. Short stretch elastic wraps, Unna boots, and CircAids may be other effective options. (See the discussion on compression therapy in the Venous Thromboembolism section.)

Débridement

To promote healing, the wound is kept clean of drainage and necrotic tissue. The usual method is to flush the area with normal saline solution or clean it with a noncytotoxic wound-cleansing agent (Saf-Clens, Biolex, Restore). If this is unsuccessful, débridement may be necessary. Débridement is the removal of nonviable tissue from wounds. Removing the dead tissue is important, particularly in instances of infection. Débridement can be accomplished by several different methods:

- Surgical débridement is the fastest method and can be performed by a physician, skilled advanced practice nurse, or wound-ostomy-continence nurse in collaboration with the physician.

- Nonselective débridement can be accomplished by applying isotonic saline dressings of fine mesh gauze to the ulcer. When the dressing dries, it is removed (dry), along with the debris adhering to the gauze. Pain management is usually necessary.

- Enzymatic débridement with the application of enzyme ointments may be prescribed to treat the ulcer. The ointment is applied to the lesion but not to normal surrounding skin. Most enzymatic ointments are covered with saline-soaked gauze that has been thoroughly wrung out. A dry gauze dressing and a loose bandage are then applied. The enzymatic ointment is discontinued when the necrotic tissue has been débrided, and an appropriate wound dressing is applied.

- Calcium alginate dressings (e.g., Kaltostat, Sorbsan, Aquacel Hydrofiber) may be used for débridement when absorption of exudate is needed. These dressings are changed when the exudate seeps through the cover dressing or at least every 7 days. The dressing can also be used on areas that are bleeding, because the material helps stop the bleeding. As the dry fibers absorb exudate, they become a gel that can be painlessly removed from the ulcer bed. Calcium alginate dressings should not be used on dry or nonexudative wounds.

- Foam dressings (e.g., Lyofoam, Allevyn, Cavi-Care) may be an option for exudative wounds because they absorb exudate into the foam, keeping the wound moist.

Arterial insufficiency may result in gangrene of the toe (digital gangrene), which usually is caused by trauma. The toe is stubbed and then turns black (see Fig. 30-15). Usually, patients with this problem are older people without adequate circulation to provide revascularization. Débridement is contraindicated in these instances. Although the toe is gangrenous, it is dry. Managing dry gangrene is preferable to débriding the toe and causing an open wound that will not heal because of insufficient circulation. If the toe were to be amputated, the lack of adequate circulation would prevent healing and might make further amputation necessary—a below-knee or an above-knee amputation. A higher-level amputation in an older adult could result in a loss of independence and possibly the need for institutional care. Dry gangrene of the toe in an older adult with poor circulation is usually left undisturbed. The nurse keeps the toe clean and dry until it separates (without creating an open wound).

Topical Therapy

A variety of topical agents can be used in conjunction with cleansing and débridement therapies to promote healing of leg ulcers. The goals of treatment are to remove devitalized tissue and to keep the ulcer clean and moist while healing takes place. The treatment should not destroy developing tissue. For topical treatments to be successful, adequate nutritional therapy must be maintained.

Wound Dressing

After the circulatory status has been assessed and determined to be adequate for healing (ABI of more than 0.5) (Mosti, Iabichella, & Partsch, 2012), surgical dressings can be used to promote a moist environment. Semiocclusive or occlusive wound dressings prevent evaporative water loss from the wound and retain warmth; these factors favor healing. When determining the appropriate dressing to apply, the following should be considered: simplicity of application, frequency of required dressing changes, ability to absorb wound drainage, expense, and patient comfort. Available options that promote the growth of granulation tissue and re-epithelialization include the hydrocolloids (e.g., Comfeel, DuoDERM CGF, Restore, Tegasorb). These materials also provide a barrier for protection because they adhere to the wound bed and surrounding tissue. Semiper-meable film dressings (e.g., Bioclusive, OpSite, Tegaderm) may be selected because they keep the wound moist and are impervious to bacteria while allowing some gas exchange. However, they may not be effective treatment for deep wounds and infected wounds.

Growth factor dressings (e.g., OASIS, becaplermin [Regranex], keratinocyte lysate) may directly provide a growth factor, or they may stimulate important growth substances within the wound. In a multicenter registry of patients with chronic, mixed wounds, there was a positive response within 2.2 weeks in 96% of wounds treated an average of 2.8 times with a platelet-rich plasma gel, which is a type of growth factor topically applied to the wounds (De Leon, Driver, Fylling, et al., 2011).

Knowledge deficit, frustration, fear, and depression can decrease the patient's and family's compliance with the prescribed therapy; therefore, patient and family education is necessary before beginning and throughout the wound care program.

Stimulated Healing

Tissue-engineered human skin equivalent (e.g., Apligraf, Graftskin) is a skin product cultured from human dermal fibroblasts and keratinocytes used in combination with ther-apeutic compression. When applied, it interacts with the patient's cells within the wound to stimulate the production of growth factors. Application is not difficult, no suturing is involved, and the procedure is painless. PriMatrix is a bio-active and regenerative extracellular matrix that binds with the patient's own cells and growth factors. PriMatrix has been used successfully for tunneling wounds, as well as wounds with exposed tendon and bone, in which Apligraf cannot be used (Karr, 2011).

Hyperbaric Oxygenation

Hyperbaric oxygenation (HBO) may be beneficial as an adjunct treatment in patients with diabetes with no signs of wound healing after 30 days of standard wound treatment. HBO is accomplished by placing the patient into a cham-ber that increases barometric pressure while the patient is breathing 100% oxygen. Treatment regimens vary from 90 to 120 minutes once daily for 30 to 90 sessions. The process by which HBO is thought to work involves several factors. The edema in the wound area is decreased because high oxygen tension facilitates vasoconstriction and enhances the ability of leukocytes to phagocytize and kill bacteria. In addition, HBO is thought to increase diffusion of oxygen to the hypoxic wound, thereby enhancing epithelial migration and improving collagen production. The two most common adverse effects of HBO are middle ear barotrauma and con-finement anxiety. Patients may also experience worsening of

shortsightedness; this is rarely permanent (O'Reilly, Linden, Fedorko, et al., 2011).

Negative Pressure Wound Therapy

Research findings suggest that negative pressure wound ther-apy using vacuum-assisted closure (VAC) devices decreases time to healing in complex wounds that have not healed in a 3-week period. Groin incisions, common in vascular surgery, may be complicated by wound dehiscence, lymphatic fistula, or infections in 5% to 10% of patients. Wound VAC ther-apy has been found to be effective in treating patients who develop postoperative groin wound infections, decreasing hospital lengths of stay, rates of graft infection, and likelihood of limb loss (Dosluoglu, Loghmanee, Lall, 2010). Ambulatory patients may be given the small, portable VAC devices that can be strapped around the waist, giving patients the freedom to perform their ADLs.

NURSING PROCESS

The Patient With Leg Ulcers

Assessment

A careful nursing history and assessment are important. The extent and type of pain are carefully assessed, as are the appearance and temperature of the skin of both legs. The quality of all peripheral pulses is assessed, and the pulses in both legs are compared. The legs are checked for edema. If the extremity is edematous, the degree of edema is deter-mined. Any limitation of mobility and activity that results from vascular insufficiency is identified. The patient's nutri-tional status is assessed, and a history of diabetes, collagen disease, or varicose veins is obtained.

Diagnosis

Nursing Diagnoses
Based on the assessment data, major nursing diagnoses may include:
- Impaired skin integrity related to vascular insufficiency
- Impaired physical mobility related to activity restric-tions of the therapeutic regimen and pain
- Imbalanced nutrition: less than body requirements, related to increased need for nutrients that promote wound healing

Collaborative Problems/Potential Complications
Potential complications may include the following:
- Infection
- Gangrene

Planning and Goals

The major goals for the patient may include restoration of skin integrity, improved physical mobility, adequate nutri-tion, and absence of complications.

Nursing Interventions

The nursing challenge in caring for these patients is great, whether the patient is in the hospital, in a long-term care facility, or at home. The physical problem is often a long-term and disabling one that causes a substantial drain on the patient's physical, emotional, and economic resources.

Restoring Skin Integrity

To promote wound healing, measures are used to keep the area clean. Cleansing requires very gentle handling, a mild soap, and lukewarm water. Positioning of the legs depends on whether the ulcer is of arterial or venous origin. If there is arterial insufficiency, the patient should be referred for evaluation for vascular reconstruction. If there is venous insufficiency, dependent edema can be avoided by elevating the lower extremities. A decrease in edema promotes the exchange of cellular nutrients and waste products in the area of the ulcer, promoting healing.

Avoiding trauma to the lower extremities is imperative in promoting skin integrity. Protective boots may be used (e.g., Rooke vascular boot); they are soft and provide warmth and protection from injury and displace tissue pressure to prevent ulcer formation. If the patient is on bed rest, it is important to relieve pressure on the heels to prevent pressure ulcerations. When the patient is in bed, a bed cradle can be used to relieve pressure from bed linens and to prevent anything from touching the legs. When the patient is ambulatory, all obstacles are moved from the patient's path so that the patient's legs are not bumped. Heating pads, hot water bottles, or hot baths are avoided, because they increase the oxygen demands and thus the blood flow demands of the already compromised tissue. The patient with diabetes suffers from neuropathy with decreased sensation, and heating pads may produce injury before the patient is aware of being burned.

Improving Physical Mobility

Generally, physical activity is initially restricted to promote healing. When infection resolves and healing begins, ambulation should resume gradually and progressively. Activity promotes arterial flow and venous return and is encouraged after the acute phase of the ulcer process. Until full activity is resumed, the patient is encouraged to move about when in bed, to turn from side to side frequently, and to exercise the upper extremities to maintain muscle tone and strength. Meanwhile, diversional activities are encouraged. Consultation with an occupational therapist may be helpful if prolonged immobility and inactivity are anticipated.

If pain limits the patient's activity, analgesic agents may be prescribed. The pain of peripheral vascular disease is typically chronic and often disabling. Analgesic agents may be taken before scheduled activities to help the patient participate more comfortably.

Promoting Adequate Nutrition

Nutritional deficiencies are common, requiring dietary alterations to remedy them. A diet that is high in protein, vitamins C and A, iron, and zinc is encouraged to promote healing. Many patients with peripheral vascular disease are older adults. Particular consideration should be given to their iron intake, because many older people are anemic. After a dietary plan has been developed that meets the patient's nutritional needs and promotes healing, diet instruction is provided to the patient and family.

Promoting Home and Community-Based Care

The self-care program is planned with the patient so that activities that promote arterial and venous circulation, relieve pain, and promote tissue integrity are encouraged. Reasons for each aspect of the program are explained to the patient and family. Leg ulcers are often chronic and difficult to heal; they frequently recur, even when the patient rigorously follows the plan of care. Long-term care of the feet and legs to promote healing of wounds and prevent recurrence of ulcerations is the primary goal. Leg ulcers increase the patient's risk of infection, may be painful, and may limit mobility, necessitating lifestyle changes. Participation of family members and home health care providers may be necessary for treatments such as dressing changes, reassessments, reinforcement of instruction, and evaluation of the effectiveness of the plan of care. Regular follow-up with a primary provider is necessary.

Evaluation

Expected patient outcomes may include:

1. Demonstrates restored skin integrity
   a. Exhibits absence of inflammation
   b. Exhibits absence of drainage; negative wound culture
   c. Avoids trauma to the legs
2. Increases physical mobility
   a. Progresses gradually to optimal level of activity
   b. Reports that pain does not impede activity
3. Attains adequate nutrition
   a. Selects foods high in protein, vitamins, iron, and zinc
   b. Discusses with family members dietary modifications that need to be made at home
   c. Plans, with the family, a diet that is nutritionally sound

Varicose Veins

Varicose veins (varicosities) are abnormally dilated, tortuous, superficial veins caused by incompetent venous valves (see Fig. 30-14). Most commonly, this condition occurs in the lower extremities, the saphenous veins, or the lower trunk, but it can occur elsewhere in the body, such as the esophagus (e.g., esophageal varices; see Chapter 49).

It is estimated that varicose veins occur in 16% to 46% of women and 12% to 40% of men with an increased incidence correlated with increased age (Fiebig, Krusche, Wolf, et al., 2010). The condition is most common in people whose occupations require prolonged standing, such as salespeople, hair stylists, teachers, nurses and ancillary medical personnel, and construction workers. A hereditary weakness of the vein wall may contribute to the development of varicosities, and it commonly occurs in several members of the same family. Varicose veins are rare before puberty. Pregnancy may cause varicosities because of hormonal effects related to decreased venous outflow, increased pressure by the gravid uterus, and increased blood volume (Bagaria & Bagaria, 2011).

Pathophysiology

Varicose veins may be primary (without involvement of deep veins) or secondary (resulting from obstruction of deep veins). A reflux of venous blood results in venous stasis. If only the superficial veins are affected, the person may have no symptoms but may be troubled by his or her appearance.

Clinical Manifestations

Symptoms, if present, may include dull aches, muscle cramps, increased muscle fatigue in the lower legs, ankle edema, and a feeling of heaviness of the legs. Nocturnal cramps are common. When deep venous obstruction results in varicose veins, the patient may develop the signs and symptoms of chronic venous insufficiency: edema, pain, pigmentation, and ulcerations. Susceptibility to injury and infection is increased.

Assessment and Diagnostic Findings

Diagnostic tests for varicose veins include the duplex ultrasound scan, which documents the anatomic site of reflux and provides a quantitative measure of the severity of valvular reflux. Venography is not routinely performed to evaluate for valvular reflux. However, when it is used, it involves injecting a radiopaque contrast agent into the leg veins so that the vein anatomy can be visualized by x-ray studies during various leg movements. CT venography can be helpful, especially if the pelvic venous structures are involved.

Prevention

The patient should avoid activities that cause venous stasis, such as wearing socks that are too tight at the top or that leave marks on the skin, crossing the legs at the thighs, and sitting or standing for long periods. Changing position frequently, elevating the legs 3 to 6 inches higher than heart level when they are tired, and getting up to walk for several minutes of every hour promote circulation. The patient is encouraged to walk 1 or 2 miles each day if there are no contraindications. Walking up the stairs rather than using the elevator or escalator is helpful, and swimming is good exercise.

Graduated compression stockings, especially knee-high stockings, are useful. The patient who is overweight should be encouraged to begin a weight reduction plan.

Medical Management

Ligation and Stripping

Surgery for varicose veins requires that the deep veins be patent and functional. The saphenous vein is ligated high in the groin, where the saphenous vein meets the femoral vein. In addition, the vein may be removed (stripped). After the vein is ligated, an incision is made 2 to 3 cm below the knee, and a metal or plastic wire is passed the full length of the vein to the point of ligation. The wire is then withdrawn, pulling (removing, stripping) the vein as it is removed. Pressure and elevation minimize bleeding during surgery.

Thermal Ablation

Thermal ablation is a nonsurgical approach using thermal energy. Radiofrequency ablation uses an electrical contact inside the vein. As the device is withdrawn, the vein is sealed. Laser ablation uses a laser fiber tip that seals the vein (decompressed). Topical gel may be used first to numb the skin along the course of the saphenous vein. To protect the surrounding tissue, several small punctures are made along the vein, and 100 to 200 mL of dilute lidocaine is delivered to the perivenous space using ultrasound guidance. The goal of this tumescent anesthesia (i.e., anesthesia that causes localized swelling) is to provide analgesia, thermal protection (the

cuff of fluid surrounds the veins and accompanying nerves), and extrinsic compression of the vein (Weiss, Weiss, Feied, et al., 2012). The saphenous vein is entered percutaneously near the knee using ultrasound guidance. A catheter is introduced into the saphenous vein and advanced to the saphenofemoral junction. The device is then activated and withdrawn, sealing the vein. Small bandages and graduated compression stockings are applied after the procedure. The patient is asked not to remove the stockings for at least 48 hours and then to rewrap the legs and wear the compression stockings while ambulatory for at least 3 weeks. Patients are ambulatory prior to being discharged from the outpatient facility and have no activity restrictions, except that swimming is discouraged for 3 weeks. Nonsteroidal anti-inflammatory medications such as ibuprofen (Motrin) are used as needed for pain. The patient is informed that bruising may occur along the course of the saphenous vein and that he or she may experience leg cramps for a few days and may find it difficult to straighten the knees for up to 1.5 weeks.

Sclerotherapy

Sclerotherapy involves injection of an irritating chemical into a vein to produce localized phlebitis and fibrosis, thereby obliterating the lumen of the vein. This treatment may be performed alone for small varicosities or may follow vein ablation, ligation, or stripping. Sclerosing is palliative rather than curative. Sclerotherapy is typically performed in an examination or procedure room and does not require sedation. After the sclerosing agent is injected, anti-embolism stockings are applied to the leg and are worn for approximately 5 days after the procedure. Graduated compression stockings are then worn for an additional 5 weeks. After sclerotherapy, walking activities are encouraged as prescribed to maintain blood flow in the leg and to dilute the sclerosing agent. Promising early studies suggest that foam sclerosant is more effective in achieving obliteration of varicose veins than liquid sclerosant; however, clinical trials continue to monitor foam sclerosant's effectiveness and it is not yet FDA approved (Nael & Rathbun, 2009).

Nursing Management

Ligation and stripping can be performed in an outpatient setting, or the patient may be admitted to the hospital on the day of surgery and discharged the next day if a bilateral procedure is to be performed and the patient is at high risk for postoperative complications. If the procedure is performed in an outpatient setting, nursing measures are the same as if the patient were hospitalized. Bed rest is discouraged, and the patient is encouraged to become ambulatory as soon as sedation has worn off. The patient is instructed to walk every hour for 5 to 10 minutes while awake for the first 24 hours if he or she can tolerate the discomfort, and then to increase walking and activity as tolerated. Graduated compression stockings are worn continuously for about 1 week after vein stripping. The nurse assists the patient to perform exercises and move the legs. The foot of the bed should be elevated. Standing and sitting are discouraged.

Promoting Comfort and Understanding

Analgesic agents are prescribed to help the patient move the affected extremities more comfortably. Dressings are inspected for bleeding, particularly at the groin, where the risk of bleeding is greatest. The nurse is alert for reported sensations of "pins and needles." Hypersensitivity to touch in the involved extremity may indicate a temporary or permanent nerve injury resulting from surgery, because the saphenous vein and nerve are close to each other in the leg.

Usually, the patient may shower after the first 24 hours. The patient is instructed to dry the incisions well with a clean towel using a patting technique rather than rubbing. Alternatively, the patient may be instructed to dry the area using a blow-dryer. Application of skin lotion is avoided until the incisions are completely healed to avoid infection. The patient is instructed to apply sunscreen or zinc oxide to the incisional area prior to sun exposure; otherwise, hyperpigmentation of the incision, scarring, or both may occur.

If the patient has undergone sclerotherapy, a burning sensation in the injected leg may be experienced for 1 or 2 days. The nurse may encourage the use of a mild analgesic medication as prescribed and walking to provide relief.

Promoting Home and Community-Based Care

Long-term venous compression is essential after discharge, and the patient needs to obtain adequate supplies of graduated compression stockings or elastic bandages. Exercise of the legs is necessary; the development of an individualized plan requires consultation with the patient and the health care team.

LYMPHATIC DISORDERS

The lymphatic system consists of a set of vessels that spread throughout most of the body, as described previously in this chapter (Anatomy of the Vascular System, Lymphatic Vessels section). The fluid drained from the interstitial space by the lymphatic system is called *lymph*. The flow of lymph depends on the intrinsic contractions of the lymph vessels, the contraction of muscles, respiratory movements, and gravity. The lymphatic system of the abdominal cavity maintains a steady flow of digested fatty food (chyle) from the intestinal mucosa to the thoracic duct. In other parts of the body, the lymphatic system's function is regional; the lymphatic vessels of the head, for example, empty into clusters of lymph nodes located in the neck, and those of the extremities empty into nodes of the axillae and the groin.

Lymphangitis and Lymphadenitis

Lymphangitis is an acute inflammation of the lymphatic channels. It arises most commonly from a focus of infection in an extremity. Usually, the infectious organism is a hemolytic streptococcus. The characteristic red streaks that extend up the arm or the leg from an infected wound outline the course of the lymphatic vessels as they drain.

The lymph nodes located along the course of the lymphatic channels also become enlarged, red, and tender (acute lymphadenitis). They can also become necrotic and form an abscess (suppurative lymphadenitis). The nodes involved most often are those in the groin, axilla, or cervical region.

Because these infections are nearly always caused by organisms that are sensitive to antibiotics, it is unusual to see abscess formation. Recurrent episodes of lymphangitis are often associated with progressive lymphedema. After acute attacks, a graduated compression stocking should be worn on the affected extremity for several months to prevent long-term edema.

Lymphedema and Elephantiasis

Lymphedema may be primary (congenital malformations) or secondary (acquired obstructions). Tissue swelling occurs in the extremities because of an increased quantity of lymph that results from obstruction of lymphatic vessels. It is especially marked when the extremity is in a dependent position. Initially, the edema is soft and pitting. As the condition progresses, the edema becomes firm, nonpitting, and unresponsive to treatment. The most common type is congenital lymphedema (lymphedema praecox), which is caused by hypoplasia of the lymphatic system of the lower extremity. This disorder is usually seen in women and first appears between 15 and 25 years of age (Raju, Furrh, & Neglen, 2012).

The obstruction may be in the lymph nodes and the lymphatic vessels. Sometimes, it is seen in the arm after an axillary node dissection (e.g., for breast cancer) and in the leg in association with varicose veins or chronic thrombophlebitis. In the latter case, the lymphatic obstruction usually is caused by chronic lymphangitis. Lymphatic obstruction caused by a parasite (filaria) is most frequently seen in the tropics. When chronic swelling is present, there may be frequent bouts of acute infection characterized by high fever and chills and increased residual edema after the inflammation has resolved. These lead to chronic fibrosis, thickening of the subcutaneous tissues, and hypertrophy of the skin. This condition, in which chronic swelling of the extremity recedes only slightly with elevation, is referred to as elephantiasis.

Medical Management

The goal of therapy is to reduce and control the edema and prevent infection. Active and passive exercises assist in moving lymphatic fluid into the bloodstream. External compression devices milk the fluid proximally from the foot to the hip or from the hand to the axilla. When the patient is ambulatory, custom-fitted graduated compression stockings or sleeves are worn; those with the highest compression strength (exceeding 40 mm Hg) are required. When the leg is affected, continuous bed rest with the leg elevated may aid in mobilizing the fluids. Manual lymphatic drainage performed by specially trained therapists is a technique designed to direct or shift the congested lymph through functioning lymphatics that have preserved drainage. Manual lymphatic drainage is incorporated in a sequential treatment approach used in combination with multilayer compression bandages, exercises, skin care, pressure gradient sleeves, and pneumatic pumps, depending on the severity and stage of the lymphedema (Rockson, 2010).

Pharmacologic Therapy

As initial therapy, the diuretic furosemide (Lasix) may be prescribed to prevent fluid overload due to mobilization of extracellular fluid. Diuretics have also been used along with elevation of the leg and the use of graduated compression stockings or sleeves. However, the use of diuretics alone has little benefit because their main action is to limit capillary filtration by decreasing the circulating blood volume. If lymphangitis or cellulitis is present, antibiotic therapy is initiated. The patient is taught to inspect the skin for evidence of infection.

Surgical Management

Surgery is performed if the edema is severe and uncontrolled by medical therapy, if mobility is severely compromised, or if infection persists. One surgical approach involves the excision of the affected subcutaneous tissue and fascia, with skin grafting to cover the defect. Another procedure involves the surgical relocation of superficial lymphatic vessels into the deep lymphatic system by means of a buried dermal flap to provide a conduit for lymphatic drainage.

Nursing Management

After surgery, the management of skin grafts and flaps is the same as when these therapies are used for other conditions. Antibiotics may be prescribed for 3 to 7 days (Winstanley, Maino, Ratner, et al., 2012). Constant elevation of the affected extremity and observation for complications are essential. Complications may include flap necrosis, hematoma or abscess under the flap, and cellulitis. The nurse instructs the patient or caregiver to inspect the dressing daily. Unusual drainage or any inflammation around the wound margin suggests infection and should be reported to the surgeon. The patient is informed that there may be a loss of sensation in the skin graft area. The patient is also instructed to avoid the application of heating pads or exposure to sun to prevent burns or trauma to the area.

CELLULITIS

Cellulitis is the most common infectious cause of limb swelling. Cellulitis can occur as a single isolated event or a series of recurrent events. It is sometimes misdiagnosed as recurrent thrombophlebitis or chronic venous insufficiency.

Pathophysiology

Cellulitis occurs when an entry point through normal skin barriers allows bacteria to enter and release their toxins in the subcutaneous tissues.

Clinical Manifestations

The acute onset of swelling, localized redness, and pain is frequently associated with systemic signs of fever, chills, and sweating. The redness may not be uniform and often skips areas. Regional lymph nodes may also be tender and enlarged.

Concept Mastery Alert

Cellulitis needs to be differentiated from lymphangitis. With cellulitis, the swelling and redness is localized and anatomically nonspecific. With lymphangitis, characteristic red streaks appear denoting the outline of the lymphatic vessels that are affected.

Medical Management

Mild cases of cellulitis can be treated on an outpatient basis with oral antibiotic therapy. If the cellulitis is severe, the patient is treated with IV antibiotics. The key to preventing recurrent episodes of cellulitis lies in adequate antibiotic therapy for the initial event and in identifying the site of bacterial entry. Cracks and fissures that occur in the skin between the toes must be examined as potential sites of bacterial entry. Other locations include drug use injection sites, contusions, abrasions, ulceration, ingrown toenails, and hangnails.

Nursing Management

The patient is instructed to elevate the affected area 3 to 6 inches above heart level and apply warm, moist packs to the site every 2 to 4 hours. Patients with sensory and circulatory deficits, such as those caused by diabetes and paralysis, should use caution when applying warm packs because burns may occur; it is advisable to use a thermometer or have a caregiver ensure that the temperature is not more than lukewarm. Education should focus on preventing a recurrent episode. The patient with peripheral vascular disease or diabetes should receive education or reinforcement about skin and foot care.

Critical Thinking Exercises

1 A 75-year-old man has been diagnosed with stenosis of his external iliac artery and is scheduled for an angiogram with a possible balloon angioplasty and stent placement. What factors would you consider when planning his postprocedure care, continuing care, and home care? If the patient is taking dabigatran (Pradaxa) for atrial fibrillation and has renal insufficiency (creatinine of 2.0 mg/dL) as a complication of diabetes, how would you address these factors in the plan of care?

2 **pq** A 72-year-old man with diabetes, hypertension, and stage III heart failure is newly admitted to a home health service after being discharged from the hospital 2 days ago for exacerbation of his heart failure. You are the home health nurse. During your assessment, you note that he has edema of his left leg (the left calf is 2 cm larger than the right calf), with hemosiderin stains on the lower one third of the calf. Further questioning reveals a previous diagnosis of left femoral DVT 2 years ago that was treated in the hospital. What are your priority assessments with this patient? What further information will you obtain from him? What additional information is needed as part of the physical examination to aid in determining the diagnosis and implementing a priority intervention?

3 **ebp** A 63-year-old man has been diagnosed with a 5.8- × 5.6-cm infrarenal aortic aneurysm and has been referred for treatment of his asymptomatic aneurysm. He was informed by the vascular provider that he needs to undergo a surgical or interventional procedure to treat this aneurysm. He tells you that he does not think he needs to have any treatment and states, "I feel fine, and if I did have a repair, I would have the endovascular approach as they don't have any problems." What is the strength of the evidence from the research literature that suggests how aortic aneurysms should be repaired? What size aneurysm requires surgical intervention? What is the strength of evidence from the research literature that compares open surgical repair with endovascular repair of aneurysms? What are the rates of complications for these methods of repair?

4 A 50-year-old man presents to the community clinic. He recently moved to the area and needs a physical examination prior to beginning a job as a truck driver. The patient is found to have a history of diabetes ("diet controlled") and has a 30-year history of smoking two packs of cigarettes per day (60-year pack-year history). Physical examination reveals blood pressure of 170/96 mm Hg, diminished femoral pulses, bilateral varicose veins, and 1+ pitting ankle edema. What additional information is needed as part of the history and physical examination? What risk factor modifications would you want to address with this patient?

Brunner Suite Resources

Explore these additional resources to enhance learning for this chapter:
- NCLEX-Style Questions and Other Resources on thePoint, http://thePoint.lww.com/Brunner13e
- Study Guide
- PrepU
- Clinical Handbook
- Handbook of Laboratory and Diagnostic Tests

References

*Asterisk indicates nursing research.

Books

Cronenwett, J. L., & Johnston, K. W. (2010). *Rutherford's vascular surgery* (7th ed., Vols. I and II). Philadelphia: Elsevier.

Mitchell, R. O. (2012). *Advanced hybrid and endovascular aortic surgery. A case-based approach.* Cincinnati: Tempus Fugit Medical, API.

Porth, C. M., & Matfin, G. (2009). *Pathophysiology: Concepts of altered health states* (8th ed.). Philadelphia: Lippincott Williams & Wilkins.

Rutherford, R. B. (2005). *Vascular surgery* (6th ed., Vols. 1 and 2). Philadelphia: W. B. Saunders.

Zierler, R. E. (2009). *Strandness's duplex scanning in vascular disorders* (4th ed.). Philadelphia: Lippincott Williams & Wilkins.

Journals and Electronic Documents

Alfirevic, Z., & Alfirevic, I. (2010). Hypercoagulable state, pathophysiology, classification and epidemiology. *Clinical Chemistry and Laboratory Medicine, 48*(Suppl. 1), S15–S26.

Arnaoutoglou, E., Kouvelos, G., Milionis, H., et al. (2011). Post-implantation syndrome following endovascular abdominal aortic aneurysm repair: Preliminary data. *Interactive Cardiovascular and Thoracic Surgery, 12,* 609–614.

Bagaria, S. J., & Bagaria, V. B. (2011, July 21). Strategies for diagnosis and prevention of venous thromboembolism during pregnancy. *Journal of Pregnancy,* Art. ID 206858, Available at: www.hindawi.com/journals

Bakst, R., Merola, J. F., Franks, A. G., et al. (2008). Raynaud's phenomenon: Pathogenesis and management. *Journal of the American Academy of Dermatology, 59,* 633–653.

Bronas, U. G., Treat-Jacobson, D., & Leon, A. S. (2011). Comparison of the effect of upper body ergometry aerobic training vs treadmill training on central cardiorespiratory improvement and walking distance in patients with claudication. *Journal of Vascular Surgery, 53*(6), 1557–1564.

Coady, M. A., Ikonomidis, J. S., Cheung, A. T., et al. (2010). Surgical management of descending thoracic aortic disease: Open and endovascular approaches. A scientific statement from the American Heart Association. *Circulation, 121,* 2780–2804.

Collins, N., & Eilender, E. (2012). Vitamin supplementation: The lingering questions in wound healing. *Ostomy Wound Management, 58*(6), 8–11.

Crowther, M. A., Ageno, W., Garcia, E., et al. (2009). Oral vitamin K versus placebo to correct excessive anticoagulation in patients receiving warfarin. *Annals of Internal Medicine, 150,* 293–300.

Czihal, M., & Hoffmann, U. (2011). Upper extremity deep venous thrombosis. *Vascular Medicine, 16*(3), 191–202.

De Leon, J. M., Driver, V. R., Fylling, C. P., et al. (2011). The clinical relevance of treating chronic wounds with an enhanced near-physiological concentration of platelet-rich plasma gel. *Advances in Skin & Wound Care, 23*(8), 357–368.

Dixon, M. (2011). Misdiagnosing aortic dissection: A fatal mistake. *Journal of Vascular Nursing, 29*(4), 139–145.

Dolinger, C., & Strider, D. V. (2010). Endovascular interventions for descending thoracic aortic aneurysms: The pivotal role of the clinical nurse in postoperative care. *Journal of Vascular Nursing, 28*(4), 147–153.

Dosluoglu, H. H., Loghmanee, C., Lall, P., et al., (2010). Management of early (<30 day) vascular groin infections using vacuum-assisted closure alone without muscle flap coverage in a consecutive patient series. *Journal of Vascular Surgery, 51*(5), 1160–1166.

Dusing, R. (2010). Optimizing blood pressure control through the use of fixed combinations. *Vascular Health and Risk Management, 6,* 321–325.

Fiebig, A., Krusche, P., Wolf, A., et al. (2010). Heritability of chronic venous disease. *Human Genetics, 127,* 669–674.

Gardner, A. W., Parker, D. E., Montgomery, P. S., et al. (2011). Efficacy of quantified home-based exercise and supervised exercise in patients with intermittent claudication. A randomized controlled trial. *Circulation, 123*(5), 491–498.

Gillespie, D. L. (2010). Venous ulcer diagnosis, treatment, and prevention of recurrences. *Journal of Vascular Surgery, 52*(14S), 8S–14S.

Gist, S., Tio-Matos, I., Falzgraf, S., et al. (2009). Wound care in the geriatric client. *Clinical Interventions in Aging, 4,* 269–287.

Gulseth, M. P., Wittkowsky, A. K., Fanikos, J., et al. (2011). Dabigatran etexilate in clinical practice: Confronting challenges to improve safety and effectiveness. *Pharmacotherapy, 31*(12), 1232–1249.

Henke, P. K., & Comerata, A. J. (2011). An update on etiology, prevention, and therapy of postthrombotic syndrome. *Journal of Vascular Surgery, 53*(5), 500–509.

Hiatt, W. R., Hirsch, A. T., Creager, M. A., et al. (2010). Effect of niacin ER/lovastatin on claudication symptoms in patients with peripheral arterial disease. *Vascular Medicine, 15*(3), 171–179.

Holbrook, A., Schulman, S., Witt, D. M., et al. (2012). Evidence-based management of anticoagulation therapy: Antithrombotic therapy and prevention of thrombus, 9th ed: American College of Chest Physicians Evidence-Based Clinical Practice Guidelines. *Chest, 141*(2 Suppl.), e152S–e184S.

Kahn, S. R. (2010). The post-thrombotic syndrome. *Hematology, 210*(1), 216–220.

Karr, J. C. (2011). Retrospective comparison of diabetic foot ulcer and venous stasis ulcer healing outcome between a dermal repair scaffold (PriMatrix) and a bilayer living cell therapy (Apligraf). *Advances in Skin & Wound Care, 24*(3), 119–125.

Keeling, A. N., Farrelly, C., Carr, J. C., et al. (2011). Technical considerations for lower limb multidetector computed tomographic angiography. *Vascular Medicine, 16*(1), 131–143.

Key, N. S., & Kasthuri, R. S. (2010). Current treatment of venous thromboembolism. *Arteriosclerosis, Thrombosis, and Vascular Biology, 30,* 372–375.

Kurlinsky, A. K., Miller, V. M., & Rooke, T. W. (2011). Acrocyanosis: The Flying Dutchman. *Vascular Medicine, 16*(4), 288–301.

Libby, P., Ridker, P. M., & Hansson, G. K. (2009). Inflammation in atherosclerosis. *Journal of the American College of Cardiology, 54*(23), 2129–2138.

Lippi, G., Favaloro, E. J., Montagnana, M., et al. (2010). C-reactive protein and venous thromboembolism: Causal or casual association? *Clinical Chemistry and Laboratory Medicine, 48*(12), 1693–1701.

Lipsky, B. A., & Hoey, C. (2009). Topical antimicrobial therapy for treating chronic wounds. *Clinical Infectious Diseases, 49*(15), 1541–1549.

*Lovell, M., Myers, K., Forbes, T. L., et al. (2011). Peripheral arterial disease: Application of the chronic care model. *Journal of Vascular Nursing, 29*(4), 147–152.

Mohler, E. R., Gornik, H. I., Gerhard-Herman, M. D., et al. (2012). ACCF/ACR/AIUM/ASE/ASN/ICAVL/SCAI/SCCT/SIR/SVM/SVS 2012 appropriate use criteria for peripheral vascular ultrasound and physiological testing part I: Arterial ultrasound and physiological testing. *Journal of the American College of Cardiology, 60,* 242–276.

Mosti, G., Iabichella, M. L., & Partsch, H. (2012). Compression therapy in mixed ulcers increases venous output and arterial perfusion. *Journal of Vascular Surgery*, 55(1), 122–128.

Mwipatayi, B. P., Thomas, S., Wong, J., et al. (2011). A comparison of covered versus bare expandable stents for the treatment of aortoiliac occlusive disease. *Journal of Vascular Surgery*, 54(6), 1561–1570.

Nael, R., & Rathbun, S. (2009). Effectiveness of foam sclerotherapy for the treatment of varicose veins. *Vascular Medicine*, 15(1), 27–32.

Olin, J. W., Allie, D. E., Belkin, M., et al. (2010). ACCF/AHA/ACR/SCAI/SIR/SVM/SVN/SVS 2010 performance measures for adults with peripheral artery disease: A report of the American College of Cardiology Foundation/American Heart Association Task Force on Performance Measures, the American College of Radiology, the Society for Cardiac Angiography and Interventions, the Society for Interventional Radiology, the Society for Vascular Medicine, the Society for Vascular Nursing, and the Society for Vascular Surgery (Writing Committee to Develop Performance Measures for Peripheral Arterial Disease). *Journal of the American College of Cardiology*, 56, 2147–2181.

Olin, J. W., & Sealove, B. A. (2010). Peripheral arterial disease: Current insight into the disease and its diagnosis and management. *Mayo Clinic Proceedings*, 85(7), 678–692.

O'Reilly, D., Linden, R., Fedorko, L., et al. (2011). A prospective, double blind, randomized, controlled clinical trial comparing standard wound care with adjunctive hyperbaric oxygen therapy (HBOT) to standard wound care only for the treatment of chronic, non-healing ulcers of the lower limb in patients with diabetes mellitus: A study protocol. *Trials*, 12, 69. Available at: www.trialsjournal.com/content/12/1/69

O'Rourke, M. F., Safar, M. E., & Dzau, V. (2010). The cardiovascular continuum extended: Aging effects on the aorta and microvasculature. *Vascular Medicine*, 15(6), 461–468.

Ortmann, J., Nuesch, E., Traupe, T., et al. (2012). Gender is an independent risk factor for distribution pattern and lesion morphology in chronic critical limb ischemia. *Journal of Vascular Surgery*, 55(1), 98–104.

Paraskevas, K. I., Mikhailidis, D. P., & Veith, F. J. (2011). Optimal statin type and dosage for vascular patients. *Journal of Vascular Surgery*, 53(3), 837–844.

Patterson, B. O., Hinchlifee, R., Loftus, I. M., et al. (2010). Indications for catheter-directed thrombolysis in the management of acute proximal deep venous thrombosis. *Arteriosclerosis, Thrombosis, and Vascular Biology*, 30, 669–674.

Pearce, W. H., Annambhotla, S., Kaufman, J. L., et al. (2012). Abdominal aortic aneurysm medication. *Medscape Reference*. Available at: emedicine.medscape.com/article/1979501-medication

Polillo, R., Brower, J., Benson, V., et al. (2011). Ultrasound-assisted thrombolysis of thrombus and pulmonary embolus. *Journal of Vascular Nursing*, 29(2), 73–80.

Powell, T., Glynn, R., Buring, J., et al. (2011). The relative importance of systolic versus diastolic blood pressure control and incident symptomatic peripheral artery disease in women. *Vascular Medicine*, 16(4), 239–246.

Prandoni, P., & Kahn, S. (2009). Post-thrombotic syndrome: Prevalence, prognostication and need for progress. *British Journal of Haematology*, 145, 286–295.

Qaseem, A., Chou, R., Humphrey, L., et al. (2011). Venous thromboembolism prophylaxis in hospitalized patients: A clinical practice guideline from the American College of Physicians. *Annals of Internal Medicine*, 155(9), 625–632.

Raju, S., Furrh, J. B., IV, & Neglen, P. (2012). Diagnosis and treatment of venous lymphedema. *Journal of Vascular Surgery*, 55(1), 141–149.

Ray, K. K., Seshasai, S. R., Erqou, S., et al. (2010). Statins and all-cause mortality in high-risk primary prevention. *Archives of Internal Medicine*, 170(12), 1024–1031.

Rice, V. H., & Stead, L. F. (2009). Nursing intervention for smoking cessation. *Cochrane Database of Systematic Reviews*, (1), CD001188. Available at: www.thecochranelibrary.com

Rivera-Bou, W. L., Cabanas, J. G., Villanueva, S. E., et al. (2012). Thrombolytic therapy in emergency medicine. *Medscape Reference*. Available at: emedicine.medscape.com/article/811234-overview

Rockson, S. G. (2010). Current concepts and future direction in the diagnosis and management of lymphatic vascular disease. *Journal of Vascular Medicine*, 15(3), 223–231.

Rundback, J. H., Nahl, D., & Yoo, V. (2011). Contrast induced nephropathy. *Journal of Vascular Surgery*, 54(2), 575–579.

Sen, U., Mishra, P., Tyagi, N., et al. (2010). Homocysteine to hydrogen sulfide or hypertension. *Cell Biochemistry and Biophysics*, 57(2–3), 49–58.

Singh, A., Khaja A., & Alpert, M. A. (2010). Cocaine and aortic dissection. *Vascular Medicine*, 15(2), 127–133.

Stillman, R. M., Pearce, W. H., Talavera, F., et al. (2012). Infrainguinal occlusive disease treatment and management. *Medscape Reference*. Available at: emedicine.medscape.com/article/460965-treatment

Suwanabol, P., Tefera, G., & Schwarze, M. L. (2010). Syndromes associated with the deep veins: Phlegmasia cerulea dolens, May-Thurner syndrome, and nutcracker syndrome. *Perspectives in Vascular Surgery and Endovascular Therapy*, 22(4), 223–230.

Van Es, J., Eerenberg, E. S., Kamphuisen, P. W., et al. (2011). How to prevent, treat, and overcome current clinical challenges of VTE. *Journal of Thrombosis and Haemostasis*, 9(Suppl. 1), 265–274.

Vardavas, C. I., & Panagiotakos, D. B. (2009). The causal relationship between passive smoking and inflammation on the development of cardiovascular disease: A review of the evidence. *Inflammation & Allergy Drug Targets*, 8(5), 328–333.

Weiss, M., Weiss, R., Feied, C. F., et al. (2012). Radiofrequency ablation therapy for varicose veins. *Medscape Reference*. Available at: emedicine.medscape.com/article/1085800-overview

Wilson, A. M., Sadrzadeh-Rafie, A. H., Myers, J., et al. (2011). Low lifetime recreational activity is a risk factor for peripheral arterial disease. *Journal of Vascular Surgery*, 54(2), 427–432.

Winstanley, D. A., Maino, K. L., Ratner, D., et al. (2012). The role of antibiotics in cutaneous surgery. *Medscape Reference*. Available at: emedicine.medscape.com/article/1127413-overview

Wong, I. K., Andriessen, A., Lee, D. T., et al. (2012). Randomized controlled trial comparing treatment outcome of two compression bandaging systems and standard care without compression in patients with leg ulcers. *Journal of Vascular Surgery*, 55(5), 1376–1385.

Zhu, T., Martinez, I., & Emmerich, J. (2009). Venous thromboembolism: Risk factors for recurrence. *Arteriosclerosis, Thrombosis, and Vascular Biology*, 29, 298–310.

Resources

American Venous Forum, www.veinforum.org
National Heart, Lung, and Blood Institute, www.nhlbi.nih.gov
Society for Vascular Nursing (SVN), www.svnnet.org
Society for Vascular Surgery (SVS), www.vascularweb.org
Society for Vascular Ultrasound (SVU), www.svunet.org
Vascular Disease Foundation, vasculardisease.org
Vascular Disease Foundation, Peripheral Arterial Disease (PAD) Coalition, vasculardisease.org/padcoalition

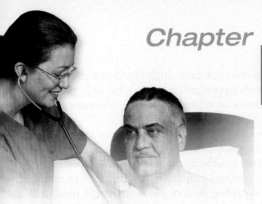

Assessment and Management of Patients With Hypertension

Learning Objectives

On completion of this chapter, the learner will be able to:

1 Define normal blood pressure and categories of abnormal pressures.
2 Identify risk factors for hypertension.
3 Explain the differences between normal blood pressure and hypertension and discuss the significance of hypertension.

4 Describe treatment approaches for hypertension, including lifestyle modifications and medication therapy.
5 Use the nursing process as a framework for care of the patient with hypertension.
6 Describe hypertensive crises and their treatment.

Glossary

dyslipidemia: abnormal blood lipid levels, including high total, low-density lipoprotein, and triglyceride levels as well as low high-density lipoprotein levels
glomerular filtration rate (GFR): flow rate of filtered fluid through the kidney, an indicator of renal function
hypertensive emergency: a situation in which blood pressure is severely elevated and there is evidence of actual or probable target organ damage
hypertensive urgency: a situation in which blood pressure is severely elevated but there is no evidence of target organ damage
isolated systolic hypertension: a condition most commonly seen in the older adult in which the

systolic pressure is greater than 140 mm Hg and the diastolic pressure is within normal limits (less than 90 mm Hg)
monotherapy: medication therapy with a single medication
primary hypertension: denotes high blood pressure from an unidentified cause; also called *essential hypertension*
rebound hypertension: blood pressure that is controlled with medication and becomes uncontrolled (abnormally high) with the abrupt discontinuation of medication
secondary hypertension: high blood pressure from an identified cause, such as renal disease

Hypertension is defined by the *Seventh Report of the Joint National Committee on Prevention, Detection, Evaluation, and Treatment of High Blood Pressure* (JNC 7) as a systolic blood pressure greater than 140 mm Hg and a diastolic pressure greater than 90 mm Hg based on the average of two or more accurate blood pressure measurements taken during two or more contacts with a health care provider (Chobanian, Bakris, Black, et al., 2003). Table 31-1 shows the classification of blood pressure established by JNC 7. The blood pressure categories, from normal to stage 2 hypertension, emphasize the direct relationship between levels of systolic and diastolic blood pressures and the risks of morbidity, all-cause mortality, and, more specifically, cardiovascular disease mortality. Although increasing levels of either systolic or diastolic pressure are risky, treatment that controls blood pressure is so effective that mortality has been found to be no different between treated hypertensive persons and normotensive persons (Barengo, Antikainen, Kastarinen, et al., 2013).

JNC 7 defines a blood pressure of less than 120/80 mm Hg diastolic as normal, 120 to 129/80 to 89 mm Hg as prehypertension, and 140/90 mm Hg or higher as hypertension (Chobanian et al., 2003) (see Table 31-1). The term *stage* is

used to define levels of hypertension; the classification system parallels that used to describe cancer progression so that both the public and health care professionals will understand that consistently higher elevations in blood pressure from prehypertension to stage 1 or 2 are associated with greater health risks. JNC 7 introduced the category of *prehypertension* to emphasize that people whose blood pressure begins to rise above 120/80 mm Hg are more likely to become hypertensive, and that even small increases in pressure are associated with an adverse risk factor profile as well as increased risk of stroke, heart attack, heart failure, and cardiovascular death (Pimenta & Oparil, 2010). To prevent or delay progression to hypertension and reduce risk, JNC 7 urged health care providers to encourage people with blood pressures in the prehypertension category to begin lifestyle modifications such as nutritional changes and exercise. JNC 7 recommended that people with stage 1 hypertension be treated with medications and be seen by their health care provider every month until their blood pressure goal is reached and subsequently about every 3 to 6 months. People with stage 2 hypertension or with other complicating conditions need to be seen more frequently.

TABLE 31-1	Classification of Blood Pressure for Adults Age 18 and Older*		
BP Classification*	**Systolic BP (mm Hg)**		**Diastolic BP (mm Hg)**
Normal	<120	and	<80
Prehypertension	120–139	or	80–89
Stage 1 hypertension	140–159	or	90–99
Stage 2 hypertension	≥160	or	≥100

BP, blood pressure.

*Based on the average of two or more properly measured, seated readings taken on each of two or more office visits.

Adapted from Chobanian, A. V., Bakris, G. L., Black, H. R., et al. (2003). Seventh Report of the Joint National Committee on Prevention, Detection, Evaluation, and Treatment of High Blood Pressure. *Hypertension, 42*(6), 1206–1252.

Hypertension

About 30% of the adults in the United States have hypertension, and the prevalence increases significantly as people get older or have other cardiovascular risk factors. Approximately 54% of persons with hypertension do not have their blood pressure under control as defined by JNC 7. The prevalence of uncontrolled hypertension varies by ethnicity, with Hispanics and African Americans having the highest prevalence at approximately 63% and 57%, respectively (Valderrama, Gillespie, King et al., 2012). A high percentage of persons with high blood pressure have **primary hypertension** (also called *essential hypertension*), which is defined as high blood pressure from an unidentified cause. The remaining small percentage, probably about 5% to 10%, have **secondary hypertension**, which occurs when a cause for the high blood pressure can be identified. These causes include renal parenchymal disease, narrowing of the renal arteries, hyperaldosteronism (mineralocorticoid hypertension), pheochromocytoma, certain medications (e.g., prednisone, epoetin alfa [Epogen]), and coarctation of the aorta (Sukor, 2011). High blood pressure can also occur with pregnancy; women who experience high blood pressure during pregnancy are at increased risk of ischemic heart disease, heart attacks, strokes, kidney disease, diabetes, and death from heart attack. (Männistö, Mendola, Väräsmäki, et al., 2013).

Hypertension is sometimes called the *silent killer* because people who have it are often symptom free. In the National Health and Nutrition Examination Survey (NHANES) conducted from 2003 to 2010, 39% of people who had pressures exceeding 140/90 mm Hg were unaware of their elevated blood pressure (Valderrama et al., 2012). Once identified, elevated blood pressure requires monitoring at regular intervals because hypertension is a lifelong condition.

Hypertension often accompanies other risk factors for atherosclerotic heart disease, such as **dyslipidemia** (abnormal blood lipid levels, including high total, low-density lipoprotein, and triglyceride levels as well as low high-density lipoprotein [HDL] levels), obesity, diabetes, metabolic syndrome, a sedentary lifestyle, and obstructive sleep apnea (Aronow, Fleg, Pepine, et al., 2011; Pedrosa, Krieger, Lorenzi-Filho, et al., 2011). The prevalence is also higher in persons who have other cardiovascular conditions, including heart failure, coronary artery disease, and a history of stroke.

Cigarette smoking does not cause high blood pressure; however, if a person with hypertension smokes, his or her risk of dying of heart disease or related disorders increases significantly (Fagard, 2009).

High blood pressure can be viewed as a sign, as a risk factor for atherosclerotic cardiovascular disease, or as a disease. As a sign, nurses and other health care professionals use blood pressure to monitor a patient's clinical status. Elevated pressure may indicate an excessive dose of vasoconstrictive medication, stress, or other problems. As a risk factor, hypertension contributes to the rate at which atherosclerotic plaque accumulates within arterial walls. As a disease, hypertension is a major contributor to death related to cardiac, cerebrovascular, renal, and peripheral vascular disease.

Prolonged blood pressure elevation gradually damages blood vessels throughout the body, particularly in target organs such as the heart, kidneys, brain, and eyes. Brain imaging research in Framingham Heart Study participants younger than 50 years has revealed early subtle brain injuries that likely predispose to cognitive decline and are directly associated with systolic blood pressure (Maillard, Seshadri, Beiser, et al., 2012). The typical outcomes of prolonged, uncontrolled hypertension are myocardial infarction, heart failure, renal failure, strokes, and impaired vision. Hypertrophy (enlargement) of the left ventricle of the heart may occur as it works to pump blood against the elevated pressure. (See Chapter 28 for discussion of assessment, diagnosis, and treatment of ventricular hypertrophy.)

Pathophysiology

Blood pressure is the product of cardiac output multiplied by peripheral resistance. Cardiac output is the product of the heart rate multiplied by the stroke volume. Each time the heart contracts, pressure is transferred from the contraction of the heart muscle to the blood and then pressure is exerted by the blood as it flows through the blood vessels. Hypertension can result from increases in cardiac output, increases in peripheral resistance (constriction of the blood vessels), or both. Increases in cardiac output are often related to an expansion in vascular volume. Although no precise cause can be identified for most cases of hypertension, it is understood that hypertension is a multifactorial condition. Because hypertension can be a sign, it is most likely to have many causes, just as fever has many causes.

For hypertension to occur, there must be a change in one or more factors affecting peripheral resistance or cardiac output. In addition, there must also be a problem with the body's control systems that monitor or regulate pressure (Fig. 31-1). More than 40 single gene mutations associated with hypertension have been identified, but most types of hypertension are thought to be polygenic (i.e., mutations in more than one gene) (Padmanabhan, Newton-Cheh, & Dominiczak, 2012). The tendency to develop hypertension is inherited; however, genetic profiles alone cannot predict who will and will not develop hypertension. In fact, researchers estimate that genetics play a role in explaining blood pressure variation between individuals in 15% to 70% of cases (Singh, Mensah, & Bakris, 2010).

Many causes of hypertension have been suggested:

- Increased sympathetic nervous system activity related to dysfunction of the autonomic nervous system

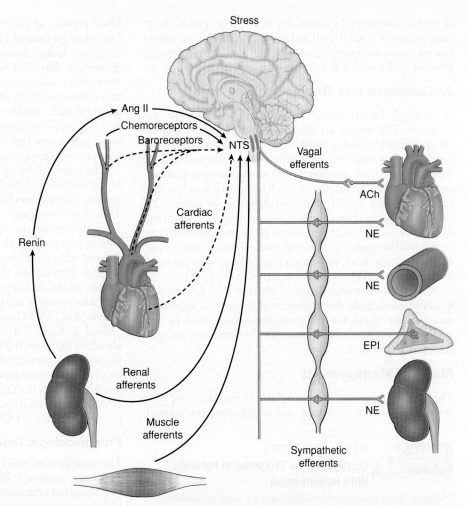

FIGURE 31-1 • Central and reflex mechanisms involved in the neural control of blood pressure. *Dotted arrows* represent inhibitory neural influences, and *solid arrows* represent excitatory neural influences on sympathetic outflow. EPI, epinephrine; NTS, nucleus tractus solitarius; NE, norepinephrine; ACh, acetylcholine. Adapted from Kaplan, N. M., & Victor, R. G. (2010). *Kaplan's clinical hypertension* (9th ed.). Philadelphia: Lippincott Williams & Wilkins.

- Increased renal reabsorption of sodium, chloride, and water related to a genetic variation in the pathways by which the kidneys handle sodium
- Increased activity of the renin–angiotensin–aldosterone system, resulting in expansion of extracellular fluid volume and increased systemic vascular resistance
- Decreased vasodilation of the arterioles related to dysfunction of the vascular endothelium
- Resistance to insulin action, which may be a common factor linking hypertension, type 2 diabetes, hypertriglyceridemia, obesity, and glucose intolerance
- Activation of the innate and adaptive components of the immune response that may contribute to renal inflammation and dysfunction (Leibowitz & Schiffrin, 2011)

 Gerontologic Considerations

Structural and functional changes in the heart, blood vessels, and kidneys contribute to increases in blood pressure that occur with aging. These changes include accumulation of atherosclerotic plaque, fragmentation of arterial elastins, increased collagen deposits, impaired vasodilation, and renal dysfunction. The result of these changes is decreased elasticity of the major blood vessels and volume expansion (Aronow et al., 2011). Consequently, the aorta and large arteries are less able to accommodate the volume of blood pumped out by the heart (stroke volume), and the energy that would have stretched the vessels instead elevates the systolic blood pressure, resulting in an elevated systolic pressure without a change in diastolic pressure. This condition, known as **isolated systolic hypertension**, is more common in older adults and is associated with significant cardiovascular and cerebrovascular morbidity and mortality (Chobanian et al., 2003).

Clinical Manifestations

Physical examination may reveal no abnormalities other than elevated blood pressure. Occasionally, retinal changes such as hemorrhages, exudates (fluid accumulation), arteriolar narrowing, and cotton-wool spots (small infarctions) occur. In severe hypertension, papilledema (swelling of the optic disc) may be seen. People with hypertension may be asymptomatic and remain so for many years. However, when specific signs and symptoms appear, they usually indicate vascular damage, with specific manifestations related to the organs served by the involved vessels. Coronary artery disease with angina and myocardial infarction are common consequences of hypertension. Left ventricular hypertrophy occurs in response to the increased workload placed on the ventricle as it contracts against higher systemic pressure. When heart damage is extensive, heart failure follows. Pathologic changes in the kidneys (indicated by increased blood urea nitrogen [BUN] and serum creatinine levels) may manifest as nocturia. Cerebrovascular involvement may lead to a transient ischemic attack (TIA) or stroke, manifested by alterations in vision or speech, dizziness, weakness, a sudden fall, or transient or permanent paralysis on one side (hemiplegia). Cerebral infarctions account for most of the strokes in patients with hypertension.

Assessment and Diagnostic Findings

A thorough health history and physical examination are necessary. The retinas are examined and laboratory studies are performed to assess possible target organ damage. Routine laboratory tests include urinalysis, blood chemistry (i.e., analysis of sodium, potassium, creatinine, fasting glucose, and total and HDL cholesterol levels), and a 12-lead electrocardiogram. Left ventricular hypertrophy can be assessed by echocardiography. Renal damage may be suggested by elevations in BUN and creatinine levels or by microalbuminuria or macroalbuminuria. Additional studies, such as creatinine clearance, renin level, urine tests, and 24-hour urine protein, may be performed (Bonow, Mann, Zipes, et al., 2012).

A risk factor assessment, as advocated by JNC 7, is needed to classify and guide the treatment of those with hypertension who are at risk for cardiovascular damage. Risk factors and cardiovascular problems related to hypertension are presented in Chart 31-1.

Medical Management

The goal of hypertension treatment is to prevent complications and death by achieving and maintaining the arterial

---

RISK FACTORS

Chart 31-1

Cardiovascular Problems in Patients With Hypertension

Major Risk Factors (in Addition to Hypertension)

- Smoking
- Dyslipidemia (elevated LDL [or total] cholesterol and/or low HDL cholesterol)*
- Diabetes*
- Impaired renal function (GFR <60 mL/min and/or microalbuminuria)
- Obesity (BMI ≥30 kg/m²)*
- Physical inactivity
- Age (>55 years for men, >65 years for women)
- Family history of cardiovascular disease (in female relative <65 years or male relative <55 years)

Target Organ Damage or Clinical Cardiovascular Disease

- Heart disease (left ventricular hypertrophy, angina or previous myocardial infarction, previous coronary revascularization, heart failure)
- Stroke (cerebrovascular accident, brain attack) or TIA
- Chronic kidney disease
- Peripheral arterial disease
- Retinopathy

*These risk factors plus hypertension, elevated triglyceride levels, and abdominal obesity are components of the metabolic syndrome.
LDL, low-density lipoprotein; HDL, high-density lipoprotein; GFR, glomerular filtration rate; BMI, body mass index; TIA, transient ischemic attack.
Adapted from Table 6 of Chobanian, A. V., Bakris, G. L., Black, H. R., et al. (2003). Seventh Report of the Joint National Committee on Prevention, Detection, Evaluation, and Treatment of High Blood Pressure. *Hypertension, 42*(6), 1206–1252.

---

blood pressure at 140/90 mm Hg or lower. JNC 7 specifies a lower goal pressure of 130/80 mm Hg for people with diabetes or chronic kidney disease, which is defined as either a reduced **glomerular filtration rate (GFR)** (flow rate of filtered fluid through the kidney, an indicator of renal function) resulting in a serum creatinine of greater than 1.3 mg/dL in women or greater than 1.5 mg/dL in men, or albuminuria of greater than 300 mg/day (Chobanian et al., 2003). The optimal management plan is one that is inexpensive, simple, and causes the least possible disruption in the patient's life.

The management options for hypertension are summarized in the treatment algorithm issued by JNC 7 (Fig. 31-2); these include lifestyle modifications and pharmacologic therapy. Table 31-2 summarizes recommended lifestyle modifications. The clinician uses the algorithm with the risk factor assessment data and the patient's blood pressure category to choose the initial and subsequent treatment plans for the patient. Research findings demonstrate that weight loss, reduced alcohol and sodium intake, and regular physical activity are effective lifestyle adaptations to reduce blood pressure (Appel, Champagne, Harsha, et al., 2003; Coxson, Cook, Joffres, et al., 2013; Hedayati, Elsayed, & Reilly, 2011; Kawano, 2010; Knight, 2012). Studies also show that diets high in fruits, vegetables, and low-fat dairy products can prevent the development of hypertension and lower elevated blood pressure (Appel, Sacks, Carey, et al., 2005). Table 31-3 shows the Dietary Approaches to Stop Hypertension (DASH) diet, which has been shown to lower blood pressure in people who follow it (Appel et al., 2003).

Pharmacologic Therapy

The medications used for treating hypertension decrease peripheral resistance, blood volume, or the strength and rate of myocardial contraction. For patients with uncomplicated hypertension and no specific indications for another medication, the recommended initial medications include diuretics, beta-blockers, or both. Patients are first given low doses of medication. If blood pressure does not fall to less than 140/90 mm Hg, the dose is increased gradually and additional medications are included as necessary to achieve control. Table 31-4 describes the various pharmacologic agents that are recommended for the treatment of hypertension. When the blood pressure is less than 140/90 mm Hg for at least 1 year, gradual reduction of the types and doses of medication is indicated. To promote adherence to the regimen, clinicians try to prescribe the simplest treatment schedule possible, ideally one pill once each day. The pill may be a single agent or two or more agents combined into a single pill (Egan, Bandyopadhyay, Shaftman, et al., 2012).

 Gerontologic Considerations

Hypertension, particularly elevated systolic blood pressure, increases the risk of death, stroke, and heart failure in people older than 50 years, and treatment reduces this risk (Chobanian et al., 2003). Like younger patients, older patients should begin treatment with lifestyle modifications. If medications are needed to achieve the blood pressure goal of less than 140/90 mm Hg, the starting dose should be the lowest available and then gradually increased with a second medication from a different class added if control is difficult to achieve. It is recommended that a diuretic be included as either the first or second treatment choice. As older adults often have other comorbid

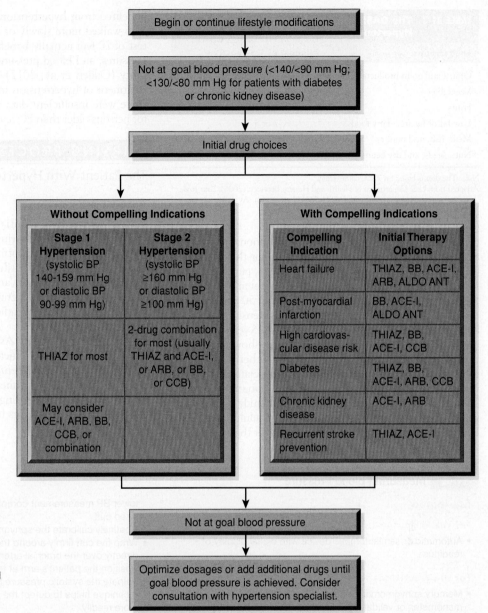

FIGURE 31-2 • Algorithm of hypertension treatment. Treatment begins with lifestyle modifications and continues with various medication regimens. ACE-I, angiotensin-converting enzyme inhibitor; ALDO ANT, aldosterone antagonist; ARB, angiotensin receptor blocker; BB, beta-blocker; BP, blood pressure; CCB, calcium channel blocker; THIAZ, thiazide diuretic. Adapted from Seventh Report of the Joint National Committee on Prevention, Detection, Evaluation, and Treatment of High Blood Pressure (JNC7). Reference card available from the National, Heart, Lung, and Blood Institute. Available at: www.nhlbi.nih.gov/guidelines/hypertension/phycard.pdf

TABLE 31-2 Lifestyle Modifications to Prevent and Manage Hypertension*

Modification	Recommendation	Goal of SBP Reduction (Range)†
Weight reduction	Maintain normal body weight (body mass index 18.5–24.9 kg/m²).	5–20 mm Hg/10 kg
Adopt DASH eating plan	Consume a diet rich in fruits, vegetables, and low-fat dairy products with a reduced content of saturated and total fat.	8–14 mm Hg
Dietary sodium reduction	Reduce dietary sodium intake to ≤100 mmol/day (2.4 g sodium or 6 g sodium chloride).	2–8 mm Hg
Physical activity	Engage in regular aerobic physical activity such as brisk walking (≥30 min/d, most days of the week).	4–9 mm Hg
Moderation of alcohol consumption	Limit consumption to ≤2 drinks (e.g., 24 oz beer, 10 oz wine, or 3 oz 80-proof whiskey) per day in most men and to ≤1 drink per day in women and lighter-weight people.	2–4 mm Hg

SBP, systolic blood pressure; DASH, Dietary Approaches to Stop Hypertension.
*For overall cardiovascular risk reduction, stop smoking.
†The effects of implementing these modifications are dose and time dependent and could be greater for some individuals.
Adapted from Chobanian, A. V., Bakris, G. L., Black, H. R., et al. (2003). Seventh Report of the Joint National Committee on Prevention, Detection, Evaluation, and Treatment of High Blood Pressure. *Hypertension, 42*(6), 1206–1252.

TABLE 31-3	The DASH (Dietary Approaches to Stop Hypertension) Diet	
Food Group		**Number of Servings/Day**
Grains and grain products		7 or 8
Vegetables		4 or 5
Fruits		4 or 5
Low-fat or fat-free dairy foods		2 or 3
Meat, fish, and poultry		≤2
Nuts, seeds, and dry beans		4 or 5 weekly

Note: The diet is based on 2,000 calories/day.
Adapted from U.S. Department of Health and Human Services. (2006). *Your guide to lowering your blood pressure with DASH: DASH eating plan.* Available at: www.nhlbi.nih.gov/health/public/heart/hbp/dash/new_dash.pdf

conditions, awareness of possible drug interactions is critical. In addition, older adults are at increased risk for the side effects of hyperkalemia and orthostatic hypotension, putting them at increased risk for falls and fractures (Aronow et al., 2011).

Compared to people between the ages of 50 and 75 years, there has been much less research on hypertension treatment and appropriate goals in persons older than 75 years. Research results have been contradictory, with some showing a reduction in morbidity and mortality, whereas other studies have found either no benefit or increased risk associated with treatment (Goodwin, 2012). One possible explanation for these discrepant results may be the health of the study participants. Odden and colleagues (2012) found that adults older than 65 years who were able to walk briskly (faster than 0.8 m/sec)

benefited from hypertension treatment. Survey participants who walked more slowly or who could not complete a walk test of 20 feet actually benefited from having elevated blood pressures, and blood pressure treatment did not reduce mortality (Odden et al., 2012). A consensus document on the treatment of hypertension in the older adult concluded that there were insufficient data to establish blood pressure goals for persons older than 80 years (Aronow et al., 2011).

NURSING PROCESS

The Patient With Hypertension

Assessment

When hypertension is initially detected, nursing assessment involves carefully monitoring the blood pressure at frequent intervals and then at routinely scheduled intervals. When the patient begins an antihypertensive treatment regimen, blood pressure assessments are needed to determine the effectiveness of medication therapy and to detect any changes in blood pressure that may indicate the need for a modification in the treatment plan.

The American Heart Association has defined the standards for blood pressure measurement, including conditions required before measurements are made, equipment specifications, and techniques for measuring blood pressure to obtain accurate and reliable readings (Pickering, Hall, Appel, et al., 2005) (Chart 31-2). Errors in measurement can occur when

(text continues on page 870)

Chart 31-2 Measuring Blood Pressure

Equipment

For the Patient at Home
- Automatic or semiautomatic device with digital display of readings

For the Practitioner
- Mercury sphygmomanometer, recently calibrated aneroid manometer, or validated electronic device
- Appropriately sized cuff

Instructions for the Patient

- Avoid smoking cigarettes or drinking caffeine for 30 minutes before blood pressure (BP) is measured.
- Sit quietly for 5 minutes before the measurement.
- Sit comfortably with the forearm supported at heart level on a firm surface, with both feet on the ground; avoid talking while the measurement is being taken.

Instructions for the Practitioner

- Select the size of the cuff based on the size of the patient. (The cuff size should have a bladder width of at least 40% of limb circumference and length at least 80% of limb circumference.) The average adult cuff is 12 to 14 cm wide and 30 cm long. Using a cuff that is too small will give a higher BP measurement, and using a cuff that is too large results in a

lower BP measurement compared to one taken with a properly sized cuff.
- Routinely calibrate the sphygmomanometer.
- Wrap the cuff firmly around the arm. Center the cuff bladder directly over the brachial artery.
- Position the patient's arm at the level of the heart.
- Palpate the systolic pressure before auscultating. This technique helps to detect the presence of an auscultatory gap more readily.
- Ask the patient to sit quietly while the BP is measured, because the BP can increase when the patient is engaged in conversation.
- Initially, record BP results of both arms and take subsequent measurements from the arm with the higher BP. Normally, the BP should vary by no more than 5 mm Hg between arms.
- Record the site where the BP was measured and the position of the patient (i.e., right arm).
- Inform the patient of his or her BP value and what it means. Emphasize the need for periodic reassessment, and encourage patients who measure BP at home to keep a written record of readings.

Interpretation

Assessment is based on the average of at least two readings. (If two readings differ by more than 5 mm Hg, additional readings are taken and an average reading is calculated from the results.)

Adapted from Pickering, T. G., Hall, J. E., Appel, L. J., et al. (2005). Recommendations for blood pressure measurement in humans and experimental animals: Part 1: Blood pressure measurement in humans: A statement for professionals from the Subcommittee of Professional and Public Education of the American Heart Association Council on High Blood Pressure Research. *Hypertension, 45*(1), 142–161.

TABLE 31-4   Medication Therapy for Hypertension

Medications	Major Action	Advantages and Contraindications	Effects and Nursing Considerations
Diuretics and Related Drugs			
Thiazide Diuretics chlorthalidone chlorothiazide (Diuril) hydrochlorothiazide indapamide methyclothiazide metolazone (Zaroxolyn)	Decrease of blood volume, renal blood flow, and cardiac output Depletion of extracellular fluid Negative sodium balance (from natriuresis), mild hypokalemia Directly affect vascular smooth muscle	Relatively inexpensive Effective orally Effective during long-term administration Mild side effects Enhance other antihypertensive medications Counter sodium retention effects of other antihypertensive medications *Contraindications:* Gout, known sensitivity to sulfonamide-derived medications, severely impaired kidney function, and history of hyponatremia	Side effects include dry mouth, thirst, weakness, drowsiness, lethargy, muscle aches, muscular fatigue, tachycardia, GI disturbance. Postural hypotension may be potentiated by alcohol, barbiturates, opioids, or hot weather. Because thiazides cause loss of sodium, potassium, and magnesium, monitor for signs of electrolyte imbalance. Encourage intake of potassium-rich foods (i.e., fruits). *Gerontologic considerations:* Risk of postural hypotension is significant because of volume depletion; measure blood pressure in 3 positions; caution patient to rise slowly.
Loop Diuretics furosemide (Lasix) bumetanide (Bumex) torsemide (Demadex)	Volume depletion Blocks reabsorption of sodium, chloride, and water in kidney	Action rapid Potent Used when thiazides fail or patient needs rapid diuresis *Contraindications:* Same as for thiazides	There is risk of volume and electrolyte depletion from the profound diuresis that can occur. Fluid and electrolyte replacement may be required. *Gerontologic considerations:* Same as for thiazides
Potassium-Sparing Diuretics amiloride (Midamor) triamterene (Dyrenium)	Blocks sodium reabsorption Acts on distal tubule independently of aldosterone	Causes potassium retention *Contraindications:* Renal disease, azotemia, severe hepatic disease, hyperkalemia	Drowsiness, lethargy, headache Monitor for hyperkalemia if given with ACE inhibitor or angiotensin receptor blocker. Diarrhea and other GI symptoms—administer medication after meals.
Aldosterone Receptor Blockers eplerenone (Inspra) spironolactone (Aldactone)	Competitive inhibitors of aldosterone binding	Indicated for patients with a history of myocardial infarction or symptomatic ventricular dysfunction *Contraindications:* Hyperkalemia and impaired renal function Eplerenone is contraindicated in diabetes with microalbuminuria.	Drowsiness, lethargy, headache Monitor for hyperkalemia if given with ACE inhibitor or angiotensin receptor blocker. Diarrhea and other GI symptoms—administer medication after meals. Avoid the use of potassium supplements or salt substitutes. Educate patients, families, and caregivers about the signs and symptoms of hyperkalemia. Spironolactone may cause gynecomastia.
Central Alpha$_2$-Agonists and Other Centrally Acting Drugs			
reserpine (Harmonyl)	Impairs synthesis and reuptake of norepinephrine	Slows pulse, which counteracts tachycardia of hydralazine *Contraindications:* History of depression, psychosis, obesity, chronic sinusitis, peptic ulcer	May cause severe depression; report manifestations, as this may require that drug be discontinued. Nasal congestion Use with caution if history of gallbladder, renal, or cardiac disease, or seizure disorder. *Gerontologic considerations:* Depression and postural hypotension is common in older adults.

(continues on page 868)

TABLE 31-4 Medication Therapy for Hypertension (continued)

Medications	Major Action	Advantages and Contraindications	Effects and Nursing Considerations
Central Alpha₂-Agonists and Other Centrally Acting Drugs			
methyldopa (Aldomet)	Dopa decarboxylase inhibitor; displaces norepinephrine from storage sites	Drug of choice for pregnant women with hypertension Useful in patients with renal failure or prostate disease Does not decrease cardiac output or renal blood flow Does not induce oliguria *Contraindications:* Liver disease	Drowsiness, dizziness Dry mouth; nasal congestion (troublesome at first but then tends to disappear) Use with caution with renal disease. *Gerontologic considerations:* May produce mental and behavioral changes in the older adult.
clonidine (Catapres) clonidine patch (Catapres-TTS)	Exact mode of action is not understood, but acts through the central nervous system, apparently through centrally mediated alpha-adrenergic stimulation in the brain, producing blood pressure reduction.	Little or no orthostatic effect; moderately potent, and sometimes is effective when other medications fail to lower blood pressure. *Contraindications:* Severe coronary artery disease, pregnancy	Dry mouth, drowsiness, sedation, and occasional headaches and fatigue. Anorexia, malaise, and vomiting with mild disturbance of liver function have been reported. Rebound or withdrawal hypertension is relatively common; monitor blood pressure when stopping medication. Common side effects include dry mouth, dizziness, sleepiness, fatigue, headache, constipation, and impotence.
guanfacine (Tenex)	Stimulates central alpha₂-adrenergic receptors	Reduces heart rate and causes vasodilation. Serious adverse reactions are uncommon; use with caution in persons with diminished liver function, recent myocardial infarction, or known cardiovascular disease.	
Beta-Blockers			
atenolol (Tenormin) betaxolol (Kerlone) bisoprolol (Zebeta) metoprolol (Lopressor) metoprolol extended release (Toprol-XL) nadolol (Corgard) propranolol (Inderal) propranolol long acting (Inderal LA) timolol (Blocadren)	Block the sympathetic nervous system (beta-adrenergic receptors), especially the sympathetics to the heart, producing a slower heart rate and lowered blood pressure	Reduce pulse rate in patients with tachycardia and blood pressure elevation Indicated for patients who also have stable angina pectoris and silent ischemia *Contraindications:* Bronchial asthma, allergic rhinitis, right ventricular failure from pulmonary hypertension, heart failure, depression, diabetes, dyslipidemia, heart block, peripheral vascular disease, heart rate <60 bpm	Mental depression manifested by insomnia, lassitude, weakness, and fatigue Avoid sudden discontinuation. Lightheadedness and occasional nausea, vomiting, and epigastric distress Check heart rate before giving. *Gerontologic considerations:* Risk of toxicity is increased for older adult patients with decreased renal and liver function. Take blood pressure in 3 positions, and observe for hypotension.
Beta-Blockers With Intrinsic Sympathomimetic Activity			
acebutolol (Sectral) penbutolol (Levatol) pindolol (Visken)	Block both cardiac beta-1 and beta-2 receptors Also have antiarrhythmic activity by slowing atrioventricular conduction	Similar to beta-blockers *Contraindications:* Similar to beta-blockers	Avoid sudden discontinuation. Withhold if bradycardia or heart block is present. Use with caution with COPD, diabetes. Similar to beta-blockers
Beta-Blocker With Cardioselective and Vasodilatory Activity			
Nebivolol (Bystolic)	Blocks beta-1 adrenergic receptors	Similar to other beta-blockers with additional capacity for vasodilation *Contraindications:* Similar to beta-blockers but with greater risk of severe bradycardia, heart block, cardiogenic shock, decompensated cardiac failure, sick sinus syndrome, severe hepatic impairment	Avoid sudden discontinuation. FDA warns that drug has not been shown to be more effective than any other beta-blocker.

Medications	Major Action	Advantages and Contraindications	Effects and Nursing Considerations
Alpha₁-Blockers			
doxazosin (Cardura) prazosin hydrochloride (Minipress) terazosin (Hytrin)	Peripheral vasodilator acting directly on the blood vessel; similar to hydralazine	Act directly on the blood vessels and are effective agents in patients with adverse reactions to hydralazine *Contraindications:* Angina pectoris and coronary artery disease; induces tachycardia if not preceded by administration of propranolol and a diuretic	Occasional vomiting and diarrhea, urinary frequency, and cardiovascular collapse, especially if given in addition to hydralazine without lowering the dose of the latter. Patients occasionally experience drowsiness, lack of energy, and weakness.
Combined Alpha- and Beta-Blockers			
carvedilol (Coreg) labetalol hydrochloride (Trandate)	Block alpha- and beta-adrenergic receptors; cause peripheral dilation and decrease peripheral vascular resistance	Fast acting No decrease in renal blood flow *Contraindications:* Asthma, cardiogenic shock, severe tachycardia, heart block	Orthostatic hypotension, tachycardia
Vasodilators			
fenoldopam mesylate (Corlopam)	Stimulates dopamine and alpha₂-adrenergic receptors	Given IV for hypertensive emergencies; use with caution in patients with glaucoma, recent stroke (brain attack), asthma, hypokalemia, or diminished liver function.	Headache, flushing, hypotension, sweating, tachycardia caused by vasodilation Observe for local reactions at the injection site.
hydralazine (Apresoline)	Decreases peripheral resistance but concurrently elevates cardiac output Acts directly on smooth muscle of blood vessels	Not used as initial therapy; used in combination with other medications Used also in pregnancy-induced hypertension *Contraindications:* Angina or coronary disease, heart failure, hypersensitivity	Headache, tachycardia, flushing, and dyspnea may occur—can be prevented by pretreating with reserpine. Peripheral edema may require diuretics. May produce lupus erythematosus–like syndrome Tachycardia, angina pectoris, ECG changes, edema
minoxidil (Loniten)	Direct vasodilatory action on arteriolar vessels, causing decreased peripheral vascular resistance; reduces systolic and diastolic pressures	Hypotensive effect more pronounced than with hydralazine No effect on vasomotor reflexes, so does not cause postural hypotension *Contraindications:* Pheochromocytoma	Take blood pressure and apical pulse before administration. Monitor intake and output and daily weights. Causes hirsutism Dizziness, headache, nausea, edema, tachycardia, palpitations
sodium nitroprusside (Nitropress) nitroglycerin	Peripheral vasodilation by relaxation of smooth muscle	Fast acting Used only in hypertensive emergencies *Contraindications:* Sepsis, azotemia, high intracranial pressure	Can cause thiocyanate and cyanide intoxication
ACE Inhibitors			
benazepril (Lotensin) captopril (Capoten) enalapril (Vasotec) enalaprilat (Vasotec IV) fosinopril (Monopril) lisinopril (Prinivil, Zestril) moexipril (Univasc) perindopril (Aceon) quinapril (Accupril) ramipril (Altace) trandolapril (Mavik)	Inhibit conversion of angiotensin I to angiotensin II Lower total peripheral resistance	Fewer cardiovascular side effects Can be used with thiazide diuretic and digitalis Hypotension can be reversed by fluid replacement. Angioedema is a rare but potentially life-threatening complication. *Contraindications:* Renal impairment, pregnancy	*Gerontologic considerations:* Require reduced dosages and the addition of loop diuretics when there is renal dysfunction
Angiotensin II Receptor Blockers Azilsartan medoxomil (Edarbi) candesartan (Atacand) eprosartan (Teveten) irbesartan (Avapro) losartan (Cozaar) olmesartan (Benicar) telmisartan (Micardis) valsartan (Diovan)	Block the effects of angiotensin II at the receptor Reduce peripheral resistance	Minimal side effects *Contraindications:* Pregnancy, lactation, renovascular disease, hypersensitivity reaction to other ARBs	Monitor for hyperkalemia.

(continues on page 870)

TABLE 31-4   Medication Therapy for Hypertension (continued)

Medications	Major Action	Advantages and Contraindications	Effects and Nursing Considerations
Calcium Channel Blockers			
Nondihydropyridines diltiazem extended release (Cardizem CD, Dilacor XR, Tiazac) diltiazem long acting (Cardizem LA)	Inhibit calcium ion influx Reduce cardiac afterload	Inhibit coronary artery spasm not controlled by beta-blockers or nitrates *Contraindications:* Sick sinus syndrome, AV block, hypotension, heart failure	Do not discontinue suddenly. Observe for hypotension. Report irregular heartbeat, dizziness, edema. Instruct on regular dental care because of potential gingivitis.
verapamil immediate release (Calan, Isoptin) verapamil long acting (Calan SR, Isoptin SR) verapamil (Covera-HS, Verelan PM)	Inhibit calcium ion influx Slow velocity of conduction of cardiac impulse	Effective antiarrhythmic Rapid IV onset Block SA and AV node channels *Contraindications:* Sinus or AV node disease, severe heart failure, severe hypotension	Administer on empty stomach or before meal. Do not discontinue suddenly. Depression may subside when medication is discontinued. To relieve headaches, reduce noise, monitor electrolytes Decrease dose for patients with liver or renal failure.
Dihydropyridines amlodipine (Norvasc) felodipine (Plendil) isradipine (Dynacirc CR) nicardipine (Cardene) nifedipine long acting (Procardia XL, Adalat CC) nisoldipine (Sular)	Inhibit calcium ion influx across membranes Vasodilatory effects on coronary arteries and peripheral arteriole Decrease cardiac work and energy consumption, increase delivery of oxygen to myocardium	Rapid action Effective by oral or sublingual route No tendency to slow SA nodal activity or prolong AV node conduction Isolated systolic hypertension *Contraindications:* None (except heart failure for nifedipine)	Administer on empty stomach. Use with caution in patients with diabetes. Small frequent meals if nausea Muscle cramps, joint stiffness, sexual difficulties may disappear when dose decreased. Report irregular heartbeat, constipation, shortness of breath, edema. May cause dizziness
clevidipine (Cleviprex)	Calcium channel antagonist causing rapid vasodilation	*Advantages:* Rapid acting with additional capacity for vasodilation; given IV *Contraindications:* Allergies to soybeans, soy products, eggs or egg products; impaired lipid metabolism as might be seen with pancreatitis and other hyperlipidemias; severe aortic stenosis	Monitor carefully for hypotension and tachycardia; there is risk of rebound hypertension, so careful monitoring after cessation of treatment is indicated.
Direct Renin Inhibitors			
aliskiren (Tekturna)	Blocks the conversion of angiotensinogen to angiotensin I by inhibiting the activity of the enzyme renin	Given once daily for mild to moderate high blood pressure with minimal side effects Headaches, dizziness, and diarrhea are most frequent side effects. Angioedema is a rare but potentially life-threatening complication. Contraindicated in pregnancy; has not been studied in persons with diminished renal function	Monitor for hyperkalemia and hypotension.

GI, gastrointestinal; ACE, angiotensin-converting enzyme; COPD, chronic obstructive pulmonary disease; FDA, U.S. Food and Drug Administration, IV, intravenous; ECG, electrocardiogram; ARBs, angiotensin receptor blockers; AV, atrioventricular; SA, sinoatrial.

the cuff is too small for the patient's arm, when the cuff is deflated too slowly (recommended rate is 2 to 3 mm Hg per second), and when an auscultatory gap is not recognized. An auscultatory gap is when the Korotkoff sounds disappear for a brief period as the cuff is being deflated. Failure to notice an auscultatory gap can result in erroneously high diastolic or low systolic pressure readings (Ogedegbe & Pickering, 2010).

A complete history is obtained to assess for other cardiovascular risk factors and for signs and symptoms that indicate target organ damage (i.e., whether specific tissues are damaged by the

elevated blood pressure). Manifestations of target organ damage may include angina; shortness of breath; alterations in speech, vision, or balance; nosebleeds; headaches; dizziness; or nocturia. The patient's partner may be helpful in identifying whether the patient may be experiencing obstructive sleep apnea.

During the physical examination, the nurse must also pay specific attention to the rate, rhythm, and character of the apical and peripheral pulses to detect the effects of hypertension on the heart and blood vessels. A thorough assessment can yield valuable information about the extent to which the hypertension has affected the body and any other personal, social, or financial factors. For example, a patient's ability to adhere to an antihypertensive medication regimen may be influenced by the patient's financial resources to buy the medication and also by a lack of health insurance (Viswanathan, Golan, Jones, et al., 2012).

Diagnosis

Nursing Diagnoses

Based on the assessment data, nursing diagnoses may include the following:

- Deficient knowledge regarding the relation between the treatment regimen and control of the disease process
- Noncompliance with therapeutic regimen related to side effects of prescribed therapy

Collaborative Problems/Potential Complications

Potential complications may include the following:

- Left ventricular hypertrophy
- Myocardial infarction
- Heart failure
- TIA
- Cerebrovascular accident (stroke or brain attack)
- Renal insufficiency and failure
- Retinal hemorrhage

Planning and Goals

The major goals for the patient include understanding of the disease process and its treatment, participation in a self-care program, and absence of complications.

Nursing Interventions

The objective of nursing care for patients with hypertension focuses on lowering and controlling the blood pressure without adverse effects and without undue cost. To achieve these goals, the nurse's role is to support and educate the patient about the treatment regimen, including making lifestyle changes, taking medications as prescribed, and scheduling regular follow-up appointments with the patient's primary provider to monitor progress or identify and treat any complications of disease or therapy.

Increasing Knowledge

The patient needs to understand the disease process and how lifestyle changes and medications can control hypertension. The nurse needs to emphasize the concept of controlling hypertension rather than curing it. The nurse can encourage the patient to consult a dietitian to help develop a plan for improving nutrient intake or for weight loss. The program usually consists of restricting sodium and fat intake, increasing intake of fruits and vegetables, and implementing regular physical activity. Explaining that it takes 2 to 3 months for the taste buds to adapt to changes in salt intake may help the patient adjust to reduced salt intake. The patient should be advised to limit alcohol intake (see Table 31-2 for specific recommendations), and tobacco should be avoided because anyone with high blood pressure is already at increased risk for heart disease, and smoking amplifies this risk.

Promoting Adherence to the Therapeutic Regimen

Deviation from the therapeutic program is a significant problem for people with hypertension and other chronic conditions requiring lifetime management. An estimated 50%

of patients discontinue their medications within 1 year of beginning to take them. Blood pressure control is achieved by only 54% (Valderrama et al., 2012). Adherence to the therapeutic regimen increases, however, when patients actively participate in self-care, including self-monitoring of blood pressure and diet, possibly because patients receive immediate feedback and have a greater sense of control. Nurse-led wellness programs that are tailored to take into account patients' behaviors and eating and exercise practices are more effective than generic programs (Walker, Pullen, Hageman, et al., 2010).

Patients with hypertension must make considerable effort to adhere to recommended lifestyle modifications (see Table 31-2) and to take regularly prescribed medications. The effort needed to follow the therapeutic plan may seem unreasonable to some, particularly when they have no symptoms without medications but do have side effects with medications. Continued education and encouragement are usually needed to enable patients to formulate an acceptable plan that helps them live with their hypertension and adhere to the treatment plan. Compromises may have to be made about some aspects of therapy to achieve higher-priority goals.

The nurse can assist with behavior change by supporting patients in making small changes with each visit that move them toward their goals. Another important factor is following up at each visit to see how the patient has progressed with the plans made at the prior visit. If the patient has had difficulty with a particular aspect of the plan, the patient and nurse can work together to develop an alternative or modification to the plan that the patient believes will be more successful. Support groups for weight control, smoking cessation, and stress reduction may be beneficial for some patients; others can benefit from the support of family and friends. The nurse assists the patient to develop and adhere to an appropriate exercise regimen, because regular activity is a significant factor in weight reduction and a blood pressure–reducing intervention in the absence of any loss in weight (Chobanian et al., 2003).

Promoting Home and Community-Based Care

Blood pressure screenings with the sole purpose of case finding are not recommended by the National High Blood Pressure Education Program because approximately 61% of people with hypertension are already aware of their blood pressure levels (Valderrama et al., 2012). If asked to participate in a blood pressure screening program, the nurse should ensure that proper blood pressure measurement technique is being used (see Chart 31-2), that the manometers used are calibrated, and that provision has been made to provide follow-up for any person identified as having an elevated blood pressure level. Adequate time should also be allowed to educate each person screened about what the blood pressure numbers mean. Each person should be given a written record of his or her blood pressure at the screening.

Educating Patients About Self-Care. The therapeutic regimen is the responsibility of the patient in collaboration with the primary provider. The nurse can help the patient achieve blood pressure control through education about managing blood pressure (see earlier education discussion), setting goal blood pressures, and providing assistance with social support. Involving family members in education programs enables them to support the patient's efforts to control hypertension. The American

Heart Association and the National Heart, Lung, and Blood Institute both provide printed and electronic patient education materials.

Providing written information about the expected effects and side effects of medications is important. When side effects occur, patients need to understand the importance of reporting them and to whom they should be reported. Patients need to be informed that **rebound hypertension** can occur if antihypertensive medications are suddenly stopped. Thus, patients should be advised to have an adequate supply of medication, particularly when traveling and in case of emergencies such as natural disasters. If traveling by airplane, patients should pack the medication in their carry-on luggage. All patients should be informed that some medications, such as beta-blockers, might cause sexual dysfunction and that other medications are available if problems with sexual function or satisfaction occur. The nurse can encourage and educate patients to measure their blood pressure at home. This practice involves patients in their own care and emphasizes that failing to take medications may result in an identifiable rise in blood pressure. Patients need to know that blood pressure varies continuously and that the range within which their pressure varies should be monitored.

Gerontologic Considerations. Adherence to the therapeutic program may be more difficult for older adults. The medication regimen can be difficult to remember, and the expense can be a challenge. **Monotherapy** (treatment with a single agent), if appropriate, may simplify the medication regimen and make it less expensive. Special care must be taken to ensure that the older adult patient understands the regimen and can see and read instructions, open the medication container, and get the prescription refilled. The older adult's family or caregivers should be included in the educational program so that they understand the patient's needs, can encourage adherence to the treatment plan, and know when and whom to call if problems arise or information is needed.

Continuing Care. Regular follow-up care is imperative so that the disease process can continue to be optimally assessed and treated, as shown in Table 31-5. A history and physical examination should be completed at each clinic visit. The history should include all data pertaining to any potential problem, specifically medication-related problems such as postural (orthostatic) hypotension (experienced as dizziness or lightheadedness on standing).

► Quality and Safety Nursing Alert

The patient and caregivers should be cautioned that antihypertensive medications might cause hypotension. Low blood pressure or postural hypotension should be reported immediately. Older adults have impaired cardiovascular reflexes and thus are more sensitive to the extracellular volume depletion caused by diuretics and to the sympathetic inhibition caused by adrenergic antagonists. The nurse educates patients to change positions slowly when moving from a lying or sitting position to a standing position. The nurse also counsels older adult patients to use supportive devices such as handrails and walkers as necessary to prevent falls that could result from dizziness.

TABLE 31-5 Recommendations for Follow-Up Based on Initial Blood Pressure Measurements for Adults Without Acute End Organ Damage

Initial BP (mm Hg)*	Follow-Up Recommended†
Normal	Recheck in 2 years
Prehypertension	Recheck in 1 year‡
Stage 1 hypertension	Confirm within 2 months‡
Stage 2 hypertension	Evaluate or refer to source of care within 1 month. For those with higher pressures (e.g., >180/100 mm Hg), evaluate and treat immediately or within 1 week, depending on clinical situation and complications

BP, blood pressure.
*If systolic and diastolic values fall into different categories, follow recommendations for shorter follow-up (e.g., 160/86 mm Hg should be evaluated or referred to source of care within 1 month).
†Modify the scheduling of follow-up according to reliable information about past BP measurements, other cardiovascular risk factors, or target organ disease.
‡Provide advice about lifestyle modifications.
Adapted from Chobanian, A. V., Bakris, G. L., Black, H. R., et al. (2003). Seventh Report of the Joint National Committee on Prevention, Detection, Evaluation, and Treatment of High Blood Pressure. *Hypertension, 42*(6), 1206–1252.

Monitoring and Managing Potential Complications

Symptoms suggesting that hypertension is progressing to the extent that target organ damage is occurring must be detected early so that appropriate treatment can be initiated. When the patient returns for follow-up care, all body systems must be assessed to detect any evidence of vascular damage. An eye examination with an ophthalmoscope is particularly important because retinal blood vessel damage indicates similar damage elsewhere in the vascular system. The patient is questioned about blurred vision, spots in front of the eyes, and diminished visual acuity. The heart, nervous system, and kidneys are also carefully assessed. Any significant findings are promptly reported to determine whether additional diagnostic studies are required. Based on the findings, medications may be changed to improve blood pressure control.

Evaluation

Expected patient outcomes may include:
1. Reports knowledge of disease management sufficient to maintain adequate tissue perfusion
   a. Maintains blood pressure at less than 140/90 mm Hg (or less than 130/80 mm Hg for people with diabetes or chronic kidney disease) with lifestyle modifications, medications, or both
   b. Demonstrates no symptoms of angina, palpitations, or vision changes
   c. Has stable BUN and serum creatinine levels
   d. Has palpable peripheral pulses
2. Adheres to the self-care program
   a. Adheres to the dietary regimen as prescribed: reduces calorie, sodium, and fat intake; increases fruit and vegetable intake
   b. Exercises regularly
   c. Takes medications as prescribed and reports any side effects
   d. Measures blood pressure routinely
   e. Abstains from tobacco and excessive alcohol intake
   f. Keeps follow-up appointments

3. Has no complications
   a. Reports no changes in vision
   b. Exhibits no retinal damage on vision testing
   c. Maintains pulse rate and rhythm and respiratory rate within normal ranges
   d. Reports no dyspnea or edema
   e. Maintains urine output consistent with intake
   f. Has renal function test results within normal range
   g. Demonstrates no motor, speech, or sensory deficits
   h. Reports no headaches, dizziness, weakness, changes in gait, or falls

 Concept Mastery Alert

Visit **thePoint** to view an Interactive Tutorial on key concepts related to hypertension.

 ## Hypertensive Crises

JNC 7 describes two classes of hypertensive crisis that require immediate intervention: hypertensive emergency and hypertensive urgency (pressures above 180 mm Hg systolic and/or above 120 mm Hg diastolic) (Chobanian et al., 2003). Hypertensive emergencies and urgencies may occur in patients whose hypertension has been poorly controlled, whose hypertension has been undiagnosed, or in those who have abruptly discontinued their medications. Once the hypertensive crisis has been managed, a complete evaluation is performed to review the patient's ongoing treatment plan and strategies to minimize the occurrence of subsequent hypertensive crises. The current recommendations for management of both hypertensive emergencies and urgencies are based on expert opinions because there are not clinical trial data comparing treatment options or identifying the impact of treatment on morbidity and mortality (Rodriguez, Kumar, & De Caro, 2010).

A **hypertensive emergency** is a situation in which blood pressures are extremely elevated and must be lowered immediately (not necessarily to less than 140/90 mm Hg) to halt or prevent damage to the target organs (Chobanian et al., 2003; Rodriguez et al., 2010). Assessment will reveal actual or developing clinical dysfunction of the target organ. Conditions associated with a hypertensive emergency include hypertension of pregnancy, acute myocardial infarction, dissecting aortic aneurysm, and intracranial hemorrhage. Hypertensive emergencies are acute, life-threatening blood pressure elevations that require prompt treatment in an intensive care setting because of the serious target organ damage that may occur. The therapeutic goals are reduction of the mean blood pressure by 20% to 25% within the first hour of treatment, a further reduction to a goal pressure of about 160/100 mm Hg over a period of up to 6 hours, and then a more gradual reduction in pressure over a period of days. The exceptions to these goals are the treatment of ischemic stroke (in which there is no evidence of benefit from immediate pressure reduction) and treatment of aortic dissection (in which the goal is to lower systolic pressure to less than 100 mm Hg if the patient can tolerate the reduction) (Chobanian et al., 2003).

The medications of choice in hypertensive emergencies are those that have an immediate effect. Intravenous vasodilators, including sodium nitroprusside (Nitropress), nicardipine hydrochloride (Cardene), clevidipine (Cleviprex), fenoldopam mesylate (Corlopam), enalaprilat, and nitroglycerin have immediate actions that are short-lived (minutes to 4 hours), and they are therefore used for initial treatment. For more information about these medications, see Table 31-4. Experts also recommend assessing the individual's fluid volume status. If there is volume depletion secondary to natriuresis caused by the elevated blood pressure, then volume replacement with normal saline can prevent large sudden drops in blood pressure when antihypertensive medications are administered (Rodriguez et al., 2010).

Hypertensive urgency describes a situation in which blood pressure is very elevated but there is no evidence of impending or progressive target organ damage (Chobanian et al., 2003). Elevated blood pressures associated with severe headaches, nosebleeds, or anxiety are classified as urgencies. In these situations, oral agents can be administered with the goal of normalizing blood pressure within 24 to 48 hours (Rodriguez et al., 2010). Oral doses of fast-acting agents such as beta-adrenergic blockers (i.e., labetalol [Trandate]), ACE inhibitors (i.e., captopril [Capoten]), or alpha₂-agonists (i.e., clonidine [Catapres]) are recommended for the treatment of hypertensive urgencies (see Table 31-4).

Extremely close hemodynamic monitoring of the patient's blood pressure and cardiovascular status is required during treatment of hypertensive emergencies and urgencies (see Chapter 25). The exact frequency of monitoring is a matter of clinical judgment and varies with the patient's condition. Taking vital signs every 5 minutes is appropriate if the blood pressure is changing rapidly; taking vital signs at 15- or 30-minute intervals in a more stable situation may be sufficient. A precipitous drop in blood pressure can occur that would require immediate action to restore blood pressure to an acceptable level.

Critical Thinking Exercises

1 **pcg** You are working as a nurse in a clinic that serves both an assisted living and skilled nursing facility. One of the patients today is a 68-year-old woman who is a new resident of the assisted living facility. When you take her blood pressure, you note that it is 210/158 mm Hg. As you talk with her, you find that she had stopped taking her medications when she moved into the assisted living facility. She tells you that she has too many other things to worry about with her recent move. What additional assessment data do you plan to gather from this patient? What is your priority plan of action?

2 **ebp** You are employed as an occupational health nurse in a manufacturing facility. A forklift operator, a 32-year-old man, presents to be treated after scraping his forearm on a piece of equipment. You find that his blood pressure is 148/98 mm Hg. What further follow-up would you recommend? Assume that this patient's blood pressure reading remains approximately the same over two additional visits to the occupational health office. What classification would then be given to his blood pressure according to JNC 7 recommendations? Discuss the evidence that supports specific strategies aimed at treating hypertension and how you would approach a discussion of recommended lifestyle modifications.

Brunner Suite Resources

Explore these additional resources to enhance learning for this chapter:
• NCLEX-Style Questions and Other Resources on thePoint, http://thePoint.lww.com/Brunner13e
• Study Guide
• PrepU
• Clinical Handbook
• Handbook of Laboratory and Diagnostic Tests

References

*Asterisk indicates nursing research.
**Double asterisk indicates classic reference.

Books

Bonow, R. O., Mann, D. L., Zipes, D. P., et al. (Eds.). (2012). *Braunwald's heart disease: A textbook of cardiovascular medicine* (9th ed.). Philadelphia: Elsevier Saunders.

Journals and Electronic Documents

**Appel, L. J., Champagne, C. M., Harsha, D. W., et al. (2003). Effects of comprehensive lifestyle modification on blood pressure control: Main results of the PREMIER clinical trial. *Journal of the American Medical Association,* 289(16), 2083–2093.

**Appel, L. J., Sacks, F. M., Carey, V. J., et al. (2005). Effects of protein, monounsaturated fat, and carbohydrate intake on blood pressure and serum lipids: Results of the OmniHeart randomized trial. *Journal of the American Medical Association,* 294(19), 2455–2464.

Aronow, W. S., Fleg, J. L., Pepine, C. J., et al. (2011). ACC/AHA 2011 expert consensus document on hypertension in the elderly: A report of the American College of Cardiology Foundation Task Force on Clinical Expert Consensus Documents. *Circulation, 123*(21), 2434–2506.

Barengo, N. C., Antikainen, R., Kastarinen, M., et al. (2013). The effects of control of systolic and diastolic hypertension on cardiovascular and all-cause mortality in a community based population cohort. *Journal of Human Hypertension,* advance online publication, 21 March 2013; doi: 10.1038/jhh.2013.22.

Chobanian, A. V., Bakris, G. L., Black, H. R., et al. (2003). The Seventh Report of the Joint National Committee on Prevention, Detection, Evaluation, and Treatment of High Blood Pressure: The JNC 7 Report (erratum in: *Journal of the American Medical Association,* 2003; 290(2), 197). *Journal of the American Medical Association,* 289(19), 2560–2572.

Coxson, P. G., Cook N. R., Joffres, M., et al. (2013). Mortality benefits from US population-wide reduction in sodium consumption: Projections from 3 modeling approaches. *Hypertension, 61*(3), 564–570.

Egan, B. M., Bandyopadhyay, D., Shaftman, S.R., et al. (2012). Initial monotherapy and combination therapy and hypertension control the first year. *Hypertension,* 59(6), 1124–1131.

Fagard, R. H. (2009). Smoking amplifies cardiovascular risk in patients with hypertension and diabetes. *Diabetes Care, 32*(Suppl. 2), S429–S431.

Goodwin, J. S. (2012). Gait speed: An important vital sign in old age. *Archives of Internal Medicine, 172*(15), 1168–1169.

Hedayati, S. S., Elsayed E. F., & Reilly, R. F. (2011). Non-pharmacological aspects of hypertension management: What are the data? *Kidney International, 79*(10), 1061–1070.

Kawano, Y. (2010). Physio-pathological effects of alcohol on the cardiovascular system: Its role in hypertension and cardiovascular disease. *Hypertension Research, 33*(3), 181–191.

Knight, J. A. (2012). Physical inactivity: Associated diseases and disorders. *Annals of Clinical & Laboratory Science, 42*(3), 320–337.

Leibowitz, A., & Schiffrin, E. L. (2011). Immune mechanisms in hypertension. *Current Hypertension Research, 13*(6), 465–472.

Maillard, P., Seshadri, S., Beiser, A., et al. (2012). Effects of systolic blood pressure on white-matter integrity in young adults in the Framingham Heart Study: A cross-sectional study. *Lancet Neurology, 11*(12), 1039–1047.

Männistö, T., Mendola, P., Vääräsmäki, M., et al. (2013). Elevated blood pressure in pregnancy and subsequent chronic disease risk. *Circulation, 127*(6), 681–690.

Odden, M. C., Peralta, C. A., Haan, M. N., et al. (2012). Rethinking the association of high blood pressure with mortality in elderly adults. *Archives of Internal Medicine, 172*(15), 1162–1168.

Ogedegbe, G., & Pickering, T. (2010). Principles and techniques of blood pressure measurement. *Cardiology Clinics, 28*(4), 571–586.

Padmanabhan, S., Newton-Cheh, C., & Dominiczak, A. F. (2012). Genetic basis of blood pressure and hypertension. *Trends in Genetics, 28*(8), 397–408.

Pedrosa, R. P., Krieger, E. M., Lorenzi-Filho, G., et al. (2011). Recent advances of the impact of obstructive sleep apnea on systemic hypertension. *Arquivos Brasileiros de Cardiologia, 97*(2), e40–e47.

Pickering, T. G., Hall, J. E., Appel, L. J., et al. (2005). Recommendations for blood pressure measurement in humans and experimental animals: Part 1: Blood pressure measurement in humans: A statement for professionals from the Subcommittee of Professional and Public Education of the American Heart Association Council on High Blood Pressure Research. *Hypertension, 45*(1), 142–161.

Pimenta, E., & Oparil S. (2010). Prehypertension: Epidemiology, consequences and treatment. *Nature Reviews Nephrology, 6*(1), 21–30.

Rodriguez, M. A., Kumar, S. K., & De Caro, M. (2010). Hypertensive crisis. *Cardiology in Review, 18*(2), 102–107.

Singh, M., Mensah, G. A., & Bakris, G. (2010). Pathogenesis and clinical physiology of hypertension. *Cardiology Clinics, 28*(4), 545–559.

Sukor, N. (2011). Secondary hypertension: A condition not to be missed. *Postgraduate Medicine, 87*(1032), 706–713.

Valderrama, A. L., Gillespie, C., King, S. K., et al. (2012). Vital signs: Awareness and treatment of uncontrolled hypertension among adults—United States, 2003–2010. *Morbidity and Mortality Weekly Report, 61*(35), 703–709.

Viswanathan, M., Golan, C. E., Jones, C. D., et al. (2012). Interventions to improve adherence to self-administered medications for chronic diseases in the United States: A systematic review. *Annals of Internal Medicine, 157*(11), 785–795.

*Walker, S. N., Pullen, C. H., Hageman, P. A., et al. (2010). Maintenance of activity and eating change after a clinical trial of tailored newsletters with older rural women. *Nursing Research, 59*(5), 311–321.

Resources

American Heart Association National Center, www.heart.org
Centers for Disease Control and Prevention (CDC), www.cdc.gov/dhdsp/
Heart and Stroke Foundation of Canada, www.heartandstroke.com
National Heart, Lung, and Blood Institute, www.nhlbi.nih.gov
World Health Association (WHO), Cardiovascular Disease Information, www.who.int/topics/cardiovascular_diseases/en

Unit 7

Hematologic Function

Case Study

A "NEAR-MISS" TRANSFUSION MISTAKE

Mr. Johnson, age 26 years, with blood type A positive, and Mr. Brown, age 72 years, with blood type B positive, are both multitrauma patients involved in the same mass casualty event. They arrive at the same emergency department (ED) in hemorrhagic shock within minutes of each other. They are both to be emergently transfused with 2 units of packed red blood cells (PRBCs). Mr. Johnson's PRBCs are sent by the blood bank to the ED first but are taken by mistake to Mr. Brown's suite for transfusion. The nurse in Mr. Brown's trauma suite verifies that the 2 units of PRBCs are not compatible with Mr. Brown and are instead meant for Mr. Johnson, averting a possible hemolytic reaction.

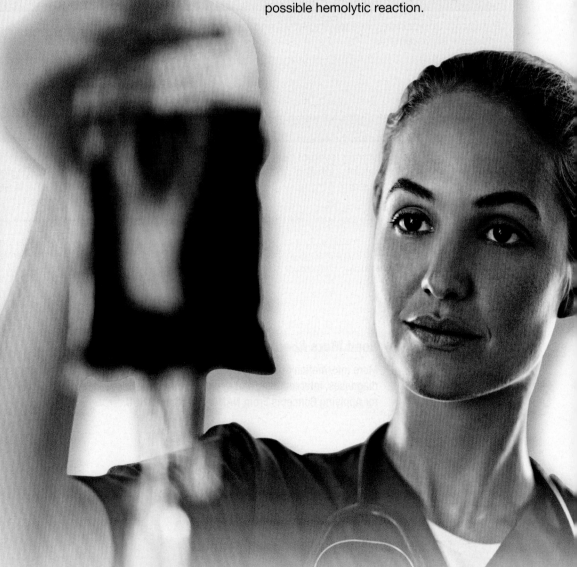

QSEN Competency Focus: *Safety*

The complexities inherent in today's health care system challenge nurses to demonstrate integration of specific interdisciplinary core competencies. These competencies are aimed at ensuring the delivery of safe, quality patient care (Institute of Medicine, 2003). The concepts from the Quality and Safety Education for Nurses (QSEN) Institute (2012) provide a framework for the knowledge, skills, and attitudes (KSAs) required for nurses to demonstrate competency in these key areas, which include *patient-centered care, interdisciplinary teamwork and collaboration, evidence-based practice, quality improvement, safety,* and *informatics.*

Safety Definition: Minimizes risk of harm to patients and providers through both system effectiveness and individual performance.

RELEVANT PRE-LICENSURE KSAs	APPLICATION AND REFLECTION
Knowledge	
Describe processes used in understanding causes of error and allocation of responsibility and accountability (such as root cause analysis and failure mode effects analysis).	What verification process did the nurse in Mr. Brown's trauma suite likely follow so that she found the potentially life-threatening error before Mr. Brown was transfused with the wrong blood type?
Skills	
Participate appropriately in analyzing errors and designing system improvements.	Think about how a "near-miss" event like this could occur. Although the nurse caring for Mr. Brown averted this error, should Mr. Brown's well-being hinge on the skill sets and diligence of one person (i.e., the nurse)? What could be done to improve the system so that this type of near-miss event does not happen again?
Attitudes	
Value vigilance and monitoring (even of own performance of care activities) by patients, families, and other members of the health care team.	Think about how you tend to react to stressful situations. Might you think about "cutting corners" and not engage in safety checks when time is of the essence? How might haste result in errors?

Cronenwett, L., Sherwood, G., Barnsteiner, J., et al. (2007). Quality and safety education for nurses. *Nursing Outlook, 55*(3), 122–131.
Institute of Medicine. (2003). *Health professions education: A bridge to quality*. Washington, DC: National Academies Press.
QSEN Institute (2012). *Competencies: Prelicensure KSAs*. Available at: qsen.org/competencies/pre-licensure-ksas

Read More About This Case

More information about this case study and the relationships between nursing diagnoses, interventions, and expected outcomes is available online. Visit thePoint for Applying Concepts From NANDA-I, NIC, and NOC.

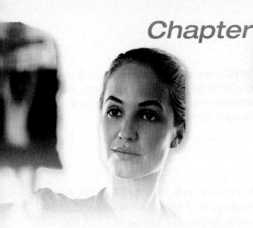

Chapter

32

Assessment of Hematologic Function and Treatment Modalities

Learning Objectives

On completion of this chapter, the learner will be able to:

1 Describe the process of hematopoiesis.
2 Describe the processes involved in maintaining hemostasis.
3 Discuss the significance of the health history to the assessment of hematologic health.
4 Describe the significance of physical assessment and diagnostic test findings to the diagnosis of hematologic dysfunction.
5 Identify therapies for blood disorders, including nursing implications for the administration of blood components.

Glossary

anemia: decreased red blood cell (RBC) count

band cell: slightly immature neutrophil

blast cell: primitive white blood cell (WBC)

cytokines: proteins produced by leukocytes that are vital to regulation of hematopoiesis, apoptosis, and immune responses

differentiation: development of functions and characteristics that are different from those of the parent stem cell

erythrocyte: a cellular component of blood involved in the transport of oxygen and carbon dioxide (*synonym*: red blood cell)

erythropoiesis: process of formation of RBCs

erythropoietin: hormone produced primarily by the kidney; necessary for erythropoiesis

fibrin: filamentous protein; basis of thrombus and blood clot

fibrinogen: protein converted into fibrin to form thrombus and clot

fibrinolysis: process of breakdown of fibrin clot

granulocyte: granulated WBC (i.e., neutrophil, eosinophil, basophil); sometimes used synonymously with neutrophil

hematocrit: percentage of total blood volume consisting of RBCs

hematopoiesis: complex process of the formation and maturation of blood cells

hemoglobin: iron-containing protein of RBCs; delivers oxygen to tissues

hemostasis: intricate balance between clot formation and clot dissolution

histiocytes: cells present in all loose connective tissue, capable of phagocytosis

left shift, or shift to the left: increased release of immature forms of WBCs from the bone marrow in response to need

leukocyte: one of several cellular components of blood involved in defense of the body; subtypes include neutrophils, eosinophils, basophils, monocytes, and lymphocytes (*synonym:* white blood cell)

leukopenia: less-than-normal amount of WBCs in circulation

lymphocyte: form of WBC involved in immune functions

lymphoid: pertaining to lymphocytes

macrophage: reticuloendothelial cells capable of phagocytosis

monocyte: large WBC that becomes a macrophage when it leaves the circulation and moves into body tissues

myeloid: pertaining to nonlymphoid blood cells that differentiate into RBCs, platelets, macrophages, mast cells, and various WBCs

myelopoiesis: formation and maturation of cells derived from myeloid stem cell

natural killer cells: immune cells that accumulate in lymphoid tissue that are potent killers of virus-infected and cancer cells

neutrophil: fully mature WBC capable of phagocytosis; primary defense against bacterial infection

nucleated RBC: immature form of red blood cell (RBC); portion of nucleus remains within the RBC

oxyhemoglobin: combined form of oxygen and hemoglobin; found in arterial blood

phagocytosis: process of cellular ingestion and digestion of foreign bodies

plasma: liquid portion of blood

plasminogen: protein converted to plasmin to dissolve thrombi and clots

platelet: a cellular component of blood involved in blood coagulation (*synonym:* thrombocyte)

red blood cell (RBC): a cellular component of blood involved in the transport of oxygen and carbon dioxide (*synonym:* erythrocyte)

reticulocytes: slightly immature RBCs, usually only 1% of total circulating RBCs

reticuloendothelial system: complex system of cells throughout the body capable of phagocytosis

serum: portion of blood remaining after coagulation occurs

stem cell: primitive cell, capable of self-replication and differentiation into myeloid or lymphoid stem cell

stroma: component of the bone marrow not directly related to hematopoiesis but serves important supportive roles in this process

(continues on page 878)

thrombin: enzyme necessary to convert fibrinogen into fibrin clot

thrombocyte: a cellular component of blood involved in blood coagulation (*synonym:* platelet)

white blood cell (WBC): one of several cellular components of blood involved in defense of the body; subtypes include neutrophils, eosinophils, basophils, monocytes, and lymphocytes (*synonym:* leukocyte)

Unlike many other body systems, the hematologic system encompasses the entire human body. Patients with hematologic disorders often have significant abnormalities in blood tests but few or no symptoms. Therefore, the nurse must have a good understanding of the pathophysiology of the patient's condition and the ability to make a thorough assessment that relies heavily on the interpretation of laboratory tests. It is equally important for the nurse to anticipate potential patient needs and to target nursing interventions accordingly. Because it is so important to the understanding of most hematologic diseases, a basic appreciation of blood cells and bone marrow function is necessary.

Anatomic and Physiologic Overview

The hematologic system consists of the blood and the sites where blood is produced, including the bone marrow and the **reticuloendothelial system** (RES). Blood is a specialized organ that differs from other organs in that it exists in a fluid state. Blood is composed of plasma and various types of cells. **Plasma** is the fluid portion of blood; it contains various proteins, such as albumin, globulin, **fibrinogen**, and other factors necessary for clotting, as well as electrolytes, waste products, and nutrients. About 55% of blood volume is plasma (Barrett, Barman, Boitano, et al., 2012).

■ Structure and Function of the Hematologic System

Blood

The cellular component of blood consists of three primary cell types (Table 32-1): **erythrocytes (red blood cells [RBCs], red cells)**, **leukocytes (white blood cells [WBCs])**, and **thrombocytes (platelets)**. These cellular components of blood normally make up 40% to 45% of the blood volume. Because most blood cells have a short lifespan, the need for the body to replenish its supply of cells is continuous; this process is termed **hematopoiesis.** The primary site for hematopoiesis is the bone marrow. During embryonic development and in other conditions, the liver and spleen may also be involved.

Under normal conditions, the adult bone marrow produces about 175 billion erythrocytes, 70 billion **neutrophils** (a mature type of WBC), and 175 billion platelets each day. When the body needs more blood cells, as in infection (when neutrophils are needed to fight the invading pathogen) or in bleeding (when more RBCs are required), the marrow increases its production of the cells required. Thus, under normal conditions, the marrow responds to increased demand and releases adequate numbers of cells into the circulation.

Blood makes up approximately 7% to 10% of the normal body weight and amounts to 5 to 6 L of volume. Circulating through the vascular system and serving as a link between body organs, blood carries oxygen absorbed from the lungs and nutrients absorbed from the gastrointestinal (GI) tract to the body cells for cellular metabolism. Blood also carries hormones, antibodies, and other substances to their sites of action or use. In addition, blood carries waste products produced by cellular metabolism to the lungs, skin, liver, and kidneys, where they are transformed and eliminated from the body.

The danger that trauma can lead to excess blood loss always exists. To prevent this, an intricate clotting mechanism is activated when necessary to seal any leak in the blood vessels. Excessive clotting is equally dangerous, because it can obstruct blood flow to vital tissues. To prevent this, the body has a fibrinolytic mechanism that eventually dissolves clots (thrombi) formed within blood vessels. The balance between these two systems—clot (thrombus) formation and clot dissolution or **fibrinolysis**—is called **hemostasis.**

Bone Marrow

The bone marrow is the site of hematopoiesis, or blood cell formation. In adults, blood cell formation is usually limited to the pelvis, ribs, vertebrae, and sternum. Marrow is one of the largest organs of the body, making up 4% to 5% of total body weight. It consists of islands of cellular components

TABLE 32-1	Blood Cells
Cell Type	**Major Function**
WBC (Leukocyte)	Fights infection
Neutrophil	Essential in preventing or limiting bacterial infection via phagocytosis
Monocyte	Enters tissue as macrophage; highly phagocytic, especially against fungus; immune surveillance
Eosinophil	Involved in allergic reactions (neutralizes histamine); digests foreign proteins
Basophil	Contains histamine; integral part of hypersensitivity reactions
Lymphocyte	Integral component of immune system
T lymphocyte	Responsible for cell-mediated immunity; recognizes material as "foreign" (surveillance system)
B lymphocyte	Responsible for humoral immunity; many mature into plasma cells to form antibodies
Plasma cell	Secretes immunoglobulin (antibody); most mature form of B lymphocyte
RBC (Erythrocyte)	Carries hemoglobin to provide oxygen to tissues; average lifespan is 120 days
Platelet (Thrombocyte)	Fragment of megakaryocyte; provides basis for coagulation to occur; maintains hemostasis; average lifespan is 10 days

WBC, white blood cell; RBC, red blood cell.

(red marrow) separated by fat (yellow marrow). As people age, the proportion of active marrow is gradually replaced by fat; however, in healthy adults, the fat can again be replaced by active marrow when more blood cell production is required. In adults with disease that causes marrow destruction, fibrosis, or scarring, the liver and spleen can also resume production of blood cells by a process known as extramedullary hematopoiesis.

The marrow is highly vascular. Within it are primitive cells called **stem cells**. The stem cells have the ability to self-replicate, thereby ensuring a continuous supply of stem cells throughout the life cycle. When stimulated to do so, stem cells can begin a process of **differentiation** into either **myeloid** or **lymphoid** stem cells (Fig. 32-1). These stem cells are committed to produce specific types of blood cells. Lymphoid stem cells produce either T or B **lymphocytes**. Myeloid stem cells differentiate into three broad cell types: erythrocytes, leukocytes, and platelets. Thus, with the exception of lymphocytes, all blood cells are derived from myeloid stem cells. A defect in a myeloid stem cell can cause problems with erythrocyte, leukocyte, and platelet production. In contrast, a defect in the lymphoid stem cell can cause problems with T or B lymphocytes, plasma cells (a more differentiated form of B lymphocyte), or natural killer (NK) cells.

The **stroma** of the marrow refers to all tissue within the marrow that is not directly involved in hematopoiesis. However, the stroma is important in an indirect manner, in that it produces the colony-stimulating factors needed for hematopoiesis. The yellow marrow is the largest component of the stroma. Other cells comprising the stroma include fibroblasts (reticular connective tissue), osteoclasts, osteoblasts (both needed for remodeling of skeletal bone), and endothelial cells.

Blood Cells

Erythrocytes (Red Blood Cells)

The normal erythrocyte is a biconcave disk that resembles a soft ball compressed between two fingers (Fig. 32-2). It has a diameter of about 8 mcm and is so flexible that it can pass easily through capillaries that may be as small as 2.8 mcm in diameter. The membrane of the red cell is very thin so that gases, such as oxygen and carbon dioxide, can easily diffuse across it; the disk shape provides a large surface area that facilitates the absorption and release of oxygen molecules.

Mature erythrocytes consist primarily of **hemoglobin**, which contains iron and makes up 95% of the cell mass. Mature erythrocytes have no nuclei, and they have many fewer metabolic enzymes than do most other cells. The presence of a large amount of hemoglobin enables the red cell to perform its principal function, which is the transport of oxygen between the lungs and tissues. Occasionally, the marrow releases slightly immature forms of erythrocytes, called **reticulocytes**, into the circulation. This occurs as a normal response to an increased demand for erythrocytes (as in bleeding) or in some disease states.

The oxygen-carrying hemoglobin molecule is made up of four subunits, each containing a heme portion attached to a globin chain. Iron is present in the heme component of the molecule. An important property of heme is its ability to bind to oxygen loosely and reversibly. Oxygen readily binds

to hemoglobin in the lungs and is carried as **oxyhemoglobin** in arterial blood. Oxyhemoglobin is a brighter red than hemoglobin that does not contain oxygen (reduced hemoglobin); thus, arterial blood is a brighter red than venous blood. The oxygen readily dissociates (detaches) from hemoglobin in the tissues, where the oxygen is needed for cellular metabolism. In venous blood, hemoglobin combines with hydrogen ions produced by cellular metabolism and thus buffers excessive acid. Whole blood normally contains about 15 g of hemoglobin per 100 mL of blood (Fischbach & Dunning, 2010).

Erythropoiesis

Erythroblasts arise from the primitive myeloid stem cells in bone marrow. The erythroblast is an immature nucleated cell that gradually loses its nucleus. At this stage, the cell is known as a reticulocyte. Further maturation into an erythrocyte entails the loss of the dark-staining material within the cell and slight shrinkage. The mature erythrocyte is then released into the circulation. Under conditions of rapid **erythropoiesis** (i.e., erythrocyte production), reticulocytes and other immature cells (e.g., **nucleated RBCs**) may be released prematurely into the circulation. This is often seen when the liver or spleen takes over as the site of erythropoiesis and more nucleated red cells appear within the circulation.

Differentiation of the primitive myeloid stem cell into an erythroblast is stimulated by **erythropoietin**, a hormone produced primarily by the kidney. If the kidney detects low levels of oxygen, as occurs when fewer red cells are available to bind oxygen (i.e., **anemia**), or with people living at high altitudes with lower atmospheric oxygen concentrations, erythropoietin levels increase. The increased erythropoietin then stimulates the marrow to increase production of erythrocytes. The entire process of erythropoiesis typically takes 5 days (Cook, Ineck, & Lyons, 2011).

For normal erythrocyte production, the bone marrow also requires iron, vitamin B_{12}, folate, pyridoxine (vitamin B_6), protein, and other factors. A deficiency of these factors during erythropoiesis can result in decreased red cell production and anemia.

Iron Stores and Metabolism. The average daily diet in the United States contains 10 to 15 mg of elemental iron, but only 0.5 to 1 mg of ingested iron is normally absorbed from the small intestine (Masters, 2012). The rate of iron absorption is regulated by the amount of iron already stored in the body and by the rate of erythrocyte production. Additional amounts of iron, up to 2 mg daily, must be absorbed by women of childbearing age to replace that lost during menstruation. Total body iron content in the average adult is approximately 3 g, most of which is present in hemoglobin or in one of its breakdown products. Iron is stored as ferritin and when required, the iron is released into the plasma, binds to transferrin, and is transported into the membranes of the normoblasts (erythrocyte precursor cells) within the marrow, where it is incorporated into hemoglobin. Iron is lost in the feces, either in bile, blood, or mucosal cells from the intestine.

The concentration of iron in blood is normally about 75 to 175 mcg/dL (13 to 31 mcmol/L) for men and 65 to 165 mcg/dL (11 to 29 mcmol/L) for women (Fischbach & Dunning,

Physiology ⋅∴⋅ Pathophysiology

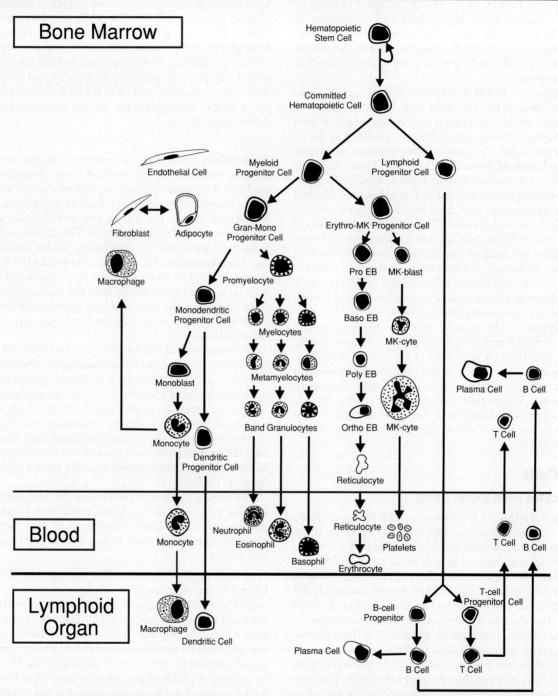

FIGURE 32-1 • Hematopoiesis and stromal stem cell differentiation. Uncommitted (pluripotent) stem cells can differentiate into myeloid or lymphoid stem cells. These stem cells then undergo a complex process of differentiation and maturation into normal cells that are released into the circulation. The myeloid stem cell is responsible not only for all nonlymphoid white blood cells but also for the production of red blood cells (RBCs) and platelets. Each step of the differentiation process depends in part on the presence of specific growth factors for each cell type. When the stem cells are dysfunctional, they may respond inadequately to the need for more cells, or they may respond excessively, and sometimes uncontrollably, as in leukemia. From Koury, M., Mahmud, N., & Rhodes, M. (2009). Origin and development of blood cells. In J. P. Greer, J. Foerster, G. M. Rodgers, & F. Paraskevas (Eds.). *Wintrobe's clinical hematology* (12th ed.). Philadelphia: Lippincott Williams & Wilkins.

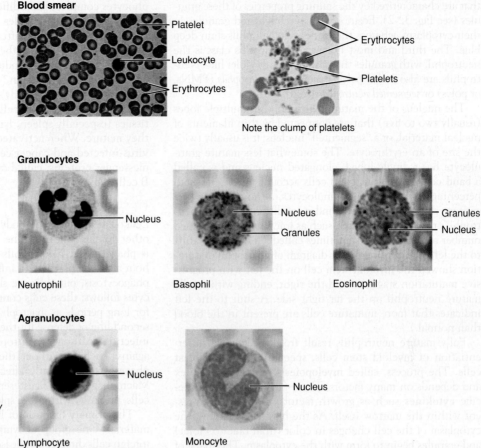

FIGURE 32-2 • Normal types of blood cells. From Cohen, B. J. (2005). *Memmler's the human body in health and disease* (10th ed.). Philadelphia: Lippincott Williams & Wilkins.

2010). With iron deficiency, bone marrow iron stores are rapidly depleted; hemoglobin synthesis is depressed, and the erythrocytes produced by the marrow are small and low in hemoglobin. Iron deficiency in the adult generally indicates blood loss (e.g., from bleeding in the GI tract or heavy menstrual flow). Lack of dietary iron is rarely the sole cause of iron deficiency anemia in adults. The source of iron deficiency should be investigated promptly, because iron deficiency in an adult may be a sign of bleeding in the GI tract or colon cancer.

Vitamin B_{12} and Folate Metabolism. Vitamin B_{12} and folate are required for the synthesis of deoxyribonucleic acid (DNA) in RBCs. Both vitamin B_{12} and folate are derived from the diet. Folate is absorbed in the proximal small intestine, but only small amounts are stored within the body. If the diet is deficient in folate, stores within the body quickly become depleted. Because vitamin B_{12} is found only in foods of animal origin, strict vegetarians may ingest little vitamin B_{12}. Vitamin B_{12} combines with intrinsic factor produced in the stomach. The vitamin B_{12}–intrinsic factor complex is absorbed in the distal ileum. People who have had a partial or total gastrectomy may have limited amounts of intrinsic factor, and therefore the absorption of vitamin B_{12} may be diminished. The effects of either decreased absorption or decreased intake of vitamin B_{12} are not apparent for 2 to 4 years.

Vitamin B_{12} and folate deficiencies are characterized by the production of abnormally large erythrocytes called *megaloblasts*. Because these cells are abnormal, many are seques-tered (trapped) while still in the bone marrow, and their rate of release is decreased. Some of these cells actually die in the marrow before they can be released into the circulation. This results in megaloblastic anemia.

Red Blood Cell Destruction

The average lifespan of a normal circulating erythrocyte is 120 days. Aged erythrocytes lose their elasticity and become trapped in small blood vessels and the spleen. They are removed from the blood by the reticuloendothelial cells, particularly in the liver and the spleen. As the erythrocytes are destroyed, most of their hemoglobin is recycled. Some hemoglobin also breaks down to form bilirubin and is secreted in the bile. Most of the iron is recycled to form new hemoglobin molecules within the bone marrow; small amounts are lost daily in the feces and urine and monthly in menstrual flow.

Leukocytes (White Blood Cells)

Leukocytes are divided into two general categories: granulocytes and lymphocytes. In normal blood, the total leukocyte count is 4,000 to 11,000 cells/mm³. Of these, approximately 60% to 80% are granulocytes and 20% to 40% are lymphocytes. Both of these types of leukocytes primarily protect the body against infection and tissue injury.

Granulocytes

Granulocytes are defined by the presence of granules in the cytoplasm of the cell. Granulocytes are divided into three main subgroups—eosinophils, basophils, and neutrophils—

that are characterized by the staining properties of these granules (see Fig. 32-2). Eosinophils have bright-red granules in their cytoplasm, whereas the granules in basophils stain deep blue. The third and most numerous cell in this class is the neutrophil, with granules that stain a pink to violet hue. Neutrophils are also called *polymorphonuclear neutrophils* (PMNs, or polys) or *segmented neutrophils* (segs).

The nucleus of the mature neutrophil has multiple lobes (usually two to five) that are connected by thin filaments of nuclear material, or a "segmented" nucleus; it is usually twice the size of an erythrocyte. The somewhat less mature granulocyte has a single-lobed, elongated nucleus and is called a **band cell.** Ordinarily, band cells account for only a small percentage of circulating granulocytes, although their percentage can increase greatly under conditions in which neutrophil production increases, such as infection. An increased number of band cells is sometimes called a **left shift** or **shift to the left.** (Traditionally, the diagram of neutrophil maturation showed the myeloid stem cell on the left with progressive maturation stages toward the right, ending with a fully mature neutrophil on the far right side. A shift to the left indicates that more immature cells are present in the blood than normal.)

Fully mature neutrophils result from the gradual differentiation of myeloid stem cells, specifically myeloid **blast cells.** The process, called **myelopoiesis,** is highly complex and depends on many factors. These factors, including specific **cytokines** such as growth factors, are normally present within the marrow itself. As the blast cell matures, the cytoplasm of the cell changes in color (from blue to violet) and granules begin to form with the cytoplasm. The shape of the nucleus also changes. The entire process of maturation and differentiation takes about 10 days (see Fig. 32-1). Once the neutrophil is released into the circulation from the marrow, it stays there for only about 6 hours before it migrates into the body tissues to perform its function of **phagocytosis** (ingestion and digestion of bacteria and particles). Neutrophils die here within 1 to 2 days. The number of circulating granulocytes found in the healthy person is relatively constant; however, in infection, large numbers of these cells are rapidly released into the circulation.

Agranulocytes

Monocytes. **Monocytes** (also called *mononuclear leukocytes*) are leukocytes with a single-lobed nucleus and a granule-free cytoplasm—hence the term *agranulocyte* (see Fig. 32-2). In normal adult blood, monocytes account for approximately 5% of the total leukocytes. Monocytes are the largest of the leukocytes. Produced by the bone marrow, they remain in the circulation for a short time before entering the tissues and transforming into **macrophages.** Macrophages are particularly active in the spleen, liver, peritoneum, and alveoli; they remove debris from these areas and phagocytize bacteria within the tissues.

Lymphocytes. Mature lymphocytes are small cells with scanty cytoplasm (see Fig. 32-2). Immature lymphocytes are produced in the marrow from the lymphoid stem cells. A second major source of production is the thymus. Cells derived from the thymus are known as T lymphocytes (or T cells); those derived from the marrow can also be T cells but are more commonly B lymphocytes (or B cells). Lym-

phocytes complete their differentiation and maturation primarily in the lymph nodes and in the lymphoid tissue of the intestine and spleen after exposure to a specific antigen. Mature lymphocytes are the principal cells of the immune system, producing antibodies and identifying other cells and organisms as "foreign." **Natural killer cells** serve an important role in the body's immune defense system. Like other lymphocytes, NK cells accumulate in the lymphoid tissues (especially spleen, lymph nodes, and tonsils), where they mature. When activated, they serve as potent killers of virus-infected and cancer cells. They also secrete chemical messenger proteins, called *cytokines,* to mobilize the T and B cells into action.

Function of Leukocytes

Leukocytes protect the body from invasion by bacteria and other foreign entities. The major function of neutrophils is phagocytosis. Neutrophils arrive at a given site within 1 hour after the onset of an inflammatory reaction and initiate phagocytosis, but they are short-lived. An influx of monocytes follows; these cells continue their phagocytic activities for long periods as macrophages. This process constitutes a second line of defense for the body against inflammation and infection. Although neutrophils can often work adequately against bacteria without the help of macrophages, macrophages are particularly effective against fungi and viruses. Macrophages also digest senescent (aging or aged) blood cells, primarily within the spleen.

The primary function of lymphocytes is to attack foreign material. One group of lymphocytes (T lymphocytes) kills foreign cells directly or releases lymphokines, substances that enhance the activity of phagocytic cells. T lymphocytes are responsible for delayed allergic reactions, rejection of foreign tissue (e.g., transplanted organs), and destruction of tumor cells. This process is known as *cellular immunity.* The other group of lymphocytes (B lymphocytes) is capable of differentiating into plasma cells. Plasma cells, in turn, produce antibodies called *immunoglobulins* (Igs), which are protein molecules that destroy foreign material by several mechanisms. This process is known as humoral immunity.

Eosinophils and basophils function in hypersensitivity reactions. Eosinophils are important in the phagocytosis of parasites. The increase in eosinophil levels in allergic states indicates that these cells are involved in the hypersensitivity reaction; they neutralize histamine. Basophils produce and store histamine as well as other substances involved in hypersensitivity reactions. The release of these substances provokes allergic reactions. (See Chapter 35 for further information on the immune response.)

Platelets (Thrombocytes)

Platelets, or thrombocytes, are not technically cells; rather, they are granular fragments of giant cells in the bone marrow called *megakaryocytes* (see Fig. 32-2). Platelet production in the marrow is regulated in part by the hormone thrombopoietin, which stimulates the production and differentiation of megakaryocytes from the myeloid stem cell.

Platelets play an essential role in the control of bleeding. They circulate freely in the blood in an inactive state, where they nurture the endothelium of the blood vessels, maintaining the integrity of the vessel. When vascular injury occurs, platelets collect at the site and are activated. They adhere to the site of injury and to each other, forming a platelet plug that temporarily stops bleeding. Substances released from platelet granules activate coagulation factors in the blood plasma and initiate the formation of a stable clot composed of **fibrin,** a filamentous protein. Platelets have a normal lifespan of 7 to 10 days (Diz-Kucukkaya, Chen, Geddis, et al., 2010).

Plasma and Plasma Proteins

After cellular elements are removed from blood, the remaining liquid portion is called *plasma.* More than 90% of plasma is water. The remainder consists primarily of plasma proteins, clotting factors (particularly fibrinogen), and small amounts of other substances such as nutrients, enzymes, waste products, and gases. If plasma is allowed to clot, the remaining fluid is called **serum.** Serum has essentially the same composition as plasma, except that fibrinogen and several clotting factors have been removed during the clotting process.

Plasma proteins consist primarily of albumin and the globulins. The globulins can be separated into three main fractions (alpha, beta, and gamma), each of which consists of distinct proteins that have different functions. Important proteins in the alpha and beta fractions are the transport globulins and the clotting factors that are made in the liver. The transport globulins carry various substances in bound form in the circulation. For example, thyroid-binding globulin carries thyroxin, and transferrin carries iron. The clotting factors, including fibrinogen, remain in an inactive form in the blood plasma until activated by the clotting cascade. The gamma-globulin fraction refers to the Igs, or antibodies. These proteins are produced by well-differentiated B lymphocytes and plasma cells. The actual fractionation of the globulins can be seen on a specific laboratory test (serum protein electrophoresis).

Albumin is particularly important for the maintenance of fluid balance within the vascular system. Capillary walls are impermeable to albumin, so its presence in the plasma creates an osmotic force that keeps fluid within the vascular space. Albumin, which is produced by the liver, has the capacity to bind to several substances that are transported in plasma (e.g., certain medications, bilirubin, and some hormones). People with impaired hepatic function may have low concentrations of albumin, with a resultant decrease in osmotic pressure and the development of edema.

Reticuloendothelial System

The RES is composed of special tissue macrophages. When released from the marrow, monocytes spend a short time in the circulation (about 24 hours) and then enter the body tissues. Within the tissues, the monocytes continue to differentiate into macrophages, which can survive for months or years. Macrophages have a variety of important functions. They defend the body against foreign invaders (i.e., bacteria and other pathogens) via phagocytosis. They remove old or damaged cells from the circulation. They stimulate the inflammatory process and present antigens to the immune system (see Chapter 35). Macrophages give rise to tissue **histiocytes,** including Kupffer cells of the liver, peritoneal macrophages, alveolar macrophages, and other components of the RES. Thus, the RES is a component of many other organs within the body, particularly the spleen, lymph nodes, lungs, and liver.

The spleen is the site of activity for most macrophages. Most of the spleen (75%) is made of red pulp; here, the blood enters the venous sinuses through capillaries that are surrounded by macrophages. Within the red pulp are tiny aggregates of white pulp, consisting of B and T lymphocytes. The spleen sequesters newly released reticulocytes from the marrow, removing nuclear fragments and other materials (e.g., denatured hemoglobin, iron) before the now fully mature erythrocyte returns to the circulation. Although a minority of erythrocytes (less than 5%) pool in the spleen, a significant proportion of platelets (20% to 40%) pool here (Henry & Longo, 2012). If the spleen is enlarged, a greater proportion of red cells and platelets can be sequestered. The spleen is a major source of hematopoiesis in fetal life. It can resume hematopoiesis later in adulthood if necessary, particularly when marrow function is compromised (e.g., in bone marrow fibrosis). The spleen has important immunologic functions as well. It forms substances called *opsonins* that promote the phagocytosis of neutrophils; it also forms the antibody immunoglobulin M (IgM) after exposure to an antigen.

Hemostasis

Hemostasis is the process of preventing blood loss from intact vessels and of stopping bleeding from a severed vessel, which requires adequate numbers of functional platelets. Platelets nurture the endothelium and thereby maintain the structural integrity of the vessel wall. Two processes are involved in arresting bleeding: primary and secondary hemostasis (Fig. 32-3).

In primary hemostasis, the severed blood vessel constricts. Circulating platelets aggregate at the site and adhere to the vessel and to one another. An unstable hemostatic plug is formed. For the coagulation process to be correctly activated, circulating inactive coagulation factors must be converted to active forms. This process occurs on the surface of the aggregated platelets at the site of vessel injury. The end result is the formation of fibrin, which reinforces the platelet plug and anchors it to the injury site. This process is referred to as secondary hemostasis. The process of blood coagulation is highly complex. It can be activated by the extrinsic pathway (also known as the tissue factor pathway) or the intrinsic pathway (also known as the contact activation pathway). Both pathways are needed for maintenance of normal hemostasis.

Many factors are involved in the reaction cascade that forms fibrin. When tissue is injured, the extrinsic pathway is activated by the release of thromboplastin from the tissue. As the result of a series of reactions, prothrombin is converted to **thrombin,** which in turn catalyzes the conversion of fibrinogen to fibrin. Clotting by the intrinsic or contact activation pathway is activated when the collagen that lines blood vessels is exposed. Clotting factors are activated sequentially until, as with the extrinsic pathway, fibrin is ultimately formed. The intrinsic pathway is slower, and this sequence is less often responsible for clotting in response to tissue injury.

Physiology Pathophysiology

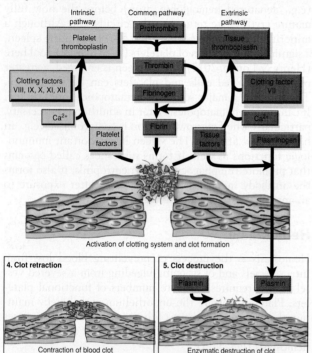

1. Vascular phase

Injury

Spasm in damaged muscle

2. Platelet phase

Platelet aggregation and adhesion

3. Coagulation phase

Intrinsic pathway

Common pathway

Extrinsic pathway

Platelet thromboplastin

Prothrombin

Tissue thromboplastin

Clotting factors VIII, IX, X, XI, XII

Thrombin

Clotting factor VII

Ca^{2+}

Fibrinogen

Ca^{2+}

Platelet factors

Fibrin

Tissue factors

Plasminogen

Activation of clotting system and clot formation

4. Clot retraction

Contraction of blood clot

5. Clot destruction

Plasmin

Plasmin

Enzymatic destruction of clot

FIGURE 32-3 • Hemostasis. When the endothelial surface of a blood vessel is injured, several processes occur. In primary hemostasis, platelets within the circulation are attracted to the exposed layer of collagen at the site of injury. They adhere to the site of injury, releasing factors that stimulate other platelets to aggregate at the site, forming an unstable platelet plug. In secondary hemostasis, based on the type of stimulus, one of two clotting pathways is initiated—the intrinsic or extrinsic pathway—and the clotting factors within that pathway are activated. The end result from either pathway is the conversion of prothrombin to thrombin. Thrombin is necessary for fibrinogen to be converted into fibrin, the stabilizing protein that anchors the fragile platelet plug to the site of injury to prevent further bleeding and permit the injuring vessel or site to heal. Modified from www.irvingcrowley.com/cls/clotting.gif

However, it is important if a noninjured vessel wall comes into contact with lipoproteins (e.g., atherosclerosis) or with bacteria, resulting in a clot that is formed for purposes other than protection from trauma or bleeding.

As the injured vessel is repaired and again covered with endothelial cells, the fibrin clot is no longer needed. The fibrin is digested via two systems: the plasma fibrinolytic system and the cellular fibrinolytic system. The substance **plasminogen** is required to lyse (break down) the fibrin. Plasminogen, which is present in all body fluids, circulates with fibrinogen and is therefore incorporated into the fibrin clot as it forms. When

the clot is no longer needed (e.g., after an injured blood vessel has healed), the plasminogen is activated to form plasmin. Plasmin digests the fibrinogen and fibrin. The breakdown particles of the clot, called *fibrin degradation products*, are released into the circulation. Through this system, clots are dissolved as tissue is repaired, and the vascular system returns to its normal baseline state.

Gerontologic Considerations

In older patients, the bone marrow's ability to respond to the body's need for blood cells (erythrocytes, leukocytes, and platelets) may be decreased. This decreased ability is a result of many factors, including diminished production of the growth factors necessary for hematopoiesis by stromal cells within the marrow or a diminished response to the growth factors (in the case of erythropoietin). In addition, in older patients, the bone marrow may be more susceptible to the myelosuppressive effects of medications. As a result of these factors, when an older person needs more blood cells, the bone marrow may not be able to increase production of these cells adequately. **Leukopenia** (a decreased number of circulating leukocytes) or anemia can result.

Assessment

Health History

A careful health history and physical assessment can provide important information related to a patient's known or potential hematologic diagnosis. Because many hematologic disorders are more prevalent in certain ethnic groups, assessments of ethnicity and family history are useful (Chart 32-1). Similarly, obtaining a nutritional history and assessing the use of prescription and over-the-counter medications, as well as herbal supplements, are important to note, because several conditions can result from nutritional deficiencies, herbs, or certain medications. Careful attention to the onset of a symptom or finding (e.g., rapid vs. gradual; persistent vs. intermittent), its severity, and any contributing factors can further differentiate potential causes. Of equal importance is assessing the impact of these findings on the patient's functional ability, manifestations of distress, and coping mechanisms.

Physical Assessment

The physical assessment should be comprehensive and include careful attention to the skin, oral cavity, lymph nodes, and spleen (Fig. 32-4). Table 32-2 highlights a general approach to the physical assessment findings in hematologic disorders (more specific findings are presented in Chapters 33 and 34).

Diagnostic Evaluation

Most hematologic diseases reflect a defect in the hematopoietic, hemostatic, or reticuloendothelial system. The defect can be quantitative (e.g., increased or decreased production of cells), qualitative (e.g., the cells that are produced

GENETICS IN NURSING PRACTICE

Chart 32-1

Hematologic Disorders

Hematologic disorders are marked by aberrations in the structure or function of the blood cells or the blood clotting mechanism. Many hematologic disorders are associated with genetic abnormalities. Some examples of these hematologic disorders are:

- Aplastic anemia
- Factor V Leiden
- Hemophilia
- Hemochromatosis
- Sickle cell disease
- Thalassemia
- Thrombotic thrombocytopenic purpura
- Von Willebrand disease

Nursing Assessments

Family History Assessment

- Collect family history information on maternal and paternal relatives from three generations of the family.
- Assess family history for other family members with histories of blood disorders that involve the blood cells or the blood clotting mechanism.

Patient Assessment

- Assess for specific symptoms of hematologic diseases, such as deep bruises and unexplained bleeding and bruising in

hemophilia or nosebleeds and swelling in the hands and feet in sickle cell disease.
- Assess for the most common symptom in hematologic diseases, which is extreme fatigue.
- Assess the blood cell counts to see if they are reduced.

Management Issues Specific to Genetics

- Inquire whether DNA mutation or other genetic testing has been performed on affected family members.
- Refer for further genetic counseling and evaluation so that family members can discuss inheritance, risk to other family members, and availability of genetic testing and gene-based interventions.
- Offer appropriate genetic information and resources.
- Assess patient's understanding of genetic information.
- Provide support to families with newly diagnosed, genetics-related hematologic disorders.
- Participate in the management and coordination of care of patients with hematologic genetic conditions and people predisposed to develop or pass on a genetic condition.

Resources

See Chapter 8, Chart 8-6 for genetic resources.

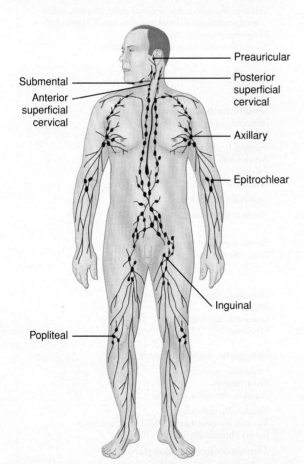

FIGURE 32-4 • Lymphatic system. *Arrows* indicate sites of lymph nodes accessible for palpation. Developed by M. Thomas & K. Morrow (2011). Veterans Administration Palo Alto Health Care System. Used with permission.

are defective in their normal functional capacity), or both. Initially, many hematologic conditions cause few symptoms, and extensive laboratory tests are often required to establish a diagnosis. For most hematologic conditions, continued monitoring via specific blood tests is required because it is very important to assess for changes in test results over time. In general, it is important to assess trends in test results because these trends help the clinician decide whether the patient is responding appropriately to interventions.

Hematologic Studies

The most common tests used are the complete blood count (CBC) and the peripheral blood smear. The CBC identifies the total number of blood cells (leukocytes, erythrocytes, and platelets) as well as the hemoglobin, **hematocrit** (percentage of blood volume consisting of erythrocytes), and RBC indices. Because cellular morphology (shape and appearance of the cells) is particularly important in accurately diagnosing most hematologic disorders, the blood cells involved must be examined. This process is referred to as the manual examination of the peripheral smear, which may be part of the CBC. In this test, a drop of blood is spread on a glass slide, stained, and examined under a microscope. The shape and size of the erythrocytes and platelets, as well as the actual appearance of the leukocytes, provide useful information in identifying hematologic conditions. Blood for the CBC is typically obtained by venipuncture.

Other common tests of coagulation are the prothrombin time (PT), replaced by the standardized test, international normalized ratio (INR), and the activated partial thromboplastin time (aPTT). The INR and aPTT serve as useful screening tools for evaluating a patient's clotting ability and monitoring the therapeutic effectiveness of

TABLE 32-2   Health History and Physical Assessment in Hematologic Disorders*

Findings	Potential Indications of Hematologic Disorder
Health History	
Prior episodes of bleeding (epistaxis, tooth, gum, hematuria, menorrhagia, hematochezia, gastrointestinal bleeding and/or ulcers)	Thrombocytopenia, coagulopathy, anemia
Prior blood clots, pulmonary emboli, miscarriages	Thrombotic disorder
Fatigue and weakness	Anemia, infection, malignancy, clonal disorders
Dyspnea, particularly dyspnea on exertion, orthopnea, shortness of breath	Anemia, infection
Prior radiation therapy (especially pelvic irradiation)	Anemia, pancytopenia, myelodysplastic syndrome, leukemia
Prior chemotherapy	Myelodysplastic syndrome, leukemia
Occupational/military exposure history; hobbies (especially benzene, Agent Orange)	Myelodysplastic syndrome, leukemia, myeloma, lymphoma
Diet history	Anemia (due to vitamin B_{12}, folate, iron deficiency)
Alcohol consumption	Anemia (effect on hematopoiesis, nutritional deficiency)
Use of herbal supplements	Platelet dysfunction
Concurrent medications	Neutropenia, anemia, hemolysis, thrombocytopenia
Family history/ethnicity	Some hematologic disorders have a higher prevalence in certain ethnic groups and families (see Chart 32-1)
Physical Assessment	
Skin	
Gray-tan or bronze skin color (especially genitalia, scars, exposed areas)	Hemochromatosis (primary or secondary)
Ruddy complexion (face, conjunctiva, hands, feet)	Polycythemia
Ecchymoses (i.e., bruises)	Thrombocytopenia, coagulopathy
Petechiae (i.e., pinpoint hemorrhagic lesions, usually more prominent on trunk or anterior aspects of lower extremities)	Severe thrombocytopenia
Rash	Variable; if pruritic, may indicate polycythemia, other nonhematologic-related disorders (see Chapter 60)
Bleeding (including around vascular lines, tubes)	Thrombocytopenia, coagulopathy
Conjunctival hemorrhage	Severe thrombocytopenia, coagulopathy
Pallor, especially in mucous membranes (including conjunctiva), nail beds	Anemia
Jaundice in mucous membranes (including conjunctiva), nail beds, palate	Hemolysis
Oral cavity	
Petechiae in the buccal mucosa, gingiva, hard palate	Severe thrombocytopenia
Ulceration of oral mucosa	Infection, leukemia
Tongue: Smooth	Pernicious anemia
Beefy red	Vitamin B_{12}/folate deficiency
Enlarged	Amyloidosis
Angular cheilosis (ulceration at corners of mouth)	Anemia
Enlarged gums; hyperplasia	Leukemia
Lymph nodes	Enlarged size, firm and fixed vs. mobile and tender	Leukemia, lymphoma
Respiratory	Increased rate and depth of respirations; adventitious breath sounds	Anemia; infection
Cardiovascular	Distended neck veins, edema, chest pain on exertion, murmurs, gallops	Severe anemia
	Hypotension (below baseline)	Polycythemia
	Hypertension (above baseline)	
Genitourinary	Hematuria	Hemolysis, thrombocytopenia
	Proteinuria	Myeloma
Musculoskeletal	Rib/sternal tenderness to palpation	Leukemia, myeloma
	Back pain; tenderness to palpation over spine, loss of height, kyphosis	Myeloma
	Pain/swelling in knees, wrists, hands	Hemophilia, sickle cell anemia
Abdominal	Enlarged spleen	Leukemia, myelofibrosis
	Enlarged liver	Myelofibrosis
	Stool positive for occult blood	Anemia, thrombocytopenia
Central nervous system	Cranial nerve dysfunction	Vitamin B_{12} deficiency
	Peripheral nerve dysfunction (especially sensory)	Vitamin B_{12} deficiency, amyloidosis, myeloma
	Visual changes, headache, alteration in mental status	Severe thrombocytopenia
Gynecologic	Menorrhagia	Thrombocytopenia, coagulopathy
Constitutional	Fever, chills, sweats, asthenia	Leukemia, lymphoma; infection

*Common findings (obtained via health history and physical assessment) that occur in patients with hematologic disorders. Note that signs and symptoms are not disease specific but are useful in guiding the nurse to establishing an etiology for the findings noted.

anticoagulant medications. In both tests, specific reagents are mixed into the plasma sample, and the time taken to form a clot is measured. For these tests to be accurate, the test tube must be filled with the correct amount of the patient's blood; either excess or inadequate blood volume within the tube can render the results inaccurate.

Bone Marrow Aspiration and Biopsy

Bone marrow aspiration and biopsy are crucial when additional information is needed to assess how a patient's blood cells are being formed and to assess the quantity and quality of each type of cell produced within the marrow. These tests are also used to document infection or tumor within the marrow. Other specialized tests can be performed on the marrow aspirate, such as cytogenetic analysis or immunophenotyping (i.e., identifying specific proteins expressed by cells), which are useful in further identifying certain malignant conditions and, in some instances, establishing a prognosis.

Normal bone marrow is in a semifluid state and can be aspirated through a special large needle. In adults, bone marrow is usually aspirated from the iliac crest and occasionally from the sternum. The aspirate provides only a sample of cells. Aspirate alone may be adequate for evaluating certain conditions, such as anemia. However, when more information is required, a biopsy is also performed. Biopsy samples are taken from the posterior iliac crest; occasionally, an anterior approach is required. A marrow biopsy shows the architecture of the bone marrow as well as its degree of cellularity.

Patient preparation includes a careful explanation of the procedure, which may be done at the patient's bedside (for a hospitalized patient) or in the outpatient setting. Some patients may be anxious, thus an antianxiety agent may be prescribed. It is always important for the physician or nurse to describe and explain to the patient the procedure and the sensations that will be experienced. The risks, benefits, and alternatives are also discussed. A signed informed consent is needed before the procedure is performed.

Before aspiration, the skin is cleansed using aseptic technique. Then, a small area is anesthetized with a local anesthetic agent through the skin and subcutaneous tissue to the periosteum of the bone. It is not possible to anesthetize the bone itself. The bone marrow needle is introduced with a stylet in place. When the needle is felt to go through the outer cortex of bone and enter the marrow cavity, the stylet is removed, a syringe is attached, and a small volume (5 mL) of blood and marrow is aspirated. Patients typically feel a pressure sensation as the needle is advanced into position. The actual aspiration always causes sharp but brief pain, resulting from the suction exerted as the marrow is aspirated into the syringe; the patient should be warned about this. Taking deep breaths or using relaxation techniques often helps ease the discomfort (Fig. 32-5).

If a bone marrow biopsy is necessary, it is best performed after the aspiration and in a slightly different location, because the marrow structure may be altered after aspiration. A special biopsy needle is used. Because these needles are large, the

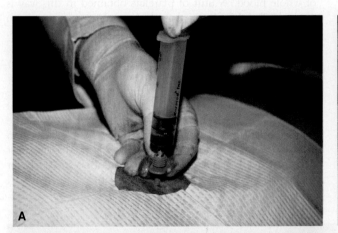

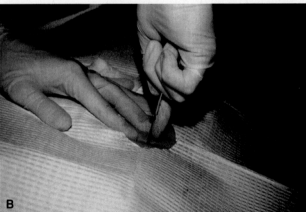

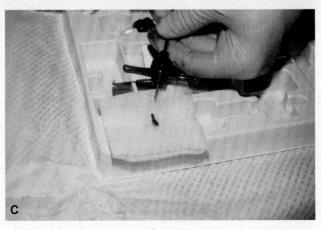

FIGURE 32-5 • Bone marrow aspiration procedure. The posterior superior iliac crest is the preferred site for bone marrow aspiration and biopsy because no vital organs or vessels are nearby. The patient is placed either in the lateral position with one leg flexed or in the prone position. The anterior iliac crest or sternum may also be used. Note that the sternum cannot be used for a marrow biopsy. **A.** Bone marrow aspiration. **B.** Inserting a Jamshidi biopsy needle. **C.** Dispensing the bone marrow core. From Farhi, D. C. (2009). *Pathology of bone marrow and blood cells* (2nd ed.). Philadelphia: Lippincott Williams & Wilkins.

skin may be punctured first with a surgical blade to make a 3- or 4-mm incision. The biopsy needle is advanced well into the marrow cavity. When the needle is properly positioned, a portion of marrow is cored out. The patient feels a pressure sensation but should not feel actual pain. The nurse should assist the patient in maintaining a comfortable position and encourage relaxation and deep breathing throughout the procedure. The patient should be instructed to inform the physician if pain occurs so that an additional anesthetic agent can be administered.

Hazards of either bone marrow aspiration or biopsy include bleeding and infection. The risk of bleeding is somewhat increased if the patient's platelet count is low or if the patient has been taking a medication (e.g., aspirin) that alters platelet function. After the marrow sample is obtained, pressure is applied to the site for several minutes. The site is then covered with a sterile dressing. Most patients have no discomfort after a bone marrow aspiration, but the site of a biopsy may ache for 1 or 2 days. Warm tub baths and a mild analgesic agent (e.g., acetaminophen [Tylenol]) may be useful. Aspirin-containing analgesic agents should be avoided it the immediate postprocedure period because they can aggravate or potentiate bleeding.

Therapeutic Approaches to Hematologic Disorders

Splenectomy

The surgical removal of the spleen (splenectomy) is a possible treatment for some hematologic disorders. For example, an enlarged spleen may be the site of excessive destruction of blood cells. In addition, some patients with grossly enlarged spleens develop severe thrombocytopenia as a result of platelets being sequestered in the spleen. Splenectomy removes the "trap," and platelet counts may normalize over time.

Laparoscopic splenectomy can be performed in selected patients, with a resultant decrease in postoperative morbidity. Postoperative complications include atelectasis, pneumonia, abdominal distention, and abscess formation. Although young children are at the highest risk after splenectomy, all age groups are vulnerable to overwhelming lethal infections and should receive the pneumococcal vaccine (Pneumovax) before undergoing splenectomy, if possible.

The patient is instructed to seek prompt medical attention if even relatively minor symptoms of infection occur. Often, patients with high platelet counts have even higher counts after splenectomy (more than 1 million/mm^3), which can predispose them to serious thrombotic or hemorrhagic problems. However, this increase is usually transient and therefore often does not warrant additional treatment.

Therapeutic Apheresis

Apheresis is a Greek word meaning "separation." In therapeutic apheresis (or pheresis), blood is taken from the patient and passed through a centrifuge, where a specific component is separated from the blood and removed (Table 32-3). The remaining blood is then returned to the patient. The entire system is closed, so the risk of bacterial contamination is low. When platelets or leukocytes are removed, the decrease in these cells within the circulation is temporary. However, the temporary decrease provides a window of time until suppressive medications (e.g., chemotherapy) can have therapeutic effects. Sometimes plasma is removed rather than blood cells—typically so that specific, abnormal proteins within the plasma are transiently lowered until a long-term therapy can be initiated.

Apheresis is also used to obtain larger amounts of platelets from a donor than can be provided from a single unit of whole blood. A unit of platelets obtained in this way is equivalent to 6 to 8 units of platelets obtained from six to eight separate donors via standard blood donation methods. Platelet donors can have their platelets apheresed as often as every 14 days. Leukocytes can be obtained similarly, typically after the donor has received growth factors (granulocyte colony-stimulating factor, granulocyte-macrophage colony-stimulating factor) to stimulate the formation of additional leukocytes and thereby increase the leukocyte count. The use of these growth factors also stimulates the release of stem cells within the circulation. Apheresis is used to harvest these stem cells (typically over a period of several days) for use in peripheral blood stem cell transplant.

TABLE 32-3	Types of Apheresis*	
Procedure	**Purpose**	**Examples of Clinical Use**
Plateletpheresis	Remove platelets	Extreme thrombocytosis, essential thrombocythemia (temporary measure); single-donor platelet transfusion
Leukapheresis	Remove WBCs (can be specific to neutrophils or lymphocytes)	Extreme leukocytosis (e.g., AML, CML) (very temporary measure); harvest WBCs for transfusion
Erythrocytapheresis (RBC exchange)	Remove RBCs	RBC dyscrasias (e.g., sickle cell disease); RBCs replaced via transfusion
Plasmapheresis (plasma exchange)	Remove plasma proteins	Hyperviscosity syndromes; treatment for some renal and neurologic diseases (e.g., Goodpasture syndrome, TTP, Guillain-Barré, myasthenia gravis)
Stem cell harvest	Remove circulating stem cells	Transplantation (donor harvest or autologous)

WBCs, white blood cells; AML, acute myeloid leukemia; CML, chronic myeloid leukemia; RBC, red blood cell; TTP, thrombotic thrombocytopenic purpura.

*Therapeutic apheresis can be used to treat a wide variety of conditions. When it is used to treat a disease that causes an increase in a specific cell type with a short life in circulation (i.e., WBCs, platelets), the reduction in those cells is temporary. However, this temporary reduction permits a margin of safety while waiting for a longer-lasting treatment modality (e.g., chemotherapy) to take effect. Apheresis can also be used to obtain stem cells for transplantation, either from a matched donor (allogenic) or from the patient (autologous).

Hematopoietic Stem Cell Transplantation

Hematopoietic stem cell transplantation (HSCT) is a therapeutic modality that offers the possibility of cure for some patients with hematologic disorders such as severe aplastic anemia, some forms of leukemia, and thalassemia. It can also provide longer remission from disease even when cure is not possible, such as in multiple myeloma. Hematopoietic stem cells may be transplanted from either allogeneic or autologous donors. For most hematologic diseases, allogeneic transplant is more effective; here, stem cells are obtained from a donor whose cells match those of the patient. In contrast, the patient's own stem cells are harvested and then used in autologous transplant. (See Chapter 15 for a detailed discussion of these procedures.)

Therapeutic Phlebotomy

Therapeutic phlebotomy is the removal of a certain amount of blood under controlled conditions. Patients with elevated hematocrits (e.g., those with polycythemia vera) or excessive iron absorption (e.g., hemochromatosis) can usually be managed by periodically removing 1 unit (about 500 mL) of whole blood. Over time, this process can produce iron deficiency, leaving the patient unable to produce as many erythrocytes. The actual procedure for therapeutic phlebotomy is similar to that for blood donation (see later discussion).

Blood Component Therapy

A single unit of whole blood contains 450 mL of blood and 50 mL of an anticoagulant, which can be processed and dispensed for administration. However, it is more appropriate, economical, and practical to separate that unit of whole blood into its primary components: erythrocytes, platelets, and plasma (leukocytes are rarely used; see later discussion). Because the plasma is removed, a unit of packed red blood cells (PRBCs) is very concentrated (hematocrit approximately 65% to 85%) (Strecker-McGraw, 2011).

Each component must be processed and stored differently to maximize the longevity of the viable cells and factors within it; thus, each individual blood component has a different storage life. PRBCs are stored at 4°C (39.2°F). With special preservatives, they can be stored safely for up to 42 days before they must be discarded (American Red Cross, 2012a; Roback, 2011). In contrast, platelets must be stored at room temperature because they cannot withstand cold temperatures, and they last for only 5 days before they must be discarded. To prevent clumping, platelets are gently agitated while stored. Plasma is immediately frozen to maintain the activity of the clotting factors within; it lasts for 1 year if it remains frozen. Alternatively, plasma can be further pooled and processed into blood derivatives, such as albumin, immune globulin, factor VIII, and factor IX. Table 32-4 describes each blood component and how it is commonly used.

Special Preparations

Factor VIII concentrate (antihemophilic factor) is a lyophilized, freeze-dried concentrate of pooled fractionated human plasma. It is used in treating hemophilia A. Factor IX concentrate (prothrombin complex) is similarly prepared and contains factors II, VII, IX, and X. It is used primarily for treatment of factor IX deficiency (hemophilia B). Factor IX concentrate is also useful in treating congenital factor VII and factor X deficiencies. Recombinant forms of factor VIII, such as Humate-P or Alphanate, are also useful. Because they contain von Willebrand factor, these agents are used in von Willebrand disease as well as in hemophilia A, particularly when patients develop factor VIII inhibitors.

Plasma albumin is a large protein molecule that usually stays within vessels and is a major contributor to plasma oncotic pressure. This protein is used to expand the blood volume of patients in hypovolemic shock and, rarely, to increase the concentration of circulating albumin in patients with hypoalbuminemia.

Immune globulin is a concentrated solution of the antibody immunoglobulin G (IgG), prepared from large pools of plasma. It contains very little immunoglobulin A (IgA) or IgM. The IV form (IVIG) is used in various clinical situations to replace inadequate amounts of IgG in patients who are at risk for recurrent bacterial infection (e.g., those with chronic lymphocytic leukemia, those receiving HSCT). It is also used in certain autoimmune disorders, such as idiopathic thrombocytopenic purpura (ITP). Albumin, antihemophilic factors, and IVIG, in contrast to all other fractions of human blood, cells, or plasma, can survive being subjected to heating at 60°C (140°F) for 10 hours to free them of the viral contaminants that may be present.

Procuring Blood and Blood Products

Blood Donation

To protect both the donor and the recipients, all prospective donors are examined and interviewed before they are allowed to donate their blood. The intent of the interview is to assess the general health status of the donor and to identify risk factors that might harm a recipient of the donor's blood. There is no upper age limit to donation. The American Red Cross (2012b) requires that donors be in good health and meet specific eligibility criteria related to medications and vaccinations, medical conditions and treatments, travel outside the United States, lifestyle and life events, and so on. Detailed information about these criteria is available on the American Red Cross Web site (see the Resources section).

All donors are expected to meet the following minimal requirements (American Red Cross, 2012b):
- Body weight should be at least 50 kg (110 lb) for a standard 450-mL donation. Donors weighing less than 50 kg donate proportionately less blood. People younger than 17 years require parental consent in some states.
- The oral temperature should not exceed 37.5°C (99.6°F).
- The pulse rate should be regular and between 50 and 100 bpm.
- The systolic arterial blood pressure should be 90 to 180 mm Hg, and the diastolic pressure should be 50 to 100 mm Hg.
- The hemoglobin level should be at least 12.5 g/dL for women and 13.5 g/dL for men.

TABLE 32-4   Blood and Blood Components Commonly Used in Transfusion Therapy*

Composition		Indications and Considerations
Whole blood	Cells and plasma, hematocrit about 40%	Volume replacement and oxygen-carrying capacity; usually used only in significant bleeding (>25% blood volume lost)
PBRCs	RBCs with little plasma (hematocrit about 75%); some platelets and WBCs remain	↑ RBC mass; symptomatic anemia: • Platelets within the unit are not functional. • WBCs within the unit may cause reaction and are not functional.
Platelets—random	Platelets (5.5×10^{10} platelets/unit), plasma; some RBCs, WBCs	Bleeding due to severe ↓ platelets Prevent bleeding when platelets <5,000–10,000/mm^3 Survival ↓ in presence of fever, chills, infection Repeated treatment leads to ↓ survival due to alloimmunization.
Platelets—single donor	Platelets (3×10^{11} platelets/unit) 1 unit is equivalent to 6–8 units of random platelets.	Used for repeated treatment: • ↓ alloimmunization risk by limiting exposure to multiple donors
Plasma	Plasma; all coagulation factors Complement	Bleeding in patients with coagulation factor deficiencies; plasmapheresis
Granulocytes	Neutrophils (>1×10^{10}/unit); some lymphocytes, RBCs, and platelets will remain within the unit.	Severe neutropenia in selected patients; controversial
Lymphocytes	Lymphocytes (number varies)	Stimulate graft-versus-host disease effect
Cryoprecipitate	Fibrinogen ≥150 mg/bag, AHF (VIII:C) 80–110 units/bag, von Willebrand factor; fibronectin	von Willebrand disease Hypofibrinogenemia Hemophilia A
AHF	Factor VIII	Hemophilia A
Factor IX concentrate	Factor IX	Hemophilia B (Christmas disease)
Factor IX complex	Factors II, VII, IX, X	Hereditary factor VII, IX, X deficiency; hemophilia A with factor VII inhibitors
Albumin	Albumin 5%, 25%	Hypoproteinemia; burns; volume expansion by 5% to ↑ blood volume; 25% leads to ↓ hematocrit
IV gamma-globulin	Immunoglobulin G antibodies	Hypogammaglobulinemia (in CLL, recurrent infections); ITP; primary immunodeficiency states
Antithrombin III concentrate (AT III)	AT III (trace amounts of other plasma proteins)	AT III deficiency with or at risk for thrombosis

PBRCs, packed red blood cells; RBCs, red blood cells; WBCs, white blood cells; ↑, increased; ↓, decreased; AHF, antihemophilic factor; IV, intravenous; CLL, chronic lymphocytic leukemia; ITP, idiopathic thrombocytopenic purpura.

*The composition of each type of blood component is described as well as the most common indications for using a given blood component. RBCs, platelets, and fresh-frozen plasma are the blood products most commonly used. When transfusing these blood products, it is important to realize that the individual product is always "contaminated" with very small amounts of other blood products (e.g., WBCs mixed in a unit of platelets). This contamination can cause some difficulties, particularly isosensitization, in certain patients.

Directed Donation

At times, friends and family of a patient wish to donate blood for that person. These blood donations are referred to as directed donations. These donations are not any safer than those provided by random donors, because directed donors may not be as willing to identify themselves as having a history of any of the risk factors that disqualify a person from donating blood. Therefore, some blood centers no longer accept directed donations.

Standard Donation

Phlebotomy consists of venipuncture and blood withdrawal. Standard precautions are used. Donors are placed in a semirecumbent position. The skin over the antecubital fossa is carefully cleansed with an antiseptic preparation, a tourniquet is applied, and venipuncture is performed. Withdrawal of 450 mL of blood usually takes less than 15 minutes. After the needle is removed, donors are asked to hold the involved arm straight up, and firm pressure is applied with sterile gauze for 2 to 3 minutes. A firm bandage is then applied. The donor remains recumbent until he or she feels able to sit up, usually within a few minutes. Donors who experience weakness or faintness should rest for a longer period. The donor then receives food and fluids and is asked to remain another 15 minutes.

The donor is instructed to leave the dressing on and to avoid heavy lifting for several hours, to avoid smoking for 1 hour, to avoid drinking alcoholic beverages for 3 hours, to increase fluid intake for 2 days, and to eat healthy meals for at least 2 weeks. Specimens from the donated blood are tested to detect infections and to identify the specific blood type (see later discussion).

Autologous Donation

A patient's own blood may be collected for future transfusion; this method is useful for many elective surgeries where the potential need for transfusion is high (e.g., orthopedic surgery). Preoperative donations are ideally collected 4 to 6 weeks before surgery. Iron supplements are prescribed during this period to prevent depletion of iron stores. Typically, 1 unit of blood is drawn each week; the number of units obtained varies with the type of surgical procedure to be performed (i.e., the amount of blood anticipated to be transfused). Phlebotomies are not performed within 72 hours of surgery. Individual blood components can also be collected.

The primary advantage of autologous transfusions is the prevention of viral infections from another person's blood. Other advantages include safe transfusion for patients with a history of transfusion reactions, prevention of alloimmunization, and avoidance of complications in patients with alloantibodies. It is the policy of the American Red Cross that autologous blood is transfused only to the donor. If the blood is not required, it can be frozen until the donor needs it in the future (for up to 10 years). The blood is never returned to the general donor supply of blood products to be used by another person.

Needless autologous donation (i.e., performed when the likelihood of transfusion is small) is discouraged because it is expensive, takes time, and uses resources inappropriately. Moreover, in an emergency situation, the autologous units available may be inadequate, and the patient may still require additional units from the general donor supply. Furthermore, although autologous transfusion can eliminate the risk of viral contamination, the risk of bacterial contamination is the same as that in transfusion from random donors.

Contraindications to donation of blood for autologous transfusion are acute infection, severely debilitating chronic disease, hemoglobin level less than 11 g/dL, unstable angina, and acute cardiovascular or cerebrovascular disease. A history of poorly controlled epilepsy may be considered a contraindication in some centers.

Intraoperative Blood Salvage

This transfusion method provides replacement for patients who cannot donate blood before surgery and for those undergoing vascular, orthopedic, or thoracic surgery. During a surgical procedure, blood lost into a sterile cavity (e.g., hip joint) is suctioned into a cell-saver machine. The whole blood or PRBCs are washed, often with saline solution; filtered; and then returned to the patient as an intravenous (IV) infusion. Salvaged blood cannot be stored, because bacteria cannot be completely removed from the blood and thus cannot be used when it is contaminated with bacteria. The use of intraoperative blood salvage has decreased the need for autologous blood donation but has not affected the need for allogeneic blood products (Ashworth & Klein, 2010; Carless, Henry, Carson, et al., 2010).

Hemodilution

This transfusion method may be initiated before or after induction of anesthesia. About 1 to 2 units of blood are removed from the patient through a venous or arterial line and simultaneously replaced with a colloid or crystalloid solution. The blood obtained is then reinfused after surgery. The advantage of this method is that the patient loses fewer erythrocytes during surgery, because the added IV solutions dilute the concentration of erythrocytes and lower the hematocrit. However, patients who are at risk for myocardial injury should not be further stressed by hemodilution. Hemodilution has been associated with adverse outcomes in patients having cardiopulmonary bypass; it has also been linked to tissue ischemia, particularly in the kidneys (Ranucci, Conti, Castelvecchio, et al., 2010).

Complications of Blood Donation

Excessive bleeding at the donor's venipuncture site is sometimes caused by a bleeding disorder but more often results from a technique error: laceration of the vein, excessive tourniquet pressure, or failure to apply enough pressure after the needle is withdrawn.

Fainting may occur after blood donation and may be related to emotional factors, a vasovagal reaction, or prolonged fasting before donation. Because of the loss of blood volume, hypotension and syncope may occur when the donor assumes an erect position. A donor who appears pale or complains of faintness should immediately lie down or sit with the head lowered below the knees. He or she should be observed for another 30 minutes.

Anginal chest pain may be precipitated in patients with unsuspected coronary artery disease. Seizures can occur in donors with epilepsy, although the incidence is very low. Both angina and seizures require further medical evaluation and treatment.

Blood Processing

Samples of the unit of blood are always taken immediately after donation so that the blood can be typed and tested. Each donation is tested for antibodies to human immunodeficiency virus (HIV) types 1 and 2, hepatitis B core antibody (anti-HBc), hepatitis C virus (HCV), human T-cell lymphotropic virus type I (anti-HTLV-I/II), hepatitis B surface antigen (HbsAG), and syphilis. Negative reactions are required for the blood to be used, and each unit of blood is labeled to certify the results. Nucleic acid amplification testing has increased the ability to detect the presence of HCV, HIV, and West Nile virus infections, because it directly tests for genomic nucleic acids of the viruses rather than for the presence of antibodies to the viruses. This testing significantly shortens the "window" of inability to detect HIV and HCV from a donated unit, further ensuring the safety of the blood; the risk of transmission of HIV or HCV is now estimated at 1 in 2 million units and 1 in 200,000 units of blood donated, respectively (Zou, Dorsey, Notari, et al., 2010). Blood is also screened for cytomegalovirus (CMV); if it tests positive for CMV, it can still be used, except in recipients who are negative for CMV and who are severely immunocompromised.

Equally important is accurate determination of the blood type. More than 200 antigens have been identified on the surface of RBC membranes. Of these, the most important for safe transfusion are the ABO and Rh systems. The ABO system identifies which sugars are present on the membrane of a person's erythrocytes: A, B, both A and B, or neither A nor B (type O). To prevent a significant reaction, the same type of PRBCs should be transfused. Previously, it was thought that in an emergency situation in which the patient's blood type was not known, type O blood could be safely transfused. This practice is no longer recommended.

The Rh antigen (also referred to as D) is present on the surface of erythrocytes in 85% of the population (Rh positive). Those who lack the D antigen are referred to as being Rh negative. PRBCs are routinely tested for the D antigen as well as ABO. Patients should receive PRBCs with a compatible Rh type.

The majority of transfusion reactions are due to clerical error where the patient is transfused an incompatible unit of blood product. Reactions (other than those due to procedural error) are most frequently due to the presence of donor leukocytes within the blood component unit (PRBCs or platelets); the recipient may form antibodies to the antigens present on these leukocytes. PRBC components typically have 1 to 3 × 10^9 leukocytes remaining in each unit. Leukocytes from the blood product are frequently filtered to diminish the likelihood of developing reactions and refractoriness to transfusions, particularly in patients who have chronic transfusion needs. The process of leukocyte filtration renders the blood component "leukocyte poor" (i.e., leukopoor). Filtration can occur at the time the unit is collected from the donor and processed, which achieves better results but is more expensive, or at the time the blood component is transfused by attaching a leukocyte filter to the blood administration tubing. Many centers advocate routinely using leukopoor filtered blood components for people who have or are likely to develop chronic transfusion requirements.

When a patient is immunocompromised, as in the case following stem cell transplant, any donor lymphocytes must be removed from the blood components. In this situation, the blood component is exposed to low amounts of radiation (25 Gy) that kill any lymphocytes within the blood component. Irradiated blood products are highly effective in preventing transfusion-associated graft-versus-host disease, which is fatal in most cases. Irradiated blood products have a shorter shelf life.

Transfusion

Administration of blood and blood components requires knowledge of correct administration techniques and possible complications. It is very important to be familiar with the agency's policies and procedures for transfusion therapy. Methods for transfusing blood components are presented in Charts 32-2 and 32-3.

Setting

Although most blood transfusions are performed in the acute care setting, patients with chronic transfusion requirements often can receive transfusions in other settings. Freestanding infusion centers, ambulatory care clinics, physicians' offices, and even patients' homes may be appropriate settings for transfusion. Typically, patients who need chronic transfusions but are otherwise stable physically are appropriate candidates for outpatient therapy. Verification and administration of the blood product are performed as in a hospital setting. Although most blood products can be transfused in the outpatient setting, the home is typically limited to transfusions of PRBCs and factor components (e.g., factor VIII for patients with hemophilia).

Chart 32-2　Transfusion of Packed Red Blood Cells

Preprocedure

1. Confirm that the transfusion has been prescribed.
2. Check that patient's blood has been typed and cross-matched.
3. Verify that patient has signed a written consent form per institution or agency policy and agrees to procedure.
4. Explain procedure to patient. Instruct patient in signs and symptoms of transfusion reaction (itching, hives, swelling, shortness of breath, fever, chills).
5. Take patient's temperature, pulse, respiration, and blood pressure to establish a baseline and auscultate lungs; assess for jugular venous distention to serve as a baseline for comparison during transfusion.
6. Use hand hygiene and wear gloves in accordance with standard precautions.
7. Use a 20-gauge or larger needle for insertion in a large vein. Use special tubing that contains a blood filter to screen out fibrin clots and other particulate matter. Do not vent blood container.

Procedure

1. Obtain packed red blood cells (PRBCs) from the blood bank *after* the IV line is started. (Institution policy may limit release to only 1 unit at a time.)
2. Double-check labels with another nurse or physician to ensure that the ABO group and Rh type agree with the compatibility record. Check to see that number and type on donor blood label and on patient's medical record are correct. Confirm patient's identification by asking the patient's name and checking the identification wristband.
3. Check blood for gas bubbles and any unusual color or cloudiness. (Gas bubbles may indicate bacterial growth. Abnormal color or cloudiness may be a sign of hemolysis.)
4. Make sure that PRBC transfusion is initiated within 30 minutes after removal of the PRBCs from blood bank refrigerator.
5. For first 15 minutes, run the transfusion slowly—no faster than 5 mL/min. Observe patient carefully for adverse effects. If no adverse effects occur during the first 15 minutes, increase the flow rate unless patient is at high risk for circulatory overload.
6. Monitor closely for 15–30 minutes to detect signs of reaction. Monitor vital signs at regular intervals per institution or agency policy; compare results with baseline measurements. Increase frequency of measurements based on patient's condition. Observe patient frequently throughout the transfusion for any signs of adverse reaction, including restlessness, hives, nausea, vomiting, torso or back pain, shortness of breath, flushing, hematuria, fever, or chills. Should any adverse reaction occur, stop infusion immediately, notify primary provider, and follow the agency's transfusion reaction standard.
7. Note that administration time does not exceed 4 hours because of increased risk of bacterial proliferation.
8. Be alert for signs of adverse reactions: circulatory overload, sepsis, febrile reaction, allergic reaction, and acute hemolytic reaction.
9. Change blood tubing after every 2 units transfused to decrease chance of bacterial contamination.

Postprocedure

1. Obtain vital signs and compare with baseline measurements.
2. Dispose of used materials properly.
3. Document procedure in patient's medical record, including patient assessment findings and tolerance to procedure.
4. Monitor patient for response to and effectiveness of procedure.

Note: Never add medications to blood or blood products; if blood is too thick to run freely, normal saline may be added to the unit. If blood must be warmed, use an in-line blood warmer with a monitoring system.

Chart 32-3 Transfusion of Platelets or Fresh-Frozen Plasma

Preprocedure

1. Confirm that the transfusion has been prescribed.
2. Verify that patient has signed a written consent form per institution policy and agrees to procedure.
3. Explain procedure to patient. Instruct patient in signs and symptoms of transfusion reaction (itching, hives, swelling, shortness of breath, fever, chills).
4. Take patient's temperature, pulse, respiration, and blood pressure to establish a baseline and auscultate breath sounds to establish a baseline for comparison during transfusion.
5. Use hand hygiene and wear gloves in accordance with standard precautions.
6. Use a 22-gauge or larger needle for placement in a large vein, if possible. Use appropriate tubing per institution policy (platelets often require different tubing from that used for other blood products).

Procedure

1. Obtain platelets or fresh-frozen plasma (FFP) from the blood bank (only *after* the IV line is started.)
2. Double-check labels with another nurse or physician to ensure that the ABO group matches the compatibility record (not usually necessary for platelets; here only if compatible platelets are ordered). Check to see that number and type on donor blood label and on patient's chart are correct. Confirm patient's identification by asking the patient's name and checking the identification wristband.
3. Check blood product for any unusual color or clumps (excessive redness indicates contamination with larger amounts of red blood cells).

4. Make sure that platelets or FFP units are administered immediately after they are obtained.
5. Infuse each unit of FFP over 30–60 minutes per patient tolerance; infuse each unit of platelets as fast as patient can tolerate to diminish platelet clumping during administration. Observe patient carefully for adverse effects, including circulatory overload. Decrease rate of infusion if necessary.
6. Observe patient closely throughout transfusion for any signs of adverse reaction, including restlessness, hives, nausea, vomiting, torso or back pain, shortness of breath, flushing, hematuria, fever, or chills. Should any adverse reaction occur, stop infusion immediately, notify primary provider, and follow the agency's transfusion reaction standard.
7. Monitor vital signs at end of transfusion per institution policy; compare results with baseline measurements.
8. Flush line with saline after transfusion to remove blood component from tubing.

Postprocedure

1. Obtain vital signs and compare with baseline measurements.
2. Dispose of used materials properly.
3. Document procedure in patient's medical record, including patient assessment findings and tolerance to procedure.
4. Monitor patient for response to and effectiveness of procedure. A platelet count may be ordered 1 hour after platelet transfusion to facilitate this evaluation.

Note: FFP requires ABO but not Rh compatibility. Platelets are not typically cross-matched for ABO compatibility. Never add medications to blood or blood products.

Pretransfusion Assessment

Patient History

The patient history is an important component of the pretransfusion assessment to determine the history of previous transfusions as well as previous reactions to transfusion. The history should include the type of reaction, its manifestations, the interventions required, and whether any preventive interventions were used in subsequent transfusions. The nurse assesses the number of pregnancies a woman has had, because a high number can increase her risk of reaction due to antibodies developed from exposure to fetal circulation. Other concurrent health problems should be noted, with careful attention to cardiac, pulmonary, and vascular disease.

Physical Assessment

A systematic physical assessment and measurement of baseline vital signs are important before transfusing any blood product. The respiratory system should be assessed, including careful auscultation of the lungs and the patient's use of accessory muscles. Cardiac system assessment should include careful inspection for any edema as well as other signs of cardiac failure (e.g., jugular venous distention). The skin should be observed for rashes, petechiae, and ecchymoses. The sclera should be examined for icterus. In the event of a transfusion reaction, a comparison of findings can help differentiate between types of reactions.

Patient Education

Reviewing the signs and symptoms of a transfusion reaction is crucial for patients who have not received a previous transfusion. Even for patients who have received prior transfusions, a brief review of the signs and symptoms of transfusion reactions is advised. Signs and symptoms of a reaction include fever, chills, respiratory distress, low back pain, nausea, pain at the IV site, or anything "unusual." Although a thorough review is very important, the nurse also reassures the patient that the blood is carefully tested against the patient's own blood (cross-matched) to diminish the likelihood of any untoward reaction. Similarly, the patient can be reassured about the very low possibility of contracting HIV from the transfusion; this fear persists among many people.

Complications

Any patient who receives a blood transfusion is at risk for developing complications from the transfusion. During patient education, the nurse explains the risks and benefits and what to expect during and after the transfusion. Patients must be informed that although it has been tested carefully, the supply of blood is not completely risk free. Nursing management is directed toward preventing complications, promptly recognizing complications if they develop, and promptly initiating measures to control complications. The following sections describe the most common or potentially severe transfusion-related complications.

Febrile Nonhemolytic Reaction

A febrile nonhemolytic reaction is caused by antibodies to donor leukocytes that remain in the unit of blood or blood component; it is the most common type of transfusion reaction. It occurs more frequently in patients who have had previous transfusions (exposure to multiple antigens from previous blood products) and in Rh-negative women who have borne Rh-positive children (exposure to an Rh-positive fetus raises antibody levels in the untreated mother).

The diagnosis of a febrile nonhemolytic reaction is made by excluding other potential causes, such as a hemolytic reaction or bacterial contamination of the blood product. The signs and symptoms of a febrile nonhemolytic transfusion reaction are chills (minimal to severe) followed by fever (more than 1°C elevation). The fever typically begins within 2 hours after the transfusion is begun. Although the reaction is not life threatening, the fever, and particularly the chills and muscle stiffness, can be frightening to the patient.

This reaction can be diminished, even prevented, by further depleting the blood component of donor leukocytes; this is accomplished by a leukocyte reduction filter. Antipyretic agents can be given to prevent fever; however, routine premedication is not advised because it can mask the beginning of a more serious transfusion reaction.

Acute Hemolytic Reaction

The most dangerous, and potentially life-threatening, type of transfusion reaction occurs when the donor blood is incompatible with that of the recipient (i.e., type II hypersensitivity reaction). Antibodies already present in the recipient's plasma rapidly combine with antigens on donor erythrocytes, and the erythrocytes are destroyed in the circulation (i.e., intravascular hemolysis). The most rapid hemolysis occurs in ABO incompatibility. Rh incompatibility often causes a less severe reaction. This reaction can occur after transfusion of as little as 10 mL of PRBCs. Although the overall incidence of such reactions is not high (1:20,000 to 1:40,000 units transfused [Leo & Pedal, 2010]), they are largely preventable. The most common causes of acute hemolytic reaction are errors in blood component labeling and patient identification that result in the administration of an ABO-incompatible transfusion.

Symptoms consist of fever, chills, low back pain, nausea, chest tightness, dyspnea, and anxiety. As the erythrocytes are destroyed, the hemoglobin is released from the cells and excreted by the kidneys; therefore, hemoglobin appears in the urine (hemoglobinuria). Hypotension, bronchospasm, and vascular collapse may result. Diminished renal perfusion results in acute renal failure, and disseminated intravascular coagulation may also occur. The reaction must be recognized promptly and the transfusion discontinued immediately (see the Nursing Management for Transfusion Reactions section).

Acute hemolytic transfusion reactions are preventable. Meticulous attention to detail in labeling blood samples and blood components and accurately identifying the recipient cannot be overemphasized. Bar coding methods can be useful safeguards in matching a patient's wristband with the label on the blood component (Pagliaro, Turdo, & Capuzzo, 2009); however, these methods are not fail proof and do not reduce the nurse's responsibility to ensure the correct blood component is transfused to the correct patient.

Allergic Reaction

Some patients develop urticaria (hives) or generalized itching during a transfusion; the cause is thought to be a sensitivity reaction to a plasma protein within the blood component being transfused. Symptoms of an allergic reaction are urticaria, itching, and flushing. The reactions are usually mild and respond to antihistamines. If the symptoms resolve after administration of an antihistamine (e.g., diphenhydramine [Benadryl]), the transfusion may be resumed. Rarely, the allergic reaction is severe, with bronchospasm, laryngeal edema, and shock. These reactions are managed with epinephrine, corticosteroids, and vasopressor support, if necessary.

Giving the patient antihistamines or corticosteroids before the transfusion may prevent future reactions. For severe reactions, future blood components are washed to remove any remaining plasma proteins. Leukocyte filters are not useful to prevent such reactions, because the offending plasma proteins can pass through the filter.

Circulatory Overload

If too much blood is infused too quickly, hypervolemia can occur. This condition can be aggravated in patients who already have increased circulatory volume (e.g., those with heart failure). PRBCs are safer to use than whole blood. If the administration rate is sufficiently slow, circulatory overload may be prevented. For patients who are at risk for, or already in, circulatory overload, diuretics are administered after the transfusion or between units of PRBCs. Patients receiving fresh-frozen plasma or even platelets may also develop circulatory overload. The infusion rate of these blood components must also be titrated to the patient's tolerance.

Signs of circulatory overload include dyspnea, orthopnea, tachycardia, and sudden anxiety. Jugular vein distention, crackles at the base of the lungs, and an increase in blood pressure can also occur. If the transfusion is continued, pulmonary edema can develop, as manifested by severe dyspnea and coughing of pink, frothy sputum.

If fluid overload is mild, the transfusion can often be continued after slowing the rate of infusion and administering diuretics. However, if the overload is severe, the patient is placed upright with the feet in a dependent position, the transfusion is discontinued, and the primary provider is notified. The IV line is kept patent with a very slow infusion of normal saline solution or a saline lock device to maintain access to the vein in case IV medications are necessary. Oxygen and morphine may be needed to treat severe dyspnea (see Chapter 29).

Bacterial Contamination

The incidence of bacterial contamination of blood components is very low; however, administration of contaminated products puts the patient at great risk. Contamination can occur at any point during procurement or processing but often results from organisms on the donor's skin. Many bacteria cannot survive in the cold temperatures used to store PRBCs, but some organisms can do so. Platelets are at greater risk of contamination because they are stored at room temperature.

Recently, blood centers have developed rapid methods of culturing platelet units, thereby diminishing the risk of using a contaminated platelet unit for transfusion.

Preventive measures include meticulous care in the procurement and processing of blood components. When PRBCs or whole blood is transfused, it should be administered within a 4-hour period, because warm room temperatures promote bacterial growth. A contaminated unit of blood product may appear normal, or it may have an abnormal color.

The signs of bacterial contamination are fever, chills, and hypotension. These manifestations may not occur until the transfusion is complete, occasionally not until several hours after the transfusion. As soon as the reaction is recognized, any remaining transfusion is discontinued (see the Nursing Management for Transfusion Reactions section). If the condition is not treated immediately with fluids and broad-spectrum antibiotics, sepsis can occur. Sepsis is treated with IV fluids and antibiotics; corticosteroids and vasopressors are often also necessary (see Chapter 14).

Transfusion-Related Acute Lung Injury

Transfusion-related acute lung injury (TRALI) is a potentially fatal, idiosyncratic reaction that is defined as the development of acute lung injury occurring within 6 hours after a blood transfusion. All blood components have been implicated in TRALI, including IVIG, cryoprecipitate, and stem cells. TRALI is the most common cause of transfusion-related death (Cherry, Steciuk, Reddy, et al., 2008).

The underlying pathophysiologic mechanism for TRALI is unknown but is thought to involve antibodies in the donor's plasma that react to the leukocytes in the recipient's blood. Occasionally, the reverse occurs, and antibodies present in the recipient's plasma agglutinate the antigens on the few remaining leukocytes in the blood component being transfused. Another theory suggests that an initial insult to the patient's vascular endothelium causes neutrophils to aggregate at the injured endothelium. Various substances within the transfused blood component (lipids, cytokines) then activate these neutrophils. Each of these pathophysiologic mechanisms can contribute to the process (Fung & Silliman, 2009). The end result of this process is interstitial and intra-alveolar edema, as well as extensive sequestration of WBCs within the pulmonary capillaries.

Onset is abrupt (usually within 6 hours of transfusion, often within 2 hours). Signs and symptoms include acute shortness of breath, hypoxia (arterial oxygen saturation [SaO_2] less than 90%; partial pressure of arterial oxygen [PaO_2] to fraction of inspired oxygen [FIO_2] ratio of less than 300), hypotension, fever, and eventual pulmonary edema. Diagnostic criteria include hypoxemia, bilateral pulmonary infiltrates (seen on chest x-ray), no evidence of cardiac cause for the pulmonary edema, and no other plausible alternative cause within 6 hours of completing transfusion. Aggressive supportive therapy (e.g., oxygen, intubation, fluid support) may prevent death.

Although TRALI can occur with the transfusion of any blood component, it is more likely to occur when plasma and, to a lesser extent, platelets are transfused. One commonly used preventive strategy involves limiting the frequency and amount of blood products transfused. Another entails obtaining plasma and possibly platelets only from men or from women who have never been pregnant (and, consequently, are less likely to have developed offending antibodies). The efficacy of this approach and its impact on the availability of these blood components remain unclear (Müller, Porcelijn, & Vlaar, 2012).

Delayed Hemolytic Reaction

Delayed hemolytic reactions usually occur within 14 days after transfusion, when the level of antibody has been increased to the extent that a reaction can occur. The hemolysis of the erythrocytes is extravascular via the RES and occurs gradually.

Signs and symptoms of a delayed hemolytic reaction are fever, anemia, increased bilirubin level, decreased or absent haptoglobin, and possibly jaundice. Rarely, there is hemoglobinuria. Generally, these reactions are not dangerous, but it is important to recognize them because subsequent transfusions with blood products containing these antibodies may cause a more severe hemolytic reaction. However, recognition is also difficult because the patient may not be in a health care setting to be tested for this reaction, and even if the patient is hospitalized, the reaction may be too mild to be recognized clinically. Because the amount of antibody present can be too low to detect, it is difficult to prevent delayed hemolytic reactions. Fortunately, the reaction is usually mild and requires no intervention.

Disease Acquisition

Despite advances in donor screening and blood testing, certain diseases can still be transmitted by transfusion of blood components (Chart 32-4).

Complications of Long-Term Transfusion Therapy

The complications that have been described represent a real risk to any patient any time a blood component is administered. However, patients with long-term transfusion requirements (e.g., those with myelodysplastic syndrome, thalassemia, aplastic anemia, sickle cell anemia) are at greater risk for infection transmission and for becoming more sensitized to donor antigens, simply because they are exposed to more units of blood and, consequently, more donors. A summary of complications associated with long-term transfusion therapy is given in Table 32-5.

Iron overload is a complication unique to people who have had long-term PRBC transfusions. One unit of PRBCs contains 250 mg of iron. Patients with chronic transfusion requirements can quickly acquire more iron than they can use, leading to iron overload. Over time, the excess iron deposits in body tissues and can cause organ damage, particularly in the liver, heart, testes, and pancreas. Promptly initiating a program of iron chelation therapy can prevent end-organ damage from iron toxicity. (See Chapter 33, Hereditary Hemochromatosis, Nursing Management, and Chapter 34, Myelodysplastic Syndrome, Nursing Management.)

Nursing Management for Transfusion Reactions

If a transfusion reaction is suspected, the transfusion must be stopped immediately and the primary provider notified. A thorough patient assessment is crucial, because many

Chart 32-4 Diseases Transmitted by Blood Transfusion

Hepatitis (Viral Hepatitis B, C)

- There is greater risk from pooled blood products and blood of paid donors than from volunteer donors.
- A screening test detects most hepatitis B and C.

AIDS (HIV and HTLV)

- Donated blood is screened for antibodies to HIV.
- Transmittal risk is estimated at 1:1.5 million per transfusion.
- People with high-risk behaviors (multiple sex partners, anal sex, IV/injection drug use) and people with signs and symptoms that suggest AIDS should not donate blood.

Cytomegalovirus (CMV)

- Transmittal risk is greater for premature newborns with CMV antibody–negative mothers and for immunocompromised recipients who are CMV negative (e.g., those with acute leukemia, organ or tissue transplant recipients).
- Blood products rendered "leukocyte reduced" help reduce transmission of virus.

Graft-Versus-Host Disease (GVHD)

- GVHD occurs only in severely immunocompromised recipients (e.g., Hodgkin disease, bone marrow transplantation).
- Transfused lymphocytes engraft in recipient and attack host lymphocytes or body tissues; signs and symptoms are fever, diffuse reddened skin rash, nausea, vomiting, diarrhea.
- Preventive measures include irradiating blood products to inactivate donor lymphocytes (no known radiation risks to transfusion recipient) and processing donor blood with leukocyte reduction filters.

Creutzfeldt-Jakob Disease (CJD)

- CJD is a rare, fatal disease that causes irreversible brain damage.
- There is no evidence of transmittal by transfusion.
- All blood donors must be screened for positive family history of CJD.
- Potential donors who spent 3 months or more in the United Kingdom or 6 months or more in Europe since 1980 cannot donate blood; blood products from a donor who develops CJD are recalled.

AIDS, acquired immunodeficiency syndrome; HIV, human immunodeficiency virus; HTLV, human T-lymphotropic virus.

---

complications have similar signs and symptoms. The following steps are taken to determine the type and severity of the reaction:

- Stop the transfusion. Maintain the IV line with normal saline solution through new IV tubing, administered at a slow rate.
- Assess the patient carefully. Compare the vital signs with baseline, including oxygen saturation. Assess the patient's respiratory status carefully. Note the presence of adventitious breath sounds; the use of accessory muscles; extent of dyspnea; and changes in mental status, including anxiety and confusion. Note any chills, diaphoresis, jugular vein distention, and reports of back pain or urticaria.
- Notify the primary provider of the assessment findings, and implement any treatments prescribed. Continue to monitor the patient's vital signs and respiratory, cardiovascular, and renal status.
- Notify the blood bank that a suspected transfusion reaction has occurred.

- Send the blood container and tubing to the blood bank for repeat typing and culture. The patient's identity and blood component identifying tags and numbers are verified.

If a hemolytic transfusion reaction or bacterial infection is suspected, the nurse does the following:

- Obtains appropriate blood specimens from the patient
- Collects a urine sample as soon as possible to detect hemoglobin in the urine
- Documents the reaction according to the institution's policy

Pharmacologic Alternatives to Blood Transfusions

Pharmacologic agents that stimulate production of one or more types of blood cells by the marrow are commonly used (Chart 32-5). Researchers continue to seek a blood substitute that is practical and safe. Manufacturing artificial blood

---

TABLE 32-5   Common Complications Resulting From Long-Term Packed Red Blood Cell Transfusion Therapy*

Complication	Manifestation	Management
Infection	Hepatitis (B, C)	May immunize against hepatitis B; treat hepatitis C; monitor hepatic function
	CMV	WBC filters to protect against CMV
Iron overload	Heart failure	Prevent by chelation therapy
	Endocrine failure (diabetes, hypothyroidism, hypoparathyroidism, hypogonadism)	
Transfusion reaction	Sensitization	Diminish by RBC phenotyping, using WBC-filtered products
	Febrile reactions	Diminish by using WBC-filtered products

CMV, cytomegalovirus; WBC, white blood cell; RBC, red blood cell.
*Patients with long-term transfusion therapy requirements are at risk not only for the transfusion reactions discussed in the text but also for the complications noted in the table. In many cases, the use of WBC-filtered (i.e., leukocyte-poor) blood products is standard for patients who receive long-term packed red blood cell transfusion therapy. An aggressive chelation program initiated early in the course of therapy can prevent problems with iron overload.

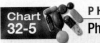

Chart
32-5 **PHARMACOLOGY**
Pharmacologic Alternatives to Blood Transfusions

Growth Factors

Recombinant technology has provided a means to produce hematopoietic growth factors necessary for the production of blood cells within the bone marrow. By increasing the body's production of blood cells, transfusions and complications resulting from diminished blood cells (e.g., infection from neutropenia) may be avoided. However, the successful use of growth factors requires functional bone marrow. Moreover, the safety of these products has been questioned, and the U.S. Food and Drug Administration is limiting their use in some patient populations.

Erythropoietin

Erythropoietin (epoetin alfa [Epogen, Procrit]) is an effective alternative treatment for patients with chronic anemia secondary to diminished levels of erythropoietin, as in chronic renal disease. This medication stimulates erythropoiesis. It also has been used for patients who are anemic from chemotherapy or zidovudine (AZT) therapy and for those who have diseases involving bone marrow suppression, such as myelodysplastic syndrome (MDS). The use of erythropoietin can also enable a patient to donate several units of blood for future use (e.g., preoperative autologous donation). The medication can be administered IV or subcutaneously, although plasma levels are better sustained with the subcutaneous route. Side effects are rare, but erythropoietin can cause or exacerbate hypertension. If the anemia is corrected too quickly or is overcorrected, the elevated hematocrit can cause headache and, potentially, seizures. Thrombosis has been noted in some patients whose hemoglobins were raised to a high level; thus, it is recommended that a target hemoglobin level of <12 g/dL be used. These adverse effects are rare except for patients with renal failure. Serial complete blood counts (CBCs) must be performed to evaluate the response to the medication. The dose and frequency of administration are titrated to the hemoglobin level.

Granulocyte Colony-Stimulating Factor (G-CSF)

G-CSF (filgrastim [Neupogen]) is a cytokine that stimulates the proliferation and differentiation of myeloid stem cells; a rapid increase in neutrophils is seen within the circulation. G-CSF is effective in improving transient but severe neutropenia after chemotherapy or in some forms of MDS. It is particularly useful in preventing bacterial infections that would be likely to occur with neutropenia. G-CSF is administered subcutaneously on a daily basis. The primary side effect is bone pain; this probably reflects the increase in hematopoiesis within the marrow. Serial CBCs should be performed to evaluate the response to the medication and to ensure that the rise in white blood cells is not excessive. The effect of G-CSF on myelopoiesis is short; the neutrophil count drops once the medication is stopped.

Granulocyte-Macrophage Colony-Stimulating Factor (GM-CSF)

GM-CSF (sargramostim [Leukine]) is a cytokine that is naturally produced by a variety of cells, including monocytes and endothelial cells. It works either directly or synergistically with other growth factors to stimulate myelopoiesis. GM-CSF is not as specific to neutrophils as is G-CSF; thus, an increase in erythroid (red blood cell) and megakaryocytic (platelet) production may also be seen. GM-CSF serves the same purpose as G-CSF. However, it may have a greater effect on macrophage function and therefore may be more useful against fungal infections, whereas G-CSF may be better used to fight bacterial infections. GM-CSF is also administered subcutaneously. Side effects include bone pain, fevers, and myalgias.

Thrombopoietin

Thrombopoietin (TPO) is a cytokine that is necessary for the proliferation of megakaryocytes and subsequent platelet formation. Nonimmunogenic second-generation thrombopoietic growth factors (romiplostim [Nplate]; eltrombopag [Promacta]) were recently approved for the treatment of idiopathic thrombocytopenic purpura.

---

is problematic, given the myriad functions of blood components. Currently, there are two types of products in development: hemoglobin-based oxygen carriers and perfluorocarbons (which have great ability to dissolve gases and thus carry oxygen indirectly) (Cabrales & Carlos Briceño, 2011; Hsia & Ma, 2012). None of these products are available for use in the United States.

Critical Thinking Exercises

1 You are caring for an 86-year-old male patient with a prior medical history of coronary artery disease, heart failure, and iron deficiency anemia. He was admitted to the cardiovascular unit with anginal symptoms and a hemoglobin of 8 mg/dL. What does his hemoglobin level suggest? How might it explain his symptoms of cardiac ischemia (i.e., angina)? He is to receive two units of PRBCs. What special considerations might be required to ensure that this patient receives safe transfusions of these units of PRBCs, particularly given his history of heart failure?

2 **ebp** A 19-year-old woman who is being followed for ITP in the hematology clinic where you work is scheduled for a laparoscopic splenectomy. You wish to administer the pneumococcal vaccine (Pneumovax) to her as part of her preoperative workup. She tells you that she has received "too many shots" and asks why she needs this particular vaccine. What is the strength of the evidence that supports administration of this vaccine to this woman?

3 **pg** You are caring for a 50-year-old male patient in the intensive care unit who is septic and receiving a transfusion of two units of PRBCs. The patient's temperature spikes to 38.5°C (101.3°F) after 25% of the second unit has been transfused. What are the possible causes of the fever? How would you differentiate the cause as sepsis versus a transfusion reaction? What are the appropriate priority nursing interventions? What are the potential causes of the transfusion reactions? How are they manifested?

Brunner Suite Resources

Explore these additional resources to enhance learning for this chapter:
 • NCLEX-Style Questions and Other Resources
on **thePoint**, http://thePoint.lww.com/Brunner13e
 • Study Guide
 • PrepU
 • Clinical Handbook
 • Handbook of Laboratory and Diagnostic Tests

References

Books

Fischbach F., & Dunning M. (2010). *A manual of laboratory and diagnostic tests* (9th ed.). Philadelphia: Wolters Kluwer Health/Lippincott Williams & Wilkins.

Roback, J. (2011). *Technical manual* (17th ed.). Bethesda, MD: AABB.

Journals and Electronic Documents

American Red Cross. (2012a). *Blood components*. Available at: www.redcross-blood.org/learn-about-blood/blood-components

American Red Cross (2012b). *Eligibility criteria by topic*. Available at: www.redcrossblood.org/donating-blood/eligibility-requirements/eligibility-criteria-topic

Ashworth, A., & Klein, A. (2010). Cell salvage as part of a blood conservation strategy in anaesthesia. *British Journal of Anaesthesia*, 105(4), 401–416.

Barrett, K. E., Barman, S. M., Boitano, S., et al. (2012). Chapter 31. Blood as a circulatory fluid & the dynamics of blood & lymph flow. In K. E. Barrett, S. M. Barman, S. Boitano, et al. (Eds.). *Ganong's review of medical physiology* (24th ed.). Available at: www.accessmedicine.com.laneproxy.stanford.edu/content.aspx?aID=56264612

Cabrales, P., & Carlos Briceño, J. (2011). Delaying blood transfusion in experimental acute anemia with a perfluorocarbon emulsion. *Anesthesiology*, 114(4), 901–911.

Carless, P., Henry, D., Carson, J., et al. (2010). Transfusion thresholds and other strategies for guiding allogeneic red blood cell transfusion. *Cochrane Database of Systematic Reviews*, (10), CD002042.

Cherry, T., Steciuk, M., Reddy, V. V., et al. (2008). Transfusion-related acute lung injury: Past, present, and future. *American Journal of Clinical Pathology*, 129(2), 287–297.

Cook, K., Ineck, B., & Lyons W. (2011). Chapter 109. Anemias. In R. L. Talbert, J. T. DiPiro, G. R. Matzke, et al. (Eds). *Pharmacotherapy: A pathophysiologic approach* (8th ed.). Available at: www.accesspharmacy.com/content.aspx?aID=7999561

Diz-Kucukkaya, R., Chen, J., Geddis A., et al. (2010). Chapter 119. Thrombocytopenia. In K. Kaushansky, M. A. Lichtman, et al. (Eds.). *Williams hematology* (8th ed.). Available at: www.accessmedicine.com.laneproxy.stanford.edu/content.aspx?aID=6238643

Fung, Y. L., & Silliman, C. C. (2009). The role of neutrophils in the pathogenesis of transfusion-related acute lung injury. *Transfusion Medicine Reviews*, 23(4), 266–283.

Henry, P. H., & Longo, D. L. (2012). Chapter 59. Enlargement of lymph nodes and spleen. In D. L. Longo, A. S. Fauci, D. L. Kasper, et al. (Eds.). *Harrison's principles of internal medicine* (18th ed.). Available at: www.accessmedicine.com.laneproxy.stanford.edu/content.aspx?aID=9113581

Hsia, C. J., & Ma, L. (2012). A hemoglobin-based multifunctional therapeutic: Polynitroxylated pegylated hemoglobin. *Artificial Organs*, 36(2), 215–220.

Leo, A., & Pedal, I. (2010). Diagnostic approaches to acute transfusion reactions. *Forensic Science, Medicine, and Pathology*, 6(2), 135–145.

Masters, S. B. (2012). Chapter 33. Agents used in anemias; hematopoietic growth factors. In B. G. Katzung, S. B. Masters, & A. J. Trevor (Eds.). *Basic & Clinical Pharmacology* (12th ed.). Available at: www.accessmedicine.com.laneproxy.stanford.edu/content.aspx?aID=55826559

Müller, M., Porcelijn, L., & Vlaar, A. (2012). Prevention of immune-mediated transfusion-related acute lung injury: From blood bank to patient. *Current Pharmaceutical Design*, 18(22), 3241–3248.

Pagliaro, P., Turdo, R., & Capuzzo, E. (2009). Patients' positive identification systems. *Blood Transfusion*, 7(4), 313–318.

Ranucci, M., Conti, D., Castelvecchio, S., et al. (2010). Hematocrit on cardiopulmonary bypass and outcome after coronary surgery in nontransfused patients. *Annals of Thoracic Surgery*, 89(1), 11–17.

Strecker-McGraw, M. (2011). Hematologic emergencies. In R. L. Humphries (Eds.). *CURRENT diagnosis & treatment emergency medicine* (7th ed.). Available at: www.accessmedicine.com.laneproxy.stanford.edu/content.aspx?aID=55756032

Zou, S., Dorsey, K. A., Notari, E. P., et al. (2010). Prevalence, incidence, and residual risk of human immunodeficiency virus and hepatitis C virus infections among United States blood donors since the introduction of nucleic acid testing. *Transfusion*, 50(7), 1408–1412.

Resources

AABB (formerly known as the American Association of Blood Banks), www.aabb.org
American Cancer Society, www.cancer.org
American Red Cross, www.redcross.org
Blood and Marrow Transplant Information Network, www.bmtinfonet.org
Myelodysplastic Syndromes Foundation, www.mds-foundation.org
National Cancer Institute Cancer Information Service, www.cancer.gov
National Hemophilia Foundation, www.hemophilia.org
National Marrow Donor Program, www.marrow.org
Oncology Nursing Society (ONS), www.ons.org

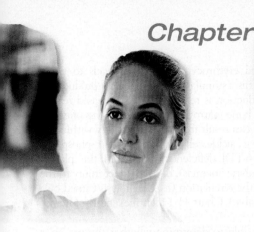

Chapter 33

Management of Patients With Nonmalignant Hematologic Disorders

Learning Objectives

On completion of this chapter, the learner will be able to:

1 Differentiate between the hypoproliferative and the hemolytic anemias and compare and contrast the physiologic mechanisms, clinical manifestations, medical management, and nursing interventions for each.
2 Use the nursing process as a framework for care of patients with anemia.
3 Use the nursing process as a framework for care of patients with sickle cell crises.

4 Discuss treatment of secondary polycythemias.
5 Describe the processes involved in neutropenia and lymphopenia and the general principles of medical and nursing management of patients with these disorders.
6 Describe the medical and nursing management of patients with bleeding and thrombotic disorders.
7 Use the nursing process as a framework for care of patients with disseminated intravascular coagulation.

Glossary

absolute neutrophil count: a calculation of the number of circulating neutrophils, derived from the total white blood cells (WBCs) and the percentage of neutrophils counted in a microscope's visual field

anemia: decreased red blood cell (RBC) count

angular cheilosis: cracking sore at corner of mouth

aplasia: lack of cellular development (e.g., of cells within the bone marrow)

cytokines: proteins produced by leukocytes that are vital to regulation of hematopoiesis, apoptosis, and immune responses

D-dimer: test to measure fibrin breakdown; considered more specific than fibrin degradation products in the diagnosis of disseminated intravascular coagulation

erythrocyte: a cellular component of blood involved in the transport of oxygen and carbon dioxide; (synonym: red blood cell [RBC])

erythroid cells: any cell that is or will become a mature RBC

erythropoietin: hormone produced primarily by the kidney; necessary for erythropoiesis

haptoglobin: blood protein synthesized by liver; binds free hemoglobin released from erythrocytes, which is then removed by the reticuloendothelial system

hemolysis: destruction of RBCs; can occur within or outside of the vasculature

hemosiderin: iron-containing pigment derived from breakdown of hemoglobin

hypochromia: pallor within the RBC caused by decreased hemoglobin content

leukemia: uncontrolled proliferation of WBCs, often immature

lymphopenia: a lymphocyte count less than 1,500/mm³

megaloblastic anemia: a type of anemia characterized by the presence of abnormally large, nucleated RBCs

microcytosis: smaller-than-normal RBCs

neutropenia: lower-than-normal number of neutrophils

normochromic: normal RBC color, indicating normal amount of hemoglobin

normocytic: normal size of RBC

oxyhemoglobin: combined form of oxygen and hemoglobin; found in arterial blood

pancytopenia: abnormal decrease in WBCs, RBCs, and platelets

petechiae: tiny capillary hemorrhages

poikilocytosis: variation in shape of RBCs

polycythemia: excess RBCs

reticulocytes: slightly immature RBCs, usually only 1% of total circulating RBCs

spherocytes: small, spherically shaped erythrocytes

thrombocytopenia: lower-than-normal platelet count

thrombocytosis: higher-than-normal platelet count

The majority of hematologic disorders are considered benign (i.e., non-malignant). Whereas many are relatively indolent, others have severe consequences and can be life threatening. Most hematologic disorders are quite complex; a thorough understanding of the underlying processes associated with the disorders can assist nurses so that they may appropriately assess, monitor, educate, and intervene with patients with hematologic disorders.

899

ANEMIA

Anemia is a condition in which the hemoglobin concentration is lower than normal; it reflects the presence of fewer than the normal number of **erythrocytes** within the circulation. As a result, the amount of oxygen delivered to body tissues is also diminished. Anemia is not a specific disease state but a sign of an underlying disorder. It is by far the most common hematologic condition.

Classification of Anemias

Anemia may be classified in several ways (Table 33-1). A physiologic approach classifies anemia according to whether the deficiency in erythrocytes is caused by a defect in their production (i.e., hypoproliferative anemia), by their destruction (i.e., hemolytic anemia), or by their loss (i.e., bleeding).

In hypoproliferative anemias, the marrow cannot produce adequate numbers of erythrocytes. Decreased erythrocyte production is reflected by a low or inappropriately normal reticulocyte count. Inadequate production of erythrocytes may result from marrow damage due to medications (e.g., chloramphenicol) or chemicals (e.g., benzene) or from a lack of factors (e.g., iron, vitamin B₁₂, folic acid, **erythropoietin**) necessary for erythrocyte formation.

In hemolytic anemias, premature destruction of erythrocytes results in the liberation of hemoglobin from the erythrocytes into the plasma; the released hemoglobin is converted in large part to bilirubin and, therefore, the bilirubin concentration rises. The increased erythrocyte destruction leads to tissue hypoxia, which in turn stimulates erythropoietin production. This increased production is reflected in an increased reticulocyte count as the bone marrow responds to the loss of erythrocytes. **Hemolysis** can result from an abnormality within the erythrocyte itself (e.g., sickle cell anemia, glucose-6-phosphate dehydrogenase [G-6-PD] deficiency) or within the plasma (e.g., immune hemolytic anemias), or from direct injury to the erythrocyte within the circulation (e.g., hemolysis caused by a mechanical heart valve). Chart 33-1 identifies causes of hemolytic anemia.

It is usually possible to determine whether the presence of anemia in a given patient is caused by destruction or by inadequate production of erythrocytes on the basis of the following factors:

- The marrow's ability to respond to decreased erythrocytes (as evidenced by an increased reticulocyte count in the circulating blood)
- The degree to which young erythrocytes proliferate in the bone marrow and the manner in which they mature (as observed on bone marrow aspirate)
- The presence or absence of end products of erythrocyte destruction within the circulation (e.g., increased bilirubin level, decreased haptoglobin level)

Clinical Manifestations

Aside from the severity of the anemia itself, several factors influence the development of anemia-associated symptoms:

TABLE 33-1 Classification of Anemias

Type of Anemia	Laboratory Findings CBC	Other
Hypoproliferative (Resulting From Defective RBC Production)		
Iron deficiency	↓ MCV, ↓ reticulocytes	↓ Iron, % saturation, ferritin ↑ TIBC
Vitamin B₁₂ deficiency (megaloblastic)	↑ MCV	↓ Vitamin B₁₂
Folate deficiency (megaloblastic)	↑ MCV	↓ Folate
Decreased erythropoietin production (e.g., from renal dysfunction)	Normal MCV	↓ Erythropoietin level ↑ Creatinine
Cancer/inflammation	Normal MCV	↑ Ferritin, % saturation ↓ Iron, TIBC ↓ Erythropoietin level (usually)
Bleeding (Resulting From RBC Loss)		
Bleeding from gastrointestinal tract, epistaxis (nosebleed), trauma, bleeding from genitourinary tract (e.g., menorrhagia)	↓ Hgb and Hct (*Note:* Hgb and Hct may be normal if measured soon after bleeding starts) ↓ MCV (normal MCV initially) ↑ Reticulocytes	↓ Iron, % saturation, ferritin (later)
Hemolytic (Resulting From RBC Destruction)		
Altered erythropoiesis (sickle cell anemia, thalassemia, other hemoglobinopathies)	↓ MCV ↑ Reticulocytes Fragmented RBCs (various shapes)	
Hypersplenism (hemolysis)	↑ MCV	
Drug-induced anemia	↑ Presence of spherocytes	
Autoimmune anemia	↑ Presence of spherocytes	
Mechanical heart valve–related anemia	Fragmented red cells	

CBC, complete blood count; RBC, red blood cell; ↓, decreased; MCV, mean corpuscular volume; %, percent; ↑, increased; TIBC, total iron-binding capacity; Hgb, hemoglobin; Hct, hematocrit.

Causes of Hemolytic Anemias

Inherited Hemolytic Anemia

Abnormal Hemoglobin

Sickle cell anemia*
Thalassemia*

Red Blood Cell Membrane Abnormality

Hereditary spherocytosis
Hereditary elliptocytosis
Acanthocytosis
Stomatocytosis

Enzyme Deficiencies

Glucose-6-phosphate dehydrogenase deficiency*

Acquired Hemolytic Anemia

Antibody Related

Iso-antibody/transfusion reaction**
Autoimmune hemolytic anemia*
Cold agglutinin disease

Not Antibody Related

Paroxysmal nocturnal hemoglobinuria
Liver disease
Uremia
Trauma
Mechanical heart valve
Microangiopathic hemolytic anemia
Infection
  Bacterial
  Parasitic
Disseminated intravascular coagulation*
Toxins
Hypersplenism*

*Discussed in text.
**Discussed in Chapter 32.

the rapidity with which the anemia has developed, the duration of the anemia (i.e., its chronicity), the metabolic requirements of the patient, other concurrent disorders or disabilities (e.g., cardiac or pulmonary disease), and complications or concomitant features of the condition that produced the anemia.

In general, the more rapidly an anemia develops, the more severe its symptoms. An otherwise healthy person can often tolerate as much as a 50% gradual reduction in hemoglobin without pronounced symptoms or significant incapacity, whereas the rapid loss of as little as 30% may precipitate profound vascular collapse in the same person. A person who has become gradually anemic, with hemoglobin levels between 9 and 11 g/dL, usually has few or no symptoms other than slight tachycardia on exertion and possibly fatigue.

People who customarily are very active or who have significant demands on their lives (e.g., a single, working mother of small children) are more likely to have symptoms, and those symptoms are more likely to be pronounced than in more sedentary people. Patients with hypothyroidism with decreased oxygen needs may be completely asymptomatic, without tachycardia or increased cardiac output, at a hemoglobin level of 10 g/dL. Similarly, patients with coexistent cardiac, vascular, or pulmonary disease may develop more pronounced

symptoms of anemia (e.g., dyspnea, chest pain, muscle pain or cramping) with a higher hemoglobin level than those without these concurrent health problems.

Finally, some anemias are complicated by various other abnormalities that do not result from the anemia but are inherently associated with these particular diseases. These abnormalities may give rise to symptoms that completely overshadow those of the anemia, as in the painful crises of sickle cell anemia.

Assessment and Diagnostic Findings

A variety of hematologic studies are performed to determine the type and cause of the anemia. In an initial evaluation, the hemoglobin, hematocrit, reticulocyte count, and red blood cell (RBC) indices, particularly the mean corpuscular volume (MCV) and red cell distribution width (RDW), are especially useful. Iron studies (serum iron level, total iron-binding capacity [TIBC], percent saturation, and ferritin), as well as serum vitamin B_{12} and folate levels, are also frequently obtained (Bryan & Zakai, 2012). Other tests include haptoglobin and erythropoietin levels. The remaining complete blood count (CBC) values are useful in determining whether the anemia is an isolated problem or part of another hematologic condition, such as **leukemia** or myelodysplastic syndrome (MDS). Bone marrow aspiration may be performed. In addition, other diagnostic studies may be performed to determine the presence of underlying chronic illness, such as malignancy, or the source of any blood loss, such as polyps or ulcers within the gastrointestinal (GI) tract. (See Chapter 32 for discussion of diagnostic tests.)

Complications

General complications of severe anemia include heart failure, paresthesias, and delirium. Patients with underlying heart disease are far more likely to have angina or symptoms of heart failure than those without heart disease. Complications associated with specific types of anemia are included in the description of each type.

Medical Management

Management of anemia is directed toward correcting or controlling the cause of the anemia; if the anemia is severe, the erythrocytes that are lost or destroyed may be replaced with a transfusion of packed red blood cells (PRBCs). The management of the various types of anemia is covered in the discussions that follow.

 ## Gerontologic Considerations

Anemia is the most common hematologic condition affecting older patients, particularly those admitted to hospitals or in long-term care facilities. The overall prevalence of anemia increases with age, from 4% to 6% in persons 65 to 69 years of age to 13% to 14% in persons older than 85 years (Bross, Soch, & Smith-Knuppel, 2010). The impact of anemia on function in older adults is significant and may include decreased mobility, increased depression, increased risk for falling (Sabol, Resnick, Galik, et al., 2010), and delirium (when hospitalized). Older adults often cannot respond to anemia as well as younger individuals, in that heart rate and cardiac output do not increase as quickly; thus, fatigue, dyspnea, and confusion may be seen more readily in the older adult who is anemic. Anemia prevalence increases markedly to almost 50% in older adults who are chronically ill and reside in community dwellings or long-term care facilities and is associated with increased mortality in these settings (Bross et al., 2010). Those with pre-existing renal or cardiac disease or who have had recent surgery are also at increased risk for mortality when anemic.

NURSING PROCESS

The Patient With Anemia

Assessment

The health history and physical examination provide important data about the type of anemia involved, the extent and type of symptoms it produces, and the impact of those symptoms on the patient's life. Weakness, fatigue, and general malaise are common, as are pallor of the skin and mucous membranes (conjunctivae, oral mucosa) (Fig. 33-1).

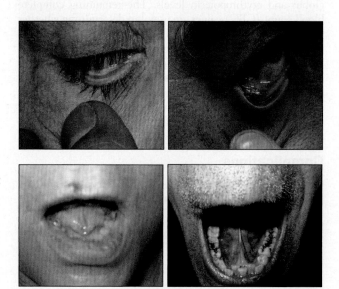

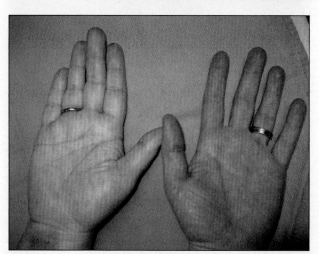

FIGURE 33-1 • Pallor seen in the patient with anemia. From Tkachuk, D. C., & Hirschman, J. V. (2007). *Wintrobe's atlas of clinical hematology* (Fig. 1.1, p. 9). Philadelphia: Lippincott Williams & Wilkins.

Jaundice may be present in patients with megaloblastic anemia or hemolytic anemia. The tongue may be smooth and red (in iron deficiency anemia) or beefy red and sore (in megaloblastic anemia); the corners of the mouth may be ulcerated (**angular cheilosis**) in both types of anemia. People with iron deficiency anemia may crave ice, starch, or dirt; this craving is known as pica. The nails may be brittle, ridged, and concave.

The health history should include a medication history, because some medications can depress bone marrow activity, induce hemolysis, or interfere with folate metabolism. An accurate history of alcohol intake, including the amount and duration, should be obtained. Family history is important, because certain anemias are inherited. It is necessary to ask about athletic endeavors, because extreme exercise can decrease erythropoiesis and erythrocyte survival.

A nutritional assessment is important, because it may indicate deficiencies in essential nutrients such as iron, vitamin B_{12}, and folate. Strict vegetarians are at risk for **megaloblastic anemias**, which are characterized by the presence of abnormally large, nucleated RBCs, if they do not supplement their diet with vitamin B_{12}. Older adults also may have a diminished intake of vitamin B_{12} or folate.

Cardiac status should be carefully assessed. When the hemoglobin level is low, the heart attempts to compensate by pumping faster and harder in an effort to deliver more blood to hypoxic tissue. This increased cardiac workload can result in such symptoms as tachycardia, palpitations, dyspnea, dizziness, orthopnea, and exertional dyspnea. Heart failure may eventually develop, as evidenced by an enlarged heart (cardiomegaly) and liver (hepatomegaly) and by peripheral edema.

Assessment of the GI system may disclose complaints of nausea, vomiting (with specific questions about the appearance of any emesis [e.g., looks like "coffee grounds"]), melena [dark stools], diarrhea, anorexia, and glossitis (inflammation of the tongue). Stools should be tested for occult blood (see Chapter 32). Women should be questioned about their menstrual periods (e.g., excessive menstrual flow, other vaginal bleeding) and the use of iron supplements during pregnancy.

Neurologic examination is also important because pernicious anemia affects the central and peripheral nervous systems. Assessment should include the presence and extent of peripheral numbness and paresthesias, ataxia, poor coordination, and confusion. Delirium can sometimes result from other types of anemia, particularly in older adults. Finally, it is important to monitor relevant laboratory test results and to note any changes over time (see Chapter 32 for further discussion).

Diagnosis

Nursing Diagnoses

Based on the assessment data, major nursing diagnoses may include:
* Fatigue related to decreased hemoglobin and diminished oxygen-carrying capacity of the blood
* Imbalanced nutrition, less than body requirements, related to inadequate intake of essential nutrients
* Ineffective tissue perfusion related to inadequate hemoglobin and hematocrit
* Noncompliance with prescribed therapy

Collaborative Problems/Potential Complications

Potential complications may include the following:

- Heart failure
- Angina
- Paresthesias
- Confusion
- Injury related to falls
- Depressed mood

Planning and Goals

The major goals for the patient may include decreased fatigue, attainment or maintenance of adequate nutrition, maintenance of adequate tissue perfusion, compliance with prescribed therapy, and absence of complications.

Nursing Interventions

Managing Fatigue

The most common symptom and complication of anemia is fatigue. Fatigue is often the symptom that has the greatest negative impact on a patient's level of functioning and consequent quality of life. Therefore, it should not be minimized. Patients often describe the fatigue from anemia as oppressive. Fatigue can be significant, yet the anemia may not be severe enough to warrant transfusion. Fatigue can interfere with a person's ability to work and to participate in activities with family and friends. Patients often lose interest in hobbies and activities, including sexual activity. The distress from fatigue is often related to a person's responsibilities and life demands as well as the amount of assistance and support received from others.

Nursing interventions can focus on assisting the patient to prioritize activities and to establish a balance between activity and rest that is acceptable to the patient. Patients with chronic anemia need to maintain some physical activity and exercise to prevent the deconditioning that results from inactivity. It is also important to assess for other conditions that can exacerbate fatigue, such as pain, depression, and sleep disturbance.

Maintaining Adequate Nutrition

Inadequate intake of essential nutrients, such as iron, vitamin B_{12}, folic acid, and protein, can cause some anemias. The symptoms associated with anemia (e.g., fatigue, anorexia) can in turn interfere with maintaining adequate nutrition. A healthy diet should be encouraged. The nurse should inform the patient that alcohol interferes with the utilization of essential nutrients and should advise moderation in the intake of alcoholic beverages (Bode, 2003; Ioannou, Dominitz, Weiss, et al., 2004) (see Chapter 5). Dietary education sessions should be individualized, involve family members, and include cultural aspects related to food preferences and food preparation. Dietary supplements (e.g., vitamins, iron, folate, protein) may be prescribed.

Equally important, the patient and family must understand the role of nutritional supplements in the proper context, because many forms of anemia are not the result of a nutritional deficiency. In such cases, even an excessive intake of nutritional supplements will not improve the anemia. A potential problem in patients with chronic transfusion requirements occurs with the indiscriminate use of iron supplements. Unless an aggressive program of chelation therapy is implemented, these people are at risk for iron overload from their transfusions (Eckes, 2011). The addition of an iron supplement only exacerbates the situation.

Maintaining Adequate Perfusion

Patients with acute blood loss or severe hemolysis may have decreased tissue perfusion from decreased blood volume or reduced circulating erythrocytes (decreased hematocrit). Lost volume is replaced with transfusions or intravenous (IV) fluids, based on symptoms and laboratory test results. Supplemental oxygen may be necessary, but it is rarely needed on a long-term basis unless there is underlying severe cardiac or pulmonary disease. The nurse monitors the patient's vital signs and pulse oximeter readings closely; other medications, such as antihypertensive agents, may need to be adjusted or withheld.

Promoting Compliance With Prescribed Therapy

For patients with anemia, medications or nutritional supplements are often prescribed to treat the condition. These patients need to understand the purpose of the medication, how to take the medication and over what time period, and how to manage any side effects of therapy. To enhance compliance, the nurse assists the patient to develop ways to incorporate the therapeutic plan into everyday activities rather than merely giving the patient a list of instructions. For example, many patients have difficulty taking iron supplements because of related GI effects. Rather than seeking assistance from a health care provider in managing the problem, some patients simply stop taking the iron.

Abruptly stopping some medications can have serious consequences, as in the case of high-dose corticosteroids to manage hemolytic anemias. Some medications, such as growth factors, are extremely expensive. Patients receiving these medications may need assistance to obtain needed insurance coverage or to explore alternative ways to obtain these medications.

Monitoring and Managing Potential Complications

A significant complication of anemia is heart failure from chronic diminished blood volume and the heart's compensatory effort to increase cardiac output. Patients with anemia should be assessed for signs and symptoms of heart failure (see Chapter 29).

In megaloblastic forms of anemia, the significant potential complications are neurologic. A neurologic assessment should be performed for patients with known or suspected megaloblastic anemia. Patients may initially complain of paresthesias in their lower extremities. These paresthesias are usually manifested as numbness and tingling on the bottom of the foot, and they gradually progress. As the anemia progresses, other signs become apparent. Position and vibration sense may be diminished; difficulty maintaining balance is not uncommon, and some patients have gait disturbances as well. Initially mild confusion may develop; it may become severe (Savage & Lindenbaum, 1995).

Evaluation

Expected patient outcomes may include:

1. Reports less fatigue
   a. Follows a progressive plan of rest, activity, and exercise
   b. Prioritizes activities
   c. Paces activities according to energy level

2. Attains and maintains adequate nutrition
   a. Eats a healthy diet
   b. Develops a meal plan that promotes optimal nutrition
   c. Maintains adequate amounts of iron, vitamins, and protein from diet or supplements
   d. Adheres to nutritional supplement therapy when prescribed
   e. Verbalizes understanding of rationale for using recommended nutritional supplements
   f. Verbalizes understanding of rationale for avoiding nonrecommended nutritional supplements
3. Maintains adequate perfusion
   a. Has vital signs within baseline for patient
   b. Has pulse oximetry (arterial oxygenation) value within normal limits
4. Absence of complications
   a. Avoids or limits activities that trigger dyspnea, palpitations, dizziness, or tachycardia
   b. Uses rest and comfort measures to alleviate dyspnea
   c. Has vital signs within baseline for patient
   d. Has no signs of increasing fluid retention (e.g., peripheral edema, decreased urine output, neck vein distention)
   e. Remains oriented to time, place, and situation
   f. Remains engaged in social situations, exhibits no signs of depression
   g. Ambulates safely, using assistive devices as necessary
   h. Remains free of injury
   i. Verbalizes understanding of importance of serial CBC measurements
   j. Maintains safe home environment; obtains assistance as necessary

Hypoproliferative Anemias

Iron Deficiency Anemia

Iron deficiency anemia typically results when the intake of dietary iron is inadequate for hemoglobin synthesis. The body can store about one fourth to one third of its iron, and it is not until those stores are depleted that iron deficiency anemia actually begins to develop. Iron deficiency anemia is the most common type of anemia in all age groups, and it is the most common anemia in the world. It is particularly prevalent in developing countries, where inadequate iron stores can result from inadequate intake of iron (seen with vegetarian diets) or from blood loss (e.g., from intestinal hookworm). Iron deficiency is also common among adults in the United States, and the most common cause is blood loss. In fact, bleeding should be considered the cause of iron deficiency anemia until proven otherwise.

The most common cause of iron deficiency anemia in men and postmenopausal women is bleeding from ulcers, gastritis, inflammatory bowel disease, or GI tumors. The most common causes of iron deficiency anemia in premenopausal women are menorrhagia (i.e., excessive menstrual bleeding) and pregnancy with inadequate iron supplementation. Patients with chronic alcoholism often have chronic blood loss from the GI tract, which causes iron loss and eventual anemia. Other causes include iron malabsorption, as is seen after gastrectomy or with celiac disease.

Clinical Manifestations

Patients with iron deficiency primarily have symptoms of anemia. If the deficiency is severe or prolonged, they may also have a smooth, sore tongue; brittle and ridged nails; and angular cheilosis. These signs subside after iron replacement therapy. The health history may be significant for multiple pregnancies, GI bleeding, and pica (Barton, Barton, & Bertoli, 2010).

Assessment and Diagnostic Findings

The definitive method of establishing the diagnosis of iron deficiency anemia is bone marrow aspiration (see Chapter 32 for further discussion of bone marrow aspiration). The aspirate is stained to detect iron, which is at a low level or even absent. However, few patients with suspected iron deficiency anemia undergo bone marrow aspiration. In many patients, the diagnosis can be established with other tests, particularly in patients with a history of conditions that predispose them to this type of anemia.

A strong correlation exists between laboratory values that measure iron stores and hemoglobin levels. After iron stores are depleted (as reflected by low serum ferritin levels), the hemoglobin level falls. The diminished iron stores cause small erythrocytes to be produced by the marrow. Therefore, as the anemia progresses, the MCV, which measures the size of the erythrocytes, also decreases. Hematocrit and RBC levels are also low in relation to the hemoglobin level. Other laboratory tests that measure iron stores are useful but not as precise as ferritin levels. Typically, patients with iron deficiency anemia have a low serum iron level and an elevated TIBC, which measures the transport protein supplying the marrow with iron as needed (also referred to as transferrin) (Fischbach & Dunning, 2010). However, other disease states, such as infection and inflammatory conditions, can also cause a low serum iron level and TIBC, as well as an elevated ferritin level. If these are suspected, measuring the soluble transferring receptor can aid in differentiating the cause of anemia. This test result will be increased in the setting of iron deficiency, but not in chronic inflammation.

Medical Management

Except in the case of pregnancy, the cause of iron deficiency should be investigated. Anemia may be a sign of a curable GI cancer or of uterine fibroid tumors. Stool specimens should be tested for occult blood. People 50 years of age or older should have a colonoscopy, endoscopy, or x-ray examination of the GI tract to detect ulcerations, gastritis, polyps, or cancer (Centers for Disease Control and Prevention [CDC], 2011). Several oral iron preparations—ferrous sulfate, ferrous gluconate, and ferrous fumarate—are available for treating iron deficiency anemia. The hemoglobin level may increase in only a few weeks, and the anemia can be corrected in a few months. Iron store replenishment takes much longer, so the patient must continue taking the iron for as long as 6 to 12 months.

Parenteral Iron Formulations

- Older formulations of parenteral iron had a high molecular weight, and the risk of hypersensitivity reactions, including anaphylaxis, was significant. Newer formulations have a low molecular weight, and the risk of anaphylaxis is markedly reduced.
- Ferric gluconate (Ferrlecit): Each 5 mL contains 62.5 mg elemental iron; 125 mg is diluted in 100 mL normal saline and infused over 1 hour, or 5 mL undiluted is given as a slow IV push injection over 5 minutes. Although the likelihood of an allergic reaction is extremely low, a test dose is often given prior to the first infusion.
- Iron sucrose (Venofer): Each 5 mL contains 100 mg elemental iron; 100–200 mg can be given undiluted as a slow IV push injection over 2–5 minutes. This procedure can be repeated as often as every 3 days for a total cumulative dose of 1,000 mg within a 2-week period.

In some cases, oral iron is poorly absorbed or poorly tolerated, or iron supplementation is needed in large amounts. In these situations, IV administration of iron may be needed. Several doses are required to replenish the patient's iron stores (Chart 33-2).

Nursing Management

Preventive education is important, because iron deficiency anemia is common in menstruating and pregnant women. Food sources high in iron include organ meats (e.g., beef or calf's liver, chicken liver), other meats, beans (e.g., black, pinto, and garbanzo), leafy green vegetables, raisins, and molasses. Taking iron-rich foods with a source of vitamin C (e.g., orange juice) enhances the absorption of iron.

The nurse helps the patient select a healthy diet. Nutritional counseling can be provided for those whose usual diet is inadequate. Patients with a history of eating fad diets or strict vegetarian diets are counseled that such diets often contain inadequate amounts of absorbable iron. The nurse encourages the patient to continue iron therapy for as long as it is prescribed even though the patient may no longer feel fatigued.

Because iron is best absorbed on an empty stomach, the patient is instructed to take the supplement an hour before meals. Iron supplements are usually given in the oral form, typically as ferrous sulfate. Most patients can use the less expensive, more standard forms of ferrous sulfate. Tablets with enteric coating may be poorly absorbed and should be avoided. Many patients have difficulty tolerating iron supplements because of GI side effects (primarily constipation, but also cramping, nausea, and vomiting). Some iron formulations are designed to limit GI side effects by the addition of a stool softener or the use of sustained-release formulations to limit nausea or gastritis. Specific education aids (Chart 33-3) can assist patients with the use of iron supplements.

If taking iron on an empty stomach causes gastric distress, the patient may need to take it with meals. However, doing so diminishes iron absorption by as much as 50%, thus prolonging the time required to replenish iron stores. Antacids or dairy products should not be taken with iron, because they greatly diminish its absorption. Polysaccharide iron complex forms are also available; they have less GI toxicity but are more expensive.

Liquid forms of iron that cause less GI distress are available. Iron replacement therapy should not cause a false-positive result on stool analyses for occult blood even though it may change the color of stool.

IV supplementation may be used when the patient's iron stores are completely depleted, the patient cannot tolerate oral forms of iron supplementation (see earlier Medical Management section), or both. The nurse needs to be aware of the type of parenteral formulation of iron ordered so that the risk of anaphylaxis may be determined. High molecular formulations are associated with a much higher incidence of anaphylaxis. Administering a test dose of low-molecular formulations of iron dextran is still recommended by many manufacturers. The nurse needs to assist the patient in understanding the need for repeated dosing to replenish iron stores or to maintain iron stores in the setting of chronic blood loss, such as dialysis, or chronic GI bleeding.

Anemias in Renal Disease

The degree of anemia in patients with end-stage renal disease varies greatly; however, in general, patients do not become significantly anemic until the serum creatinine level exceeds 3 mg/100 mL. The symptoms of anemia are often the most disturbing of the patient's symptoms. If untreated, the hematocrit usually falls to between 20% and 30%, although in rare cases it may fall to less than 15% (Lowrie, Kirkwood, & Pollack, 2012). The erythrocytes are normal in appearance.

This type of anemia is caused by both a mild shortening of erythrocyte lifespan and a deficiency of erythropoietin (necessary for erythropoiesis). As renal function decreases, erythropoietin, which is produced by the kidney, also decreases. Because erythropoietin is also produced outside the kidney, some erythropoiesis continues, even in patients whose kidneys have been removed. However, the number of RBCs produced is small, and the degree of erythropoiesis is inadequate.

Patients undergoing long-term hemodialysis lose blood into the dialyzer and therefore may become iron deficient.

**Chart
33-3** **PATIENT EDUCATION**

Taking Oral Iron Supplements

- Take iron on an empty stomach (1 hour before or 2 hours after a meal), preferably with orange juice or other forms of vitamin C. Iron absorption is reduced with food, especially dairy products.
- To prevent gastrointestinal distress, the following schedule may work better if more than one tablet a day is prescribed: Start with only one tablet per day for a few days, then increase to two tablets per day, then three tablets per day. This method permits the body to adjust gradually to the iron.
- Increase the intake of vitamin C (citrus fruits and juices, strawberries, tomatoes, broccoli) to enhance iron absorption.
- Eat foods high in fiber to minimize problems with constipation.
- Remember that stools will become dark in color.
- To prevent staining the teeth with a liquid preparation, use a straw or place a spoon at the back of the mouth to take the supplement. Rinse the mouth thoroughly afterward.

Folic acid deficiency develops because this vitamin passes into the dialysate. Therefore, patients who receive hemodialysis and who have anemia should be evaluated for iron and folate deficiency and treated appropriately.

The availability of recombinant erythropoietin (epoetin alfa [Epogen, Procrit], darbepoetin alfa [Aranesp]) has dramatically altered the management of anemia in end-stage renal disease (or associated with myelosuppressive chemotherapy for cancer) by decreasing the need for RBC transfusion, with its associated risks. Erythropoietin, in combination with oral or IV iron supplementation, can raise and maintain hematocrit levels significantly. However, recombinant erythropoietin use is not without risk. Studies suggest that the use of recombinant erythropoietin is associated with increased cardiovascular events, stroke, increased risk of tumor progression or recurrence, and increased mortality, particularly when the hemoglobin level exceeds 13 g/dL (Aapro, Jelkmann, Constantinescu, et al., 2012; Palmer, Navaneethan, Craig, et al., 2012). The U.S. Food and Drug Administration (FDA, 2011) has therefore placed restrictions on the use of these agents, which include using the lowest possible dose needed to avoid red cell transfusion, limiting their use to raise the hemoglobin to a level not greater than 12 g/dL, and prohibiting their use when the aim of chemotherapy is curative. When using recombinant erythropoietin, the hemoglobin must be checked at least monthly (more frequently until a maintenance dose is established) and the dose titrated to ensure the hemoglobin level does not exceed 12 g/dL.

■ Anemia of Chronic Disease

The term *anemia of chronic disease* is a misnomer in that only the chronic diseases of inflammation, infection, and malignancy cause this type of anemia (Ganz, 2010). Many chronic inflammatory diseases are associated with a **normochromic, normocytic** anemia (i.e., the erythrocytes are normal in color and size). These disorders include rheumatoid arthritis; severe, chronic infections; and many cancers. It is therefore imperative that the "chronic disease" be diagnosed when this form of anemia is identified so that it can be appropriately managed.

The anemia is usually mild to moderate and nonprogressive. It develops gradually over 6 to 8 weeks and then stabilizes at a hematocrit seldom less than 25% (Davis & Littlewood, 2012). The hemoglobin level rarely falls below 9 g/dL, and the bone marrow has normal cellularity with increased stores of iron as the iron is diverted from the serum. Erythropoietin levels are low, perhaps because of decreased production, and iron use is blocked by **erythroid cells** (cells that are or will become mature erythrocytes). A moderate shortening of erythrocyte survival also occurs.

Most of these patients have few symptoms and do not require treatment for the anemia. With successful treatment of the underlying disorder, the bone marrow iron is used to make erythrocytes and the hemoglobin level rises. These patients do not benefit from additional iron supplementation.

Increasing evidence suggests that inflammation may have a significant role in the development of anemia in older adults (Vanasse & Berliner, 2010). Higher-than-normal levels of inflammatory **cytokines** (proteins) are found in the older adult population, such as tumor necrosis factor and interleukin 6, which may also be associated with anemia (Fulop, Larbi, Witkowski, et al., 2010). This proinflammatory state may predispose older adults to frailty, manifested by weight loss, decreased mobility, generalized weakness, and poor balance; frailty is strongly associated with the anemia of inflammation (Vanasse & Berliner, 2010). As in renal disease, erythropoietin levels may not rise appropriately in response to decreased hemoglobin.

■ Aplastic Anemia

Aplastic anemia is a rare disease caused by a decrease in or damage to marrow stem cells, damage to the microenvironment within the marrow, and replacement of the marrow with fat. Stem cell damage is caused by the body's T cells mediating an inappropriate attack against the bone marrow, resulting in bone marrow **aplasia** (i.e., markedly reduced hematopoiesis). Therefore, in addition to severe anemia, significant neutropenia and thrombocytopenia also occur.

Pathophysiology

Aplastic anemia can be congenital or acquired, but most cases are idiopathic (i.e., without apparent cause) (National Heart, Lung, and Blood Institute [NHLBI], 2010). Infections and pregnancy can trigger it, or it may be caused by certain medications, chemicals, or radiation damage. Agents that may produce marrow aplasia include benzene and benzene derivatives (e.g., airplane glue, paint remover, dry-cleaning solutions). Certain toxic materials, such as inorganic arsenic, glycol ethers, plutonium, and radon, have also been implicated as potential causes.

Clinical Manifestations

The manifestations of aplastic anemia are often insidious. Complications resulting from bone marrow failure may occur before the diagnosis is established. Typical complications are infection and the symptoms of anemia (e.g., fatigue, pallor, dyspnea). Purpura (bruising) may develop later and should trigger a CBC and hematologic evaluation if these were not performed initially. If the patient has had repeated throat infections, cervical lymphadenopathy may be seen. Other lymphadenopathies and splenomegaly sometimes occur. Retinal hemorrhages are common.

Assessment and Diagnostic Findings

In many situations, aplastic anemia occurs when a medication or chemical is ingested in toxic amounts. However, in a few people, it develops after a medication has been taken at the recommended dosage. This may be considered an idiosyncratic reaction in those who are highly susceptible, possibly caused by a genetic defect in the medication biotransformation or elimination process. A bone marrow aspirate shows an extremely hypoplastic or even aplastic (very few to no cells) marrow replaced with fat.

Medical Management

It is presumed that the T lymphocytes of patients with aplastic anemia destroy the stem cells and consequently impair the production of erythrocytes, leukocytes, and platelets (Young, Scheinberg, & Calado, 2008). Despite its severity, aplastic anemia can be treated in most people. Those who are younger than 60 years, who are otherwise healthy, and who have a compatible donor can be cured of the disease with hematopoietic stem cell transplant (HSCT). In others, the disease can be managed with immunosuppressive therapy, commonly using a combination of antithymocyte globulin (ATG) and cyclosporine or androgens. ATG, a purified gamma-globulin solution, is obtained from horses or rabbits immunized with human T lymphocytes. Side effects during the infusion are common and include fever and chills. The sudden onset of a rash or bronchospasm may herald anaphylaxis and requires prompt management (see Chapters 38 and 72). Serum sickness, as evidenced by fever, rash, arthralgias, and pruritus, may develop in some patients; it may take weeks to resolve (Gupta, Eapen, Brazauskas, et al., 2010).

Immunosuppressants prevent the patient's lymphocytes from destroying the stem cells. If relapse occurs (i.e., the patient becomes pancytopenic again), reinstitution of the same immunologic agents may induce another remission. Corticosteroids are not very useful as immunosuppressive agents in the long term, because patients with aplastic anemia are particularly susceptible to the development of bone complications from corticosteroids (e.g., aseptic necrosis of the head of the femur).

Supportive therapy plays a major role in the management of aplastic anemia. Any offending agent is discontinued. The patient is supported with transfusions of PRBCs and platelets as necessary. Death usually is caused by hemorrhage or infection.

Nursing Management

Patients with aplastic anemia are vulnerable to problems related to erythrocyte, leukocyte, and platelet deficiencies. They should be assessed carefully for signs of infection and bleeding. Specific interventions are delineated in the Neutropenia and Thrombocytopenia sections. Nurses must also monitor for side effects of therapy, particularly for hypersensitivity reaction while administering ATG. If patients require long-term cyclosporine therapy, they should be monitored for long-term effects, including renal or liver dysfunction, hypertension, pruritus, visual impairment, tremor, and skin cancer. They should also be informed that the metabolism of ATG is altered by many other medications; thus, each new prescription needs careful assessment for drug–drug interactions. Patients also need to understand the importance of not abruptly stopping their immunosuppressive therapy.

■ Megaloblastic Anemias

In the anemias caused by deficiencies of vitamin B_{12} or folic acid, identical bone marrow and peripheral blood changes occur because both vitamins are essential for normal DNA synthesis. In either case, the erythrocytes that are produced are abnormally large and called *megaloblastic red cells*. Other cells derived from the myeloid stem cell (nonlymphoid leukocytes, platelets) are also abnormal. A bone marrow analysis reveals hyperplasia (abnormal increase in the number of

cells), and the precursor erythroid and myeloid cells are large and bizarre in appearance. However, many of these abnormal erythroid and myeloid cells are destroyed within the marrow, so the mature cells that do leave the marrow are actually fewer in number. Thus, **pancytopenia** (a decrease in all myeloid stem cell–derived cells) can develop. In advanced stages of disease, the hemoglobin value may be as low as 4 to 5 g/dL, the leukocyte count 2,000 to 3,000/mm^3, and the platelet count less than 50,000/mm^3 (Primack & Mahaniah, 2011). Those cells that are released into the circulation are often abnormally shaped. The neutrophils are hypersegmented. The platelets may be abnormally large. The erythrocytes are abnormally shaped, and the shapes may vary widely (**poikilocytosis**). Because the erythrocytes are very large, the MCV is very high, usually exceeding 110 mcm^3.

Pathophysiology

Folic Acid Deficiency

Folic acid is stored as compounds referred to as folates. The folate stores in the body are much smaller than those of vitamin B_{12} and can become depleted within 4 months when the dietary intake of folate is deficient (Green, 2010). Folate is found in green vegetables and liver. Thus, folate deficiency occurs in people who rarely eat uncooked vegetables. Alcohol increases folic acid requirements, and, at the same time, patients with alcoholism usually have a diet that is deficient in the vitamin. Folic acid requirements are also increased in patients with chronic hemolytic anemias and in women who are pregnant, because the need for erythrocyte production is increased in these conditions. Some patients with malabsorptive diseases of the small bowel, such as celiac disease, may not absorb folic acid normally (Green, 2010).

Vitamin B_{12} Deficiency

A deficiency of vitamin B_{12} can occur in several ways. Inadequate dietary intake is rare but can develop in strict vegetarians who consume no meat or dairy products. Faulty absorption from the GI tract is more common. This occurs in conditions such as Crohn's disease or after ileal resection, bariatric surgery, or gastrectomy. Chronic use of proton pump inhibitors to reduce gastric acid production can also inhibit B_{12} absorption, as can the use of the drug metformin (Glucophage) in managing diabetes (Langan & Zawistoski, 2011). Another cause is the absence of intrinsic factor; in this particular context, the resultant anemia is called *pernicious anemia*. Intrinsic factor is normally secreted by cells within the gastric mucosa; it binds with dietary vitamin B_{12} and travels with it to the ileum, where the vitamin is absorbed. Without intrinsic factor, orally consumed vitamin B_{12} cannot be adequately absorbed, and erythrocyte production is eventually diminished. Even if adequate vitamin B_{12} and intrinsic factor are present, a deficiency may occur if disease involving the ileum or pancreas impairs absorption. Pernicious anemia, which tends to run in families, is primarily a disorder of adults, particularly older adults.

The body normally has large stores of vitamin B_{12}, so years may pass before the deficiency results in anemia. Because the body compensates so well, the anemia can be severe before the patient becomes symptomatic. Patients with pernicious anemia have a higher incidence of gastric cancer than the general population; these patients may benefit from having endoscopies at regular intervals to screen for early gastric cancer (Annibale, Lahner, & Fave, 2011).

Clinical Manifestations

Symptoms of folic acid and vitamin B_{12} deficiencies are similar, and the two anemias may coexist. However, the neurologic manifestations of vitamin B_{12} deficiency do not occur with folic acid deficiency, and they persist if vitamin B_{12} is not replaced. Therefore, careful distinction between the two anemias must be made. Serum levels of both vitamins can be measured. In the case of folic acid deficiency, even small amounts of folate increase the serum folate level, sometimes to normal. Measuring the amount of folate within the red cell itself (red cell folate) is therefore a more sensitive test in determining true folate deficiency.

After the body stores of vitamin B_{12} are depleted, the patient may begin to show signs and symptoms of the anemia. However, because the onset and progression of the anemia are so gradual, the body can compensate well until the anemia is severe, so the typical manifestations of anemia (weakness, listlessness, fatigue) may not be apparent initially. The hematologic effects of vitamin B_{12} deficiency are accompanied by effects on other organ systems, particularly the GI tract and nervous system. Patients with pernicious anemia develop a smooth, sore, red tongue and mild diarrhea. They are extremely pale, particularly in the mucous membranes. They may become confused; more often, they have paresthesias in the extremities (particularly numbness and tingling in the feet and lower legs). They may have difficulty maintaining their balance because of damage to the spinal cord, and they also lose position sense (proprioception). These symptoms are progressive, although the course of illness may be marked by spontaneous partial remissions and exacerbations. Without treatment, patients can die after several years, usually from heart failure secondary to anemia.

Assessment and Diagnostic Findings

The classic method of determining the cause of vitamin B_{12} deficiency is the Schilling test, in which the patient receives a small oral dose of radioactive vitamin B_{12}, followed in a few hours by a large, nonradioactive parenteral dose of vitamin B_{12} (this aids in renal excretion of the radioactive dose). If the oral vitamin is absorbed, more than 8% is excreted in the urine within 24 hours; therefore, if no radioactivity is present in the urine (i.e., the radioactive vitamin B_{12} stays within the GI tract), the cause is GI malabsorption of the vitamin B_{12}. Conversely, if radioactivity is detected in the urine, the cause of the deficiency is not ileal disease or pernicious anemia. Later, the same procedure is repeated, but this time intrinsic factor is added to the oral radioactive vitamin B_{12}. If radioactivity is now detected in the urine (i.e., the vitamin B_{12} was absorbed from the GI tract in the presence of intrinsic factor), the diagnosis of pernicious anemia can be made. The Schilling test is useful only if the urine collections are complete; therefore, the nurse must promote the patient's understanding and adherence to this collection (Fischbach & Dunning, 2010).

Other methods of establishing the diagnosis are now more commonly used. Although it is possible to measure methyl-

malonic acid levels in vitamin B_{12} deficiency, these levels also increase in the setting of renal insufficiency. Furthermore, it is expensive to measure these levels, which also limits the utility of the test. A more useful, easier test is the intrinsic factor antibody test (Fischbach & Dunning, 2010). A positive test indicates the presence of antibodies that bind the vitamin B_{12}–intrinsic factor complex and prevent it from binding to receptors in the ileum, thus preventing its absorption. Although this test is not specific for pernicious anemia alone, it can aid in the diagnosis.

Medical Management

Folate deficiency is treated by increasing the amount of folic acid in the diet and administering 1 mg of folic acid daily. Folic acid is administered intramuscularly only to people with malabsorption problems. Although many multivitamin preparations now contain folic acid, additional supplements may be necessary because the amount may be inadequate to fully replace deficient body stores. Patients who abuse alcohol should receive folic acid as long as they continue to consume alcohol.

Vitamin B_{12} deficiency is treated by vitamin B_{12} replacement. Vegetarians can prevent or treat deficiency with oral supplements with vitamins or fortified soy milk. When the deficiency is due to the more common defect in absorption or the absence of intrinsic factor, replacement is by monthly intramuscular injections of vitamin B_{12}. A small amount of an oral dose of vitamin B_{12} can be absorbed by passive diffusion, even in the absence of intrinsic factor; however, large doses are required if vitamin B_{12} is to be replaced orally (Annibale et al., 2011).

As vitamin B_{12} is replaced, the reticulocyte count rises within 1 week, and in several weeks the blood counts are all normal (Andres, Fothergill, & Mecili, 2010). The tongue feels better and appears less red in several days. However, the neurologic manifestations require more time for recovery; if there is severe neuropathy, the patient may never recover fully. To prevent recurrence of pernicious anemia, vitamin B_{12} therapy must be continued for life.

Nursing Management

Assessment of patients who have or are at risk for megaloblastic anemia includes inspection of the skin, mucous membranes, and tongue. Mild jaundice may be apparent and is best seen in the sclera without using fluorescent lights. Vitiligo (patchy loss of skin pigmentation) and premature graying of the hair are often seen in patients with pernicious anemia. Because of the neurologic complications associated with these anemias, a careful neurologic assessment is important, including tests of position, vibration sense, and cognitive function.

The nurse needs to pay particular attention to ambulation and should assess the patient's gait and stability, as well as the need for assistive devices (e.g., canes, walkers) and for assistance in managing daily activities. Of particular concern is ensuring safety when position sense, coordination, and gait are affected. Physical and occupational therapy referrals may be needed. If sensation is altered, the patient needs to be instructed to avoid excessive heat and cold.

Because mouth and tongue soreness may limit nutritional intake, the nurse advises the patient to eat small amounts of bland, soft foods frequently. The nurse also may explain that other nutritional deficiencies, such as alcohol-induced anemia, can induce neurologic problems.

Promoting Home and Community-Based Care

The patient must be taught about the chronicity of the disorder and the need for monthly vitamin B_{12} injections or daily oral vitamin B_{12} even in the absence of symptoms. If parenteral replacement is used, many patients can be taught to self-administer their injections. The gastric atrophy associated with pernicious anemia increases the risk for gastric carcinoma, so the patient needs to understand that ongoing medical follow-up and screening are important.

Hemolytic Anemias

In hemolytic anemias, the erythrocytes have a shortened lifespan; thus, their number in the circulation is reduced. Fewer erythrocytes result in decreased available oxygen, causing hypoxia, which in turn stimulates an increase in erythropoietin release from the kidney. The erythropoietin stimulates the bone marrow to compensate by producing new erythrocytes and releasing some of them into the circulation somewhat prematurely as **reticulocytes**. If the red cell destruction persists, the hemoglobin is broken down excessively; about 80% of the heme is converted to bilirubin, conjugated in the liver, and excreted in the bile (Barrett, Barman, Boitano, et al., 2012).

The mechanism of erythrocyte destruction varies, but all types of hemolytic anemia share certain laboratory features: the reticulocyte count is elevated, the fraction of indirect (unconjugated) bilirubin is increased, and the supply of **haptoglobin** (a binding protein for free hemoglobin) is depleted as more hemoglobin is released. As a result, the plasma haptoglobin level is low. If the marrow cannot compensate to replace the erythrocytes destroyed in the circulation, the anemia will progress.

Hemolytic anemia has various forms. Inherited forms include sickle cell anemia, thalassemia and thalassemia major, G-6-PD deficiency, and hereditary spherocytosis. Acquired forms include autoimmune hemolytic anemia, non–immune-mediated paroxysmal nocturnal hemoglobinuria, microangiopathic hemolytic anemia, and heart valve hemolysis, as well as anemias associated with hypersplenism.

■ *Sickle Cell Anemia*

Sickle cell anemia is a severe hemolytic anemia that results from inheritance of the sickle hemoglobin (HbS) gene, which causes the hemoglobin molecule to be defective. HbS acquires a crystal-like formation when exposed to low oxygen tension. The oxygen level in venous blood can be low enough to cause this change; consequently, the erythrocyte containing HbS loses its round, pliable, biconcave disk shape and becomes dehydrated, rigid, and sickle shaped (Fig. 33-2). These long, rigid erythrocytes can adhere to the endothelium of small vessels; when they adhere to each other, blood flow to a region or an organ may be reduced. If ischemia or infarction results, the patient may have pain, swelling, and fever. The sickling process takes time; if the erythrocyte is again

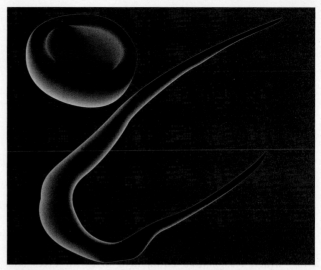

FIGURE 33-2 • A normal red blood cell (*upper left*) and a sickled red blood cell.

exposed to adequate amounts of oxygen before the membrane becomes too rigid (e.g., when it travels through the pulmonary circulation), it can revert to a normal shape. For this reason, the "sickling crises" are intermittent. Cold can aggravate the sickling process, because vasoconstriction slows the blood flow. Oxygen delivery can also be impaired by an increased blood viscosity, with or without occlusion due to adhesion of sickled cells; in this situation, the effects are seen in larger vessels, such as arterioles.

The *HbS* gene is inherited in people of African descent and to a lesser extent in people from the Middle East, the Mediterranean area, and aboriginal tribes in India. Sickle cell anemia is the most severe form of sickle cell disease. This form of the disease is found in about 1 in 500 African American live births and 1 in 36,000 live Hispanic live births (NHLBI, 2011). Less severe forms include sickle cell hemoglobin C (SC) disease, sickle cell hemoglobin D (SD) disease, and sickle cell beta-thalassemia. The clinical manifestations and management are the same as for sickle cell anemia. The term *sickle cell trait* refers to the carrier state for SC diseases; it is the most benign type of SC disease, in that less than 50% of the hemoglobin within an erythrocyte is HbS. One in twelve African Americans have sickle cell trait (NHLBI, 2011). However, if two people with sickle cell trait have children, the children may inherit two abnormal genes and will have sickle cell anemia. (Refer to Chapter 8 for additional discussion of genetic diseases.)

Clinical Manifestations

Symptoms of sickle cell anemia vary and are only somewhat based on the amount of HbS. Symptoms and complications result from chronic hemolysis or thrombosis. Sickled cells are rapidly hemolyzed and thus have a very short lifespan of 10 to 20 days (Franco, Lohman, Silberstein, et al., 1998). Anemia is always present; usually, hemoglobin values range between 7 and 10 g/dL. Jaundice is characteristic and is usually obvious in the sclerae. The bone marrow expands in childhood in a compensatory effort to offset the anemia, sometimes leading to enlargement of the bones of the face and skull. The chronic anemia is associated with tachycardia, cardiac murmurs, and often an enlarged heart (cardiomegaly). Dysrhythmias and heart failure may occur in adults.

Virtually any organ may be affected by thrombosis, but the primary sites involve those areas with slower circulation, such as the spleen, lungs, and central nervous system. All tissues and organs are vulnerable to microcirculatory interruptions by the sickling process and therefore are susceptible to hypoxic damage or ischemic necrosis. Patients with sickle cell anemia are unusually susceptible to infection, particularly pneumonia and osteomyelitis. Complications of sickle cell anemia include infection, stroke, renal failure, impotence, heart failure, and pulmonary hypertension (Table 33-2).

Sickle Cell Crisis

There are three types of sickle cell crisis in the adult population. The most common is the very painful *acute vaso-occlusive crisis*, which results from entrapment of erythrocytes and leukocytes in the microcirculation, causing tissue hypoxia, inflammation, and necrosis due to inadequate blood flow to a specific region of tissue or organ. When perfusion is resumed, substances are released (e.g., free radicals, free plasma hemoglobin) that cause oxidative damage to the vessel. In turn, the endothelium of the vessel becomes dysfunctional and vasculopathy develops (Johnson & Telen, 2008). *Aplastic crisis* results from infection with the human parvovirus. The hemoglobin level falls rapidly and the marrow cannot compensate, as evidenced by an absence of reticulocytes. *Sequestration crisis* results when other organs pool the sickled cells. Although the spleen is the most common organ responsible for sequestration in children, most children with sickle cell anemia have had a splenic infarction by 10 years of age, and the spleen is then no longer functional (autosplenectomy). In adults, the common organs involved in sequestration are the liver and, more seriously, the lungs.

Acute Chest Syndrome

Acute chest syndrome is manifested by fever, respiratory distress (tachypnea, cough, wheezing), and new infiltrates seen on the chest x-ray. These signs often mimic infection, which is often the cause. However, the infectious etiology appears to be atypical bacteria such as *Chlamydia pneumoniae* and *Mycoplasma pneumoniae* as well as viruses such as respiratory syncytial virus and parvovirus. Other causes include pulmonary fat embolism, pulmonary infarction, and pulmonary thromboembolism. Seventy-five percent of patients who develop acute chest syndrome had a painful vaso-occlusive crisis, usually lasting an average of 2.5 days prior to developing symptoms of acute chest syndrome (Laurie, 2010). Medical management includes red cell transfusion, antimicrobial therapy, bronchodilators, inhaled nitric oxide therapy, and possibly mechanical ventilation. Although this syndrome can rapidly progress to acute respiratory distress syndrome and death, prompt and aggressive intervention can result in a favorable outcome.

Pulmonary Hypertension

Pulmonary hypertension is a common sequela of sickle cell disease, and often the cause of death (Wahl & Vichinsky, 2010). Diagnosing pulmonary hypertension is difficult because clinical symptoms rarely occur until damage is irreversible. Pulse oximetry measurements are typically normal, and breath sounds are clear to auscultation until the disease has progressed to later stages. Pulmonary artery pressures are elevated above baseline but typically much lower than that seen in idiopathic or hereditary pulmonary hypertension. Screening patients with sickle cell disease with Doppler echocardiography may be useful in identifying those with elevated pulmonary artery pressures (Parent, Bachir, Inamo, et al., 2011). High levels of the amino-terminal form of

TABLE 33-2	Complications in Sickle Cell Anemia*		
Organ Involved	**Mechanisms***	**Diagnostic Findings**	**Signs and Symptoms**
Spleen	Primary site of sickling → infarctions → ↓ phagocytic function of macrophages	Autosplenectomy; ↑ infection (especially pneumonia, osteomyelitis)	Abdominal pain; fever, signs of infection
Lungs	Infection	Pulmonary infiltrate	Chest pain; dyspnea
	Infarction → ↑ pulmonary pressure → pulmonary hypertension	↑ sPLA₂[†]	Chest pain; dyspnea
Central nervous system	Infarction	Cerebrovascular accident (stroke)	Weakness (if severe); learning difficulties (if mild)
Kidney	Sickling → damage to renal medulla	Hematuria; inability to concentrate urine; renal failure	Dehydration
Heart	Anemia	Tachycardia; cardiomegaly → heart failure	Weakness, fatigue, dyspnea
Bone	↑ Erythroid production	Widening of medullary spaces and cortical thinning	Ache, arthralgias
	Infarction of bone	Osteosclerosis → avascular necrosis	Bone pain, especially hips
Liver	Hemolysis	Jaundice and gallstone formation; hepatomegaly	Abdominal pain
Skin and peripheral vasculature	↑ Viscosity/stasis → infarction → skin ulcers	Skin ulcers; ↓ wound healing	Pain
Eye	Infarction	Scarring, hemorrhage, retinal detachment	↓ Vision; blindness
Penis	Sickling → vascular thrombosis	Priapism → impotence	Pain, impotence

→, leading to; ↓, decreased; ↑, increased; sPLA₂, secretory phospholipase A₂.
*Problems encountered in sickle cell anemia vary and are the result of a variety of mechanisms, as depicted in this table. Common physical findings and symptoms are also variable.
[†]Elevated sPLA₂ levels can predict impending acute chest syndrome [see text]).

brain natriuretic peptide can serve as a useful biomarker for pulmonary hypertension in this patient population and as an independent predictor of mortality (Wahl & Vichinsky, 2010). Although changes are not evident on chest x-ray, computed tomography of the chest often demonstrates microvascular pulmonary occlusion and diminished perfusion of the lung.

Assessment and Diagnostic Findings

The patient with sickle cell trait usually has a normal hemoglobin level, a normal hematocrit, and a normal blood smear. In contrast, the patient with sickle cell anemia has a low hematocrit and sickled cells on the smear. The diagnosis is confirmed by hemoglobin electrophoresis.

Prognosis

Patients with sickle cell anemia are usually diagnosed in childhood because they become anemic in infancy and begin to have sickle cell crises at 1 or 2 years of age. Some children die in the first years of life, typically of infection, but antibiotic use and parent education strategies have greatly improved the outcomes for these children. Despite current management strategies, the average life expectancy is still suboptimal, typically in the fifth decade. Young adults often live with multiple, often severe, complications from their disease. In some patients, the symptoms and complications diminish by 30 years of age. Currently, there is no way to predict which patients will fall into this subgroup.

Medical Management

Treatment for sickle cell anemia is the focus of continued research. However, aside from the equally important aggressive management of symptoms and complications, there are few primary treatment modalities for sickle cell diseases.

Hematopoietic Stem Cell Transplant

HSCT may cure sickle cell anemia. However, this treatment modality is available to only a small subset of affected patients, because of either the lack of a compatible donor or because severe organ damage (e.g., renal, liver, lung) that may be already present in the patient is a contraindication for HSCT (see Chapter 15).

Pharmacologic Therapy

Hydroxyurea (Hydrea) is a chemotherapy agent that is effective in increasing fetal hemoglobin (i.e., hemoglobin F) levels in patients with sickle cell anemia, thereby decreasing the formation of sickled cells. Patients who receive hydroxyurea appear to have fewer painful episodes of sickle cell crisis, a lower incidence of acute chest syndrome, and less need for transfusions. However, whether hydroxyurea can prevent or reverse actual organ damage remains unknown. Side effects of hydroxyurea include chronic suppression of leukocyte formation, teratogenesis, and potential for later development of a malignancy. Patient response to this agent varies significantly. The incidence and severity of side effects are also highly variable within a dose range. Adherence to taking this medication as prescribed is a common problem.

Arginine has antisickling properties and enhances the availability of nitric oxide, the most potent vasodilator,

resulting in decreased pulmonary artery pressure. Arginine may be useful in managing pulmonary hypertension and acute chest syndrome, but patients may develop resistance, diminishing its effectiveness (Natarajan, Townes, & Kutlar, 2010).

Transfusion Therapy

RBC transfusions have been shown to be highly effective in several situations: in an acute exacerbation of anemia (e.g., aplastic crisis, severe vaso-occlusive crisis), in the prevention of severe complications from anesthesia and surgery, in improving the response to infection (when it results in exacerbated anemia), in the case of acute chest syndrome and multiorgan failure, and in thwarting the evolution of a stroke or an acute neurologic defect. Transfusions are also effective in diminishing episodes of sickle cell crisis in pregnant women, although such transfusions do not improve fetal survival. Chronic transfusion therapy may be effective in preventing or managing complications from sickle cell disease by keeping the HbS level to less than 30%. The hemoglobin level is usually kept below 11 to keep blood viscosity low (Natarajan et al., 2010).

The risk of complications from transfusion is important to consider. These complications include iron overload, which necessitates chelation therapy (see Chapter 34, Myelodysplastic Syndromes, Nursing Management); poor venous access, which necessitates a vascular access device (and its attendant risk of infection or thrombosis); infections (particularly hepatitis); and especially alloimmunization (an immune response to antigens from donor cells) from repeated transfusions. Although iron overload is likely, the majority of iron deposition is within the liver; unlike patients with transfusion-dependent thalassemia, where other organs are affected by iron deposition, cardiac, thyroid, and pituitary dysfunction are not seen in patients with sickle cell anemia and iron overload (Inati, Khoriaty, & Musallam, 2011). Another complication from transfusion is increased blood viscosity without reduction in the concentration of hemoglobin S. Exchange transfusion (in which the patient's own blood is removed and replaced via transfusion) may be performed to diminish the risk of increasing the viscosity excessively; the objective is to reduce the patient's own blood volume with transfused (non-sickled) packed red cells to a target hemoglobin of 10 gm/dL (Kato & Gladwin, 2005). Finally, it is important to consider the significant financial cost of an aggressive transfusion and chelation program.

Patients with sickle cell anemia may require daily folic acid replacements to maintain the supply required for increased erythropoiesis from hemolysis. Infections must be treated promptly with appropriate antibiotics; infection, particularly pneumococcal infection can be serious (Natarajan et al., 2010). These patients should receive pneumococcal and annual influenza vaccinations.

Acute chest syndrome is managed by prompt initiation of antibiotic therapy. Incentive spirometry has been shown to decrease the incidence of pulmonary complications significantly. In severe cases, bronchoscopy may be required to identify the source of pulmonary disease. Hydration is important but must be carefully monitored. Corticosteroids may also be useful. Transfusions reverse the hypoxia and decrease the level of secretory phospholipase A_2. Pulmonary function should be monitored regularly to detect pulmonary hypertension early, when therapy (hydroxyurea, arginine, transfusions, or HSCT) may have a positive impact.

Because repeated blood transfusions are necessary, patients may develop multiple autoantibodies, making cross-matching difficult. In this patient population, a hemolytic transfusion reaction (see Chapter 32) may mimic the signs and symptoms of a sickle cell crisis. The classic distinguishing factor is that with a hemolytic transfusion reaction, the patient becomes *more* anemic after being transfused. These patients need very close observation. Further transfusion is avoided if possible until the hemolytic process abates. If possible, the patient is supported with corticosteroids (prednisone), or intravenous immunoglobulin (IVIG), erythropoietin (epoetin alfa [Epogen]).

Supportive Therapy

Supportive care is equally important. Pain is a significant issue. The incidence of painful sickle cell crises is highly variable; many patients have pain on a daily basis. The severity of the pain may not be enough to cause the patient to seek assistance from health care providers but severe enough to interfere with the ability to work and function within the family unit. Acute pain episodes tend to be self-limited, lasting hours to days. If the patient cannot manage the pain at home, intervention is frequently sought in an urgent care facility or emergency department. Studies suggest that patients have pain in an average of three to four different sites; furthermore, the pain experienced may be acute or chronic or both (Smith & Scherer, 2010; Wilkie, Molokie, Boyd-Seal, et al.,

2010). The most commonly reported sites of pain include the back (lower or upper), hip, lower and upper extremities, and knees. Wilkie and colleagues (2010) found that patients with sickle cell disease reported their pain was more severe than that experienced in individuals with cancer or during labor and childbirth (Chart 33-4).

Adequate hydration is important during a painful sickling episode. Oral hydration is acceptable if the patient can maintain adequate fluid intake; IV hydration with dextrose 5% in water (D_5W) or dextrose 5% in 0.25 normal saline solution ($3 \text{ L/m}^2/24 \text{ h}$) may be required for a sickle crisis. Supplemental oxygen may also be needed.

The use of medication to relieve acute pain is important. Aspirin is very useful in diminishing mild to moderate pain; it also diminishes inflammation and potential thrombosis (due to its ability to decrease platelet adhesion). Nonsteroidal anti-inflammatory drugs (NSAIDs) are useful for moderate pain or in combination with opioid analgesics. Although no tolerance develops with NSAIDs, a "ceiling effect" does develop whereby an increase in dosage does not increase analgesia. NSAID use must be carefully monitored, because these medications can precipitate renal dysfunction. When opioid analgesic agents are used, morphine is the medication of choice for acute pain. Patient-controlled analgesia is frequently used in the acute care setting. (See Chapter 12 for a discussion of pain management.)

Chronic pain increases in incidence as the patient ages and is caused by continued complications from the sickling (e.g., avascular necrosis of the hip). Recent data suggest that

---

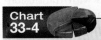

NURSING RESEARCH PROFILE

Chart 33-4

Barriers to Pain Management in Patients With Sickle Cell Disease

Wilkie, D., Molokie, R., Boyd-Seal, D., et al. (2010). Patient-reported outcomes: Descriptors of nociceptive and neuropathic pain and barriers to effective pain management in adult outpatients with sickle cell disease. *Journal of the National Medical Association, 102*(1), 18–27.

Purpose

Despite the frequent nature of recurrent pain episodes in adults with sickle cell disease (SCD), little is known about the actual characteristics of these pain episodes. Adherence to prescribed analgesic medications is pivotal to adequate pain management in the outpatient setting. Yet patients may have barriers that interfere with such adherence. The purpose of this study was twofold: (1) to describe the sensory pain characteristics of adults with SCD and (2) to describe the barriers and analgesic use by these patients.

Design

A convenience sample of 145 adults with SCD and a history of prior SCD-related pain within the past 12 months consented to participate. These participants were all receiving outpatient treatment in the same outpatient SCD clinic in a midwestern city. Participants completed a demographic questionnaire, the McGill Pain Questionnaire, and Barriers Questionnaire, and provided a list of currently used analgesic medications (e.g., acetaminophen, nonsteroidal anti-inflammatory agents, opioids, and adjuvant drugs [membrane stabilizing drugs and antidepressants]).

Findings

Patients reported having pain in an average of 3.6 unique anatomic locations. At the time of data collection, 27% reported moderate and 19% severe pain levels. Only 52% were satisfied with their pain level. Eighty percent of patients described their pain as constant or steady, whereas 43% described it as transient or brief. Analgesics used included acetaminophen (72%) and ibuprofen (57%); codeine with acetaminophen (66%) or morphine (immediate release, 24% or injection, 28%). Adjuvant drugs were rarely used. Distress from side effects (constipation and nausea) was identified as a frequent barrier to the use of analgesics, as was the belief that one could become addicted to pain medication (85%). An interesting finding was that the pain-quality descriptors selected were similar to those used in describing neuropathic pain. Pain composite scores were higher in this study population than that published in patients with cancer or women during childbirth.

Nursing Implications

Most clinicians presume that pain related to SCD relates to crisis. Data from this study suggest that adults living with SCD cope with pain on a much more frequent basis and that the pain is not always episodic in nature. Nurses should assess patients with SCD for attitudinal barriers to using analgesics, particularly opioids, for pain management and should more aggressively manage opioid-related side effects. Finally, many participants in this study reported a neuropathic component to their pain, which suggests that there is a need to alter pain management approaches to incorporate those more effective for managing neuropathic pain into the pain management plan for patients with SCD.

these patients may also have neuropathic pain, including possible allodynia (i.e., pain elicited from a stimulus that does not normally cause pain) and hyperalgesia (i.e., increased pain sensitivity) (Wilkie et al., 2010). Smith and Scherer (2010) suggest that neuropathic pain may result from prior episodes of nociceptive pain and may not develop until adulthood. Further research is needed to better understand this type of pain and appropriate management methods in this population. With chronic pain management, the principal goal is to maximize functioning; pain may not be completely eliminated without sacrificing function. This concept may be difficult for patients to accept; they may need repeated explanations and support from nonjudgmental health care providers. Nonpharmacologic approaches to pain management are crucial in this setting. Examples include physical and occupational therapy, physiotherapy (including the use of heat, massage, and exercise), cognitive and behavioral intervention (including distraction, relaxation, and motivational therapy), and support groups.

Another significant issue for patients with sickle cell disease is fatigue, and its cause is multifactorial. Fatigue is due to hypoxia, which in turn is due to low levels of normal hemoglobin and decreased oxygen affinity of sickled hemoglobin. The hemolysis occurring in sickle cell disease and resultant anemia is associated with **oxyhemoglobin** desaturation due to acute splenic sequestration or to infection (Ameringer & Smith, 2011). These patients can also develop tissue hypoxia when the hematocrit approaches more normal levels (35% to 45%), as the blood viscosity may become increased to the point where blood flow through small capillaries and arterioles is compromised.

The vascular endothelium becomes inflamed from the sickled red cells and resultant hypoxia. These endothelial changes induce oxidative stress, which in turn amplifies the inflammatory response (Ameringer & Smith, 2011). Inflammatory cytokines are increased in patients with sickle cell anemia and are known to decrease muscle strength, decrease exercise capacity, increase resting energy expenditure, and decrease rapid eye movement stage of sleep—all exacerbating fatigue. Fatigue is further increased in the setting of pain, stress, depression, and anxiety.

Working with patients who have multiple episodes of severe pain and fatigue can be challenging. Health care providers must realize that patients with sickle cell disease face a lifelong experience with severe, unpredictable pain and fatigue. These disrupt the patient's level of functioning, including social functioning, and may result in a feeling of helplessness. Patients with inadequate social support systems may have more difficulty coping with these issues.

NURSING PROCESS

The Patient With Sickle Cell Crisis

Assessment

The patient is asked to identify factors that precipitated previous crises and measures taken to prevent and manage crises. If a sickle cell crisis is suspected, the nurse needs to determine whether the pain currently experienced is the same as or different from the pain typically encountered in crisis.

Pain levels should always be monitored using a pain intensity scale, such as a 0-to-10 scale. The quality of the pain (e.g., sharp, dull, burning), the frequency of the pain (constant vs. intermittent), and factors that aggravate or alleviate the pain are included in this assessment. A similar assessment should be made of the patient's fatigue, including the impact of fatigue on current lifestyle, quality of life, and the extent that fatigue exacerbates pain and interferes with sleep.

Because the sickling process can interrupt circulation in any tissue or organ, with resultant hypoxia and ischemia, a careful assessment of all body systems is necessary. Particular emphasis is placed on pain, swelling, and fever. All joint areas are carefully examined for pain and swelling. The abdomen is assessed for pain and tenderness because of the possibility of splenic infarction.

The cardiopulmonary systems must be assessed carefully, including auscultation of breath sounds, measurement of oxygen saturation levels, and signs of cardiac failure, such as the presence and extent of dependent edema, an increased point of maximal impulse, and cardiomegaly (as seen on a chest x-ray). The patient is assessed for signs of dehydration by a history of fluid intake and careful examination of mucous membranes, skin turgor, urine output, and serum creatinine and blood urea nitrogen values.

A careful neurologic examination is important to elicit symptoms of cerebral hypoxia. However, ischemic findings on magnetic resonance imaging (MRI) or Doppler studies may precede findings on the physical examination. MRI and Doppler studies may be used for early diagnosis and may result in improved patient outcome because therapy can be initiated promptly.

Because patients with sickle cell anemia are susceptible to infections, they are assessed for the presence of any infectious process. Particular attention is given to examination of the chest, long bones, and femoral head, because pneumonia and osteomyelitis are especially common. Leg ulcers, which may be infected and slow to heal, are common (Fig. 33-3).

The extent of anemia and the ability of the marrow to replenish erythrocytes are assessed by the hemoglobin level, hematocrit, and reticulocyte counts; these are compared with the patient's baseline values. The patient's current and past history of medical management is also obtained, particularly chronic transfusion therapy, hydroxyurea use, and prior treatment for infection.

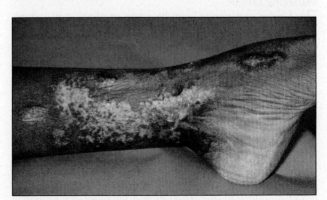

FIGURE 33-3 • Chronic skin ulcers seen in a patient with sickle cell anemia. From Tkachuk, D. C., & Hirschman, J. V. (2007). *Wintrobe's atlas of clinical hematology* (Fig. 1.71, p. 36). Philadelphia: Lippincott Williams & Wilkins.

Diagnosis

Nursing Diagnoses

Based on the assessment data, major nursing diagnoses may include:

- Acute pain and fatigue related to tissue hypoxia due to agglutination of sickled cells within blood vessels
- Risk for infection
- Risk for powerlessness related to illness-induced helplessness
- Deficient knowledge regarding sickle crisis prevention

Collaborative Problems/Potential Complications

Potential complications may include the following:

- Hypoxia, ischemia, infection, and poor wound healing leading to skin breakdown and ulcers
- Dehydration
- Cerebrovascular accident (CVA, stroke)
- Anemia
- Acute and chronic renal failure
- Heart failure, pulmonary hypertension, and acute chest syndrome
- Impotence
- Poor compliance
- Substance abuse related to poorly managed chronic pain

Planning and Goals

The major goals for the patient are relief of pain, decreased incidence of crisis, enhanced sense of self-esteem and power, and absence of complications.

Nursing Interventions

Managing Pain

Acute pain during a sickle cell crisis can be severe and unpredictable. The patient's subjective description and rating of pain on a pain scale must guide the use of analgesic agents. Any joint that is acutely swollen should be supported and elevated until the swelling diminishes. Relaxation techniques, breathing exercises, and distraction are helpful for some patients. After the acute painful episode has diminished, aggressive measures should be implemented to preserve function. Physical therapy, whirlpool baths, and transcutaneous electrical nerve stimulation (TENS) are examples of such modalities.

Managing Fatigue

The fatigue experienced can be acute or chronic in nature. Assisting the patient to find an appropriate balance between exercise and rest can be a useful strategy. Patients will need to develop strategies to cope with daily life demands in the setting of chronic fatigue. Maximizing nutrition, hydration, healthy sleep cycles, and diminishing tissue hypoxia can all serve to minimize fatigue. Research is needed to better understand fatigue in this patient population as well as to delineate the most effective ways to ameliorate it.

Preventing and Managing Infection

Nursing care focuses on monitoring patients for signs and symptoms of infection. Prescribed antibiotics should be initiated promptly, and patients should be assessed for signs of dehydration. If patients are to take prescribed oral antibiotics at home, they must understand the importance of completing the entire course of antibiotic therapy.

Promoting Coping Skills

This illness can leave the patient feeling powerless and with decreased self-esteem because its acute exacerbations often result in chronic health problems. These feelings can be exacerbated by inadequate management of pain and fatigue, and enhancing management of pain and fatigue can be extremely useful in establishing a therapeutic relationship based on mutual trust. Nursing care that focuses on the patient's strengths rather than deficits can enhance effective coping skills. Providing the patient with opportunities to make decisions about daily care may increase the patient's feelings of control. The patient needs to understand the rationale for and importance of compliance with a therapeutic medication regimen.

Minimizing Deficient Knowledge

Patients with sickle cell anemia benefit from understanding what situations can precipitate a sickle cell crisis and the steps they can take to prevent or diminish such crises. Keeping warm and providing adequate hydration can be effective in diminishing the occurrence and severity of attacks.

If hydroxyurea is prescribed for a woman of childbearing age, she should be informed that the drug can cause congenital harm to unborn children and advised about pregnancy prevention.

Monitoring and Managing Potential Complications

Management measures for many of the potential complications have been described in previous sections. Other measures follow.

Leg Ulcers. Leg ulcers require careful management and protection from trauma and contamination. Referral to a wound-ostomy-continence nurse may facilitate healing and assist with prevention. If leg ulcers fail to heal, skin grafting may be necessary. Scrupulous aseptic technique is warranted to prevent nosocomial infections.

Priapism Leading to Impotence. Male patients may develop sudden, painful episodes of priapism (persistent penile erection). The patient is taught to empty his bladder at the onset of the attack, exercise, and take a warm bath. If an episode persists longer than 3 hours, medical attention, which consists of IV hydration, administration of analgesic agents, and possible penile intracavernosal aspiration, is recommended. Repeated episodes may lead to extensive vascular thrombosis, resulting in impotence.

Chronic Pain and Substance Abuse. Many patients have considerable difficulty coping with chronic pain and repeated episodes of sickle cell crisis and may find it difficult to adhere to a prescribed treatment plan. Some patients with sickle cell anemia develop problems with substance abuse. This results from inadequate management of acute pain during episodes of crisis, which then promotes mistrust of the health care system and (from the patient's perspective) the need to seek care from other sources. Prevention is the best way to manage this problem (Benjamin, Dampier, Jacox, et al., 1999). Receiving care from a single provider over time is much more beneficial than receiving care from rotating physicians and staff in an emergency department. When crises occur, the staff in the emergency department should be in contact with the patient's primary provider so that optimal management can be achieved. The patient should be assessed for hyperalgesia as a potential cause for increased drug-seeking behavior. An established pattern of substance abuse is very difficult to manage, but continuity of care and establishing written contracts with the patient can be useful.

Promoting Home and Community-Based Care

Educating Patients About Self-Care. Because patients with sickle cell anemia are typically diagnosed as children, parents participate in the initial education. As the child ages, educational interventions prepare the child to assume more responsibility for self-care. Most families can learn about vascular access device management and chelation therapy. Nurses in outpatient facilities or home care nurses may need to provide follow-up care for patients with vascular access devices.

Continuing Care. The illness trajectory of sickle cell anemia is highly varied, with unpredictable episodes of complications and crises. Care is often provided on an emergency basis, especially for some patients with pain management problems (see previous section). All health care providers who provide services to patients with sickle cell disease and their families need to communicate regularly with each other. The home care nurse is in an excellent position to serve as coordinator and facilitator between health care providers in a variety of settings so that the care of these patients is optimized (Lee, Askew, Walker, et al., 2012). Patients need to learn which parameters are important for them to monitor and how to monitor them. Guidelines should also be given regarding when it is appropriate to seek urgent care.

Evaluation

Expected patient outcomes may include:

1. Control of pain and fatigue
   a. Uses analgesic agents to control acute pain
   b. Uses relaxation techniques, breathing exercises, and distraction to help relieve pain and fatigue
2. Absence of infection
   a. Has normal temperature
   b. Has leukocyte count within normal range (4,500/mm^3 to 11,000/mm^3)
   c. Identifies importance of continuing antibiotics at home (if applicable)
3. Expresses improved sense of control
   a. Participates in goal setting and in planning and implementing daily activities
   b. Participates in decisions about care
4. Increases knowledge about disease process
   a. Identifies situations and factors that can precipitate sickle cell crisis
   b. Describes lifestyle changes needed to prevent crisis
   c. Describes the importance of warmth, adequate hydration, and prevention of infection in preventing crisis
5. Absence of complications

■ *Thalassemia*

The thalassemias are a group of hereditary anemias characterized by **hypochromia** (an abnormal decrease in the hemoglobin content of erythrocytes), extreme **microcytosis** (smaller-than-normal erythrocytes), destruction of blood elements (hemolysis), and variable degrees of anemia. The thalassemias occur worldwide, but the highest prevalence is found in people of Mediterranean, African, and Southeast Asian ancestry (Weatherall, 2010).

Thalassemias are associated with defective synthesis of hemoglobin; the production of one or more globulin chains within the hemoglobin molecule is reduced. When this occurs, the imbalance in the configuration of the hemoglobin causes it to precipitate in the erythroid precursors or the erythrocytes themselves. This increases the rigidity of the erythrocytes and thus the premature destruction of these cells.

Thalassemias are classified into two major groups according to which hemoglobin chain is diminished: alpha or beta. The alpha-thalassemias occur mainly in people from Asia and the Middle East, and the beta-thalassemias are most prevalent in people from Mediterranean regions but also occur in those from the Middle East or Asia. However, due to extensive immigration, the prevalence of either type of thalassemia is no longer limited to geographic distribution (Weatherall, 2010). The alpha-thalassemias are milder than the beta forms and often occur without symptoms; the erythrocytes are extremely microcytic, but the anemia, if present, is mild.

The severity of beta-thalassemia varies depending on the extent to which the hemoglobin chains are affected. Patients with mild forms have microcytosis and mild anemia. If left untreated, severe beta-thalassemia (i.e., thalassemia major or Cooley's anemia) can be fatal within the first few years of life. HSCT offers a chance of cure, but when this is not possible, the disease is usually treated with transfusion of PRBCs. Patients may now survive into their 60s or 70s if they have mild forms of the disease (Taher, Musallam, Karimi, et al., 2010). Patient education during the reproductive years should include preconception counseling about the risk of thalassemia major in offspring. (See Chapter 8 for discussion of genetic counseling and evaluation services.)

Thalassemia major is characterized by severe anemia, marked hemolysis, and ineffective erythropoiesis. With early regular transfusion therapy, growth and development through childhood are facilitated. Organ dysfunction due to iron overload results from the excessive amounts of iron in multiple PRBC transfusions. Regular chelation therapy (see Myelodysplastic Syndromes section in Chapter 34) can reduce the complications of iron overload and prolong the life of these patients. This disease is potentially curable by HSCT if the procedure can be performed before significant liver damage occurs (i.e., during childhood) (Higgs, Engel, & Stamatoyannopoulos, 2012). Death is often due to heart failure (Kremastinos, Farmakis, Aessopos, et al., 2010).

■ *Glucose-6-Phosphate Dehydrogenase Deficiency*

The G-6-PD gene is the source of the abnormality in this disorder; this gene produces an enzyme within the erythrocyte that is essential for membrane stability. A few patients have inherited an enzyme that is so defective that they have a chronic hemolytic anemia; however, the most common type of defect results in hemolysis only when the erythrocytes are stressed by certain situations, such as fever or the use of certain medications. African Americans and people of Greek or Italian origin are those primarily affected by this disorder. The type of deficiency found in the Mediterranean population is more severe than that in the African American population, resulting in greater hemolysis and sometimes in life-threatening anemia. All types of G-6-PD deficiency are inherited as X-linked defects; however, women may also develop the disease as one of the X chromosomes is inactivated in each cell of the female embryo. Thus, a female heterozygous for this deficiency would have half red cells normal for the enzyme and half deficient for it. Although those deficient cells are at risk for hemolysis, symptoms may be mild overall because the normal erythrocytes would not be subject to hemolysis. In the United States, about 12% of African American males are affected. The deficiency is also common in those of Asian ancestry and in certain Jewish populations (Van Solinge & van Wijk, 2010).

Oxidant drugs have hemolytic effects for people with G-6-PD deficiency, particularly the antibacterial agents nitrofurantoin (Macrodantin) and dapsone, the antimalarial agent primaquine, as well as other medications that include phenazopyridine (Pyridium), rasburicase, (Elitek), methylthioninium chloride (methylene blue), and tolonium chloride (toluidine blue). Other medications that may be tried, but whose effectiveness is questionable, include other antimalarial agents such as chloroquine (Aralen), the sulfonamide trimethoprim–sulfamethoxazole (Bactrim, Septra), other antibacterial drugs such as moxifloxacin (Avelox) and chloramphenicol (Chloromycetin), as well as other medications that include tamsulosin (Flomax), glyburide (DiaBeta, Micronase), furosemide (Lasix), NSAIDs, and the street drug amyl nitrite ("poppers") (Youngster, Arcavi, Schechmaster, et al., 2010). In affected people, a severe hemolytic episode can also result from ingestion of fava beans, menthol, tonic water, and some Chinese herbs such as *Coptis chinensis* (chuen lien), *Calculus bovis* (neu huang), and thorn roses (leh mei hua) (Chan, 1996).

Clinical Manifestations

Patients are asymptomatic and have normal hemoglobin levels and reticulocyte counts most of the time. However, several days after exposure to an offending medication, they may develop pallor, jaundice, and hemoglobinuria (i.e., hemoglobin in the urine). The reticulocyte count increases, and symptoms of hemolysis develop. Special stains of the peripheral blood may then disclose Heinz bodies (degraded hemoglobin) within the erythrocytes. Hemolysis is often mild and self-limited. However, in the more severe Mediterranean type of G-6-PD deficiency, spontaneous recovery may not occur.

Assessment and Diagnostic Findings

The diagnosis is made by a screening test for the deficiency or by a quantitative assay of G-6-PD.

Medical Management

The treatment is to arrest the source and stop the offending medication. Transfusion is necessary only in the severe hemolytic state, which is more commonly seen in the Mediterranean variety of G-6-PD deficiency.

Nursing Management

Patients are educated about the disease and given a list of medications and substances to avoid. If hemolysis develops, nursing interventions are the same as for hemolysis from other causes. Patients should be instructed to wear Medic-Alert bracelets that identify that they have G-6-PD deficiency. Genetic counseling may be indicated (see Chapter 8).

■ Immune Hemolytic Anemia

Hemolytic anemias can result from exposure of the erythrocyte to antibodies. Alloantibodies (i.e., antibodies against the host, or "self") result from the immunization of a person with foreign antigens (e.g., the immunization of an Rh-negative person with Rh-positive blood). Alloantibodies tend to be of the immunoglobulin G (IgG) type and cause immediate destruction of the sensitized erythrocytes, either within the blood vessel (intravascular hemolysis) or within the liver. An example of alloimmune hemolytic anemia in adults is anemia that results from a hemolytic transfusion reaction.

Autoantibodies may develop for many reasons. In many instances, the person's immune system is dysfunctional and falsely recognizes its own erythrocytes as foreign and produces antibodies against them. This mechanism is seen in people with chronic lymphocytic leukemia (CLL). Another mechanism is a deficiency in suppressor lymphocytes, which normally prevent antibody formation against a person's own antigens. The erythrocytes are sequestered in the spleen and destroyed by the macrophages outside the blood vessel (extravascular hemolysis).

Autoimmune hemolytic anemias can be classified based on the body temperature involved when the antibodies react with the RBC antigen. Warm-body antibodies are the most common (80%) and bind to erythrocytes most actively in warm conditions (37°C [98.6°F]); cold-body antibodies react in cold conditions (0°C [32°F]) (Packman, 2010). Autoimmune hemolytic anemia is associated with other disorders in most cases (e.g., medication exposure, lymphoma, CLL, other malignancy, collagen vascular disease, autoimmune disease, infection). In idiopathic autoimmune hemolytic states, the reason why the immune system produces the antibodies is not known. This primary form affects patients of all ages and both genders equally, whereas the incidence of secondary forms is greater in people older than 45 years and in females.

Clinical Manifestations

Clinical manifestations vary and usually reflect the degree of anemia. The hemolysis may range from very mild, in which the patient's marrow compensates adequately and the patient is asymptomatic, to so severe that the resultant anemia is life threatening. Most patients complain of fatigue and dizziness. Splenomegaly is the most common physical finding; hepatomegaly, lymphadenopathy, and jaundice are also common.

Assessment and Diagnostic Findings

Laboratory tests show a low hemoglobin level and hematocrit, most often with an accompanying increase in the reticulocyte count. Erythrocytes appear abnormal; **sphero-cytes** (small, spherically shaped erythrocytes) are common. The serum bilirubin level is elevated, and if the hemolysis is severe, the haptoglobin level is low or absent. The Coombs test (also referred to as the direct antiglobulin test), which detects antibodies on the surface of erythrocytes, shows a positive result.

Medical Management

Any possible contributing medication should be immediately discontinued. The treatment consists of high doses of corticosteroids until hemolysis decreases; this is particularly effective in treating warm-antibody–induced hemolytic anemia (Packman, 2010). Corticosteroids decrease the macrophage's ability to clear the antibody-coated erythrocytes. If the hemoglobin level returns toward normal, usually after several weeks, the corticosteroid dose can be lowered or, in some cases, tapered and discontinued. However, corticosteroids rarely produce a lasting remission. In severe cases, blood transfusions may be required. Because the antibody may react with all possible donor cells, careful blood typing is necessary, and the transfusion should be administered slowly and cautiously (Packman, 2010).

Splenectomy (i.e., removal of the spleen) may be performed if corticosteroids do not produce a remission, because it removes the major site of erythrocyte destruction. If neither corticosteroid therapy nor splenectomy is successful, immunosuppressive agents may be administered. The two immunosuppressive agents most frequently used are cyclophosphamide (Cytoxan), which has a more rapid effect but more toxicity, and azathioprine (Imuran), which has a less rapid effect but less toxicity. The synthetic androgen danazol (Danocrine) can be useful in some patients, particularly in combination with corticosteroids. If corticosteroids or immunosuppressive agents are used, the taper must be gradual to prevent a rebound "hyperimmune" response and exacerbation of the hemolysis. Monoclonal antibodies (e.g., rituximab [Rituxan]) can also be effective for some patients, although this is a non-FDA approved indication and the long-term efficacy is not well known (Lechner & Jäger, 2010). Immunoglobulin administration is effective in about one third of patients, but the effect is transient and the medication is expensive. Transfusions may be necessary if the anemia is severe; it may be extremely difficult to cross-match samples of available units of PRBCs with that of the patient.

▶ Quality and Safety Nursing Alert

Cross-matching blood when antibodies are present can be difficult. If imperfectly cross-matched RBCs must be transfused, the nurse should begin the infusion very slowly (10 to 15 mL over 20 to 30 minutes) and monitor the patient very closely for signs and symptoms of a hemolytic transfusion reaction.

For patients with cold-antibody hemolytic anemia, no treatment may be required other than to advise the patient to keep warm; relocation to a warm climate may be advisable. However, in other situations, the hemolysis may warrant more aggressive interventions as described previously.

Nursing Management

Patients may have great difficulty understanding the pathologic mechanisms underlying the disease and may need repeated explanations in terms they can understand. Patients who have had a splenectomy should be vaccinated against pneumococcal infections (e.g., with Pneumovax) and informed that they are permanently at greater risk for infection. Patients receiving long-term corticosteroid therapy, particularly those with concurrent diabetes or hypertension, need careful monitoring. They must understand the need for the medication and the importance of never abruptly discontinuing it. A written explanation and a tapering schedule should be provided, and adjustments based on hemoglobin levels should be emphasized. Similar education should be provided when immunosuppressive agents are used. Corticosteroid therapy is not without significant risk, and patients need to be monitored closely for complications (see Table 52-5: Corticosteroid therapy and implications for nursing practice).

■ *Hereditary Hemochromatosis*

Hemochromatosis is a genetic condition in which excess iron is absorbed from the GI tract. Normally, the GI tract absorbs 1 to 2 mg of iron daily, but in those with hereditary hemochromatosis, this rate increases significantly. The excess iron is deposited in various organs, particularly the liver, myocardium, testes, thyroid, and pancreas. Eventually, the affected organs become dysfunctional. Although hereditary hemochromatosis is diagnosed in 0.5% of the population in the United States (i.e., more than 1 million people), the actual prevalence is unknown because it is not always diagnosed (Friedman, 2012). The genetic defect associated with hemochromatosis is most commonly seen as a specific mutation (C282Y homozygosity) of the *HFE* gene. Despite the high prevalence of the genetic mutation, the actual expression of the disease is much lower; the reason for this discrepancy is unclear. The actual prevalence of hemochromatosis is lower among Asian Americans, African Americans, Latinos, and Pacific Islanders and higher in people of European descent (Friedman, 2012). Women are less often affected than men because women lose iron through menses.

Clinical Manifestations

Often there is no evidence of tissue damage until middle age, because the accumulation of iron in body organs occurs gradually. Symptoms of weakness, lethargy, arthralgia, weight loss, and loss of libido are common and occur earlier in the illness trajectory. The skin may appear hyperpigmented from melanin deposits (and occasionally **hemosiderin**, an iron-containing pigment) or appear bronze in color. Cardiac dysrhythmias and cardiomyopathy can occur, with resulting dyspnea and edema. Endocrine dysfunction is manifested as hypothyroidism, diabetes, and hypogonadism (testicular atrophy, diminished libido, and impotence). Cirrhosis is common in later stages of the disease, shortens life expectancy, and is a risk factor for hepatocellular carcinoma (Villanueva, Newell, & Hoshida, 2010).

Assessment and Diagnostic Findings

Diagnostic laboratory findings include an elevated serum iron level and high transferrin saturation (more than 60% in men, more than 50% in women). CBC values are typically normal. The definitive diagnostic test for hemochromatosis was formerly the liver biopsy, but testing for the associated genetic mutation (i.e., C282Y homozygosity) is now more commonly used. While not all individuals with this genetic mutation will develop severe consequences of iron overload, 60% to 80% of these individuals will develop abnormal iron tests during their lifetime (Allen, 2010).

Medical Management

Therapy involves the removal of excess iron via therapeutic phlebotomy (removal of whole blood from a vein). Each unit of blood removed results in a decrease of 200 to 250 mg of iron. The objective is to reduce the serum ferritin to less than 50 mcg/L and the transferrin saturation to 50% or less (Friedman, 2012). To achieve this, frequent phlebotomy is required, at 1 to 2 units weekly initially. Phlebotomy is then necessary only every 1 to 4 months until the serum ferritin levels are maintained at 50 mcg/L. After 1 to 3 years, the frequency of phlebotomy can often be further reduced to prevent reaccumulation of iron deposits. The goal is to maintain an iron saturation of less than 50% and a serum ferritin of less than 100 mcg/L. Aggressive removal of excess iron can prevent end-organ dysfunction, particularly liver cirrhosis and its complications (e.g., ascites, hemorrhage, hepatocellular carcinoma) (Allen, 2010).

Nursing Management

Patients with hemochromatosis often limit their dietary intake of iron, although this is not effective; however, they should be advised to refrain from taking any additional iron supplements. In addition, vitamin C intake should be limited because it enhances iron absorption (Allen, 2010). These patients must avoid any additional insults to the liver, such as alcohol abuse. Serial screening tests for hepatoma (e.g., through monitoring alpha-fetoprotein) are important. Other body systems should be monitored for signs of organ dysfunction, particularly the endocrine and cardiac systems, so that appropriate management can be implemented quickly (Sheahan & O'Connell, 2009). Because patients with hemochromatosis require frequent phlebotomies, problems with venous access are common. Children of patients who are homozygous for the *HFE* gene mutation should be screened for the mutation as well. Patients who are heterozygous for the *HFE* gene do not develop the disease but need to be advised that they can transmit the gene to their children.

POLYCYTHEMIA

Polycythemia refers to an increased volume of RBCs. The term is used when the hematocrit is elevated (more than 55% in males, more than 50% in females). Dehydration (decreased volume of plasma) can cause an elevated hematocrit but not typically to the level to be considered polycythemia. Polycythemia is classified as either primary or secondary. Primary polycythemia, also called *polycythemia vera*, is a clonal disorder that is discussed in Chapter 34.

Secondary Polycythemia

Secondary polycythemia is caused by excessive production of erythropoietin. This may occur in response to a reduced amount of oxygen, which acts as a hypoxic stimulus, as in heavy cigarette smoking, chronic obstructive pulmonary disease (COPD), or cyanotic heart disease, or in nonpathologic conditions such as living at a high altitude. It can also result from certain hemoglobinopathies (e.g., hemoglobin Chesapeake), in which the hemoglobin has an abnormally high affinity for oxygen or from genetic mutations (e.g., von Hippel-Lindau) that cause abnormally high erythropoietin levels and thus increased erythropoiesis (Patnaik & Tefferi, 2009). Secondary polycythemia can also occur from neoplasms (e.g., renal cell carcinoma) that stimulate erythropoietin production.

Medical Management

When secondary polycythemia is mild, treatment may not be necessary; when treatment is necessary, it involves treating the primary condition. If the cause cannot be corrected (e.g., by treating the COPD or improving pulmonary function with smoking cessation), therapeutic phlebotomy may be necessary in symptomatic patients to reduce blood viscosity and volume as well as when the hematocrit is significantly elevated.

NEUTROPENIA

Neutropenia (a neutrophil count of less than 2,000/mm³) results from decreased production of neutrophils or increased destruction of these cells (Chart 33-5). Neutrophils are essential in preventing and limiting bacterial infection. A patient with neutropenia is at increased risk for infection from both exogenous and endogenous sources. (The GI tract and skin are common endogenous sources.) The risk of infection is based not only on the severity of the neutropenia but also

---

Chart 33-5 Causes of Neutropenia

Decreased Production of Neutrophils

- Aplastic anemia, due to medications or toxins
- Metastatic cancer, lymphoma, leukemia
- Myelodysplastic syndromes
- Chemotherapy
- Radiation therapy

Ineffective Granulocytopoiesis

- Megaloblastic anemia

Increased Destruction of Neutrophils

- Hypersplenism
- Medication induced*
- Immunologic disorders (e.g., systemic lupus erythematosus)
- Viral disease (e.g., infectious hepatitis, mononucleosis)
- Bacterial infections

*Formation of antibody to medication, leading to a rapid decrease in neutrophils.

Chart 33-6

RISK FACTORS

Development of Infection and Bleeding in Patients With Hematologic Disorders

Risk of Infection

- *Severity of neutropenia:* Risk of infection is proportional to severity of neutropenia.
- *Duration of neutropenia:* Increased duration leads to increased risk of infection.
- *Nutritional status:* Decreased protein stores lead to decreased immune response and anergy.
- *Deconditioning:* Decreased mobility leads to decreased respiratory effort, leading to increased pooling of secretions.
- *Lymphocytopenia; disorders of lymphoid system (chronic lymphocytic leukemia, lymphoma, myeloma):* Decreased cell-mediated and humoral immunity
- *Invasive procedures:* Break in skin integrity leads to increased opportunity for organisms to enter blood system.
- *Hypogammaglobulinemia:* Decreased antibody formation
- *Poor hygiene:* Increased organisms on skin and mucous membranes, including perineum
- *Poor dentition; mucositis:* Decreased endothelial integrity leads to increased opportunity for organisms to enter blood system.
- *Antibiotic therapy:* Increased risk for superinfection, often fungal
- *Certain medications:* See text.

Risk of Bleeding

- *Severity of thrombocytopenia:* Risk increases when platelet count decreases; usually not a significant risk until platelet count is <10,000/mm^3, or <50,000/mm^3 when invasive procedure is performed.
- *Duration of thrombocytopenia:* Risk increases when duration increases (e.g., risk is less when duration is transient after chemotherapy than when duration is permanent with poor marrow production).
- *Sepsis:* Mechanism unknown; appears to cause increased platelet consumption.
- *Increased intracranial pressure:* Increased blood pressure leads to rupture of blood vessels.
- *Liver dysfunction:* Decreased synthesis of clotting factors
- *Renal dysfunction:* Decreased platelet function
- *Dysproteinemia:* Protein coats surface of platelet, leading to decreased platelet function; protein causes increased viscosity, which leads to increased stretching of capillaries and thus increased bleeding.
- *Alcohol abuse:* Suppressive effect on marrow leads to decreased platelet production and decreased ability to function; decreased liver function results in decreased production of clotting factors.
- *Splenomegaly:* Increased platelet destruction; spleen traps circulating platelets
- *Concurrent medications:* See text.

---

on its duration. The actual number of neutrophils, known as the **absolute neutrophil count** (ANC), is determined by a simple mathematical calculation using data obtained from the CBC and differential (see Chapter 15). The risk of infection increases proportionately with the decrease in neutrophil count. The risk is significant when the ANC is less than 1,000/mm^3, is high when it is less than 500/mm^3, and is almost certain when it is less than 100/mm^3 (Dale, 2010). The risk of developing infection also increases with the length of time during which neutropenia persists, even if it is somewhat mild. Conversely, even a severe neutropenia may not result in infection if the duration of the neutropenia is brief, as is often seen after chemotherapy (Chart 33-6).

Clinical Manifestations

There are no definite symptoms of neutropenia until the patient develops an infection. A routine CBC with differential, as obtained after chemotherapy treatment, can reveal neutropenia before the onset of infection.

 Quality and Safety Nursing Alert

Patients with neutropenia often do not exhibit classic signs of infection. Fever is the most common indicator of infection, yet it is not always present, particularly if the patient is taking corticosteroids.

Medical Management

Treatment of the neutropenia varies depending on its cause. If the neutropenia is medication induced, the offending agent is stopped immediately, if possible. Treatment of an underlying neoplasm can temporarily make the neutropenia worse, but with bone marrow recovery, treatment may actually improve it. Corticosteroids may be used if the cause is an immunologic disorder. The use of growth factors such as granulocyte colony-stimulating factor or granulocyte-macrophage colony-stimulating factor can be effective in increasing neutrophil production when the cause of the neutropenia is decreased production. Withholding or reducing the dose of chemotherapy or radiation therapy may be required when the neutropenia is caused by these treatments; however, in the case of potentially curative therapy, administration of growth factor is considered to be preferable so that the maximum antitumor effect can be achieved by maintaining the chemotherapy regimen as originally planned (Miller, 2010).

If the neutropenia is accompanied by fever, the patient is considered to have an infection and usually is admitted to the hospital. Cultures of blood, urine, and sputum, as well as a chest x-ray, are obtained. To ensure adequate therapy against the infectious organisms, broad-spectrum antibiotics are initiated as soon as the cultures are obtained, although the antibiotics may be changed after culture and sensitivity results are available.

Nursing Management

Nurses in all settings have a crucial role in assessing the severity of neutropenia and in preventing and managing complications, which most often include infections. Patient education is equally important, particularly in the outpatient setting, so that the patient can implement appropriate self-care measures and know when and how to seek medical care (Chart 33-7).

Chart 33-7

HOME CARE CHECKLIST
The Patient at Risk for Infection

At the completion of home care education, the patient or caregiver will be able to:	PATIENT	CAREGIVER
• Describe consequences of alterations in neutrophils, lymphocytes, immunoglobulins, or their sources.	✔	✔
• Verbalize the reason for being at risk for infection.	✔	✔
• Identify signs and symptoms of infection.	✔	✔
• Demonstrate how to monitor for signs of infection.	✔	✔
• Describe to whom, how, and when to report signs of infection.	✔	✔
• Identify appropriate behaviors to take to prevent infection. • Maintain good hand hygiene technique, total body hygiene, and skin integrity. • Avoid cleaning birdcages and litter boxes; consider avoiding garden work (soil), fresh flowers in stagnant water. • Maintain a high-calorie, high-protein diet, with fluid intake of 3,000 mL daily (unless fluids are restricted). • Avoid people with infections and crowds. • Perform deep breathing; use incentive spirometer every 4 hour while awake if mobility is restricted. • Provide adequate lubrication with gentle vaginal manipulation during sexual intercourse; avoid anal intercourse.	✔	
• Describe appropriate actions to take should infection occur.	✔	✔

Patients at risk for neutropenia should have blood drawn for a CBC with differential; the frequency is based on the suspected severity and duration of the neutropenia. To assess the severity of neutropenia and the risk of infection, nurses must assess patients' ANC (see Chapter 15 for formula). Nursing interventions related to neutropenia are delineated in Chapter 34.

LYMPHOPENIA

Lymphopenia (a lymphocyte count less than 1,500/mm^3) can result from ionizing radiation, long-term use of corticosteroids, uremia, infections (particularly viral infections), some neoplasms (e.g., breast and lung cancers, advanced Hodgkin disease), and some protein-losing enteropathies (in which the lymphocytes within the intestines are lost) (Kipps, 2010). When lymphopenia is mild, it is often without sequelae; when severe, it can result in bacterial infections (due to low B lymphocytes) or in opportunistic infections (due to low T lymphocytes).

BLEEDING DISORDERS

Failure of normal hemostatic mechanisms can result in bleeding, which may be severe. This bleeding is commonly provoked by trauma; however, in certain circumstances, it can occur spontaneously. When the source is platelet or coagulation factor abnormalities, the site of bleeding can be anywhere in the body. When the source is vascular abnormalities, the site of bleeding may be more localized. Some patients have simultaneous defects in more than one hemostatic mechanism.

The bone marrow may be stimulated to increase platelet production (thrombopoiesis). This may be a reactive response, as in a compensatory response to significant bleeding, or a more general response to increased hematopoiesis,

as in iron deficiency anemia. Sometimes, the increase in platelets does not result from increased production but from a loss in platelet pooling within the spleen. The spleen typically holds about one third of the circulating platelets at any time. If the spleen is absent (e.g., splenectomy), the platelet reservoir is also lost, and an abnormally high number of platelets enters the circulation. In time, the rate of thrombopoiesis slows to reestablish a more normal platelet level.

Clinical Manifestations

Signs and symptoms of bleeding disorders vary according to the type of defect. A careful history and physical examination can be useful in determining the source of the hemostatic defect. Abnormalities of the vascular system give rise to local bleeding, usually into the skin. Because platelets are primarily responsible for stopping bleeding from small vessels, patients with platelet defects develop **petechiae**, often in clusters; these are seen on the skin and mucous membranes but also occur throughout the body (Fig. 33-4). Bleeding from platelet disorders can be severe. Unless the platelet disorder is severe, bleeding can often be stopped promptly when local pressure is applied; it does not typically recur when the pressure is released.

In contrast, coagulation factor defects do not tend to cause superficial bleeding, because the primary hemostatic mechanisms are still intact. Instead, bleeding occurs deeper within the body (e.g., subcutaneous or intramuscular hematomas, hemorrhage into joint spaces). External bleeding diminishes very slowly when local pressure is applied; it often recurs several hours after pressure is removed. For example, severe bleeding may start several hours after a tooth extraction. Risk factors for bleeding are listed in Chart 33-6.

Medical Management

Management varies based on the underlying cause of the bleeding disorder. If bleeding is significant, transfusions of

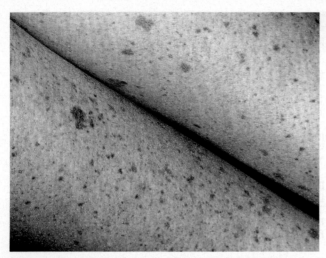

FIGURE 33-4 • Petechiae in a patient with idiopathic thrombocytopenic purpura. From Craft, N., Fox, L. P., Goldsmith, L. A., et al. (2011). *VisualDx: Essential adult dermatology.* Philadelphia: Lippincott Williams & Wilkins.

blood products are indicated. The specific blood product used is determined by the underlying defect and the extent of the blood loss. If fibrinolysis is excessive, hemostatic agents such as aminocaproic acid (Amicar) can be used to inhibit this process. This agent must be used with caution, because excessive inhibition of fibrinolysis can result in thrombosis. A patient scheduled for an invasive procedure, including a dental extraction, may need a transfusion prior to the procedure to minimize the risk of excessive bleeding.

Nursing Management

Patients who have bleeding disorders or who have the potential for development of such disorders as a result of disease or therapeutic agents must be educated to observe themselves carefully and frequently for signs of bleeding (Chart 33-8). They need to understand the importance of avoiding activities that increase the risk of bleeding, such as contact sports. It is necessary to examine the skin for petechiae and ecchymoses (bruises) and the nose and gums for bleeding.

Hospitalized patients are monitored for bleeding by testing all drainage and excreta (feces, urine, emesis, and gastric drainage) for occult blood as well as obvious blood. Outpatients are often given fecal occult blood screening cards to detect occult blood in stools.

Secondary Thrombocytosis

Increased platelet production is the primary mechanism of secondary, or reactive, **thrombocytosis**. The platelet count is above normal, but, in contrast to essential thrombocythemia (see Chapter 34), an increase of more than 1 million/mm^3 is rare. Platelet function is normal; the platelet survival time is normal or decreased. Consequently, symptoms associated with hemorrhage or thrombosis are rare (Kaushansky, 2010). Many disorders or conditions can cause a reactive increase in platelets, including infection, chronic inflammatory disorders, iron deficiency, malignant disease, acute hemorrhage, and splenectomy. Treatment is aimed at the underlying disorder. With successful management, the platelet count usually returns to normal.

Thrombocytopenia

Thrombocytopenia (low platelet level) can result from various factors: decreased production of platelets within the bone marrow, increased destruction of platelets, or increased consumption of platelets (e.g., the use of platelets in clot formation). Causes and treatments are summarized in Table 33-3.

Clinical Manifestations

Bleeding and petechiae usually do not occur with platelet counts greater than 50,000/mm^3, although excessive bleeding can follow surgery or other trauma. When the platelet count drops to less than 20,000/mm^3, petechiae can appear, along with nasal and gingival bleeding, excessive menstrual bleeding, and excessive bleeding after surgery or dental extractions. When the platelet count is less than 5,000/mm^3,

Chart 33-8	**HOME CARE CHECKLIST** The Patient at Risk for Bleeding		
At the completion of home care education, the patient or caregiver will be able to:		**PATIENT**	**CAREGIVER**
• Describe the source and function of platelets and clotting factors.		✔	✔
• Verbalize the rationale for being at risk for bleeding.		✔	✔
• Identify medications and other substances to avoid (e.g., aspirin-containing medications, alcohol).		✔	✔
• Demonstrate how to monitor for signs of bleeding.		✔	✔
• Describe to whom, how, and when to report signs of bleeding.		✔	✔
• Notify health care professional before having dental work or other invasive procedures.		✔	✔
• Describe appropriate ways to prevent bleeding (avoid the use of suppositories, enemas, tampons; avoid constipation, vigorous sexual intercourse, anal sex; avoid contact sports; avoid or limit aggressive manual labor; use only electric razor for shaving and a soft-bristled toothbrush for teeth brushing).		✔	✔
• Demonstrate appropriate actions to take should bleeding occur.		✔	✔

TABLE 33-3   Causes and Management of Thrombocytopenia

Cause	Management
Decreased Platelet Production	
Hematologic malignancy, especially acute leukemias	Treat leukemia; platelet transfusion.
MDS	Treat MDS; platelet transfusion.
Metastatic involvement of bone marrow from solid tumors	Treat solid tumor.
Aplastic anemia	Treat underlying condition.
Megaloblastic anemia	Treat underlying anemia.
Toxins	Remove toxin.
Medications (e.g., sulfa drugs, methotrexate)	Stop medication.
Infection (especially septicemia, viral infection, tuberculosis, chronic hepatitis C)	Treat infection.
Chronic alcohol abuse	Refrain from alcohol consumption.
Chemotherapy	Delay or decrease dose; platelet transfusion.
Chronic liver disease	Treat underlying disease.
Radiation (e.g., pelvic irradiation)	Platelet transfusion
Delayed engraftment after stem cell transplantation	Platelet transfusion
Increased Platelet Destruction	
Due to antibodies:	Treat condition.
ITP	
Lupus erythematosus	
Malignant lymphoma	
CLL	Treat CLL and/or treat as ITP.
Medications	Stop medication.
Due to infection:	Treat infection.
Bacteremia/sepsis	
Postviral infection	
Sequestration of platelets in an enlarged spleen	If thrombocytopenia is severe, splenectomy may be needed.
Increased Platelet Consumption	
DIC	Treat underlying condition triggering DIC; administer heparin, aminocaproic acid (EACA), blood products
Major bleeding	Transfusion support, surgery if appropriate
Severe pulmonary embolism/severe thrombosis	Treat clot.
Intravascular devices (intra-aortic balloon pump, cardiac assist devices)	Transfusion support as needed
Extracorporeal circulation (hemofiltration, extracorporeal lung assist)	Transfusion support as needed

MDS, myelodysplastic syndrome; ITP, idiopathic thrombocytopenic purpura; CLL, chronic lymphocytic leukemia; DIC, disseminated intravascular coagulation.

spontaneous, potentially fatal central nervous system or GI hemorrhage can occur. If the platelets are dysfunctional as a result of disease (e.g., MDS) or medications (e.g., aspirin), the risk of bleeding may be much greater even when the actual platelet count is not significantly reduced, because the function of the platelets is altered.

Assessment and Diagnostic Findings

A platelet deficiency that results from decreased production (e.g., leukemia, MDS) can usually be diagnosed by examining the bone marrow via aspiration and biopsy. Numerous genetic causes of thrombocytopenia have been discovered, including autosomal dominant, autosomal recessive, and X-linked mutations. If platelet destruction is the cause of thrombocytopenia, the marrow shows increased megakaryocytes and normal or even increased platelet production as the body attempts to compensate for the decreased platelets in circulation. Hepatitis B or C can cause thrombocytopenia; thus, the patient should be screened for these diseases.

An important cause to exclude is pseudothrombocytopenia. Here, platelets aggregate and clump in the presence of ethylenediaminetetraacetic acid (EDTA), the anticoagulant present in the tube used for CBC collection. This clumping is seen in 0.8% of the population (Froom & Barak, 2011). A manual examination of the peripheral smear can easily determine platelet clumping as the cause of thrombocytopenia; newer cell counter machines can also detect this.

Medical Management

The management of secondary thrombocytopenia is usually treatment of the underlying disease. If platelet production is impaired, platelet transfusions may increase the platelet count and stop bleeding or prevent spontaneous hemorrhage. If excessive platelet destruction occurs, transfused platelets are also destroyed, and the platelet count does not increase. The most common cause of excessive platelet destruction is immune thrombocytopenic purpura (ITP) (see the following discussion). In some instances, splenectomy can be a useful therapeutic intervention, but often it is not an option. For example, in patients in whom the enlarged spleen is due to portal hypertension related to cirrhosis, splenectomy may cause more bleeding disorders.

Nursing Management

When selecting nursing interventions for a particular patient, the nurse considers the cause of the thrombocytopenia, the likely duration of it, and the overall condition of the patient. Education is important, as are interventions to promote patient safety, particularly fall prevention in the older adult or patient who is frail. The interventions for a patient with thrombocytopenia are the same as those for a patient with cancer who is at risk for bleeding (see Chart 15-7 in Chapter 15).

Immune Thrombocytopenic Purpura

ITP is a disease that affects people of all ages, but it is more common among children and young women. Other names for the disorder are idiopathic thrombocytopenic purpura and immune thrombocytopenia. Primary ITP occurs in isolation; secondary ITP often results from autoimmune diseases (e.g., antiphospholipid antibody syndrome, viral infections, human immunodeficiency virus [HIV] infections, and various drugs). Primary ITP is defined as a platelet count less than 100×10^9/L with an inexplicable absence of a cause for thrombocytopenia (Rodeghiero, Stasi, Gernsheimer, et al., 2009).

Pathophysiology

ITP is an autoimmune disorder characterized by a destruction of normal platelets by an unknown stimulus (Neunert, Lim, Crowther, et al., 2011). Antiplatelet antibodies develop in the blood and bind to the patient's platelets. These antibody-bound platelets are then ingested and destroyed by the reticuloendothelial system (RES) or tissue macrophages. The body attempts to compensate for this destruction by increasing platelet production within the marrow. This compensatory mechanism may not be effective as thrombopoietin levels are not elevated in patients with ITP, and as such, platelet production may be diminished.

As stated previously, viral illness (e.g., hepatitis) may lead to ITP. Medications (e.g., sulfa drugs), as well as diseases such as systemic lupus erythematosus or conditions such as pregnancy, can also induce ITP.

Clinical Manifestations

Many patients have no symptoms, and the low platelet count is an incidental finding (often less than 30,000/mm³; less than 5,000/mm³ is not uncommon). Common physical manifestations are easy bruising, heavy menses, and petechiae on the extremities or trunk (see Fig. 33-4). Patients with simple bruising or petechiae ("dry purpura") tend to have fewer complications from bleeding than those with bleeding from mucosal surfaces, such as the GI tract (including the mouth) and pulmonary system (e.g., hemoptysis), which is termed *wet purpura*. Patients with wet purpura have a greater risk of intracranial bleeding than do those with dry purpura. Despite low platelet counts, the platelets are young and very functional. They adhere to endothelial surfaces and to one another, so spontaneous bleeding does not always occur. Thus, treatment may not be initiated unless bleeding becomes severe or life threatening, or the platelet count is extremely low (less than 30,000/mm³) (Wong & Rose, 2012).

Assessment and Diagnostic Findings

A careful history and physical assessment must be obtained to exclude causes of the thrombocytopenia and identify evidence of bleeding. Patients should be tested for hepatitis C and HIV, if not previously done to rule out these potential causes. If a bone marrow aspirate is performed, an increase in megakaryocytes may be seen. The severity of the thrombo-

cytopenia is highly variable, but a platelet count that is less than 20,000/mm³ is a common finding. Some patients are found to be infected with *Helicobacter pylori,* and eradicating the infection may improve platelet counts (Franchini, Vescovi, Garofano, et al., 2012). It is unclear why *H. pylori* and ITP are correlated, but possible causes are that *H. pylori* may trigger an autoimmune reaction or that it binds to von Willebrand factor (vWF), both of which may result in accelerated platelet demise.

Medical Management

The primary goal of treatment is a "safe" platelet count (i.e., platelets adequate to maintain hemostasis). Because the risk of bleeding typically does not increase until the platelet count is less than 30,000/mm³, a patient whose count exceeds 30,000/mm³ to 50,000/mm³ may be carefully observed without additional intervention. However, if the count is less than 30,000/mm³ or if bleeding occurs, the goal is to improve the patient's platelet count rather than to cure the disease. The decision to treat should not be made merely on the basis of the patient's platelet count but, more importantly, on the severity of bleeding (if any), likely treatment-related side effects, and the patient's lifestyle, activity level, and overall preference. A person with a sedentary lifestyle can tolerate a low platelet count more safely than one with a more active lifestyle; however, increasing age is also associated with increased bleeding risk (Fogarty, 2009).

Treatment for ITP usually involves several approaches. If the patient is taking a medication known to be associated with ITP (e.g., quinine, sulfa-containing medications), then that medication must be stopped immediately. The mainstay of short-term therapy is the use of immunosuppressive agents. These agents block the binding receptors on macrophages so that the platelets are not destroyed. The American Society of Hematology recommends administering the corticosteroid prednisone at a dose of 1 mg per kilogram of body weight for 21 days and then tapering the dose until the patient is off the medication (Neunert et al., 2011). Because of the associated side effects, patients cannot take high doses of corticosteroids indefinitely. Platelet counts typically begin to rise within a few days after institution of corticosteroid therapy. The platelet count tends to drop once the corticosteroid dose is tapered, but it often can remain at an adequate level. The immunosuppressant azathioprine (Imuran) may also be indicated, particularly when some form of "maintenance" therapy is needed to maintain the platelet count. The rise in platelet counts is slower with azathioprine (Provan, Stasi, Newland, et al., 2010).

IVIG is also commonly used to treat ITP. It is effective in binding the receptors on the macrophages; however, high doses are required, the drug is very expensive, and the effect is transient. Splenectomy is an alternative treatment and results in a sustained normal platelet count approximately 50% of the time, although many patients can maintain a "safe" platelet count of more than 30,000/mm³ after removal of the spleen. Even those who do respond to splenectomy may have recurrences of severe thrombocytopenia months or years later. Patients who have undergone splenectomy are permanently at risk for sepsis and should receive pneumococcal (Pneumovax), *Haemophilus influenzae* type B, and meningococcal vaccines, preferably 2 to 3 weeks before the splenectomy is performed. The pneumococcal vaccine should be repeated at intervals of 5 to 10 years.

Other management options include certain monoclonal antibodies (e.g., rituximab). This agent may increase platelet counts for up to 1 year in 20% to 35% of those treated, but when that response is lost, the platelet count may not fall so low as to warrant additional therapy.

Infrequently, the chemotherapy agent vincristine (Oncovin) is used. Vincristine appears to work by blocking the receptors on the macrophages and therefore inhibiting platelet destruction; it may also stimulate thrombopoiesis.

Another approach to the management of chronic ITP involves the use of anti-D (WinRho) in patients who are Rh (D) positive. The actual mechanism of action is unknown. One theory is that the anti-D binds to the patient's erythrocytes, which are in turn destroyed by the body's macrophages. The receptors in the RES may become saturated with the sensitized erythrocytes, diminishing removal of antibody-coated platelets. Anti-D produces a transient decreased hematocrit and increased platelet count in many, but not all, patients with ITP. Anti-D appears to be most effective in children with ITP and least effective in patients who have undergone splenectomy.

In addition, two thrombopoietin receptor agonists have been approved for use in steroid-refractory ITP. Romiplostim (Nplate) is administered weekly as a subcutaneous injection; eltrombopag (Promacta) is given orally. The timing of taking eltrombopag is somewhat complex, as the drug metabolism is altered with food and many medications. Side effects include headache, blistering of the oral mucosa, and ecchymoses. If either of these drugs is tapered, a rebound thrombocytopenia can occur; thus, careful monitoring and plans to resume or start alternative therapy should be established (Provan et al., 2010).

Despite extremely low platelet counts, platelet transfusions are usually avoided. Transfusions tend to be ineffective because the patient's antiplatelet antibodies bind with the transfused platelets, causing them to be destroyed. Platelet counts can actually drop further after platelet transfusion. Occasionally, transfusion of platelets may protect against catastrophic bleeding in patients with severe wet purpura. Aminocaproic acid—a fibrinolytic enzyme inhibitor that slows the dissolution of clots—may be useful for patients with significant mucosal bleeding refractory to other treatments.

Nursing Management

Nursing care includes an assessment of the patient's lifestyle to determine the risk of bleeding from activity. A careful medication history is also obtained, including use of over-the-counter medications, herbs, and nutritional supplements. The nurse must be alert for sulfa-containing medications and others that alter platelet function (e.g., aspirin-based or other NSAIDs). The nurse assesses for any history of recent viral illness and reports of headache or visual disturbances, which could be initial symptoms of intracranial bleeding. Patients who are admitted to the hospital with wet purpura and low platelet counts should have a neurologic assessment incorporated into their routine vital sign measurements. All

injections or rectal medications should be avoided, and rectal temperature measurements should not be performed, because they can stimulate bleeding.

Studies of patients with ITP have demonstrated a significant increase in fatigue compared to those without the disease (Newton, Reese, Watson, et al., 2011) that was not associated with the duration of the disease, corticosteroid use, bleeding episodes, and low platelet count. Nurses should explore the extent the patient experiences fatigue and offer strategies to ameliorate this problem.

Patient education addresses signs of exacerbation of disease (e.g., petechiae, ecchymoses), how to contact appropriate health care personnel, the name and type of medication inducing ITP (if appropriate), current medical treatment (medications, side effects, tapering schedule if relevant), and the frequency of monitoring the platelet count. The patient is instructed to avoid all agents that interfere with platelet function, including herbal therapies and over-the-counter medications. The patient should avoid constipation, the Valsalva maneuver (e.g., straining at stool), and vigorous flossing of the teeth. Electric razors should be used for shaving, and soft-bristled toothbrushes should replace stiff-bristled ones. The patient may also be counseled to refrain from vigorous sexual intercourse when the platelet count is less than $10,000/mm^3$. Patients who are receiving corticosteroids long term are at risk for complications including osteoporosis, proximal muscle wasting, cataract formation, and dental caries (see Table 52-5). Bone mineral density should be monitored, and these patients may benefit from calcium and vitamin D supplementation and bisphosphonate therapy to prevent significant bone disease.

Platelet Defects

Quantitative platelet defects (i.e., thrombocytopenia, thrombocytosis) are relatively common; however, qualitative defects can also occur. With qualitative defects, the number of platelets may be normal but the platelets do not function normally. In the past, the bleeding time was most commonly used to evaluate platelet function. Now, a platelet function analyzer is often used; this method is particularly valuable for rapid and simple screening. Examining the platelet morphology (via peripheral smear evaluation) can also be useful in assessing potential qualitative defects. In this situation, platelets are often hypogranular and pale, and may be larger than normal.

Aspirin may induce a platelet disorder. Even small amounts of aspirin reduce normal platelet aggregation, and the prolonged bleeding time lasts for several days after aspirin ingestion. Although this does not cause bleeding in most people, patients with a coagulation disorder (e.g., hemophilia) or thrombocytopenia can have significant bleeding after taking aspirin, particularly if invasive procedures or trauma have occurred.

NSAIDs can also inhibit platelet function, but the effect is not as prolonged as with aspirin (about 4 days vs. 7 to 10 days). Other causes of platelet dysfunction include end-stage renal disease, possibly from metabolic products affecting platelet function; MDS; multiple myeloma (due to abnormal

Chart 33-9

PHARMACOLOGY

Medications and Substances That Impair Platelet Function

Anesthetic Agents

Cocaine
Halothane (Fluothane)
Local anesthetic agents

Antibiotics

Aminoglycosides
Beta-lactam antibiotics
  Penicillins
  Cephalosporins
Nitrofurantoin
Sulfonamides

Anticoagulation and Antiplatelet Agents

Antithrombin agents
Dipyridamole (Persantine)
Fibrinolytic agents
Heparin
  Unfractionated heparin
  Low-molecular-weight heparins
Ticlopidine (Ticlid)

Anti-Inflammatory Agents (Nonsteroidal)

Aspirin
Colchicine (Colcrys)
Ibuprofen (Advil, Motrin)
Indomethacin (Indocin)
Naproxen (Aleve)

Antineoplastic Agents

Carmustine (BCNU)
Daunorubicin (Cerubidine)
Mithramycin (Mithracin)
Vinblastine (Velban)
Vincristine (Oncovin)

Cardiovascular/Respiratory Drugs

Angiotensin-converting enzyme inhibitors
Angiotensin receptor blockers
Beta-blockers
Calcium channel blockers
Clofibrate (Atromid-S)
Diuretics
  Ethacrynic acid (Edecrin)
  Furosemide (Lasix)

Hydralazine (Apresoline)
Methylxanthines
  Aminophylline
  Theophylline (Theo-Dur)
Nitrates
  Isosorbide (Isordil)
Phentolamine (Regitine)
Prostacyclin
Quinidine

Food and Food Additives

Caffeine
Chinese black tree fungus
Clove
Cumin
Ethanol (i.e., alcohol)
Fish oils
Garlic
Ginger
Onion extract
Turmeric

Plasma Expanders

Dextrans
Hydroxyethyl starch (HES)

Psychotropic Agents

Phenothiazines
Tricyclic antidepressants
  Doxepin (Sinequan)
  Imipramine (Tofranil)

Miscellaneous

Antihistamines
Contrast agents
Glyceryl guaiacolate (cough syrup base)
Heroin
Hydroxychloroquine (Plaquenil; Quineprox)
Vitamin E

Herbal Supplements

Feverfew
Gingko
Ginseng
Kava kava

---

protein interfering with platelet function); cardiopulmonary bypass; herbal therapy; and other medications (Chart 33-9).

Clinical Manifestations

Bleeding may be mild or severe. Its extent is not necessarily correlated with the platelet count or with tests that measure coagulation (prothrombin time [PT], activated partial thromboplastin time [aPTT]). However, if results from one of these tests are abnormal and the results from the other two are normal, that may help determine the specific etiology of the bleeding disorder (Kaushansky, 2010; Seligsohn, 2012). For example, an elevated PT in the setting of a normal aPTT

and platelet count may suggest factor VII deficiency, whereas an elevated partial thromboplastin time (PTT) in the setting of a normal PT and platelet count may suggest hemophilia or von Willebrand disease (vWD). Ecchymoses are common, particularly on the extremities. Patients with platelet dysfunction may be at risk for significant bleeding after trauma or invasive procedures (e.g., biopsy, dental extraction).

Medical Management

If the platelet dysfunction is caused by medication, its use should be stopped, if possible, particularly when bleeding occurs. If platelet dysfunction is marked, bleeding can often be prevented by transfusion of normal platelets before invasive procedures. Antifibrinolytic agents (e.g., aminocaproic acid) may be required to prevent significant bleeding after such procedures (Seligsohn, 2012).

Nursing Management

Patients with significant platelet dysfunction need to be instructed to avoid substances that can diminish platelet function, such as certain over-the-counter medications, some herbal therapies, nutritional supplements, and alcohol. They also need to inform their health care providers (including dentists) of the underlying condition before any invasive procedure is performed so that appropriate steps can be initiated to diminish the risk of bleeding.

Hemophilia

Two inherited bleeding disorders—hemophilia A and hemophilia B—are clinically indistinguishable, although they can be distinguished by laboratory tests. Hemophilia A is caused by a genetic defect that results in deficient or defective factor VIII. Hemophilia B (also called *Christmas disease*) stems from a genetic defect that causes deficient or defective factor IX. Hemophilia is a relatively common disease; hemophilia A occurs in 1 of every 10,000 births and is four times more common than hemophilia B (Berntorp & Shapiro, 2012). Both types of hemophilia are inherited as X-linked traits, so almost all affected people are males; females can be carriers but are almost always asymptomatic. The disease occurs in all ethnic groups (Berntop & Shapiro, 2012).

Hemophilia is recognized in early childhood, usually in the toddler age group. However, patients with mild hemophilia may not be diagnosed until they experience severe trauma (e.g., a high school football injury) or surgery.

Clinical Manifestations

Hemophilia is manifested by hemorrhages into various parts of the body; these hemorrhages can be severe and can occur even after minimal trauma. The frequency and severity of the bleeding depend on the degree of factor deficiency as well as the intensity of the precipitating trauma. For example, patients with a mild factor VIII deficiency (i.e., 6% to 50% of normal levels) rarely develop hemorrhage spontaneously; hemorrhage tends to occur secondary to trauma. In contrast, spontaneous hemorrhages, particularly hemarthroses and hematomas, can frequently occur in patients with severe factor VIII deficiency (i.e., less than 1% of normal levels). These patients require frequent factor VIII replacement therapy (Fijnvandraat, Cnossen, Leebeek, et al., 2012).

About 75% of all bleeding in patients with hemophilia occurs into joints. The most commonly affected joints are the knees, elbows, ankles, shoulders, wrists, and hips. Patients often note pain in a joint before they are aware of swelling and limitation of motion. Recurrent joint hemorrhages can result in damage so severe that chronic pain, ankylosis (fixation), or arthropathy of the joint occurs (Fig. 33-5). Patients with severe factor deficiency can become crippled by the joint damage before they become adults. Bleeding

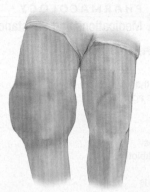

FIGURE 33-5 • Bleeding into the knee in a person with hemophilia.

can be superficial as hematomas or as deep hemorrhages into muscle or subcutaneous tissue. With severe factor VIII deficiency, hematomas can occur without known trauma and progressively extend in all directions. When the hematomas occur within muscle, particularly in the extremities, peripheral nerves can be compressed. Over time, this compression results in decreased sensation, weakness, and atrophy of the area involved.

Bleeding is not limited to the joints and muscles. Spontaneous hematuria and GI bleeding can occur. Bleeding is also common in mucous membranes, such as the nasal passages, and in soft tissues. The most dangerous site of hemorrhage is in the head (intracranial or extracranial). Any head trauma requires prompt evaluation and treatment. Surgical procedures typically result in excessive bleeding at the surgical site. Because clot formation is poor, wound healing is also poor. Bleeding is most commonly associated with dental extraction.

Medical Management

Recombinant forms of factor VIII and X concentrates are available and decrease the need for using factor concentrates, or, more infrequently, fresh-frozen plasma. Patients are given concentrates when they are actively bleeding; it is crucial to initiate treatment as soon as possible so that bleeding complications can be avoided. Prophylactic use of these factors as a preventive measure before traumatic procedures (e.g., lumbar puncture, dental extraction, surgery) is an important strategy in preventing bleeding in the setting of severe factor VIII deficiency (Berntorp & Shapiro, 2012). A systematic review demonstrated the efficacy of prophylactic factor administration in preserving joint function in children, but the efficacy of its use in adults to diminish bleeding and related complications is not as well demonstrated (Iorio, Marchesini, Marcucci, et al., 2011).

Between 15% and 30% of patients with hemophilia A and between 2% and 5% of patients with hemophilia B develop antibodies (inhibitors) to factor concentrates (Franchini & Lippi, 2009; Iorio, Halimeh, Holzhauer, et al., 2010). Although one third of such inhibitors are transient, their effects can be significant and induce partial or complete refractoriness to factor replacement, thus resulting in a markedly increased risk of bleeding. Patients may require plasmapheresis or concurrent immunosuppressive therapy, particularly in the setting of significant bleeding. Occasionally, tolerance to the antibody can be induced by repeated daily exposure to factor VIII, but it may take months or longer for tolerance to develop. Treatment success is optimal when antibody titers remain low; thus, it is important to identify rising titers and act promptly. Activated prothrombin complex concentrates can also be used to control bleeding by improving fibrin clot stability (Dai, Bevan, Rangarajan, et al., 2011). However, efficacy is unpredictable, and if infused too quickly, effective hemostasis is not achieved and bleeding persists; thrombosis is also a possible sequela. Patients with severe factor deficiency should be screened for antibodies, particularly before major surgery. Recombinant factor VIIa is approved by the FDA for patients with acquired antibodies to factors VIII and IX, but treatment is expensive, requires frequent administration because of its short half-life, and is not always successful.

Aminocaproic acid inhibits fibrinolysis and therefore stabilizes the clot; it is very effective as an adjunctive measure after oral surgery and in treating mucosal bleeding. Another agent—desmopressin (DDAVP)—induces a significant but transient rise in factor VIII levels; the mechanism for this response is unknown. In patients with mild forms of hemophilia A, desmopressin is extremely useful, significantly reducing the amount of blood products required. However, desmopressin is not effective in patients with severe factor VIII deficiency.

Nursing Management

Most patients with hemophilia are diagnosed as children. They often require assistance in coping with the condition because it is chronic, places restrictions on their lives, and is an inherited disorder that can be passed to future generations. From childhood, patients are helped to cope with the disease and to identify the positive aspects of their lives. They are encouraged to be self-sufficient and to maintain independence by preventing unnecessary trauma that can cause acute bleeding episodes and temporarily interfere with normal activities. As they work through their feelings about the condition and progress to accepting it, they can assume more and more responsibility for maintaining optimal health.

Patients with mild factor deficiency may not be diagnosed until adulthood if they do not experience significant trauma or surgery as children. These patients need extensive education about activity restrictions and self-care measures to diminish the chance of hemorrhage and complications of bleeding. The nurse should emphasize safety at home and in the workplace.

Patients and family members are instructed how to administer the factor concentrate at home at the first sign of bleeding so that bleeding is minimized and complications avoided. The use of prophylactic factor replacement can be very effective in diminishing the morbidity associated with repeated bleeding. However, this method requires administration of these factors as often as two to three times each week (Mannucci, 2012). Nurses can be instrumental in assisting patients to consider that the potential benefits from maintaining this prophylactic therapy outweighs the disadvantage that it is time-consuming.

Patients with hemophilia are instructed to avoid agents that interfere with platelet aggregation, such as aspirin, NSAIDs, some herbal and nutritional supplements (e.g.,

chamomile, nettle, alfalfa), and alcohol. This restriction applies to over-the-counter medications such as cold remedies. Dental hygiene is very important as a preventive measure because dental extractions are hazardous. Applying pressure to a minor wound may be sufficient to control bleeding if the factor deficiency is not severe. Nasal packing should be avoided, because bleeding frequently resumes when the packing is removed. Splints and other orthopedic devices may be useful in patients with joint or muscle hemorrhages. All injections should be avoided; invasive procedures (e.g., endoscopy, lumbar puncture) should be minimized or performed after administration of appropriate factor replacement. Patients with hemophilia should carry or wear medical identification (e.g., Medic-Alert bracelets). In addition, patients or families should have a written emergency plan that includes what to do in specific situations as well as names and phone numbers of emergency contacts.

During hemorrhagic episodes, the extent of bleeding must be assessed carefully. Patients who are at risk for significant compromise (e.g., bleeding into the respiratory tract or brain) warrant close observation and systematic assessment for emergent complications (e.g., respiratory distress, altered level of consciousness). If the patient has had recent surgery, the nurse frequently and carefully assesses the surgical site for bleeding. Frequent monitoring of vital signs is needed until the nurse is certain that there is no excessive postoperative bleeding.

Analgesic agents are commonly required to alleviate the pain associated with hematomas and hemorrhage into joints. Many patients report that warm baths promote relaxation, improve mobility, and lessen pain. However, during bleeding episodes, heat is avoided because it can accentuate bleeding; applications of cold are used instead.

Although the formulation of heat-solvent or detergent-treated factor concentrates has rendered factor VIII and IX preparations free of viruses such as HIV and hepatitis C, many patients have already been exposed to these infections through previous transfusions (Berntorp & Shapiro, 2012). These patients and their families may need assistance in coping with the diagnosis and the consequences of these infections.

Genetic testing and counseling should be provided to female carriers so that they can make informed decisions regarding having children and managing pregnancy (see Chapter 8).

 Gerontologic Considerations

With improved therapy, the average lifespan of the patient with hemophilia continues to rise. Several unique challenges are seen in this patient population. The older adult patient with hemophilia was likely managed with blood component transfusion, at least early in life. Thus, hepatitis B and C infection are very common in this population, particularly hepatitis C. HIV is also common (Siboni, Mannucci, Gringeri, et al., 2009); patients with HIV or hepatitis C are at increased risk for liver disease, which can be fatal. Intracranial hemorrhage is the third most common cause of death after HIV and hepatitis and may not result from trauma. The major cause of morbidity in these patients is joint disease; arthropathy is often common in four or more joints. Pain management can be challenging, because the use of NSAIDs is contraindicated due to the increased risk of bleeding.

The likelihood of acquiring inhibitors, especially hemophilia A inhibitors, increases with age. Therefore, these patients are not only at increased risk of bleeding but also of thrombosis (Kruse-Jarres, 2011).

Although patients with hemophilia less commonly have concomitant cardiovascular disease, it is difficult to manage when it is present. Coronary bypass graft surgery is extremely high risk, as are stent placements. Antiplatelet therapy (including aspirin) can be challenging in those with severe hemophilia. Close coordination of care with a hematologist can improve outcomes.

Von Willebrand Disease

Usually inherited as a dominant trait, vWD is a common bleeding disorder that affects males and females equally. The prevalence of this disease is estimated to be 1% to 2% of the population (National Hemophilia Foundation, 2011). The disease is caused by a deficiency of vWF, which is neces-

sary for factor VIII activity. vWF is also necessary for platelet adhesion at the site of vascular injury. Although synthesis of factor VIII is normal, its half-life is shortened; therefore, factor VIII levels commonly are mildly low (15% to 50% of normal).

There are three types of vWD. Type 1, the most common, is characterized by decreases in structurally normal vWF. Type 2 shows variable qualitative defects based on the specific vWF subtype involved. Type 3 is very rare (less than 5% of cases) and is characterized by a severe vWF deficiency as well as significant deficiency of factor VIII. Figure 33-6 depicts the abnormal differences in clotting found in hemophilia and vWD.

Clinical Manifestations

Bleeding tends to be mucosal. Patients commonly have recurrent nosebleeds, easy bruising, heavy menses, prolonged bleeding from cuts, and postoperative bleeding. Massive soft tissue or joint hemorrhages are not often seen, unless the patient has severe type 3 vWD. As the laboratory values fluctuate (see the following Assessment and Diagnostic Findings section), so does the bleeding. For example, a careful history of prior bleeding may show little problem with postoperative

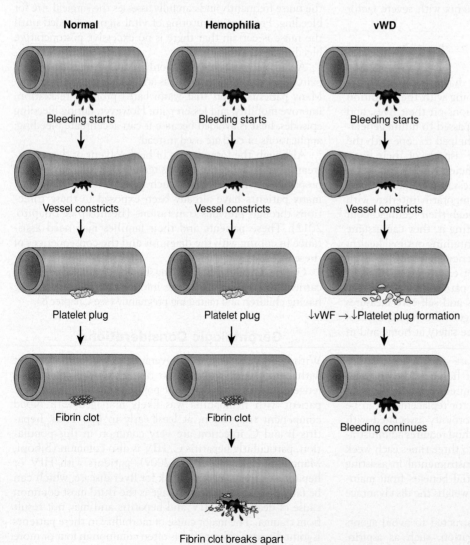

FIGURE 33-6 • Differences in bleeding. Normal, hemophilia, and Von Willebrand disease (vWD).

bleeding on one occasion but significant bleeding from a dental extraction at another time.

Assessment and Diagnostic Findings

Laboratory test results show a normal platelet count but a prolonged bleeding time and a slightly prolonged aPTT. These defects are not static, and laboratory test results can vary widely within the same patient over time. Thus, it is crucial to review these values over time rather than rely on a single measurement. More important tests include the ristocetin cofactor, or vWF collagen binding assay, which measures vWF activity. Other tests include vWF antigen, factor VIII, and, for patients with suspected type 2 defects, vWF multimers, which measure specific subtypes of vWF.

Medical Management

The goal of treatment is to replace the deficient protein (e.g., vWF or factor VIII) at the time of spontaneous bleeding or prior to an invasive procedure to prevent subsequent bleeding. Desmopressin (DDAVP), a synthetic vasopressin analogue, can be used to prevent bleeding associated with dental or surgical procedures or to manage mild bleeding after surgery in those individuals with mild vWD, although it is often ineffective in treating those with type 3 vWD (Castaman, 2011). DDAVP provides a transient increase in factor VIII coagulant activity and may also correct the bleeding time. It can be administered as an IV infusion or intranasally. With major surgery or invasive procedures, IV administration is preferable. DDAVP is contraindicated in patients with unstable coronary artery disease, because it can induce platelet aggregation and cause acute coronary syndrome (ACS) (Castaman, 2011). Side effects include headache, facial flushing, tachycardia, hyponatremia, and, rarely, seizures.

Replacement products include Humate-P and Alphanate, which are commercial concentrates of vWF and factor VIII. The dosage and frequency of administration of these agents depend on the patient's factor VIII levels and the extent of bleeding. Treatment may be necessary for up to 7 to 10 days after major surgery and 3 to 4 days postpartum. In patients with severe type 3 vWD, the prophylactic administration of these replacement agents has been very successful in preventing or limiting spontaneous bleeding. Antibody formation to these products usually occurs only in patients with type 3 vWD, after administration of high doses.

Other agents may be effective in reducing bleeding. Aminocaproic acid is useful in managing mild forms of mucosal bleeding. Estrogen–progesterone compounds may diminish the extent of menses. Platelet transfusions are useful when there is significant bleeding. Herbs and medications that interfere with platelet function (e.g., aspirin) should be avoided.

ACQUIRED COAGULATION DISORDERS

Liver Disease

With the exception of factor VIII, most blood coagulation factors are synthesized in the liver. Therefore, hepatic

dysfunction (due to cirrhosis, tumor, or hepatitis; see Chapter 49) can result in diminished amounts of the factors needed to maintain coagulation and hemostasis. Prolongation of the PT, unless it is caused by vitamin K deficiency, may indicate severe hepatic dysfunction. Although bleeding is usually minor (e.g., ecchymoses), these patients are also at risk for significant bleeding, related especially to trauma or surgery. Transfusion of fresh-frozen plasma may be required to replace clotting factors and to prevent or stop bleeding. Patients may also have life-threatening hemorrhage from peptic ulcers or esophageal varices. In these cases, replacement with fresh-frozen plasma, PRBCs, and platelets is usually required.

Vitamin K Deficiency

The synthesis of many coagulation factors depends on vitamin K. Vitamin K deficiency is common in malnourished patients. Prolonged use of some antibiotics decreases the intestinal flora that produce vitamin K, depleting vitamin K stores. Administration of vitamin K (phytonadione [Mephyton]), either orally or as a subcutaneous injection, can correct the deficiency quickly; adequate synthesis of coagulation factors is reflected by normalization of the PT.

Complications of Anticoagulant Therapy

Anticoagulants are used in the treatment or prevention of thrombosis. These agents, particularly warfarin (Coumadin) or unfractionated heparin, can cause bleeding, particularly if their use is not carefully monitored. Because the PT levels can vary from one laboratory to another, the World Health Organization (WHO) developed a standardized system for reporting PT results by using an international sensitivity index for the reagent used in an individual lab. This test, known as the INR (international normalized ratio), is now used to monitor the efficacy of anticoagulants that were measured by the PT. If the INR or aPTT is longer than desired and bleeding has not occurred, the medication can be stopped or the dose decreased. Vitamin K is administered as an antidote for warfarin toxicity. Protamine sulfate is rarely needed for heparin toxicity, because the half-life of heparin is very short; furthermore, it is not as effective when used to correct the effects of low-molecular-weight heparins (LMWHs) (Van Veen, Maclean, Hampton, et al., 2011). With significant bleeding, fresh-frozen plasma is needed to replace the vitamin K–dependent coagulation factors.

Disseminated Intravascular Coagulation

Disseminated intravascular coagulation (DIC) is not a disease but a sign of an underlying condition. DIC may be triggered by sepsis, trauma, cancer, shock, abruptio placentae, toxins, allergic reactions, and other conditions. The severity of DIC is variable, but it is potentially life threatening.

Physiology · · · · · Pathophysiology

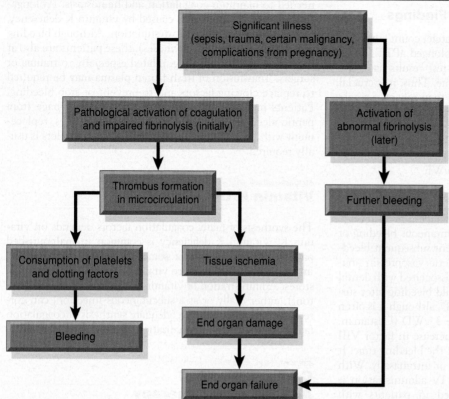

FIGURE 33-7 • Pathophysiology of disseminated intravascular coagulation.

Pathophysiology

In DIC, normal hemostatic mechanisms are altered. The inflammatory response generated by the underlying disease initiates the process of inflammation and coagulation within the vasculature. The natural anticoagulant pathways within the body are simultaneously impaired, and the fibrinolytic system is suppressed so that a massive amount of tiny clots forms in the microcirculation. Initially, the coagulation time is normal. However, as the platelets and clotting factors form microthrombi, coagulation fails. Thus, the paradoxical result of excessive clotting is bleeding (Fig. 33-7).

The clinical manifestations of DIC are primarily reflected in compromised organ function or failure. Decline in organ function is usually a result of excessive clot formation (with resultant ischemia to all or part of the organ) or, less often, of bleeding. The excessive clotting triggers the fibrinolytic system to release fibrin degradation products, which are potent anticoagulants, furthering the bleeding. The bleeding is characterized by low platelet and fibrinogen levels; prolonged PT, aPTT, and thrombin time; and elevated fibrin degradation products and **D-dimers**.

The mortality rate can exceed 80% in patients who develop severe DIC with ischemic thrombosis, frank hemorrhage, and multiple organ dysfunction syndrome (MODS). Identification of patients who are at risk for DIC and recognition of the early clinical manifestations of this syndrome can result in prompt medical intervention, which may improve the prognosis. However, the primary prognostic factor is the ability to treat the underlying condition that precipitated DIC.

Clinical Manifestions

Patients with frank DIC may bleed from mucous membranes, venipuncture sites, and the GI and urinary tracts. The bleeding can range from minimal occult internal bleeding to profuse hemorrhage from all orifices. Patients typically develop MODS, and they may exhibit renal failure as well as pulmonary and multifocal central nervous system infarctions as a result of microthromboses, macrothromboses, or hemorrhages.

During the initial process of DIC, the patient may have no new symptoms—the only manifestation being a progressive decrease in the platelet count. As the thrombosis becomes more extensive, the patient exhibits signs and symptoms of thrombosis in the organs involved. Then, as the clotting factors and platelets are consumed to form these thrombi, bleeding occurs. Initially, the bleeding is subtle, but it can develop into frank hemorrhage. Signs and symptoms depend on the organs involved and are listed in Chart 33-10.

Assessment and Diagnostic Findings

Clinically, the diagnosis of DIC is often established by laboratory tests that reflect consumption of platelets and clotting factors (i.e., drop in platelet count, an elevation in fibrin degradation products and D-dimer, an increase in PT and aPTT, and a low fibrinogen level) (Table 33-4). Although each of these tests is useful in establishing the diagnosis of DIC, the specificity of each individual parameter is not great, although D-dimer levels are more accurate than fibrin

ASSESSMENT
Assessing for Thrombosis and Bleeding in Disseminated Intravascular Coagulation

System	Signs and Symptoms of Microvascular Thrombosis	Signs and Symptoms of Microvascular and Frank Bleeding
Integumentary (skin)	↓ Temperature, sensation; ↑ pain; cyanosis in extremities, nose, earlobes; focal ischemia, superficial gangrene	Petechiae, including periorbital and oral mucosa; bleeding: gums, oozing from wounds, previous injection sites, around catheters (IVs, tracheostomies); epistaxis; diffuse ecchymoses; subcutaneous hemorrhage; joint pain
Circulatory	↓ Pulses; capillary filling time >3 s	Tachycardia
Respiratory	Hypoxia (secondary to clot in lung); dyspnea; chest pain with deep inspiration; ↓ breath sounds over areas of large embolism	High-pitched bronchial breath sounds; tachypnea; ↑ consolidation; signs and symptoms of acute respiratory distress syndrome
Gastrointestinal	Gastric pain; "heartburn"	Hematemesis (heme⊕ nasogastric output); melena (heme⊕ stools → tarry stools → bright-red blood from rectum); retroperitoneal bleeding (abdomen firm and tender to palpation; distended; ↑ abdominal girth)
Renal	↓ Urine output; ↑ creatinine, ↑ blood urea nitrogen	Hematuria
Neurologic	↓ Alertness and orientation; ↓ pupillary reaction; ↓ response to commands; ↓ strength and movement ability	Anxiety; restlessness; ↓ mentation, altered level of consciousness; headache; visual disturbances; conjunctival hemorrhage

*heme⊕, positive for hemoglobin.
Note: Signs of microvascular thrombosis are the result of an inappropriate activation of the coagulation system, causing thrombotic occlusion of small vessels within all body organs. As the clotting factors and platelets are consumed, signs of microvascular bleeding appear. This bleeding can quickly extend into frank hemorrhage. Treatment must be aimed at the disorder underlying the disseminated intravascular coagulation; otherwise, the stimulus for the syndrome will persist.

degradation products. The International Society on Thrombosis and Haemostasis has developed a highly sensitive and specific scoring system using the platelet count, fibrin degradation products, PT, and fibrinogen level to diagnose DIC (Levi & Meijers, 2011) (Table 33-5). This system is also useful in predicting the severity of the disease over time and subsequent mortality.

Medical Management

The most important factor in managing DIC is treating the underlying cause; until the cause is controlled, the DIC will persist. Correcting the secondary effects of tissue ischemia by improving oxygenation, replacing fluids, correcting electrolyte imbalances, and administering vasopressor medica-

tions is also important. If serious hemorrhage occurs, the depleted coagulation factors and platelets may be replaced to reestablish the potential for normal hemostasis and thereby diminish bleeding. However, decisions to provide transfusion support should not be solely based on the laboratory results, but on the extent of hemorrhage. Cryoprecipitate is given to replace fibrinogen and factors V and VII; fresh-frozen plasma is administered to replace other coagulation factors (Hook & Abrams, 2011).

A controversial treatment strategy is to interrupt the thrombosis process through the use of heparin infusion. Heparin may inhibit the formation of microthrombi and thus permit perfusion of the organs (skin, kidneys, or brain) to resume. Heparin use was traditionally reserved for patients in whom thrombotic manifestations predominated or in

---

TABLE 33-4 Laboratory Values Commonly Found in Disseminated Intravascular Coagulation*

Test	Function Evaluated	Normal Range	Changes in DIC
Platelet count	Platelet number	150,000–450,000/mm³	↓
Prothrombin time (PT)	Extrinsic pathway	11–12.5 seconds	↑
Partial thromboplastin time (activated)(aPTT)	Intrinsic pathway	23–35 seconds	↑
Thrombin time (TT)	Clot formation	8–11 seconds	↑
Fibrinogen	Amount available for coagulation	170–340 mg/dL	↓
D-dimer	Local fibrinolysis	0–250 ng/mL	↑
Fibrin degradation products (FDPs)	Fibrinolysis	0–5 mcg/mL	↑
Euglobulin clot lysis	Fibrinolytic activity	≥2 h	≤1 h

DIC, disseminated intravascular coagulation; ↓, decreased; ↑, increased.
*Because DIC is a dynamic condition, the laboratory values measured will change over time. Therefore, a progressive increase or decrease in a given laboratory value is likely to be more important than the actual value of a test at a single point in time.

TABLE 33-5   Scoring System for Disseminated Intravascular Coagulation

Laboratory Test	0	1	2	3
Platelet count	>100,000/mm³	>50,000/mm³, <100,000/mm³	<50,000/mm³	
Fibrin degradation products	No increase		Moderate increase	Strong increase
Prothrombin time (upper limit of normal)	<3 seconds	>3 seconds, <6 seconds	>6 seconds	
Fibrinogen	>100 mg/dL	<100 mg/dL		

Note: 5 or more is compatible with overt disseminated intravascular coagulation.
Adapted from www.isth.org/members/group_content_view.asp?group=100346&id=159221&hhSearchTerms=DIC

whom extensive blood component replacement failed to halt the hemorrhage or increased fibrinogen and other clotting levels. In the absence of bleeding, prophylactic doses of unfractionated heparin or LMWH are recommended to prevent venous thromboembolism (VTE). Therapeutic doses may be used when severe thrombosis predominates. The effectiveness of heparin can be determined by observing for normalization of the plasma fibrinogen concentration and diminishing signs of bleeding. Fibrinolytic inhibitors, such as aminocaproic acid, may be used with heparin. Recombinant activated protein C (APC; drotrecogin alfa [Xigris]), formerly used to treat some cases of DIC, is no longer an FDA-approved agent.

Nursing Management

Nurses need to be aware of which patients are at risk for DIC. Sepsis and acute promyelocytic leukemia are common causes of DIC. Patients need to be assessed thoroughly and frequently for signs and symptoms of thrombi and bleeding and monitored for any progression of these signs (see Chart 33-10). Lab values must be monitored frequently, not only for the actual result but to note trends over time as well as the rate of change in values.

Chart 33-11 describes care of the patient with DIC. Assessment and interventions should target potential sites of end-organ damage. As organs become ischemic from microthrombi, organ function diminishes; the kidneys, lungs, brain, and skin are particularly vulnerable. Lack of renal perfusion may result in acute tubular necrosis and renal failure, sometimes requiring dialysis. Placement of a large-bore dialysis catheter is extremely hazardous for this patient population and should be accompanied by adequate platelet and plasma transfusions. Hepatic dysfunction is also relatively common, reflected in altered liver function tests, depleted albumin stores, and diminished synthesis of clotting factors. Respiratory function warrants careful monitoring and aggressive measures to diminish alveolar compromise. Suctioning should be performed as gently as possible to diminish the risk of additional bleeding. Central nervous system involvement can be manifested as headache, visual changes, and alteration in level of consciousness.

Thrombotic Disorders

Several conditions can alter balance within the normal hemostasis process, causing excessive thrombosis that may be arterial (due to platelet aggregation) or venous (comprised of platelets, red cells, and thrombin). Abnormalities that predispose a person to thrombotic events include decreased clotting inhibitors within the circulation (which enhances coagulation), altered hepatic function (which may decrease production of clotting factors or clearance of activated coagulation factors), lack of fibrinolytic enzymes, and tortuous or atherosclerotic vessels (which promote platelet aggregation). Thrombosis may occur as an initial manifestation of an occult malignancy or as a complication from a preexisting cancer. It can also be caused by more than one predisposing factor. Several inherited or acquired deficiency conditions, including hyperhomocysteinemia, antithrombin (AT) deficiency, protein C deficiency, protein S deficiency, APC resistance, and factor V Leiden deficiency, can predispose a patient to repeated episodes of thrombosis; they are referred to as hypercoagulable states or thrombophilia. Those disorders that are inherited should trigger the need for familial genetic testing for the disorder (see Chapter 8); acquired disorders do not warrant familial testing.

Conditions that may result from thrombosis include ACS (see Chapter 27), CVA (ischemic stroke, see Chapter 67), and peripheral arterial occlusive disease (see Chapter 30). Anticoagulation therapy is necessary. The duration of therapy varies with the location and extent of the thrombosis, precipitating events (e.g., trauma, immobilization), and concurrent risk factors (e.g., the use of oral contraceptives or cigarettes, obesity, tortuous blood vessels, history of thrombotic events; Table 33-6). A recent study found that taking aspirin after completing standard anticoagulation therapy for treating VTE reduced the risk of recurrent thrombosis (Becattini, Agnelli, Poggio, et al., 2011). With some conditions, or with repeated thrombosis, lifelong anticoagulant therapy is necessary.

Hyperhomocysteinemia

Homocysteine can promote platelet aggregation. Increased plasma levels of homocysteine are a significant risk factor for venous thrombosis (e.g., deep vein thrombosis [DVT], pulmonary embolism [PE]) and arterial thrombosis (e.g., ischemic stroke, ACS). Hyperhomocysteinemia can be hereditary, or it can result from a nutritional deficiency of folate and, to a lesser extent, of vitamins B_{12} and B_6, because these vitamins are cofactors in homocysteine metabolism. For unknown reasons, people who are older and those with renal failure may also have elevated levels of homocysteine in the absence of nutritional deficiencies of these vitamins. Although a simple fasting measurement of plasma homocysteine can serve as a useful screening test, people with genetically inherited

Chart
33-11

PLAN OF NURSING CARE

The Patient With Disseminated Intravascular Coagulation

NURSING DIAGNOSIS: Risk for deficient fluid volume related to bleeding
GOALS: Hemodynamic status maintained; urine output ≥30 mL/h

Nursing Interventions	Rationale	Expected Outcomes
1. Avoid procedures/activities that can increase intracranial pressure (e.g., coughing, straining to have a bowel movement).	1. Prevents intracranial bleeding	• Level of consciousness (LOC) stable • Central venous pressure 5–12 cm H$_2$O, systolic blood pressure ≥70 mm Hg • Urine output ≥30 mL/h • Decreased bleeding • Decreased oozing • Decreased ecchymoses • Amenorrhea • Absence of oral and bronchial bleeding • Oral mucosa clean, moist, intact
2. Monitor vital signs closely, including neurologic checks: 　a. Monitor hemodynamics. 　b. Monitor abdominal girth. 　c. Monitor urine output.	2. Identifies signs of hemorrhage/shock quickly	
3. Avoid medications that interfere with platelet function if possible (e.g., aspirin, nonsteroidal anti-inflammatory drugs, beta-lactam antibiotics).	3. Decreases problems with platelet aggregation and adhesion	
4. Avoid rectal probes, rectal medications.	4. Decreases risk of rectal bleeding	
5. Avoid intramuscular injections.	5. Decreases risk of intramuscular bleeding	
6. Monitor amount of external bleeding carefully: 　a. Monitor number of dressings, percentage of dressing saturated; time to saturate a dressing is more objective than "dressing saturated a moderate amount." 　b. Assess suction output, all excreta for frank or occult blood. 　c. Monitor pad counts in women with vaginal bleeding. 　d. Females may receive progesterone to prevent menses.	6. 　a. Provides accurate, objective assessment of extent of bleeding 　b. Identifies presence of or quantifies extent of bleeding 　c. Quantifies extent of bleeding 　d. Decreases chance for gynecologic source of hemorrhage	
7. Use low pressure with any suctioning.	7. Prevents excessive trauma that could cause bleeding	
8. Administer oral hygiene carefully. 　a. Avoid lemon-glycerin swabs, hydrogen peroxide, commercial mouthwashes. 　b. Use sponge-tipped swabs, salt/baking soda (bicarbonate of soda) mouth rinses.	8. Prevents excessive trauma that could cause bleeding. Glycerin and alcohol (in commercial mouthwashes) will dry mucosa, increasing risk for bleeding.	
9. Avoid dislodging any clots, including those around IV sites and injection sites.	9. Prevents excessive bleeding at sites	

NURSING DIAGNOSIS: Risk for impaired skin integrity related to ischemia or bleeding
GOALS: Skin integrity remains intact; oral mucosa remains intact

Nursing Interventions	Rationale	Expected Outcomes
1. Assess skin, with particular attention to bony prominences, skin folds.	1. Prompt identification of any area at risk for skin breakdown or showing early signs of breakdown can facilitate prompt intervention and thus prevent complications.	• Skin integrity remains intact; skin is warm, and of normal color. • Oral mucosa is intact, pink, moist, without bleeding.
2. Reposition carefully; use pressure-reducing mattress.	2–4. Meticulous skin care and the use of measures to prevent pressure on bony prominences decrease the risk of skin trauma.	
3. Perform careful skin care every 2 hours, emphasizing dependent areas, all bony prominences, perineum.		
4. Use lamb's wool between digits, around ears, as needed.		
5. Use prolonged pressure after injection or procedure when such measures must be performed (at least 5 minutes).	5. Initial platelet plug is very unstable and easily dislodged, which can lead to increased bleeding.	
6. Perform oral hygiene carefully (see earlier discussion).	6. Meticulous care is needed to decrease trauma, bleeding, and risk of infection.	

(continues on page 934)

PLAN OF NURSING CARE

Chart 33-11

The Patient With Disseminated Intravascular Coagulation (continued)

NURSING DIAGNOSIS: Risk for imbalanced fluid volume related to excessive blood and/or factor component replacement
GOALS: Absence of edema; absence of crackles; intake not greater than output

Nursing Interventions	Rationale	Expected Outcomes
1. Auscultate breath sounds every 2–4 hours.	1. Crackles can develop quickly.	• Breath sounds clear
2. Monitor extent of edema.	2. Fluid may extend beyond intravascular system.	• Absence of edema • Intake does not exceed output
3. Monitor volume of IVs, blood products; decrease volume of IV medications if indicated.	3. Helps prevent fluid overload	• Weight stable
4. Administer diuretics as prescribed.	4. Decreases fluid volume	

NURSING DIAGNOSIS: Ineffective tissue perfusion related to microthrombi
GOALS: Neurologic status remains intact; absence of hypoxemia; peripheral pulses remain intact; skin integrity remains intact; urine output remains ≥30 mL/h

Nursing Interventions	Rationale	Expected Outcomes
1. Assess neurologic, pulmonary, integumentary systems.	1. Initial signs of thrombosis can be subtle.	• Arterial blood gases, O_2 saturation, pulse oximetry, LOC within normal limits
2. Monitor response to heparin therapy.	2. Assure anticoagulation effectiveness that may prevent formation of additional thromboses.	• Breath sounds clear • Absence of edema
3. Assess extent of bleeding.	3. Objective measurements of all sites of bleeding are crucial to accurately assess extent of blood loss.	• Intake does not exceed output • Weight stable
4. Monitor fibrinogen levels.	4. Response to heparin is most accurately reflected in fibrinogen level.	
5. Stop aminocaproic acid (EACA) if symptoms of thrombosis occur.	5. EACA should be used only in setting of extensive hemorrhage not responding to replacement therapy.	

NURSING DIAGNOSIS: Anxiety related to uncertainty or possible death
GOALS: Fears verbalized/identified; realistic hope maintained

Nursing Interventions	Rationale	Expected Outcomes
1. Identify previous coping mechanisms, if possible; encourage patient to use them as appropriate.	1. Identifying previous stressful situations can aid in recall of successful coping mechanisms.	• Previously used coping strategies identified and tried, to extent patient is able to do so
2. Explain all procedures and their rationale in terms that patient and family can understand.	2. Decreased knowledge and uncertainty can increase anxiety.	• Patient indicates understanding of procedures and situation as condition permits.
3. Assist family in supporting patient.	3. Family can be useful in assisting patient to use coping strategies and to maintain hope.	
4. Use services from behavioral medicine, chaplain as needed.	4. Additional professional intervention may be necessary, particularly if previous coping mechanisms are maladaptive or ineffective. Spiritual dimension should be supported.	

hyperhomocysteinemia and those who are vitamin B_6 deficient may have normal or minimally elevated levels (Anderson & Weitz, 2010). A more sensitive method involves obtaining a second measurement 4 hours after the patient consumes methionine; the hyperhomocysteinemia is found twice as often when this method is used. In hyperhomocysteinemia, the endothelial lining of the vessel walls is denuded, which can precipitate thrombus formation. Research findings

do not support that taking folic acid, vitamin B_6, and vitamin B_{12} supplements are effective in decreasing risk of recurrent venous or arterial thromboembolism, although patients with hyperhomocysteinemia are frequently counseled to take these supplements (Anderson & Weitz, 2010). Smoking causes low levels of vitamin B_6 and B_{12} and folate; thus, homocysteine levels rise. Patients need to be encouraged to refrain from smoking (Cacciapuoti, 2011).

TABLE 33-6	Risk Factors for Thrombosis	
Acquired	**Inherited**	**Mixed/Unknown**
Advanced age	Antithrombin	Activated protein
Antiphospholipid antibody	deficiency	C resistance
syndrome	Factor V	↑ Factor VII
Atrial fibrillation	Leiden	↑ Factor VIII
Diabetes	Factor XII	↑ Factor IX
Drugs (e.g., cocaine, ergot)	deficiency	↑ Factor XI
Estrogen use	Protein C	↓ Fibrinolytic
Hypertension	deficiency	activity
Inflammatory bowel disease	Protein S	↑ Homocysteine
Immobility	deficiency	
Lupus anticoagulant	Prothrombin	
Major surgery	20210a	
Myeloproliferative disease		
Nephrotic syndrome		
Obesity		
Paralysis		
Pregnancy/postpartum		
period		
Prior superficial vein		
thrombosis		
Trauma/fracture		

↑, increased; ↓, decreased.

Note: Risk factors for first, unprovoked venous thromboembolism. Note that the factor levels that are increased are procoagulant proteins.

Adapted from Bauer, K. (2010). Duration of anticoagulation: Applying the guidelines and beyond. *Hematology. The Education Program of the American Society of Hematology, 2010,* 210–215.

Antithrombin Deficiency

AT is a protein that inhibits thrombin and certain coagulation factors, and it may also play a role in diminishing inflammation within the endothelium of blood vessels. AT deficiency is a hereditary condition that can cause venous thrombosis, particularly when the AT level is less than 60% of normal. Patients with AT deficiency rarely develop thrombosis before puberty. By 50 years of age, half of patients with AT deficiency have venous thrombosis (Patnaik & Moll, 2008). The most common sites for thrombosis are the deep veins of the leg and the mesentery. Recurrent thrombosis often occurs, particularly as the patient ages. Patients tend to exhibit heparin resistance; thus, they may require greater amounts of heparin to achieve adequate anticoagulation. Patients with AT deficiency should be encouraged to have their family members tested for the deficiency.

AT deficiency can also be acquired by four mechanisms: accelerated consumption of AT (as in DIC), reduced synthesis of AT (as in hepatic dysfunction), increased excretion of AT (as in nephrotic syndrome), and medication induced (e.g., estrogens, L-asparaginase) (Johnson, Khor, & Van Cott, 2012).

Protein C Deficiency

Protein C is a vitamin K–dependent enzyme synthesized in the liver; when activated, it inhibits coagulation. When levels of protein C are deficient, the risk of thrombosis increases, and thrombosis can often occur spontaneously. People who are deficient in protein C are often without symptoms until their 20s; the risk of having a thrombotic

event then increases (Khor & Van Cott, 2010). A rare but significant complication of anticoagulation management in patients with protein C deficiency is warfarin-induced skin necrosis. This complication appears to result from progressive thrombosis in the capillaries within the skin. The extent of the necrosis can be extreme. Prompt cessation of warfarin, treatment with vitamin K, and infusions of heparin and fresh-frozen plasma are crucial to arrest the pathophysiologic process and reverse the effects of the warfarin. Treatment with purified protein C concentrate is sometimes indicated.

Protein S Deficiency

Protein S is another natural anticoagulant normally produced by the liver. APC requires protein S to inactivate certain clotting factors. When the level of protein S is deficient, this inactivation process is diminished, and the risk of thrombosis can be increased. Like patients with protein C deficiency, those with protein S deficiency have a greater risk of recurrent venous thrombosis early in life, as early as 15 years of age. More than 50% of these thromboses are spontaneous (Seligsohn & Lubetsky, 2010). Thromboses most commonly occur in the axillary, mesenteric, and cerebral veins. Warfarin-induced skin necrosis is possible. Acquired protein S deficiency can also occur. Pregnancy, DIC, liver disease, nephritic syndrome, HIV infection, and the use of L-asparaginase have all been associated with reduced protein S levels.

Activated Protein C Resistance and Factor V Leiden Mutation

APC resistance is a common condition that can occur with other hypercoagulable states. APC is an anticoagulant, and resistance to APC increases the risk of venous thrombosis. A molecular defect in the factor V gene has been identified in most (90%) patients with APC resistance. This factor V Leiden mutation is the most common cause of inherited hypercoagulability in Caucasians, but its incidence appears to be much lower in other ethnic groups (Anderson & Weitz, 2010). Factor V Leiden mutation synergistically increases the risk of thrombosis in patients with other risk factors (e.g., the use of oral contraceptives, hyperhomocysteinemia, increased age). People who are homozygous for the factor V Leiden mutation are at extremely high risk of thrombosis (i.e., 80-fold increased risk) and therefore need anticoagulation for life. In contrast, those who are heterozygous for the mutation have a 4- to 8-fold increased chance of developing a thrombus; thus, these patients may need anticoagulation for only several months after a thrombotic event (Cacciapuoti, 2011).

Acquired Thrombophilia

Acquired thrombophilias are types of clotting disorders that do not have inherited/genetic causes.

Etiology

Acquired thrombophilias result in inappropriate clot formation, typically caused by either an excess in antibodies that cause clotting or because of an increase in clotting factors.

Antiphospholipid Syndrome

Antibodies to phospholipids are common acquired causes of thrombophilia (i.e., hypercoagulable states); up to 5% of the general population may have this disorder. These antibodies reduce levels of annexin V, a protein that binds phospholipids and has anticoagulant activity (Ruiz-Irastorza, Crowther, Branch, et al., 2010). The most common of these phospholipid antibodies are either lupus or anticardiolipin antibodies, although a third type of antibody to B_2-glycoprotein may also be implicated. Antiphospholipid syndrome is classified as primary or secondary, with a reaction secondary to a preexisting autoimmune disease—with systemic lupus erythematosus being the most common disease implicated. Primary antiphospholipid syndrome is associated with certain infections (hepatitis C, HIV, syphilis, malaria) or certain medications (e.g., antibiotics, quinine [Qualaquin], hydralazine [Apresoline], procainamide [Pronestyl], cocaine); a genetic predisposition to this syndrome has been postulated but not yet proven. Antiphospholipid antibodies are associated with repeated miscarriages and felt to be a significant cause of stroke. Most thrombotic events are venous, but arterial thrombosis can occur in up to one third of the cases. Patients who persistently test positive for any of these antibodies and who have had a thrombotic event are at significant risk of recurrent thrombosis (greater than 50%); if all three types of antibodies are found, the risk of thrombosis is markedly increased, even if the patient receives anticoagulant therapy (Ruiz-Irastora et al., 2010). Recurrent thromboses tend to be of the same type—that is, venous thrombosis after an initial venous thrombosis, arterial thrombosis after an initial arterial thrombosis. Thrombi typically occur in large vessels. Therapy varies, based on the type of syndrome (e.g., secondary forms may be treated with immunosuppressive therapy), history of prior thrombosis, and location of thrombosis (venous versus arterial); arterial thrombosis often necessitates adding low-dose aspirin to some form of heparin (see later discussion).

Malignancy

Another common acquired cause of thrombophilia is cancer, particularly stomach, pancreatic, lung, and ovarian cancers. The type of thrombosis that results is unusual. Rather than DVT or PE, the thrombosis occurs in unusual sites, such as the portal, hepatic, or renal vein or the inferior vena cava. Migratory superficial thrombophlebitis or nonbacterial thrombotic endocarditis can also occur. In these patients, anticoagulation can be difficult to manage, and the thrombosis can progress despite standard doses of anticoagulants. LMWH appears to be a more effective anticoagulant than warfarin in treating this patient population (Piatek, O'Connell, & Liebman, 2012).

Medical Management

The primary method of treating thrombotic disorders is anticoagulation. However, in thrombophilic conditions, when to treat (prophylaxis or not) and how long to treat (lifelong or not) can be controversial. Anticoagulation therapy is not without risks; the most significant risk is bleeding. The most common anticoagulant medications are identified in the following section.

Pharmacologic Therapy

Along with administering anticoagulant therapy, concerns include minimizing any risk factors that predispose a patient to thrombosis. When risk factors (e.g., immobility after surgery, pregnancy) cannot be avoided, prophylactic anticoagulation may be necessary.

Unfractionated Heparin Therapy

Heparin is a naturally occurring anticoagulant that enhances AT III and inhibits platelet function. To prevent thrombosis, heparin is typically given as a subcutaneous injection two or three times daily. To treat thrombosis, heparin is usually administered IV. The therapeutic effect of heparin is monitored by serial measurements of the aPTT; the dose is adjusted to maintain the range at 1.5 to 2.5 times the laboratory control. Oral forms are being evaluated in clinical trials (Sattari & Lowenthal, 2011).

Heparin-Induced Thrombocytopenia. Heparin-induced thrombocytopenia (HIT) is a significant complication of heparin-based therapy. HIT involves the formation of antibodies against the heparin–platelet complex. HIT may occur in as many as 5% of patients receiving heparin (Lassila, Antovic, Armstrong, et al., 2011). The type of heparin used, duration of heparin therapy (beyond 4 days), and surgery (especially if it requires use of cardiopulmonary bypass) appear to be risk factors for developing HIT. Bovine preparations are more likely to lead to HIT than porcine preparations, and LMWH formulations carry a lower risk. Neither the dose nor the route of administration (IV vs. subcutaneous) is a risk. Women appear to be at a higher risk and young adults are at a very low risk for developing the disorder for reasons that are not clear (Cuker, 2011). A decline in platelet count is a hallmark sign that typically occurs after 4 to 14 days of heparin therapy; therefore, the platelet count should be monitored in any patient beginning heparin therapy. The platelet count can drop significantly, usually by 50% of baseline. The antibodies typically disappear in 2 to 3 months.

Affected patients are at increased risk for thrombosis, either venous, arterial, or both, and the thrombosis can range from DVT to ACS or CVA, or to ischemic damage to an extremity, necessitating amputation. The risk of fatal thrombosis was once very high (as much as 30%) but has dropped significantly with expeditious treatment (Jang & Hursting, 2005).

Heparin-associated thrombocytopenia (previously known as HIT-1) is actually more common than HIT. The platelet count declines slightly (rarely less than $100,000/mm^3$) within 2 to 3 days after heparin is initiated and returns to a normal level within 4 days after the heparin is stopped). There is no associated thrombosis.

Treatment for HIT includes prompt cessation of heparin (including any heparin-coated catheters) and initiation of an alternative means of anticoagulation. If the heparin is stopped without providing additional anticoagulation, the patient is at increased risk for developing new thrombi. Two inhibitors of thrombin—lepirudin (Refludan) and argatroban—are FDA-approved anticoagulants for the treatment of HIT. Oral anticoagulation with warfarin is contraindicated because it initially promotes thrombosis in the microvasculature by depleting protein C, which can lead to ischemia and gangrenous limbs (Warkentin, 2010). Once the platelet count has recovered, transitioning to treatment with warfarin is possible. Individuals who develop thrombosis in the setting of HIT should receive anticoagulation for 3 to 6 months; the duration of anticoagulation in the absence of thrombosis is less well studied (Cuker, 2011). Patients need to be aware of their risk for reactivation of the disorder should they be exposed to any amount of heparin within 3 to 4 months after diagnosis. This time frame is thought to be sufficient to remove anti-heparin-platelet antibodies from the circulation by the RES.

Low-Molecular-Weight Heparin Therapy

LMWHs (e.g., dalteparin [Fragmin], enoxaparin [Lovenox]) are special forms of heparin that have more selective effects on coagulation. Based on their biochemical properties, LMWHs have a longer half-life and a less variable anticoagulant response than unfractionated heparin. These differences permit LMWHs to be safely administered only once or twice daily, without the need for laboratory monitoring for dose adjustments. The incidence of HIT is much lower when an LMWH is used; however, LMWH is 100% cross-reactive with HIT antibodies and therefore contraindicated in HIT. In certain conditions, the use of an LMWH has allowed anticoagulation therapy to be moved entirely to the outpatient setting. Many cases of uncomplicated DVT are being managed outside the hospital. LMWHs are also used as "bridge therapy" when patients receiving anticoagulation therapy (warfarin) require a major invasive procedure such as surgery. In this situation, warfarin is stopped 2 to 3 days preoperatively, and an LMWH is used in its place until the procedure is performed. After the procedure, warfarin therapy is resumed. If the LMWH is resumed after the procedure, it is discontinued when a therapeutic level of warfarin is achieved.

Warfarin (Coumadin) Therapy

Coumarin anticoagulants (warfarin [Coumadin]) are antagonists of vitamin K and therefore interfere with the synthesis of vitamin K–dependent clotting factors. Coumarin anticoagulants bind to albumin, are metabolized in the liver, and have an extremely long half-life. Typically, a patient with a venous thromboembolus is initially treated with both heparin (either unfractionated or an LMWH) and warfarin. When the INR reaches the desired therapeutic range, the heparin is stopped. The dosage required to maintain the therapeutic range (typically an INR of 2.0 to 3.0) varies widely among patients and even within the same patient, depending on the diagnosis and the rationale for anticoagulation. Frequent monitoring of the INR is extremely important so that the dosage of warfarin can be adjusted as needed.

Warfarin is affected by many medications; consultation with a pharmacist is important to assess the extent to which concurrently administered medications, herbs, and nutritional supplements may interact with warfarin. It is also affected by many foods, so patients need dietary instruction and may benefit from consultation with a dietitian. In particular, foods with high vitamin K content antagonize the effects of warfarin. Some of these foods include spinach, broccoli, and lettuce. Patients need not avoid such foods but do need

to maintain consistent intake; for example, eating a salad daily as opposed to weekly will diminish the antagonistic effect (although will likely necessitate a higher dose of warfarin). Chart 33-12 lists agents that interact with warfarin.

Dabigatran (Pradaxa) Therapy

Dabigatran is a new oral direct thrombin inhibitor that has been approved by the FDA to reduce the risk of CVA and embolism in patients with atrial fibrillation (Mangiafico & Mangiafico, 2012). It appears to be as efficacious as warfarin but has the advantage of not needing frequent INR monitoring and dose adjustment. However, it still carries a risk of bleeding (which can be severe) and is considerably more expensive. Moreover, dabigatran must remain in its original packaging, because the potential for product breakdown and loss of potency is high if it becomes moist (Boehringer Ingelheim Pharmaceuticals, 2012). Therefore, this medication cannot be stored in a medication cassette (pillbox), which may limit its use in older adults or those with other issues limiting their ability to adhere to medication regimens.

Nursing Management

Patients with thrombotic disorders should avoid activities that lead to circulatory stasis (e.g., immobility, crossing the legs). Exercise, especially ambulation, should be performed frequently throughout the day, particularly during long trips by car or plane. Anti-embolism stockings are often prescribed, and patients usually need assistance in learning how to use them properly. Surgery further increases the risk of thrombosis. Medications that alter platelet aggregation, such as low-dose aspirin or clopidogrel (Plavix), may be prescribed. Some patients require lifelong therapy with anticoagulants such as warfarin. No evidence supports the use of bed rest as a therapeutic intervention in people with DVT or PE (Kahn, Shrier, & Kearon, 2008).

Patients with thrombotic disorders, particularly those with thrombophilia, should be assessed for concurrent risk factors for thrombosis and should avoid them if possible. For example, the use of tobacco and nicotine products should be avoided. In many instances, younger patients with thrombophilia may not require prophylactic anticoagulation; however, with concomitant risk factors (e.g., pregnancy), increasing age, or subsequent thrombotic events, prophylactic or long-term anticoagulation therapy may be required. Being able to provide the health care provider with an accurate health history can be extremely useful and can help guide the selection of appropriate therapeutic interventions. Patients need to understand risk factors for thrombosis and what they can do to diminish or reduce them, such as avoiding smoking, using alternative forms of contraception, increasing mobility, and maintaining a healthy weight. Patients with hereditary disorders should encourage their siblings and children to be tested for the disorder.

When a patient with a thrombotic disorder is hospitalized, frequent assessments should be performed for signs and symptoms of beginning thrombus formation, particularly in the legs (DVT) and lungs (PE). Ambulation or range-of-motion exercises as well as the use of anti-embolism stockings should be initiated promptly to decrease stasis. Prophylactic anticoagulants or antiplatelet agents should be initiated for those at risk for thrombosis.

Chart 33-12

PHARMACOLOGY
Agents That Interact With Warfarin (Coumadin)

Although warfarin (Coumadin), an anticoagulant medication, is commonly used to treat and prevent thrombosis, many drug–drug and drug–food interactions are associated with its use. A careful medication history (including over-the-counter medications, herbs, and other substances, such as vitamins and minerals) is important when oral anticoagulation therapy is prescribed. Consultation with a pharmacist is recommended to assess the extent to which concurrent medications may affect the anticoagulant and for appropriate dosage adjustments. The following list contains a few examples of agents that interact with warfarin.

Agents That Inhibit Warfarin Function

Azathioprine (Imuran)
Barbiturates
Carbamazepine (Tegretol)
Cholestyramine (Questran)
Corticosteroids
Cyclosporine (Sandimmune)
Dicloxacillin (Dynapen)
Digitalis
Estrogens
Ethanol (Alcohol)
Glutethimide (Doriden)
Griseofulvin (Grisovin)
Haloperidol (Haldol)
Herbal medicines: coenzyme Q, ginseng, St. John's wort, Cat's claw
Nafcillin
Oral contraceptives
Phenytoin (Dilantin) (long term)
Rifampin (Rifadin)
Spironolactone (Aldactone)
Sucralfate (Carafate)
Trazodone (Desyrel)

Agents That Potentiate Warfarin Function

Acetaminophen (Tylenol)
Allopurinol (Zyloprim)
Amiodarone
Anabolic steroids
Anti-inflammatory agents, including nonsteroidal anti-inflammatory drugs

Antimalarial agents
Aspirin
Broad-spectrum antibiotics
Chloral hydrate
Chloramphenicol
Cimetidine (Tagamet)
Colchicine (Colcrys)
Clofibrate (Atromid-S)
Chlorpromazine (Thorazine)
Danazol (Danocrine)
Disulfiram (Antabuse)
Erythromycin (E-Mycin)
Ethacrynic acid (Edecrin)
Feprazone (Prenazone)
Fluconazole (Diflucan)
Herbal medicines: danshen, devil's claw, dong quai, feverfew, garlic, gingko, ginseng, papain
Vitamin C (in very large doses)
Vitamin E (in very large doses)
Green tea
Isoniazid (INH)
Lovastatin (Mevacor)
Mefenamic acid (Ponstel)
Methotrexate (MTX)
Metronidazole (Flagyl)
Miconazole (Monistat)
Omeprazole (Prilosec)
Oral hypoglycemic agents
Oxyphenbutazone (Tandearil)
Phenytoin (Dilantin) (short term)
Probenecid (Benemid)
Propranolol (Inderal)
Propylthiouracil (PTU)
Quinidine
Quinine
Salicylates
Sulfinpyrazone (Anturane)
Sulfonamides (long acting)
Tamoxifen (Nolvadex)
Thyroxine
Triclofos
Tricyclic antidepressants

Critical Thinking Exercises

1 **ebp** You are caring for a 32-year-old woman who has had repeated hospitalizations for sickle cell crisis. What is the evidence that indicates which factors should be assessed to determine the patient's educational, coping, and pain management needs? What is the strength of that evidence? Identify the evidence base that supports concepts that you will incorporate into the patient's discharge plan.

2 A 63-year-old man presents to the emergency department (ED) with unilateral swelling and pain of the left lower extremity, which is diagnosed as a DVT. He reports this is the third time he has had a VTE. How would you determine if he is at risk for having a hypercoagulable disorder? What would you include in your health history to assist you? How would you respond if he asks you if he will "ever get off Coumadin"? What would you include in your patient education to aid him in adhering to lifelong anticoagulation?

3 **pq** You are caring for an 18-year-old male patient who presents to the ED with a fractured femur. As you begin to assess this patient, he tells you that he has hemophilia. What further questions would you elicit in your health history? How does this condition impact how you prioritize your care of this patient? How would you assess the patient's risk of bleeding?

Brunner Suite Resources

Explore these additional resources to enhance learning for this chapter:
• NCLEX-Style Questions and Other Resources on **thePoint**, http://thePoint.lww.com/Brunner13e
• Study Guide
• PrepU
• Clinical Handbook
• Handbook of Laboratory and Diagnostic Tests

References

*Asterisk indicates nursing research.
**Double asterisk indicates classic reference.

Books

**Benjamin, L., Dampier, C., Jacox, A., et al. (1999). Guidelines for the management of acute and chronic pain in sickle-cell disease. *APS clinical practice guideline series (No. 1)*. Glenville, IL: American Pain Society.

Dale, D. (2010). Neutropenia. In: M. Lichtman, T. Kipps, E. Beutler, et al. (Eds.). *Williams hematology* (8th ed.). New York: McGraw-Hill Medical.

Fischbach F., & Dunning M. (2010). *A manual of laboratory and diagnostic tests* (9th ed.). Philadelphia: Wolters Kluwer Health/Lippincott Williams & Wilkins.

Friedman, L. S. (2012). Liver, biliary tract, & pancreas disorders. In: S. J. McPhee, M. A. Papadakis, & M. W. Rabow (Eds.). *CURRENT medical diagnosis & treatment*. New York: McGraw-Hill Medical.

Ganz, T. (2010). Anemia of chronic disease. In: M. Lichtman, T. Kipps, E. Beutler, et al. (Eds.). *Williams hematology* (8th ed.). New York: McGraw-Hill Medical.

Green, R. (2010). Folate, cobalamin, and megaloblastic anemias. In: M. Lichtman, T. Kipps, E. Beutler, et al. (Eds.). *Williams hematology* (8th ed.). New York: McGraw-Hill Medical.

Kaushansky, K. (2010). Reactive thrombocytosis. In: M. Lichtman, T. Kipps, E. Beutler, et al. (Eds.). *Williams hematology* (8th ed.). New York: McGraw-Hill Medical.

Kipps, T. (2010). Lymphocytosis and lymphocytopenia. In: M. Lichtman, T. Kipps, E. Beutler, et al. (Eds.). *Williams hematology* (8th ed.). New York: McGraw-Hill Medical.

Natarajan, K., Townes, T., & Kutlar, A. (2010). Disorders of hemoglobin structure: Sickle cell anemia and related abnormalities. In: M. Lichtman, T. Kipps, E. Beutler, et al. (Eds.). *Williams hematology* (8th ed.). New York: McGraw-Hill Medical.

Packman, C. (2010). Hemolytic anemia resulting from immune injury. In: M. Lichtman, T. Kipps, E. Beutler, et al. (Eds.). *Williams hematology* (8th ed.). New York: McGraw-Hill Medical.

Seligsohn U., & Lubetsky A. (2010). Hereditary thrombophilia. In: M. Lichtman, T. Kipps, E. Beutler, et al. (Eds.). *Williams hematology* (8th ed.). New York: McGraw-Hill Medical.

Van Solinge, W. W., & van Wijk, R. (2010). Disorders of red cells resulting from enzyme abnormalities. In: M. Lichtman, T. Kipps, E. Beutler, et al. (Eds.). *Williams hematology* (8th ed.). New York: McGraw-Hill Medical.

Weatherall, D. (2010). The thalassemias: Disorders of globin synthesis. In: M. Lichtman, T. Kipps, E. Beutler, et al. (Eds.). *Williams hematology* (8th ed.). New York: McGraw-Hill Medical.

Journals and Electronic Documents

Aapro, M., Jelkmann, W., Constantinescu, S., et al. (2012). Effects of erythropoietin receptors and erythropoiesis-stimulating agents on disease progression in cancer. *British Journal of Cancer, 106*(7), 1249–1258.

Allen, K. (2010). Hereditary hemochromatosis—diagnosis and management. *Australian Family Physician, 39*(12), 938–941.

Ameringer, S., & Smith, W. (2011). Emerging biobehavioral factors of fatigue in sickle cell disease. *Journal of Nursing Scholarship, 43*(1), 22–29.

Anderson, J., & Weitz, J. (2010). Hypercoagulable states. *Clinics in Chest Medicine, 31*(4), 659–673.

Andres, E., Fothergill, H., & Mecili, M. (2010). Efficacy of oral cobalamin (vitamin B12) therapy. *Expert Opinion on Pharmacotherapy, 11*(2), 249–256.

Annibale, B., Lahner, E., & Fave, G. (2011). Diagnosis and management of pernicious anemia. *Current Gastroenterology Reports, 13*(6), 518–524.

Barrett, K., Barman, S., Boitano, S., et al. (2012). Blood as a circulatory fluid & the dynamics of blood & lymph flow. In: K. E. Barrett, S. M. Barman, S. Boitano, et al. (Eds.). *Ganong's review of medical physiology* (24th ed.). New York: McGraw-Hill. Available at: www.accessmedicine.com.laneproxy.stanford.edu/content.aspx?aID=56264612

Barton, J., Barton, J. C., & Bertoli, L. (2010). Pica associated with iron deficiency or depletion: Clinical and laboratory correlates in 262 non-pregnant adult patients. *BMC Blood Disorders, 10*, 9.

Becattini, C., Agnelli, G., Poggio, R., et al. (2011). Aspirin after oral anticoagulants for prevention of recurrence in patients with unprovoked venous thromboembolism. The WARFASA study. *Blood, 118*(21), 543.

Berntorp, E., & Shapiro, A. (2012). Modern haemophilia care. *Lancet, 379*(9824), 1447–1456.

Bode, C. (2003). Effect of alcohol consumption on the gut. *Best Practice & Research Clinical Gastroenterology, 17*(4), 575–592.

Boehringer Ingelheim Pharamceuticals. (2012). *Pradaxa product information*. Available at: bidocs.boehringer-ingelheim.com/BIWebAccess/ViewServlet.ser?docBase=renetnt&folderPath=/Prescribing%20Information/PIs/Pradaxa/Pradaxa.pdf

Bross, M., Soch, K., & Smith-Knuppel, T. (2010). Anemia in older persons. *American Family Physician, 82*(5), 480–487.

Bryan, L., & Zakai, N. (2012). Why is my patient anemic? *Hematology Oncology Clinics of North America, 26*(2), 205–230.

Cacciapuoti, F. (2011). Some considerations about the hypercoagulable states and their treatments. *Blood Coagulation & Fibrinolysis, 22*(3), 155–159.

Castaman, G. (2011). Treatment of von Willebrand disease with FVIII/vWF concentrates. *Blood Transfusion, 9*(Suppl. 2), s9–s13.

Centers for Disease Control and Prevention. (2011). *Colorectal cancer screening guidelines*. Available at: www.cdc.gov/cancer/colorectal/basic_info/screening/guidelines/htm

Chan, T. (1996). Glucose-6-phosphate dehydrogenase deficiency: A review. *Hong Kong Journal of Paediatrics, 1*(1), 23–30.

Cuker, A. (2011). Heparin-induced thrombocytopenia: Present and future. *Journal of Thrombosis & Thrombolysis, 31*(3), 353–366.

Dai, L., Bevan, R., Rangarajan, S., et al. (2011). Stabilization of fibrin clots by activated prothrombin complex concentrate and tranexamic acid in FVIII inhibitor plasma. *Haemophilia, 17*(5), e944–e948.

Davis, S., & Littlewood, T. (2012). The investigation and treatment of secondary anaemia. *Blood Reviews, 26*(2), 65–71.

Eckes, E. (2011). Chelation therapy for iron overload: Nursing practice implications. *Journal of Infusion Nursing, 34*(6), 374–380.

Fijnvandraat, K., Cnossen, M. H., Leebeek, F. W., et al. (2012). Diagnosis and management of haemophilia. *British Medical Journal, 344*, e2707.

Fogarty, P. (2009). Chronic immune thrombocytopenia in adults: Epidemiology and clinical presentation. *Hematology Oncology Clinics of North America, 23*(6), 1213–1221.

Franchini, M., & Lippi, G. (2009). Recent improvements in the clinical treatment of coagulation factor inhibitors. *Seminars in Thrombosis and Hemostasis, 35*(8), 806–813.

Franchini, M., Vescovi, P., Garofano, M., et al. (2012). Heliobacter pylori-associated idiopathic thrombocytopenia purpura: A narrative review. *Seminars in Thrombosis and Hemostasis, 38*(5), 463–468.

**Franco, R., Lohman, J., Silberstein, E., et al. (1998). Time-dependent changes in the density and hemoglobin F content of biotin-labeled sickle cells. *Journal of Clinical Investigation, 101*(12), 2730–2740.

Froom, P., & Barak, M. (2011). Prevalence and course of pseudothrombocytopenia in outpatients. *Clinical Chemistry and Laboratory Medicine, 49*(1), 111–114.

Fulop, T., Larbi, A., Witkowski, J., et al. (2010). Aging, frailty and age-related diseases. *Biogerontology, 11*(5), 547–563.

Gupta, V., Eapen, M., Brazauskas, R., et al. (2010). Impact of age on outcomes after bone marrow transplantation for acquired aplastic anemia using HLA-matched sibling donors. *Heamatologica, 95*(12), 2119–2125.

Higgs, D., Engel, J., & Stamatoyannopoulos, G. (2012). Thalassemia. *Lancet, 379*(9813), 373–383.

Hook, K., & Abrams, C. (2011). The loss of homeostasis in hemostasis: New approaches in treating and understanding acute disseminated in disseminated intravascular coagulation in critically ill patients. *Clinical and Translational Science, 5*(1), 85–92.

Inati, A., Khoriaty, E., & Musallam, K. (2011). Iron in sickle-cell disease: What have we learned over the years? *Pediatric Blood & Cancer, 56*(2), 182–190.

Ioannou, G., Dominitz, J., Weiss, N., et al. (2004). The effect of alcohol consumption on the prevalence of iron overload, iron deficiency, and iron deficiency anemia. *Gastroenterology, 126*(5), 1293–1301.

Iorio, A., Halimeh, S., Holzhauer, S., et al. (2010). Rate of inhibitor development in previously untreated hemophilia A patients treated with plasma-derived or recombinant factor VIII concentrates: A systematic review. *Journal of Thrombosis and Hemostasis, 8*(6), 1256–1265.

Iorio, A., Marchesini, E., Marcucci, M., et al. (2011). Clotting factor concentrates given to prevent bleeding and bleeding-related complications in people with hemophilia A or B. *Cochrane Database of Systematic Reviews, (9)*, CD003429.

Jang, I., & Hursting, M. (2005). When heparins promote thrombosis: Review of heparin-induced thrombocytopenia. *Circulation, 111*(20), 2671–2683.

Johnson, C., & Telen, M. (2008). Adhesion molecules and hydroxyurea in he pathophysiology of sickle cell disease. *Haematologica, 93*(4), 481–485.

Johnson, N., Khor, B., & Van Cott, E. (2012). Advances in laboratory testing for thrombophilia. *American Journal of Hematology, 87*(Suppl. 1), S108–S112.

Kahn, S., Shrier, I., & Kearon, C. (2008). Physical activity in patients with deep venous thrombosis: A systematic review. *Thrombosis Research, 122*(6), 763–773.

Kato, G. J., & Gladwin, M. T. (2005). Sickle cell disease. In: J. B. Hall, G. A. Schmidt, & L. D. Wood (Eds.). *Principles of critical care* (3rd ed.). New York: McGraw-Hill Medical. Available at: www.accessmedicine.com.laneproxy.stanford.edu/content.aspx?aID=2282146

Khor, B., & Van Cott, E. (2010). Laboratory tests for protein C deficiency. *American Journal of Hematology, 85*(6), 440–442.

Kremastinos, D., Farmakis, D., Aessopos, A., et al. (2010). Beta-thalassemia cardiomyopathy: History, present considerations, and future perspectives. *Circulation. Heart Failure, 3*(3), 451–458.

Kruse-Jarres, R. (2011). Current controversies in the formation and treatment of alloantibodies to factor VIII in congenital hemophilia A. *American Society of Hematology Educational Program, 2011*, 407–412.

Langan, R., & Zawistoski, K. (2011). Update on vitamin B12 deficiency. *American Family Physician, 83*(12), 1425–1430.

Lassila, R., Antovic, J., Armstrong, E., et al. (2011). Practical viewpoints on the diagnosis and management of heparin-induced thrombocytopenia. *Seminars in Thrombosis and Hemostasis, 37*(3), 328–334.

Laurie, G. (2010). Acute chest syndrome in sickle cell disease. *Internal Medicine Journal, 40*(5), 372–376.

Lechner, K., & Jäger, U. (2010). How I treat autoimmune hemolytic anemias in adults. *Blood, 116*(11), 1831–1838.

Lee, L., Askew, R., Walker, J., et al. (2012). Adults with sickle cell disease: An interdisciplinary approach to home care and self-care management with a case study. *Home Healthcare Nurse, 30*(3), 172–183.

Levi, M., & Meijers, J. (2011). DIC: Which laboratory tests are most useful. *Blood Reviews, 25*(1), 33–37.

Lowrie, E., Kirkwood, G., & Pollack, M. (2012). *Chapter 19: Anemia in patients with chronic renal failure and in patients undergoing chronic hemodialysis.* Available at: http://msl1.mit.edu/ESD10/kidneys/HndbkHTML/ch19.htm

Mangiafico, R., & Mangiafico, M. (2012). Emerging anticoagulant therapies for atrial fibrillation: New options, new challenges. *Current Medicinal Chemistry, 19*(47), 4688–4698.

Mannucci, P. (2012). The role of natural VWF/FVIII complex concentrates in contemporary haemophilia care: A guideline for the next decade. *Haemophilia, 18*(Suppl. 2), 2–7.

Miller, K. (2010). Using a computer-based risk assessment tool to identify risk for chemotherapy-induced febrile neutropenia. *Clinical Journal of Oncology Nursing, 14*(1), 87–91.

National Heart, Lung, and Blood Institute. (2010). *What is aplastic anemia?* Available at: www.nhlbi.nih.gov/health/health-topics/topics/aplastic/

National Heart, Lung, and Blood Institute. (2011). *Who is at risk for sickle cell anemia?* Available at: www.nhlbi.nih.gov/health/health-topics/topics/sca/atrisk.html

National Hemophilia Foundation. (2011). *What is von Willebrand disease?* Available at: www.hemophilia.org/NHFWeb/MainPgs/MainNHF.aspx?menuid=182&contentid=47&rptname=bleeding

Neunert, C., Lim, W., Crowther, M., et al. (2011). The American Society of Hematology 2011 evidence-based practice guideline for immune thrombocytopenia. *Blood, 117*(16), 4190–4207.

Newton, J., Reese, J., Watson, S., et al. (2011). Fatigue in adult patients with primary immune thrombocytopenia. *European Journal of Hematology, 86*(5), 420–429.

Palmer, S., Navaneethan, S., Craig, J., et al. (2012). Meta-analysis: Erythropoiesis-stimulating agents in patients with chronic kidney disease. *Annals of Internal Medicine, 153*(1), 23–33.

Parent, F., Bachir, D., Inamo, J., et al. (2011). A hemodynamic study of pulmonary hypertension in sickle cell disease. *New England Journal of Medicine, 365*(1), 44–53.

Patnaik, M., & Moll, S. (2008). Inherited antithrombin deficiency: A review. *Haemophilia, 14*(6), 1229–1239.

Patnaik, M., & Tefferi, A. (2009). The complete evaluation of erythrocytosis: Congenital and acquired. *Leukemia, 23*(5), 834–844.

Piatek, C., O'Connell, C., & Liebman, H. (2012). Treating venous thromboembolism in patients with cancer. *Expert Reviews of Hematology, 5*(2), 201–209.

Primack, B. A., & Mahaniah, K. J. (2011). Anemia. In: J. E. South-Paul, S. C. Matheny, & E. L. Lewis (Eds.). *CURRENT diagnosis & treatment in family medicine* (3rd ed.). New York: McGraw-Hill Medical. Available at: www.accessmedicine.com.laneproxy.stanford.edu/content.aspx?aID=8153552

Provan, D., Stasi, R., Newland, A., et al. (2010). International consensus report on the investigation and management of primary immune thrombocytopenia. *Blood, 115*(2), 168–186.

Rodeghiero, F., Stasi, R., Gernsheimer, T., et al. (2009). Standardization of terminology, definitions, and outcome criteria in immune thrombocytopenic purpura of adults and children: Report from an international working group. *Blood, 113*(11), 2386–2393.

Ruiz-Irastorza, G., Crowther, M., Branch, W., et al. (2010). Antiphospholipid syndrome. *Lancet, 376*(9751), 1498–1509.

*Sabol, V., Resnick, B., Galik, E., et al. (2010). Anemia evaluation and management in nursing home residents. *Western Journal of Nursing Research, 32*(4), 447–461.

Sattari, M., & Lowenthal, D. (2011). Novel oral anticoagulants in development: Dabigatran, rivaroxaban, and apixaban. *American Journal of Therapeutics, 18*(4), 332–328.

**Savage, D., & Lindenbaum, J. (1995). Neurological complications of acquired cobalamin deficiency: Clinical aspects. *Bailliere's Clinical Haematology, 8*(3), 657–678.

Seligsohn, U. (2012). Treatment of inherited platelet disorders. *Haemophilia, 18*(Suppl. 4), 161–165.

Sheahan, O., & O'Connell, E. (2009). Hereditary haemochromatosis: Patient support and education. *Nursing Standard, 24*(3), 49–56.

Siboni, S., Mannucci, P., Gringeri, A., et al. (2009). Health status and quality of life of elderly persons with severe hemophilia born before the advent of modern replacement therapy. *Journal of Thrombosis and Hemostasis, 7*(3), 780–786.

Smith, W., & Scherer, M. (2010). Sickle-cell pain: Advances in epidemiology and etiology. *Hematology. The Educational Program of the American Society of Hematology, 2010*, 409–415.

Taher, A., Musallam, K., Karimi, et al. (2010). Overview on practices in thalassemia intermedia management aiming for lowering complication rates across a region of endemicity: The OPTIMAL CARE study. *Blood, 115*(10), 1886–1892.

U.S. Food and Drug Administration. (2011). *Information on erythropoiesis-stimulating agents (ESA) epoetin alfa (marketed as Procrit, Epogen), darbepoetin alfa (marketed as Aranesp).* Available at: www.fda.gov/drugs/drugsafety/postmarketdrugsafetyinformationforpatientsandproviders/ucm109375.htm

Vanasse, G., & Berliner, N. (2010). Anemia in elderly patients: An emerging problem for the 21st century. *Hematology. The Educational Program of the American Society of Hematology, 2010*, 271–275.

Van Veen, J., Maclean, R., Hampton, K., et al. (2011). Protamine reversal of low molecular weight heparin: Clinically effective? *Blood Coagulation & Fibrinolysis, 22*(7), 565–570.

Villanueva, A., Newell, P., & Hoshida, Y. (2010). Inherited hepatocellular carcinoma. *Best Practice & Research. Clinical Gastroenterology, 24*(5), 725–734.

Wahl, S., & Vichinsky, E. (2010). Pulmonary hypertension in hemolytic anemias. *F1000 Medicine Reports, 11*(2), pii: 10.

Warkentin, T. (2010). Agents for the treatment of heparin-induced thrombocytopenia. *Hematology Oncology Clinics of North America, 24*(4), 755–775.

*Wilkie, D., Molokie, R., Boyd-Seal, D., et al. (2010). Patient-reported outcomes: Descriptors of nociceptive and neuropathic pain and barriers to effective pain management in adult outpatients with sickle cell disease. *Journal of the National Medical Association, 102*(1), 18–27.

Wong, E., & Rose, M. (2012). Why does my patient have thrombocytopenia? *Hematology Oncology Clinics of North America, 26*(2), 231–252.

Young, N., Scheinberg, P., & Calado, R. (2008). Aplastic anemia. *Current Opinion in Hematology, 15*(3), 162–168.

Youngster, I., Arcavi, L., Schechmaster, R., et al. (2010). Medications and glucose-6-phosphate dehydrogenase deficiency: An evidence-based review. *Drug Safety, 33*(9), 713–726.

Resources

AABB (American Association of Blood Banks), www.aabb.org

Alternative Medicine Foundation, www.amfoundation.org

American Hemochromatosis Society, www.americanhs.org

American Pain Society (APS), www.ampainsoc.org

American Red Cross, www.redcross.org

American Society for Blood and Marrow Transplantation (ASBMT), www.asbmt.org

Aplastic Anemia and MDS International Foundation, www.aamds.org/aplastic

APS Foundation of America (antiphospholipid antibody syndrome), www.apsfa.org

G6PD Deficiency, g6pddeficiency.org

ITP Support Association (immune thrombocytopenic purpura), www.itpsupport.org.uk/

MedlinePlus (information on drug–herb interaction), www.nlm.nih.gov/medlineplus/druginfo/herb_All.html

National Heart, Lung, and Blood Institute, Sickle Cell Anemia, www.nhlbi.nih.gov/health/dci/Diseases/Sca/SCA_WhatIs.html

National Marrow Donor Program, www.marrow.org

Platelet Disorder Support Association (PDSA), www.pdsa.org

Sickle Cell Disease Association of America (SCDAA), www.sicklecelldisease.org

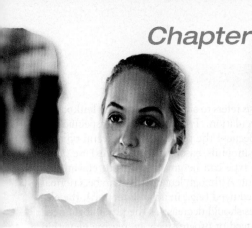

Chapter

34

Management of Patients With Hematologic Neoplasms

Learning Objectives

On completion of this chapter, the learner will be able to:

1 Distinguish between hematologic clonal disorders and frank malignancy.
2 Compare the leukemias in terms of their incidence, physiologic alterations, clinical manifestations, management, and prognosis.

3 Use the nursing process as a framework for care of patients with acute leukemia.
4 Compare the myeloproliferative disorders in terms of their incidence, clinical manifestations, management, complications, and prognosis.
5 Describe nursing management of patients with lymphoma or multiple myeloma.

Glossary

absolute neutrophil count: a calculation of the number of circulating neutrophils, derived from the total white blood cells (WBCs) and the percentage of neutrophils counted in a microscope's visual field
angiogenesis: formation of new blood vessels
apoptosis: programmed cell death
blast cell: primitive leukocyte
clonality (clone): proliferation from same cell of origin so that descendent cells are identical to the cell of origin
cytokines: proteins produced by leukocytes that are vital to regulation of hematopoiesis, apoptosis, and immune responses
erythrocyte sedimentation rate: laboratory test that measures the rate of settling of red blood cells (RBCs); elevation is indicative of inflammation; also called the *sed rate*
granulocyte: granulated WBC (neutrophil, eosinophil, basophil); term sometimes used as synonymous with neutrophil
hematopoiesis: complex process of the formation and maturation of blood cells
indolent neoplasm: a slow-growing cancer that often remains localized or causes few symptoms
leukocyte: one of several cellular components of blood involved in defense of the body; subtypes include neutrophils, eosinophils, basophils, monocytes, and lymphocytes (*synonym:* white blood cell [WBC])
leukemia: uncontrolled proliferation of WBCs, often immature

leukopenia: less-than-normal amount of WBCs in circulation
lymphadenopathy: enlargement of a lymph node or lymph nodes
lymphocyte: type of WBC involved in immune functions
lymphoid: pertaining to lymphocytes
lysis: destruction of cells
monocyte: large WBC that becomes a macrophage when it leaves the circulation and moves into body tissues
myeloid: pertaining to nonlymphoid blood cells that differentiate into RBCs, platelets, macrophages, mast cells, and various WBCs
neutropenia: lower-than-normal number of neutrophils
neutrophil: fully mature WBC capable of phagocytosis; primary defense against bacterial infection
nucleated red blood cell (RBC): immature form of RBC; portion of nucleus remains within the RBC
pancytopenia: abnormal decrease in WBCs, RBCs, and platelets
petechiae: tiny capillary hemorrhages
phagocytosis: process of cellular ingestion and digestion of foreign bodies
polycythemia: excess RBCs
splenomegaly: enlargement of the spleen
stem cell: primitive cell, capable of self-replication and differentiation into myeloid or lymphoid stem cell
thrombocytopenia: lower-than-normal platelet count
thrombocytosis: higher-than-normal platelet count
white blood cell (WBC): *synonym:* leukocyte

Hematopoiesis is characterized by a rapid, continuous turnover of blood cells. Normally, production of specific blood cells from their **stem cell** precursors is carefully regulated according to the body's needs. If the mechanisms that control the production of these cells are disrupted, the cells can proliferate excessively, as seen in the development of hematologic neoplasms. As is true with nonmalignant hematologic disorders, the pathophysiologic processes that undergird the development of hematologic neoplasms are complex. Understanding these processes and the rationale for treatments is

941

important so that nurses may appropriately assess, monitor, educate, and intervene with patients with hematologic neoplasms.

Hematopoietic malignancies are often classified by the cells involved. **Leukemia** is a neoplastic proliferation of one particular cell type (granulocytes, **monocytes** [i.e., precursor to macrophages], **lymphocytes** [type of **white blood cell (WBC)** or leukocyte involved in immune functions], or infrequently erythrocytes or megakaryocytes). The defect originates in the hematopoietic stem cell, the myeloid, or the lymphoid stem cell. The lymphomas are neoplasms of lymphoid tissue, usually derived from B lymphocytes. Multiple myeloma is a malignancy of the most mature form of B lymphocyte—the plasma cell.

CLONAL STEM CELL DISORDERS

When some hematologic neoplasms develop, hematopoietic control mechanisms may be in place to continue to produce adequate numbers of normal blood cells. These are commonly referred to as **indolent neoplasms,** where the increased numbers of cells produced from a culprit clone all have the same genotype (see Chapter 8 for further discussion of genotypes). However, at some time, the control mechanisms may fail and the "indolent" **clone** may then evolve into a more aggressive clone.

Not all malignancies arise from an indolent neoplasm, however. Rather, they may evolve directly from a change in the stem cell. Similarly, not all indolent neoplasms will eventually evolve into a malignancy. Nonetheless, such evolution is possible for virtually any clonal disorder. Figure 34-1 illustrates this concept for myeloid stem cell disorders. Similar neoplastic conditions are derived from disorders within the lymphoid stem cell disorder (Greaves & Maley, 2012). (Refer to later discussions about specific diseases noted in Fig. 34-1).

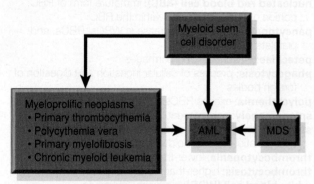

FIGURE 34-1 • The development of myeloid neoplasms. Changes within the myeloid stem cell can cause the development of neoplasms that are either proliferative or, in the case of myelodysplastic syndrome, dysplastic. Although any indolent neoplasm can evolve into a malignant condition (e.g., acute myeloid leukemia [AML]), in most instances this will not occur. For example, the incidence of evolution from primary thrombocythemia is very low, yet it is much higher when from primary myelofibrosis. The actual incidence of evolution continues to change as therapy before more effective, as in the case of chronic myeloid leukemia. Note that AML can arise directly from the altered myeloid stem cell; it need not evolve from an existing indolent neoplasm. Similar events occur with lymphoid malignancy development.

LEUKEMIA

The term *leukocytosis* refers to an increased level of **leukocytes** (WBCs) in the circulation. Typically, only one specific cell type is increased. Because the proportions of several types of leukocytes (e.g., eosinophils, basophils, monocytes) are small, an increase in one type can be great enough to elevate the total leukocyte count. Although leukocytosis can be a normal response to increased need (e.g., in acute infection), the elevation in leukocytes should decrease as the physiologic need decreases. A prolonged or progressively increasing elevation in leukocytes is abnormal and should be evaluated. A significant cause of persistent leukocytosis is hematologic malignancy (i.e., leukemia).

The common feature of the leukemias is an unregulated proliferation of leukocytes in the bone marrow. In acute forms (or late stages of chronic forms), the proliferation of leukemic cells leaves little room for normal cell production. There can also be a proliferation of cells in the liver and spleen (extramedullary hematopoiesis). With acute forms, there can be infiltration of leukemic cells in other organs, such as the meninges, lymph nodes, gums, and skin. The cause of leukemia is not fully known, but there is some evidence of genetic and viral influences. Bone marrow damage from radiation exposure or from chemicals such as benzene and alkylating agents (e.g., melphalan [Alkeran]) can cause leukemia (Liesveld & Lichtman, 2010).

The leukemias are commonly classified according to the stem cell line involved, either **lymphoid** (referring to stem cells that produce lymphocytes) or **myeloid** (referring to stem cells that produce nonlymphoid blood cells). They are also classified as either acute or chronic, based on the time it takes for symptoms to evolve and the phase of cell development that is halted (i.e., with few leukocytes differentiating beyond that phase).

In acute leukemia, the onset of symptoms is abrupt, often occurring within a few weeks. Leukocyte development is halted at the blast phase and thus most leukocytes are undifferentiated cells or blasts. Acute leukemia can progress rapidly, with death occurring within weeks to months without aggressive treatment.

In chronic leukemia, symptoms evolve over a period of months to years, and the majority of leukocytes produced are mature. Chronic leukemia progresses more slowly; the disease trajectory can extend for years.

Acute Myeloid Leukemia

Acute myeloid leukemia (AML) results from a defect in the hematopoietic stem cell that differentiates into all myeloid cells: monocytes, **granulocytes** (e.g., **neutrophils**, basophils, eosinophils), erythrocytes, and platelets. Any age group can be affected, although it infrequently occurs before age 55 years, and the incidence rises with age, with a peak incidence at age 67 years (National Cancer Institute [NCI], 2011). AML is the most common nonlymphocytic leukemia.

The prognosis is highly variable. Patient age is a significant factor; patients who are younger may survive for 5 years or more after diagnosis of AML. However, patients who are older than 60 years, have a more undifferentiated form of AML, have central nervous system (CNS) involvement, or have a systemic infection at the time of diagnosis tend to have a worse prognosis. The 5-year survival rate for patients with AML who are 50 years of age or younger is 43%; it drops to 19% for those between 50 and 64 years, and drops to 1.6% for those older than 75 years (NCI, 2011). The development of AML in people with preexisting myelodysplastic syndrome (MDS) or myeloproliferative disorders (refer to later discussions in this chapter) or in those who previously received alkylating agents for cancer (secondary AML) is associated with a much worse prognosis. Secondary AML tends to be more resistant to treatment, resulting in a much shorter duration of remission. With treatment, patients with secondary AML survive an average of less than 1 year, with death usually a result of infection or hemorrhage. Patients receiving transfusion and antimicrobial support alone to treat AML also usually survive less than 1 year, dying of infection or bleeding.

Clinical Manifestations

AML develops without warning, with symptoms typically occurring over a period of weeks. Signs and symptoms result from insufficient production of normal blood cells. Fever and infection result from **neutropenia** (low neutrophil count); weakness and fatigue, dyspnea on exertion, and pallor from anemia; and petechiae, ecchymoses, and bleeding tendencies from thrombocytopenia. The proliferation of leukemic cells within organs leads to a variety of additional symptoms: pain from an enlarged liver or spleen, hyperplasia of the gums, and bone pain from expansion of marrow (Fig. 34-2). **Petechiae** (pinpoint red or purple hemorrhagic spots on the skin) or ecchymoses (bruises) are common on the skin (see Fig. 33-4 in Chapter 33); occasionally, leukemic infiltrates are also seen (Fig. 34-3). Leukemic cells can also infiltrate the gingiva or synovial spaces of joints. **Lymphadenopathy** (enlargement of lymph nodes) or **splenomegaly** (enlargement of the spleen) is rare. Fevers may occur and are not always due to infection.

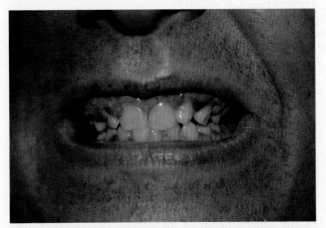

FIGURE 34-2 • Gingival infiltration of leukemic cells in a patient with acute myeloid leukemia. From Greer, J. P., Foerster, J., Rodgers, G. M., et al. (2009). *Wintrobe's clinical hematology* (12th ed., p. 1680, Fig. 72.8). Philadelphia: Lippincott Williams & Wilkins.

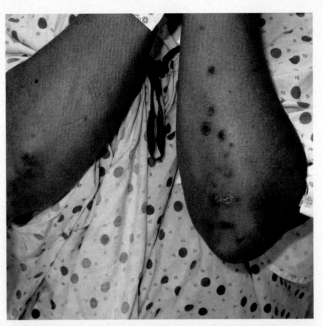

FIGURE 34-3 • Leukemia cutis. Infiltration of leukemic cells in skin on extensor surface of forearms. Reproduced with permission from Stedman's Medical Dictionary. Copyright ©2008 Lippincott Williams & Wilkins.

Assessment and Diagnostic Findings

The complete blood count (CBC) shows a decrease in both erythrocytes and platelets. Although the total leukocyte count can be low, normal, or high, the percentage of normal cells is usually vastly decreased. A bone marrow analysis shows an excess of immature **blast cells** (immature leukocytes) (more than 20%), which is the hallmark of the diagnosis. AML can be further classified into seven different subgroups, based on cytogenetics, histology, and morphology of the blasts. The actual prognosis varies somewhat between subgroups and with the extent of cytogenetic abnormalities and genetic mutations, yet the clinical course and treatment differ substantially with only one subtype. Patients with acute promyelocytic leukemia (APL, or AML-M3) often have significantly more problems with bleeding, in that they have underlying coagulopathy and a higher incidence of disseminated intravascular coagulation (DIC) (Franchini, Di Minno, & Coppola, 2010).

Medical Management

Despite advances in understanding of the biology of AML, substantive advances in treatment response rates and survival rates have not occurred for decades, with the exception of advances made in treating APL (see later discussion). Even for patients with subtypes that have not benefited from advances in treatment, cure is still possible. The overall objective of treatment is to achieve complete remission, in which there is no evidence of residual leukemia in the bone marrow. Attempts are made to achieve remission by the aggressive administration of chemotherapy, called *induction therapy*, which usually requires hospitalization for several weeks. Induction therapy typically involves high doses of cytarabine (Cytosar, Ara-C) and daunorubicin (Cerubidine) or mitoxantrone (Novantrone) or idarubicin (Idamycin);

sometimes etoposide (VP-16, VePesid) is added to the regimen. The choice of agents is based on the patient's physical status and history of prior antineoplastic treatment. Older patients (especially those older than 70 years) tend to not tolerate standard therapy. Lower-intensity therapy (using low doses of cytarabine or other agents) may extend survival without significant increase in toxicity (Kantarjian, Thomas, Dmoszynska, et al., 2012).

Treatment of APL revolves around induction therapy using the differentiating agent all-trans retinoic acid (ATRA), which induces the promyelocytic blast cells to differentiate, thereby deterring the blasts from proliferating. ATRA is typically combined with a conventional chemotherapeutic agent, usually an anthracycline drug. This regimen yields a very high response rate, and cure is possible (Stein & Tallman, 2012).

The aim of induction therapy is to eradicate the leukemic cells; however, this is also accompanied by the eradication of normal types of myeloid cells. Thus, the patient becomes severely neutropenic (an **absolute neutrophil count** [ANC; a precise calculation of the number of circulating neutrophils] of 0 is not uncommon), anemic, and thrombocytopenic (a platelet count of less than 5,000/mm³ is common). During this time, the patient is typically very ill, with bacterial, fungal, and occasionally viral infections; bleeding; and severe mucositis, which causes diarrhea and an inability to maintain adequate nutrition. Management consists of administering blood products (packed red blood cells [PRBCs] and platelets) and promptly treating infections. The use of granulocytic growth factors, either granulocyte colony-stimulating factor (G-CSF; filgrastim [Neupogen]) or granulocyte-macrophage colony-stimulating factor (GM-CSF; sargramostim [Leukine]), can shorten the period of significant neutropenia by stimulating the bone marrow to produce leukocytes more quickly; these agents do not appear to increase the risk of producing more leukemic cells (NCI, 2012a).

When the patient has recovered from the induction therapy (i.e., the neutrophil and platelet counts have returned to normal and any infection has resolved), consolidation, (post-remission) therapy is administered to eliminate any residual leukemia cells that are not clinically detectable and reduce the chance for recurrence. Multiple treatment cycles of various agents are used, usually containing some form of cytarabine. Frequently, the patient receives one cycle of treatment that is almost the same as, if not identical to, the induction treatment but at lower dosages, therefore resulting in less toxicity (Burnett, 2012).

Another aggressive treatment option is hematopoietic stem cell transplantation (HSCT). When a suitable tissue match can be obtained, the patient embarks on an even more aggressive regimen of chemotherapy (sometimes in combination with radiation therapy), with the treatment goal of destroying the hematopoietic function of the patient's bone marrow. The patient is then "rescued" with the infusion of the donor stem cells to reinitiate blood cell production. Patients who undergo HSCT have a significant risk of infection, graft-versus-host disease (in which the donor's lymphocytes [graft] recognize the patient's body as "foreign" and set up reactions to attack the foreign host), and other complications. The most appropriate use and timing of HSCT remain unclear. Patients with a poorer prognosis may benefit from early HSCT; those with a good prognosis may not need transplant at all. (See Chapter 15 for a discussion of nursing management in HSCT.)

Another important option for the patient to consider is supportive care alone. In fact, supportive care may be the only option if the patient has significant comorbidity, such as extremely poor cardiac, pulmonary, renal, or hepatic function, and/or is older and frail. In such cases, aggressive antileukemia therapy is not used; occasionally, hydroxyurea (Hydrea) or low-doses of cytarabine may be used briefly to control the increase of blast cells. Patients are more commonly supported with antimicrobial therapy and transfusions as needed. This treatment approach provides the patient with some additional time outside the hospital; however, death frequently occurs within months, typically from infection or bleeding. (Refer to Chapter 16 for a discussion of end-of-life care.)

Complications

Complications of AML include bleeding and infection, which are the major causes of death. The risk of bleeding correlates with the level and duration of platelet deficiency (**thrombocytopenia**). The low platelet count can cause ecchymoses (bruises) and petechiae. Major hemorrhages also may develop when the platelet count drops to less than 10,000/mm³. The most common bleeding sources include gastrointestinal (GI), pulmonary, vaginal, and intracranial. For undetermined reasons, fever and infection also increase the likelihood of bleeding. DIC is common, particularly in patients with APL (Franchini et al., 2010). A very high WBC count (greater than $100,000 \times 10^9/L$) can cause stasis within the cerebral or pulmonary circulation.

Because of the lack of mature and normal granulocytes that help fight infection, patients with leukemia are prone to infection. The likelihood of infection increases with the degree and duration of neutropenia; neutrophil counts that persist at less than 100/mm³ dramatically increase the risk of systemic infections. As the duration of severe neutropenia increases, the patient's risk of developing fungal infections also increases. Fungal infections remain difficult to treat despite the development of new antifungal agents, particularly if the patient has persistent neutropenia (Neofytos, Lu, Hatfield-Seung, et al., 2013).

Massive leukemic cell destruction from chemotherapy results in the release of intracellular electrolytes and fluids into the systemic circulation. Increases in uric acid levels, potassium, and phosphate are seen; this process is referred to as tumor **lysis** (cell destruction) syndrome (see Chapter 15). The increased uric acid and phosphorus levels make the patient vulnerable to renal stone formation and renal colic, which can progress to acute renal failure. Hyperkalemia and hypocalcemia can lead to cardiac dysrhythmias; hypotension; neuromuscular effects such as muscle cramps, weakness, and spasm/tetany; confusion; and seizures. Patients require a high fluid intake, and prophylaxis with allopurinol (Zyloprim) to prevent crystallization of uric acid and subsequent stone formation. If necessary, uric acid degradation can be promoted by the administration of the enzyme rasburicase (Elitek) (Cortes, Moore, Maziarz, et al., 2010).

GI problems may result from the infiltration of abnormal leukocytes into the abdominal organs and from the toxicity of the chemotherapeutic agents. Anorexia, nausea, vomiting, diarrhea, and severe mucositis are common. Because of the profound myelosuppressive effects of chemotherapy, significant neutropenia and thrombocytopenia typically result in serious infection and increased risk of bleeding.

Nursing Management

Nursing management of the patient with acute leukemia is presented at the end of the discussion of leukemia in this chapter.

Chronic Myeloid Leukemia

Chronic myeloid leukemia (CML) arises from a mutation in the myeloid stem cell. Normal myeloid cells continue to be produced, but there is a pathologic increase in the production of forms of blast cells. Therefore, a wide spectrum of cell types exists within the blood, from blast forms to mature neutrophils. Because there is an uncontrolled proliferation of cells, the marrow expands into the cavities of long bones, such as the femur, and cells are also formed in the liver and spleen (extramedullary hematopoiesis), resulting in enlargement of these organs that is sometimes painful. In 90% to 95% of patients with CML, a section of deoxyribonucleic acid (DNA) is missing from chromosome 22 (the Philadelphia chromosome [Ph1]); it is translocated onto chromosome 9 (Gambacorti-Passerini, Antolini, Mahon, et al., 2011). The specific location of these changes is on the BCR gene on chromosome 22 and the ABL gene on chromosome 9. When these two genes fuse (BCR-ABL gene), they produce an abnormal protein (a tyrosine kinase protein) that causes leukocytes to divide rapidly. This BCR-ABL gene is present in virtually all patients with this disease (American Cancer Society [ACS], 2013).

CML accounts for 10% to 15% of all leukemias; it is uncommon in people younger than 20 years; the incidence increases with age (mean age is 65 years) (ACS, 2013). Due to marked advances in treatment, patients diagnosed with CML in the chronic phase have an overall median life expectancy well exceeding 5 years; in one multicenter study, those patients who were in complete cytogenetic remission from treatment had no difference in survival compared to the general population (Gambacorti-Passerini et al., 2011). During the chronic phase, patients have few symptoms and complications from the disease itself and problems with infections and bleeding are rare. However, if the disease transforms to the acute phase (blast crisis), the disease becomes more difficult to treat.

Clinical Manifestations

The clinical picture of CML varies. Patients may be asymptomatic, and leukocytosis is detected by a CBC performed for some other reason. The leukocyte count commonly exceeds 100,000/mm^3. Patients with extremely high leukocyte counts may be short of breath or slightly confused because of decreased perfusion to the lungs and brain from leukostasis (the excessive volume of leukocytes inhibits blood flow through the capillaries). The patient may have an enlarged, tender spleen, and occasionally the liver may also be enlarged and tender. Some patients have insidious symptoms, such as malaise, anorexia, and weight loss. Lymphadenopathy is rare. There are three stages in CML: chronic, transformation, and accelerated or blast crisis. Patients develop more symptoms and complications as the disease progresses.

Medical Management

Advances in understanding the pathology of CML at a molecular level have led to dramatic changes in treatment. An oral formulation of a tyrosine kinase inhibitor, imatinib mesylate (Gleevec), works by blocking signals within the leukemia cells that express the BCR-ABL protein, thus preventing a series of chemical reactions that cause the cell to grow and divide. Imatinib therapy appears to be most useful in the chronic phase of the illness. It can induce complete remission at the cellular and even molecular level. Imatinib is metabolized by the cytochrome P450 pathway, which means that drug–drug interactions are common. In particular, antacids and grapefruit juice may limit drug absorption, and large doses of acetaminophen can cause hepatotoxicity. Other tyrosine kinase inhibitors (dasatinib [Sprycel] or nilotinib [Tasigna]) are also approved for primary therapy; each has a slightly (but importantly) different toxicity profile. For instance, dasatinib is very myelosuppressive, and its use carries a significant risk for pleural effusion and for causing a prolonged QT interval; nilotinib has more cardiotoxic effects, including dysrhythmias and risk for sudden death (Tinsley, 2010).

In those instances where imatinib (at conventional doses) does not elicit a molecular remission, or when that remission is not maintained, other treatment options may be considered. The dosage of imatinib can be increased (with increased toxicity), or another inhibitor of BCR-ABL (e.g., dasatinib or nilotinib) or HSCT can be used.

CML is a disease that can potentially be cured with HSCT in otherwise healthy patients who are younger than 65 years. However, with the development of tyrosine kinase inhibitors, the timing of transplant has come into question. Patients who receive such transplants while still in the chronic phase of the illness tend to have a greater chance for cure than those who receive them in the acute phase. The use of tyrosine kinase therapy may decrease the need for transplantation in CML. (See Chapter 15 for more information on tyrosine kinase inhibitors and HSCT.)

The transformation phase can be insidious or rapid; it marks the process of evolution (or transformation) to the acute form of leukemia (blast crisis). In the transformation phase, the patient may complain of bone pain and may report fevers (without any obvious sign of infection) and weight loss. Even with chemotherapy, the spleen may continue to enlarge. The patient may become more anemic and thrombocytopenic; an increased basophil level is detected by the CBC.

In the acute form of CML (blast crisis), treatment may resemble induction therapy for acute leukemia, using the same medications as for AML or acute lymphocytic leukemia (ALL). Patients whose disease evolves into a "lymphoid" blast crisis are more likely to be able to reenter a chronic phase after induction therapy. For those whose disease evolves into AML, therapy has been largely ineffective in achieving a second chronic phase. However, an increased dose of imatinib or dasatinib can be effective in the later stages of CML. Life-threatening infections and bleeding occur frequently in this phase.

In rare instances, when a purely palliative approach is desired, the therapeutic approach focuses on reducing the leukocyte count to a more normal level but does not alter cytogenetic changes. This goal can be achieved by using oral chemotherapeutic agents, typically hydroxyurea or busulfan (Myleran). In the case of an extreme leukocytosis at diagnosis (e.g., leukocyte count greater than 300,000/mm^3), a more emergent treatment may be required. In this instance, leukapheresis (in which the patient's blood is removed and separated, with the leukocytes withdrawn and the remaining blood returned to the patient) can temporarily reduce the number of leukocytes. An anthracycline chemotherapeutic agent (e.g., daunorubicin [Cerubidine]) may also be used to bring the leukocyte count down quickly to a safer level, where more conservative therapy can then be instituted.

Nursing Management

Advances in treatment of CML have changed the trajectory of the disease, from life threatening and likely fatal to being a chronic illness. However, nurses need to understand that the effectiveness of the drugs used to treat CML is based on the ability of the patient to adhere to the medication regimen as prescribed. For example, one study found that response to treatment was not achieved when adherence to taking the medication was less than 80% (Marin, Bazeos, Mahon, et al., 2010). In another study, patients were found to both unintentionally and intentionally not adhere to their medication regimen, from respectively either forgetting to take a dose or due to side effects of the medication (Eliasson, Clifford, Barber, et al., 2011). Most patients were not informed of the consequences of not taking their medication and did not perceive missing doses as jeopardizing the efficacy of treatment. This highlights the importance of nurses educating patients and assisting them to identify methods that help them remember to take their medication, to manage side effects, and to obtain prescription renewals on time. Furthermore, nurses must encourage patients to raise issues of concern that interfere with their adherence to their prescribed therapy.

Acute Lymphocytic Leukemia

ALL results from an uncontrolled proliferation of immature cells (lymphoblasts) derived from the lymphoid stem cell. The cell of origin is the precursor to the B lymphocyte in approximately 75% of ALL cases; T-lymphocyte ALL occurs in approximately 25% of cases. The *BCR-ABL* translocation (see earlier CML discussion) is found in 20% of ALL blast cells. ALL is most common in young children, with boys affected more often than girls; the peak incidence is 4 years of age. After 15 years of age, it is relatively uncommon, until age 50 when the incidence again rises (Pui, 2010).

ALL is very responsive to treatment; complete remission rates are approximately 85% for adults (ACS, 2010a). Increasing age appears to be associated with diminished survival; the 5-year event-free survival rate is more than 80% for children with ALL but drops to 35% for adults between 20 and 49 years of age and to 25% for adults between 50 and 64 years of age (NCI, 2011). If relapse occurs, resumption of induction therapy can often achieve a second complete remission. Moreover, HSCT may be successful even after a second relapse, particularly in certain subsets of patients (e.g., those with Philadelphia chromosome–positive ALL [Ph+ ALL]).

Clinical Manifestations

Immature lymphocytes proliferate in the marrow and impede the development of normal myeloid cells. As a result, normal hematopoiesis is inhibited, resulting in reduced numbers of granulocytes, erythrocytes, and platelets. Leukocyte counts may be either low or high, but there always is a high proportion of immature cells. Manifestations of leukemic cell infiltration into other organs are more common with ALL than with other forms of leukemia and include pain from an enlarged liver or spleen and bone pain. The CNS is frequently a site for leukemic cells; thus, patients may exhibit cranial nerve palsies or headache and vomiting because of meningeal involvement. Other extranodal sites include the testes and breasts.

Medical Management

The goal of treatment is to obtain remission without excess toxicity and with a rapid hematologic recovery so that additional therapy can be administered if needed. Due to the heterogeneity of the disease, treatment plans are based on genetic markers of the disease as well as risk factors of the patient, primarily age. Because ALL frequently invades the CNS, preventive intrathecal chemotherapy is also a key part of the treatment plan. Cranial irradiation is infrequently used as a preventative measure (Robinson, 2011).

Treatment protocols for ALL tend to be complex, using a wide variety of chemotherapeutic agents and complicated administration schedules. The expected outcome of treatment is complete remission. Lymphoid blast cells are typically very sensitive to corticosteroids and to vinca alkaloids; therefore, these medications are an integral part of the initial induction therapy. The corticosteroid dexamethasone is preferred to prednisone, as it is more toxic to lymphoid cells and has better CNS penetration (Bassan & Hoelzer, 2011). Typically, an anthracycline is included, sometimes with asparaginase (Elspar). Once a patient is in remission, special testing (immunophenotyping, immunoglobulin gene rearrangements, T-cell receptor genes, molecular testing) is done to look for residual leukemia cells; these tests can detect as little as one ALL cell among 10,000 to 100,000 normal cells. This minimal residual disease testing is useful as a prognostic indicator. Based on these results and the rapidity in which remission is achieved, a consolidation regimen ensues, using different combinations and dosages of the drugs used in induction therapy; the goal of consolidation is to improve outcomes in those patients at high risk for relapse. If relapse occurs, the goal is to reinitiate treatment to again obtain a remission and then move quickly to HSCT (Campana, 2010).

In the adult with ALL, the role of HSCT is controversial, however. When feasible, HSCT may be used for intensification therapy. Transplantation can improve long-term disease-free survival, although the risks of death or long-term morbidity are associated with the procedure. More frequently, transplantation is reserved for patients whose disease relapses after chemotherapy or those who are at high risk for relapse.

Despite its complexity, treatment can be provided in the outpatient setting in some circumstances until severe complications develop. Tyrosine kinase inhibitors (e.g., imatinib) appear effective in patients with Ph+ ALL; these can be used alone or in combination with conventional chemotherapy. Monoclonal antibodies, in which the antibody specific to the antigen expressed on the ALL blast cell is selected for treatment, are also under study (Bassan & Hoelzer, 2011).

Patients with ALL can experience some unique adverse effects from treatment. The use of corticosteroids to treat ALL increases the patient's susceptibility to infection; viral infections are common. Avascular necrosis can occur in patients treated with corticosteroid-based chemotherapy, as well as with transplantation. Patients treated with asparaginase are at increased risk for thrombosis. Hepatic toxicity is also common and may necessitate cessation of supportive drugs, such as proton pump inhibitors and certain antibacterial and antifungal drugs. However, patients with ALL tend to have a better response to treatment than do patients with AML (NCI, 2012a, 2012b).

Nursing Management

Nursing management of the patient with acute leukemia is presented at the end of the leukemia section in this chapter.

Chronic Lymphocytic Leukemia

CLL is a common malignancy of older adults; the average age at diagnosis is 72 years (ACS, 2010b). CLL is the most common form of leukemia in the United States and Europe, affecting more than 120,000 people. It is rarely seen in Native Americans and infrequently among persons of Asian descent. A family history of CLL may be the most important risk factor for developing the disease (Lanasa, 2010). Veterans of the Vietnam War who were exposed to Agent Orange may be at risk for developing this disease, but there is no definitive link to other pesticides or chemical exposure (ACS, 2010b). On average, most patients with CLL survive more than 20 years, although some patients may survive for shorter time periods (e.g., 2 to 4 years) (Parker & Strout, 2011).

Pathophysiology

CLL is typically derived from a malignant clone of B lymphocytes (T-lymphocyte CLL is rare). In contrast to the acute forms of leukemia, most leukemia cells in CLL are fully mature. One possible mechanism that can explain this oncogenesis is that these cells can escape **apoptosis** (programmed cell death), resulting in an excessive accumulation of the cells in the marrow and circulation. The disease is classified into three or four stages (two classification systems are in use). In the early stage, an elevated lymphocyte count is seen; it can exceed 100,000/mm³.

Because the lymphocytes are small, they can easily travel through the small capillaries within the circulation, and the pulmonary and cerebral complications of leukocytosis (as seen with myeloid leukemias) are not typically found in CLL. However, when it takes less than 12 months for the absolute number of lymphocytes to double (lymphocyte doubling time), a more aggressive disease course may ensue.

More sophisticated prognostic markers (i.e., tests that gauge the overall prognosis) are now used for patients with CLL. Beta-2 microglobulin, a protein found on the surface of lymphocytes, can be measured in the serum; an elevated level correlates with more advanced clinical stage and poorer prognosis. Immunophenotyping not only helps establish the diagnosis but also the prognosis; other special cytogenetic analyses (e.g., fluorescence in situ hybridization [FISH]) are also used to guide prognosis and therapy.

Autoimmune complications can occur at any stage, as either autoimmune hemolytic anemia or idiopathic thrombocytopenic purpura. In the autoimmune process, the reticuloendothelial system destroys the body's own erythrocytes or platelets. Patients with CLL also have a greater risk for developing other cancers, typically bone, lung, and skin. Roughly 10% of patients will experience a gradual transformation of their disease to one that becomes refractory to chemotherapy (prolymphocytoid transformation). Slightly fewer patients will experience a sudden transformation to a very aggressive lymphoma (Richter's transformation) markedly increased lymphadenopathy, splenomegaly, worsening B symptoms (fever, night sweats, weight loss), average survival only 6 months (Sagatys & Zhang, 2012).

Clinical Manifestations

Many patients are asymptomatic and are diagnosed incidentally during routine physical examinations or during treatment for another disease. An increased lymphocyte count (lymphocytosis) is always present. The erythrocyte and platelet counts may be normal or, in later stages of the illness, decreased. Enlargement of lymph nodes (lymphadenopathy) is common; this can be severe and sometimes painful (Fig. 34-4). The spleen can also be enlarged (splenomegaly).

Patients with CLL can develop "B symptoms," a constellation of symptoms including fevers, drenching sweats (especially at night), and unintentional weight loss. T-cell function is impaired and may be the cause of tumor progression and increased susceptibility to second malignancies and infections (Lanasa, 2010). Life-threatening infections are particularly common with advanced disease. Viral infections, such as herpes zoster, can become widely disseminated. Defects in the complement system are also seen, which results in increased risk of developing infection with encapsulated organisms (e.g., *Haemophilus influenzae*).

Medical Management

A major paradigm shift has occurred in CLL therapy. In the past, there appeared to be no survival advantage in treating CLL in its early stages. However, with the advent of newer treatment modalities and of more sensitive means of determining prognosis, achieving a complete remission and eradicating even minimal residual disease results in improved survival (Gibben & O'Brien, 2011). As a result, treatment may be initiated sooner in the illness trajectory; clinical trials are ongoing to assess for an advantage in survival with this approach.

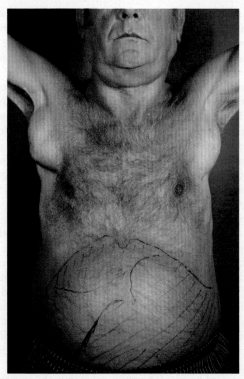

FIGURE 34-4 • Massive lymphadenopathy in a patient with chronic lymphocytic leukemia. Note the enlarged liver and spleen as well. From Tkachuk, D. C., & Hirschman, J. V. (2007). *Wintrobe's atlas of clinical hematology* (p. 154, Fig. 5.1). Philadelphia: Lippincott Williams & Wilkins.

If treatment is not initiated early in the course of the illness, it can begin when symptoms are severe (drenching night sweats, painful lymphadenopathy) or when the disease progresses to later stages (with resultant anemia and thrombocytopenia).

The chemotherapy agents fludarabine (Fludara) and cyclophosphamide (Cytoxan) are often given in combination with the monoclonal antibody rituximab (Rituxan). This regimen can result in remission that lasts for 5 years in 70% of patients (Gibben & O'Brien, 2011). The major side effect of fludarabine is prolonged bone marrow suppression, manifested by prolonged periods of neutropenia, lymphopenia, and thrombocytopenia, which puts patients at risk for such infections as *Pneumocystis jiroveci*, *Listeria*, mycobacteria, herpes viruses, and cytomegalovirus. Another alkylating agent, bendamustine (Trenda) is also effective, particularly when combined with rituximab (Gibben & O'Brien, 2011). The monoclonal antibody alemtuzumab (Campath) is often used in combination with other chemotherapeutic agents when the disease is refractory to fludarabine, the patient has very poor prognostic markers, or it is necessary to eradicate residual disease after initial treatment. Alemtuzumab targets the CD52 antigen commonly found on CLL cells, and it is effective in clearing the marrow and circulation of these cells without affecting the stem cells. Because CD52 is present on both B and T lymphocytes, patients receiving alemtuzumab are at significant risk for infection; prophylactic use of antiviral agents and antibiotics (e.g., trimethoprim–sulfamethoxazole [Bactrim, Septra]) is important and needs to continue for several months after treatment ends. Bacterial infections are common in patients with CLL, and intravenous treatment with immunoglobulin may be given to selected patients with recurrent infection.

The role of HSCT is unclear. Due to the older age of most patients with CLL, transplantation may not be an option, particularly if significant comorbidities exist. The efficacy of transplantation in patients with a specific cytogenetic abnormality (del 17p) is being evaluated in clinical studies (Gibben & O'Brien, 2011).

NURSING PROCESS

The Patient With Acute Leukemia

Assessment

Although the clinical picture varies with the type of leukemia as well as with the treatment implemented, the health history may reveal a range of subtle symptoms reported by the patient before the problem is detectable on physical examination. If the patient is hospitalized, assessments should be performed daily, or more frequently as warranted. Because the physical findings may be subtle initially, a thorough, systematic assessment incorporating all body systems is essential. For example, a dry cough, mild dyspnea, and diminished breath sounds may indicate a pulmonary infection. However, the infection may not be seen initially on the chest x-ray; the absence of neutrophils delays the inflammatory response against the pulmonary infection, thus delaying radiographic changes. When serial assessments are performed, current findings are compared with previous findings to evaluate improvement or worsening. Specific body system assessments are delineated in the neutropenic and bleeding precautions found in Chart 15–7 in Chapter 15.

The nurse also must closely monitor the results of laboratory studies. Flow sheets and spreadsheets are particularly useful in tracking the leukocyte count, ANC, hematocrit, platelet, creatinine and electrolyte levels, and coagulation and hepatic function tests. Culture results need to be reported immediately so that appropriate antimicrobial therapy can begin or be modified.

Diagnosis

Nursing Diagnoses

Based on the assessment data, major nursing diagnoses may include:

- Risk for infection and/or bleeding
- Risk for impaired skin integrity related to toxic effects of chemotherapy, alteration in nutrition, and impaired mobility
- Impaired gas exchange
- Impaired tissue integrity related to damaged mucous membranes due to changes in epithelial lining of the GI tract from chemotherapy or prolonged use of antimicrobial medications
- Imbalanced nutrition: less than body requirements related to hypermetabolic state, anorexia, mucositis, pain, and nausea
- Acute pain and discomfort related to mucositis, leukocyte infiltration of systemic tissues, fever, and infection
- Hyperthermia related to tumor lysis or infection
- Fatigue and activity intolerance related to anemia, infection, inadequate nutrition, and deconditioning

- Impaired physical mobility due to anemia, malaise, discomfort, and protective isolation
- Risk for excess fluid volume related to renal dysfunction, hypoproteinemia, and need for multiple intravenous medications and blood products
- Diarrhea due to altered GI flora, mucosal denudation, and prolonged use of broad-spectrum antibiotics and chemotherapy agents
- Risk for deficient fluid volume related to potential for diarrhea, bleeding, infection, and increased metabolic rate
- Self-care deficit due to fatigue, malaise, and protective isolation/prolonged hospitalization
- Anxiety due to knowledge deficit and uncertainty about future
- Disturbed body image related to change in appearance, function, and roles
- Grieving related to anticipatory loss and altered role functioning
- Risk for spiritual distress
- Deficient knowledge about disease process, treatment, complication management, and self-care measures

Collaborative Problems/Potential Complications

Potential complications may include the following:

- Infection
- Bleeding/DIC
- Renal dysfunction
- Tumor lysis syndrome
- Nutritional depletion
- Mucositis
- Depression and anxiety

Planning and Goals

The major goals for the patient may include absence of complications and pain, attainment and maintenance of adequate nutrition, activity tolerance, ability to provide self-care and to cope with the diagnosis and prognosis, positive body image, and an understanding of the disease process and its treatment.

Nursing Interventions

Preventing or Managing Infection and Bleeding

The nursing interventions related to diminishing the risk of infection and bleeding are delineated in Chart 15-7 in Chapter 15.

Managing Mucositis

Although emphasis is placed on the oral mucosa, the entire GI mucosa can be altered, not only by the effects of chemotherapy but also from prolonged administration of antibiotics. (See Chapter 15 for assessment and management of mucositis.)

Improving Nutritional Intake

The disease process can increase the patient's metabolic rate and nutritional requirements. Nutritional intake is often reduced because of pain and discomfort associated with stomatitis. Encouraging or providing mouth care before and after meals and administering analgesic agents before eating can help increase intake. If oral anesthetic agents are used, the patient must be warned to chew with extreme care to avoid inadvertently biting the tongue or buccal mucosa.

Nausea should not interfere with nutritional intake, because appropriate antiemetic therapy is highly effective. However, nausea can result from antimicrobial therapy, so some antiemetic therapy may still be required after the chemotherapy has been completed.

Small, frequent feedings of foods that are soft in texture and moderate in temperature may be better tolerated. Low-microbial diets may be prescribed (avoiding uncooked fruits or vegetables and those without a peelable skin), although there is little evidence to support this intervention (Jubelirer, 2011). Nutritional supplements are frequently used. Daily body weight (as well as intake and output measurements) is useful in monitoring fluid status. Both calorie counts and more formal nutritional assessments are useful. Parenteral nutrition may be required to maintain adequate nutrition.

Easing Pain and Discomfort

Recurrent fevers are common in acute leukemia; at times, they are accompanied by shaking chills (rigors), which can be severe. Myalgias and arthralgias can result. Acetaminophen (Tylenol) is typically given to decrease fever, but it also increases diaphoresis. Sponging with cool water may be useful, but cold water or ice packs should be avoided because the heat cannot dissipate from constricted blood vessels. Bedclothes need frequent changing as well. Gentle back and shoulder massage may provide comfort.

Mucositis can also cause significant discomfort. In addition to oral hygiene practices, patient-controlled analgesia can be effective in controlling the pain (see Chapter 12). With the exception of severe mucositis, less pain is associated with acute leukemia than with many other forms of cancer. However, the amount of psychological suffering that the patient must endure can be immense. Patients often benefit from active listening and possible referral for professional counseling.

Because patients with acute leukemia require hospitalization for extensive nursing care (either during induction or consolidation therapy or during resultant complications), sleep deprivation frequently results. Nurses need to implement creative strategies that permit uninterrupted sleep for at least a few hours while still administering necessary medications on time.

Decreasing Fatigue and Deconditioning

Fatigue is a common and oppressive symptom. Nursing interventions should focus on assisting the patient to establish a balance between activity and rest. Patients with acute leukemia need to maintain some physical activity and exercise to prevent the deconditioning that results from inactivity. The use of a high-efficiency particulate air (HEPA) filter mask can permit the patient to ambulate outside the room despite severe neutropenia. Stationary bicycles may also be set up in the room; however, many patients lack the motivation or stamina to use them. At a minimum, patients should be encouraged to sit up in a chair while awake rather than staying in bed; even this simple activity can improve the patient's tidal volume and enhance circulation. Physical therapy can also be beneficial.

Maintaining Fluid and Electrolyte Balance

Febrile episodes, bleeding, and inadequate or overly aggressive fluid replacement can alter the patient's fluid status. Similarly, persistent diarrhea, vomiting, and long-term use of certain antimicrobial agents can cause significant deficits in electrolytes. Intake and output need to be measured accurately, and daily weights should also be monitored. The patient should be assessed for signs of dehydration as well as fluid overload, with particular attention to pulmonary status and the development of dependent edema. Laboratory test results, particularly electrolytes, blood urea nitrogen, creatinine, and hematocrit, should be monitored and compared with previous results. Replacement of electrolytes, particularly potassium and magnesium, is commonly required. Patients receiving amphotericin or certain antibiotics are at increased risk for electrolyte depletion.

Improving Self-Care

Because hygiene measures are so important in this patient population, they must be performed by the nurse when the patient cannot do so. However, the patient should be encouraged to do as much as possible to preserve mobility and function as well as self-esteem. Patients may have negative feelings because they can no longer care for themselves. Empathetic listening is helpful, as is realistic reassurance that these deficits are temporary. As the patient recovers, the nurse assists him or her to resume more self-care. Patients are usually discharged from the hospital with a vascular access device (e.g., Hickman catheter, peripherally inserted central catheter [PICC]), and coordination with appropriate home care services is needed for catheter management.

Managing Anxiety and Grief

Being diagnosed with acute leukemia can be extremely frightening. In many instances, the need to begin treatment is emergent, and the patient has little time to process the fact that he or she has the illness before making decisions about therapy. Providing emotional support and discussing the uncertain future are crucial. The nurse also needs to assess how much information the patient wants to have regarding the illness, its treatment, and potential complications. This desire should be reassessed at intervals, because needs and interest in information change throughout the course of the disease and treatment. Priorities must be identified so that procedures, assessments, and self-care expectations are adequately explained even to those who do not wish extensive information.

Many patients exhibit depressive symptoms and begin to grieve for their losses, such as normal family functioning, professional roles and responsibilities, and social roles, as well as physical functioning. The nurse can assist the patient to identify the source of the grief and encourage him or her to allow time to adjust to the major life changes produced by the illness. Role restructuring, in both family and professional life, may be required. Again, when possible, encouraging the patient to identify options and to take time making important decisions is helpful.

Discharge from the hospital can also provoke anxiety. Although most patients are eager to go home, they may lack confidence in their ability to manage potential complications and to resume their normal activity. Close communication between nurses across care settings can reassure patients that they will not be abandoned.

Encouraging Spiritual Well-Being

Because acute leukemia is a serious, potentially life-threatening illness, the nurse may offer support to enhance the patient's spiritual well-being. The patient's spiritual and religious practices should be assessed and pastoral services offered. Throughout the patient's illness, the nurse assists the patient to maintain hope. However, that hope should be realistic and will certainly change over the course of the illness. For example, the patient may initially hope to be cured, but with repeated relapses and a change to hospice or palliative care, the same patient may hope for a quiet, dignified death. (Refer to Chapter 16 for a discussion of end-of-life care.)

Promoting Home and Community-Based Care

Educating Patients About Self-Care. Most patients cope better when they understand what is happening to them. Based on their literacy level, and interest, educating the patient and family should begin with a focus on the disease (including some pathophysiology), its treatment, and certainly the resulting significant risk of infection and bleeding (see Chapter Charts 33-7 and 33-8 in Chapter 33).

Although management of a vascular access device can be taught to most patients or family members, this care is typically performed by a home care agency or outpatient clinic nursing staff. Patients and family members do need basic education regarding management of the vascular access device, particularly with regard to prevention of infections.

Continuing Care. Shortened lengths of hospital stay and outpatient care have significantly altered care for patients with acute leukemia. In many instances, when the patient is clinically stable but still requires parenteral antibiotics or blood products, these procedures can be performed in an outpatient setting. Nurses in these various settings must communicate regularly. They need to inform the patient about which parameters are important to monitor, how to monitor them, and to give the patient specific instructions about when to seek care from the physician or other health care provider. The primary provider is often responsible for monitoring the patient who is cured or in sustained remission, and the transition from specialty care to primary care requires careful coordination and sharing of relevant information.

The patient and family need to have a clear understanding of the disease, the prognosis, and how to monitor for complications or recurrence. The nurse ensures that this information is provided. Should the patient no longer respond to therapy, it is important to respect the patient's choices about treatment, including measures to prolong life and other end-of-life measures. Advance directives, including living wills, provide patients with some measure of control during terminal illness.

Most patients in this stage choose to be cared for at home, and families often need support when considering this option. Coordination of home care services and instruction can help alleviate anxiety about managing the patient's care in the home. As the patient becomes weaker, the caregivers must assume more of the patient's care. In addition, caregivers often need to be encouraged to take care of themselves, allowing time for rest and accepting emotional support (Chart 34-1). Hospice staff can assist in providing respite for family members as well as care for the patient. Patients and families also need assistance to cope with changes in their roles and responsibilities. Anticipatory grieving is an essential task during this time (see Chapter 16).

In patients with acute leukemia, death typically occurs from infection or bleeding. Family members need to have information about these complications and the measures to take should

NURSING RESEARCH PROFILE

Chart 34-1

Expressed Needs of Family Caregivers for Patients With Leukemia

Tamayo, G., Broxson, A., Munsell, M., et al. (2010). Caring for the caregiver. *Oncology Nursing Forum*, *37*(1), E50–E57.

Purpose

With changing health care delivery systems, care is delivered in the outpatient setting with increasing frequency, leaving the patient and caregiver to manage many aspects of illness and treatment at home. Although some studies have explored the physical and emotional demands placed on caregivers of patients with other illnesses, caregivers of patients with leukemia have not yet been studied. The purpose of this descriptive cross-sectional study was (1) to describe the quality of life and well-being of caregivers of leukemia patients receiving chemotherapy treatment in the outpatient setting and (2) to identify strategies to promote quality of life and well-being for the caregiver.

Design

A convenience sample of 194 caregivers was asked to complete the following questionnaires: Caregiver Quality-of-Life Cancer Scale (measuring burden, disruptiveness, financial concerns, and positive adaptation), Caregiver Well-Being Scale (measuring attendance to physical needs, expression of feelings, self-security, and requisite activities of living [household tasks and maintenance, family support, time for self or leisure activities, maintenance of functions outside the home]), and an investigator-developed Learning Needs Questionnaire (e.g., medication administration, managing medication-related side effects, and other symptoms).

Results

Participants were primarily middle-aged female spouses of patients with cancer, many of whom were working outside the home (43%). Burden was the highest concern, followed by disruptiveness. Expression of feelings, attendance to physical needs, household maintenance, and family support were all identified as important factors of caregiver well-being. Receiving additional education regarding medication and relevant side effects and symptoms of disease were all rated as very important by more than 70% of the sample. Responding to an open-ended question asking what nurses could do to improve caregivers' quality of life elicited five themes: communication, improved schedule coordination, ensure family has adequate support, provide education, and demonstrate a positive attitude and compassion.

Nursing Implications

This study highlights the importance of addressing caregiver needs—educational, psychological, and pragmatic—so that their quality of life and sense of well-being might be enhanced. Like the patient, caregivers have significant educational needs, particularly regarding symptom management and medication administration. Meeting these needs is crucial so that caregivers can better assist patients in managing the complex care involved in living with leukemia.

---

either occur. Many family members cannot cope with the care required when a patient begins to bleed actively. It is important to delineate alternatives to keeping the patient at home, such as inpatient hospice units. Should another option be sought, family members who may feel guilty that they could not keep the patient at home will require support from the nurse.

Evaluation

Expected patient outcomes may include:

1. Shows no evidence of infection
2. Experiences no bleeding
3. Has intact oral mucous membranes
    a. Participates in oral hygiene regimen
    b. Reports no discomfort in mouth
4. Attains optimal level of nutrition
    a. Maintains weight with increased food and fluid intake
    b. Maintains adequate protein stores (e.g., albumin, prealbumin)
5. Reports satisfaction with pain and comfort levels
6. Has less fatigue and increased activity
7. Maintains fluid and electrolyte balance
8. Participates in self-care
9. Copes with anxiety and grief
    a. Discusses concerns and fears
    b. Uses stress management strategies appropriately
    c. Participates in decisions regarding end-of-life care (as appropriate)
    d. Discusses hope for peaceful death (as appropriate)
10. Absence of complications

MYELODYSPLASTIC SYNDROMES

The MDS are a group of clonal disorders of the myeloid stem cell that cause dysplasia (abnormal development) in one or more types of cell lines. The most common feature of MDS—dysplasia of the erythrocytes—is manifested as a macrocytic anemia; however, the leukocytes (myeloid cells, particularly neutrophils) and platelets can also be affected. Although the bone marrow is actually hypercellular, many of the cells within it die before being released into the circulation. Therefore, the actual number of cells in the circulation is typically lower than normal. In MDS, the cells do not function normally. The neutrophils have diminished ability to destroy bacteria by **phagocytosis**; platelets are less able to aggregate and are less adhesive than usual. The result of these defects is an increased risk of infection and bleeding, even when the actual number of circulating cells may not be excessively low.

Primary MDS tends to be a disease of people older than 70 years. Because the initial findings are so subtle, the disease may not be diagnosed until later in the illness trajectory, if at all. Thus, the actual incidence of MDS is not known. Thirty percent of cases evolve into AML; this type of leukemia tends to be resistant to standard therapy (Shukron, Vainstein, Kündgen, et al., 2012).

Secondary MDS can occur at any age and results from prior toxic exposure to chemicals, including chemotherapeutic medications (particularly alkylating agents or topoisomerase inhibitors). Secondary MDS has a poorer prognosis than does primary MDS, as it tends to be resistant to treatment, has more cytogenetic abnormalities associated with it, and evolves into AML more frequently (Bhatia & Deeg, 2011).

Clinical Manifestations

The manifestations of MDS can vary widely. Many patients are asymptomatic, with the illness being discovered incidentally when a CBC is performed for other purposes. Other patients have profound symptoms and complications from the illness. Fatigue is often present, with varying levels of intensity and frequency. Neutrophil dysfunction puts the person at risk for recurrent pneumonias and other infections. Because platelet function can also be altered, bleeding can occur. These problems may persist in a fairly steady state for months, even years. Over time, the marrow may fail to provide enough cells that can be supported with transfusion or growth factors; this is called *bone marrow failure*. MDS may also progress over time; as the dysplasia evolves into a leukemic state, the complications increase in severity.

Assessment and Diagnostic Findings

The CBC typically reveals a macrocytic anemia; leukocyte and platelet counts may be diminished as well. Serum erythropoietin levels and the reticulocyte count may be inappropriately low. If the disease evolves into AML, more immature blast cells are noted on the CBC.

The official diagnosis of MDS is based on the results of a bone marrow aspiration and biopsy. The clinical trajectory of these syndromes varies widely; thus, the nurse must understand the risk stratification category of each patient. Those patients with low-risk disease have a much longer survival (as much as 10 years or more) compared to untreated patients with high-risk disease (where survival is usually less than 12 months) (Garcia-Manero & Fenaux, 2011). Cytogenetic analysis of the bone marrow is important in determining the overall prognosis, risk of evolution into AML, and method of treatment. (See Chapter 32 for discussion of bone marrow biopsy.)

Medical Management

HSCT is the only cure for MDS but is not often a viable option for most patients due to the presence of comorbidity or age. Patients with low-risk disease are often treated with the use of erythroid-stimulating agents (epoetin alfa [Procrit], or darbopoetin alfa [Aranesp]). Lenalidomide (Revlimid) is extremely effective in treating patients who have a specific cytogenetic/chromosomal abnormality (e.g., the deletion of 5q). Traditionally, chemotherapy has been used, particularly in patients with more aggressive forms of the illness, although with disappointing results (Garcia-Manero & Fenaux, 2011). Patients frequently need repeated transfusions (red blood cells [RBCs], platelets, or both) throughout the illness trajectory to maintain adequate hemoglobin and platelet levels (termed *transfusion dependence*).

In patients with high-risk disease, the goal of treatment is to improve survival and decrease the likelihood that the disease transforms into AML. Azacitidine (Vidaza) and decitabine (Dacogen) have demonstrated utility in meeting these goals; in a key study, azacitidine was shown to delay transformation to AML and to improve transfusion dependence and survival in this group of patients (Fenaux, Mufti, Hellstrom-Lindberg, et al., 2009). Patients with hypocellular marrows may respond well to immunosuppressive therapy using antithymocyte globulin (Garcia-Manero & Fenaux, 2011).

For most patients with MDS, transfusions of RBCs may be required to control the anemia and its symptoms. These patients can develop iron overload from the repeated transfusions; this risk can be diminished with prompt initiation of chelation therapy (see following Nursing Management section). Some patients may require ongoing platelet transfusions to prevent significant bleeding. Over time, these patients often have suboptimal increases in the platelet count after platelets are transfused. Infections need to be managed aggressively and promptly. The administration of G-CSF may be useful in some patients with infections and severe neutropenia, but it is not typically used to prevent infection.

Because MDS tends to occur in older adults, other concurrent chronic health conditions may limit treatment options. Secondary MDS and MDS that evolves into AML tend to be refractory to conventional therapy for leukemia.

Nursing Management

Caring for patients with MDS can be challenging because the illness is unpredictable. As with other hematologic conditions, some patients (especially those with no symptoms) have difficulty perceiving that they have a serious illness that can place them at risk of life-threatening complications. At the other extreme, many patients have tremendous difficulty coping with the uncertain trajectory of the illness and fear that the illness will evolve into AML. Thus, it is important for patients to understand their unique risk of the disease transforming to AML and to recognize that, for most patients, MDS is a chronic illness.

Patients with MDS need extensive education about infection risk, measures to avoid it, signs and symptoms of developing infection, and appropriate actions to take should such symptoms occur. Instruction should also be given regarding the risk of bleeding. They may need assistance in devising strategies to live with recurrent fatigue. Patients with MDS who are hospitalized may require neutropenic precautions.

Laboratory values need to be monitored closely to anticipate the need for transfusion and to determine response to treatment with growth factors. Patients with chronic transfusion requirements often benefit from the insertion of a vascular access device for this purpose. Those individuals receiving chemotherapy need extensive education regarding treatment side effects (and how to manage them) and treatment schedules. Patients receiving growth factors or chelation therapy need instruction about these medications, their side effects, and administration techniques, if self-administered.

Chelation therapy is a process that is used to remove excess iron acquired from chronic transfusions. Iron is bound to the chelating agent and then excreted in the urine. Because chelation therapy removes only a small amount of iron with each treatment, patients with chronic iron overload from RBC transfusions need to continue chelation therapy as long as the iron overload exists, potentially for the rest of their lives.

Renal and liver dysfunction are possible, so serum creatinine and liver function tests should be monitored and the medication held until the laboratory results return to baseline; the medication is typically resumed at a reduced dose. Patients should also have baseline and annual auditory and eye examinations, because hearing loss and visual changes can occur with chelation treatment.

MYELOPROLIFERATIVE NEOPLASMS

Polycythemia Vera

Polycythemia vera (sometimes called *P vera*), or primary **polycythemia**, is a proliferative disorder of the myeloid stem cells. The bone marrow is hypercellular, and the erythrocyte, leukocyte, and platelet counts in the peripheral blood are often elevated. However, erythrocyte elevation predominates; the hematocrit can exceed 60%. This phase can last for an extended period of 10 to 20 years or more (Malak, Labopin, Saint-Martin, et al., 2012). Over time, the spleen resumes its embryonic function of hematopoiesis and enlarges. In some instances, the bone marrow may become fibrotic, with a resultant inability to produce as many cells; this process is referred to as the "burnt out" or "spent" phase of the disease. The disease may then evolve into myeloid metaplasia with myelofibrosis, MDS, or AML; this form of AML is usually refractory to standard treatment. The median age at onset is 65 years and is more common in males than in females. With treatment, median survival exceeds 10 years. Death typically results from thrombosis, hemorrhage, or, more rarely, evolution to AML (Kundranda, Tibes, & Mesa, 2012).

Clinical Manifestations

Patients typically have a ruddy complexion and splenomegaly. Symptoms result from increased blood volume and may include headache, dizziness, tinnitus, fatigue, paresthesias, and blurred vision. Symptoms also result from increased blood viscosity and may include angina, claudication, dyspnea, and thrombophlebitis, particularly if the patient has atherosclerotic blood vessels. For this reason, blood pressure is often elevated. Uric acid may be elevated as well, resulting in gout and renal stone formation. Another common problem is generalized pruritus, which may be caused by histamine release due to an increased number of basophils. Erythromelalgia, a burning sensation in the fingers and toes, may be reported and is only partially relieved by cooling.

Assessment and Diagnostic Findings

Diagnosis is based on an elevated erythrocyte mass, a normal oxygen saturation level, and often an enlarged spleen. Other factors useful in establishing the diagnosis include elevated leukocyte and platelet counts. The erythropoietin level is not as low as would be expected with an elevated hematocrit; it is typically normal or only slightly low. Causes of secondary erythrocytosis should not be present (see later discussion).

The mutation of the enzyme JAK2 causes an erythrocyte hypersensitivity to the effects of erythropoietin. Although a mutation in JAK2 is found in the majority of people with polycythemia vera, it is not specific for the disease. Those with other hematologic disorders (essential thrombocythemia [ET] and myelofibrosis) also have this mutation.

Complications

Patients with polycythemia vera are at increased risk for thromboses that may result in cerebrovascular accidents (strokes) or myocardial infarctions; thrombotic complications are the most common cause of death. Patients older than 60 years of age, or those with concurrent diabetes, hypertension, a prior history of thrombosis, and an elevated platelet count (exceeding 1 million) (Tefferi, 2011). Bleeding is also a complication, possibly because the platelets are often very large and somewhat dysfunctional. The bleeding can be significant and can occur in the form of nosebleeds, ulcers, frank GI bleeding, hematuria, and intracranial hemorrhage.

Medical Management

The objective of management is to reduce the high RBC count and reduce the risk of thrombosis. Phlebotomy is an important part of therapy (Fig. 34-5). It involves removing enough blood (initially 500 mL once or twice weekly) to reduce blood viscosity and to deplete the patient's iron stores, thereby rendering the patient iron deficient and consequently unable to continue to manufacture hemoglobin excessively. Many patients are managed by routine phlebotomy on an intermittent basis, with the target of maintaining the hematocrit less than 45%.

Chemotherapeutic agents (e.g., hydroxyurea) can be used to suppress marrow function, thereby controlling blood counts. Patients receiving hydroxyurea appear to have a lower incidence of thrombotic complications than those treated by phlebotomy alone, but they may have increased risk of developing leukemia (Tefferi & Vainchenker, 2011). Anagrelide (Agrylin), which inhibits platelet aggregation, has been used to control the **thrombocytosis** (abnormally high platelet count) associated with polycythemia vera.

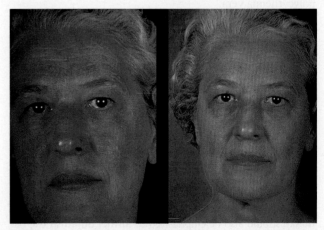

FIGURE 34-5 • Phlebotomy can markedly reduce the plethora seen in polycythemia vera. This is evidenced here by a marked reduction in facial rubor in a patient with polycythemia vera. From Turgeon, M. L. (2012). *Clinical hematology: Theory & procedures* (5th ed., p. 373, Fig. 21.10). Philadelphia: Lippincott Williams & Wilkins.

However, many patients have difficulty tolerating the medication; it can cause significant side effects, including headache, fluid retention, cardiac dysrhythmias, and heart failure. Furthermore, some studies suggest that anagrelide may be leukemogenic (i.e., may cause leukemia) and is associated with increased risk of arterial thromboses and bleeding; thus, its use has declined significantly (Squizzato, Romualdi, & Middeldorp, 2011).

Interferon alfa-2b (Intron) is also very effective in controlling blood counts in this disorder. However, it may be difficult for patients to tolerate because of its frequent side effects (e.g., flulike syndrome, depression) and cost. Currently, it is more commonly used in younger patients or in those whose disease has become resistant to hydroxyurea (Tefferi & Vainchenker, 2011).

Pruritus is very common, occurring in up to 70% of patients with polycythemia vera (Saini, Patnaik & Tefferi, 2010) and is one of the most distressing symptoms of this disease. It is triggered by contact with temperature change, alcohol consumption, or, more typically, exposure to water of any temperature but seems to be worse with exposure to hot water. Antihistamines, including histamine-2 blockers, are not particularly effective in controlling itching (Saini et al., 2010). Interferon alfa-2b is the most effective treatment for managing the pruritus associated with polycythemia vera; selective serotonin uptake inhibitors (e.g., paroxetine) are also effective (Tefferi & Vainchenker, 2011).

The use of aspirin to prevent thrombotic complications is controversial. High-dose aspirin may be associated with an increase in risk of bleeding and no decrease in risk of thrombosis. In contrast, low-dose aspirin decreases the risk of significant thrombotic complications but does not increase the risk of significant bleeding; therefore, it is now recommended as antithrombotic prophylaxis. Aspirin is also useful in reducing the pain associated with erythromelalgia. Aggressive management of atherosclerosis is also important in diminishing the risk of thrombosis, by treating hypertension and hyperlipidemia. Allopurinol (Zyloprim) is used to prevent gouty attacks in patients with elevated uric acid concentrations; such attacks are common in patients with polycythemia vera.

Nursing Management

The nurse's role is primarily that of educator. Risk factors for thrombotic complications, particularly smoking, obesity, and poorly controlled hypertension and diabetes, should be assessed, and the patient should be instructed about the signs and symptoms of thrombosis. To reduce the likelihood of deep vein thrombosis (DVT), sedentary behavior, crossing the legs, and wearing tight or restrictive clothing (particularly stockings) should be discouraged. Patients with a history of significant bleeding are usually advised to avoid high-dose aspirin and aspirin-containing medications, because these medications alter platelet function. Minimizing alcohol intake should also be emphasized to further diminish the risk of bleeding. The patient needs to be instructed to avoid iron supplements, including those within over-the-counter multivitamin supplements, because the iron can further stimulate RBC production. For pruritus, the nurse may recommend bathing in tepid or cool water and avoiding vigorous toweling off after bathing. Cocoa butter or oatmeal-based lotions and bath products or baking soda dissolved in bathwater may also be effective.

Essential Thrombocythemia

ET, also called *primary thrombocythemia*, is a stem cell disorder within the bone marrow. A mutation of the JAK2 protein promotes cell proliferation and resistance to cell death and a hypersensitivity to erythropoietin and thrombopoietin; it is found in 50% of patients with ET (Spivak, 2010). Thus, a marked increase in platelet production occurs, with the platelet count consistently greater than 450,000/mm^3. Platelet size may be abnormal, but platelet survival is typically normal. Occasionally, the increase in platelets (i.e., thrombocythemia) is accompanied by an increase in erythrocytes, leukocytes, or both; however, these cells are not increased to the extent that they are in polycythemia vera, CML, or myelofibrosis.

The exact cause of ET is unknown. Unlike other myeloproliferative disorders, it rarely evolves into acute leukemia. This disease affects women twice as often as men and tends to occur later in life (median age at diagnosis is 65 to 70 years). Survival does not appear to differ from the general population (Tefferi, 2011).

Clinical Manifestations

Many patients with ET are asymptomatic; the illness is diagnosed as the result of finding an elevated platelet count on a CBC. Symptoms occur most often when the platelet count exceeds 1 million/mm^3; however, they do not always correlate with the extent to which the platelet count is elevated. When symptoms do occur, they result primarily from vascular occlusion. This occlusion can occur in large arterial vessels (cerebrovascular, coronary, or peripheral arteries) and deep veins, as well as in the microcirculation. Microvascular vaso-occlusive manifestations are most frequently seen in the form of erythromelalgia. More common forms of venous thromboembolism include DVT and pulmonary embolism.

Headaches are the most common neurologic manifestations; other manifestations include transient ischemic attacks and diplopia. The spleen may also be enlarged but usually not to a significant extent. The toxic effects of platelet substances (e.g., beta-thromboglobulin, platelet factor 4) include painful burning, warmth, and redness in a localized distal area of the extremities.

In addition, because the platelets can be dysfunctional, minor or major hemorrhage may occur. Bleeding is commonly limited to recurrent skin manifestations (ecchymoses, hematomas, epistaxis, gum bleeding), although significant GI bleeding is also possible. Intracranial hemorrhage is also possible and often occurs after developing an intracranial thrombosis (Miller & Farquharson, 2010). Bleeding typically does not occur unless the platelet count exceeds 1.5 million/mm^3. It results from a deficiency in von Willebrand factor as the platelet count increases.

Assessment and Diagnostic Findings

The diagnosis of ET is made by ruling out other potential disorders—either other myeloproliferative disorders or underlying illnesses that cause a reactive or secondary thrombocytosis (see later discussion). Iron deficiency should be excluded, because a reactive increase in the platelet count often accompanies this deficiency. Occult malignancy should be excluded. The CBC shows markedly large and abnormal platelets; the platelet count is persistently elevated (greater than 450,000/mm^3). An analysis of the JAK2 protein is very useful, whereas an analysis of the bone marrow (by aspiration and biopsy) may not be particularly useful.

Complications

Complications include inappropriate formation of thrombi and hemorrhage; no data reliably predict their development. A study of 891 patients diagnosed with ET identified the following as risk factors for developing major thrombotic complications (including arterial thrombosis): 60 years of age or older, the presence of cardiovascular risk factors (hypertension, smoking, and diabetes), a platelet count exceeding 1 million/mm^3, and a history of prior thrombotic events. In contrast, only male gender was found to be a risk factor for the development of venous thrombosis in these patients (Carobbio, Thiele, Passamonti, et al., 2011).

Major bleeding tends to occur when the platelet count is very high (greater than 1.5 million/mm^3) and there is a prior history of major bleeding. In contrast, patients who are younger than 40 years, have no previous history of a thrombotic or hemorrhagic event, and have platelet counts less than 1 million/mm^3 are considered to be at low risk for developing thrombotic or hemorrhagic complications (Tefferi, 2011).

Medical Management

The management of ET is highly controversial. A careful assessment of risk factors, particularly the platelet count, history of peripheral vascular disease, tobacco use, atherosclerosis, diabetes, sleep apnea, and prior thrombotic events, are all considered in developing the treatment plan.

In younger patients with no risk factors, low-dose aspirin therapy may be sufficient to prevent thrombotic complications. However, the use of aspirin can increase the risk of hemorrhagic complications and is typically a contraindication in patients with a history of GI bleeding. Aspirin can relieve the neurologic symptoms (e.g., headache), erythromelalgias, and visual symptoms of ET.

In older patients and in those with concurrent risk factors, more aggressive measures may be necessary. Hydroxyurea is effective in lowering the platelet count. This agent is taken orally and causes minimal side effects other than dose-related **leukopenia** (low WBC count). (Its potential for leukogenesis diminishes its utility in younger patients with risk factors.) The medication anagrelide is more specific in lowering the platelet count than hydroxyurea but has more side effects and may not be as effective. Severe headaches cause many patients to stop taking the medication. Tachycardia and chest pain may also occur, and anagrelide is contraindicated in patients with concurrent cardiac problems. Anagrelide is also carcinogenic.

Interferon alfa-2b has been shown to lower platelet counts by inhibiting megakaryocyte differentiation (Beer, Erber, Campbell, et al., 2011). The medication is administered subcutaneously at varying frequency, most commonly three times per week. Significant side effects, such as fatigue, weakness, memory deficits, dizziness, anemia, and liver dysfunction, limit its usefulness. Moreover, it may not be effective in protecting from thrombotic complications. A new, pegylated formulation of interferon alfa-2b may have less toxicity and longer duration of action, requiring less frequent injections (Beer et al., 2011).

Rarely, the occlusive symptoms require immediate reduction in the platelet count. When necessary, plateletpheresis (see Chapter 32) can reduce the amount of circulating platelets, but only transiently. The extent to which symptoms and complications (e.g., thromboses) are reduced by pheresis is unclear.

Nursing Management

Patients with ET need to be educated about the risks of hemorrhage and thrombosis. The patient is informed about signs and symptoms of thrombosis, particularly the neurologic manifestations, such as visual changes, numbness, tingling, and weakness. Risk factors for thrombosis are assessed, such as obesity, hypertension, hyperlipidemia, and smoking; measures to diminish these risk factors are encouraged. Patients taking aspirin should be informed about the importance of taking this medication as well as the increased risk of bleeding. Patients who are at risk for bleeding should be instructed about medications (e.g., aspirin, nonsteroidal anti-inflammatory agents [NSAIDs]) and other substances (e.g., alcohol) that can alter platelet function. Patients taking interferon are taught to self-administer the medication and manage side effects. Patients taking hydroxyurea should have CBCs monitored regularly; the dosage is adjusted based on the platelet and WBC count.

Primary Myelofibrosis

Primary myelofibrosis, also known as agnogenic myeloid metaplasia or myelofibrosis with myeloid metaplasia, is a chronic myeloproliferative disorder that arises from neoplastic transformation of an early hematopoietic stem cell. The disease is characterized by marrow fibrosis or scarring, extramedullary hematopoiesis (typically involving the spleen and the liver), leukocytosis, thrombocytosis, and anemia. Some patients have diminished leukocyte, platelet, and erythrocyte counts (i.e., **pancytopenia**). Patients with myelofibrosis have increased **angiogenesis** (formation of new blood vessels) within the marrow. Early forms of blood cells (including **nucleated RBC**s [immature RBCs] and megakaryocyte fragments) are frequently found in the circulation. The cause is unknown but appears to evolve from a prior myeloproliferative disorder (i.e., polycythemia vera, ET) in 25% of cases (Stein & Moliterno, 2010). As with ET and polycythemia vera, mutations of the JAK2 protein are seen (Spivak, 2010).

Myelofibrosis is the rarest of the classic myeloproliferative diseases (ET, polycythemia vera, myelofibrosis). It is a disease of the older adult, with a median age at diagnosis of 65 to 70 years, and is more common in males. Symptoms may result from an often massively enlarged spleen, causing discomfort and early satiety; other signs and symptoms include profound

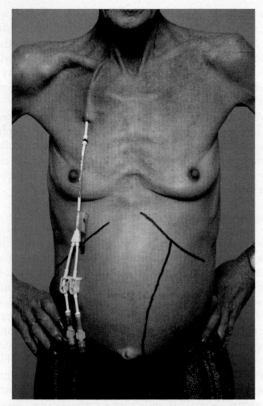

FIGURE 34-6 • Cachexia, severe wasting, and massively enlarged liver and spleen (hepatosplenomegaly) are seen in advanced myeloproliferative disorders, particularly myelofibrosis. (Note also the lack of adequate dressing over the patient's vascular access device.) From Tkachuk, D. C., & Hirschman, J. V. (2007). *Wintrobe's atlas of clinical hematology* (p. 111, Fig. 4.1). Philadelphia: Lippincott Williams & Wilkins.

fatigue, pruritus, bone pain, weight loss, infection and bleeding (from pancytopenia), and cachexia (Fig. 34-6). Arterial or venous thrombosis can occur but is less frequent than that found in polycythemia vera or ET. Average survival ranges from 3 to 10 years based on the occurrence of such adverse prognostic indicators as anemia, leukocytosis, presence of blast cells in the circulation, poor-risk cytogenetic results, and profound splenomegaly (Stein & Moliterno, 2010). Common causes of death are heart or liver failure, portal hypertension, complications of marrow failure, and transformation to AML. AML is especially difficult to treat successfully in these situations.

Medical Management

HSCT is a useful treatment modality in younger, otherwise healthy people. For patients who are not candidates for transplantation, medical management is directed toward palliation, reducing symptoms related to cytopenias, splenomegaly, and hypermetabolic state. Although one third of anemic patients respond to the combination of an androgen plus a corticosteroid, the primary treatment remains PRBC transfusion. Because of the prolonged requirement for these transfusions, iron overload is a common problem. Iron chelation therapy should be initiated in patients in whom survival is expected to exceed a few years. Hydroxyurea is often used to control high leukocyte and platelet counts and to reduce the size of the spleen. Thalidomide or lenalidomide may be

useful in improving anemia; however, these drugs are not as effective in improving thrombocytopenia or in reducing an enlarged spleen. Newly developed JAK2 inhibitors are being evaluated in patients with myelofibrosis; these agents appear to markedly reduce the massive splenomegaly and improve pruritus and occasionally anemia, but they do not reduce fibrosis within the marrow (Tibes & Mesa, 2011).

Splenectomy may also be used to control the significant problems that result from a massively enlarged spleen. The mortality rate associated with this procedure is 7% (Stein & Moliterno, 2010). Furthermore, a reactive thrombocytosis and leukocytosis can develop because the cells are no longer sequestered out of the circulation. The decision to undergo splenectomy warrants careful consideration of the advantages and disadvantages.

Nursing Management

Splenomegaly can be profound in patients with myelofibrosis, with enlargement of the spleen that may extend to the pelvic rim. This condition is extremely uncomfortable and can severely limit nutritional intake. Analgesic agents are often ineffective. Methods to reduce the size of the spleen are usually more effective in controlling pain. Splenomegaly, coupled with a hypermetabolic state, results in weight loss (often severe) and muscle wasting. Patients benefit from very small, frequent meals of foods that are high in calories and protein. Weakness, fatigue, and altered body image are other significant problems. Energy conservation methods and active listening are important nursing interventions. The patient needs to be educated about signs and symptoms of infection, bleeding, and thrombosis, as well as appropriate interventions if these occur. Ensuring that the patient takes steps to decrease risks associated with developing thrombosis (e.g., smoking; obesity; or poorly controlled hyperlipidemia, hypertension, or diabetes) can also be effective.

LYMPHOMA

The lymphomas are neoplasms of cells of lymphoid origin. These tumors usually start in lymph nodes but can involve lymphoid tissue in the spleen, GI tract (e.g., the wall of the stomach), liver, or bone marrow (see Fig. 35-1 in Chapter 35). They are often classified according to the degree of cell differentiation and the origin of the predominant malignant cell. Lymphomas can be broadly classified into two categories: Hodgkin lymphoma and non-Hodgkin lymphoma (NHL).

Hodgkin Lymphoma

Hodgkin lymphoma is a relatively rare malignancy that has a high cure rate. It is somewhat more common in men than in women and has two peaks of incidence: one in the early 20s and the other after 55 years of age. Disease occurrence has a familial pattern: First-degree relatives have a higher-than-normal frequency of disease, but the actual incidence of this pattern is low. No increased incidence for non-blood relatives (e.g., spouses) has been documented. Hodgkin lymphoma is seen more commonly in patients receiving chronic immunosuppressive therapy (e.g., for renal transplant) and also in veterans of the military who were exposed to the herbicide Agent Orange. The 5-year survival rate is 88%; it is more than 92% for those younger than 45 years (Leukemia & Lymphoma Society, 2012).

Pathophysiology

Unlike other lymphomas, Hodgkin lymphoma is unicentric in origin in that it initiates in a single node. The disease spreads by contiguous extension along the lymphatic system. The malignant cell of Hodgkin lymphoma is the Reed-Sternberg cell, a gigantic tumor cell that is morphologically unique and thought to be of immature lymphoid origin (Fig. 34-7). It is the pathologic hallmark and essential diagnostic criterion. However, the tumor is very heterogeneous and may actually contain few Reed-Sternberg cells. Repeated biopsies may be required to establish the diagnosis.

The cause of Hodgkin lymphoma is unknown, but a viral etiology is suspected. Although fragments of the Epstein-Barr virus have been found in some Reed-Sternberg cells, the precise role of this virus in the development of Hodgkin lymphoma remains unknown. Other viruses may also be implicated, including human immunodeficiency virus (HIV) and herpesvirus 8. The incidence of developing Hodgkin lymphoma is also higher in patients with immunoglobulin A (IgA) or certain types of immunoglobulin G (IgG) deficiency (Shapiro, 2011).

Hodgkin lymphoma is customarily classified into five subgroups based on pathologic analyses that reflect the natural history of the malignancy and suggest the prognosis. For example, when lymphocytes predominate, with few Reed-Sternberg cells and minimal involvement of the lymph nodes, the prognosis is much more favorable than when the lymphocyte count is low and the lymph nodes are virtually replaced by tumor cells of the most primitive type. Most patients with Hodgkin lymphoma have the types currently designated as "nodular sclerosis" or "mixed cellularity." The nodular sclerosis type tends to occur more often in young women, at an earlier stage but with a worse prognosis, than the mixed cellularity subgroup, which occurs more commonly in men and causes more constitutional symptoms but has a better prognosis.

Clinical Manifestations

Hodgkin lymphoma usually begins as an enlargement of one or more lymph nodes on one side of the neck. The individual nodes are painless and firm but not hard. The most common sites for lymphadenopathy are the cervical, supraclavicular, and mediastinal nodes; involvement of the iliac or inguinal nodes or spleen is much less common. A mediastinal mass may be seen on chest x-ray; occasionally, the mass is large enough to compress the trachea and cause dyspnea. Pruritus is common; it can be extremely distressing, and the cause is unknown. Some patients experience brief but severe pain after drinking alcohol, usually at the site of the tumor. Again, the cause of this is unknown.

All organs are vulnerable to invasion by tumor cells. The symptoms result from compression of organs by the tumor, such as cough and pulmonary effusion (from pulmonary infiltrates), jaundice (from hepatic involvement or bile duct obstruction), abdominal pain (from splenomegaly or retroperitoneal adenopathy), or bone pain (from skeletal involvement). Herpes zoster infections are common. A cluster of constitutional symptoms has important prognostic implications. Referred to as B symptoms, they include fever (without chills), drenching sweats (particularly at night), and unintentional weight loss of more than 10% of body weight. B symptoms are found in 40% of patients and are more common in advanced disease (Shenoy, Maggioncalda, Malik, et al., 2011).

A mild anemia is the most common hematologic finding. The leukocyte count may be elevated or decreased. The platelet count is typically normal, unless the tumor has invaded the bone marrow, suppressing hematopoiesis. The **erythrocyte sedimentation rate** (ESR) and the serum copper level are sometimes used to assess disease activity; elevations may reflect increases in disease activity. Patients with Hodgkin lymphoma have impaired cellular immunity, as evidenced by an absent or decreased reaction to skin sensitivity tests (e.g., *Candida*, mumps). Infections, including viral infections, are common (Fig. 34-8).

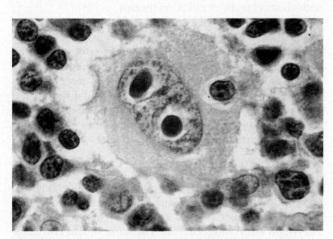

FIGURE 34-7 • Reed-Sternberg cell. Reed-Sternberg cells are large, abnormal lymphocytes that may contain more than one nucleus. These cells are found in Hodgkin lymphoma. From Porth, C. M., & Matfin, G. (2009). *Pathophysiology: Concepts of altered health states* (8th ed, p. 312). Philadelphia: Lippincott Williams & Wilkins.

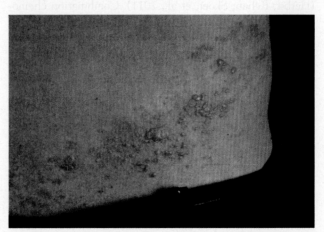

FIGURE 34-8 • Herpes zoster is a common complication in patients with lymphoproliferative disease, such as Hodgkin lymphoma here. Zoster infections are also common in patients on chronic steroid use for hematologic conditions and some chemotherapy regimens. From Tkachuk, D. C., & Hirschman, J. V. (2007). *Wintrobe's atlas of clinical hematology* (p. 207, Fig. 5.152). Philadelphia: Lippincott Williams & Wilkins.

Assessment and Diagnostic Findings

Because many manifestations are similar to those occurring with infection, diagnostic studies are performed to rule out an infectious origin of the disease. The diagnosis is made by means of an excisional lymph node biopsy and the finding of the Reed-Sternberg cell. Once the diagnosis is confirmed and the histologic type is established, it is necessary to assess the extent of the disease—a process referred to as staging.

During the health history, the patient is assessed for any B symptoms. Physical examination requires a careful, systematic evaluation of all palpable lymph node chains (see Fig. 32-4 in Chapter 32), as well as the size of the spleen and liver. A chest x-ray and a computed tomography (CT) scan of the chest, abdomen, and pelvis are crucial to identify the extent of lymphadenopathy within these regions. A positron emission tomography (PET) scan may be the most sensitive imaging test in identifying residual disease and is now being evaluated for its predictive value in this disease (Kobe, Dietlein, Kriz, et al., 2010). Laboratory tests include CBC, platelet count, ESR, and liver and renal function studies. A bone marrow biopsy is performed if there are signs of marrow involvement, and some physicians routinely perform bilateral biopsies; it is thought that unilateral biopsies may sometimes yield false-negative results. Bone scans may be performed.

Medical Management

The goal in the treatment of Hodgkin lymphoma is cure. Treatment is determined primarily by the stage of the disease, not the histologic type; however, extensive research is ongoing to target treatment regimens to histologic subtypes or prognostic features. Treatment of limited-stage Hodgkin lymphoma commonly involves a short course (2 to 4 months) of chemotherapy followed by radiation therapy to the specific involved area. This strategy has reduced the amount of radiation dosage, with subsequent decrease in long-term side effects (particularly second malignancies and late cardiovascular events) without decreasing the likelihood of controlling the disease; a recent systematic review of treatment for early-stage Hodgkin disease supported this treatment regimen (Herbst, Rehan, Skoet, et al., 2011). Combination chemotherapy with doxorubicin (Adriamycin), bleomycin (Blenoxane), vinblastine (Velban), and dacarbazine (DTIC), referred to as ABVD, is considered the standard treatment for more advanced disease (stages III and IV and all stages with B symptoms). Other combinations of chemotherapy may afford higher response rates but result in more toxicity (Borchmann & Engert, 2010).

In addition, chemotherapy is often successful in obtaining remission even when relapse occurs. Transplantation is used for advanced or refractory disease. Revised treatment approaches are aimed at diminishing the risk of complications without sacrificing the potential for cure (Bartlett, 2010).

Because most patients diagnosed with Hodgkin lymphoma are either cured or experience prolonged remissions, and thus live for many years post diagnosis, much is now known about the long-term effects of chemotherapy and radiation therapy. The development of complications may not occur for years after treatment; therefore, long-term surveillance is crucial. In large population-based studies of Hodgkin lymphoma survivors, the estimated risk of developing a second cancer was

---

> **Chart 34-2** **Potential Long-Term Complications of Therapy for Hodgkin Lymphoma**
>
> Immune dysfunction
> Herpes infections (zoster and varicella)
> Pneumococcal sepsis
> Secondary cancers:
>   Acute myeloid leukemia
>   Myelodysplastic syndromes
>   Non-Hodgkin lymphoma
>   Solid tumors (especially bone and soft tissue, lung, breast)
>   Thyroid cancer
> Hypothyroidism
> Thymic hyperplasia
> Hypothyroidism
> Pericarditis (acute or chronic)
> Cardiovascular toxicity (coronary artery disease, myocardial infarction, congestive heart failure, valvular heart disease, peripheral arterial disease)
> Pneumonitis (acute or chronic)
> Dyspnea on exertion
> Abnormalities in senses of taste, smell, and touch
> Abnormal balance, tremors, or weakness
> Avascular necrosis
> Osteoporosis
> Growth retardation in children
> Infertility
> Decreased libido
> Dental caries
> Dry mouth
> Dysphagia

Note: The complications delineated in this chart can be generalized to other patients receiving cancer chemotherapy beyond Hodgkin lymphoma.

between 18% and 26% (Baxi & Matasar, 2010). Hematologic malignancies are the most common; AML has a relative risk of 82.5%, lymphoma of 16.5%. Solid tumors can also occur; bone and soft tissue cancers have a relative risk of 12%, lung cancer of 6%, and breast cancer of 6%. Cardiovascular toxicity is the second leading cause of death after malignancy. Chart 34-2 lists long-term potential complications associated with chemotherapy or radiation therapy.

Quality-of-life (QOL) studies reveal long-term issues in Hodgkin lymphoma survivors (Baxi & Matasar, 2010). Compared to matched controls, individuals reported lower general health, vitality, sexual function, mental health, and physical functioning. Fatigue was a long-lasting effect of treatment that did not diminish over time. Mental fatigue was also higher compared with controls. Challenges related to employment and in obtaining health insurance or mortgages were also reported (Baxi & Matasar, 2010).

Nursing Management

The potential development of a second malignancy should be addressed with the patient when initial treatment decisions are made. However, patients should also be told that Hodgkin lymphoma is often curable. The nurse should encourage patients to reduce other factors that increase the risk of developing second cancers, such as use of tobacco and alcohol and exposure to environmental carcinogens and excessive sunlight. Screening for late effects of treatment (see Chart 34-2) is necessary. In addition, the nurse should provide education about relevant self-care strategies and disease management.

Non-Hodgkin Lymphomas

The NHLs are a heterogeneous group of cancers that originate from the neoplastic growth of lymphoid tissue. As in CLL, the neoplastic cells are thought to arise from a single clone of lymphocytes; however, in NHL, the cells may vary morphologically. Most NHLs involve malignant B lymphocytes; only 5% involve T lymphocytes. In contrast to Hodgkin lymphoma, the lymphoid tissues involved are largely infiltrated with malignant cells. The spread of these malignant lymphoid cells occurs unpredictably, and true localized disease is uncommon. Lymph nodes from multiple sites may be infiltrated, as may sites outside the lymphoid system (extranodal tissue; Fig. 34-9).

NHL is the seventh most common type of cancer diagnosed in the United States; incidence rates have almost doubled in the past 35 years. The incidence increases with each decade of life; the median age at diagnosis is 65 years (ACS, 2010c). Although no common etiologic factor has been identified, the incidence of NHL has increased in people with immunodeficiencies or autoimmune disorders; prior treatment for cancer; prior organ transplant; viral infections

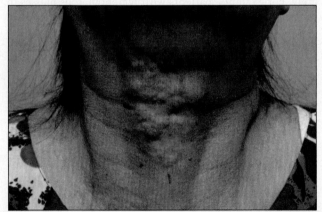
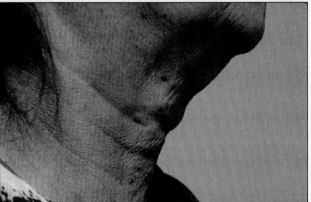

FIGURE 34-9 • Any extranodal location can be a site for diffuse B-cell lymphoma, such as the thyroid, as shown here. From Tkachuk, D. C., & Hirschman, J. V. (2007). *Wintrobe's atlas of clinical hematology* (p. 183, Fig. 5.87). Philadelphia: Lippincott Williams & Wilkins.

TABLE 34-1	Types of Lymphomas*	
Indolent	**Aggressive**	**Highly Aggressive**
Follicular	Diffuse large cell	Burkitt
Small lymphocytic	Mantle cell	Lymphoblastic

Marginal zone:
  MALT
  Splenic
  Nodal
		AIDS-related B cell

Lymphoplasmacytic:
  Waldenstrom's
  macroglobulinemia		

MALT, mucosa-associated lymphoidal tissue; AIDS, acquired immunodeficiency syndrome.
*Major types of lymphomas, many of which are indolent in nature. Table does not present an all-inclusive list.

(including Epstein-Barr virus and HIV); and exposure to pesticides, solvents, dyes, or defoliating agents, including Agent Orange. The prognosis varies greatly among the more than 30 subtypes of NHL. For example, diffuse large B-cell lymphoma, the most common form, accounts for 30% of all newly diagnosed lymphomas (80% of all aggressive types); 5-year survival rates are 26% to 73%. Follicular lymphoma, the second most common form, accounts for 20% of all new cases (70% of all indolent [less-aggressive] types); 5-year survival is 70%, and median survival is 8 to 10 years (Kallab, 2011). A recent study found that individuals who consumed more than 40 grams of alcohol weekly and were obese had a worse prognosis for both diffuse large B-cell lymphoma and follicular lymphoma (Geyer, Morton, Habermann, et al., 2010). Smoking was also associated with a worse prognosis and based on duration of smoking and cigarette consumption (number smoked per day and pack-year history). In addition, those who recently quit smoking had a worse prognosis than those who quit a longer time ago. Table 34-1 lists some of the more common lymphomas.

Clinical Manifestations

Symptoms are highly variable, reflecting the diverse nature of the NHLs. Lymphadenopathy is most common; however, in indolent types of lymphomas, the lymphadenopathy can wax and wane. With early-stage disease, or with the types that are considered indolent, symptoms may be virtually absent or very minor, and the illness typically is not diagnosed until it progresses to a later stage, when the patient is symptomatic. At these stages (III or IV), lymphadenopathy is distinctly noticeable. One third of patients with NHLs have B symptoms (fever, drenching night sweats, and unintentional weight loss). Lymphomatous masses can compromise organ function. For example, a mass in the mediastinum can cause respiratory distress; abdominal masses can compromise the ureters, leading to renal dysfunction; and splenomegaly can cause abdominal discomfort, nausea, early satiety, anorexia, and weight loss. Involvement of the CNS with lymphoma is becoming increasingly common (Norden, Hochberg, & Hochberg, 2012).

Assessment and Diagnostic Findings

The actual diagnosis of NHL is categorized into a highly complex classification system based on histopathology, immunophenotyping, and cytogenetic analyses of the malignant cells. The specific histopathologic type of the disease has important prognostic implications. Treatment also varies and is based on these features. Indolent types tend to have small cells that are distributed in a circular or follicular pattern. Aggressive types tend to have large or immature cells distributed through the nodes in a diffuse pattern. Staging is typically based on data obtained from CT and PET scans, bone marrow biopsies, and occasionally cerebrospinal fluid analysis. The stage is based on the site of disease and its spread to other sites. For example, in stage I disease, only one area of involvement is detected; thus, stage I disease is highly localized and may respond well to localized therapy (e.g., radiation therapy). In contrast, in stage IV, disease at least one extranodal site is detected.

Although stage of disease is important, often it is not an accurate predictor of prognosis. Two prognostic classification systems have been developed that are particularly useful in the older patient population: the International Prognostic Index (IPI) and, for follicular lymphomas, the Follicular Lymphoma International Prognostic Index (FLIPI). Age, performance status, lactate dehydrogenase levels, stage of disease, and extranodal involvement are scored to determine risk of failure or death from disease. Based on the IPI, 5-year overall survival rates range from 73% (low risk) to 26% (high risk) (ACS, 2010d).

Medical Management

Treatment is determined by the classification of disease, the stage of disease, prior treatment (if any), and the patient's ability to tolerate therapy. Tolerance to therapy is largely dictated by renal, hepatic, and cardiac function; the presence of concurrent diseases; functional status; and age. If the disease is not aggressive and is localized, radiation alone may be the treatment of choice. With aggressive types of NHL, aggressive combinations of chemotherapeutic agents are used; R-CHOP—the combination of the monoclonal antibody rituximab (Rituxan) with conventional chemotherapy (cyclophosphamide [Cytoxan], doxorubicin, vincristine, and prednisone)—is now considered standard treatment for common lymphomas (National Comprehensive Cancer Network [NCCN], 2012). CNS involvement is common with some aggressive forms of NHL; in this situation, cranial radiation or intrathecal chemotherapy is used in addition to systemic chemotherapy. Survival is very low when relapse occurs after being treated with rituximab-based regimens or with transplantation (Zwick, Murawski, & Pfreundschuh, 2010).

There is no standard therapy for follicular lymphoma (Rummel, 2010). "Watchful waiting," where therapy is delayed until symptoms develop, has often been used in those with indolent disease. More recently, immunotherapy (e.g., rituximab) is being used, often in combination with conventional chemotherapy. Radiopharmaceutical agents (e.g., ibritumomab tiuxetan [Zevalin] or tositumomab/iodine-131 [Bexxar]) are also used, although they cause technical difficulties with administration due to the radioactivity of the agent. More aggressive treatment (often R-CHOP or rituximab plus bendamustine [Levact]) may provide a longer duration of remission in which additional treatment is not needed. Unfortunately, in most situations, relapse is commonly seen in patients with low-grade lymphomas. Treatment after relapse is controversial; HSCT may be considered for patients younger than 60 years (see Chapter 15).

Nursing Management

Lymphoma is a highly complex constellation of diseases. When caring for patients with lymphoma, it is extremely important for the nurse to know the specific disease type, stage of disease, treatment history, and current treatment plan. Most of the care for patients with Hodgkin lymphoma or NHL takes place in the outpatient setting, unless complications occur (e.g., infection, respiratory compromise due to mediastinal mass). The most commonly used treatment methods are chemotherapy (often combined with a monoclonal antibody) and radiation therapy. Chemotherapy causes systemic side effects (e.g., myelosuppression, nausea, hair loss, risk of infection), whereas radiation therapy causes specific side effects that are limited to the area being irradiated. For example, patients receiving abdominal radiation therapy may experience nausea and diarrhea but not hair loss. Regardless of the type of treatment, all patients may experience fatigue.

The risk of infection is significant for these patients, not only from treatment-related myelosuppression but also from the defective immune response that results from the disease itself. Patients need to be educated to minimize the risks of infection, to recognize signs of possible infection, and to contact their primary provider if such signs develop (see Chart 15-7 in Chart 15–7).

Additional complications depend on the location of the lymphoma. Therefore, the nurse must know the tumor location so that assessments can be targeted appropriately. For example, patients with lymphomatous masses in the upper chest should be assessed for superior vena cava obstruction or airway obstruction, if the mass is near the bronchus or trachea.

Many lymphomas can be cured with current treatments. However, as survival rates increase, the incidence of second malignancies, particularly AML or MDS, also increases. Therefore, survivors should be screened regularly for the development of second malignancies (see Chart 34-1). A review of QOL studies found that lymphoma survivors reported worse physical QOL but comparable mental health when compared to the general population. QOL was rated higher in those survivors who were younger, male, employed, had a higher educational level, and met public health exercise guidelines (Arden-Close, Pacey & Eiser, 2010).

MULTIPLE MYELOMA

Multiple myeloma is a malignant disease of the most mature form of B lymphocyte—the plasma cell. Plasma cells secrete immunoglobulins, which are proteins necessary for antibody production to fight infection. Myeloma is the second most common hematologic cancer in the United States. The median 5-year survival rate for newly diagnosed patients is 39% (Leukemia and Lymphoma Society, 2012). Currently, prognosis is based on two simple markers: serum albumin (presumed to be a negative acute-phase reactant) and serum beta-2 microglobulin (presumed to be an indirect measure of tumor burden, defined as an approximation of the amount of cancer or the number of cancer cells in the body). Using this system, patients with a good prognosis have a median survival of 62 months, whereas those with a poor prognosis have a median survival of

29 months. Methods to incorporate cytogenetic analyses and the presence or absence of specific DNA sequences are ongoing (Munshi, Anderson, Bergsagel, et al., 2011).

Pathophysiology

In multiple myeloma, the malignant plasma cells produce an increased amount of a specific immunoglobulin that is nonfunctional. Functional types of immunoglobulin are still produced by nonmalignant plasma cells, although in lower-than-normal quantity. The specific immunoglobulin secreted by the myeloma cells is detectable in the blood or urine and is referred to as the monoclonal protein, or M protein. This protein serves as a useful marker to monitor the extent of disease and the patient's response to therapy. It is commonly measured by serum or urine protein electrophoresis, or free light chain assay (Fig. 34-10). The patient's total protein level is also typically elevated because of the production of M protein. Malignant plasma cells also secrete certain substances to stimulate the creation of new blood vessels (i.e., angiogenesis) to enhance the growth of these clusters of plasma cell. Occasionally, the plasma cells infiltrate other tissue, in which case they are referred to as plasmacytomas. Plasmacytomas can occur in the sinuses, spinal cord, and soft tissues.

Clinical Manifestations

The classic presenting symptom of multiple myeloma is bone pain, usually in the back or ribs. Bone pain is reported by two thirds of all patients at diagnosis (Roodman, 2011). The bone pain associated with myeloma increases with movement and decreases with rest; patients may report that they

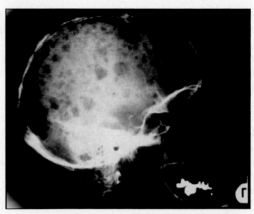

FIGURE 34-11 • Lytic lesions seen in the skull in a patient with multiple myeloma. From Tkachuk, D. C., & Hirschman, J. V. (2007). *Wintrobe's atlas of clinical hematology* (p. 164, Fig. 5.29). Philadelphia: Lippincott Williams & Wilkins.

have less pain on awakening but more during the day. In myeloma, a substance secreted by the plasma cells, osteoclast activating factor, and other substances such as interleukin-6 (IL-6) are involved in stimulating osteoclasts. Both mechanisms appear to be involved in the process of bone breakdown. Thus, lytic lesions as well as osteoporosis may be seen on bone x-rays; these lesions do not visualize on bone scans. The bone destruction can be severe enough to cause vertebral collapse and fractures, including spinal fractures, which can impinge on the spinal cord and result in spinal cord compression (Fig. 34-11).

If the bone destruction is fairly extensive, excessive ionized calcium is lost from the bone and enters the serum; hypercalcemia may therefore develop and is frequently manifested by excessive thirst, dehydration, constipation, altered mental status, confusion, and perhaps coma. Renal failure may also occur; the configuration of the circulating immunoglobulin molecule (particularly the shape of lambda light chains) can damage the renal tubules. Renal impairment occurs in 20% to 40% of patients at the time of diagnosis and can worsen when the disease becomes refractory to treatment (Palumbo & Anderson, 2011).

> ### ▶ Quality and Safety Nursing Alert
>
> **Any older adult whose chief complaint is back pain and who has an elevated total protein level should be evaluated for possible myeloma.**

As more and more malignant plasma cells are produced, the marrow has less space for erythrocyte production, and anemia may develop. This anemia is also caused to a great extent by a diminished production of erythropoietin by the kidney. In the late stage of the disease, a reduced number of leukocytes and platelets may also be seen because the bone marrow is infiltrated by malignant plasma cells.

Infection is a concern. Infections occur most commonly within the first 2 months of beginning therapy and usually with advanced, refractory disease. In multiple myeloma, in contrast to other hematologic malignancies, the incidence of infection does not appear to be related to the extent of neutropenia. Infections occurring at the beginning of treatment

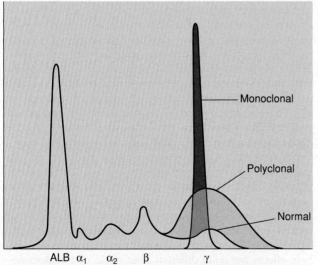

ALB α_1 α_2 β γ

FIGURE 34-10 • Abnormal serum protein electrophoresis patterns contrasted with a normal pattern. Polyclonal peaks are characterized by a broad-based increase in immunoglobulin (Ig) by myriad reactive plasma cells and indicate a benign reactive process. In contrast, a narrow spike indicates homogeneity of the Ig secreted by a single clone of plasma cells. M spikes are seen in monoclonal gammopathies of undetermined significance or in plasma malignancies (myeloma, Waldenstrom's macroglobulinemia). From Turgeon, M. (2012). *Clinical hematology theory & procedures* (5th ed., p. 347, Fig. 20.7). Philadelphia: Lippincott Williams & Wilkins.

are often caused by *Streptococcus pneumoniae, H. influenzae, and Escherichia coli;* those that occur when the disease is advanced or in the setting of renal failure are most often caused by gram-negative bacilli or *Staphylococcus aureus* (Gay & Palumbo, 2010). Infection is frequently the cause of death from multiple myeloma.

Neurologic manifestations can also occur. Spinal cord compression is the most common, and other neurologic symptoms may be present (see Chapter 15 for care of oncologic emergencies). When the M protein is immunoglobulin M (IgM), peripheral neuropathy is more likely. Nerve root compression, the presence of intracranial neoplastic cells, and meningeal involvement are quite rare.

When plasma cells secrete excessive amounts of immunoglobulin, the serum viscosity can increase. Hyperviscosity may be manifested by bleeding from the nose or mouth, headache, blurred vision, paresthesias, or heart failure. Thromboembolic events (blood clots) may occur in patients with myeloma; the incidence is thought to be 3% to 10% and may increase substantially when high doses of corticosteroids are used to treat the disease (Gay & Palumbo, 2010).

Assessment and Diagnostic Findings

An elevated monoclonal protein level in the serum (via serum protein electrophoresis), urine (via urine protein electrophoresis), or light chain (via serum free light chain analysis) is a major criterion in the diagnosis of multiple myeloma. Evidence of end organ damage is necessary to establish the diagnosis, using the acronym *CRAB* (elevated *c*alcium, *r*enal insufficiency, *a*nemia, and/or *b*one lesions). The diagnosis of myeloma is confirmed by bone marrow biopsy; the presence of more than 10% plasma cells is the hallmark diagnostic criterion. Because the infiltration of the marrow by these malignant plasma cells is not uniform, the plasma cells may not be increased in a given sample (a false-negative result).

Medical Management

There is no cure for multiple myeloma. Even autologous HSCT is considered to extend remission rather than provide a cure. However, for many patients, it is possible to control the illness and maintain their level of functioning quite well for several years or longer. For those who are not candidates for HSCT, chemotherapy is the primary treatment. Pharmacotherapeutic advances have resulted in significant improvement in response rates; corticosteroids, particularly dexamethasone (Decadron), are often combined with other agents (e.g., melphalan [Alkeran], cyclophosphamide [Cytoxan], thalidomide [Thalomid], lenalidomide [Revlimid], and bortezomib [Velcade]).

Radiation therapy is very useful in strengthening the bone at a specific lesion, particularly one at risk for bone fracture or spinal cord compression. It is also useful in relieving bone pain and reducing the size of plasma cell tumors that occur outside the skeletal system. However, because it is a nonsystemic form of treatment, it does not diminish the source of the bone conditions (i.e., the production of malignant plasma cells). Therefore, radiation therapy is typically used in combination with systemic treatment such as chemotherapy.

When lytic lesions result in vertebral compression fractures, vertebroplasty is often performed. This procedure is performed under fluoroscopy. A hollow needle is positioned within the fractured vertebra, and when the precise location is confirmed, an orthopedic cement is infiltrated into the vertebra to stabilize the fracture and strengthen the vertebra. For most patients, relief from pain is almost immediate. This procedure may be enhanced by concomitant kyphoplasty—the use of a special inflatable balloon inserted into the vertebra to increase the height of the vertebra prior to injecting the cement.

Some bisphosphonates, such as pamidronate (Aredia) and zoledronic acid (Zometa), have been shown to strengthen bone in multiple myeloma by diminishing survival of osteoclasts, thus controlling bone pain and potentially preventing bone fracture. These agents are also effective in managing and preventing hypercalcemia. Some evidence suggests that bisphosphonates may activate an antimyeloma immune response, inducing myeloma cell death and reducing tumor burden (Terpos, Moulopoulos, & Dimopoulos, 2011). Osteonecrosis of the jaw is an infrequent but serious complication that can arise in patients treated long-term with bisphosphonates; the mandible or maxilla are affected. Careful assessment for this complication should be conducted and a thorough evaluation of the patient's dentition should be performed prior to initiating bisphosphonate therapy, including panoramic dental x-rays. Necessary repairs, including those to ensure that dentures fit properly, should also be performed.

When patients have signs and symptoms of hyperviscosity, plasmapheresis may be used to lower the immunoglobulin level. Symptoms may be more useful than serum viscosity levels in determining the need for this intervention.

Recent advances in the understanding of the process of angiogenesis have resulted in new therapeutic options. Thalidomide (Thalomid), initially used as an antiemetic, has significant antimyeloma effects. It inhibits **cytokines** (regulatory proteins produced by leukocytes) necessary for new vascular generation, such as vascular endothelial growth factor, and for myeloma cell growth and survival, such as IL-6 and tumor necrosis factor, by boosting the body's immune response against the tumor and by creating favorable conditions for apoptosis (programmed cell death) of the myeloma cells. Fatigue, dizziness, constipation, rash, and peripheral neuropathy are commonly encountered in patients treated with thalidomide, whereas myelosuppression is not. There is also an increased incidence of DVT; prophylactic anticoagulation should be used to prevent this complication. Strategies to achieve this may range from administration of low-dose aspirin to anticoagulation with warfarin (Coumadin) or low-molecular-weight heparins (e.g., enoxaparin [Lovenox]) (Mateos, 2010). Thalidomide is contraindicated in pregnancy because of associated severe birth defects. Thus, the patient must be counseled and agree to use approved methods of birth control prior to taking this drug. The thalidomide analog lenalidomide (Revlimid) is also effective in treating myeloma. Side effects are quite different from those of thalidomide—myelosuppression and venous thromboembolism are common, whereas sedation, neuropathy (including peripheral neuropathy), and constipation are not. However, the drug is excreted by the kidneys, so careful monitoring of renal function is required, and dose reduction may be necessary. Thalidomide also requires concomitant anticoagulation, particularly when used in combination with dexamethasone (Gay & Palumbo, 2010).

The use of a proteasome inhibitor, bortezomib (Velcade), is included for initial therapy as well as for use in refractory disease. When combined with other medications, it can overcome resistance to those agents (Chen, Frezza, Schmitt, et al., 2011). Side effects include transient thrombocytopenia, orthostatic hypotension, nausea and vomiting, skin rash, neuropathy, and asthenia (i.e., weakness, malaise, fatigue). Because neuropathy is potentially serious, the dosage needs to be decreased as soon as the neuropathy begins to interfere with function; however, new dosing schedules (weekly administration rather than twice weekly) seem to markedly reduce this problem. Bortezomib is metabolized by the cytochrome P450 pathway, which means that a careful review of concurrent medications for drug–drug interaction is crucial.

Gerontologic Considerations

The incidence of multiple myeloma increases with age; the disease rarely occurs in patients younger than 40 years. Because of the increasing older population, more patients are seeking treatment for this disease. Back pain, which is often a presenting symptom, should be closely investigated in older patients. HSCT is an option that can prolong remission and potentially cure some patients, but it is unavailable to many older people because of concurrent diminished organ function (e.g., kidney, lung, liver, heart) associated with aging. Palliation and hospice care may be the best option in preserving QOL (Chart 34-3; see Chapter 16 for further discussion). Newer treatment options can be successfully used in the older patient but may require dose adjustments to diminish treatment-related toxicity.

Nursing Management

Pain management is very important in patients with multiple myeloma. NSAIDs can be very useful for mild pain or can be administered in combination with opioid analgesics. Because NSAIDs can cause gastritis and renal dysfunction, renal function must be carefully monitored and patients assessed for gastritis; many patients are unable to use NSAIDs due to concurrent renal insufficiency.

Promoting Home and Community-Based Care

Educating Patients About Self-Care

The patient needs to be educated about activity restrictions (e.g., lifting no more than 10 pounds, the use of proper body mechanics). Braces are occasionally needed to support the spinal column.

The patient also needs to be instructed about the signs and symptoms of hypercalcemia. Maintaining mobility and hydration are important to diminish exacerbations of this complication; however, the primary cause is the disease itself. Renal function must also be monitored closely. Renal failure can become severe, and dialysis may be needed. Maintaining high urine output (3 L/day) can be very useful in preventing or limiting this complication.

Because antibody production is impaired, infections, particularly bacterial infections, are common and can be life threatening. The patient needs to be instructed in appropriate

---

Chart 34-3   **ETHICAL DILEMMA**

Can Comfort Care at End of Life Equate to Assisted Suicide or Active Euthanasia?

Case Scenario

Working in a hospice unit, you are the primary nurse for a 77-year-old man with a terminal diagnosis of multiple myeloma. He has a several-week history of intractable pain, nausea, and vomiting despite attempts to change his medication prescriptions. The hospice center physician, the patient, and the patient's family members meet with you for a family conference. All agree that they wish the patient to die peacefully without pain and suffering. The patient is placed on a midazolam (Versed) and morphine intravenous drip that you titrate to achieve relief of symptoms. The patient dies peacefully within 72 hours of you starting this new medication regimen.

Discussion

There is a great deal of discomfort among both clinicians and laymen around what constitutes comfort care (i.e., palliative care) at end of life and what may constitute either assisted suicide or euthanasia. Although the American Nurses Association (ANA) clearly does not advocate that nurses participate in either assisted suicide (ANA, 1994b) or euthanasia (ANA, 1994a), and avows that nurses should not participate in acts that intentionally cause patient death (ANA, 2001), the ANA does advocate that nurses provide competent palliative care at end of life that preserves each individual patient's dignity and autonomy (ANA, 2010).

Analysis

• Would you describe your role in this case as complicit in assisted suicide, active euthanasia, or providing palliation? What distinction, if any, might there be among these three acts?

• Describe how the ethical principles of autonomy, beneficence, and nonmaleficence may intersect or be at odds with each other in this case (see Chart 3–3 in Chapter 3).

• Note that the ANA (2001) *Code of Ethics* clearly states that nurses should not *intentionally* cause a patient's death. What were your "intentions" in this case? How might intentionality be instrumental in making this act of titrating medications that provided palliation morally defensible? Is this nursing intervention morally defensible according to the principle of double effect (see Chart 3–3 in Chapter 3)?

References

American Nurses Association. (1994a). *Position statement on active euthanasia*. Available at: www.nursingworld.org/MainMenuCategories/EthicsStandards/Ethics-Position-Statements/prteteuth14450.html

American Nurses Association. (1994b). *Position statement on assisted suicide*. Available at: www.nursingworld.org/MainMenuCategories/EthicsStandards/Ethics-Position-Statements/prtetsuic14456.html

American Nurses Association. (2001). *Code of ethics for nurses with interpretive statements*. Washington, DC: American Nurses Publishing, American Nurses Foundation/American Nurses Association.

American Nurses Association. (2010). *Position statement on registered nurses' roles and responsibilities in providing expert care and counseling at the end of life*. Available at: http://www.nursingworld.org/MainMenuCategories/EthicsStandards/Ethics-Position-Statements/etpain14426.pdf

Resources

See Chapter 3, Chart 3-6 for ethics resources.

TABLE 34-2 Peripheral Neuropathy

Type of Neuropathy	Manifestations	Nursing Intervention/Patient Education
Sensory	Hypoesthesia	Warn patient to avoid extreme temperatures (e.g., bathwater).
		Inspect feet for trauma, potential infection.
		Use loose-fitting stockings.
	Paresthesia (tingling)	Gentle massage
		Gentle ROM exercises
	Hyperalgesia(pain)	Gentle massage (cocoa butter or menthol-based cream/lotion)
	Toes and fingers	Apply lidocaine 5% patch to affected area every 12 hours.
	Soles of feet/palms	Consider gabapentin (Neurontin), tricyclic antidepressants (e.g., amitriptyline [Elavil]).
Motor	Muscle cramps	Maximize hydration, ambulation. (Quinine is not recommended.)
	Tremor	
	↓ Strength in distal muscles	
	Gait disturbance	Encourage the use of appropriate footwear.
	↓ Fine motor function	Consider ambulatory aides (e.g., walker).
	(e.g., handwriting,	Remove scatter rugs; perform a home safety evaluation.
	buttoning clothes)	PT referral
		OT referral (if severe limitations)
Autonomic Nervous System	Orthostatic hypotension	Warn patient to avoid abrupt position change.
		Maximize hydration.
		Consider adjusting antihypertensive medications, diuretics.
	Bradycardia	Assess/warn patient for impact (fatigue, impairment in function).
		Consider adjusting drugs that cause bradycardia (e.g., calcium channel blockers, beta-blockers, alpha-/beta-adrenergic blockers, digoxin).
		Explore the use of activity to increase heart rate.
	Sexual dysfunction	Explore alternative means of sexual activity beyond intercourse.
		Consider the use of erectile dysfunction medication.
	Constipation	Maximize fluid intake, fiber.
		Use stool softeners, laxatives.

ROM, range of motion; ↓, decreased; PT, physical therapy; OT, occupational therapy.
Note: Peripheral neuropathy can be classified into three main categories. Within each category, specific manifestations are delineated as well as relevant nursing interventions. If the neuropathy is related to myeloma therapy, it is crucial to promptly stop the potentially offending medication. It is also important to reduce the impact from other predisposing factors. For example, diabetes should be well controlled and alcohol consumption reduced.

infection prevention measures and should be advised to contact the primary provider immediately if fever or other signs and symptoms of infection develop. The patient should receive pneumococcal and influenza vaccines. Prophylactic antibiotics are often used, particularly when patients are treated with steroid-containing regimens. The antiviral agent acyclovir (Zovirax) is recommended when patients are treated with bortezomib-based regimens to diminish the potential development of viral infection, such as herpes zoster.

Continuing Care

Many newer medications are associated with higher risks of thromboembolism formation, particularly when used concurrently with corticosteroids. Other risk factors include decreased mobility, obesity, prior thromboembolic events, diabetes, cardiac or renal disease, and the presence of a vascular access device (e.g., PICC). It is important to maintain mobility and to use strategies that enhance venous return (e.g., anti-embolism stockings, avoid crossing the legs).

A significant toxicity associated with the use of thalidomide or bortezomib for multiple myeloma is peripheral neuropathy, as noted previously. The neuropathy is primarily sensory, but motor or autonomic nervous system neuropathy is also seen (Delforge, Bladé, Dimopoulos, et al., 2010) (Table 34-2). Painful neuropathy can be quite disabling and may interfere with the patient's ability to perform normal activities of daily living. Other risk factors for peripheral neuropathy (e.g., diabetes, vitamin deficiencies, viral infection, or excessive alcohol consumption) should be aggressively managed. The nurse needs to assess for symptoms related to peripheral neuropathy and make assessments of the home for safety. Sensation (touch,

temperature, pain, vibration, proprioception), ankle reflexes, distal muscle strength, and blood pressure should be evaluated (Delforge et al., 2010). Patients should be educated to report any symptoms of peripheral neuropathy and to not minimize such symptoms, because prompt cessation of therapy can prevent the neuropathy from progressing. Resuming treatment with a lower dosage and at a longer interval between dosing may diminish the worsening of peripheral nerve damage.

Critical Thinking Exercises

1 **ebp** You are working in a hematology-oncology clinic. The laboratory reports a critical laboratory result for one of your patients with possible MDS. The leukocyte count is 1,800/mm^3 with 40% neutrophils. What other laboratory results would be important to review or consider? The patient is also anemic (hemoglobin 8.2 g/dL), and platelets are 65,000/mm^3. What observations will you include in your assessment of this patient? Determine the extent to which this patient is neutropenic. What medical treatments would you anticipate? How would you educate the patient about neutropenic precautions? What evidence exists to support your educational interventions? What is the strength of that evidence?

2 **ebp** A 78-year-old woman with multiple myeloma is admitted to your unit with an L2 vertebral fracture and acute renal failure (serum creatinine 4.3 mg/dL). During your admission assessment, you learn that she has been managing her pain by taking six to eight tablets of

200-mg ibuprofen (Motrin) daily in place of her morphine because she "doesn't like the constipation" associated with the morphine and "doesn't want to get addicted." How did this change in pain management impact her current renal function? What is the evidence for opioid addiction in the setting of malignant bone disease? How would you incorporate these findings into your education plan? What other medical interventions might you anticipate being ordered? What other parameters would you include in your physical assessment? What other nursing interventions would you employ in caring for this woman?

3 **PG** You are caring for a 48-year-old man newly diagnosed with AML who has just completed induction chemotherapy. He is now febrile, with a temperature of 38.5°C (101.3°F), pulse 112/min, respirations 28/min, and blood pressure 108/62 mm Hg. His has lost 1 kg of body weight. You assess him and note that his breath sounds are clear, and his abdomen is soft with active bowel sounds. He has multiple petechiae over his lower extremities, chest, and back, accompanied by some scattered purpura. He has multiple open lesions on his buccal mucosa and complains of painful dysphagia, loose stools, and headache. His CBC shows a WBC of $0.4/mm^3$, hemoglobin of 6.8 g/dL, and platelets of $4,000/mm^3$. The microbiology lab calls you to report a positive blood culture. You notice that the report suggests the organism is not sensitive to his current antibiotic regimen. What additional observations will you include in your assessment? What other laboratory and radiographic information will you include in your assessment? How will you prioritize your care for this gentleman?

Brunner Suite Resources

Explore these additional resources to enhance learning for this chapter:
• NCLEX-Style Questions and Other Resources on thePoint, http://thePoint.lww.com/Brunner13e
• Study Guide
• PrepU
• Clinical Handbook
• Handbook of Laboratory and Diagnostic Tests

References

*Asterisk indicates nursing research.

Books

Liesveld, J. L., & Lichtman, M. A. (2010). Chapter 89. Acute myelogenous leukemia. In K. Kaushansky, M. A. Lichtman, E. Beutler, et al. (Eds.). *Williams hematology* (8th ed.). New York: McGraw-Hill.
Pui, C. (2010). Acute lymphoblastic leukemia. In K. Kaushansky, M. A. Lichtman, E. Beutler, et al. (Eds.). *Williams hematology* (8th ed.). New York: McGraw-Hill.

Journals and Electronic Documents

Leukemia
American Cancer Society. (2010a). *Treating leukemia—acute lymphocytic (ALL) in adults.* Revised 10/29/2010. Available at: www.cancer.org/Cancer/Leukemia-AcuteLymphocyticALLinAdults/DetailedGuide
American Cancer Society. (2010b). *What is leukemia—chronic lymphocytic (CLL)?* Available at: www.cancer.org/Cancer/Leukemia-ChronicLymphocyticCLL/DetailedGuide/leukemia-chronic-lymphocytic-what-is-cll

American Cancer Society. (2013). *Do we know what causes chronic myeloid leukemia?* Available at: www.cancer.org/cancer/leukemia-chronicmyeloidcml/detailedguide/leukemia-chronic-myeloid-myelogenous-what-causes
Bassan, R., & Hoelzer, D. (2011). Modern therapy of acute lymphoblastic leukemia. *Journal of Clinical Oncology, 29*(5), 532–543.
Burnett, A. (2012). New induction and postinduction strategies in acute myeloid leukemia. *Current Opinion in Hematology, 19*(2), 76–81.
Campana, D. (2010). Minimal residual disease in acute lymphoblastic leukemia. *Hematology: American Society of Hematology Education Program, 2010*(1), 7–12.
Cortes, J., Moore, J., Maziarz, R., et al. (2010). Control of plasma uric acid in adults at risk for tumor lysis syndrome: Efficacy and safety of rasburicase alone and rasburicase followed by allopurinol compared with allopurinol alone—results of a multicenter phase III study. *Journal of Clinical Oncology, 28*(27), 4207–4213.
Eliasson, L., Clifford, S., Barber, N., et al. (2011). Exploring chronic myeloid leukemia patients' reasons for not adhering to the oral anticancer drug imatinib as prescribed. *Leukemia Research, 35*(5), 626–630.
Franchini, M., Di Minno, M., & Coppola, A. (2010). Disseminated intravascular coagulation in hematologic malignancies. *Seminars in Thrombosis & Hemostasis, 36*(4), 388–403.
Gambacorti-Passerini, C., Antolini, L., Mahon, F. X., et al. (2011). Multicenter independent assessment of outcomes in chronic myeloid leukemia patients treated with imatinib. *Journal of the National Cancer Institute, 103*(7), 553–561.
Gibben, J., & O'Brien, S. (2011). Update on therapy of chronic lymphocytic leukemia. *Journal of Clinical Oncology, 29*(5), 544–550.
Greaves, M., & Maley, C. (2012). Clonal evolution in cancer. *Nature, 481*(7381), 306–313.
Jubelirer, S. J. (2011). The benefit of the neutropenic diet: Fact or fiction? *Oncologist, 16*(5), 704–707.
Kantarjian, H. M., Thomas, X. G., Dmoszynska, A., et al. (2012). Multicenter, randomized, open-label, phase III trial of decitabine versus patient choice, with physician advice, of either supportive care or low-dose cytarabine for the treatment of older patients with newly diagnosed acute myeloid leukemia. *Journal of Clinical Oncology, 30*(21), 2670–2677.
Lanasa, M. (2010). Novel insights into the biology of CLL. *Hematology: American Society of Hematology Education Program, 2010*(1), 70–76.
Leukemia and Lymphoma Society. (2012). *Facts and Statistics.* Available at: www.lls.org/#/diseaseinformation/getinformationsupport/faststastics
Marin, D., Bazeos, A., Mahon, F., et al. (2010). Adherence is the critical factor for achieving molecular responses in patients with chronic myeloid leukemia who achieve complete cytogenetic responses on imatinib. *Journal of Clinical Oncology, 28*(14), 2381–2388.
National Cancer Institute. (2011). *Cancer statistics: Acute myeloid leukemia.* Available at: seer.cancer.gov/faststats/selections.php?#Output
National Cancer Institute. (2012a). *General information about adult acute myeloid leukemia.* Available at: www.cancer.gov/cancertopics/pdq/treatment/adultAML/healthprofessional
National Cancer Institute. (2012b). *Treatment for untreated adult ALL.* Available at: www.cancer.gov/cancertopics/pdq/treatment/adultALL/HealthProfessional/Page5#Section_87
Neofytos, D., Lu, K., Hatfield-Seung, A., et al. (2013). Epidemiology, outcomes, and risk factors of invasive fungal infections in adult patients with acute myelogenous leukemia after induction chemotherapy. *Diagnostic Microbiology and Infectious Disease, 75*(2), 144–149.
Parker, T., & Strout, M. (2011). Chronic lymphocytic leukemia: Prognostic factors and impact on treatment. *Discovery Medicine, 11*(57), 115–123.
Robinson, L. (2011). Late effects of acute lymphoblastic leukemia therapy in patients diagnosed at 0–20 years of age. *Hematology: American Society of Hematology Education Program, 2011*(1), 238–242.
Sagatys, A., & Zhang, L. (2012). Clinical and laboratory prognostic indicators in chronic lymphocytic leukemia. *Cancer Control, 19*(1), 18–25.
Stein, E., & Tallman, M. (2012). Provocative pearls in diagnosing and treating acute promyelocytic leukemia. *Oncology, 26*(7), 636–641.
*Tamayo, G., Broxson, A., Munsell, M., et al. (2010). Caring for the caregiver. *Oncology Nursing Forum, 37*(1), E50–E57.
Tinsley, S. (2010). Safety profiles of second-line tyrosine kinase inhibitors in patients with chronic myeloid leukemia. *Journal of Clinical Nursing, 19*(9–10), 1207–1218.

Myelodysplastic Syndromes
Bhatia, R., & Deeg, H. J. (2011). Treatment-related myelodysplastic syndrome: Molecular characteristics and therapy. *Current Opinion in Hematology, 18*(2), 77–82.

Fenaux, P., Mufti, G., Hellstrom-Lindberg, et al. (2009). Efficacy of azacitidine compared with that of conventional care regimens in the treatment of higher-risk myelodysplastic syndromes: A randomized, open-label, phase III study. *Lancet Oncology, 10*(3), 223–232.

Garcia-Manero, G., & Fenaux, P. (2011). Hypomethylating agents and other novel strategies in myelodysplastic syndromes. *Journal of Clinical Oncology, 29*(5), 516–523.

Malak, S., Labopin, M., Saint-Martin, C., et al. (2012). French group of familial myeloproliferative disorders. *Blood Cell, Molecules, & Diseases, 49*(3–4), 170–176.

Other Myeloid Clonal Disorders (Polycythemia Vera, Essential Thrombocythemia, Myelofibrosis)

Beer, P., Erber, W., Campbell, P., et al. (2011). How I treat essential thrombocythemia. *Blood, 117*(5), 1472–1482.

Carobbio, A., Thiele, J., Passamonti, F., et al. (2011). Risk factors for arterial and venous thrombosis in WHO-defined essential thrombocythemia: An international study of 891 patients. *Blood, 117*(22), 5857–5859.

Kundranda, M., Tibes, R., & Mesa, R. (2012). Transformation of a chronic myeloproliferative neoplasm to acute myelogenous leukemia: Does anything work? *Current Hematological Reports, 7*(1), 78–86.

Miller, T., & Farquharson, M. (2010). Essential thrombocythemia and its neurological complications. *Practical Neurology, 10*(4), 195–201.

Saini, K., Patnaik, M., & Tefferi, A. (2010). Polycythemia vera–associated pruritis and its management. *European Journal of Clinical Investigation, 40*(9), 828–834.

Shukron, O., Vainstein, V., Kündgen, A., et al. (2012). Analyzing transformation of myelodysplastic syndrome to secondary acute myeloid leukemia using a large patient database. *American Journal of Hematology, 87*(9), 853–860.

Spivak, J. (2010). Narrative review: Thrombocytosis, polycythemia vera, and JAK2 mutations: The phenotypic mimicry of chronic myeloproliferation. *Annals of Internal Medicine, 152*(5), 300–306.

Squizzato, A., Romualdi, E., & Middeldorp, S. (2011). Antiplatelet drugs for polycythaemia vera and essential thrombocythaemia. *Cochrane Database of Systematic Reviews, (2), CD006503.

Stein, B. L., & Moliterno, A. R. (2010). Primary myelofibrosis and the myeloproliferative neoplasms: The role of individual variation. *Journal of the American Medical Association, 303*(24), 2513–2518.

Tefferi, A. (2011). Annual clinical updates in hematological malignancies: A continuing medical education series: Polycythemia vera and essential thrombocythemia: 2011 update on diagnosis, risk-stratification, and management. *American Journal of Hematology, 86*(3), 292–301.

Tefferi, A., & Vainchenker, W. (2011). Myeloproliferative neoplasms: Molecular pathophysiology, essential clinical understanding, and treatment strategies. *Journal of Clinical Oncology, 29*(5), 573–582.

Tibes, R., & Mesa, R. (2011). Myeloproliferative neoplasms 5 years after discovery of JAK2V617F: What is the impact of JAK2 inhibitor therapy? *Leukemia & Lymphoma, 52*(7), 1178–1187.

Lymphoma

American Cancer Society. (2010c). *What are the key statistics about non-Hodgkin lymphoma?* Available at: www.cancer.org/Cancer/non-hodgkinLymphoma/DetailedGuide/non-hodgkin-lymphoma-key-statistics

American Cancer Society. (2010d). *Early detection, diagnosis, and staging topics.* Last revised 1/26/12. Available at: www.cancer.org/cancer/non-hodgkinlymphoma/detailedguide/non-hodgkin-lymphoma-survival-rates

Arden-Close, E., Pacey, A., & Eiser, C. (2010). Health-related quality of life in survivors of lymphoma: A systematic review and methodological critique. *Leukemia & Lymphoma, 51*(4), 628–640.

Bartlett, N. (2010). The present: Optimizing therapy—too much or too little? *Hematology: American Society of Hematology Educational Program, 2010,* 108–114.

Baxi, S., & Matasar, M. (2010). State-of-the-art issues in Hodgkin's lymphoma survivorship. *Current Oncology Reports, 12*(6), 366–373.

Borchmann, P., & Engert, A. (2010). The past: What we have learned in the last decade. *Hematology: American Society of Hematology Educational Program, 2010,* 101–107.

Geyer, S., Morton, L., Habermann, T., et al. (2010). Smoking, alcohol use, obesity, and overall survival from non-Hodgkin lymphoma: A population-based study. *Cancer, 116*(12), 2993–3000.

Herbst, C., Rehan, F., Skoet, N., et al. (2011). Chemotherapy alone versus chemotherapy plus radiotherapy for early stage Hodgkin lymphoma. *Cochrane Database of Systematic Reviews, (2), CD007110.

Kallab, A. (2011). *Diffuse large cell lymphoma.* Available at: emedicine.medscape.com/article/202969-overview#aw2aab6c18aa

Kobe, C., Dietlein, M., Kriz, J., et al. (2010). The role of PET in Hodgkin's lymphoma and its impact on radiation oncology. *Expert Review of Anticancer Therapy, 10*(9), 1419–1428.

National Comprehensive Cancer Network. (2012). NCCN non-Hodgkin's lymphomas version 3.2012. *NCCN clinical practice guidelines in oncology, 2012. National Comprehensive Cancer Network, Inc.* Available at: www.nccn.org

Norden, A., Hochberg, E., & Hochberg, F. (2012). *Secondary involvement of the central nervous system by non-Hodgkin lymphoma.* In A. Freedman (Ed.). *UpToDate.* Available at: www.uptodate.com

Rummel, M. (2010). Reassessing the standard of care in indolent lymphoma: A clinical update to improve clinical practice. *Journal of the National Comprehensive Cancer Network, 8*(Suppl. 6), S1–S14.

Shapiro, R. (2011). Malignancies in the setting of primary immunodeficiency: Implications for hematologists/oncologists. *American Journal of Hematology, 86*(1), 48–55.

Shenoy, P., Maggioncalda, A., Malik, N., et al. (2011). Incidence patterns and outcomes for Hodgkin lymphoma patients in the United States. *Advances in Hematology, 2011,* 725219. Epub 2010 Dec 16. PMID: 21197477.

Zwick, C., Murawski, N., & Pfreundschuh, M. (2010). Rituximab in high-grade lymphoma. *Seminars in Hematology, 47*(2), 148–155.

Multiple Myeloma

Chen, D., Frezza, M., Schmitt, S., et al. (2011). Bortezomib as the first proteasome inhibitor anticancer drug: Current status and future perspectives. *Current Cancer Drug Targets, 11*(3), 2239–2253.

Delforge, M., Bladé, J., Dimopoulos, M., et al. (2010). Treatment-related peripheral neuropathy in multiple myeloma: The challenge continues. *Lancet Oncology, 11*(11), 1086–1095.

Gay, F., & Palumbo, A. (2010). Management of disease and treatment-related complications in patients with multiple myeloma. *Medical Oncology, 27*(Suppl. 1), S43–S52.

Mateos, M. (2010). Management of treatment-related adverse events in patients with multiple myeloma. *Cancer Treatment Reviews, 36*(Suppl. 2), S24–S32.

Munshi, N., Anderson, K., Bersagel, L., et al. (2011). Consensus recommendations for risk stratification in multiple myeloma: A report of the International Myeloma Workshop Consensus Panel 2. *Blood, 117*(18), 4696–4700.

Palumbo, A., & Anderson, K. (2011). Multiple myeloma. *New England Journal of Medicine, 364*(11), 1046–1060.

Roodman, G. (2011). Osteoblast function in myeloma. *Bone, 48*(1), 135–140.

Terpos, E., Moulopoulos, L., & Dimopoulos, M. (2011). Advances in imaging and the management of myeloma bone disease. *Journal of Clinical Oncology, 29*(14), 1907–1915.

Resources

Alternative Medicine Foundation, www.amfoundation.org
American Cancer Society, www.cancer.org
American Pain Society, www.ampainsoc.org
American Society for Blood and Marrow Transplantation (ASBMT), www.asbmt.org
APS Foundation of America (antiphospholipid antibody syndrome), www.apsfa.org
Blood and Marrow Transplant Information Network, www.bmtinfonet.org
International Myeloma Foundation, www.myeloma.org
Leukemia and Lymphoma Society, www.lls.org
Lymphoma Research Foundation, www.lymphoma.org
MedlinePlus (information on drug–herb interaction), www.nlm.nih.gov/medlineplus/druginfo/herb_All.html
Myelodysplastic Syndromes Foundation (MDS), www.mds-foundation.org
National Cancer Institute, www.cancer.gov
National Heart, Lung, and Blood Institute, www.nhlbi.nih.gov
National Marrow Donor Program, www.marrow.org
Oncology Nursing Society (ONS), www.ons.org

Unit
8
Immunologic Function

AN IMMUNOSUPPRESSED PATIENT WITH A HISTORY OF ORAL INFECTIONS

Mrs. Baker is a 67-year-old grandmother who has severe rheumatoid arthritis and provides day care for her three preschool-aged grandchildren. She has been taking prednisone, 10 mg daily for 6 months, as part of a treatment plan that also includes nonsteroidal anti-inflammatory drugs and disease-modifying antirheumatic drugs. Although her primary provider has tried to taper the prednisone, Mrs. Baker experiences a painful flare-up of her rheumatoid arthritis and symptoms of steroid withdrawal each time the dose is reduced. Mrs. Baker states that when her symptoms flare, she takes an extra dose of prednisone. She has had oral candidal disease twice in the preceding 3 months and has had frequent upper respiratory tract infections.

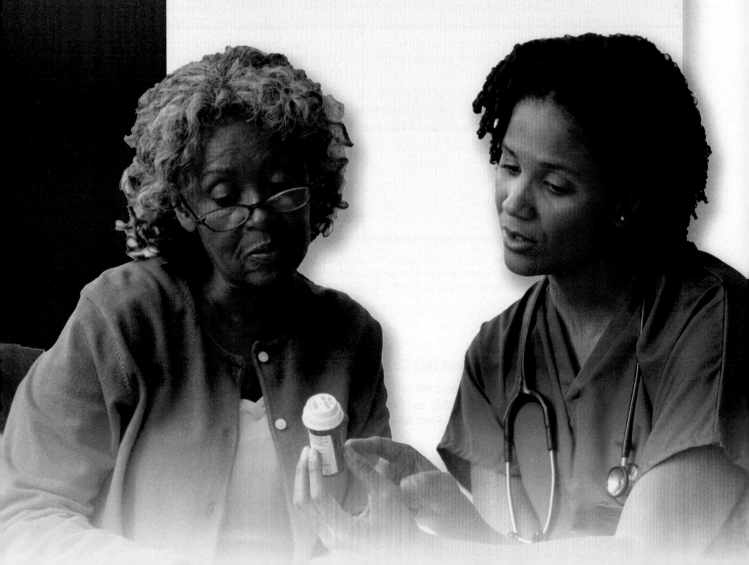

QSEN Competency Focus: *Evidence-Based Practice*

The complexities inherent in today's health care system challenge nurses to demonstrate integration of specific interdisciplinary core competencies. These competencies are aimed at ensuring the delivery of safe, quality patient care (Institute of Medicine, 2003). The concepts from the Quality and Safety Education for Nurses (QSEN) Institute (2012) provide a framework for the knowledge, skills, and attitudes (KSAs) required for nurses to demonstrate competency in these key areas, which include *patient-centered care, interdisciplinary teamwork and collaboration, evidence-based practice, quality improvement, safety*, and *informatics*.

Evidence-Based Practice Definition: Integrate best current evidence with clinical expertise and patient/family preferences and values for delivery of optimal health care.

RELEVANT PRE-LICENSURE KSAs	APPLICATION AND REFLECTION
Knowledge	
Explain the role of evidence in determining best clinical practice.	Based upon current best practices, critique Mrs. Baker's use of medications to treat her rheumatoid arthritis. Discuss how Mrs. Baker's self-tapering of dosages of prednisone may affect her rheumatoid arthritis and her bouts of oral candidiasis and upper respiratory tract infections.
Skills	
Question rationale for routine approaches to care that result in less-than-desired outcomes or adverse events.	Identify how you might begin a conversation with Mrs. Baker about her satisfaction with her current therapeutic regimen. What resources might you mobilize for her so that her outcomes may improve?
Attitudes	
Value the need for continuous improvement in clinical practice based on new knowledge.	Reflect on your attitudes toward patients with chronic diseases with unpredictable clinical trajectories, such as rheumatoid arthritis. Do you tend to think that patients with chronic diseases must inevitably have more episodic illnesses, such as oral infections and upper respiratory infections?

Cronenwett, L., Sherwood, G., Barnsteiner, J., et al. (2007). Quality and safety education for nurses. *Nursing Outlook, 55*(3), 122–131.
Institute of Medicine. (2003). *Health professions education: A bridge to quality.* Washington, DC: National Academies Press.
QSEN Institute. (2012). *Competencies: Prelicensure KSAs.* Available at: qsen.org/competencies/pre-licensure-ksas

Read More About This Case

More information about this case study and the relationships between nursing diagnoses, interventions, and expected outcomes is available online. Visit thePoint for Applying Concepts From NANDA-I, NIC, and NOC.

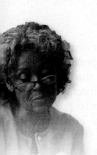
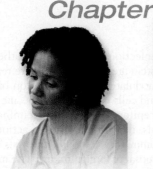

35

Assessment of Immune Function

Learning Objectives

On completion of this chapter, the learner will be able to:

1 Describe the body's general immune responses.
2 Discuss the stages of the immune response.
3 Differentiate between cellular and humoral immune responses.

4 Describe the effects of selected variables on function of the immune system.
5 Use assessment parameters for determining the status of patients' immune function.

Glossary

agglutination: clumping effect occurring when an antibody acts as a cross-link between two antigens

antibody: a protein substance developed by the body in response to and interacting with a specific antigen

antigen: substance that induces the production of antibodies

antigenic determinant: the specific area of an antigen that binds with an antibody combining site and determines the specificity of the antigen–antibody reaction

apoptosis: programmed cell death that results from the digestion of deoxyribonucleic acid by end nucleases

B cells: cells that are important for producing a humoral immune response

cellular immune response: the immune system's third line of defense, involving the attack of pathogens by T cells

complement: series of enzymatic proteins in the serum that, when activated, destroy bacteria and other cells

cytokines: generic term for nonantibody proteins that act as intercellular mediators, as in the generation of immune response

cytotoxic T cells: lymphocytes that lyse cells infected with virus; also play a role in graft rejection

epitope: any component of an antigen molecule that functions as an antigenetic determinant by permitting the attachment of certain antibodies

genetic engineering: emerging technology designed to enable replacement of missing or defective genes

helper T cells: lymphocytes that attack foreign invaders (antigens) directly

humoral immune response: the immune system's second line of defense; often termed the antibody response

immune response: the coordinated response of the components of the immune system to a foreign agent or organism

immune system: the collection of organs, cells, tissues, and molecules that mediate the immune response

immunity: the body's specific protective response to a foreign agent or organism; resistance to disease, specifically infectious diseases

immunopathology: study of diseases resulting in dysfunctions within the immune system

immunoregulation: complex system of checks and balances that regulates or controls immune responses

interferons: proteins formed when cells are exposed to viral or foreign agents; capable of activating other components of the immune system

lymphokines: substances released by sensitized lymphocytes when they come in contact with specific antigens

memory cells: cells that are responsible for recognizing antigens from previous exposure and mounting an immune response

natural killer (NK) cells: lymphocytes that defend against microorganisms and malignant cells

null lymphocytes: lymphocytes that destroy antigens already coated with the antibody

opsonization: the coating of antigen–antibody molecules with a sticky substance to facilitate phagocytosis

phagocytic cells: cells that engulf, ingest, and destroy foreign bodies or toxins

phagocytic immune response: the immune system's first line of defense, involving white blood cells that have the ability to ingest foreign particles

stem cells: precursors of all blood cells; reside primarily in bone marrow

suppressor T cells: lymphocytes that decrease B-cell activity to a level at which the immune system is compatible with life

T cells: cells that are important for producing a cellular immune response

Immunity is the body's specific protective response to a foreign agent or organism. The **immune system** functions as the body's defense mechanism against invasion and allows a rapid response to foreign substances in a specific manner. Genetic and cellular responses result. Any qualitative or quantitative change in the components of the immune system can produce profound effects on the integrity of the human organism. Immune function is affected by a variety of factors, such as central nervous system integrity; general physical and emotional status; medications; dietary patterns; and the stress of illness, trauma, or surgery (Yermal, Witek-Janusek, Peterson, et al., 2010). Dysfunctions involving the immune system occur across the lifespan. Many are genetically based; others are acquired. Immune memory is a property of the immune system that provides protection against harmful microbial agents despite the timing of re-exposure to the agent. Tolerance is the mechanism by which the immune system is programmed to eliminate foreign substances such as microbes, toxins, and cellular mutations but maintains the ability to accept self-antigens. Some credence is given to the concept of surveillance, in which the immune system is in a perpetual state of vigilance, screening and rejecting any invader that is recognized as foreign to the host. The term **immunopathology** refers to the study of diseases that result from dysfunctions within the immune system. Disorders of the immune system may stem from excesses or deficiencies of immunocompetent cells, alterations in the function of these cells, immunologic attack on self-antigens, or inappropriate or exaggerated responses to specific antigens (Table 35-1).

Growing numbers of patients with primary immune deficiencies live to adulthood, and many others acquire immune disorders during their adult years. Thus, nurses in many practice settings need to understand how the immune system functions as well as immunopathologic processes. In addition, knowledge about assessment and care of people with immunologic disorders enables nurses to make appropriate management decisions.

Anatomic and Physiologic Overview

Anatomy of the Immune System

The immune system is composed of an integrated collection of various cell types, each with a designated function in defending against infection and invasion by other organisms. Supporting this system are molecules that are responsible for the interactions, modulations, and regulation of the system. These molecules and cells participate in specific interactions with immunogenic **epitopes** (antigenic determinants) present on foreign materials, initiating a series of actions in a host, including the inflammatory response, the lysis of microbial agents, and the disposal of foreign toxins. The major components of the immune system include central and peripheral organs, tissues, and cells (Fig. 35-1).

Bone Marrow

The white blood cells (WBCs) involved in immunity are produced in the bone marrow (Fig. 35-2). Like other blood cells, lymphocytes are generated from **stem cells** (undifferentiated cells). There are two types of lymphocytes—B lymphocytes (**B cells**) and T lymphocytes (**T cells**) (Fig. 35-3).

Lymphoid Tissues

The spleen, composed of red and white pulp, acts somewhat like a filter. The red pulp is the site where old and injured red blood cells (RBCs) are destroyed. The white pulp contains concentrations of lymphocytes. The lymph nodes, which are

TABLE 35-1	Immune System Disorders
Disorder	**Description**
Autoimmunity	Normal protective immune response paradoxically turns against or attacks the body, leading to tissue damage
Hypersensitivity	Body produces inappropriate or exaggerated responses to specific antigens
Gammopathies	Overproduction of immunoglobulins
Immune deficiencies	
Primary	Deficiency results from improper development of immune cells or tissues; usually congenital or inherited
Secondary	Deficiency results from some interference with an already developed immune system; usually acquired later in life

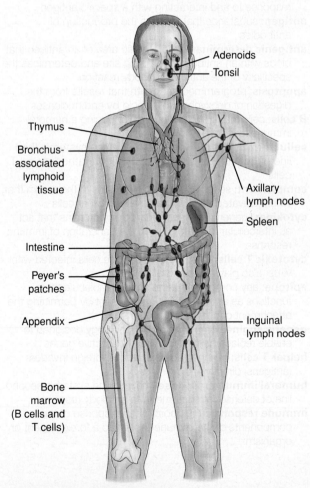

FIGURE 35-1 • Central and peripheral lymphoid organs, tissues, and cells. Adapted from Porth, C. M., & Matfin, G. (2009). *Pathophysiology: Concepts of altered health states* (8th ed., p. 371). Philadelphia: Lippincott Williams & Wilkins.

Labels on figure: Adenoids, Tonsil, Thymus, Bronchus-associated lymphoid tissue, Axillary lymph nodes, Spleen, Intestine, Peyer's patches, Appendix, Inguinal lymph nodes, Bone marrow (B cells and T cells)

Physiology ·:·:· Pathophysiology

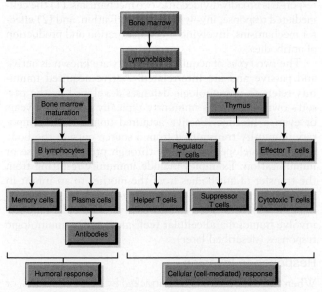

FIGURE 35-2 • Development of cells of the immune system.

connected by lymph channels and capillaries, are distributed throughout the body. They remove foreign material from the lymph system before it enters the bloodstream. The lymph nodes also serve as centers for immune cell proliferation. The remaining lymphoid tissues contain immune cells that defend the body's mucosal surfaces against microorganisms (Levinson, 2010).

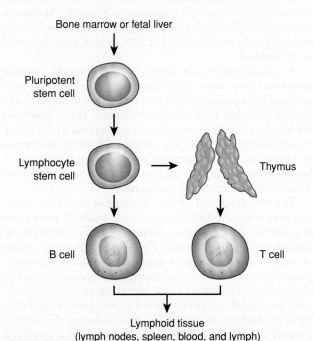

FIGURE 35-3 • Lymphocytes originate from stem cells in the bone marrow. B lymphocytes mature in the bone marrow before entering the bloodstream, whereas T lymphocytes mature in the thymus, where they also differentiate into cells with various functions. Redrawn from Porth, C. M., & Matfin, G. (2009). *Pathophysiology: Concepts of altered health states* (8th ed., p. 362). Philadelphia: Lippincott Williams & Wilkins.

Function of the Immune System

The basic function of the immune system is to remove foreign antigens such as viruses and bacteria to maintain homeostasis. There are two general types of immunity: natural (innate) and acquired (adaptive). Natural immunity or nonspecific immunity is present at birth. Acquired or specific immunity develops after birth. Each type of immunity has a distinct role in defending the body against harmful invaders, but the various components are usually interdependent (Levinson, 2010).

Natural Immunity

Natural immunity, which is nonspecific, provides a broad spectrum of defense against and resistance to infection. It is considered the first line of host defense following antigen exposure, because it protects the host without remembering prior contact with an infectious agent (Abbas & Lichtman, 2011). Responses to a foreign invader are very similar from one encounter to the next, regardless of the number of times the invader is encountered. Natural (innate) immunity co-coordinates the initial response to pathogens through the production of cytokines and other effector molecules, which either activate cells for control of the pathogen (by elimination) or promote the development of the acquired **immune response**. The cells involved in this response are monocytes, macrophages, dendrite cells, **natural killer (NK) cells**, basophils, eosinophils, and granulocytes. The early events in this process are critical in determining the nature of the adaptive immune response. Natural immune mechanisms can be divided into two stages: immediate (generally occurring within 4 hours after exposure) and delayed (occurring between 4 and 96 hours after exposure) (Haynes, Soderberg, & Fauci, 2012).

White Blood Cell Action

The cellular response is key to the effective initiation of the immune response. WBCs, or leukocytes, participate in both the natural and the acquired immune responses. Granular leukocytes, or granulocytes (so called because of granules in their cytoplasm), fight invasion by foreign bodies or toxins by releasing cell mediators, such as histamine, bradykinin, and prostaglandins, and engulfing the foreign bodies or toxins. Granulocytes include neutrophils, eosinophils, and basophils.

Neutrophils (polymorphonuclear leukocytes) are the first cells to arrive at the site where inflammation occurs. Eosinophils and basophils, other types of granulocytes, increase in number during allergic reactions and stress responses. Nongranular leukocytes include monocytes or macrophages (referred to as histocytes when they enter tissue spaces) and lymphocytes. Monocytes also function as **phagocytic cells**, engulfing, ingesting, and destroying greater numbers and quantities of foreign bodies or toxins than granulocytes do. Lymphocytes, consisting of B cells and T cells, play major roles in humoral and cell-mediated immune responses. About 60% to 70% of lymphocytes in the blood are T cells, and about 10% to 20% are B cells (Abbas & Lichtman, 2011).

Inflammatory Response

The inflammatory response is a major function of the natural immune system that is elicited in response to tissue injury or invading organisms. Chemical mediators assist this response by minimizing blood loss, walling off the invading organism, activating phagocytes, and promoting formation of fibrous scar tissue and regeneration of injured tissue. The inflammatory response (discussed further in Chapter 6) is facilitated by physical and chemical barriers that are part of the human organism.

Physical and Chemical Barriers

Activation of the natural immunity response is enhanced by processes inherent in physical and chemical barriers. Physical surface barriers include intact skin, mucous membranes, and cilia of the respiratory tract, which prevent pathogens from gaining access to the body. The cilia of the respiratory tract, along with coughing and sneezing responses, filter and clear pathogens from the upper respiratory tract before they can invade the body further. Chemical barriers, such as mucus, acidic gastric secretions, enzymes in tears and saliva, and substances in sebaceous and sweat secretions, act in a nonspecific way to destroy invading bacteria and fungi. Viruses are countered by other means, such as interferon (see discussion later in chapter).

Immune Regulation

Regulation of the immune response involves balance and counterbalance. Dysfunction of the natural immune system can occur when the immune components are inactivated or when they remain active long after their effects are beneficial. A successful immune response eliminates the responsible antigen. If an immune response fails to develop and clear an antigen sufficiently, the host is considered to be immunocompromised or immunodeficient. If the response is overly robust or misdirected, allergies, asthma, or autoimmune disease results. The immune system's recognition of one's own cells or tissues as "foreign" rather than as self is the basis of many autoimmune disorders (Porth & Matfin, 2009). Despite the fact that the immune response is critical to the prevention of disease, it must be well controlled to curtail immunopathology. Most microbial infections induce an inflammatory response mediated by T cells and cytokines, which, in excess, can cause tissue damage. Therefore, regulatory mechanisms must be in place to suppress or halt the immune response. This is mainly achieved by the production of cytokines and transformation of growth factor that inhibits macrophage activation. In some cases, T-cell activation is so overwhelming that these mechanisms fail, and pathology develops. Ongoing research on **immunoregulation** holds the promise of preventing graft rejection and aiding the body in eliminating cancerous or infected cells (Kumar, Abbas, Fausto, et al., 2010; Vergati, Intrivici, Huen, et al., 2010).

Although natural immunity can effectively combat infections, many pathogenic microbes have evolved that resist natural immunity. Acquired immunity is necessary to defend against these resistant agents.

Acquired Immunity

Acquired (adaptive) immunity usually develops as a result of prior exposure to an antigen through immunization (vaccination) or by contracting a disease, both of which generate a protective immune response. Weeks or months after exposure to the disease or vaccine, the body produces an immune response that is sufficient to defend against the disease on re-exposure. In contrast to the rapid but nonspecific natural immune response, this form of immunity relies on the recognition of specific foreign antigens. The acquired immune response is broadly divided into two mechanisms: (1) the cell-mediated response, involving T-cell activation, and (2) effector mechanisms, involving B-cell maturation and production of antibodies.

The two types of acquired immunity are known as active and passive and are interrelated. Active acquired immunity refers to immunologic defenses developed by the person's own body. This immunity typically lasts many years or even a lifetime. Passive acquired immunity is temporary immunity transmitted from a source outside the body that has developed immunity through previous disease or immunization. Examples include immunity resulting from the transfer of antibodies from the mother to an infant in utero or through breast-feeding or receiving injections of immune globulin. Active and passive acquired immunity involve humoral and cellular (cell-mediated) immunologic responses (described later).

Response to Invasion

When the body is invaded or attacked by bacteria, viruses, or other pathogens, it has three means of defense:
- The phagocytic immune response
- The humoral or antibody immune response
- The cellular immune response

The first line of defense, the **phagocytic immune response**, primarily involves the WBCs (granulocytes and macrophages), which have the ability to ingest foreign particles and destroy the invading agent; eosinophils are only weakly phagocytic. Phagocytes also remove the body's own dying or dead cells. Cells in necrotic tissue that are dying release substances that trigger an inflammatory response. **Apoptosis,** or programmed cell death, is the body's way of destroying worn-out cells such as blood or skin cells or cells that need to be renewed.

A second protective response, the **humoral immune response** (sometimes called the **antibody response**), begins with the B lymphocytes, which can transform themselves into plasma cells that manufacture antibodies. These antibodies are highly specific proteins that are transported in the bloodstream and attempt to disable invaders. The third mechanism of defense, the **cellular immune response**, also involves the T lymphocytes, which can turn into special cytotoxic (or killer) T cells that can attack the pathogens.

The structural part of the invading or attacking organism that is responsible for stimulating antibody production is called an **antigen** (or an immunogen). For example, an antigen can be a small patch of proteins on the outer surface of a microorganism. Not all antigens are naturally immunogenic; some must be coupled to other molecules to stimulate the immune response. A single bacterium or large molecule, such as a diphtheria or tetanus toxin, may have several antigens, or markers, on its surface, thus inducing the body to produce a number of different antibodies. Once produced, an antibody is released into the bloodstream and carried to the attacking organism. There, it combines with the antigen, binding with it like an interlocking piece of a jigsaw puzzle (Fig. 35-4). There are four well-defined stages in an immune response: recognition, proliferation, response, and effector (Fig. 35-5).

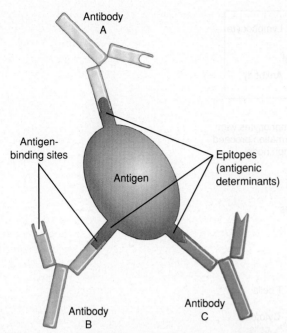

FIGURE 35-4 • Complement-mediated immune responses. Redrawn from Porth, C. M., & Matfin, G. (2009). *Pathophysiology: Concepts of altered health states* (8th ed., p. 361). Philadelphia: Lippincott Williams & Wilkins.

Recognition Stage

Recognition of antigens as foreign, or non-self, by the immune system is the initiating event in any immune response. Recognition involves the use of lymph nodes and lymphocytes for surveillance. Lymph nodes are widely distributed internally throughout the body and in the circulating blood, as well as externally near the body's surfaces. They continuously discharge small lymphocytes into the bloodstream. These lymphocytes patrol the tissues and vessels that drain the areas served by that node. Lymphocytes recirculate from the blood to lymph nodes and from the lymph nodes back into the bloodstream in a continuous circuit. The exact way in which they recognize antigens on foreign surfaces is not known; however, recognition is thought to depend on specific receptor sites on the surface of the lymphocytes. Macrophages play an important role in helping the circulating lymphocytes process the antigens. Both macrophages and neutrophils have receptors for antibodies and complement; as a result, they coat microorganisms with antibodies, complement, or both, thereby enhancing phagocytosis.

In a streptococcal throat infection, for example, the streptococcal organism gains access to the mucous membranes of the throat. A circulating lymphocyte moving through the tissues of the throat comes in contact with the organism. The lymphocyte recognizes the antigens on the microbe as different (non-self) and the streptococcal organism as antigenic (foreign). This triggers the second stage of the immune response—proliferation.

Proliferation Stage

The circulating lymphocytes containing the antigenic message return to the nearest lymph node. Once in the node, these sensitized lymphocytes stimulate some of the resident T and B lymphocytes to enlarge, divide, and proliferate. T lymphocytes differentiate into cytotoxic (or killer) T cells, whereas B lymphocytes produce and release antibodies. Enlargement of the lymph nodes in the neck in conjunction with a sore throat is one example of the immune response.

Response Stage

In the response stage, the differentiated lymphocytes function in either a humoral or a cellular capacity. This stage begins with the production of antibodies by the B lymphocytes in response to a specific antigen. The cellular response stimulates the resident lymphocytes to become cells that attack microbes directly rather than through the action of antibodies. These transformed lymphocytes are known as cytotoxic (killer) T cells.

Viral rather than bacterial antigens induce a cellular response. This response is manifested by the increasing number of T lymphocytes (lymphocytosis) seen in the blood tests of people with viral illnesses such as infectious mononucleosis. (Cellular immunity is discussed in further detail later in this chapter.) Most immune responses to antigens involve both humoral and cellular responses, although one usually predominates. For example, during transplant rejection, the cellular response involving T cells predominates, whereas in the bacterial pneumonias and sepsis, the humoral response involving B cells plays the dominant protective role (Chart 35-1).

Effector Stage

In the effector stage, either the antibody of the humoral response or the cytotoxic (killer) T cell of the cellular response reaches and connects with the antigen on the surface of the foreign invader. This initiates activities involving interplay of antibodies (humoral immunity), complement, and action by the cytotoxic T cells (cellular immunity).

Humoral Immune Response

The humoral response is characterized by the production of antibodies by B lymphocytes in response to a specific antigen. Whereas B lymphocytes are responsible for the production of antibodies, both the macrophages of natural immunity and the special T lymphocytes of cellular immunity are involved in recognition.

Chart 35-1 **Comparison of Cellular and Humoral Immune Responses**

Humoral Responses (B Cells)

- Bacterial phagocytosis and lysis
- Anaphylaxis
- Allergic hay fever and asthma
- Immune complex disease
- Bacterial and some viral infections

Cellular Responses (T Cells)

- Transplant rejection
- Delayed hypersensitivity (tuberculin reaction)
- Graft-versus-host disease
- Tumor surveillance or destruction
- Intracellular infections
- Viral, fungal, and parasitic infections

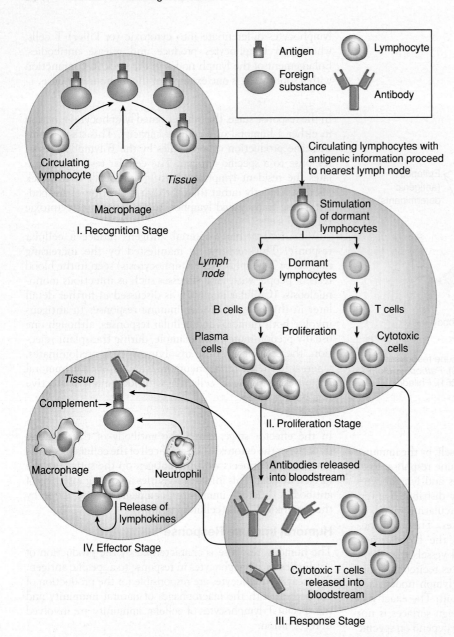

FIGURE 35-5 • Stages of the immune response. **I.** In the *recognition stage,* antigens are recognized by circulating lymphocytes and macrophages. **II.** In the *proliferation stage,* the dormant lymphocytes proliferate and differentiate into cytotoxic (killer) T cells or B cells responsible for formation and release of antibodies. **III.** In the *response stage,* the cytotoxic T cells and the B cells perform cellular and humoral functions, respectively. **IV.** In the *effector stage,* antigens are destroyed or neutralized through the action of antibodies, complement, macrophages, and cytotoxic T cells.

Antigen Recognition

Several theories explain the mechanisms by which B lymphocytes recognize the invading antigen and respond by producing antibodies. It is known that B lymphocytes recognize and respond to invading antigens in more than one way.

The B lymphocytes respond to some antigens by directly triggering antibody formation; however, in response to other antigens, they need the assistance of T cells to trigger antibody formation. With the help of macrophages, the T lymphocytes are believed to recognize the antigen of a foreign invader. The T lymphocyte picks up the antigenic message, or "blueprint," of the antigen and returns to the nearest lymph node with that message. B lymphocytes stored in the lymph nodes are subdivided into thousands of clones, which are stimulated to enlarge, divide, proliferate, and differentiate into plasma cells capable of producing specific antibodies to the antigen. Other B lymphocytes differentiate into B-lymphocyte clones with a memory for the antigen. These memory cells are responsible

for the more exaggerated and rapid immune response in a person who is repeatedly exposed to the same antigen.

Role of Antibodies

Antibodies are large proteins, called *immunoglobulins,* that consist of two subunits, each containing a light and a heavy peptide chain held together by a chemical link composed of disulfide bonds. Each subunit has one portion that serves as a binding site for a specific antigen and another portion that allows the antibody molecule to take part in the complement system.

Antibodies defend against foreign invaders in several ways, and the type of defense used depends on the structure and composition of both the antigen and the immunoglobulin. The antibody molecule has at least two combining sites, or Fab fragments (Fig. 35-6). One antibody can act as a crosslink between two antigens, causing them to bind or clump together. This clumping effect, referred to as **agglutination,**

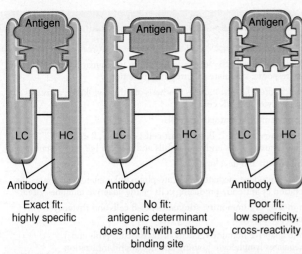

Exact fit:
highly specific

No fit:
antigenic determinant
does not fit with antibody
binding site

Poor fit:
low specificity,
cross-reactivity

FIGURE 35-6 • Antigen–antibody binding.(*Left*) A highly specific antigen–antibody complex. (*Center*) No match and, therefore, no immune response. (*Right*) Poor fit or match with low specificity; antibody reacts to antigen with similar characteristics, producing cross-reactivity. LC, light chain; HC, heavy chain.

helps clear the body of the invading organism by facilitating phagocytosis. Some antibodies assist in removal of offending organisms through **opsonization.** In this process, the antigen–antibody molecule is coated with a sticky substance that also facilitates phagocytosis.

Antibodies also promote the release of vasoactive substances, such as histamine and slow-reacting substances, two of the chemical mediators of the inflammatory response. Antibodies do not function in isolation; rather, they mobilize other components of the immune system to defend against the invader.

The body can produce five different types of immunoglobulin (Ig). Each of the five types, or classes, is identified by a specific letter of the alphabet, IgA, IgD, IgE, IgG, and IgM. Classification is based on the chemical structure and biologic role of the individual immunoglobulin. Major characteristics of the immunoglobulins are summarized in Chart 35-2. The normal laboratory values for the three major Igs (IgA, IgG and IgM) can be found in Table 39-1 in Chapter 39; see also Appendix A on thePoint.

Antigen–Antibody Binding

The portion of the antigen involved in binding with the antibody is referred to as the **antigenic determinant.** The most efficient immunologic responses occur when the antibody and antigen fit like a lock and key. Poor fit can occur with an antibody that was produced in response to a different antigen. This phenomenon is known as cross-reactivity. For example, in acute rheumatic fever, the antibody produced against *Streptococcus pyogenes* in the upper respiratory tract may cross-react with the patient's heart tissue, leading to heart valve damage.

Cellular Immune Response

The T lymphocytes are primarily responsible for cellular immunity. Stem cells continuously migrate from the bone marrow to the thymus gland, where they develop into T cells. Despite the partial degeneration of the gland at puberty, T cells continue to develop in the thymus gland. Several types of T cells exist, each with designated roles in the defense

---

Chart 35-2   Major Characteristics of the Immunoglobulins

IgG (75% of Total Immunoglobulin)

• Appears in serum and tissues (interstitial fluid)
• Assumes a major role in bloodborne and tissue infections
• Activates the complement system
• Enhances phagocytosis
• Crosses the placenta

IgA (15% of Total Immunoglobulin)

• Appears in body fluids (blood, saliva, tears, and breast milk, as well as pulmonary, gastrointestinal, prostatic, and vaginal secretions)
• Protects against respiratory, gastrointestinal, and genitourinary infections
• Prevents absorption of antigens from food
• Passes to neonate in breast milk for protection

IgM (10% of Total Immunoglobulin)

• Appears mostly in intravascular serum
• Appears as the first immunoglobulin produced in response to bacterial and viral infections
• Activates the complement system

IgD (0.2% of Total Immunoglobulin)

• Appears in small amounts in serum
• Possibly influences B-lymphocyte differentiation, but role is unclear

IgE (0.004% of Total Immunoglobulin)

• Appears in serum
• Takes part in allergic and some hypersensitivity reactions
• Combats parasitic infections

Ig, immunoglobulin

against bacteria, viruses, fungi, parasites, and malignant cells. T cells attack foreign invaders directly rather than by producing antibodies.

Cellular reactions are initiated, with or without the assistance of macrophages, by the binding of an antigen to an antigen receptor located on the surface of a T cell. The T cells then carry the antigenic message, or blueprint, to the lymph nodes, where the production of other T cells is stimulated. Some T cells remain in the lymph nodes and retain a memory for the antigen. Other T cells migrate from the lymph nodes into the general circulatory system and ultimately to the tissues, where they remain until they either come in contact with their respective antigens or die (Abbas & Lichtman, 2011).

Types of T Lymphocytes

T cells include effector T cells, suppressor T cells, and memory T cells. The two major categories of effector T cells— helper T cells (also referred to as CD4+ cells) and cytotoxic T cells (also referred to as CD8+ cells)—participate in the destruction of foreign organisms. T cells interact closely with B cells, indicating that humoral and cellular immune responses are not separate, unrelated processes but rather are branches of the immune response that interact.

Helper T cells are activated on recognition of antigens and stimulate the rest of the immune system. When activated,

TABLE 35-2 Cytokines of Innate and Adaptive Immunity

Cytokines	Source	Biologic Activity
Interleukin 1 (IL-1)	Macrophages, endothelial cells, some epithelial cells	Wide variety of biologic effects; activates endothelium in inflammation; induces fever and acute-phase response; stimulates neutrophil production
Interleukin 2 (IL-2)	CD4+, CD8+ T cells	Growth factor for activated T cells; induces synthesis of other cytokines; activates cytotoxic T lymphocytes and NK cells
Interleukin 3 (IL-3)	CD4+ T cells	Growth factor for progenitor hematopoietic cells
Interleukin 4 (IL-4)	CD4+ T_H2 cells, mast cells	Promotes growth and survival o f T, B, and mast cells; causes T_H2 cell differentiation; activates B cells and eosinophils and induces IgE-type responses
Interleukin 5 (IL-5)	CD4+ T_H2 cells	Induces eosinophil growth and development
Interleukin 6 (IL-6)	Macrophages, endothelial cells, T lymphocytes	Stimulates the liver to produce mediators of acute-phase inflammatory response; also induces proliferation of antibody-producing cells by the adaptive immune system
Interleukin 7 (IL-7)	Bone marrow stromal cells	Primary function in adaptive immunity; stimulates pre-B cells and thymocyte development and proliferation
Interleukin 8 (IL-8)	Macrophages, endothelial cells	Primary function in adaptive immunity; chemoattracts neutrophils and T lymphocytes; regulates lymphocyte homing and neutrophil infiltration
Interleukin 10 (IL-10)	Macrophages, some T-helper cells	Inhibitor of activated macrophages and dendritic cells; decreases inflammation by inhibiting T_H1 cells and release of interleukin 12 from macrophages
Interleukin 12 (IL-12)	Macrophages, dendritic cells	Enhances NK cell cytotoxicity in innate immunity; induces T_H1 cell differentiation in adaptive immunity
Type I interferons (IFN-α, IFN-β)	Macrophages, fibroblasts	Inhibit viral replication, activate NK cells, and increase expression of MHC-I molecules on virus-infected cells
Interferon-γ (IFN-γ)	NK cells, CD4+ and CD8+ T lymphocytes	Activates macrophages in both innate immune responses and adaptive cell-mediated immune responses; increases expression of MHC I and II and antigen processing and presentation
Tumor necrosis factor-α (TNF-α)	Macrophages, T cells	Induces inflammation, fever, and acute-phase response; activates neutrophils and endothelial cells; kills cells through apoptosis
Chemokines	Macrophages, endothelial cells, T lymphocytes	Large family of structurally similar cytokines that stimulate leukocyte movement and regulate the migration of leukocytes from the blood to the tissues
Granulocyte-monocyte CSF (GM-CSF)	T cells, macrophages, endothelial cells, fibroblasts	Promotes neutrophil, eosinophil, and monocyte maturation and growth; activates mature granulocytes
Granulocyte CSF (G-CSF)	Macrophages, fibroblasts, endothelial cells	Promotes growth and maturation of neutrophils consumed in inflammatory reactions
Monocyte CSF (M-CSF)	Macrophages, activated T cells, endothelial cells	Promotes growth and maturation of mononuclear phagocytes

NK, natural killer; T_H2, T-helper type 2; IgE, immunoglobulin E; T_H1, T-helper type 1; MHC, major histocompatibility complex; CSF, colony-stimulating factor.
Adapted from Porth, C. M., & Matfin, G. (2009). *Pathophysiology: Concepts of altered health states* (8th ed.). Philadelphia: Lippincott Williams & Wilkins.

helper T cells secrete **cytokines,** which attract and activate B cells, cytotoxic T cells, NK cells, macrophages, and other cells of the immune system. Separate subpopulations of helper T cells produce different types of cytokines and determine whether the immune response will be the production of antibodies or a cell-mediated immune response. Helper T cells also produce **lymphokines,** one category of cytokines (Table 35-2).

Cytotoxic T cells (killer T cells) attack the antigen directly by altering the cell membrane and causing cell lysis (disintegration) and by releasing cytolytic enzymes and cytokines. Lymphokines can recruit, activate, and regulate other lymphocytes and WBCs. These cells then assist in destroying the invading organism. Delayed-type hypersensitivity is an example of an immune reaction that protects the body from antigens through the production and release of lymphokines (see later discussion).

Suppressor T cells have the ability to decrease B-cell production, thereby keeping the immune response at a level that is compatible with health (e.g., sufficient to fight infection adequately without attacking the body's healthy tissues). **Memory cells** are responsible for recognizing antigens from previous exposure and mounting an immune response (Table 35-3).

Null Lymphocytes and Natural Killer Cells

Null lymphocytes and NK cells are other lymphocytes that assist in combating organisms. These cells are distinct from B cells and T cells and lack the usual characteristics of those cells. **Null lymphocytes,** a subpopulation of lymphocytes, destroy antigens already coated with antibody. These cells have special receptor sites on their surface that allow them to connect with the end of antibodies; this is known as antibody-dependent, cell-mediated cytotoxicity.

NK cells are a class of lymphocytes that recognize infected and stressed cells and respond by killing these cells and by secreting macrophage-activating cytokine. The helper T cells contribute to the differentiation of null and NK cells.

Complement System

Circulating plasma proteins, known as **complement,** are made in the liver and activated when an antibody connects with its antigen. Complement plays an important role in the defense against microbes. Destruction of an invading or attacking organism or toxin is not achieved merely by the binding of the antibody and antigens; it also requires activation of complement, the arrival of killer T cells, or the attraction of

TABLE 35-3 Lymphocytes Involved in Immune Responses

Type of Immune Response	Cell Type	Function
Humoral	B lymphocyte	Produces antibodies or immunoglobulins (IgA, IgD, IgE, IgG, IgM)
Cellular	T lymphocyte	
	Helper T	Attacks foreign invaders (antigens) directly
		Initiates and augments inflammatory response
	Helper T$_1$	Increases activated cytotoxic T cells
	Helper T$_2$	Increases B-cell [BG8]antibody production
	Suppressor T	Suppresses the immune response
	Memory T	Remembers contact with an antigen and on subsequent exposures mounts an immune response
	Cytotoxic T (killer T)	Lyses cells infected with virus; plays a role in graft rejection
Nonspecific	Non-T or non-B lymphocyte Null cell	Destroys antigens already coated with antibody
	Natural killer cell (granular lymphocyte)	Defends against microorganisms and some types of malignant cells; produces cytokines

macrophages. Complement has three major physiologic functions: defending the body against bacterial infection, bridging natural and acquired immunity, and disposing of immune complexes and the by-products associated with inflammation (Porth & Matfin, 2009).

The proteins that comprise complement interact sequentially with one another in a cascading effect. The complement cascade is important to modifying the effector arm of the immune system. Activation of complement allows important events, such as removal of infectious agents and initiation of the inflammatory response, to take place. These events involve active parts of the pathway that enhance chemotaxis of macrophages and granulocytes, alter blood vessel permeability, change blood vessel diameters, cause cells to lyse, alter blood clotting, and cause other points of modification. These macrophages and granulocytes continue the body's defense by devouring the antibody-coated microbes and by releasing bacterial products.

The complement cascade may be activated by any of three pathways: classic, lectin, and alternative. The classic pathway is triggered after antibodies bind to microbes or other antigens and is part of the humoral type of adaptive immunity. The lectin pathway is activated when a plasma protein (mannose-binding lectin) binds to terminal mannose residue on the surface glycoproteins of microbes. The alternative pathway is triggered when complement proteins are activated on microbial surfaces. This pathway is part of natural immunity.

Complement components, prostaglandins, leukotrienes, and other inflammatory mediators all contribute to the recruitment of inflammatory cells, as do chemokines, a group of cytokines. The activated neutrophils pass through the vessel walls to accumulate at the site of infection, where they phagocytize complement-coated microbes (Abbas & Lichtman, 2011). This response is usually therapeutic and can be lifesaving if the cell attacked by the complement system is a true foreign invader. However, if that cell is part of the human organism, the result can be devastating disease and even death. Many autoimmune diseases and disorders characterized by chronic infection are thought to be caused in part by continued or chronic activation of complement, which in turn results in chronic inflammation. The RBCs and platelets have complement receptors and, as a result, play an important role in the clearance of immune complexes that consist of antigen, antibody, and components of the complement system (Abbas & Lichtman, 2011).

Immunomodulators

Antimicrobial agents and vaccines have yielded considerable therapeutic success and the immune system usually works effectively; however, many infectious diseases remain difficult clinical challenges. Treatment success may be compromised by defects of the immune system; in this case, enhancement of the host immune response may be therapeutically beneficial. An immunomodulator (also known as a biologic response modifier) affects the host via direct or indirect effects on one or more components of the immunoregulatory network. Interferons, colony-stimulating factors, and monoclonal antibodies (MoAbs) are examples of agents used to help enhance the immune system (Liles, 2009).

Interferons

Interferon, one type of biologic response modifier, is a nonspecific viricidal protein that is naturally produced by the body and is capable of activating other components of the immune system. Interferons continue to be investigated to determine their roles in the immune system and their potential therapeutic effects in disorders characterized by disturbed immune responses. These substances have antiviral and antitumor properties. In addition to responding to viral infection, interferons are produced by T lymphocytes, B lymphocytes, and macrophages in response to antigens. They are thought to modify the immune response by suppressing antibody production and cellular immunity. They also facilitate the cytolytic role of macrophages and NK cells. Interferons are used to treat immune-related disorders (e.g., multiple sclerosis) and chronic inflammatory conditions (e.g., chronic hepatitis). Research continues to evaluate the effectiveness of interferons in treating cancers (Lapka & Franson, 2010) and acquired immunodeficiency syndrome.

Colony-Stimulating Factors

Colony-stimulating factors are a group of naturally occurring glycoprotein cytokines that regulate production, differentiation, survival, and activation of hematopoietic cells. Erythropoietin stimulates RBC production. Thrombopoietin plays a key regulatory role in the growth and differentiation of bone marrow cells. Interleukin 5 (IL-5) stimulates the growth and survival of eosinophils and basophils. Stem cell factor and IL-3 serve as stimuli for multiple hematopoietic cell lines. Granulocyte colony-stimulating factor, granulocyte-macrophage colony-stimulating factor, and macrophage colony-stimulating factor all serve as growth factors for specific cell lines. These cytokines have attracted considerable interest for their potential role in immunomodulation (Kumar et al., 2010).

Monoclonal Antibodies

MoAbs have become available through technologic advances, enabling investigators to grow and produce targeted antibodies for specific pathologic organisms. This type of specificity allows MoAbs to destroy pathologic organisms and spare normal cells. The specificity of MoAbs depends on identifying key antigen proteins that are present on the surface of tumors, but not on normal tissues. When the MoAb attaches to the cell surface antigen, it blocks an important signal transduction pathway for communication between the malignant cells and the extracellular environment. The results may include an inability to initiate apoptosis, reproduce, or invade surrounding tissues. To date, more than 1,000 tumor antigens have been identified (Lapka & Franson, 2010). (See Chapter 15 for a discussion on the use of MoAbs in cancer.)

Advances in Immunology

Genetic Engineering

One of the more remarkable evolving technologies is **genetic engineering,** which uses recombinant deoxyribonucleic acid (DNA) technology. Two facets of this technology exist. The first permits scientists to combine genes from one type of organism with genes of a second organism. This type of technology allows cells and microorganisms to manufacture proteins, monokines, and lymphokines, which can alter and enhance immune system function. The second facet of recombinant DNA technology involves gene therapy. If a particular gene is abnormal or missing, experimental recombinant DNA technology may be capable of restoring normal gene function. For example, a recombinant gene is inserted onto a virus particle. When the virus particle splices its genes, the virus automatically inserts the missing gene and theoretically corrects the genetic anomaly. Extensive research into recombinant DNA technology and gene therapy is ongoing (Abbas & Lichtman, 2011).

Stem Cells

Stem cells are capable of self-renewal and differentiation; they continually replenish the body's entire supply of both RBCs and WBCs. Some stem cells, described as totipotent cells, have tremendous capacity to self-renew and differentiate. Embryonic stem cells, described as pluripotent, give rise to numerous cell types that are able to form tissues. Research has shown that stem cells can restore an immune system that has been destroyed (Ko, 2012). Stem cell transplantation has been carried out in humans with certain types of immune dysfunction, such as severe combined immunodeficiency; clinical trials using stem cells are under way in patients with

a variety of disorders having an autoimmune component, including systemic lupus erythematosus, rheumatoid arthritis, scleroderma, and multiple sclerosis. Research with embryonic stem cells has enabled investigators to make substantial gains in developmental biology, gene therapy, therapeutic tissue engineering, and the treatment of a variety of diseases (Ko, 2012). However, along with these remarkable opportunities, many ethical challenges arise, which are largely based on concerns about safety, efficacy, resource allocation, and human cloning.

Assessment of the Immune System

An assessment of immune function begins during the health history and physical examination. Areas to be assessed include nutritional status; infections and immunizations; allergies; disorders and disease states, such as autoimmune disorders, cancer, and chronic illnesses; surgeries; medications; and blood transfusions. In addition to inspection of general characteristics, palpation of the lymph nodes and examinations of the skin, mucous membranes, and respiratory, gastrointestinal, musculoskeletal, genitourinary, cardiovascular, and neurosensory systems are performed (Chart 35-3).

Health History

The history should note the patient's age along with information about past and present conditions and events that may provide clues to the status of the patient's immune system.

Gender

There are differences in the immune system functions of men and women. For example, many autoimmune diseases have a higher incidence in females than in males, a phenomenon believed to be correlated with sex hormones. Sex hormones have long been recognized for their role in reproductive function; in the past two decades, research has revealed that these hormones are integral signaling modulators of the immune system. Sex hormones play definitive roles in lymphocyte maturation, activation, and synthesis of antibodies and cytokines. In autoimmune disease, expression of sex hormones is altered, and this change contributes to immune dysregulation (Munoz-Cruz, 2011).

Gerontologic Considerations

Immunosenescence is a complex route in which the aging process stimulates changes in the immune system (Miller, 2009). As the immune system undergoes age-associated alterations, its response to infections progressively deteriorates. The capacity for self-renewal of hematopoietic stem cells diminishes. There is a notable decline in the total number of phagocytes, coupled with an intrinsic reduction in their activity. The cytotoxicity of NK cells decreases, contributing to a decline in humoral immunity (Brunner, Herndler-Brandstetter, Weinberger, et al., 2011; Buchholtz, Neuenhahn, & Busch, 2011; Swain & Nikolich-Zugich, 2009). Acquired immunity may be negatively affected; the efficacy of vaccines is frequently decreased in older adults. Natural immunity continues to function reasonably well but diminishes with age. However, inflammatory cytokines increase with age (Masoro & Austad, 2011).

ASSESSMENT

Assessing for Immune Dysfunction

Be alert for the following signs and symptoms:

Respiratory System

- Changes in respiratory rate
- Cough (dry or productive)
- Abnormal lung sounds (wheezing, crackles, rhonchi)
- Rhinitis
- Hyperventilation
- Bronchospasm

Cardiovascular System

- Hypotension
- Tachycardia
- Dysrhythmia
- Vasculitis
- Anemia

Gastrointestinal System

- Hepatosplenomegaly
- Colitis
- Vomiting
- Diarrhea

Genitourinary System

- Frequency and burning on urination
- Hematuria
- Discharge

Musculoskeletal System

- Joint mobility, edema, and pain

Skin

- Rashes
- Lesions
- Dermatitis
- Hematomas or purpura
- Edema or urticaria
- Inflammation
- Discharge

Neurosensory System

- Cognitive dysfunction
- Hearing loss
- Visual changes
- Headaches and migraines
- Ataxia
- Tetany

The incidence of autoimmune diseases also increases with age, possibly from a decreased ability of antibodies to differentiate between self and non-self. Failure of the surveillance system to recognize mutant or abnormal cells also may be responsible, in part, for the high incidence of cancer associated with increasing age.

Age-related changes in many body systems also contribute to impaired immunity (Table 35-4). For example, postmenopausal females are at a greater risk for urinary tract infections due to residual urine, urinary incontinence, and estrogen deficiency (Torine, 2011). Secondary changes, including malnutrition and poor circulation, as well as the breakdown of

TABLE 35-4 Age-Related Changes in Immunologic Function

Body System	Changes	Consequences
Immune	Impaired function of B and T lymphocytes Failure of lymphocytes to recognize mutant or abnormal cells Decreased antibody production Failure of immune system to differentiate "self" from "non-self" Suppressed phagocytic immune response	Suppressed responses to pathogenic organisms with increased risk for infection Increased incidence of cancers Anergy (lack of response to antigens applied to the skin [allergens]) Increased incidence of autoimmune diseases Absence of typical signs and symptoms of infection and inflammation Dissemination of organisms usually destroyed or suppressed by phagocytes (e.g., reactivation or spread of tuberculosis)
Gastrointestinal	Decreased gastric secretions and motility Decreased phagocytosis by the liver's Kupffer cells Altered nutritional intake with inadequate protein intake	Proliferation of intestinal organisms resulting in gastroenteritis and diarrhea Increased incidence and severity of hepatitis B; increased incidence of liver abscesses Suppressed immune response
Urinary	Decreased kidney function and changes in lower urinary tract function (enlargement of prostate gland, neurogenic bladder); altered genitourinary tract flora	Urinary stasis and increased incidence of urinary tract infections
Pulmonary	Impaired ciliary action due to exposure to smoke and environmental toxins	Impaired clearance of pulmonary secretions; increased incidence of respiratory infections
Integumentary	Thinning of skin with less elasticity; loss of adipose tissue	Increased risk of skin injury, breakdown, and infection
Circulatory	Impaired microcirculation	Stasis and pressure ulcers
Neurologic function	Decreased sensation and slowing of reflexes	Increased risk of injury, skin ulcers, abrasions, and burns

natural mechanical barriers such as the skin, place the aging immune system at even greater disadvantage against infection.

The effects of the aging process and psychological stress interact, with the potential to negatively influence immune integrity (Masoro & Austad, 2011). Consequently, continual assessment of the physical and emotional status of older adults is imperative, because early recognition and management of factors influencing immune response may prevent or mitigate the high morbidity and mortality seen with illness in the older adult population (Brunner et al., 2011; Swain & Nikolich-Zugich, 2009).

Nutrition

The relationship of infection to nutritional status is a key determinant of health. Traditionally, this relationship focused on the effect of nutrients on host defenses and the effect of infection on nutritional needs. This has expanded in scope to encompass the role of specific nutrients in acquired immune function—the modulation of inflammatory processes and the virulence of the infectious agent itself. Iron and the immune system are linked in homeostasis and pathology, thus making it essential for maximum function (Ward, Crichton, Taylor, et al., 2011). The list of nutrients affecting infection, immunity, inflammation, and cell injury has expanded from traditional proteins to several vitamins, multiple minerals, and, more recently, specific lipid components of the diet (Takagi, Matsui, Ohno, et al., 2009). Vitamin D deficiency has been associated with increased risk of common cancers, autoimmune diseases, and inflammatory disorders (DiRosa, Malaguarnera, Nicoletti, et al., 2011). The role of micronutrients and fatty acids on the response of cells and tissues to hypoxic and toxic damage has been recognized, suggesting that there is another dimension to the relationship. Micronutrients such as zinc may have widespread negative effects on the immune response, which can be reversed by supplementation (Mocchegiani, Malavolta, Costarelli, et al., 2010).

The effects exerted by polyunsaturated fatty acids on immune system functions are under investigation. Studies suggest that these elements play a role in diminishing the incidence and severity of inflammatory disorders. Recent studies suggest that diets high in olive oil are not as immunosuppressive as diets rich in fish oil. The contribution of immune modulation by lipids to the high risk of infectious complications associated with the use of parenteral nutrition is unclear; however, a recent meta-analysis revealed that the use of glutamine-supplemented parenteral nutrition decreased the incidence of infections postoperatively (Wang, Jiang, Nolan, et al., 2010).

Depletion of protein reserves results in atrophy of lymphoid tissues, depression of antibody response, reduction in the number of circulating T cells, and impaired phagocytic function. As a result, susceptibility to infection is greatly increased. During periods of infection or serious illness, nutritional requirements may be further altered, potentially contributing to depletion of protein, fatty acid, vitamin, and trace elements and causing even greater risk of impaired immune response and sepsis. Nutritional intake that supports a competent immune response plays an important role in reducing the incidence of infections; patients whose nutritional status is compromised have a delayed postoperative recovery and often experience more severe infections and delayed wound healing. The nurse must assess the patient's nutritional status, caloric intake, and quality of foods ingested. There is evidence that nutrition plays a role in the development of cancer and that diet and lifestyle can alter the risk of cancer development as well as other chronic diseases (Strasser, Van, & Jatoi, 2011). The nurse must assume a proactive role in ensuring the best possible nutritional intake for all patients as a vital step in preventing disease and poor outcomes (DeBusk, Sierpina & Kreitzer, 2011).

Infection and Immunization

The patient is asked about childhood and adult immunizations, including vaccinations to provide protection against influenza, pneumococcal disease (Pneumovax), pertussis, herpes simplex, and the usual childhood diseases (e.g., measles, mumps). Herpes simplex virus infections have a significant impact on health, causing a wide range of diseases (e.g., oral and genital herpes). Education about the importance of adhering to the recommended schedule for these vaccines should be initiated. Known past or present exposure to tuberculosis is assessed, and the dates and results of any tuberculin tests (purified protein derivative [PPD] test) and chest x-rays are documented. Recent exposure to any infections and the exposure dates are elicited. The nurse must assess whether the patient has been exposed to any sexually transmitted infections (STIs) or bloodborne pathogens such as hepatitis B, C, and D viruses and human immunodeficiency virus (HIV). A history of STIs such as gonorrhea, syphilis, human papillomavirus infection, and chlamydia can alert the nurse that the patient may have been exposed to HIV or hepatitis. A history of past and present infections and the dates and types of treatments, along with a history of any multiple persistent infections, fevers of unknown origin, lesions or sores, or any type of drainage, as well as the response to treatment, are obtained.

Allergy

The patient is asked about any allergies, including types of allergens (e.g., pollens, dust, plants, cosmetics, food, medications, vaccines, latex), the symptoms experienced, and seasonal variations in occurrence or severity in the symptoms. A history of testing and treatments, including prescribed and over-the-counter medications that the patient has taken or is currently taking for these allergies and the effectiveness of the treatments, is obtained. All medication and food allergies are listed on an allergy alert sticker and placed on the front of the patient's health or medical record to alert others. Continued assessment for potential allergic reactions in the patient is vital. (See Chapter 38 for more information on allergies.)

Disorders and Diseases

Autoimmune Disorders

Autoimmune disorders affect people of both genders of all ages, ethnicities, and social classes. Autoimmune disorders are a group of disorders that can affect almost any cell or tissue in the body (Porth & Matfin, 2009). As mentioned previously, they tend to be more common in women because estrogen tends to enhance immunity. Androgen, on the other

GENETICS IN NURSING PRACTICE

Immunologic Disorders

An immunologic disorder is a disorder of an individual's immune system, which is a network of cells, tissues, and organs that work together to defend the body against attacks by foreign invaders such as bacteria, parasites, and fungi that can cause infection. A number of immunologic disorders are caused by a genetic abnormality. Some examples of immunologic disorders caused by a genetic abnormality include:

- Asthma
- Ataxia telangiectasia
- Autoimmune polyglandular syndrome
- Burkitt lymphoma
- Diabetes, type 1
- DiGeorge syndrome
- Familial Mediterranean fever
- Severe combined immunodeficiency

Nursing Assessments

Family History Assessment

- Collect a family history for both maternal and paternal relatives for three generations.
- Assess family history for other family members with histories of immunologic disorders.

Patient Assessment

- Assess for symptoms of autoimmune disease such as fatigue and mild rashes to rare, serious warning signs such as seizures.

- Assess for symptoms such as changes in respiratory status associated with asthma (e.g., wheezing, or airway hyperresponsiveness; mucosal edema; and mucus production).
- Assess for symptoms of immunodeficiency disorders in which a patient's resistance to disease becomes dangerously low.

Management Issues Specific to Genetics

- Inquire as to whether genetic testing has been performed on affected family members. For example, genetic testing is done for DiGeorge syndrome (also known as 22q11.2 deletion syndrome) to look for a defect in chromosome 22.
- Refer for further genetic counseling and evaluation so that family members can discuss inheritance, risk to other family members, and availability of genetic testing and gene-based interventions.
- Offer appropriate genetic information and resources.
- Assess the patient's understanding of genetic information.
- Provide support to families with newly diagnosed, genetics-related immunologic disorders.
- Participate in management and coordination of care of patients with genetics-related immunologic disorders and other genetic conditions.

Resources

See Chapter 8, Chart 8-6 for genetic resources.

---

hand, tends to be immunosuppressive. Autoimmune diseases are a leading cause of death by disease in females of reproductive age.

The patient is asked about any autoimmune disorders, such as lupus erythematosus, rheumatoid arthritis, multiple sclerosis, or psoriasis. The onset, severity, remissions and exacerbations, functional limitations, treatments that the patient has received or is currently receiving, and effectiveness of the treatments are described. The occurrence of different autoimmune diseases within a family strongly suggests a genetic predisposition to more than one autoimmune disease (Brooks, 2010) (Chart 35-4).

Neoplastic Disease

If there is a history of cancer in the family, more information is obtained, including the type of cancer, age at onset, and relationship (maternal or paternal) of the patient to the affected family members. Dates and results of any cancer screening tests for the patient are documented.

A history of cancer in the patient is also obtained, along with the type of cancer, date of diagnosis, and treatment modalities used. Immunosuppression contributes to the development of cancers; however, cancer itself is immunosuppressive, as is the treatment for cancer. Large tumors can release antigens into the blood, and these antigens combine with circulating antibodies and prevent them from attacking the tumor cells. Furthermore, tumor cells may possess special blocking factors that coat tumor cells and prevent their destruction by killer T lymphocytes. During the early development of tumors, the body may fail to recognize the tumor

antigens as foreign and subsequently fail to initiate destruction of the malignant cells. Hematologic cancers, such as leukemia and lymphoma, are associated with altered production and function of WBCs and lymphocytes.

All treatments that the patient has received or is currently receiving, such as radiation or chemotherapy, are recorded in the health history. In addition, the nurse should elicit information related to complementary or alternative modalities that have been used and the response to these efforts. Radiation destroys lymphocytes and decreases the ability to mount an effective immune response. The size and extent of the irradiated area determine the extent of immunosuppression. Whole-body irradiation may leave the patient totally immunosuppressed. Chemotherapy also affects bone marrow function, destroying cells that contribute to an effective immune response and resulting in immunosuppression (Sompayrac, 2012; VanDyne, 2011).

Chronic Illness and Surgery

The health assessment includes a history of chronic illness, such as diabetes, renal disease, chronic obstructive pulmonary disease (COPD), or fibromyalgia. The onset and severity of illnesses, as well as treatment that the patient is receiving for the illness, are obtained. Chronic illness may contribute to immune system impairments in various ways. Renal failure is associated with a deficiency in circulating lymphocytes. In addition, immune defenses may be altered by acidosis and uremic toxins. In diabetes, an increased incidence of infection has been associated with vascular insufficiency, neuropathy, and poor control of serum glucose levels.

Recurrent respiratory tract infections are associated with COPD as a result of altered inspiratory and expiratory function and ineffective airway clearance. Additionally, a history of organ transplantation or surgical removal of the spleen, lymph nodes, or thymus is noted, because these conditions may place the patient at risk for impaired immune function (Orlando, 2010).

Special Problems

Conditions such as burns and other forms of injury and infection may contribute to altered immune system function. Major burns cause impaired skin integrity and compromise the body's first line of defense. Loss of large amounts of serum occurs with burn injuries and depletes the body of essential proteins, including immunoglobulins. The physiologic and psychological stressors associated with surgery or injury stimulate cortisol release from the adrenal cortex; increased serum cortisol also contributes to suppression of normal immune responses (Jeckel, Lopes, Berleze, et al., 2010).

Medications and Blood Transfusions

A list of past and present medications is obtained. In large doses, antibiotics, corticosteroids, cytotoxic agents, salicylates, nonsteroidal anti-inflammatory drugs, and anesthetic agents can cause immune suppression (Table 35-5).

A history of blood transfusions is obtained, because previous exposure to foreign antigens through transfusion may be associated with abnormal immune function. Additionally, although the risk of HIV transmission through blood transfusion is extremely low in patients who received a transfusion after 1985 (when testing of blood for HIV was initiated in the United States), a small risk remains.

The patient is also asked about use of herbal agents and over-the-counter medications. Because many of these products have not been subjected to rigorous testing, their effects have not been fully identified. It is important, therefore, to ask patients about their use of these substances, to document their use, and to educate patients about untoward effects that may alter immune responsiveness.

TABLE 35-5 Selected Medications and Effects on the Immune System

Drug Classification (and Examples)	Effects on the Immune System
Antibiotics (in large doses)	Bone Marrow Suppression
ceftriaxone (Rocephin)	Eosinophilia, hemolytic anemia, hypoprothrombinemia, neutropenia, thrombocytopenia
cefuroxime sodium (Ceftin)	Eosinophilia, hemolytic anemia, hypoprothrombinemia, neutropenia, thrombocytopenia
chloramphenicol (Chloromycetin)	Leukopenia, aplastic anemia
dactinomycin (Cosmegen)	Agranulocytosis, neutropenia
fluoroquinolones (Cipro, Levaquin, Tequin)	Hemolytic anemia, methemoglobinemia, eosinophilia, leukopenia, pancytopenia
gentamicin sulfate (Garamycin)	Agranulocytosis, granulocytosis
macrolides (erythromycin, azithromycin [Zithromax], clarithromycin [Biaxin])	Neutropenia, leukopenia
penicillins	Agranulocytosis
streptomycin	Leukopenia, neutropenia, pancytopenia
vancomycin (Vancocin, Vancoled)	Transient leukopenia
Antithyroid Drugs	
propylthiouracil (PTU)	Agranulocytosis, leukopenia
Nonsteroidal Anti-Inflammatory Drugs (NSAIDs) (in large doses)	Inhibit Prostaglandin Synthesis or Release
Aspirin	Agranulocytosis
COX-2 inhibitors (celecoxib [Celebrex])	Anemia, allergy, no major other adverse affects to the immune system
ibuprofen (Advil, Motrin)	Leukopenia, neutropenia
indomethacin (Indocid, Indocin)	Agranulocytosis, leukopenia
Phenylbutazone	Pancytopenia, agranulocytosis, aplastic anemia
Adrenal Corticosteroids	Immunosuppression
Prednisone	
Antineoplastic Agents (cytotoxic agents)	Immunosuppression
cyclophosphamide (Cytoxan)	Leukopenia, neutropenia
mechlorethamine HCl (Mustargen)	Agranulocytosis, neutropenia
cyclosporine (Neoral)	Leukopenia, inhibits T-lymphocyte function
Antimetabolites	Immunosuppression
Pyrimidine antagonist (Fluorouracil [5-FU])	Leukopenia, eosinophilia
Folic acid antagonist (Methotrexate)	Leukopenia, aplastic bone marrow
Purine antagonist (Mercaptopurine[(6-MP])	Leukopenia, pancytopenia

COX, cyclo-oxygenase.
Adapted from Karch, A. (2012). *2012 Lippincott's nursing drug guide.* Philadelphia: Lippincott Williams & Wilkins.

Lifestyle Factors

Like any other body system, the functions of the immune system are interrelated with other body systems. Poor nutritional status, smoking (Nakata, Swanson, & Caruso, 2010), excessive consumption of alcohol, illicit drug use, STIs, and occupational or residential exposure to environmental radiation and pollutants have been associated with impaired immune function and are assessed in a detailed patient history (Chart 35-5). Although factors that are not consistent with a healthy lifestyle are predominately responsible for ineffective immune function, positive lifestyle factors can also negatively affect immune function and require assessment. For example, rigorous exercise or competitive exercise—usually considered a positive lifestyle factor—can be a physiologic stressor and cause negative effects on immune response (Walsh, Gleeson, Shephard, et al., 2011). This outcome is compounded if the person also faces stressful environmental conditions while undergoing exercise. Given the cumulative impact of various environmental stressors on the immune system, every effort should be made to minimize the person's exposure to stressors other than the exercise performed (Walsh et al., 2011).

Psychoneuroimmunologic Factors

Patient assessment must also address psychoneuroimmunologic factors. The bidirectional pathway between the brain and immune system is referred to as psychoneuroimmunology (Matthews & Janusek, 2011). The immune response is regulated and modulated in part by neuroendocrine influences. Lymphocytes and macrophages have receptors that can respond to neurotransmitters and endocrine hormones. Lymphocytes can produce and secrete adrenocorticotropic hormone and endorphinlike compounds. Cells in the brain, especially in the hypothalamus, can recognize prostaglandins, interferons, and interleukins, as well as histamine and serotonin, all of which are released during the inflammatory process. Like all other biologic systems functioning to maintain homeostasis, the immune system is integrated with other psychophysiologic processes and is regulated and modulated by the brain. These relationships may have immunologic consequences.

Conversely, the immune processes can affect neural and endocrine function, including behavior. Growing evidence indicates that a measurable immune system response can be positively influenced by biobehavioral strategies such as relaxation and imagery techniques, biofeedback, humor, hypnosis, and conditioning (Bennett & Lengacher, 2009). Therefore, the assessment should address the patient's general psychological status and the patient's use of and response to these strategies.

Physical Assessment

During the physical examination (see Chart 35-3), the skin and mucous membranes are assessed for lesions, dermatitis, purpura (subcutaneous bleeding), urticaria, inflammation, or any discharge. Any signs of infection are noted. The patient's temperature is recorded, and the patient is observed for chills and sweating. The anterior and posterior cervical, supraclavicular, axillary, and inguinal lymph nodes are palpated for enlargement; if palpable nodes are detected, their location, size, consistency, and reports of tenderness

---

Chart 35-5

NURSING RESEARCH PROFILE
Nurses, Smoking, and Immunity

Nakata, A., Swanson, N. G., & Caruso, C. C. (2010). Nurses, smoking, and immunity: A review. *Rehabilitation Nursing, 35*(5), 198–205.

Purpose

Occupational exposure to biologic, chemical, physical, and psychosocial hazards is an expected but potentially dangerous component of the nursing profession. The addition of cigarette smoking by nurses places them at a higher risk for adverse events, such as improper immune system functioning. The purpose of this study was to look at a review of the literature pertaining to studies on the effects of cigarette smoking, as well as secondhand smoke exposure, on the immune system in rehabilitation nurses in the United States.

Design

A review of the literature was conducted using the following key words: immune system, nurse, secondhand smoke, smoking, and smoking cessation. Articles were included on the prevalence of smoking in nurses, factors affecting the rate of smoking in nurses, cigarette smoking and immunity, secondhand smoke exposure and immunity, and smoking cessation and immunity.

Findings

Smoking is the leading cause of premature death in the United States despite recent decreases in prevalence rates.

The underlying causes of smoking in nurses, however, have not changed: work stress and poor work environment. These stressors predispose nurses to smoking. Smoking causes an increased white blood cell count (indicating inflammation), elevated T cells (with decreased function), decreased antibody production (Immunoglobulin [Ig]G, IgA, IgM), increased IgE (allergic response), and decreased natural killer (NK) cells (increased risk for infection) in the immune system. These findings were also suggested, although to a lesser extent, for secondhand smoke. The effects of secondhand smoke are particularly important in fetuses, neonates, infants, and children and can cause lifelong immune alterations. Cessation has been shown to help regain some of the immune function that was lost due to smoking. Within 1 to 6 months, the NK cells and immunoglobulin levels increase and T cells diminish.

Nursing Implications

Smoking cessation is extremely effective in decreasing mortality due to primary and secondhand smoke. This is true for the nurses themselves, as well as the patients who smoke. Education on the effects of smoking (increased risk of cancer, cardiac disease, stroke and pulmonary dysfunction) may deter the smoking behavior and prevent relapse after smoking cessation has occurred. An important issue raised: How can nurses advocate smoking cessation with patients when they are not following their own advice?

on palpation are noted. Joints are assessed for tenderness, swelling, increased warmth, and limited range of motion. The patient's respiratory, cardiovascular, genitourinary, gastrointestinal, and neurosensory systems are evaluated for signs and symptoms indicative of immune dysfunction. Any functional limitations or disabilities the patient may have are also assessed.

Diagnostic Evaluation

A series of blood tests and skin tests, as well as bone marrow biopsy, may be performed to evaluate the patient's immune competence. Specific laboratory and diagnostic tests are discussed in greater detail along with individual disease processes in subsequent chapters in this unit. Selected laboratory and diagnostic tests used to evaluate immune competence are summarized in Chart 35-6.

Nursing Management

The nurse needs to be aware that patients undergoing evaluation for possible immune system disorders experience not only physical pain and discomfort with certain types of diagnostic procedures but also many psychological reactions. It is the nurse's role to counsel, educate, and support patients throughout the diagnostic process. Many patients may be extremely anxious about the results of diagnostic tests and the possible implications of those results for their employment, insurance, and personal relationships. This is an ideal time for the nurse to provide counseling and education, should these interventions be warranted.

Chart 35-6 Selected Tests for Evaluating Immunologic Status

Various laboratory tests may be performed to assess immune system activity or dysfunction. The studies assess leukocytes and lymphocytes, humoral immunity, cellular immunity, phagocytic cell function, complement activity, hypersensitivity reactions, specific antigen–antibodies, or human immunodeficiency virus infection.

Humoral (Antibody-Mediated) Immunity Tests

- B-cell quantification with monoclonal antibody
- In vivo immunoglobulin synthesis with T-cell subsets
- Specific antibody response
- Total serum globulins and individual immunoglobulins (electrophoresis, immunoelectrophoresis, single radial immunodiffusion, nephelometry, and isohemagglutinin techniques)

Cellular (Cell-Mediated) Immunity Tests

- Total lymphocyte count
- T-cell and T-cell-subset quantification with monoclonal antibody
- Delayed hypersensitivity skin test
- Cytokine production
- Lymphocyte response to mitogens, antigens, and allogenic cells
- Helper and suppressor T-cell functions

Critical Thinking Exercises

1 A 75-year-old man presents to his primary provider. This is his fourth visit for bronchitis in the past 5 months, and he has been on three different antibiotics without resolution of his symptoms. What diagnostic tests would you expect to be ordered? What is the rationale for these tests? What further assessment data would you want to obtain from this patient?

---

2 **ebp** A 32-year-old woman is admitted to the hospital for a hip replacement due to avascular necrosis from chronic steroid use as treatment for her juvenile rheumatoid arthritis. Describe how her altered immune function would affect the care that you provide. Develop an evidence-based education plan for the patient and her family before hospital discharge. Discuss the criteria used to assess the strength of the evidence for your education plan.

---

3 **pq** A 74-year-old man with emphysema presents with an acute exacerbation of pneumonia. Antibiotics and corticosteroids are prescribed. What are your priority nursing observations and assessments? Identify priorities for patient education appropriate for the new prescription of steroids.

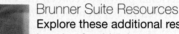

Brunner Suite Resources

Explore these additional resources to enhance learning for this chapter:
- NCLEX-Style Questions and Other Resources on **thePoint**, http://thePoint.lww.com/Brunner13e
- Study Guide
- PrepU
- Clinical Handbook
- Handbook of Laboratory and Diagnostic Tests

References

*Asterisk indicates nursing research.

Books

Abbas, A. K., & Lichtman, A. H. (2011). *Basic immunology, functions and disorders of the immune system* (3rd ed.). Philadelphia: W. B. Saunders.

Haynes, B. F., Soderberg, K. A., & Fauci, A.S. (2012). Introduction to the immune system. In: D. L. Longo, A. S. Fauci, D. L. Kasper, et al. (Eds.). *Harrison's principles of internal medicine* (18th ed.). New York: McGraw-Hill Medical.

Karch, A. (2012). *2012 Lippincott's nursing drug guide.* Philadelphia: Lippincott Williams & Wilkins.

Ko, M. S. H. (2012). Stem cell biology. In: D. L. Longo, A. S. Fauci, D. L. Kasper, et al. (Eds.). *Harrison's principles of internal medicine* (18th ed.). New York: McGraw-Hill Medical.

Kumar, V., Abbas, A. K., Fausto, N., et al. (2010). *Robbins and Cotran pathologic basis of disease* (8th ed.). Philadelphia: W. B. Saunders.

Lapka, D. V., & Franson, P. J. (2010). Biologics and targeted therapies. In: J. Eggert (Ed.): *Cancer basics.* Pittsburgh: Oncology Nursing Society.

Levinson, W. (2010). *Review of medical microbiology and immunology* (11th ed.). New York: McGraw-Hill Medical.

Liles, W. C. (2009). *Immunomodulators.* In: G. L. Mandell, J. E. Bennett, & R. Dolin (Eds.). *Principles and practices of infectious diseases* (7th ed.). Philadelphia: Elsevier/Churchill Livingstone.

Masoro, E. J., & Austad, S. N. (2011). *Handbook of the biology of aging* (7th ed.). London: Academic Press.

Miller, C. A. (2009). *Nursing for wellness in older adults* (5th ed.). Philadelphia: Lippincott Williams & Wilkins.

Porth, C. M., & Matfin, G. (2009). *Pathophysiology: Concepts of altered health states* (8th ed.). Philadelphia: Lippincott Williams & Wilkins.

Sompayrac, L. (2012). *How the immune system works* (4th ed.). Malden, MA: Blackwell.

Journals and Electronic Documents

Bennett, M. P., & Lengacher C. (2009). Humor and laughter may influence health IV. Humor and immune function. *Evidence-Based Complementary and Alternative Medicine, 6*(2), 159–164.

Brooks, W. H. (2010). X chromosome inactivation and autoimmunity. *Clinical Review of Allergy & Immunology, 39*(1), 20–29.

Brunner, S., Herndler-Brandstetter, D., Weinberger, B., et al. (2011). Persistent viral infections and immune aging. *Ageing Research Reviews, 10*(3), 362–369.

Buchholz, V. R., Neuenhahn, M., & Busch, D. H. (2011). CD8+ T cell differentiation in the aging immune system: Until the last clone standing. *Current Opinions in Immunology, 23*(4), 549–554.

DeBusk, R., Sierpina, V. S., & Kreitzer, M. J. (2011). Applying functional nutrition for chronic disease prevention and management: Bridging nutrition and functional medicine in the 21st century healthcare. *Explore: The Journal of Science and Healing, 7*(1), 55–57.

DiRosa, M., Malaguarnera, M., Nicoletti, F., et al. (2011). Vitamin D3: A helpful immune-modulator. *Immunology, 134*(2), 123–139.

Jeckel, C. M. M., Lopes, R. P., Berleze, M. C., et al. (2010). Neuroendocrine and immunological correlates of chronic stress in "strictly healthy" populations. *Neuroimmunomodulation, 17*(1), 9–18.

Matthews, H. L., & Janusek, L. W. (2011). Epigenetics and psychoneuroimmunology: Mechanisms and models. *Brain and Behavioral Immunology, 25*(1), 25–39.

Mocchegiani, E., Malavolta, M., Costarelli, L., et al. (2010). Zinc, metallothioneins, and immunosenescence. *Proceedings of the Nutrition Society, 69*(3), 290–299.

Munoz-Cruz, S. (2011). Non-reproductive effects of sex-steroids: Their immune-regulatory role. *Current Topics in Medicinal Chemistry, 11*(13), 1714–1727.

*Nakata, A., Swanson, N. G., & Caruso, C. C. (2010). Nurses, smoking, and immunity: A review. *Rehabilitation Nursing, 35*(5), 198–205.

Orlando, G. (2010). Finding the right time for weaning off immunosuppression in solid organ transplant recipients. *Expert Reviews in Clinical Immunology, 6*(6), 879–892.

Strasser, F., Van, D. B., & Jatoi, A. (2011). An overview of the European Society of Medical Oncology (ESMO) symposium on cancer and nutrition 2009: From cancer prevention to nutrition support to alleviating suffering in patients with advanced cancer. *Supportive Cancer Care, 19*(12), 1895–1898.

Swain, S. L., & Nikolich-Zugich, J. (2009). Key research opportunities in immune system aging. *Journal of Gerontology, 64A*(2), 183–186.

Takagi, A., Matsui, M., Ohno, S., et al. (2009). Highly efficient antiviral CD8+ T cell induction by peptides coupled to the surface of liposomes. *Clinical & Vaccine Immunology, 16*(10), 1383–1392.

*Torine L. A. (2011). Urinary tract infection: Diabetic women's strategies for prevention. *British Journal of Nursing, 20*(13), 791–796.

VanDyne, E. A. (2011). Issues in chemotherapy. *Pediatric Review, 32*(2), 86–87.

Vergati, M., Intrivici, C., Huen, N. Y., et al. (2010). Strategies for cancer vaccine development. *Journal of Biomedicine & Biotechnology.* Doi:10.1155/2010/596432. Epub 2010 Jul 11.

Walsh, N. P., Gleeson, M., Shephard, R. J., et al. (2011). Position statement. Part one: Immune function and exercise. *Exercise & Immunology Review, 17,* 6–63.

*Wang, Y., Jiang, Z. M., Nolan, M. T., et al. (2010). The impact of glutamine dipeptide-supplemented parenteral nutrition on outcomes of surgical patients: A meta-analysis of randomized clinical trials. *Journal of Enteral & Parenteral Nutrition, 34*(5), 521–529.

Ward, R. J., Crichton, R. R., Taylor, D. L., et al. (2011). Iron and the immune system. *Journal of Neural Transmission, 118*(3), 315–328.

*Yermal, S. J., Witek-Janusek, L., Peterson, J., et al. (2010). Perioperative pain, psychological distress, and immune function in men undergoing prostatectomy for cancer of the prostate. *Biological Research for Nursing, 11*(4), 351–362.

Resources

Centers for Disease Control and Prevention, www.cdc.gov

National Institute of Allergy and Infectious Diseases, www3.niaid.nih.gov/

National Institutes of Health, Health Information, www.nih.gov/health/infoline.htm

U.S. Department of Health and Human Services, www.hhs.gov

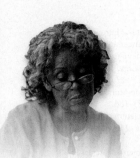
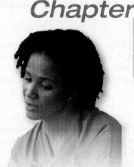

Management of Patients With Immunodeficiency Disorders

Learning Objectives

On completion of this chapter, the learner will be able to:

1 Compare the different types of primary immunodeficiency disorders and their causes, clinical manifestations, potential complications, and treatment modalities.

2 Describe the nursing management of the patient with immunodeficiency disorders.
3 Identify the essential educational needs for a patient with an immunodeficiency disorder.

Glossary

agammaglobulinemia: disorder marked by an almost complete lack of immunoglobulins or antibodies

angioneurotic edema: condition marked by development of urticaria and an edematous area of skin, mucous membranes, or viscera (i.e., angioedema)

ataxia: loss of muscle coordination

ataxia-telangiectasia: autosomal recessive disorder affecting T- and B-cell immunity primarily seen in children and resulting in a degenerative brain disease

hypogammaglobulinemia: lack of one or more of the five immunoglobulins; caused by B-cell deficiency

immunocompromised host: person with a secondary immunodeficiency and associated immunosuppression

panhypoglobulinemia: general lack of immunoglobulins in the blood

severe combined immunodeficiency disease: disorder involving a complete absence of humoral and cellular immunity resulting from an X-linked or autosomal genetic abnormality

telangiectasia: vascular lesions caused by dilated blood vessels

thymic hypoplasia: T-cell deficiency that occurs when the thymus gland fails to develop normally during embryogenesis; also known as DiGeorge syndrome

Wiskott-Aldrich syndrome: immunodeficiency characterized by thrombocytopenia and the absence of T and B cells

Immunodeficiency disorders may be caused by a defect in or a deficiency of phagocytic cells, B lymphocytes, T lymphocytes, or the complement system. The specific symptoms and their severity, age at onset, and prognosis depend on the immune system components affected and their degree of functional impairment. Regardless of the underlying cause, the cardinal symptoms of immunodeficiency include chronic or recurrent and severe infections, infections caused by unusual organisms or by organisms that are normal body flora, poor response to standard treatment for infections, and chronic diarrhea. In addition, the patient is susceptible to a variety of secondary disorders, including autoimmune disease and lymphoreticular malignancies (Fischer, 2012; Marodi & Casanova, 2009).

Immunodeficiencies may be acquired spontaneously or as a consequence of medical treatment. These disorders can be classified as either primary or secondary and by the affected components of the immune system. Primary immunodeficiency diseases are genetic in origin and result from intrinsic defects in the cells of the immune system. In contrast, secondary immunodeficiencies result from external factors such as infection. Effective nursing care reflects knowledge of the immune system, potential secondary disorders, relevant assessment parameters, and strategies for symptom management, as well as sensitivity and responsiveness to the educational needs of the patient and caregiver.

PRIMARY IMMUNODEFICIENCIES

Primary immunodeficiencies represent inborn errors of immune function that predispose people to frequent, severe infections; autoimmunity; and cancer. Advances in medical treatment have meant that patients with primary immunodeficiencies live longer, thus increasing their overall risk of developing cancer (Rezaei, Hedayat, Aghamohammadi, et al., 2011). The type of malignancy depends on the immunodeficiency, the patient's age, and possible viral infection, which suggests that different pathogenic mechanisms are implicated in each case. Non-Hodgkin lymphomas account for the majority of cancers. The primary immunodeficiencies known to be associated with increased incidence of malignancy are common variable immunodeficiency (CVID), immunoglobulin A (IgA) deficiency, and deoxyribonucleic acid repair disorders. More recently, investigators have shown that severe combined immunodeficiency disease (SCID) and Wiskott-Aldrich syndrome (WAS; thrombocytopenia and the absence of T and B cells) may also lead to cancer (Fischer, 2012). People with various primary immunodeficiencies, who are predisposed to cancer, exhibit immune deficits that also increase their susceptibility to fungal infections. A number of yeasts, molds, and fungi may cause infections in patients with chronic granulomatous disease, SCID, chronic mucocutaneous candidiasis, and CVID; these infections may occasionally be the presenting clinical manifestation of a primary immunodeficiency. If the immune condition is misdiagnosed or mistreated, it can lead to significant morbidity and mortality (Fischer, 2012).

The majority of primary immunodeficiencies are diagnosed in infancy, with a male-to-female ratio of 5 to 1. However, a large fraction of primary immunodeficiencies are not diagnosed until adolescence or early adulthood, when the gender distribution equalizes. Diagnosis at this stage frequently is confounded by frequent use of antibiotics that mask symptoms. On occasion, adults present with clinical episodes of infectious diseases that are beyond the scope of normal immunocompetence. Examples include infections that are unusually persistent, recurrent, or resistant to treatment and those involving unexpected dissemination of disease or atypical pathogens. To date, many immunodeficiencies of genetic origin have been identified (Savides & Shaker, 2010).

Common primary immunodeficiencies include disorders of humoral immunity (affecting B-cell differentiation or antibody production), T-cell defects, combined B- and T-cell defects, phagocytic disorders, and complement deficiencies. These disorders may involve one or more components of the immune system. Symptoms of immune deficiency disorders are related to the deficient component (Table 36-1). Major signs and symptoms include multiple infections despite aggressive treatment, infections with unusual or opportunistic organisms, failure to thrive or poor growth, and a positive family history (Fischer, 2012).

TABLE 36-1 Selected Primary Immunodeficiency Disorders

Immune Component	Disorder	Major Symptoms	Treatment
Phagocytic cells	Hyperimmunoglobulinemia E syndrome	Bacterial, fungal, and viral infections; deep-seated cold abscesses	Antibiotic therapy and treatment for viral and fungal infections Granulocyte-macrophage colony-stimulating factor; granulocyte colony-stimulating factor
B lymphocytes	Sex-linked agammaglobulinemia (Bruton's disease)	Severe pyogenic infections soon after birth Bacterial infections, infection with *Giardia lamblia*	Passive pooled plasma or gamma-globulin IVIG Metronidazole (Flagyl) Quinacrine HCl (Atabrine)
	Common variable immunodeficiency	Pernicious anemia Chronic respiratory infections	Vitamin B$_{12}$ Antimicrobial therapy
	IgA deficiency	Predisposition to recurrent infections, adverse reactions to blood transfusions or immunoglobulin, autoimmune diseases, hypothyroidism	None
	IgC$_2$ deficiency	Heightened incidence of infectious diseases	Pooled immunoglobulin
T lymphocytes	Thymic hypoplasia (DiGeorge syndrome)	Recurrent infections; hypoparathyroidism, hypocalcemia, tetany, convulsions, congenital heart disease, possible renal abnormalities; abnormal facies	Thymus graft
	Chronic mucocutaneous candidiasis	*Candida albicans* infections of mucous membrane, skin, and nails; endocrine abnormalities (hypoparathyroidism, Addison's disease)	Antifungal agents: *Topical:* miconazole *Oral:* clotrimazole, ketoconazole *IV:* amphotericin B
B and T lymphocytes	Ataxia-telangiectasia	Ataxia with progressive neurologic deterioration, telangiectasia (vascular lesions), recurrent infections; malignancies	Antimicrobial therapy; management of presenting symptoms; fetal thymus transplant, IVIG
	Nezelof's syndrome	Severe infections, malignancies	Antimicrobial therapy; IVIG, bone marrow transplantation; thymus transplantation; thymus factors
	Wiskott-Aldrich syndrome	Thrombocytopenia, resulting in bleeding, infections; malignancies	Antimicrobial therapy; splenectomy with continuous antibiotic prophylaxis; IVIG and bone marrow transplantation
	Severe combined immunodeficiency disease	Overwhelming severe fatal infections soon after birth (also includes opportunistic infections)	Antimicrobial therapy; IVIG and bone marrow transplantation
Complement system	Angioneurotic edema	Episodes of edema in various parts of the body, including respiratory tract and bowels	Pooled plasma, androgen therapy
	Paroxysmal nocturnal hemoglobinuria	Lysis of erythrocytes due to lack of decay-accelerating factor on erythrocytes	None

IVIG, intravenous immunoglobulin; Ig, immunoglobulin.

Phagocytic Dysfunction

Pathophysiology

A variety of primary defects of phagocytes may occur; almost all of them are genetic in origin and affect the natural (innate) immune system. In some types of phagocytic disorders, the neutrophils are impaired so that they cannot exit the circulation and travel to sites of infection. As a result, the person cannot initiate a normal inflammatory response against pathogenic organisms. In some disorders, the neutrophil count may be very low; in others, it may be very high because the neutrophils remain in the vascular system. Phagocytic cell disorders are characterized by disease-specific infections, such as chronic granulomatous disease (Abbas & Lichtman, 2011).

Clinical Manifestations

In phagocytic cell disorders, there is an increased incidence of bacterial and fungal infections caused by organisms that are normally nonpathogenic. People with these disorders may also develop fungal infections from *Candida* organisms and viral infections from herpes simplex or herpes zoster. These patients experience recurrent cutaneous abscesses, chronic eczema, bronchitis, pneumonia, chronic otitis media, and sinusitis. In one rare type of phagocytic disorder, hyperimmunoglobulinemia E syndrome (formerly known as Job syndrome), white blood cells cannot initiate an inflammatory response to infectious organisms. This results in recurrent bacterial infections of the skin and lung; abnormalities of the connective tissue, skeleton, vascular system, and dentition; and extremely elevated levels of IgE (Rezaei et al., 2011).

Although patients with phagocytic cell disorders may be asymptomatic, severe neutropenia may present and may be accompanied by deep and painful mouth ulcers, gingivitis, stomatitis, and cellulitis. Death from overwhelming infection occurs in about 10% of patients with severe neutropenia. Chronic granulomatous disease, another type of primary phagocytic disorder, produces recurrent or persistent infections of the soft tissues, lungs, and other organs; these are resistant to aggressive treatment with antibiotics (McPhee, Papadakis, & Rabow, 2012).

Assessment and Diagnostic Findings

Diagnosis is based on the history, signs, and symptoms (see Chart 35-3 in Chapter 35), and laboratory analysis by the nitroblue tetrazolium reductase test, which indicates the cytocidal (causing death of cells) activity of the phagocytic cells. A history of recurrent infection and fever, including the treatment given, is an important key to diagnosis; timely intervention can prevent morbidity and mortality (Al-Muhsen, 2010). Failure of an infection to resolve with the usual treatment is an important indicator. Warning signs of primary immunodeficiency disorders are summarized in Figure 36-1.

Medical Management

Patients with neutropenia continue to be at increased risk for developing severe infections despite substantial advances in supportive care. Epidemiologic shifts occur periodically and

must be detected early because they influence prophylactic, empiric, and specific strategies for medical management. Attention to infection control practices is important, especially with the emergence of multidrug-resistant organisms. Although prophylactic drug treatment effectively prevents some bacterial and fungal infections, it must be used with caution because it has been implicated in the emergence of resistant organisms. The choices for empiric therapy include combination regimens and monotherapy. Specific choices depend on local factors (epidemiology, susceptibility/resistance patterns, availability, cost). Home and inpatient settings are also available, and the selection of setting depends on the patient's risk category.

Although granulocyte transfusions are used as a medical treatment, they are seldom successful because of the short half-life of these cells. Treatment with granulocyte-macrophage colony-stimulating factor or granulocyte colony-stimulating factor may prove successful, because these proteins draw nonlymphoid stem cells from the bone marrow and hasten their maturation. Cell therapy, which refers to the provision of living cells to patients for the prevention of human disease, may be effective. (The infusion of blood and blood products is the best-established and most widely practiced form of cell therapy.)

Hematopoietic stem cell transplantation (HSCT), another form of cell therapy, has proven to be a successful curative modality (Devine, Tierney, Schmit-Pokorny, et al., 2010). The stem cells may be from embryos or adults. Toxicity and reduced efficacy are frequent limitations of HSCT; however, the use of prophylactic antibiotics has helped to decrease associated mortality (Subramanian, 2011). (See Chapter 15 for further discussion of HSCT.)

Another emerging therapy involves the use of cells as vehicles for the delivery of genes or gene products. Gene therapy has had many adverse effects; the first studies in human participants revealed numerous toxicities with this therapy. Knowledge of these toxicities is being used in planning further studies to increase tolerability (Barese & Dunbar, 2011).

B-Cell Deficiencies

Pathophysiology

Two types of inherited B-cell deficiencies exist. The first type results from lack of differentiation of B-cell precursors into mature B cells. As a result, plasma cells are absent, and the germinal centers from all lymphatic tissues disappear, leading to a complete absence of antibody production against invading bacteria, viruses, and other pathogens. This syndrome is called X-linked **agammaglobulinemia** (Bruton's disease), because all antibodies disappear from the patient's plasma. B cells in the peripheral blood and IgG, IgM, IgA, IgD, and IgE are low or absent. Infants born with this disorder suffer from severe infections starting soon after birth. Males are at a high risk for having X-linked agammaglobulinemia if they have an affected male relative. More than 10% of patients with X-linked agammaglobulinemia are hospitalized for infection when they are younger than 6 months of age; the prognosis depends on prompt recognition and treatment (Levinson, 2010).

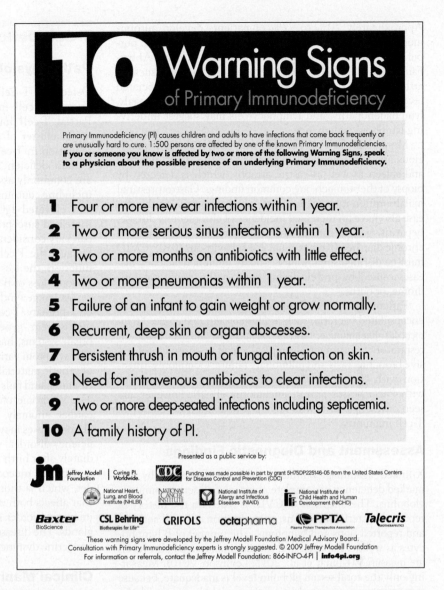

FIGURE 36-1 • The 10 warning signs of primary immune deficiency. These warning signs were developed by the Jeffrey Modell Foundation Medical Advisory Board. Consultation with Primary Immunodeficiency experts is strongly suggested. © 2009 Jeffrey Modell Foundation. Used with permission.

Autosomal agammaglobulinemia refers to a rare instance in which normal hypogammaglobulinemia of infancy is prolonged. It can result from mutations in a variety of genes whose products are required for differentiation of B cells. However, IgG levels do rise eventually. Periodic immunologic assessment is needed to differentiate transient hypogammaglobulinemia from other forms of antibody deficiency.

The second type of B-cell deficiency results from a lack of differentiation of B cells into plasma cells. Only diminished antibody production occurs with this disorder. Although plasma cells are the most vigorous producers of antibodies, affected patients have normal lymph follicles and many B lymphocytes that produce some antibodies. This syndrome, called **hypogammaglobulinemia**, is a frequently occurring immunodeficiency. It is also referred to as CVID; this disorder encompasses a variety of defects ranging from IgA deficiency, in which only the plasma cells that produce IgA are absent, to the other extreme, in which there is severe **panhypoglobulinemia** (general lack of immunoglobulins in the blood) (Abbas & Lichtman, 2011).

CVID is the most common primary immunodeficiency seen in adults; it can occur in either gender. Although it usually presents within the first two decades of life, most patients are diagnosed as adults because CVID often goes unrecognized prior to adulthood. Several T- and B-cell defects have been described; however, the underlying cause is still unknown—the etiology is believed to be multifactorial. Patients usually have normal B-cell lymphocyte counts, but the cells are clinically diverse and immature. Although they can recognize antigens and mount a response, their ability to become memory B cells and mature plasma cells is impaired.

Clinical Manifestations

Infants with X-linked agammaglobulinemia usually become symptomatic after the natural loss of maternally transmitted immunoglobulins, which occurs at about 5 to 6 months of age. Symptoms of recurrent pyogenic infections usually occur by that time.

Besides recurrent infection, patients with CVID are at increased risk for autoimmune disease, granulomatous disease, and malignancy, indicating that CVID is a disease of abnormal immune regulation as well as of immunodeficiency.

Approximately 20% to 22% of patients develop autoimmune diseases, notably autoimmune thrombocytopenic purpura and autoimmune hemolytic anemia (Kumar, Abbas, Fausto, et al., 2010). Other autoimmune diseases, such as arthritis and hypothyroidism, frequently occur. Associated fever, weight loss, anemia, thrombocytopenia, splenomegaly, lymphadenopathy, and lymphocytosis may suggest underlying lymphoid malignancy.

More than 50% of patients with CVID develop pernicious anemia. Lymphoid hyperplasia of the small intestine and spleen as well as gastric atrophy, which is detected by biopsy of the stomach, are common findings. Gastrointestinal malabsorption may occur. Young adults who develop the disease also have an increased incidence of chronic lung disease, hepatitis, gastric cancer, and malabsorption that results in chronic diarrhea (Kumar et al., 2012; Levinson, 2010). CVID must be distinguished from secondary immunodeficiency diseases caused by protein-losing enteropathy, nephrotic syndrome, or burns.

Patients with CVID are susceptible to infections with encapsulated bacteria, such as *Haemophilus influenzae*, *Streptococcus pneumoniae*, and *Staphylococcus aureus*. Frequent respiratory tract infections typically lead to chronic progressive bronchiectasis and pulmonary failure. Commonly, infection with *Giardia lamblia* occurs. Opportunistic infections with *Pneumocystis jiroveci* pneumonia (PCP), however, are seen only in patients who have a concomitant deficiency in T-cell immunity.

Assessment and Diagnostic Findings

X-linked agammaglobulinemia may be diagnosed by the marked deficiency or complete absence of all serum immunoglobulins. The diagnosis of CVID is based on the history of repeated bacterial infections, quantification of B-cell activity, and reported signs and symptoms. The number of B lymphocytes as well as the total and specific immunoglobulin levels are measured (Kumar et al., 2012; Levinson, 2010). Measuring only the total serum globulin level is inadequate, because a compensatory overproduction of one globulin may mask the loss of another globulin or the deficiency of a globulin that is present in very low amounts. Antibody titers to confirm successful childhood vaccination are determined by specific serologic tests. Previous successful childhood immunization indicates that B cells were functioning adequately earlier in life. If the patient exhibits signs and symptoms suggestive of pernicious anemia, hemoglobin and hematocrit levels are also obtained. Biopsies of the small intestine, spleen, and stomach may also be obtained to assess for lymphoid hyperplasia.

Medical Management

Patients with primary phagocytic disorders may be treated with intravenous immunoglobulin (IVIG) (Chart 36-1). Its administration is an essential part of the prevention and treatment of complications of CVID (Kumar et al., 2010). The use of subcutaneous immunoglobulin has also shown efficacy with easier administration for patients (Wasserman, Melamed, Nelson, et al., 2011). Antibody replacement therapy is recommended for severe, recurrent infections. Other interventions aimed at overcoming the immunologic defects in CVID are being studied (Keogh & Parker, 2011).

T-Cell Deficiencies

Pathophysiology

Defects in T cells lead to opportunistic infections. Most primary T-cell immunodeficiencies are genetic in origin. Partial T-cell immunodeficiencies constitute a heterogeneous cluster of disorders characterized by an incomplete reduction in T-cell number or activity. Unlike severe T-cell immunodeficiencies, however, partial immunodeficiencies are commonly associated with hyperimmune dysregulation, including autoimmune disorders, inflammatory diseases, and elevated IgG production (Fischer, 2012). Although increased susceptibility to infection is common, symptoms can vary considerably depending on the type of T-cell defect. Because the T cells play a regulatory role in immune system function, the loss of T-cell function is usually accompanied by some loss of B-cell activity.

DiGeorge syndrome, or **thymic hypoplasia**, is an example of a primary T-cell immunodeficiency. This rare, complex, multisystem genetic abnormality, which affects multiple organ systems, has been mapped to chromosomes 10 or 22. The symptom variation is a result of differences in the amount of genetic material affected. T-cell deficiency occurs when the thymus gland fails to develop normally during embryogenesis. The syndrome often manifests in the neonatal period as a cardiac anomaly, although hypocalcemic tetany and facial abnormalities may also occur. It is one of the few immunodeficiency disorders with symptoms that manifest almost immediately after birth (Fischer, 2012).

Chronic mucocutaneous candidiasis is a rare T-cell disorder, which is thought to be an autosomal recessive disorder that affects both males and females. It is considered an autoimmune disorder involving the thymus and other endocrine glands. The disease causes extensive morbidity resulting from endocrine dysfunction.

Clinical Manifestations

Infants born with DiGeorge syndrome have hypoparathyroidism with resultant hypocalcemia resistant to standard therapy, congenital heart disease, cleft lip and palate, dysmorphic facial features, and possibly renal abnormalities. These infants are susceptible to yeast, fungal, protozoan, and viral infections and are particularly susceptible to childhood diseases (chickenpox, measles, rubella), which are usually severe and may be fatal. Infection with *Candida albicans* is almost universal in patients with severe deficiencies in T-cell–mediated immunity. Many affected infants are also born with congenital heart defects, which can result in heart failure. The most frequent presenting sign in patients with DiGeorge syndrome is hypocalcemia that is resistant to standard therapy. It usually occurs within the first 24 hours of life (Fischer, 2012; Fomin, Pastorino, Kim, et al., 2010).

The initial presentation of chronic mucocutaneous candidiasis may be a result of either chronic candidal infection or idiopathic endocrinopathy. The disease is characterized by persistent or recurrent candidal infections of the skin, nails, and mucous membranes or by a variable combination of endocrine failure as well as immunodeficiency (Kumar et al., 2010). Patients may survive to the second or

Chart 36-1

PHARMACOLOGY

Managing an Intravenous Immunoglobulin Infusion

Intravenous immunoglobulin (IVIG) has become an important treatment for a variety of disease states that are characterized by deficient production of antibodies. It may have other indications but is commonly used for the treatment of DiGeorge syndrome, common variable immunodeficiency disease, severe combined immunodeficiency disease, Wiskott-Aldrich syndrome, and idiopathic thrombocytopenic purpura. Previously available only for intramuscular injection, immunoglobulin can now be administered for replacement therapy as an IV infusion in greater, more effective doses without painful side effects, and it can safely be given in outpatient as well as inpatient settings. Variables affecting the risk and intensity of adverse events associated with the administration of IVIG include patient age, underlying condition, history of migraine, and cardiovascular and/or renal disease; dose, concentration, and rate of infusion; and specific data related to the precise lot of the product. The nurse must assess all of these variables before starting the IVIG infusion and during the infusion process. He or she must anticipate adverse effects if any of these variables are present (Shelton, Griffin, & Goldman, 2006).

How Supplied

Immunoglobulin is supplied in a 5% solution or a lyophilized powder with a reconstituting diluent prepared from Cohn fraction II obtained from pools of 1,000–20,000 donors. Currently, a number of different IV preparations are approved for use and have been shown to be effective and safe by the U.S. Food and Drug Administration.

Dosage

The optimal dose is determined by the patient's response. In most instances, an IV dose of 200–800 mg/kg of body weight is administered every 3–4 weeks to ensure adequate serum levels of immunoglobulin G (IgG).

Adverse Effects

- Complaints of flank and back pain, shaking chills, flushing, dyspnea, and tightness in the chest; headache, fever, muscle cramps, nausea/vomiting, and local reaction at the infusion site
- Serious conditions, including aseptic meningitis, renal failure, thromboembolic events, Stevens-Johnson syndrome, and anaphylaxis. Anaphylactic reactions typically occur 30–60 minutes after the start of the infusion. The potential increases as the dose of IVIG increases.
  - Hypotension (possible with severe reactions)
  - Transfusion-related acute lung injury
  - Elevated blood urea nitrogen/creatinine

Guidelines for Nursing Management

- Pretreatment assessments should be performed before each infusion.
- Obtain height and weight before treatment to verify accurate dosing.
- Assess baseline vital signs before, during, and after treatment. An elevated temperature at the beginning of treatment may be an indication to delay the infusion to avoid misinterpretation as a reaction to the infusion.
- Premedicate with acetaminophen and diphenhydramine as prescribed 30 minutes before the start of the infusion.
- Understand that long-term tolerance of an older IVIG product does not necessarily imply tolerance to a newer product, even if it is technically superior. Caution should be exercised when changing IVIG products, because they are not biologically equivalent.
- Be aware that corticosteroids may be used to prevent possible severe reactions in patients who are perceived to be at risk.
- Administer the IV infusion at a slow rate, not to exceed 3 mL/min, usually at 100–200 mL/h.
- Continually assess the patient for adverse reactions; be especially aware of complaints of a tickle or lump in the throat as the precursor to laryngospasm that precedes bronchoconstriction.
- Stop the infusions at the first sign of reaction, and initiate the institutional protocol to be followed in this emergent situation.
- Be aware that patients with low gamma-globulin levels have more severe reactions than those with normal levels (e.g., patients who receive gamma-globulin for thrombocytopenia or Kawasaki disease).
- Keep in mind that patients who have an IgA deficiency have IgE antibodies to IgA, which requires administration of plasma or immunoglobulin replacement from IgA-deficient patients. Because all IV immunoglobulin preparations contain some IgA, they may cause an anaphylactic reaction in patients with IgE anti-IgA antibodies.
- Recognize that the pharmacokinetics of IgG differ when smaller doses are given more frequently, as is commonly done with subcutaneous regimens. Differences include lower peaks and higher troughs, which may be preferable for some patients.
- Remember that the risk of transmission of hepatitis, human immunodeficiency virus, or other known viruses is extremely low.

---

third decade of life. Problems may include hypocalcemia and tetany secondary to hypofunction of the parathyroid glands (see Chapter 13). Hypofunction of the adrenal cortex (Addison's disease) is the major cause of death in these patients; it may develop suddenly and without any history of previous symptoms.

Assessment and Diagnostic Findings

Prompt diagnosis is necessary for appropriate management. A comprehensive immunologic laboratory analysis is necessary. Findings in children with DiGeorge syndrome include cardiac and nutritional abnormalities (failure to thrive), and opportunistic skin infections (Martin-Nalda, Soler-Palacin, Espanol, et al., 2011).

Medical Management

Patients with T-cell deficiency should receive prophylaxis for PCP. General care includes management of hypocalcemia and correction of cardiac abnormalities. Hypocalcemia is controlled by oral calcium supplementation in conjunction with administration of vitamin D or parathyroid hormone. Congenital heart disease frequently results in heart failure, and these patients may require immediate surgical intervention in a tertiary care center. Transplantation of fetal thymus, postnatal thymus, or human leukocyte antigen (HLA)-matched bone marrow has been used for permanent reconstitution of T-cell immunity (Hagin & Reisner, 2010). In DiGeorge syndrome, attention must be given to cardiac, nutritional, and developmental needs (Martin-Nalda et al.,

2011). IVIG may be used if an antibody deficiency exists. This therapy may also be used to control recurrent infections. T-cell function improves with age and often is normal by 5 years of age. Prolonged survival has been reported after spontaneous remission of immunodeficiency, which occurs in some patients.

Combined B-Cell and T-Cell Deficiencies

Pathophysiology

T-cell and B-cell immune deficiencies comprise a heterogeneous group of disorders, all characterized by profound impairment in the development or function of the cellular, the humoral, or both parts of the immune system. A variety of inherited (autosomal recessive and X-linked) conditions fit this description. These conditions are typified by disruption of the normal communication system of B cells and T cells and impairment of the immune response, and they appear early in life (Fischer, 2012).

Ataxia-telangiectasia is an autosomal recessive neurodegenerative disorder characterized by cerebellar **ataxia** (loss of muscle coordination), **telangiectasia** (vascular lesions caused by dilated blood vessels), and immune deficiency. The immunologic defects reflect abnormalities of the thymus. The disorder is characterized by some degree of T-cell deficiency, which becomes more severe with advancing age. In 40% of patients, a selective IgA deficiency exists. In addition, IgG and IgE deficiencies have been identified. Immunodeficiency is manifested by recurrent and chronic sinus and pulmonary infections, leading to bronchiectasis. Frequent causes of death are chronic pulmonary disease and malignancy. Although lymphomas are most common, other carcinomas occur. The disease is also associated with neurologic, vascular, endocrine, hepatic, and cutaneous abnormalities (Levinson, 2010).

Severe combined immunodeficiency disease is a disorder in which both B cells and T cells are missing. Consequently, both cell-mediated and humoral functions are affected. In addition, SCID is marked by susceptibility to serious fungal, bacterial, and viral infections. It refers to a wide variety of congenital and hereditary immunologic defects characterized by early onset of infections, defects in both B-cell and T-cell systems, lymphoid aplasia, and thymic dysplasia. It is one of the most common causes of primary immunodeficiencies. Inheritance of this disorder can be X-linked, autosomal recessive, or sporadic. The exact incidence of SCID is unknown; it is recognized as a rare disease in most population groups, with an incidence of about 1 case in 1,000,000. This illness occurs in all racial groups and both genders.

Wiskott-Aldrich syndrome, a variation of SCID, is an inherited immunodeficiency caused by a variety of mutations in the gene encoding the WAS protein. It is characterized by frequent infections, thrombocytopenia with small platelets, eczema, and increased risk of autoimmune disorders and malignancies. Vasculitides and autoimmune hemolytic anemia are the two most common autoimmune manifestations and often cause considerable morbidity and mortality.

The prognosis is poor, because most affected patients develop overwhelming fatal infections.

Clinical Manifestations

The onset of ataxia and telangiectasia occurs in the first 4 years of life. Many patients, however, remain symptom free for 10 years or longer. As the patient approaches the second decade of life, chronic lung disease, cognitive impairment, neurologic symptoms, and physical disability become severe. Long-term survivors develop progressive deterioration of immunologic and neurologic functions. Some affected patients have lived until the fifth decade of life. The primary causes of death in these patients are overwhelming infection and lymphoreticular or epithelial cancer.

The onset of symptoms occurs within the first 3 months of life in most patients with SCID. Symptoms include respiratory infections and pneumonia, thrush, diarrhea, and failure to thrive. Many of these infections are resistant to treatment. Shedding of viruses such as respiratory syncytial virus or cytomegalovirus from the respiratory and gastrointestinal tracts is persistent. Maculopapular and erythematous skin rashes may occur. Vomiting, fever, and a persistent rash are also common manifestations (Geha & Natarangelo, 2011).

Medical Management

Treatment of ataxia-telangiectasia includes early management of infections with antimicrobial therapy, management of chronic lung disease with postural drainage and physical therapy, and management of other presenting symptoms. Other treatments include transplantation of fetal thymus tissue and IVIG administration (see Chart 36-1).

Treatment options for SCID include stem cell and bone marrow transplantation. HSCT is the definitive therapy for SCID; the best outcome is achieved if the disease is recognized and treated early in life. Improvements continue in the use of HSCT to treat patients with SCID as well as other primary immunodeficiencies. The ideal donor is an HLA-identical sibling. Evidence demonstrates that transplantation of allogeneic hematopoietic stem cells can cause an enhanced improvement over time. Other treatment options include administration of IVIG or thymus-derived factors and thymus gland transplantation. Gene therapy has been used and is still in the developmental stages (Kasztalska, Ciebiada, Cebula-Obrzut, et al., 2011). For the most common forms of combined immune deficiency, gene therapy can lead to immune reconstitution in most patients; however, a minority derives minimal clinical benefit, and some have suffered severe adverse effects, including death (Barese & Dunbar, 2011). As treatment improves, an increasing number of patients who previously would have died in infancy are living to adulthood. Newborn screening is proposed as a means to make a prompt diagnosis and initiate treatment in all affected infants (Lin, Epport, Azen, et al., 2009).

Nursing Management

Many patients require immunosuppression to ensure engraftment of depleted bone marrow during transplantation procedures. For this reason, nursing care must be

NURSING RESEARCH PROFILE

Chart 36-2
Hand Hygiene Monitoring and Infection Control Practices

Waltman. P. A., Schenk, L. K., Martin, T. M., et al. (2011). Effects of student participation in hand hygiene monitoring on knowledge and perception of infection control practices. *Journal of Nursing Education, 50*(4), 216–221.

Purpose

The Centers for Disease Control and Prevention (CDC) established guidelines in 2002 to reduce the rates of infections in health care settings. The purpose of this study was to describe the effect that participation in hand hygiene monitoring of health care workers had on retention of knowledge of infection control principles, opinions about handwashing, and hand hygiene practices among baccalaureate nursing students.

Design

The investigators used an exploratory descriptive survey design. Three data collection tools (Knowledge of Infection Control, Handwashing Opinions Survey, and Hand Hygiene Practice Survey) were administered to the students (N = 75) after participation in an educational session delivered by infection control personnel, a skills training session, and a study of health care workers in patient care areas of a tertiary hospital.

Findings

Results from the Hand Hygiene Practice Survey revealed that 92% of the students identified handwashing as the most effective infection control factor. Lack of clean facilities (41%) was identified as a deterrent to handwashing, and 18% felt that alcohol-based hand rubs would cause skin irritation and dryness. More than 40% of students viewed a poster reminder negatively. The majority of students felt that the hand hygiene class and the monitoring activity would influence their hand hygiene practice. This activity helped to raise awareness of a nurse's accountability for infection control in 70% of the participants; overall feedback about the project was positive.

Nursing Implications

A multidimensional approach to learning can facilitate a nursing student's compliance with the CDC's *Guideline for Hand Hygiene in Health-Care Settings* (CDC, 2002). This activity also helped to highlight the importance of evidence-based practice in nursing care by actively involving the students in nursing research. In turn, this will reinforce the link between practice and research among nursing students.

meticulous. Appropriate infection control precautions and thorough hand hygiene are essential (Chart 36-2). Institutional policies and procedures related to protective care must be followed scrupulously until definitive evidence demonstrates that precautions are unnecessary. Continual monitoring of the patient's condition is critical, so early signs of impending infection may be detected and treated before they seriously compromise the patient's status. It also is imperative that nurses appropriately apply standard precautions (previously known as universal precautions), which have become one of the first-line tools for decreasing transmission of disease, whether from nurse to patient, patient to patient, or patient to nurse. Standard precautions are based on the principle that all blood and body fluids, secretions, and excretions may contain transmissible infectious agents. Some of the key elements of standard precautions include performing hand hygiene, as mentioned previously; using appropriate personal protective equipment, depending on the expected type of exposure; and using safe injection practices (Dixon, 2011).

Deficiencies of the Complement System

The complement system is an integral part of the immune system, and deficiencies in normal levels of complement result in increased susceptibility to infectious diseases and immune-mediated disorders. Improved techniques to identify the individual components of the complement system have led to a steady increase in the number of deficiencies identified.

Hereditary **angioneurotic edema** results from the deficiency of C1 esterase inhibitor, which opposes the release of inflammatory mediators. The clinical picture of this autosomal dominant disorder includes recurrent attacks of edema formation in the subcutaneous tissue, gastrointestinal tract, and upper airway (Antoniu, 2011). Although the disease is mild in childhood and becomes more severe after puberty, first episodes have been reported later in life. Food allergy has often been linked to this disorder, although recent evidence has implicated a C1 esterase inhibitor deficiency. The fluctuations in hormone levels at the beginning of adolescence, in the perimenopausal period, during pregnancy, and during the use of oral contraceptives can precipitate edematous attacks that usually disappear after the onset of menopause. Fresh-frozen plasma has been used as well as other treatment options (Antoniu, 2011).

Paroxysmal nocturnal hemoglobinuria is an acquired clonal stem cell disorder resulting from a somatic mutation in the hematopoietic stem cell. An absent glycosylphosphatidylinositol (GPI)-anchored receptor prevents several proteins from binding to the erythrocyte membrane. These include the complement-regulatory proteins—CD55 and CD59—the absence of which results in enhanced complement-mediated lysis. Clinical manifestations may be indolent or life threatening. The disorder is characterized by hemoglobinuria that increases during sleep, as well as intravascular hemolysis, cytopenia, infections, bone marrow hyperplasia, and a high incidence of life-threatening venous thrombosis, which occurs most commonly in the abdominal and cerebral veins. Severe fatigue, abdominal pain, and esophageal spasm may also be present. Leukopenia, thrombocytopenia, and episodic crises are common. Severe infection can occur as a result of aplastic bone marrow and splenic thrombosis. Laboratory diagnosis can include specialized tests, such as the sucrose hemolysis test, Ham acid hemolysis test, and fluorescent-activated cell analysis. A coagulation profile is also indicated.

SECONDARY IMMUNODEFICIENCIES

Secondary immunodeficiencies are more common than primary immunodeficiencies and frequently occur as a result of underlying disease processes or the treatment of these disorders. The immune system can be affected by a variety of intrinsic factors, including immunosuppressive agents, harsh environmental conditions, hereditary disorders other than primary immunodeficiencies, and acquired metabolic disorders that cause secondary immunodeficiencies. Common causes of secondary immunodeficiencies include chronic stress, burns, uremia, diabetes, autoimmune disorders, viruses, exposure to immunotoxic medications and chemicals, and substance and alcohol misuse. Perhaps the best-known secondary immunodeficiency results from human immunodeficiency virus infection, which causes acquired immunodeficiency syndrome (AIDS); however, the most prevalent cause of immunodeficiency worldwide is severe malnutrition. AIDS, the most common secondary disorder, is discussed in detail in Chapter 37.

In secondary immunodeficiencies, abnormalities of the immune system affect both natural and acquired immunity, may be subtle, and are usually heterogeneous in their clinical manifestations. Patients with secondary immunodeficiencies are known as **immunocompromised hosts**.

Medical Management

Medical management of secondary immunodeficiencies includes diagnosis and treatment of the underlying disease process. Treatment of the primary condition often results in improvement of the affected immune components (McPhee et al., 2012). Factors that contribute to immunosuppression are identified and infection is treated. Additional treatment includes HSCT, monoclonal antibody therapy, IVIG, and anticoagulation therapy as indicated. HSCT may be curative (Kasztalska et al., 2011; McPhee et al., 2012).

NURSING MANAGEMENT OF PATIENTS WITH IMMUNODEFICIENCIES

Nursing management includes assessment, patient education, selected interventions, and supportive care. Assessment of the patient for infection and timely initiation of treatment are essential. Nursing care of patients with primary and secondary immunodeficiencies depends on the underlying cause of the immunodeficiency, the type of immunodeficiency, and its severity. Because immunodeficiencies result in a compromised immune system and pose a high risk for infection, careful assessment of the patient's immune status is essential. The assessment focuses on the history of past infections, particularly the type and frequency of infection; methods of and response to past treatments; signs and symptoms of any current skin, respiratory, oral, gastrointestinal, or genitourinary infection; and measures taken by the patient to prevent infection. The nurse assesses and monitors the patient for signs and symptoms of infection (Chart 36-3).

Many patients develop oral manifestations and need education about promoting good dental hygiene to diminish the

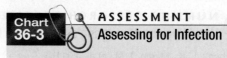

Chart 36-3

ASSESSMENT

Assessing for Infection

Be alert for the following signs and symptoms:

- Fever with or without chills
- Cough with or without sputum
- Shortness of breath
- Difficulty breathing
- Difficulty swallowing
- White patches in the oral cavity
- Swollen lymph nodes
- Nausea with or without vomiting
- Persistent diarrhea
- Frequency, urgency, or pain on urination
- Change in the character of the urine
- Lesions on the face, lips, or perianal area
- Redness, swelling, or drainage from skin lesions
- Persistent vaginal discharge with or without perianal itching
- Persistent abdominal pain

Adapted from Weber, J. & Kelley, J. (2010). *Health assessment in nursing.* (4th ed.) Philadelphia: Lippincott Williams & Wilkins.

oral discomfort and complications that frequently result in inadequate nutritional intake. Involving patients in their daily oral assessment and care helps them become proactive in preventing complications. To implement individualized care strategies, the nurse provides patients with the skills to promote health and limit the incidence of disease.

Because the inflammatory response may be blunted, the patient is observed for subtle and unusual signs and changes in physical status. Vital signs and the development of pain, neurologic signs, cough, and skin and oral lesions are monitored and reported immediately. Pulse rate and respiratory rate should be counted for a full minute, because subtle changes can signal deterioration in the patient's clinical status. Auscultation of the breath sounds is important to detect changes in respiratory status that signal an existing or impending infection. Any unusual response to treatment or a significant change in the patient's clinical condition must be promptly reported to the primary provider (Weber & Kelley, 2010).

The nurse continuously monitors laboratory values for changes indicative of infection. Culture and sensitivity reports from wound drainage, lesions, sputum, stool, urine, and blood are monitored to identify pathogenic organisms and appropriate antimicrobial therapy. Changes in laboratory results and subtle changes in clinical status must be reported to the primary provider, because the immunocompromised patient may fail to develop typical signs and symptoms of infection.

Assessment also focuses on nutritional status, stress level and coping skills, the use of alcohol, drugs, or tobacco, and general hygiene practices—all of which may affect immune function. Strategies that the patient has used to reduce the risk of infection are identified and evaluated for their appropriateness and effectiveness (Dudek, 2010). Other aspects of nursing care are directed toward reducing the patient's risk for infection; assisting with medical measures aimed at improving immune status and treating infection; achieving optimal nutritional status; and maintaining respiratory, bowel, and bladder function. The patient's ability to demonstrate good hand hygiene must be assessed, and the patient is encouraged to cough and perform deep-breathing exercises at regular intervals. Educating the patient about good dental hygiene measures reduces the potential for oral lesions, as do instructions on measures to protect the integrity of the skin. Attention to strict aseptic technique when performing invasive procedures, such as dressing changes, venipunctures, and bladder catheterizations, is essential. Other aspects of nursing care include assisting the patient to manage stress, to incorporate lifelong patterns of physiologic safety, and to adopt behaviors that strengthen immune system function.

Gene defects that cause many of the currently recognized immunodeficiency disorders are being identified, and genetic testing is becoming available for many of these disorders. Although this testing is rarely indicated in the initial workup for immunodeficiency (Fischer, 2012), nurses should be aware of and knowledgeable about it. Some deficiencies can be diagnosed by phenotype and functional assays. Genetic testing can establish or confirm a suspected diagnosis of some primary immune deficiencies. In addition, it also may predict future disease risk prior to the onset of clinical signs and symptoms and guide clinicians in selecting the most appropriate therapeutic options (Fischer, 2012). Genetic testing is not typically required in CVID because known genetic defects cause only a small number of cases of CVID, and results would not alter treatment. To perform genetic testing, informed consent from the patient or legal guardian is necessary. It can be accomplished using whole blood samples and mouth swab samples. (See Chapter 8.)

If the patient is a candidate for any of the newer or experimental therapies (gene therapy, bone marrow transplantation, immunomodulators such as interferon-γ), the patient and family must be informed about the potential risks and benefits of the treatment regimen. A major role of the nurse is to develop and maintain a knowledge base in these evolving treatment modalities in order to help the patient and family understand the treatment options and cope with the uncertainties of treatment outcomes.

Promoting Home and Community-Based Care

Educating Patients About Self-Care

The patient and caregivers require education about the signs and symptoms that indicate infection and about the potential for occurrence of atypical symptoms secondary to underlying immunosuppression. Patients should be made aware that their temperature may not be elevated to indicate an infection. They must be informed of the need for continuous monitoring for subtle changes in the patient's physical health status and of the importance of seeking immediate health care if changes are detected. Patients should be advised that they know themselves best; therefore, whenever they experience a symptom that is not typical for them, they should contact their primary provider, who will determine and initiate appropriate therapy. Education needs to be provided about prophylactic medication regimens, including dosage, indications, times, actions, potential interactions, and side effects. Patients and their families are also instructed about the importance of continuing treatment regimens without interruption and incorporating these routines into their daily living patterns. The patient is educated about the importance of avoiding others with infections and avoiding crowds, and about other ways to prevent infection (Chart 36-4).

Chart 36-4

HOME CARE CHECKLIST
Infection Prevention for the Patient With Immunodeficiency

At the completion of home care education, the patient or caregiver will be able to:	PATIENT	CAREGIVER
• Identify signs and symptoms of infection to report to the primary provider, such as fever; chills; wet or dry cough; breathing problems; white patches in the mouth; swollen glands; nausea; vomiting; persistent abdominal pain; persistent diarrhea; problems with urination or changes in the character of the urine; red, swollen, or draining wounds; sores or lesions on the body; persistent vaginal discharge with or without itching; and severe fatigue.	✔	✔
• Demonstrate correct hand hygiene procedure.	✔	✔
• State rationale for thorough hand hygiene before eating, after using the bathroom, and before and after performing health care procedures.	✔	✔
• State rationale for the use of cream and emollients to prevent or manage dry, chafed, or cracked skin.	✔	✔
• Demonstrate recommended personal hygiene in bathing and foot care to prevent bacterial and fungal diseases.	✔	✔
• State rationale for avoiding contact with people who have known illness or who have recently been vaccinated.	✔	✔
• Verbalize understanding of ways to maintain a nutritious diet and adequate calories.	✔	✔
• State the reason for avoiding the eating of raw fruits and vegetables, cooking all foods thoroughly, and immediately refrigerating all leftover food.	✔	✔
• Identify the rationale for frequent cleaning of kitchen and bathroom surfaces with disinfectant.	✔	✔
• Identify rationale and benefits of avoiding alcohol, tobacco, and unprescribed medications.	✔	✔
• State rationale for taking prescribed medications as directed.	✔	✔
• Verbalize ways to cope with stress successfully, plans for regular exercise, and rationale for obtaining adequate rest.	✔	✔

Chart 36-5 **HOME CARE CHECKLIST**
Home Infusion of Intravenous Immunoglobulin

At the completion of home care education, the patient or caregiver will be able to:	PATIENT	CAREGIVER
• Identify the benefits and expected outcome of intravenous immunoglobulin (IVIG).	✔	✔
• Demonstrate how to check for patency of the IV access device.	✔	✔
• Demonstrate how to prepare IVIG.	✔	✔
• Demonstrate how to infuse IVIG.	✔	✔
• Demonstrate how to clean and maintain IV equipment.	✔	✔
• Identify side effects and adverse effects of IVIG.	✔	✔
• State rationale for prophylactic use of acetaminophen (Tylenol) and diphenhydramine (Benadryl) before treatment begins.	✔	✔
• State the rationale for prehydration on the day before infusion.	✔	✔
• Verbalize understanding of emergency measures for anaphylactic shock.	✔	✔

The patient who is to receive IVIG at home will need information about the expected benefits and outcomes of the treatment as well as expected adverse reactions and their management (Chart 36-5). Patients who can perform self-infusion at home must be instructed in sterile technique, medication dosages, administration rate, and detection and management of adverse reactions (Shelton et al., 2006).

Continuing Care

Encouraging the patient and family to be active partners in managing the immunodeficiency is the key to successful outcomes and a favorable prognosis. The patient must recognize that all health-related instructions are lifelong, that follow-up with all scheduled appointments is essential, and that it is the patient's responsibility to notify the primary provider of any early signs or symptoms of infection, however subtle they may be. If the patient's treatment includes IVIG and the patient or family cannot administer treatment, a referral for home care or an infusion service is warranted.

Critical Thinking Exercises

1 **ebp** As a staff nurse in the intensive care unit, you are asked by a senior nursing student about the reasoning behind wound precautions on a patient with methicillin-resistant *Staphylococcus aureus*. Identify why the infection control measures are indicated. Describe the evidence base for the infection control measures you identified and the criteria used to evaluate the strength of that evidence.

2 A young man comes to the clinic for a possible recurrence of an infected leg wound. He is concerned because he has been on antibiotics for this same infection eight times in the past year. Identify the 10 warning signs of primary immune deficiency that you would consider when responding to this situation.

3 **pg** Identify the priorities, approach, and techniques you would use to perform a comprehensive admission

assessment on a 45-year-old female patient for whom IVIG has been prescribed. How would your priorities, approach, and techniques differ if the IVIG is to be administered in the home?

Brunner Suite Resources

Explore these additional resources to enhance learning for this chapter:
• NCLEX-Style Questions and Other Resources on thePoint, http://thePoint.lww.com/Brunner13e
• Study Guide
• PrepU
• Clinical Handbook
• Handbook of Laboratory and Diagnostic Tests

References

*Asterisk indicates nursing research.
**Double asterisk indicates classic reference.

Books

Abbas, A. K., & Lichtman, A. H. (2011). *Basic immunology: Functions and disorders of the immune system* (3rd ed.). Philadelphia: W. B. Saunders.

Dudek, S. G. (2010). *Nutrition essentials for nursing practice* (6th ed.). Philadelphia: Lippincott Williams & Wilkins.

Fischer, A. (2012). *Primary immune deficiency diseases.* In: D. Longo, A. Fauci, D. Kasper, et al. (Eds.). *Harrison's principles of internal medicine* (18th ed.). New York: McGraw-Hill Medical.

Geha, R., & Natarangelo, L. (2011). *Case studies in immunology* (6th ed.). New York: Garland Publishing.

Kumar, V., Abbas, A. K., Fausto, N. et al. (2010). *Robbins and Cotran pathologic basis of disease* (8th ed.). Philadelphia: W. B. Saunders.

Levinson, W. (2010). Congenital immunodeficiencies. In: *Review of medical microbiology and immunology.* New York: McGraw-Hill Medical.

McPhee, S. J., Papadakis, M. A., & Rabow, M. W. (2012). *Current medical diagnosis and treatment* (51st ed.). Stamford, CT: Appleton & Lange.

Weber, J., & Kelley, J. (2010). *Health assessment in nursing* (4th ed.). Philadelphia: Lippincott Williams & Wilkins.

Journals and Electronic Documents

Al-Muhsen, S. Z. (2010). Gastrointestinal and hepatic manifestations of primary immune deficiency disease. *Saudi Journal of Gastroenterology, 16*(2), 66–74.

Antoniu, S. A. (2011). Therapeutic approaches in hereditary angioedema. *Clinical Review of Allergy & Immunology, 41*(1), 114–122.

Barese, C. N., & Dunbar, C. E. (2011). Contributions of gene marking to cell and gene therapies. *Human Gene Therapy, 22*(6), 659–668.

**Centers for Disease Control and Prevention (CDC). (2002). Guideline for hand hygiene in health care settings. *MMWR: Morbidity and Mortality Weekly Report, 51*(RR-16), 1–56.

Devine, H., Tierney, K., Schmit-Pokorny, K., et al. (2010). Mobilization of hemopoietic stem cells for use in autologous transplantation. *Clinical Journal of Oncology Nursing, 14*(2), 212–222.

Dixon, R. E. (2011). Control of health-care-associated infections, 1961–2011. *Morbidity & Mortality Weekly Surveillance Summaries, 60*(Suppl. 4), 58–63.

Fomin, A. B., Pastorino, A. C., Kim, C. A., et al. (2010). DiGeorge syndrome: A not so rare disease. *Clinics (sao Paulo, Brazil), 65*(9), 865–869.

Hagin, D., & Reisner, Y. (2010). Haploidentical bone marrow transplantation in primary immune deficiency: Stem cell selection and manipulation. *Immunology & Allergy Clinics of North America, 30*(1), 45–62.

Kasztalska, K., Ciebiada, M., Cebula-Obrzut, B., et al. (2011). Intravenous immunoglobulin replacement therapy in the treatment of patients with common variable immunodeficiency disease: An open-label prospective study. *Clinical Drug Investigation, 31*(5), 299–307.

Keogh, B., & Parker, A. E. (2011). Toll-like receptors as targets for immune disorders. *Trends in Pharmacologic Science, 32*(7), 435–442.

Lin, M., Epport, K., Azen, C., et al. (2009). Long-term neurocognitive function of pediatric patients with severe combined immune deficiency (SCID): Pre-and post-hematopoietic stem cell transplant (HSCT). *Journal of Clinical Immunology, 29*(2), 231–237.

Marodi, L., & Casanova, J. L. (2009). Novel primary immunodeficiencies relevant to internal medicine: Novel phenotypes. *Journal of Internal Medicine, 266*(6), 502–506.

Martin-Nalda, A. Soler-Palacin, P., Espanol B. T., et al. (2011). Spectrum of primary immunodeficiencies in a tertiary hospital over a period of 10 years. *Anales de Pediatria, 74*(2), 74–83.

Rezaei, N., Hedayat, M., Aghamohammadi, A., et al. (2011). Primary immunodeficiency diseases associated with increased susceptibility to viral infections and malignancies. *Journal of Allergy & Clinical Immunology, 127*(6), 1329–1341.

Savides, C., & Shaker, M. (2010). More than just infections: An update on primary immune deficiencies. *Current Opinions in Pediatrics, 22*(5), 647–654.

Shelton, B., Griffin, J., & Goldman, F. (2006). Immune globulin IV therapy: Optimizing care of patients in the oncology setting. *Oncology Nursing Forum, 33*(5), 911–921.

Subramanian, A. K. (2011). Antimicrobial prophylaxis regimens following transplantation. *Current Opinions in Infectious Disease, 24*(4), 344–349.

*Waltman, P. A., Schenk, L. K., & Martin, T. M. (2011). Effects of student participation in hand hygiene monitoring on knowledge and perception of infection control practices. *Journal of Nursing Education, 50*(4), 216–221.

Wasserman, R. L., Melamed, I., Nelson, R. P., et al. (2011). Pharmacokinetics of subcutaneous IgPro20 in patients with immunodeficiency. *Clinical Pharmacokinetics, 50*(6), 405–414.

Resources

Centers for Disease Control and Prevention, www.cdc.gov
Immune Deficiency Foundation (IDF), www.primaryimmune.org
National Institute of Allergy and Infectious Diseases (NIAID), www.niaid.nih.gov
National Institutes of Health, www.nih.gov
National Library of Medicine, www.nlm.nih.gov
National Primary Immunodeficiency Resource Center/Jeffrey Modell Foundation, www.info4pi.org
U.S. Department of Health and Human Services, www.hhs.gov
U.S. Food and Drug Administration, www.fda.gov

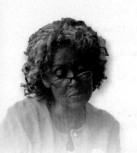
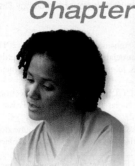

Management of Patients With HIV Infection and AIDS

Learning Objectives

On completion of this chapter, the learner will be able to:

1 Describe the modes of transmission of human immunodeficiency virus (HIV) infection and prevention strategies.
2 Describe the host viral interaction during primary infection with HIV.
3 Explain the pathophysiology associated with the clinical manifestations of HIV and acquired immunodeficiency syndrome (AIDS).
4 Describe the gerontologic considerations related to HIV/AIDS.
5 Describe the clinical management of patients with HIV/AIDS.
6 Use the nursing process as a framework for care of the patient with HIV/AIDS.

Glossary

alpha-interferon: protein substance that the body produces in response to infection
B-cell lymphoma: common malignancy in patients with HIV/AIDS
candidiasis: yeast infection of skin or mucous membrane
CCR5: along with the CD4+ receptor, this cell surface molecule is used by HIV to fuse with the host's cell membranes
EIA (enzyme immunoassay): a blood test that can determine the presence of antibodies to HIV in the blood or saliva; a variant of this test is called **enzyme-linked immunosorbent assay (ELISA)**. Positive results must be validated, usually with Western blot test
HIV-1: retrovirus isolated and recognized as the etiologic agent of HIV disease
HIV-2: retrovirus identified in 1986 in patients with AIDS in western Africa
HIV encephalopathy: degenerative neurologic condition characterized by a group of clinical presentations including loss of coordination, mood swings, loss of inhibitions, and widespread cognitive dysfunctions; formerly referred to as AIDS dementia complex (ADC)
human papillomavirus (HPV): viruses that cause various warts, including plantar and genital warts; some strains of HPV can also cause cervical cancer
immune reconstitution inflammatory syndrome (IRIS): a syndrome that results from rapid restoration of pathogen-specific immune responses to opportunistic infections; most often occurs after starting antiretroviral therapy
Kaposi's sarcoma: malignancy that involves the epithelial layer of blood and lymphatic vessels
latent reservoir: the integrated HIV provirus within the CD4+ T cell during the resting memory state; does not express viral proteins and is invisible to the immune system and antiviral medications
Mycobacterium avium **complex (MAC):** opportunistic infection caused by mycobacterial organisms that commonly causes a respiratory illness but can also infect other body systems

opportunistic infection: illness caused by various organisms, some of which usually do not cause disease in people with normal immune systems
p24 antigen: blood test that measures viral core protein; accuracy of test is limited because the p24 antibody binds with the antigen and makes it undetectable
peripheral neuropathy: disorder characterized by sensory loss, pain, muscle weakness, and wasting of muscles in the hands or legs and feet
Pneumocystis pneumonia or *Pneumocystis jiroveci* pneumonia (PCP): common opportunistic lung infection caused by an organism; based on its structure, believed to be a fungus
polymerase chain reaction: a sensitive laboratory technique that can detect and quantify HIV in a person's blood or lymph nodes
primary infection: 4- to 7-week period of rapid viral replication immediately following infection; also known as acute HIV infection
progressive multifocal leukoencephalopathy: opportunistic infection that infects brain tissue and causes damage to the brain and spinal cord
protease inhibitor: medication that inhibits the function of protease, an enzyme needed for HIV replication
provirus: viral genetic material in the form of deoxyribonucleic acid (DNA) that has been integrated into the host genome. When it is latent in human cells, HIV is in a proviral form.
retrovirus: a virus that carries genetic material in ribonucleic acid (RNA) instead of DNA and contains reverse transcriptase
reverse transcriptase: enzyme that transforms single-stranded RNA into a double-stranded DNA
viral load test: measures the quantity of HIV RNA in the blood
viral set point: amount of virus present in the blood after the initial burst of viremia and the immune response that follows
wasting syndrome: involuntary weight loss consisting of both lean and fat body mass
Western blot assay: a blood test that identifies antibodies to HIV and is used to confirm the results of an EIA or ELISA test

Advances have been made in treating human immunodeficiency virus (HIV) infection and acquired immunodeficiency syndrome (AIDS); however the epidemic remains a critical public health issue in communities across the country and around the world. Prevention, early detection, and ongoing treatment remain important aspects of care for persons living with HIV infection or AIDS, sometimes referred to as PLWHA. Nurses in all settings encounter people who have HIV infection and AIDS. Nurses need a solid understanding of the pathophysiology, knowledge of the physical and psychological consequences associated with the diagnosis, and expert assessment and clinical management skills to provide optimal care for people with HIV infection and AIDS.

In the late 1980s, the U.S. Food and Drug Administration (FDA) approved the first antiretroviral agent to treat HIV infection, and the first randomized controlled trial of primary prophylaxis of *Pneumocystis jiroveci* pneumonia (PCP; formerly *Pneumocystis carinii* pneumonia) appeared in the literature. Antiretroviral therapy (ART) for the treatment of HIV infection has improved steadily since the advent of combination therapy in 1996. Drug therapy offers new mechanisms of action, improvements in potency and activity (including those against multidrug-resistant viruses), dosing convenience, and tolerability (Panel on Antiretroviral Guidelines for Adults and Adolescents, 2011). Although damage to the immune system can be significant, survival rates have increased dramatically, and HIV/AIDS has evolved into a chronic disease.

HIV Infection and AIDS

Since AIDS was first identified more than 30 years ago, remarkable progress has been made in improving the length and quality of life for people living with HIV disease. During the first decade, progress was associated with the recognition and treatment of opportunistic diseases and introduction of prophylaxis against **opportunistic infections**. The second decade witnessed progress in the development of highly active antiretroviral drug therapies (HAART) as well as continuing progress in the treatment of opportunistic infections. The third decade has focused on issues of adherence to ART, development of second-generation combination medications that affect different stages of the viral life cycle, and

continued need for an effective vaccine. The HIV antibody test, an enzyme immunoassay (EIA; or a variant of this test called *enzyme-linked immunosorbent assay* [ELISA]), became available in 1984, allowing early diagnosis of the infection before onset of symptoms. Since then, HIV infection has been best managed as a chronic disease, most appropriately in an outpatient care setting, whereas AIDS may involve acute conditions that require hospital treatment.

Epidemiology

The case definition of AIDS has been revised a number of times (1985, 1987, and 1993). All 50 states, the District of Columbia, U.S. dependencies and possessions, and independent nations in free association with the United States report AIDS cases to the Centers for Disease Control and Prevention (CDC) using a uniform surveillance case definition and case report form (CDC, 2011a). In 2008, the CDC revised a single case definition of HIV infection. The new case definition is intended for public health surveillance and not as a guide for clinical diagnosis (CDC, 2008) and is presented in Table 37-1. In 2010, President Obama introduced the *National HIV/AIDS Strategy* to address three public health goals for HIV/AIDS treatment and prevention that included (1) reducing the number of people who become infected with HIV, (2) increasing access to care and optimizing health outcomes for people living with HIV, and (3) reducing HIV-related health disparities (White House, 2010).

According to the CDC (2011b), 1.2 million people in the United States are living with HIV, 1 in 5 are unaware that they are infected, and the rate of new infections has remained relatively stable at 50,000 Americans becoming infected each year. Gay, bisexual, and other men who have sex with men remain the population most affected and account for 2% of the population but 61% of the new infections. Young black men who have sex with men were the only risk group to experience significant increases in new HIV infections from 2006 to 2009. Blacks, irrespective of sexual behavior or gender, continue to experience the most severe burden of HIV (CDC, 2011b). New HIV infections continue to impact all age groups, including older persons. Behaviors, rather than age or gender, are the contributing factor to becoming infected with HIV.

As a result of an immense global response, the number of new HIV infections globally declined 19% over the

TABLE 37-1	Surveillance Case Definition for HIV Infection Among Adults and Adolescents	
Stage	**Laboratory Evidence**	**Clinical Evidence**
1	Laboratory confirmation of HIV infection AND CD4+ T-lymphocyte count ≥500 mcL OR CD4+ T-lymphocyte percentage ≥29	None required (but no AIDS-defining condition)
2	Laboratory confirmation of HIV infection AND CD4+ T-lymphocyte count 200–499 mcL OR CD4+ T-lymphocyte percentage of 14–28	None required (but no AIDS-defining condition)
3 (AIDS)	Laboratory confirmation of HIV infection AND CD4+ T-lymphocyte count <200 mcL OR CD4+ T-lymphocyte percentage <14	OR documentation of an AIDS-defining condition (with laboratory confirmation of HIV infection)
State unknown	Laboratory confirmation of HIV infection AND no information on CD4+ T-lymphocyte count or CD4+ T-lymphocyte percentage	AND no information on presence of AIDS-defining condition

Adapted from Centers for Disease Control and Prevention. (2008). Revised surveillance case definitions for HIV infection among adults, adolescents, and children aged <18 months and for HIV infection and AIDS among children aged 18 months to <13 years—United States, 2008. *MMWR: Morbidity and Mortality Weekly Report Recommendations and Reports, 57*(RR 10), 1–8.

past decade; in 15 high-burden countries, HIV prevalence declined more than 25% among those aged 15 to 24 years; access to ART in low- and middle-income countries increased from only 400,000 people receiving such therapy in 2003 to 5.25 million by the end of 2009 (comprising 35% of those estimated to be in need); AIDS-related deaths dropped by 19% globally over the period from 2004 to 2009 alone; and 53% of pregnant women living with HIV had access to antiretroviral medicines to prevent transmission of HIV to their infants, up from 45% in 2008. The World Health Organization (WHO, 2011a) *Global Health Sector Strategy on HIV/ AIDS 2011–2015* is the guide for the health sectors' response to HIV epidemics in order to achieve universal access to HIV prevention, diagnosis, treatment, care and support. The strategy reaffirms global goals and targets for the health sector response to HIV, identifies strategic directions to guide national responses, and outlines recommended country actions and the WHO's contributions within each strategic direction (WHO, 2011b).

HIV Transmission

Inflammation and breaks in the skin or mucosa result in the increased probability that an HIV exposure will lead to infection. Human immunodeficiency virus type 1 (**HIV-1**) is transmitted in body fluids (blood, seminal fluid, vaginal secretions, amniotic fluid, and breast milk) that contain free virions and infected CD4+ T cells. Higher amounts of HIV and infected cells in the body fluid are associated with the probability that the exposure will result in infection. Mother-to-child transmission of HIV-1 may occur in utero, at the time of delivery, or through breast-feeding, but most perinatal infections are thought to occur after exposure during delivery. HIV is not transmitted through casual contact (Chart 37-1).

Blood and blood products can transmit HIV to recipients. However, the risk associated with transfusions has been virtually eliminated as a result of voluntary self-deferral, completion of a detailed health history, extensive testing, heat treatment of clotting factor concentrates, and more effective virus inactivation methods. Donated blood is tested for antibodies to HIV-1, human immunodeficiency virus type 2 (**HIV-2**), and **p24 antigen**; in addition, since 1999, nucleic acid amplification testing (NAT) has been performed.

 ### Gerontologic Considerations

Approximately one quarter of people living with HIV are older than 50 years. This group of HIV-infected adults face

Chart 37-1 ⚠	RISK FACTORS

Risks Associated With HIV Infection and AIDS

- Sharing infected injection drug use equipment
- Having sexual relations with infected individuals (both male and female)
- Infants born to mothers with HIV infection and/or who are breast-fed by HIV-infected mothers
- People who received organ transplants, HIV-infected blood, or blood products (especially between 1978 and 1985)

Adapted from Eliopoulos, C. (2010). *Gerontological nursing* (7th ed.). Philadelphia: Lippincott Williams & Wilkins.

unique health challenges stemming from age-related changes, side effects of long-term treatment, and comorbidities (Eliopoulos, 2010; Fauci, Hodes, & Whitescarver, 2010). The characteristics of older people living with HIV infection reflect those of others in their country of origin who have HIV infection.

Several factors put older adults at risk for HIV infection:
- Many older adults are sexually active but do not use condoms, viewing them only as a means of unneeded birth control.
- Many older adults do not consider themselves at risk for HIV infection.
- Older gay men, who grew up and lived in an era when disclosure of their sexual orientation was not acceptable and who have lost long-time partners, may begin new relationships with younger men.
- Older adults may be intravenous (IV) drug users.
- Older adults may have received HIV-infected blood through organ transplants or transfusions before 1985.
- Normal age-related changes include a reduction in immune system function, which puts the older adult at greater risk for infections, cancers, and autoimmune disorders. Many older adults also experience the loss of loved ones, resulting in depression and bereavement, factors that are associated with depressed immune function.

Prevention of HIV Infection

Until an effective vaccine is developed, nurses need to prevent HIV infection by educating how to eliminate or reduce risky behaviors (see Chart 37-1).

Preventive Education

Evidence-based programs are used to educate the public regarding safer sexual practices to decrease the risk of transmitting HIV infection to sexual partners (Chart 37-2). The CDC (2011c), through the HIV/AIDS Prevention Research Synthesis Project, identified evidence-based behavioral interventions that can be applied in a number of settings. Other than abstinence, consistent and correct use of condoms (Chart 37-3) is the only effective method to decrease the risk of sexual transmission of HIV infection. When latex male condoms are used consistently and correctly during vaginal or anal intercourse, they are highly effective in preventing the sexual transmission of HIV (CDC, 2011d). Non-latex condoms made of natural materials such as lambskin are available for people with latex allergy but will not protect against HIV infection. A male condom should be used for oral contact with the penis, and a dental dam (a flat piece of latex used by dentists to isolate a tooth for treatment) or an altered condom can be used for oral contact with the vagina or rectum. The polyurethane female condom, which is an effective contraceptive, provides a physical barrier that prevents exposure to genital secretions containing HIV, such as semen and vaginal fluid, and is controlled by the woman (see Chapter 56).

Finding effective woman-controlled methods and interventions that prevent risky behaviors that lead to HIV infection are important (Coffman & Kugler, 2012). Nonoxynol-9 (N-9) was widely advocated to reduce the risk of HIV infection until

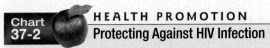

HEALTH PROMOTION

Protecting Against HIV Infection

Chart 37-2

All patients should be advised to:

- Abstain from sharing sexual fluids (semen and vaginal fluid).
- Reduce the number of sexual partners to one.
- Always use latex condoms. If the patient is allergic to latex, nonlatex condoms should be used; however, they will not protect against HIV infection.
- Not reuse condoms.
- Avoid using cervical caps or diaphragms without using a condom as well.
- Always use dental dams for oral–genital or anal stimulation.
- Avoid anal intercourse, because this practice may injure tissues.
- Avoid manual–anal intercourse ("fisting").
- Not ingest urine or semen.
- Avoid sharing needles, razors, toothbrushes, sex toys, or blood-contaminated articles.

All patients should be educated about nonpenetrative sexual activities, such as body massage, social kissing (dry), mutual masturbation, fantasy, and sex films.

Patients who are HIV seropositive should also be advised to:

- Inform previous, present, and prospective sexual and drug-using partners of their HIV-positive status. If the patient is concerned for his or her safety, advise the patient that many states have established mechanisms through the public health department in which professionals are available to notify exposed people.
- Avoid having unprotected sex with another HIV-seropositive person. Cross-infection with that person's HIV can increase the severity of infection.
- Avoid donating blood, plasma, body organs, or sperm.

PATIENT EDUCATION

The Correct Way to Use a Male Condom

Chart 37-3

1. Put on a new condom before any kind of sex.
2. Hold the condom by the tip to squeeze out the air.

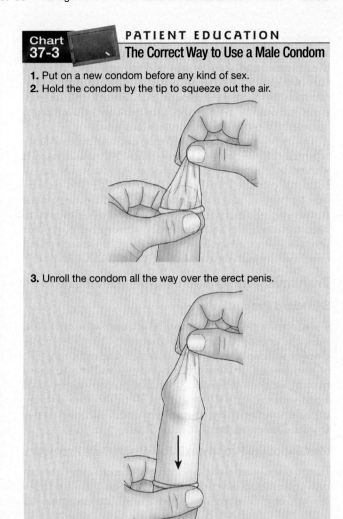

3. Unroll the condom all the way over the erect penis.

4. Have sex.
5. Hold the condom so it cannot come off the penis.
6. Pull out.
7. Use a new condom if you want to have sex again or if you want to have sex in a different place (e.g., in the anus and then in the vagina).

Note: Keep condoms cool and dry. Never use skin lotions, baby oil, petroleum jelly, or cold cream with condoms. The oil in these products will cause the condom to break. Products made with water (such as K-Y jelly or glycerin) are safer to use.

a clinical trial conducted with almost 1,000 female commercial sex workers in African countries revealed that those who used N-9 intravaginally along with condoms were 50% more likely to be infected with HIV than those who did not use the N-9 gel (Van Damme, Ramjee, Alary, et al. 2002). Results of another clinical trial found a significant reduction in HIV infection for women who inserted a microbicide gel containing tenofovir into the vagina twice (within 12 hours before and after vaginal intercourse) (Karim, Karim, & Frohlich, et al., 2010).

Two clinical trials have reported that male circumcision reduced the risk of female-to-male sexual transmission by roughly 60% (WHO, 2011b). As a result, the WHO and UNAIDS (the Joint United Nations Programme on HIV/AIDS) recommended circumcision as an effective strategy to reduce the risk of HIV acquisition in men.

Total abstinence from addictive drugs might not be a realistic short-term goal; therefore, working with drug users to assist them to increase their healthy behaviors might be more realistic. Needle exchange programs are available in some locations so that IV/injection drug users can obtain sterile drug equipment at no cost. Needle exchange programs do not promote increased drug use; on the contrary, they have been found to decrease the incidence of blood-borne infections in people who inject drugs (CDC, 2010a). Nurses should refer clients to needle exchange programs in their neighborhood whenever available. In the absence of needle exchange programs, IV drug users should be instructed on methods to clean their syringes and advised to avoid sharing drug use equipment. Drug users interested

in treatment programs should be referred to those programs. The CDC (2010a) has developed a toolkit to address reducing HIV transmission in those who use drugs and their support network.

Related Reproductive Education

Because HIV infection in women often occurs during the childbearing years, family planning issues need to be addressed. Attempts to achieve pregnancy by couples in which only one partner has HIV (known as discordant couples) expose the unaffected partner to the virus. Efforts at artificial insemination using processed semen from an HIV-infected partner continue. Studies are needed, because HIV has been found in the spermatozoa of patients with HIV infection, and it is possible that HIV can replicate in the male germ cell. Women considering pregnancy need to have accurate information about the risks of transmitting HIV infection to themselves, their partner, and their future children, and about the benefits of taking antiretroviral agents to reduce perinatal HIV transmission. Women in resource-rich settings who are HIV positive should be instructed not to breast-feed their infants, because HIV is transmitted through breast milk.

Hormonal contraceptives including daily oral pills and long-acting injectables are used by more than 140 million women worldwide (Heffron, Donnell, Rees, et al., 2012). The use of hormonal contraceptives had twice the risk of HIV-1 acquisition for women, and transmission rates from female to male partners was also higher (Heffron et al., 2012). Nurses need to educate women who take hormonal contraceptives to prevent pregnancy about using condoms to prevent HIV infection and other sexually transmitted infections (STIs) (CDC, 2010b).

Transmission to Health Care Providers

Standard Precautions

To reduce the risk of exposure of health care workers to HIV, the CDC developed standard precautions (Chart 37-4). Specifically, standard precautions are designed to reduce the risk of transmission of bloodborne pathogens and of pathogens from moist body substances. Standard precautions are used when working with all patients in all health care settings, regardless of their diagnosis or presumed infectious status (Siegel, Rhinehart, Jackson, et al., 2007).

Postexposure Prophylaxis for Health Care Providers

Postexposure prophylaxis in response to the exposure of health care personnel to infected blood or other body fluids reduces the risk of HIV infection. The CDC recommends that all health care providers who have sustained a significant exposure to HIV be counseled and offered psychosocial support and anti-HIV postexposure prophylaxis medication as appropriate (Chart 37-5). Guidelines for treatment of health care workers with possible occupational exposure to HIV are available from the CDC (2011e). The phone number for the Health Resources and Service Administration (HRSA) Postexposure Prophylaxis Hotline is listed in the Resources section at the end of this chapter; the hotline is answered by a health care provider.

Vaccination

Two vaccine types that could be developed include a therapeutic vaccine for those who are already infected with HIV and a preventative vaccine. The Scientific Strategic Plan of the Global HIV Vaccine Enterprise (2010) provides an international framework to speed the development, execution, and analysis of HIV vaccine trials, to better integrate preclinical and clinical research, to more effectively capitalize on scientific advances from other fields, and to bring new researchers and funders to the global effort to develop a safe and effective HIV vaccine. As a result of this enterprise, vaccine development has accelerated throughout the world, although the goal is still elusive.

Pathophysiology

Because HIV is an infectious disease, it is important to understand how HIV-1 integrates itself into a person's immune system and how the immune response plays a role in the course of HIV disease. This knowledge is also essential for understanding medication therapy and vaccine development.

Viruses are intracellular parasites. HIV belongs to a group of viruses known as **retroviruses**, which carry their

---

Chart 37-4 Recommendations for Standard Precautions

1. **Hand hygiene:** Use after touching blood, body fluids, secretions, excretions, or contaminated items; immediately after removing gloves; and between patient contacts.
2. **Personal protective equipment:**
   - *Gloves:* Use for touching blood, body fluids, secretions, excretions, and contaminated items, and for touching mucous membranes and nonintact skin.
   - *Gown:* Use during procedures and patient care activities when contact of clothing/exposed skin with blood or body fluids, secretions, and excretions is anticipated.
   - *Mask, eye protection (goggles), face shield*:* Use during procedures and patient care activities likely to generate splashes or sprays of blood, body fluids, and secretions, especially suctioning or endotracheal intubation.
3. **Soiled patient care equipment:** Handle in a manner that prevents transfer of microorganisms to others and to the environment; wear gloves if visibly contaminated; and perform hand hygiene.
4. **Environmental control:** Develop procedures for routine care, cleaning, and disinfection of environmental surfaces, especially frequently touched surfaces in patient care areas.
5. **Textiles and laundry:** Handle in a manner that prevents transfer of microorganisms to others and to the environment.
6. **Needles and other sharps:** Do not recap, bend, break, or hand manipulate used needles; if recapping is required, use a one-handed scoop technique only; use safety features when available; and place used sharps in a puncture-resistant container.
7. **Patient resuscitation:** Use mouthpiece, resuscitation bag, and other ventilation devices to prevent contact with mouth and oral secretions.
8. **Patient placement:** Prioritize for single-patient room if patient is at increased risk for transmission, is likely to contaminate the environment, does not maintain appropriate hygiene, or is at increased risk for acquiring infection or developing adverse outcome following infection.
9. **Respiratory hygiene/cough etiquette** (source containment of infectious respiratory secretions in symptomatic patients, beginning at initial point of encounter, such as triage and reception areas in emergency departments and physician offices): Instruct symptomatic people to cover mouth and nose when sneezing or coughing, use tissues and dispose in no-touch receptacle, observe hand hygiene after soiling of hands with respiratory secretions, and wear surgical mask if tolerated.

*During aerosol-generating procedures on patients with suspected or proven infections transmitted by respiratory aerosols (e.g., severe acute respiratory syndrome, wear a fit-tested N95 or higher respirator in addition to gloves, gown, and face/eye protection.

From Centers for Disease Control and Prevention (2007). 2007 Guideline for Isolation Precautions: Preventing Transmission of Infectious Agents in Healthcare Settings. Available at: www.cdc.gov/hicpac/2007ip/2007ip_part1.html

Chart 37-5 Postexposure Prophylaxis for Health Care Providers

The average risk for HIV transmission to health care providers after a percutaneous exposure to HIV-infected blood is estimated to be approximately 0.3%; after a mucous membrane exposure, the risk is approximately 0.09%. If you sustain an occupational exposure to HIV, take the following actions immediately:

- Alert your supervisor/nursing faculty, and initiate the injury-reporting system used in the setting.
- Identify the source patient, who may need to be tested for HIV, hepatitis B, and hepatitis C. State laws will determine whether written informed consent must be obtained from the source patient before his or her testing. OraQuick® rapid testing should be used if possible if the HIV status of the source patient is unknown, because results can be available within 20 minutes.
- Report as quickly as possible to the employee health services, the emergency department, or other designated treatment facility. This visit should be documented in the health care worker's confidential medical record.
- Give consent for baseline testing for HIV, hepatitis B, and hepatitis C. Confidential HIV testing can be performed up to 72 hours after the exposure but should be performed as soon as the health care worker can give informed consent for baseline testing.
- Get postexposure prophylaxis for HIV in accordance with Centers for Disease Control and Prevention guidelines. Start the prophylaxis medications within 2 hours after exposure. Make sure that you are being monitored for symptoms of toxicity. Practice safer sex until follow-up testing is complete. Continue the HIV medications for the full 4 weeks after exposure. The majority of HIV exposures will warrant a combination of antiretroviral agents. Combinations that may be prescribed for postexposure prophylaxis include zidovudine (ZDV) and lamivudine (3TC) or emtricitabine (FTC); stavudine (d4T) and 3TC or FTC; and tenofovir (TDF) and 3TC or FTC.
- Follow up with postexposure testing at 1 month, 3 months, and 6 months, and perhaps 1 year.
- Document the exposure in detail for your own records as well as for the employer.
- Take the psychosocial support offered or seek support outside of the employment setting.

From Centers for Disease Control and Prevention. (2011e). *Occupational HIV transmission and prevention among health care workers.* Available at: www.cdc.gov/hiv/resources/factsheets/PDF/hcw.pdf

Physiology :·:··· Pathophysiology

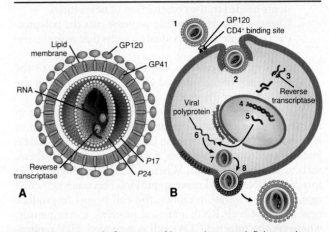

FIGURE 37-1 • A. Structure of human immunodeficiency virus type 1 (HIV-1). A glycoprotein envelope surrounds the virus, which carries its genetic material in ribonucleic acid (RNA). Knobs, consisting of proteins GP120 and GP41, protrude from the envelope. These proteins are essential for binding the virus to the CD4+ T lymphocyte. **B.** Life cycle of HIV-1: *(1)* Attachment of the HIV virus to a CD4+ receptor; *(2)* internalization and uncoating of the virus with viral RNA and reverse transcriptase; *(3)* reverse transcription, which produces a mirror image of the viral RNA and double-stranded deoxyribonucleic acid (DNA) molecule; *(4)* integration of viral DNA into host DNA using the integrase enzyme; *(5)* transcription of the inserted viral DNA to produce viral messenger RNA; *(6)* translation of viral messenger RNA to create viral polyprotein; *(7)* cleavage of viral polyprotein into individual viral proteins that make up the new virus; and *(8)* assembly and release of the new virus from the host cell. Redrawn from Porth, C., & Matfin, G. (2009). *Pathophysiology: Concepts of altered health states* (7th ed.). Philadelphia: Lippincott Williams & Wilkins.

genetic material in the form of ribonucleic acid (RNA) rather than deoxyribonucleic acid (DNA). As shown in Figure 37-1A, HIV consists of a viral core containing the viral RNA, surrounded by an envelope consisting of protruding glycoproteins.

All viruses target specific cells. HIV targets cells with CD4 receptors, which are expressed on the surface of T lymphocytes, monocytes, dendritic cells, and brain microglia. Mature T cells (T lymphocytes) are composed of two major subpopulations that are defined by cell surface receptors of CD4 or CD8. Approximately two thirds of peripheral blood T cells are CD4+, and approximately one third are CD8+. Most people have about 700 to 1,000 CD4+ cells/mm³, but a level as low as 500 cells/mm³ can be considered within normal limits. During acute/recent infection, most varieties of HIV-1 use the chemokine receptor **CCR5** (R5 virus) for entry to T cells

in addition to the CD4+ receptor, which suggests that the R5 variant is preferred to a different variant (CXCR4) but the preferred coreceptor can shift over the course of infection.

The HIV life cycle is complex (see Fig. 37-1B) and consists of the following steps (Porth & Matfin, 2009):

1. *Attachment:* In this first step, the GP120 and GP41 glycoproteins of HIV bind with the host's uninfected CD4+ receptor and chemokine coreceptors, usually CCR5, which results in fusion of HIV with the CD4+ T-cell membrane.
2. *Uncoating:* Only the contents of HIV's viral core (two single strands of viral RNA and three viral enzymes: reverse transcriptase, integrase, and protease) are emptied into the CD4+ T cell.
3. *DNA synthesis:* HIV changes its genetic material from RNA to DNA through action of **reverse transcriptase**, resulting in double-stranded DNA that carries instruction for viral replication.
4. *Integration:* New viral DNA enters the nucleus of the CD4+ T cell and through action of integrase is blended with the DNA of the CD4+ T cell, resulting in permanent, lifelong infection. Prior to this, the uninfected person has been only exposed to, not infected with, HIV. With this step, HIV infection is permanent.
5. *Transcription:* When the CD4+ T cell is activated, the double-stranded DNA forms single-stranded messenger RNA (mRNA), which builds new viruses.

6. *Translation:* The mRNA creates chains of new proteins and enzymes (polyproteins) that contain the components needed in the construction of new viruses.
7. *Cleavage:* The HIV enzyme protease cuts the polyprotein chain into the individual proteins that make up the new virus.
8. *Budding:* New proteins and viral RNA migrate to the membrane of the infected CD4+ T cell, exit from the cell, and start the process all over.

In resting (nondividing) CD4+ cells, HIV can survive in a latent state as an integrated **provirus** that produces few or no viral particles. These resting CD4+ T cells can be stimulated to produce new particles if something activates them, such as another infection. When a T cell that harbors this integrated DNA (also known as provirus) becomes activated against HIV or other microbes, the cell begins to produce new copies of both RNA and viral proteins. Consequently, whenever the infected CD4+ cell is activated, HIV replication and budding occur, which can destroy the host cell. Newly formed HIV released into the blood can infect other CD4+ cells (see Fig. 37-1B).

A mutation of CCR5 that is common in Caucasians, but not other ethnic groups, has been identified. About 1% of Caucasians lack functional CCR5 and are highly protected against HIV infection even if exposed (although protection is not absolute); about 18% are not markedly protected against infection but, if infected, demonstrate significantly slower rates of disease progression.

HIV-1 mutates quickly, at a relatively constant rate, with about 1% of the virus's genetic material changing annually. HIV-1 exhibits substantial genetic diversity, and several different genotypes of HIV-1 exist throughout the world. There is a major group (group M), which consists of subtypes A through L, and a more diverse collection of outliers, which has been referred to as groups N and O. Subtype B HIV-1 viruses predominate in the Western world; this genetic variation is one of the major reasons why effective vaccine development has been such a challenge.

Stages of HIV Infection

There are three stages of HIV infection based on clinical history, physical examination, laboratory evidence (CDC, 2008), signs and symptoms, and associated infections and malignancies. The staging system is outlined in Table 37-1.

The period from infection with HIV to the development of HIV-specific antibodies is known as **primary infection**, or stage 1. Initially, there is a period during which those who are HIV positive test negative on the HIV antibody blood test, although they are infected and highly infectious, because their viral loads are very high. About 40% to 80% of patients develop clinical symptoms of a nonspecific viral illness (e.g., fever, fatigue, or rash) lasting 1 to 2 weeks (CDC, 2008). After 2 to 3 weeks, antibodies to the glycoproteins of the HIV envelope can be detected in the sera of people infected with HIV, but most of these antibodies lack the ability to totally control the virus. By the time neutralizing antibodies can be detected, HIV-1 is firmly established in the host.

Primary infection is characterized by high levels of viral replication, widespread dissemination of HIV throughout the body, and destruction of CD4+ T cells, which leads to dramatic drops in CD4+ T-cell counts (normally 500 to 1,500 cells/mm³ of blood). The host responds to the HIV infection through a CD4+ T-cell response that causes other immune cells, such as CD8+ lymphocytes, to increase their killing of infected, virus-producing cells. The body produces antibody molecules in an effort to contain the free HIV particles (outside cells) and assist in their removal. During this stage, the virus is widely disseminated in lymphoid tissue, and a **latent reservoir** within resting memory CD4+ T cells is created.

The amount of virus in the body after the initial immune response subsides is referred to as the **viral set point**, which results in an equilibrium between HIV levels and the immune response that may be elicited. This can last for years and is inversely correlated with disease prognosis; that is, the higher the viral set point, the poorer the prognosis. After the viral set point is reached, a chronic stage persists in which the immune system cannot eliminate the virus despite its best efforts. This set point varies greatly from patient to patient and dictates the subsequent rate of disease progression; on average, 8 to 10 years can pass before a major HIV-related complication develops. In this prolonged, chronic stage, patients feel well and have few, if any, symptoms. Apparent good health continues because CD4+ T-cell levels remain high enough to preserve immune defensive responses, but over time, the number of CD4+ T cells continues to decrease.

Stage 2 occurs when CD4 T-lymphocyte cells are between 200 and 499 and when the count drops below 200 cells/mm³ of blood; at this point, the person is considered to have AIDS. For surveillance purposes, HIV disease progression is classified from less to more severe; once a case is classified into a surveillance severity stage, it cannot be reclassified into a less severe stage even if the CD4 T-lymphocytes increase, which often occurs when a person receives medications to treat HIV infection. A stage 3 classification has implications for services (e.g., disability benefits, housing, and food stamps), because these programs are often linked to an AIDS diagnosis. The CDC's 2008 definition also emphasizes CD4+ percentages, which are less subject to variation on repeated measurements than the absolute CD4+ T-cell count.

Assessment and Diagnostic Findings in HIV Infection

During the first stage of HIV infection, the patient may be asymptomatic or may exhibit various signs and symptoms such as fatigue or skin rash. Patients who are in later stages of HIV infection may have a variety of symptoms related to their immunosuppressed state. Several screening tests are used to diagnose HIV infection, and others are used to determine the stage and severity of the infection. Table 37-2 identifies common blood tests.

HIV Antibody Tests

The staging system requires laboratory evidence of HIV infection in order to diagnose HIV or AIDS (see Table 37-1). Since 2006, the CDC has endorsed efforts to increase HIV testing in order to identify the estimated 25% of persons infected with HIV who are unaware of their infection. Such efforts have included streamlining the consent

TABLE 37-2 **Selected Laboratory Tests for Diagnosing and Tracking HIV and Assessing Immune Status**

Test	Findings in HIV Infection
EIA	Antibodies are detected, resulting in positive results and marking the end of the window period.
Western blot	Also detects antibodies to HIV; used to confirm EIA
Viral load	Measures HIV RNA in the plasma
CD4/CD8	These are markers found on lymphocytes. HIV kills CD4+ cells, which results in a significantly impaired immune system.
OraQuick®	In-home HIV test

HIV, human immunodeficiency virus; EIA, enzyme immunoassay; RNA, ribonucleic acid.

process and expanding opt-out testing to all health care settings, especially STI clinics. The following are specific recommendations from the CDC (2010b) that apply to testing for HIV infection:

- HIV screening is recommended for all persons who seek evaluation and treatment for STIs.
- HIV testing must be voluntary and free of coercion. Patients must not be tested without their knowledge.
- HIV screening after notifying the patient that an HIV test will be performed (unless the patient declines) is recommended in all health care settings.
- Specific signed consent for HIV testing should not be required. In most settings, general informed consent for medical care is considered sufficient to encompass informed consent for HIV testing.
- The use of rapid HIV tests should be considered, especially in clinics where a high proportion of patients do not return for HIV test results.
- Positive screening tests for HIV antibody must be confirmed by a supplemental test before the diagnosis of HIV infection can be established.
- Providers should be alert to the possibility of acute HIV infection and perform a viral load test in addition to an antibody test for HIV, if indicated. Persons suspected of recently acquired HIV infection should be referred for immediate consultation with an infectious disease specialist.

Although these guidelines are already in effect in most states, they have not been implemented in others because they violate the states' existing HIV confidentiality laws.

Stigma around HIV persists. When the result of the HIV antibody test is received, it is carefully explained to the patient in private (Chart 37-6). All test results are kept confidential. Education and counseling about the test result and about preventing transmission are essential. The patient's psychological response to a positive test result may include feelings of panic, depression, and hopelessness. The social and interpersonal consequences of a positive test result can be devastating. The patient may lose his or her sexual partner, housing, and health insurance because of disclosure. He or she may experience discrimination in employment as well as social ostracism. For these reasons and others, patients who test positive may need ongoing counseling as well as referrals for social, financial, medical, and psychological support services. They must be connected to health care services to

Chart 37-6 **HIV Test Results: Implications for Patients**

Interpretation of Positive Test Results

- Antibodies to HIV are present in the blood (the patient has been infected with the virus, and the body has produced antibodies).
- HIV is active in the body, and the patient can transmit the virus to others.
- Despite HIV infection, the patient does not necessarily have AIDS.
- The patient is not immune to HIV (the antibodies do not indicate immunity).

Interpretation of Negative Test Results

- Antibodies to HIV are not present in the blood at this time, which can mean that the patient has not been infected with HIV or, if infected, the body has not yet produced antibodies (window period—may be between 3 weeks and 6 months).
- The patient should continue taking precautions. The test result does not mean that the patient is immune to the virus, nor does it mean the patient is not infected; it just means that the body may not have produced antibodies yet.

evaluate their stage of HIV infection and determine if treatment is indicated. Patients whose test results are seronegative may develop a false sense of security, possibly resulting in continued high-risk behaviors or feelings that they are immune to the virus. These patients may need ongoing counseling to help modify high-risk behaviors and to encourage returns for repeated testing. Other patients may experience anxiety regarding the uncertainty of their status.

When a person is infected with HIV, the immune system responds by producing antibodies against the virus, usually within 3 to 12 weeks after infection. In 1985, the FDA licensed an HIV-1 antibody assay that uses approximately 5 to 7 mL of blood. Samples are tested using two different laboratory techniques to determine the presence of antibodies to HIV. The **EIA (enzyme immunoassay)** test, or a variant of this called **ELISA (enzyme-linked immunosorbent assay)**, identifies antibodies directed specifically against HIV. The **Western blot assay** is used to confirm seropositivity when the EIA result is positive. Adults whose blood contains antibodies for HIV are infected. Continued work on the sensitivity of these antibody tests has reduced the length of time before antibodies are measurable.

In addition to the HIV-1 antibody assay, additional rapid testing techniques are now available. Using less than a drop of blood, the OraQuick ADVANCE® Rapid HIV-1 Antibody Test quickly (approximately 20 minutes) and reliably (99.6% accuracy) detects antibodies to HIV-1. This test is used when a delay in testing would seriously affect treatment, such as in labor and delivery rooms or in emergency departments when the HIV status of a sexual abuser is unknown. OraQuick ADVANCE® is the first FDA-approved home-based test for HIV antibodies.

Viral Load Tests

Target amplification methods quantify HIV RNA or DNA levels in the plasma and have replaced p24 antigen capture assays. Target amplification methods include reverse transcriptase–**polymerase chain reaction** (RT-PCR) and nucleic acid sequence–based amplification. A widely used **viral load test** measures plasma HIV RNA levels. Currently, these tests are used to track viral load and response to treatment of HIV infection. RT-PCR is also used to detect HIV in high-risk sero-negative people before antibodies are measurable, to confirm a positive EIA result, and to screen neonates. HIV culture or quantitative plasma culture and plasma viremia are additional tests that measure viral burden, but they are used infrequently. Viral load is a better predictor of the risk of HIV disease progression than the CD4+ count. The lower the viral load, the longer the time to AIDS diagnosis and the longer the survival time.

Treatment of HIV Infection

Protocols on how and when to start treatment for HIV infection change often. The U.S. Department of Health and Human Services Panel on Antiretroviral Guidelines for Adults and Adolescents (2011) is composed of HIV specialists from across the country that meet at least once a year to review the latest scientific evidence. The CD4 count serves as the major laboratory indicator of immune function, is one of the key factors in deciding whether to initiate ART and prophylaxis for opportunistic infections, and is the strongest predictor of subsequent disease progression and survival (Panel on Antiretroviral Guidelines, 2011). The major goals for initiating ART are to (1) reduce HIV-associated morbidity and prolong the duration and quality of survival, (2) restore and preserve immunologic function, (3) maximally and durably suppress plasma HIV viral load, and (4) prevent HIV transmission (Panel on Antiretroviral Guidelines, 2011). The decision about when to start ART is earlier now, with the goal of reducing the HIV-associated inflammation that impacts multiple body systems. Currently, treatment is recommended when CD4 counts are between 350 mm^3 and 500 mm^3; however, some clinicians think that treatment should be started with even higher CD4 counts. Clinicians, in partnership with patients, make treatment decisions based on a number of factors, including the willingness of the patient to adhere to the lifelong treatment regimen.

ART targets different stages of the HIV life cycle (see Fig. 37-1). The number of antiretroviral agents (Table 37-3) and the rapid evolution of new information have introduced extraordinary complexity into the treatment of HIV infection. Drugs from established classes such as nucleoside/nucleotide reverse transcriptase inhibitors (NRTIs) or non-nucleoside reverse transcriptase inhibitors (NNRTIs), which both interfere with the change of viral RNA into viral DNA through the action of blocking reverse transcriptase and **protease inhibitors**, continue to serve as the mainstays of ART. In 2008, the integrate inhibitor raltegravir (Isentress) and the CCR5 antagonist maraviroc (Selzentry), a novel entry inhibitor, were approved and joined the other fusion inhibitors such as enfuvirtide (T-20), which inhibits attachment or entry of HIV into the CD4+ T cell. The Panel on Antiretroviral Guidelines (2011) provides clear directions regarding which medications should be prescribed.

To achieve sustained viral suppression, patients must take more than one antiretroviral medication. Some pharmaceutical companies have combined two to three agents into one tablet or capsule, such as Kaletra (lopinavir and ritonavir) and Atripla (efavirenz, emtricitabine, and tenofovir disoproxil fumarate), for once-a-day use. Simplifying treatment regimens and decreasing the number of medications that must be taken each day increase patients' adherence to therapy.

In the majority of patients, ART leads to sustained reductions in HIV replication as measured by viral loads, a rise in CD4+ T-cell counts with reconstitution of immune function, and significant reductions in morbidity and mortality.

Although antiretroviral regimens have become less complex, side effects create barriers to adherence and inadequate dosing can lead to viral resistance. It is difficult to predict patients' adherence to medication regimens, but a positive relationship between the patient and health care provider is associated with better adherence. Individualized plans of care that consider housing and social support issues, in addition to health indicators, are essential. Self-reported adherence measures can distinguish clinically meaningful patterns of medication-taking behaviors; therefore, nurses should assess if patients can describe how they are taking their ART. Factors associated with nonadherence include active substance abuse, depression, and lack of social support. Gender, race, pregnancy, and history of past substance use have not been associated with nonadherence (Panel on Antiretroviral Guidelines, 2011). Chart 37-7 summarizes strategies that health care providers can encourage to promote treatment regimen adherence. Every health care encounter should be used as an opportunity to briefly review the treatment regimen, identify any new issues, and reinforce successful behaviors.

Regular laboratory tests are used to evaluate whether ART is effective for a specific patient. An adequate CD4 response for most patients on ART is an increase in CD4 count in the range of 50 mm^3 to 150 mm^3 per year, generally with an accelerated response in the first 3 months (Panel on Antiretroviral Guidelines, 2011). Viral load should be measured at baseline and on a regular basis thereafter because viral load is the most important indicator of response to ART. For most individuals who are adherent to their ART regimens and who do not harbor resistance mutations to the prescribed drugs, viral suppression is generally achieved in 12 to 24 weeks, even though it may take longer in some patients (Panel on Antiretroviral Guidelines, 2011).

Adverse effects associated with all HIV treatment regimens include hepatotoxicity, nephrotoxicity, and osteopenia, along with increased risk of cardiovascular disease and myocardial infarction (see Table 37-3). Many of the antiretroviral agents that prolong life may simultaneously cause fat redistribution syndrome and metabolic alterations such as dyslipidemia and insulin resistance, which put the patient at risk for early-onset heart disease and diabetes. The fat redistribution syndrome (lipodystrophy) consists of lipoatrophy (localized subcutaneous fat loss in the face, arms, legs, and buttocks) and lipohypertrophy (central visceral fat [lipomata] accumulation in the abdomen, although possibly in the breasts, dorsocervical region [buffalo hump], and within the muscle and liver). These changes can disturb the body image of people living with HIV/AIDS (Gagnon & Holmes, 2011) and may be a reason they decline or stop ART (Chart 37-8).

Facial wasting, characterized as a sinking of the cheeks, eyes, and temples caused by the loss of fat tissue under the skin, may be treated by injectable fillers such as poly-L-lactic acid (Sculptra) (Fig. 37-2). Hepatotoxicity associated with certain protease inhibitors may limit the use of these agents, especially in patients with underlying liver dysfunction (Panel on Antiretroviral Guidelines, 2011).

TABLE 37-3 Antiretroviral Agents*

Generic Name (Abbreviation) and Trade Names (Italic)	Food Interactions	Adverse Effects
Nucleoside Reverse Transcriptase Inhibitors (NRTIs)		
abacavir (ABC) *Ziagen* *Trizivir (ABC/ZDV/3TC)* *Epzicom (ABC/3TC)*	Take without regard to meals. Alcohol increases abacavir levels 41%. Abacavir has no effect on alcohol.	Hypersensitivity reaction, which can be fatal; symptoms may include fever, rash, nausea, vomiting, malaise or fatigue, loss of appetite, and respiratory symptoms such as sore throat, cough, shortness of breath.
didanosine (ddI) *Videx* *Videx EC*	Levels decrease 55%; take half hour before or 2 hours after meals.	Pancreatitis, peripheral neuropathy, nausea, diarrhea, lactic acidosis with fatty degeneration of the liver (rare but potentially life-threatening toxicity associated with the use of NRTIs)
emtricitabine (FTC) *Emtriva* *Truvada (FTC/TDF)*	Take without regard to meals.	Minimal toxicity, lactic acidosis with hepatic steatosis (rare but potentially life-threatening toxicity with the use of NRTIs)
lamivudine (3TC) *Epivir* *Combivir (3TC/ZDV)* *Trizivir (ABC/3TC/ZDV)*	Take without regard to meals.	Minimal toxicity, lactic acidosis with hepatic steatosis (rare but potentially life-threatening toxicity with the use of NRTIs)
stavudine (d4T) *Zerit*	Take without regard to meals.	Peripheral neuropathy, lipodystrophy, rapidly progressive ascending neuromuscular weakness (rare), pancreatitis, lactic acidosis with hepatic steatosis (higher incidence with d4T than with other NRTIs), hyperlipidemia
tenofovir disoproxil fumarate (TDF) *Viread* *Truvada (FTC/TDF)*	Take without regard to meals.	Asthenia, headache, diarrhea, nausea, vomiting, and flatulence; kidney insufficiency; lactic acidosis with hepatic steatosis (rare but potentially life-threatening toxicity with the use of NRTIs)
zalcitabine (ddC) *Hivid*	Take without regard to meals.	Peripheral neuropathy, stomatitis, lactic acidosis with hepatic steatosis (rare but potentially life-threatening toxicity with the use of NRTIs), pancreatitis
Zidovudine (AZT or ZDV) *Retrovir* *Combivir (3TC/AZT)* *Trizivir (ABC/3TC/AZT)*	Take without regard to meals.	Bone marrow suppression; macrocytic anemia or neutropenia; gastrointestinal (GI) intolerance, headache, insomnia, asthenia; lactic acidosis with hepatic steatosis (rare but potentially life-threatening toxicity with use of NRTIs)
Non-Nucleoside Reverse Transcriptase Inhibitors		
delavirdine (DLV) *Rescriptor*	Take without regard to meals.	Rash (rare cases of Stevens-Johnson syndrome have been reported), increased transaminase levels, headaches
efavirenz (EFV) *Sustiva*	High-fat/high-caloric meals increase peak plasma concentrations of capsules by 39% and tablets by 79%; take on an empty stomach.	Rash (rare cases of Stevens-Johnson syndrome have been reported), central nervous system symptoms (dizziness, somnolence, insomnia, abnormal dreams, confusion, abnormal thinking, impaired concentration, amnesia, agitation, depersonalization, hallucinations, and euphoria), increased transaminase levels, false-positive cannabinoid test, teratogenic in monkeys
nevirapine (NVP) *Viramune*	Take without regard to meals.	Rash including Stevens-Johnson syndrome, symptomatic hepatitis including fatal hepatic necrosis has been reported. Single dose used in developing countries to prevent vertical transmission.
etravirine (ETR) *Intelence*	Take after a meal with water.	Serious side effects of this medication include severe skin rash. Mild to moderate rash occurs in the 2nd week of therapy and generally resolves within 1–2 weeks of continued therapy. Nausea, diarrhea, abdominal pain, vomiting, fatigue, peripheral neuropathy, headache, high blood pressure
Protease Inhibitors		
amprenavir (APV) *Agenerase*	High-fat meal decreases blood concentration 21%; can be taken with or without food, but high-fat meal should be avoided.	GI intolerance, nausea, vomiting, diarrhea, rash, oral paresthesias, hyperlipidemia, transaminase elevation, hyperglycemia, fat maldistribution, possible increased bleeding episodes in patients with hemophilia
atazanavir (ATV) *Reyataz*	Administration with food increases bioavailability. Should be taken with food; avoid taking with antacids.	Indirect hyperbilirubinemia; prolonged PR interval (some patients experience asymptomatic 1st-degree AV block); use with caution in patients with underlying conduction defects or on concomitant medications that can cause PR prolongation; hyperglycemia; fat maldistribution; possible increased bleeding episodes in patients with hemophilia
fosamprenavir (FPV) *Lexiva*	Take without regard to meals.	Skin rash (19%), diarrhea, nausea, vomiting, headache, hyperlipidemia, transaminase elevation, hyperglycemia, fat maldistribution, possible increased bleeding episodes in patients with hemophilia
indinavir (IDV) *Crixivan*	For unboosted IDV: Should be taken 1 hour before or 2 hours after meals; may take with skim milk or low-fat meal. For RTV-boosted IDV: Can be taken with or without food.	Nephrolithiasis, GI intolerance, nausea, indirect hyperbilirubinemia, hyperlipidemia, headache, asthenia, blurred vision, dizziness, rash, metallic taste, thrombocytopenia, alopecia, hemolytic anemia, hyperglycemia, fat maldistribution, possible increased bleeding episodes in patients with hemophilia

(continues on page 1008)

TABLE 37-3 Antiretroviral Agents* (continued)

Generic Name (Abbreviation) and Trade Names (Italic)	Food Interactions	Adverse Effects
lopinavir + ritonavir (LPV/RTV) *Kaletra*	Should be taken with food.	GI intolerance, nausea, vomiting, diarrhea, asthenia, hyperlipidemia (especially hypertriglyceridemia), elevated serum transaminase, hyperglycemia, fat maldistribution, possible increased bleeding episodes in patients with hemophilia
nelfinavir (NFV) *Viracept*	Should be taken with food if possible; may improve tolerability.	Diarrhea, hyperlipidemia, hyperglycemia, fat maldistribution, possible increased bleeding episodes in patients with hemophilia, serum transaminase elevation
ritonavir (RTV) *Norvir*	Should be taken with food if possible; may improve tolerability.	GI intolerance, nausea, vomiting, diarrhea, paresthesias (circumoral and extremities), hyperlipidemia (especially hypertriglyceridemia), hepatitis, asthenia, taste perversion, hyperglycemia, fat maldistribution, possible increased bleeding in patients with hemophilia. Lower doses used as a booster.
saquinavir (SQV) *Invirase*	No food restrictions identified	GI intolerance, nausea, diarrhea, abdominal pain and dyspepsia, headache, hyperlipidemia, elevated transaminase enzymes, hyperglycemia, fat maldistribution, possible increased bleeding episodes in patients with hemophilia. Take with RTV as booster, if prescribed.
tipranavir (TPV) *Aptivus*	Take with food.	Serious liver problems, bleeding on the brain, rash, increased cholesterol and triglyceride levels, and changes in body fat; women taking birth control pills that contain estrogen may be more likely to develop a rash. Individuals with hemophilia may have increased bleeding. Take with RTV, if prescribed.
darunavir (DRV) *Prezista*	No food restrictions identified	Diarrhea, nausea, headache, coldlike symptoms (including runny nose or sore throat), inflammation of the liver, abnormal liver function tests, severe skin rash, fever, and abnormally high cholesterol and triglyceride levels have been reported. Take with RTV.
Fusion Inhibitors		
enfuvirtide (T-20) *Fuzeon*	Injected subcutaneously, so meals are not an issue.	Local injection site reactions—almost 100% of patients (pain, erythema, induration, nodules and cysts, pruritus, ecchymosis); increased rate of bacterial pneumonia; hypersensitivity reaction—symptoms may include rash, fever, nausea, vomiting, chills, rigors, hypotension, or elevated serum transaminases; may recur on challenge
Maraviroc (MVC) *Selzentry*	Take with or without food; requires CCR5 tropism blood test before starting.	Cough, fever, dizziness, headache, lowered blood pressure, nausea, bladder irritation; possible liver problems and cardiac events; an increased risk for some infections; a slight increase in cholesterol levels
Integrase Strand Transfer Inhibitor		
raltegravir (RAL) *Isentress*	No food restrictions identified	Diarrhea, nausea, headache, and fever have been reported.
Multiclass Combination Products		
efavirenz + emtricitabine + tenofovir disoproxil fumarate (EFV/FTC/TDF) *Atripla*		

*This information changes often. Check the U.S. Food and Drug Administration Web site (www.fda.gov/oashi/aids/virals.html) and www.aidsinfo.nih.gov/DrugsNew/Default.aspx?MenuItem=Drugs for current information when caring for people with HIV/AIDS.

 Concept Mastery Alert

Nurses must recognize the differences among common laboratory tests used to diagnose and assess HIV infection and guide therapy. For example, the EIA is a diagnostic screening test that determines the presence of antibodies to HIV. The RT-PCR test, which measures viral load, is used along with the CD4 count, which indicates the level of immune dysfunction, to assess the stage and severity of HIV infection. The CD4 count indicates the level of immune dysfunction. It is important to assess the extent of damage to the immune system before initiation of ART and/or prophylactic treatment for opportunistic infections.

Drug Resistance

Drug resistance can be broadly defined as the ability of pathogens to withstand the effects of medications that are intended to be toxic to them. There are two major components of antiretroviral drug resistance: (1) transmission of drug-resistant HIV at the time of initial infection and (2) selective drug resistance in patients who are receiving nonsuppressive regimens. Genotypic and phenotypic resistance assays are used to assess viral strains and inform selection of treatment strategies. No definitive data support using one type of resistance assay over another (i.e., genotypic vs. phenotypic); however, in most situations, genotypic testing is preferred because of the faster turnaround time, lower cost, and enhanced

HOME CARE CHECKLIST

Chart 37-7 Adhering to Medication Therapy for HIV

At the completion of home care education, the patient or caregiver will be able to:	PATIENT	CAREGIVER
• Verbalize knowledge of each medication name.	✔	✔
• State the action of each medication.	✔	✔
• State the correct times that medications are to be taken.	✔	✔
• Identify special guidelines to follow when taking medications (e.g., with meals, on an empty stomach, medications that are not to be taken together).	✔	✔
• Demonstrate methods of keeping track of the medication regimen and storage of the prescribed medications, and use reminders such as beepers and/or pillboxes.	✔	✔
• Identify specific laboratory tests, such as viral load, that are necessary to monitor the effectiveness of the prescribed medication regimen.	✔	✔
• List expected side effects of each medication.	✔	✔
• Identify side effects that should be reported to health care providers.	✔	✔
• Explain the importance of and necessity for adherence with prescribed medication regimen.	✔	✔
• Demonstrate correct administration of intramuscular, subcutaneous, or IV medications.	✔	✔
• Demonstrate correct use and safe disposal of needles, syringes, and other IV equipment.	✔	✔
• Discuss with health care providers any problems that the patient is having with side effects and adherence.	✔	✔
• Discuss episodes of nonadherence to the medication regimen.	✔	✔

sensitivity for detecting mixtures of wild-type and resistant virus. Resistance testing appears to be a useful tool in selecting active drugs when changing ART for virologic failure in persons with HIV RNA greater than 1,000 mL. In persons with levels greater than 500 mL but less than 1,000 mL, testing may be unsuccessful but should still be considered. Drug-resistance testing is not usually recommended in persons with a plasma viral load greater than 500 mL because resistance

assays cannot be consistently performed given low HIV RNA levels (Panel on Antiretroviral Guidelines, 2011).

Immune Reconstitution Inflammatory Syndrome

Immune reconstitution inflammatory syndrome (IRIS) results from rapid restoration of pathogen-specific immune responses to opportunistic infections that cause either the deterioration of a treated infection or new presentation of a

NURSING RESEARCH PROFILE

Chart 37-8 Body Changes From Lipodystrophy in Women

Gagnon, M., & Holmes, D. (2011). Bodies in mutation: Understanding lipodystrophy among women living with HIV/AIDS. *Research and Theory for Nursing Practice: An International Journal, 25*(1), 23–38.

Purpose

Lipodystrophy syndrome has been associated with HIV infection and the use of antiretroviral therapy (ART). The objective of this qualitative study was to highlight the experiences of women with lipodystrophy from ART who go through a body transformation process and the challenges they face as they move progressively from one bodily state to another.

Design

This study used grounded theory principles to describe the basic social process that emerged from the data. Researchers conducted individual interviews with 19 women living with HIV/AIDS in Montreal, Canada.

Findings

Three phases of the basic social process emerged and were called the *bodily transformation process.* Phase one was labeled

normalization, phase two was problematization, and phase three was pathologization. During the first phase, women did not associate the signs of lipodystrophy as abnormal but rather as normal body changes associated with factors such as lack of exercise, diet, aging, or menopause. Phase two was characterized by body changes becoming problematic, and the women could no longer interpret them as part of an ordinary transformation. They explained that moment as understanding that something was terribly wrong with their bodies. Phase three was characterized by the understanding that the physical changes associated with lipodystrophy were probably irreversible even if ART was stopped. Women reported feelings of powerlessness, hopelessness, betrayal, anger, and despair and stigma during the final phase.

Nursing Implications

The findings of this study suggest that although ART prolongs life, the changes associated with treatment might impact adversely on the quality of life for women. The potential changes associated with lipodystrophy need to be shared with women before they begin ART. Nurses have a professional responsibility to act as advocates and educators.

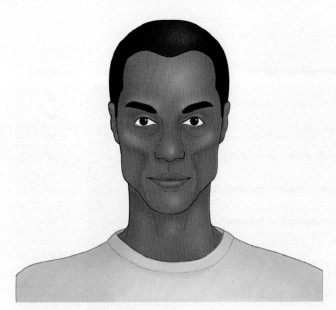

FIGURE 37-2 • Facial lipoatrophy.

subclinical infection. This syndrome typically occurs during the initial months after beginning ART and is associated with a wide spectrum of pathogens, most commonly mycobacteria, herpes viruses, and deep fungal infections (New York State Department of Health, 2009). IRIS is characterized by fever, respiratory and/or abdominal symptoms, and worsening of the clinical manifestations of an opportunistic infection or the appearance of new manifestations. IRIS is treated with anti-inflammatory medications such as cortisone. The nurse should be alert to the possibility of IRIS, especially in the 3-month period after treatment with ART is initiated, because this syndrome is associated with significant morbidity and patients often require hospital admission.

Clinical Manifestations

Patients with HIV/AIDS experience a number of symptoms related to the disease, side effects of treatment, and other comorbidities, including pancreatitis, hepatitis, and cardiometabolic abnormalities (Merlin, Cen, Praestgaard, et al., 2012). The clinical manifestations of HIV/AIDS are widespread and may involve virtually any organ system. Diseases associated with HIV infection and AIDS result from infections, malignancies, or the direct effect of HIV on body tissues. Nurses need to understand the causes, signs and symptoms, and interventions, including self-care strategies that can enhance the quality of life for patients throughout the illness. Symptom assessment tools can be used to assess patients' symptom intensity and severity. People with HIV/AIDS use a variety of self-care strategies to minimize common symptoms, which can arise from HIV disease, comorbidities, or the effects of medications used to treat HIV and opportunistic infections.

Respiratory Manifestations

Shortness of breath, dyspnea (labored breathing), cough, chest pain, and fever are associated with various opportunistic infections, such as those caused by *P. jiroveci*, *Mycobacterium avium-intracellulare*, cytomegalovirus (CMV), and *Legionella* species.

Pneumocystis Pneumonia

The most common life-threatening infection in those living with AIDS is ***Pneumocystis*** **pneumonia (PCP)**, caused by *P. jiroveci* (formerly *P. carinii*) (Durham & Lashley, 2010). Without prophylactic therapy (discussed later), most people infected with HIV will develop PCP. The clinical presentation of PCP in HIV infection is generally less acute than in people who are immunosuppressed as a result of other conditions. Patients with HIV infection initially develop nonspecific signs and symptoms, such as nonproductive cough, fever, chills, shortness of breath, dyspnea, and occasionally chest pain. Arterial oxygen concentrations in patients who are breathing room air may be mildly decreased, indicating minimal hypoxemia.

If left untreated, PCP eventually progresses and causes significant pulmonary impairment and, ultimately, respiratory failure. A few patients have a dramatic onset and a fulminating course involving severe hypoxemia, cyanosis, tachypnea, and altered mental status. Respiratory failure can develop within 2 to 3 days after the initial appearance of symptoms.

PCP can be diagnosed definitively by identifying the organism in lung tissue or bronchial secretions. This is accomplished by such procedures as sputum induction, bronchoalveolar lavage, and transbronchial biopsy (by fiberoptic bronchoscopy).

Mycobacterium avium Complex

Mycobacterium avium **complex (MAC)** disease is a common opportunistic infection in people with AIDS who have severe immune depression. MAC comprises a group of acidfast bacilli (mycobacteria) that includes *M. avium*, *Mycobacterium intracellulare*, and *Mycobacterium scrofulaceum*. MAC usually causes respiratory infection but is also commonly found in the gastrointestinal tract, lymph nodes, and bone marrow. Most patients with AIDS who have T-cell counts lower than 100 cells/mm³ have widespread disease at diagnosis and are debilitated. MAC infections are associated with rising mortality rates (Durham & Lashley, 2010).

Tuberculosis

In those who are HIV negative with latent tuberculosis (TB) infection, the *lifetime* risk of developing active TB disease is 5% to 10%, whereas in those who are HIV positive with latent TB, the *annual* risk is 10%. TB can develop in the lungs as well as in extrapulmonary sites such as the central nervous system (CNS), bone, pericardium, stomach, peritoneum, and scrotum. The CD4 T-cell count influences both the occurrence and clinical picture of active TB disease (Durham & Lashley, 2010). Important issues related to the use of ART in patients with active TB disease include when to start ART, significant pharmacokinetic drug interactions with rifamycins, the additive toxicities associated with antiretroviral and TB drugs, the development of IRIS with TB after ART initiation, and the need for treatment support including directly observed therapy and the integration of HIV and TB care and treatment (Panel on Antiretroviral Guidelines, 2011).

Gastrointestinal Manifestations

The gastrointestinal manifestations of HIV infection and AIDS include loss of appetite, nausea, vomiting, oral and esophageal candidiasis, and chronic diarrhea. Diarrhea is a problem in 50% to 60% of AIDS patients (Durham & Lashley, 2010). Gastrointestinal symptoms may be related to the direct effect of HIV on the cells lining the intestines. Some of the enteric pathogens that occur most frequently, identified by stool cultures or intestinal biopsy, are *Cryptosporidium muris*, *Salmonella* species, *Isospora belli*, *Giardia lamblia*, CMV, *Clostridium difficile*, and *M. avium-intracellulare*. In patients with AIDS, the effects of diarrhea can be devastating in terms of profound weight loss (more than 10% of body weight), fluid and electrolyte imbalances, perianal skin excoriation, weakness, and inability to perform the usual activities of daily living.

Candidiasis

Candidiasis, a fungal infection, occurs in almost all patients with AIDS and immune depression (Durham & Lashley, 2010). Oral candidiasis is characterized by creamy-white patches in the oral cavity and, if left untreated, can progress to involve the esophagus and stomach. Associated signs and symptoms include difficult and painful swallowing and retrosternal pain. Some patients also develop ulcerating oral lesions and are particularly susceptible to dissemination of candidiasis to other organs such as the vagina.

Wasting Syndrome

AIDS **wasting syndrome** includes involuntary weight loss consisting of both lean and fat mass (Lutz & Przytulski, 2011). The distinction between cachexia (wasting) and malnutrition, or between cachexia and simple weight loss, is important, because the metabolic derangement seen in wasting syndrome may not be modified by nutritional support alone.

Anorexia, diarrhea, gastrointestinal malabsorption, and lack of nutrition in chronic disease all contribute to wasting syndrome. Progressive tissue wasting, however, may occur with only modest gastrointestinal involvement and without diarrhea. Tumor necrosis factor (TNF) and interleukin 1 (IL-1) are cytokines that play important roles in AIDS-related wasting syndrome. Both act directly on the hypothalamus to cause anorexia. TNF causes inefficient use of lipids by reducing enzymes that are needed for fat metabolism, whereas IL-1 triggers the release of amino acids from muscle tissue. People with AIDS generally experience increased protein metabolism in relation to fat metabolism, which results in significant decreases in lean body mass due to muscle and protein breakdown. Hypertriglyceridemia can reach levels that require treatment with antilipid medications (Lutz & Przytulski, 2011).

Oncologic Manifestations

Those with HIV/AIDS are at greater risk of developing certain cancers. These include Kaposi's sarcoma (KS), lymphoma (especially non-Hodgkin lymphoma and primary CNS lymphoma), and invasive cervical cancer (Durham & Lashley, 2010). KS and lymphoma are discussed next. Cervical carcinoma is described later in the Gynecologic Manifestations section.

Kaposi's Sarcoma

Kaposi's sarcoma, the most common HIV-related malignancy, is a disease that involves the endothelial layer of blood and lymphatic vessels. In people with AIDS, epidemic KS is most often seen among men who have sex with men. AIDS-

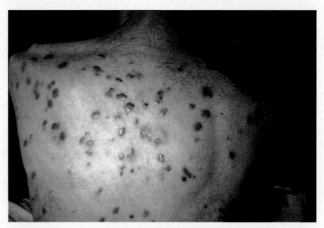

FIGURE 37-3 • Lesions of the AIDS-related Kaposi's sarcoma. Whereas some patients may have lesions that remain flat, others experience extensively disseminated, raised lesions with edema. From DeVita, V. T., Jr., Hellman, S., & Rosenberg, S. (Eds.). (1993). *AIDS: Etiology, diagnosis, treatment, and prevention* (4th ed.). Philadelphia: Lippincott Williams & Wilkins.

related KS exhibits a variable and aggressive course, ranging from localized cutaneous lesions to disseminated disease involving multiple organ systems. Cutaneous signs may be the first manifestation of HIV; they can appear anywhere on the body and are usually brownish pink to deep purple. They may be flat or raised and surrounded by ecchymoses (hemorrhagic patches) and edema (Fig. 37-3). Rapid development of lesions involving large areas of skin is associated with extensive disfigurement. The location and size of some lesions can lead to venous stasis, lymphedema, and pain. Ulcerative lesions disrupt skin integrity and increase discomfort and susceptibility to infection. The most common sites of visceral involvement are the lymph nodes, gastrointestinal tract, and lungs. Involvement of internal organs may eventually lead to organ failure, hemorrhage, infection, and death.

Diagnosis of KS is confirmed by biopsy of suspected lesions. Prognosis depends on the extent of the tumor, the presence of other symptoms of HIV infection, and the CD4+ count. Death may result from tumor progression. More often, however, it results from other complications of HIV infection.

B-Cell Lymphomas

B-cell lymphomas are the second most common malignancy occurring in people with AIDS. Lymphomas associated with AIDS usually differ from those occurring in the general population. Patients with AIDS are typically much younger than the usual population affected by non-Hodgkin lymphoma. In addition, AIDS-related lymphomas tend to develop outside the lymph nodes, most commonly in the brain, bone marrow, and gastrointestinal tract. These types of lymphomas are characteristically of a higher grade, indicating aggressive growth and resistance to treatment. The course of AIDS-related lymphomas includes multiple sites of organ involvement and complications related to opportunistic infections. Although aggressive combination chemotherapy is frequently successful in the treatment of non-Hodgkin lymphoma that is not associated with HIV infection, treatment is less successful in people with AIDS because of severe hematologic toxicity and complications of opportunistic infections that can occur from treatment.

Neurologic Manifestations

The advent of ART greatly lowered the incidence of HIV dementia and increased the survival of people with HIV-associated neurocognitive disorders; however, cognitive changes persist. HIV-related brain changes have profound effects on cognition, including motor function, executive function, attention, visual memory, and visuospatial function (Al-Khindi, Zakzanis, & van Gorp, 2011). Neurologic dysfunction results from direct effects of HIV on nervous system tissue, opportunistic infections, primary or metastatic neoplasm, cerebrovascular changes, metabolic encephalopathies, or complications secondary to therapy. Immune system response to HIV infection in the CNS includes inflammation, atrophy, demyelination, degeneration, and necrosis.

Peripheral Neuropathy

Peripheral neuropathy is the most common neurologic symptom at any stage of HIV infection and may occur in a variety of patterns, with distal sensory polyneuropathy or distal symmetric polyneuropathy the most frequently occurring type. It can lead to significant pain and functional impairment, and patients use a variety of self-care strategies to control the symptom (Nicholas, Voss, Wantland, et al., 2010) that may be associated with ART.

HIV Encephalopathy

HIV encephalopathy was formerly referred to as AIDS dementia complex (Chart 37-9). It is a clinical syndrome that is characterized by a progressive decline in cognitive, behavioral, and motor functions as a direct result of HIV

infection. HIV has been found in the brain and cerebrospinal fluid (CSF) of patients with HIV encephalopathy. The brain cells infected by HIV are predominantly the CD4+ cells of monocyte-macrophage lineage. HIV infection is thought to trigger the release of toxins or lymphokines that result in cellular dysfunction, inflammation, or interference with neurotransmitter function rather than cellular damage.

Signs and symptoms may be subtle and difficult to distinguish from fatigue, depression, or the adverse effects of treatment for infections and malignancies. Early manifestations include memory deficits, headache, difficulty concentrating, progressive confusion, psychomotor slowing, apathy, and ataxia. Later stages include global cognitive impairments, delay in verbal responses, a vacant stare, spastic paraparesis, hyperreflexia, psychosis, hallucinations, tremor, incontinence, seizures, mutism, and death.

Confirming the diagnosis of HIV encephalopathy can be difficult. Extensive neurologic evaluation includes a computed tomography scan, which may indicate diffuse cerebral atrophy and ventricular enlargement. Other tests that may detect abnormalities include magnetic resonance imaging, analysis of CSF through lumbar puncture, and brain biopsy.

Cryptococcus neoformans

A fungal infection, *Cryptococcus neoformans* is another common opportunistic infection among patients with AIDS, and it causes neurologic disease. Cryptococcal meningitis is characterized by symptoms such as fever, headache, malaise, stiff neck, nausea, vomiting, mental status changes, and seizures. Diagnosis is confirmed by CSF analysis.

Chart 37-9 Care of the Patient With HIV Encephalopathy

Altered Thought Processes

- Assess mental status and neurologic functioning.
- Monitor for medication interactions, infections, electrolyte imbalance, and depression.
- Frequently orient the patient to time, place, person, reality, and the environment.
- Use simple explanations.
- Instruct the patient to perform tasks in incremental steps.
- Provide memory aids (clocks and calendars).
- Provide memory aids for medication administration.
- Post activity schedule.
- Give positive feedback for appropriate behavior.
- Educate caretakers about orienting patient to time, place, person, reality, and the environment.
- Encourage the patient to designate a responsible person to assume power of attorney.

Disturbed Sensation

- Assess sensory impairment.
- Decrease amount of stimuli in the patient's environment.
- Correct inaccurate perceptions.
- Provide reassurance and safety if the patient displays fear.
- Provide a secure and stable environment.
- Educate caregivers about recognizing inaccurate sensory perceptions.
- Provide caregivers techniques to correct inaccurate perceptions.
- Instruct the patient and caregivers to report any changes in the patient's vision to the patient's health care provider.

Risk for Injury

- Assess the patient's level of anxiety, confusion, or disorientation.
- Assess the patient for delusions or hallucinations.
- Remove potentially dangerous objects from the patient's environment.
- Structure the environment for safety (ensure adequate lighting, avoid clutter, provide bed rails if needed).
- Supervise smoking.
- Do not let the patient drive a car if confusion is present.
- Instruct the patient and caregiver in home safety.
- Provide assistance as needed for ambulation and in getting in and out of bed.
- Pad headboard and side rails if the patient has seizures.

Self-Care Deficits

- Encourage activities of daily living within the patient's level of ability.
- Encourage independence, but assist if the patient cannot perform an activity.
- Demonstrate any activity that the patient is having difficulty accomplishing.
- Monitor food and fluid intake.
- Weigh patient weekly.
- Encourage the patient to eat, and offer nutritious meals, snacks, and adequate fluids.
- If patient is incontinent, establish a routine toileting schedule.
- Educate caregivers about meeting the patient's self-care needs.

Progressive Multifocal Leukoencephalopathy

Progressive multifocal leukoencephalopathy (PML) is a demyelinating CNS disorder that affects the oligodendroglia. Clinical manifestations often begin with mental confusion and rapidly progress to include blindness, aphasia, muscle weakness, paresis (partial or complete paralysis), and death. ART has greatly reduced the threat of mortality associated with this disorder.

Other Neurologic Disorders

Other common infections involving the nervous system include *Toxoplasma gondii*, CMV, and *Mycobacterium tuberculosis* infections. Additional neurologic manifestations include both central and peripheral neuropathies. Vascular myelopathy is a degenerative disorder that affects the lateral and posterior columns of the spinal cord, resulting in progressive spastic paraparesis, ataxia, and incontinence.

Depressive Manifestations

Individuals infected with HIV demonstrate higher rates of depression than the general population (Thames, Becker, & Marcotte, et al., 2011). The causes of depression are multifactorial and may include a history of preexisting mental illness, neuropsychiatric disturbances, and psychosocial factors. Depression also occurs in people with HIV infection in response to the physical symptoms, including pain and weight loss, stigma, and the lack of someone to talk with about their concerns. People with HIV/AIDS who are depressed may experience irrational guilt and shame, loss of self-esteem, feelings of helplessness and worthlessness, and suicidal ideation and may tend to overestimate disability in their daily functioning (Vance, Ross, Moneyham, et al., 2010).

Integumentary Manifestations

Cutaneous manifestations are associated with HIV infection and the accompanying opportunistic infections and malignancies. KS (described earlier) and opportunistic infections such as herpes zoster and herpes simplex are associated with painful vesicles that disrupt skin integrity. Molluscum contagiosum is a viral infection characterized by deforming plaque formation. Seborrheic dermatitis is associated with an indurated, diffuse, scaly rash involving the scalp and face. Patients with AIDS may also exhibit a generalized folliculitis associated with dry, flaking skin or atopic dermatitis, such as eczema or psoriasis. Many patients treated with the antibacterial agent trimethoprim–sulfamethoxazole (TMP-SMZ) develop a drug-related rash that is pruritic with pinkish-red macules and papules (Karch, 2012). Patients with any of these rashes experience discomfort and are at increased risk for infection from disrupted skin integrity.

Gynecologic Manifestations

Persistent, recurrent vaginal candidiasis may be the first sign of HIV infection in women. Past or present genital ulcers are a risk factor for the transmission of HIV infection. Women with HIV infection are more susceptible to genital ulcers and venereal warts and have increased rates of incidence and recurrence of these conditions. Ulcerative STIs such as chancroid, syphilis, and herpes are more severe in women with HIV infection. **Human papillomavirus (HPV)** causes venereal warts and is a risk factor for cervical intraepithelial neoplasia, a cellular change that is frequently a precursor to cervical cancer. Women with HIV are 10 times more likely to develop cervical intraepithelial neoplasia than those not infected with HIV. Women who are HIV seropositive and have cervical carcinoma present at a more advanced stage of disease and have more persistent and recurrent disease and a shorter interval to recurrence and death than women without HIV infection.

A significant percentage of women who require hospitalization for pelvic inflammatory disease have HIV infection. Women with HIV are at increased risk for pelvic inflammatory disease, and the associated inflammation may potentiate the transmission of HIV infection. Moreover, women with HIV infection appear to have a higher incidence of menstrual abnormalities, including amenorrhea or bleeding between periods, than do women without HIV infection. The failure of health care providers to consider HIV infection in women may lead to a later diagnosis, thereby denying these patients appropriate treatment.

Medical Management

Treatment of Opportunistic Infections

Guidelines for the treatment of opportunistic infections should be consulted for the most current recommendations (National Institutes of Health [NIH], 2009). Despite the availability of antiretroviral medications, opportunistic infections continue to cause considerable morbidity and mortality for three main reasons: (1) many patients are unaware of their HIV infection and present with an opportunistic infection as the initial indicator of their disease, (2) some patients are aware of their HIV infection but do not take antiretroviral agents because of psychosocial or economic factors, and (3) others receive prescriptions for antiretroviral medications but fail to attain adequate virologic and immunologic response as a result of issues related to adherence, pharmacokinetics, or unexplained biologic factors (NIH, 2009).

Laboratory tests should indicate immune function has improved with initiation of ART, resulting in faster resolution of the opportunistic infection. This has been most clearly shown for opportunistic infections for which effective therapy does not exist, such as cryptosporidiosis, microsporidiosis, and PML. These conditions may resolve or at least stabilize after the institution of ART as well as resolution of lesions of KS (NIH, 2009).

Pneumocystis Pneumonia

TMP-SMZ (Bactrim, Cotrim, Septra) is the treatment of choice for PCP; it is as effective as parenteral pentamidine isethionate (Pentacarinat) and more effective than other regimens. Oral outpatient therapy using TMP-SMZ is highly effective among patients with mild to moderate PCP. Adjunctive corticosteroids should be started as early as possible and within 72 hours after starting PCP therapy. There are many alternative therapeutic regimens based on the disease severity (Durham & Lashley, 2010). The recommended duration of therapy for PCP is 21 days (NIH, 2009). Adverse effects, in addition to hypotension, include impaired glucose metabolism leading to the development of diabetes from damage to the pancreas, kidney damage, hepatic dysfunction, and neutropenia.

Mycobacterium avium Complex

Adults and adolescents who are infected with HIV should receive chemoprophylaxis against disseminated MAC disease if they have a CD4+ count less than 50 cells/mcL. Azithromycin (Zithromax) or clarithromycin (Biaxin) are the preferred prophylactic agents. If azithromycin or clarithromycin cannot be tolerated, rifabutin (Mycobutin) is an alternative prophylactic agent for MAC disease, although drug interactions may make this agent difficult to use (Durham & Lashley, 2010; NIH, 2009). Secondary prophylaxis for disseminated MAC may be discontinued in patients who have sustained increases in CD4 counts (greater than 100 cells/mm³; longer than 3 months) in response to HAART, have completed 12 months of MAC therapy, and have no signs or symptoms attributable to MAC.

Cryptococcal Meningitis

Cryptococcosis among patients with HIV infection most commonly occurs as a subacute meningitis or meningoencephalitis with fever, malaise, and headache. Current primary therapy for cryptococcal meningitis is IV amphotericin B with or without oral flucytosine (5-FC, Ancobon) or fluconazole (Diflucan). Serious potential adverse effects of amphotericin B include anaphylaxis, kidney and hepatic impairment, electrolyte imbalances, anemia, fever, and severe chills (NIH, 2009).

Cytomegalovirus Retinitis

Retinitis caused by CMV is a leading cause of blindness in patients with AIDS. Oral valganciclovir (Valcyte), IV ganciclovir (Cytovene), IV ganciclovir followed by oral valganciclovir, IV foscarnet (Foscavir), IV cidofovir (Vistide), and a ganciclovir intraocular implant coupled with valganciclovir are all effective treatments for CMV retinitis (NIH, 2009). A common adverse reaction to ganciclovir is severe neutropenia, which limits the concomitant use of zidovudine (AZT, Compound S, Retrovir). Common adverse reactions to foscarnet are nephrotoxicity, including acute kidney failure, and electrolyte imbalances, including hypocalcemia, hyperphosphatemia, and hypomagnesemia, which can be life threatening. Other common adverse effects include seizures, gastrointestinal disturbances, anemia, phlebitis at the infusion site, and low back pain. Possible bone marrow suppression (producing a decrease in white blood cell and platelet counts), oral candidiasis, and liver and kidney impairments require close monitoring.

Other Infections

Oral acyclovir (Zovirax), famciclovir (Famvir), or valacyclovir (Valtrex) may be used to treat infections caused by herpes simplex or herpes zoster (Karch, 2012). Esophageal or oral candidiasis is treated topically with clotrimazole (Mycelex) oral troches or nystatin suspension. Chronic refractory infection with candidiasis (thrush) or esophageal involvement is treated with ketoconazole (Nizoral) or fluconazole (Diflucan).

Prevention of Opportunistic Infections

TMP-SMZ is an antibacterial agent used to treat various organisms causing infection. It also confers cross-protection against toxoplasmosis and some common respiratory bacterial infections. People with HIV infection who have a T-cell count of less than 200 cells/mm³ should receive chemoprophylaxis with TMP-SMZ to prevent PCP (Durham & Lashley, 2010). PCP prophylaxis can be safely discontinued in patients who are responding to ART with a sustained increase in T lymphocytes.

Antidiarrheal Therapy

Although many forms of diarrhea respond to treatment, it is not unusual for this condition to recur and become a chronic problem for the patient with HIV infection. Therapy with octreotide acetate (Sandostatin), a synthetic analogue of somatostatin, has been shown to effectively manage chronic severe diarrhea. High concentrations of somatostatin receptors have been found in the gastrointestinal tract and in other tissues. Somatostatin inhibits many physiologic functions, including gastrointestinal motility and intestinal secretion of water and electrolytes.

Chemotherapy

Kaposi's Sarcoma

Management of KS is usually difficult because of the variability of symptoms and the organ systems involved. KS is rarely life threatening except when there is pulmonary or gastrointestinal involvement. The treatment goals are to reduce symptoms by decreasing the size of the skin lesions, to reduce discomfort associated with edema and ulcerations, and to control symptoms associated with mucosal or visceral involvement. No one treatment has been shown to increase survival. Radiation therapy is effective as a palliative measure to relieve localized pain due to tumor mass (especially in the legs) and for KS lesions that are in sites such as the oral mucosa, conjunctiva, face, and soles of the feet.

Interferon is known for its antiviral and antitumor effects. Patients with cutaneous KS treated with **alpha-interferon** have experienced tumor regression and improved immune system function. Interferon alfa-2b (Intron) is approved for use in AIDS-related KS (Lapka & Franson, 2010). Alpha-interferon is administered by the IV, intramuscular, or subcutaneous routes. Patients may self-administer interferon at home or receive it in an outpatient setting.

Lymphoma

Successful treatment of AIDS-related lymphomas has been limited because of the rapid progression of these malignancies. Combination chemotherapy and radiation therapy regimens may produce an initial response, but it is usually short-lived. Because standard regimens for non-AIDS lymphomas have been ineffective, it has been suggested that AIDS-related lymphomas should be studied as a separate group in clinical trials.

Antidepressant Therapy

Treatment for depression in people with HIV infection involves psychotherapy integrated with pharmacotherapy. If depressive symptoms are severe and of sufficient duration, treatment with antidepressants may be initiated. Antidepressants such as imipramine (Tofranil), desipramine (Norpramin), and fluoxetine (Prozac) may be used, because these medications also alleviate the fatigue and lethargy that are associated with depression.

A psychostimulant such as methylphenidate (Ritalin) may be used in low doses in patients with neuropsychiatric impairment. Electroconvulsive therapy may be an option for patients with severe depression who do not respond to pharmacologic interventions.

Nutrition Therapy

Alterations in lipid metabolism are associated with HIV infection and ART. One study suggested that those with HIV infection had higher rates of metabolic syndrome (Woods, Wanke, Ling, et al., 2009). Malnutrition increases the risk of infection and the incidence of opportunistic infections. Nutrition therapy should be part of the overall management plan and should be tailored to meet the nutritional needs of the patient, whether by oral diet, enteral tube feedings, or parenteral nutritional support, if needed. As with all patients, a healthy diet is essential for the patient with HIV infection. For all patients with AIDS who experience unexplained weight loss, calorie counts should be obtained to evaluate nutritional status and initiate appropriate therapy. The goal is to maintain the ideal weight and, when necessary, to increase weight.

Appetite stimulants have been successfully used in patients with AIDS-related anorexia. Megestrol acetate (Megace), a synthetic oral progesterone preparation, promotes significant weight gain and inhibits cytokine IL-1 synthesis. In patients with HIV infection, it increases body weight primarily by increasing body fat stores. Dronabinol (Marinol), which is a synthetic tetrahydrocannabinol (THC), the active ingredient in marijuana, has been used to relieve nausea and vomiting associated with cancer chemotherapy. After beginning dronabinol therapy, almost all patients with HIV infection experience a modest weight gain. The effects on body composition are unknown.

Oral supplements may be used when the diet is deficient in calories and protein. Ideally, oral supplements should be lactose free (many people with HIV infection are intolerant to lactose), high in calories and easily digestible protein, low in fat with the fat easily digestible, palatable, inexpensive, and tolerated without causing diarrhea. Nutritional supplements have been developed specifically for people with HIV infection and AIDS. Parenteral nutrition is the final option because of its prohibitive cost and associated risks, including possible infection.

Complementary and Alternative Modalities

People with HIV infection, including those who use illicit drugs, report substantial use of complementary and alternative medicine (CAM) (Merenstein, Hu, & Robison, et al., 2010). Combined with traditional therapies, CAM may improve the patient's overall well-being. However, there can be adverse drug–drug interactions between certain CAM therapies (e.g., St. John's wort) and some ART.

CAM can be divided into four categories:

- Spiritual or psychological therapies may include humor, hypnosis, faith healing, guided imagery, and positive affirmations.
- Nutritional therapies may include vegetarian or macrobiotic diets; vitamin C or beta-carotene supplements; and turmeric, which contains curcumin, a food spice

supplement. Chinese herbs, such as traditional herbal mixtures, are also used, in addition to compound Q (a Chinese cucumber extract) and *Momordica charantia* (bitter melon), which is given as an enema.
- Drug and biologic therapies include medications and other substances not approved by the FDA. Examples are *N*-acetylcysteine, pentoxifylline (Trental), and 1-chloro-2,4-dinitrobenzene. Also included in this category are oxygen therapy, ozone therapy, and urine therapy.
- Treatment with physical forces and devices may include acupuncture, acupressure, massage therapy, reflexology, therapeutic touch, yoga, and crystals.

Although there is insufficient research on the effects of CAM, a growing body of literature reports benefits for modalities involving nutrition, exercise, psychosocial treatment, and Chinese medicine.

Many patients who use these therapies do not report use of CAM to their health care providers. To obtain a complete health history, the nurse should ask about the patient's use of alternative therapies. Patients may need to be encouraged to report their use of CAM to their primary provider. Problems may arise, for example, when patients are using CAM while participating in clinical drug trials; alternative therapies can have significant adverse side effects, making it difficult to assess the effects of the medications in the clinical trial. The nurse needs to become familiar with the potential adverse side effects of these therapies. The nurse who suspects that CAM is causing a side effect needs to discuss this with the patient, the alternative therapy provider, and the primary provider. The nurse needs to view CAM with an open mind and try to understand the importance of this treatment to the patient. This approach will improve communication with the patient and reduce conflict.

Supportive Care

Patients who are weak and debilitated as a result of chronic illness associated with HIV infection typically require many kinds of supportive care. Nutritional support may be as simple as providing assistance in obtaining or preparing meals. For patients with more advanced nutritional impairment resulting from decreased intake, wasting syndrome, or gastrointestinal malabsorption associated with diarrhea, parenteral feedings may be required. Imbalances that result from nausea, vomiting, and profuse diarrhea often necessitate IV fluid and electrolyte replacement.

Management of skin breakdown associated with KS, perianal skin excoriation, or immobility entails thorough and meticulous skin care that involves regular turning, cleansing, and applications of medicated ointments and dressings. To combat pain associated with skin breakdown, abdominal cramping, peripheral neuropathy, or KS, the nurse administers analgesic agents at regular intervals around the clock. Relaxation and guided imagery may help reduce pain and anxiety.

Pulmonary symptoms, such as dyspnea and shortness of breath, may be related to infection, KS, or fatigue. For patients with these symptoms, oxygen therapy, relaxation training, and energy conservation techniques may be effective. Patients with severe respiratory dysfunction may require mechanical ventilation. Before mechanical ventilation is instituted, the procedure is explained to the patient and the caregiver. If the patient decides to forego mechanical ventilation, his or her wishes should be followed. Ideally, the patient has prepared an advance directive identifying preferences for treatments and end-of-life care, including hospice care. If the patient has not identified preferences in advance, treatment options are described so that the patient can make informed decisions and have those wishes respected.

Nurses should anticipate that patients as well as family and friends will need support and time to share concerns. In some family systems, more than one person might be living with HIV/AIDS.

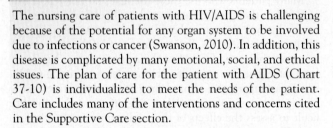

NURSING PROCESS

The Patient With HIV/AIDS

The nursing care of patients with HIV/AIDS is challenging because of the potential for any organ system to be involved due to infections or cancer (Swanson, 2010). In addition, this disease is complicated by many emotional, social, and ethical issues. The plan of care for the patient with AIDS (Chart 37-10) is individualized to meet the needs of the patient. Care includes many of the interventions and concerns cited in the Supportive Care section.

Assessment

Nursing assessment includes identification of potential risk factors, including a history of risky sexual practices or IV/injection drug use. The patient's physical status and psychological status are assessed. All factors affecting immune system functioning are thoroughly explored. A number of instruments exist for active symptom assessment (Durham & Lashley, 2010).

Nutritional Status
Nutritional status is assessed by obtaining a dietary history and identifying factors that may interfere with oral intake, such as anorexia, nausea, vomiting, oral pain, or difficulty swallowing. In addition, the patient's ability to purchase and prepare food is assessed. Weight history (i.e., changes over time), anthropometric measurements, and blood urea nitrogen (BUN), serum protein, albumin, and transferrin levels provide objective measurements of nutritional status.

Skin Integrity
The skin and mucous membranes are inspected daily for evidence of breakdown, ulceration, or infection. The oral cavity is monitored for redness, ulcerations, and the presence of creamy-white patches indicative of candidiasis. Assessment of the perianal area for excoriation and infection in patients with profuse diarrhea is important. Wounds are cultured to identify infectious organisms.

Respiratory Status
Respiratory status is assessed by monitoring the patient for cough, sputum production (i.e., amount and color), shortness of breath, orthopnea, tachypnea, and chest pain. The presence and quality of breath sounds are investigated. Other measures of pulmonary function include chest x-ray results, arterial blood gas values, pulse oximetry, and pulmonary function test results.

Neurologic Status
Neurologic status is determined by assessing level of consciousness; orientation to person, place, and time; and memory lapses. Mental status is assessed as early as possible to provide a baseline. The patient is also assessed for sensory deficits (visual changes, headache, or numbness and tingling in the extremities), motor involvement (altered gait, paresis, or paralysis), and seizure activity.

Fluid and Electrolyte Balance
Fluid and electrolyte status is assessed by examining the skin and mucous membranes for turgor and dryness. Dehydration may be indicated by increased thirst, decreased urine output, postural hypotension, weak and rapid pulse, and urine specific gravity of 1.025 or more. Electrolyte imbalances, such as decreased serum sodium, potassium, calcium, magnesium, and chloride, typically result from profuse diarrhea. The patient is assessed for signs and symptoms of electrolyte deficits, including decreased mental status, muscle twitching, muscle cramps, irregular pulse, nausea and vomiting, and shallow respirations.

Knowledge Level
The patient's level of knowledge about the disease and the modes of disease transmission are evaluated. In addition, the level of knowledge of family (biologic and family of choice) and friends is assessed. The patient's psychological reaction to the diagnosis of HIV infection or AIDS is important to explore. Reactions vary among patients and may include denial, anger, fear, shame, withdrawal from social interactions, and depressive symptoms. It is often helpful to gain an understanding of how the patient has dealt with illness and major life stresses in the past. The patient's resources for support are also identified.

Diagnosis

Nursing Diagnoses
The list of potential nursing diagnoses is extensive because of the complex nature of HIV/AIDS. However, based on the assessment data, major nursing diagnoses may include the following:

- Impaired skin integrity related to cutaneous manifestations of HIV infection, excoriation, and diarrhea
- Diarrhea related to enteric pathogens or HIV infection
- Risk for infection related to immunodeficiency
- Activity intolerance related to weakness, fatigue, malnutrition, impaired fluid and electrolyte balance, and hypoxia associated with pulmonary infections
- Altered thought processes related to shortened attention span, impaired memory, confusion, and disorientation associated with HIV encephalopathy
- Ineffective airway clearance related to infection, increased bronchial secretions, and decreased ability to cough related to weakness and fatigue
- Acute and chronic pain related to impaired perianal skin integrity secondary to diarrhea, KS, and peripheral neuropathy
- Imbalanced nutrition: less than body requirements related to decreased oral intake
- Social isolation related to stigma of the disease, withdrawal of support systems, isolation procedures, and fear of infecting others

(continues on page 1021)

PLAN OF NURSING CARE
Care of the Patient With AIDS

Chart 37-10

NURSING DIAGNOSIS: Diarrhea related to enteric pathogens or HIV infection
GOAL: Resumption of usual bowel habits

Nursing Interventions	Rationale	Expected Outcomes

1. Assess patient's normal bowel habits.
2. Assess for diarrhea: frequent, loose stools; abdominal pain or cramping, volume of liquid stools, and exacerbating and alleviating factors.
3. Obtain stool cultures, and administer antimicrobial therapy as prescribed.
4. Initiate measures to reduce hyperactivity of bowel.
  a. Maintain food and fluid restrictions as prescribed. Suggest BRAT diet (*b*ananas, *r*ice, *a*pplesauce, *t*ea and *t*oast).
  b. Discourage smoking.
 	
  c. Avoid bowel irritants such as fatty or fried foods, raw vegetables, and nuts. Offer small, frequent meals.
5. Administer anticholinergic antispasmodics and opioids or other medications as prescribed.
6. Maintain fluid intake of at least 3 L/day unless contraindicated.
	1. Provides baseline for evaluation
	2. Detects changes in status, quantifies loss of fluid, and provides basis for nursing measures
	
	3. Identifies pathogenic organism; therapy targets specific organism
	4. Promotes bowel rest, which may decrease acute episodes
	  a. Reduces stimulation of bowel
	
	  b. Eliminates nicotine, which acts as bowel stimulant
	  c. Prevents stimulation of bowel and abdominal distention and promotes adequate nutrition
	5. Decreases intestinal spasms and motility
	
	6. Prevents hypovolemia
		• Exhibits return to normal bowel patterns
		• Reports decreasing episodes of diarrhea and abdominal cramping
		• Identifies and avoids foods that irritate the gastrointestinal tract
		• Takes appropriate therapy as prescribed
		• Exhibits normal stool cultures
		• Maintains adequate fluid intake
		• Maintains body weight and reports no additional weight loss
		• States rationale for avoiding smoking
		• Enrolls in program to stop smoking
		• Uses medication as prescribed
		• Maintains adequate fluid status
		• Exhibits normal skin turgor, moist mucous membranes, adequate urine output, and absence of excessive thirst

---

NURSING DIAGNOSIS: Risk for infection related to immunodeficiency
GOAL: Absence of infection

Nursing Interventions	Rationale	Expected Outcomes

1. Monitor for infection: fever, chills, and diaphoresis; cough; shortness of breath; oral pain or painful swallowing; creamy-white patches in oral cavity; urinary frequency, urgency, or dysuria; redness, swelling, or drainage from wounds; vesicular lesions on face, lips, or perianal area.
2. Educate patient or caregiver about need to report possible infection.
3. Monitor white blood cell (WBC) count and differential.
4. Obtain cultures of wound drainage, skin lesions, urine, stool, sputum, mouth, and blood as prescribed. Administer antimicrobial therapy as prescribed.
5. Instruct patient in ways to prevent infection.
  a. Clean kitchen and bathroom surfaces with disinfectants.
  b. Clean hands thoroughly after exposure to body fluids.
  c. Avoid exposure to others' body fluids or sharing eating utensils.
  d. Turn, cough, and deep breathe, especially when activity is decreased.
  e. Maintain cleanliness of perianal area.
  f. Avoid handling pet excreta or cleaning litter boxes, birdcages, or aquariums.
  g. Cook meat and eggs thoroughly.
6. Maintain aseptic technique when performing invasive procedures such as venipunctures, bladder catheterizations, and injections.
	1. Allows for early detection of infection, essential for prompt initiation of treatment. Repeated and prolonged infections contribute to patient's debilitation.
	
	2. Allows early detection of infection
	
	3. Elevated WBC count possibly associated with infection
	4. Assists in determining offending organism to initiate appropriate treatment
	
	5. Minimizes exposure to infection and transmission of HIV infection to others
	
	6. Prevents hospital-acquired infections
		• Identifies reportable signs and symptoms of infection
		• Reports signs and symptoms of infection if present
		• Exhibits and reports absence of fever, chills, and diaphoresis
		• Exhibits normal (clear) breath sounds without adventitious breath sounds
		• Maintains weight
		• Reports adequate energy level without excessive fatigue
		• Reports absence of shortness of breath and cough
		• Exhibits pink, moist oral mucous membranes without fissures or lesions
		• Takes appropriate therapy as prescribed
		• Experiences no infection
		• States rationale for strategies to avoid infection
		• Modifies activities to reduce exposure to infection or infectious persons
		• Practices "safer sex"
		• Avoids sharing eating utensils and toothbrush
		• Exhibits normal body temperature
		• Uses recommended techniques to maintain cleanliness of skin, skin lesions, and perianal area
		• Has others handle pet excreta and cleanup
		• Uses recommended cooking techniques

(continues on page 1018)

Chart 37-10

PLAN OF NURSING CARE

Care of the Patient With AIDS (continued)

NURSING DIAGNOSIS: Ineffective airway clearance related to *Pneumocystis* pneumonia, increased bronchial secretions, and decreased ability to cough related to weakness and fatigue

GOAL: Improved airway clearance

Nursing Interventions	Rationale	Expected Outcomes

1. Assess and report signs and symptoms of altered respiratory status, tachypnea, the use of accessory muscles, cough, color and amount of sputum, abnormal breath sounds, dusky or cyanotic skin color, restlessness, confusion, or somnolence.	1. Indicates abnormal respiratory function	• Maintains normal airway clearance:
		  • Respiratory rate <20 breaths/min
		  • Unlabored breathing without the use of accessory muscles and flaring nares (nostrils)
		  • Skin color pink (without cyanosis)
		  • Alert and aware of surroundings
		  • Arterial blood gas values normal
		  • Normal breath sounds without adventitious breath sounds

2. Obtain sputum sample for culture as prescribed. Administer antimicrobial therapy as prescribed.	2. Aids in identification of pathogenic organisms	• Begins appropriate therapy • Takes medication as prescribed
3. Provide pulmonary care (cough, deep breathing, postural drainage, and vibration) every 2–4 hours.	3. Prevents stasis of secretions and promotes airway clearance	• Reports improved breathing • Maintains clear airway • Coughs and takes deep breaths every 2–4 hours as recommended
4. Assist patient in attaining semi- or high Fowler's position.	4. Facilitates breathing and airway clearance	• Demonstrates appropriate positions and practices postural drainage every 2–4 hours
5. Encourage adequate rest periods.	5. Maximizes energy expenditure and prevents excessive fatigue	• Reports reduced breathing difficulty when in semi- or high Fowler's position

6. Initiate measures to decrease viscosity of secretions.
  a. Maintain fluid intake of at least 3 L/day unless contraindicated.
  b. Humidify inspired air as prescribed.
  c. Consult with physician concerning the use of mucolytic agents delivered through nebulizer or intermittent positive pressure breathing treatment.
	6. Facilitates expectoration of secretions; prevents stasis of secretions	• Practices energy-conserving strategies and alternates rest with activity
		• Demonstrates reduction in thickness (viscosity) of pulmonary secretions
		• Reports increased ease in coughing up sputum

7. Perform tracheal suctioning as needed.	7. Removes secretions if patient is unable to do so	• Uses humidified air or oxygen as prescribed and indicated
8. Administer oxygen therapy as prescribed.	8. Increases availability of oxygen	• Indicates need for assistance with removal of pulmonary secretions
9. Assist with endotracheal intubation; maintain ventilator settings as prescribed.	9. Maintains ventilation	• Understands need for and cooperates with endotracheal intubation and the use of a mechanical ventilator • Verbalizes concerns about respiratory difficulty, intubation, and mechanical ventilation

NURSING DIAGNOSIS: Imbalanced nutrition: less than body requirements related to decreased oral intake

GOAL: Improvement of nutritional status

Nursing Interventions	Rationale	Expected Outcomes
1. Assess nutritional status with height, weight, age; blood urea nitrogen, serum protein, albumin, transferrin, hemoglobin, and hematocrit levels; and cutaneous anergy.	1. Provides objective measurement of nutritional status	• Identifies factors limiting oral intake, and uses resources to promote adequate dietary intake • Reports increased appetite • States understanding of nutritional needs
2. Obtain dietary history, including likes and dislikes and food intolerances.	2. Defines need for nutritional education; helps individualize interventions	• Identifies ways to reduce factors that limit oral intake
3. Assess factors that interfere with oral intake.	3. Provides basis and directions for interventions	• Rests before meals • Eats in pleasant, odor-free environment
4. Consult with dietitian to determine patient's nutritional needs.	4. Facilitates meal planning	• Arranges meals to coincide with visitors' visits

PLAN OF NURSING CARE

Chart 37-10

Care of the Patient With AIDS (continued)

Nursing Interventions	Rationale	Expected Outcomes

5. Reduce factors limiting oral intake.
  a. Encourage patient to rest before meals.
  b. Plan meals so that they do not occur immediately after painful or unpleasant procedures.
  c. Encourage patient to eat meals with visitors or others when possible.
  d. Encourage patient to prepare simple meals or to obtain assistance with meal preparation if possible.
  e. Serve small, frequent meals: 6/day.
  f. Limit fluids 1 hour before meals and with meals.
6. Instruct patient in ways to supplement nutrition: consume protein-rich foods (meat, poultry, fish) and carbohydrates (pasta, fruit, breads).
7. Consult with physician and dietitian about alternative feeding (enteral or parenteral nutrition).
8. Consult with social worker or community liaison about financial assistance if patient cannot afford food.
	5. Addresses factors limiting intake.
	  a. Minimizes fatigue, which can decrease appetite
	  b. Decreases noxious stimuli
	
	  c. Limits social isolation
	
	  d. Limits energy expenditure
	
	  e. Prevents overwhelming patient
	  f. Reduces satiety
	6. Provides additional proteins and calories
	
	7. Provides nutritional support if patient is unable to take sufficient amounts by mouth
	8. Increases availability of resources and nutrition
		• Reports increased dietary intake
		• Uses oral hygiene before meals
		• Takes analgesic agents before meals as prescribed
		• Identifies ways to increase protein and caloric intake
		• Identifies foods high in protein and calories
		• Consumes foods high in protein and calories
		• Reports decreased rate of weight loss
		• Maintains adequate caloric intake
		• States rationale for enteral or parenteral nutrition if needed
		• Demonstrates skill in preparing alternate sources of nutrition

NURSING DIAGNOSIS: Deficient knowledge related to means of preventing HIV transmission
GOAL: Increased knowledge concerning means of preventing disease transmission

Nursing Interventions	Rationale	Expected Outcomes

1. Instruct patient, family, and friends about routes of transmission of HIV.
 	
2. Instruct patient, family, and friends about means of preventing transmission of HIV.
  a. Avoid sexual contact with multiple partners, and use precautions if sexual partner's HIV status is not certain.
 	
  b. Use condoms during sexual intercourse (vaginal, anal, oral–genital); avoid mouth contact with the penis, vagina, or rectum; avoid sexual practices that can cause cuts or tears in the lining of the rectum, vagina, or penis.
  c. Avoid sex with sex workers and others at high risk.
 	
  d. Do not use IV/injection drugs; if addicted and unable or unwilling to change behavior, use clean needles and syringes.
 	
  e. Women who may have been exposed to HIV through sexual or drug practices should consult with a physician before becoming pregnant; consider the use of antiretroviral agents if pregnant.
	1. Knowledge about disease transmission can help prevent spread of disease; may also alleviate fears.
	2. Reduces transmission risk
	
	  a. The risk of infection increases with the number of sexual partners, male or female, and sexual contact with those who engage in high-risk behaviors.
	  b. Risk of HIV transmission is reduced.
	
	  c. Many sex workers are infected with HIV through sexual contact with multiple partners or IV/injection drug use.
	  d. Clean needles and syringes are the only way to prevent HIV transmission for those who continue to use drugs. Taking precautions is important for those who are antibody positive to prevent transmitting HIV.
	  e. HIV can be transmitted from mother to child in utero; the use of antiretroviral agents during pregnancy significantly reduces perinatal transmission of HIV.
		• Patient, family, and friends state means of transmission
		• Reports and demonstrates practices to reduce exposure of others to HIV
		• Demonstrates knowledge of safer sexual practices
		• Identifies means of preventing disease transmission
		• States that sexual partners are informed about patient's positive HIV status in blood
		• Avoids IV/injection drug use and sharing of drug equipment with others

(continues on page 1020)

PLAN OF NURSING CARE

Care of the Patient With AIDS (continued)

NURSING DIAGNOSIS: Social isolation related to stigma of the disease, withdrawal of support systems, isolation procedures, and fear of infecting others

GOAL: Decreased sense of social isolation

Nursing Interventions	Rationale	Expected Outcomes
1. Assess patient's usual patterns of social interaction. 2. Observe for behaviors indicative of social isolation, such as decreased interaction with others, hostility, noncompliance, sad affect, and stated feelings of rejection or loneliness. 3. Provide instruction concerning modes of transmission of HIV. 4. Assist patient to identify and explore resources for support and positive mechanisms for coping (e.g., contact with family, friends, AIDS task force). 5. Allow time to be with patient other than for medications and procedures. 6. Encourage participation in diversional activities such as reading, television, or handcrafts.	1. Establishes basis for individualized interventions 2. Promotes early detection of social isolation, which may be manifested in several ways 3. Provides accurate information, corrects misconceptions, and alleviates anxiety 4. Enables mobilization of resources and supports 5. Promotes feelings of self-worth and provides social interaction 6. Provides distraction	• Shares with others the need for valued social interaction • Demonstrates interest in events, activities, and communication • Verbalizes feelings and reactions to diagnosis, prognosis, and life changes • Identifies modes of transmission of HIV • States ways of preventing transmission of HIV to others while maintaining contact with valued friends and relatives • Reveals HIV/AIDS diagnosis to others when appropriate • Identifies resources (i.e., family, friends, and support groups) • Uses resources when appropriate • Accepts offers of assistance and support • Reports decreased sense of isolation • Maintains contacts with those of importance to him or her • Develops or continues hobbies that effectively serve as diversion or distraction

COLLABORATIVE PROBLEMS: Opportunistic infections; impaired breathing; wasting syndrome and fluid and electrolyte imbalances; adverse reaction to medications

GOAL: Absence of complications

Nursing Interventions	Rationale	Expected Outcomes
Opportunistic Infections 1. Monitor vital signs. 2. Obtain laboratory specimens, and monitor test results. 3. Instruct the patient and caregiver about signs and symptoms of infection and the need to report them early.	1. Changes in vital signs such as increases in pulse rate, respirations, blood pressure, and temperature may indicate infection. 2. Smears and cultures can identify causative agents such as bacteria, fungi, and protozoa, and sensitivity studies can identify antibiotics or other medications effective against the causative agent. 3. Early recognition of symptoms facilitates prompt treatment and avoids extra complications.	• Exhibits stable vital signs • Experiences control of infection • Identifies signs and symptoms correctly and experiences no complications • Identifies signs and symptoms that are reportable to the physician • Takes medications as prescribed
Impaired Breathing 1. Monitor respiratory rate and pattern. 2. Auscultate the chest for breath sounds and abnormal lung sounds. 3. Monitor pulse rate, blood pressure, and oxygen saturation levels.	1. Rapid shallow breathing, diminished breath sounds, and shortness of breath may indicate respiratory failure resulting in hypoxia. 2. Crackles and wheezes may indicate fluid in the lungs, which disrupts respiratory function and alters the blood's oxygen-carrying capacity. 3. Changes in pulse rate, blood pressure, and oxygen levels may indicate the development of respiratory or cardiac failure.	• Maintains stable respiratory rate and pattern within the normal limits • Exhibits no adventitious lung sounds; normal breath sounds • Has stable pulse rate and blood pressure within normal limits, and exhibits no evidence of hypoxia • Oxygen saturation levels within acceptable range

PLAN OF NURSING CARE
Care of the Patient With AIDS (continued)

Nursing Interventions	Rationale	Expected Outcomes
Wasting Syndrome and Fluid and Electrolyte Disturbances		
1. Monitor weight and laboratory values for nutritional status.	1. Weight loss, malnutrition, and anemia are common in HIV infection and increase risk of superinfection.	• Maintains stable weight
		• Eats a nutritious diet
2. Monitor intake and output and laboratory values for fluid and electrolyte imbalance (potassium, sodium, calcium, phosphorus, magnesium, and zinc).	2. Chronic diarrhea, inadequate oral intake, vomiting, and profuse sweating deplete electrolytes. Small intestine inflammation may impair the absorption of fluids and electrolytes.	• Attains and maintains hemoglobin, hematocrit, and ferritin levels within normal limits
		• Sustains fluid and electrolyte balance within normal limits
3. Monitor for and report signs and symptoms of dehydration.	3. Fluid loss results in decreased circulating volume leading to tachycardia, dry skin and mucous membranes, poor skin turgor, elevated urine specific gravity, and thirst. Early detection allows early treatment.	• Exhibits no signs and symptoms of dehydration
Reactions to Medications		
1. Monitor for medication interactions.	1. People with HIV infection receive many medications for HIV and for disease complications. Early detection of medication interactions is necessary to prevent complications.	• Experiences no serious side effects or complications from medications
		• Correctly describes medication regimen and complies with therapy, including adaptations in eating routines and type of food used with prescribed medications
2. Monitor for and promptly report side effects from antiretroviral agents.	2. Side effects from antiretroviral agents can be life threatening. Serious side effects include anemia, pancreatitis, peripheral neuropathy, mental confusion, and persistent nausea and vomiting. Corrective measures need to be instituted.	
3. Instruct the patient and caregiver in the medication regimen.	3. Knowledge of the medication purpose, correct administration, side effects, and strategies to manage or prevent side effects promotes safety and greater compliance with treatment.	

• Grieving related to changes in lifestyle and roles and unfavorable prognosis
• Deficient knowledge related to HIV infection, means of preventing HIV transmission, and self-care

Collaborative Problems/Potential Complications
Possible complications may include the following:
• Opportunistic infections
• Impaired breathing or respiratory failure
• Wasting syndrome and fluid and electrolyte imbalance
• Adverse effects of medications

Planning and Goals

Goals for the patient may include achievement and maintenance of skin integrity, resumption of usual bowel patterns, absence of infection, improved activity tolerance, coherent thought processes, improved airway clearance, increased comfort, improved nutritional status, increased socialization, expression of grief, increased knowledge regarding disease prevention and self-care, and absence of complications.

Nursing Interventions

Promoting Skin Integrity
The skin and oral mucosa are assessed routinely for changes in appearance, location and size of lesions, and evidence of

infection and breakdown. The patient is encouraged to maintain a balance between rest and mobility whenever possible. Patients who are immobile are assisted to change position at least every 2 hours and more often as needed. Devices such as alternating-pressure mattresses and low-air-loss beds are used to prevent skin breakdown. Patients are encouraged to avoid scratching, to use nonabrasive, nondrying soaps, and to apply nonperfumed skin moisturizers to dry skin. Regular oral care is also encouraged.

Medicated lotions, ointments, and dressings are applied to affected skin surfaces as prescribed. Adhesive tape is avoided. Skin surfaces are protected from friction and rubbing by keeping bed linens free of wrinkles and avoiding tight or restrictive clothing. Patients with foot lesions are advised to wear cotton socks and shoes that do not cause the feet to perspire. Antipruritic, antibiotic, and analgesic agents are administered as prescribed.

The perianal region is assessed frequently for impairment of skin integrity and infection. The patient is instructed to keep the area as clean as possible. The perianal area is cleaned after each bowel movement with nonabrasive soap and water to prevent further excoriation and breakdown of the skin and infection. If the area is very painful, soft cloths or cotton sponges may be less irritating than washcloths. In addition, sitz baths or gentle irrigation may facilitate cleaning and promote comfort. The area is dried thoroughly after cleaning. Topical lotions or ointments may be prescribed to promote healing. Wounds are cultured if infection is suspected so that the appropriate antimicrobial treatment can be initiated. Debilitated patients may require assistance in maintaining hygienic practices.

Promoting Usual Bowel Patterns

Bowel patterns are assessed for diarrhea. The nurse monitors the frequency and consistency of stools and the patient's reports of abdominal pain or cramping associated with bowel movements. Factors that exacerbate frequent diarrhea are also assessed. The quantity and volume of liquid stools are measured to document fluid volume losses. Stool cultures are obtained to identify pathogenic organisms.

The patient is counseled about ways to decrease diarrhea. The primary provider may recommend restriction of oral intake to rest the bowel during periods of acute inflammation associated with severe enteric infections. As the patient's dietary intake is increased, foods that act as bowel irritants, such as raw fruits and vegetables, popcorn, carbonated beverages, spicy foods, and foods of extreme temperatures, should be avoided. Small, frequent meals help to prevent abdominal distention. Medications, such as anticholinergic agents, antispasmodic agents, or opioids, can be prescribed to decrease diarrhea by reducing intestinal spasms and motility. Administering antidiarrheal agents on a regular schedule may be more beneficial than administering them on an as-needed basis. Antibiotics and antifungal agents may also be prescribed to combat pathogens identified by stool cultures. Assessment of the patient's self-care strategies is essential.

Preventing Infection

The patient and caregivers are instructed to monitor for signs and symptoms of infection: fever; chills; night sweats; cough with or without sputum production; shortness of breath; difficulty breathing; oral pain or difficulty swallowing; creamy-white patches in the oral cavity; unexplained weight loss; swollen lymph nodes; nausea; vomiting; persistent diarrhea; frequency, urgency, or pain on urination; headache; visual changes or memory lapses; redness, swelling, or drainage from skin wounds; and vesicular lesions on the face, lips, or perianal area. The nurse also monitors laboratory test results that indicate infection, such as the white blood cell count and differential. Cultures of specimens from wound drainage, skin lesions, urine, stool, sputum, mouth, and blood are obtained to identify pathogenic organisms and the most appropriate antimicrobial therapy.

Improving Activity Tolerance

Activity tolerance is assessed by monitoring the patient's ability to ambulate and perform activities of daily living. Patients may be unable to maintain their usual levels of activity because of weakness, fatigue, shortness of breath, dizziness, and neurologic involvement. Assistance in planning daily routines that maintain a balance between activity and rest may be necessary. In addition, patients benefit from instructions about energy conservation techniques, such as sitting while washing or preparing meals. Personal items that are frequently used should be kept within the patient's reach.

Measures such as relaxation and guided imagery may be beneficial because they decrease anxiety, which contributes to weakness and fatigue.

Collaboration with other members of the health care team may uncover other factors associated with increasing fatigue and strategies to address them. For example, if fatigue is related to anemia, administering epoetin alfa (Epogen) as prescribed may relieve fatigue and increase activity tolerance.

Maintaining Coherent Thought Processes

The patient is assessed for alterations in mental status that may be related to neurologic involvement, metabolic abnormalities, infection, side effects of treatment, and coping mechanisms. Manifestations of neurologic impairment may be difficult to distinguish from psychological reactions to HIV infection, such as anger and depression.

If the patient experiences altered mental or cognitive status, family and support network members are instructed to speak to the patient in simple, clear language and give the patient sufficient time to respond to questions. Reorientation to surroundings and location is conducted as needed. The patient's support network is encouraged to orient the patient to the daily routine by talking about what is taking place during daily activities and providing the patient with a regular daily schedule for medication administration, grooming, meal times, bedtimes, and awakening times. Posting the schedule in a prominent area (e.g., on the refrigerator), providing nightlights for the bedroom and bathroom, and planning safe leisure activities allow the patient to maintain a regular routine in a safe manner. Activities that the patient previously enjoyed are encouraged. These should be easy to accomplish and fairly short in duration. The nurse encourages the social support network to remain calm and not to argue with the patient while protecting the patient from injury. Around-the-clock supervision may be necessary, and strategies can be implemented to prevent the patient from engaging in potentially dangerous activities, such as driving, using the stove, or mowing the lawn. Strategies for improving or maintaining functional abilities and for providing a safe environment are used for patients with HIV encephalopathy and other cognitive impairments (see Chart 37-9).

Improving Airway Clearance

Respiratory status, including rate, rhythm, the use of accessory muscles, and breath sounds, as well as mental status and skin color, must be assessed at least daily. Any cough and the quantity and characteristics of sputum are documented. Sputum specimens are analyzed for infectious organisms. Pulmonary therapy (coughing, deep breathing, postural drainage, percussion, and vibration) is provided as often as every 2 hours to prevent stasis of secretions and to promote airway clearance. Because of weakness and fatigue, many patients require assistance in attaining a position (such as a high Fowler's or semi-Fowler's position) that facilitates breathing and airway clearance. Adequate rest is essential to minimize energy expenditure and prevent excessive fatigue. The fluid volume status is evaluated so that adequate hydration can be maintained. Unless contraindicated because of kidney or cardiac disease, daily intake of 3 L of fluid is encouraged. Humidified oxygen may be prescribed, and nasopharyngeal or tracheal suctioning, intubation, and mechanical ventilation may be necessary to maintain adequate ventilation.

Relieving Pain and Discomfort

The patient is assessed for the quality and severity of pain associated with impaired perianal skin integrity, the lesions of KS, and peripheral neuropathy. In addition, the effects of pain on elimination, nutrition, sleep, affect, and communication are explored, along with exacerbating and relieving factors. Cleaning the perianal area, as described previously, can promote comfort. Topical anesthetic medications or ointments may be prescribed. The use of soft cushions or foam pads may increase comfort while sitting. The patient is instructed to avoid foods that act as bowel irritants. Antispasmodic and antidiarrheal medications may be prescribed to reduce the discomfort and frequency of bowel movements. If necessary, systemic analgesic agents may also be prescribed. Pain from KS is frequently described as a sharp, throbbing pressure, and heaviness, if lymphedema is present. Pain management may include the use of nonsteroidal anti-inflammatory drugs (NSAIDs) and opioids plus nonpharmacologic approaches such as relaxation techniques. When NSAIDs are administered to patients who are receiving zidovudine, hepatic and hematologic status must be monitored (Karch, 2012).

The patient with pain related to peripheral neuropathy frequently describes it as burning, numbness, and "pins and needles." Pain management approaches may include opioids, tricyclic antidepressants, and anti-embolism stockings to equalize pressure. Tricyclic antidepressants can be helpful in controlling the symptoms of neuropathic pain (Karch, 2012). They also potentiate the actions of opioids and can be used to relieve pain without increasing the dose of the opioid.

Improving Nutritional Status

Nutritional status is assessed by monitoring weight; dietary intake; and serum albumin, BUN, protein, and transferrin levels. The patient is also assessed for factors that interfere with oral intake, such as anorexia, oral and esophageal candidal infection, nausea, pain, weakness, fatigue, and lactose intolerance (Dudek, 2010). Based on the results of assessment, the nurse can implement specific measures to facilitate oral intake. The dietitian is consulted to determine the patient's nutritional requirements.

Control of nausea and vomiting with antiemetic medications administered on a regular basis may increase the patient's dietary intake. Inadequate food intake resulting from pain caused by oral lesions or a sore throat may be managed by administering prescribed opioids and viscous lidocaine (the patient is instructed to rinse the mouth and swallow). Additionally, the patient is encouraged to eat foods that are easy to swallow and to avoid spicy or sticky food items and foods that are excessively hot or cold. Oral hygiene before and after meals is encouraged. If fatigue and weakness interfere with intake, the nurse encourages the patient to rest before meals. If the patient is hospitalized, meals should be scheduled so that they do not occur immediately after painful or unpleasant procedures. The patient with diarrhea and abdominal cramping is encouraged to avoid foods that stimulate intestinal motility and abdominal distention, such as fiber-rich foods or lactose, if the patient is intolerant to

lactose. The patient is instructed about ways to enhance the nutritional value of meals. Adding eggs, butter, or fortified milk (milk to which powdered skim milk has been added to increase the caloric content) to gravies, soups, or milkshakes can provide additional calories and protein. High-calorie, nutritional foods such as puddings, powders, milkshakes, and nutritional supplements may also be useful (Dudek, 2010). Patients who cannot maintain their nutritional status through oral intake may require enteral feedings or parenteral nutrition.

Decreasing the Sense of Isolation

People with AIDS are at risk for double stigmatization. They have what society refers to as a "dreaded disease," and they may have a lifestyle that differs from what is considered acceptable by many people. Many people with AIDS are young adults at a developmental stage that is associated with establishing intimate relationships, personal goals, and career goals, as well as having and raising children. Their focus changes as they are faced with a chronic disease. In addition, they may reveal hidden lifestyles or behaviors to family, friends, coworkers, and health care providers. As a result, people with HIV infection may be overwhelmed with emotions such as anxiety, guilt, shame, and fear. They also may be faced with multiple losses, such as loss of financial security, normal roles and functions, self-esteem, privacy, ability to control bodily functions, ability to interact meaningfully with the environment, and sexual functioning as well as rejection by sexual partners, family, and friends. Some patients may harbor feelings of guilt because of their lifestyle or because they may have infected others in current or previous relationships. Other patients may feel anger toward sexual partners who transmitted the virus to them. Infection control measures used in the hospital or at home may further contribute to the patient's emotional isolation. Any or all of these stressors may cause the patient with AIDS to withdraw both physically and emotionally from social contact.

Nurses are in a key position to provide an atmosphere of acceptance and understanding for people with AIDS and their social networks. The patient's usual level of social interaction is assessed as early as possible to provide a baseline for monitoring changes in behaviors that suggest social isolation (e.g., decreased interaction with staff or family, hostility, nonadherence). Patients are encouraged to express feelings of isolation and loneliness, with the assurance that these feelings are not unique or abnormal.

Providing information about how to protect themselves and others may help patients avoid social isolation. Patients, family, and friends must be reassured that HIV is not spread through casual contact. Education of ancillary personnel, nurses, and physicians helps reduce factors that might contribute to patients' feelings of isolation. Patient care conferences that address the psychosocial issues associated with HIV/AIDS may help sensitize the health care team to patients' needs.

Coping With Grief

The nurse can help the patient verbalize feelings and explore and identify resources for support and mechanisms for coping, especially when the patient is grieving anticipated losses. The patient is encouraged to maintain contact with family, friends, and coworkers and to use local or national AIDS support groups and hotlines. If possible, losses are identified and addressed. The patient is encouraged to continue usual activities whenever possible. Consultations with mental health counselors are useful for many patients and their families.

Improving Knowledge of HIV

The patient and family are educated about HIV infection, means of preventing HIV transmission, and appropriate self-care measures. Information about the purpose of the medications, their correct administration, side effects, and strategies to manage or prevent side effects is provided. The patient is instructed to avoid others with active infections, such as upper respiratory infections.

Monitoring and Managing Potential Complications

Opportunistic Infections. Patients who are severely immunosuppressed are at risk for opportunistic infections. Therefore, anti-infective agents may be prescribed and laboratory tests obtained to monitor their effect. Signs and symptoms of opportunistic infections, including fever, malaise, difficulty breathing, nausea or vomiting, diarrhea, difficulty swallowing, and any occurrences of swelling or discharge, should be reported as treated as indicated.

Respiratory Failure. Impaired breathing is a major complication that increases the patient's discomfort and anxiety and may lead to respiratory and cardiac failure. The respiratory rate and pattern are monitored, and the lungs are auscultated for abnormal breath sounds. The patient is instructed to report shortness of breath and increasing difficulty in carrying out usual activities. Pulse rate and rhythm, blood pressure, and oxygen saturation are monitored. Suctioning and oxygen therapy may be prescribed to ensure an adequate airway and to prevent hypoxia. Mechanical ventilation may be necessary for the patient who cannot maintain adequate ventilation as a result of pulmonary infection, fluid and electrolyte imbalance, or respiratory muscle weakness. Arterial blood gas values are used to guide ventilator settings. If the patient is intubated, methods must be established to allow communication with the nurse and others. The patient receiving mechanical ventilation will require support to cope with the stress associated with intubation and ventilator assistance. The possible need for mechanical ventilation in the future should be discussed early in the course of the disease, when the patient is able to make known his or her preferences about treatment. The use of mechanical ventilation should be consistent with the patient's decisions about end-of-life treatment. (Further discussion of end-of-life care can be found in Chapter 16.)

Wasting Syndrome. Wasting syndrome and fluid and electrolyte disturbances, including dehydration, are common complications of untreated HIV infection. The patient's nutritional and electrolyte status is evaluated by monitoring weight gains or losses, skin turgor, ferritin levels, hemoglobin and hematocrit values, and electrolyte levels. Fluid and electrolyte status is monitored on an ongoing basis; fluid intake and output and urine specific gravity may be monitored daily if the patient is hospitalized with complications. The skin is assessed for dryness and adequate turgor. Vital signs are monitored for decreased systolic blood pressure or increased pulse rate on sitting or standing. Signs and symptoms of electrolyte disturbances, such as muscle cramping,

weakness, irregular pulse, decreased mental status, nausea, and vomiting, are documented and reported to the physician. Serum electrolyte values are monitored, and abnormalities are reported.

The nurse helps the patient select foods that will replenish electrolytes, such as oranges and bananas (potassium) and cheese and soups (sodium) (Dudek, 2010). A fluid intake of 3 L or more per day, unless contraindicated, is encouraged to replace fluid lost with diarrhea, and measures to control diarrhea are initiated. If fluid and electrolyte imbalances persist, the nurse administers IV fluids and electrolytes as prescribed. Effects of parenteral therapy are monitored.

Side Effects of Medications. Adverse effects are of concern in patients who receive many medications to treat HIV infection or its complications. Many medications can cause severe toxic effects. Patients and their caregivers need to know which signs and symptoms of side effects should be reported immediately to their primary provider (see Table 37-3).

In addition to medications used to treat HIV infection, other medications that may be required include opioids, tricyclic antidepressants, and NSAIDs for pain relief; medications for treatment of opportunistic infections; antihistamines (diphenhydramine [Benadryl]) for relief of pruritus; acetaminophen (Tylenol) or aspirin for management of fever; and antiemetic agents for control of nausea and vomiting. Concurrent use of these medications can cause many drug interactions, resulting in hepatic and hematologic abnormalities. Therefore, careful monitoring of laboratory test results is essential.

During each contact with the patient, it is important for the nurse to ask not only about side effects but also about how well the patient is managing the medication regimen. The nurse may be able to assist the patient in organizing and planning the medication schedule to promote adherence to the treatment regimen.

Promoting Home and Community-Based Care

Educating Patients About Self-Care. Patients, families, and friends are educated about the routes of transmission of HIV. As discussed earlier, the nurse discusses precautions the patient can use to avoid transmitting HIV sexually (see Charts 37-2 and 37-3) or through sharing of body fluids, especially blood. Patients and their families or caregivers must receive instructions about how to prevent disease transmission, including handwashing techniques and methods for safely handling and disposing of items soiled with body fluids. Clear guidelines about avoiding and controlling infection, keeping regular health care appointments, symptom management, nutrition, rest, and exercise are necessary. The importance of personal and environmental hygiene is emphasized. Caregivers are taught many of the guidelines (standard precautions) described in Chart 37-4. Kitchen and bathroom surfaces should be cleaned regularly with disinfectants to prevent growth of fungi and bacteria. Patients with pets are encouraged to have another person clean areas soiled by animals, such as birdcages and litter boxes. If this is not possible, patients should use gloves to clean the area and then wash their hands afterward. Patients are advised to avoid exposure to others who are sick or who have been recently vaccinated. The importance of avoiding smoking, excessive alcohol, and over-the-counter and street drugs is emphasized. Patients who are HIV positive or who inject drugs are instructed not to donate blood. IV/injection drug users who are unwilling to stop using drugs are advised to avoid sharing drug equipment with others.

Caregivers in the home are taught how to administer medications, including IV preparations. The medication regimens used for patients with HIV infection and AIDS are often complex and expensive. Patients receiving combination therapies for treatment of HIV infection and its complications require careful education about the importance of taking medications as prescribed and explanations and assistance in fitting the medication regimen into their lives (see Chart 37-7). If the patient requires enteral or parenteral nutrition, instruction is provided to the patient and family about how to administer nutritional therapies at home. Home care nurses provide ongoing education and support for the patient and family.

Continuing Care. Many people with AIDS remain in their community and continue their usual daily activities, whereas others can no longer work or maintain their independence. Families or caregivers may need assistance in providing supportive care. Many community-based organizations provide a variety of services for people living with HIV infection and AIDS; nurses can help identify these services.

Community health nurses, home care nurses, and hospice nurses are in an excellent position to provide the support and guidance that is so often needed in the home setting. As hospital costs continue to rise and insurance coverage continues to decline, the complexity of home care increases. Home care nurses are key to the safe and effective administration of parenteral antibiotics, chemotherapy, and nutrition in the home.

During home visits, the nurse assesses the patient's physical and emotional status and home environment. The patient's adherence to the therapeutic regimen is assessed, and strategies are suggested to assist with adherence. The patient is assessed for progression of disease and for adverse side effects of medications. Previous education is reinforced, and the importance of keeping follow-up appointments is stressed.

Complex wound care or respiratory care may be required in the home. Patients and families are often unable to meet these skilled care needs without assistance. Nurses may refer patients to community programs that offer a range of services for patients, friends, and families, including help with housekeeping, hygiene, and meals; transportation and shopping; individual and group therapy; support for caregivers; telephone networks for the homebound; and legal and financial assistance. These services are typically provided by both professionals and nonprofessional volunteers. A social worker may be consulted to identify sources of financial support, if needed.

Home care and hospice nurses are increasingly called on to provide physical and emotional support to patients and families as patients with AIDS enter the terminal stages of disease. This support takes on special meaning when people with AIDS lose friends and when family members fear the disease or feel anger concerning the patient's lifestyle. The nurse encourages the patient and family to discuss end-of-life decisions and to ensure that care is consistent with those decisions, all comfort measures are employed, and the patient is treated with dignity at all times.

Evaluation

Expected patient outcomes may include:
1. Maintains skin integrity
2. Resumes usual bowel habits
3. Experiences no infections
4. Maintains adequate level of activity tolerance
5. Maintains usual thought processes
6. Maintains effective airway clearance
7. Experiences increased sense of comfort and less pain
8. Maintains adequate nutritional status
9. Experiences decreased sense of social isolation
10. Progresses through grieving process
11. Reports increased understanding of AIDS and participates in self-care activities as possible
12. Remains free of complications

Detailed outcomes are included in the plan of nursing care for a patient with AIDS (see Chart 37-10).

 Concept Mastery Alert

For further review, visit the Point to view an interactive tutorial on HIV and AIDS.

Emotional and Ethical Concerns

Nurses in all settings are called on to provide care for patients with HIV infection. In doing so, they encounter not only the physical challenges of this epidemic but also emotional and ethical concerns. The concerns raised by health care professionals involve issues such as fear of infection, responsibility for giving care, values clarification, confidentiality, developmental stages of patients and caregivers, and poor prognostic outcomes.

Many patients with HIV infection have engaged in "stigmatized" behaviors. Because these behaviors challenge some traditional religious and moral values, nurses may feel reluctant to care for these patients. In addition, health care providers may still have fear and anxiety about disease transmission despite education concerning infection control and the low incidence of transmission to health care providers (see Chart 37-5). Nurses are encouraged to examine their personal beliefs and to use the process of values clarification to approach controversial issues (Chart 37-11). The American Nurses Association's Code of Ethics for Nurses (2008) can also be used to help resolve ethical dilemmas that might affect the quality of care given to patients with HIV infection and AIDS.

Nurses are responsible for protecting the patient's right to privacy by safeguarding confidential information. Inadvertent disclosure of confidential patient information may result in personal, financial, and emotional hardships for the patient. The controversy surrounding confidentiality concerns the circumstances in which information may be disclosed to others. Health care team members need accurate patient information to conduct assessment, planning, implementation, and evaluation of patient care. Failure to disclose HIV status could compromise the quality of patient care. Sexual partners of patients infected with HIV should know about the potential for infection and the need to engage in safer sex practices,

ETHICAL DILEMMA

Chart 37-11 Under What Circumstances May a Nurse Refuse to Care for a Patient?

Case Scenario

You are a charge nurse in the emergency department (ED) of a community hospital. A 52-year-old male patient with a known history of being positive for HIV presents to the ED with a 4-day history of nausea and incontinent diarrhea. He complains of "feeling woozy" when he tries to stand up and appears emaciated. According to his male partner, who holds his durable power of attorney for health care, he has lost significant weight over the past month. The nurse assigned to care for him tells you, "I bet he now has AIDS. I don't agree with his lifestyle with that partner of his—it disgusts me that he is gay. He brought this upon himself. I go to church every Sunday, and my religious faith tells me that I should not have anything to do with him. And to top it off, with his incontinence, I could get infected too if I were to come in contact with his waste. I'm not going to take care of him—give me another assignment."

Discussion

The American Nurses Association (ANA) clearly stipulates that nurses have an obligation to "provide fair and equal treatment to all patients" (ANA, 2010, p. 5) and also stipulates in its *Code of Ethics* that nurses must provide fair and equitable treatment to "every individual, unrestricted by considerations of social or economic status, personal attributes, or the nature of the health problem" (ANA, 2001, p. 7).

Analysis

*   Does a nurse have the right to refuse treating a patient? What if a nurse refuses to treat a patient because he or she believes

that by doing so the nurse may suffer harm or it may conflict with tenets of his or her religious beliefs?

*   There are several statements that the staff nurse in this case makes with regard to this patient assignment. Analyze each of these in turn. Does the staff nurse demonstrate respect for the patient's autonomy? Is she adhering to the ethical principles of beneficence and nonmaleficence? What about distributive justice? (See Chart 3-3 in Chapter 3.)
*   What might be the legal implications of the staff nurse refusing this assignment? As the charge nurse, how would you act to ensure that applicable hospital policies are adhered to, that you do not permit any type of negligent or other potentially criminal act to occur, and that the patient and his partner receive just and equitable health care?

References

American Nurses Association. (2001). *Code of ethics for nurses with interpretive statements*. Washington, DC: American Nurses Publishing, American Nurses Foundation/American Nurses Association.

American Nurses Association. (2010). *Position statement on the nurse's role in ethics and human rights: Protecting and promoting individual worth, dignity, and human rights in practice settings*. Available at: www.nursingworld.org/MainMenu Categories/EthicsStandards/Ethics-Position-Statements

Resources

See Chapter 3, Chart 3-6 for ethics resources.

---

as well as the possible need for testing and health care. Nurses are advised to discuss concerns about confidentiality with nurse administrators and to consult professional nursing organizations such as the Association of Nurses in AIDS Care and legal experts in their state to identify the most appropriate course of action.

AIDS has had a high mortality rate, but advances in ART have demonstrated promise in slowing or controlling disease progression. Most nurses in the United States have never faced an epidemic in which so many young and middle-aged adults experience serious illness and may die during the usual course of the disease process. Nurses may struggle with the value and meaning of their professional roles as they witness repeated instances of deterioration. Exposure to many deaths among patients at the same developmental stage as many nurses can create stress. Contributing to this stress are personal fears of contagion or disapproval of the patient's lifestyle and behaviors. Unlike cancer or other diseases, AIDS is associated with controversies challenging our legal and political systems as well as religious and personal beliefs.

Many strategies have been used by nurses to cope with the stress associated with caring for patients with AIDS. Education and provision of up-to-date information help to alleviate apprehension and prepare nurses to deliver safe, high-quality patient care. Interdisciplinary meetings allow participants to support one another and provide comprehensive patient care. Staff support groups give nurses an opportunity to solve problems and explore values and feelings about caring for patients with AIDS and their families; they also provide a forum for

grieving. Other sources of support include nursing administrators, peers, and spiritual advisors.

Critical Thinking Exercises

1 ebp A 53-year-old man who has sex with men wants to reduce the risk of HIV infection. What is the best evidence for counseling this patient? What is the evidence base on safer sex and strategies to reduce risk? How would your approach differ if the man was using IV/injection drugs? What is the evidence base on strategies to reduce risk from use of IV/injection drugs? What is the evidence about the effectiveness of needle exchange programs? How would you determine the strength of the evidence and how would you present information to him?

2 pg A 28-year-old woman who is bleeding from a gunshot wound presents to the emergency department. She is intoxicated and combative. What are the first three actions the nurse should take?

3 You are making a home visit to a patient with AIDS who is exhibiting some incoherent thought. Describe the aspects of the home environment that you would assess to ensure safety and adequate care. Describe the nursing plan of care to promote adherence with ART and other medications since the patient is taking multiple different medications many times during the day.

Brunner Suite Resources
Explore these additional resources to enhance learning for this chapter:
• NCLEX-Style Questions and Other Resources on thePoint, http://thePoint.lww.com/Brunner13e
• Study Guide
• PrepU
• Clinical Handbook
• Handbook of Laboratory and Diagnostic Tests

References

*Asterisk indicates nursing research.
**Double asterisk indicates classic reference.

Books

American Nurses Association. (2008). *Guide to the code of ethics for nurses: Interpretation and application.* Silver Spring, MD: Author.

Dudek, S. G. (2010). *Nutrition essentials for nursing practice* (6th ed.). Philadelphia: Lippincott Williams & Wilkins.

Durham, J. D., & Lashley, F. R. (2010). *The person with HIV/AIDS: Nursing perspectives.* New York: Springer.

Eliopoulos, C. (2010). *Gerontological nursing* (7th ed.). Philadelphia: Lippincott Williams & Wilkins.

Karch, A. M. (2012). *2012 Lippincott's nursing drug guide.* Philadelphia: Lippincott Williams & Wilkins.

Lapka, D. V., & Franson, P. J. (2010). Biologics and targeted therapies. In J. Eggert (Ed.): *Cancer basics.* Pittsburgh: Oncology Nursing Society.

Lutz, C., & Przytulski, K. (2011). *Nutrition and diet therapy* (5th ed.). Philadelphia: F. A. Davis.

Porth, C. M., & Matfin, G. (2009). *Pathophysiology: Concepts of altered health states* (8th ed.). Philadelphia: Lippincott Williams & Wilkins.

Swanson, B. (2010). *ANAC's core curriculum for HIV/AIDS nursing* (3rd ed.). Sudbury, MA: Jones & Bartlett.

Journals and Electronic Documents

Al-Khindi, T., Zakzanis, K., & van Gorp, W. (2011). Does antiretroviral therapy improve HIV-associated cognitive impairment? A quantitative review of the literature. *Journal of the International Neuropsychological Society, 17*(6), 956–969.

Centers for Disease Control and Prevention. (2008). Revised surveillance case definitions for HIV infection among adults, adolescents, and children aged <18 months and for HIV infection and AIDS among children aged 18 months to <13 years—United States, 2008. *MMWR: Morbidity and Mortality Weekly Report Recommendations and Reports, 57*(RR 10), 1–8.

Centers for Disease Control and Prevention. (2010a). *Toolkit for implementing comprehensive HIV prevention programs for people who use drugs.* Available at: www.cdc.gov/globalaids/Resources/prevention/docs/Toolkit-for-Implementing-Programs-for-People-Who-Use-Drugs.pdf

Centers for Disease Control and Prevention. (2010b). *Sexually transmitted diseases: Treatment guidelines, 2010. HIV infection: Detection, counseling, and referral.* Available at: www.cdc.gov/std/treatment/2010/hiv.htm

Centers for Disease Control and Prevention. (2011a). *HIV surveillance report, 2009* (Vol. 21). Available at: www.cdc.gov/hiv/topics/surveillance/resources/reports/

Centers for Disease Control and Prevention. (2011b). *HIV in the United States: Fact sheet.* Available at: www.cdc.gov/hiv/statistics/basics/ataglance.html

Centers for Disease Control and Prevention. (2011c). *Compendium of evidence-based HIV behavioral intervention.* Available at: www.cdc.gov/hiv/topics/research/prs/evidence-based-interventions.htm

Centers for Disease Control and Prevention. (2011d). *Condoms and STDs: Fact sheet for public health personnel.* Available at: www.cdc.gov/condomeffectiveness/latex.htm

Centers for Disease Control and Prevention. (2011e). *Occupational HIV transmission and prevention among health care workers.* Available at: www.cdc.gov/hiv/resources/factsheets/PDF/hcw.pdf

Coffman, D. L., & Kugler, K. C. (2012). Causal mediation of a human immunodeficiency virus prevention intervention. *Nursing Research, 61*(3), 224–230.

Fauci, A., Hodes, R., & Whitescarver, J. (2010). *NIH statement on National HIV/AIDS and Aging Awareness Day.* Sept 18, 2010. Available at: www.niaid.nih.gov/news/newsreleases/2010/Pages/HIVagingday10.aspx

Gagnon, M., & Holmes, D. (2011). Bodies in mutation: Understanding lipodystrophy among women living with HIV/AIDS. *Research and Theory for Nursing Practice: An International Journal, 25*(1), 23–38.

Global HIV Vaccine Enterprise. (2010). *Comprehensive new framework to speed and enhance HIV vaccine research released.* Available at: www.vaccineenterprise.org/sites/default/files/Enterprise%20Scientific%20Strategic%20Plan%20Announcement.pdf

Heffron, R., Donnell, D., Rees, H., et al. (2012). Use of hormonal contraceptives and risk of HIV-1 transmission: A prospective cohort study. *Lancet Infectious Diseases, 12*(1), 19–26.

Karim, Q., Karim, S., Frohlich, J., et al. (2010). Effectiveness and safety of tenofovir gel, an antiretroviral microbicide for the prevention of HIV infection in women. *Science, 329*(2), 1168–1174.

Merenstein, D., Hu, H., Robison, E., et al. (2010). Relationship between complementary/alternate treatment use and illicit drug use among a cohort of women with, or at risk for, HIV infection. *Journal of Alternative and Complementary Medicine, 16*(9), 989–993.

Merlin, J., Cen, L., Praestgaard, A., et al. (2012). Pain and physical and psychological symptoms in ambulatory HIV patients in the current treatment era. *Journal of Pain and Symptom Management, 43*(3), 638–645.

National Institutes of Health, Centers for Disease Control and Prevention, and HIV Medicine Association of the Infectious Diseases Society of America. (2009). *Guidelines for prevention and treatment of opportunistic infections in HIV-infected adults and adolescents.* Available at: aidsinfo.nih.gov/contentfiles/Adult_OI.pdf

New York State Department of Health AIDS Institute. (2009). *Immune reconstitution inflammatory syndrome (IRIS) in HIV-infected patients.* Available at: www.hivguidelines.org/wp-content/uploads/2009/08/IMMUNE-RECONSTITUTION-INFLAMMATORY.pdf

*Nicholas, P., Voss, J., Wantland, D., et al. (2010). Prevalence, self-care behaviors, and self-care activities for peripheral neuropathy symptoms of HIV/AIDS. *Nursing and Health Sciences, 12*(1), 119–126.

Panel on Antiretroviral Guidelines for Adults and Adolescents. (2013). *Guidelines for the use of antiretroviral agents in HIV-1-infected adults and adolescents.* U.S. Department of Health and Human Services. Available at: aidsinfo.nih.gov/ContentFiles/AdultandAdolescentGL.pdf

Siegel, J. D., Rhinehart, E., Jackson, M., et al. (2007). *Guideline for isolation precautions: Preventing transmission of infectious agents in healthcare settings.* Available at: www.cdc.gov/ncidod/dhqp/gl_isolation.html

Thames, A. D., Becker, B. W., Marcotte, T. D. (2011). Depression, cognition, and self-appraisal of functional abilities in HIV: An examination of subjective appraisal versus objective performance. *Clinical Neuropsychologist, 25*(2):224–243.

Van Damme, L., Ramjee, G., Alary, M. et al. (2002). Effectiveness of COL-1492, a nonoxynol-9 vaginal gel, on HIV-1 transmission in female sex workers: a randomised controlled trial. *Lancet, 360*(9338), 971–977.

Vance, D. E., Ross, J. A., Moneyham, L., et al. (2010). A model of cognitive decline and suicidal ideation in adults aging with HIV. *Journal of Neuroscience Nursing, 42*(3), 150–156.

White House. (2010). *National HIV/AIDS strategy for the United States.* Available at: www.whitehouse.gov/sites/default/files/uploads/NHAS.pdf

Woods, M., Wanke, C., Ling, P., et al. (2009). Metabolic syndrome and serum fatty acid patterns in serum phospholipids in hypertriglyceridemic persons with human immunodeficiency virus. *American Journal of Clinical Nutrition, 89*(4), 1180–1187.

World Health Organization. (2011a). *Global health sector strategy on HIV/AIDS 2011–2015.* Available at: whqlibdoc.who.int/publications/2011/9789241501651_eng.pdf

World Health Organization. (2011b). *Joint strategic action framework to accelerate the scale-up of voluntary medical male circumcision for HIV prevention in eastern and southern Africa: 2012–2016.* Joint United Nations Programme on HIV/AIDS (UNAIDS). Available at: whqlibdoc.who.int/unaids/2011/JC2251E_eng.pdf

Resources

AIDS Community Research Initiative of America (ACRIA), www.acria.org
AIDS Education and Training Centers (AETCs) Program (regional, national, and international training opportunities), www.aidsetc.org
American Red Cross, www.redcross.org

Antiretroviral medication information Web sites: www.AIDSmeds.com; www.projectinform.org; www.sfaf.org; hivinsite.ucsf.edu/; www.amfAR.org; www.natap.org; www.thebody.com

Centers for Disease Control and Prevention, HIV/AIDS Prevention Research Synthesis Project, www.cdc.gov/hiv/topics/research/prs/evidence-based-interventions.htm; www.cdc.gov

Gay Men's Health Crisis Network (GMHC), www.gmhc.org

Health Resources and Service Administration (HRSA), National Clinician's Postexposure Prophylaxis Hotline (health care providers only), 1-888-HIV-4911

Health Resources and Service Administration (HRSA), National HIV Telephone Consultation Service, 1-800-933-3413

International AIDS Vaccine Initiative (AVI), www.iavi.org

International Partnership for Microbicides, www.ipmglobal.org

National Association of People with AIDS (NAPWA), www.napwa.org

National Institutes of Health, Glossary of HIV/AIDS-Related Terms, aidsinfo.nih.gov/contentfiles/GlossaryHIVrelatedTerms_English.pdf

National Institutes of Health, HIV/AIDS Treatment, Prevention, and Research, www.aidsinfo.nih.gov

National Pediatric and Family HIV Resource Center, www.womenchildrenhiv.org

Office of Minority Health Resource Center, www.minorityhealth.hhs.gov

Pharmaceutical Research and Manufacturers of America (PhRMA), www.phrma.org

POZ, *Health, Life, & HIV*. Published by Smart+Strong, 500 Fifth Avenue, Suite 320, New York, NY 10110

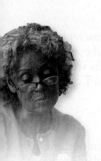
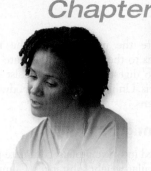

Assessment and Management of Patients With Allergic Disorders

Learning Objectives

On completion of this chapter, the learner will be able to:

1 Explain the physiologic events involved with allergic reactions.
2 Describe the types of hypersensitivity.
3 Describe the management of patients with allergic disorders.

4 Describe measures to prevent and manage anaphylaxis.
5 Use the nursing process as a framework for care of the patient with allergic rhinitis.
6 Discuss the different allergic disorders according to type.

Glossary

allergen: substance that causes manifestations of allergy

allergy: inappropriate and often harmful immune system response to substances that are normally harmless

anaphylaxis: rapid clinical response to an immediate immunologic reaction between a specific antigen and antibody

angioneurotic edema: condition characterized by urticaria and diffuse swelling of the deeper layers of the skin (i.e., angioedema)

antibody: protein substance developed by the body in response to and interacting with a specific antigen

antigen: substance that induces the production of antibodies

antihistamine: medication that opposes the action of histamine

atopic dermatitis: type I hypersensitivity involving inflammation of the skin evidenced by itching, redness, and a variety of skin lesions

atopy: term often used to describe immunoglobulin E–mediated diseases (i.e., atopic dermatitis, asthma, and allergic rhinitis) with a genetic component

B lymphocytes: cells that are important in producing circulating antibodies

bradykinin: a substance that stimulates nerve fibers and causes pain

eosinophil: granular leukocyte

erythema: diffuse redness of the skin

hapten: incomplete antigen

histamine: substance in the body that causes increased gastric secretion, dilation of capillaries, and constriction of the bronchial smooth muscle

hypersensitivity: abnormal heightened reaction to a stimulus of any kind

immunoglobulins: a family of closely related proteins capable of acting as antibodies

leukotrienes: a group of chemical mediators that initiate the inflammatory response

mast cells: connective tissue cells that contain heparin and histamine in their granules

prostaglandins: unsaturated fatty acids that have a wide assortment of biologic activity

rhinitis: inflammation of the nasal mucosa

serotonin: chemical mediator that acts as a potent vasoconstrictor and bronchoconstrictor

T lymphocytes: cells that can cause graft rejection, kill foreign cells, or suppress production of antibodies

urticaria: hives

The human body is bombarded by a host of potential invaders—allergens as well as microbial organisms—that constantly threaten its defenses. After penetrating those defenses, these allergens and organisms, if allowed to continue unimpeded, disrupt the body's enzyme systems and destroy its vital tissues. To protect against these agents, the body is equipped with an elaborate defense system.

The epithelial cells that coat the skin and make up the lining of the respiratory, gastrointestinal, and genitourinary tracts provide the first line of defense against microbial invaders. The structure and continuity of these surfaces

and their resistance to penetration are initial deterrents to invaders.

One of the most effective defense mechanisms is the body's capacity to equip itself rapidly with antibodies individually designed to meet each new invader—namely, specific protein antigens. Antibodies react with antigens in a variety of ways: (1) by coating the antigens' surfaces if they are particular substances, (2) by neutralizing the antigens if they are toxins, and (3) by precipitating the antigens out of solution if they are dissolved. The antibodies prepare the antigens so that the phagocytic cells of the blood and the tissues can dispose of them. However, although this system is normally protective, in some cases the body produces inappropriate or exaggerated responses to specific antigens, and the result is an allergic or hypersensitivity disorder.

ALLERGIC ASSESSMENT

Physiologic Overview

An allergic reaction is a manifestation of tissue injury resulting from interaction between an antigen and an antibody. **Allergy** is an inappropriate and often harmful response of the immune system to normally harmless substances, called **allergens** (e.g., dust, weeds, pollen, dander). Chemical mediators released in allergic reactions may produce symptoms that range from mild to life threatening.

In allergic reactions the body encounters allergens that are types of **antigens**, usually proteins that the body's defenses recognize as foreign, and a series of events occurs in an attempt to render the invaders harmless, destroy them, and remove them from the body. When lymphocytes respond to the antigens, **antibodies** (protein substances that protect against antigens) are produced.

Antibodies combine with antigens in a special way, which has been likened to keys fitting into a lock. Antigens (the keys) fit only certain antibodies (the locks). Hence, the term *specificity* refers to the specific reaction of an antibody to an antigen. There are many variations and complexities in these patterns.

Function of Immunoglobulins

Antibodies that are formed by lymphocytes and plasma cells in response to an immunogenic stimulus constitute a group of serum proteins called **immunoglobulins**. Grouped into five classes (IgE, IgD, IgG, IgM, and IgA), immunoglobulins can be found in the lymph nodes, tonsils, appendix, and Peyer's patches of the intestinal tract or circulating in the blood and lymph. These antibodies are capable of binding with a wide variety of antigens. Immunoglobulins of the IgE class are involved in allergic disorders and some parasitic infections. IgE-producing cells are located in the respiratory and intestinal mucosa. Two or more IgE molecules bind together to an allergen and trigger **mast cells** or basophils to release chemical mediators, such as histamine, serotonin, kinins, slow-reacting substances of anaphylaxis, and the neutrophil factor, which produces allergic skin reactions, asthma, and hay fever. **Atopy** refers to IgE-mediated diseases, such as allergic rhinitis, that have a genetic component. (See Chapter 35 for more information on immunoglobulins.)

Role of B Cells

B cells, or **B lymphocytes**, are programmed to produce one specific antibody. On encountering a specific antigen, B cells stimulate production of plasma cells, the site of antibody production. The result is the outpouring of antibodies for the purpose of destroying and removing the antigens.

Role of T Cells

T cells, or **T lymphocytes**, assist the B cells. T cells secrete substances that direct the flow of cell activity, destroy target

cells, and stimulate the macrophages. The macrophages present the antigens to the T cells and initiate the immune response. They also digest antigens and assist in removing cells and other debris. Unlike a specific antibody, a T cell does not bind free antigens.

Function of Antigens

Antigens are divided into two groups: complete protein antigens and low-molecular-weight substances. Complete protein antigens, such as animal dander, pollen, and horse serum, stimulate a complete humoral response. (See Chapter 35 for a discussion of humoral immunity.) Low-molecular-weight substances, such as medications, function as **haptens** (incomplete antigens), binding to tissue or serum proteins to produce a carrier complex that initiates an antibody response. In an allergic reaction, the production of antibodies requires active communication between cells. When the allergen is absorbed through the respiratory tract, gastrointestinal tract, or skin, allergen sensitization occurs. Macrophages process the antigen and present it to the appropriate cells. These cells mature into allergen-specific secreting plasma cells that synthesize and secrete antigen-specific antibodies.

Function of Chemical Mediators

Mast cells, which are located in the skin and mucous membranes, play a major role in IgE-mediated immediate hypersensitivity. When mast cells are stimulated by antigens, powerful chemical mediators are released, causing a sequence of physiologic events that result in symptoms of immediate hypersensitivity (Fig. 38-1). There are two types of chemical mediators: primary and secondary. Primary mediators are preformed and are found in mast cells or basophils. Secondary mediators are inactive precursors that are formed or released in response to primary mediators. Table 38-1 summarizes the actions of primary and secondary chemical mediators.

Primary Mediators

Histamine

Histamine, which is released by mast cells, plays an important role in the immune response. Its effects, which are greatest within about 15 minutes after antigen contact, include erythema; localized edema in the form of wheals; pruritus; contraction of bronchial smooth muscle, resulting in wheezing and bronchospasm; dilation of small venules and constriction of larger vessels; and increased secretion of gastric and mucosal cells, resulting in diarrhea (Porth & Matfin, 2009). Histamine action results from stimulation of histamine-1 (H_1) and histamine-2 (H_2) receptors. H_1 receptors are found predominantly on bronchiolar and vascular smooth muscle cells; H_2 receptors are found on gastric parietal cells.

Certain medications are categorized by their action at these receptors. Diphenhydramine (Benadryl) is an example of an **antihistamine**, a medication that displays an affinity for H_1 receptors. Cimetidine (Tagamet) and ranitidine (Zantac) target H_2 receptors to inhibit gastric secretions in peptic ulcer disease.

Eosinophil Chemotactic Factor of Anaphylaxis

Eosinophil chemotactic factor of anaphylaxis affects movement of **eosinophils** (granular leukocytes) to the site of

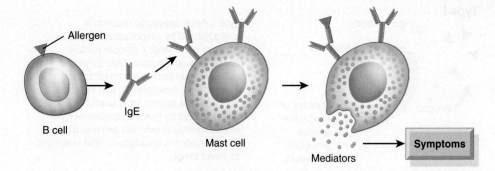

FIGURE 38-1 • Allergen triggers the B cell to make immunoglobulin E (IgE) antibody, which attaches to the mast cell. When that allergen reappears, it binds to the IgE and triggers the mast cell to release its chemicals. Courtesy of U.S. Department of Health and Human Services, National Institutes of Health.

allergens. It is preformed in the mast cells and is released from disrupted mast cells.

Platelet-Activating Factor

Platelet-activating factor is responsible for initiating platelet aggregation and leukocyte infiltration at sites of immediate hypersensitivity reactions. It also causes bronchoconstriction and increased vascular permeability (Porth & Matfin, 2009).

Prostaglandins

Prostaglandins produce smooth muscle contraction as well as vasodilation and increased capillary permeability (Porth & Matfin, 2009). The fever and pain that occur with inflammation in allergic responses are caused in part by the prostaglandins.

Secondary Mediators

Leukotrienes

Leukotrienes are chemical mediators that initiate the inflammatory response. Many manifestations of inflammation can be attributed in part to leukotrienes. In addition, leukotrienes cause smooth muscle contraction, bronchial constriction, mucus secretion in the airways, and the typical wheal-and-flare

reactions of the skin. Compared with histamine, leukotrienes are 100 to 1,000 times more potent in causing bronchospasm.

Bradykinin

Bradykinin is a substance that has the ability to cause increased vascular permeability, vasodilation, hypotension, and contraction of many types of smooth muscle, such as the bronchi. Increased permeability of the capillaries results in edema. Bradykinin stimulates nerve cell fibers and produces pain.

Serotonin

Serotonin acts as a potent vasoconstrictor and causes contraction of bronchial smooth muscle.

Hypersensitivity

Although the immune system defends the host against infections and foreign antigens, immune responses can themselves cause tissue injury and disease. **Hypersensitivity** is a reflection of excessive or aberrant immune response to any type of stimulus (Abbas & Lichtman, 2011). It usually does not occur with the first exposure to an allergen. Rather, the reaction follows a re-exposure after sensitization, or buildup of antibodies, in a predisposed person. To promote understanding

TABLE 38-1 **Chemical Mediators of Hypersensitivity**	
Mediators	**Action**
Primary Mediators	
Preformed and Found in Mast Cells or Basophils	
Histamine (preformed in mast cells)	Vasodilation
	Smooth muscle contraction, increased vascular permeability, increased mucus secretions
Eosinophil chemotactic factor of anaphylaxis (preformed in mast cells)	Attracts eosinophils
Platelet-activating factor (requires synthesis by mast cells, neutrophils, and macrophages)	Smooth muscle contraction
	Incites platelets to aggregate and release serotonin and histamine
Prostaglandins (chemically derived from arachidonic acid; require synthesis by cells)	D and F series → bronchoconstriction
	E series → bronchodilation
	D, E, and F series → vasodilation
Basophil kallikrein (preformed in mast cells)	Frees bradykinin, which causes bronchoconstriction, vasodilation, and nerve stimulation
Secondary Mediators	
Inactive Precursors Formed or Released in Response to Primary Mediators	
Bradykinin (derived from precursor kininogen)	Smooth muscle contraction, increased vascular permeability, stimulates pain receptors, increased mucus production
Serotonin (preformed in platelets)	Smooth muscle contraction, increased vascular permeability
Heparin (preformed in mast cells)	Anticoagulant
Leukotrienes (derived from arachidonic acid and activated by mast cell degranulation) C, D, and E or slow-reacting substance of anaphylaxis	Smooth muscle contraction, increased vascular permeability

Adapted from Menzies, F. M., Shepherd, M. C., Nibbs, R. J., & Nelson, S. M. (2011). The role of mast cells and their mediators in reproduction, pregnancy and labour. *Human Reproduction Update, 17*(3), 383–396; and Porth, C. M., & Matfin G. (2009). *Pathophysiology: Concepts of altered health states* (8th ed.). Philadelphia: Lippincott Williams & Wilkins.

Type I

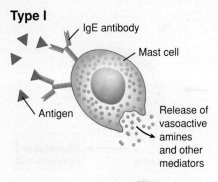

Type I. An anaphylactic reaction is characterized by vasodilation, increased capillary permeability, smooth muscle contraction, and eosinophilia. Systemic reactions may involve laryngeal stridor, angioedema, hypotension, and bronchial, GI, or uterine spasm; local reactions are characterized by hives. Examples of type I reactions include extrinsic asthma, allergic rhinitis, systemic anaphylaxis, and reactions to insect stings.

Type II

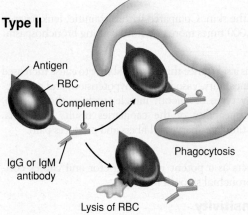

Type II. A cytotoxic reaction, which involves binding either the IgG or IgM antibody to a cell-bound antigen, may lead to eventual cell and tissue damage. The reaction is the result of mistaken identity when the system identifies a normal constituent of the body as foreign and activates the complement cascade. Examples of type II reactions are myasthenia gravis, Goodpasture syndrome, pernicious anemia, hemolytic disease of the newborn, transfusion reaction, and thrombocytopenia.

Type III

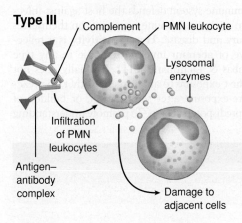

Type III. An immune complex reaction is marked by acute inflammation resulting from formation and deposition of immune complexes. The joints and kidneys are particularly susceptible to this kind of reaction, which is associated with systemic lupus erythematosus, serum sickness, nephritis, and rheumatoid arthritis. Some signs and symptoms include urticaria, joint pain, fever, rash, and adenopathy (swollen glands).

Type IV

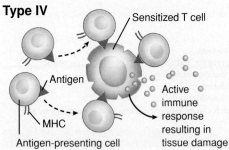

Type IV. A delayed, or cellular, reaction occurs 1 to 3 days after exposure to an antigen. The reaction, which results in tissue damage, involves activity by lymphokines, macrophages, and lysozymes. Erythema and itching are common; a few examples include contact dermatitis, graft-versus-host disease, Hashimoto's thyroiditis, and sarcoidosis.

FIGURE 38-2 • Four types of hypersensitivity reactions. Ig, immunoglobulin; PMN, polymorphonuclear; RBC, red blood cell.

of the immunopathogenesis of disease, hypersensitivity reactions have been classified into four specific types of reactions (Fig. 38-2). Most allergic reactions are either type I or type IV hypersensitivity reactions.

Anaphylactic (Type I) Hypersensitivity

The most severe hypersensitivity reaction is **anaphylaxis**. An unanticipated severe allergic reaction that is rapid in

onset, anaphylaxis is characterized by edema in many tissues, including the larynx, and is often accompanied by hypotension, bronchospasm, and cardiovascular collapse in severe cases. Type I or anaphylactic hypersensitivity is an immediate reaction beginning within minutes of exposure to an antigen. Primary chemical mediators are responsible for the symptoms of type I hypersensitivity because of their effects on the skin, lungs, and gastrointestinal tract. If chemical mediators continue to be released, a delayed reaction may occur and may last for up to 24 hours.

Clinical symptoms are determined by the amount of the allergen, the amount of mediator released, the sensitivity of the target organ, and the route of allergen entry. Type I hypersensitivity reactions may include both local and systemic anaphylaxis.

Cytotoxic (Type II) Hypersensitivity

Type II, or cytotoxic, hypersensitivity occurs when the system mistakenly identifies a normal constituent of the body as foreign. This reaction may be the result of a cross-reacting antibody, possibly leading to cell and tissue damage.

Type II hypersensitivity reactions are associated with several disorders. For example, in myasthenia gravis, the body mistakenly generates antibodies against normal nerve ending receptors. In Goodpasture syndrome, it generates antibodies against lung and renal tissue, producing lung damage and renal failure.

Immune Complex (Type III) Hypersensitivity

Type III, or immune complex, hypersensitivity involves immune complexes that are formed when antigens bind to antibodies. These complexes are cleared from the circulation by phagocytic action. If these type III complexes are deposited in tissues or vascular endothelium, two factors contribute to injury: the increased amount of circulating complexes and the presence of vasoactive amines. As a result, there is an increase in vascular permeability and tissue injury.

Delayed-Type (Type IV) Hypersensitivity

Type IV, or delayed-type, hypersensitivity, also known as cellular hypersensitivity, occurs 24 to 72 hours after exposure to an allergen. It is mediated by sensitized T cells that cause cell and tissue damage (Port & Matfin, 2009). Symptoms include itching, erythema, and raised lesions.

Assessment

A comprehensive allergy history and a thorough physical examination provide useful data for the diagnosis and management of allergic disorders. An allergy assessment form is useful for obtaining and organizing pertinent information (Chart 38-1).

The degree of difficulty and discomfort experienced by the patient because of allergic symptoms and the degree of improvement in those symptoms with and without treatment are assessed and documented. The relationship of symptoms to exposure to possible allergens is noted.

Diagnostic Evaluation

Diagnostic evaluation of the patient with allergic disorders commonly includes blood tests, smears of body secretions, skin tests, and the radioallergosorbent test (RAST). Results of laboratory blood studies provide supportive data for various diagnostic possibilities; however, they are not the major criteria for the diagnosis of allergic disease.

Complete Blood Count With Differential

The white blood cell (WBC) count is usually normal except with infection. Eosinophils, which are granular leukocytes, normally make up 0% to 3% of the total number of WBCs (Fischbach & Dunning, 2009). A level between 5% and 15% is nonspecific but does suggest allergic reaction. Higher percentages of eosinophils are considered to represent moderate to severe eosinophilia. Moderate eosinophilia is defined as 15% to 40% eosinophils and may be found in patients with allergic disorders.

Eosinophil Count

An actual count of eosinophils can be obtained from blood samples or smears of secretions (Fischbach & Dunning, 2009). During symptomatic episodes, smears obtained from nasal secretions, conjunctival secretions, and sputum of patients with allergies usually reveal eosinophils, indicating an active allergic response.

Total Serum Immunoglobulin E Levels

High total serum IgE levels support the diagnosis of allergic disease (Fischbach & Dunning, 2009). However, a normal IgE level does not exclude the diagnosis of an allergic disorder. IgE levels are not as sensitive as the paper radioimmunosorbent test (PRIST), the enzyme immunoassay (EIA), or a variant of this test known as enzyme-linked immunosorbent assay (ELISA).

Skin Tests

Skin testing entails the intradermal injection or superficial application (epicutaneous) of solutions at several sites. Depending on the suspected cause of allergic signs and symptoms, several different solutions may be applied at separate sites. These solutions contain individual antigens representing an assortment of allergens most likely to be implicated in the patient's disease. Positive (wheal-and-flare) reactions are clinically significant when correlated with the history, physical findings, and results of other laboratory tests.

The results of skin tests complement the data obtained from the history. They indicate which of several antigens are most likely to provoke symptoms and indicate the intensity of the patient's sensitization. The dosage of the antigen (allergen) injected is also important. Most patients are hypersensitive to more than one allergen. Under testing conditions, they may not react (although they usually do) to the specific allergens that induce their attacks.

In cases of doubt about the validity of the skin tests, a RAST or a provocative challenge test may be performed. If a skin test is indicated, there is a reasonable suspicion that a specific allergen is producing symptoms in a patient with allergies. However, several precautionary steps must be observed before skin testing with allergens is performed:

- Testing is not performed during periods of bronchospasm.
- Epicutaneous tests (scratch or prick tests) are performed before other testing methods, in an effort to minimize the risk of systemic reaction.
- Emergency equipment must be readily available to treat anaphylaxis.

Chart 38-1

ASSESSMENT

Allergy Assessment Form

Name _____ Age _____ Sex _____ Date _____

I. Chief complaint: _____

II. Present illness: _____

III. Collateral allergic symptoms: _____

    Eyes: Pruritus _____   Burning _____   Lacrimation _____

               Swelling _____   Injection _____   Discharge _____

    Ears: Pruritus _____   Fullness _____   Popping _____

               Frequent infections _____

    Nose: Sneezing _____   Rhinorrhea _____   Obstruction _____

               Pruritus _____   Mouth breathing _____

               Purulent discharge _____

    Throat: Soreness _____ Postnasal discharge _____

               Palatal pruritus _____ Mucus in the morning _____

    Chest: Cough _____   Pain _____   Wheezing _____

               Sputum _____   Dyspnea _____

               Color _____   Rest _____

               Amount _____   Exertion _____

    Skin: Dermatitis _____   Eczema _____   Urticaria _____

IV. Family allergies: _____

V. Previous allergic treatment or testing: _____

    Prior skin testing: _____

    Medications: Antihistamines   Improved _____   Unimproved _____

                      Bronchodilators   Improved _____   Unimproved _____

                      Nose drops   Improved _____   Unimproved _____

                      Hyposensitization   Improved _____   Unimproved _____

                        Duration _____

                        Antigens _____

                        Reactions _____

                      Antibiotics   Improved _____   Unimproved _____

                      Corticosteroids   Improved _____   Unimproved _____

VI. Physical agents and habits: _____

                              Bothered by:

    Tobacco for _____ years   Alcohol _____   Air-conditioning _____

    Cigarettes _____ packs/day   Heat _____   Muggy weather _____

    Cigars _____ per day   Cold _____   Weather changes _____

    Pipes _____ per day   Perfumes _____   Chemicals _____

    Never smoked _____   Paints _____   Hair spray _____

    Bothered by smoke _____   Insecticides _____   Newspapers _____

                                Cosmetics _____   Latex _____

VII. When symptoms occur: _____

    Time and circumstances of 1st episode: _____

    Prior health: _____

    Course of illness over decades: progressing _____ regressing _____

    Time of year: _____   Exact dates: _____

        Perennial _____

        Seasonal _____

        Seasonally exacerbated _____

    Monthly variations (menses, occupation): _____

    Time of week (weekends vs. weekdays): _____

    Time of day or night: _____

    After insect stings: _____

VIII. Where symptoms occur: _____

    Living where at onset: _____

    Living where since onset: _____

    Effect of vacation or major geographic change: _____

    Symptoms better indoors or outdoors: _____

    Effect of school or work: _____

    Effect of staying elsewhere nearby: _____

    Effect of hospitalization: _____

    Effect of specific environments: _____

    Do symptoms occur around: _____

        old leaves _____ hay _____ lakeside _____ barns _____

        summer homes _____ damp basement _____ dry attic _____

        lawn mowing _____ animals _____ other _____

Chart 38-1

ASSESSMENT
Allergy Assessment Form (continued)

Do symptoms occur after eating:

   cheese _____ mushrooms _____ beer _____ melons _____

   bananas _____ fish _____ nuts _____ citrus fruits _____

   other foods (list) _____

Home: city _____ rural _____

         house _____ age _____

         apartment _____ basement _____ damp _____ dry _____

         heating system _____

         vacuum cleaner system _____ use of HEPA filter _____

         pets (how long) _____ dog _____ cat _____ other _____

Bedroom:	Type	Age	*Living room:*	Type	Age
Pillow	___	___	Rug	___	___
Mattress	___	___	Matting	___	___
Blankets	___	___	Furniture	___	___
Quilts	___	___			
Furniture	___	___			

   Anywhere in home symptoms are worse: _____

IX. What does patient think makes symptoms worse? _____

X. Under what circumstances is patient free of symptoms? _____

XI. Summary and additional comments: _____

Types of Skin Tests

The methods of skin testing include prick skin tests, scratch tests, and intradermal skin testing (Fig. 38-3). After negative prick or scratch tests, intradermal skin testing is performed with allergens that are suggested by the patient's history to be problematic. The back is the most suitable area of the body for skin testing because it permits the performance of many tests. A multitest applicator with multiple test heads is commercially available for simultaneous administration of antigens by multiple punctures at different sites. A negative response on a skin test cannot be interpreted as an absence of sensitivity to an allergen. Such a response may occur with insufficient sensitivity of the test or with the use of an inappropriate allergen in testing. Therefore, it is essential to observe the patient undergoing skin testing for an allergic reaction even if the previous response was negative.

Interpretation of Skin Test Results

Familiarity with and consistent use of a grading system are essential. The grading system used should be identified on a skin test record for later interpretation. A positive reaction, evidenced by the appearance of an urticarial wheal (round, reddened skin elevation) (Fig. 38-4), localized **erythema** (diffuse

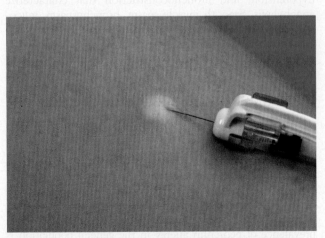

FIGURE 38-3 • Intradermal testing. A 0.5- or 1-mL sterile syringe with a 26/27-gauge intradermal needle is used to inject 0.02 to 0.03 mL of intradermal allergen. The needle is inserted with the bevel facing upward and the syringe parallel to the skin. The skin is penetrated superficially, and a small amount of the allergen solution is injected to create a bleb (raised area) approximately 5 mm in diameter. A separate sterile syringe and needle are used for each injection. From Taylor, C., Lillis C., LeMone, P., & Lynn, P. (2011). *Fundamentals of nursing: The art and science of nursing care* (7th ed.). Philadelphia: Lippincott Williams & Wilkins.

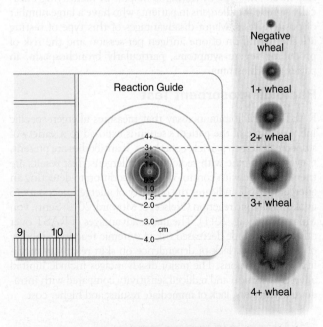

FIGURE 38-4 • Interpretation of reactions: Negative = wheal soft with minimal erythema; 1+ = wheal present (5 to 8 mm) with associated erythema; 2+ = wheal (7 to 10 mm) with associated erythema; 3+ = wheal (9 to 15 mm), slight pseudopodia possible with associated erythema; 4+ = wheal (12 mm+) with pseudopodia and diffuse erythema.

redness) in the area of inoculation or contact, or pseudopodia (irregular projection at the end of a wheal) with associated erythema is considered indicative of sensitivity to the corresponding antigen. False-positive results may occur because of improper preparation or administration of allergen solutions.

 Quality and Safety Nursing Alert

Corticosteroids and antihistamines, including over-the-counter allergy medications, suppress skin test reactivity and should be stopped 48 to 96 hours before testing, depending on the duration of their activity. False-positive results may occur because of improper preparation or administration of allergen solutions.

Interpretation of positive or negative skin tests must be based on the history, physical examination, and other laboratory test results. The following guidelines are used for the interpretation of skin test results:
- Skin tests are more reliable for diagnosing atopic sensitivity in patients with allergic rhinoconjunctivitis than in patients with asthma (Bachert, Claeys, Tomassen, et al., 2010).
- Positive skin tests correlate highly with food allergy.
- The use of skin tests to diagnose immediate hypersensitivity to medications is limited, because metabolites of medications, not the medications themselves, are usually responsible for causing hypersensitivity.

Provocative Testing

Provocative testing involves the direct administration of the suspected allergen to the sensitive tissue, such as the conjunctiva, nasal or bronchial mucosa, or gastrointestinal tract (by ingestion of the allergen), with observation of target organ response. This type of testing is helpful in identifying clinically significant allergens in patients who have a large number of positive tests. Major disadvantages of this type of testing are the limitation of one antigen per session and the risk of producing severe symptoms, particularly bronchospasm, in patients with asthma.

Radioallergosorbent Test

RAST is a radioimmunoassay that measures allergen-specific IgE. A sample of the patient's serum is exposed to a variety of suspected allergen particle complexes. If antibodies are present, they will combine with radiolabeled allergens. Test results are then compared with control values. In addition to detecting an allergen, RAST indicates the quantity of allergen necessary to evoke an allergic reaction (Nelson & Moward, 2010; Senti, von Moos, & Kündig, 2011). The major advantages of RAST over other tests include decreased risk of systemic reaction, stability of antigens, and lack of dependence on skin reactivity modified by medications. The major disadvantages include limited allergen selection and reduced sensitivity compared with intradermal skin tests, lack of immediate results, and higher cost.

ALLERGIC DISORDERS

There are two types of IgE-mediated allergic reactions: atopic and nonatopic disorders. Although the underlying immunologic reactions of the two types of disorders are the same, the predisposing factors and manifestations are different. The atopic disorders are characterized by a hereditary predisposition and production of a local reaction to IgE antibodies, which manifests in one or more of the following three atopic disorders: allergic rhinitis, asthma, and atopic dermatitis/eczema. The nonatopic disorders lack the genetic component and organ specificity of the atopic disorders (Porth & Matfin, 2009). Latex allergy (see later discussion) may be a type I or type IV hypersensitivity reaction, although true latex allergy is considered to be a type I hypersensitivity reaction (Adkinson, Busse, Bochner, et al., 2009; American Academy of Allergy, Asthma, & Immunology [AAAAI], 2011). Contact dermatitis is considered to be a type IV hypersensitivity reaction.

Anaphylaxis

Anaphylaxis is a clinical response to an immediate (type I hypersensitivity) immunologic reaction between a specific antigen and an antibody. The reaction results from a rapid release of IgE-mediated chemicals, which can induce a severe, life-threatening allergic reaction. It is estimated that between 33 and 43 million people in the United States are at risk for anaphylaxis (Arnold & Williams, 2011; Munn, 2009; Solensky, 2011).

Pathophysiology

Anaphylaxis is caused by the interaction of a foreign antigen with specific IgE antibodies found on the surface membrane of mast cells and peripheral blood basophils. The subsequent release of histamine and other bioactive mediators causes activation of platelets, eosinophils, and neutrophils. Histamine, prostaglandins, and inflammatory leukotrienes are potent vasoactive mediators that are implicated in the vascular permeability changes, flushing, urticaria, angioedema, hypotension, and bronchoconstriction that characterize anaphylaxis. Smooth muscle spasm, bronchospasm, mucosal edema and inflammation, and increased capillary permeability result. These systemic changes characteristically produce clinical manifestations within seconds or minutes after antigen exposure (Arnold & Williams, 2011; Solensky, 2011). Closely related to anaphylaxis is a nonallergenic anaphylaxis (anaphylactoid) reaction, which is described in Chart 38-2.

Substances that most commonly cause anaphylaxis include foods, medications, insect stings, and latex (Chart 38-3). Antibiotics and radiocontrast agents cause the most serious anaphylactic reactions, producing reactions in about 1 of every 5,000 exposures. Penicillin is the most common cause of anaphylaxis and accounts for about 75% of fatal anaphylactic reactions in the United States each year. The actual prevalence of penicillin allergy in the general population is unknown; however, the incidence of self-reported penicillin allergy ranges from 1% to 10%. It has been reported that 80% to 90% of those patients with self-reported penicillin allergy have no evidence of IgE antibodies to penicillin on skin testing (Adkinson et al., 2009; Solensky, 2011).

The diagnosis of risk of anaphylaxis is determined by prick and intradermal skin testing. Skin testing of patients who

Nonallergenic Anaphylaxis (Anaphylactoid Reaction)

Closely resembling anaphylaxis is an anaphylactoid reaction, which is caused by the release of mast cell and basophil mediators triggered by non–immunoglobulin E (IgE)-mediated events. This nonallergenic anaphylaxis reaction may occur with medications, food, exercise, or cytotoxic antibody transfusions. The reaction may be local or systemic. Local reactions usually involve urticaria and angioedema at the site of the antigen exposure. Although possibly severe, nonallergenic anaphylaxis reactions are rarely fatal. Systemic reactions occur within about 30 minutes after exposure and involve cardiovascular, respiratory, gastrointestinal, and integumentary organ systems. For the most part, the treatment of nonallergenic anaphylaxis reaction is identical to that of anaphylaxis.

Adapted from Holgate, S. T., Church, M., Bromid, D., et al. (2011). *Allergy*. Philadelphia: Elsevier Health Sciences.

have clinical symptoms consistent with a type I, IgE-mediated reaction has been recommended (Adkinson et al., 2009).

Clinical Manifestations

Anaphylactic reactions produce a clinical syndrome that affects multiple organ systems. Reactions may be categorized as mild, moderate, or severe. The time from exposure to the antigen to onset of symptoms is a good indicator of the severity of the reaction—the faster the onset, the more severe the reaction. The severity of previous reactions does not determine the severity of subsequent reactions, which could be the same or more or less severe. The severity depends on the degree of allergy and the dose of allergen (Holgate, Church, Bromid, et al., 2011; Peakman & Vergani, 2009; Solensky, 2011).

Mild systemic reactions consist of peripheral tingling and a sensation of warmth, possibly accompanied by a sensation of fullness in the mouth and throat. Nasal congestion, periorbital

Common Causes of Anaphylaxis

Foods

Peanuts, tree nuts (e.g., walnuts, pecans, cashews, almonds), shellfish (e.g., shrimp, lobster, crab), fish, milk, eggs, soy, wheat

Medications

Antibiotics, especially penicillin and sulfa antibiotics, allopurinol, radiocontrast agents, anesthetic agents (lidocaine, procaine), vaccines, hormones (insulin, vasopressin, adrenocorticotropic hormone), aspirin, nonsteroidal anti-inflammatory drugs

Other Pharmaceutical/Biologic Agents

Animal serums (tetanus antitoxin, snake venom antitoxin, rabies antitoxin), antigens used in skin testing

Insect Stings

Bees, wasps, hornets, yellow jackets, ants (including fire ants)

Latex

Medical and nonmedical products containing latex

swelling, pruritus, sneezing, and tearing of the eyes can also be expected. Onset of symptoms begins within the first 2 hours after exposure.

Moderate systemic reactions may include flushing, warmth, anxiety, and itching in addition to any of the milder symptoms. More serious reactions include bronchospasm and edema of the airways or larynx with dyspnea, cough, and wheezing. The onset of symptoms is the same as for a mild reaction.

Severe systemic reactions have an abrupt onset with the same signs and symptoms described previously. These symptoms progress rapidly to bronchospasm, laryngeal edema, severe dyspnea, cyanosis, and hypotension. Dysphagia (difficulty swallowing), abdominal cramping, vomiting, diarrhea, and seizures can also occur. Cardiac arrest and coma may follow.

Prevention

Strict avoidance of potential allergens is an important preventive measure for the patient at risk for anaphylaxis. Those at risk for anaphylaxis from insect stings should avoid areas populated by insects and should use appropriate clothing, insect repellent, and caution to avoid further stings.

If avoidance of exposure to allergens is impossible, an auto-injector system for epinephrine will be prescribed. The patient should be instructed to carry and administer epinephrine to prevent an anaphylactic reaction in the event of exposure to the allergen. People who are sensitive to insect bites and stings, those who have experienced food or medication reactions, and those who have experienced idiopathic or exercise-induced anaphylactic reactions should always carry an emergency kit that contains epinephrine. The EpiPen Auto-Injector is a commercially available first aid device that delivers premeasured doses of 0.3 mg (EpiPen) or 0.15 mg (EpiPen Jr.) of epinephrine (Karch, 2012). The auto-injector system requires no preparation, and the self-administration technique is not complicated. The patient must be given an opportunity to demonstrate the correct technique for use; an EpiPen training device can be used for educating about the correct technique. Verbal and written information about the emergency kit, as well as strategies to avoid exposure to threatening allergens, must also be provided.

Screening for allergies before a medication is prescribed or first administered is an important preventive measure. A careful history of any sensitivity to suspected antigens must be obtained before administering any medication, particularly in parenteral form, because this route is associated with the most severe anaphylaxis. Nurses caring for patients in any setting (hospital, home, outpatient diagnostic testing sites, long-term care facilities) must assess patients' risks for anaphylactic reactions. Patients are asked about previous exposure to contrast agents used for diagnostic tests and any allergic reactions, as well as reactions to any medications, foods, insect stings, and latex. People who are predisposed to anaphylaxis should wear medical identification such as a bracelet or necklace, which names allergies to medications, food, and other substances.

People who are allergic to insect venom may require venom immunotherapy, which is used as a control measure and not a cure. The most common serious allergic reactions to insect stings are from the Hymenoptera family, which includes honeybees, fire ants, and wasps (Tracy, 2011). Immunotherapy administered after an insect sting is very effective in reducing the risk of anaphylaxis from future stings (Arcangelo & Peterson, 2013; Peakman & Vergani, 2009; Tracy, 2011). Insulin-allergic patients with diabetes and those who are allergic to penicillin may require desensitization. Desensitization is based on controlled anaphylaxis, with a gradual release of mediators. Patients who undergo desensitization are cautioned to avoid lapses in therapy, because this may lead to the reappearance of the allergic reaction when the use of the medication is resumed.

Medical Management

Management depends on the severity of the reaction. Initially, respiratory and cardiovascular functions are evaluated. If the patient is in cardiac arrest, cardiopulmonary resuscitation (CPR) is instituted (Neumar, Otto, Link, et al., 2010). Supplemental oxygen is provided during CPR or if the patient is cyanotic, dyspneic, or wheezing. Epinephrine, in a 1:1,000 dilution, is administered subcutaneously in the upper extremity or thigh and may be followed by a continuous intravenous infusion. Most adverse events associated with administration of epinephrine (i.e., adrenaline) occur when the dose is excessive or is given intravenously. Patients at risk for adverse effects include older patients and those with hypertension, arteriopathies, or known ischemic heart disease.

Antihistamines and corticosteroids may also be administered to prevent recurrences of the reaction (Goroll & Mulley, 2009; Tracy, 2011) and to treat urticaria (Schaefer, 2011) and angioedema. Intravenous fluids (e.g., normal saline solution), volume expanders, and vasopressor agents are administered to maintain blood pressure and normal hemodynamic status. In patients with episodes of bronchospasm or a history of bronchial asthma or chronic obstructive pulmonary disease, aminophylline and corticosteroids may also be administered to improve airway patency and function. (See Chapter 14 for management of anaphylactic shock.)

Patients who have experienced anaphylactic reactions and received epinephrine should be transported to the local emergency department for observation and monitoring because of the risk for a "rebound" or delayed reaction 4 to 10 hours after the initial allergic reaction. Patients with severe reactions are monitored closely for 12 to 14 hours in a facility that can provide emergency care, if needed. Because of the potential for recurrence, patients with even mild reactions must be informed about this risk (Arnold & Williams, 2011; Munn, 2009).

Nursing Management

If a patient is experiencing an allergic response, the nurse's initial action is to assess the patient for signs and symptoms of anaphylaxis. The nurse assesses the airway, breathing pattern, and vital signs. The patient is observed for signs of increasing edema and respiratory distress. Prompt notification of the rapid response team and/or the provider is required. Rapid initiation of emergency measures

(intubation, administration of emergency medications, insertion of intravenous lines, fluid administration, and oxygen administration) are important to reduce the severity of the reaction and to restore cardiovascular function. The nurse documents the interventions used and the patient's vital signs and response to treatment.

The patient who has recovered from anaphylaxis needs an explanation of what occurred, instruction about avoiding future exposure to antigens, and how to administer emergency medications to treat anaphylaxis. The patient must be instructed about antigens that should be avoided and about other strategies to prevent recurrence of anaphylaxis. All patients who have experienced an anaphylactic reaction should receive a prescription for preloaded syringes of epinephrine. The nurse instructs the patient and family in their use and has the patient and family demonstrate correct administration (Chart 38-4).

Allergic Rhinitis

Allergic **rhinitis** (hay fever, seasonal allergic rhinitis) is the most common form of respiratory allergy, which is presumed to be mediated by an immediate (type I hypersensitivity) immunologic reaction and is among the top 10 reasons for visits to primary providers (Lambert, 2009; Mayhew, 2009; Wallengren, 2011). It affects about 31 million Americans and results in approximately 20 million primary care visits each year (Shoup, 2011). Symptoms are similar to those of viral rhinitis (see Chapter 22) but are usually more persistent and demonstrate seasonal variation; rhinitis is considered to be the allergic form if the symptoms are caused by an allergen-specific IgE-mediated immunologic response. However, a sizable proportion of patients with rhinitis have mixed rhinitis, or coexisting allergic and nonallergic rhinitis (Shoup, 2011). The proportion of patients with the allergic form of rhinitis increases with age. It often occurs with other conditions, such as allergic conjunctivitis, sinusitis, and asthma (Dykewicz & Hamilos, 2010). If symptoms are severe, allergic rhinitis may interfere with sleep, leisure, and school or work activities (Lambert, 2009; Shoup, 2011). If left untreated, many complications may result, such as allergic asthma, chronic nasal obstruction, chronic otitis media with hearing loss, and anosmia (absence of the sense of smell). Early diagnosis and adequate treatment are essential to reduce complications and relieve symptoms.

Because allergic rhinitis is induced by airborne pollens or molds, it is characterized by the following seasonal occurrences:
* Early spring—tree pollen (oak, elm, poplar)
* Early summer—rose pollen (rose fever), grass pollen (Timothy, Redtop)
* Early fall—weed pollen (ragweed)

Each year, attacks begin and end at about the same time. Airborne mold spores require warm, damp weather. Although there is no rigid seasonal pattern, these spores appear in early spring, are rampant during the summer, then taper off and disappear by the first frost in areas that experience dramatic seasonal temperature variation. In temperate areas that do not experience freezing temperatures, these allergens, especially mold, can persist throughout the year.

Chart 38-4

PATIENT EDUCATION

Self-Administration of Epinephrine

1. After removing the EpiPen autoinjector from its carrying tube, grasp the unit with the orange tip (injecting end) pointing downward. Form a fist around the unit with the orange tip down; with your other hand, remove the blue safety release cap.

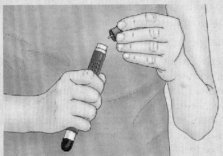

2. Hold the black tip near outer thigh. Swing and **jab firmly** into the outer thigh until a click is heard with the device perpendicular (90-degree angle) to the thigh. Do NOT inject into buttocks.

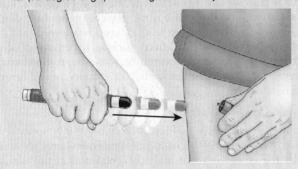

3. Hold firmly against the thigh for approximately 10 seconds. Remove the unit from the thigh, and massage the injection area for 10 seconds. Call 911 and seek immediate medical attention. Carefully place the used EpiPen, needle-end first, into the device storage tube without bending the needle. Screw on the storage tube completely, and take it with you to the hospital emergency room.

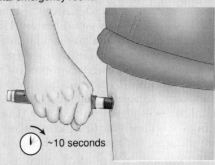

~10 seconds

Pathophysiology

Sensitization begins by ingestion or inhalation of an antigen. On re-exposure, the nasal mucosa reacts by the slowing of ciliary action, edema formation, and leukocyte (primarily eosinophil) infiltration. Histamine is the major mediator of allergic reactions in the nasal mucosa. Tissue edema results from vasodilation and increased capillary permeability.

Clinical Manifestations

Typical signs and symptoms of allergic rhinitis include sneezing and nasal congestion; clear, watery nasal discharge; and nasal itching. Itching of the throat and soft palate is common. Drainage of nasal mucus into the pharynx results in multiple attempts to clear the throat and results in a dry cough or hoarseness. Headache, pain over the paranasal sinuses, and epistaxis can accompany allergic rhinitis. The symptoms of this chronic condition depend on environmental exposure and intrinsic host responsiveness. Allergic rhinitis can affect quality of life by also producing fatigue, loss of sleep, and poor concentration (Lambert, 2009; Shoup, 2011).

Assessment and Diagnostic Findings

Diagnosis of seasonal allergic rhinitis is based on history, physical examination, and diagnostic test results. Diagnostic tests include nasal smears, peripheral blood counts, total serum IgE, epicutaneous and intradermal testing, RAST, food elimination and challenge, and nasal provocation tests. Results indicative of allergy as the cause of rhinitis include increased IgE and eosinophil levels and positive reactions on allergen testing. False-positive and false-negative responses to these tests, particularly skin testing and provocation tests, may occur (Bernstein, Li, Bernstein, et al., 2008).

Medical Management

The goal of therapy is to provide relief from symptoms. Therapy may include one or all of the following interventions: avoidance therapy, pharmacologic therapy, and immunotherapy. Verbal instructions must be reinforced by written information. Knowledge of general concepts regarding assessment and therapy in allergic diseases is important so that the patient can learn to manage certain conditions as well as prevent severe reactions and illnesses.

Avoidance Therapy

In avoidance therapy, every attempt is made to remove the allergens that act as precipitating factors. Simple measures and environmental controls are often effective in decreasing symptoms. Examples include the use of air conditioners, air cleaners, humidifiers, and dehumidifiers; removal of dust-catching furnishings, carpets, and window coverings; removal of pets from the home or bedroom; the use of pillow and mattress covers that are impermeable to dust mites; and a smoke-free environment (Distler, 2011; Lambert, 2009; Shoup, 2011). Additional measures include changing clothing when coming in from outside, showering to wash allergens from hair and skin, and using a Neti Pot (an over-the-counter nasal irrigation device) or saline nasal spray to reduce allergens in the nasal passages (Thornton, Alston, Dye, et al., 2011). Because multiple allergens are often implicated, multiple measures to avoid exposure to allergens are often necessary (Distler, 2011; Shoup, 2011). High-efficiency particulate air (HEPA) purifiers and vacuum cleaner filters may also be used to reduce allergens in the environment. Research suggests that multiple avoidance strategies tailored to a person's risk factors can reduce the severity of symptoms, the number of work or school days missed because of symptoms, and the number of unscheduled health care visits for treatment (Distler, 2011). In many cases, it is impossible to avoid exposure to all environmental allergens, so pharmacologic therapy or immunotherapy is needed.

Pharmacologic Therapy

Antihistamines

Antihistamines, now classified as H_1 receptor antagonists (or H_1 blockers), are used in the management of mild allergic disorders. H_1 blockers bind selectively to H_1 receptors, preventing the actions of histamines at these sites. They do not prevent the release of histamine from mast cells or basophils. The H_1 antagonists have no effect on H_2 receptors, but they do have the ability to bind to nonhistaminic receptors. The ability of certain antihistamines to bind to and block muscarinic receptors underlies several of the prominent anticholinergic side effects of these medications.

Oral antihistamines, which are readily absorbed, are most effective when given at the first occurrence of symptoms, because they prevent the development of new symptoms. The effectiveness of these medications is limited to certain patients with hay fever, vasomotor rhinitis, **urticaria** (hives), and mild asthma. They are rarely effective in other conditions or in any severe conditions.

Antihistamines are the major class of medications prescribed for the symptomatic relief of allergic rhinitis. The major side effect is sedation, although H_1 antagonists are less sedating than earlier antihistamines (Arcangelo & Peterson, 2013; Karch, 2012). Additional side effects include nervousness, tremors, dizziness, dry mouth, palpitations, anorexia, nausea, and vomiting. Antihistamines are contraindicated during the third trimester of pregnancy; in nursing mothers and newborns; in children and older people; and in patients whose conditions may be aggravated by muscarinic blockade (e.g., asthma, urinary retention, open-angle glaucoma, hypertension, prostatic hyperplasia).

Second-generation or nonsedating H_1 receptor antagonists are newer types of antihistamines. Unlike first-generation H_1 receptor antagonists, they do not cross the blood–brain barrier and do not bind to cholinergic, serotonergic, or alpha-adrenergic receptors (Karch, 2012). They bind to peripheral rather than central nervous system H_1 receptors, causing less sedation. Examples of these medications are loratadine (Claritin), cetirizine (Zyrtec), and fexofenadine (Allegra). Selected H_1 antihistamines are shown in Table 38-2.

Antihistamines may also be combined with decongestants to reduce the nasal congestion associated with allergies. Most combination products are available as over-the-counter (nonprescription) medications; examples are loratadine/pseudoephedrine (Claritin-D) and cetirizine/pseudoephedrine (Zyrtec-D). Decongestants can cause an increase in blood pressure; therefore, patients with a history of hypertension should be cautioned about long-term use of any medication that contains decongestants.

Adrenergic Agents

Adrenergic agents, which are vasoconstrictors of mucosal vessels, are used topically in nasal (Afrin) and ophthalmic (Alphagan P) formulations in addition to the oral route (pseudoephedrine [Sudafed]) (Karch, 2012). The topical route (drops and sprays) causes fewer side effects than oral administration; however, the use of drops and sprays should be limited to a few days to avoid rebound congestion. Adrenergic nasal decongestants are applied topically to the nasal mucosa for the relief of nasal congestion. They activate the alpha-adrenergic receptor sites on the smooth muscle of the nasal mucosal blood vessels, reducing local blood flow, fluid exudation, and mucosal edema. Topical ophthalmic drops are used for symptomatic relief of eye irritations caused by allergies. Potential side effects include hypertension, dysrhythmias, palpitations, central nervous system stimulation, irritability, tremor, and tachyphylaxis (acceleration of hemodynamic status).

Mast Cell Stabilizers

Intranasal cromolyn sodium (NasalCrom) is a spray that acts by stabilizing the mast cell membrane, thus reducing the release of histamine and other mediators of the allergic response. In addition, it inhibits macrophages, eosinophils, monocytes, and platelets involved in the immune response (Arcangelo & Peterson, 2013). Cromolyn interrupts the physiologic response to nasal antigens, and it is used prophylactically (before exposure to allergens) to prevent the onset of symptoms and to treat symptoms once they occur. It is also used therapeutically in chronic allergic rhinitis. This spray is as effective as antihistamines but is less effective than intranasal corticosteroids in the treatment of seasonal allergic rhinitis. The patient must be informed that the beneficial effects of the medication may take a week or so to manifest. The medication is of no benefit in the treatment of nonallergic rhinitis. Adverse effects (e.g., sneezing, local stinging and burning sensations) are usually mild.

Corticosteroids

Intranasal corticosteroids are indicated in more severe cases of allergic and perennial rhinitis that cannot be controlled by more conventional medications such as decongestants, antihistamines, and intranasal cromolyn. Examples of these medications include beclomethasone (Beconase, Vancenase), budesonide (Rhinocort), dexamethasone (Aeroseb-Dex), flunisolide (Nasalide), fluticasone (Cutivate, Flonase), and triamcinolone (Nasacort).

Because of their anti-inflammatory actions, corticosteroids are equally effective in preventing or suppressing the major symptoms of allergic rhinitis. These medications are administered by metered-spray devices. If the nasal passages are blocked, a topical decongestant may be used to clear the

TABLE 38-2 Selected H₁ Antihistamines

H₁ Antihistamine	Contraindications	Major Side Effects	Nursing Implications and Patient Education
First-Generation H₁ Antihistamines (Sedating)			
Diphenhydramine (Benadryl)	Allergy to any antihistamines Third trimester of pregnancy Lactation Use cautiously with narrow-angle glaucoma, asthma, stenosing peptic ulcer, benign prostatic hyperplasia (BPH) or bladder neck obstruction, first and second trimester of pregnancy, older patients, hypertension.	Drowsiness, confusion, dizziness, dry mouth, nausea, vomiting, photosensitivity, urinary retention	Administer with food if gastrointestinal (GI) upset occurs. Caution patients to avoid alcohol, driving, or engaging in any hazardous activities until central nervous system (CNS) response to medication is stabilized. Suggest sucking on sugarless lozenges or ice chips for relief of dry mouth. Encourage the use of sunscreen and hat while outdoors. Assess for urinary retention; monitor urinary output.
Chlorpheniramine (Chlor-Trimeton)	Allergy to any antihistamines Third trimester of pregnancy Lactation Use cautiously with narrow-angle glaucoma, asthma, stenosing peptic ulcer, BPH or bladder neck obstruction, first and second trimester of pregnancy, older patients, hypertension.	Drowsiness, sedation, and dizziness, although less than other sedating agents; confusion, dry mouth, nausea, vomiting, urinary retention, epigastric distress, thickening of bronchial secretions	Caution patients to avoid alcohol, driving, or engaging in any hazardous activities until CNS response to medication is stabilized. Suggest sucking on sugarless lozenges or ice chips for relief of dry mouth. Recommend the use of a humidifier.
Hydroxyzine (Atarax)	Allergy to hydroxyzine or cetirizine (Zyrtec), pregnancy, lactation, hypertension	Drowsiness; dry mouth; involuntary motor activity, including tremor and seizures	Caution patients to avoid alcohol, driving, or engaging in any hazardous activities until CNS response to medication is stabilized. Suggest sucking on sugarless lozenges or ice chips for relief of dry mouth. Instruct patients to report tremors.
Second-Generation H₁ Antihistamines (Nonsedating)			
Cetirizine (Zyrtec)	Allergy to any antihistamines Narrow-angle glaucoma Asthma Stenosing peptic ulcer BPH or bladder neck obstruction Lactation Hypertension	Dry nasal mucosa, thickening of bronchial secretions	Can be taken without regard to meals. Instruct patients to use caution if driving or performing tasks that require alertness. Recommend the use of a humidifier.
Desloratadine (Clarinex)	Allergy to loratadine (Alavert, Claritin) Lactation Use cautiously with renal or hepatic impairment, pregnancy, hypertension.	Somnolence, nervousness, dizziness, fatigue, dry mouth	Can be taken without regard to meals. Suggest sucking on sugarless lozenges or ice chips for relief of dry mouth. Recommend the use of a humidifier.
Loratadine (Alavert, Claritin)	Allergy to any antihistamines Narrow-angle glaucoma Asthma Stenosing peptic ulcer BPH or bladder neck obstruction Hypertension	Headache, nervousness, dizziness, depression, edema, increased appetite	Instruct patients to take on empty stomach (1 hour before or 2 hours after meals or food). Instruct patients to avoid alcohol and to use caution if driving or performing tasks that require alertness. Suggest sucking on sugarless lozenges or ice chips for relief of dry mouth. Recommend the use of a humidifier.
Fexofenadine (Allegra)	Allergy to any antihistamines Pregnancy Lactation Use cautiously with hepatic or renal impairment, older patients, hypertension.	Fatigue, drowsiness, GI upset	Should not be administered within 15 minutes of ingestion of antacids. Instruct patients to use caution if driving or performing tasks that require alertness. Recommend the use of a humidifier.
Levocetirizine (Xyzal)	Hypersensitivity to any antihistamines End-stage renal disease Hemodialysis Use cautiously with pregnancy, lactation, older patients.	Drowsiness, GI disturbance, headache	Can be taken without regard to meals. Instruct patients to use caution if driving or performing tasks that require alertness. Recommend the use of a humidifier.

Adapted from Karch, A. M. (2012). *Lippincott's nursing drug guide*. Philadelphia: Lippincott Williams & Wilkins.

passages before the administration of the intranasal corticosteroid. Patients must be aware that full benefit may not be achieved for several days to 2 weeks. Adverse effects of intranasal corticosteroids are mild and include drying of the nasal mucosa and burning and itching sensations caused by the vehicle used to administer the medication. Systemic effects are more likely with dexamethasone. Recommended use of this medication is limited to 30 days. Beclomethasone, budesonide, flunisolide, fluticasone, and triamcinolone are

deactivated rapidly after absorption, so they do not achieve significant blood levels. Because corticosteroids suppress host defenses, they must be used with caution in patients with tuberculosis or untreated bacterial infections of the lungs. Patients taking corticosteroids are at risk for infection and suppression of typical manifestations of inflammation, because host defenses are compromised. Inhaled corticosteroids do not affect the immune system to the same degree as systemic corticosteroids (i.e., oral corticosteroids). Because corticosteroids are inhaled into the upper respiratory tract, tuberculosis or untreated bacterial infections of the lungs may become apparent and progress. Whenever possible, patients with tuberculosis or other bacterial infections of the lungs should avoid inhaled corticosteroids.

Oral and parenteral corticosteroids are used when conventional therapy has failed and symptoms are severe and of short duration (Karch, 2012). They can control symptoms of allergic reactions such as hay fever, medication-induced allergies, and allergic reactions to insect stings. Because the response to corticosteroids is delayed, these agents have little or no value in acute therapy for severe reactions such as anaphylaxis.

 Quality and Safety Nursing Alert

Patients who receive high-dose or long-term corticosteroid therapy must be cautioned not to stop taking the medication suddenly. Doses are tapered when discontinuing this medication to avoid adrenal insufficiency.

The patient is also instructed about side effects, which include fluid retention, weight gain, hypertension, gastric irritation, glucose intolerance, and adrenal suppression. Further discussion of corticosteroids is provided in Chapter 52, Table 52-4.

Leukotriene Modifiers

As discussed previously, leukotrienes have many effects on the inflammatory cycle. Leukotriene modifiers, such as zileuton (Zyflo), zafirlukast (Accolate), and montelukast (Singulair), block the synthesis or action of leukotrienes and prevent the signs and symptoms associated with asthma (Table 38-3).

Leukotriene modifiers are for long-term use, and patients should be advised to take their medication daily. Patients take appropriate "rescue" medications for symptom exacerbation but continue to take the leukotriene modifier on a daily basis. The National Asthma Education and Prevention Program (NAEPP) suggests using a leukotriene modifier in conjunction with an inhaled corticosteroid for mild persistent asthma (National Heart, Lung, and Blood Institute, 2007).

Immunotherapy

Allergen desensitization (allergen immunotherapy, hyposensitization) is primarily used to treat IgE-mediated diseases by injections of allergen extracts. Immunotherapy, also referred to as allergy vaccine therapy, involves the

Chart 38-5 Immunotherapy: Indications and Contraindications

Indications

- Allergic rhinitis, conjunctivitis, or allergic asthma
- History of a systemic reaction to Hymenoptera and specific immunoglobulin E antibodies to Hymenoptera venom
- Desire to avoid the long-term use, potential adverse effects, or costs of medications
- Lack of control of symptoms by avoidance measures or the use of medications

Contraindications

- The use of beta-blocker or angiotensin-converting enzyme inhibitor therapy, which may mask early signs of anaphylaxis
- Presence of significant pulmonary or cardiac disease or organ failure
- Inability of the patient to recognize or report signs and symptoms of a systemic reaction
- Nonadherence of the patient to other therapeutic regimens and nonlikelihood that the patient will adhere to the immunization schedule (often weekly for an indefinite period)
- Inability to monitor the patient for at least 30 minutes after administration of immunotherapy
- Absence of equipment or adequate personnel to respond to allergic reaction if one occurs

administration of gradually increasing quantities of specific allergens to the patient until a dose is reached that is effective in reducing disease severity from natural exposure (Fitzhugh & Lockey, 2011; Goroll & Mulley, 2009; Grateau & Duruöz, 2010). This type of therapy provides an adjunct to symptomatic pharmacologic therapy and can be used when avoidance of allergens is not possible. Specific immunotherapy has been used in the treatment of allergic disorders for many years. Goals of immunotherapy include reducing the level of circulating IgE, increasing the level of blocking antibody IgG, and reducing mediator cell sensitivity. Immunotherapy has been most effective for ragweed pollen; however, treatment for grass, tree pollen, cat dander, and house dust mite allergens has also been effective. Indications and contraindications for immunotherapy are presented in Chart 38-5.

Correlation of a positive skin test with a positive allergy history is an indication for immunotherapy if the allergen

TABLE 38-3 Leukotriene Modifiers		
Leukotriene Modifier	**Available Formulations**	**Frequency of Dosing**
Leukotriene-Receptor Antagonists		
Zafirlukast (Accolate)	Tablets: 10 mg; 20 mg	Taken twice a day
Montelukast (Singulair)	Tablets: 10 mg Chewable tablets: 4 mg; 5 mg Granules: 4 mg/packet	Taken once a day in PM
Leukotriene-Receptor Inhibitors		
Zileuton (Zyflo CR)	Tablets: 600 mg extended release	Taken twice a day within 1 hour after morning and evening meals

cannot be avoided. The benefit of immunotherapy has been fairly well established in instances of allergic rhinitis and bronchial asthma that are clearly due to sensitivity to one of the common pollens, molds, or household dust. Unlike antiallergy medication, allergen immunotherapy has the potential to alter the allergic disease course after 3 to 5 years of therapy. Because it may prevent progression or development of asthma or multiple or additional allergies, it is also considered to be a potential preventive measure (Fitzhugh & Lockey, 2011; Goroll & Mulley, 2009). The patient must understand what to expect and the importance of continuing therapy for several years before immunotherapy is accomplished. When skin tests are performed, the results are correlated with symptoms; treatment is based on the patient's needs rather than on the results of skin tests.

The most common method of treatment is the serial injection of one or more antigens that are selected in each particular case on the basis of skin testing. This method provides a simple and efficient technique for identifying IgE antibodies to specific antigens. Specific treatment consists of injecting extracts of the allergens that cause symptoms in a particular patient. Injections begin with very small amounts and are gradually increased, usually at weekly intervals, until a maximum tolerated dose is attained. Maintenance booster injections are administered at 2- to 4-week intervals, frequently for a period of several years, before maximum benefit is achieved, although some patients will note early improvement in their symptoms. Long-term benefit seems to be related to the cumulative dose of vaccine given over time (Fitzhugh & Lockey, 2011). Immunotherapy should not be initiated during pregnancy; for patients who have been receiving immunotherapy before pregnancy, the dosage should not be increased during pregnancy.

Although severe systemic reactions are rare, the risk of systemic and potentially fatal anaphylaxis exists. It tends to occur most frequently at the induction or "up-dosing" phase. Therefore, the patient must be monitored after administration of immunotherapy. Because of the risk of anaphylaxis, injections should not be administered by a lay person or by the patient. The patient must remain in the office or clinic for at least 30 minutes after the injection and is observed for possible systemic symptoms. If a large, local swelling develops at the injection site, the next dose should not be increased, because this may be a warning sign of a possible systemic reaction.

▶ *Quality and Safety Nursing Alert*

Because the injection of an allergen may induce systemic reactions, such injections are administered only in a setting where epinephrine is immediately available (i.e., primary provider's office, clinic).

Therapeutic failure is evident when a patient does not experience a decrease of symptoms within 12 to 24 months, fails to develop increased tolerance to known allergens, and cannot decrease the use of medications to reduce symptoms. Potential causes of treatment failure include misdiagnosis of allergies, inadequate doses of allergen, newly developed allergies, and inadequate environmental controls.

NURSING PROCESS

The Patient With Allergic Rhinitis

Assessment

The examination and history of the patient reveal sneezing, often in paroxysms; thin and watery nasal discharge; itching eyes and nose; lacrimation; and occasionally headache. The health history includes a personal or family history of allergy. The allergy assessment identifies the nature of antigens, seasonal changes in symptoms, and medication history. The nurse also obtains subjective data about how the patient feels just before symptoms become obvious, such as the occurrence of pruritus, breathing problems, and tingling sensations. In addition to these symptoms, hoarseness, wheezing, hives, rash, erythema, and edema are noted. Any relationship between emotional problems or stress and the triggering of allergy symptoms is assessed.

Diagnosis

Nursing Diagnoses

Based on the assessment data, major nursing diagnoses may include:

- Ineffective breathing pattern related to allergic reaction
- Deficient knowledge about allergy and the recommended modifications in lifestyle and self-care practices
- Ineffective coping with chronicity of condition and need for environmental modifications

Collaborative Problems/Potential Complications

Potential complications may include the following:

- Anaphylaxis
- Impaired breathing
- Nonadherence to the therapeutic regimen

Planning and Goals

The goals for the patient may include restoration of normal breathing pattern, increased knowledge about the causes and control of allergic symptoms, improved coping with alterations and modifications, and absence of complications.

Nursing Interventions

Improving Breathing Pattern

The patient is instructed and assisted to modify the environment to reduce the severity of allergic symptoms or to prevent their occurrence. The patient is instructed to reduce exposure to people with upper respiratory tract infections. If an upper respiratory infection occurs, the patient is encouraged to take deep breaths and to cough frequently to ensure adequate gas exchange and prevent atelectasis. The patient is instructed to seek medical attention, because the presence of allergy symptoms along with an upper respiratory tract infection may compromise adequate lung function. Adherence to medication schedules and other treatment regimens is encouraged and reinforced.

Promoting Understanding of Allergy and Allergy Control

Instruction includes strategies to minimize exposure to allergens and explanation about desensitization procedures and correct use of medications. The nurse informs and reminds the patient of the importance of keeping appointments for desensitization procedures, because dosages are usually adjusted on a weekly basis, and missed appointments may interfere with the dosage adjustment.

Patients need to understand the difference between rescue medications for allergy exacerbation and seasonal flares (e.g., antihistamines) and medications used for allergy control throughout the year (e.g., inhaled corticosteroids, leukotriene modifiers). Patients also need to understand that medications for allergy exacerbation and seasonal flares should be used only when the allergy is apparent. Continued use of these medications when not required can cause tolerance to the medication, with the result that the medication will not be effective when needed.

Coping With a Chronic Disorder

Although allergic reactions are infrequently life threatening, they require constant vigilance to avoid allergens and modification of the lifestyle or environment to prevent recurrence of symptoms. Allergic symptoms are often present year-round and create discomfort and inconvenience for the patient. Although patients may not feel ill during allergy seasons, they often do not feel well, either. The need to be alert for possible allergens in the environment may be tiresome, placing a burden on the patient's ability to lead a normal life. Stress related to these difficulties may in turn increase the frequency or severity of symptoms. To assist the patient in adjusting to these modifications, the nurse must have an appreciation of the difficulties encountered by the patient. The patient is encouraged to verbalize feelings and concerns in a supportive environment and to identify strategies to deal with them effectively.

Monitoring and Managing Potential Complications

Anaphylaxis and Impaired Breathing. Respiratory and cardiovascular functioning can be significantly altered during allergic reactions by the reaction itself or by the medications used to treat reactions. The respiratory status is evaluated by monitoring the respiratory rate and pattern and by assessing for breathing difficulties or abnormal lung sounds. The pulse rate and rhythm and blood pressure are monitored to assess cardiovascular status regularly or any time the patient reports symptoms such as itching or difficulty breathing. In the event of signs and symptoms suggestive of anaphylaxis, emergency medications and equipment must be available for immediate use.

Nonadherence to the Therapeutic Regimen. Knowledge about the treatment regimen does not ensure adherence. Having the patient identify potential barriers and explore acceptable solutions for effective management of the condition (e.g., installing tile floors rather than carpet, not gardening in the spring) can increase adherence to the treatment regimen.

Promoting Home and Community-Based Care

Educating Patients About Self-Care. The patient is instructed about strategies to minimize exposure to allergens, the actions and adverse effects of medications, and the correct use of medications. The patient should know the name, dose, frequency, actions, and side effects of all medications taken.

Instruction about strategies to control allergic symptoms is based on the needs of the patient as determined by the results of tests, the severity of symptoms, and the motivation of the patient and family to deal with the condition. Suggestions for patients who are sensitive to dust and mold in the home are given in Chart 38-6. Additional nursing strategies for allergy management are presented in Chart 38-7.

If the patient is to undergo immunotherapy, the nurse reinforces the primary provider's explanation regarding the purpose and procedure. Instructions are given regarding the series of injections, which usually are administered initially every week and then at 2- to 4-week intervals. These instructions include remaining in the primary provider's office or the clinic for at least 30 minutes after the injection so that emergency treatment can be given if the patient has a reaction; avoiding rubbing or scratching the injection site; and continuing with the series for the period of time required. In addition, the patient and family are instructed about emergency treatment of severe allergic symptoms.

Because antihistamines may produce drowsiness, the patient is cautioned about this and other side effects applicable to the medication. Operating machinery, driving a car, and performing activities that require intense concentration should be postponed. The patient is also informed about the dangers of drinking alcohol when taking antihistamines, because they tend to exaggerate the effects of alcohol.

The patient must be aware of the effects caused by overuse of the sympathomimetic agents in nose drops or sprays, because a condition referred to as rhinitis medicamentosa may result. After topical application of the medication, a rebound period occurs in which the nasal mucous membranes become more edematous and congested than they were before the medication was used. Such a reaction encourages the use of more medication, and a cyclic pattern results. The topical agent must be discontinued immediately and completely to correct this problem.

 Concept Mastery Alert

In rhinitis medicamentosa, the rebound reaction from overuse of sympathomimetic nose drops or sprays worsens the congestion, causing the patient to use more of the medication and thus leads to more nasal congestion. This condition should not be confused with a patient developing tolerance to the drug.

Continuing Care. Follow-up telephone calls to the patient are often reassuring to the patient and family and provide an opportunity for the nurse to answer any questions. The patient is reminded to keep follow-up appointments and informed about the importance of continuing with treatment. The importance of participating in health promotion activities and health screening is also emphasized.

Evaluation

Expected patient outcomes may include:
1. Exhibits normal breathing patterns
   a. Demonstrates lungs clear on auscultation
   b. Exhibits absence of adventitious breath sounds (crackles, rhonchi, wheezing)
   c. Has a normal respiratory rate and pattern
   d. Reports no complaints of respiratory distress (shortness of breath, difficulty on inspiration or expiration)

Chart 38-6	HOME CARE CHECKLIST
	Allergy Management

At the completion of home care education, the patient or caregiver will be able to:	PATIENT	CAREGIVER
• Verbalize how to maintain a dust-free environment by removing drapes, curtains, and venetian blinds and replacing them with pull shades; covering the mattress with a hypoallergenic cover that can be zipped; and removing rugs and replacing them with wood flooring or linoleum.	✔	✔
• Identify rationale for washing the floor and dusting and vacuuming daily.	✔	✔
• Identify rationale for replacing stuffed furniture with wood pieces that can easily be dusted.	✔	✔
• State rationale for wearing a mask whenever cleaning is being done.	✔	✔
• Identify rationale for avoiding the use of tufted bedspreads, stuffed toys, and feather pillows and replacing them with washable cotton material.	✔	✔
• State rationale for avoiding the use of any clothing that causes itching.	✔	✔
• Verbalize ways to reduce dust in the house as a whole by using steam or hot water for heating and using air filters or air-conditioning.	✔	✔
• Verbalize ways to reduce exposure to pollens or molds by identifying seasons of the year when pollen counts are high; wearing a mask at times of increased exposure (windy days and when grass is being cut); and avoiding contact with weeds, dry leaves, and freshly cut grass.	✔	✔
• State rationale for seeking air-conditioned areas at the height of the allergy season.	✔	✔
• State rationale for avoiding sprays and perfumes.	✔	✔
• State rationale for the use of hypoallergenic cosmetics.	✔	
• State rationale for taking prescribed medications as ordered.	✔	✔
• Identify specific foods that may cause allergic symptoms. (Examples of foods that can cause allergic reactions are fish, nuts, eggs, and chocolate.)	✔	✔
• Develop a list of foods to avoid.	✔	✔

Chart 38-7	Selected Nursing Strategies for Allergy Management

- Identify the patient's known allergens (e.g., medications, foods, insects, environmental allergens).
- Describe the patient's typical allergic reaction and its severity.
- Document the patient's allergies (e.g., medications, foods, insects, environmental allergens) in the patient's medical record.
- Post allergy alerts appropriately.
- Encourage the patient to wear a medical alert band and to carry information about allergies at all times.
- Monitor the patient closely after administration of new medications and exposure to new foods, contrast agents, latex, and other allergens.
- Investigate potential for allergic reactions with all new medications through consultation with the pharmacist.
- Instruct the patient to question all medications and new foods.
- Identify early manifestations of allergic reactions.
- Administer emergency treatment for allergic reactions.
- Monitor the patient's response and status for 12–14 hours after a severe allergic reaction.
- Educate the patient and family about emergency home management of allergic reaction.
- Educate the patient and family about avoidance measures to reduce risk of exposure to allergens.

2. Demonstrates knowledge about allergy and strategies to control symptoms
   a. Identifies causative allergens, if known
   b. States methods of avoiding allergens and controlling indoor and outdoor precipitating factors
   c. Removes from the environment items that retain dust
   d. Wears a dampened mask if dust or mold may be a problem
   e. Avoids smoke-filled rooms and dust-filled or freshly sprayed areas
   f. Uses air-conditioning for a major part of the day when allergens are high
   g. Takes antihistamines as prescribed; participates in hyposensitization program, if applicable
   h. Describes name, purpose, side effects, and method of administration of prescribed medications
   i. Identifies when to seek immediate medical attention for severe allergic responses
   j. Describes activities that are possible, including ways to participate in activities without activating the allergies
3. Adapts to the inconveniences of an allergy
   a. Relates the emotional aspects of the allergic response
   b. Demonstrates the use of measures to cope positively with allergy
4. Demonstrates absence of complications
   a. Exhibits vital signs within normal limits
   b. Reports no symptoms or episodes of anaphylaxis (urticaria, itching, peripheral tingling, fullness in

the mouth and throat, flushing, difficulty swallowing, coughing, wheezing, or difficulty breathing)
  c. Demonstrates correct procedure to self-administer emergency medications to treat severe allergic reaction
  d. Correctly states medication names, dose and frequency of administration, and medication actions
  e. Correctly identifies side effects and untoward signs and symptoms to report to primary provider
  f. Discusses acceptable lifestyle changes and solutions for identified potential barriers to adherence to treatment and medication regimen

Contact Dermatitis

Contact dermatitis, a type IV delayed hypersensitivity reaction, is an acute or chronic skin inflammation that results from direct skin contact with chemicals or allergens. There are four basic types: allergic, irritant, phototoxic, and photoallergic (Table 38-4). Eighty percent of cases are caused by excessive exposure to or additive effects of irritants (e.g., soaps, detergents, organic solvents). Skin sensitivity may develop after brief or prolonged periods of exposure, and the clinical picture may appear hours or weeks after the sensitized skin has been exposed.

Clinical Manifestations

Symptoms include itching, burning, erythema, skin lesions (vesicles), and edema, followed by weeping, crusting, and finally drying and peeling of the skin. In severe responses, hemorrhagic bullae may develop. Repeated reactions may be accompanied by thickening of the skin and pigmentary changes. Secondary invasion by bacteria may develop in skin that is abraded by rubbing or scratching. Usually, there are no systemic symptoms unless the eruption is widespread.

Assessment and Diagnostic Findings

The location of the skin eruption and the history of exposure aid in determining the condition. However, in cases of obscure irritants or an unobservant patient, the diagnosis can be extremely difficult, often involving many trial-and-error procedures before the cause is determined. Patch tests on the skin with suspected offending agents may clarify the diagnosis. The patch test most commonly used is the Thin-layer Rapid Use Epicutaneous (T.R.U.E.) test (Nelson & Moward, 2010).

Atopic Dermatitis

Atopic dermatitis is a type I immediate hypersensitivity disorder characterized by inflammation and hyperreactivity of the skin. Other terms used to describe this skin disorder include *atopic eczema, atopic dermatitis*, and atopic dermatitis/eczema syndrome (AEDS). In a revised classification system developed to clarify terminology, AEDS includes both allergic and nonallergic disorders (Nelson & Moward, 2010). Currently, *atopic dermatitis* is the most commonly used term and will be used for the purpose of this discussion.

Atopic dermatitis affects 15% to 20% of children and 1% to 3% of adults in developed countries (Goroll & Mulley, 2009). Most patients have significant elevations of serum IgE and peripheral eosinophilia. Pruritus and hyperirritability of

TABLE 38-4	Types, Testing, and Treatment of Contact Dermatitis			
Type	**Etiology**	**Clinical Presentation**	**Diagnostic Testing**	**Treatment**
Allergic	Results from contact of skin and allergenic substance; has a sensitization period of 10–14 days	Vasodilation and perivascular infiltrates on the dermis Intracellular edema Usually seen on dorsal aspects of hand	Patch testing (contraindicated in acute, widespread dermatitis)	Avoidance of offending material Aluminum acetate (Burow's Solution, Domeboro Powder) or cool water compress Systemic corticosteroids (prednisone) for 7–10 days Topical corticosteroids for mild cases Oral antihistamines to relieve pruritus
Irritant	Results from contact with a substance that chemically or physically damages the skin on a nonimmunologic basis; occurs after first exposure to irritant or repeated exposures to milder irritants over an extended time	Dryness lasting days to months Vesiculation, fissures, cracks Hands and lower arms most common areas	Clinical picture Appropriate negative patch tests	Identification and removal of source of irritation Application of hydrophilic cream or petrolatum to soothe and protect Topical corticosteroids and compresses for weeping lesions Antibiotics for infection and oral antihistamines for pruritus
Phototoxic	Resembles the irritant type but requires sun and a chemical in combination to damage the epidermis	Similar to irritant dermatitis	Photo-patch test	Same as for allergic and irritant dermatitis
Photoallergic	Resembles allergic dermatitis but requires light exposure in addition to allergen contact to produce immunologic reactivity	Similar to allergic dermatitis	Photo-patch test	Same as for allergic and irritant dermatitis

Adapted from Karch, A. M. (2012). *Lippincott's nursing drug guide*. Philadelphia: Lippincott Williams & Wilkins.

the skin are the most consistent features of atopic dermatitis and are related to large amounts of histamine in the skin. Excessive dryness of the skin with resultant itching is related to changes in lipid content, sebaceous gland activity, and sweating. In response to stroking of the skin, immediate redness appears on the skin. Pallor follows in 15 to 30 seconds and persists for 1 to 3 minutes. Lesions develop secondary to the trauma of scratching and appear in areas of increased sweating and hypervascularity. Atopic dermatitis is chronic, with remissions and exacerbations. This condition has a tendency to recur, with remission from adolescence to 20 years of age.

Nurses should be aware that atopic dermatitis is often the first step in a process that leads to asthma and allergic rhinitis (Brozek, Bousquet, Baena-Cagnani, et al., 2010). It is the result of interactions between susceptibility genes, the environment, defective function of the skin barrier, and immunologic responses.

Medical Management

Treatment of patients with atopic dermatitis must be individualized. Guidelines for treatment include decreasing itching and scratching by wearing cotton fabrics; washing with a mild detergent; humidifying dry heat in winter; maintaining room temperature at 20°C to 22.2°C (68°F to 72°F); using antihistamines such as diphenhydramine (Benadryl); and avoiding animals, dust, sprays, and perfumes. Keeping the skin moisturized with daily baths to hydrate the skin and the use of topical skin moisturizers is encouraged. Topical corticosteroids are used to prevent inflammation, and any infection is treated with antibiotics to eliminate *Staphylococcus aureus* when indicated. The use of immunosuppressive agents, such as cyclosporine (Neoral, Sandimmune), tacrolimus (Prograf, Protopic), and pimecrolimus (Elidel), may be effective in inhibiting T cells and mast cells involved in atopic dermatitis (Nijhawan, Matiz, & Jacob, 2009). Research is needed to assess the effectiveness and the adverse side effects of medications used to treat atopic dermatitis.

Nursing Management

Patients who experience atopic dermatitis and their families require assistance and support from the nurse to cope with the disorder. The symptoms are often disturbing to the patient and disruptive to the family. The appearance of the skin may affect the patient's self-esteem and his or her willingness to interact with others. Instructions and counseling about strategies to incorporate preventive measures and treatments into the lifestyle of the family may be helpful.

The patient and family need to be aware of signs of secondary infection and of the need to seek treatment if infection occurs. The nurse also educates the patient and family about the side effects of medications used in treatment.

Dermatitis Medicamentosa (Drug Reactions)

Dermatitis medicamentosa, a type I hypersensitivity disorder, is the term applied to skin rashes associated with certain medications. Although people react differently to each medication, certain medications tend to induce eruptions of similar types. Rashes are among the most common adverse reactions to medications and occur in approximately 2% to 3% of hospitalized patients (Karch, 2012).

In general, drug reactions appear suddenly, have a particularly vivid color, manifest with characteristics that are more intense than the somewhat similar eruptions of infectious origin, and, with the exception of bromide and the iodide rashes, disappear rapidly after the medication is withdrawn (Karch 2012). Rashes may be accompanied by systemic or generalized symptoms. On discovery of a medication allergy, patients are warned that they have a hypersensitivity to a particular medication and are advised not to take it again. Patients should carry information identifying the hypersensitivity with them at all times.

Skin eruptions related to medication therapy suggest more serious hypersensitivities. Frequent assessment and prompt reporting of the appearance of any eruptions are important so that early treatment can be initiated. Some cutaneous drug reactions may indicate involvement of other organs and are known as complex drug reactions. Patients who suspect that a new rash may be caused by a drug allergy (newly prescribed medications, especially antibiotics such as penicillin or sulfa medications) should stop taking the medication immediately and contact their prescribing clinician, who will determine whether the medication and the rash are related.

Urticaria and Angioneurotic Edema

Urticaria (hives) is a type I hypersensitive allergic reaction of the skin that is characterized by the sudden appearance of pinkish, edematous elevations that vary in size and shape, itch, and cause local discomfort. They may involve any part of the body, including the mucous membranes (especially those of the mouth), the larynx (occasionally with serious respiratory complications), and the gastrointestinal tract.

Each hive remains for a few minutes to several hours before disappearing. For hours or days, clusters of these lesions may come, go, and return episodically. If this sequence continues for longer than 6 weeks, the condition is called *chronic urticaria*.

Angioneurotic edema (i.e., angioedema) involves the deeper layers of the skin, resulting in more diffuse swelling rather than the discrete lesions characteristic of hives. On occasion, this reaction covers the entire back. The skin over the reaction may appear normal but often has a reddish hue. The skin does not pit on pressure, as ordinary edema does. The regions most often involved are the lips, eyelids, cheeks, hands, feet, genitalia, and tongue; the mucous membranes of the larynx, bronchi, and gastrointestinal canal may also be affected, particularly in the hereditary type (see discussion in the following section). Swellings may appear suddenly, in a few seconds or minutes, or slowly in 1 or 2 hours. In the latter case, their appearance is often preceded by itching or burning sensations. Seldom does more than a single swelling appear at one time, although one may develop while another is disappearing. Infrequently, swelling recurs in the same region. Individual lesions usually last 24 to 36 hours. On rare occasions, swelling may recur with remarkable regularity at intervals of 3 to 4 weeks.

Several frequently prescribed medications, such as angiotensin-converting enzyme inhibitors and penicillin, may cause angioedema. The nurse needs to be aware of all medications the patient is taking and be alert to the potential of angioedema as a side effect.

Hereditary Angioedema

Hereditary angioedema is a rare, potentially life-threatening condition that affects approximately 1 in 50,000 people (Sardana & Craig, 2011). It is inherited as an autosomal dominant trait (Adkinson et al., 2009; Sardana & Craig, 2011). Although not an immunologic disorder in the usual sense, this condition is included because of its resemblance to allergic angioedema and because of the potential seriousness of the condition. Symptoms are caused by edema of the skin, the respiratory tract, or the digestive tract. Attacks may be precipitated by trauma, or they may seem to occur spontaneously.

Clinical Manifestations

When skin is involved, the swelling usually is diffuse, does not itch, and usually is not accompanied by urticaria. Gastrointestinal edema may cause abdominal pain severe enough to suggest the need for surgery. Typically, attacks last 1 to 4 days and are harmless; however, attacks can occasionally affect the subcutaneous and submucosal tissues in the region of the upper airway and can be associated with respiratory obstruction and asphyxiation.

Medical Management

Attacks usually subside within 3 to 4 days, but during this time the patient should be observed carefully for signs of laryngeal obstruction, which may necessitate tracheostomy as a lifesaving measure. Epinephrine, antihistamines, and corticosteroids are usually used in treatment, although their success is limited.

Cold Urticaria

Familial atypical cold urticaria (FACU) and acquired cold urticaria (ACU) are fairly newly described diseases within the spectrum of physical urticaria induced by temperature exposure. FACU is an autosomal dominant condition, inherited from one affected parent, and symptoms usually begin at birth (Grateau & Duruöz, 2010). ACU most frequently affects young adults between 18 and 25 years of age and is commonly associated with the more common physical urticarias. Why a cold stimulus causes the activation of mast cells and subsequent release inflammatory mediators and histamine is unknown. Most cases are idiopathic (Dyall-Smith, 2011).

Clinical Manifestations

Patients with cold urticaria break out in hives (i.e., urticaria) when exposed to cold. The urticaria may be prompted by exposure to cold weather or cold water or after coming in contact with cold objects. In some patients, holding an ice cube in the hand can spark the reaction. The clinical manifestations typically last for 5 to 6 years in ACU.

The condition is diagnosed by physical testing. Ice cube provocation testing involves applying an ice cube to the skin of the forearm for 1 to 5 minutes. A positive test results in development of urticaria at the site in a patient with ACU. Clinical manifestations of FACU can be precipitated by the patient merely entering a 4°C (39°F) room.

Medical Management

Prevention involves avoidance of cold stimuli. Treatment involves bed rest, warmth, and corticosteroids to treat an acute attack (Dyall-Smith, 2011; Grateau & Duruöz, 2010). All patients with any form of cold urticaria should carry an EpiPen for emergency use because hives can progress to anaphylaxis.

Food Allergy

IgE-mediated food allergy, a type I hypersensitivity reaction, occurs in about 2% of the adult population; it is thought to occur in people who have a genetic predisposition combined with exposure to allergens early in life through the gastrointestinal or respiratory tract or nasal mucosa. More than 170 foods have been reported to cause IgE-mediated reactions (Boyce, Assa'ad, Burks, et al., 2010). Researchers have also identified a second type of food allergy—a non–IgE-mediated food allergy syndrome in which T cells play a major role.

Almost any food can cause allergic symptoms. Any food can contain an allergen that results in anaphylaxis. The most common offenders are seafood (lobster, shrimp, crab, clams, fish), legumes (peanuts, peas, beans, licorice), seeds (sesame, cottonseed, caraway, mustard, flaxseed, sunflower), tree nuts, berries, egg white, buckwheat, milk, and chocolate. Peanut and tree nut (e.g., cashew, walnut) allergies are responsible for the most severe food allergy reactions (Fitzharris & Sinclair, 2011; Johnson & Daitch, 2011). Pregnant and breast-feeding women who are aware of a family history of allergy (an unborn infant's mother, father, or sibling with asthma, eczema, hay fever, or other allergy) should avoid peanuts and peanut-containing foods during pregnancy as a precaution (Boyce et al., 2010; Johnson & Daitch, 2011).

One of the dangers of food allergens is that they may be hidden in other foods and not apparent to people who are susceptible to the allergen. For example, peanuts and peanut butter are often used in salad dressings and Asian, African, and Mexican cooking and may result in severe allergic reactions, including anaphylaxis. Previous contamination of equipment with allergens (e.g., peanuts) during preparation of another food product (e.g., chocolate cake) is enough to produce anaphylaxis in people with severe allergy.

Clinical Manifestations

The clinical symptoms are classic allergic symptoms (urticaria, dermatitis, wheezing, cough, laryngeal edema, angioedema) and gastrointestinal symptoms (itching; swelling of lips, tongue, and palate; abdominal pain; nausea; cramps; vomiting; and diarrhea).

Assessment and Diagnostic Findings

A careful diagnostic workup is required in any patient with suspected food hypersensitivity. Included are a detailed allergy history, a physical examination, and pertinent diagnostic tests. Skin testing is used to identify the source of symptoms and assists in identifying specific foods as causative agents.

Medical Management

Therapy for food hypersensitivity includes elimination of the food responsible for the hypersensitivity (Chart 38-8). Pharmacologic therapy is necessary for patients who cannot avoid exposure to offending foods and for patients with multiple food sensitivities not responsive to avoidance measures. Medication therapy involves the use of H_1 blockers, antihistamines, adrenergic agents, corticosteroids, and cromolyn sodium. All patients with food allergies, especially seafood and nuts, should have an EpiPen device prescribed. Another essential aspect of management is educating patients and family members about how to recognize and manage the early stages of an acute anaphylactic reaction (Boyce et al., 2010). Many food allergies disappear with time, particularly in children. About one third of proven allergies disappear in 1 to 2 years if the patient carefully avoids the offending food. However, peanut allergy has been reported to persist throughout adulthood in some people (Johnson & Daitch, 2011).

Nursing Management

In addition to participating in management of the allergic reaction, the nurse focuses on preventing future exposure of the patient to the food allergen. If a severe allergic or anaphylactic reaction to food allergens has occurred, the nurse must instruct the patient and family about strategies to prevent its recurrence (Chart 38-8). Patients' food allergies should be noted on their medical records, because there may be risk of allergic reactions not only to food but also to some medications containing similar substances (Fitzharris & Sinclair, 2011).

Latex Allergy

Latex allergy—the allergic reaction to natural rubber proteins—has been implicated in rhinitis, conjunctivitis, contact dermatitis, urticaria, asthma, and anaphylaxis. Once hospitals and outpatient facilities mandated the use of powdered latex gloves to prevent transmission of infections, some health care workers began to experience adverse reactions (Palosuo, Antoniadou, Gottrup, et al., 2011; Pollart, Warniment & Mori, 2009). Recently, the prevalence has been steadily declining, possibly because of the use of nonpowdered latex and latex-free gloves (Mayo Foundation for Medical Education and Research, 2011).

Natural rubber latex is derived from the sap of the rubber tree (*Hevea brasiliensis*). The conversion of the liquid rubber latex into a finished product entails the addition of more than 200 chemicals. The proteins in the natural rubber latex (Hevea proteins) or the various chemicals that are used in the manufacturing process are thought to be the source of the allergic reactions. Not all objects composed of latex have the same ability to stimulate an allergic response. For example, the antigenicity of latex gloves can vary widely depending on the manufacturing method used.

Those at risk include health care workers, patients with atopic allergies or multiple surgeries, people working in factories that manufacture latex products, females, and patients with spina bifida. Because more food handlers, hairdressers, automobile mechanics, and police wear latex gloves, they are at risk for latex allergy. In 2008, the Occupational and Safety Health Administration (OSHA) estimated that 8% to 12% of health care workers are latex sensitive (OSHA, 2010). Patients are at risk for anaphylactic reactions as a result of contact with latex during medical treatments, especially surgical procedures. Food that has been handled by people wearing latex gloves may stimulate an allergic response. Cross-reactions have been reported in people who are allergic to certain food products, such as kiwis, bananas, pineapples, mangoes, passion fruit, avocados, and chestnuts (AAAAI, 2011; Mayo Foundation for Medical Education and Research, 2011).

Routes of exposure to latex products can be cutaneous, percutaneous, mucosal, parenteral, or aerosol. Allergic

Chart 38-8	**HOME CARE CHECKLIST** Managing Food Allergies		
At the completion of home care education, the patient or caregiver will be able to:		**PATIENT**	**CAREGIVER**
• Verbalize understanding of the need to maintain an allergen-free diet.		✔	✔
• Demonstrate reading of food labels to identify hidden allergens in food.		✔	✔
• Identify ways to manage an allergen-free diet when eating away from home.		✔	✔
• State the need to wear medical identification bracelet or necklace.		✔	✔
• List symptoms of food allergy.		✔	✔
• Demonstrate emergency administration of epinephrine.		✔	✔
• State the importance of replacing epinephrine when outdated.		✔	✔
• State the importance of prompt treatment of allergic reactions and health care follow-up.		✔	✔

TABLE 38-5 **Selected Products Containing Natural Rubber Latex and Latex-Free Alternatives**

Products Containing Latex	Examples of Latex-Safe Alternatives*
Hospital Environment	
Ace bandage (brown)	Ace bandage, white all cotton
Adhesive bandages, Band-Aid dressing, Telfa	Cotton pads and plastic or silk tape, Active Strips (3M), DuoDERM
Anesthesia equipment	Neoprene anesthesia kit (King)
Blood pressure cuff, tubing, and bladder	Clean Cuff, single-use nylon or vinyl blood pressure cuffs or wrap with stockinette or apply over clothing
Catheters	All-silicone or vinyl catheters
Catheter leg bag straps	Velcro straps
Crutch axillary pads and hand grips, tips	Cover with cloth, tape
ECG pads	Baxter, Red Dot 3M ECG pads
Elastic compression stockings	Kendall SCD stockings with stockinette
Gloves	Derma Prene, neoprene, polymer, or vinyl gloves
IV catheters	Jelco, Deseret IV catheters
IV rubber injection ports	Cover Y-sites and ports; do not puncture. Use three-way stopcocks on plastic tubing.
Levin tube	Salem sump tube
Medication vials	Remove rubber stopper.
Penrose drains	Jackson-Pratt, Zimmer Hemovac drains
Prepackaged enema kits	Therevac, Fleet Ready-to-Use
Pulse oximeters	Nonin oximeters
Resuscitation bags	Laerdal, Puritan Bennett, *certain* Ambu
Stethoscope tubing	PVC tubing; cover with latex-free stockinette
Suction tubing	PVC (Davol, Laerdal)
Syringes—single use (Monoject, BD)	Terumo syringes, Abbott PCA Abboject
Tapes	Dermicel, Micropore
Theraband	New Thera-band Exercisers, plastic tubing
Thermometer probes	Diatek probe covers
Tourniquets	X-Tourn straps (Avcor)
Home Environment	
Balloons	Mylar balloons
Condoms, diaphragms	Polyurethane products, Durex Avanti and Reality products (female condom)
Diapers, incontinence pads	Huggies, Always, *some* Attends
Feminine hygiene pads	Kimberly-Clark products
Wheelchair cushions	ROHO cushions, Sof Care bed/chair cushions

ECG, electrocardiogram; IV, intravenous; PVC, polyvinyl chloride.
*Confirmation is essential to verify that all items are latex free before using, especially if risk of latex allergy is present.

reactions are more likely with parenteral or mucous membrane exposure but can also occur with cutaneous contact or inhalation. The most frequent source of exposure is cutaneous, which usually involves the wearing of natural latex gloves. The powder used to facilitate putting on latex gloves can become a carrier of latex proteins from the gloves; when the gloves are put on or removed, the particles become airborne and can be inhaled or settle on skin, mucous membranes, or clothing. Mucosal exposure can occur from the use of latex condoms, catheters, airways, and nipples. Parenteral exposure can occur from intravenous lines or hemodialysis equipment. In addition to latex-derived medical devices, many household items also contain latex. Examples of medical and household items containing latex and a list of alternative products are found in Table 38-5. It is estimated that more than 40,000 medical devices and nonmedical products contain latex. Chemical additives used in the manufacture of nonlatex gloves and other items have been associated with allergic symptoms, although these otherwise have a low potential to stimulate an allergic response (AAAAI, 2011; Mayo Foundation for Medical Education and Research, 2011).

Clinical Manifestations

Several different types of reactions to latex are possible (Table 38-6). Irritant contact dermatitis, a nonimmunologic response, may be caused by mechanical skin irritation or an alkaline pH associated with latex gloves. Common symptoms of irritant dermatitis include erythema and pruritus. These symptoms can be eliminated by changing the brand of gloves or by using powder-free gloves. The use of hand lotion before donning latex gloves can worsen the symptoms, because lotions may leach latex proteins from the gloves, thus increasing skin exposure and the risk of developing true allergic reactions (AAAAI, 2011; Mayo Foundation for Medical Education and Research, 2011).

Delayed hypersensitivity to latex, a type IV reaction mediated by T cells in the immune system, is localized to the area of exposure and is characterized by symptoms of contact dermatitis, including vesicular skin lesions, papules, pruritus, edema, erythema, and crusting and thickening of the skin. These symptoms usually appear on the back of the hands. This reaction is thought to be caused by chemicals that are used in the manufacturing of latex products. It is the most common allergic reaction to latex. Although usually not life threatening, delayed hypersensitivity reactions often require major changes in the patient's home and work environment to avoid further exposure. People who are sensitized to latex are at increased risk for development of type I allergic reactions (AAAAI, 2011; Holgate et al., 2011).

Immediate hypersensitivity, a type I allergic reaction, is mediated by the IgE mast cell system (Menzies, Shepherd, Nibbs, et al., 2011). Symptoms can include rhinitis, conjunctivitis,

TABLE 38-6	Types of Reactions to Latex			
Type of Reaction	**Cause**		**Signs/Symptoms**	**Treatment**
Irritant contact dermatitis	Damage to skin because of irritation and loss of epidermoid skin layer; not an allergic reaction. Can be caused by excessive use of soaps and cleansers, repeated handwashing, inadequate hand drying, mechanical irritation (e.g., sweating, rubbing inside powdered gloves), exposure to chemicals added during the manufacturing of gloves, and alkaline pH of powdered gloves. Reaction may occur with first exposure, is usually benign, and is not life threatening.		*Acute:* Redness, edema, burning, discomfort, itching *Chronic:* Dry, thickened, cracked skin	Referral for diagnostic testing Avoidance of exposure to irritant Thorough washing and drying of hands Use of powder-free gloves with more frequent changes of gloves Changing glove types Use of water- or silicone-based moisturizing creams, lotions, or topical barrier agents Avoidance of oil- or petroleum-based skin agents with latex products, because they cause breakdown of the latex product
Allergic contact dermatitis	Delayed hypersensitivity (type IV) reaction. Usually affects only area in contact with latex; reaction is usually to chemical additives used in the manufacturing process rather than to latex itself. Cause of reaction is T-cell–mediated sensitization to additives of latex. Reaction is not life threatening and is far more common than a type I reaction. Slow onset; occurs 18–24 hours after exposure. Resolves within 3–4 days after exposure. More severe reactions may occur with subsequent exposures.		Pruritus, erythema, swelling, crusty thickened skin, blisters, other skin lesions	Referral for diagnosis (patch tests) and treatment Thorough washing and drying of hands Use of water- or silicone-based moisturizing creams, lotions, or topical barrier agents Avoidance of oil- or petroleum-based products unless they are latex compatible Avoidance of identified causative agent, because continued exposure to latex products in presence of breaks in skin may contribute to latex protein sensitization
Latex allergy	Type I IgE-mediated immediate hypersensitivity to plant proteins in natural rubber latex. In sensitized people, antilatex IgE antibody stimulates mast cell proliferation and basophil histamine release. Exposure can be through contact with the skin, mucous membranes, or internal tissues, or through inhalation of traces of powder from latex gloves. Severe reactions usually occur shortly after parenteral or mucous membrane exposure. People with any type I reaction to latex are at high risk for anaphylaxis. Local swelling, redness, edema, itching, and systemic reactions, including anaphylaxis, occur within minutes after exposure.		Rhinitis, flushing, conjunctivitis, urticaria, laryngeal edema, bronchospasm, asthma, severe vasodilation angioedema, anaphylaxis, cardiovascular collapse, death	Immediate treatment of reaction with epinephrine, fluids, vasopressors, and corticosteroids, and airway and ventilator support, with close monitoring for recurrence for next 12–14 hours Prompt referral for diagnostic evaluation Treatment and diagnostic evaluation in latex-free environment Assessment of all patients for symptoms of latex allergy Educating patients and family members about the disorder and the importance of preventing future reactions by avoiding latex (e.g., wearing medical identification, carrying EpiPen)

IgE, immunoglobulin E.

asthma, and anaphylaxis. The term *latex allergy* is usually used to describe the type I reaction. Clinical manifestations have a rapid onset and can include urticaria, wheezing, dyspnea, laryngeal edema, bronchospasm, tachycardia, angioedema, hypotension, and cardiac arrest.

Localized itching, erythema, or local urticaria within minutes after exposure to latex is often the initial symptom. Symptoms of subsequent reactions can include generalized urticaria, angioedema, rhinitis, conjunctivitis, asthma, and anaphylactic shock minutes after dermal or mucosal exposure to latex. An increasing number of people who are allergic to latex experience severe reactions characterized by generalized urticaria, bronchospasm, and hypotension.

Assessment and Diagnostic Findings

The diagnosis of latex allergy is based on the history and diagnostic test results (OSHA, 2010; Pollart et al., 2009). Sensitization is detected by skin testing, RAST, EIA, or ELISA, or the level of Hevea latex-specific IgE antibody in the serum. Testing for the chemicals found in the rubber production that makes latex is performed using the patch test. Skin patch testing is the preferred method for patients with contact allergies. The T.R.U.E. test and other skin tests should be performed only by clinicians who have expertise in their administration and interpretation and who have the necessary equipment available to treat local or systemic allergic reactions to the reagent. Nasal challenge and dipstick tests may be useful in the future as screening tests for latex allergy.

Medical Management

The best treatment available for latex allergy is the avoidance of latex-based products, although avoidance is often difficult because of the widespread use of such products. Patients who have experienced an anaphylactic reaction to latex should be instructed to wear medical identification. Antihistamines and an emergency kit containing epinephrine should be provided to these patients, along with instructions about emergency management of latex allergy symptoms. Patients should be counseled to notify all health care workers, as well as local paramedic and ambulance companies, about their allergy. Warning labels can be attached to car windows to alert police and paramedics about the driver's or passenger's latex allergy in case of a motor vehicle crash. People with latex allergy should be provided with a list of alternative products and referred to local support groups; they are also urged to carry their own supply of nonlatex gloves.

People with type I latex sensitivity may be unable to continue to work if a latex-free work environment is not possible. This may occur with surgeons, dentists, operating room personnel, or intensive care nurses. Occupational implications for employees with type IV latex sensitivity are usually easier to manage by changing to nonlatex gloves and avoiding direct contact with latex-based medical equipment. Although latex-specific immunotherapy has been attempted, this method of treatment remains experimental.

Nursing Management

The nurse can assume a pivotal role in the management of latex allergies in both patients and staff. All patients should be asked about latex allergy, although special attention should be given to those at particularly high risk (e.g., patients with spina bifida, patients who have undergone multiple surgical procedures). Every time an invasive procedure must be performed, the nurse should consider the possibility of latex allergies. Nurses working in operating rooms, intensive care units, short procedure units, and emergency departments need to pay particular attention to latex allergy. (See Fig. 17-1 in Chapter 17 for a latex allergy assessment form.)

Although the type I reaction is the most significant of the reactions to latex, care must be taken in the presence of irritant contact dermatitis and delayed hypersensitivity reaction to avoid further exposure of the person to latex. Patients with latex allergy are advised to notify their health care providers and to wear medical identification. Patients must become knowledgeable about what products contain latex and what products are safe, nonlatex alternatives. They must also become knowledgeable about signs and symptoms of latex allergy and emergency treatment and self-injection of epinephrine in case of allergic reaction.

Nurses can be instrumental in establishing and participating in multidisciplinary committees to address latex allergy and to promote a latex-free environment. Latex allergy protocols and education of staff about latex allergy and precautions are important strategies to reduce this growing problem and to ensure assessment and prompt treatment of those affected by allergy to latex.

Critical Thinking Exercises

1 **ebp** You are a nurse working in an allergy clinic. Your nurse manager asks you to investigate the evidence for nursing assessment of patients with allergies. Identify the essential components of an evidence-based assessment form to be used in an adult outpatient allergy clinic. Describe the strength of the evidence and criteria used to assess its strength.

2 An 18-year-old man has recently developed food allergies. Describe the nursing plan of care. What specific interventions and nursing management strategies are indicated? Develop a plan of patient education for him, and identify outcomes measures to assess the effectiveness of the education.

3 **pq** A 65-year-old woman is scheduled for an outpatient procedure. She reports that she has experienced an episode of hives and itching during a dental procedure in the past. She also reports that she has had to use emergency epinephrine on several occasions in the past because of severe allergic reactions caused by bee stings. List the top three interventions and nursing management strategies that would be indicated if she develops a severe allergic reaction.

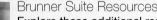

Brunner Suite Resources

Explore these additional resources to enhance learning for this chapter:
• NCLEX-Style Questions and Other Resources on **thePoint**, http://thePoint.lww.com/Brunner13e
• Study Guide
• PrepU
• Clinical Handbook
• Handbook of Laboratory and Diagnostic Tests

References

Books

Abbas, A. K., & Lichtman, A. H. (2011). *Basic immunology: Functions and disorders of the immune system*. Philadelphia: W. B. Saunders.
Adkinson, N. F., Busse, W. W., Bochner, B. S., et al. (Eds.). (2009). *Middleton's allergy: Principles and practice* (7th ed.). Philadelphia: Elsevier.
Arcangelo, V. P., & Peterson, A. (Eds.). (2013). *Pharmacotherapeutics for advanced practice: A practical approach* (3rd ed.). Philadelphia: Lippincott Williams & Wilkins.
Fischbach, F., & Dunning, M. B. (2009). *A manual of laboratory and diagnostic tests* (8th ed.). Philadelphia: Lippincott Williams & Wilkins.
Goroll, A. G., & Mulley, A. G. (2009). *Primary care medicine: Office evaluation and management of the adult patient*. Philadelphia: Lippincott Williams & Wilkins.
Holgate, S. T., Church, M., Bromid, D., et al. (2011). *Allergy*. Philadelphia: Elsevier Health Sciences.
Karch, A. M. (2012). *Lippincott's nursing drug guide*. Philadelphia: Lippincott Williams & Wilkins.
National Heart, Lung, and Blood Institute. (2007). Managing exacerbations of asthma. In National Asthma Education and Prevention Program (NAEPP). *Expert panel report 3: Guidelines for the diagnosis and management of asthma*. Bethesda, MD: Author.
Peakman, M., & Vergani, D. (2009). *Basic and clinical immunology* (2nd ed.). Philadelphia: Churchill Livingstone.
Porth, C. M., & Matfin G. (2009). *Pathophysiology: Concepts of altered health states* (8th ed.). Philadelphia: Lippincott Williams & Wilkins.
Wynne, A. L., Woo, T. M., & Olyaei, A. J. (2011). *Pharmacotherapeutics for nurse practitioner prescribers*. Philadelphia: F. A. Davis.

Journals & Electronic Documents

American Academy of Allergy, Asthma, & Immunology. (2011). *Latex allergy: Tips to remember*. Available at: www.aaaai.org/conditions-and-treatments/Library/At-a-Glance/Latex-Allergy.aspx
Arnold, J. J., & Williams, P. M. (2011). Anaphylaxis: Recognition and management. *American Family Physician, 84*(10), 1111–1118.
Bachert, C., Claeys, S. E. M., Tomassen, P., et al. (2010). Rhinosinusitis and asthma: A link for asthma severity. *Current Allergy and Asthma Reports, 10*(3), 194–201.
Bernstein, I. L., Li, J. T., Bernstein, D. I., et al. (2008). Allergy diagnostic testing: An updated practice parameter. *Annals of Allergy, Asthma & Immunology, 100*(Suppl. 3), S1–S148.
Boyce, J. A., Assa'ad, A., Burks, A. W., et al. (2010). Guidelines for the diagnosis and management of food allergy in the United States: Report of the NIAID-sponsored expert panel. *Journal of Allergy & Clinical Immunology, 126*(6 Suppl.), S1–S58.
Brozek, J. L., Bousquet, J., Baena-Cagnani, C. E., et al. (2010). Allergic Rhinitis and its Impact on Asthma (ARIA) guidelines: 2010 revision. *Journal of Allergy and Clinical Immunology, 126*(3), 466–476.

Distler, J. W. (2011). Environmental allergens: Diagnosis and management of IgE-mediated disorders. *American Journal for Nurse Practitioners, 9*(10), 15–24.

Dykewicz, M. S., & Hamilos, D. L. (2010). Rhinitis and sinusitis. *Journal of Allergy and Clinical Immunology, 125*(2), S103–S115.

Dyall-Smith, D. (2011). Familial cold autoinflammatory syndrome. *DermNet NZ.* Available at: dermnetnz.org/systemic/fcas.html

Fitzharris, P., & Sinclair, J. (2011). Food allergy. *British Medical Journal, 342*(7796), 933.

Fitzhugh, D. J., & Lockey, F. (2011). Allergen immunotherapy: A history of the first 100 years. *Current Opinion in Allergy & Clinical Immunology, 11*(6), 554–559.

Grateau, G., & Duruöz, M. T. (2010). Autoinflammatory conditions: When to suspect? How to treat? *Best Practice & Research Clinical Rheumatology, 24*(2), 401–411.

Johnson, K., & Daitch, L. (2011). Peanut allergy awareness. *Clinician Reviews, 21*(12), 28–38.

Lambert, M. (2009). Practice parameters for managing allergic rhinitis. *American Family Physician, 80*(1), 79–85.

Mayhew, M. (2009). Management of rhinitis. *Journal for Nurse Practitioners, 5*(1), 54–55.

Mayo Foundation for Medical Education and Research. (2011). *Latex allergy.* Available at: www.mayoclinic.com/health/latex-allergy/DS00621

Menzies, F. M., Shepherd, M. C., Nibbs, R. J., & Nelson, S. M. (2011). The role of mast cells and their mediators in reproduction, pregnancy and labour. *Human Reproduction Update, 17*(3), 383–396.

Munn, Z. (2009). *Anaphylaxis: Management.* Joanna Briggs Institute. Available at: ezproxy.villanova.edu/login?url=http://search.proquest.com/docview/1907 00633?accountid=14853

Nelson, J., & Moward, C. M. (2010). Allergic contact dermatitis: Patch testing beyond the TRUE test. *Journal of Clinical and Aesthetic Dermatology, 3*(10), 36–41.

Neumar, R. W., Otto, C. W., Link, M. S., et al. (2010). Adult advanced cardiovascular life support: 2010 American Heart Association guidelines for cardiopulmonary resuscitation and emergency cardiovascular care. *Circulation, 122,* S729–S767.

Nijhawan, R. I., Matiz, C., & Jacob, S. E. (2009). Contact dermatitis: From basics to allergodromes. *Pediatric Annals, 38*(2), 99–108.

Occupational Safety and Health Administration. (2010). *Latex allergy.* Available at: www.osha.gov/SLTC/latexallergy/

Palosuo, T., Antoniadou, I., Gottrup, F., & Phillips, P. (2011). Latex medical gloves: Time for a reappraisal. *International Archives of Allergy and Immunology, 156*(3), 234–246.

Pollart, S., Warniment, C., & Mori, T. (2009). Latex allergy. *American Family Physician, 80*(12), 1419–1420.

Sardana, N., & Craig, T. J. (2011). Recent advances in management and treatment of hereditary angioedema. *Pediatrics, 128*(6), 1173.

Schaefer, P. (2011). Urticaria: Evaluation and treatment. *American Family Physician, 83*(9), 1078–1080.

Senti, G., von Moos, S., & Kündig, T. M. (2011). Epicutaneous allergen administration: Is this the future of allergen-specific immunotherapy? *Allergy, 66*(6), 798–809.

Shoup, J. (2011). Management of adult rhinosinusitis. *Nurse Practitioner, 36*(11), 22–26.

Solensky, R. (2011). Allergy to penicillins. *UpToDate.* Available at: novanet. villanova.edu/tag.410a947e4dc4e533.render.userLayoutRootNode. uP?uP_root=root&uP_sparam=activeTab&activeTab=u59l1s13&uP_ tparam=frm&frm=

Thornton, K., Alston, M., Dye, H., et al. (2011). Are saline irrigations effective in relieving chronic rhinosinusitis symptoms? A review of the evidence. *Journal for Nurse Practitioners, 7*(8), 680–688.

Tracy, J. M. (2011). Diagnosis of *Hymenoptera* venom allergy. *UpToDate.* Available at: novanet.villanova.edu/tag.410a947e4dc4e533.render.user LayoutRootNode.uP?uP_root=root&uP_sparam=activeTab&activeTab= u59l1s13&uP_tparam=frm&f

Wallengren, J. (2011). Identification of core competencies for primary care of allergy patients using a modified Delphi technique. *BMC Medical Education, 11,* 12. Available at: www.biomedcentral.com/1472–6920/11/12

Resources

American Academy of Allergy, Asthma, and Immunology (AAAAI), www.aaaai.org

American College of Allergy, Asthma, and Immunology (ACAAI), www.acaai.org

Asthma and Allergy Foundation of America (AAFA), www.aafa.org

Centers for Disease Control and Prevention (CDC), www.cdc.gov

Food Allergy Research Education (FARE), www.foodallergy.org

MD Junction, Urticaria Support Group, www.mdjunction.com/urticaria

National Institute of Allergy and Infectious Diseases, www.niaid.nih.gov

Occupational Safety and Health Administration (OSHA), www.osha.gov

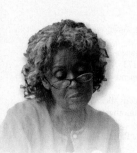
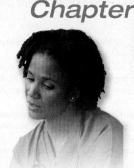

39

Assessment and Management of Patients With Rheumatic Disorders

On completion of this chapter, the learner will be able to:

1 Explain the pathophysiology of rheumatic diseases.
2 Describe the assessment and diagnostic findings seen in patients with rheumatic diseases or disorders.
3 Use the nursing process as a framework for the care of patients with rheumatic disorders.

4 Describe the systemic effects of a connective tissue disease.
5 Devise an education plan for the patient with newly diagnosed rheumatic disease.
6 Identify modifications in interventions to accommodate changes in patients' functional ability that may occur with disease progression.

ankylosis: fixation or immobility of a joint
arthritis: inflammation of a joint
arthroplasty: replacement of a joint
cytokines: cell signaling proteins
exacerbation: period when disease symptoms occur or increase
osteophyte: a bony outgrowth or protuberance; bone spur
pannus: proliferation of newly formed synovial tissue infiltrated with inflammatory cells

remission: period when disease symptoms are reduced or absent
rheumatic diseases: numerous disorders affecting skeletal muscles, bones, cartilage, ligaments, tendons, and joints
rheumatoid arthritis: autoimmune disease of unknown origin
subchondral bone: bony plate that supports the articular cartilage
tophi: accumulation of crystalline deposits in articular surfaces, bones, soft tissue, and cartilage

R**heumatic diseases** encompass autoimmune, degenerative, inflammatory, and systemic conditions that affect the joints, muscles, and soft tissues of the body. Rheumatic diseases most commonly manifest the clinical features of **arthritis** (inflammation of a joint) and pain. There are more than 100 types of rheumatic diseases. The problems caused by rheumatic diseases include limitations in mobility and activities of daily living, pain, fatigue, altered self-image, and sleep disturbances, as well as systemic effects that can lead to organ failure and death. An understanding of rheumatic diseases and their effects on a patient's function and well-being is essential to developing an appropriate plan of nursing care.

Rheumatic Diseases

An estimated 50 million (22%) adults have self-reported arthritis or other rheumatologic disease. Approximately 21 million (9% of all adults) have arthritis-attributable activity limitation. By 2030, an estimated 67 million (25%) adults will have arthritis or a rheumatologic condition, and an estimated 25 million adults (37%) will report arthritis-attributable activity limitations (Cheng, Hootman, Murphy, et al.,

2010). Arthritis and other rheumatologic diseases and the physical limitations that occur with them are becoming more prominent and a larger public health issue.

Rheumatologic disease processes affect males and females of all ages and ethnic groups. Some disorders are more likely to occur at a particular time of life or to affect one gender more often than the other. In general, women are two to nine times more commonly affected by rheumatologic diseases than men (Oliver & Silman, 2009). The onset of these conditions may be acute or insidious, with a course possibly marked by periods of **remission** (a period when disease symptoms are reduced or absent) and **exacerbation** (a period when symptoms occur or increase). Treatment can be simple, aimed at localized relief, or it can be complex, directed toward relief of systemic effects. Permanent changes and disability may result from these disorders.

Nurses need to understand the classification of rheumatic diseases. One system is to classify disease as either monoarticular (affecting a single joint) or polyarticular (affecting multiple joints). Another system is to classify the disease as either inflammatory or noninflammatory. Conditions that may secondarily affect the musculoskeletal structure are also considered in disease classification.

Pathophysiology

Each of the rheumatologic diseases exhibits unique pathophysiologic features. Three distinct characteristics of pathophysiology include inflammation, autoimmunity, and degeneration.

Inflammation

Inflammation is a complex physiologic process mediated by the immune system that occurs in response to harmful stimuli like damaged cells or pathogens (also known as antigens). Inflammation is meant to protect the body from insult by removing the triggering antigen or event. In response to a triggering episode, the antigen stimulus activates the body's immune system to form antibodies like monocytes and T lymphocytes (also referred to as T cells). Next, the immunoglobulin antibodies form immune complexes with antigens. Phagocytosis of the immune complexes is initiated, generating an inflammatory reaction (joint effusion, pain, and edema) (Fig. 39-1). Phagocytosis produces chemicals such as leukotrienes and prostaglandins. Leukotrienes contribute to the inflammatory process by attracting other white blood cells to the area. Prostaglandins act as modifiers to inflammation. In some cases, they increase inflammation; in other cases, they decrease it. Leukotrienes and prostaglandins produce enzymes such as collagenase that break down collagen, which is a vital part of a normal joint. The release of these enzymes in the joint causes edema and proliferation of synovial membrane. In patients with chronic inflammation, the immune response can deviate from normal. Instead of resolution of swelling and joint pain once the triggering event has subsided, **pannus** (proliferation of newly formed synovial tissue infiltrated with inflammatory cells) formation occurs. Destruction of the joint's cartilage and erosion of bone soon follow.

The immunologic inflammatory process begins when antigens are presented to T lymphocytes, leading to a proliferation of T and B cells. B cells (also referred to as plasma cells) are a source of antibody-forming cells. In response to specific antigens, plasma cells produce and release antibodies. Antibodies combine with corresponding antigens to form pairs, or immune complexes. The immune complexes build up and are deposited in synovial tissue or other organs in the body, triggering the inflammatory reaction that can ultimately damage the involved tissue.

Autoimmunity

A hallmark of rheumatologic diseases is autoimmunity, where the body mistakenly recognizes its own tissue as a foreign pathogen (antigen). Autoimmunity leads to destruction of tissue via the same inflammatory process as discussed earlier, along with chronic and long-standing pain. Although focused in the joints, inflammation and autoimmunity also involve other areas. The blood vessels (vasculitis and arteritis), lungs, heart, and kidneys may be affected by the autoimmunity and inflammation. (See Chapter 35 more information on autoimmune disease.) A large group of genes, called *human leukocyte antigen* (HLA) genes, has been linked to the immune response and the development of multiple rheumatologic diseases (Clancy & Hasthorpe, 2011).

Degeneration

In degenerative rheumatic diseases, inflammation also occurs, but as a secondary process. Although the cause of degeneration of the articular cartilage is poorly understood, the process is known to be metabolically active and therefore is more accurately called *degradation*. One theory of degradation is that genetic or hormonal influences, mechanical factors, and prior joint damage cause cartilage failure. Degradation of cartilage ensues, and increased mechanical stress on bone ends

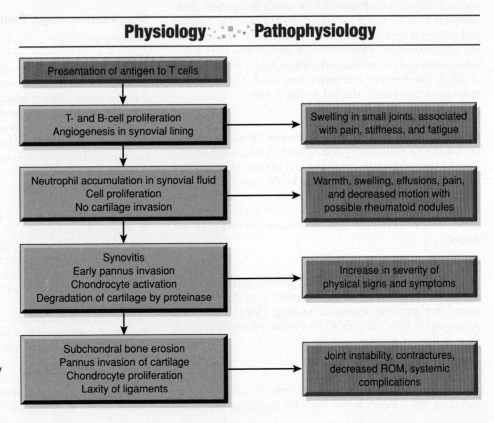

Physiology ⋯⋯ Pathophysiology

Presentation of antigen to T cells

T- and B-cell proliferation
Angiogenesis in synovial lining
→ Swelling in small joints, associated with pain, stiffness, and fatigue

Neutrophil accumulation in synovial fluid
Cell proliferation
No cartilage invasion
→ Warmth, swelling, effusions, pain, and decreased motion with possible rheumatoid nodules

Synovitis
Early pannus invasion
Chondrocyte activation
Degradation of cartilage by proteinase
→ Increase in severity of physical signs and symptoms

Subchondral bone erosion
Pannus invasion of cartilage
Chondrocyte proliferation
Laxity of ligaments
→ Joint instability, contractures, decreased ROM, systemic complications

FIGURE 39-1 • Pathophysiology and associated physical signs of rheumatoid arthritis. ROM, range of motion.

causes stiffening of bone tissue. Another theory is that bone stiffening occurs and results in increased mechanical stress on cartilage, which in turn initiates the processes of degradation. (See Chapter 40 for more information on the structure and function of the articular system.)

Clinical Manifestations

The most common symptom in the rheumatic diseases is pain. Other common symptoms include joint swelling, limited movement, stiffness, weakness, and fatigue.

Assessment and Diagnostic Findings

Assessment begins with a general health history, which includes the onset of symptoms and how they evolved, family history, past health history, and any other contributing factors. Because many of the rheumatic diseases are chronic conditions, the health history should also include information about the patient's perception of the problem, previous treatments and their effectiveness, the patient's support systems, and the patient's current knowledge base and the source of that information. A complete health history is followed by a complete physical assessment (see Chapter 5).

Assessment for rheumatic diseases combines the physical examination with a functional assessment. Inspection of the patient's general appearance occurs during initial contact. Gait, posture, and general musculoskeletal size and structure are observed. Gross deformities and abnormalities in movement are noted. The symmetry, size, and contour of other connective tissues, such as the skin and adipose tissue, are also noted and recorded. Chart 39-1 outlines the important areas for consideration during the physical assessment. The functional assessment is a combination of history (what the patient reports that he or she can and cannot do) and examination (observation of activities, in which the patient demonstrates what he or she can and cannot do, such as dressing and getting in and out of a chair). Observation also includes the adaptations and adjustments the patient may have made (sometimes without awareness)—for example, with shoulder or elbow involvement, the person may bend over to reach a fork rather than raising the fork to the mouth.

Laboratory Studies

In Table 39-1, some of the most common laboratory studies are listed with their corresponding normal ranges and significance. Many of the tests require special laboratory techniques and may not be performed in every health care facility. The primary provider determines which tests are necessary based on symptoms, stage of disease, cost, and likely benefit. In some instances, tests are used to monitor the course of the disease.

Other Diagnostic Studies

Imaging studies commonly used for patients with rheumatic diseases include x-ray studies, computed tomography (CT) scans, and magnetic resonance imaging (MRI) scans, and arthrography. (See Chapter 40 for further information about these and other diagnostic studies.)

Medical Management

A treatment program involving an interdisciplinary team, including the patient, is the basis for managing rheumatic diseases (Lesko, Young, & Higham, 2010). The chronic nature of most of these diseases mandates that the patient understands the disease, has the information necessary to make good self-management decisions, and is presented with a therapeutic program that is compatible with his or her lifestyle (Palmer & El Miedany, 2010). How rheumatologic diseases are managed over time is based on the patient's report of symptoms and self-assessment (Ovayolu, Ovayolu & Karadag, 2012). Table 39-2 outlines goals and strategies for care of the patient with rheumatic diseases.

Pharmacologic Therapy

Medications are used with the rheumatic diseases to manage symptoms, to control inflammation, and, in some instances, to modify the disease. Useful medications include the salicylates, nonsteroidal anti-inflammatory drugs (NSAIDs), and both biologic and nonbiologic disease-modifying antirheumatic drugs (DMARDs). As their name suggests, DMARDs have the ability to alter disease progression and stop or decrease further tissue damage. Nonbiologic DMARDs are thought to reduce proinflammatory **cytokines** (cell signaling proteins) and increase anti-inflammatory cytokines (Firth & Critchley, 2011). Biologic DMARDs, in contrast, have been specifically engineered to target a certain cell or molecule within the immune system to treat the specific rheumatologic condition. Specific biologic DMARDs target tumor necrosis factor alpha (TNF-α), B cells, T cells, interleukin 1 (IL-1), and interleukin 6 (IL-6). Table 39-3 reviews commonly used medications.

Controlling the inflammation related to the disease process helps manage pain, but this is often a delayed response. Nonopioid medications are often used for pain management, especially early in the treatment program, until other measures can be instituted.

Nonpharmacologic Pain Management

Nonpharmacologic methods of pain management are important. Heat applications are helpful in relieving pain, stiffness, and muscle spasm. Superficial heat may be applied in the form of warm tub baths or showers and warm moist compresses. Paraffin baths (dips), which offer concentrated heat, are helpful to patients with wrist and small-joint involvement. Maximum benefit is achieved within 20 minutes after application. More frequent use for shorter lengths of time is most beneficial. Therapeutic exercises can be carried out more comfortably and effectively after heat has been applied.

Devices such as braces, splints, and assistive devices for ambulation (e.g., canes, crutches, walkers) ease pain by limiting movement or stress from putting weight on painful joints. Acutely inflamed joints can be rested by applying splints to limit motion. Splints also support the joint to relieve spasm. Canes and crutches can relieve stress from inflamed and painful weight-bearing joints while promoting safe ambulation. Cervical collars may be used to support the weight of the head and limit cervical motion. A metatarsal bar or special pads may be put into the patient's shoes if foot pain or deformity is present. A combination of methods may be required, because different methods often work better at different times.

Exercise and Activity

The ongoing nature of most rheumatic diseases makes it important to maintain and, when possible, improve joint

Chart 39-1   Assessing for Rheumatic Disorders

In addition to the head-to-toe assessment or systems review, the following are important areas of consideration to be noted when performing the complete physical assessment of a patient with a known or suspected rheumatic disorder.

Manifestation	Significance
Skin (inquire and inspect)	
Rash, lesions	Associated with systemic lupus erythematosus (SLE) vasculitis, adverse effect of medication
Increased bruising	Associated with several rheumatic diseases and adverse effect of medication
Erythema	Sign of inflammation
Thinning	Adverse effect of medication
Warmth	Sign of inflammation
Photosensitivity	Associated with SLE, dermatomyositis, adverse effect of medication
Hair (inquire and inspect)	
Alopecia or thinning	Associated with rheumatic diseases or adverse effect of medication
Eye (inquire and inspect)	
Dryness, grittiness	Associated with Sjögren's syndrome (commonly occurring with rheumatoid arthritis [RA] and SLE)
Decreased acuity or blindness	Associated with temporal arteritis, medication complications
Cataracts	Adverse effect of medication
Decreased peripheral vision	Adverse effect of medication
Conjunctivitis, uveitis	Associated with ankylosing spondylitis and Reiter's syndrome
Ear (inquire)	
Tinnitus	Adverse effect of medication
Decreased acuity	Adverse effect of medication
Mouth (inquire and inspect)	
Buccal, sublingual lesions	Associated with vasculitis, dermatomyositis, adverse effect of medication
Altered sense of taste	Adverse effect of medication
Dryness	Associated with Sjögren's syndrome
Dysphagia	Associated with myositis
Difficulty chewing	Associated with decreased range of motion of jaw
Chest (inspect and inquire)	
Pleuritic pain	Associated with RA and SLE
Decreased chest expansion	Associated with ankylosing spondylitis
Activity intolerance (dyspnea)	Associated with pulmonary hypertension in scleroderma
Cardiovascular system (inquire, inspect, palpate)	
Blanching of fingers on exposure to cold	Associated with Raynaud's phenomenon
Peripheral pulses	Deficit may indicate vascular involvement or edema associated with medication effect or rheumatic diseases, especially SLE or scleroderma
Abdomen (inquire and palpate)	
Altered bowel habits	Associated with scleroderma, spondylosis, ulcerative colitis, decreased physical mobility, medication effect
Nausea, vomiting, bloating, and pain	Adverse effect of medication
Weight change (measure)	Associated with RA (decreased), adverse effect of medication (increased or decreased)
Genitalia (inquire and inspect)	
Dryness, itching	Associated with Sjögren's syndrome
Abnormal menses	Adverse effect of medication
Altered sexual performance	Fear of pain (or of pain caused by partner) and limitation of motion may affect sexual mobility.
Hygiene	Poor hygiene may be related to limitations in activities of daily living.
Urethritis, dysuria	Associated with ankylosing spondylitis and Reiter's syndrome
Lesions	Associated with vasculitis
Neurologic (inquire and inspect)	
Paresthesias of extremities; abnormal reflex pattern	Nerve compressions (e.g., carpal tunnel syndrome, spinal stenosis)
Headaches	Associated with temporal arteritis, adverse effect of medication
Musculoskeletal (inspect and palpate)	
Joint redness, warmth, swelling, tenderness, deformity—location of first joint involved, pattern of progression, symmetry, acute versus chronic nature	Signs of inflammation
Joint range of motion	Decreased range of motion may indicate severity or progression of disease.
Surrounding tissue findings	
Muscle atrophy, subcutaneous nodules, popliteal cyst	Extra-articular manifestations
Muscle strength (grip)	Muscle strength decreases with increased disease activity.

TABLE 39-1 Common Blood Studies for Rheumatic Diseases

Test	Normal Value	Significance
Serum		
Creatinine Metabolic waste excreted through the kidneys	0.7–1.4 mg/dL (62–124 mcmol/L)	Increase may indicate kidney damage in SLE, scleroderma, and polyarteritis.
Erythrocyte Count Measures circulating erythrocytes	Men: 4,600,000–6,200,000/cu mm (4.6–6.2 × 10^{12}/L) Women: 4,200,000–5,400,000/cu mm (4.2–5.4 × 10^{12}/L)	Decrease can be seen in RA, SLE.
Erythrocyte Sedimentation Rate (ESR) Measures the rate at which RBCs settle out of unclotted blood in 1 hour	Westergren: Men under 50 yr: <15 mm/h Men over 50 yr: <20 mm/h Women under 50 yr: <25 mm/h Women over 50 yr: <30 mm/h	Increase is usually seen in inflammatory connective tissue diseases. An increase indicates rising inflammation, resulting in clustering of RBCs, which makes them heavier than normal. The higher the ESR, the greater the inflammatory activity.
Hematocrit Measures the size, capacity, and number of cells present in blood	Men: 42%–52% Women: 35%–47%	Decrease can be seen in chronic inflammation (anemia of chronic disease); also, blood loss through GI bleed.
White Blood Cell Count Measures circulating leukocytes	4,500–11,000 cells/mm^3	Decrease may be seen in SLE.
VDRL (Venereal Disease Research Laboratory) Measures antibody to syphilis	Nonreactive	False-positive results are sometimes found with SLE.
Uric Acid Measures level of uric acid in serum	2.5–8 mg/dL (0.15–0.5 mmol/L)	Increase is seen with gout.
Serum Immunology		
Antinuclear Antibody (ANA) Measures antibodies that react with a variety of nuclear antigens If antibodies are present, further testing determines the type of ANA circulating in the blood (anti-DNA, anti-RNP).	Negative A few healthy adults have a positive ANA.	Positive test is associated with SLE, RA, scleroderma, Raynaud's disease, Sjögren's syndrome, necrotizing arteritis. The higher the titer, the greater the inflammation. The pattern of immunofluorescence (speckled, homogeneous, or nucleolar) helps determine the diagnosis.
Anti-DNA, DNA Binding Titer measurement of antibody to double-stranded DNA	Negative	High titer is seen in SLE; increases in titer may indicate increase in disease activity.
Complement Levels—C3, C4 Complement is a protein substance that binds with antigen–antibody complexes for the purpose of lysis. When the number of complexes increases markedly, complement is used for lysis, thus depleting the amount available in the blood.	C3: 80–170 mg/dL (0.8–1.7 g/L) C4: 18–51 mg/dL (180–510 mg/dL)	Decrease may be seen in RA and SLE. Decrease indicates autoimmune and inflammatory activity.
C-Reactive Protein (CRP) Shows presence of abnormal glycoprotein due to inflammatory process	<1 mg/dL (<10 mg/L)	A positive reading indicates active inflammation. Test is often positive for RA and SLE.
Immunoglobulin Electrophoresis Measures the values of immunoglobulins	IgA: 80–400 mg/dL (0.8–4 g/L) IgG: 600–1,800 mg/dL (6–18 g/L) IgM: 55–250 mg/dL (0.55–2.5 g/L)	Increased levels are found in people who have autoimmune disorders.
Rheumatoid Factor (RF) Determines the presence of abnormal antibodies seen in connective tissue disease	Negative	Positive titer >1:80 Present in 80% of those with RA Positive RF may also suggest SLE, Sjögren's syndrome, or mixed connective tissue disease. The higher the titer (number at right of colon), the greater the inflammation.
Tissue Typing		
HLA-B27 Antigen Measures presence of HLA antigens, which are used for tissue recognition	Negative	Found in 80%–90% of those with ankylosing spondylitis and Reiter's syndrome

SLE, system lupus erythematosus; RBCs, red blood cells; GI, gastrointestinal; RA, rheumatoid arthritis; DNA, deoxyribonucleic acid; RNP, ribonucleoprotein; IgA, immunoglobulin A; IgG, immunoglobulin G; IgM, immunoglobulin M; HLA, human leukocyte antigen.

Adapted from Fischbach, F., & Dunning, M. B. (2009). *A manual of laboratory and diagnostic tests* (8th ed.). Philadelphia: Lippincott Williams & Wilkins.

TABLE 39-2	**Management Goals and Strategies for Rheumatic Diseases**
Goals	**Management Strategies**
Suppress inflammation and the autoimmune response	Optimize pharmacologic therapy (anti-inflammatory and disease-modifying agents).
Control pain	Protect joints; ease pain with splints, thermal modalities, relaxation techniques.
Maintain or improve joint mobility	Implement exercise programs for joint motion, muscle strengthening, weight loss as appropriate, and overall health.
Maintain or improve functional status	Make use of adaptive devices and techniques.
Increase patient's knowledge of disease process	Provide and reinforce patient education.
Promote self-management by patient adherence with the therapeutic regimen	Emphasize compatibility of therapeutic regimen and lifestyle.

mobility and overall functional status. Changes in gait as well as joint limitations commonly require referral for rehabilitation therapy (Del Din, Carraro, Sawacha, et al., 2011; Durmus, Altay, Ersoy, et al., 2010). An individualized exercise program is crucial to movement. Table 39-4 summarizes the exercises appropriate for patients with rheumatic diseases. Appropriate programs of exercise have been shown to decrease pain and improve function (Breedland, van Scheppingen, Leijsma, et al., 2011; Hurley, Hanson, & Sheaff, 2011; Miller, 2012). A mild analgesic agent may be suggested before exercise for a patient starting a program of exercise. Other strategies for decreasing pain include muscle relaxation techniques, imagery, self-hypnosis, and distraction; acute or prolonged pain associated with exercise should be reported to a health care provider for evaluation. A weight reduction program may be recommended to relieve stress on painful joints (Zychowicz, Pope, & Graser, 2010).

The major challenge for the patient and the health care provider is the need to adjust all aspects of treatment according to the activity of the disease. Especially for the patient with an active diffuse connective tissue disease, such as rheumatoid arthritis (RA) or systemic lupus erythematosus (SLE), activity levels may vary from day to day and even within a single day.

Sleep

Short-term use of low-dose antidepressant medications, such as amitriptyline (Elavil), may be prescribed to reestablish adequate sleep patterns and improve pain management (McPhee, Papadakis, & Rabow, 2012). Patients need restful sleep so they can cope with pain, minimize physical fatigue, and deal with the changes related to having a chronic disease. In patients with acute disease, sleep time is frequently reduced and fragmented by prolonged awakenings. Stiffness, depression, and medications may also compromise the quality of sleep and increase daytime fatigue. A sleep-inducing routine, medication, and comfort measures may help improve the quality of sleep.

Education about sleep hygiene strategies may help promote restorative sleep. These strategies include establishing

a set time to sleep and a regular wake-up time, creating a quiet sleep environment with a comfortable room temperature, avoiding factors that interfere with sleep (e.g., the use of alcohol and caffeine), using relaxation exercises, and getting out of bed and engaging in another activity (e.g., reading) if unable to sleep.

Nursing Management

Chart 39-2 details the nursing diagnoses, interventions, and expected outcomes for the patient with a rheumatic disorder.

 Gerontologic Considerations

The various rheumatologic disease conditions in the older adult pose unique challenges. These challenges relate to disability, cognitive changes, comorbid conditions, and diagnosis. Musculoskeletal problems are the most frequently reported conditions in older adults (Miller, 2012) and will be seen more frequently by health professionals in the coming years along with associated disability, especially among frail older adults.

Comorbid conditions pose a unique challenge in diagnosing rheumatologic disease in older adults because they have the potential to mask or alter presenting symptoms (McPhee et al., 2012). The frequency, pattern of onset, clinical features, severity, and effects on function of the rheumatic disease in older patients may be different in very old patients. In addition, other medical conditions may take precedence over the rheumatic disease, which commonly becomes a secondary diagnosis and concern. Decreased vision and altered balance, often present in older people, may be problematic if rheumatic disease in the lower extremities affects locomotion. The combination of decreased hearing and visual acuity, memory loss, and depression contributes to failure to follow the treatment regimen in older adult patients as well (Miller, 2012). Special techniques for promoting patient safety, self-management, and strategies such as memory aids for medications may be necessary.

Behavioral clues such as gait patterns, guarding and joint flexion may aid the nurse in assessing the patient's pain when cognitive impairment is present (Tsai, Kuo, Beck, et al., 2011). Older adults, especially men, may also neglect to communicate their pain unless elicited by the provider (Shea & McDonald, 2011). Pain, in general, in this population has been associated with sleep disturbances, which can exacerbate all other medical conditions (Chen, Hayman, Shmerling, et al., 2011).

Older adults have an increased risk of osteoporosis (Bultink, 2012). Pain, loss of mobility, diminished self-image, and increasing morbidity can result from progressive osteoporosis. Therefore, diagnosis and treatment of osteoporosis should not be overlooked in this population. Pharmacologic therapy (including analgesic agents), exercise, postural assistance, modification of activities of daily living, and psychological support are useful components of the treatment program for the older adult.

Identifying the effects of the rheumatic disease on the patient's lifestyle, independence, and psychological status is important and can improve the quality of life for older people (Stamp & Jordan, 2011). Depressed mood is routinely found in those suffering from chronic joint disease (Gleicher, Croxford,

TABLE 39-3　Medications Used in Rheumatic Diseases

Medication	Action, Use, and Indication	Nursing Considerations
Salicylates		
Acetylated: aspirin *Nonacetylated:* choline trilisalicylate (Arthropan, Trilisate), salsalate (Disalcid), sodium salicylate	*Action:* Anti-inflammatory, analgesic, antipyretic Acetylated salicylates are platelet aggregation inhibitors. Anti-inflammatory doses will produce blood salicylate levels of 20–30 mg/dL.	Administer with meals to prevent gastric irritation. Assess for tinnitus, gastric intolerance, GI bleeding, and purpura. Monitor for possible confusion in the older adult.
Nonsteroidal Anti-inflammatory Drugs (NSAIDs)		
diclofenac (Voltaren), diflunisal (Dolobid), etodolac (Lodine), flurbiprofen (Ansaid), ibuprofen (Motrin), indomethacin (Indocin), ketoprofen (Orudis, Oruvail), meclofenamate (Meclomen), meloxicam (Mobic), nabumetone (Relafen), naproxen (Naprosyn), oxaprozin (Daypro), piroxicam (Feldene), sulindac (Clinoril), tolmetin sodium (Tolectin) *COX-2 enzyme blockers:* celecoxib (Celebrex)	*Action:* Anti-inflammatory, analgesic, antipyretic, platelet aggregation inhibitor Anti-inflammatory effect occurs 2–4 weeks after initiation. All NSAIDs are useful for short-term treatment of acute gout attack. NSAIDs are an alternative to salicylates for first-line therapy in several rheumatic diseases. *Action:* Inhibit only COX-2 enzymes, which are produced during inflammation, and spare COX-1 enzymes, which can be protective to the stomach	Administer NSAIDs with food. Monitor for GI, CNS, cardiovascular, renal, hematologic, and dermatologic adverse effects. Avoid salicylates; use acetaminophen for additional analgesia. Watch for possible confusion in older adults. Monitoring is the same as for other NSAIDs. Increased risk of cardiovascular events, including myocardial infarction and stroke Appropriate for older adults and patients who are at high risk for gastric ulcers
Disease-Modifying Antirheumatic Drugs (DMARDs)		
Antimalarials: hydroxychloroquine (Plaquenil), chloroquine (Aralen)	*Action:* Anti-inflammatory, inhibit lysosomal enzymes Slow acting; onset may take 2–4 months. Useful in RA and SLE	Administer concurrently with NSAIDs. Assess for visual changes, GI upset, skin rash, headaches, photosensitivity, bleaching of hair. Emphasize need for ophthalmologic examinations (every 6–12 months).
Gold-containing compounds: aurothioglucose (Solganal), gold sodium thiomalate (Myochrysine), auranofin (Ridaura)	*Action:* Inhibits T- and B-cell activity, suppresses synovitis during active stage of rheumatoid disease Slow acting; onset may take 3–6 months. IM preparations are given weekly for about 6 months, then every 2–4 weeks.	Administer concurrently with NSAIDs. Assess for stomatitis, diarrhea, dermatitis, proteinuria, hematuria, bone marrow suppression (decreased WBCs and/or platelets), CBC, and urinalysis with every other injection.
sulfasalazine (Azulfidine)	*Action:* Anti-inflammatory, reduces lymphocyte response, inhibits angiogenesis Useful in RA, seronegative spondyloarthropathies	Administer concurrently with NSAIDs. Do not use in patients with allergy to sulfa medications or salicylates. Emphasize adequate fluid intake. Assess for GI upset, skin rash, headache, liver abnormalities, anemia.
penicillamine (Cuprimine, Depen)	*Action:* Anti-inflammatory, inhibits T-cell function, impairs antigen presentation Slow acting; onset may take 2–3 months. Useful in RA and systemic sclerosis	Administer concurrently with NSAIDs. Assess for GI irritation, decreased taste, skin rash or itching, bone marrow suppression, proteinuria with CBC, and urinalysis every 2–4 weeks.
Immunosuppressives: methotrexate (Rheumatrex), azathioprine (Imuran), cyclophosphamide (Cytoxan)	*Action:* Immune suppression, affect DNA synthesis and other cellular effects Have teratogenic potential; azathioprine and cyclophosphamide reserved for more aggressive or unresponsive disease Methotrexate is gold standard for RA treatment; also useful in SLE.	Assess for bone marrow suppression, GI ulcerations, skin rashes, alopecia, bladder toxicity, increased infections. Monitor CBC, liver enzymes, creatinine every 2–4 weeks. Advise patient of contraceptive measures because of teratogenicity.
cyclosporine (Neoral)	*Action:* Immune suppression by inhibiting T lymphocytes Used for severe, progressive RA, unresponsive to other DMARDs Used in combination with methotrexate	Assess slow dose titration upward until response noted or toxicity occurs. Assess for toxic effects, such as bleeding gums, fluid retention, hair growth, tremors. Monitor blood pressure and creatinine every 2 weeks until stable.
Immunomodulators		
Pyrimidine synthesis inhibitor: leflunomide (Arava)	*Action:* Has antiproliferative and anti-inflammatory effects; used in moderate to severe RA May be used alone or in combination with other DMARDs (except methotrexate)	Long half-life; requires loading dose followed by daily administration. Assess for diarrhea, hair loss, skin rash, mouth sores. Monitor liver function tests. Contraindicated in pregnancy and breast-feeding Administered orally

Medication	Action, Use, and Indication	Nursing Considerations
TNF blocking agents: adalimumab (Humira), certolizumab pegol (Cimzia), etanercept (Enbrel), infliximab (Remicade), golimumab (Simponi)	*Action:* Biologic response modifier that binds to TNF, a cytokine involved in inflammatory and immune responses. Used in moderate to severe RA. Can be used alone or with methotrexate or other nonbiologic DMARDs. Humira is administered every 1–2 weeks, and Enbrel is administered twice a week.	Patient should be tested for tuberculosis before beginning this medication. Educate patient about subcutaneous self-injection of adalimumab (Humira) or etanercept (Enbrel). Infliximab (Remicade) is administered by IV line over 2 hours or more. Medication must be refrigerated. Monitor for injection site reactions. Educate patient about increased risk for infection and to withhold medication if fever occurs.
T-cell costimulation modulator: abatacept (Orencia)	*Action:* Blocks one of the pathways needed to fully activate T cells, decreasing inflammatory and immunologic responses. Used in moderate to severe RA unresponsive to TNF inhibitors. Used with methotrexate or DMARDs other than TNF inhibitors or anakinra.	Administered IV initially, then transitions to subcutaneous dosage once weekly. Educate patient about subcutaneous self-injections administered daily. Monitor for injection site reactions. Educate patient about increased risk of infection and to withhold medication if fever occurs.
B-cell production blocker: rituximab (Rituxan)	*Action:* Binds to B-lymphocyte CD20 surface antigens. Used in refractory RA in patients with inadequate response to TNF antagonist. Given with methotrexate.	Administered IV every 2 weeks. Premedicate with acetaminophen, antihistamine, and glucocorticoid. Educate patient about increased risk of infection.
Human IL-1 receptor antagonist: anakinra (Kineret)	*Action:* Blocks IL-1 receptors, decreasing inflammatory and immunologic responses. Used in moderate to severe RA. Can be used alone or with methotrexate or DMARDs other than TNF blocking agents.	Administered daily by subcutaneous injection. Educate patient about subcutaneous self-injections administered daily. Medication must be refrigerated. Monitor for injection site reactions. Educate patient about increased risk of infection and to withhold medication if fever occurs.
Human IL-6 receptor antagonist: tocilizumab (Actemra)	*Action:* Binds to and inhibits IL-6 receptors, decreasing inflammatory and immunologic responses. Can be used alone or with methotrexate or in combination with other nonbiologic DMARDs.	Administered IV every 4 weeks. Educate patient about increased risk of infection.
Corticosteroids prednisone, prednisolone, hydrocortisone	*Action:* Anti-inflammatory. Used for shortest duration and at lowest dose possible to minimize adverse effects. Useful for unremitting RA, SLE, polymyalgia rheumatica, myositis, arteritis Fast acting; onset in days Intra-articular injections useful for joints unresponsive to NSAIDs	*Assess for toxicity:* Cataracts, GI irritation, hyperglycemia, hypertension, fractures, avascular necrosis, hirsutism, psychosis. Joints most amenable to injections include ankles, knees, hips, shoulders, and hands. Repeated injections can cause joint damage.
Topical Analgesics capsaicin (Zostrix)	*Action:* Analgesic	Instruct patient to apply sparingly, avoid areas of open skin, and avoid contact with eyes and mucous membranes. Wash hands carefully after application. Assess for local skin irritation.

GI, gastrointestinal; CNS, central nervous system; COX, cyclo-oxygenase; RA, rheumatoid arthritis; SLE, systemic lupus erythematosus; IM, intramuscular; WBCs, white blood cells; CBC, complete blood count; TNF, tumor necrosis factor; IV, intravenous; IL-1, interleukin 1; IL-6, interleukin 6.

Hochman, et al., 2011). The body image and self-esteem of the older adult with rheumatic disease, combined with underlying depression, may interfere with the use of assistive devices such as canes (Vriezekolk, Eijsbouts, Evers, et al., 2010). The use of adaptive equipment such as long-handled reachers or tongs may be viewed by the older adult as evidence of aging rather than as a means of increasing independence.

Because most rheumatologic diseases involve pain, especially with joints, some older adults may consider their symptoms as inevitable consequences of aging. In fact, many older

people expect and accept the immobility and self-care problems related to the rheumatic diseases and do not seek help, thinking that nothing can be done.

The older adult usually has a lifelong pattern of dealing with the stresses of daily life. Depending on the success of that pattern, the older adult can often maintain a positive attitude and self-esteem when faced with a rheumatic disease, especially if support is available. Previous stress management strategies are assessed. If these strategies have been effective, the patient is encouraged and supported in their use. If they

TABLE 39-4   Exercise to Promote Mobility

Type of Exercise	Purpose	Recommended Performance	Precautions
Range of motion	Maintain flexibility and joint motion	Active or active/self-assisted at least daily	Reduce number of repetitions when inflammation is present.
Isometric exercise	Improve muscle tone, static endurance, and strength; prepare for dynamic and weight-bearing exercises	Perform at 70% of maximal voluntary contraction daily.	Monitor blood pressure; isometric exercises may increase blood pressure and decrease blood flow to muscles.
Dynamic exercise	Maintain or increase dynamic strength and endurance; increase muscle power; enhance synovial blood flow; promote strength of bone and cartilage	Start with repetitions against gravity and add progressive resistance; perform 2–3 days per week.	May increase biomechanical stress on unstable or misaligned joints
Aerobic exercise	Improve cardiovascular fitness and endurance	Perform 3–5 days per week for 20–30 minutes of moderate-intensity exercise.	Progress slowly as activity tolerance and fitness improve.
Pool exercise	Water supports or resists movement; warm water may provide muscle relaxation.	Provide buoyant medium for performance of dynamic or aerobic exercise	Heated swimming pool; deep water to minimize joint compression; nonslip footwear for safety and comfort. Receive appropriate instruction in a program designed for people with arthritis.

Adapted from Firestein, G. S., Panayi, G. S., & Willheim, F. A. (2006). *Rheumatoid arthritis*. Oxford, UK: Oxford University Press.

were ineffective, the nurse assists the patient in identifying alternative strategies, encourages the use of new strategies, and assesses their effectiveness (Vriezekolk et al., 2010).

Pharmacologic treatment of rheumatic disease in older patients is more difficult than in younger patients. If therapeutic medications have an effect on the senses (hearing, cognition), this effect is intensified in the older adult. The cumulative effect of medications, in general, is accentuated because of the physiologic changes of aging. For example, decreased renal function in the older adult alters the metabolism of certain medications, such as NSAIDs. Older adults are more prone to side effects associated with the use of multiple-drug therapy (Stamp & Jordan, 2011).

Partly because of the more frequent contact of older adults with health care providers for a variety of health issues, overtreatment or inappropriate treatment is possible. Complaints of pain may be met with a prescription for an opioid analgesic agent rather than instructions for rest, the use of an assistive device, and local comfort measures such as heat or cold. Acetaminophen may be appropriate and worth trying before other medications that pose a greater chance of side effects. NSAIDs can be used; however, long-term use can increase the risks of peptic ulcers. NSAIDs are used in conjunction with a proton pump inhibitor (i.e., omeprazole [Prilosec]) to decrease the likelihood of ulcer formation (Dhillon, 2011). Intra-articular corticosteroid injections, with their usually rapid relief of symptoms, may be requested by the patient who is unaware of the consequences of too-frequent use of this treatment. In addition, exercise programs may not be instituted or may be ineffective because the patient expects results to occur quickly or fails to appreciate the effectiveness of a program of exercise. In fact, strength training is encouraged in the older adult with chronic diseases (Hurley et al., 2011).

Diffuse Connective Tissue Diseases

Diffuse connective tissue disease refers to a group of systemic disorders that are chronic in nature and are characterized by diffuse inflammation and degeneration in the connective tissues. These disorders share similar clinical features and may affect some of the same organs. The characteristic clinical course is one of exacerbations and remissions. Although diffuse connective tissue diseases have unknown causes, they are thought to be the result of immunologic abnormalities. They include RA, SLE, scleroderma, polymyositis, and polymyalgia rheumatica (PMR), giant cell arteritis.

■ *Rheumatoid Arthritis*

Rheumatoid arthritis is an autoimmune disease of unknown origin that affects 1% of the population worldwide, with a female-to-male ratio between 2:1 and 4:1, suggesting that there may be a link between RA and sex hormones (Oliver & Silman, 2009). In the United States, the lifetime risk of developing RA is 2.4% (Crowson, Matteson, Myasoedova, et al., 2011).

Pathophysiology

The exact mechanism of action for the etiology of RA is unknown. Research has, however, identified that the autoimmune reaction (see Fig. 39-1) originates in the synovial tissue. It is hypothesized that both environmental factors, such as cigarette smoking, and genetic factors coalesce to produce inflammatory and destructive synovial fluid, starting in the more distal joints (Ferraccioli & Gremese, 2011; Rojas-Serrano, Perez, Garcia, et al., 2011). This RA synovium breaks down collagen, causing edema, proliferation of the synovial membrane, and ultimately pannus formation. Pannus destroys cartilage and erodes the bone. The consequence is loss of articular surfaces and joint motion. Muscle fibers undergo degenerative changes. Tendon and ligament elasticity and contractile power are lost.

The RA inflammatory process has also been implicated in other disease processes (i.e., arteriosclerosis) (Clancy & Hasthorpe, 2011). It is hypothesized that the RA disease process somehow interferes with the production of high-density lipoprotein cholesterol, which is the form of cholesterol

(text continues on page 1065)

Chart 39-2

PLAN OF NURSING CARE
Care of the Patient With a Rheumatic Disorder

NURSING DIAGNOSIS: Acute and chronic pain related to inflammation and increased disease activity, tissue damage, fatigue, or lowered tolerance level
GOAL: Improvement in comfort level; incorporation of pain management techniques into daily life

Nursing Interventions	Rationale	Expected Outcomes
1. Provide variety of comfort measures: a. Application of heat or cold b. Massage, position changes, rest c. Foam mattress, supportive pillow, splints d. Relaxation techniques, diversional activities	1. Pain may respond to nonpharmacologic interventions such as joint protection, exercise, relaxation, and thermal modalities.	• Identifies factors that exacerbate or influence pain response • Identifies and uses pain management strategies • Verbalizes decrease in pain • Reports signs and symptoms of side effects in timely manner to prevent additional problems
2. Administer anti-inflammatory, analgesic, and slow-acting antirheumatic medications as prescribed.	2. Pain of rheumatic disease responds to individual or combination medication regimens.	• Verbalizes that pain is characteristic of rheumatic disease
3. Individualize medication schedule to meet patient's need for pain management.	3. Previous pain experiences and management strategies may be different from those needed for persistent pain.	• Establishes realistic pain relief goals • Verbalizes that pain often leads to the use of nontraditional and unproven self-treatment methods
4. Encourage verbalization of feelings about pain and chronicity of disease.	4. Verbalization promotes coping.	• Identifies changes in quality or intensity of pain
5. Educate patient about pathophysiology of pain and rheumatic disease, and assist patient to recognize that pain often leads to unproven treatment methods.	5. Knowledge of rheumatic pain and appropriate treatment may help patient avoid unsafe, ineffective therapies.	
6. Assist in identification of pain that leads to the use of unproven methods of treatment.	6. The impact of pain on an individual's life often leads to misconceptions about pain and pain management techniques.	
7. Assess for subjective changes in pain.	7. The individual's description of pain is a more reliable indicator than objective measurements such as change in vital signs, body movement, and facial expression.	

NURSING DIAGNOSIS: Fatigue related to increased disease activity, pain, inadequate sleep/rest, deconditioning, inadequate nutrition, and emotional stress/depression
GOAL: Incorporates as part of daily activities strategies necessary to modify fatigue

Nursing Interventions	Rationale	Expected Outcomes
1. Provide instruction about fatigue. a. Describe relationship of disease activity to fatigue. b. Describe comfort measures while providing them. c. Develop and encourage a sleep routine (warm bath and relaxation techniques that promote sleep). d. Explain importance of rest for relieving systematic, articular, and emotional stress. e. Explain how to use energy conservation techniques (pacing, delegating, setting priorities). f. Identify physical and emotional factors that can cause fatigue.	1. The patient's understanding of fatigue will affect his or her actions. a. The amount of fatigue is directly related to the activity of the disease. b. Relief of discomfort can relieve fatigue. c. Effective bedtime routine promotes restorative sleep. d. Different kinds of rest are needed to relieve fatigue and are based on patient need and response. e. A variety of measures can be used to conserve energy. f. Awareness of the various causes of fatigue provides the basis for measures to modify the fatigue.	• Self-evaluates and monitors fatigue pattern • Verbalizes the relationship of fatigue to disease activity • Uses comfort measures as appropriate • Practices effective sleep hygiene and routine • Makes use of various assistive devices (splints, canes) and strategies (bed rest, relaxation techniques) to ease different kinds of fatigue • Incorporates time management strategies in daily activities • Uses appropriate measures to prevent physical and emotional fatigue • Has an established plan to ensure well-paced, therapeutic activity schedule • Adheres to therapeutic program • Follows a planned conditioning program • Consumes a nutritious diet consisting of the five major groups and recommended daily allowance of vitamins and minerals
2. Facilitate development of appropriate activity/rest schedule.	2. Alternating rest and activity conserves energy while allowing most productivity.	
3. Encourage adherence to the treatment program.	3. Overall control of disease activity can decrease the amount of fatigue.	
4. Refer to and encourage a conditioning program.	4. Deconditioning resulting from lack of mobility, understanding, and disease activity contributes to fatigue.	

(continues on page 1064)

Chart 39-2

PLAN OF NURSING CARE

Care of the Patient With a Rheumatic Disorder (continued)

Nursing Interventions	Rationale	Expected Outcomes
5. Encourage adequate nutrition, including source of iron from food and supplements.	**5.** A nutritious diet can help counteract fatigue.	

NURSING DIAGNOSIS: Impaired physical mobility related to decreased range of motion, muscle weakness, pain on movement, limited endurance, lack of or improper use of ambulatory devices
GOAL: Attains and maintains optimal functional mobility

Nursing Interventions	Rationale	Expected Outcomes
1. Encourage verbalization regarding limitations in mobility.	**1.** Mobility is not necessarily related to deformity. Pain, stiffness, and fatigue may temporarily limit mobility. The degree of mobility is not synonymous with the degree of independence. Decreased mobility may influence a person's self-concept and lead to social isolation.	• Identifies factors that interfere with mobility • Describes and uses measures to prevent loss of motion • Identifies environmental (home, school, work, community) barriers to optimal mobility • Uses appropriate techniques and/or assistive equipment to aid mobility • Identifies community resources available to assist in managing decreased mobility

2. Assess need for occupational or physical therapy consultation.
  a. Emphasize range of motion of affected joints.
  b. Promote the use of assistive ambulatory devices.
  c. Explain the use of safe footwear.
  d. Use individual appropriate positioning/posture.
	2. Therapeutic exercises, proper footwear, and/or assistive equipment may improve mobility. Correct posture and positioning are necessary for maintaining optimal mobility.	

3. Assist to identify environmental barriers.	**3.** Furniture and architectural adaptations may enhance mobility.	

4. Encourage independence in mobility and assist as needed.
  a. Allow ample time for activity.
  b. Provide rest period after activity.
  c. Reinforce principles of joint protection and work simplification.
	4. Changes in mobility may lead to a decrease in personal safety.	

5. Initiate referral to community health agency.	**5.** The degree of mobility may be slow to improve or may not improve with intervention.	

NURSING DIAGNOSIS: Readiness for enhanced self-care related to contractures, fatigue, or loss of motion
GOAL: Performs self-care activities independently or with the use of resources

Nursing Interventions	Rationale	Expected Outcomes
1. Assist patient to identify self-care deficits and factors that interfere with ability to perform self-care activities.	**1.** The ability to perform self-care activities is influenced by the disease activity and the accompanying pain, stiffness, fatigue, muscle weakness, loss of motion, and depression.	• Identifies factors that interfere with the ability to perform self-care activities • Identifies alternative methods for meeting self-care needs • Uses alternative methods for meeting self-care needs • Identifies and uses other health care resources for meeting self-care needs

2. Develop a plan based on the patient's perceptions and priorities on how to establish and achieve goals to meet self-care needs, incorporating joint protection, energy conservation, and work simplification concepts.
  a. Provide appropriate assistive devices.
  b. Reinforce correct and safe use of assistive devices.
  c. Allow patient to control timing of self-care activities.
  d. Explore with the patient different ways to perform difficult tasks or ways to enlist the help of someone else.
	2. Assistive devices may enhance self-care abilities. Effective planning for changes must include the patient, who must accept and adopt the plan.	

PLAN OF NURSING CARE

Care of the Patient With a Rheumatic Disorder (continued)

Nursing Interventions	Rationale	Expected Outcomes
3. Consult with community health care agencies when individuals have attained a maximum level of self-care yet still have some deficits, especially regarding safety.	3. Individuals differ in ability and willingness to perform self-care activities. Changes in ability to care for self may lead to a decrease in personal safety.	

NURSING DIAGNOSIS: Disturbed body image related to physical and psychological changes and dependency imposed by chronic illness
GOAL: Adapts to physical and psychological changes imposed by the rheumatic disease

Nursing Interventions	Rationale	Expected Outcomes
1. Help patient identify elements of control over disease symptoms and treatment. 2. Encourage patient's verbalization of feelings, perceptions, and fears. a. Help to assess present situation and identify problems.	1. The individual's self-concept may be altered by the disease or its treatment. 2. The individual's coping strategies reflect the strength of his or her self-concept.	• Verbalizes an awareness that changes taking place in self-concept are normal responses to rheumatic disease and other chronic illnesses • Identifies strategies to cope with altered self-concept

NURSING DIAGNOSIS: Ineffective coping related to actual or perceived lifestyle or role changes
GOAL: Use of effective coping behaviors for dealing with actual or perceived limitations and role changes

Nursing Interventions	Rationale	Expected Outcomes

1. Identify areas of life affected by disease. Answer questions and dispel possible myths.
  a. Assist to identify past coping mechanisms.
  b. Assist to identify effective coping mechanisms.
2. Develop plan for managing symptoms and enlisting support of family and friends to promote daily function.
	1. The effects of disease may be more or less manageable once identified and explored reasonably.
	
	2. By taking action and involving others appropriately, patient develops or draws on coping skills and community support.
		• Names functions and roles affected and not affected by disease process
		• Describes therapeutic regimen and states actions to take to improve, change, or accept a particular situation, function, or role

COLLABORATIVE PROBLEMS: Complications secondary to effects of medications
GOAL: Absence or resolution of complications

Nursing Interventions	Rationale	Expected Outcomes
1. Perform periodic clinical assessment and laboratory evaluation. 2. Provide education about correct self-administration, potential side effects, and importance of monitoring. 3. Counsel regarding methods to reduce side effects and manage symptoms. 4. Administer medications in modified doses as prescribed if complications occur.	1. Skillful assessment helps detect early symptoms of side effects of medications. 2. The patient needs accurate information about medications and potential side effects to avoid or manage them. 3. Appropriate identification and early intervention may minimize complications. 4. Modifications may help minimize side effects or other complications.	• Adheres to monitoring procedures and experiences minimal side effects • Takes medication as prescribed and lists potential side effects • Identifies strategies to reduce or manage side effects • Reports that side effects or complications have subsided

responsible for decreasing cellular lipids and, therefore, is considered antiatherosclerotic. RA inflammatory processes have also been implicated in arterial wall stiffness and endothelial dysfunction.

The nervous system is also affected by the RA inflammatory process. The synovial inflammation can compress the adjacent nerve, causing neuropathies and paresthesias. Axonal degeneration and neuronal demyelination are also possible due to the infiltration of polymorphonuclear leukocytes, eosinophils, and mononuclear cells, causing necrotizing or occlusive vasculitis (Ramos-Remus, Duran-Barragan, & Castillo-Ortiz, 2012).

Clinical Manifestations

The initial clinical manifestations of RA include symmetric joint pain and morning joint stiffness lasting longer than 1 hour. Over the course of the disease, clinical manifestations of RA vary, usually reflecting the stage and severity of the disease. Symmetric joint pain, swelling, warmth, erythema, and lack of function are classic symptoms. Palpation of the joints reveals spongy or boggy tissue. Often, fluid can be aspirated from the inflamed joint. Characteristically, the pattern of joint involvement begins in the small joints of the hands, wrists, and feet (Klippel, Stone, Crofford, et al., 2008; McPhee et al., 2012). As the disease progresses, the knees, shoulders, hips, elbows, ankles, cervical spine, and temporomandibular joints are affected. The onset of symptoms is usually acute. Symptoms are usually bilateral and symmetric.

In the early stages of disease, even before the presentation of bony changes, limitation in function can occur when there is active inflammation in the joints. Joints that are hot, swollen, and painful are not easily moved. The patient tends to guard or protect these joints by immobilizing them. Immobilization for extended periods can lead to contractures, creating soft tissue deformity.

Deformities of the hands (e.g., ulnar deviation and swan neck deformity) and feet are common in RA (see Fig. 40-6 in Chapter 40). The deformity may be caused by misalignment resulting from swelling, progressive joint destruction, or the subluxation (partial dislocation) that occurs when one bone slips over another and eliminates the joint space. Deformities of RA differ from those seen with osteoarthritis (OA), such as Heberden's and Bouchard's nodes.

RA is a systemic disease with multiple extra-articular features. Most common are fever, weight loss, fatigue, anemia, lymph node enlargement, and Raynaud's phenomenon (cold- and stress-induced vasospasm causing episodes of digital blanching or cyanosis). Rheumatoid nodules may be noted in patients with more advanced RA, and they develop at some time in the course of the disease in about 20% of patients (McPhee et al., 2012). These nodules are usually nontender and movable in the subcutaneous tissue. They usually appear over bony prominences such as the elbow, are varied in size, and can disappear spontaneously. Nodules occur only in people who have rheumatoid factor. The nodules often are associated with rapidly progressive and destructive disease. Other extra-articular features include arteritis, neuropathy, pericarditis, splenomegaly, and Sjögren's syndrome (dry eyes and dry mucous membranes).

Assessment and Diagnostic Findings

Several assessment findings are associated with RA: rheumatoid nodules, joint inflammation detected on palpation, and laboratory findings. The history and physical examination focuses on manifestations such as bilateral and symmetric stiffness, tenderness, swelling, and temperature changes in the joints. The patient is also assessed for extra-articular changes; these often include weight loss, sensory changes, lymph node enlargement, and fatigue. Symptoms and examination findings are often recorded using a Disease Activity Score-28 (DAS28) form to evaluate disease activity and help guide treatment decisions (Firth, 2011b).

Rheumatoid factor is present in about 80% of patients with RA, but its presence alone is not diagnostic of RA, and its absence does not rule out the diagnosis. Antibodies to cyclic citrullinated peptide (anti-CCP) have a specificity of approximately 95% at detecting RA (McPhee et al., 2012). The erythrocyte sedimentation rate (ESR) and C-reactive protein (CRP) tend to be significantly elevated in the acute phases of RA and are therefore useful in monitoring active disease and disease progression. The red blood cell count and

C4 complement component are decreased. Antinuclear antibody (ANA) test results may also be positive (Firth, 2011a). Arthrocentesis shows synovial fluid that is cloudy, milky, or dark yellow and contains numerous inflammatory components, such as leukocytes and complement.

X-rays show bony erosions and narrowed joint spaces. X-rays of the hands and feet should be performed at baseline to help establish the diagnosis of RA and then every 3 years to monitor the progression of the disease (Lesko et al., 2010).

Medical Management

The goal of treatment at all phases of the RA disease process is to decrease joint pain and swelling, achieve clinical remission, decrease the likelihood of joint deformity, and minimize disability. Initial treatment delays have been implicated in greater long-term joint deformity (Lesko et al., 2010). Aggressive and early treatment regimens are warranted.

Early Rheumatoid Arthritis

Once the diagnosis of RA is made, treatment should begin with either a nonbiologic or biologic DMARD. In the past, a step-wise approach starting with NSAIDs was the standard of care. However, evidence clearly documenting the benefits of early DMARD treatment has changed national guidelines for management (Firth, 2011b). Now it is recommended that treatment with the nonbiologic DMARDs (methotrexate [Rheumatrex], antimalarial agents, leflunomide [Arava], or sulfasalazine [Azulfidine]) begin within 3 months of disease onset. At this time, methotrexate is the initial nonbiologic DMARD used for patients with RA. After initiating treatment, patients generally report a beneficial effect within 2 to 6 weeks and tolerate the medication relatively well (McPhee et al., 2012). Research suggests that methotrexate combined with low-dose prednisone improves patient outcome compared to the use of methotrexate alone for early RA (Bakker, Jacobs, Walsing, et al., 2012).

Another treatment approach for RA is the use of biologic DMARDs. These agents have been specifically engineered to target the most prominent proinflammatory mediators in RA—TNF-α, B cells, T cells, IL-1, and IL-6 (Firth & Critchley, 2011; Klippel et al., 2008) (see Table 39-3). Biologic DMARDs are the first targeted therapy for RA. Clinical evidence suggests that biologic DMARDs work more quickly and show a greater delay in radiologic disease progression when compared to nonbiologic DMARDs (Klippel et al., 2008). The biologic DMARDs are more expensive and have fewer years of usage with the RA population. Therefore, they tend to be reserved for patients with persistent moderate-to-severe RA who have not responded adequately to synthetic DMARDs (McPhee et al., 2012).

NSAIDs and specifically the cyclo-oxygenase 2 (COX-2) enzyme blockers are used for pain and inflammation relief. NSAIDs, such as ibuprofen (Motrin) and naproxen (Naprosyn), are commonly prescribed because of their low cost and analgesic properties. They must be used, however, with caution in long-term chronic diseases because of the possibility of gastric ulcers (Dhillon, 2011). Several COX-2 enzyme blockers have been approved for treatment of RA. Cyclooxygenase is an enzyme that is involved in the inflammatory process. COX-2 medications block the enzyme involved in inflammation (COX-2) while leaving intact the enzyme involved in protecting the stomach lining (COX-1). As a result, COX-2 enzyme blockers are less likely to cause gastric irritation and ulceration than other NSAIDs; however, they are associated with increased risk of cardiovascular disease and must be used with caution (Dhillon, 2011; Karch, 2012). The nurse should be aware that no NSAIDs, not even the COX-2 inhibitors, prevent erosions or alter disease progression and, consequently, are medications useful only for symptom relief.

Additional analgesia may be prescribed for periods of extreme pain. Opioid analgesic agents are avoided because of the potential for continuing need for pain relief. Nonpharmacologic pain management techniques (e.g., relaxation techniques, heat and cold applications) are taught (Firth, 2011b).

Moderate, Erosive Rheumatoid Arthritis

For moderate, erosive RA, a formal program with occupational and physical therapy is prescribed to educate the patient about principles of joint protection, pacing activities, work simplification, range of motion, and muscle-strengthening exercises (Firth, 2011a). The patient is encouraged to participate actively in the management program. The medication program is reevaluated periodically, and appropriate changes are made if indicated. Cyclosporine (Neoral), an immunosuppressant, may be added to enhance the disease-modifying effect of methotrexate (Klippel et al., 2008). Combination therapy using one nonbiologic DMARD and one biologic DMARD is common.

Persistent, Erosive Rheumatoid Arthritis

For persistent, erosive RA, reconstructive surgery and corticosteroids are often used. Reconstructive surgery is indicated when pain cannot be relieved by conservative measures and the threat of loss of independence is eminent (Woo, Kim, Chung, et al., 2011). Surgical procedures include synovectomy (excision of the synovial membrane), tenorrhaphy (suturing of a tendon), arthrodesis (surgical fusion of the joint), and **arthroplasty** (surgical repair and replacement of the joint). Surgery is not performed during exacerbations.

Systemic corticosteroids are used when the patient has unremitting inflammation and pain or needs a "bridging" medication while waiting for the slower DMARDs (e.g., methotrexate) to begin taking effect. Low-dose corticosteroid therapy is prescribed for the shortest time necessary to minimize side effects (McPhee et al., 2012). Single large joints that are severely inflamed and fail to respond promptly to the measures outlined previously may be treated by local injection of a corticosteroid.

Advanced, Unremitting Rheumatoid Arthritis

For advanced, unremitting RA, immunosuppressive agents are prescribed because of their ability to affect the production of antibodies at the cellular level. These include high-dose methotrexate, cyclophosphamide (Cytoxan), and azathioprine (Imuran). However, these medications are highly toxic and can produce bone marrow suppression, anemia, gastrointestinal disturbances, severe birth defects, and rashes (Karch, 2012).

The U.S. Food and Drug Administration (FDA) has approved a medical device for use in treating patients with more severe and long-standing RA who have had no response to or are intolerant of DMARDs. The device, a protein A immunoadsorption column (Prosorba), is used in 12 weekly, 2-hour apheresis treatments to bind immunoglobulin G (IgG) (i.e., circulating immune complex). This treatment offers a limited duration of relief, has many side effects, and is therefore limited to the treatment of patients with severe RA (American College of Rheumatology Subcommittee, 2002).

For most patients with RA, the emotional and possible financial burden of the disease can lead to depressive symptoms and sleep deprivation (Chamberlain, 2011; Vriezekolk et al., 2010). The patient may require the short-term use of low-dose antidepressant medications, such as amitriptyline (Elavil), paroxetine (Paxil), or sertraline (Zoloft), to reestablish an adequate sleep pattern and manage depressive symptoms. Patients may benefit from referrals for talk therapy or group support.

Nutrition Therapy

Patients with RA frequently experience anorexia, weight loss, and anemia. A dietary history identifies usual eating habits and food preferences. Food selection should include the five major groups (grains, vegetables, fruits, dairy, and protein), with emphasis on foods high in vitamins, protein, and iron for tissue building and repair. For the patient who is extremely anorexic, small, frequent feedings with increased protein supplements may be prescribed. Supplemental vitamins and minerals may also be prescribed as needed (Klippel et al., 2008). Certain medications (i.e., oral corticosteroids) used in RA treatment stimulate the appetite and, when combined with decreased activity, may lead to weight gain. Therefore, patients may need to be counseled about eating a healthy, calorie-restricted diet.

Nursing Management

Nursing care of the patient with RA follows the basic plan of care presented earlier (see Chart 39-2). The most common issues for the patient with RA include pain, sleep disturbance, fatigue, altered mood, and limited mobility (Chamberlain, 2011). The patient with newly diagnosed RA needs information about the disease to make daily self-management decisions and cope with having a chronic disease.

Monitoring and Managing Potential Complications

Medications used for treating RA may cause serious and adverse effects. The primary provider bases the prescribed medication regimen on clinical findings and past medical history, and then, with the help of the nurse, monitors for side effects using periodic clinical assessments and laboratory testing. The nurse, who can be available for consultation between physician visits, works to help the patient recognize and deal with these side effects (see Table 39-3). Medication may need to be stopped or the dose reduced. If the patient experiences an increase in symptoms while the complication is being resolved or a new medication is being initiated, the nurse's counseling regarding symptom management may relieve potential anxiety and distress (Chamberlain, 2011).

Promoting Home and Community-Based Care

Educating Patients About Self-Care

Patient education is an essential aspect in nursing care of the patient with RA to enable the patient to maintain as much independence as possible, to take medications accurately and safely, and to use adaptive devices correctly. Patient education focuses on the disorder itself, the possible changes related to the disorder, the therapeutic regimen prescribed to treat it, and the potential side effects of medications. Patients undergoing

Chart 39-3

NURSING RESEARCH PROFILE
Presurgical Admission Education in Rheumatoid Arthritis

Johansson, K., Kataajistoo, J., & Salantera, S. (2010). Pre-admission education in surgical rheumatology nursing: Towards greater patient empowerment. *Journal of Clinical Nursing, 19*(21), 2980–988.

Purpose

Rheumatoid arthritis (RA) is a chronic, progressive, inflammatory disease that can cause disability through joint erosion and bone deformities. In many instances, surgical correction is required. The purpose of this study was to compare the effectiveness of two types of presurgical admission education: measuring effects of knowledge and empowerment.

Design

This was a quasi-experimental study using a pre-post-test design for 59 patients undergoing hip arthroplasty for RA. Two randomized groups were formed: one receiving written material only, and one receiving written material and a telephone encounter 2 to 4 weeks prior to admission. Data were collected using the Orthopedic Patient Knowledge Questionnaire (OPKQ) and the Modified Empowerment Questionnaire (MEQ)

prior to preadmission education, at admission (following the intervention), and at discharge.

Findings

There were no statistically significant differences in patient knowledge between the two groups, except at discharge, where the educational materials–only group showed increased knowledge. However, patients receiving the education via telephone scored higher in patient empowerment, with patients reporting that they were better able to make choices and receive support for their concerns, and that the counseling provided them was suitable.

Nursing Implications

Written educational materials seem appropriate for preadmission patient education. With regard to patient empowerment, however, the education received via telephone may be more beneficial. Talking with patients, especially when using empowering educational techniques, is an important part of current nursing practice.

surgery need education as well (Chart 39-3). The nurse works with the patient and family on strategies to maintain independence, function, and safety in the home (Ovayolu et al., 2012) (Chart 39-4).

The patient and family are encouraged to verbalize their concerns and ask questions. Because RA commonly affects young women, major concerns may be related to the effects of the disease on childbearing potential, caring for family, or work responsibilities. The patient with a chronic illness may seek a "cure" or have questions about alternative therapies. A recent systematic review of complementary and alternative medicine (CAM) examined the efficacy of herbal medicine, acupuncture, T'ai chi, and biofeedback in the treatment for RA and OA. Although acupuncture treatment for pain management showed some promise, in all modalities the evidence was ambiguous. There is not enough evidence of the effec-

tiveness of CAM, and more rigorous research is needed (Ernst & Posadzki, 2011).

Pain, fatigue, and depressive symptoms can interfere with the patient's ability to learn and should be addressed before instruction is initiated (Vriezekolk et al., 2010). Various educational strategies may then be used, depending on the patient's previous knowledge base, interest level, degree of comfort, social or cultural influences, and readiness to learn (Lesko et al., 2010). The nurse educates the patient about basic disease management and necessary adaptations in lifestyle. Some types of aerobic exercise and strength training should be discussed (Hurley et al., 2011). Because suppression of inflammation and autoimmune responses requires the use of anti-inflammatory, disease-modifying antirheumatic, and immunosuppressive agents, the patient is taught about prescribed medications, including type, dosage, rationale,

Chart 39-4

HOME CARE CHECKLIST
The Patient With Rheumatoid Arthritis

At the completion of home care education, the patient or caregiver will be able to:	PATIENT	CAREGIVER
• Explain the nature of the disease and principles of disease management.	✔	✔
• Describe the medication regimen (name of medications, dosage, schedule of administration, precautions, potential side effects, and desired effects).	✔	✔
• Identify monitoring procedures and strategies that should be implemented.	✔	✔
• Identify sources of additional information, if necessary.	✔	✔
• Demonstrate accurate and safe self-administration of medications.	✔	
• Describe and demonstrate the use of pain management techniques.	✔	✔
• Demonstrate the use of joint protection techniques in activities of daily living.	✔	✔
• Demonstrate ability to perform self-care activities independently or with assistive devices.	✔	
• Demonstrate a safe exercise program.	✔	
• Demonstrate a relaxation technique.	✔	

potential side effects, self-administration, and required monitoring procedures. If hospitalized, the patient is encouraged to practice new self-management skills with support from caregivers and significant others. The nurse then reinforces disease management skills during each patient contact. Barriers are assessed, and measures are taken to promote adherence to medications and the treatment program (Palmer & El Miedany, 2010).

Continuing Care

Depending on the severity of the disease and the patient's resources and supports, referral for home care may be warranted. For example, the patient who is an older adult or frail, has RA that limits function significantly, and lives alone may need referral for home care.

The impact of RA on everyday life is not always evident when the patient is seen in the hospital or in an ambulatory care setting. The increased frequency with which nurses see patients in the home provides opportunities for recognizing problems and implementing interventions aimed at improving the quality of life of patients with RA.

During home visits, the nurse has the opportunity to assess the home environment and its adequacy for patient safety and management of the disorder. Adherence to the treatment program can be more easily monitored in the home setting, where physical and social barriers to adherence are more readily identified. For example, a patient who also has diabetes and requires insulin may be unable to fill the syringe accurately or unable to administer the insulin because of impaired joint mobility. Appropriate adaptive equipment needed for increased independence is often identified more readily when the nurse sees how the patient functions in the home. Any barriers to adherence are identified, and appropriate referrals are made.

For patients at risk for impaired skin integrity, the home care nurse can closely monitor skin status and also educate, provide, or supervise the patient and family in preventive skin care measures. The nurse also assesses the patient's need for assistance in the home and supervises home health aides, who may meet many of the needs of the patient with RA. Referrals to physical and occupational therapists may be made as problems are identified and limitations increase (Firth, 2011a). A home care nurse may visit the home to make sure the patient can function as independently as possible despite mobility problems and can safely manage treatments, including pharmacotherapy. The patient and family should be informed about support services such as Meals on Wheels and local Arthritis Foundation chapters.

Because many of the medications used to suppress inflammation are injectable, the nurse may administer the medication to the patient or educate about self-injection. These frequent contacts allow the nurse to reinforce other disease management techniques.

The nurse also assesses the patient's physical and psychological status, adequacy of symptom management, and adherence to the management plan. Patients should know which type of rheumatic disease they have, not just that they have "arthritis" or "arthritis of the knee." The importance of attending follow-up appointments is emphasized to the patient and family, and they should be reminded about the importance of participating in other health promotion activities and health screening.

Systemic Lupus Erythematosus

SLE is an inflammatory, autoimmune disorder that affects nearly every organ in the body. The overall incidence of SLE is estimated to be 1.8 to 7.6 per 100,000 persons (Centers for Disease Control and Prevention [CDC], 2012a). The lifetime risk of developing SLE is 0.91% for women and 0.21% for men (Crowson et al., 2011). It occurs 6 to10 times more frequently in women than in men and occurs more in African American populations than among Caucasians (CDC, 2012a). It also appears to affect African American women at an earlier stage in life (before 40 years) than in Caucasians (after 40 years) (Pons-Estel, Alarcón, Scofield, et al., 2010). The focus here is on SLE; however, there are three other forms of lupus: discoid lupus (which primarily affects the skin on the face), drug-induced lupus (which rarely includes some brain or kidney effects and has a clearer pathophysiology), and neonatal lupus (which is passed to the newborn during childbirth and usually resolved by 6 months of age) (Klippel et al., 2008).

Pathophysiology

SLE starts with the body's immune system inaccurately recognizing one or more components of the cell's nucleus as foreign, seeing it as an antigen. The immune system starts to develop antibodies to the nuclear antigen. In particular, B cells begin to overproduce antibodies with the help of multiple cytokines such as B-lymphocyte stimulator (BLyS), which is overexpressed in SLE (Navarra, Guzmán, Gallacher, et al., 2011). The antibodies and antigens form antigen–antibody complexes and have the propensity to get trapped in the capillaries of visceral structures. The antibodies also act to destroy host cells. It is thought that those two mechanisms are responsible for the majority of the clinical manifestations of this disease process (McPhee et al., 2012). It is hypothesized that the immunoregulatory disturbance is brought about by some combination of four distinct factors: genetic, immunologic, hormonal, and environmental (Bernknop, Rowley, & Bailey, 2011).

Research into the genetic origins of SLE has thus far revealed that multiple genes are likely implicated in the development of SLE. In support of this theory, research with homozygous twins has shown a higher incidence of SLE, especially considering that the prevalence of SLE was low in other family members (Bernknop et al., 2011). The large majority of SLE cases, however, remain sporadic and unrelated to family medical history.

Given the overwhelming numbers of women with SLE as compared to men, it is hypothesized that female sex hormones also play a role in the predisposition to SLE. In addition, women who used oral contraceptive medication, had an earlier onset of menarche, or used hormone replacement therapy post menopause have an increased incidence of SLE (Bernknop et al., 2011).

Although genetics and hormones likely play a role in the predisposition of SLE, it is hypothesized that an exogenous or environmental trigger is implicated in the onset of the disease process (Klippel et al., 2008). These triggers may include exposure to a virus or sunlight or brought about by stress or diet.

Certain medications, such as hydralazine (Apresoline), procainamide (Pronestyl), isoniazid (INH), chlorpromazine (Thorazine), and some antiseizure medications, have been implicated in chemical or drug-induced SLE (Klippel et al., 2008).

Clinical Manifestations

SLE is an autoimmune, systemic disease that can affect any body system. The disease process involves chronic states where symptoms are minimal or absent and acute flares where symptoms and lab results are elevated. Systemic symptoms include fever, malaise, weight loss, and anorexia. The mucocutaneous, musculoskeletal, renal, nervous, cardiovascular, and respiratory systems are most commonly involved. Less commonly affected are the gastrointestinal tract and liver as well as the ocular system.

Some type of cutaneous system manifestation is experienced in 80% to 90% of patients with SLE (Klippel et al., 2008). Four of the 11 criteria used for diagnosing SLE by the American College of Rheumatology involve the cutaneous system (Tan, Cohen, Fries, et al., 1982). The most familiar skin manifestation (occurring in less than 50% of patients with SLE) is an acute cutaneous lesion consisting of a butterfly-shaped erythematous rash across the bridge of the nose and cheeks (McPhee et al., 2012) (Fig. 39-2). Several other skin manifestations may occur in patients with SLE, including subacute cutaneous lupus erythematosus, which involves papulosquamous or annular polycyclic lesions, and a discoid rash, which is a chronic rash with erythematous papules or plaques and scaling and can cause scarring and pigmentation changes. In some cases, the only skin involvement may be a discoid rash. In some patients with SLE, the initial skin involvement is the precursor to more systemic involvement. The lesions often worsen during exacerbations (flares) of the systemic disease and possibly are provoked by sunlight or artificial ultraviolet light (Klippel et al., 2008). Oral ulcers, which may accompany skin lesions, may involve the buccal mucosa or the hard palate, occur in crops, and are often associated with exacerbations. Other cutaneous manifestations include splinter hemorrhages, alopecia, and Raynaud's phenomenon.

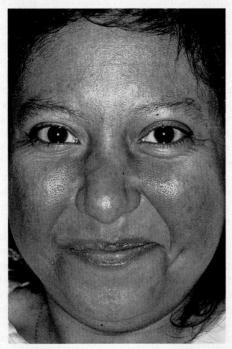

FIGURE 39-2 • The characteristic butterfly rash of systemic lupus erythematosus.

Joint symptoms, with arthralgias and/or arthritis (synovitis), occur in more than 90% of patients with SLE and are commonly the earliest manifestation of the disease process (McPhee et al., 2012). Joint swelling, tenderness, and pain on movement are also common. Frequently, these are accompanied by morning stiffness.

The cardiac system is also commonly affected in SLE. Pericarditis is the most common cardiac manifestation, occurring in 6% to 45% of patients (Klippel et al., 2008). Patients may present with substernal chest pain that is aggravated by movement or inspiration. Symptoms can be acute and severe or last for weeks at a time. Other cardiac symptoms may involve myocarditis, hypertension, cardiac dysrhythmias, and valvular incompetence (McPhee et al., 2012). Women who have SLE are also at risk for early-onset atherosclerosis.

Nephritis as a result of SLE, also referred to as lupus nephritis, occurs due to a buildup of antibodies and immune complexes that cause damage to the nephrons (Gigante, Gasperini, Afeltra, et al., 2011). Serum creatinine levels and urinalysis are used in screening for renal involvement. Early detection allows for prompt treatment so that renal damage can be prevented. Renal involvement may lead to hypertension, which also requires careful monitoring and management (see Chapter 31).

Central nervous system involvement is widespread, encompassing the entire range of neurologic disease. The varied and frequent neuropsychiatric presentations of SLE are now widely recognized and include psychosis, cognitive impairment, seizures, peripheral and cranial neuropathies, transverse myelitis, and strokes (McPhee et al., 2012). These are generally demonstrated by subtle changes in behavior patterns or cognitive ability.

Assessment and Diagnostic Findings

Diagnosis of SLE is based on a complete history, physical examination, and blood tests. In addition to the general assessment performed for any patient with a rheumatic disease, assessment for known or suspected SLE has special features. The skin is inspected for erythematous rashes. Cutaneous erythematous plaques with an adherent scale may be observed on the scalp, face, or neck. Areas of hyperpigmentation or depigmentation may be noted, depending on the phase and type of disease. The patient should be questioned about skin changes (because these may be transitory) and specifically about sensitivity to sunlight or artificial ultraviolet light. The scalp should be inspected for alopecia and the mouth and throat for ulcerations reflecting gastrointestinal involvement.

Cardiovascular assessment includes auscultation for pericardial friction rub, possibly associated with myocarditis and accompanying pleural effusions. The pleural effusions and infiltrations, which reflect respiratory insufficiency, are demonstrated by abnormal lung sounds. Papular, erythematous, and purpuric lesions developing on the fingertips, elbows, toes, and extensor surfaces of the forearms or lateral sides of the hand that may become necrotic suggest vascular involvement.

Joint swelling, tenderness, warmth, pain on movement, stiffness, and edema may be detected on physical examination. The joint involvement is often symmetric and similar to that found in RA.

Criteria for Classifying Systemic Lupus Erythematosus

The American College of Rheumatology has established criteria for the classification of systemic lupus erythematosus (SLE) involving these 11 distinct elements:

- Malar rash
- Discoid rash
- Photosensitivity
- Oral ulcers
- Arthritis
- Serositis
- Kidney disease
- Neurologic disease
- Hematologic disorder
- Immunologic disorder
- Positive antinuclear antibody

The diagnosis of SLE is generally made if 4 of the 11 criteria are present, either serially or simultaneously.

Adapted from Tan, E. M., Cohen, A. S., Fries, J. F., et al. (1982). The 1982 revised criteria for the classification of systemic lupus erythematosus. *Arthritis and Rheumatism*, 25(11), 1271–1277.

The neurologic assessment is directed at identifying and describing any central nervous system changes. The patient and family members are asked about any behavioral changes, including manifestations of neurosis or psychosis. Signs of depression are noted, as are reports of seizures, chorea, or other central nervous system manifestations.

The American College of Rheumatology has established criteria for the classification of SLE involving 11 distinct elements (Tan et al., 1982), which are listed in Chart 39-5. The diagnosis of SLE is generally made if 4 of the 11 criteria are present, either serially or simultaneously.

The ANA is positive in more than 95% of patients with SLE, indicating exceptional specificity (Bernknop et al., 2011). Other laboratory tests include anti-DNA (antibody that develops against the patient's own DNA), anti-dsDNA (antibody against DNA that is highly specific to SLE, which helps differentiate it from drug-induced lupus), and anti-Sm (antibody against Sm, which is a specific protein found in the nucleus). Other blood work includes a complete blood count, which may reveal anemia, thrombocytopenia, leukocytosis, or leukopenia (Klippel et al., 2008).

Medical Management

SLE can be life threatening, but advances in its treatment have led to improved survival and reduced morbidity (Bernknop et al., 2011). Acute disease requires interventions directed at controlling increased disease activity or exacerbations that can involve any organ system. Disease activity is a composite of clinical and laboratory features that reflect active inflammation secondary to SLE. Management of the more chronic condition involves periodic monitoring and recognition of meaningful clinical changes requiring adjustments in therapy.

The goals of treatment include preventing progressive loss of organ function, reducing the likelihood of acute disease, minimizing disease-related disabilities, and preventing complications from therapy. Management of SLE involves regular monitoring to assess disease activity and therapeutic effectiveness.

Pharmacologic Therapy

The mainstay of SLE treatment is based on pain management and nonspecific immunosuppression. Therapy includes NSAIDs, corticosteroids, antimalarial agents, and cytotoxic agents. Each of these medications has potentially serious side effects, including organ damage.

The FDA recently approved belimumab (Benlysta) for the treatment of SLE (Phung, 2011). Belimumab is a human antibody that specifically recognizes and binds to BLyS. BLyS acts to stimulate B cells to produce antibodies against the body's own nuclei, which is an integral part of the disease process in SLE. Belimumab acts to render BLyS inactive, preventing it from binding to B-cell surfaces and stimulating B-cell activity. This action then halts the production of unnecessary antibodies and decreases disease activity in SLE (Navarra et al., 2011). Research suggests that belimumab reduces disease activity and flares in patients with SLE (Phung, 2011). Live vaccines are contraindicated while taking this medication, and caution should be used with all concurrent medications given the short duration that belimumab has been available.

Corticosteroids are another medication used topically for cutaneous manifestations, in low oral doses for minor disease activity, and in high doses for major disease activity. Intravenous administration of corticosteroids is an alternative to traditional high-dose oral administration. One of the most important risk factors associated with the use of corticosteroids in SLE is osteoporosis and fractures. In fact, osteopenia is reported in 25% to 74% and osteoporosis in 1.4% to 68% of patients with SLE (Bultink, 2012).

Antimalarial medications are effective for managing cutaneous, musculoskeletal, and mild systemic features of SLE. The NSAIDs used for minor clinical manifestations are often used in conjunction with corticosteroids in an effort to minimize corticosteroid requirements (McPhee et al., 2012).

Immunosuppressive agents (alkylating agents and purine analogues) are used because of their effect on overall immune function. These medications are generally reserved for patients who have serious forms of SLE that have not responded to conservative therapies. Such medications include cyclophosphamide, azathioprine, mycophenolic acid (Myfortic), and methotrexate, which are contraindicated in pregnancy and have been used most frequently in SLE nephritis (Bernknop et al., 2011). Anti-TNF therapy has also been considered in refractory SLE but is still controversial (Campar, Farinha, & Vasconcelos, 2011).

Nursing Management

Nursing care of the patient with SLE is based on the fundamental plan presented earlier in the chapter (see Chart 39-2). The most common nursing diagnoses include fatigue, impaired skin integrity, body image disturbance, and deficient knowledge for self-management decisions. The disease or its treatment may produce dramatic changes in appearance and considerable distress for the patient. The changes and the unpredictable course of SLE necessitate expert assessment skills and nursing care with sensitivity to the psychological reactions of the patient. In particular, patients with SLE report feelings of depression and anxiety as well as difficulty coping with the disease and the financial strain associated with it

(Beckerman, 2011). The patient may benefit from participation in support groups, which can provide disease information, daily management tips, and social support. Because sun and ultraviolet light exposure can increase disease activity or cause an exacerbation, patients should be instructed to avoid exposure or to protect themselves with sunscreen and clothing.

Because of the increased risk of involvement of multiple organ systems, patients should understand the need for routine periodic screenings as well as health promotion activities. A dietary consultation may be indicated to ensure that the patient is knowledgeable about dietary recommendations, given the increased risk of cardiovascular disease, including hypertension and atherosclerosis. The nurse educates the patient about the importance of continuing prescribed medications and addresses the changes and potential side effects that are likely to occur with their use. The patient is reminded of the importance of monitoring because of the increased risk of systemic involvement, including renal and cardiovascular effects.

Due to the immunosuppression associated with systemic corticosteroid usage, the nurse must watch for signs and symptoms of infection, especially with acutely ill patients. Some research suggests that initiation of antibiotic therapy longer than 24 hours after onset of infection symptoms in the patient with SLE can increase mortality (Feng, Lin, Yu, et al., 2010).

■ Sjögren's Syndrome

Sjögren's syndrome is a systemic autoimmune disease that progressively affects the lacrimal and salivary glands of the body. More than 90% of patients affected are women, and the onset tends to begin between 45 and 55 years of age (Klippel et al., 2008). Sjögren's syndrome very commonly manifests in conjunction with other autoimmune diseases such as RA or SLE.

Pathophysiology

B-cell–mediated antibodies infiltrate the exocrine glands, leading to gland dysfunction and gland destruction (Martel, Gondran, Launay, et al., 2011). This phenomenon seems to be somewhat regulated by genetics (HLA subtype). There also appears to be environmental triggers such as viruses. Given the clinical makeup and antibodies present, it may also be that Sjögren's disease is a subtype of SLE (Klippel et al., 2008).

Clinical Manifestations

The most common symptoms involve dry eyes (sicca syndrome) and dry mouth (xerostomia). Some patients will complain that their eyes feel "gritty," as if there is sand present. The patient's eyes will exhibit increased redness and lack of tearing. These ocular symptoms can also lead to increased levels of anxiety and depression (Li, Gong, Sun, et al., 2011). The mouth will have dry and sticky mucous membranes. The reduced saliva production may lead to difficulty swallowing, although one study suggested that 96% of patients with Sjögren's syndrome had functional swallowing (Rogus-Pulia & Logemann, 2011).

Sjögren's syndrome can also exhibit symptoms in many other organ systems. Vasculitis can manifest with palpable purpura on the skin (Scofield, 2011). Optic neuritis, trigeminal neuralgia, and sensory neuropathy may be present, with symptoms such as burning pain in the extremities, numbness, vertigo, arthralgia, and/or myalgia (Gono, Kawaguchi, Katsumata, et al., 2011). Raynaud's phenomenon, which involves blood vessel spasms leading to decreased circulation to the toes, fingers, nose and ears, is noted in 13% to 62% of patients (Klippel et al., 2008). Symptoms such as cough, dyspnea, and abdominal pain may also occur.

Assessment and Diagnostic Findings

The classification criteria for diagnosis of Sjögren's syndrome identifies six distinct indices (Vitali, Bombardieri, Jonsson, et al., 2002):

- Ocular symptoms
- Positive ocular tests (evaluating tear production and corneal and conjunctival damage)
- Oral symptoms
- Histopathology evaluation (of salivary glands)
- Salivary gland involvement
- Autoantibodies

Laboratory tests include antibodies to ribonucleoprotein particles (Ro[SS-A] and/or La[SS-B]), which act as antigens in this disease process. Other laboratory indices are also useful in diagnosing Sjögren's syndrome. Rheumatoid factor is present in 50% to 70% of patients (Martel et al., 2011). ANA, circulating DNA (cDNA), anti-CCP, and anticentromere antibody (ACA) are all potentially present in Sjögren's syndrome and in some cases may act as markers for disease activity (Bartoloni, Ludovini, Alunno, et al., 2011; Haga, Andersen, & Peen, 2011; Kitagawa, Shibasaki, & Toya, 2012). Some research also suggests that salivary samples may be able to diagnose this disease (Ching, Burbelo, Gonzalez-Begne, et al., 2011).

For vasculitis manifestations, a skin biopsy can yield useful information such as leukocytoclastic vasculitis found on histological examination (Scofield, 2011). If neurologic symptoms are present, nerve conduction studies, MRI, electroencephalograms, and cerebrospinal fluid testing may be used to aid in diagnosis and treatment planning (Gono et al., 2011).

Medical Management

There is no cure for Sjögren's syndrome, and treatment is aimed at symptom management. Artificial tears, drops such as pilocarpine (Piloptic), and ocular ointments such as topical cyclosporine are used for dry eyes. Tears normally drain through the lacrimal puncta to the nose, which can render artificial tears ineffective. Therefore, punctum plugs have become very important management tools (Egrilmez, Aslan, Karabulut, et al., 2011). Systemic cholinergic agents such as cevimeline (Evoxac) are also used regularly (Ramos-Casals, Tzioufas, Stone, et al., 2010). The use of biologic DMARDs such as rituximab (Rituxan) and nonbiologic DMARDs such as hydroxychloroquine (Plaquenil) are sometimes used, but evidence regarding their effectiveness is limited (Ramos-Casals et al., 2010; Yavuz, Asfuroğlu, Bicakcigil, et al., 2011).

Nursing Management

Nursing care is based on the fundamental plan of nursing care presented earlier (see Chart 39-2). The most frequent nursing diagnoses for the patient with Sjögren's syndrome are altered skin integrity, self-care deficit, and deficient knowledge of self-management techniques.

The nurse is in the unique position to reinforce the treatment regimen with the patient, especially involving the ocular treatments to avoid sequelaelike eye infections secondary to the dry eyes. Special attention must also be given to the psychological disturbances associated with the syndrome.

■ Scleroderma

Scleroderma is a compilation of autoimmune diseases affecting the connective tissue of the skin, blood vessel walls, and internal organs. There are two general types: localized (affecting only the cutaneous system) and systemic (routinely referred to as systemic sclerosis and affecting multiple organ systems). Scleroderma is a rare disease affecting 286 patients per million population (Klippel et al., 2008). Similar to other autoimmune diseases, women are affected three to five times more than men, and onset occurs typically between the ages of 30 and 50 years. Scleroderma has a variable course with remissions and exacerbations.

Pathophysiology

The pathogenesis is poorly understood. Scleroderma commonly begins with skin involvement. Mononuclear cells cluster on the skin and stimulate lymphokines to stimulate procollagen. Insoluble collagen is formed and accumulates excessively in the tissues. Initially, the inflammatory response causes edema, with a resulting taut, smooth, and shiny skin appearance. The skin then undergoes fibrotic changes, leading to loss of elasticity and movement. Eventually, the tissue degenerates and becomes nonfunctional. This chain of events, from inflammation to degeneration, also occurs in blood vessels, major organs, and body systems (Klippel et al., 2008). Both genetics and environmental factors can influence the disease process.

Clinical Manifestations

Scleroderma starts insidiously with Raynaud's phenomenon and swelling in the hands. Raynaud's phenomenon is observed in 90% to 98% of patients with scleroderma and can precede the official scleroderma diagnosis for years (Haustein, 2011). The skin and subcutaneous tissues become increasingly hard and rigid and cannot be pinched up from the underlying structures. Wrinkles and lines are obliterated. The skin is dry because sweat secretion over the involved region is suppressed. The extremities stiffen and lose mobility. The condition spreads slowly; for years, these changes may remain localized in the hands and the feet. The face appears masklike, immobile, and expressionless, and the mouth becomes rigid.

The changes within the body, although not visible directly, are vastly more important than the visible changes. The left ventricle of the heart is involved, resulting in heart failure. The esophagus hardens, interfering with swallowing. The lungs become scarred, impeding respiration. Digestive disturbances occur because of hardening (sclerosing) of the intestinal mucosa. Progressive kidney failure may occur.

The patient may manifest a variety of symptoms referred to as the CREST syndrome. *CREST* stands for calcinosis (calcium deposits in the tissues), *Raynaud's phenomenon, esophageal hardening and dysfunction, sclerodactyly (scleroderma of the digits), and telangiectasia (capillary dilation that forms a vascular lesion) (McPhee et al., 2012).

Assessment and Diagnostic Findings

Assessment focuses on the sclerotic changes in the skin, contractures in the fingers, and color changes or lesions in the fingertips. Assessment of systemic involvement requires a systems review with special attention to gastrointestinal, pulmonary, renal, and cardiac symptoms (Haustein, 2011). Limitations in mobility and self-care activities should be assessed, along with the impact the disease has had (or will have) on body image.

There is no one conclusive diagnostic test used to diagnose scleroderma. High-resolution CT is used to diagnose the presence of pulmonary hypertension (Pandey, Wilcox, Mayo, et al., 2010). Echocardiography identifies pericardial effusion (often present with cardiac involvement). Echocardiograms show some promise as well in detecting vascular changes in the early stages of the disease process (Cusmà Piccione, Bagnato, Zito, et al., 2011). Esophageal studies demonstrate decreased motility in most patients with scleroderma. Blood tests may detect ANAs, indicating a connective tissue disorder and possibly distinguishing the subgroup (diffuse or limited) of scleroderma. A positive ANA test result is common in patients with scleroderma (Klippel et al., 2008).

Medical Management

Treatment of scleroderma depends on the clinical manifestations. All patients require counseling, during which realistic individual goals may be determined. Support measures include strategies to decrease pain and limit disability. A moderate exercise program is encouraged to prevent joint contractures. Patients are advised to avoid extreme temperatures and to use lotion to minimize skin dryness.

Pharmacologic Therapy

No medication regimen is effective in modifying the disease process in scleroderma, but various medications are used to treat organ system involvement. Calcium channel blockers and other antihypertensive agents may provide improvement in symptoms of Raynaud's phenomenon. Anti-inflammatory medications can be used to control arthralgia, stiffness, and general musculoskeletal discomfort. Proton pump inhibitors are used for symptoms of gastric reflux. Aspirin and HMG-CoA (3-hydroxy-3-methylglutaryl coenzyme A) reductase inhibitors (statins) are used to help reduce cardiovascular risk factors. Given the propensity toward digital ulcers due to Raynaud's phenomenon and the potential for pulmonary hypertension, vasoactive medications such as epoprostenol (Flolan), bosentan (Tracleer), and sildenafil (Viagra) are used. Immunosuppressive agents such as cyclophosphamide and methotrexate have been used to improve skin and lung function. The antifibrotic agent imatinib mesylate is used to decrease fibrosis in various organs. Ultraviolet A irradiation is sometimes used to decrease the synthesis of collagen in dermal fibrosis and improve skin symptoms (Haustein, 2011).

Nursing Management

Nursing care of the patient with scleroderma is based on the fundamental plan of nursing care presented earlier (see Chart 39-2). The most common nursing diagnoses are impaired skin integrity; self-care deficits; imbalanced nutrition: less than body requirements; and disturbed body image. The patient with advanced disease may also have impaired gas exchange, decreased cardiac output, impaired swallowing, and constipation.

Providing meticulous skin care and preventing the effects of Raynaud's phenomenon are major nursing challenges. Patient education must include the importance of avoiding cold temperatures and protecting the fingers with mittens in cold weather and when shopping in the frozen food section of the grocery store. Warm socks and properly fitting shoes are helpful in preventing ulcers. Careful, frequent inspection for early ulcers is important. Smoking cessation is critical.

■ *Polymyositis*

Polymyositis is a group of diseases that are termed *idiopathic inflammatory myopathies* (Klippel et al., 2008). They are rare conditions, with an incidence estimated at 5 to 10 cases per million adults per year.

Pathophysiology

Polymyositis is classified as autoimmune because autoantibodies are present. However, these antibodies do not cause damage to muscle cells, indicating only an indirect role in tissue damage. The pathogenesis is multifactorial, and a genetic predisposition is likely. Drug-induced disease is rare. Some evidence suggests a viral link.

Clinical Manifestations

The onset ranges from sudden with rapid progression to very slow and insidious. Proximal muscle weakness is typically a first symptom. Muscle weakness is usually symmetric and diffuse. Dermatomyositis, a related condition, is most commonly identified by an erythematous smooth or scaly lesion found over the joint surface.

Assessment and Diagnostic Findings

A complete history and physical examination help exclude other muscle-related disorders. As with other diffuse connective tissue disorders, no single test confirms polymyositis. An electromyogram is performed to rule out degenerative muscle disease. A muscle biopsy may reveal inflammatory infiltrate in the tissue. Serum studies indicate increased muscle enzyme activity.

Medical Management

Management involves high-dose corticosteroid therapy initially, followed by a gradual dosage reduction over several months as muscle enzyme activity decreases. Patients who do not respond to corticosteroids require the addition of an immunosuppressive agent. Plasmapheresis, lymphapheresis, and total-body irradiation have been used if there is no response to corticosteroids and immunosuppressive

medications. The antimalarial agent hydroxychloroquine may be effective for skin rashes. Physical therapy is initiated slowly, with range-of-motion exercises to maintain joint mobility, followed by gradual strengthening exercises (Klippel et al., 2008).

Nursing Management

Nursing care is based on the fundamental plan of nursing care presented earlier (see Chart 39-2). The most frequent nursing diagnoses for the patient with polymyositis are impaired physical mobility, fatigue, self-care deficit, and deficient knowledge of self-management techniques.

Patients with polymyositis may have symptoms similar to those of other inflammatory diseases. However, proximal muscle weakness is characteristic, making activities such as combing the hair, reaching overhead, and using stairs difficult. Therefore, the use of assistive devices may be recommended, and referral to occupational or physical therapy may be warranted.

■ *Polymyalgia Rheumatica and Giant Cell Arteritis*

PMR involves stiffness of muscles and pain in the neck, shoulder, and pelvic girdle. GCA is a form of vasculitis affecting the medium-sized and large arteries of the body (Klippel et al., 2008). GCA is also sometimes referred to as temporal arteritis because the majority of arteries affected are extracranial branches of the carotid artery. It is widely agreed, however, that both PMR and GCA represent a spectrum of one disease (McPhee et al., 2012). Both primarily affect individuals older than 50 years and are associated with the same HLA haplotype genetic markers. PMR and GCA occur predominately in Caucasians and often in first-degree relatives. PMR has an annual incidence rate of 52 cases per 100,000 people older than 50 years. GCA varies by geographic location and has the highest incidence in Scandinavian countries (Klippel et al., 2008). PMR is two to three times more common than GCA (Ji, Liu, Sundquist, et al., 2010).

Pathophysiology

The underlying mechanism of action involved with PMR and GCA is unknown. It is clear, however, that the immune system is abnormally activated in both disease processes with increases in circulating monocytes that produce IL-1 and IL-6. These circulating monocytes make the endothelial linings of blood vessels more vulnerable to vasculitis (Klippel et al., 2008). Immunoglobulin deposits in the walls of inflamed temporal arteries suggest that an autoimmune process is at work.

Clinical Manifestations

PMR is characterized by severe proximal muscle discomfort with mild joint swelling. Severe aching in the neck, shoulder, and pelvic muscles is common. Stiffness is noticeable most often in the morning and after periods of inactivity. This stiffness can become so severe that patients struggle putting on a coat or combing their hair. Systemic features include low-grade fever, weight loss, malaise, anorexia, and depression.

Because PMR usually occurs in people 50 years and older, it may be confused with, or dismissed as, an inevitable consequence of aging.

GCA may cause headaches, changes in vision, and jaw claudication. These symptoms should be evaluated immediately because of the potential for a sudden and permanent loss of vision if the condition is left untreated (Belliveau & Ten Hove, 2011). PMR and GCA have a self-limited course, lasting several months to several years (Klippel et al., 2008).

There is a possible link between cancer risk and PMR and GCA. In one study, there was a 19% overall excess incidence of cancer in patients with GCA and PMR, with skin cancer and myeloid leukemia being most frequent (Ji et al., 2010). However, another study examining cancer risk in a smaller cohort of patients with biopsy-proven GCA found no increased risk for malignancy (Hill, Cole, Rischmueller, et al., 2010).

Assessment and Diagnostic Findings

Assessment focuses on musculoskeletal tenderness, weakness, and decreased function. Careful attention should be directed toward assessing the head (for changes in vision, headaches, and jaw claudication). An MRI scan may be used in the assessment of extra-articular synovitis in patients with PMR, regardless of symptoms (Cimmino, Parodi, Zampogna, et al., 2011).

Often, diagnosis is difficult because of the lack of specificity of tests. A markedly high ESR is a screening test but is not definitive. CRP level and platelet count also provide valuable data. In fact, simultaneous elevation in the ESR and CRP have a sensitivity of 88% and a specificity of 98% in making the diagnosis of GCA when coupled with clinical findings (Belliveau & Ten Hove, 2011). Diagnosis of both GCA and PMR is more likely to be made by eliminating other potential diagnoses. The dramatic and immediate response to treatment with corticosteroids is considered by some to be diagnostic.

In the case of GCA, biopsy of the temporal artery is the definitive diagnostic tool (Goslin & Chung, 2011). High-resolution MRI is an alternative or adjunct to the traditional temporal artery biopsy (Belliveau & Ten Hove, 2011).

Medical Management

The treatment for patients with PMR (without GCA) is moderate doses of corticosteroids (Cimmino, Parodi, Montecucco, et al., 2011). Longer durations of corticosteroid treatment are required with patients who have higher baseline inflammatory markers (Mackie, Hensor, Haugeberg, et al., 2010). NSAIDs are sometimes administered in mild disease. The treatment for patients with GCA is rapid initiation of and strict adherence to a regimen of corticosteroids. This is essential to avoid the complication of blindness. Aspirin is a useful adjunctive treatment that also helps reduce the risk of visual loss (Belliveau & Ten Hove, 2011).

Nursing Management

Nursing care of the patient with PMR is based on the fundamental plan of nursing care presented earlier (see Chart 39-2).

The most common nursing diagnoses are pain and deficient knowledge of the medication regimen.

A management concern is that the patient will take the prescribed medication, frequently corticosteroids, until symptoms improve and then discontinue the medication. The decision to discontinue the medication should be based on clinical and laboratory findings and the prescription. Nursing implications are related to helping the patient prevent and monitor adverse effects of medications (e.g., infections, diabetes, gastrointestinal problems, and depression) and adjust to those side effects that cannot be prevented (e.g., increased appetite and altered body image).

> ### ▶ Quality and Safety Nursing Alert
>
> The nurse must emphasize to the patient the need for continued adherence to the prescribed medication regimen to avoid complications of GCA, such as blindness.

The loss of bone mass with corticosteroid use increases the risk of osteoporosis in this already at-risk population. Interventions to promote bone health, such as adequate dietary calcium and vitamin D, measurement of bone mineral density, weight-bearing exercise, smoking cessation, and reduction of alcohol consumption if indicated, should be emphasized.

Osteoarthritis (Degenerative Joint Disease)

OA is a noninflammatory degenerative disorder of the joints. It is the most common form of joint disease and is routinely referred to as degenerative joint disease. OA is classified as either primary (idiopathic), with no prior event or disease related to the OA, or secondary, resulting from previous joint injury or inflammatory disease, similar to RA (McPhee et al., 2012). Unlike most of the disease processes discussed in this chapter, the pathophysiology of primary OA does not involve autoimmunity or inflammation. It can occur as an end result of an autoimmune disorder where joint destruction occurs. Another distinguishing characteristic of OA is that it is limited to the affected joints; there are no systemic symptoms associated with it.

OA often begins in the third decade of life and peaks between the fifth and sixth decades. By 40 years of age, 90% of the population has degenerative joint changes in their weight-bearing joints, even though clinical symptoms are usually absent (McPhee et al., 2012). Women, especially those who are Hispanic or African American, are more commonly affected. Prevalence of OA is between 50% and 80% in older adults, and over the past two decades, the prevalence of knee pain itself has increased substantially (Nguyen, Zhang, Zhu, et al., 2011). Although OA is usually thought of as a disease of aging, it also affects younger patients and results in significant losses in work-related productivity and higher costs (Dibonaventura, Gupta, McDonald, et al., 2011).

Pathophysiology

All joints consist of bone, particularly **subchondral bone** to which the articular cartilage is attached. This articular

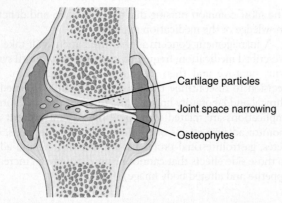

FIGURE 39-3 • Joint space narrowing and osteophytes (bone spurs) are characteristic of degenerative changes in joints.

cartilage is a lubricated, smooth tissue that protects the bone from damage with physical activity. Between the articular cartilage of the bones forming the joint is a space (called the *joint space*) that allows for movement. To aid in fluidity, each joint contains synovial fluid to help lubricate and protect the joint's movement. With OA, the articular cartilage breaks down, leading to progressive damage to the underlying bone and eventual formation of **osteophytes** (bone spurs) that protrude into the joint space. The result is that the joint space is narrowed, leading to decreased joint movement and the potential for more damage. Consequently, the joint can progressively degenerate (Fig. 39-3). Understanding of OA pathophysiology has been greatly expanded beyond what was previously thought of as simply "wear and tear" related to aging (Wang, Shen, Jin, et al., 2011). The basic degenerative process in the joint exemplified in OA is presented in Figure 39-4. In addition to the degeneration, an infectious arteritis can occur. (See Chapter 42 for discussion of septic [infectious] arthritis.)

Risks factors for the disease and its progression include older age, female gender, and obesity. In addition, certain occupations (e.g., those requiring laborious tasks), engaging in sport activities, and a history of previous injuries, muscle weakness, genetic predisposition, and certain diseases can also place patients at risk for joint destruction. The most prominent modifiable risk factor for OA is obesity. In fact, both quality and quantity of life are reduced with OA, especially when obesity and OA are combined (Caban-Martinez, Lee, Fleming, et al., 2011; Losina, Walensky, Reichmann, et al. 2011). A program of diet and exercise can help minimize symptoms of OA in patients who are obese (Brosseau, Wells, Tugwell, et al., 2011).

Clinical Manifestations

The main clinical manifestations of OA are pain, stiffness, and functional impairment. The joint pain is usually aggravated by movement or exercise and relieved by rest. If morning stiffness is present, it is usually brief, lasting less than 30 minutes. Onset is routinely insidious, progressing over multiple years.

On physical examination, the affected joint may be enlarged with a decreased range of motion. Although OA occurs most often in weight-bearing joints (hips, knees, cervical and lumbar spine), the proximal interphalangeal (PIP)

Physiology ⋅⋅⋅ Pathophysiology

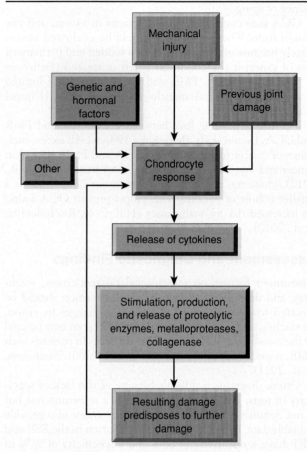

FIGURE 39-4 • Pathophysiology of osteoarthritis.

and distal interphalangeal (DIP) joints are also often involved causing bony enlargements of the DIP (Heberden's nodes) and PIP (Bouchard's nodes) joints. Crepitus may be palpated, especially over the knee. Joint effusion, a sign of inflammation, is usually mild. No systemic manifestations are found.

Assessment and Diagnostic Findings

Blood tests and examination of joint fluid are not useful in the diagnosis of OA but are occasionally ordered to rule out an autoimmune cause for the joint pain, such as RA. X-rays may show a narrowing of the joint space; osteophyte formation; and dense, thickened subchondral bone (McPhee et al., 2012).

Medical Management

The goals of management are to decrease pain and stiffness and to maintain or, when possible, improve joint mobility. Exercise, especially in the form of cardiovascular aerobic exercise and lower extremity strength training, have been found to prevent OA progression and decrease symptoms of OA (Esser & Bailey, 2011). Along with exercise, weight loss, which in turn decreases excess load on the joint, can also be extremely beneficial (Losina et al., 2011). Occupational and physical therapy can help the patient adopt self-management strategies.

Wedged insoles, knee braces, and other modalities are being evaluated as possible therapies aimed at treating the abnormalities in biomechanics found in OA (Waller, Hayes, Block, et al., 2011). The use of orthotic devices (e.g., splints, braces) and walking aids (e.g., canes) can improve pain and function by decreasing force on the affected joint (Walker, 2011).

Patients with arthritis often use CAM therapies, such as massage, yoga, pulsed electromagnetic fields, transcutaneous electrical nerve stimulation (TENS), and music therapy. These may also include herbal and dietary supplements, other special diets, acupuncture, acupressure, wearing copper bracelets or magnets, and participation in T'ai chi. Research is under way to determine the effectiveness of many of these treatments. To date, no definitive evidence has been found regarding their efficacy (Ernst & Posadzki, 2011).

Pharmacologic Therapy

Pharmacologic management of OA is directed toward symptom management and pain control. Selection of medication is based on the patient's needs, the stage of disease, and the risk of side effects. Medications are used in conjunction with nonpharmacologic strategies. In most patients with OA, the initial analgesic therapy is acetaminophen. Some patients respond to the nonselective NSAIDs, and patients who are at increased risk for gastrointestinal complications, especially gastrointestinal bleeding, have been managed effectively with COX-2 enzyme blockers. However, COX-2 enzyme blockers must be used with caution because of the associated risk of cardiovascular disease. Other medications that may be considered are the opioids and intra-articular corticosteroids. Topical analgesic agents such as capsaicin (Capsin, Zostrix) and methylsalicylate are also used (Klippel et al., 2008; Walker, 2011)

Other therapeutic approaches include glucosamine and chondroitin. Although it has been suggested that these substances modify cartilage structure, studies have not shown them to be effective (Stuber, Sajko, & Kristmanson, 2011). Viscosupplementation, the injection of gel-like substances (hyaluronates) into a joint (intra-articular), is thought to supplement the viscous properties of synovial fluid. These viscosupplements aim to prevent loss of cartilage and repair chondral defects (Waller et al., 2011).

Surgical Management

In moderate to severe OA, when pain is severe or because of loss of function, surgical intervention may be used. The procedures most commonly used are osteotomy (to alter the distribution of weight within the joint) and arthroplasty. In arthroplasty, diseased joint components are replaced (see Chapter 41). Rehabilitation with physical therapy that is initiated within the first 24 hours is associated with decreased hospital length of stay and improved balance and gait function (Labraca, Castro-Sánchez, Matarán-Peñarrocha, et al., 2011).

Nursing Management

Pain management and optimal functional ability are major goals of nursing intervention. With those goals in mind, nursing management of the patient with OA includes pharmacologic and nonpharmacologic approaches as well as education. The patient's understanding of the disease process and symptom pattern is critical to the plan of care. Because patients with OA usually are older, they may have other health problems. Commonly they are overweight, and they may have a sedentary lifestyle. Weight loss and exercise are important approaches to pain and disability improvement (Walker, 2011). A referral for physical therapy or to an exercise program for people with similar problems can be very helpful. Canes or other assistive devices for ambulation should be considered, and any stigma about the use of these devices should be explored. Exercises such as walking should be begun in moderation and increased gradually. Patients should plan their daily exercise for a time when the pain is least severe or plan to use an analgesic agent, if appropriate, before exercising. Adequate pain management is important for the success of an exercise program. Open discussion regarding the use of CAM therapies is important to maintain safe and effective practices for patients looking for relief.

Spondyloarthropathies

The spondyloarthropathies are another category of systemic inflammatory disorders of the skeleton. The spondyloarthropathies include ankylosing spondylitis (AS), reactive arthritis (formerly known as Reiter's syndrome), and psoriatic arthritis. Spondyloarthritis is also associated with inflammatory bowel diseases such as Crohn's disease (regional enteritis) and ulcerative colitis (Dougados & Baeten, 2011).

These rheumatic diseases share several clinical features. The inflammation tends to occur peripherally at the sites of attachment—at tendons, joint capsules, and ligaments. Periosteal inflammation may be present. Many patients have arthritis of the sacroiliac joints. Onset tends to occur during young adulthood, with the disease affecting men more often than women. There is a strong tendency for these conditions to occur in families. Frequently, the HLA-B27 genetic marker is found. In addition, more than one of these conditions can be found simultaneously in the same person or another family member (Dougados & Baeten, 2011).

As with other inflammatory conditions, patients with spondyloarthropathies have an increased risk for cardiovascular disease. One study found that patients with AS had enzyme and endothelial changes consistent with atherosclerosis (Cece, Yazgan, Karakas, et al., 2011). These findings may be related to a state of chronic systemic inflammation and an increase in traditional cardiac risk factors, such as lack of exercise due to increased pain (Mathieu, Motreff, & Soubrier, 2010; Taylan, Sari, Kozaci, et al. 2012).

■ Ankylosing Spondylitis

AS is a chronic and inflammatory disease of the spine. It is more prevalent in males than in females and is usually diagnosed in the second or third decade of life. The disease is also more severe in males, and significant systemic involvement is likely.

AS affects the cartilaginous joints of the spine and surrounding tissues, making them rigid, decreasing mobility, and leading to kyphosis (a stooped position) (Del Din et al., 2011). This kyphosis can, in turn, lead to decreased stability and balance (Durmus et al., 2010). Back pain is the characteristic feature. The back pain can be so severe that it may mask symptoms of a cervical fracture, which can lead to neurologic problems if left untreated (Anwar, Al-Khayer, Joseph, et al., 2011). Occasionally, the large synovial joints, such as the hips, knees, or shoulders, may be involved.

AS also exhibits systemic effects. Uveitis occurs in 20% to 25% of patients with AS and may be a presenting feature (Wendling, Paccou, Berthelot, et al., 2011). Another potential complication of AS is the risk of osteoporosis, which appears to be related to the inflammatory process as well as bone turnover and low vitamin D levels (Arends, Spoorenberg, Bruyn, et al., 2011). Other complications involve atrioventricular conduction defects, aortic insufficiency, and pulmonary fibrosis (McPhee et al., 2012). As the disease progresses, ankylosis of the entire spine may occur, leading to respiratory compromise and further complications.

■ Reactive Arthritis (Reiter's Syndrome)

The disease process involved in reactive arthritis is called *reactive* because the arthritis occurs after an infection, primarily gastrointestinal or genitourinary (Curry, Riddle, Gormley, et al., 2010; Edrees, 2012). It mostly affects young adult males and is characterized primarily by urethritis, arthritis, and conjunctivitis. Dermatitis and ulcerations of the mouth and penis may also be present. Low back pain is common.

■ Psoriatic Arthritis

Psoriatic arthritis is an inflammatory arthritis associated with the skin disease psoriasis. In fact, research has suggested that between 10% and 20% of people with psoriasis will eventually develop psoriatic arthritis (Langham, Langham, Goertz, et al., 2011). Psoriasis is the most common autoimmune disease in the United States, affecting 2% to 3% of the population (Langham et al., 2011). Psoriatic arthritis onset occurs between 30 and 50 years of age and affects equal numbers of men and women (Snyder, 2010).

Pathogenesis of the disease process is hypothesized to start in the skin with an exaggerated immune response to environmental factors and then spreads to the joints in genetically susceptible individuals (Prodanovich, Ricotti, Glick, et al., 2010). Although these patients test negative for rheumatoid factor, levels of TNF-α are elevated (Snyder, 2010). Psoriatic arthritis is characterized by synovitis, polyarthritis, and spondylitis. The arthritis is usually symmetric with "sausage" appearance of fingers and toes (McPhee et al., 2012).

Medical Management

Medical management of spondyloarthropathies focuses on treating pain and maintaining mobility by suppressing inflammation. For the patient with AS, good body positioning and posture are essential so that if **ankylosis** (fixation) does occur, the patient is in the most functional position. Maintaining

range of motion with regular exercise and a muscle-strengthening program is especially important and has been linked with higher quality of life for the patient (Aytekin, Caglar, Ozgonenel, et al., 2012).

Pharmacologic Management

NSAIDs and corticosteroids often produce marked improvement in back, skin, and joint symptoms. Sulfasalazine and methotrexate may help with peripheral joint disease. Methotrexate is also used to control psoriasis. More recently, anti-TNF therapy, such as etanercept (Enbrel) has been used effectively in all three conditions (Edrees, 2012; Prodanovich et al., 2010).

Surgical Management

With advanced AS and subsequent debilitating kyphosis, an osteotomy of the spine can be done. One study showed that an average correction of 45 degrees in the cervical spine was obtained and that quality of life also improved (Kiaer & Gehrchen, 2010). Surgical management may also include total joint replacement (see Chapter 41).

Nursing Management

Major nursing interventions in the spondyloarthropathies are related to symptom management and maintenance of optimal functioning. Affected patients are primarily young men. Their major concerns are often related to prognosis and job modification, especially among those who perform physical work. Patients may also express concerns about leisure and recreational activities.

Metabolic and Endocrine Diseases Associated With Rheumatic Disorders

Metabolic and endocrine diseases may be associated with rheumatic disorders. These include biochemical abnormalities (amyloidosis and scurvy), endocrine diseases (diabetes and acromegaly), immunodeficiency diseases (human immunodeficiency virus infection, acquired immunodeficiency syndrome), and some inherited disorders (hypermobility syndromes). However, the most common conditions are the crystal-induced arthropathies, in which crystals such as monosodium urate (gout) or calcium pyrophosphate (calcium pyrophosphate dihydrate disease or pseudogout) are deposited within joints and other tissues (McPhee et al., 2012).

■ Gout

Gout is the most common form of inflammatory arthritis. More than 3 million Americans self-report the diagnosis of gout (CDC, 2012c). The prevalence is reported to be about 2% and appears to be on the rise. Men are three to four times more likely to be diagnosed with gout than women. The incidence of gout increases with age, body mass index, alcohol consumption, hypertension, and diuretic use (Bhole, de Vera, Rahman, et al., 2010; Zychowicz et al., 2010). Evidence links the consumption of fructose-rich beverages with the risk of gout for both men and women (Choi, Willett, & Curhan,

2010; Greener, 2011). Patients with gout have an increased risk of cardiovascular disease. In one study, for example, gout was implicated as an independent risk factor for acute myocardial infarction in older women (De Vera, Rahman, Bhole, et al., 2010). Comorbid conditions such as hypertension, dyslipidemia, diabetes, OA, and kidney disease may be present in patients with gout (Greener, 2011).

Given that the incidence of gout increases with age, its management can be complicated by other medical conditions, medications, and age-related changes (Stamp & Jordan, 2011).

Pathophysiology

Gout is caused by hyperuricemia (increased serum uric acid). Uric acid is a by-product of purine metabolism; purines are basic chemical compounds found in high concentrations in meat products. Urate levels are affected by diet, medications, overproduction in the body, and inadequate excretion by the kidneys. Hyperuricemia (serum concentration greater than 6.8 mg/dL) can, but does not always, cause urate crystal deposition (Gonzalez, 2012). However, as uric acid levels increase, the risk becomes greater. The initial cause for the gout attack occurs when macrophages in the joint space phagocytize urate crystals. Through a series of immunologic steps, interleukin 1 beta is secreted, increasing the inflammation. This process is exacerbated by the presence of free fatty acids. Both alcohol and consumption of a large meal, especially with red meat, can lead to increases in free fatty acid concentrations; they also are implicated as triggers to acute gout attacks (Gonzalez, 2012).

With repeated attacks, accumulations of sodium urate crystals, called **tophi**, are deposited in peripheral areas of the body, such as the great toe, the hands, and the ear. Renal urate lithiasis (kidney stones), with chronic renal disease secondary to urate deposition, may develop.

Primary hyperuricemia may be caused by severe dieting or starvation, excessive intake of foods that are high in purines (shellfish, organ meats), or heredity. In secondary hyperuricemia, gout is a clinical feature secondary to any of a number of genetic or acquired processes, including conditions in which there is an increase in cell turnover (leukemia, multiple myeloma, some types of anemias, psoriasis) and an increase in cell breakdown. Altered renal tubular function, either as a major action or as an unintended side effect of certain pharmacologic agents (e.g., diuretics such as thiazides and furosemide), low-dose salicylates, or ethanol can contribute to uric acid underexcretion (Klippel et al., 2008). The finding of urate crystals in the synovial fluid of asymptomatic joints suggests that factors other than crystals may be related to the inflammatory reaction. Recovered monosodium urate crystals are coated with immunoglobulins that are mainly IgG. IgG enhances crystal phagocytosis, thereby demonstrating immunologic activity (Klippel et al., 2008).

Clinical Manifestations

Manifestations of the gout syndrome include acute gouty arthritis (recurrent attacks of severe articular and periarticular inflammation), tophi (crystalline deposits accumulating in articular tissue, osseous tissue, soft tissue, and cartilage), gouty nephropathy (renal impairment), and uric acid urinary calculi. Four stages of gout can be identified: asymptomatic hyperuricemia, acute gouty arthritis, intercritical gout, and chronic tophaceous gout (Zychowicz et al., 2010). The subsequent development of gout is directly related to the duration and magnitude of the hyperuricemia. Therefore, the commitment to lifelong pharmacologic treatment of hyperuricemia is deferred until there is an initial attack of gout.

For hyperuricemic people who are going to develop gout, acute arthritis is the most common early clinical manifestation. The metatarsophalangeal joint of the big toe is the most commonly affected joint (90% of patients) (Porth & Matfin, 2009; Zychowicz et al., 2010). The tarsal area, ankle, or knee may also be affected. Less commonly, the wrists, fingers, and elbows may be affected. Trauma, alcohol ingestion, dieting, medications, surgical stress, or illness may trigger the acute attack. The abrupt onset often occurs at night, awakening the patient with severe pain, redness, swelling, and warmth of the affected joint. Early attacks tend to subside spontaneously over 3 to 10 days even without treatment. The attack is followed by a symptom-free period (the intercritical stage) until the next attack, which may not come for months or years. However, with time, attacks tend to occur more frequently, involve more joints, and last longer.

Tophi (seen in chronic tophaceous gout) are generally associated with more frequent and severe inflammatory episodes. Higher serum concentrations of uric acid are also associated with more extensive tophus formation. Tophi most commonly occur in the synovium, olecranon bursa, subchondral bone, infrapatellar and Achilles tendons, and subcutaneous tissue on the extensor surface of the forearms and overlying joints. They have also been found in the aortic walls, heart valves, nasal and ear cartilage, eyelids, cornea, and sclera. Joint enlargement may cause a loss of joint motion. Uric acid deposits may cause renal stones and kidney damage.

Medical Management

A definitive diagnosis of gouty arthritis is established by polarized light microscopy of the synovial fluid of the involved joint. Uric acid crystals are seen within the polymorphonuclear leukocytes in the fluid.

Acute attacks are managed with colchicine (Colcrys) (oral or parenteral), an NSAID such as indomethacin (Indocin), or a corticosteroid (Shamim, Shaheen, Muhammad Asif, et al., 2011). Management of hyperuricemia, tophi, joint destruction, and renal disorders is usually initiated after the acute inflammatory process has subsided. Once the acute attack has subsided, uric acid lowering therapy should be considered. Xanthine oxidase inhibitors, such as allopurinol (Zyloprim) and febuxostat (Uloric), are the agents of choice. In fact, taking allopurinol reduced the occurrence of gout flares by 20% in one study (Rothenbacher, Primatesta, Ferreira, et al., 2011). Given the role of IL-1 in the pathogenesis of gout, some experts suggest that there may be a role for anakinra (Kineret), an IL-1 receptor antagonist in the management of acute gout (McPhee et al., 2012).

Management between gout attacks needs to include lifestyle changes such as avoiding purine-rich foods, weight

TABLE 39-5 **Common Medications Used to Treat Gout**

Medication	Actions and Use	Nursing Implications
colchicine (Colcrys)	Lowers the deposition of uric acid and interferes with leukocyte infiltration, thus reducing inflammation; does not alter serum or urine levels of uric acid; used in acute and chronic management	*Acute management:* Administer when attack begins; dosage increased until pain is relieved or diarrhea develops. *Chronic management:* Causes gastrointestinal upset in most patients.
probenecid (Benemid)	Uricosuric agent; inhibits renal reabsorption of urates and increases the urinary excretion of uric acid; prevents tophi formation	Be alert for nausea and rash.
allopurinol (Zyloprim), febuxostat (Uloric)	Xanthine oxidase inhibitors; interrupt the breakdown of purines before uric acid is formed; inhibit xanthinoxidase because uric acid formation is blocked	Monitor for side effects, including bone marrow depression, vomiting, and abdominal pain.

Adapted from Karch, A. (2012). *Lippincott's nursing drug guide*. Philadelphia: Lippincott Williams & Wilkins.

loss, decreasing alcohol consumption, and avoiding certain medications. Uricosuric agents, such as probenecid (Benemid) or sulfinpyrazone (Anturane), may be indicated in patients with frequent acute attacks. Uricosuric medications correct hyperuricemia and dissolve deposited urate (Gonzalez, 2012; Greener, 2011; Zychowicz et al., 2010). Corticosteroids may also be used in patients who have no response to other therapy. In patients with refractory chronic gout who are not controlled with the regimens mentioned earlier, pegloticase (Krystexxa), a newly approved urate-lowering agent not yet commonly used, has been shown to be effective in lowering uric acid levels (Sundy, Baraf, Yood, et al., 2011). Specific treatment is based on the serum uric acid level, 24-hour urinary uric acid excretion, and renal function (Table 39-5).

Nursing Management

Severe dietary restriction is not necessary; however, the nurse encourages the patient to restrict consumption of foods high in purines, especially organ meats, and to limit alcohol intake. Maintenance of normal body weight should be encouraged. In an acute episode of gouty arthritis, pain management with prescribed medications is essential, along with avoidance of factors that increase pain and inflammation, such as trauma, stress, and alcohol. Medication adherence is critical; therefore, counseling needs to be initiated by the nurse when appropriate. Between acute episodes, the patient feels well and may abandon preventive behaviors, which may result in an acute attack. Acute attacks are most effectively treated if therapy is begun early (Greener, 2011).

Fibromyalgia

Fibromyalgia is a chronic pain syndrome that involves chronic fatigue, generalized muscle aching, stiffness, sleep disturbances, and functional impairment (Arnold, Clauw, & McCarberg, 2011). It is estimated to affect more than 5 million Americans, representing 2% to 5% of the general population, with women affected more than men (Ryan, 2011). Between 25% and 65% of patients with fibromyalgia have other rheumatologic conditions such as RA, SLE, and AS (CDC, 2012b).

Pathophysiology

The amplified pain experienced by patients with fibromyalgia is neurogenic in origin (Clauw, Arnold, & McCarberg, 2011). Specifically, the central nervous system's ascending and descending pathways (that regulate and moderate pain processing) function abnormally, causing central amplification of pain signals (Clauw et al., 2011). Some scientists describe this as if the "volume control setting" for pain were abnormally high (Clauw et al., 2011). Therefore, stimulation that may not normally elicit pain, such as touch, may do so. In addition, there are a number of predisposing factors to pain, including anxiety, depression, physical trauma, emotional stress, and viral infection (Ryan, 2011).

Assessment and Diagnostic Findings

The American College of Rheumatology established preliminary diagnostic criteria and symptom severity indices for fibromyalgia (Wolfe, Clauw, Fitzcharles, et al., 2010). These criteria emphasize the regions of pain, rather than specific points, and take into account the fatigue, cognitive symptoms, and unrefreshed sleep that patients with fibromyalgia also tend to experience (Wolfe et al., 2010).

Medical Management

Treatment consists of attention to the specific symptoms reported by the patient. NSAIDs may be used to treat the diffuse muscle aching and stiffness. Tricyclic antidepressants and sleep hygiene measures are used to improve or restore normal sleep patterns (Roizenblatt, Neto, & Tufik, 2011). Cognitive behavioral therapy is also useful in improving sleep and attentional dysfunction (Miró, Lupiáñez, Martínez, et al., 2011). In addition, selective serotonin reuptake inhibitors and anticonvulsants have been effective in preliminary reports (Ryan, 2011). Individualized programs of exercise are used to decrease muscle weakness and discomfort and to improve the general deconditioning that occurs in affected patients (Busch, Webber, Brachaniec, et al., 2011). There has also been some promising research in CAM therapies, such as acupuncture, massage, homeopathy, hydrotherapy, craniosacral therapy, and myofascial therapy (Castro-Sánchez, Matarán-Peñarrocha, Arroyo-Morales, et al., 2011; Castro-Sánchez,

Matarán-Peñarrocha, Sánchez-Labraca, et al., 2011; Terry, Perry, & Ernst, 2012).

Nursing Management

Typically, patients with fibromyalgia have endured their symptoms for a long period of time. They may feel as if their symptoms have not been taken seriously. Nurses need to pay special attention to supporting these patients and providing encouragement as they begin their program of therapy. Patient support groups may be helpful. Careful listening to patients' descriptions of their concerns and symptoms is essential to help them make the changes that are necessary to improve their quality of life (Eide, Sibbern, & Johannessen, 2011; Ryan, 2011).

Miscellaneous Disorders

The last category in the classification of the rheumatic diseases is aptly labeled miscellaneous disorders because it contains a mix of disorders that are frequently associated with arthritis and other conditions. These include the direct consequences of trauma (including internal derangement and loose bodies of joints), pancreatic disease (related to avascular necrosis or osteonecrosis), sarcoidosis (a multisystem disorder particularly of the lymph nodes and lungs), and palindromic rheumatism (an uncommon variety of recurring and acute arthritis and periarthritis that in some may progress to RA but is characterized by symptom-free periods of days to months). Other conditions include villonodular synovitis, chronic active hepatitis, and drug-related rheumatic syndromes. The nursing interventions related to these varied conditions are specific to the multisystemic problems experienced by the patient. However, the musculoskeletal components should not be neglected or overlooked. Further information about these rare disorders can be found in specialty references.

Critical Thinking Exercises

1 A 44-year-old mother with two children was recently diagnosed with RA. She is skeptical about taking the prescribed "weird-named" medications, especially because her symptoms "aren't that bad." What type of education can you provide about RA's pathogenesis and disease progression? What are the principles of treatment for RA? What educational tools can you use to promote patient adherence to the medication regimen?

2 **ebp** An 83-year-old retired veteran has been diagnosed with AS. He now has significant pain and kyphosis, as well as difficulty with balance when walking. He also has hypertension and hypercholesterolemia. What is the evidence base for available assessments to assist in a more comprehensive evaluation of this patient? Identify the criteria used to evaluate the strength of the evidence for the practices you have identified.

3 **pq** Your patient is a 62-year-old economist and amateur bird enthusiast who routinely hikes the local nature preserves to look for his favorite species. Over the past 6 months, he has had to cancel three of his hikes because of gout flares. He voices his frustration at missing his favorite activity because of his medical condition. Identify the priorities, approach, and techniques you would use to perform a comprehensive admission assessment of this patient. How would your priorities, approach, and techniques differ if the patient were from a culture different from your own?

Brunner Suite Resources
Explore these additional resources to enhance learning for this chapter:
• NCLEX-Style Questions and Other Resources on thePoint, http://thePoint.lww.com/Brunner13e
• Study Guide
• PrepU
• Clinical Handbook
• Handbook of Laboratory and Diagnostic Tests

References

*Asterisk indicates nursing research.
**Double asterisk indicates classic reference.

Books

Karch, A. (2012). *Lippincott's nursing drug guide*. Philadelphia: Lippincott Williams & Wilkins.

Klippel, J. H., Stone, J. H., Crofford, L. J., & White, P. (Eds.). (2008). *Primer on the rheumatic diseases* (13th ed.). New York: Springer.

Miller, C. A. (2012). *Nursing for wellness in older adults* (6th ed.). Philadelphia: Lippincott Williams & Wilkins.

McPhee, S. J., Papadakis, M. A., & Rabow, M. W. (2012). *Current medical diagnosis and treatment* (51st ed.). Stamford, CT: Appleton & Lange.

Porth, C. M., & Matfin, G. (2009). *Pathophysiology: Concepts of altered health status* (8th ed.). Philadelphia: Lippincott Williams & Wilkins.

Journals and Electronic Documents

**American College of Rheumatology Subcommittee. (2002). Guidelines for the management of rheumatoid arthritis. *Arthritis and Rheumatism*, 46(2), 328–346.

Anwar, F., Al-Khayer, A., Joseph, G., et al. (2011). Delayed presentation and diagnosis of cervical spine injuries in long-standing ankylosing spondylitis. *European Spine Journal*, 20(3), 403–407.

Arends, S., Spoorenberg, A., Bruyn, G., et al. (2011). The relation between bone mineral density, bone turnover markers, and vitamin D status in ankylosing spondylitis patients with active disease: A cross-sectional analysis. *Osteoporosis International*, 22(5), 1431–1439.

Arnold, L. M., Clauw, D. J., & McCarberg, B. H. (2011). Improving the recognition and diagnosis of fibromyalgia. *Mayo Clinic Proceedings*, 86(5), 457–464.

Aytekin, E., Caglar, N., Ozgonenel, L., et al. (2012). Home-based exercise therapy in patients with ankylosing spondylitis: Effects on pain, mobility, disease activity, quality of life, and respiratory functions. *Clinical Rheumatology*, 31(1), 91–97.

Bakker, M. F., Jacobs, J. W. G., Walsing, P. W. J, et al. (2012). Low-dose prednisone inclusion in a methotrexate-based tight control strategy for early rheumatoid arthritis. *Annals of Internal Medicine*, 156(3), 329–339.

Bartoloni, E., Ludovini, V., Alunno, A., et al. (2011). Increased levels of circulating DNA in patients with systemic autoimmune diseases: A possible marker of disease activity in Sjögren's syndrome. *Lupus*, 20(9), 928–935.

Beckerman, N. L. (2011). Living with lupus: A qualitative report. *Social Work in Health Care*, 50(4), 330–343.

Belliveau, M. J., & Ten Hove, M. (2011). Giant cell arteritis. *CMAJ: Canadian Medical Association Journal, 183*(5), 581.

Bernknop, A., Rowley, K., & Bailey, T. (2011). A review of systemic lupus erythematosus and current treatment options. *Formulary, 46*(5), 178–194.

Bhole, V., de Vera, M., Rahman, M. M., et al. (2010). Epidemiology of gout in women: Fifty-two-year followup of a prospective cohort. *Arthritis and Rheumatism, 62*(4), 1069–1076.

Breedland, I., van Scheppingen, Leijsma, M., et al. (2011). Effects of a group-based exercise and educational program on physical performance and disease self-management in rheumatoid arthritis: A randomized controlled study. *Physical Therapy, 91*(6), 879–893.

Brosseau, L., Wells, G. A., Tugwell, P., et al. (2011). Ottawa panel evidence-based clinical practice guidelines for the management of osteoarthritis in adults who are obese or overweight.*Physical Therapy, 91*(6), 843–861.

Bultink, I. E. M. (2012). Osteoporosis and fractures in systemic lupus erythematosus. *Arthritis Care & Research, 64*(1), 2–8.

Busch, A. J., Webber, S. C., Brachaniec, M., et al. (2011). Exercise therapy for fibromyalgia. *Current Pain and Headache Reports, 15*(5), 358–367.

Caban-Martinez, A., Lee, D. J., Fleming, L. E., et al. (2011). Arthritis, occupational class, and the aging US workforce. *American Journal of Public Health, 101*(9), 1729–1734.

Campar, A., Farinha, F., & Vasconcelos, C. (2011). Refractory disease in systemic lupus erythematosus. *Autoimmunity Reviews, 10*(11), 685–692.

Castro-Sánchez, A. M., Matarán-Peñarrocha, G. A., Arroyo-Morales, M., et al. (2011). Effects of myofascial release techniques on pain, physical function, and postural stability in patients with fibromyalgia: A randomized controlled trial. *Clinical Rehabilitation, 25*(9), 800–813.

Castro-Sánchez, A., Matarán-Peñarrocha, G., Sánchez-Labraca, N., et al. (2011). A randomized controlled trial investigating the effects of craniosacral therapy on pain and heart rate variability in fibromyalgia patients. *Clinical Rehabilitation, 25*(1), 25–35.

Cece, H., Yazgan, P., Karakas, E., et al. (2011). Carotid intima-media thickness and paraoxonase activity in patients with ankylosing spondylitis. *Clinical & Investigative Medicine, 34*(4), E225–E225.

Centers for Disease Control and Prevention. (2012a). *Systemic lupus erythematous (SLE or lupus): Prevalence and incidence.* Available at: www.cdc.gov/arthritis/basics/lupus.htm

Centers for Disease Control and Prevention. (2012b). *Fibromyalgia: Background.* Available at: www.cdc.gov/arthritis/basics/fibromyalgia.htm

Centers for Disease Control and Prevention. (2012c). *Gout: Background.* Available at: www.cdc.gov/arthritis/basics/gout.htm

Chamberlain, V. (2011). Patients with inflammatory arthritis: An opportunity for community nurses. *British Journal of Community Nursing, 16*(6), 268–273.

Chen, Q., Hayman, L. L., Shmerling, R. H., et al. (2011). Characteristics of chronic pain associated with sleep difficulty in older adults: The maintenance of balance, independent living, intellect, and zest in the elderly (MOBILIZE) Boston study. *Journal of the American Geriatrics Society, 59*(8), 1385–1392.

Cheng, Y. J., Hootman, J. M., Murphy, L. B., et al. (2010). Prevalence of doctor-diagnosed arthritis and arthritis-attributable activity limitation—United States, 2007–2009. *MMWR: Morbidity and Mortality Weekly Report, 59*(39), 1261–1265. Available at: www.cdc.gov/mmwr/preview/mmwrhtml/mm5939a1.htm

Ching, K. H., Burbelo, P. D., Gonzalez-Begne, M., et al. (2011). Salivary anti-Ro60 and anti-Ro52 antibody profiles to diagnose Sjogren's syndrome. *Journal of Dental Research, 90*(4), 445–449.

Choi, H. K., Willett, W., & Curhan, G. (2010). Fructose-rich beverages and risk of gout in women. *Journal of the American Medical Association, 304*(20), 2270–2278.

Cimmino, M. A., Parodi, M., Montecucco, C., et al. (2011). The correct prednisone starting dose in polymyalgia rheumatica is related to body weight but not to disease severity. *BMC Musculoskeletal Disorders, 12*(1), 94–94.

Cimmino, M. A., Parodi, M., Zampogna, G., et al. (2011). Polymyalgia rheumatica is associated with extensor tendon tenosynovitis but not with synovitis of the hands: A magnetic resonance imaging study. *Rheumatology, 50*(3), 494–499.

Clancy, J., & Hasthorpe, H. (2011). Pathophysiology of rheumatoid arthritis: Nature or nurture? *Primary Health Care, 21*(9), 29–36.

Clauw, D. J., Arnold, L. M., & McCarberg, B. H. (2011). The science of fibromyalgia. *Mayo Clinic Proceedings, 86*(9), 907–911.

Crowson, C. S., Matteson, E. L., Myasoedova, E., et al. (2011). The lifetime risk of adult-onset rheumatoid arthritis and other inflammatory autoimmune rheumatic diseases. *Arthritis and Rheumatism, 63*(3), 633–639.

Curry, J. A., Riddle, M. S., Gormley, R. P., et al. (2010). The epidemiology of infectious gastroenteritis related reactive arthritis in U.S. military personnel: A case-control study. *BMC Infectious Diseases, 10*, 266–266.

Cusmà Piccione, M., Bagnato, G., Zito, C., et al. (2011). Early identification of vascular damage in patients with systemic sclerosis. *Angiology, 62*(4), 338–343.

De Vera, M. A., Rahman, M. M., Bhole, V., et al. (2010). Independent impact of gout on the risk of acute myocardial infarction among elderly women: A population-based study. *Annals of the Rheumatic Diseases, 69*(6), 1162–1164.

Del Din, S., Carraro, E., Sawacha, Z., et al. (2011). Impaired gait in ankylosing spondylitis. *Medical & Biological Engineering & Computing, 49*(7), 801–809.

Dhillon, S. (2011). Naproxen/Esomeprazole fixed-dose combination: For the treatment of arthritic symptoms and to reduce the risk of gastric ulcers. *Drugs & Aging, 28*(3), 237–248.

Dibonaventura, M. D., Gupta, S., McDonald, M., et al. (2011). Evaluating the health and economic impact of osteoarthritis pain in the workforce: Results from the National Health and Wellness Survey. *BMC Musculoskeletal Disorders, 12*(83), 1–9.

Dougados, M., & Baeten, D. (2011). Spondyloarthritis. *Lancet, 377*(9783), 2127–2137.

Durmus, B., Altay, Z., Ersoy, Y., et al. (2010). Postural stability in patients with ankylosing spondylitis. *Disability & Rehabilitation, 32*(14), 1156–1162.

Edrees, A. (2012). Successful use of etanercept for the treatment of Reiter's syndrome: A case report and review of the literature. *Rheumatology International, 32*(1), 1–3.

Egrilmez, S., Aslan, F., Karabulut, G., et al. (2011). Clinical efficacy of the SmartPlug™ in the treatment of primary Sjogren's syndrome with keratoconjunctivitis sicca: One-year follow-up study. *Rheumatology International, 31*(12), 1567–1570.

*Eide, H., Sibbern, T., & Johannessen, T. (2011). Empathic accuracy of nurses' immediate responses to fibromyalgia patients' expressions of negative emotions: An evaluation using interaction analysis. *Journal of Advanced Nursing, 67*(6), 1242–1253.

Ernst, E., & Posadzki, P. (2011). Complementary and alternative medicine for rheumatoid arthritis and osteoarthritis: An overview of systematic reviews. *Current Pain and Headache Reports, 15*(6), 431–437.

Esser, S., & Bailey, A. (2011). Effects of exercise and physical activity on knee osteoarthritis. *Current Pain and Headache Reports, 15*(6), 423–430.

Feng, P., Lin, S., Yu, C., et al. (2010). Inadequate antimicrobial treatment for nosocomial infection is a mortality risk factor for systemic lupus erythematous patients admitted to intensive care unit. *American Journal of the Medical Sciences, 340*(1), 64–68.

Ferraccioli, G., & Gremese, E. (2011). Pathogenetic, clinical and pharmaco-economic assessment in rheumatoid arthritis (RA). *Internal & Emergency Medicine, 6*, 11–15.

Firth, J. (2011a). Rheumatoid arthritis: Diagnosis and multidisciplinary management. *British Journal of Nursing, 20*(18), 1179.

Firth, J. (2011b). Rheumatoid arthritis: Treating to target with disease-modifying drugs. *British Journal of Nursing, 20*(19), 1240.

Firth, J., & Critchley, S. (2011). Treating to target in rheumatoid arthritis: Biologic therapies. *British Journal of Nursing, 20*(20), 1284–1291.

Gigante, A., Gasperini, M. L., Afeltra, A., et al. (2011). Cytokines expression in SLE nephritis. *European Review for Medical and Pharmacological Sciences, 15*(1), 15–24.

Gleicher, Y., Croxford, R., Hochman, J., et al. (2011). A prospective study of mental health care for comorbid depressed mood in older adults with painful osteoarthritis. *BMC Psychiatry, 11*, 147–147.

Gono, T., Kawaguchi, Y., Katsumata, Y., et al. (2011). Clinical manifestations of neurological involvement in primary Sjögren's syndrome. *Clinical Rheumatology, 30*(4), 485–490.

Gonzalez, E. B. (2012). An update on the pathology and clinical management of gouty arthritis. *Clinical Rheumatology, 31*(1), 13–21.

Goslin, B. J., & Chung, M. H. (2011). Temporal artery biopsy as a means of diagnosing giant cell arteritis: Is there over-utilization? *American Surgeon, 77*(9), 1158–1160.

Greener, M. (2011). For an effective management of gout. *Nurse Prescribing, 9*(7), 342–346.

Haga, H., Andersen, D. T., & Peen, E. (2011). Prevalence of IgA class antibodies to cyclic citrullinated peptide (anti-CCP) in patients with primary Sjögren's syndrome, and its association to clinical manifestations. *Clinical Rheumatology, 30*(3), 369–372.

Haustein, U. (2011). Systemic sclerosis—an update. *Laboratory Medicine, 42*(9), 562–572.

Hill, C. L., Cole, A., Rischmueller, M., et al. (2010). Risk of cancer in patients with biopsy-proven giant cell arteritis. *Rheumatology, 49*(4), 756–759.

Hurley, B. F., Hanson, E. D., & Sheaff, A. K. (2011). Strength training as a countermeasure to aging muscle and chronic disease. *Sports Medicine, 41*(4), 289–306.

Ji, J., Liu, X., Sundquist, K., et al. (2010). Cancer risk in patients hospitalized with polymyalgia rheumatica and giant cell arteritis: A follow-up study in Sweden. *Rheumatology (Oxford, England), 49*(6), 1158–1163.

*Johansson, K., Kataajistoo, J., & Salantera, S. (2010). Pre-admission education in surgical rheumatology nursing: Towards greater patient empowerment. *Journal of Clinical Nursing, 19*(21), 2980–2988.

Kiaer, T., & Gehrchen, M. (2010). Transpedicular closed wedge osteotomy in ankylosing spondylitis: Results of surgical treatment and prospective outcome analysis. *European Spine Journal, 19*(1), 57–64.

Kitagawa, T., Shibasaki, K., & Toya, S. (2012). Clinical significance and diagnostic usefulness of anti-centromere antibody in Sjögren's syndrome. *Clinical Rheumatology, 31*(1), 105–112.

Labraca, N. S., Castro-Sánchez, A. M., Matarán-Peñarrocha, G. A., et al. (2011). Benefits of starting rehabilitation within 24 hours of primary total knee arthroplasty: Randomized clinical trial. *Clinical Rehabilitation, 25*(6), 557–566.

Langham, S., Langham, J., Goertz, H., et al. (2011). Large-scale, prospective, observational studies in patients with psoriasis and psoriatic arthritis: A systematic and critical review. *BMC Medical Research Methodology, 11*, 32–32.

Lesko, M., Young, M., & Higham, R. (2010). Managing inflammatory arthritides: Role of the nurse practitioner and physician assistant. *Journal of the American Academy of Nurse Practitioners, 22*(7), 382–392.

Li, M., Gong, L., Sun, X., et al. (2011). Anxiety and depression in patients with dry eye syndrome. *Current Eye Research, 36*(1), 1–7.

Losina, E., Walensky, R. P., Reichmann, W. M., et al. (2011). Impact of obesity and knee osteoarthritis on morbidity and mortality in older Americans. *Annals of Internal Medicine, 154*(4), 217–226.

Mackie, S. L., Hensor, E. M. A., Haugeberg, G., et al. (2010). Can the prognosis of polymyalgia rheumatica be predicted at disease onset? Results from a 5-year prospective study. *Rheumatology (Oxford, England), 49*(4), 716–722.

Martel, C., Gondran, G., Launay, D., et al. (2011). Active immunological profile is associated with systemic Sjögren's syndrome. *Journal of Clinical Immunology, 31*(5), 840–847.

Mathieu, S., Motreff, P., & Soubrier, M. (2010). Spondyloarthropathies: An independent cardiovascular risk factor? *Joint, Bone, Spine, 77*(6), 542–545.

Miró, E., Lupiáñez, J., Martínez, M. P., et al. (2011). Cognitive-behavioral therapy for insomnia improves attentional function in fibromyalgia syndrome: A pilot, randomized controlled trial. *Journal of Health Psychology, 16*(5), 770–782.

Navarra, S. V., Guzmán, R. M., Gallacher, A. E., et al. (2011). Efficacy and safety of belimumab in patients with active systemic lupus erythematosus: A randomised, placebo-controlled, phase 3 trial. *Lancet, 377*(9767), 721–731.

Nguyen, U. D. T., Zhang, Y., Zhu, Y., et al. (2011). Increasing prevalence of knee pain and symptomatic knee osteoarthritis: Survey and cohort data. *Annals of Internal Medicine, 155*(11), 725–732.

Oliver, J. E., & Silman, A. J. (2009). Why are women predisposed to autoimmune rheumatic diseases? *Arthritis Research & Therapy, 11*(5), 252–252.

*Ovayolu, O. U., Ovayolu, N., & Karadag, G. (2012). The relationship between self-care agency, disability levels and factors regarding these situations among patients with rheumatoid arthritis. *Journal of Clinical Nursing, 21*(1), 101–110.

Palmer, D., & El Miedany, Y. (2010). Biological nurse specialist: Goodwill to good practice. *British Journal of Nursing, 19*(8), 477–480.

Pandey, A. K., Wilcox, P., Mayo, J. R., et al. (2010). Predictors of pulmonary hypertension on high-resolution computed tomography of the chest in systemic sclerosis: A retrospective analysis. *Canadian Association of Radiologists Journal, 61*(5), 291–296.

Phung, O. J. (2011). Belimumab: A B-lymphocyte stimulator inhibitor for systemic lupus erythematosus. *Formulary, 46*(4), 118–129.

Pons-Estel, G. J., Alarcón, G. S., Scofield, L., et al. (2010). Understanding the epidemiology and progression of systemic lupus erythematosus. *Seminars in Arthritis and Rheumatism, 39*(4), 257–268.

Prodanovich, S., Ricotti, C., Glick, B. P., et al. (2010). Etanercept: An evolving role in psoriasis and psoriatic arthritis. *American Journal of Clinical Dermatology, 11*, 3–9.

Ramos-Casals, M., Tzioufas, A. G., Stone, J. H., et al. (2010). Treatment of primary Sjögren syndrome: A systematic review. *Journal of the American Medical Association, 304*(4), 452–460.

Ramos-Remus, C., Duran-Barragan, S., & Castillo-Ortiz, J. (2012). Beyond the joints. *Clinical Rheumatology, 31*(1), 1–12.

Rogus-Pulia, N., & Logemann, J. A. (2011). Effects of reduced saliva production on swallowing in patients with Sjögren's syndrome. *Dysphagia, 26*(3), 295–303.

Roizenblatt, S., Neto, N. S., & Tufik, S. (2011). Sleep disorders and fibromyalgia. *Current Pain and Headache Reports, 15*(5), 347–357.

Rojas-Serrano, J., Pérez, L., García, C., et al. (2011). Current smoking status is associated to a non-ACR 50 response in early rheumatoid arthritis. A cohort study. *Clinical Rheumatology, 30*(12), 1589–1593.

Rothenbacher, D., Primatesta, P., Ferreira, A., et al. (2011). Frequency and risk factors of gout flares in a large population-based cohort of incident gout. *Rheumatology (Oxford, England), 50*(5), 973–981.

Ryan, S. (2011). Fibromyalgia: An overview and comparison of treatment options. *British Journal of Nursing, 20*(16), 991–995.

Scofield, R. H. (2011). Vasculitis in Sjögren's syndrome. *Current Rheumatology Reports, 13*(6), 482–488.

Shamim, T., Shaheen, G., Muhammad Asif, H., et al. (2011). Management of acute gout: A review article. *Internet Journal of Pain, Symptom Control, and Palliative Care, 8*(2), doi: 10.5580/23e2.

*Shea, M., & McDonald, D. D. (2011). Factors associated with increased pain communication by older adults. *Western Journal of Nursing Research, 33*(2), 196–206.

Snyder, R. A. (2010). Psoriatic arthritis: A dermatologist's perspective. *American Journal of Clinical Dermatology, 11*, 19–22.

Stamp, L. K., & Jordan, S. (2011). The challenges of gout management in the elderly. *Drugs & Aging, 28*(8), 591–603.

Stuber, K., Sajko, S., & Kristmanson, K. (2011). Efficacy of glucosamine, chondroitin, and methylsulfonylmethane for spinal degenerative joint disease and degenerative disc disease: A systematic review. *Journal of the Canadian Chiropractic Association, 55*(1), 47–55.

Sundy, J. S., Baraf, H. S., Yood, R., et al. (2011). Efficacy and tolerability of pegloticase for the treatment of chronic gout in patients refractory to conventional treatment: Two randomized controlled trials. *Journal of the American Medical Association, 306*(7), 711–720.

**Tan, E. M., Cohen, A. S., Fries, J. F., et al. (1982). The 1982 revised criteria for the classification of systemic lupus erythematosus. *Arthritis and Rheumatism, 25*(11), 1271–1277.

Taylan, A., Sari, I., Kozaci, D., et al. (2012). Evaluation of various endothelial biomarkers in ankylosing spondylitis. *Clinical Rheumatology, 31*(1), 23–28.

Terry, R., Perry, R., & Ernst, E. (2012). An overview of systematic reviews of complementary and alternative medicine for fibromyalgia. *Clinical Rheumatology, 31*(1), 55–66.

Tsai, P., Kuo, Y., Beck, C., et al. (2011). Non-verbal cues to osteoarthritic knee and/or hip pain in elders. *Research in Nursing & Health, 34*(3), 218–227.

**Vitali, C., Bombardieri, S., Jonsson, R., et al. (2002). Classification criteria for Sjögren's syndrome: A revised version of the European criteria proposed by the American-European Consensus Group. *Annals of the Rheumatic Diseases, 61*(6), 554–558.

Vriezekolk, J., Eijsbouts, A., Evers, A., et al. (2010). Poor psychological health status among patients with inflammatory rheumatic diseases and osteoarthritis in multidisciplinary rehabilitation: Need for a routine psychological assessment. *Disability & Rehabilitation, 32*(10), 836–844.

Walker, J. (2011). Effective management strategies for osteoarthritis. *British Journal of Nursing, 20*(2), 81–85.

Waller, C., Hayes, D., Block, J. E., et al. (2011). Unload it: The key to the treatment of knee osteoarthritis. *Knee Surgery, Sports Traumatology, Arthroscopy: Official Journal of the ESSKA, 19*(11), 1823–1829.

Wang, M., Shen, J., Jin, H., et al. (2011). Recent progress in understanding molecular mechanisms of cartilage degeneration during osteoarthritis. *Annals of the New York Academy of Sciences, 1240*, 61–69.

Wendling, D., Paccou, J., Berthelot, J., et al. (2011). New onset of uveitis during anti-tumor necrosis factor treatment for rheumatic diseases. *Seminars in Arthritis and Rheumatism, 41*(3), 503–510.

Wolfe, F., Clauw, D. J., Fitzcharles, M., et al. (2010). The American College of Rheumatology preliminary diagnostic criteria for fibromyalgia and measurement of symptom severity. *Arthritis Care & Research, 62*(5), 600–610.

Woo, Y. K., Kim, K. W., Chung, J. W., et al. (2011). Average 10.1-year follow-up of cementless total knee arthroplasty in patients with rheumatoid arthritis. *Canadian Journal of Surgery, 54*(3), 179–184.

Yavuz, S., Asfuroğlu, E., Bicakcigil, M., et al. (2011). Hydroxychloroquine improves dry eye symptoms of patients with primary Sjogren's syndrome. *Rheumatology International, 31*(8), 1045–1049.

Zychowicz, M. E., Pope, R. S., & Graser, E. (2010). The current state of care in gout: Addressing the need for better understanding of an ancient disease. *Journal of the American Academy of Nurse Practitioners, 22*, 623–636.

Resources

American College of Rheumatology and Association of Rheumatology Health Professionals, www.rheumatology.org
American Fibromyalgia Syndrome Association (AFSA), www.afsafund.org
Arthritis Foundation, www.arthritis.org
Centers for Disease Control and Prevention, www.cdc.gov
Lupus Foundation of America, www.lupus.org
National Institute of Arthritis and Musculoskeletal and Skin Diseases, National Institutes of Health, www.niams.nih.gov
Scleroderma Foundation, www.scleroderma.org
Sjögren's Syndrome Foundation, www.sjogrens.org
Spondylitis Association of America, www.spondylitis.org

Index

Page numbers followed by c indicate charts; those followed by f indicate figures; those followed by t indicate tables.

Features Index

HEALTH PROMOTION

HOME CARE CHECKLIST

NURSING RESEARCH PROFILE